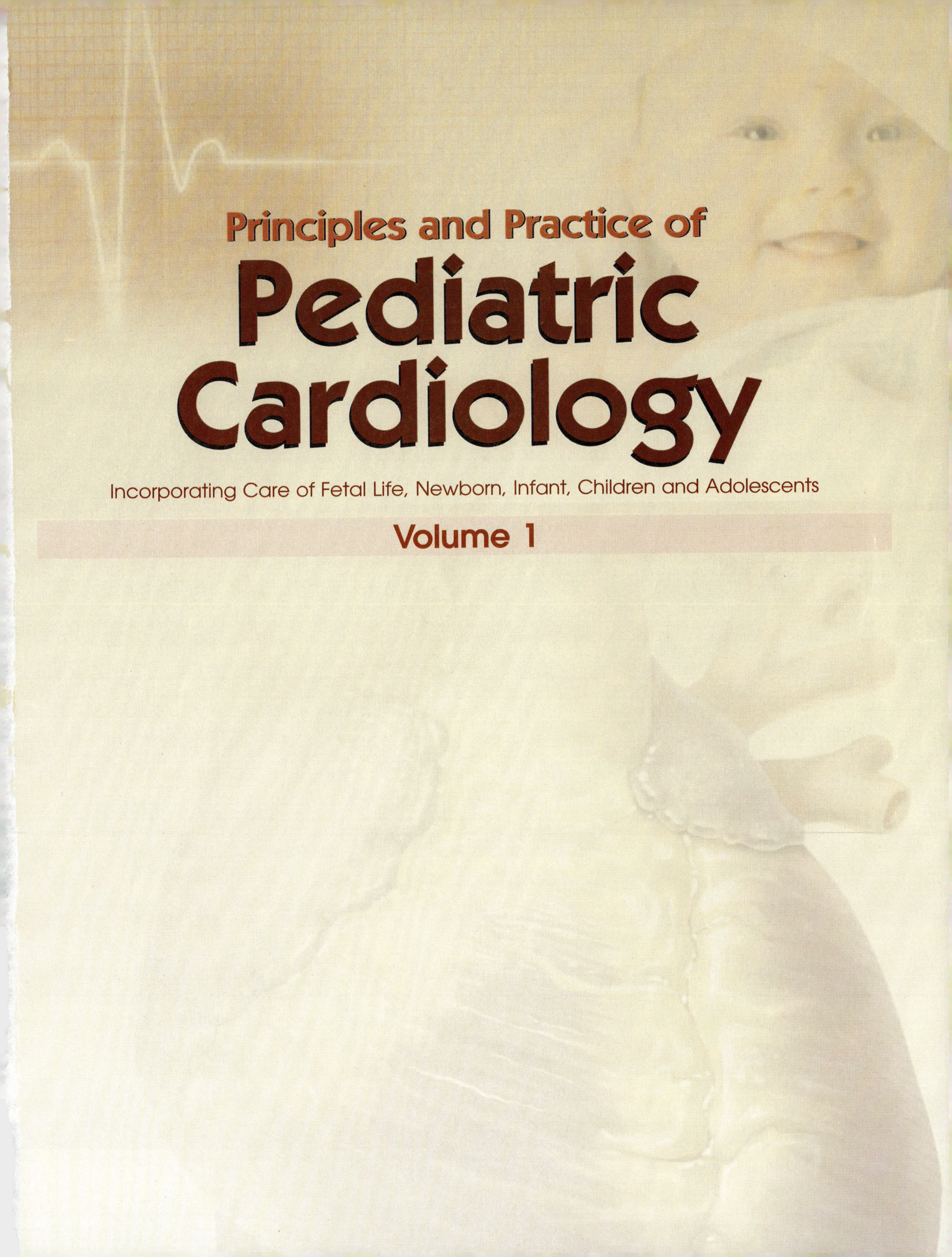

Principles and Practice of

Pediatric Cardiology

Incorporating Care of Fetal Life, Newborn, Infant, Children and Adolescents

Volume 1

Principles and Practice of

Pediatric Cardiology

Incorporating Care of Fetal Life, Newborn, Infant, Children and Adolescents

Volume 1

KC Verma

MBBS, DCH, MD, DM (Cardiology), FICP (USA), FRST M&H (Lond), FCSI (India)

Senior Consulting Heart Specialist and
Formerly Professor in Cardiovascular and Thoracic Unit
Govt. Medical College, Jammu (J&K)

CBS

CBS Publishers & Distributors Pvt Ltd

New Delhi • Bengaluru • Chennai • Kochi • Kolkata • Mumbai
Hyderabad • Nagpur • Patna • Pune • Vijayawada

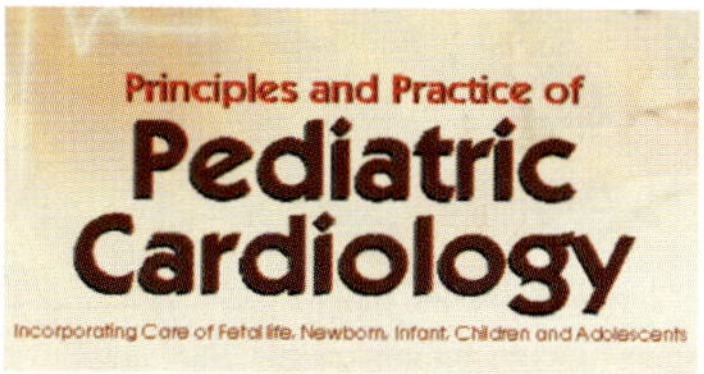

Volume 1

ISBN: 978-81-239-2639-1

First Edition: 2016

Published by Satish Kumar Jain and produced by Varun Jain for
CBS Publishers & Distributors Pvt Ltd
4819/XI Prahlad Street, 24 Ansari Road, Daryaganj, New Delhi 110 002, India.
Ph: 23289259, 23266861, 23266867 Fax: 011-23243014 Website: www.cbspd.com
e-mail: delhi@cbspd.com; cbspubs@airtelmail.in.
Corporate Office: 204 FIE, Industrial Area, Patparganj, Delhi 110 092
Ph: 4934 4934 Fax: 4934 4935 e-mail: publishing@cbspd.com; publicity@cbspd.com

Branches

- **Bengaluru:** Seema House 2975, 17th Cross, K.R. Road, Banasankari 2nd Stage, Bengaluru 560 070, Karnataka
  Ph: +91-80-26771678/79 Fax: +91-80-26771680 e-mail: bangalore@cbspd.com
- **Chennai:** No. 7, Subbaraya Street, Shenoy Nagar, Chennai 600 030, Tamil Nadu
  Ph: +91-44-26680620, 26681266 Fax: +91-44-42032115 e-mail: chennai@cbspd.com
- **Kochi:** Ashana House, 39/1904, AM Thomas Road, Valanjambalam, Ernakulam 682 016, Kochi, Kerala
  Ph: +91-484-4059061-65,67 Fax: +91-484-4059065 e-mail: kochi@cbspd.com
- **Kolkata:** No. 6/B, Ground Floor, Rameswar Shaw Road, Kolkata-700014 (West Bengal), India
  Ph: +91-33-2289-1126, 2289-1127, 2289-1128 e-mail: kolkata@cbspd.com
- **Mumbai:** 83-C, Dr E Moses Road, Worli, Mumbai-400018, Maharashtra
  Ph: +91-22-24902340/41 Fax: +91-22-24902342 e-mail: mumbai@cbspd.com

Representatives

- **Hyderabad** 0-9885175004
- **Nagpur** 0-9021734563
- **Patna** 0-9334159340
- **Pune** 0-9623451994
- **Vijayawada** 0-9000660880

Printed at RP Printers

to

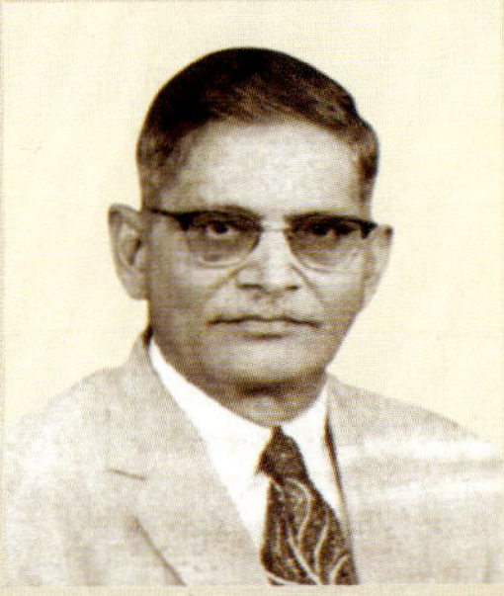

ST Achar MD, FRCP **(1902–1968)**

Dr ST Achar was born on the 11th september 1902 and he retired from service on the 10th september 1965. He entered Madras Medical College Services in 1928 after a brilliant academic career (MBBS First class and first rank 1927; first in the competitive examination for entry into service 1928). In 1948, he was selected to organize the Pediatric of the Madras Medical College occupying the first chair in pediatric in India. Under his chairmanship, this department was upgraded into a full-fledged All India Institute of Pediatrics in 1957 with Dr Achar as its first Director. His main scientific published work had been on pediatric nutritional problems on childhood cirrhosis and on diarrhoeal disorders and had earned for him nation-wide recognition and international reputation. By his hard work and dedication, he gained international fame. He was visiting Lecturer in USA in 1959 and was delegate to the World International Pediatric Congress in 1950 (Zurich) and read his resereach papers in various conferences in 1956 (Copenhagen), 1959 (Montreal), 1965 (Tokyo). He had laid down his office in September 1965 after 37 years of official service. In recognition to his scientific contributions and abilities, the Indian Council of Medical Research had selected him as Emeritus Medical Scientist to do research work in any institution of his choice for five years—an honour conferred for the first time by the council on retired persons unfortunately, he could not complete this mission as he passed away in june 1968.

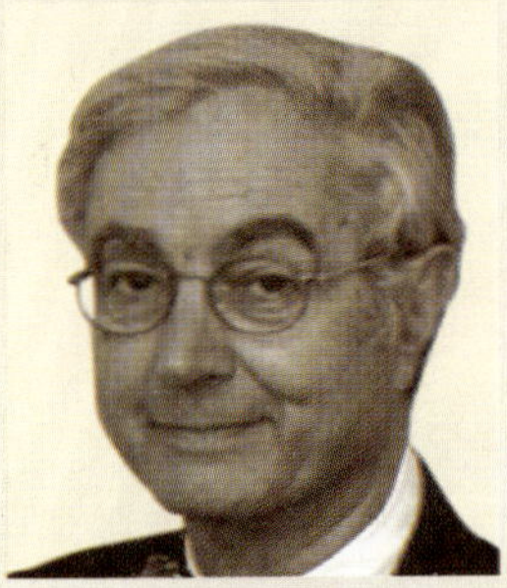

Alexander Nadas (1913–2000)

Dr Alexander Sandor Nadas of Harvard was described as the Father of Paediatric Cardiology. Dr Alexander Sandor Nadas, who trained generations of pediatric cardiologists at Children's Hospital in Boston and at Harvard Medical School, died on Tuesday at his home in Needham, Mass. He was 86.

Dr Nadas, a long-time former resident of Wellesley, Mass, retired in 1982 as chairman emeritus of the hospital's department of cardiology and in 1984 as professor emeritus of pediatrics at the medical school. He had been associated with Children's Hospital since 1949 and was credited with helping build the department's national and international renown for the care of children with heart disease. Harvard Medical School and Children's Hospital honored Dr. Nadas in 1989 by establishing a professorship in his name. And, just days before he died, the American Heart Association gave him its Paul Dudley White Award for his work as a pediatric cardiologist.

Dr Nadas's research centered on cardiovascular physiology and the physiology of congenital heart disease in children. He was the author of hundreds of clinical research papers, and wrote four editions of a textbook for medical students, Pediatric Cardiology, first published in 1957 by WB Saunders.

Preface

This book in its general section deals with brief account of **Anatomy and physiology** including **foetal circulation** of the cardiovascular system.

Examination of heart patient, with physical techniques of history taking, recording of symptoms and signs of heart disease along with thorough bodily examination of a patient has been lucidly detailed in this book.

As this book progresses in its chapters, it discusses the **latest innovations in both non-invasive and invasive techniques** such as cardiovascular imaging, stress testing, CMRI and cardiac CT, Holter study, nuclear evaluation of cardiac functions, echocardiography (transthoracic, transesophageal and intracardiac), cardiac catheterization and angiography.

Subject of **Cardiac arrhythmia** in children which is difficult to understand by both the postgraduates of general medicine and cardiac fellows has been made easy to grasp its fundamentals of diagnosis and treatment with both invasive and minimally invasive techniques.

A brief description of diagnosis and management of **rheumatic fever**, acute and chronic rheumatic valvular dysfunctions, infective endocarditis, pericardial diseases and cardiac tumors, emerging problems of metabolic syndrome, juvenile atherosclerosis, thyroid hormone disorders, mitral valve prolapse, sudden death syndrome and common cardio-pulmonary emergencies has been included skilfully.

This manuscript deals with **congenital heart diseases in younger age group of patients**, which carry maximum burden in cardiology and the author has been able to review its chapter with utmost care and construct its format in such a way that it could be understood with ease and comprehension by the readers of pediatric cardiology.

Heart failure remains as one of the leading causes of deaths in children and is often found to be the terminal event of various congenital and acquired heart ailments, particularly in malnourished patients in tropical and subtropical regions of the world including Indian subcontinent. This chapter has been written with simple text describing both types of systolic and diastolic heart failures supported with self-explanatory illustrations.

With the progress in the field of **interventional cardiology**, most of cardiac defects are being managed with the application of percutaneous catheter techniques in the closure of congenital intracardiac defects with occluders, ablation of foci of cardiac arrhythmias, AV and semilunar valve placement and percutaneous coronary interventions. The author has been able to mention a brief account of this technology.

Currently **medical genomics and stem cell technolgy** have revolutionized the management of various cardiovascular diseases by regenerating the damaged myocardium due to blocked blood supply of coronary vessels and peripheral arteries by advanced atherosclerosis. With the help of genetic engineering and genomic formulations, the scientists have been able to manufacture almost all the damaged tissues of the body. The author has been able to describe a brief review in this context and certainly this will evoke a healthy response among both the geneticists and medical workers, particularly with the recent introduction of **leadless pacemaker** and genetically prepared **pacing cellular system** in the management of cardiac arrhythmias.

Since large number of young adults are taking parts in different **sports** activities, it is therefore important for a specialised doctor in sport medicine to conduct a thorough examination before their selection into a particular sport. Some of them may be having congenital or acquired cardiovascular disorders and are therefore not fit for such exercising activities. The author, therefore, has made a comprehensive review guiding sports doctors in their final selection.

Robotic cardiac surgery in the management of various congenital and acquired cardiac defects and ***in utero* interventions** with minimal invasion, lesser operative time and least discomfort are becoming the popular techniques of the present time and author of this book, therefore has been able to attach a brief review of the subject in separate chapters.

Since we are living in a tropical country and systemic invasion by various viral and bacterial infections and parasitic infestations lead to high morbidity and mortality with cardiorespiratory failure particularly among the malnourished children. The author, therefore, thought it proper to add a brief review of **tropical cardiology.**

Many patients live at distance places from their consulting cardiologist and only way to approach them in hour of emergency, is through the mode of telecommunication, i.e. **"Telemedicine"**. Therefore, a brief review in this subject has been attached for the benefit of the pediatric patients.

This book in its present format and contents is considered as a treasure house of knowledge of cardiology and would certainly act as a ready reckoner to the budding cardiologist, cardiac fellows, junior and senior residents of general medicine for their understanding of the anatomical and physiological basis of cardiovascular system.and various newer non-invasive and invasive methodologies employed in the assessment and management of different cardiovascular disorders.

KC Verma

Acknowledgements

I am very grateful to my wife Dr Mrs Urmil Kanta Verma, Formerly Professor in Department of Blood Transfusion Medicine and Pathology for providing me a perfect congenial atmosphere and all material and moral support needed for writing such a specialised book on Pediatric Cardiology. I also appreciate the support of my grand daughter, Adwita Verma by posing as a physical model in chapter "Yogic exercises in children and adolescents".

Under the perfect guidance of Production manager, Vice-President and CMD of CBSP&D, New Delhi, contributions and hard work rendered by various individuals with respect to its perfect designing, typesetting, preparation of thousands of figures and line diagrams, which itself was a big challenging task, is joyfully acknowledged.

KC Verma

Contents

History of Pediatric Cardiology in India

Historically, pediatric cardiology as a subspeciality has its origin from the main discipline of General Pediatrics. The American Heart Association started a subgroup called council on rheumatic fever (1945) which later became council on cardiovascular diseases in young and accommodated congenital heart diseases (CHD) in 1950. Pediatric cardiology received its formal recognition as subspeciality, first time in 1961 internationally in India, cardiology chapter was founded as a subspeciality group of IAP in 1990. Pediatric Cardiology Society of India was founded much later in year 1997.

The main burden of structural heart diseases belongs to neonatal and infant population. Conversely, acquired heart diseases including acute rheumatic fever, rheumatic heart diseases, Kawasaki disease, myocardial diseases and rhythm disorders also influence children below 18 years of age. Hence, pediatrician have the role of diagnosing the specific defect as well as the care of such children. Despite all its virtues, pediatric cardiology is lagging behind, particularly at suburban and rural areas where even simple diagnostic modalities are not available. With growing number of institutions dealing with pediatric cardiac patients, the sensitization towards the problem is increasing. This cannot be directly converted into therapeutic advantage for the simple reason that majority of the population is poor and below poverty line. Therefore, the upcoming private cardiac set up may not meet the enormity of demand amongst economically deprived India. Pediatricians, with growing awareness about cardiac ailments can play a pivotal role in its management.

In 1931, Dr Robert Gross operated and closed a patent ductus arteriosus. Six years later in 1945 Dr Blalock performed the well-known Blalock-Taussig shunt. The amount of clinical and pathological data accumulated so fast that Dr Taussig could write a whole book devoted to congenital cardiac anomalies in 1947. The first comprehensive textbook in pediatric cardiology, written by Dr Alexander Nadas came out in 1956, 30 years after Dr Morses' book. Pediatric cardiology as a speciality was established.

The first formal department of cardiology in India was established by Dr Vythilingam in 1957 at Vellore. First doctor who completed her training in pediatric cardiology is Dr S Padmavati. She spent a year with Dr Helen Taussig and settled in Delhi in late fifties. Dr S Padmavati, however worked as a cardiologist predominantly looking after adults and did not have access to surgical management of cardiac patients. Although senior, the late Dr.Vythilingam completed a year's training with Dr Taussig in 1961. The availability of surgical help allowed her to look after both adult as well as pediatric patients. The birth of the speciality of pediatric cardiology in India took place at Vellore under Dr Reev Betz who started the first cardiothoracic surgery department at Vellore in 1949. Dr T Thomas and Dr Gopinath joined Dr Betz subsequently and initiated the first open heart surgery programs in 1960.

A well-known, dedicated and most efficient late Prof (Dr) R K Tandon, after completing his two years training in pediatric cardiology, joined All India Institute of Medical Sciences, New Delhi in 1963, established himself as a full time teacher and pediatric cardiologist, supported by Dr Savitri Srivastava. Other pediatricians who obtained excellent training in pediatric cardiology were Dr Vishnu Jain of Patna worked with Dr Vlad and Dr Ed Lambert at Buffalo, Dr Bachu Edibam Master of Jamshedpur got her training with Dr Keith in Toronto and Dr SK Sanyal who trained with Dr Norman Talner and settled at Safdarjung Hospital in Delhi. Unfortunately they did not have access to surgical help and the former two predominantly worked as pediatricians and could not continue as pediatric cardiologists. Dr Sanyal, however, went back to USA . Dr IP Sukumar spent two years with Dr Keith in 1972–73 and took over the responsibility of pediatric cardiology at Vellore. Two others who had formal training in pediatric cardiology were Dr PS Rao who went back to USA and late Dr PS Bidwai who joined PGI Chandigarh and remained active as a full time pediatric cardiologist. Subsequently, however, many others have now joined the speciality but after a considerable gap. The speciality is becoming more popular and now we have some pediatric cardiology Board Certified specialist from USA.

With the growth of therapeutic interventions, Pediatric Cardiology has become more attractive and nonsurgical dependant. The Pediatric Cardiologist has not to wait for a surgical colleagues for relieving obstructions like pulmonic stenosis, aortic stenosis and coarctation of aorta. They can dilate distally located peripheral pulmonic stenosis which is not only difficult but at times impossible for a surgeon to reach. Atrial septal defect, PDA and some VSDs can be closed without operation. Coil embolization of collaterals, pulmonary and coronary arteriovenous fistulae and shunts is being done routinely at many centres in India, pediatric cardiology has become a speciality rather than remaining a subspeciality. A separate training programme and an examination for certifying the specialist has started.

With the revised recommendations, the pediatric patients entering into most of the Indian clinics are up to 18 years rather than 13 years previously. In the USA, pediatric age has further increased up to 21 years. In well established pediatric cardiology/cardiothoracic centres in India, one may not surprise patients in the age range of 25–30 years entering into such clinics with regular follow-up program managed with either occluder devices, embolization techniques or surgically operated at much younger age groups.

Follow-up care, of adult congenital heart diseases like ASD secundum, PDA, coarctation of aorta and pulmonary stenosis, tetralogy of Fallot (adult tetralogy), milder form of VSD (muscular variety), congenital cardiac arrhythmias including congenital complete heart block, is becoming a big challenge in future for both Indian pediatric cardiologist and pediatric cardiac surgeon.

On 5th March, 2015 at Mumbai, Indian pediatric cardiologist with the help of pediatric cardiac surgeons, have been able to fit permanent pacemaker in the heart of premature baby during 20th minutes after birth, born at 34th weeks, weighing 1.5 kg and whose diagnosis of complete heart block was established at 28th weeks of intrauterine life. This is considered to be the world's smallest baby with permanent cardiac pacemaker said the doctors. Earlier too, permanent pacemakers have been fitted by Mumbai pediatric cardiologists in smaller babies weighing 1.6/1.5 kg during 15th minutes and two days old in Feb. and July 2012, respectively.

Over the past one decade or so, the work of pediatric cardiologist has changed very significantly. Till recently, discipline of pediatrics has shown further split into neonatal cardiology and pediatric cardiology subdivisions.

The main departments of pediatric cardiology have now trained specialists dealing exclusively with clinical work, diagnostic hemodynamic studies, interventionists, echo and Doppler experts, electrophysiologists, pathologists and more recently molecular cardiologists.

In the USA and other developed countries of the world, fetal and neonatal pediatric cardiologists with their *in utero* approach, are now managing most of the critical cardiac defects like severe aortic stenosis, fetus to fetus transfusion syndrome, hypoplastic left heart syndrome, hydrop fetalis with congestive heart failure and critical RVOT obstructions. Moreover, fetal cardiac arrhythmias are being managed with timely and appropriate fetal pharmacotherapy. Hopefully, Indian pediatric cardiologists would be able to develop such facility sooner in their respective centres of excellence.

Finally, with deep sense of gratitude I, owe my sincere respect to the dedicated, past and present pediatric cardiologists and pediatric cardiac surgeons of India, who with their untiring efforts has brought this speciality to a reputable developmental stage.

KC Verma

1

Fetal Circulation and Physiological Alterations after Birth

FETAL CIRCULATION

Blood flow patterns, oxygenation and fetal gas exchange after birth occurs in the lungs, and oxygenated blood returns to the left atrium and ventricle to be ejected into the systemic circulation. In the fetus, gas exchange occurs in the placenta, and the fetal lungs do not transfer O_2 or CO_2. So that, this oxygenated blood returning to the venous circulation from the placenta might reach the systemic arterial circulation and unoxygenated venous blood from the body return to the placenta for oxygenation and CO_2 removal. The fetal circulation has several shunts in addition, preferential streaming of venous return occurs to offset the disadvantages of the mixing of oxygenated and unoxygenated blood. The patterns of blood flow into and out of the fetal heart.

These data are from studies in chronically instrumented close-to-term fetal lambs, because no truly quantitative information is available on the human or nonhuman primate fetal circulations. The fetal circulation is arranged in parallel, rather than in series, the right ventricle delivering the majority of its output to the placenta for oxygenation, and the left ventricle delivering the majority of its output to the heart, brain, and upper part of the body However, there is mixing of the streams at the atrial and

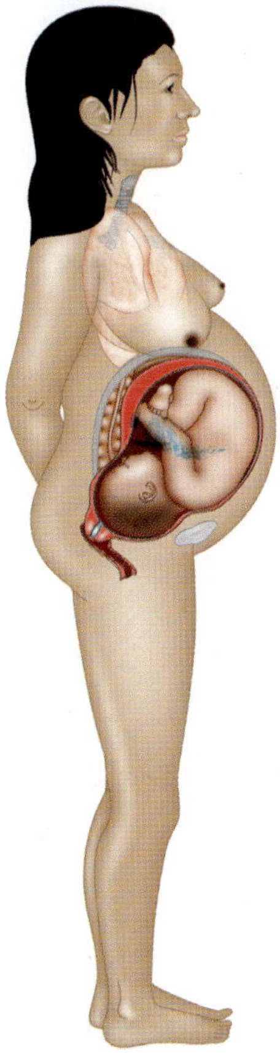

Fig. 1.1A: *Diagram showing a pregnant woman with full term fetus in her womb*

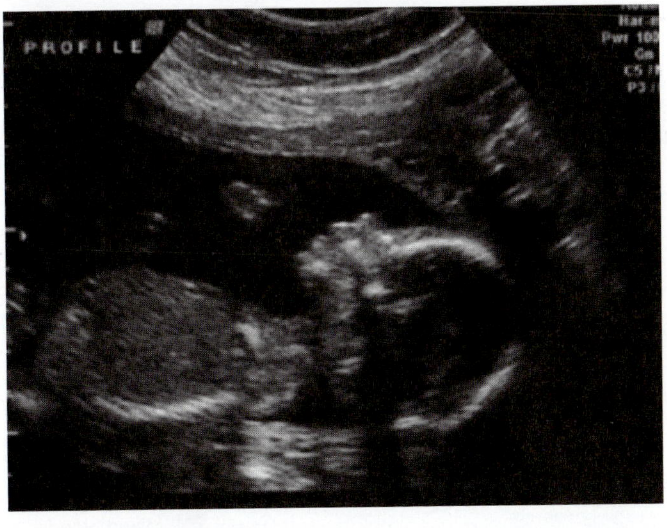

Fig. 1.1B: *Fetal ultrasonography shows fully developed fetus after 30 weeks of gestation*

great vessel level which diverts blood from the immature lungs to the placenta for oxygen exchange. This parallel circulation permits fetal survival despite a wide variety of complex cardiac lesions. Normally, blood returning from the placenta via the umbilical venous return splits in the liver; some of it goes into the hepatic veins and the portal system of the liver, while the remainder (slightly over half) passes through the ductus venosus into the inferior vena cava near its junction with the right atrium. In the right atrium, the blood from the inferior vena cava is divided into two streams by the crista dividends. About 40% of the blood returning from the inferior vena cava (27% of the combined ventricular output) passes across the foramen ovale into the left atrium where it with the pulmonary venous return from the lung, passing through the mitral valve into the left ventricle. This blood is then pumped out the ascending aorta where it supplies the coronary, carotid, and subclavian arteries, with approximately a third of this stream (10% of combined ventricular output) passing across the aortic arch into the descending aorta (Fig. 1.3).

The majority of blood returning from the inferior vena cava joins the superior vena caval drainage and coronary sinus return before passing through the tricuspid valve into the right ventricle and pulmonary artery. Because the fluid-filled lungs and constricted pulmonary arterioles offer a high resistance to flow, most of the blood, almost 90%, passes not to the lungs, but through the open ductus arteriosus into the low resistance descending aorta and placenta.

The oxygen content of the blood in the fetus is considerably lower than that in the neonate or child, because of the lower efficiency of the placenta compared with the lung as an organ for oxygen exchange blood

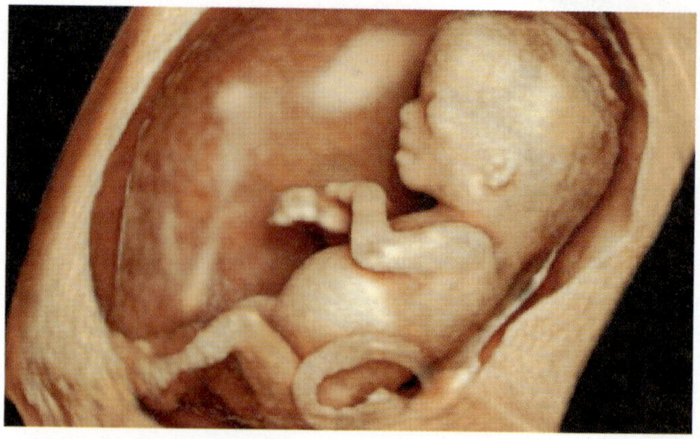

Fig. 1.2: *3D ultrasonographic scan reveal hair and facial features of unborn babies. These three dimensional scan of baby while still in the womb is some of the most detailed ever achieved, revealing details including hair, skin texture and even facial expressions*

returning from the placenta via the umbilical veins has the highest pO_2 (32–35 torr; oxygen saturation, 70%). The blood that passes into the left ventricle has already mixed with the less saturated vena caval and pulmonary venous return, lowering the pO_2 to 26–28 torr (oxygen saturation about 65%) before its distribution to the ascending aorta and upper half of the body.

The umbilical venous return destined for the right ventricle mixes with the superior vena caval return (PO_2, 12–14 torr; oxygen saturation, 40%), reducing the oxygen content of blood passing into the right ventricle, main pulmonary artery, and descending aorta to about 20–22 torr (oxygen saturation, 50–55%). Thus, blood with the highest

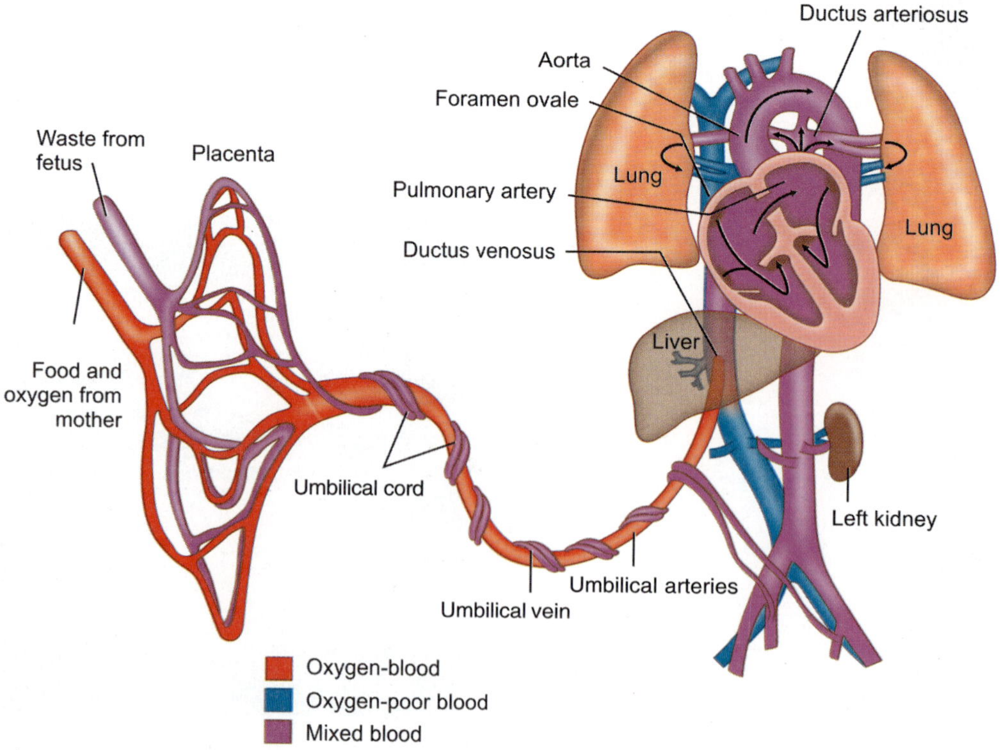

Fig. 1.3: *Showing placental and fetal heart circulation*

oxygen content is diverted to the coronary arteries and brain, and that with the lowest oxygen content is diverted to the placenta, increasing the efficiency of oxygen pickup. An additional fetal adaptation to oxygen transport at low oxygen saturations is the presence of high levels fetal hemoglobin with its high affinity for oxygen and its low pO_2 (partial pressure of oxygen at the point where 50% of the hemoglobin is oxidized) of approximately 18 or 19 torr. This leftward shift of the oxygen association curve facilitates oxygen uptake at the relatively low pO_2 levels of the placental vasculature (Table 1.1).

The wide communication between the atria allows for equalization of pressures in the atria; similarly, the patency of the ductus arteriosus results in equalization of pressures in the aorta and pulmonary artery. Because atrial and great vessel pressures are equal, in the absence of pulmonic or aortic stenosis, the ventricular pressures are equal also, with a systolic pressure of approximately 70 mm, using amniotic pressure as zero (Table 1.2).

It has been shown that the fetus has a limited ability to adjust cardiac output. The primary determinants of cardiac output are heart rate, filling pressure (preload), resistance against which the ventricles eject (after load), and myocardial contractility. It has been known that there are spontaneous changes in heart rate associated with electrocortical activity as well as with the sleep state and fetal activity. Using continuous measurements of left and right ventricular output, utilizing electromagnetic flow probes, Rudolph and Heymann have shown that spontaneous increases in heart rate are associated with increasing ventricular output, whereas decreases in heart rate result in a considerable fall of both right and left ventricular output. By electrically pacing the right atrium above the resting level of 160–180, the left ventricular output eventually increases to about 15% above resting levels. Decreasing the heart rate by 50% by vagal stimulation caused a fall in output of approximately 30%. Contrary to the significant effects of increasing or decreasing heart rate on fetal cardiac output, increasing preload (even to levels as high as a right atrial pressure of 20 mm Hg) produces only very small increases in ventricular output, suggesting that the fetal ventricle normally functions near the top of its function curve and has little reserve to increase cardiac output. Increasing the work of the heart by increasing afterload (by inflating a balloon in the fetal descending aorta or by methoxamine) produces a dramatic fall in right ventricular output, suggesting that the fetal heart is very sensitive to increases in afterload.

Morphometric studies on the fetal myocardium have demonstrated a significant decrease in myofibrillar content per tissue volume, suggesting that the fetal myocardium has much less contractile tissue than the adult. The active tension produced in excised strips of fetal myocardium was less than that produced by adult myocardium, possibly because of the myofibrillar content, a reduced content of sarcoplasmic reticulum and/or the T-tubule system.

Table 1.1: *Changes in neonatal circulation*

Structure	*Prenatal function*	*Postnatal function*
Ductus arteriosus	Right to left shunt	Initially bidirectional, 24–48 hours later left to right shunt. Functional closure by 8 hours. Anatomical closure by 3 months
Foramen ovale	Shunting of blood from IVC through RA into LA	Right to left shunt may occasionally persist and remain patent in 25% of cases; but mainly the dominant shunt is from left to right as left atrial pressure is higher than the right
Ductus venosus	Shunting of blood from umbilical vein into IVC	Obliterates to form ligamentum venosum

Table 1.2: *Blood pressure and pulse rates of children (at different ages)*

	Pulse rate (per min)		*BP (in mm of Hg)*	
	Average	*Range*	*Systolic*	*Diastolic*
Newborn	120	70–170	86	60
1 year	120	80–160	86	60
2 years	120	80–130		
4 years	110	80–120		
6 years	100	76–116	90	60
8 years	90	70–110	96	64
10 years	90	70–110	100	64
12 years	90	65–105	110	70

All of the above data suggest that the fetal myocardium is structurally and functionally immature compared with that of the older child or adult. The fetal heart appears to work at the peak of its ventricular function curve, with increases in preload causing little or no change in cardiac output, and increases in afterload resulting in a marked depression. The limited ability of the fetal heart to respond to stress seems to be mediated primarily through increasing the heart rate.

The structure, hemodynamics, and myocardial function of the fetal circulation have significant consequences in the neonate with congenital heart disease:

1. The parallel circulation, with connections at the atrial and great vessel level, allows a wide variety of cardiac malformations to provide adequate transport of blood to the placenta to pickup oxygen and deliver it to the tissues.
2. The right ventricle performs approximately two-thirds of the cardiac work before birth. This is reflected in the size and thickness of the right ventricle before and after birth and may explain why left-sided defects are poorly tolerated after birth, compared with right-sided lesions.
3. Because the normal flow across the aortic isthmus is small (10% of ventricular output), the aortic isthmus is especially vulnerable to small changes in intracardiac flow from various congenital defects. This may account for the relatively, high incidence of narrowing (coarctation of the aorta) or atresia (interrupted aortic arch) in this region.
4. Because the pulmonary flow *in utero* is very small compared with that immediately after birth, anomalies preventing normal pulmonary return (total anomalous pulmonary return, mitral stenosis, etc) may be masked *in utero* when pulmonary venous return is so low anyway.
5. The low levels of circulating oxygen before birth (pO_2 26–28 torr in the ascending aorta and 20–22 torr in the descending aorta) may account for the relative level of comfort of infants with cyanotic heart disease who may be quite active and comfortable, and may feed well with an arterial pO_2 of 20–25, a level that would lead to cerebral and cardiac anoxia, acidosis, and death within a few minutes for the older child or adult.
6. The limited ability of the fetal myocardium to respond to stress makes the hemodynamic consequences of congenital heart disease after birth that much more difficult to tolerate.
7. Birth is a time of stress for the left ventricle. Because of the switch from parallel to serial circulation, there is an increased amount of blood to pump. The ductus arteriosus may, at least briefly, shunt left to right. The work of respiration must be assumed. Of greater importance is the loss of the incubator effect of the uterus; the body metabolism and the circulation must adapt to maintaining body temperature. The possible role of the thyroid in these events has been noted.

Transitional Circulation

Within a few moments of birth, profound changes must occur as the newborn rapidly switches from the placenta to the lung as the organ of respiration. Failure of anyone of a complex series of pulmonary or cardiac events that take place within minutes of birth leads to generalized hypoxemia and brain damage or death (Figs 1.4 to 1.6).

Soon after the onset of spontaneous respiration, the placenta is removed from the circulation, either by clamping the umbilical cord or, more naturally, by constriction of the umbilical arteries. This suddenly increases the systemic resistance as the lower-resistance

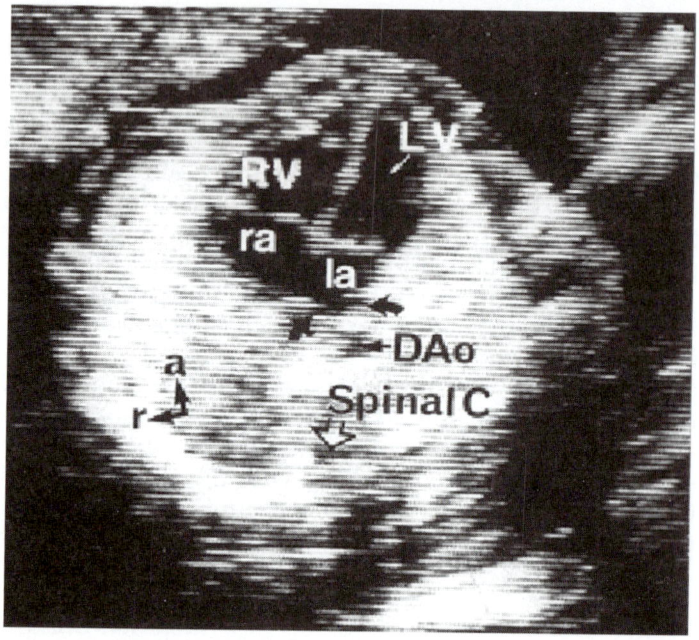

Fig 1.4: *Fetal 4C echocardiographic view obtained from a transverse section through the fetal thorax showing DAo = descending aorta, spinal C = spinal canal. The curved black arrows indicate pulmonary veins entering into left atrium*

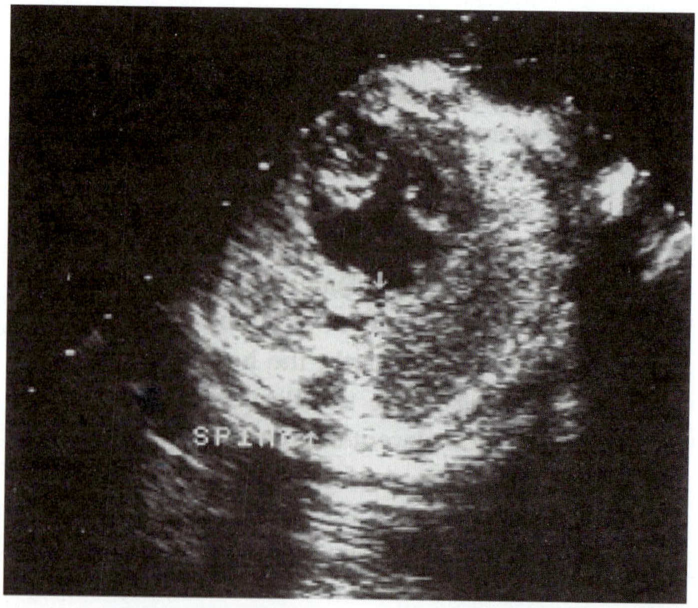

Fig 1.5: *Transverse thoracic echocardiography section in fetus with right atrial isomerism,common atrium,double inlet left ventricle through common A-V valve*

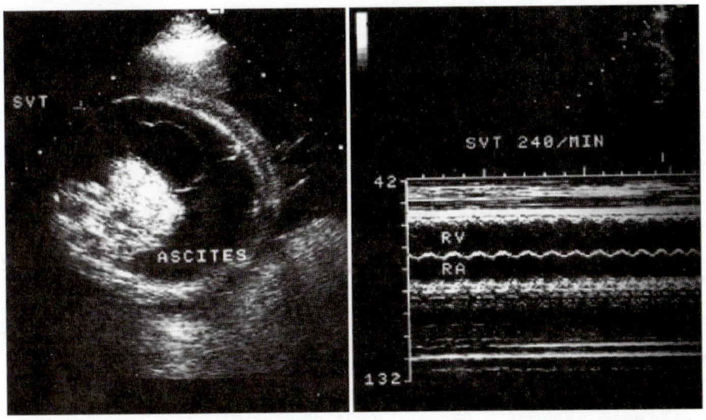

Fig. 1.6: *Transverse section per abdomen echocardiogram of the fetus showing severe form of fetal hydrops (left) secondary to heart failure due to sustained atrioventricular reentry tachycardia which is demonstrated by the M-mode recording of the fetal heart rate (right) with 1.1 AV conduction*

placenta is excluded from the circulation. At approximately the same time, the onset of spontaneous respiration expands the lungs and brings oxygen to the pulmonary alveoli. Reduction in the pulmonary vascular resistance results both from simple physical expansion of the vessels and from the chemoreflex vasodilatation of the pulmonary arterioles caused by the high level of oxygen in the alveolar gas.

This sudden increase in systemic vascular resistance and drop in pulmonary vascular resistance causes a reversal of the *flow* through the ductus arteriosus and an increase in pulmonary *flow*. Before birth the relative pulmonary and systemic resistances cause 90% of the blood to go through the ductus arteriosus into the descending aorta; by a few minutes after birth 90% goes to the pulmonary arteries, with the pulmonary blood *flow* increasing from 35 mL/kg/min to 160–200 mL/kg/min.

The rapid drop in systemic venous return to the inferior vena cava as the umbilical venous *flow* is cut-off, as well as the increase in pulmonary venous return as the pulmonary

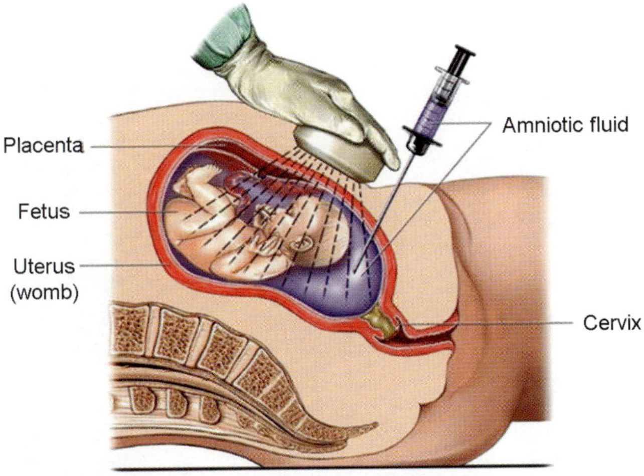

Fig. 1.7: *Placement of fetus in intrauterine cavity relation to surrounding structures including amniotic sac and placental attachment*

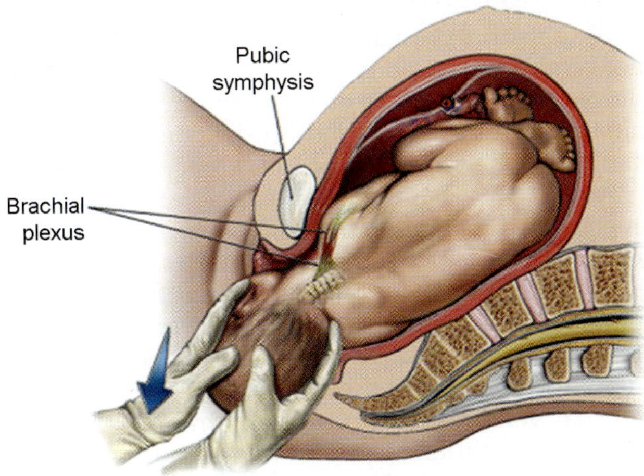

Fig. 1.8: *Pervaginal normal delivery of the baby*

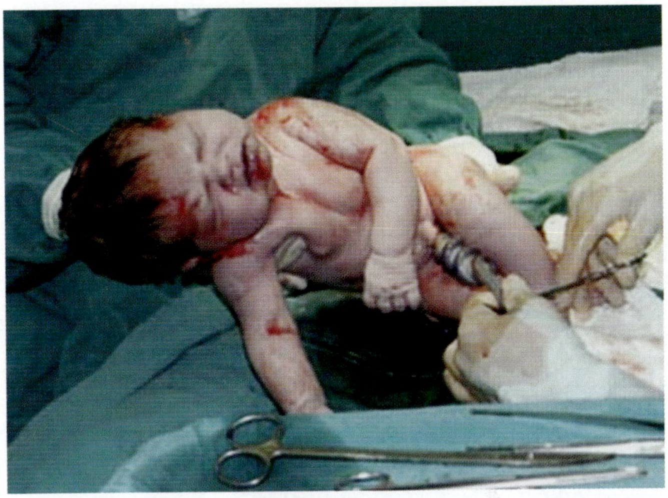

Fig. 1.9: *Mildly cyanosed baby soon after difficult delivery*

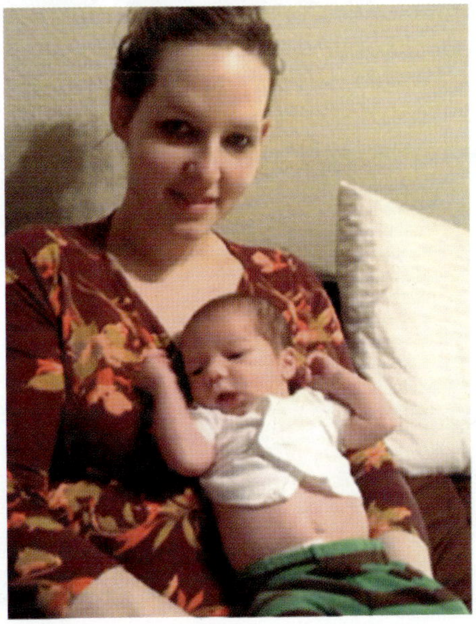

Fig. 1.10: *Healthy baby in the lap of the mother who is facing post-placental life with altered hemodynamics*

blood *flow* increases, causes the left atrial pressure to rise and the right atrial pressure to fall. When left atrial pressure exceeds right atrial pressure, the flap valve of the foramen ovale closes against the edge of the crista dividends, eliminating left-to-right or right-to-left shunting.

There have been questions in the past regarding how much these marked circulatory changes are influenced by the mechanical changes in the lung parenchyma due to the onset of ventilation, how much by the vasodilatory effects of oxygen, and how much by the increase in systemic vascular resistance, with constriction of the umbilical vessels removing the low-resistance placenta from the circulation. Tietel, using monitored fetal sheep near term, found that ventilation alone caused dramatic changes in the central *flow* patterns, attributable to a large decrease in pulmonary vascular resistance and an associated increase in pulmonary blood *flow*. Ventilation alone increased the pulmonary venous return from 8% of combined ventricular output to 31%, whereas right ventricular output (which had formerly ejected 90% to the ductus arteriosus) was reduced to less than 50%. Oxygenation further changed the flow patterns so that more than 90% of the flow from the main pulmonary artery went to the lungs rather than through the ductus arteriosus. Umbilical cord occlusion had few additional effects.

Usually, the ductus arteriosus remains patent for several hours or days after birth. Initially, the pulmonary vascular resistance exceeds systemic vascular resistance so that there is a small right-to-left (pulmonary artery-to-aorta) shunt with some systemic desaturation to the lower half of the body. Anything that increases the pulmonary vascular resistance, such as acidosis, hypoxemia, polycythemia, or lung disease, may exacerbate or prolong the normal transient right-to-left shunt. Within a few hours of birth, however, in the normal child, the pulmonary vascular resistance has fallen lower than systemic vascular resistance, resulting in a small "physiologic" left-to-right (aorta-to-pulmonary artery) shunt. Normally, within 10–15 hours of birth, the ductus arteriosus has closed, although permanent structural closure may not take place for another 2–3 weeks (Figs 1.11 to 1.14).

The mechanism of closure of the ductus arteriosus is not completely understood. It has been clear for some time that oxygen plays a role. Coceani and Olley' have shown that prostaglandins of the E series are responsible for maintaining patency of the ductus arteriosus during fetal life.

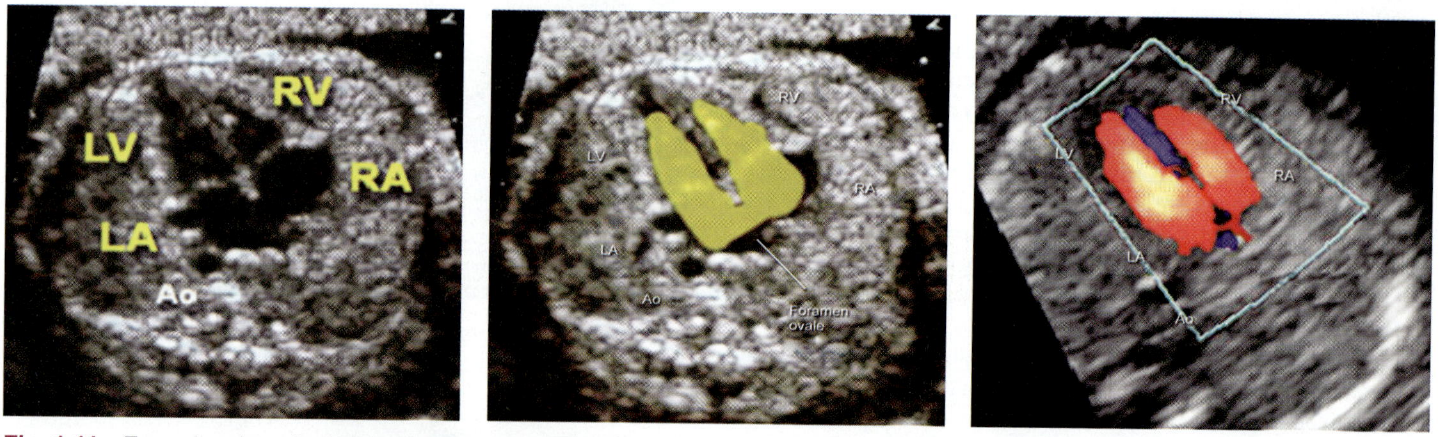

Fig. 1.11: *Four-chamber view in real-time (left) and color Doppler. During diastole, flow is visualized entering from both the right and left atria (RA, LA) into the right and left ventricles (RV, LV) and the flows are separated by the interatrial and interventricular septum*

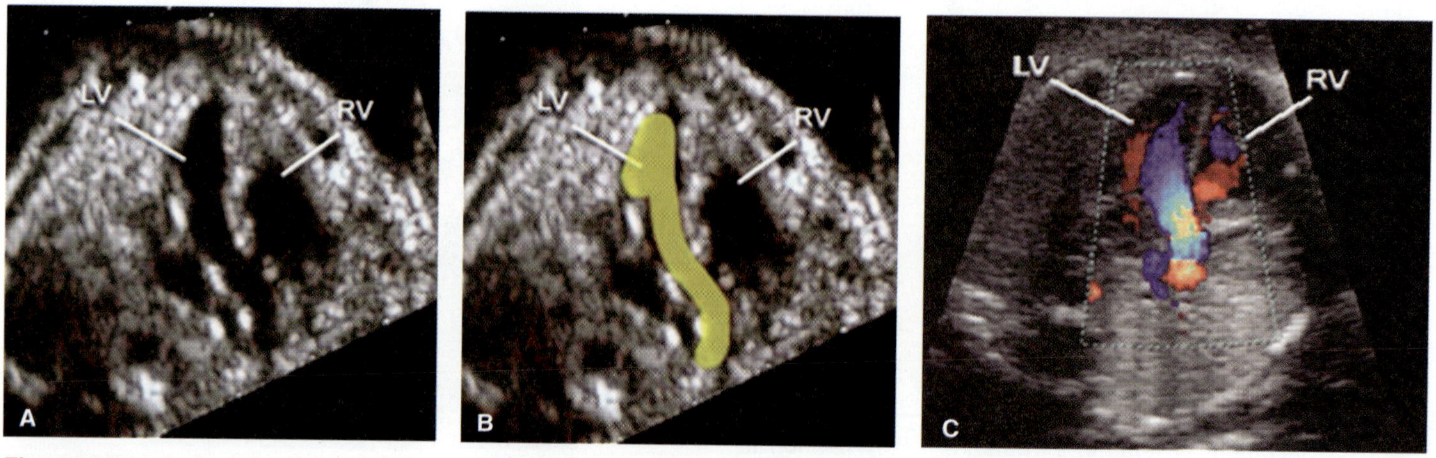

Fig. 1.12A to C: *Five-chamber view in real-time (A) using color Doppler (B). The aorta, arising from the left ventricle, is seen and color shows the laminar flow across the aortic valve during systole (C)*

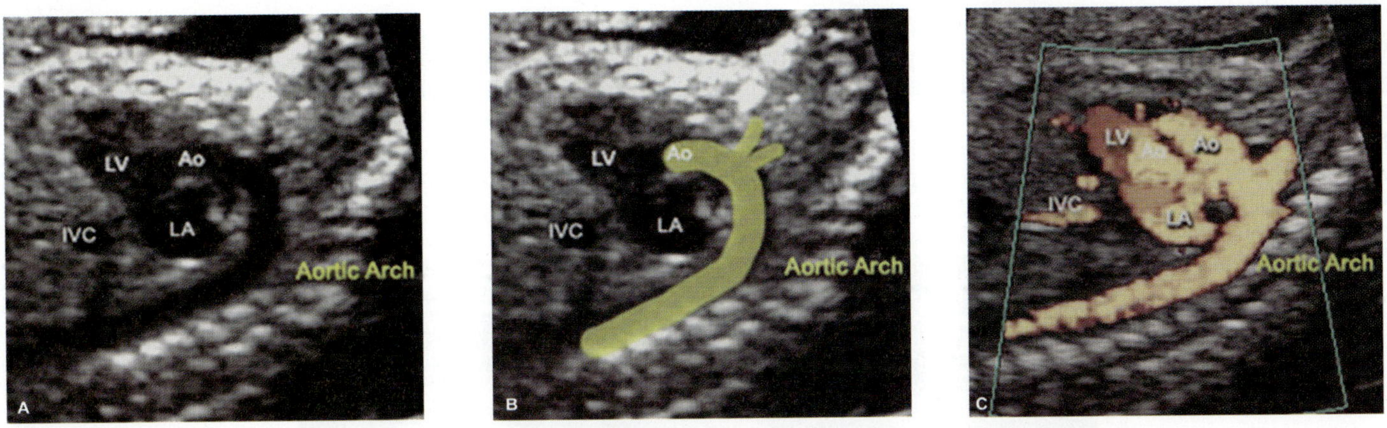

Fig. 1.13: *(A,B) Aortic arch; (C) color Doppler imaging of the aortic arch*

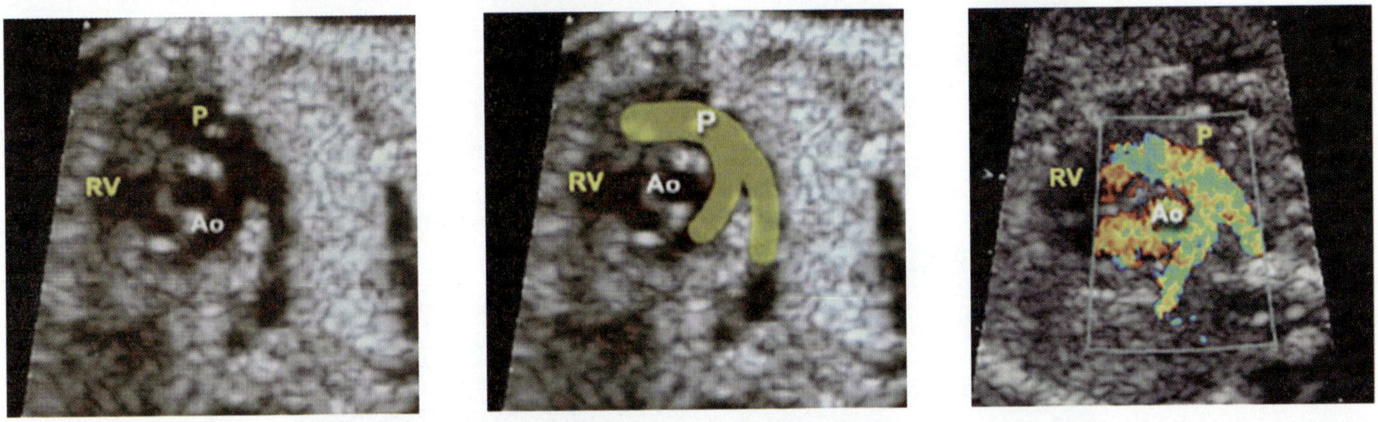

Fig. 1.14: *Five-chamber view in real-time (left) using color Doppler (right). The pulmonary vein, arising from the right ventricle*

It has been possible to keep the ductus open for days, weeks, or months, or even longer in infants with congenital heart disease, by infusion of exogenous prostaglandins E, and it has been possible to close the ductus arteriosus in about 80% of preterm infants weighing less than 1,750 gm with indomethacin, a nonselective prostaglandin synthetase inhibitor.

Clyman and coworkers observed a decrease in the ability of the ductus arteriosus to dilate and contract within a few hours of postnatal ductal constriction, before the loss of an anatomically patent lumen, in both human newborns and full-term lambs. They postulated that this change reflects early ischemic damage to the inner muscle wall. Fay and Cook proposed that irreversibility reflects a mechanical restraint imposed by cellular necrosis, with a loss of intact endothelium leading to constriction from opposing walls until an anatomic lumen is eliminated. The etiology of the necrosis is unknown but it has been postulated that it is caused by interruption of luminal blood flow.

Although some hypoxemia is present soon after birth, because of right-to-left shunting through the ductus arteriosus over the first few hours of life, with continued vasodilatation and improved ventilation/perfusion ratios, the normal arterial pO_2 gradually increases from 50 torr at 10 minutes to 62 at 1 hour and 75–83 between 3 hours and 2 days of age. With continued vasodilatation the pulmonary pressure gradually falls to about 30 torr within approximately 48 hours. Although further falls in the pulmonary vascular resistance continue for several weeks, the transition to adult circulation is virtually completed within the first few days of life.

Compromised Systemic Blood Flow (Fig. 1.18)

Presentation of lesions such as hypoplastic left heart syndrome, critical aortic stenosis or severe coarctation of the aorta is characterized by inadequate systemic blood flow. Typically, these infants present on the second or third day of life, as the duct constricts, with cool peripheries. weak or absent arterial pulses (femoral pulses in the case of isolated coarctation of the aorta) and hepatomegaly. Dyspnea and tachypnea occur because of progressive metabolic acidosis secondary to hypoxia, but also because pulmonary venous congestion, increased pulmonary blood flow. or both. may accompany these lesions. Emergency treatment will include intravenous infusion of prostaglandin E to maintain ductal patency, as adequate systemic blood flow is likely to be dependent on continuing pulmonary artery-to-aorta flow via the duct. Inadequate systemic blood flow may become manifest less acutely beyond the neonatal period because of the lesions such as dilated cardiomyopathy, acute viral myocarditis, incessant tachyarrhythmia or left ventricular infarction secondary to anomalous origin of the left coronary artery from the pulmonary trunk.

Congenital diseases of the heart and vasculature are the most common birth defects, occurring in approximately eight per 1,000 live births. Some patients with congenital heart defects (CHDs) remain asymptomatic for many years; others survive to adulthood, thanks to the impressive progress in medical and surgical management made in recent decades. This relatively high incidence, coupled with improved management, has resulted in a large adult population of these patients: it has been estimated that almost one million adults with CHDs are currently living in the United States. A broad range of clinicians must now become more knowledgeable about the care of these patients, including issues such as endocarditis prophylaxis (Figs 1.15 to 1.18).

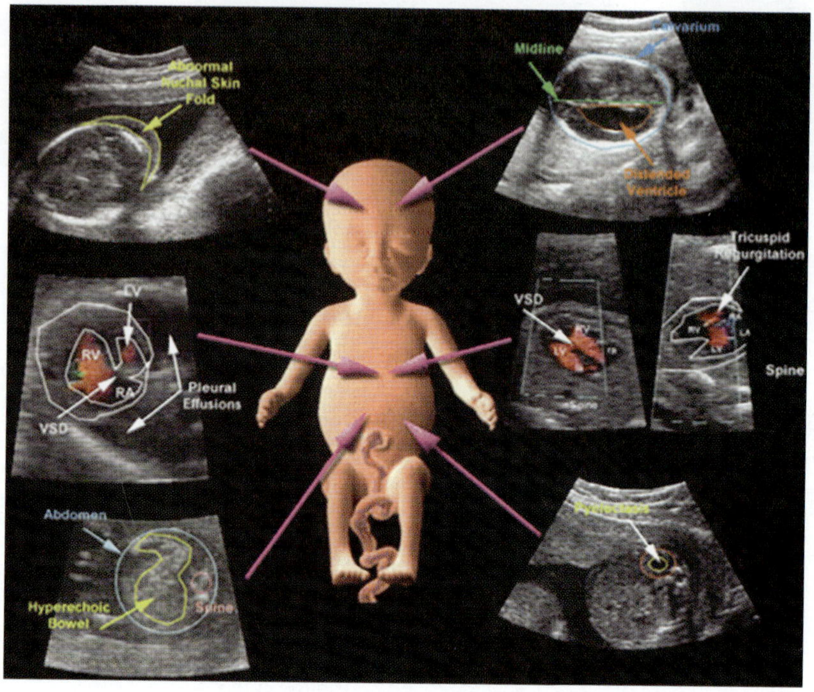

Fig. 1.15: *Genetic ultrasound is a technique in which fetuses are examined for anatomical defects that have been associated with an increased risk for Down syndrome. The reason that this concept was developed because of the number of physical features identified in children with this condition*

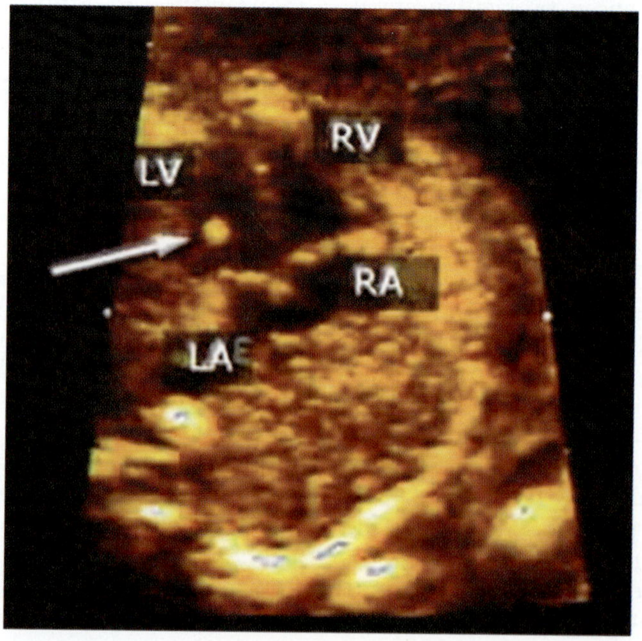

Fig. 1.16: *Four-chamber view. Note the white arrow pointing the echogenic foci in the left ventricule. Echogenic foci are usually of no pathological significance and in more than 90% of cases the resolve by the third trimester or during pregnancy. However, they are sometimes associated with cardiac defects and chromosomal abnormalities. For isolated hyperechogenic foci, the risk for trisomy 21 may be three-times the background maternal age and gestation-related risk*

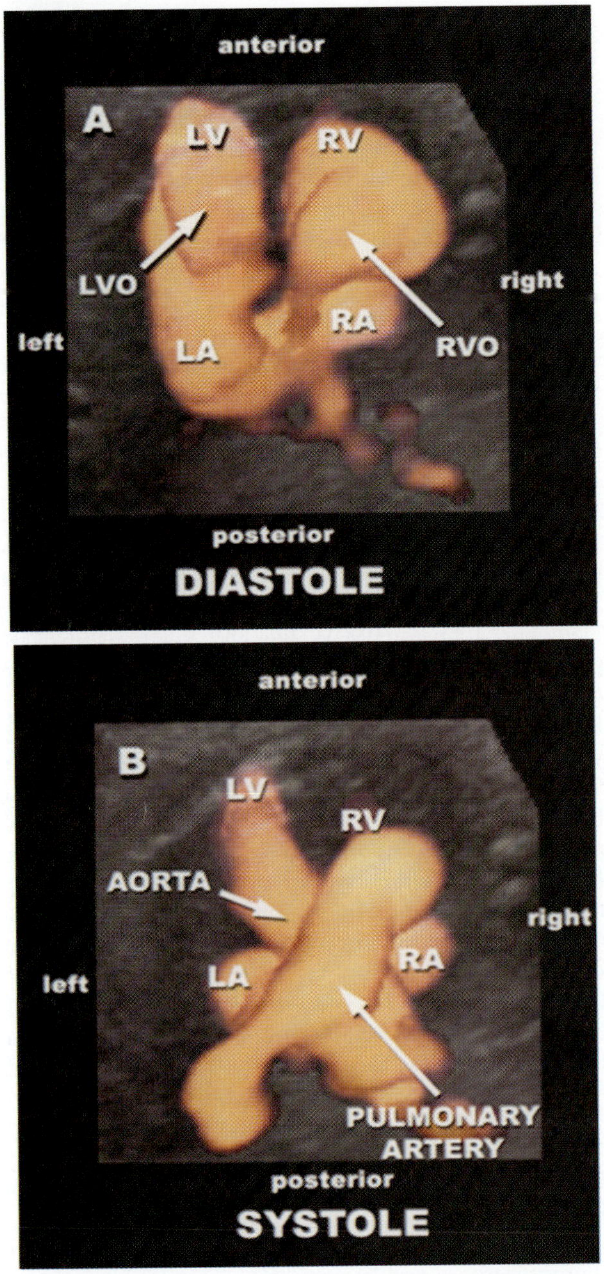

Fig. 1.17: *Four dimensional ultrasonography. Volume-rendered image of the outflow tracts during diastole (panel A) and systole (panel B). The volume was acquired with power Doppler imaging. Note the right and left ventricular outlets (RVO and LVO) clearly visualized at the end of diastole, before opening of the aortic and pulmonary valves. Panel B shows the normal criss-crossing of the atrioventricular valves during systole*

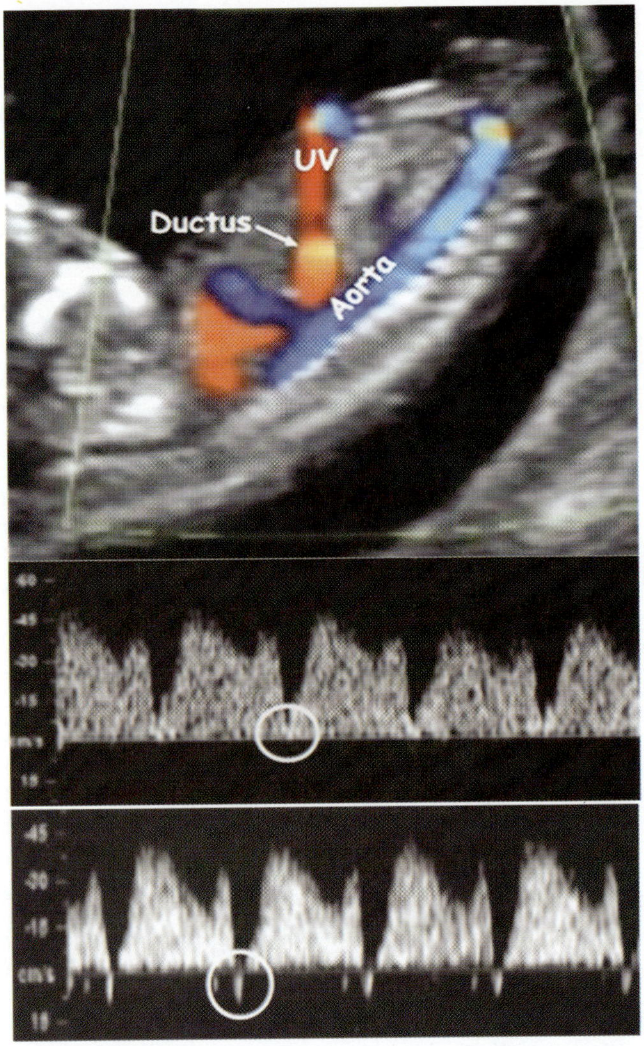

Fig. 1.18: *(Upper) shows ductus venosus in color flow (middle) positive a-wave and (bottom) reversed a-wave. The incidence of reversed ductus venosus a-wave is related to NT and CRL as well as aneuploidy, being more common when the NT is high and the CRL is low. Therefore, it is not possible to give simple numbers by which the presence of normal flow will reduce the risk for trisomy 21 and the presence of reversed a-wave will increase the risk. The FMF software firstly calculates a risk based on maternal age, fetal NT and maternal serum free (β-hCG) and PAPP-A. If the risk is more than 1 in 50 and ductus venosus flow is normal the risk does not change. If the risk is 1 in 50 to 1 in 1,000 and the ductus venosus flow is normal the risk is usually reduced. If there is reversed a-wave, the risk is always increased. In addition, there is an increased risk for cardiac defects and therefore such patients should have a follow-up specialist fetal cardiac scan*

BIBLIOGRAPHY

1. Rudolph AM, Heymann MA: Circulatory changes during growth in the fetal lamb. *Circ Res* 26:289–299, 1970.
2. Edelstone DI, Rudolph AM, Heymann MA: Liver and ductus venosus blood flows in fetal lambs in utero. *Circ Res* 42:426–433, 1978.
3. Edelstone DI, Rudolph AM, Heymann MA: Effects of hypoxemia and decreasing umbilical flow on liver and ductus venosus blood flows in fetal lambs. *Am J Physiol* 238:H656–H663, 1980.
4. Bristow J, Rudolph AM, Itskovitz J, Barnes RJ: Hepatic oxygen and glucose metabolism in the fetal lamb. *J Clin Invest* 71:1–15, 1983.

5. Edelstone DI, Rudolph AM: Preferential streaming of ductus venosus blood to the brain and heart in fetal lambs. *Am J Physiol* 237:H724–H729, 1979.
6. Reuss ML, Rudolph AM, Heymann MA: Selective distribution of microspheres injected into the umbilical veins and inferior venae cavae of fetal sheep. *Am J Obstet Gynecol* 141:427–431, 19S1.
7. Bristow J, Rudolph AM, Itskovitz J: A preparation for studying liver blood flow, oxygen consumption, and metabolism in the fetal lambs in utero. *J Dev Physiol* 3:255–266, 1981.
8. Heymann MA, Creasy RK, Rudolph AM: Quantitation of blood flow patterns in the fetal lamb in utero. In *Proceedings of the Sir Joseph Barcroft Centenary Symposium: Foetal and Neonatal Physiology*. Cambridge, Cambridge University Press, 1973, pp 129–135.
9. Sahn DJ, Lange LW, Allen HD, et al.: Quantitative real-time cross-sectional echocardiography in the developing normal human fetus and newborn. *Circulation* 62:588–597, 1980.
10. Reed KL, Meijboom EJ, Sahn DJ, et al.: Cardiac Doppler flow velocities in human fetuses. *Circulation* 73:41+46, 1986.
11. Peeters LLH, Sheldon RE, Jones MD Jr, et al.: Blood flow to fetal organs as a function of arterial oxygen content. *Am J Obstet Gynecol* 135:637–646, 1979.
12. Sheldon RE, Peeters LLH, Jones MD Jr, et al.: Redistribution of cardiac output and oxygen delivery in the hypoxemic fetal lamb. *Am J Obstet Gynecol* l35:I071–1078, 1979.
13. Heymann MA, Rudolph AM: Effects of increasing preload on right ventricular output in fetal lambs in utero (abstract). *Circulation* 48:IV –37, 1973.
14. Friedman WF: The intrinsic physiologic properties of the developing heart. In Friedman WF, Lesch M, Sonnenblick EH (eds): *Neonatal Heart Disease*. New York, Grune and Stratton, 1973, pp 21–49.
15. Kirkpatrick SE, Pitlick PT, Naliboff JB, Friedman WF: Frank-Starling relationship as an important determinant of fetal cardiac output. *Am J Physiol* 231:495–500, 1976.
16. Gilbert RD: Control offetal cardiac output during changes in blood volume. *Am J Physiol* 238:H80–H86, 1980.
17. Gilbert RD: Effects of after load and baro-receptors on cardiac function in fetal sheep. *J Dev Physiol* 4:299–309, 1982.
18. Sheldon CA, Friedman WF, Sybers HD: Scanning electron microscopy of fetal and neonatal lamb cardiac cells. *J Mol Cell Cardiol* 8:853–862, 1976.
19. Friedman WF, Pool PE, Jacobowitz D, et al.: Sympathetic innervation of the developing rabbit heart. *Circ Res* 23:25–32, 1968.
20. Lebowitz EA, Novick JS, Rudolph AM: Development of myocardial sympathetic innervation in the fetal Iamb. *Pediatr Res* 6:887–893, 1972.
21. Lipp JM, Rudolph AM: Sympathetic nerve development in the rat and guinea pig heart. *Bio Neonate* 21:76–82, 1972.
22. Barrett CT, Heymann MA, Rudolph AM: Alpha and beta adrenergic function in fetal sheep. *Am J Obstet Gynecol* 112:1114–1121, 1972.
23. Rudolph AM, Heymann MA: Cardiac out-put in the fetal lamb: the effects of spontaneous and induced changes of heart rate on right and left ventricular output. *Am J Obstet Gynecoll* 24:183–192, 1976.
24. Vapaavouri EK, Shinebourne EA, Wil-liams RL, et al.: Development of cardiovascular responses to autonomic blockade in intact fetal and neonatal lambs. *Bio Neonate* 22:177–188, 1973.
25. Downing SE, Talner NS, Gardner TM: Ventricular function in the newborn lamb. *Am J Physiol* 208:931–937, 1965.
26. Fisher DJ, Heymann MA, Rudolph AM: Myocardial oxygen and carbohydrate consumption in fetal lambs in utero and in adult sheep. *Am J Physiol* 238:H399-H405, 1980.
27. Berman W Jr, Goodlin RC, Heymann MA, Rudolph AM: Relationships between pressure and flow in the umbilical and uterine circulations of the sheep. *Circ Res* 38:262–266, 1976.
28. PapHe L, Rudolph AM, Heymann MA: Autoregulation of cerebral blood flow in the preterm fetal lamb. *Pediatr Res* 19:159–161, 1985.
29. Shinebourne EA, Vapaavouri EK, Wil-liams RL, et al.: Development of baro-reflex activity in unanesthetized fetal and neonatal Iambs. *Circ Res* 31:710–718, 1972.
30. Maloney JE, Cannata JP, Dowling MH, et al.: Baroreflex activity in conscious fetal and newborn lambs. *Bio Neonate* 31:340–350, 1977.
31. Dawes GS, Johnston BM, Walker DW: Relationship of arterial pressure and heart rate in fetal, newhorn, and adult sheep. *J Physiol (Lond)* 309:405–417, 1980.
32. Biscoe TJ, Purves MJ, Sampson SR: Types of nervous activity which may be recorded from the carotid sinus nerve in the sheep foetus. *J Physiol (Lond)* 202:1–23, 1969.
33. Ponte J, Purves MJ: Types of afferent nervous activity which may be measured in the vagus nerve of the sheep foetus. *J Physiol (Lond)* 229:51–76, 1973.
34. Itskovitz J, LaGamma EF, Rudolph AM: Baroreflex control of the circulation in chronically instrumented fetal lambs. *Circ Res* 52:589–596, 1983.
35. Dawes GS, Duncan LB, Lewis BV, et al.: Cyanide stimulation of the systemic arterial chemoreceptors in fetal lambs. *J Physiol (Lond)* 201:117–128,1969.
36. Goodlin RC, Rudolph AM: Factors asso-ciated with initiation of breathing. In Ho-dari AA, Mariona FG (eds): *Proceedings of the International Symposium on Physiological Biochemistry of the Fetus*. Springfield, IL, Charles C Thomas, 1972, pp 294–318.
37. Itskovitz J, Rudolph AM: Denervation of arterial chemoreceptors and baroreceptors in fetal lambs in utero. *Am J Physiol* 242:H916–H920, 1982.
38. Zink J, Van Petten GR: Noradrenergic control of blood vessels in the premature lamb fetus. *Bio Neonate* 39:61–69, 1981.
39. Cheng JB, Cornett LE, Goldfien A, Roberts JM: Decreased concentration of myocardial alpha-adrenoceptors with increasing age in fetal Iambs. *Br J Pharmacol 70:515–517,* 1980.
40. Cheng JB, Goldfien A, Cornett LE, Roberts JM: Identification of 3-adrenergic receptors using (3H)dihydroalprenolol in fetal sheep heart: direct evidence of qualitative similarity to the receptors in adult sheep heart. *Pediatr Res* 15:1083–1087, 1981.
41. Whitsett JA, Pollinger J, Matz S: 3-Adrenergic receptors and catecholamine sensitive adenylate cyclase in developing rat ventricular myocardium: effect of thyroid status. *Pediatr Res* 16:463–469, 1982.
42. Nuwayhid B, Brinkman CR III, Su C, et al.: Systemic and pulmonary hemodynamic responses to adrenergic and

cholinergic agonists during fetal development. *Bio Neonate* 26:301–317, 1975.

43. Harris WH, Van Petten GR: Development of cardiovascular responses to nor-adrenaline, normetanephrine and metanephrine in the unanesthetised fetus. *Can J Physiol Pharmacol* 57:242–250, 1979.
44. Assali NS, Brinkman CR III, Woods JR Jr, et al.: Development of neurohumoral control of fetal, neonatal, and adult cardiovascular functions. *Am J Obstet Gynecol* 129:748–759, 1977.
45. Wyse DG, Van Petten GR, Harris WH: Responses to electrical stimulation, nor-adrenaline, seratonin, and vasopressin in the isolated ear artery of the developing lamb and ewe. *Can J Physiol Pharmacol* 55:1000–1006, 1977.
46. Harris WH, Van Petten GR: Development of cardiovascular responses to sympathomimetic amines and autonomic blockade in the unanesthetised fetus. *Can J Physiol Pharmacol* 56:400–409, 1978.
47. Walker AM, Cannata J, Dowling MH, et al.: Sympathetic and parasympathetic control of heart rate in uoonesthetised fetal and newborn lambs. *Bio Neonate* 33:135–143, 1978.
48. Comline RS, Silver lA, Silver M: Factors responsible for the stimulation of the adrenal medulla during asphyxia in the fetal lamb. *J Physiol (Lond)* 178:211–238, 1965.
49. Jones CT, Robinson RD: Plasma catecholamines in fetal and adult sheep. *J Physiol (Lond)* 248:15–33, 1975.
50. Lewis AB, Evans WN, Sischo W: Plasma catecholamine responses to hypoxemia in fetal Iambs. *Bio Neonate* 41:115–122, 1982.
51. Lorijn RWH, Longo LD: Norepinephrine elevation in the fetal lamb: oxygen consumption and cardiac output. *Am J Physiol* 239:R115-RI22, 1980.
52. Smith FGJr, Lupu AN, Barajas L, et al.: The renin-angiotensin system in the fetal lamb. *Pediatr Res* 8:611–620, 1974.
53. Broughton-Pipkin F, Lumbers ER, Mott JC: Factors influencing plasma renin and angiotensin II in the conscious pregnant ewe and its foetus. *J Physiol (Lond)* 243:619–636, 1974.
54. Iwamoto HS, Rudolph AM: Effects of endogenous angiotensin II on the fetal circulation. *J Dev Physiol* 283–293, 1979.
55. Iwamoto HS, Rudolph AM, Keil LC, Hey-mann MA: Hemodynamic responses of the sheep fetus to vasopressin infusion. *Circ Res* 44:430–436, 1979.
56. Carver JG, Mott JC: Renin substrate in plasma of unanesthetized pregnant ewes and their fetal lambs. *J Physiol (Lond)* 276:395–402, 1978.
57. Iwamoto HS, Rudolph AM: Effects of angiotensin II on the blood flow and its distribution in fetal Iambs. *Circ Res* 48:183-188, 1982.
58. Omini C, Vigano T, Marini A, et al.: Angiotensin II: A releaser of PGI2 from fetal and newborn rabbit lungs. *Prostaglandins* 25:901–910, 1983.
59. Drummond WH, Rudolph AM, Keil LC, et al.: Arginine vasopressin and prolactin after hemorrhage in the fetal lamb. *Am J Physiol* 238:E214–E219, 1980.
60. Rurak DW: Plasma vasopressin levels during hypoxaemia and the cardiovascular effects of exogenous vasopressin in fetal and adult sheep. *J Physiol (Lond)* 277:341–357, 1978.
61. Challis JRG, Dilley SR, Robinson JS, Thorburn GD: Prostaglandins in the circulation of the fetal lamb. *Prostagtandins* 11:1041–1052, 1976.
62. Challis JRG, Patrick JE: The production of prostaglandins and thromboxanes in the feto-placental unit and their effects on the developing fetus. *Semin Perinatal* 4:23–33, 1980.
63. Mitchell MD, Flint AP, Bibby J, et al.: Plasma concentrations of prostaglandins during late human pregnancy: influence of normal and pretel'm labor. *J Clin Endocrinol Metab* 46:947–951, 1978.
64. Terragno NA, Terragno A, McGiff JC: Role of prostaglandins in blood vessels. *Semin Perinatal* 4:85–90, 1980.
65. Novy MJ, Piasecki G, Jackson BT: Effect of prostaglandins E, and F2 alpha on umbilical blood flow and fetal hemodynamics. *Prostaglandins* 5:543–555, 1974.
66. Berman W Jr, Goodlin RC, Heymann MA, Rudolph AM: Effects of pharmacologic agents on umbilical blood flow in fetal lambs in utero. *Bio Neonate* 33:225–235, 1978.
67. Cassin S: Role of prostaglandins and thromboxanes in the control of the pulmonary circulation in the fetus and newborn. *Semin Perinatol* 4:101–107, 1980.
68. Tripp ME, Heymann MA, RudIJlph AM: Hemodynamic effects of prostaglandin Eon lambs in utero. In Coceani F, Olley PM (eds): Prostagtandin and Perinatal Medicine: Advances in Prostagtandin and Thromboxane Research. New York, Raven.

2 Anatomy and Physiology of the Cardiovascular System

1. ANATOMY OF CARDIOVASCULAR SYSTEM

The heart is a midline, valvular, muscular pump that is cone-shaped and the size of a fist. It weighs 300 gm in adults and lies in the middle mediastinum of the thorax. The inferior (diaphragmatic) surface sits on the central tendon of the diaphragm, and the base faces posteriorly and lies immediately anterior to the esophagus and descending aorta. The base comprises mainly the left atrium, with a small portion of right atrium. The left surface (left ventricle) and right surface (right atrium) are related laterally to the phrenic nerve and the lung, respectively. The anterior surface of the heart lies behind the sternum and the costal cartilages. The constituent parts of the anterior and inferior surfaces are largely dictated by the position of the interventricular septum.

The interventricular septum bulges to the right because the wall of the left ventricle is a much thicker (10 mm) than that of the right ventricle (3–5 mm). It also lies obliquely across the heart, almost in the coronal plane, such that the anterior surface of the heart is two-thirds right entricle and one-third left ventricle; the proportions are reversed on muscles of the four chambers and the four valves are attached to and supported by a figure-of-eight-shaped fibrous skeleton comprising a fibrous body and extensions (fila coronaria) that surround the valves. This skeleton both divides and electrically separates the atria from the ventricles is the remnant of the atrioventricular (AV) cushions, and forms the thinner, membranous part of the interventricular septum. (Figs 2.1, 2.2, 2.7a, b, c, d and 2.12)

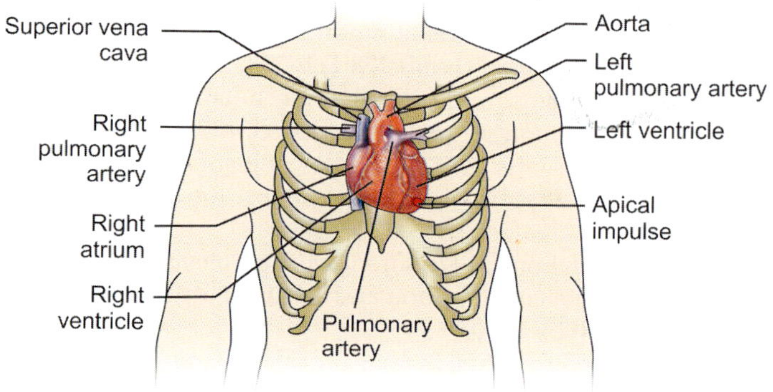

Fig. 2.1: *Illustration showing various anatomical structures of the heart as observed from outside*

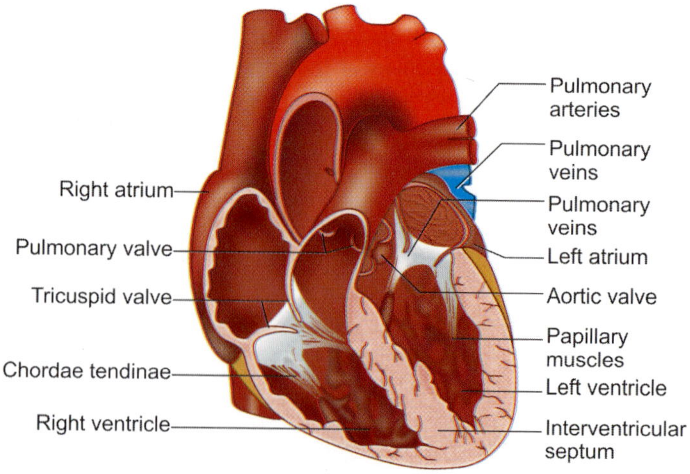

Fig. 2.2: *Illustration showing anatomical placement of various chambers, valves and great vessels of heart*

PERICARDIUM

The pericardium holds and protects the heart but provides sufficient potential space for filling and emptying of the chambers. The outer layer is the tough fibrous pericardium which blends with the adventitia of the aorta, the pulmonary trunk, the superior vena cava and the central tendon of the diaphragm. Within this, there are two layers of serous pericardium: (1) a visceral layer, lining the heart (2) a parietal layer, lining the inner surface of the fibous pericardium. These two layers of serous pericardium are continuous with each other as they reflect off the major vessels behind and above the heart. The reflection between the pulmonary veins is termed the 'oblique sinus of the heart'. The plane between the superior vena cava and the pulmonary veins posteriorly, and the aorta and the pulmonary trunk anteriorly, made by the folding of the heart, is termed the 'transverse sinus of the heart' (Fig. 2.3)

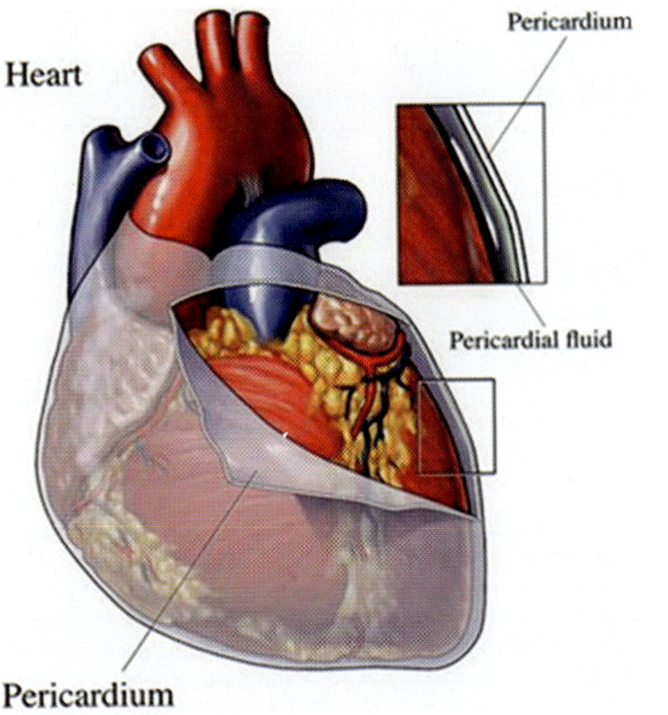

Fig. 2.3: *Anatomical features cut section of pericardium surrounded by neighboring structures*

Features of the Chambers (Figs 2.2 and 2.4)

Right Atrium

The inferior vena cava passes through the diaphragm at the level of T8 and immediately enters the right atrium, which lacks a true valve. In the fetus, however, there is tissue present that forms a valve, and which guides the blood into the foramen ovale. The superior vena cava enters the superior aspect of the chamber. The fossa ovalis (a remnant of the septum primum) and its overhanging limbus (a remnant of the septum secundum) lie on the smooth, interatrial part of the chamber, which is developed from the sinus venosus. This smooth area is separated from the muscular part with its musculi pectinati by the crista terminalis internally and the sulcus terminalis externally. The muscular part originated from the fetal atrium and is represented in the mature heart as the right auricle. Between the opening of the inferior vena cava and the AV orifice lies the opening of the coronary sinus, which is protected by a small valve that prevents regurgitation into the coronary sinus during atrial contraction. The AV node lies between this orifice and the septal cusp of the tricuspid valve.

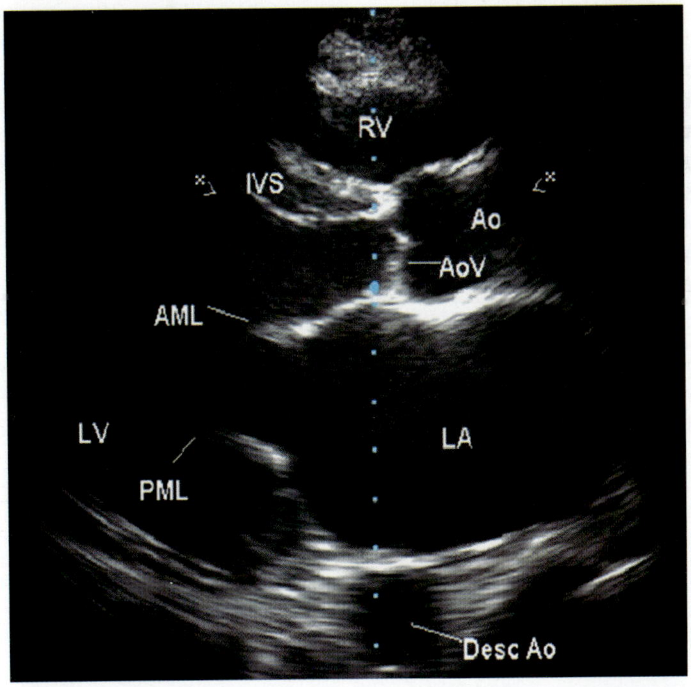

Fig. 2.4: *Transthoracic echo scan taken in long-axis view showing different chambers of the heart aorta: RV: right ventricle; LV: left ventricle; IVS: interventricular septum; Ao: aorta; AoV: aortic valve; LA: left atrium; PML: posterior mitral leaflet; AML: anterior mitral leaflet; Desc Ao: descending aorta. The mitral valve is widely open and aortic valve is closed*

Right Ventricle

Blood enters the right ventricle via the tricuspid valve, which has anterior, septal and posterior (lying inferior) cusps attached to papillary muscles by fibrous chordae tendineae. The ventricular wall is normally 3–5 mm thick and is raised internally by interweaving strands of muscle (trabeculae carneae). Some of this muscle joins the anterior papillary muscle, low on the anterior septal wall, as the septomarginal trabecula (moderator band) and carries part of the right bundle branch of conducting tissue. Blood passes upward to leave this chamber via the smooth conus arteriosus (infundibulum) and the pulmonary valve, which has two anterior cusps and one posterior cusp.

Left Atrium

The left atrium is a box-shaped chamber that lies at the base of the heart and receives blood from the lungs via four large valveless pulmonary veins into the four quadrants of the chamber. The terminology and development of the smooth and muscular parts of the left atrium correspond to those of the right atrium.

Left Ventricle

Blood enters the left ventricle via the mitral valve, which has larger anterior and smaller posterior cusps, each with chordae tendineae and papillary muscle. The muscle wall is about 10 mm thick and is roughened by trabeculae carneae. The smooth outflow tract is the aortic vestibule, corresponding to the membranous part of the interventricular septum, leading to the aortic valve with its two posterior cusps and one anterior cusp (APAP-aortic posterior anterior posterior). The relationship of these cusps to the ostia of the coronary arteries is described below. The trabeculated pattern of the musculi pectinati and the trabeculae carneae is an efficient means of gaining power without excessively thickening the wall of the chamber. A single papillary muscle has separate chordae tendineae to two adjacent valvular cusps, which helps draw them together and prevents valvular eversion during systole.

CONDUCTING SYSTEM OF THE HEART (Fig. 2.5)

Specialized cardiac muscle fibers form the: sinoatrial node (in the right atrial wall between the opening of the superior vena cava and the auricle).

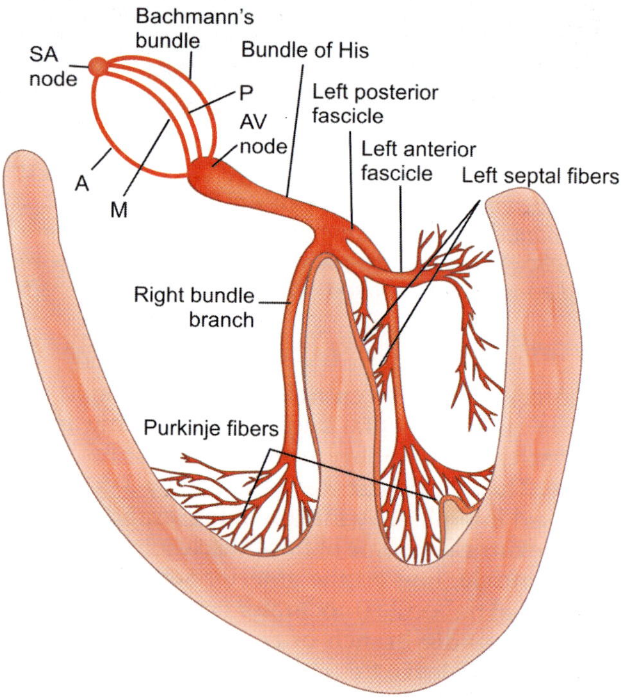

Fig. 2.5: *Diagrammatic depiction of different structures of conducting system in human as indicated on the diagram*

AV Node

AV bundle arising from the AV node and descending in the interventricular septum. Contractions originating from the sinoatrial node (pacemaker) spread through the atrial walls to reach the AV node, and then to the left and right bundles. The plexus of Purkinje fibers allows spread of excitation to the ventricular walls. Further autonomic nervous control is via cardiac branches from each of the cervical sympathetic ganglia and thoracic ganglia T 1–5; parasympathetic fibers arise from the superior and inferior cardiac branches of the vagus and from the recurrent laryngeal nerve. All autonomic nerves pass via the superficial and deep cardiac plexuses on the lateral and medial aspects of the aortic arch.

BLOOD SUPPLY TO THE HEART

The ostia of the coronary arteries arise in the aortic sinuses above the attachment of the base of the relevant cusp; the right from the anterior sinus and the left from the left posterior sinus. (Figs 2.6, 2.10 a, b, c, d, 2.8 and 2.11 a, b)

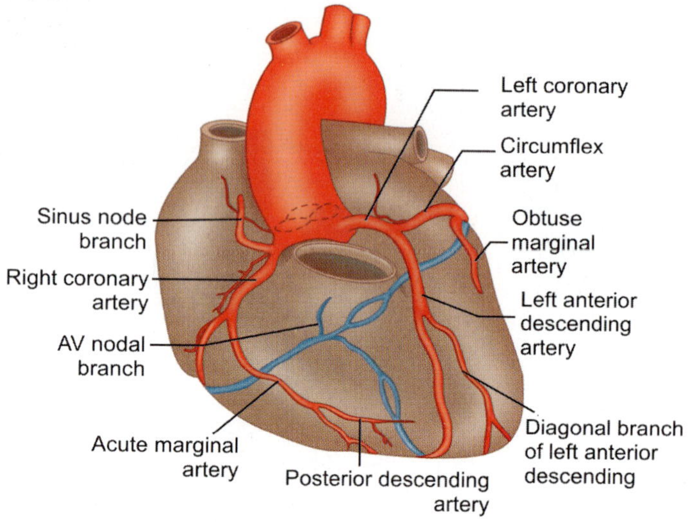

Fig. 2.6: *Shows blood supply of the heart through coronary arterial system and tries to explain as to how the coronary arteries originate from the ascending aorta to supply the heart with oxygenated blood. The demand for fresh, oxygenated blood is substantial for the heart. Like brain cells, the cells that work collectively to form the structure of the heart will not live for very long (respirate anaerobically) without oxygen*

Right Coronary Artery

The right coronary artery passes from its origin anteriorly between the right atrial appendage and the pulmonary trunk to enter first the right anterior AV groove and then the right posterior AV groove, where it anastomoses with the circumflex branch of the left coronary artery. In 90% of individuals, it gives off the posterior interventricular branch as it reaches the posterior interventricular groove on the inferior surface of the heart; this anastomoses with the termination of the anterior interventricular artery (left coronary) in the groove.

Left Coronary Artery

The left coronary artery arises from the left posterior aortic sinus and passes anteriorly between the left atrial appendage and the pulmonary trunk, to lie in the left anterior AV groove. Here, it divides into the: circumflex artery and anterior interventricular artery.

The circumflex artery continues first in the anterior and in the posterior AV grooves, and anastomoses with the terminal branches of the right coronary artery. The anterior interventricular artery (often termed the 'anterior descending artery').

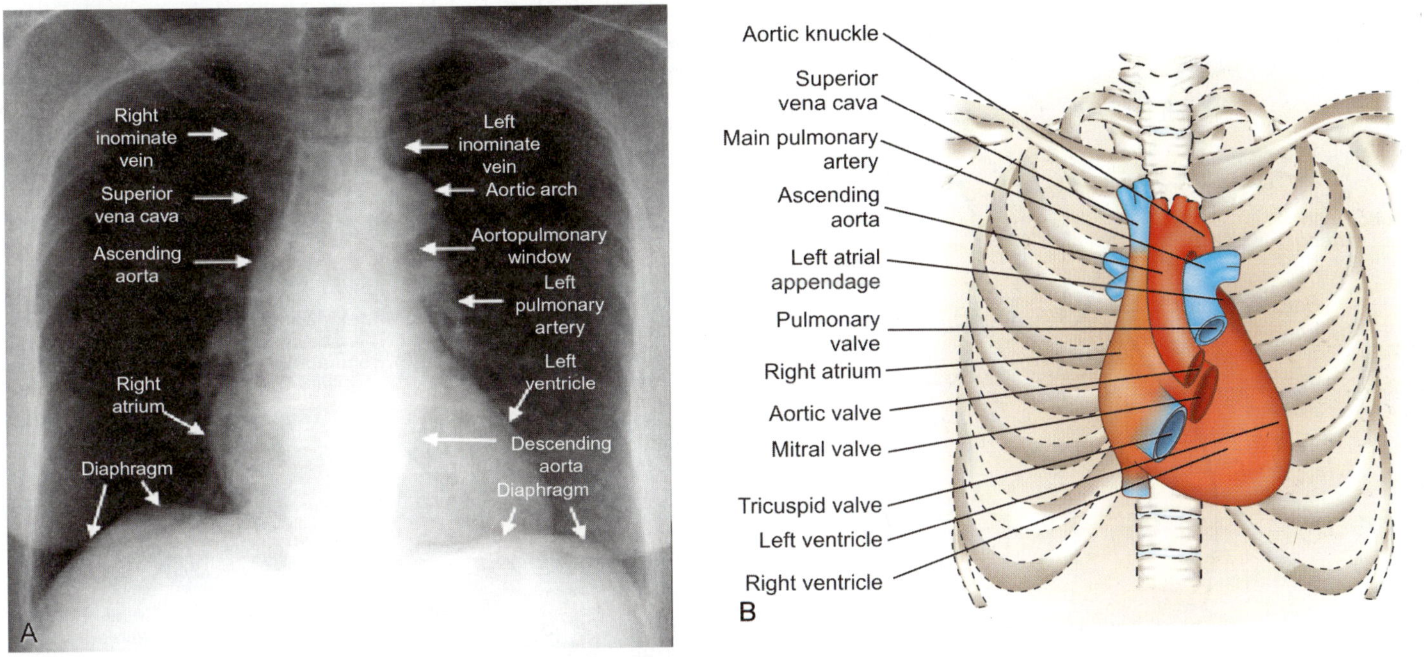

Fig. 2.7A and B: *(Left and right panels) photograph of X-ray chest (PA view) and illustration showing various anatomical structures of heart and its great vessels (shown written with arrows on skiagram)*

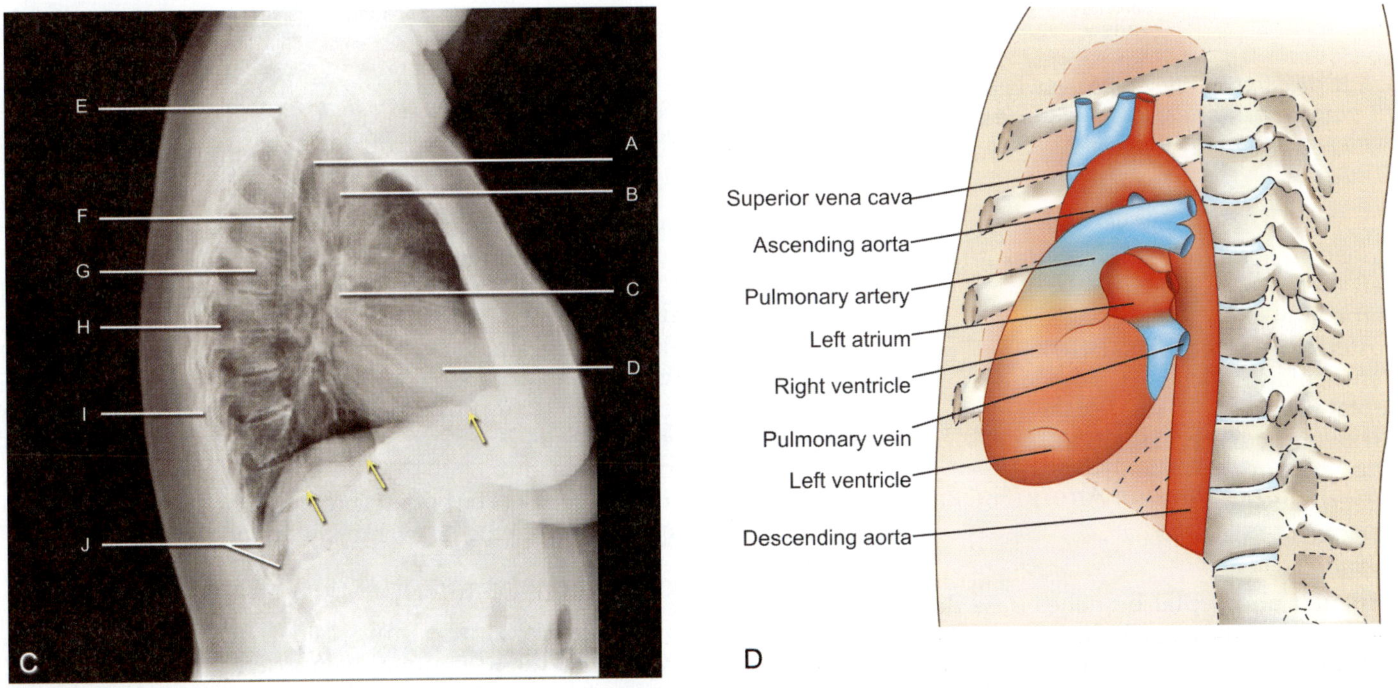

Fig. 2.7C and D: *(Left and right panels) photograph of X-ray chest (PA view) and illustration showing various anatomical structures of heart and its great vessels shown written with arrows on skiagram). Structures that should be demonstrated on the left lateral chest radiograph include: esophagus (A), trachea (B), lung hili (C), heart silhouette (D), lung apices (E), scapulae (F), thoracic vertebra (G), thoracic intervertebral foramen (H), superimposed posterior ribs (I), costophrenic angles (J), and diaphragm (yellow arrows)*

Branches of the Coronary Artery System

Right Coronary Artery

Left atrial

- Right conus
- Sinoatrial nodal (60% of individuals)

Right atrial

- Right marginal
- Posterior interventricular (90%)
- Ventricular branches, septal branches
- Atrioventricular nodal (90%).

Smaller branches to the right ventricle

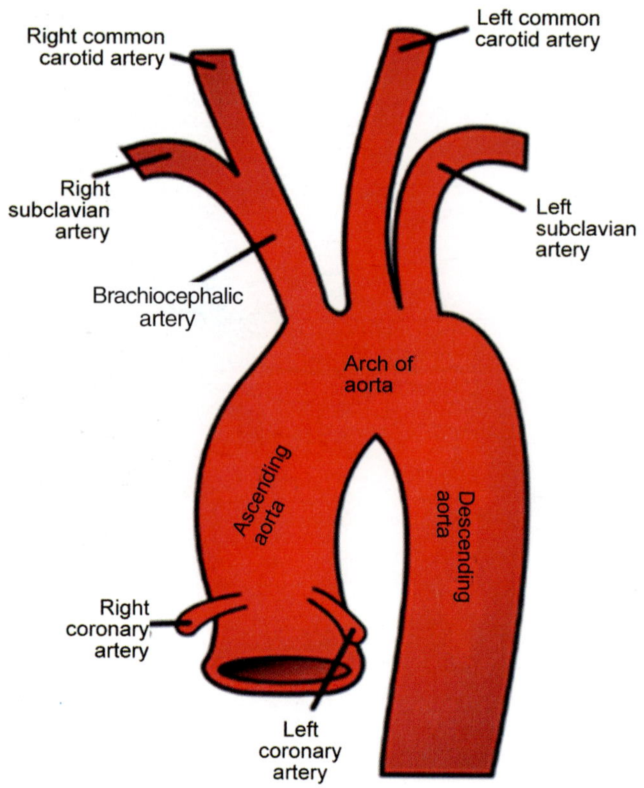

Fig. 2.8: *Illustration shows ascending aorta, emerging left and right coronary arteries, arch of aorta with its branches and descending aorta*

Left Coronary Artery (Fig. 2.6)

- Sinoatrial nodal (40%) circumflex artery
- Left marginal
- Left conus
- Posterior interventricular (10%)
- Ventricular branches
- Septal branches
- Atrioventricular nodal (10%).

Anterior Interventricular Artery (Fig. 2.10C)

Left conus

Diagonal

Ventricular and septal branches pass down in the same groove, around the apex of the heart and anastomoses with the terminal branches of the posterior interventricular artery. The 10% of individuals in whom most of the both ventricles and the septum are supplied by the left coronary artery are said to have left cardiac dominance. There is parallel collateral communication between the right and the left coronary systems.

VENOUS DRAINAGE OF THE HEART

The veins of the heart are more variable than arteries. Drainage of the left and right ventricles starts with the great cardiac vein in the anterior interventricular groove. It passes to the left in the anterior AV groove, where it collects the left marginal vein and, as it runs in the posterior AV groove, is joined by the oblique vein of the left atrium, the posterior ventricular vein and, finally the middle cardiac vein, which lies in the posterior interventricular groove and drains the left and right ventricles posteriorly (Figs 2.9 and 2.11B).

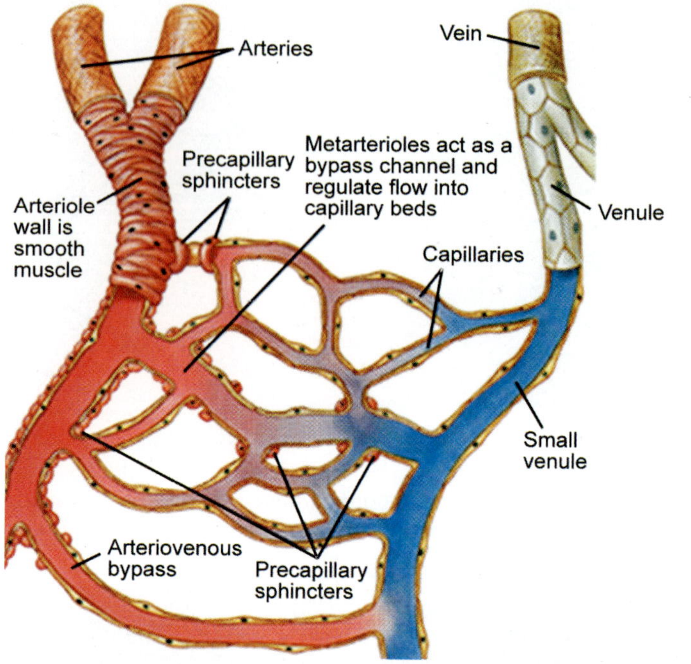

Fig. 2.9: *Showing blood circulating through various arteriovenus and capillary system of the body*

The confluence of these veins is the 3 cm long coronary sinus, lying in the posterior AV groove just before the coronary sinus enters the right atrium via the left of the entry of the inferior vena cava, it is usually joined by the small cardiac vein, which drains the right atrium and right ventricle. The small cardiac vein sometimes drains directly into the right atrium. A couple of anterior cardiac veins drain the anterior aspect of the right ventricle and right atrium before crossing the right coronary artery to enter the right atrium. In addition, 20–30% of all drainage is in the venae cordis minimae (The besian veins), which drain directly into the chambers of the heart, mostly on the right side.

PHYSIOLOGY OF THE NORMAL HEART

The normally functioning heart provides sufficient oxygenated blood containing nutrients, metabolites and hormones to meet moment-by-moment metabolic needs and to preserve a constant internal milieu. Its two essential characteristics are contractility and rhythmicity. In the regulation of these, the nervous system and neurohumoral effects modulate relationships between venous return, outflow resistance, frequency of contraction and inotropic state; there are also intrinsic cardiac autoregulatory mechanisms.

Electrical Events

It shows the impulse-generating and impulse-conducting system of the normal heart. The cardiac cycle begins with

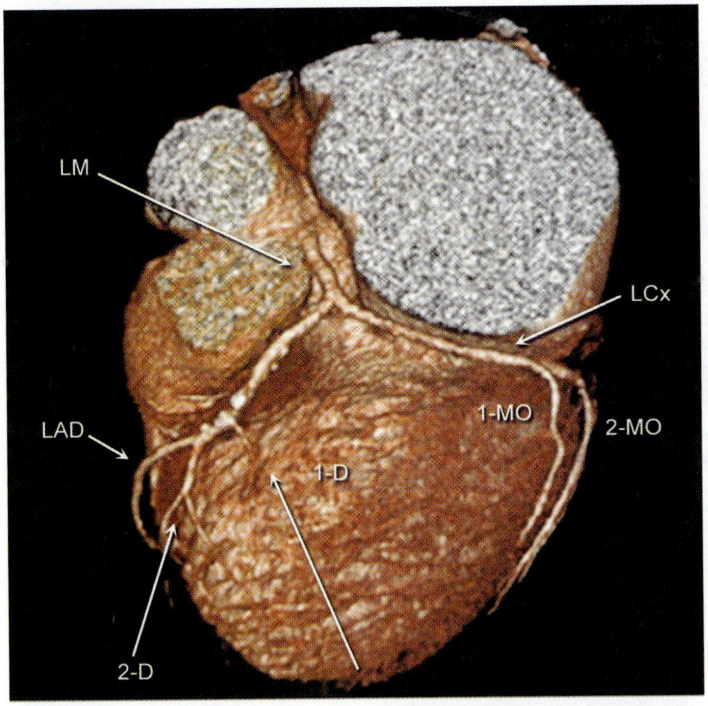

Fig. 2.10A: *Coronary CT angiographic results in patient with a dilated left atrium and atrial fibrillation with mean heart rate of 73 beats per minute at coronary CT angiographic acquisition. Volume-rendered CT image (left anterior oblique view with cranial angulation) shows the arteries: left main (LM), left anterior descending (LAD), first diagonal (1-D), second diagonal (2-D), left circumflex (LCx), and first and second marginal obtuse branches (1-MO, 2-MO)*

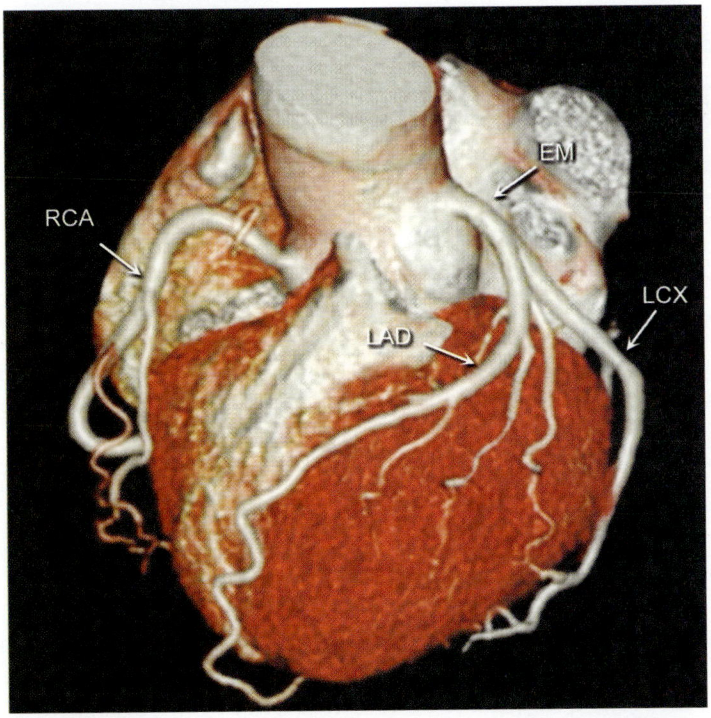

Fig 2.10B: *MDCT showing anatomical location coronary arteries of heart as depicted on the scan*

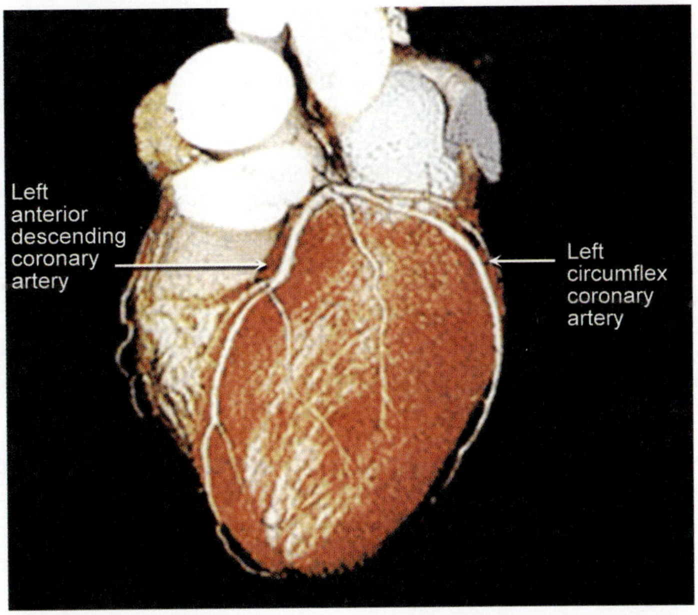

Fig. 2.10C: *A cardiac computed tomography angiogram showing left anterior descending and left circumflex coronary arteries*

depolarization of the sinoatrial node in the upper right atrium and spread of the action potential through the atria, resulting in atrial systole. The connective tissue of the atrioventricular (AV) groove prevents cell-cell conduction of the electrical impulse from atrium to ventricle, permitting this only through the specialized cells of the AV node. This region of slow conductance delays cells and maintain a diastolic intracellular potential of about –90 mV, but depolarize spontaneously. The sinoatrial node has the fastest inherent depolarization rate and normally determines the heart rate. When this does not function, pacemaker tissue in the AV node, bundle of His or Purkinje system assumes this role, but the heart rate is then considerably slower.

Mechanical Events

After the P-wave of the ECG, and coinciding with atrial systole, a waves appear in left and right atrial pressure tracings and the jugular venous pulse. Atrial contraction increases ventricular filling by about 10%. The onset of the ventricular contraction coincides with the peak wave of the R-wave of the ECG, and the rapid increase in intraventricular pressure closes the mitral and tricuspid valves. This produces the first heart sound. When ventricular pressure exceed those in the pulmonary artery and aorta, the outflow valves open and ventricular ejection follows. As the strength of the ventricular contraction declines, the aortic and pulmonary valves close, coinciding with the end of the T-wave of the ECG and the dicrotic notch seen in both pressure tracings. Aortic closure slightly precedes pulmonary closure, resulting in the two components of the second heart sound. A third heart sound coinciding with the subsequent period of early rapid diastolic filling is also usually audible in children and young adults.

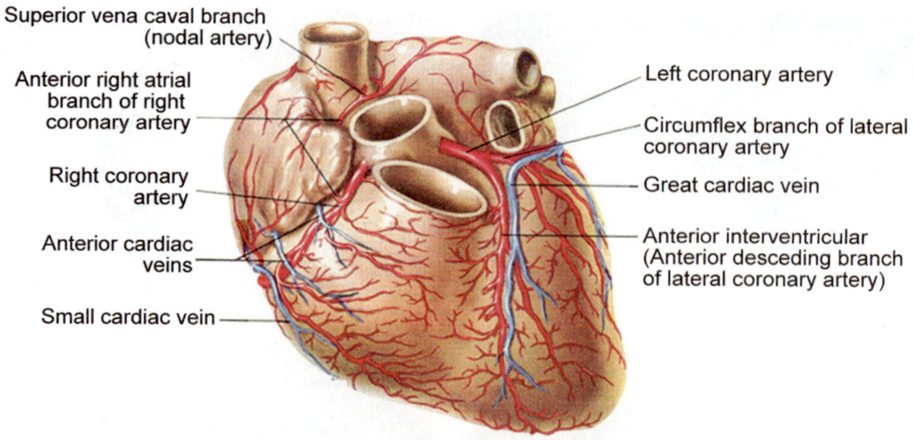

Fig. 2.11A: *Coronary arterial and venous system in sternocostal aspect of the heart*

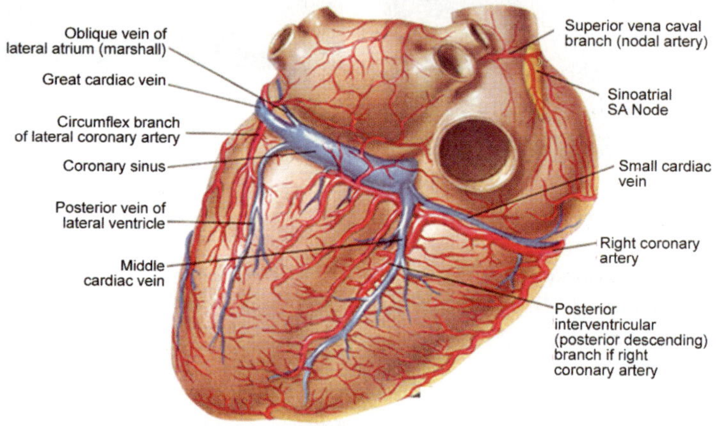

Fig. 2.11B: *Coronary arterial and venous system in diaphragmatic aspect of the heart*

II. BIOCHEMISTRY AND PHYSIOLOGY OF CARDIAC MUSCLE (Figs 2.13 to 2.17 and 2.19)

The synchronous contraction of cardiac myocytes during ventricular systole generates the power required to pump blood out of the heart. Conversely, myocyte relaxation and the passive properties of the ventricles during diastole (dependent largely on the properties of the extracellular matrix) determine the filling of the heart between beats. Several interacting regulatory processes operate to ensure that cardiac performance is finely tuned to match circulatory requirements. This contribution provides an overview of the mechanisms that regulate cardiac contractility, dysfunction of which is implicated in disease states such as heart failure.

Cardiac Myocyte Structure

The sarcolemmal membrane of cardiac myocytes has invaginations that form an extensive T-tubule network, regions of which lie in close apposition with the sarcoplasmic reticulum. The sarcoplasmic reticulum is the major intracellular store of calcium, the central regulator of cardiac contractility. The fundamental contractile unit, the sarcomere, is formed from contractile myofibrils, which comprise interdigitating thin filaments (actin and regulatory proteins, tropomyosin and troponin-C, I and T) and thick filaments (myosin). Interspersed between the myofibrils are numerous mitochondria, which generate the energy (ATP) to fuel contraction.

Excitation-Contraction Coupling

Electrical excitation of the myocyte initiates a dramatic transient increase in intracellular calcium concentration (the so called calcium transient). The events that couple sarcolemmal depolarization to elevation of calcium and initiation of contraction are known as excitation-contraction coupling. During each heart beat, the depolarization wave spreads across the sarcolemma and T-tubule system, and initiates calcium influx through voltage-gated L-type calcium channels. This calcium influx or calcium current (l_{ca}) initiates further release of calcium from the sarcoplasmic reticulum (calcium-induced calcium release). The elementary unit of sarcoplasmic reticulum calcium release, the calcium spark, represents calcium released locally from the opening of a few calcium release channels. According to the local control theory of excitation-contraction coupling, the cell calcium transient represents the spatial and temporal summation of individual calcium

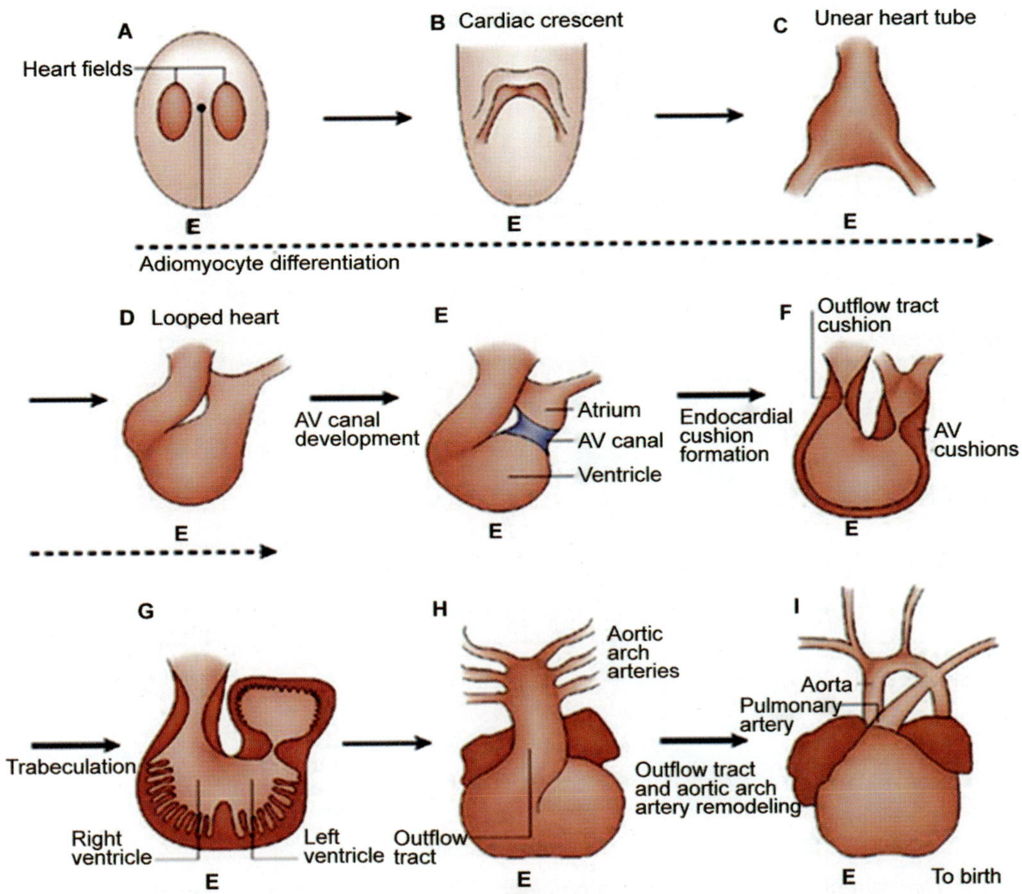

Fig. 2.12: *The principal stages of cardiac development are shown in the figure, highlighting the processes that involve notch. The primary heart fields (part A) are two bilateral regions of mesoderm that are specified shortly after gastrulation and contain the precursors of many cardiac lineages. These two heart fields then converge at the midline of the embryo to form the cardiac crescent (part B) and then the heart tube (part C), which consists of an endothelial tube surrounded by a single layer of myocardial cells. This tube then elongates and undergoes a rightward looping (part D), gaining additional cells from a second group of progenitor cells that originate in the pharynx, known as the secondary heart field. The heart is remodeled from a linear tube into a structure that contains four distinct chambers via a complex series of steps. This involves formation of the atrioventricular (AV) canal, which forms a boundary between the presumptive atrial and the ventricular regions of the heart tube (part E), the formation of endocardial cushions (the outflow tract and AV cushions), which will act as the precursors of the four major heart valves (the aortic, pulmonic, tricuspid and mitral valves; part F), the development of trabeculae within the walls of each of the heart chambers (right and left ventricle; part G), the septation of the atria and ventricles, and remodelling of the outflow tract to form the aorta and the pulmonary artery (parts H–I). The approximate stages of mouse development in embryonic days (E) are indicated for each part. All structures are viewed from their ventral aspect, with the top of the page representing cranial-anterior, and the bottom of the page representing caudal-posterior*

sparks. The contractile machinery is switched on by binding of calcium to troponin-C on the thin filament, which enables projections (SI heads) on the myosin molecules to interact with actin filaments, forming cross-bridges. This energy requiring process involves ATP hydrolysis by myosin ATPase. Repetitive cross-bridge cycles of attachment and detachment continue as long as the cytosolic calcium concentration is high. The power stroke generated by the cross-bridge cycle is responsible for force generation or muscle shortening. Cross bridge interactions show cooperativity; that is, force-generating cross-bridges promote further binding of more cross-bridges, which effectively amplifies the calcium signal. Relaxation is governed by the cytoplasmic calcium concentration, consequent dissociation of calcium from troponin-C, and switching off of the actomyosin interaction. This involves active transport of calcium back into the sarcoplasmic reticuum (via sarcoplasmic reticulum Ca^{2+}-ATPase) and extrusion across the sarcolemma, by both the Na^{+}-Ca^{2+}. exchanger and the sarcolemmal ATPase. Mitochondria can also accumulate calcium, particularly when cytosolic levels become excessively high (e.g. during severe ischemia). The events that comprise excitation-contraction coupling influence the size and kinetics of the calcium transient. An abnormally low calcium transient may lead to depressed contractility. Reduction in sarcoplasmic reticulum Ca^{2+} ATPase activity is characteristic of heart failure and is generally accompanied by diastolic calcium overload; this may contribute to delayed relaxation and diastolic dysfunction, triggering of ventricular arrhythmias, and

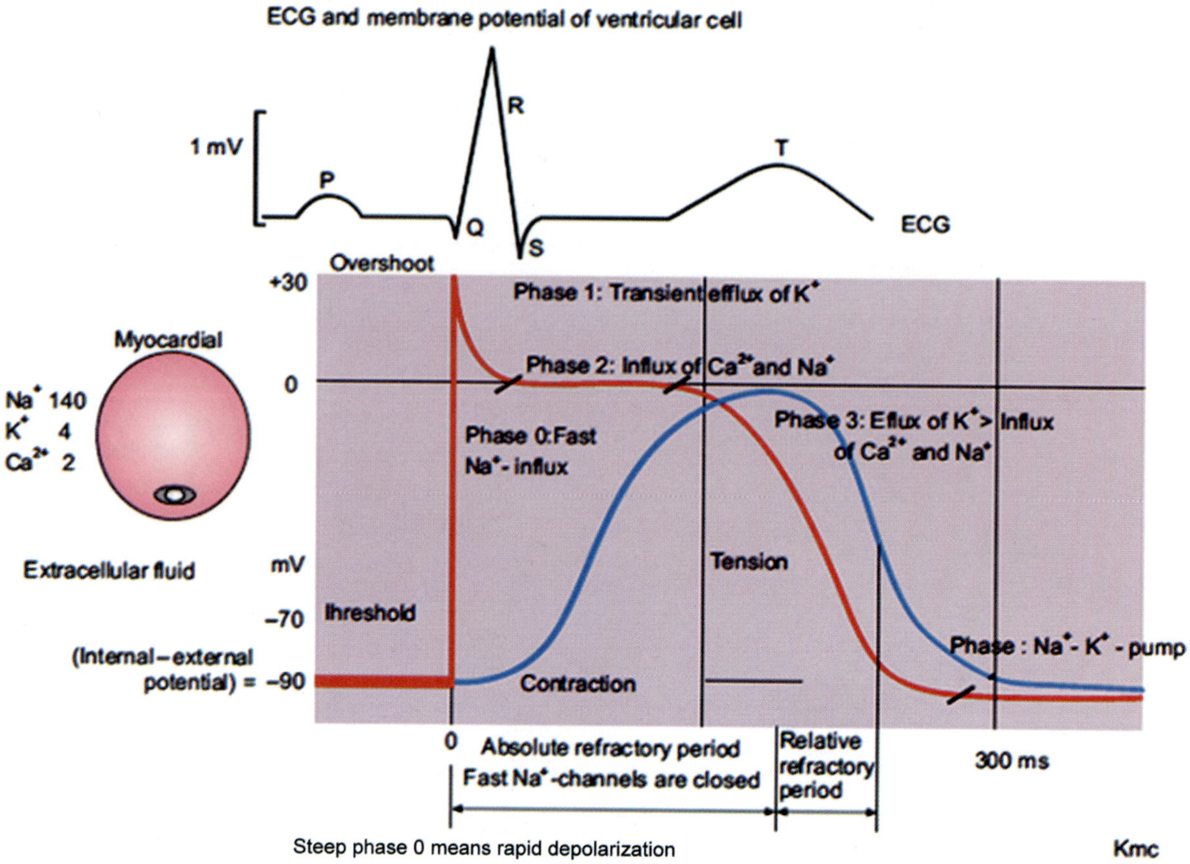

Fig. 2.13: *Diagram showing corelationship between EKG, and membrane potential of ventricular cell*

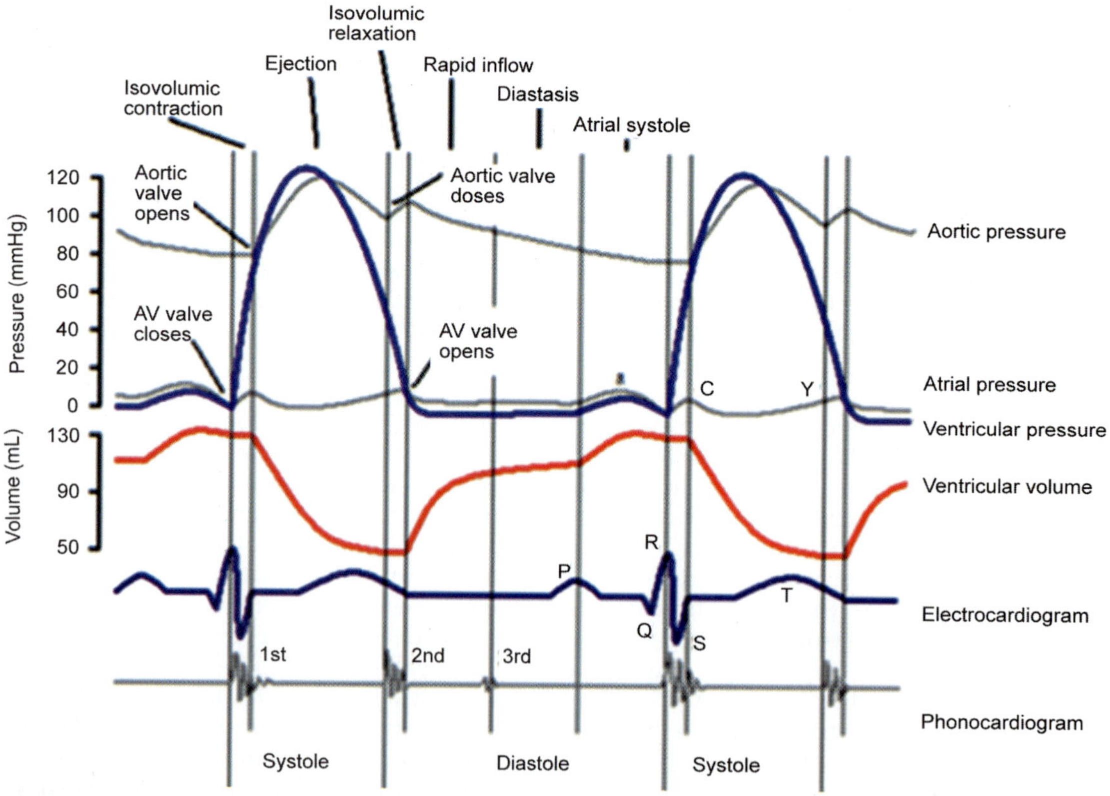

Fig. 2.14: *Illustration showing corelationship between electrocardiogram, LV hemodynamics, phonocardiogram and left ventricular volumes during cardiac cycle*

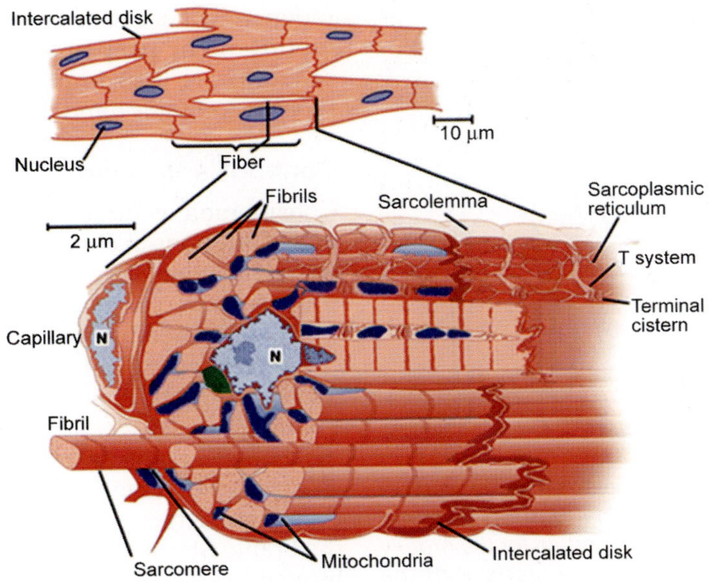

Fig. 2.15: *The muscle fibrils are surrounded by numerous and elongated mitochondria since the heart needs energy supply continously. The muscle fibers branch and interdigitate. They lie parallel to one another but at the end of each muscle fibers there are extensive folds of the cell membrane that are called as intercalated disks.The intercalated disks act as gap junctions that is very permeable and allow almost free diffusion of ions. They always occur at the Z lines, i.e. the dark middle section of the light (I) band of the muscle. They provide a strong union between fibers, maintaining cell-to-cell cohesion, so that the pull of one contractile cell can be transmitted along its axis to the next.The heart muscle thus acts as a syncytium, i.e. a multinucleated mass. Therefore when one of the cells is excited, the action potential spreads from cell to cell through the latticework interconnections fast and the syncytium as a whole contracts. The heart is divided into the atrial and ventricular syncytium separated by the fibrous annulus at the AV junction. The action potential has to travel through the specialized conducting system that pierces the fibrous tissue. This division of the heart into two functional syncytiums allow the atria to contract a short time before the ventricles, which is important for the effectiveness of the heart as a pump. The T system in cardiac muscle is located at the Z-lines rather than at the A-I junction, where it is located in mammalian skeletal muscle. The T system of transverse tubules, which is continuous with the sarcolemma of the muscle fiber, forms a grid perforated by the individual muscle fibrils. It provides a path for the rapid transmission of the action potential from the cell membrane to all the fibrils in the muscle. The sarcoplasmic reticulum is an important store of Ca^{2+} and also participates in muscle metabolism*

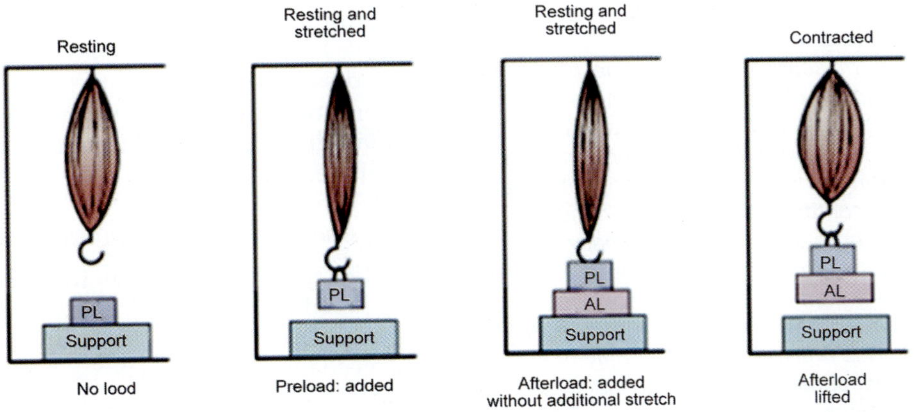

Fig. 2.16: *Showing in A, the muscle is relaxed and bears no weight. For the intact left ventricle, this situation is analogous to the relaxed ventricle after ejection; when the aortic valve is closed and the mitral valve is about to open (isovolumic relaxation). In B, the resting muscle is stretched by a preload, which represents the end of diastolic filling of the left ventricle (end-diastolic volume). In C, the resting muscle is still stretched by the preload, but an afterload has been added without allowing the muscle to be further stretched. In the intact heart, this is analogos to the isovolumetric contraction, when the ventricular is contracted, with the mitral valve closed, but the aortic valve has not yet opened because the ventricle has not developed enough intraventricular pressure to open it. In D, the ventricle has contracted (isotonic contraction) and lifted the afterload. In the intact heart, this situation represents the left ventricular ejection into the aorta. During ejection, the afterload is represented by aortic and intraventricular pressures, which are virtually equal to each other. In cardiac muscle, force generation and its control by Ca^{2+} are also very similar to skeletal muscle, although cardiac muscle is more/less dependent on the release of Ca^{2+} from the SR, and the mechanism of x release is different Force generation and its control by Ca^{2+} are also very similar to skeletal muscle, although cardiac muscle is less dependent on the release of Ca^{2+} from the SR, and the mechanism of SR Ca^{2+} release is different*

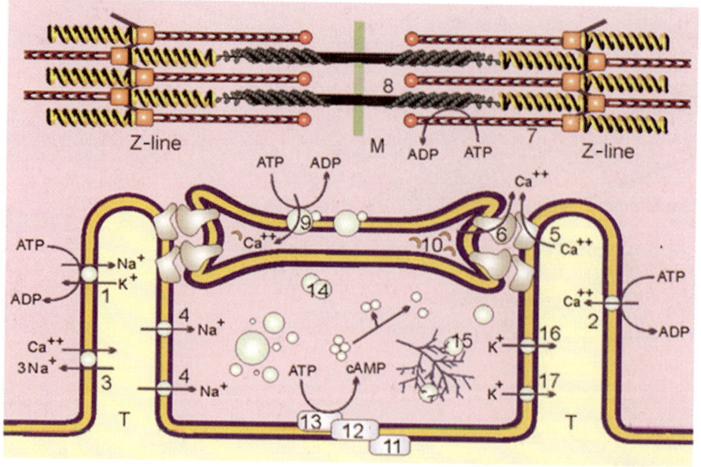

Fig. 2.17: *Cardiac muscle. In cardiac muscle and some types of smooth muscle, the cells are in electrical contact through communicating gap junctions. These are important for the orderly spread of excitation through the heart. This starts with the spontaneous depolarization of the specialized pacemaker cells in the sinoatrial node, spreads via the atria to the atrioventricular node and thence to the conducting fibers in the Bundle of His (in the intraventricular septum) and the Purkinje system. These cells finally activate the bulk of the ventricular muscle in the chamber walls, in each case through direct electrical contacts. Catecholamine hormones such as adrenalin are released during frightening or stressful situations. They increase the force and frequency of cardiac contractions by binding to beta-1 receptors,which are protein molecules protruding from the outer face of the cardiac sarcolemma. These activate G-proteins within the membrane, which in turn activate the enzyme adenyl cyclase on the inner face of the sarcolemma. Adenyl cyclase produces 3'5' cyclic AMP, which is an important second messenger controlling numerous intracellular activities. Cyclic AMP activates protein kinase A which phosphorylates many intracellular enzymes, temporarily modifying their properties.*

Cardiac muscle contains muscarinic acetylcholine receptors. These are also linked to adenyl cyclase (via inhibitory G-proteins) and to a potassium ion channel in the cardiac sarcolemma. Acetylcholine reduces the levels of cyclic AMP and increases potassium currents, promoting slower, less forceful beats. Many types of smooth muscle also contain gap junctions and muscarinic acetylcholine receptors, but here acetylcholine normally leads to contraction. Depending on the type of smooth muscle, catecholamines may produce either contraction (alpha-receptors linked to intracellular calcium stores), or relaxation (beta-receptors linked to adenyl cyclase). This relaxation is apparently mediated by the cyclic AMP-dependent phosphorylation and inactivation of the enzyme myosin light chain kinase, which plays a central role in smooth muscle contraction. Vascular smooth muscle redistributes the blood supply during exercise, and visceral smooth muscle empties the gut in stressful or frightening situations. In contrast to all this, the force of contraction in voluntary muscle is unaffected by circulating hormones

chronic changes in cell structure (e.g. altered gene expression) as a result of activation of downstream calcium-dependent signaling pathways. Upregulation of Na^+-Ca^{2+} exchanger activity may, to some extent, compensate for reduced sarcoplasmic reticulum Ca^{2+} ATPase activity. Independent of excitation-contraction coupling, changes in myofilament properties (e.g. their responsiveness to calcium) are also implicated in heart failure, ischemia reperfusion injury and hypertrophic cardiomyopathy.

Contractile Reserve

Considerable contractile reserve is normally available to meet variations in circulatory demand. Recruitment of this contractile reserve involves changes in the cytosolic calcium transient and/or myofilament responsiveness to calcium, and is regulated by the following factors.

Frank-Starling relationship: An increase in myocyte length (brought about by increased ventricular diastolic volume) increases contractile force. The major underlying mechanism is increased myofilament responsiveness to calcium, but length-dependent release of autocrine/paracrine factors may also be involved. At a cellular level, the Frank- Starling response is thought to be maintained in human heart failure ECG though myocyte strech may be a limiting factor in a heart that is dilated and stiff.

Heart rate-an increased heart rate enhances contractile force primarily as the result of an increase in sarcolemmal calcium influx per unit time, and consequent increased loading of the sarcoplasmic reticulum with calcium. The failing human heart exhibits a greatly blunted force-frequency relationship.

Autonomic control-sympathetic activation, involving catecholamine release, has both positive inotropic and chronotropic effects via beta-adrenoceptors. These actions are antagonized by parasympathetic release of acetylcholine. The inotropic effect of beta-stimulation results from an increase in the intracellular calcium transient caused by increases in l_{ca} and sarcoplasmic reticulum calcium release beta-stimulation also accelerates relaxation by stimulating sarcoplasmic reticulum calcium lower uptake, promoting faster dissociation of calcium from the myofilaments, and accelerating cross-bridge cycling. Reduced responsiveness to beta-adrenergic stimulation is a fundamental feature of human heart failure.

Autocrinelparacrine Regulation

Cardiac myocytes are in intimate contact with the endothelial cells of the coronary microvasculature, which are ideally positioned to sense and transduce local signals (e.g. mechanical forces, hypoxia, hormones) in the perfusing blood. Coordinated release of factors such as nitric oxide, endothelin-I and angiotensin II by these endothelial cells allows local regulation of contractile function. Some of these factors are also generated by cardiac myocytes themselves, particularly in pathological settings. Nitric oxide has direct actions on cardiac myocytes, independent of its vasodilator effects. These include: acceleration of myocyte relaxation and reduction in diastolic tone, resulting from a reduction in myofilament calcium responsiveness small positive inotropic and chronotropic effects damping down' of responses to beta-adrenergic stimulation. Release of nitric oxide in response to increased preload or increased shear (e.g. during exercise) may optimize cardiac pump function through increased inotropy and improved ventricular filling and coronary perfusion. Abnormal nitric oxide bioactivity (either excessively low or excessively high) contributes to contractile dysfunction in conditions such as cardiac hypertrophy, heart failure and myocarditis.

Endothelin-1

It is a potent vasoconstrictor and positive inotrope that acts by increasing both the calcium transient and myofilament calcium responsiveness. Endothelin-l may stimulate release of angiotensin II, which has similar actions and may therefore amplify the effects of endothelin-l. Stretch induced release of these peptides is suggested to contribute to length-dependent increases in contractile force. Production of endothelin-l is increased during myocardial ischemia and in heart failure. Likewise, increased angiotensin II production through increased local angiotensin-converting enzyme activity is the cardinal feature of hypertrophy and heart failure. Increased production of these peptides has several detrimental effects, including slowed ventricular relaxation, diastolic dysfunction as a result of increased fibrosis, and promotion of inappropriate hypertrophy and ventricular remodeling.

THE CARDIAC CYCLE

It describes the cycle of pressure and volume changes that result in sequential atrial and ventricular contraction. Events on both sides of the heart are similar. At resting heart rates systole (when ventricles contract) lasts for one-third of the cycle and diastole (when there is muscular relaxation and filling) for two-thirds.

The electrical activity of the heart initiates contraction of the atria and ventricles in sequence. The events described below apply to the left side of the heart (Fig. 2.18).

Mid-diastole: The AV valves are open. Atrial pressure is higher than ventricular pressure and blood flows from the atria into the ventricles.

Late diastole atrial contraction occurs adding 20% to ventricular filling.

Systole: Ventricular contraction increases ventricular pressure. When this exceeds atrial pressure the AV valve shuts. This is known as isovolumetric contraction.

Ejection: When ventricular pressure exceeds aortic pressure the aortic valve opens and blood is ejected.

Late systole: Ventricular muscle starts to relax and ventricular pressures fall below aortic pressure. Initially blood continues to be ejected because of the momentum imparted to it. At the end of systole blood flows back toward the ventricle causing the aortic valve to close. Blood is accommodated by the distension of the elastic aorta, which eventually recoils propelling blood toward the arteries. The volume of blood in the ventricle at the end of systole is the end-systolic volume.

Early diastole: All the valves are closed. There is ventricular relaxation and falling ventricular pressure. This is known as isovolumetric relaxation. Eventually ventricular pressure is less than atrial pressure, the AV valve opens and blood flows from the atrium to the ventricle. Similar changes occur on the right side of the heart. Pulmonary artery pressure is lower than aortic pressure, so right ventricular ejection precedes left ventricular ejection. Right ventricular ejection will go on for longer because the pulmonary circulation offers less resistance to blood flow than the systemic circulation and so the pulmonary valve closes after the aortic valve.

Clinical Implications

1. Loss of the contribution to ventricular filling by atrial contraction, e.g. in atrial fibrillation, can adversely affect cardiac function in failing hearts.
2. The active force needed for ejection of blood from the ventricle is greater for a large ventricle than a small one. This is explained by the Law of Laplace, which states for a sphere $P = 2T/R$. Thus, ventricular cardiac

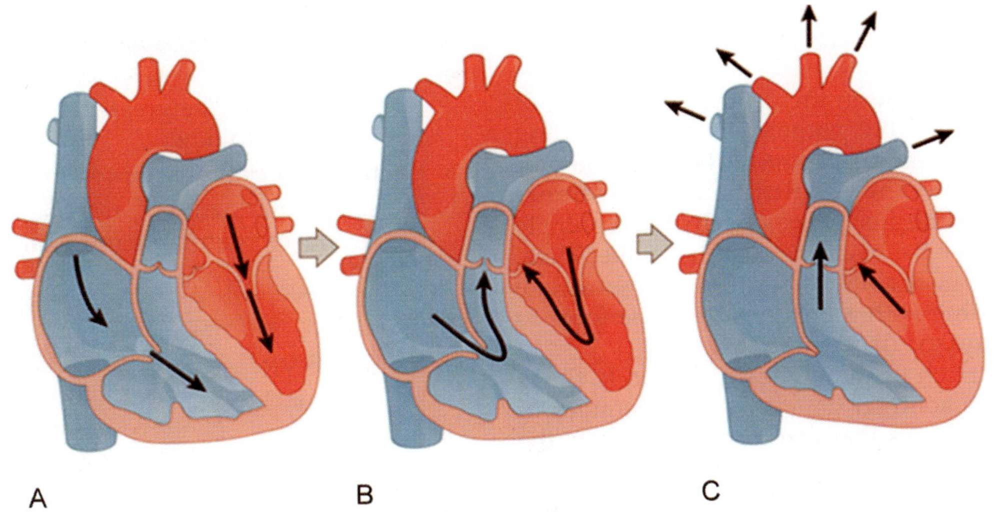

Fig. 2.18: *Cardiac cycle. (A) During a relaxation phase (diastole), blood returning from the large veinsflows into the atria and ventricles.(B) Brief period of atrial systole forces blood out of the atria into the ventricles when atrioventricular (AV) valves open and (C) then ventricular systole pumps blood into the large arteries when semilunar valves open*

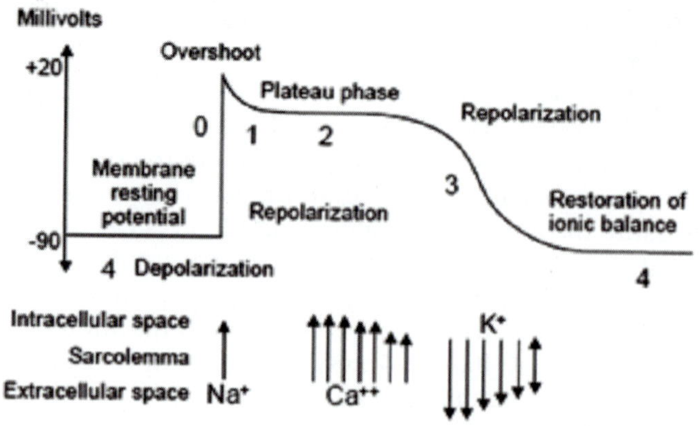

Fig. 2.19: *Showing cardiac action potential of cardiac cell*

muscle must generate a greater tension when the heart is dilated compared with a normal sized heart to produce the same intraventricular pressure.

3. Tachycardia can cause ischemia by reducing the time for ventricular filling and coronary blood flow.
4. Cardiac output = stroke volume (liters) × heart rate (beats/min). Bradycardia can reduce CO and cause hypotension.

Regulation of Stroke Volume and Cardiac Output

1. Cardiac output (CO) is the volume of blood pumped by the ventricle/min:
   Cardiac output = stroke volume × heart rate
   It ranges from 4 to 7 L/min in a normal adult at rest and can increase up to 17 L/min during exercise. CO is normally indexed to body surface area to allow comparisons of 'normal' CO between patients of different height and weight.
2. Stroke volume is the volume of blood ejected by the ventricle/heartbeat. It is the end-diastolic volume minus the end-systolic volume. Normally, 70–80 mL for a 70 kg man at rest. Factors governing stroke volume include preload, afterload and the contractility of the cardiac muscle.

Preload

This is the volume of blood in the ventricle at the end of diastole, i.e. the end-diastolic volume. The Frank Starling Law of the heart describes the relationship between the end-diastolic volume and the resulting stroke volume. According to starling, the greater the stretch of the ventricle in diastole the greater the resulting stroke volume. Thus, the heart has an intrinsic ability to control its own stroke volume by responding with a greater contractile force to the stimulus of increased diastolic stretch.

The degree of stretch of the myocardial muscle fibers when they begin to contract determines the number of actinmyosin cross bridges that can form that affects the degree of myocardial contraction achieved.

End-diastolic pressure is easier to measure than end-diastolic volume. For a compliant ventricle the two are related and end-diastolic pressure is used as a measure of preload. However, with reduced ventricular compliance (e.g. after a myocardial infarction) the pressure will be increased relative to the volume and end-diastolic pressure will overestimate preload. Preload gives information/about the filling pressure of the heart. It does not give any information about/blood volume.

Clinical Implications

1. End-diastolic pressure in the RV is nearly equal to central venous pressure (CVP), which is the pressure within the right atrium and great veins of the thorax. It can be measured via a central venous catheter, using a manometer or transducer. Thus, the filling pressures of the right side of the heart can be determined.
2. When resuscitating a hypotensive patient it should be ensured that they have an adequate preload, i.e. adequately filled with fluids before commencing inotropes or vasopressors. The CVP will not give any information on the filling pressures of the left side of the heart because the lungs are situated between the right and left sides of the heart. Pulmonary hypertension as a result of lung disease, mitral stenosis, left ventricular failure or increased pulmonary blood flow from right to left shunts will exacerbate the discrepancy. If either the RV or LV becomes selectively damaged, filling pressures on the two sides of the heart will differ. The pulmonary capillary wedge pressure (PCWP) is taken as a measure of end-diastolic pressure in the LV. This can only be measured with a pulmonary artery flotation catheter.

Afterload

This is the force that opposes ventricular muscle contraction, i.e. the ventricular wall tension that must develop to eject blood from the ventricle.

Afterload is increased by:

1. Anatomical obstruction, e.g. aortic stenosis. Increased systemic vascular resistance (SVR).
2. Decreased distensibility of the vascular system.
3. Enlarged ventricle (Laplace).
4. Increased blood viscosity, which is largely dependent on haematocrit. The greater the viscosity, the greater the resistance to flow.
5. Decreased intrathoracic pressure
6. Increased afterload will increase the workload of the heart and oxygen consumption and reduce stroke volume.

Afterload is reduced by:

1. Reduced SVR
2. Vasodilator drugs
3. Anemia
4. Increased intrathoracic pressure.

Clinical Implications

1. SVR accounts for about 95% of the resistance to ejection and is used clinically to estimate afterload.

2. Blood pressure although convenient to measure is a poor reflection of afterload and gives no information about volume and flow to organs.
3. Peripheral vasodilator drugs can improve the stroke volume of failing hearts by reducing afterload and ventricular work. Vasodilators also reduce preload via venous dilatation.

Contractility

This is the effective pumping ability of the heart muscle and is increased by.

1. Increased sympathetic activity. Inotropes.
2. Increased preload.
3. Increased afterload-the Anrep effect.
4. Increased heart rate-the Bowditch effect.

Contractility is reduced by:

1. Decreased filling.
2. Hypoxia and hypercapnia (although both will cause sympathetic stimulation)
3. Acidosis and alkalosis.
4. Electrolyte disturbances.
5. Drugs, e.g. antiarrhythmics.

Clinical Implications

The ejection fraction is often used as an indirect index of contractility:

1. Ejection fraction = (end-diastolic volume – end-systolic volume)/end-diastolic volume. The normal value is more than 60%.
2. The drugs which affect the contractility would also influence the ejection fraction.

Ventricular Interdependence

Both ventricles share a common septum. Studies have shown that about 20–40% of the right systolic pressure and volume outflow result from left ventricular contraction.

1. If right ventricular end-diastolic volume increases, this shifts the septum toward the LV decreasing left ventricular diastolic compliance.
2. Right ventricular volumes can increase with pulmonary hypertension.

MYOCARDIAL OXYGEN SUPPLY AND DEMAND

When myocardial oxygen demand exceeds supply myocardial ischemia occurs.

The coronary circulation receives 5% of the CO. It has a high oxygen consumption and therefore a high oxygen extraction from the blood of about 70%. Increased demand must be met by increased coronary blood flow. Hypoxia and adenosine are the most potent coronary artery vasodilators.

Factors Affecting Oxygen Supply

Coronary blood flow which is dependent on:

1. Coronary perfusion pressure (aortic end-diastolic pressure-left ventricular end-diastolic pressure).
2. *Length of diastole:* At a heart rate of 70 beats/min diastole occupies two-thirds of the cardiac cycle. At maximum heart rates, the cardiac cycle shortens, but diastolic filling is shortened to a greater extent than systole so that it only occupies one-half of the cycle. Perfusion of the coronary arteries occurs during diastole, a tachycardia will reduce the time for coronary perfusion and ischemia can occur. (Table 2.1)
3. *Coronary vessel caliber:* It is reduced by atherosclerosis. Chronic ischemia allows some development of a collateral circulation. However, sudden occlusion of a vessel by thrombus results in cell death in the area supplied by that vessel unless protected by collateral circulation.
4. *Blood viscosity:* Oxygen content of the blood which can be calculated using.
5. Oxygen content of blood = oxygen carried by Hb + oxygen dissolved in blood = (*1.39 × Hb × saturation%) + 0.0025 × PaO_2
   where *1.39 is the Hufner constant. The volumes of oxygen carried by 1 g Hb. Figures vary according to whether it is measured *in vitro* or *in vivo.* The values 1.39 and 1.34 are the most commonly quoted ones, respectively.

Factors Affecting Oxygen Demand

1. Myocardial contractility and wall tension-contractile work accounts for the majority of myocardial oxygen

Table 2.1: *Normal hemodynamic data*

Site	*Systolic pressure (mmHg)*	*Diastolic pressure (mmHg)*	*Mean pressure (mmHg)*
Right artium	a up to 7 v up to 5	X up to 3 y up to 3	Less than 5
		End pressure before	Not applicable
Right ventricule	up to 25	a up to 3 End pressure on a up to 7	
Pulmonary artery	up to 25	Up to 15	Up to 18
Left atrium (direct or indirect wedge)	a upto 12 v up to 10	x up to 7 Y up to 7	Up to 10
Left ventricle	120	End pressure up to 7 End pressure on a up to 12	Not applicable

consumption. There is a transmural gradient of wall tension that is greatest in the subendocardial region and least in the subpericardial region. Thus, energy requirements are greatest in the subendocardial region and may account for why the subendocardial region is more prone to ischemia. Ischemic myocardial metabolism results in the progressive loss of high-energy phosphates and progressive accumulation of catabolites. The transition from reversible to irreversible cell injury is likely to be influenced by metabolic rate.

2. *Heart rate:* Greater the heart rate more is the oxygen consumption.

ARRHYTHMIAS

The electrical activity of the heart initiates contraction of the atria and ventricles in sequence. All cardiac myocytes have an inherent rhythmicity because of an unstable membrane potential. However, the sinoatrial (SA) node acts as the pacemaker of the heart as its intrinsic rate is faster than the rest of the heart.

The electrical impulse travels across the atria to the atrioventricular (AV) node where transmission of the impulse is delayed, then rapidly down the bundle of His and Purkinje fibers to the ventricular muscle. Delay of transmission of the impulse at the AV node allows the ventricles to fill before they contract. Rapid impulse conduction down the Purkinje fibers allows simultaneous contraction of all the ventricular muscle fibers.

The principal mechanisms underlying arrhythmias are:

1. Conduction impairment-either slowed/blocked conduction, e.g. heart block or an abnormal pathway of conduction, e.g. Wolf-Parkinson-White syndrome.
2. Re-entrant circuits.
3. Enhanced automaticity-damaged myocytes develop an unstable membrane potential.
4. Pathological after potentials-damaged myocardium may generate spontaneous after potentials after the action potential.

Cardiac arrhythmias are more common with:

- Hypoxia/hypercapnia
- Electrolyte disturbances
- Pre-existing cardiac disease
- Certain drugs, e.g. inotropic drugs
- Certain procedures, e.g. central line insertion where the catheter may directly irritate the heart muscle.

Tissue Oxygenation

The function of the cardiorespiratory system is to deliver adequate oxygen to the tissues. Oxygen diffuses down a concentration gradient at the respiratory, membrane and is then transported in the blood to the tissues. Most of the oxygen is bound to hemoglobin and a small amount is dissolved in the plasma.

Oxygen delivery (DO_2) is given by:

$$DO_2 = CO \times \text{arterial oxygen content}$$

Thus, oxygen delivery is dependent on adequate CO, hemoglobin concentration and saturation. Delivery of oxygen is controlled by the metabolic demand of the tissues.

Oxygen consumption is given by Fick's equation:

$$VO_2 = CO \times (CaO_2 - CvO_2),$$

where VO_2 is oxygen consumption, CO is cardiac output, CaO_2 is arterial oxygen content and CvO_2 is venous oxygen content. Increases in demand are met by increases in blood flow and oxygen extraction. There is capillary recruitment thus increasing microvascular blood flow and increased extraction of oxygen from the blood thus reducing the mixed venous oxygen saturation (SvO_2). The saturation of mixed venous blood can be used to give information about tissue oxygenation although it needs to be interpreted with other clinical data. It can be measured continuously via an oximetric pulmonary artery flotation catheter or by blood sampling from an ordinary pulmonary artery flotation catheter.

If oxygen delivery becomes reduced, the metabolic demands of the tissues are initially maintained by increased extraction resulting in a reduced SvO_2. However, a critcal point is reached at which anaerobic tissue respiration occurs and VO_2 falls. SvO_2 never falls to zero as there is an inability to extract all of the oxygen from the blood. However, SvO_2 is a measure of global oxygenation and does not reflect oxygenation in individual organs. The normal range for SvO_2 is 68–77%.

Causes of decreased SvO_2 are:

1. Low CO
2. Increased oxygen consumption, e.g. fever, exercise thyrotoxicosis. Decreased Hb.
3. Low saturation.

Causes of increased SvO_2 are:

1. Persistently wedged pulmonary artery flotation catheter (common cause).
2. High CO sepsis, burns.
3. Low VO_2, e.g. carbon monoxide methemoglobin, sepsis, hypothermia cyanide toxicity.

Clinical Implications

1. If oxygen delivery decreases then oxygen extraction usually increases to compensate. However, in sepsis it appears that there is a decreased ability to extract oxygen.
2. In patients with cardiac failure therapy may be titrated to SvO_2 as SvO_2 relates directly to CO.

Peripheral Circulation

The main determinants of blood flow are peripheral resistance and the pressure gradient. Given by Poiseuille's equation.

$$Q = \frac{\pi r^4 (P_i - P_o)}{8 \mu L}$$

Q = The flow rate (cm^3/s or m^3/s)

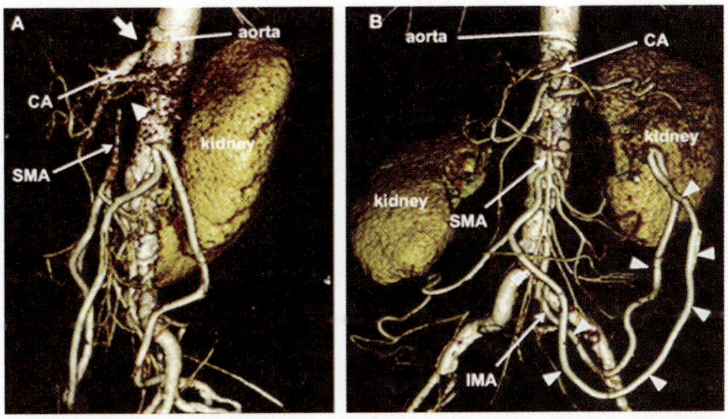

Fig. 2.20A and B: *Volume-rendered CT angiograms demonstrate the normal anatomy of the celiac axis. The left gastric artery (arrow) is seen to arise from the celiac axis*

r = The radius of the tube (cm or m)
P_o = The outlet fluid pressure (dynes/cm^2 or Pa)
P_i = The inlet fluid pressure (dynes/cm^2 or Pa)
μ = The dynamic viscosity of the fluid (poise or Pa.s)
L = The length of the tube (cm or m)

Different tissues have different functions and this requires specialized vascular control. The kidney, brain and heart regulate their own tissue blood flow. Thus, blood flow remains constant usually between a mean arterial blood pressure of 60–140 mmHg. This is known as autoregulation (Figs 2.20 and 2.21).

Distribution of CO at rest:

- Liver 25%
- Kidneys 22%
- Brain 20%
- Heart 5%
- Rest 14%.

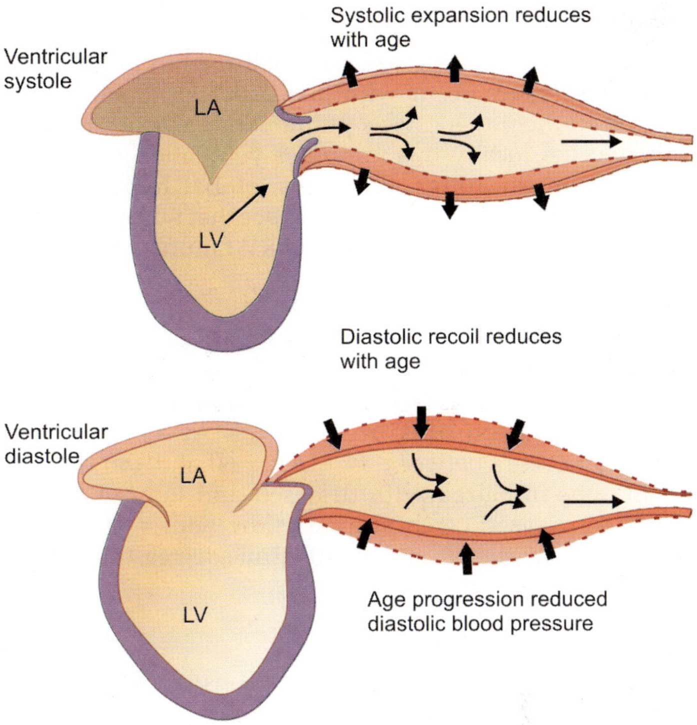

Fig. 2.21: *Diagram showing that as the age advanced. There is reduction of systolic expansion, thereby increasing systolic blood pressure and correspondingly there is reduction of diastolic recoil, resulting into decrease in diastolic blood pressure*

This will alter under different circumstances, e.g. exercise and trauma.

Coronary Circulation (Fig. 2.6)

Coronary oxygen extraction can increase to 90% in heavy exercise, but oxygen delivery mainly increased by increased blood flow.

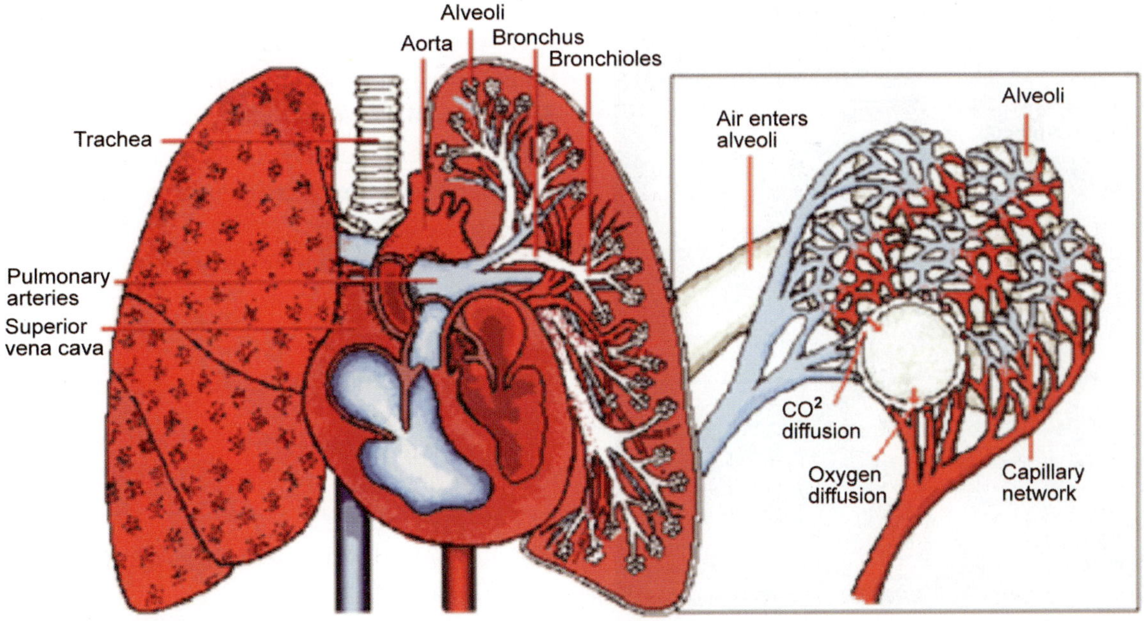

Fig. 2.22: *Pulmonary function system: exchange of O_2 and CO_2 between the atmosphere and the cells of the body*

Pulmonary Circulation (Fig. 2.22)

Low vascular resistance so only small rises in pulmonary vascular pressure occur with increased pulmonary flow hypoxia in the lungs causes pulmonary vasoconstriction. If this occurs locally this improves ventilation perfusion matching in the lungs. However, global hypoxia will increase pulmonary vascular resistance that will reduce RV ejection and can eventually lead to RV failure.

Cerebral Circulation (Fig. 2.24)

Blood flow normally 50 mL / 100 g/min.
Blood flow is affected by:
CO_2-hypercapnia increases CBF; hypocapnia decreases CBF cerebral perfusion pressure CPP = MAP–CVP. Autoregulation occurs between an MAP = 60 and 140 mmHg but may be impaired with diseased and injured brains hypoxia-increased cerebral blood flow with a $PO_2 < 6.7$ drugs, e.g. vasodilators and hypothermia decreases cerebral blood flow.

Renal Circulation (Fig. 2.23)

Autoregulation occurs to maintain a constant renal blood flow. However, in hemorrhage this is overridden with vasoconstriction and redistribution of blood away from the cortex.

Skeletal Muscle

Metabolic vasodilatation occurs during exercise. During strenuous exercise muscle blood flow accounts for up to 80–90% of CO and oxygen extraction increases from 25 to 30% at rest up to 80–90%. Extraction is facilitated by the presence of myoglobin in the fibers. During strenuous exercise anaerobic glycolysis predominates with the production of lactic acid. Post-exercise hyperemia reverses the oxygen debt and washes out the accumulated lactic acid and other vasodilator substances.

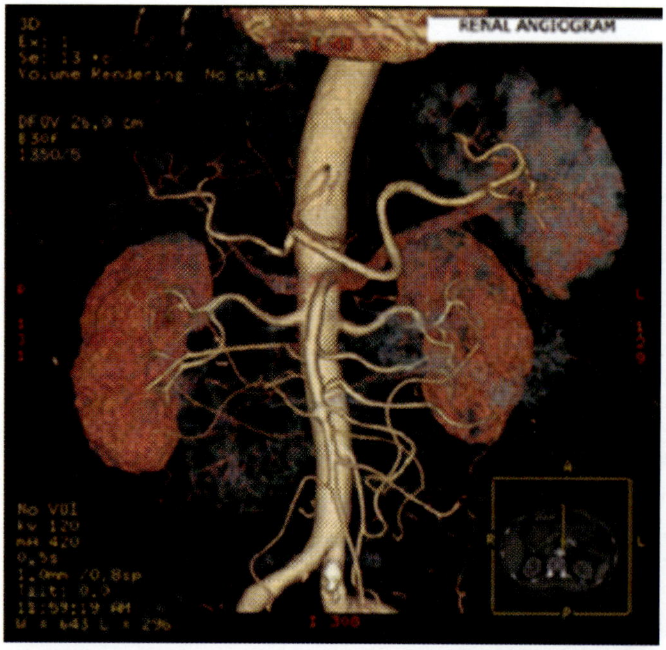

Fig. 2.23: *An MD computed tomographic renal angiogram with left-sided renal artery stenosis*

Abbreviations, normal valves and equations used in this chapter

BSA = body surface area
CO = cardiac output
CI = cardiac index
CVP = central venous pressure
EF = ejection fraction
EDV = end-diastolic volume
ESV = end-systolic volume
Hb = haemoglobin
JVP = jugular venous pressure
LAP = left atrial pressure
LV = left ventricle
LVEDP = left ventricular end-diastolic pressure
LVF = left ventricular failure
L VSWI = left ventricular stroke work index
MAP = mean arterial pressure
MI = myocardial infarction
$PaCO_2$ = partial pressure of carbon dioxide in arterial blood
PA = pulmonary artery
PAFC = pulmonary artery flotation catheter
PaO_2 = partial pressure of oxygen in arterial blood
PAP = pulmonary artery pressure
PCWP = pulmonary capillary wedge pressure
PVR = pulmonary vascular resistance
PEEP = positive end-expiratory pressure
PVR = pulmonary vascular resistance
RV = right ventricle
RAP = right atrial pressure
RVEDP = right ventricular end-diastolic pressure
SA node = sino-atrial node
SaO_2 = percentage oxygen saturation
SVO_2 = mixed venous oxygen saturation
SV,= stroke volume
SVR = Systemic vascular resistance

Normal values

CO = 4–6 L/min
CI = 2.5–3.6 L/min/m^2
CVP = 0–8 cmH_2O
EF = normally> 60%
EDV = 75 + 15 mL/m^2
ESV = 25 ±8 mL/m^2
Hb = 13–17 g/dL (men); 12–16 g/dL (women)
LVSWI = 40–80 g/m^2
PCWP = 6–15 mmHg
PVR = 20–120 dyne s/cm^2

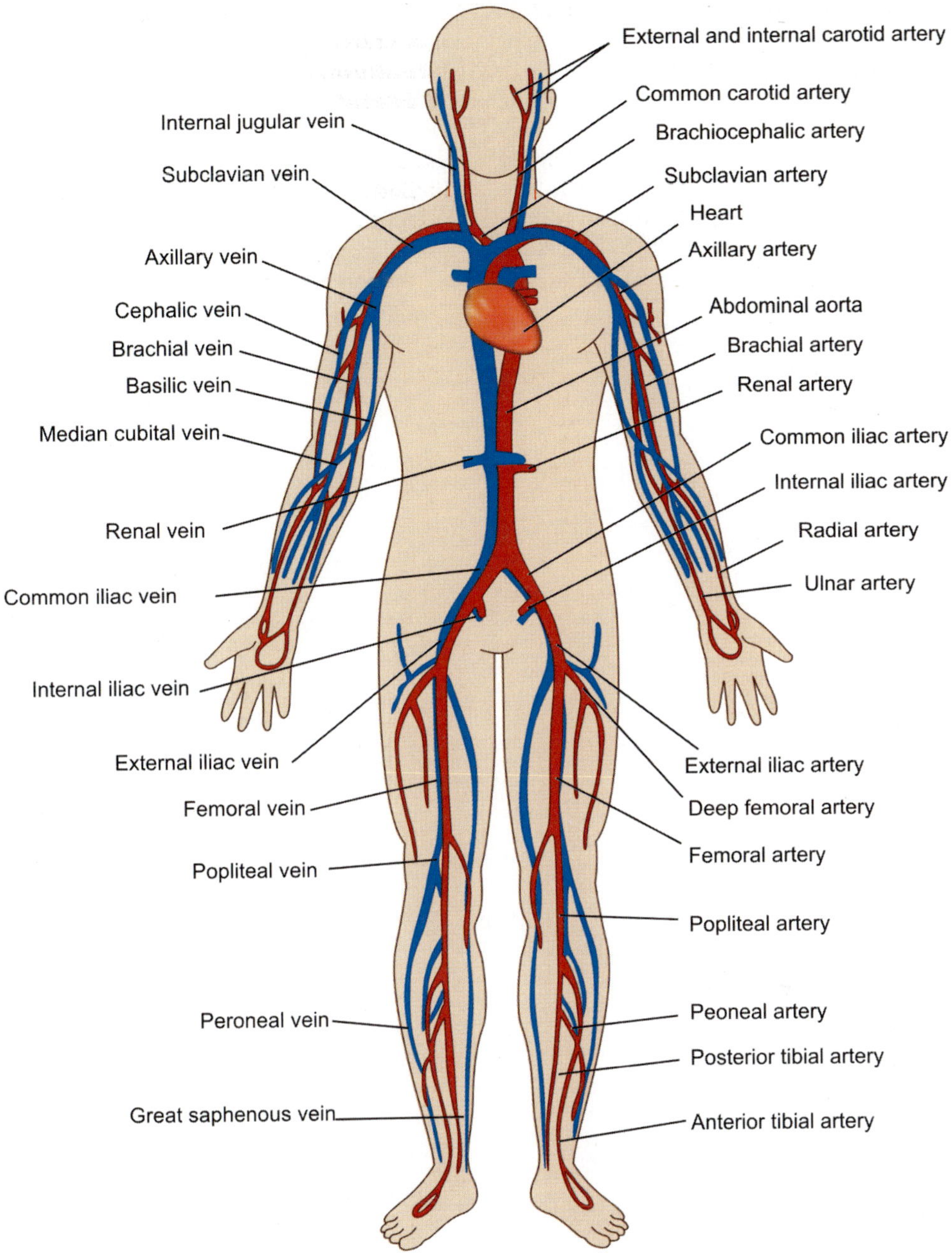

Fig. 2.24: *Circulatory system of the human body*

RAP = 1–7 mmHg
SV = 80 mL
Stroke work = 60–80 g
SVR = 1000–1500 dyne s/cm^2

Normal Valves and Equations

CO = SV (litres) × heart rate (beats/min)
Cardiac index = CO corrected for body size = CO (l/min)/BSA (m^2)
EF = left ventricular SV as a fraction of ED V = EDV - ESV/EDV
PVR = (mean PAP – LAP × 80)/CO
Stroke work = work done by the ventricle (usually left) = SV (mL) × (MAP – PCWP) × 0.0136
Stroke work index = stroke work/BSA
SVR = [MAP – CVP × 80/CO (80 is correction factor)]

BIBLIOGRAPHY

1. Pinsky MR. Applied Cardiovascular Physiology. Berlin: Springer, 1997.
2. Priebe HJ, Skarvan K. Cardiovascular Physiology. London: BMJ Pub!., 1995.
3. Lichtwarck-Aschoff M, Beale R, Pfeiffer UJ. Central venous pressure, pulmonary artery occlusion pressure, intrathoracic blood volume, and right ventricular end-diastolic volume as indicators of cardiac preload. *Crit Care* 1996;11:180–8.

4. Santamore WP, Dell'Talia LJ. Ventricular interdependence: significant left ventricular contributions to right ventricular systolic function. *Prog Cardiovasc Dis* 1998:40;289–308.
5. Boyden PA. Cellular electrophysiologic basis of cardiac arrhythmias. *Am] Cardiol 1996;* 78: 4–11.
6. Edwards JD. Practical application of oxygen transport principles. *Crit Care Med* 1990; 18: S45–8.
7. Blaufarb IS, Sonnenblick EH. The renin -angiotensin system in left ventricular remodelling. Am J *Cardiol* 1996; 77:8C–16C.
8. Bers DM. Calcium Fluxes Involved in Control of Cardiac Myocyte Contraction. *Circ Res* 2000;87:275–81.
9. Bers DM. Excitation-Contraction Coupling and Cardiac Contractile Force. Dordrecht: Kluwer Academic, 1992.
10. Marks AR. Cardiac Intracellular Calcium Release Channels. Rolen Heart Failure. *Circ Res* 2000;87:8–11.
11. Opie LH. The Heart. Physiology from Cell to Circulation. 3rd ed. Philadelphia: Uppincott-Raven, 1998.
12. Shah A M. Paracrine Modulation of Heart Cell Function by En Cells. *Cardiovasc Res* 1996; 31: 847–67.
13. Solaro R J, Rarick HM. Troponin and Tropomyosin. Proteins that on and Tune in the Activity of Cardiac Myofilaments. *Circ Res* 183: 471–80.

3 History Taking, Signs, Symptoms and Investigations in a Heart Patient—Overview

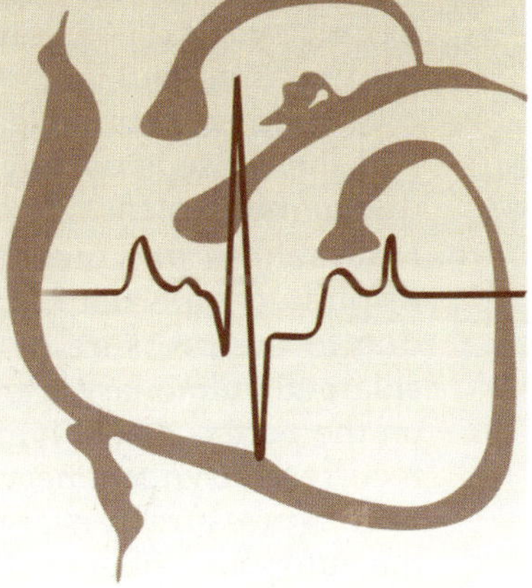

In order to arrive at an accurate diagnosis of heart disease among children and adolescents, it is important for the pediatric physician/cardiologist to follow the set clinical procedures of extracting accurate clinical history, thorough clinical examination supported with basic biochemical investigation. This provisional diagnosis is further confirmed with the help of specialized invasive techniques such as (cardiac catheterization and angiocardiography) and noninvasive tests like echocardiography, CMRI and MD/CT. The following are the different clinical and investigative steps which could help pediatric physician/ cardiologist to arrive at a correct diagnosis (Fig. 3.1).

I. HISTORY TAKING

Bedside History

A painstaking and problem-oriented history taking is often helpful in the diagnosis. Family history and attention to pertinent symptomatology in the various age groups such as cyanosis, poor feeding, tachypnea and orthopnoea, cyanotic spells, squatting, growth retardation, easy fatigability, recurrent pneumonia and congestive failure may offer clues for the presence of heart disease.

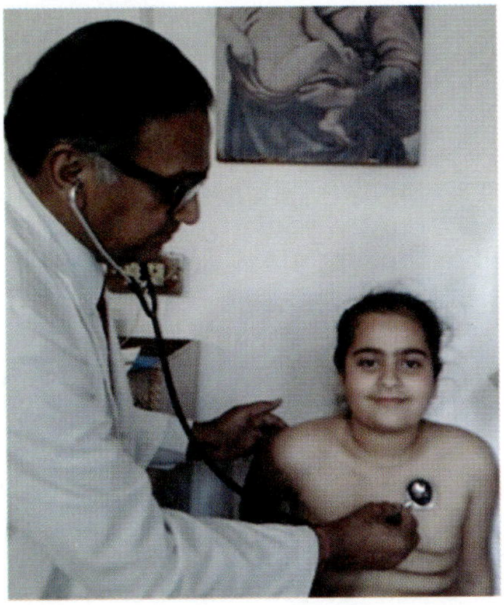

Fig. 3.1: *Doctor in conducting physical examination in a young child*

It is necessary to establish whether the disease is congenital or acquired. This can be achieved by a good history and a well conducted physical examination. The presence of a murmur especially below the age of 1 year, cyanosis and parasternal murmurs are suggestive of congenital heart disease. Even apical murmurs do not exclude the presence of congenital heart disease and have to be carefully evaluated.

History of Rheumatic Fever

1. Chorea twitches, or clumsiness for a few months in childhood? Epistaxis? Frequent sore throats? Tonsillectomy and adenoidectomy?
2. Growing pains (i.e. nocturnal pains or aches in the legs)? (Arthritis or other joint involvement in day time suggests rheumatic fever).
3. Was the diagnosis of rheumatic fever based merely on signs of fever and murmur? or were actually red swollen, painful joints and rash?
4. What therapy was given aspirin, steroids, prophylactic penicillin, prolonged bed rest?
5. Is there a family history of rheumatic fever? (This is almost as suggestive of a rheumatic origin of a patient's murmur as a history of rheumatic fever in the patient).

History of Rheumatic Heart Disease

1. Murmurs heard on previous examination (school, operation, hospitalization, insurance, military service).
2. Carditis with Caray-Coombs murmur.
3. Results of cardiac catheterization? When and where was it done?

Complications of Rheumatic Heart Disease

1. In the presence of mitral disease:
   a. Hemoptysis? Is it mixed or pure? Quantity, color, frequency? (If this occurs with dyspnea or pleuritic pain, consider pulmonary infarction. If it arises from the submucosal bronchial veins, the blood is dark, and the cause is usually raised left atrial pressure due to mitral stenosis).
   b. Hoarseness of voice: Without obvious upper respiratory infection? The cardio-vocal syndrome, due to the pressure of a large left atrium on an enlarged pulmonary artery, which in turn may press on the peribronchial lymph nodes to compress the recurrent laryngeal nerve. Dysphagia may be due to both pressure by a large left atrium and stretch of the autonomic fibers to the esophagus.
   c. Winter bronchitis or wheezing?
   d. Ruptured chordae tendinae (suggested by sudden worsening of dyspnea orthopnea, or paroxysmal nocturnal dyspnea (PND)?
   e. Embolic phenomena: Hematuria, pleurisy, unilateral weakness? Sudden loss of vision or loss in one visual field of one eye.
2. In the presence of aortic stenosis: Angina, exertional syncope, or dyspnoea (a classic triad)?
3. In the presence of aortic regurgitation nocturnal: Angina (but is a sign of vasospastic angina if no AR)? Awareness of large pulsations in arms, neck, or cheek.
4. Epilepsy (increased incidence with mitral stenosis)?
5. Possible infective endocarditis:
   a. Fever and night sweats (enough to require change of pajamas)?
   b. Tooth extraction or cleaning or other possible causes of bacteremia?
   c. Prolonged treatment with penicillin or other antibiotic?
   d. Embolic phenomena, hematuria, back pain, splinter hemorrhages, petechiae, tender finger pads, or cerebrovascular accident (unilateral weakness, paralysis or speech difficulty)?
   e. Seagull murmur usually is indicative of aortic valvulitis
6. Rheumatic nodules over joints and occipit (Figs 3.2 and 3.3).

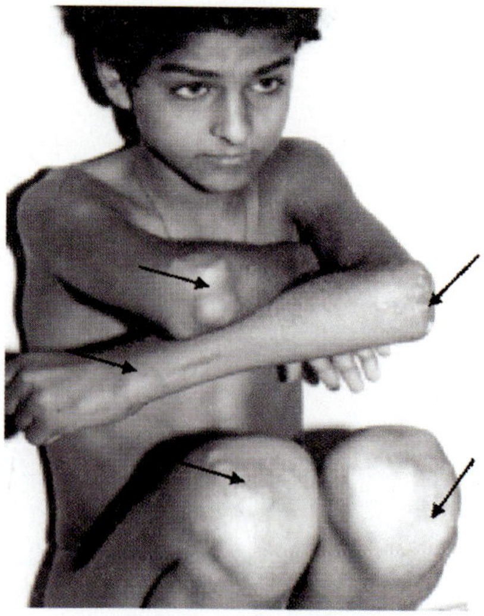

Fig. 3.2: *Showing multiple rheumatic nodules over both elbow, wrist and knee joints in active rheumatic fever*

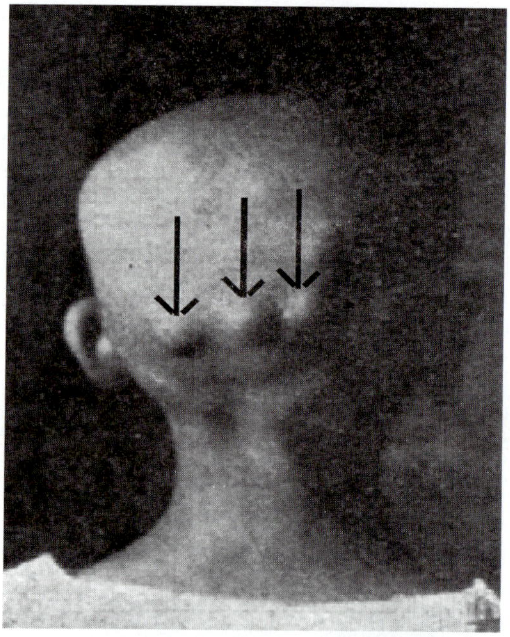

Fig. 3.3: *Rheumatic nodules over the occipit of a young child with acute rheumatic fever*

Could It be a Congenital Heart Disease?

To be asked if patient is an infant:

1. Growth and development? High birth weight suggests transposition of the great vessels.
2. Mother's pregnancy:
   a. Stilbestrol in pregnancy has been linked to transposition of great vessels
   b. Viral illness.
   c. Diabetes in pregnancy suggests transposition of great vessels combined with high birth weight.
3. Frequent pneumonias?
4. Excessive sweating? Asthmatic attacks in new born?
5. Has mother been aware of infant's heart beating against chest wall or the vibrations or a thrill?

To be asked if patient is a child or adult

1. **Mother's pregnancy:** Rubella in first trimester?
2. **Family history:** Congenital heart disease or murmur in family (Fig. 3.4)?
3. **Cyanosis:** When did it begin? (Cyanosis either from birth or within a few days of birth, suggests of TGV). Delayed for years and associated with palpitations suggests Ebstein's anomaly, especially if present with little DOE. If delayed until adolescence of middle age, suggests atrial septal defect with Eisenmenger's reaction or syndrome. Does it occur with crying,

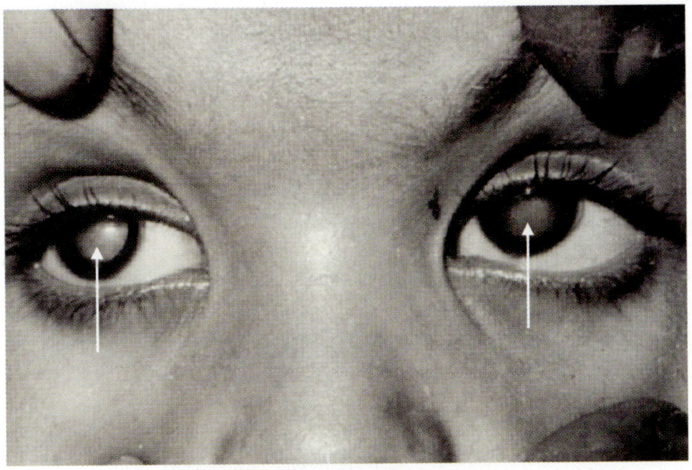

Fig. 3.4: *Showing bilateral congenital cataracts in congenital Rubella syndrome with PDA (arrows)*

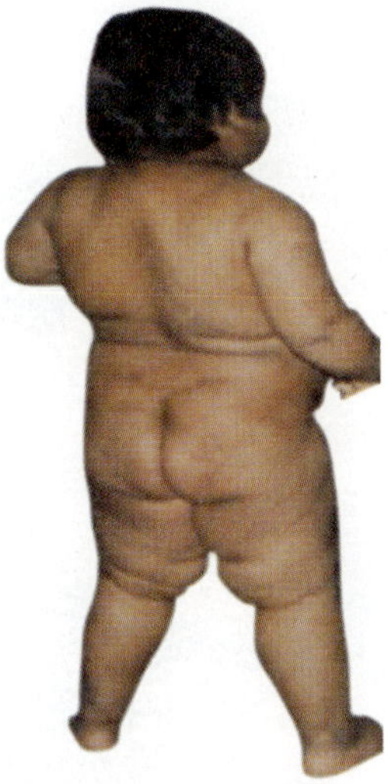

Fig. 3.5: *Truncal obesity and moon face in cushing syndrome*

feeding, or warm bath or only with syncope? (Suggests tetralogy of Fallot). Differential cyanosis and clubbing suggests patent ductus arteriosus with Eisenmenger's syndrome, especially if there is unexpectedly little DOE. Frequent phlebotomies?

4. **Syncope or faintness?** Do these signs occur on exposure to cold or only during effort or excitement? (Suggests primary pulmonary hypertension). With straining, after a long sleep and with cyanosis? (Suggests tetralogy of Fallot or complete atrio-ventricular block). Only with effort? (Suggests severe aortic stenosis, pulmonary stenosis, or primary pulmonary hypertension).
5. Angina? (Suggests severe aortic or pulmonary stenosis).
6. Exact day the murmur was first heard? (Stenotic murmurs are heard in newborn nursery; left-to-right shunt murmurs are often delayed a few weeks). Was it discovered by a physician who had seen the patient before or by a physician seeing the patient for the first time?

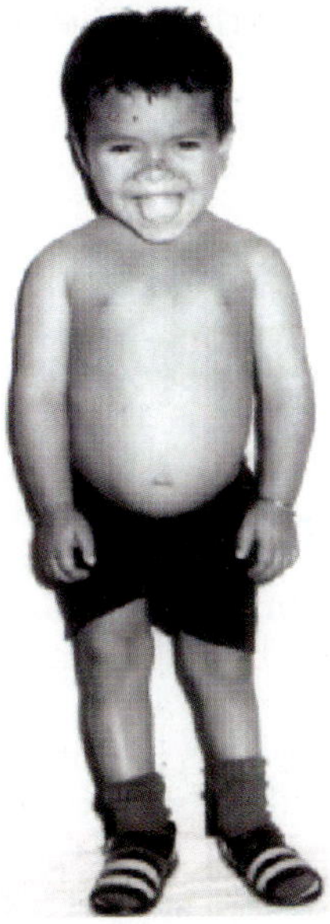

Fig. 3.6: *Stunted physical growth with rough skin and hoarseness of voice in a child with congenital hypothyroidism*

7. Squatting or knee-chest position frequent? (Suggests decreased pulmonary flow due to tetralogy or fallot or more rarely, due to tricuspid atresia).
8. Headaches, epistaxis, leg fatigue or aches after exercise, cold legs, or claudication? (Suggests aortic coarctation. Epistaxis alone suggests rheumatic fever).
9. When and where was cardiac catheterization done?
10. Dysphagia? (Consider coarctation, with the right subclavian artery passing behind the esophagus).
11. Awareness of pulsations in the neck? (Consider coarctation, aortic regurgitation, thyrotoxicosis, or the venous pulsations or gaint A-waves in primary pulmonary hypertension or severe pulmonary stenosis).
12. Strokes? (Consider emboli from endoardial fibro-elastosis if patient is an infant, or emboli from idiopathic cardiomyopathy if patient is a child. May be due to paradoxical emboli or cerebral abscess if patient is cyanotic. Somnolence with cyanosis suggests cerebral abscess).
13. Hoarseness of voice? (Suggests primary pulmonary hypertension or large patent ductus arteriosus).
14. Surgery When, where and by whom? What were the symptomatic results?
15. Mental retardation? (Consider Down's syndrome or supravalvular aortic stenosis)
16. Swelling, pain, warmth, and tenderness of lower extremities? (Hypertrophic osteoarthropathy suggests patent ductus arteriosus with Eisenmenger's syndrome).
17. Recurrent bleeding from the nose, lips, or mouth with hemoptysis or melena, multiple cerebral symptoms such as dizziness and visual disturbances, and a family history of epistaxis (this complex of symptoms comprises hereditary hemorrhagic telangiectasis or Rendu-Osler-Weber disease and suggests a pulmonary

arteriovenous fistula, especially if the patient is cyanotic).

18. Weakness and incoordination? (Suggests the cardiomyopathy of Friedreich's ataxia or muscular dystrophy),

Splinter Hemorrhages

Splinter hemorrhages are tiny lines that run vertically under nails. Splinter hemorrhage is a nonspecific finding and can be associated with subacute bacterial endocarditis, scleroderma, trichinosis, Systemic lupus erythematosus (SLE), rheumatoid arthritis, psoriatic nails, antiphospholipid syndrome, and trauma. At first they are usually plum-colored, but then darken to brown orblack in a couple of days. In certain conditions (in particular, infective endocarditis), clots can migrate from the affected heart valve and find their way into various parts of the body. If this happens in the finger, it can cause damage to the capillaries resulting in a splinter hemorrhage.

There are a number of other causes for splinter hemorrhages. They could be due to hitting the nail ("trauma"), a sign of inflammation in blood vessels all around the body ("systemic vasculitis"), or they could be where a bit of cholesterol has got lodged in the finger's capillaries. Even if a patient does have infective endocarditis, probably 5 in every 6 patients won't have splinter hemorrhages (Figs 3.7 and 3.8).

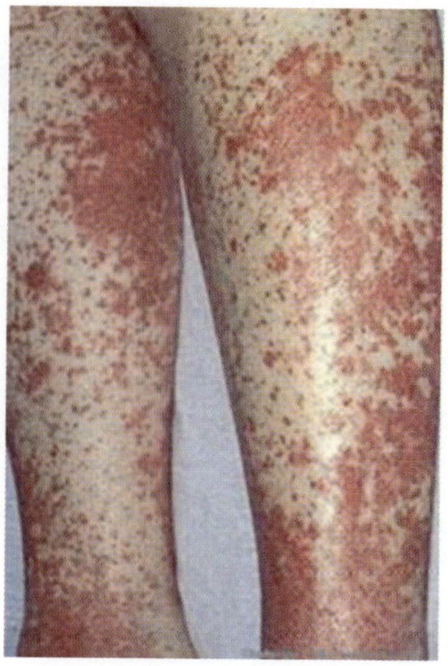

Fig. 3.8: *Ecchymosis over the legs in an adolescent patient with consumption of anticoagulants after corrective surgery*

Cardiac Syndrome X (Angina with Normal Coronary Arteries) (Figs 3.9, 3.10 and 3.13)

Cardiac syndrome X (not to be confused with metabolic syndrome X, or metabolic syndrome) is the name given to a clinical condition which produces angina-like chest pain, often with signs of cardiac ischemia (i.e. poor blood flow in the heart muscle) in the absence of coronary artery disease. The chief characteristics of cardiac syndrome X (CSX) are as follows:

- Angina-line chest pain during exertion (Fig. 3.9)

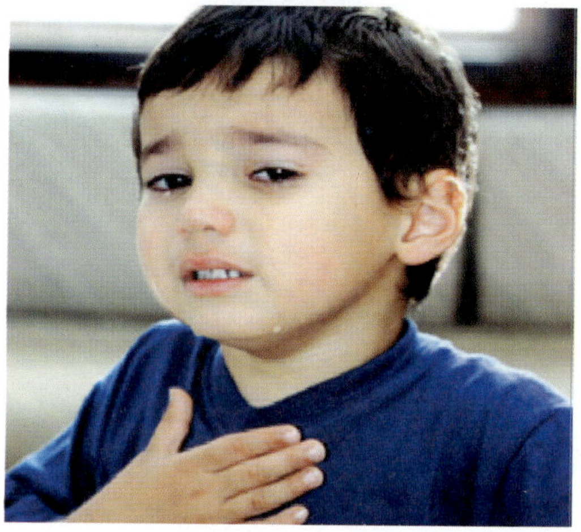

Fig. 3.9: *A young child crying with chest pain*

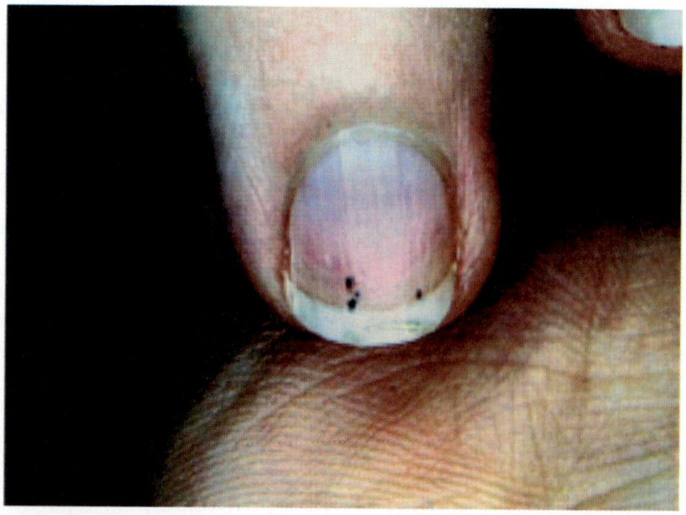

Fig. 3.7: *Thumb showing splinter hemorrhage under nails in patient with infective endocarditis*

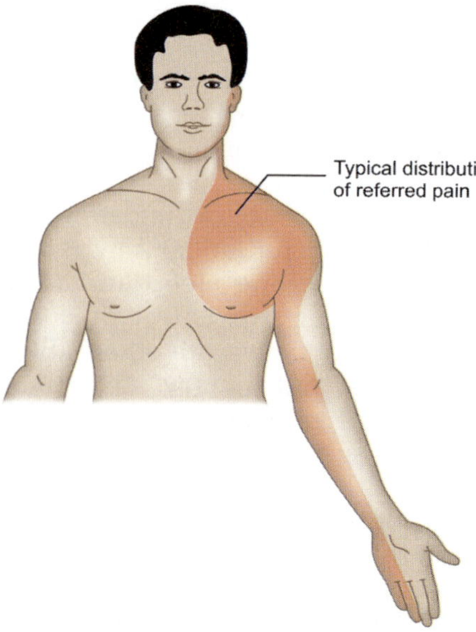

Fig. 3.10: *Classical radiating pain of angina pectoris (marked in red)*

- Characteristic ECG changes during exercise testing (Fig. 3.12)
- Normal coronary arteries on cardiac catheterization
- No inducible coronary artery spasm during catheterization

What is the cause of CSX?

Nobody knows for sure, but there are two major working theories. The first holds that CXS is caused by a poorly-defined disorder of the tiny arteries in the heart muscle (arteries too small to be seen during catheterization). The second suggests a certain "hypersensitivity" to cardiac pain. It is certainly possible (and even likely) that many patients with CSX have both of these proposed abnormalities.

Type of personality

While CSX can affect anyone, by far it is seen most often in younger (i.e. premenopausal) women. Further, doctors generally believe there is a strong association between CSX and certain "psychiatric disorders", such as panic attacks (**Note:** Dr Rich is one of those who believes that most patients with panic attacks are not suffering primarily from a psychiatric disorder, but instead have one of the dysautonomias. The dysautonomias can certainly lead to anxiety and depression, but such associated conditions are most often secondary, and not primary. CSX has also been linked to other dysautonomia syndromes, such as fibromyalgia and inappropriate sinus tachycardia, raising the possibility that some patients with CSX might have a disorder of the small blood vessels within the heart muscle secondary to autonomic dysfunction).

Diagnosis in CSX

There is no test that definitively "proves" that a patient has CSX. Indeed, the diagnosis is made primarily by excluding all other causes of chest pain. However, several tests can be helpful in making the diagnosis. These include:

1. Exercise testing, which usually reproduces the pain and shows changes on the ST segments of the ECG.

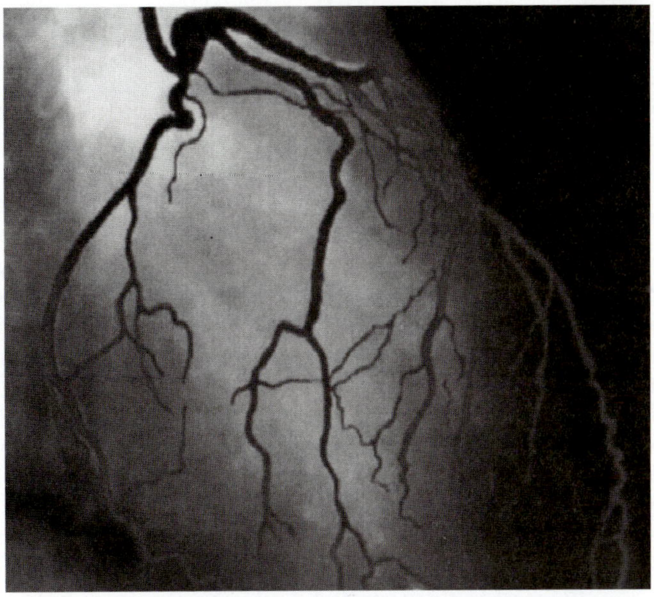

Fig. 3.11: *Angiogram showing normal coronary vessels in patient with chest pain in syndrome X with positive TMT results*

2. Cardiac catheterization, which shows normal visible coronary arteries and no inducible spasm (Fig. 3.11).
3. MRI scanning has been used in research centers to demonstrate abnormal blood flow in the heart muscle in patients with CSX after various provocative testing (such as adenosine or dobutamine infusions.) MRI scanning is not routinely done to make a diagnosis, but has offered the strongest evidence to date that patients with CSX have a true physiological abnormality associated with their chest pain.

How significant is CSX?

Fortunately, most patients with CSX appear to have a very good prognosis. Long-term follow-up studies have not shown an increased statistical risk for these patients to

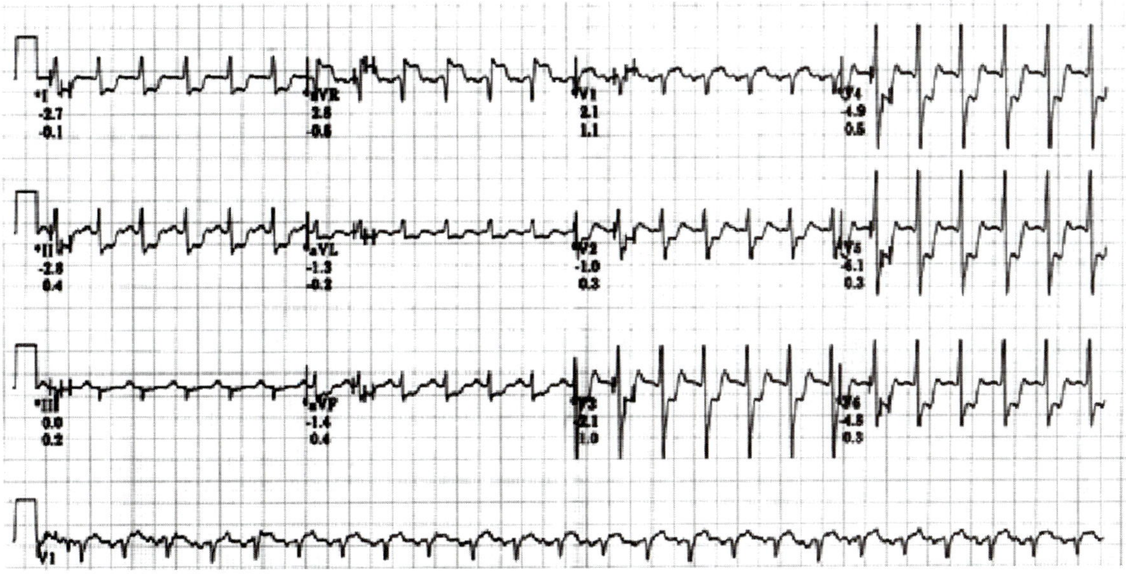

Fig. 3.12: *Showing ST depression in leads 1, 11, aVF and V3-V6 strongly positive TMT in a patient with cardiac syndrome X*

develop heart attacks or cardiomyopathy (i.e. heart muscle disease and heart failure.)

How is CSX treated?

Since CSX does not appear to be associated with long-term cardiac disease, the chief goals of therapy are:

1. Reassurance
2. Pain control.

Pain control can often be achieved by using one or more of the following drugs: nitrates, calcium channel blockers, beta-blockers, or imipramine. Usually, patients are given nitrates to take as needed for chest pain. Calcium channel blockers are usually added if nitrates are insufficient. Those patients who display an increase in sympathetic tone (i.e. those who have signs of inappropriate sinus tachycardia) often respond well to beta-blockers. Finally, if none of these drugs (alone or in combination) are effective, a trial of imipramine can be used.

Intermittent Claudication

Intermittent claudication (Latin: *claudicatio intermittens*) is a clinical diagnosis given for muscle pain (ache, cramp, numbness or sense of fatigue), classically in the calf muscle, which occurs during exercise and is relieved by a short period of rest. Claudication derives from the Latin verb *claudicare*, "to limp".

Signs

One of the hallmarks of arterial claudication is that it occurs intermittently. It disappears after a brief rest and the patient can start walking again until the pain recurs. The following signs are general signs of atherosclerosis of the lower extremity arteries:

- Cyanosis
- Atrophic changes like loss of hair, shiny skin
- Decreased temperature
- Decreased pulse
- Redness when limb is returned to a "dependent" position all the "P's"
- Increase in pallor
- Decrease in pulses
- Perishing cold
- Pain
- Paresthesia
- Paralysis.

Causes (Fig. 3.14)

Most commonly, intermittent (or vascular or venous) claudication is due to peripheral arterial disease which implies significant atherosclerotic blockages resulting in arterial insufficiency. It is distinct from neurogenic claudication, which is associated with lumbar spinal stenosis.

Epidemiology

Atherosclerosis affects up to 10% of the Western population older than 65 years and for intermittent claudication this number is around 5%. Intermittent claudication most commonly manifests in men older than 50 years.

Peripheral, Venous Congestion or Pseudo-Right Heart Failure Possibilities

1. Peripheral edema: Maximum and minimum weight? Reasons for any weight gain or loss.
2. Ascites: If this occurs before or simultaneously with orthopnea or dyspnea, consider tamponade?
3. Upper abdominal pain, especially on exercise? (This suggests increased stretch of liver capsule due to hepatomegaly).

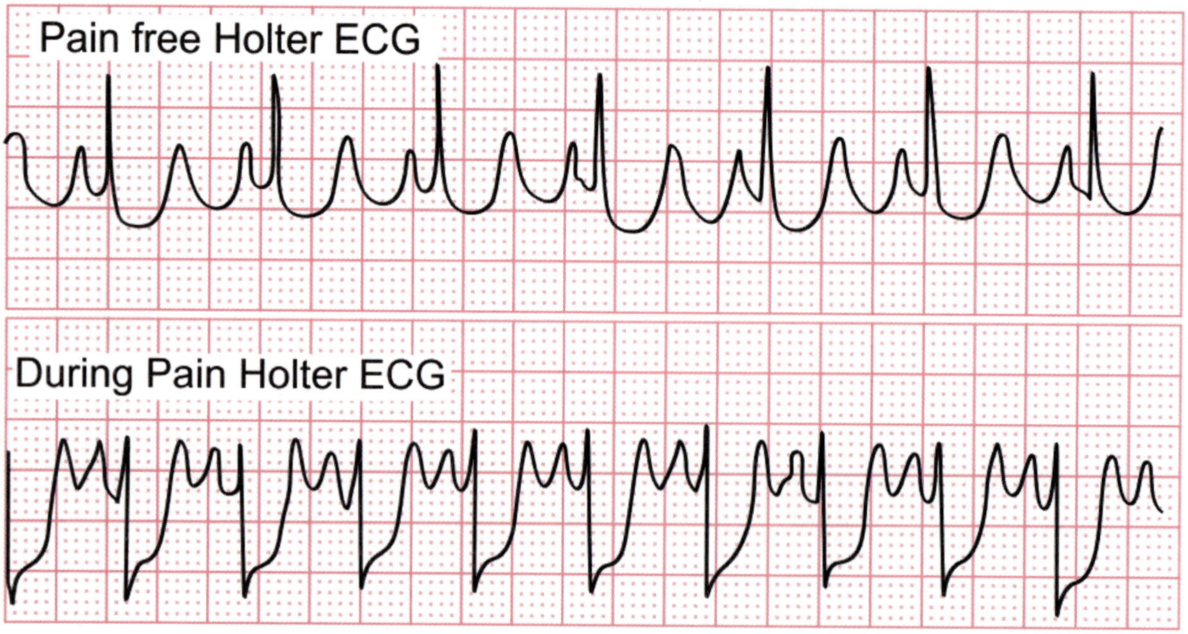

Fig. 3.13: *ECG taken at rest (upper panel) and marked ST segment depression (lower panel) during chest pain in patient with unstable angina pectoris*

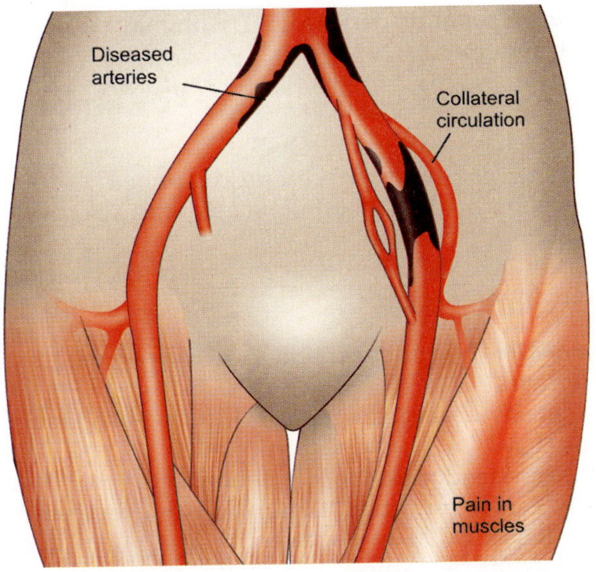

Fig. 3.14: *Diseased illiac vessels with collateral circulation in patient with intermittent claudication in his both legs*

4. Bending or stooping discomfort? (Suggests hepatomegaly).
5. Positive hepatojugular reflux.

Low output state possibilities

1. Weakness and fatigue? Do these occur only in the morning (depression)? Is afternoon nap necessary? If these signs occur only in the afternoon, they suggest low blood sugar or hypothyroidism. Is the patient on drugs that would cause weakness (i.e. digitalis, diuretics, beta-blockers, or tranquilizers)? Is there only psychoneurotic basis (relationship to family, spouse, work supervisor)? Is the patient taking a contraceptive pill, diphenylhydantoin, and spironolactone?
2. Coldness of extremities? For how long?
3. Excessive perspiration? (A common sign of failure in infants). If recent in an adult and not due to hyperthyroidism or neurosis; it suggests severe failure. With warm hands, it suggests thyrotoxicosis; with cold hands it suggests psychoneurosis or heart failure.
4. Insomnia due to hyperpnea on going to sleep or dozing. It should be asked to his wife or closely associated family member.
5. Nocturia with polyuria.

Possibilities of fixed output state

1. Syncope, faintness or dizzines.
2. Chest pain tightness, pressure or discomfort. Could it be a high out put failure?
   a. Anemia
      i. Has the patient ever been told he has anemia? Pins and needles? Bleeding from menorrhagia, hemorrhoids, or ulcers? Is anemia being treated?
      ii. Bone marrow or metabolic disorders; upper GIT surgery in the past (leading to B_{12} deficiency), sickle cell disease in self or family, contact with lead or radiation?
   b. Thyrotoxicosis
   c. Beriberi.

Exploring hypertensive heart disease

1. When was the patient first told? Under what circumstances was it discovered?
2. Has treatment been taken regularly? What drugs in what dosage have been taken?
3. Has there been a previous kidney infection or nephritis, or back injury in sport or accident?
4. Frequency of urination or nocturia, polyuria kidney X-rays, renal calculi, gout, severe diabetes?
5. Family history of hypertension. At what age, the patient was told?
6. Coarctation of aorta; cold legs or intermittent claudication, nose bleeds, shoulder girdle pains? Have angiograms been done?
7. Pheochromocytoma: Flushing with pounding headaches, dizziness sweating, palpitations, nausea, chest pain and paresthesia? Weight loss? Elevated blood sugar?
8. Cushing syndrome hirsutism, corticosteroid intake, easy bruising slow wound healing, acne, muscle weakness, kidney stones, emotional unstability or depression
9. Past blood pressure reading? Visual problems, convulsions, strokes, headaches, dyspnea on exertion, orthopnea, PND or epistaxis.
10. Known X-ray or EKG abnormalities.
11. Amount of success of medical or surgical therapy?
12. Side effects of treatment: Muscle aches and pains weakness, sleepiness, postural hypotension, nausea, nasal stuffiness, impotence or palpitation?

Enquiring for cor pulmonale

1. Chronic obstructive pulmonary disease: Pulmonary function tests? Easier to breathe leaning forward? Smoking history? Chronic cough and sputum.
2. Asthma, wheezing, or dyspnea relieved by bronchodilators?
3. Ever worked in a soft or hard coal mine?
4. Pulmonary emboli? History of phlebitis? Marked diuresis with diuretics? On contraceptive pills? Ever sudden dyspnea at rest with palpitations pleurisy, faintness, cold sweat, or hemoptysis. Recurrent stabbing groin pains. Recent trauma or surgery? Pregnancy or long automobile trip?
5. History of lung infiltrate or tuberculosis?
6. Bilateral rales over the bases of the chest.

Cardiac chamber enlargement possibilities

1. Trepopnea (certain positions in bed cause discomfort).
2. Palpitations or awareness of heart beat.
3. Has patient been told of an enlarged heart? When was he first told? If yes, was it after an ECG or X-ray or echocardiogram? Where and when done?
4. Has an X-ray examination been done? When and where was first and last one done?

How about past cardiac surgery?

1. Date and place of surgery? Type of operation or prosthesis? Name of surgeon?
2. Heart failure or other cardiac symptoms present before surgery? Which symptoms were present, and for how long?
3. Was patient catheterized before or after surgery? Was he told about the results of the studies?
4. Complications after surgery: Embolic phenomenon, infections or other?
5. What treatment was given after surgery (anti-coagulants, digitalis, diuretics)? For how long?

Pericarditis, Effusion Constriction or Tamponade Possibilities (Fig. 3.15)

History of chest trauma, recent heart surgery? (The postcardiotomy syndrome, fever, pleurisy, pericarditis and polyserositis may occur as long as 2 months after heart surgery). Myocardial infarction (Dressler's syndrome, which is the same as postcardiotomy syndrome but follows myocardial infarction, now extremely rare), radiation to chest in past few months, uremia, metastatic cancer, lymphoma, leukemia, myxedema, scleroderma, lupus, rheumatoid arthritis, and contact with tuberculosis, or recent viral infection is patient taking drugs that would produce lupus erythematosus syndrome procainamide, hydralazine, penicillin, isoniazid? Is he on drug, like minoxidil?

Symptoms of Pericarditis

1. Chest pain on exertion, swallowing, or deep breathing?
2. Joint symptoms? (With facial rash suggests possible lupus erythematosus; with rash on limbs or body, rheumatic fever).
3. Past history of pericarditis? (In about one-fourth of cases idiopathic pericarditis is recurrent).
4. Epigastric pain for 1–3 days before the chest pain? (This is the initial manifestation in one-third of patients with acute idiopathic pericarditis). Pain may occur alone in the abdomen).

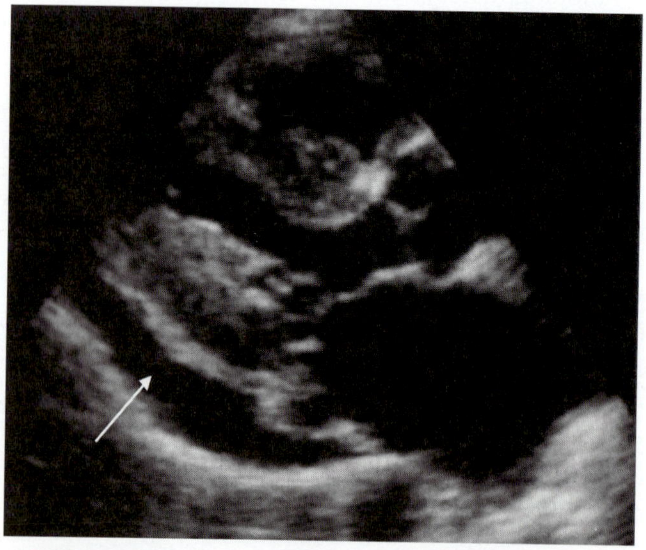

Fig. 3.15: *Echo scan in parasternal long-axis view showing pericardial effusion (arrow)*

Symptoms of Tamponade

1. Dyspnoea on exertion (DOE).
2. Edema or ascites preceding dyspnoea? Abdominal swelling before or simultaneous with edema (highly suggestive of tamponade)?
3. Does DOE stop immediately when the patient stops moving (rare sign)?

Myocarditis? endocarditis? and other heart disease possibilities

1. Acute myocarditis: Recent influenza—like illness with myalgia?
2. Infective endocarditis: Has patient ever been told about it or cardiac murmur? Drug addiction, fevers, surgical or dental cause of bacteremia, prolonged penicillin treatment hematuria, back pain, petechiae, strokes? (Fig. 3.13A)
3. "Collagen" disease: Raynaud's phenomenon, dysphagia, arthritis, or arthralgias tight skin epistaxis, rash in sunlight?
4. Ankylosing spondylitis: Pain in the hip or sciatic region, or low back pain? Does the pain awaken patient in the early morning hours? Morning back stiffness? pain increased on coughing?
5. Carcinoid heart disease: Diarrhea, bronchospasm, flushing of the upper chest and head that lasts from minutes to days?
6. Parasitic disease (Trichinosis or Chagas' disease): Consumption of special meat preparation? Foreign travel.
7. Hypophosphatemia: High intake of phosphorus-binding antacids, aluminum hydroxide gel? Acute alcohol excess?
8. Atrial myxoma: Embolic phenomena, recurrent fevers, arthralgias, or skin lesions of a vasculitis type? Paresthesias in hands? Pulsations in neck (giant "a waves, as in tricuspid stenosis)?
9. Syncope or faintness on changing body position?
10. Hemochromatosis: History of diabetes especially if patient is insulin resistant? Skin colour changes? Liver failure and enlargement symptoms; upper abdominal pain, sexual impotence, or gynecomastia? Frequent transfusions?
11. Sarcoidosis: Syncope (due to complete atrioventricular block)? Known bundle branch block? Abnormal chest radiograph? Cough? Kidney stones or eye symptoms (uveitis)?
12. Hypertrophic subaortic stenosis family history of sudden death? Angina or syncope after but not during exercise intermittent murmur? Do symptoms become worse on digitalis?
13. Amyloid heart disease: Postural hypertension with peripheral neuropathy? Skin lesions, especially if there is bleeding on scratching?
14. Syphilitic aortic regurgitation or aneurysm? History of venereal disease or positive serology?

15. Hoarseness due to recurrent laryngeal nerve compression by aneurysm.
16. Traumatic tricuspid regurgitation may not cause cardiac symptoms for upto 3 years after the accident.

NEW YORK HEART ASSOCIATION FUNCTIONAL AND THERAPEUTIC CLASSIFICATION

This functional classification refers to fatigue, dyspnea or angina. The original classification is too long to grasp and a simplified one follows:

Class 1: The patient is asymptomatic, or symptoms occur on extraordinary exertion (there is no class, or classification for a patient with a normal heart).
Class 2: Symptoms occur on ordinary exertion.
Class 3: Symptoms occur on less than ordinary exertion.
Class 4: Symptoms occur even at rest.

Note: The functional classification is easily remembered if one simply remembers the words ordinary exertion, because class 1 simply adds extra in front of ordinary class 2 adds no words in front of ordinary, and class 3 adds less than in front of ordinary.

The therapeutic classification:
It also refers only to patients with abnormal heart.
Class A: No restriction
Class B: Severe effort restricted
Class C: Ordinary effort moderately restricted
Class D: Ordinary effort markedly restricted
Class E: Confined to chair.

Enquiring about the Symptoms of the Heart Disease

The nature of the underlying physiological disturbances can often be assessed from the symptoms:

1. Raised pulmonary venous pressure
   (a) Dyspnea
   (b) Orthopnea
   (c) Paroxysmal nocturnal dyspnea
   (d) Cough
   (e) Hemoptysis.
2. Inadequate coronary blood flow: Angina pectoris.
3. Congestive cardiac failure: Ankle swelling, hepatic pain.
4. Right to left intracardiac shunt:
   (a) Cyanosis
   (b) Dyspnea
   (c) Squatting
   (d) Syncopal attacks.

Symptoms resulting from a raised pulmonary venous pressure (Fig. 3.22).

Dyspnea

Definition

Dyspnea is an uncomfortable and inappropriate awareness of respiration. Dyspnea can result from several physiological disturbances, the most frequent cause in cardiac disease being a high pulmonary venous pressure.

Mechanism

Any rise in pressure in the left atrium and pulmonary veins is transmitted to the pulmonary capillaries, increasing the transudation of fluid from the capillaries into the interstitial tissues of the lung. The lungs then offer more resistance to inflation and deflation and the greater muscular effort required gives the patient the sensation of dyspnea. Frank pulmonary edema represents the extreme situation when severe elevation of the pulmonary venous pressure forces large amounts of fluid into the alveoli.

Types

Orthopnea and paroxysmal nocturnal dyspnea describe specific forms of dyspnea arising from a high pulmonary venous pressure. The presence of either or both is evidence that the patient's dyspnea is caused by a high pulmonary venous pressure.

Orthopnea

Definition

It may be defined as respiratory difficulty while lying flat and relieved while sitting up.

Mechanism

In normal subjects the volume of blood in the lungs is increased by lying flat, right atrial filling pressure is increased and the increased filling of the right atrium and ventricle is passed on into the lungs. The pulmonary blood volume is already large in patients with a high pulmonary venous pressure and the further volume change on lying flat adds to the stiffness of the lungs.

Paroxysmal Nocturnal Dyspnea

It is that kind of acute dyspnea in which the patient feels uncomfortable during awakening from sleep.

Description

Acute dyspnea, awakening the patient from sleep, forcing him to sit upright or stand out of bed for relief. A dry cough and wheeze are commonly present during the attack, which passes off gradually after 10–20 minutes.

Mechanism

During the night the circulation of blood volume increases in heart failure as interstitial fluid returns to the blood, and the pulmonary venous pressure may build up to high levels. The reduced awareness during sleep allows high levels to be reached before dyspnea awakens the patient.

Acute Pulmonary Edema

Description

Dyspnea is acute and is accompanied by cough and a copious white or pink frothy sputum. There is cyanosis, perspiration, tachycardia, raised systemic blood pressure and wide spread crepitation over the lungs.

Mechanism

When levels of pressure of 40 mmHg are exceeded in the pulmonary veins, the osmotic pressure of the plasma is overcome and fluid transits from the lungs capillaries into the alveoli in large quantities. Rupture of pulmonary capillaries from the high pressures produces pink expectorated sputum.

Gradation of Dyspnea

Useful information about the severity of heart disease is obtained by grading the severity of dyspnea. The following workable categories have been found useful in clinical practice.

Grade 1 (Mild dyspnea): When undertaking unusual exertion (running, walking, scrubbing).
Grade 2 (Moderate): Walking on the level causes dyspnea.
Grade 3 (Severe): Unable to continue walking even slowly on the level.
Grade 4 (Gross): The slight effort induces severe breathlessness. The patient is practically confined to bed by dyspnea. A history of nocturnal dyspnea or acute pulmonary edema places the patient in the severe grade, irrespective of the effort tolerance.

Cough

Two types of cough may be caused by a high pulmonary venous pressure: dry cough during exertion. Cough, producing expectoration along with wheezing.

Mechanism

The bronchial venous return is mainly drained into the pulmonary veins, so that when the pulmonary venous pressure rises during exertion there is engorgement of the bronchial mucosa. This activates the cough reflex resulting in a troublesome dry cough. Chronic elevation of the bronchial venous pressure results in an edematous mucosa offering less resistance to infection and prone to repeated attacks of bronchitis.

Hemoptysis (Coughing out of Blood)

As a result of the high venous pressure a bronchial vein may rupture and cause a small or large hemoptysis.

Diseases associated with a raised pulmonary venous pressure.

Left Ventricular Failure

The high filling pressure required for the failing left ventricle results in an increased pressure in the left atrium and the pulmonary veins which in turn leads to left ventricular failure.

Obstruction to Blood Flow from the Lungs

The pressure in the pulmonary veins proximal to any obstruction is high, e.g. mitral stenosis, left atrial myxoma.

Symptoms of an Inadequate Coronary Blood Flow

Angina Pectoris (Fig. 3.10)

Four major characteristics are:

1. **Quality:** A crushing pain or a tight constricting sensation.
2. **Site:** Pain is maximum behind the sternum or across the front of the chest.
3. **Radiation:** Radiates into the shoulders, the neck, jaw and the fingers and through to the back of the chest.
4. **Relation to exertion:** Pain is experienced during exertion. When exertion is discontinued, the pain wears off in 2–3 minutes, pain may also be provoked by anger or excitement.

Symptoms of Right to Left Intracardiac Shunts

Central cyanosis (Fig. 3.39–3.42)

Blue discoloration of skin, nail beds and mucous membrane which is more marked on exertion or during crying. Central cyanosis in congenital heart disease implies that blood low in oxygen content reaches the systemic arteries without first passing through the lungs.

Dyspnea

Breathlessness on exertion is present with all right to left intracardiac shunts. The reduced oxygen content of the arterial blood causes breathlessness by stimulating the chemoreceptors of the carotid body and the respiratory centre.

Squatting characteristic posture of children who crawl on their heels when breathless, particularly after exertion. Squatting is most commonly seen in Fallot's tetralogy but is not specific to this condition, being occasionally seen in other forms of cyanotic congenital heart disease. By squatting the arterial oxygen saturation is improved during the compression of the great vessels of the lower extremities particularly over the femoral vessels thereby decreasing the input of the right ventricle and raising the systemic blood pressure, hence both leading to better oxygenation in a squatting posture. However, precise mechanism is not known.

Syncopal Attacks (Fig. 3.16)

Sudden attacks of loss of consciousness are common in children suffering from Fallot's tetralogy, during the attack

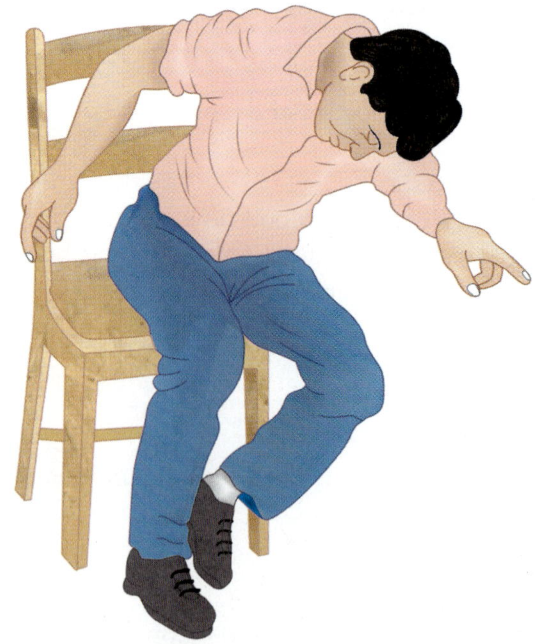

Fig: 3.16: *Model acting to reproduce syncopal attack,becoming temporarily unconcious, toneless and tendency to fall on the ground as shown in this picture*

the child has a pallid cyanosis and profound desaturation of the arterial blood at a normal blood pressure. These attacks occur with emotion, stress, being particularly common in hospital and may be due to spasm of the infundibulum of the right ventricle. The blood flow is then greatly reduced through the lungs most of the blood passing across the ventricular septal defect into the aorta. Cerebral anoxia produces syncope and if the attack is prolonged death may also occur (Fig. 3.17, 3.20, 3.21 and 3.23).

Symptoms of Congestive Heart Failure

1. Ankle Swelling (Fig. 3.18 and 3.19)

An excess of tissue fluid follows abnormal retention of sodium and water by the kidneys in heart failure, and this tissue fluid tends to localize under the influence of gravity into the most dependent parts of the body. Thus the ambulant patient develops swelling of the feet and legs

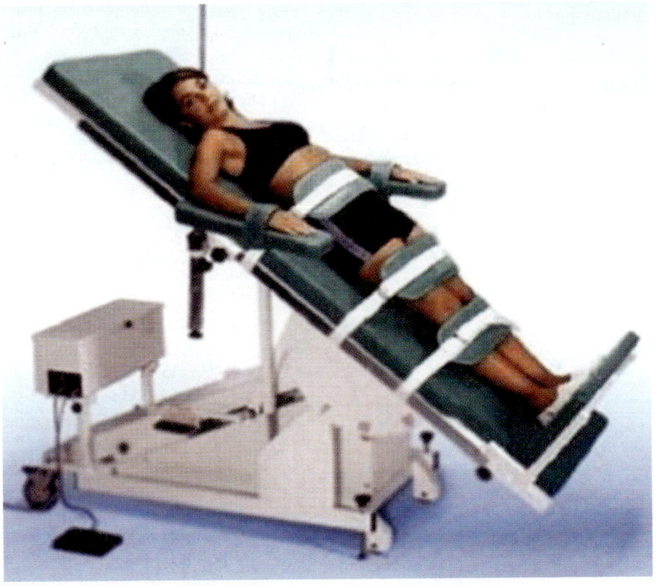

Fig. 3.17: *Young girl performing head upon tilt test (HUTT) for recurrent syncope*

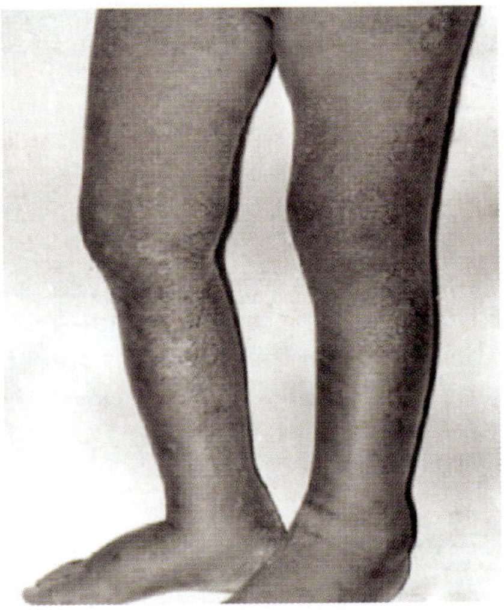

Fig. 3.18: *Edema of ankles and lower legs in patient with congestive cardiac failure*

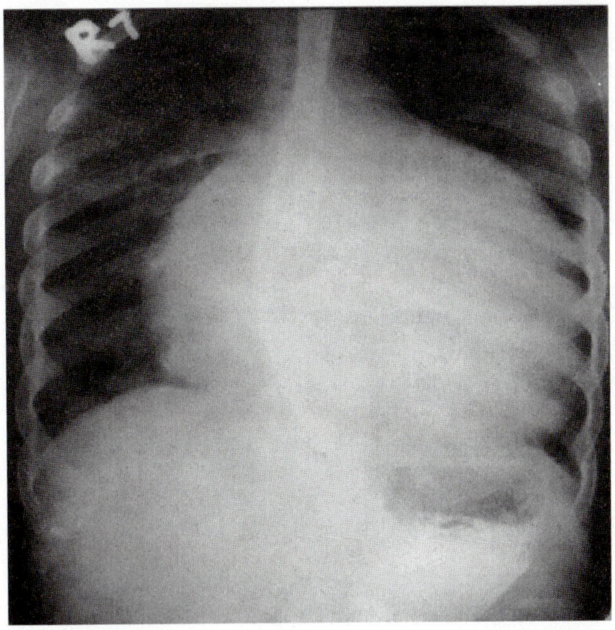

Fig. 3.19: *Chest X-ray of patient with gross diffuse cardiomegaly who presented with grade 4 type of dyspnea*

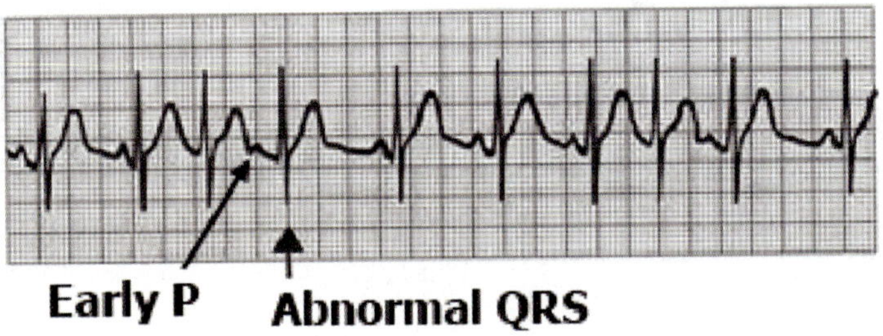

Fig. 3.20: *ECG showing features of atrial ectiopics (arrow)*

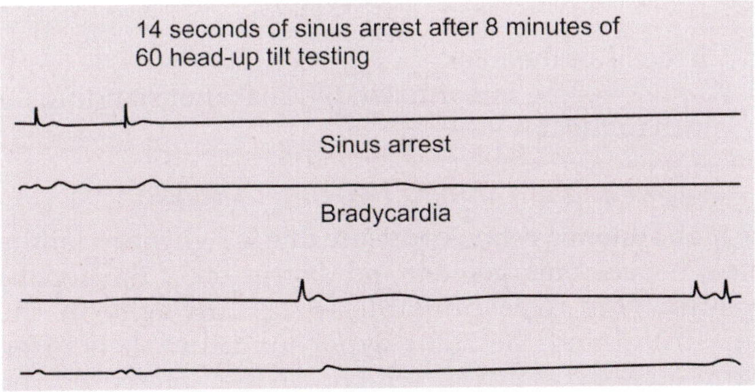

Fig. 3.21: *ECG showing depicting 14 sec sinus arrest and critical bradycardia in positive head up tilt test for investigation of cardiogenic syncope*

which is most marked in the evenings, whereas the patient confined to bed has a pad of edema overlying the sacrum. Edema over the ankles due to CCF should be differentiated from other causes such as:

1. Renal disease
2. Deficient lymphatic drainage of legs
3. Deep vein thrombosis of the legs or severe varicose veins.

Table 3.1: *Cardiovascular causes of syncope*
Neurally mediated (vasovagal)
Situational
• Micturition
• Defecation
• Postprandial
• Swallowing
• Coughing
• Sneezing
Glossopharyngeal neuralgia
Orthostatic syncope
Carotid sinus syncope
• Cardioinhibitory
• Vasodepressor
• Mixed
Mechanical
• Aortic stenosis
• Hypertrophic cardiomyopathy
• Left atrial myxoma
• Mitral stenosis
• Pulmonic stenosis
• Pulmonary hypertension or embolism
• Right atrial myxoma
• Myocardial infarction
• Cardiac tamponade
Electrical
• Second- and third-degree atrioventricular block
Sick sinus syndrome (Figs 3.21 and 3.23)
• Supraventricular tachycardia
• Ventricular tachycardia
• Torsade de pointes
• Pacemaker malfunction

4. Cirrhosis of the liver
5. Ankle swelling in normal individual after standing for much of the day.

2. Abdominal Pain Due to Hepatic Distension

The high systemic venous pressure due to right heart failure causes hepatic enlargement and distension of the hepatic capsule. This is responsible for a dull ache in the epigastrium and the right hypochondrium. It is often aggravated by exertion which, further increases the systemic venous pressure.

3. Ascites (Fig. 3.22)

It is also one of the features of right heart failure.

Symptoms of low cardiac output

Fatigue: A low cardiac out has the effect of producing a constant feeling of fatigue, presumably related to the poor blood supply to muscles and other organs. However, the symptom of tiredness is so usual in all types of illness, including psychological illness, that it cannot be regarded as reliable evidence of a low cardiac output.

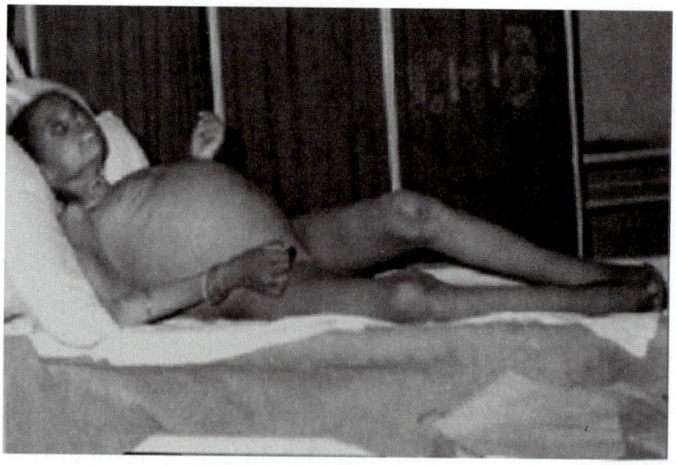

Fig. 3.22: *Photograph of a young patient showing generalized edma of the body, ascites and semiconcious state of mind in severe form of heart failure*

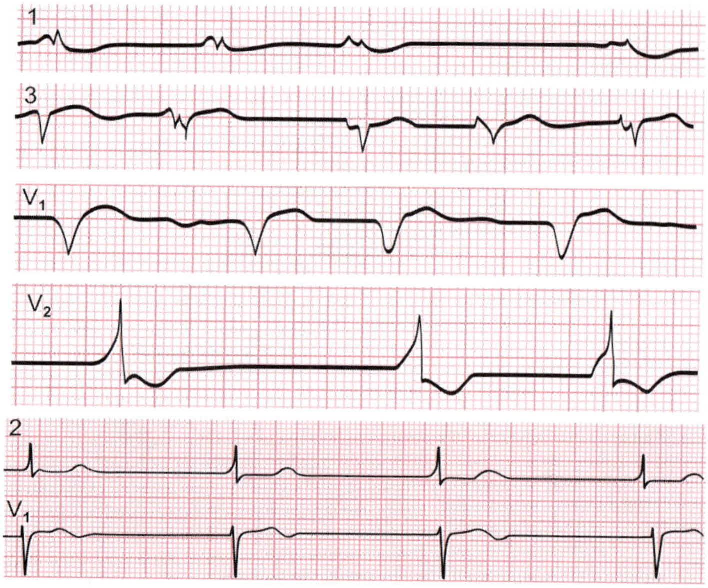

Fig: 3.23: *ECG trace shows features of sick sinus syndrome with A-V nodal rhythm with retrograde conduction at rate of 31 beats/min*

Dyspnea

The tissue anoxia of low cardiac output may lead to mild dyspnea.

Symptoms of cardiac arrhythmia

Palpitations: Palpitation is a frequently used term for any increased beats of the heart. Occasional extra beats are described as the heart "Seeming to miss a beat", or as the heart "turning over in the chest". The sudden onset of faster heart rate may represent the onset of an attack of paroxysmal tachycardia or of atrial fibrillation.

Cardiac Syncope

Definition

Syncope resulting from the sudden cessation of cerebral blood flow when there is an arrest of the cardiac pumping action.

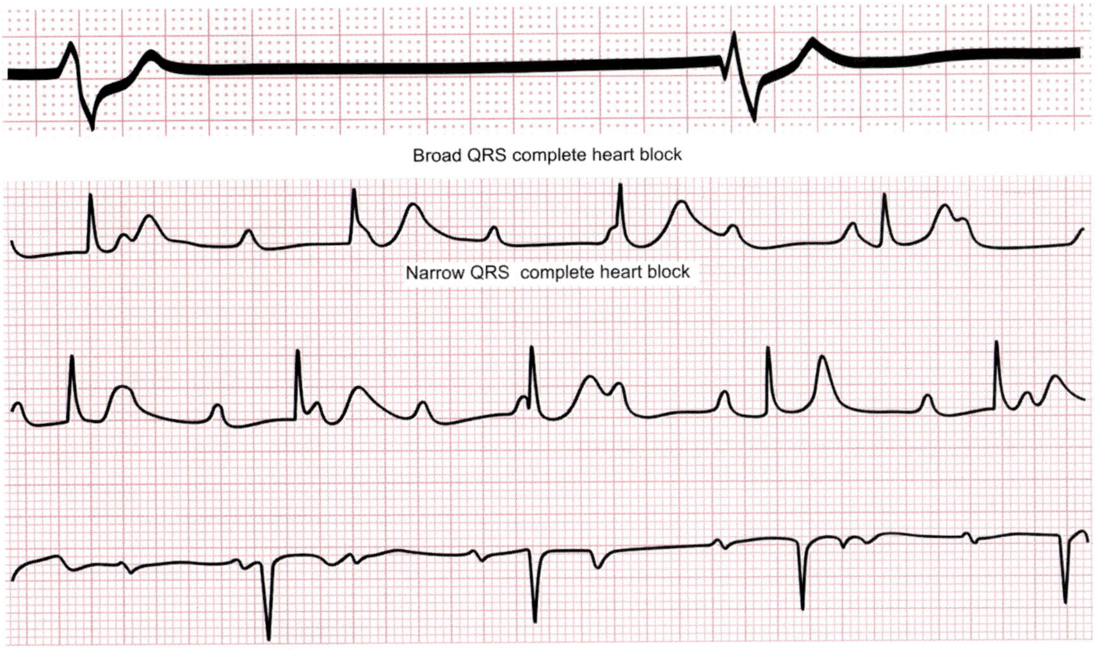

Fig. 3.24: *ECG showing narrow and wide QRS complex in two patients suffering from aquired and congenital complete heart block respectively presenting as syncopal attacks*

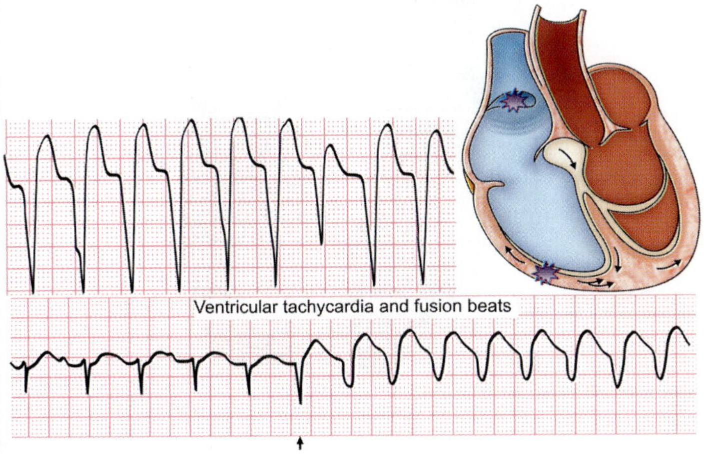

Fig. 3.25: *ECG showing ventricular tachycardia (upper panel) and fusion beat as indicated (↓lower panel) and diagram showing the genesis of fusion beats (↑upper right panel)*

Description

There is an abrupt loss of consciousness with extreme pallor. The pupils dilate and epileptiform convulsions may occur. When efficient cardiac pumping action returns there is abrupt restoration of consciousness, accompanied by a red flush of the skin as blood flows into vessels widely dilated by the accumulation of metabolites during the brief period of circulatory arrest.

Causes

1. **Complete heart block** (Stokes Adams attack): Short episodes of cardiac arrest or of ventricular fibrillation are particularly frequent at the onset of complete heart block before the ventricular pacemaker has become well established (Fig. 3.26).
2. **Severe aortic stenosis:** The syncope of severe aortic stenosis during exertion is a result of brief attacks of ventricular arrhythmias in some patients
3. **Paroxysmal tachycardia:** Occasionally the cardiac output is so reduced at the onset of fast arrhythmia that syncope results.
4. **Left atrial thrombus, and left atrial myxoma:** Impaction of these structures in the mitral valve orifice is a rare cause of syncope.

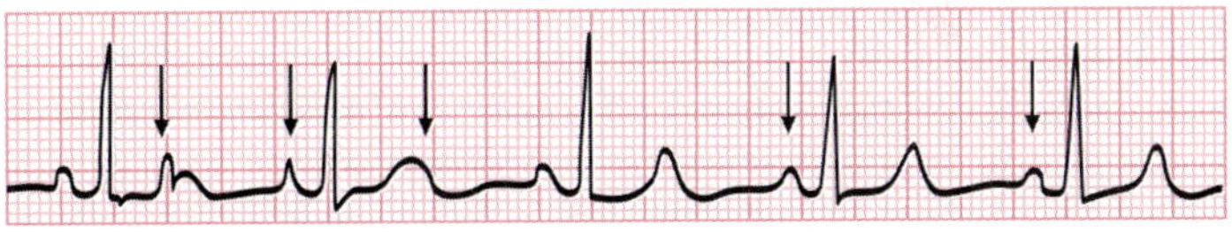

Fig. 3.26: *ECG showing complete heart block presenting as syncopal attacks*

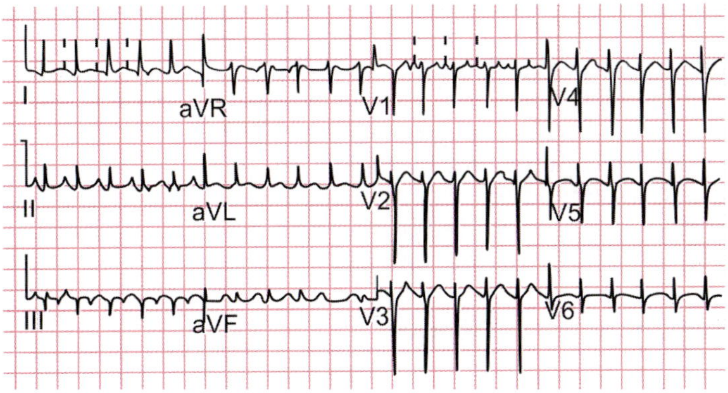

Fig. 3.27: *ECG showing features of focal atrial tachycardia with 1:1 conduction. Note the narrow, regular tachycardia. The P-waves are marked with arrows (long-RP interval), and the P-wave morphology differs from that of sinus rhythm*

Balance Problems

Other names: Dizziness, unsteadiness, light-headedness. **Description:** Inability to walk or stand without holding on to something to maintain balance some causes related to cardiovascular disease: can be seen after stroke, or due to general weakness caused by low cardiac output or low blood pressure. Some causes related to other disorders can be seen with several neurological problems or with inner ear problems, as well as to numerous general medical problems significance: many significant medical problems can cause problems with balance. This symptom always needs to be carefully evaluated by a physician.

II. GENERAL PHYSICAL EXAMINATION

Physical Characteristic

Chronic severe heart failure may cause emaciation, and cyanotic congenital heart disease may be responsible for stunted growth and poor development. Obesity aggravates the effect of cardiac disease (Figs 3.5 and 3.6).

Anatomical abnormalities: Anatomical defects. Absence or hypoplasia of one or both upper limbs are associated with intracardiac defects such as ASD or VSD (Holt-Oram syndrome).

Genetic Abnormalities

(Figs 3.31, 3.33, 3.34, 3.36 and 3.38)

Many genetically determined disorders are easily recognized from their effects on the general body configuration. The cardiac malformations commonly associated with specific genetic defects are listed below.

Chromosome Disorders

Mongolism: Endocardial cushion defects. Turner's syndrome (XO) coarctation of the aorta pulmonary stenosis.

Single Gene Disorders (Fig. 3.28)

Marfan syndrome: Aortic ectasia, dissecting aneurysm of the aorta. Hereditary hemorrhagic telangiectasia, pulmonary arteriovenous fistulae, neurofibromatosis pheochromocytoma, polydactyly common atrium, atrial septal defect etc. Stigmata indicating rubella infection lesions such as mental deficiency, nerve deafness and cataract in a child suggest that the mother was infected during early pregnancy by rubella. In such cases, there is a strong likelihood of congenital heart disease, the common cardiac lesions produced by the virus being patent ductus arteriosus (Figs 3.4, 3.29 and 3.30).

Pulmonary Valve Stenosis

Pulmonary Artery Branch Stenosis

Thoracic deformity

Massive enlargement of the heart in infancy can produce a permanent deformity of the overlying chest wall with a forward bulge of the precordium to the left of the sternum.

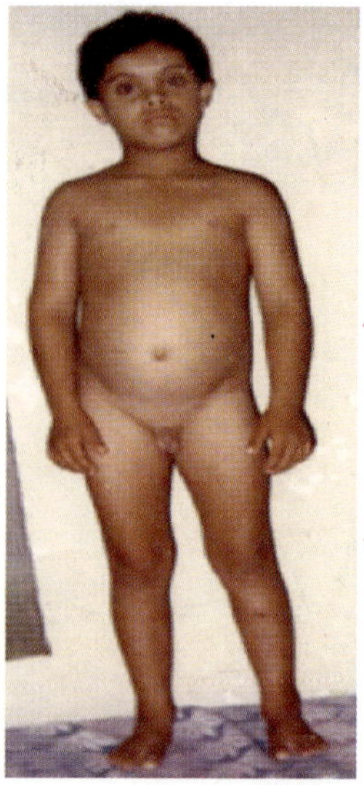

Fig. 3.28: *Physical features of mongolism associated with VSD*

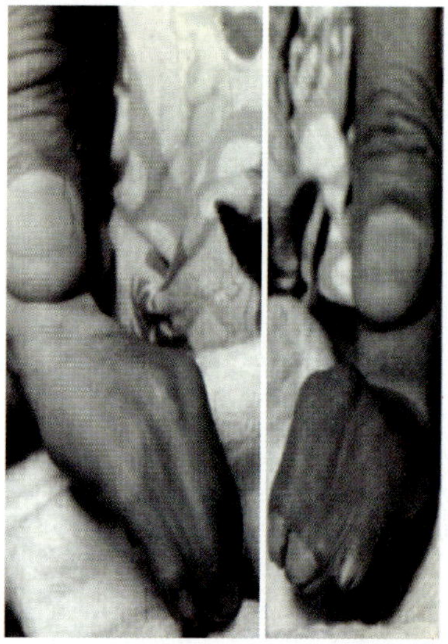

Fig. 3.29: *Bilateral syndactylism in a child with Aperts syndrome*

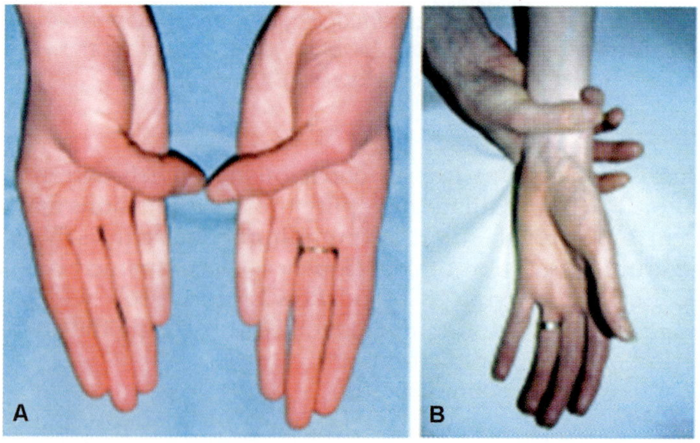

Fig. 3.30: *Arachnodactyly. (A) Steinberg thumb sign. Entire thumb nail protrudes beyond ulnar border of hand. (B) Walker-Murdoch wrist sign. Thumb and 5th finger can overlap around wrist. Both signs must be present to diagnose arachnodactyly according to the Ghent Marfan diagnostic criteria*

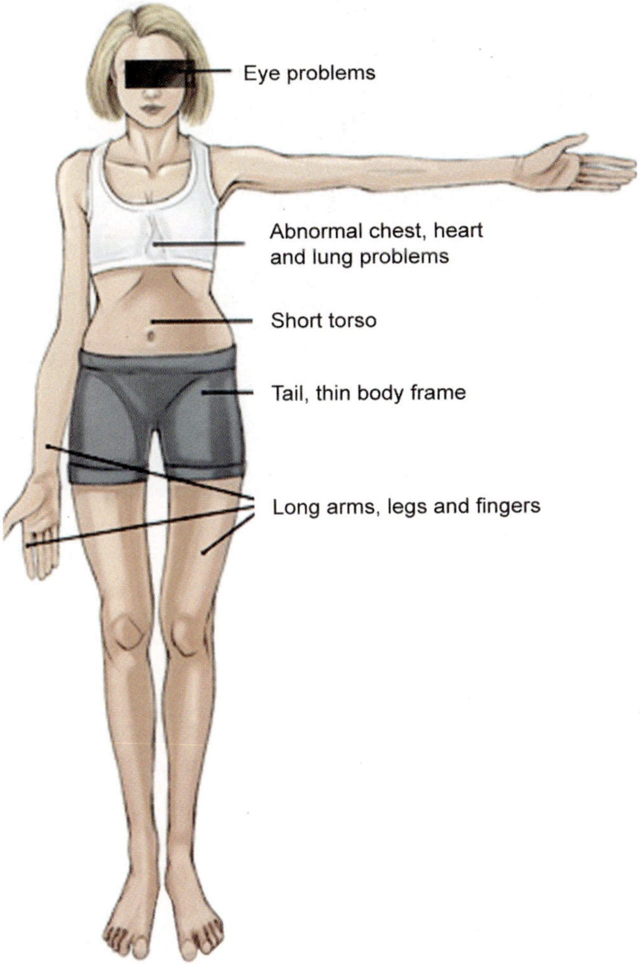

Fig. 3.31: *Physical parameters of Marfan syndrome*

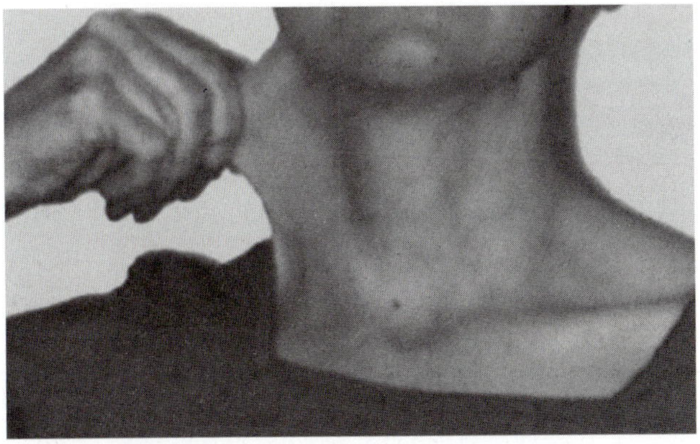

Fig. 3.32: *Feature of cutus hyperelastica. The vascular type III is considered one of the more serious forms of Ehlers-Danlos syndrome because blood vessels and organs are fragile and prone to tearing (rupture)*

Pulmonary hypertension complicating a left to right intracardiac to right intracardiac shunt may result in an abnormally rounded configuration of the front of the chest in children. Pectus excavatum type of chest deformity may also be associated with high incidence of MVP and ASD[2]

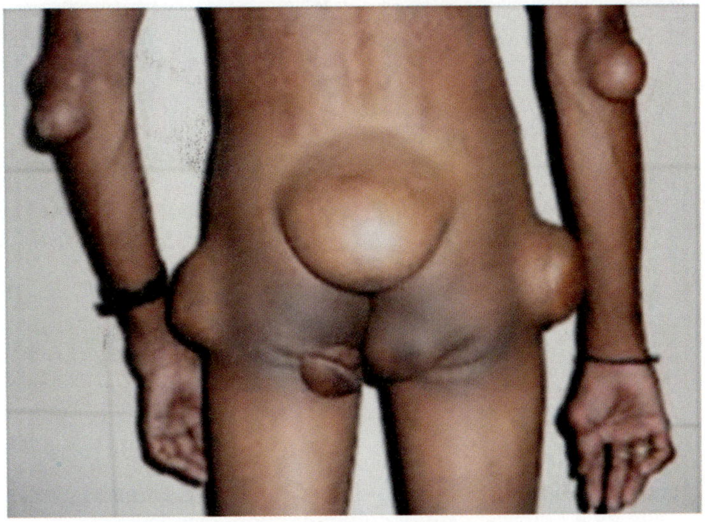

Fig. 3.33: *Multiple swellings due to giant tuberous xanthomas over extensor aspects of limbs and buttocks*

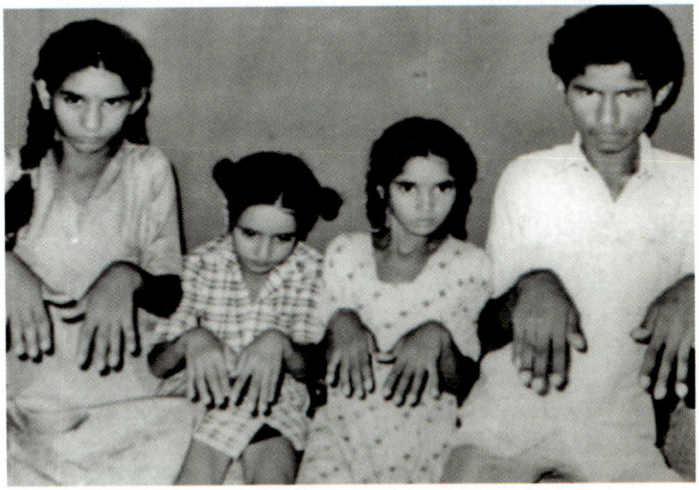

Fig. 3.34: *Photograph showing hereditary transmitted bilateral congenital clubbing among all the members of the family*

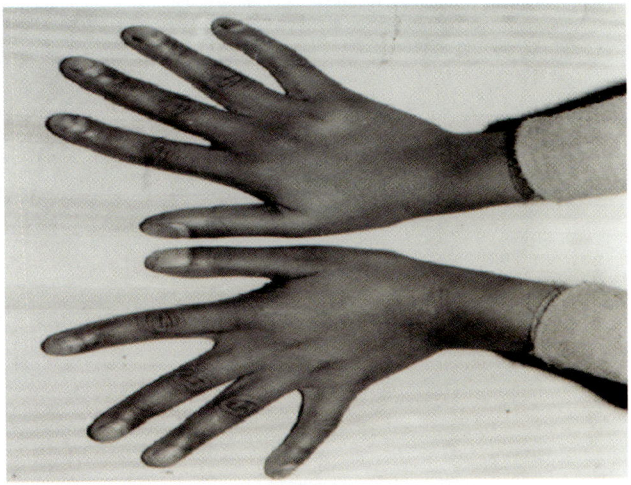

Fig. 3.35: *Bilateral clubbing of fingers in infective endocarditis in patient with chronic rheumatic valvular dysfunction*

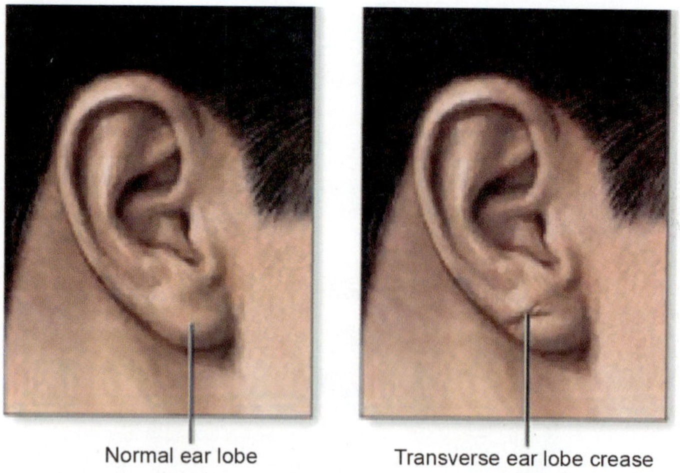

Fig. 3.36: *Showing normal ear lobe crease (left) and transverse crease as a physical sign of coronary artery disease(right)*

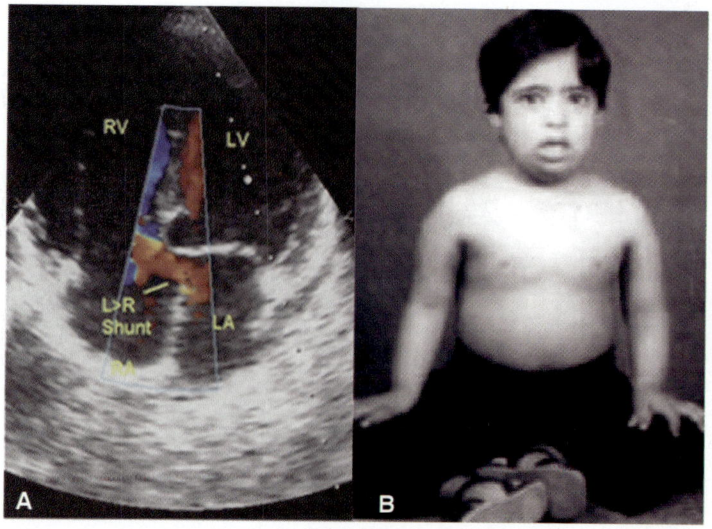

Fig. 3.38: *(A) Color flow apical 4C views in dual scan showing large septum primum defect with almost single dilated atrium, dilated LV with gross mitral regurgitation in patient with endocardial cushion defect. (B) Stunted growth,polydactylism and chest deformity in a child with endocardial cushion defect*

Malar flush (Fig. 3.37)
Patients with a chronic low cardiac output have a dusky flush of the cheeks. This color is the result of dilated capillaries in the dermis, in which the circulation of blood is slow, and is most commonly seen in mitral stenosis complicated by pulmonary hypertension.

Cyanosis

A blue discoloration of the skin and mucous membranes caused by 5.0 gm or more of reduced hemoglobin per 100 mL of blood in the skin capillaries.

Peripheral Cyanosis

There is a slow circulation of blood to the cyanosed part and, because the blood is in prolonged contact with the tissues, the extraction of oxygen is more complete than normal. The blood in the capillaries thus has an increased proportion of reduced hemoglobin. Vasoconstriction due to cold or as compensation for a low cardiac output is the usual cause of peripheral cyanosis, which is best seen in the lobes of the ears, the nose and the fingers.

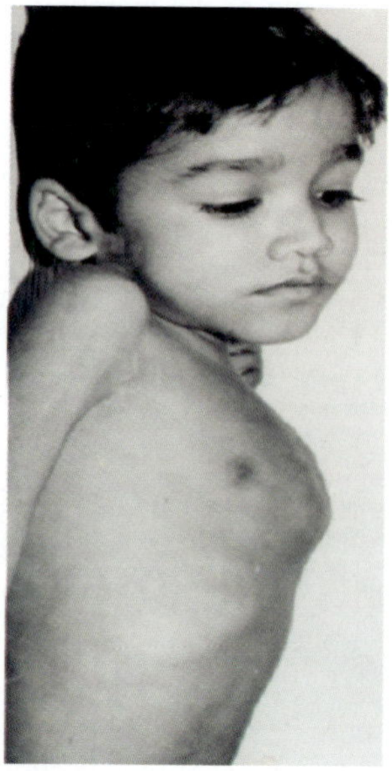

Fig. 3.37: *Pigeon-shaped chest deformity in a child with VSD*

Central Cyanosis (Figs 3.39–3.42)

Definition
Central cyanosis is defined as cyanosis caused by a reduced oxygen saturation of the systemic arterial blood.

Clinical features
The following features accompany central cyanosis and distinguish it from peripheral cyanosis.

Finger clubbing: Warm mucous membranes, blue tongue, lips and conjunctiva. Polycythemia is present with abnormally raised hemoglobin and haematocrit. Arteries

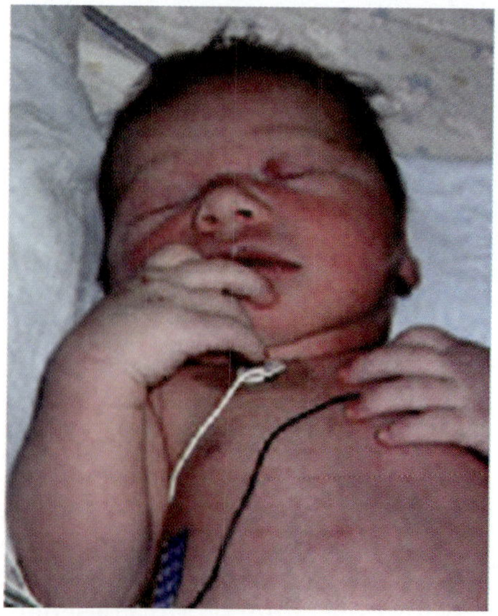

Fig. 3.39: *Cyanosis in a child with congenital heart*

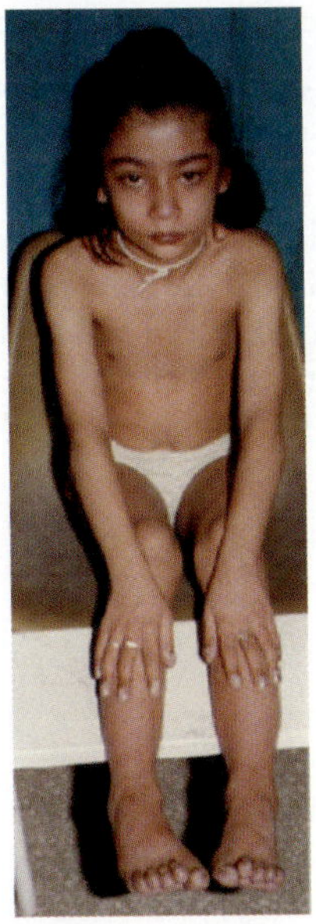

Fig. 3.40: *Central cyanosis in a child with R-L shunt*

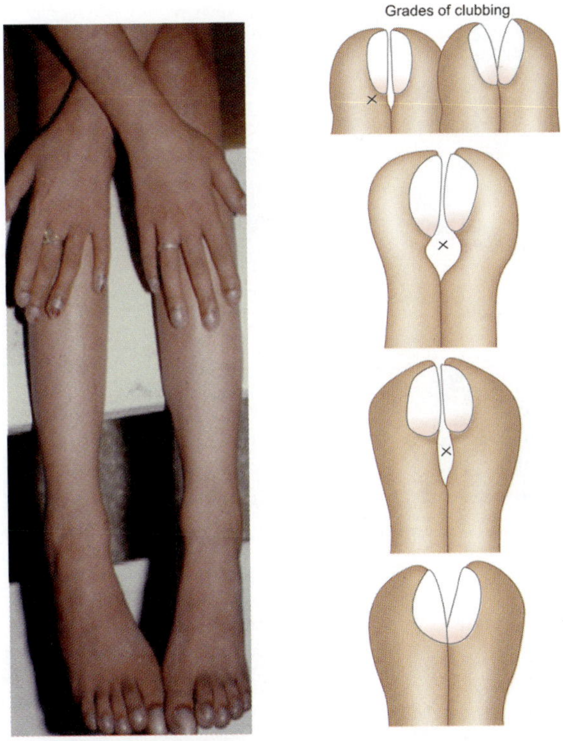

Fig. 3.41: *Bilateral digital clubbing and central cyanosis in patient with Fallot's tetralogy (left) and graphic representation of various grades of digital clubbing (right)*

blood, obtained by needle puncture from a peripheral artery, is desaturated, this is the absolute differentiating test in doubtful cases.

Causes

Cardiac disease: Venous blood entering the left heart without passing through the lungs, i.e. right to left shunting of blood through abnormal communication in the heart.

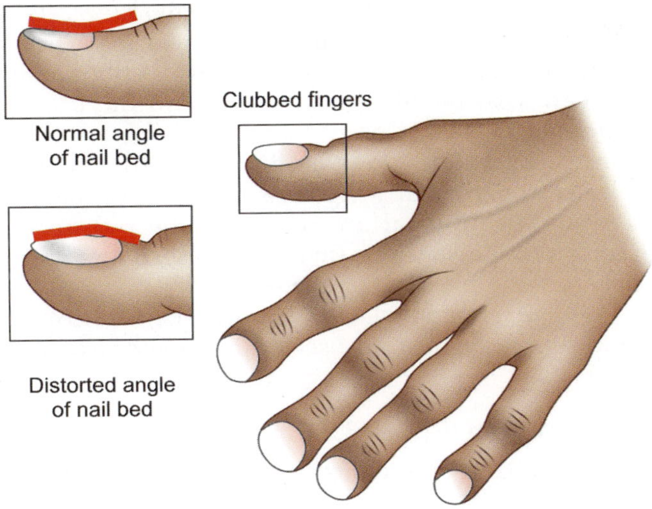

Fig. 3.42: *Features of clubbing of fingers*

Pulmonary disease

Inadequate oxygenation of the blood as the blood passes through the lungs. The breathing of oxygen for a few minutes increases the oxygen tension in the alveoli of the lungs thus compensating for poor lung functions. Cyanosis due to lung disease is markdely improved with O_2 therapy while cyanosis caused by a right to left intracardiac shunt is little affected.

Differential cyanosis

Definition: Cyanosis is more intense in the feet than in the hands when both are warm.

Cause: Differential cyanosis implies that the oxygen content of the arterial blood in the legs is lower than in the arms. Blood low in oxygen will pass from the pulmonary artery through a persistent ductus arteriosus only when there is severe pulmonary hypertension. The presence of differentials cyanosis is therefore, diagnostic of persistent ductus arteriosus with pulmonary hypertension.

Clubbing of the fingers

Stages

1. Obliteration of the normal angle between the finger nail and skin on the dorsum of the finger by an increase in the soft tissues underneath the nail bed.
2. The nail becomes curved longitudinally.
3. Swelling of soft tissues of the terminal phalanges gives a drum stick appearance to the digits.

Causes: The exact stimulus producing finger clubbing is not known. Heart disease finger clubbing is due to cyanotic heart disease, bacterial endocarditis or left atrial myxoma. However, rarely it may be of a heredito-familial.

Abnormal pulse

Description: The patient notices an area in or on the body where an unusual or a vigorous pulsation can be seen or felt. Some *causes related to* cardiovascular disease: Abnormal pulsations can be related to vascular disease, such as an aneurysm (an abnormal dilation or "ballooning" of an artery). Abnormal pulsations in the abdomen, in particular, are often indicative of an aortic aneurysm. A "bounding" pulse can also be felt in patients who have aortic insufficiency (a "leaky" aortic valve).

Some causes related to other disorders: Any condition that leads to particularly vigorous pumping of the heart can create an unusual awareness of the pulse. Such conditions include anemia, thyroid disease, hypertension, anxiety, or other medical problems.

Significance: A persistent abnormal pulsation can indicate significant medical disease, and should be reported to a doctor.

Abdominal Pain (Fig. 3.43)

Description: Pain or discomfort in or around the abdominal area.

Causes related to cardiovascular disease: Vascular disease can cause abdominal pain in several ways. Blockage or partial blockage (due to atherosclerosis) of arteries supplying the vital organs can cause those organs to become ischemic, and therefore painful. This type of pain is usually greater after a meal. An aneurysm of the abdominal aorta can cause pain, especially if the aneurysm begins to tear or rupture. This pain is often very severe, and sudden in onset. It is a medical emergency.

Causes related to other disorders: Numerous disorders of abdominal organs—stomach, intestines, bowel, liver, spleen, gallbladder, reproductive organs—can cause pain.

Significance: Vascular disease involving the abdominal blood vessels is always a significant, and potentially dangerous, medical problem. A ruptured or torn abdominal aortic aneurysm is often fatal. Many non-cardiovascular diseases causing pain in abdominal organs are also medically significant. Any unexplained abdominal pain that is severe, frequent, prolonged or persistent needs to be evaluated by a physician.

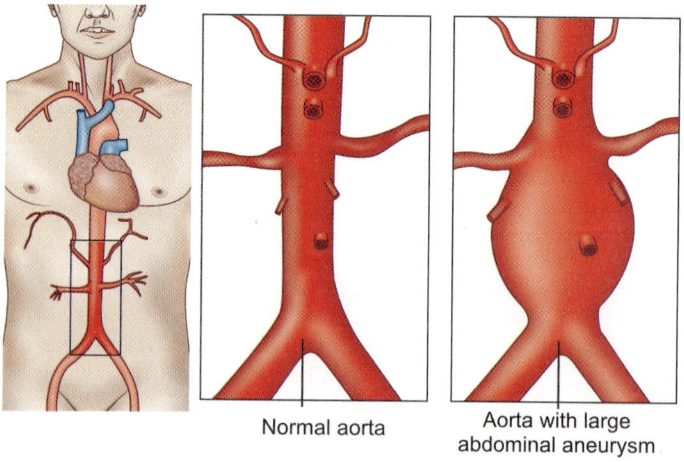

Fig. 3.43: *Diagram (left) showing normal thoracic and abdominal aorta and aneurysmal dilatation of thoracic and abdominal aorta as a cause of abdominal pain and abnormal pulsations (right)*

The Arterial Pulse (Figs 3.44–3.50)

The brachial arterial pulse is larger and more convenient for detailed study than the radial. For maximum information, the palpating finger should compress the vessel with just sufficient force to collapse the lumen in diastole. The rise in pressure with each heart beat forcibly expands the wall against the finger. The brachial pulse is analyzed under four headings (rate, rhythm, amplitude and wave form).

The carotid pulse is also examined and other arterial pulses are compared with each other.

Rate

1. An abnormally fast pulse may represent:
   (a) Sinus tachycardia (sinoatrial node remains in control), e.g. excitement, fever, exertion, thyrotoxicosis, hemorrhage.
   (b) Arrhythmia (an ectopic focus in the heart has taken over the pacemaking function from the sinoatrial node), e.g. paroxysmal atrial tachycardia, atrial flutter, atrial fibrillation, ventricular tachycardia.

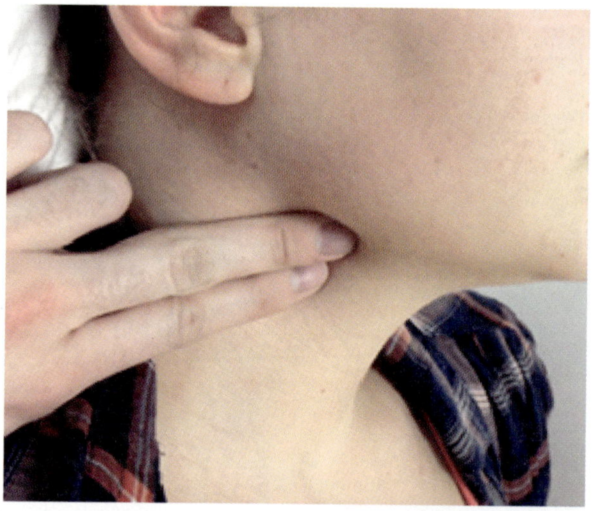

Fig. 3.44: *Palpation of carotid arteries in a young child*

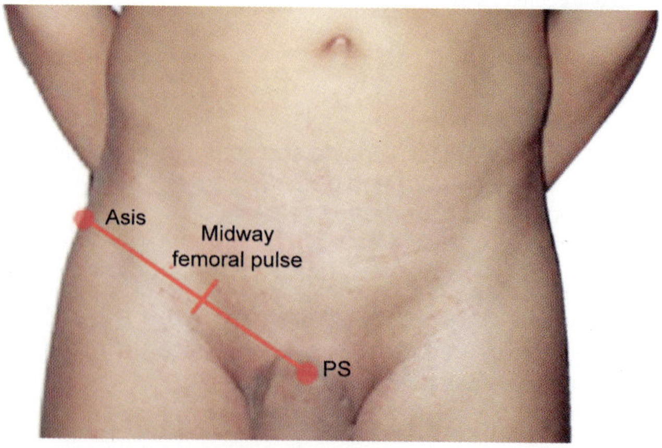

Fig. 3.45: *The femoral pulse is palpable at the mid-inguinal point, halfway between the pubic symphysis (PS) and the anterior superior iliac spine (ASIS)*

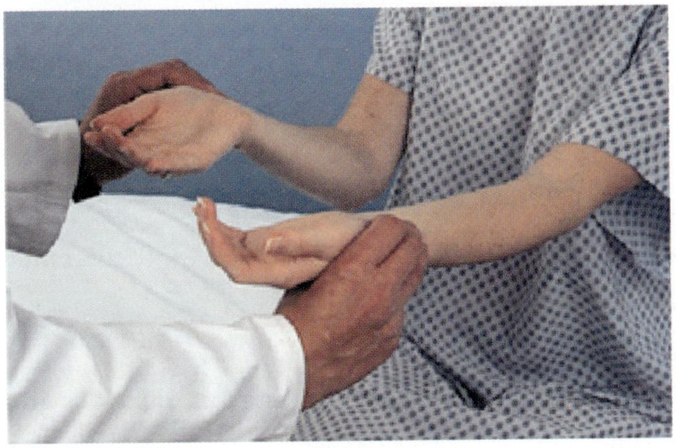

Fig. 3.46: *The radial pulse is palpable over the lateral wrist*

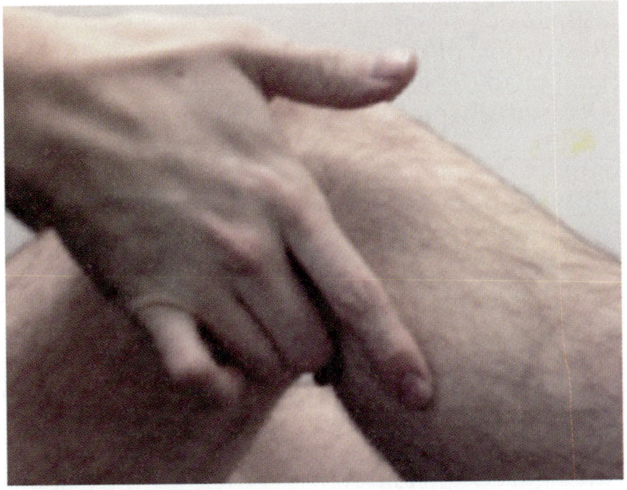

Fig. 3.47: *The popliteal pulse is palpable in the popliteal fossa whilst holding the bent knee with both hands*

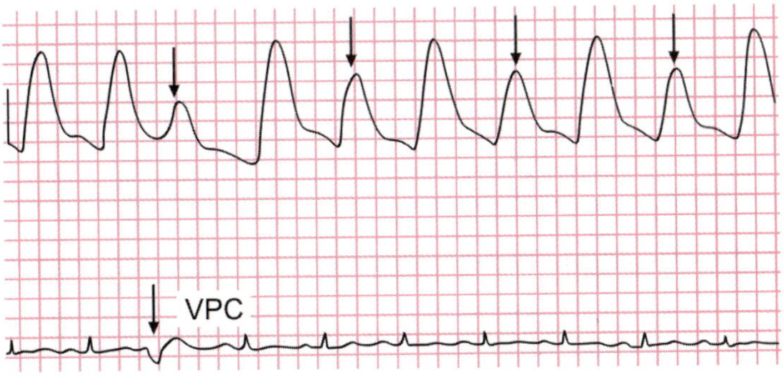

Fig. 3.48: *Hemodynamic study shows an alternating pulse-arterial pressure recording in severe left ventricular failure. After the second beat a ventricular premature beat triggers an episode of alternating pulse*

2. An abnormally slow pulse may represent:
   (a) Sinus bradycardia (sinoatrial node remains in control), e.g. trained athletes, increased intracranial pressure, jaundice.
   (b) Arrhythmia (a pulse rate below 40 beats per minute usually means complete heart block).

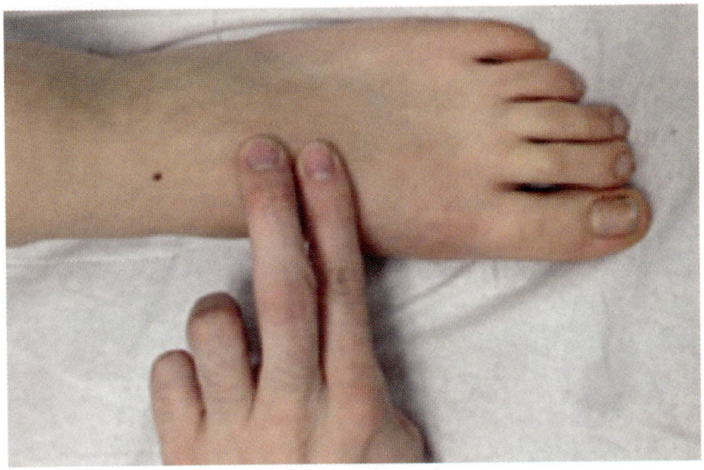

Fig. 3.49: *The dorsalis pedis pulse is palpable over the foot, lateral to the path taken by the extensor hallicus longus (the muscle which supplies the big toe)*

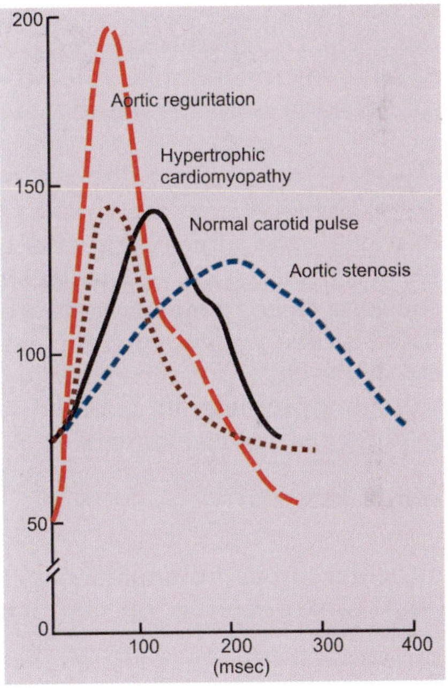

Fig. 3.50: *The normal carotid arterial pulse recording compared with recordings in hypertrophic cardiomyopathy, aortic regurgitation and aortic stenosis. Note the very rapid upstroke of the pulse in hypertrophic cardiomyopathy and aortic regurgitation compared with the slow upstroke in aortic stenosis. The pulse pressure in aortic regurgitation is widened because of the exaggerated systolic peak and the diastolic collapse*

Rhythm

The normal pulse is regular apart from a slight speeding up on inspiration and slowing on expiration most obvious in younger individuals (sinus arrhythmia). Complete irregularity indicates atrial fibrillation, but both sinus rhythm with multiple extrasystoles and atrial flutter with changing block can simulate atrial fibrillation.

During exercise, a patient with atrial fibrillation, the irregularity of the pulse is accentuated, atrial extrasystoles, disappear so that, the pulse become regular. In atrial flutter, regular degree of AV block becomes established, and the pulse becomes regular (Figs 3.24–3.27).

Amplitude

The amplitude of the pulse is judged by the movement of the palpating finger produced by the arrival of the pulse wave. A large amplitude pulse means that the pressure wave is large, i.e. there is a large difference between systolic and diastolic blood pressures.

Large Amplitude Pulse

Cause

1. Leakage of blood from the aorta in aortic valve regurgitation
2. Persistent ductus arteriosus and arteriovenous fistula
3. Increased flow of blood from aorta through dilated arterioles
4. Thyrotoxicosis and other high output states
5. Increased left ventricular volume
6. Complete heart block
7. Rigidity of aorta, i.e. atherosclerosis
   Increased left ventricular stroke volume—heart block rigidity of the aorta—atherosclerosis.

Mechanism

The rapid escape of blood from the aorta in the first two groups results in a low pressure in the arterial system by the end of diastole and the large left ventricular stroke volume ejected into the aorta causes a high systolic pressure.

The very large stroke volume of complete heart block gives an abnormally large pressure peak in the aorta. A normal stroke volume produces an abnormal great pressure rise when the aorta has lost its elasticity.

Small Amplitude Pulse

Causes

Low left ventricular stroke volume (shock, tachycardia, mitral stenosis). Obstruction to left ventricular ejection (aortic stenosis).

Mechanism

In the low cardiac output states, the volume of blood ejected into the aorta with each beat is small and the pressure rise also tends to be small.

Obstruction to left ventricular ejection reduces the speed of blood flow into the aorta during systole, thereby producing a smaller and slower than normal pressurize in aortic stenosis.

Pulse Varying In Amplitude

Pulses alternans

Description

The amplitude of the pulse wave, in a patient in sinus rhythm, is large and small alternately.

Mechanism

Usually, in a patient with heart, failure, an episode of alternans is initiated by an extrasystole. In the succeeding pause there is excessive filling of the left ventricle and the next ventricular contraction is powerful and prolonged because of the large volume to be expelled. The period available for diastolic filling of the ventricle prior to the next beat is therefore short and the contraction less forceful.

Significance

Pulsus alternans is good evidence of left ventricular failure.

Pulsus Paradoxus

Description

A marked accentuation of the normal decrease in the amplitude of the arterial pulse during quiet inspiration.

Causes

1. Increased inspiratory effort (laryngeal stridor, severe asthma)
2. Restriction of diastolic filling of the heart (cardiac tamponade, constrictive pericarditis)
3. Occasionally present in right ventricular failure.

Mechanism

1. **Pulsus paraadoxus in asthma:** The powerful inspiratory effort to overcome airway obstruction considerably increases the capacity of the lung vessels and thereby reduces the flow of blood out of the lungs to the left heart. The systemic arterial pulse pressure is then diminished during inspiration.
2. **Pulsus paradoxus in tamponade:** When the diastolic volume of the heart is limited by a pericardial effusion or a rigid pericardium, the normal increased filling of the right atrium and right ventricle during inspiration leaves less available volume for the left atrium and the left ventricle. Left ventricular stroke volume is reduced during inspiration and pulsus paradoxus is produced.
3. **Pulsus paradoxus in right ventricular failure:** If the failing right ventricle does not increase its output during inspiration the normal increase in the capacity of the lung vessels will restrict the flow out of the lungs into the left heart and the left ventricular stroke output will decrease resulting into formation of pulsus paradoxus.

Pulse Varying in Waveforms

The shape of the pressure wave is of diagnostic value as many abnormalities of the circulation produce characteristic changes in the form of the pulse wave which are readily detected by palpation. The normal brachial pulse has a smooth fairly sharp upstroke, a momentarily sustained peak and a quick downstroke. The dicrotic notch, representing aortic valve closure, cannot be detected clinically, but the other features are readily analysed.

Anacrotic pulse (Plateau pulse, slow rising pulse).

Description

The upstroke is slow with often a distinct notch on it. The time taken to reach the peak is prolonged and the entire pulse wave is of small amplitude.

Causes

Aortic valve stenosis: The rate of ejection of blood into the aorta is decreased so that the ejection is prolonged and the amplitude of the pulse is diminished.

Water Hammer Pulse (Collapsing Pulse)

Description

The upstroke is more abrupt and steep than normal. The peak is reached early, is not sustained and the downstroke is also rapid. The amplitude is usually abnormally large. The examiner's finger appreciates the sharper than normal upstroke rather than the downstroke and experiences a sharp tap with each pulse beat.

Causes

The sharp upstroke represents the rapid ejection of blood into an empty arterial system and the rapid downstroke indicates abnormally fast escape of blood from the arteries during diastole. A water hammer or bounding pulse is found in:

1. Aortic valve regurgitation
2. Persistent ductus arteriosus
3. Systemic arteriovenous fistula
4. Pregnancy
5. Fever
6. Thyrotoxicosis
7. Anemia
8. Anoxic lung disease.

Pulses Bisferiens

Description

The upstroke is sharp to a high peak, the pressure then falls and rises again to a second peak of about the same height as the first peak before falling off. The amplitude of the pulse wave is large and the palpating finger experiences two distinct impulses with each pulse beat.

Causes

This wave form indicates combined stenosis and incompetence of the aortic valve, both lesions being severe. The exact mechanism producing pulsus bisferiens is unknown.

Dicrotic Pulse

Description

A secondary pressure wave follows the dicrotic notch (later than the second peak of the bisferiens pulse) so that two impulses are felt with each pulse beat and may give the impression that the heart rate is twice as fast as it really is.

Causes

The normal very small secondary pressure wave produced by aortic valve closure is accentuated during its transmission to the peripheral arteries when the tone of the arterial system is low, classically in typhoid fever.

Carotid Pulse

Carotid arterial pulsation is normally visible in the neck.

1. **Invisible carotid pulsation:** Small pulse pressure, e.g. aortic stenosis.
2. **Prominent carotid pulsation:** Large pulse pressure, e.g. aortic regurgitation, persistent ductus arteriosus, heart block, excitement, or loss of elascity of the aorta, e.g. atheroma of the aorta and coarctation of the aorta.

Comparison of the Pulses

The radial pulses are compared one with the other and with the femoral pulses. The pulsations of both carotid arteries are also compared.

1. **Unequal or delayed radial pulsation on one side indicates obstruction**
   (a) At origin of a subclavian artery, e.g. atheromatous plaque; involvement of the origin by an aortic aneurysm and origin of a subclavian artery below a coarctation of the aorta.
   (b) Distal to origin of subclavian artery, e.g. subclavian or brachial embolus.
2. **Femoral pulses small or delayed compared with radial pulses**
   (a) Coarctation of the aorta (obstruction to blood flow in the thoracic aorta)
   (b) Saddle embolus.
3. **Unequal carotid pulses**
   Atheroma of innominate or common carotid arteries, aortic arch syndrome and dissecting aneurysm, the blood pressure.
   The blood pressure depends primarily on the
   1. Cardiac output
   2. Peripheral resistance
   3. Elasticity of the aorta, the blood volume
4. **Blood viscosity.**

Blood Pressure

(a) **The systolic blood pressure** is the peak pressure achieved during the ejection of blood from the ventricle into the aorta.

(b) **The diastolic blood pressure** varies with the peripheral resistance. If there is a rapid escape of blood from the aorta there will be a low pressure at the end of diastole. In the absence of anatomical leaks (persistent ductus arteriosus, arteriovenous fistula), the peripheral resistance is governed by the arterioles, vasodilatation lowering the diastolic pressure.

Measurement

An inflatable cuff firmly bound to the upper arm and connected to a mercury column is used for measurement of the arterial pressure in the arm. For accurate results, the width of the **sphygmomanometer cuff** must be appropriate to the circumference of the arm. A cuff 5 inches in width is correct for a normal-sized adult and smaller cuffs are necessary for the children since a large cuff gives a falsely low reading. The systolic pressure is the highest pressure at which successive sounds are heard when auscultating over the brachial artery, and the diastolic pressure is taken at the point when sounds abruptly become dull and muffled (Fig. 3.51).

Doppler technique may be employed when pulses are weak. Such as in pulseless disease. In the adult, top normal pressure should probably be taken to be about 120/80 mmHg. Whereas in infants and children one may apply the rule that by age 1 year the systolic pressure is about 90 mmHg and increases by 5 mmHg about every 3 years, so that by the age of 13 or 14, it has a reached to adult level.

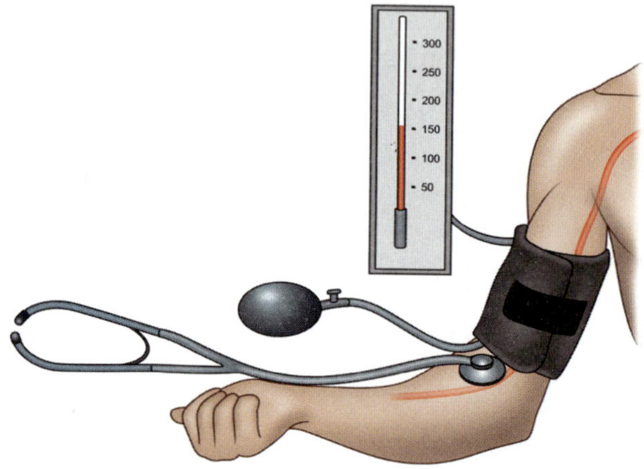

Fig. 3.51: *Showing application of Sphygmomanometer a common instrument for measuring systolic and diastolic blood pressure in human body*

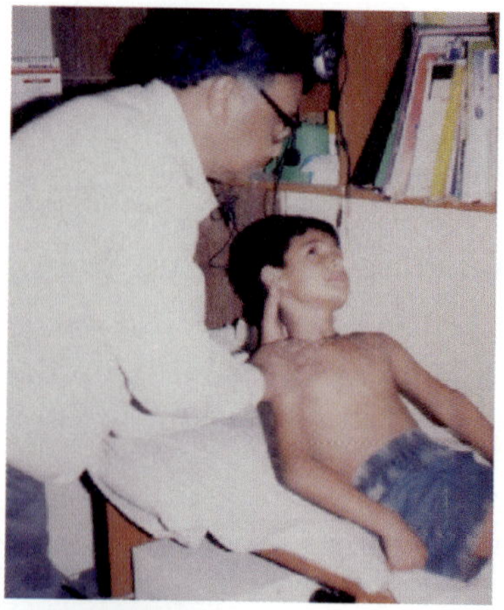

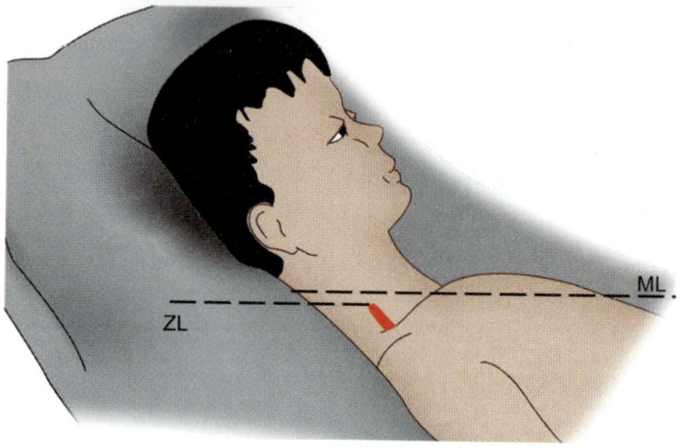

Fig. 3.52 (Top and bottom): *Doctor (author) is examining neck vein of a young child for distension and pulsations of carotid vessels at 45° angle with the bed*

The Jugularvenous (JV) Pressure

Measurement (Figs 3.52–3.57)

The patient is placed at an angle of 45° with the head supported on a pillow and the pulsations of the internal jugular vein in the neck are usually visible. The internal jugular vein is collapsed except for its lower part where the pressure from the right atrium keeps it distended. The right atrial pressure fluctuates throughout the cardiac cycle and the changing level of distension of the internal jugular vein imparts a gentle undulation to the skin of the neck which is readily distinguishable from the single sharp movement produced by carotid arterial pulsation. The vertical distance in centimeters between the top of this undulation and the sternal angle is called the jugular venous pressure and is a measurement of the pressure in the right atrium. The external jugular vein is often partially kinked and obstructed near the root of the neck and is a less reliable measure of the right atrial pressure. The jugular venous pulse is analyzed for height above the sternal angel and for wave form. The normal mean pressure is 0–2 cm above sternal angle and the wave form reveals "a" and "v" waves of approximately equal height. Many other workers refer the figure of 4.6 cm at 45° inclination.

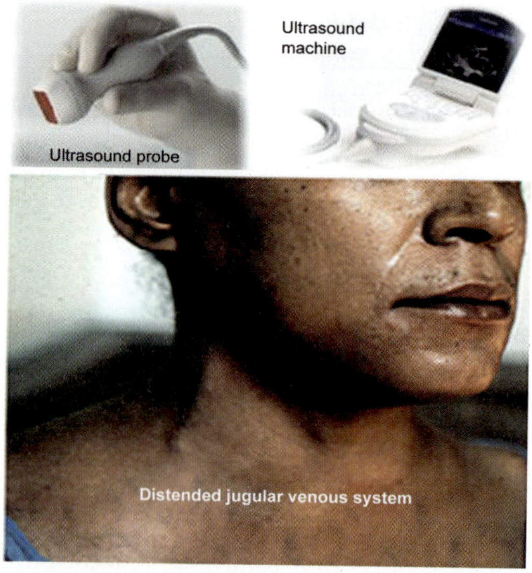

Fig. 3.53: *Looking at the neck veins for hours together has been a favorite passtime of our cardiology ancestors. Thanks to those sharp intellect, that has led us to this height of cardiovascular revolution. Measuring JV pressure by itself was considered a big science. Putting a patient in 45°, marking the sternal angle, identify the oscillating venous column, measuring the vertical distance, etc. Now in 2010, with bedside hand-held echo (one can rapidly rule out an elevated central venous pressure by imaging the jugular vein directly)*

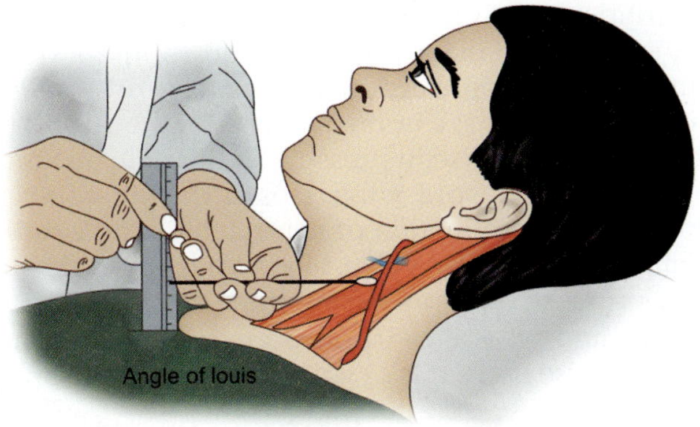

Fig: 3.54: *Method of measurement of jugular venous pressure at angle of Louis*

Causes of a Raised Mean Jugular Venous Pressure

1. High right ventricular filling pressure:
   (a) Right ventricular failure: Failing right ventricle requires a diastolic pressure as high as 4.0 mmHg to maintain a cardiac output of 4.0 liters per minute. The whole circulation adjusts to maintain a high right atrial filling pressure under these circumstances.
   (b) High output states: A slight increase in right atrial filling pressure is required even in normal hearts for the right ventricle to maintain a high cardiac output.
   (c) Increased blood volume (over transfusion, acute nephritis): Until the blood vessels dilate to accommodate the increased volume there is an increased venous return and a raised right atrial pressure.

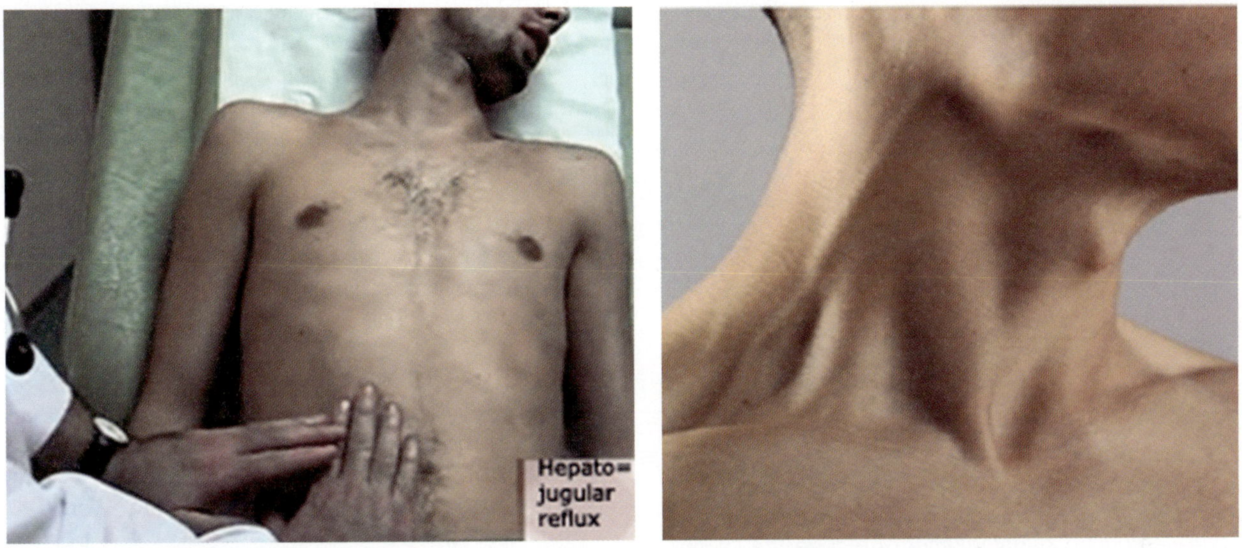

Fig. 3.55: *Doctor is pressing over the liver area and looking for distension of neck veins to demonstrate hepatojugular reflux in an adolescent with congestive heart failure (left) and engorged jugular vein in intractable heart failure (right)*

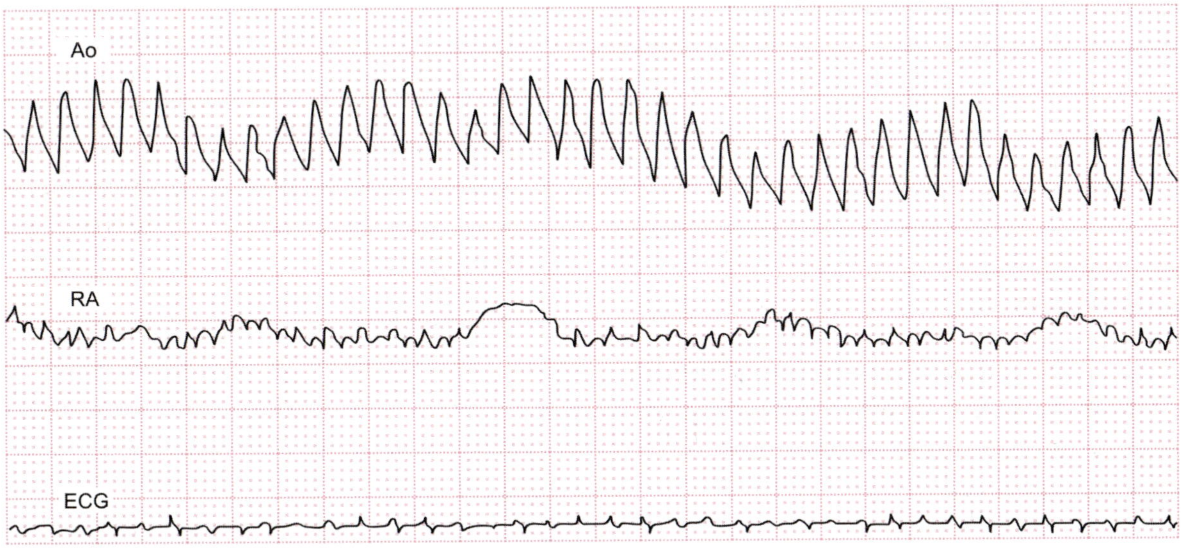

Fig. 3.56: *Paradoxical pulse and Kussmaul's sign. Pericardial effusion (evidenced by the small voltage deflexions on the ECG which has caused tamponade. Respiratory fluctuations in the aortic (Ao) and right atrial (RA) pressure signals are seen. During inspiration aortic pressure falls markedly (paradoxical pulse) and right atrial pressure rises (Kussmaul's sign)*

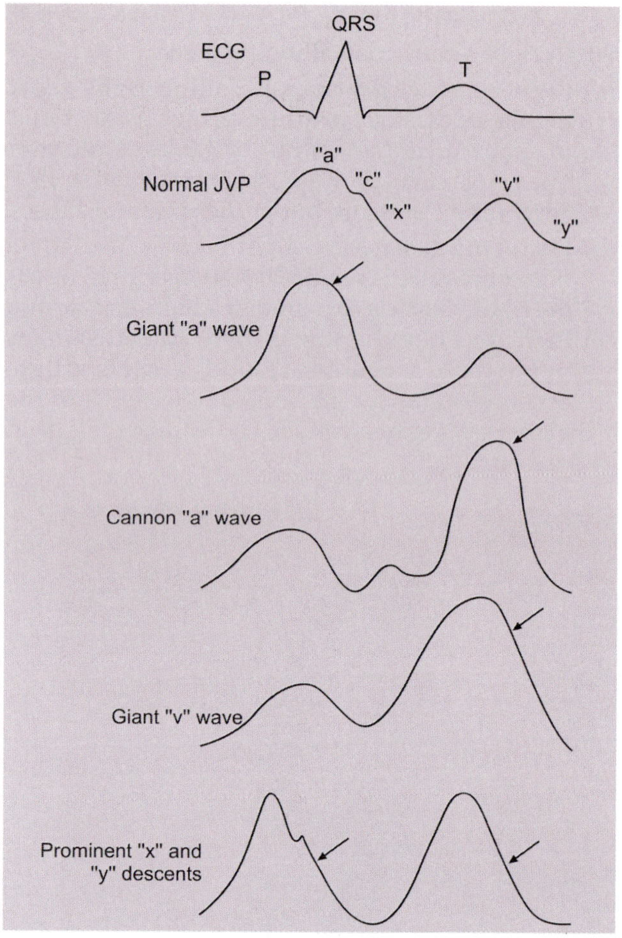

Fig. 3.57: *The jugularvenous pulse (JVP). Electrical events always precede mechanical events. Thus, the P-wave of the ECG (representing atrial depolarization) and the QRS complex (representing ventricular depolarization) precede the "a" wave and the "v" wave of the JVP, respectively*

(d) Restriction of relaxation of the heart in diastole: Normal filling of the heart is impeded during diastole in tamponade and in constrictive pericarditis.

2. Obstruction to blood flow from right atrium to right ventricle (tricuspid stenosis, right atrial myxoma): A high right atrial pressure serves to maintain the blood flow across the obstructed region.
3. Superior vena cava obstruction (involvement by or retrosternal thyroid gland enlargement): The distended veins do not pulsate which distinguishes this cause of an elevated venous pressure.
4. Loss of negative intrathoracic pressure (emphysema, pleural effusion, pneumothorax): Any rise in pressure within the thorax is transmitted to the right atrium.

Abnormalities of Waveform in the Jugular-Venous Pulse

Normal

Two peaks ("a" and "v") and two troughs ("x" and "y") are seen during each cardiac cycle. The waves are timed by relating them to the carotid pulse. The "a" wave precedes the carotid arterial pulse and is the pressure wave of right atrial systole. A fall in pressure follows, the x descent, during which the right atrium relaxes. The "v" wave is the positive pressure wave immediately after the carotid pulse and represents the rise in pressure in the right atrium as it fills with the tricuspid valve closed during ventricular systole. At the termination of ventricular systole with the opening of the tricuspid valve, blood leaves the right atrium and its pressure falls, producing the y descent.

The "a" and "v" waves are of approximately equal height and do not rise more than 2 cm above the sternal angle.

Abnormalities of the "a" Wave

1. Large a wave (powerful right atrial contraction): This implies an increase resistance to blood flow from right atrium to right ventricle. The resistance may be at valve level (tricuspid stenosis, tricuspid atresia), or the right ventricle may offer more resistance to filing when its walls are hypertrophied (pulmonary stenosis, pulmonary hypertension).
2. Absent a wave noncoordinated concretion of the right atrium), i.e. atrial fibrillation.

Abnormalities of the "v" Wave

Large v waves indicate considerable reflux of blood into the right atrium during ventricular systole, i.e. tricuspid regurgitation (TR).

Abnormalities of the "x" Descent

It is absent in atrial fibrillation. Accentuated in tamponade and in some cases of constrictive pericarditis. During ventricular systole, blood is ejected from the heart into the pulmonary artery and into the aorta. The decrease in volume of the ventricles with the rigid pericardial sac creates more volume available for filling of the right atrium from the great veins.

Abnormalities of the "y" Descent

1. *Sharp y descent:* The higher the venous pressure the more abrupt is the fall in pressure when the tricuspid valve opens, provided there is no obstruction to flow from the right atrium into the right ventricle.
2. *Slow y descent:* This provides evidence of obstruction to flow from right atrial into right ventricle and is found in tricuspid steosis or when there is tumor mass within the right atrium.

Cannon Waves

Large venous pressure waves synchronous with the carotid pulse, produced by atrial contraction against a closed tricuspid valve. A cannon waves therefore implies atrial contraction coinciding with ventricular systole.

Causes of Cannon Waves

Regular fast cannon waves are found in paroxysmal nodal tachycardia. Occasional irregular cannon waves are also encountered in **complete heart block.** Cannon waves are only seen when atrial and ventricular systole happen to coincide.

Respiratory Variation and Kussmaul's Sign

The mean jugularvenous pressure normally falls with inspiration, passively following the intrathoracic pressure. In some patients with decreased RV compliance, the relative height of the "a" wave will increase with inspiration even though the mean venous pressure falls. This is considered to be related to an enhancement in the force of atrial contraction with atrial distention caused by the ventilatory increase in the venous return. Subjects with a marked decrease in RV compliance, such as those with constrictive pericarditis (Figs 3.58–3.61).

In the later, there is a rise in the mean height of the jugular venous pulse during inspiration, This is known as Kussmaul's sign and is observed approximately 40% of the patients with constrictive pericarditis. Kussmaul's sign is generally not seen in patients with pericardial tamponade or massive pericardial effusion.

Normal Precordial Activity

The palpable apical impulse in a normal subject is produced by an anterior movement of the left ventricle during early systole. As isovolumic intraventricular pressure rises, the left ventricle rotates in a counter clockwise direction on its long axia as the cardiac apex lifts and makes contact with the left anterior chest wall. Following aortic valve opening and the first half of ejection, the LV chamber moves away from the chest wall and continues to diminish in size until systole is completed. Thus, the impulse felt or recorded on the precordium is made up of an early outward thrust followed by retraction during the last part of systole; normal palpable cardiac activity occurs only during the first half of systole.

The retraction wave can be seen but is not felt. Diastolic events, such as the LV rapid filling phase or left atrial contraction, are normally not palpable.

In angiographic studies, the interventricular septum (composed mostly of LV muscle) and the anteroseptal aspect of the left ventricle makes contact with the inner thoracic cage to form the palpable apical impulse. The true anatomical LV apex is actually slightly lower and more lateral than the palpable apical impulse.

How to Examine the Precordium?

For optimal precorial examination, it is important for the examiner and patient to be relaxed. The room should be comfortably warm. Clothing and undergarments must be removed to allow wider inspection and palpation of the chest. Because the examiner must be prepared, for example, to count intercostal spaces, measure the distance of the precordial impulse from the sternum or axillary line, and chest exposure should be maximal. The patient should be lying comfortably, in the supine position or with the thorax elevated no more than 30°. Perloff suggests that the 30° position is preferable because precordial examination in this position may bring out abnormalities more often than when the patient is lying supine. In a given patient, cardiovascular diseases should routinely be examined in the left lateral decubitus position; the subject should be instructed to turn on his or her left side at a 45–60° angle with the examining table, elevating the left arm over the head so that the examiner may have unobstructed access to the left precordium.

I. INSPECTION (Figs 3.58–3.61)

Careful inspection of the chest is useful in the precordial examination, particularly after preliminary palpation has identified the site of the apical beat or any other impulses that may be present. Retraction movements, which may be more obvious than outward motion are quite prominent in severe degrees of LV enlargement. Tangential lighting with the examining lamp or a pen torch may accentuate visible movements on the chest wall (Fig. 3.58).

II. PALPATION

The physician should be standing comfortably at the patient's right side. Both the palm of the hand and the ventral aspect of the proximal metacarpals and fingers should be used for palpation. One must learn which aspect the hand has the best sense of touch, it is advisable to use the pads of the fingers for precise localization and assessment of LV and RV activity. The palm and proximal metacarpals are usually best used to localize palpable cardiac motion as well as to detect precordial thrills. Varying pressure with the hand should be applied once a precordial impulse has been identified. High frequency sounds, such as an increased S1, and opening snap, or a transmitted thrill, are best localized with the hand firmly applied to the chest. However, the subtle, low frequency motion of a palpable **S3 or S4** or double systolic apical impulse will be felt only with light pressure of the fingers and may be totally obscured if the examination is not performed correctly. In most normal subjects, parasternal activity is not usually detectable. However, in young or thin people, a gentle shock or tap at the lower left

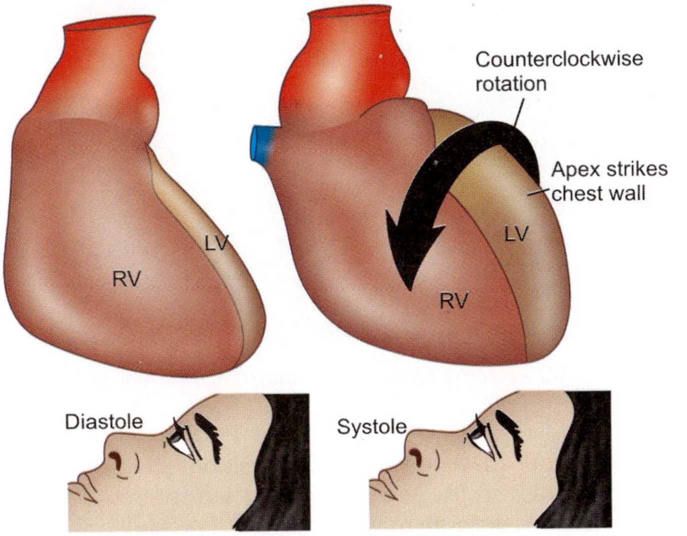

Fig. 3.58: *Diagrammatic demonstration of apical movements in syslole and diastole during cardiac cycle*

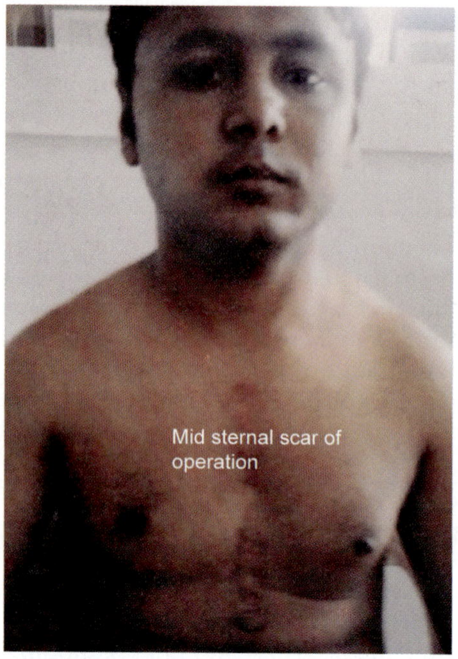

Fig 3.59: *Photograph of 20-years-old male had bicuspid aortic stenosis with AR with LVH. He was successfully operated with AVR and regular follow-up for more than 6 years maintained good health*

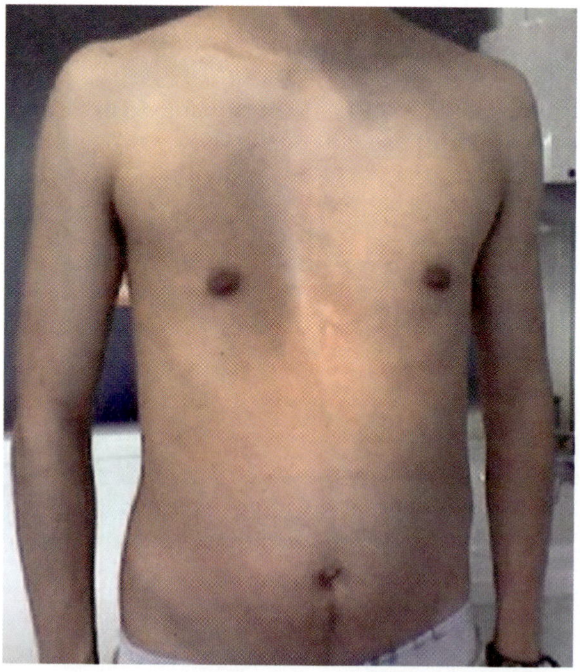

Fig. 3.60: *Pectus excavatum deformity of chest in VSD*

sternal border may be felt, and, occasionally, a pulmonary artery impulse in the second to third left intercostal space adjacent to the sternum may be detected. Forceful, unstained, or high amplitude parasternal motion is always an abnormal finding (Figs 3.62–3.64).

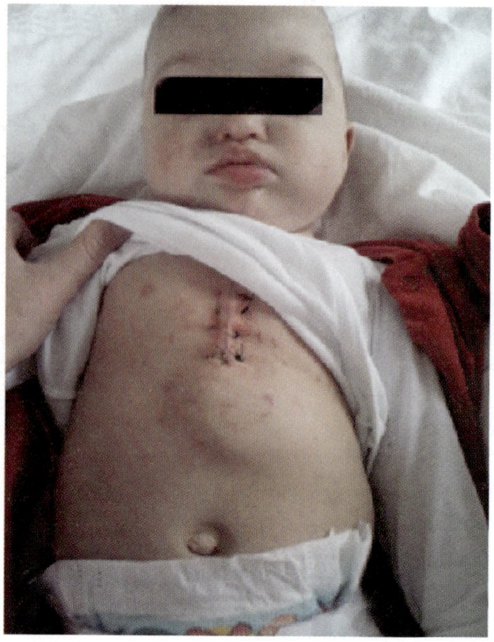

Fig. 3.61: *Dual chamber pacemaker with epicardial electrodes implanted through a median sternotomy in a newborn with complete heart block*

Point of Maximum Impulse (PMI) (Table 3.2)

Many textbooks use he term for PMI the same as the apical beat. Although not ideal, this expression is so frequently used that it has become acceptable to many.

Nevertheless, it should be recognized that the terms PMI and apical impulse are not necessarily synonymous. In some patients, the most prominent, "maximal", impulse may actually reflect ectopic LV motion, RV activity, or a vascular impulse.

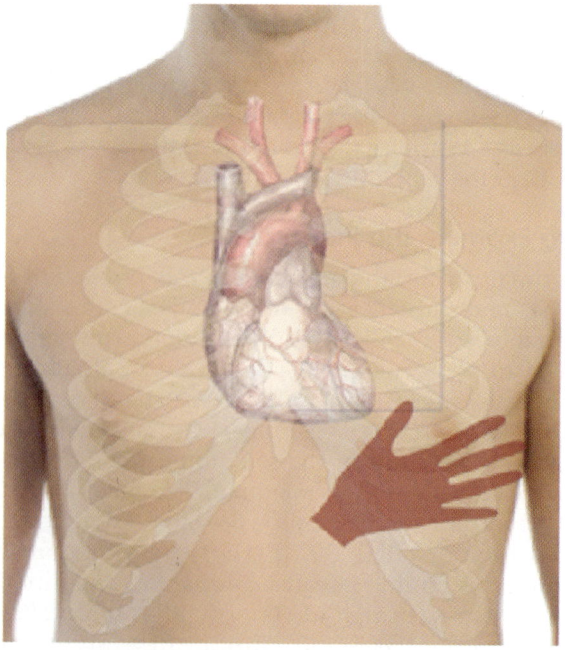

Fig. 3.62: *The apex beat is the lowest, most lateral point where the heartbeat can be felt*

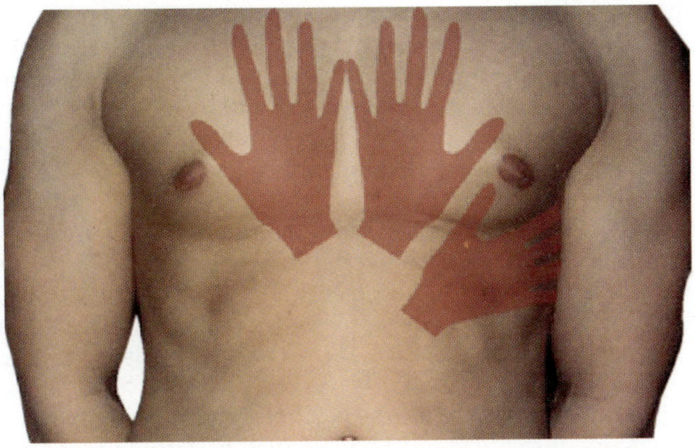

Fig. 3.63: *Heaves and thrills can be detected by placing the hand flat against either side of the sternum and over the apex of the heart*

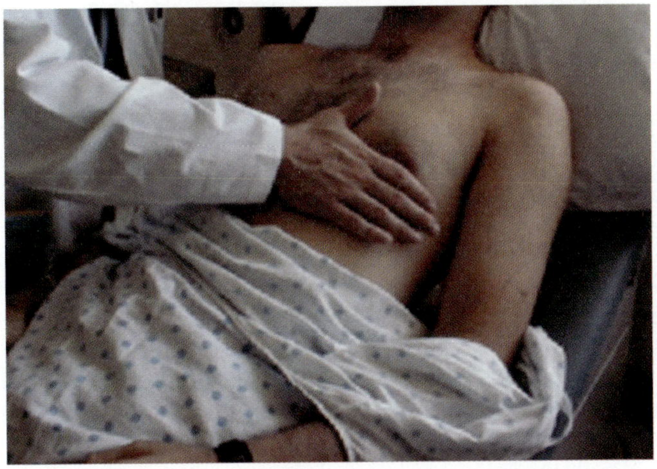

Fig. 3.64: *Method of palpation for thrill*

Other Palpable Events

In a subject with suspected cardiac disease, the examiner should explore the entire precordium with firm pressure of the hand and proximal fingers, separating the aortic, pulmonic, lower sternal and apical regions. In this way, the unexpected vascular impulse, such as a dilated or aneurysmal ascending aorta or pulmonary artery, may be detected. Particular attention should be given to the upper sternal area, to the manubrium, and to the adjacent first to second intercostal spaces below the medial aspect of the clavicles. Aortic pulsations and systolic thrills are often found there. If a patient has coronary artery disease, particularly with a prior myocardial infection, careful examination for ectopic impulse should be carried out. These typically occur medial and superior to the ectopic impulse. The use of the entire palm and proximal metacarpals will help to detect the diffuse lift of a very large left or right ventricle. At times, the entire anterior precordium will move in systole. This technique is also suited for detection of thrills and palpable heart sounds.

Assessment of the Apical Cardiac Impulse

The assessment of the apical cardiac impulse should include analysis of the following headings:

- Location
- Size
- Force
- Duration
- Contour.

In addition, there should be visual inspection of the chest for the presence of prominent retraction waves as well as for systolic and diastolic events. Timing of precordial events is best carried out by simultaneously palpating the carotid arterial pulse with the left hand. Some find that concomitant auscultation of **S1 and S2 is** useful for timing purposes.

Table 3.2: *Clinical classification and causes of precordial impulses*

Site of impulse	*Sustained*	*Hyperdynamic*	*Late systole*
1. Parasternal area	Pressure overload: Pulmonary hypertension Cor pulmonale Mitral stenosis Pulmonary emboli Cardiomyopathy	Hyperkinetic circulatory states in young subjects Volume overload: Atrial septal defect Tricuspid regurgitation	Severe mitral regurgitation
2. LV (apical beat)	Pressure overload: Hypertension aortic stenosis	Hyperkinetic circulatory states	LV dyssynergy HOCM
	Chronic or severe Volume overload: LV dilatation, especially with decreased ejection fraction LV dysfunction LV Aneurysm	Thin chest wall Pectus excavatum Volume overload: Aortic regurgitation Mitral regurgitation Ventricular septal defect	Mitral valve prolapse (uncommon)

Application of the stethoscope chest piece directly on the apical impulse can help to identify systole.

It is desirable to use held end expiration for the RV examination. Firm pressure, using the heel of the hand with the wrist turned upward, is advisable. The lower sternum and adjacent third through fifth rib and left interspaces should be examined in this manner. The examining hand and fingers should be carefully observed, as low amplitude RV activity is often found in epigastric region with the extended fingers oriented superiorly; the patient should be instructed to hold his breath in end-inspiration and careful palpation for the descending right ventricle is performed. This technique is particularly useful in patients with an increased antero-posterior diameter, obesity, or chronic obstructive lung disease.

Characteristics of the normal apical impulse

1. A gentle, nonsustained tap
2. An early systolic anterior motion that ends before the last third of systole
3. Location within 10 cm of the midsternal line in the fourth or fifth left intercostal space
4. A palpable area less than 2–2.5 cm^2 and detectable in only 1 intercostal space
5. RV motion that is not normally palpable
6. Diastolic events that are normally palpable
7. Complete absence in some older individuals.

Location

To identify the site of the apical impulse on the thorax with respect to both the longitudinal and the horizontal axes of the patient.

To note in which intercostal space the PMI or apical beat is located; occasionally a large heart will result in detectable precordial activity in two or even three intercostal spaces. Localize the apical impulse with reference to the mid-clavicular line, distance from the midsternum or relationship to the left anterior axillary line.

Size

If the apical impulse is larger than normal, it is useful to note the area of contact with the chest. Any area greater than 2–2.5 cm^2 in the supine position, or greater than 3 cm in the left decubitus position, represents cardiac enlargement.

Force or amplitude

Is the apical beat a soft, unimpressive impulse? or does it lift the examining fingers off the chest well? Is the anterior or outward excursion greater than normal? Consistent with a hyperdynamic or hyperkinetic PMI? An increase in force is consistent with LV hypertrophy with preserved systolic functions. Assessment of the force of contraction is the most subjective and least quantifiable aspect of precordial examination.

Duration

The duration of the systoli outward motion is probably the most important feature of the precordial examination, although cardiomegaly or hypertrophy can exist in the presence of a brief "normal" outward movement, or even when the PMI is absent, truly sustained LV impulse in the supine or 30° elevation position is distinctly abnormal. Such findings suggest a pressure overstressed ventricle (e.g. aortic stenosis, hypertension or an LV chamber with a depressed ejection fraction and a substantially dilated cavity. A study by "Conn" demonstrated that a sustained apex impulse in the supine position was highly correlated with an increase in angiographically determined LV mass, and this observation was actually more sensitive than the electrocardiogram (ECG) in the diagnosis of LV hypertrophy.

The critical point to assess is whether or not the impulse "stays up" into the second half of systole. Timing that uses simultaneous auscultation of S1 and S2 is essential in making this observation. With practice, one can be quite accurate in assessing the actual duration of the apical impulse. Simple observation of movement of the chest piece of the stethoscope resting on the PMI may be helpful.

Left Lateral Decubitus Position

It is unclear whether LV impulse that becomes sustained when the patient is turned into left lateral position which is of normal duration in the supine position, has the same specificity for LV enlargement as a sustained impulse (LV heave) that is present when the patient is lying flat. Since the left decubitus position causes the heart to approximate the chest wall more closely, many experts feels that the observation of a prolonged impulse in this position has little diagnostic value. Some believe that a definite sustained impulse in the left lateral position is highly indicative of true LV dilatation. False positives may occur, however, echocardiography is recommended in equivocal cases.

Contour

The normal apical impulse is a brief, nonsustained anterior motion in early systole. A sustained LV movement is the most common abnormality of contour, but occasionally other different types are also recorded.

A Double Systolic Impulse or Bifid Impulse

It may be seen in hypertrophic obstructive cardiomyopathy (IHSS) and occasionally in some patients with severe LV dyssynergy or LV aneurysm in coronary artery disease. Presystolic distention is commonly found in the left lateral position in subjects who have decreased LV compliance, complicated from coronary artery disease, hypertensive heart disease, or aortic valve disease. Palpable diastolic events, such as an S3 or a pericardial knock, also fall into the general category of contour variations.

Palpable "a" Wave (Presystolic Distention)

Palpable a waves are usually detected in the left posture. The apical beat is carefully localized, and varying pressure is applied with the pads of the fingers at the site of the LV impulse. A double early systolic impulse is noted, feeling like a "shelf or ridge" on the upstroke of the beat. Usually, this low amplitude finding will best be felt when finger pressure is light; firm pressure with the fingers may make the finding more difficult or impossible to feel. On occasion, this presystolic distention can be quite prominent. The palpable a wave reflects a high LV end-diastolic pressure and decrease LV compliance. It is important observation because it documents a definite abnormality that usually implies LV hypertrophy and increased chamber stiffness. The audibility of the S4 does not correlate with palpability; presystolic distention may be detectable when the S4 is quite soft. Occasionally, one may not be able to hear an S4 at all, even though it is palpable; this is because the frequency of the diastolic filling event is extremely low (usually less than 60 cycles per second).

Palpable S3

The S3 is less often palpable than an S4. It is most often observed in severe mitral regurgitation or in a markedly dilated cardiomyopathic ventricle. As with S4, palpation is greater enhanced in the left decubitus position. The S4, appears as a brief outward motion in early systole, gently tapping the examining finger pads but not displacing the fingers, since it is usually not forceful.

Palpable S4

A palpable S4 is related to decreased LV compliance usually as a result of hypertrophy without dilatation or ischemia with increased, diastolic stiffness. A palpable S4 is always associated with LV end-diastolic pressure that is elevated, sometimes strikingly so, although early and mid-diastolic pressure is often normal in hypertensive heart disease, coronary artery disease, and occasionally, in congestive cardiomyopathy. The implications of a palpable S4 are quite different from those of a palpable S3 in the former case, LV systolic function is usually well preserved and the ejection fraction is normal. A palpable S3 (in the absence of significant mitral regurgitation) is associated with high LV filling pressures, as in dilated ventricle, and decreased systolic function.

Palpable Right Ventricle (S3 and S4)

The pathophysiology of palpable S3 and S4 generated in the right ventricle is similar to that in the left heart. Compliance changes (RV hypertrophy secondary to pulmonary hypertension) may result in a palpable RV S4. Increased blood flow across the tricuspid valve may produce a prominent S3. Tricus- pid regurgitation is a good example. A large left-to-right shunt and atrial septal defect may also occasionally produce a palpable RV S3. In severe RV dysfunction, an S3 may be heard and felt. Classically, RV events are marked by inspiratory augmentation and expiratory attenuation or disappearance.

Other Causes of Palpable Cardiovascular Activity

In addition to the tactile precordial phenomena related to LV and RV systolic and diastolic events palpable precordial activity is occasionally detectable as a result of vascular pulsations or ectopic LV wall motion abnormalities.

Palpable Cardiovascular Events

Aorta

When either the ascending aorta or the aortic arch is enlarged or dilated, palpable systolic pulsations may be detected. Thus, with aortic aneurysms, diffuse aortic dilatation, or aortic dissection, a systolic impulse may be felt in the right first or second intercostal space, in the right or left sternoclavicular junction, or in the suprasternal areas. Dilatation or enlargement of the brachiocephalic vessels may also cause prominent vascular pulsations at the superstermal notch or above the clavicles.

Pulmonary Artery

Dilatation or enlargement of the pulmonary artery is usually associated with pulmonary hypertension, which itself may resuit from hyperkinetic; high flow states or from increased pulmonary vascular resistance. Idiopathic dilatation of the pulmonary artery results in an enlarged proximal pulmonary artery segment. All these conditions may produce a palpable systolic impulse in the second to third left intercostal space just to the left of the sternal edge. This is easily detectable in thin subjects.

Left Ventricular Ectopic Impulse

Focal wallmotion abnormalities or a big LV aneurysms may produce systolic impulses that are detectable at sites away from the LV apical beat, usually medial and superior to the apical area. With anteroseptal LV scarring or dyskinesis, the ectopic impulse may be found at the lower parasternal edge and thus may simulate RV activity.

Palpable Heart Sounds and Murmurs

Loud sounds such as an increased S1, A2 or P2 are often readily palpable. An opening snap is commonly palpable in mitral stenosis, as a loud S1, on occasion the diagnosis of this valve lesion can be made prior to using the stethoscope. Ejection clicks may be easily felt: the aortic ejection sound is detected at the LV apex, while a pulmonic ejection sound is palpable at the upper left sternal border.

Thrills

Any loud murmur may be transmitted to the chest wall, where it can produce a vibratory sensation to the examining hand. These palpable murmurs or thrills correlate with a murmur intensity of grade IV/VI or greater. Such murmurs may be felt at the apex (mitral regurgitation, hypertrophic obstructive cardiomyopathy) left sternal border (ventricular septal defect) or cardiac base (pulmonic stenosis, aortic stenosis). Obviously, in thin subjects the likelihood of a thrill is greater than in muscular or bulky patients. A diastolic thrill may occasionally be felt usually a the apex with the subject in the lateral decubitus position in mitral stenosis, or at the lower left sternal border in acute aortic regurgitation secondary to a perforated or ruptured aortic cusp.

III. PERCUSSION

Under ordinary circumstances, percussion is neither necessary nor useful. When a PMI cannot be identified, however, the technique may help establish the presence or absence of cardiomegaly and will identify the approximate left border of the heart. In patients with a large pericardial effusion, the apex beat may actually be detected inside the lateral border of the cardiac silhouette, as determined by percussion (Figs 3.65–3.66).

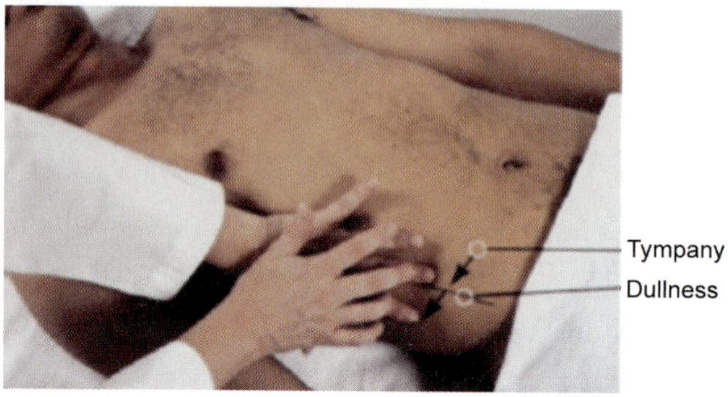

Fig 3.65: *Method of percussion over lower lung and liver areas for fluid and enlargement in patient with heart failure*

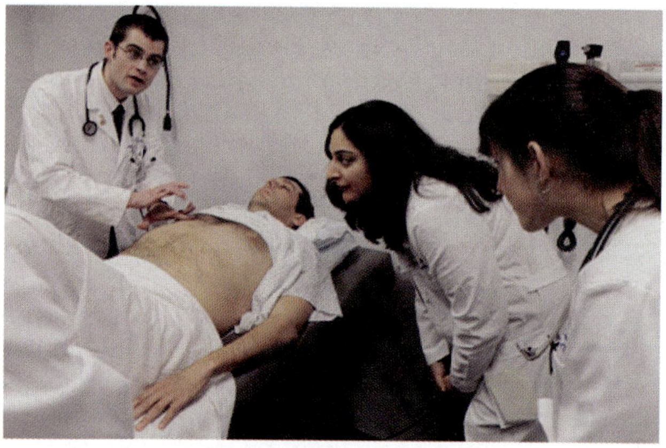

Fig. 3.66: *Senior resident in cardiology is demonstrating to the medical students the clinical technique of percussion on the chest of one of the patient admitted to the medical college hospital*

IV. AUSCULTATION

Stethoscope

The chest piece should have a diaphragm and a bell. High frequency sounds and murmurs are heard better with the diaphragm, e.g. opening snap, aortic diastolic murmur. The bell transmits low frequency sounds better, e.g. gallop sounds, mitral diastolic murmur. The bell should be applied very lightly to the chest when listening for these low frequency sounds (Figs 3.67–3.94)

New visual, amplified stethoscope for hearing impaired clinicians. Properly diagnosing patients using a stethoscope requires good hearing to discern the murmurs from normal heart sounds. Yet, many doctors and nurses suffer from poor hearing, making it difficult to auscultate their patients, seriously hampering their ability to perform a basic screening. The cardionics Vi scope aims to solve that problem by providing both amplification of the audio signal

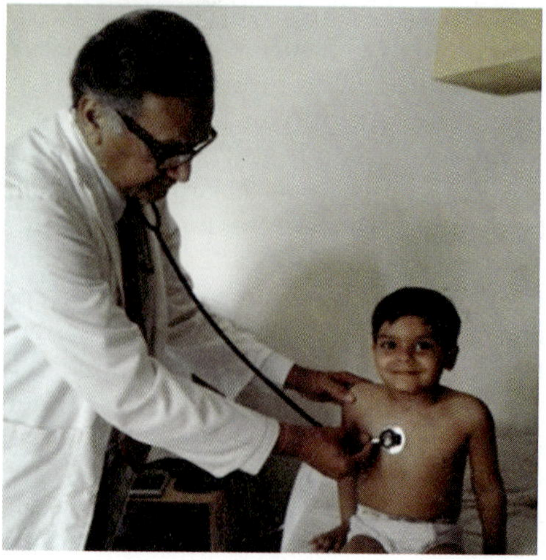

Fig. 3.67: *Cardiologist is examining a young child with traditional litman stethoscope*

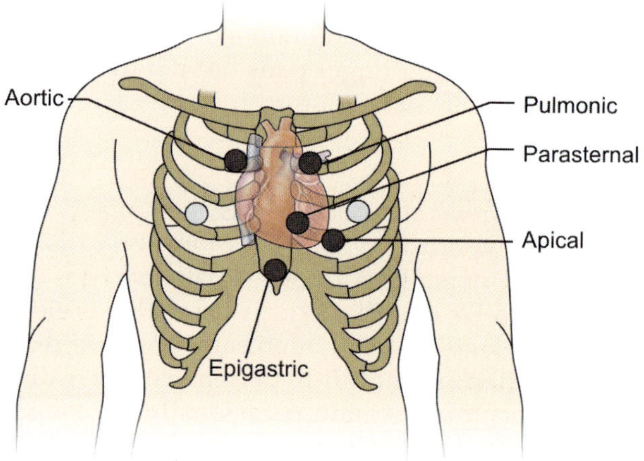

Fig. 3.68: *Conventional area of auscultation*

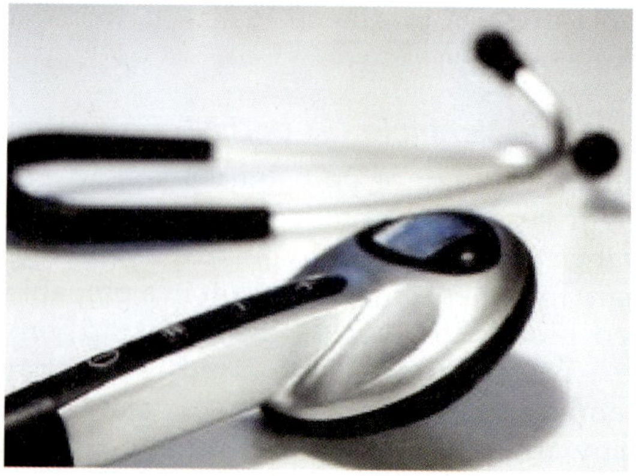

Fig. 3.69: *Conventional stethoscope used by the doctors for auscultation*

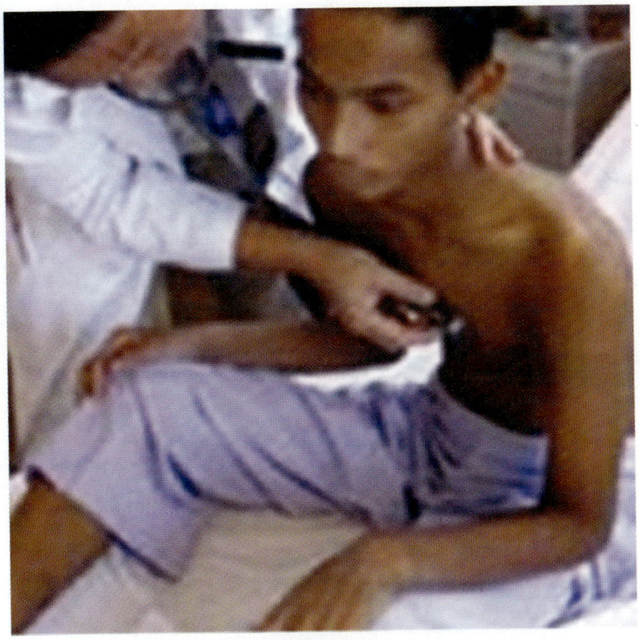

Fig. 3.70: *Method of auscultation while sitting and leaning forward posture for augmentation of aortic and pulmonary events*

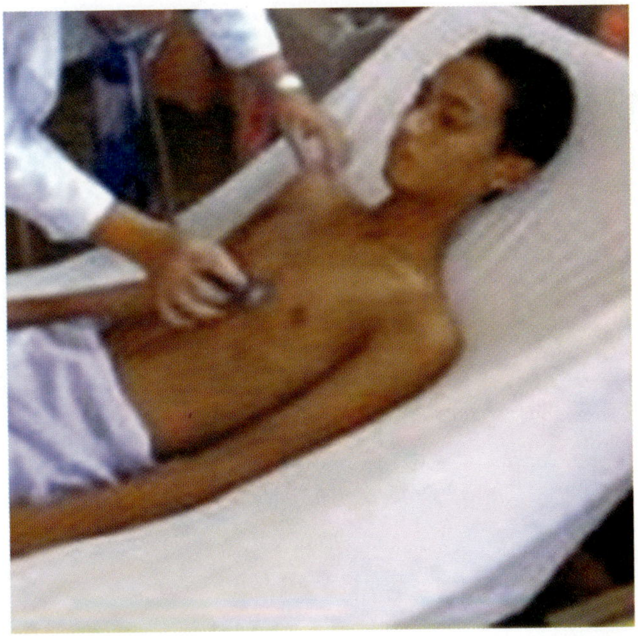

Fig. 3.71: *Method of auscultation for mitral and tricuspid defects*

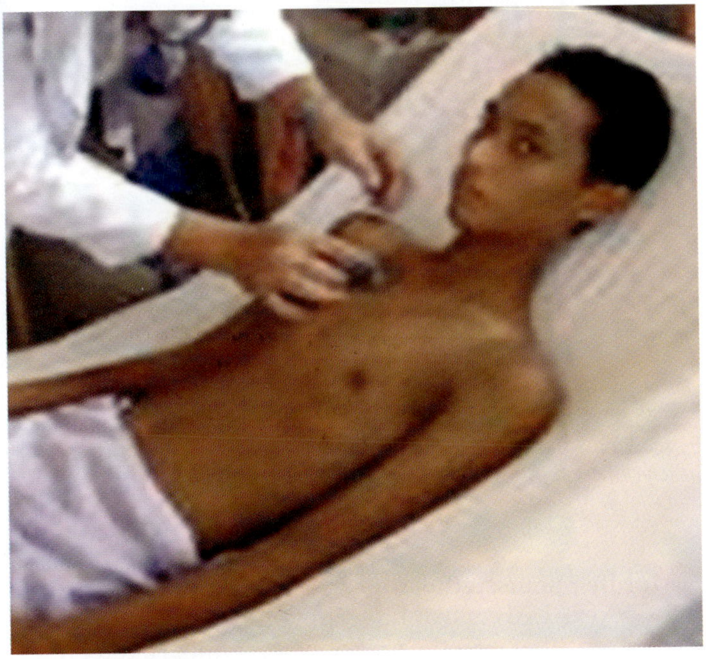

Fig. 3.72: *Method of auscultation for aortic defects*

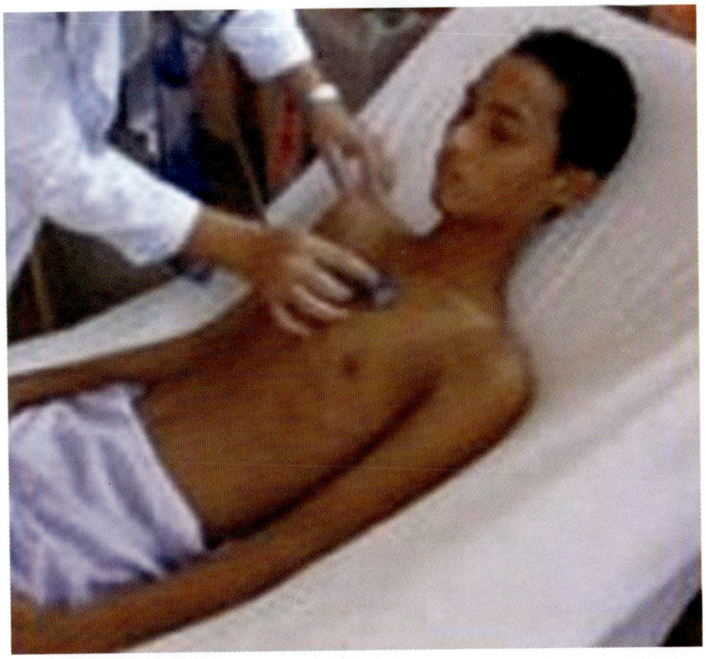

Fig. 3.73: *Method of auscultation for pulmonary valve*

and a visual display of the phonocardiogram or phonopneumogram. The device is compatible with in-the-ear or open fit behind-the-ear hearing aids, offering the ability to boost the signal 30 times over a conventional stethoscope. Visualization assists the listener in identifying the position of clicks, rubs, knocks, snaps or murmurs in the cardiac cycle. Murmurs such as aortic stenosis, aortic regurgitation or mitral regurgitation are clearly seen. Pediatric sounds including atrial septal defect, ventricular septal defect and primary pulmonary hypertension are easily identified. How it works: simply place the stethoscope on the chest and as the sounds are detected, the phonocardiogram of heart sounds will be displayed on the screen. Sounds can be downloaded to the ViScope-100 software for storage and recall. With a resolution of 1024 × 768 pixels, the software allows the trace to be enlarged for a better view. Calipers allow measurement of events such as the opening snap of mitral stenosis

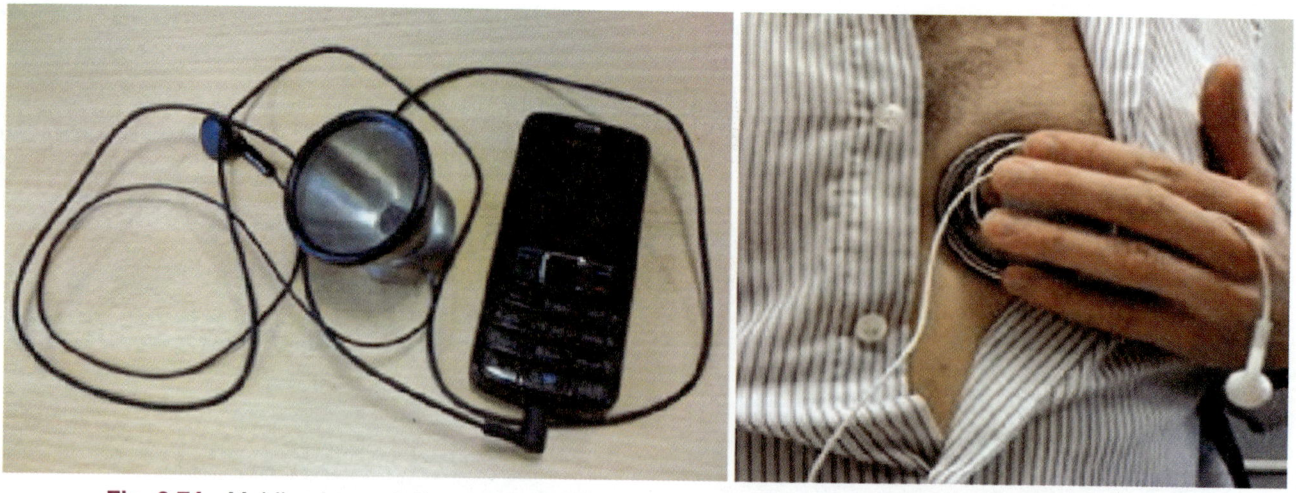

Fig. 3.74: *Mobile phone stethoscopes (left) and its applicability over the chest of the patient (right)*

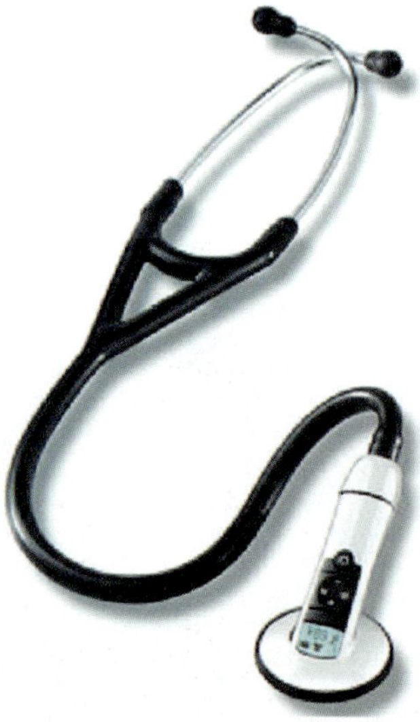

Fig. 3.75: *3M Littmann scope-to-scope teleauscultation system for remote diagnosis*

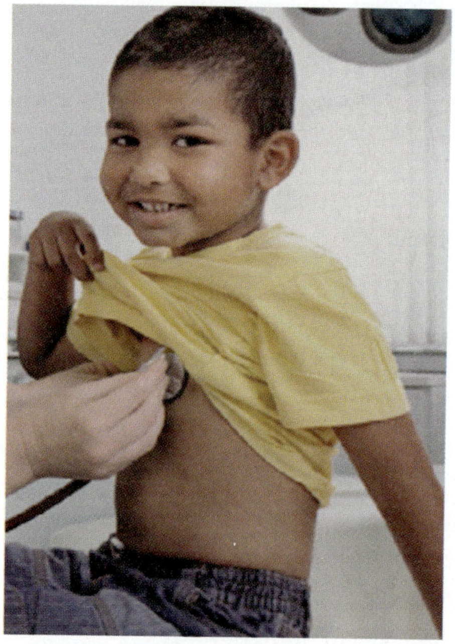

Fig. 3.77: *Auscultation in sitting position over left parasternal area in a young child with VSD*

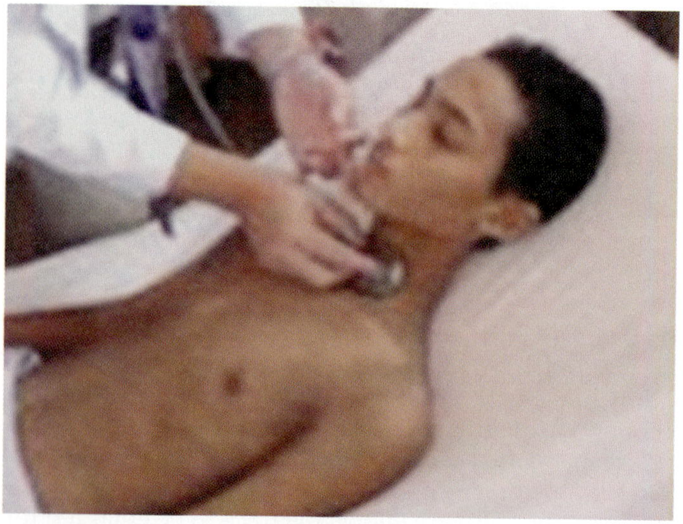

Fig. 3.76: *Auscultation of suprasternal areas of both sides for transmission of aortic stenosis murmur*

Mobile phone stethoscopes: A team of researchers from the Oxford University have developed a new kind of stethoscope that uses the microphone input of a cell phone. The rudimentary stethoscope is basically a cell phone with an external microphone attached to the base of an egg-cup to focus and collect the sounds. The phonocardiograms recorded can be analyzed by a computer to filter out distortion and noise and process the signal to identify heart rate and abnormal heart sounds. So far, the stethoscope has been tested with an iPhone 3G and a nokia 3100 classic. Surprisingly, the nokia 3100 classic outperformed a 3M Littmann electronic stethoscope in detecting heart rate. According to oxford, an android version of the phonocardiogram processing software is also in the works.

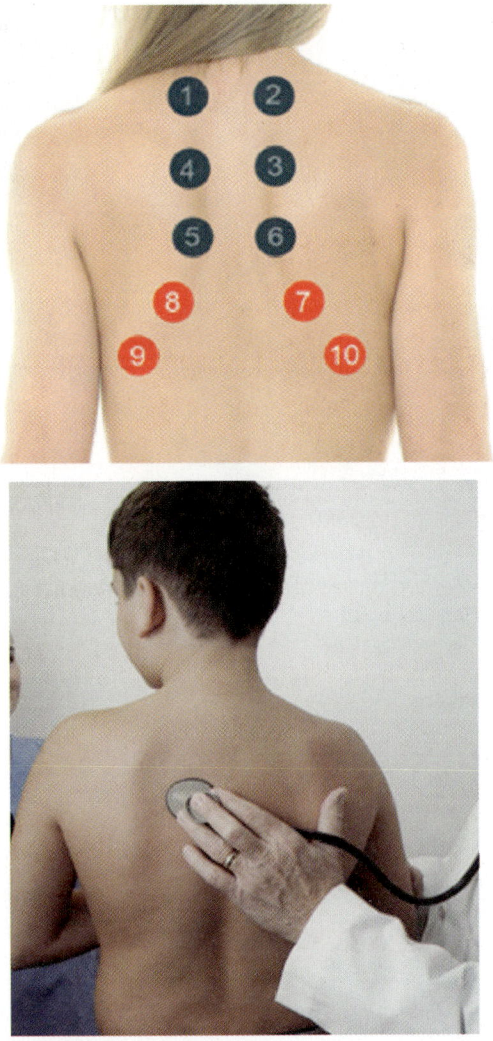

Fig. 3.78: *Auscultation of the lung bases (zones 1–10) shown (top) should be performed in a thorough cardiovascular examination (bottom)*

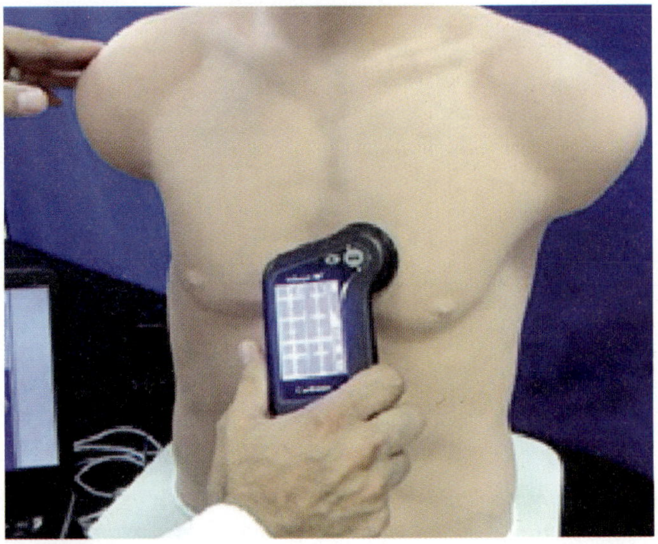

Fig. 3.79: *New visual, amplified stethoscope for hearing impaired clinicians*

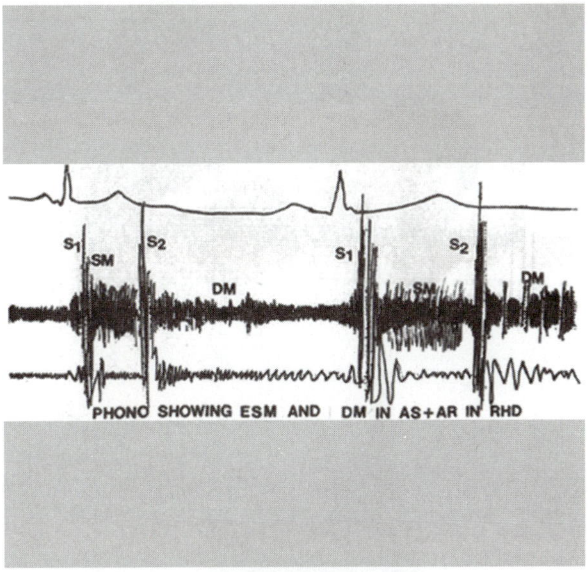

Fig. 3.80: *ECG monitored phonogram showing ejection systolic murmur (SM) of aortic stenosis and long diastolic murmur of aortic regurgitation*

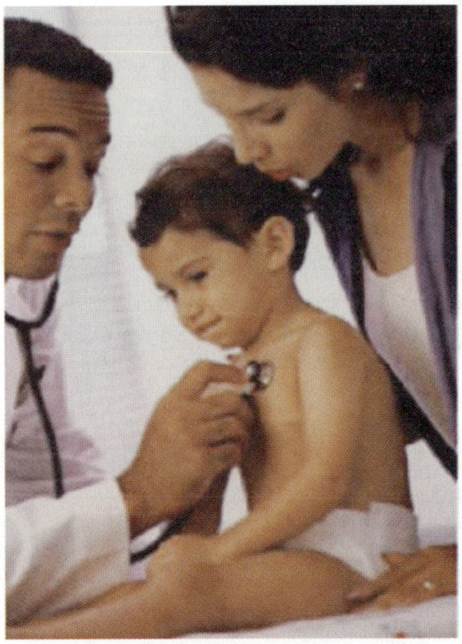

Fig. 3.81: *Auscultation in sitting position over left infraclavicular area in a young child with pulmonic stenosis*

A New Littmann Scope-to-Scope Tele-auscultation System

It allows physicians to remotely listen to patients using a stethoscope as though they're on-site. Using bluetooth connectivity, the system transfers in real-time audio gathered on one Littmann Model 3200 stethoscope to another anywhere in the world. It is truly amazing how the stethoscope, from being a medical diagnostic device, has moved to also become a communication and telemedicine device.

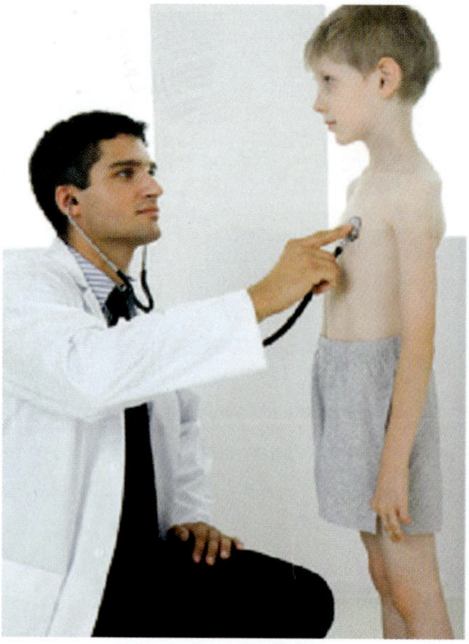

Fig. 3.82: *Auscultation in standing position over apical area in a young child with mitral valve prolapse*

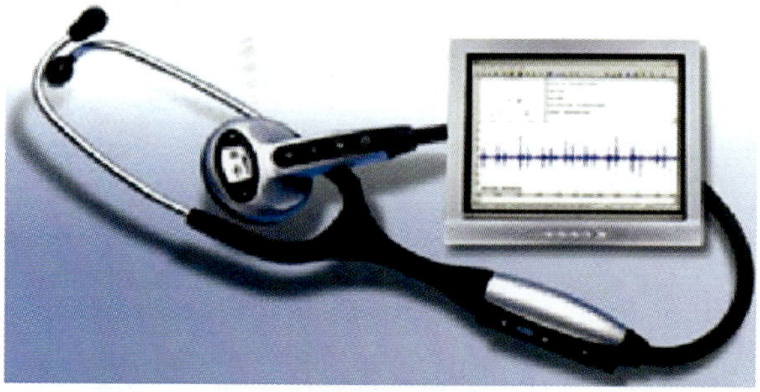

Fig. 3.83: *Heart murmur detection software designed to support physicians in analyzing cardiac sounds for the identification and classification of suspected murmurs*

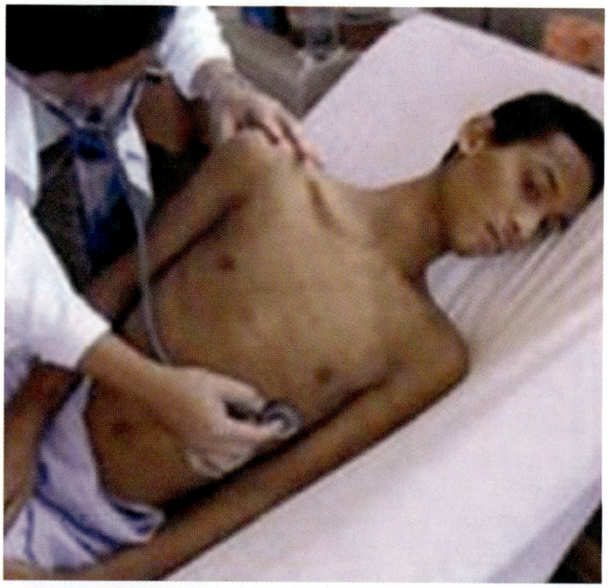

Fig. 3.84: *Method of auscultation lying left lateral position for augmentation of apical events*

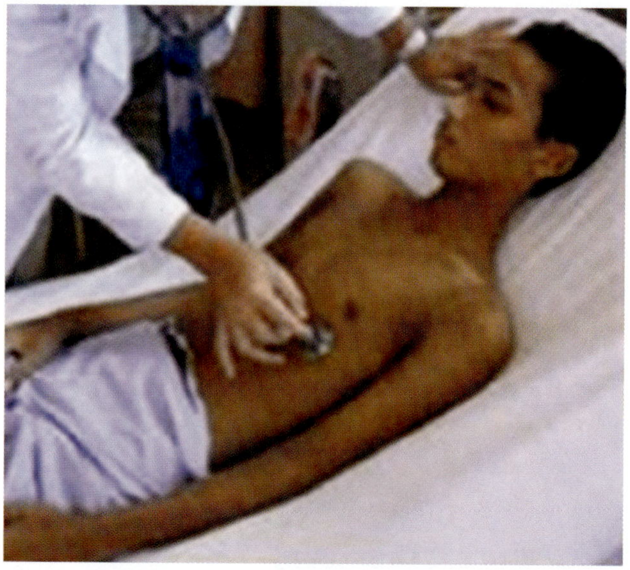

Fig. 3.85: *Method of auscultation lying supine in the bed at 45° position for apical events*

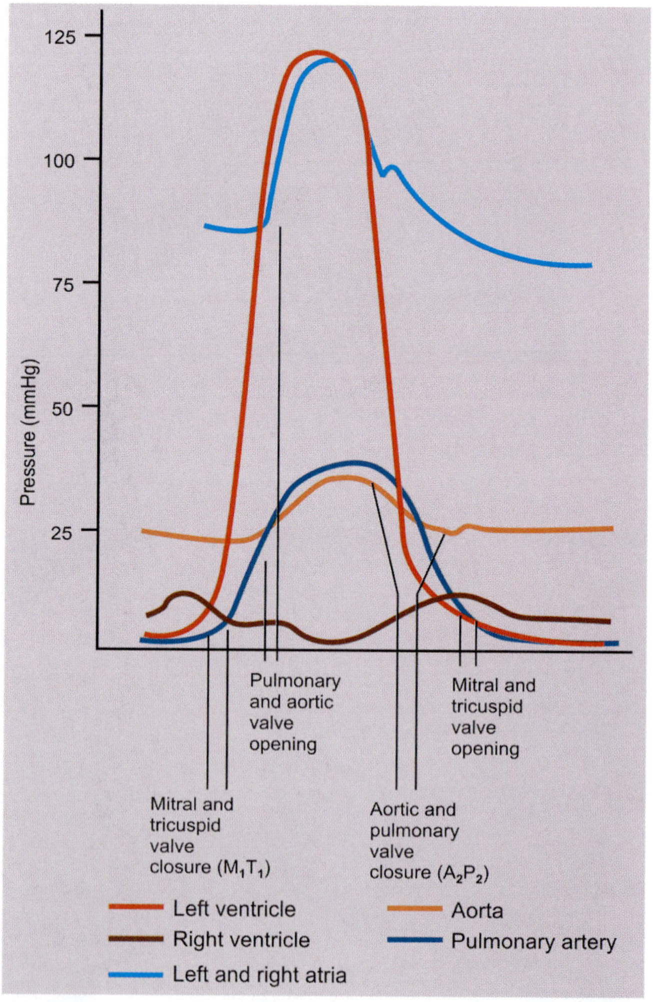

Fig. 3.86: *Intracardiac tracings of LV, RV, RA, LA, aorta and pulmonary artery demonstrating opening and closure of mitral and tricuspid valve (M1-T1) and opening and closure of aortic and pulmonary valves (A2- P2) in cardiac cycle of normal person*

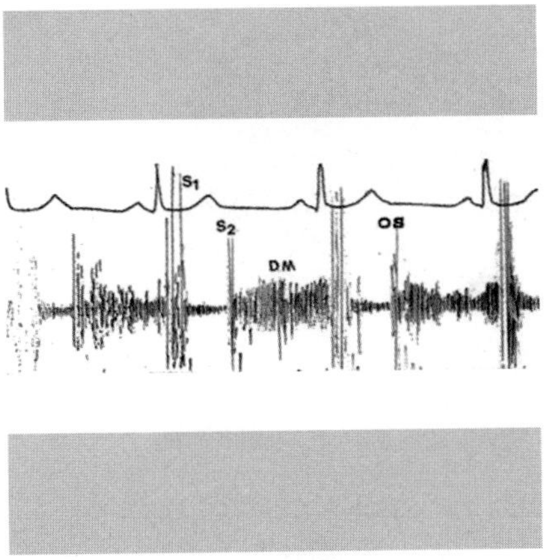

Fig. 3.87: *ECG monitored phnogram showing loud first heart sound (S1) daiastolic murmur (DM) and narrow split second heart sound (S2) and opening snap (OS) in a patient with mitral stenosis*

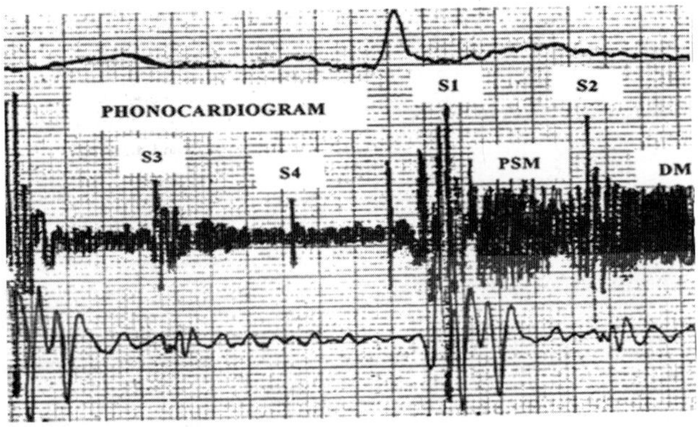

Fig 3.88: *ECG monitored phonogram showing heart sounds (S1–S4) pansystolic murmur (PSM) and diastolic murmur (DM) in mitral stenosis and regurgitation*

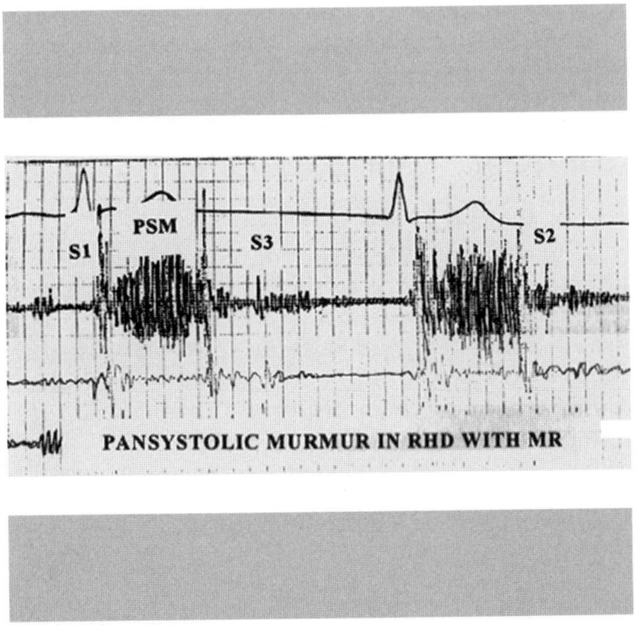

Fig. 3.89: *ECG monitored phonogram showing pansystolic murmur (PSM) in mitral regurgitation (MR) with S3*

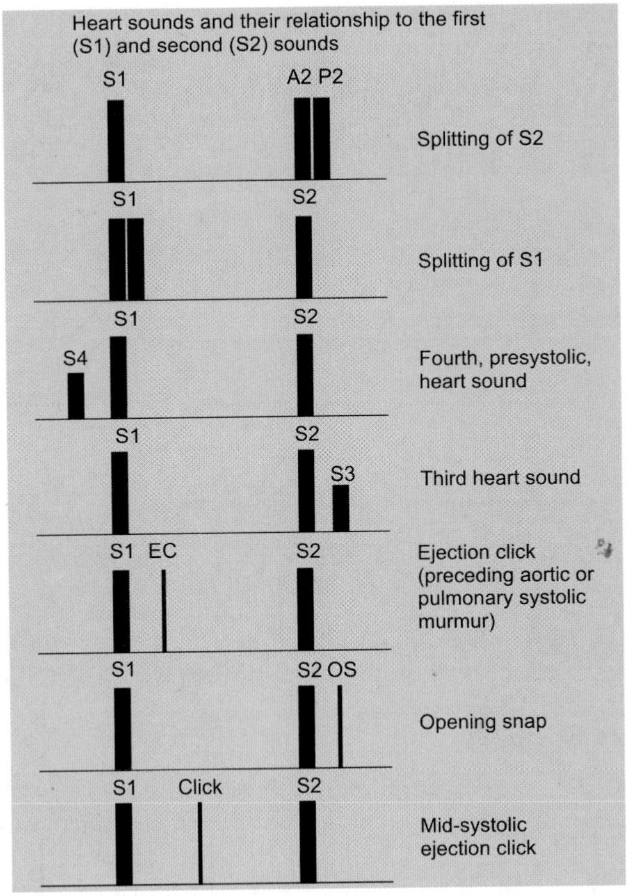

Fig. 3.90: *Diagrammatic representation of various types of ejection clicks, sounds and their splitting, along with opening snap at different timings of human cardiac cycle*

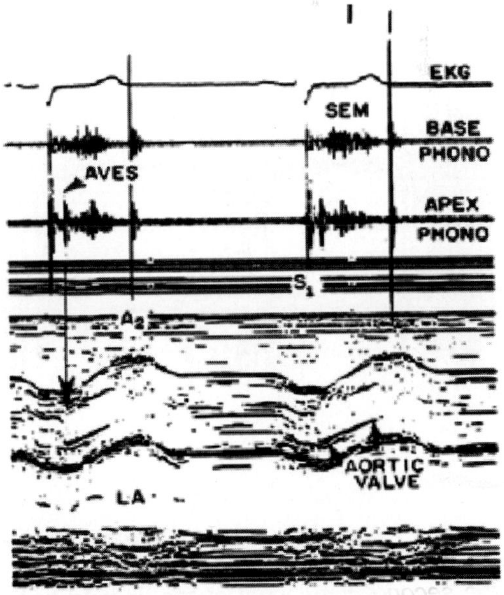

Fig. 3.91: *Base and apex phonocardiograms (PHONO) recorded simultanously with the aortic valve echocardiogram in patient with valvular aortic stenosis. A prominent aortic valvular ejection sound (AVES) is recorded at the apex and is coincident with the maximal excursion of the aortic valve in early systole It is followed by a crescendo-decrescendo SEM that ends well before a loud A2. LA, left atrium; EKG, electrocardiogram*

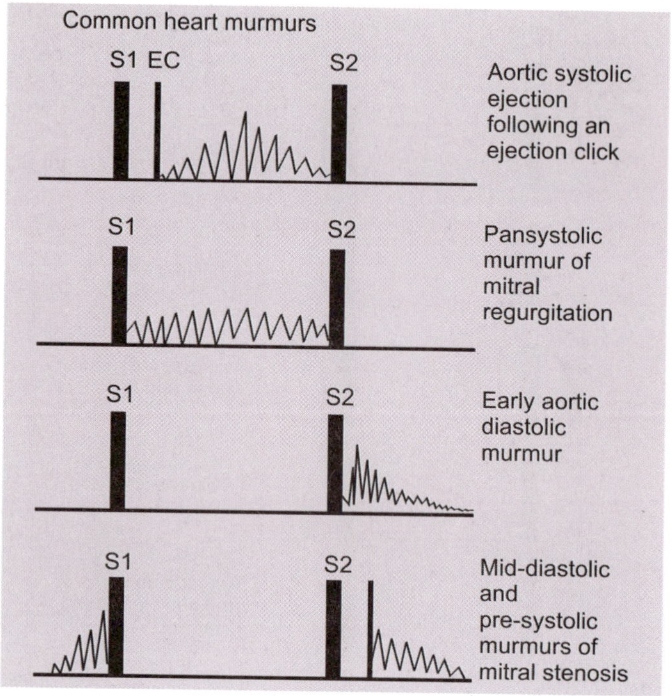

Fig. 3.92: *Graphic representation of common heart murmurs in clinical practice*

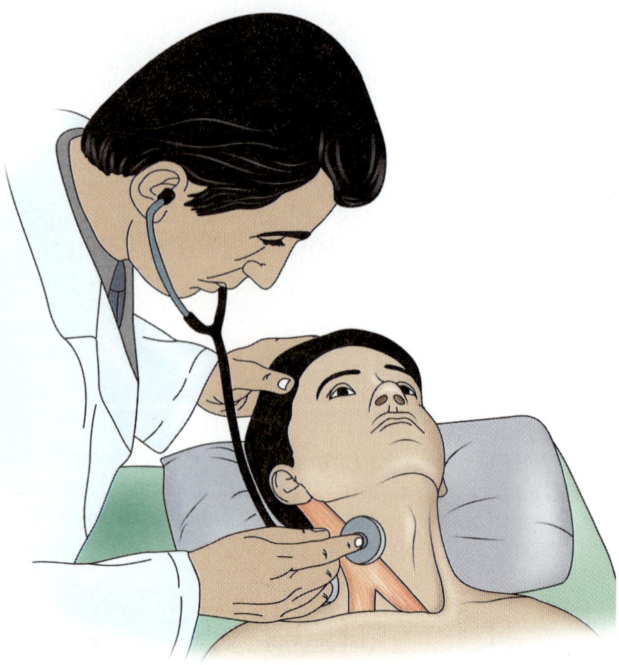

Fig. 3.94: *Auscultation over the neck for carotid artery stenosis and venus hum*

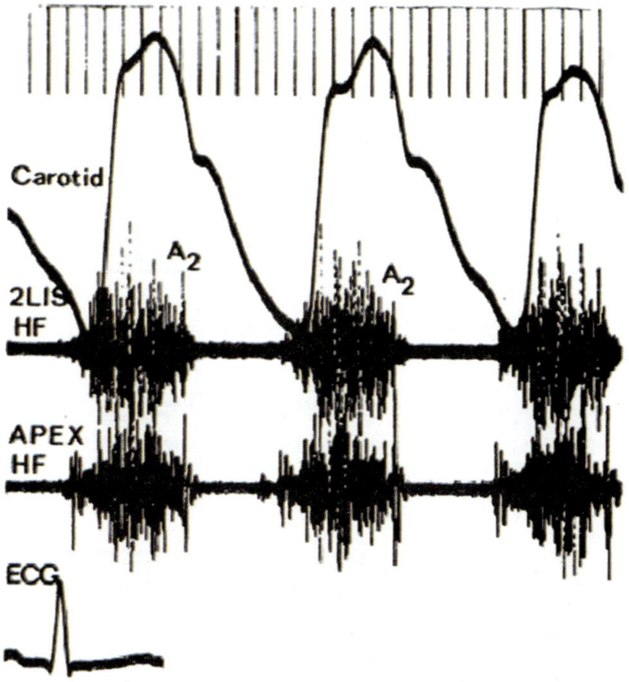

Fig. 3.93: *A loud, diamond-shaped murmur of pulmonary stenosis. Note that the murmur of pulmonary stenosis extends through to the second component of the second heart sound (pulmonary closure)*

- Allows clinicians to provide world-class patient care by hearing internal sounds of the body clearly across data networks in real-time, from anywhere in the world
- Uses the bluetooth enabled Littmann model 3200 electronic stethoscope
- Offers a user-friendly design and phenomenal sound quality
- Requires one-time software set-up that takes only a few minutes to complete
- At the patient site, the scope-to-scope software digitally captures heart sound with a state-of-the-art sound sensor, wirelessly transfers the sound to software using the Bluetooth® enabled Littmann® Model 3200 electronic stethoscope, and sends the sound across the internet securely
- At the consultant site, the sound is delivered to the eartips of the consultant who hears the patient's internal sounds as if the patient were in the room.

Site of auscultation

The site of maximum intensity of a sound of murmur is important in deciding its origin but it cannot be taken as reliable clinical observation, e.g. the murmur of aortic stenosis is frequently loudest at the apex. The diagnosis of the basic defect accounting for a murmur is considerably more accurate when the murmur is also analyzed for

- Timing
- Quality
- Direction of selective propagation
- Influence of respiration.

Mitral events

Loudest in the region of the apex beat heard with the patient turned on the left side and with the breath held in expiration

Table 3.3: *Heart murmurs in congenital heart diseases*

Description of murmurs	*Disease*
Continuous murmur with thrill	1. PDA 2. Tetralogy of Fallot 3. Venous hum 4. Pulmonary arteriovenous fistula.
Pansystolic murmur	Ventricular septal defect Plateua throughout systole, loud, harsh in the 3rd and 4th left intercostal space close the left lower sternal border. P2 heard in pulmonary area with normal split—if not obscured by the murmur. Systolic thrill in most cases (80%).
Mid or late systolic murmur with thrill	Pulmonary stenosis Murmur in 2nd left intercostal space. Thrill may be present. P2 single or may be split in moderate stenosis. In severe cases, P2 may not be heard.
Ejection systolic murmur (moderate or harsh)	Fallot's tetralogy Systolic murmur in the 3rd or 4th left intercostal space in 25% of cases the murmur is in the 2nd left intercostal space due to valvular stenosis shorter than the murmur of the pulmonary stenosis. Murmur fainter or absent when the pulmonary valv is much narrowed. The murmur is lower down in the cases of infundibular stenosis. The murmur is abscent in pulmonary atresia, P2 is single and loud in 20% of cases. Thrill not common in infancy.
Systolic murmur of loud intensity, wide splitting of P2	Atrial septal defect Moderate or faint systolic murmur in 2nd left intercostal space with widely split P2. Apical diastolic murmur is an indication of rapid inflow at the begining of diastole, occurs in larger defects of ASD and VSD. Associated systolic thrill indicates pulmonary stenosis.
Loud, harsh, systolic murmur with a thrill in the 1st and 2nd right interspace	Congenital aortic stenosis Loud, harsh, systolic murmur in aortic area ending before 2nd sound; systolic thrill present over the aortic area and transmitted to the neck over the carotids.

(heart nearest chest wall with increased flow through valve on expiration).

Tricuspid Events

Localized to the 4th left intercostal space at the sternal edge. Accentuated by inspiration (increased flow across valve during inspiration).

Aortic Events

Systolic murmur loud in the aortic area, at the cardiac apex and over the carotid arteries in the neck.

Regurgitant murmur loudest in 3rd and 4th left intercostals spaces at the sternal edge with the patient leaning forward in expiration (direction of the turbulent jet).

Pulmonary Events

Loudest in the pulmonary area and usually localized to it. Accentuated during inspiration. Low pressures in the right heart produce soft noises which are not conducted widely, but become louder with the increased blood flow into the lungs with inspiration.

THE HEART SOUNDS

The sudden tensing of a heart valve produces vi brations to both the valve and chordae tendineae and papillary muscles attached to the valve. Many of the vibrations so produced are within the acoustic range of the ear, and the normal and abnormal heart sounds are the audible vibrations produced in this way from the four valves of the heart (Table 3.3).

First Heart Sound (S1)

Normal

The sudden tensing of the mitral and tricuspid valves at the onset of ventricular systole produces the first heart sound. With the onset of ventricular systole, the left ventricular pressure rapidly exceeds the left atrial pressure. The mitral valve cusps are therefore thrust into the left atrium until suddenly held in apposition by the papillary muscles and chordae tendineae. The tricuspid valve is also closed by the rising pressure in the right ventricle within 20 msec of mitral valve closure and the sounds produced by these two valves are heard as a single sound, i.e. the first heart sound (SI).

Table 3.4: *Heart sounds and their causes*

Heart sounds	*Causes*
S_1: This results from contraction of the ventricles and closure of AV valves and opening of the semilunar valves	
	1. The heart beats force fully in exerciseor excitement, feveror anemia
	2. Mitral stenosis when it is "booming"
Decreased in intensity	1. Pericardial effusion
	2. Constrictive pericarditis
	3. When P-R interval is prolonged in acute rheumatic fever
	4. Myocarditis.
Varying in intensity	Congenital heart block
Splitting of first heart sound	1. Normal in healthy children
	2. Bundle branch block
S_2: This results from the closure of the semilunar valves	
Wide splitting of second heart sound	1. In children mild degree of splitting of S2 is normal
	2. Right bundle branch block (splitting increased with inspiration)
	3. Any condition where there is increased flow of blood to the right ventricle (ASD, VSD, anomalous venous drainage) in ASD both the factors are operative so that there is a wide splitting of S2
Single P_2	1. Tetralogy of fallot
	2. Severe type of pulmonary stenosis/pulmonary atresia
S_3: This results from the vibrations of the heart during rapid filling of the ventricles	
	It is heard at the apex and latter in the cardiac cycle in about 20% of the normal children and about 30% among children with rheumatic carditis
S_4: This results from the high atrial pressurewave which is reflected back from the ventricles	
	1. Left ventricle stress
	2. Systemic hypertension, ischemic heart disease and aortic stenosis

Loud S1

Mechanism

At the commencement of ventricular systole the valves are already almost in apposition as blood flowing into the ventricles has practically ceased. If the cusps still wide apart at the onset of ventricular systole with slack chordae, an abnormally loud first sound is produced when they are abruptly tensed.

Causes

Mitral stenosis, tricuspid stenosis: High cardiac output states (the flow of blood through the valve in late diastole remains high, keeping the cusps wide open); short PR interval (atrial contraction maintains a high flow of blood through the valve in late diastole, keeping the mitral and tricuspid valves wide apart).

Soft S1

Mechanism

If the valve cusps are rigid and incapable of much movement, or if the cusps are already close together before the onset of ventricular systole, the first heart sound is soft.

Causes

Calcification or fibrosis of the mitral valve cusps in some of the patients with mitral stenosis limit valve movement. The valve cusps are nearly closed before the onset of ventricular systole when the PR interval is long, i.e. in 1st degree heart block.

The varying PR interval of complete heart block has the effect of modifying the intensity of the first heart sound from loud, when the interval is short, to soft when the PR interval is long.

Splitting of S1

Normally the tricuspid valve closes within 0.02 sec of the mitral valve and only one sound is heard. Asynchronous contraction of the ventricles in bundle branch block particularly right bundle branch block, may produce appreciable splitting of the first heart sound.

Ejection Clicks

An ejection click is a short, high frequency clicking occurring shortly after the first heart sound and it arises from abnormal semilunar valves or from dilated great vessels.

Mechanism

When the ventricular pressures exceed the aortic and pulmonary artery pressures in early systole, the normal aortic and pulmonary valve cusps open widely against the vessel wall so that there is no obstruction to flow. Fusion of the cusps of these valves prevents their full opening and the abrupt arrest of the valve dome in a semiopen position produces a high pitched sound soon after the first heart sound.

Ejection clicks can also arise from the ejection of blood into a dilated aortic root or into a dilated pulmonary artery.

Types of Ejection Clicks

Aortic ejection click, arising from an abnormal aortic valve or from a dilated aorta. This click is loudest at the apex and at the lower left sternal edge.

Pulmonary ejection click, arising from an abnormal pulmonary valve or from a dilated pulmonary artery. A pulmonary ejection click is loudest at the pulmonary area and often heard only during expiration.

Causes

- Aortic click
- Aortic valve stenosis
- Bicuspid aortic valve (a bicuspid valve cannot open completely)
- Dilated ascending aorta, e.g. systemic hypertension
- Pulmonary click
- Pulmonary valve stenosis
- Pulmonary hypertension (dilated main pulmonary artery).

Second Heart Sound (S2)

Normal

The vibrations produced by closure of the aortic and pulmonary valves give rise to the second heart sound. The aortic valve closes at the end of left ventricular systole when the left ventricular pressure falls below the aortic pressure and the pulmonary valve closes at the end of right ventricular systole.

In expiration, both valves close almost simultaneously and the sound is single. During inspiration the systemic venous return to the right ventricle is increased, and right ventricular systole is prolonged. Accordingly pulmonary valve closure is delayed and the second heart sound becomes split during inspiration into an aortic component (A2) and a pulmonary component (P2) which accompanies A2 by 0.04 sec or more.

Normal splitting of the second heart sound on inspiration is usual at all ages, but is most frequent in the younger subjects. It is best heard in the pulmonary area.

Loud S2

When the sound splits on inspiration it is possible to determine which of the valve closure sounds is loud.

A2 is loud in systemic hypertension (more forceful closures of the aortic valve). P2 is loud in pulmonary hypertension. P2 is soft and not heard at the cardiac apex unless there is pulmonary hypertension.

Wide Splitting of S2

This is heard when pulmonary valve closure is delayed either because of prolonged right ventricular systole (pulmonary stenosis) or delay in onset of right ventricular systole (right bundle-branch block).

Splitting of S2

A constant gap between A2 and P2 throughout all phases of respiration is the characteristic feature of an atrialseptal defect (ASD). When the defect is large the right and left atria act as one common chamber and the increased return of blood to the right atrium during inspiration increased blood flow equally to both right and left ventricles. It therefore results into the prolongation of both right and left ventricular systole and the gap between A2 and P2 does not alter.

Reversed Splitting S2 (Table 3.4)

Description

In reversed splitting, second heart sound is single on inspiration and clearly split into two components during expiration.

Table 3.5: *Reversed splitting of S2*

Delayed A2
• Delayed electric activation of the left ventricle • Complete left bundle branch block • RV paced beats • RV ectopic beats
Prolonged LV mechanical systole
• Compete left bundle branch block • LV outflow tract obstruction • Hypertensive cardiovascular disease • Arteriosclerotic heart disease • Chronic ischemic heart disease • Angina pectoris
Decreased impedance of the systemic vascular bed (increasead hangout)
• Poststenotic dilation of the aorta as a result of aortic stenosis or regurgitation • Patent ductus arteriosus
Early P2
• Early electric—activation of the right ventricle • Wolf-Parkinson-White's syndrome type B

Mechanism

Reversed splitting implies that the aortic valve closes after the pulmonary valve. This occurs when left ventricular systole is prolonged or when the left ventricle contracts after the right ventricle.

Causes

Myocardial ischaemia or infarction, aortic stenosis, coarctation of the aorta (increased resistance to ejection) and large persistent ductus arteriosus (increase in left ventricular volume load). Left bundle branch block (delay in a activation of the left ventricle).

Opening Snap (OS)

It is a short, high-pitched, clicking sound closely following the second heart sound (0.06–0.12 sec), heard loudest medial to the apex or at the lower left sternal border.

Mechanism

The sound is heard in mitral stenosis provided the fused valve cusps retain pliability. When the left ventricular pressure falls below the left atrial pressure, the mobile valve is pushed downward into the left ventricular cavity until it suddenly tightens in its most fully open position with a high pitched snapping sound.

Causes

Mitral stenosis: The opening snap is absent if the valve pliability is reduced by calcification or fibrosis.

Tricuspid stenosis: A tricuspid opening snap is only occasionally present and is difficult clinically to differentiate it from a mitral snap. A low frequency, soft thud, late after the second sound, and heard at the apex (left ventricular 3rd sound) or at the tricuspid area (right ventricular 3rd sound).

Third Heart Sound (LVS3)

Mechanism

During the rapid inflow phase of early diastole the left ventricle elongates. The apex moving downward and the mitral valve ring upward. This phase of rapid ventricular filling ends when the mitral valve cusps are suddenly drawn taut stretched between the apex and the mitral valve ring by the papillary muscles and chordae tendinae.

The vibrations produced may be audible as 3rd heart sound which occurs about 0.16 sec after A2 at the end of the rapid ventricular filling phase. Similarly, rapid filling of the right ventricle may produce a 3rd heart sound from tautening of the tricuspid valve.

Causes

Physiological 3rd heart sound heard at the apex in most children and in few young adults. The early filling phase of the ventricle is more rapid due to altered myocardial tone and the raised filling pressure.

Abnormally large flow in the filling phase

(mitral incompetence, aortic incompetence, ventricular septal defect, persistent ductus arteriosus) result into left ventricular third heart sound.

Causes of right ventricular 3rd sound (RVS3)

1. Right ventricular failure
2. Constrictive pericarditis.

This sound has a different mechanism and is of higher pitch and earlier than the usual 3rd sound (0.1 sec, after A2). Sudden restriction of filling of the ventricle by the rigid pericardium plays some part in this.

Fourth Heart Sound (Atria Sound) (S4)

A low frequency, soft sound preceding the first heart sound.

Mechanism

This sound is heard when the left or right atrium contracts more forcefully than normal. A high atrial pressure wave reflected back from the ventricle tenses the mitral or tricuspid valve to produce the 4th heart sound. The sound is presystolic in timing, coincides with atrial systole and is heard when a ventricle is under stress.

Causes of a left ventricular 4th sound

Left ventricular stress, systemic hypertension, ischaemic heart disease, aortic stenosis.

Causes of a right ventricular 4th sound

Right ventricular stress, pulmonary hypertension, embolism, pulmonary stenosis.

Gallop Rhythm

The presence of a third or fourth heart sound (or both) in addition to the usual first and second sounds is referred to as a gallop rhythm. By convention the term is used to imply a pathological condition. However, physiological 3rd sound of the young is not called a gallop.

Summation Gallop

At faster heart rate, an inaudible 4th sound may be superimposed on a normally inaudible 3rd sound, the more commonly in families in which a first-degree relative has been born with a heart defect. In addition, hypertrophic cardiomyopathy, a primary muscle disorder of the heart, is an inherited autosomal dominant condition that may result in sudden unexpected death, especially during or after vigorous exercise, in young people. Obtaining a history of this condition or of sudden unexplained death in young people with first-degree relatives who have a heart defect entails a search for hypertrophic cardiomyopathy, which may be silent Physical examination of a child includes an assessment of general appearance, color, respiratory effort, and vital signs, including heart rate, respiratory rate, and blood pressure. The vital signs should be evaluated by comparing them with age-established norms. The neck should be evaluated for prominence of vessels and abnormal pulsation and listened to for bruits. The chest should be auscultated for abnormal breath sounds. The pulses in the arms and legs should be checked. If the pulses are not equal, then coarctation of the aorta may be present and extremity blood pressures should be obtained (Tables 3.2 and 3.5).

Examination of the heart begins with observation and palpation of the chest for abnormal impulses and thrills. Auscultation begins with listening for the normal sounds of the valves closing and for S1 and S2. It is important not to focus on murmurs initially. Atrial septal defect accounts for about one third of the congenital defects first detected in adulthood. This is because the characteristic murmur, a pulmonary flow murmur, also is one of the most common childhood innocent murmurs. The key to diagnosis is appreciating the wide fixedly split-second heart sound resulting from right volume overload. This will not be easily appreciated if the clinician focuses on murmurs before defining the heart sounds. Gallop sounds also may be present, signaling difficulty in keeping up with the demands placed on the heart. Conversely, isolated S3 gallop sounds may be heard in healthy adolescents.

When murmurs are heard, they should be defined by the following characteristics:

Timing—when during the cardiac cycle they occur.

Location—where in the heart they may originate, keeping in mind that vibrations are transmitted in both directions along a column of blood.

Quality or pitch—how they sound, which is important in differentiating normal flow murmurs from abnormal.

Intensity or loudness—not necessarily defining the severity, but changes in intensity may help to determine the type of murmur being heard.

Table 3.6: *Heart murmurs (acquired heart disease)*

Description of murmur	*Disease*
Mitral systotic	1. In mitral insufficiency (apex, blowing-conduction to axilla or inferior angle of scapula. 2. In any myocarditis. 3. In endocardial fibrucelastosis.
Mitral presystolic	Mitral stenosis, presystolic, crescendo leading to an accentuated Ist sound
Mitral mid-diastolic	In rheumatic heart disease of some standing but not yet full blown picture of mitral stenosis; Ist sound accentuated.
Mitral early diastolic	Short, faint, with a 3rd sound occurs in 30% of acute rheumatic fever and disappears during convalescence.
Aortic diastolic	Occurs in 10% of children with acute rheumatic fever, collapsing pulse, etc only later on. Decrescendo, often faint and best heard down the left sternal border with breath held at the end of expiration.
Pulmonary diastolic	Same features as aortic diastolic best heard in congenital hearts and severe anemia. Also right ventricle hypertrophy and prominent pulmonary artery with pulsating hilar shadows.

Ejection or nonejection clicks—presence or absence Innocent murmurs are murmurs produced by normal flow. Changing the flow should therefore change the intensity of the murmur. Characteristically, maneuvers that decrease the flow of blood returning to the heart through the venous system will decrease the intensity of flow murmurs, suggesting that the murmur is flow related or innocent. Changing the child's position from supine to sitting, then to standing, and finally to squatting during the examination will change the flow and is useful in helping to define innocent murmurs. The child may be asked to push out the abdomen or bear down to perform a valsalva maneuver, which reduces venous blood flow to the heart and the intensity of innocent murmurs. An examiner can coax even a young toddler into doing this by placing a hand on the child's abdomen and asking the child to push it out.

The following are the classic types of innocent or flow murmurs:

Still's Murmurs

These murmurs are low-pitched sounds heard at the lower left sternal area. They are musical or have a relatively pure tone in quality or may be squeaky. These most commonly occur between age 3 and adolescence. Because they are low pitched, they are heard best with the bell of the stethoscope. They are related to flow, and they can change with position alteration and then can decrease or disappear with the valsalva maneuver. No clicks are present. Pulmonary flow murmurs. These are high-pitched, harsher murmurs heard at the upper left sternal border. Because they are high pitched, they are heard best with the diaphragm of the stethoscope. They are flow dependent and also will change with position alteration and decrease or disappear with the valsalva maneuver. These murmurs originate from the right ventricular outflow tract and radiate along the pulmonary arteries and thus may be well heard in the back and axilla bilaterally. They are differentiated from pulmonic stenosis by their quality and from valvar pulmonic stenosis by the absence of an ejection click. Pulmonary flow murmurs can occur at any age, but they are common particularly in adolescents or in children with pectus excavatum. They are prominent in high-flow situations, such as when a child has a fever or is anemic, because flow increases in these situations. In infants, these sounds may be most prominent in the back or axilla because turbulence occurs when the blood flows from the larger main pulmonary artery to the smaller, less well-developed distal pulmonary arteries. In fetal life, the main pulmonary artery transports about 90% of the blood to the ductus arteriosus and only about 10% to the distal pulmonary arteries. The main pulmonary artery is thus large, whereas the distal pulmonary arteries are relatively smaller and come off at more acute angles than they do later as the child's chest grows. An analogy from nature would be the noise that is created as a large stream narrows into smaller streams. This innocent murmur has been termed "benign peripheral pulmonary stenosis of the newborn" to differentiate it from true anatomic obstructions to distal pulmonary arteries that occur in pathological conditions such as congenital rubella syndrome.

Systemic flow murmurs (supraclavicular systemic bruits). These are harsh high-pitched murmurs caused by normal blood flow into the aorta and into the head and neck vessels and are heard best high up in the chest and above the clavicles. They are also heard best with the diaphragm of the stethoscope. No ejection click is associated with these murmurs. They are transmitted to the arch vessels and are heard when listening over the carotid arteries of the neck. It has been said that because of these sounds "all children have carotid bruits"; however, the sounds differ in quality from true carotid bruits and are not associated with aortic outflow pathology.

Venous hums: These are low-pitched continuous murmurs made by blood returning from the great veins to the heart. They are heard best with the bell of the stethoscope. By changing the position of the patient's head or by pressing in the area of the major neck veins, the flow may be changed and these murmurs will change or disappear. Having the child look down or to the side while listening will often make these murmurs or sounds disappear. They are differentiated from the murmurs of patent ductus arteriosus in that they are louder in diastole, when maximal flow occurs in the venous system, and are often heard bilaterally. Venous hums are sensitive to posture and head and neck position, whereas the murmur of patent ductus is not. Although an ECG is usually part of the evaluation and may be helpful, further testing is not needed in the overwhelming majority of infants and children to distinguish between normal or pathological hearts. It has been shown that a competent pediatric cardiologist can determine with a high degree of certainty whether there is heart disease. Because of the characteristics of the sounds and the maneuvers that can be used to facilitate identifying them as flow-related phenomenon, these murmurs can be correctly identified without further testing. After concluding that the murmur or murmurs (a child may have more than one kind) are innocent, the practitioner should explain the findings to the parents and child. The practitioner should emphasize during the discussion that murmurs simply mean sounds or noises and that in and of themselves they are not synonymous with abnormalities of the heart. The clinician should stress that although a large percentage of infants and children have murmurs, less than 1% are born with the congenital heart defects that are the most common cause of heart disease in children. Parents should not be promised that their children will outgrow these murmurs because this is not necessarily true; adults can have innocent murmurs as well. Assurances should be given that because the heart is normal, whether or not the murmur disappears or changes is of no consequence. In addition, because flow changes the murmur, with growth and the changing configuration of chest and heart dynamics, murmurs may change, disappear, and reappear at various times—further evidence that the murmurs are indeed flow related and innocent.

Blood flow through the cardiac chambers is normally systematically streamlined, murmurs are produced when there is turbulence of the blood flow. The origin of murmurs is determined by the application of the following parameters:

1. Timing in the cardiac cycle
2. Site of maximal intensity and conduction
3. Loudness and quality
4. Influence of respiration
5. Timing in cardiac cycle.

Systolic murmurs occur during ventricular systole. Diastolic murmurs occurs in ventricular diastole. Continuous murmurs are heard throughout the cardiac cycle.

Systolic murmurs (pansystolic, ejection and late systotic).

Grading and Types of Murmurs

Murmurs are graded on a four point or, more commonly, a six-point scale. A common six-point scale is:

Grade 1 – Audible with difficulty
Grade 2 – Faint but recognizable
Grade 3 – Moderate intensity
Grade 4 – Loud
Grade 5 – Louder, but still needing a stethoscope
Grade 6 – Audible without a stethoscope.

Pansystolic Murmur (Fig. 3.92)

The murmur beings with the first heart sound and remains of uniform intensity throughout systole up to the second heart sound.

A pansystolic murmur is caused by a "leaking ventricle" (mitral incompetence tricuspid incompetence, ventricular septal defect). Blood escapes from the ventricle as soon as it begins to contract (1st sound) and continues to escape until the pressures equalize between the ventricle and the atrium (just after 2nd sound). Left ventricular pressure exceeds left atrial pressure throughout systole from the first heart sound until after A2 and blood escapes through the mitral valve into the left atrium giving rise to a murmur throughout systole).

A pansystolic murmur is heard in the following conditions:

- **Mitral incompetence:** The murmur is maximal at the apex, loudest on expiration and conducted into the axial.
- **Tricuspid incompetence:** The murmur is maximal at the lower left sternal edge and becomes louder during inspiration.
- **Ventricular septal defect:** The murmur is classically loud and rasping in quality, maximal at the lower left sternal edge and loudest on expiration.

Ejection Murmur

There is a short gap between the 1st heart sound and the beginning of the murmur. The murmur begins slowly, reaches highest intensity in midsystole and ends before the second heart sound. An ejection systolic murmur arises at the aortic or pulmonary valves when the blood flow through them is turbulent. This may be caused by narrowing of the valve orifice (aortic stenosis, pulmonary stenosis) or by a greatly increased flow through an orifice of normal size (high cardiac output states, left to right shunts). The murmur begins when the aortic or pulmonary valve opens, reaches its maximum with top most flow in midsystole and becomes soft again toward the end of systole. An ejection murmur must cease when flow across the valve ceases, that is, before the end of second sound which indicates closure of that valve.

Late Systolic Murmur

This murmur likely to start well after the first heart sound and thereafter increases in intensity up to the second sound. It is characteristic of mild mitral regurgitation when the greatest regurgitant flow occurs in late systole as seen in mitral valve prolapse.

Diastolic Murmurs

Early diastolic (regurgitant): The murmur begins immediately after the second sound and is loudest at its onset but may extend throughout diastole. High frequency and blowing in quality, the murmur is maximal usually in the 3rd and 4th intercostal spaces close to the sternum, and may also be heard in the aortic area and at apex.

A leaking aortic or pulmonary valve allows blood to flow back into the ventricle as soon as the valve closes (2nd sound), and is loudest at the beginning when the aortic or pulmonary artery pressure is highest, becoming softer as the pressure falls in diastole.

An early diastolic murmur is heard in either aortic valve regurgitation or pulmonary valve regurgitation usually as a result of pulmonary hypertension.

The murmurs of aortic and pulmonary regurgitation are so similar that differentiation is made on other evidence such as, a water hammer pulse favoring aortic incompetence, and evidence of pulmonary hypertension suggesting pulmonary incompetence.

Mid-Diastolic Murmur

The diastolic murmur begins some time after the 2nd heart sound. Delayed diastolic murmur is a more accurate description than mid-diastolic since the murmur may be short or may extend throughout the remainder of diastole. It is characteristically low pitched rumbling in character.

The murmur from a stenosed mitral or tricuspid valve begins with the resumption of flow through valve at the end of isometric relaxation of the ventricle. The opening snap indicates the end of isometric relaxation and is followed by the murmur, loudest at its onset when the atrial pressure is greatest, becoming softer as the pressure gradient between atrium and ventricle falls during diastole. The length of the murmur is determined by the time taken for the left atrial pressure to equalize with left ventricular pressure. When stenosis is severe the left atrial pressure does not fall to the left ventricular diastolic level in the time available and the diastolic murmur persists up to the first heart sound.

Causes of a Mid-diastolic and Flow Murmurs

Mitral stenosis: Murmur is maximal at the apex.
Tricuspid stenosis: Murmur maximal at the lower left sternal edge and becoming louder during inspiration. Increased blood flow across normal mitral and tricuspid valve (flow murmurs). Flow murmurs are low pitched, usually short and occur at the time when blood flow through the valve is rapid, that is, around mid-diastole. Mitral flow murmurs are present when there is an increased flow across that valve due to a left to right intracardiac shunt (ventricular septal defect, persistent ductus arteriosus) or due to a generalized high cardiac output states (thyrotoxicosis, anemia, systemic arteriovenous fistula). Tricuspid flow murmurs are usually the result of an increased flow over the tricuspid valve resulting from an atrial septal defect.

Presystolic Murmur

This murmur begins in late diastole and is at its loudest just before the first heart sound.

The presystolic murmur is the result of atrial systole due to flow of blood through a narrowed mitral or tricuspid valve. Atrial systole causes an increase in blood flow across the valve just before the first heart sound, provided the PR interval is normal. There is no presystolic murmur if atrial contraction is absent as in atrial fibrillation.

Causes

- **Mitral stenosis:** Murmur maximal at the apex.
- **Tricuspid stenosis:** Murmur maximal at the lower left sternal edge and louder during inspiration.

Austin Flint Murmur

A presystolic murmur or a low rumbling diastolic murmur maximal at the apex and indistinguishable from the murmur of mitral stenosis.

This murmur is heard when there is free regurgitation at the aortic valve. The regurgitant stream impinges on the anterior cusp of the mitral valve and tends to hold it closed. Under these circumstances the diastolic murmur of mitral stenosis can be produced by a normal mitral valve.

Continuous Murmurs

A continuous murmur extends uninterrupted from systole into diastole and is often heard throughout all phases of the cardiac cycle.

When a communication exists between two parts of the circulation, one of which is at a higher pressure than the other throughout the cardiac cycle, blood flows uninterruptedly which results into a continuous murmur.

Causes

1. **Escape of blood from aorta:** Persistent ductus arteriosus. Blood flow through the ductus is maximal towards the end of systole when aortic pressure is highest. The murmur is heard below the left clavicle and is loudest in late systole.
2. **Pulmonary atresia:** Blood flows from high pressure aortic bronchial arteries into the lungs. Again loudest in systole, often heard below the right left clavicles or in the interscapular region at the back.
3. **Ruptured aortic sinus of valsalva:** Coronary artenovenous fistula and any other large systemic arteriovenous fistula.
4. **Blood flowing from a high to a low pressure region in the lungs.**

Pulmonary Artery Branch Stenosis

Pulmonary Arteriovenous Fistula

A venous hum

It is common in children; mimics a continuous murmur and is caused by blood flowing through the great veins in the neck and the innominate veins. It can be distinguished from the murmur of a persistent ductus arteriosus by the following features; variations in posture and placing the head in different positions markedly affect the venous hum. Light pressure on the neck reduces venous return from the jugular veins and may abolish the venous hum.

Pericardial Friction Rub

This is a superficial sound produced by the rubbing together of inflamed surfaces of the pericardium. It may be heard anywhere over the precardium and usually has two components during each "cardiac cycle". It is often soft, localised to one small area, and the rub can be abolished by a pericardial effusion separating the inflamed surfaces. The superficial quality and timing of the sound, which is confined neither to systole nor diastole, distinguishes it from a murmur. It is commonly found in pericarditis of different etiology.

Site of maximal intensity and conduction of the murmur.

This is helpful in identifying the origin of murmurs but is unreliable if used in isolation from the other features, e.g. Aortic systolic murmurs are often loudest at the apex and aortic diastolic murmurs are loudest at the 4th left interspace close to the sternum.

Loudness and Quality

The loudness of a murmur correlates poorly with the severity of the lesion producing it. A very loud murmur may be produced by turbulent blood flow through a small ventricular septal defect whereas the murmur is softer with larger defects. Similarly, the loudness of a mitral pansystolic murmur is a poor guide to the severity of the regurgitation. The quality or pitch of a murmur aids in its identification.

High pitched murmurs indicate a stream of blood under high pressure (aortic incompetence, mitral incompetence). Low-pitched murmurs are indicative of a turbulent blood flow under low pressure (mitral stenosis, diastolic flow murmurs).

Influence of Respiration

With inspiration, the negative pressure in the thorax sucks more blood into the right atrium from the superior and inferior venae cavae. The blood flowing across the tricuspid and pulmonary valves is, therefore, increased during inspiration and increases the intensity of pulmonary and tricuspid murmurs, making this a useful clinical sign. Inspiration also brings the lung over the heart, which tends to make all sounds less well heard on the chest wall and this at times leads to confusion.

In general, right-sided events are louder or unchanged on inspiration and left-sided events are louder on expiration.

III. INVESTIGATIONS REQUIRED IN ESTABLISHING DIAGNOSIS

X-ray chest: The interpretation of chest films requires lot of experience and proper technique. It is difficult to obtain a satisfactory film in the newborn and young in fants. Likewise, a film taken in expiration may produce a false picture of cardiac enlargement, or suggestive of congenital heart disease because of the large thymic and cardiac silhouttee. Dark films may create difficulties in detection of pulmonary vascularity. It is also worth while remembering that the cardiothoracic ratio is 55 per in infants. After this age period a cardiothoracic ratio of 50% or less can be taken as normal. For a proper evaluation at least four views: posterior, anterior, lateral and oblique views may be necessary. In addition, these views of the chest may have to be supplemented with a barium swallow (Fig. 3.96).

ECG: The electrocardiogram is an important diagnostic aid in the evaluation of the cardiovascular system and is a must for the diagnosis of arrhythmias. The basic facts and the interpretation of ECG are considered separately in ECG chapter (Fig. 3.95).

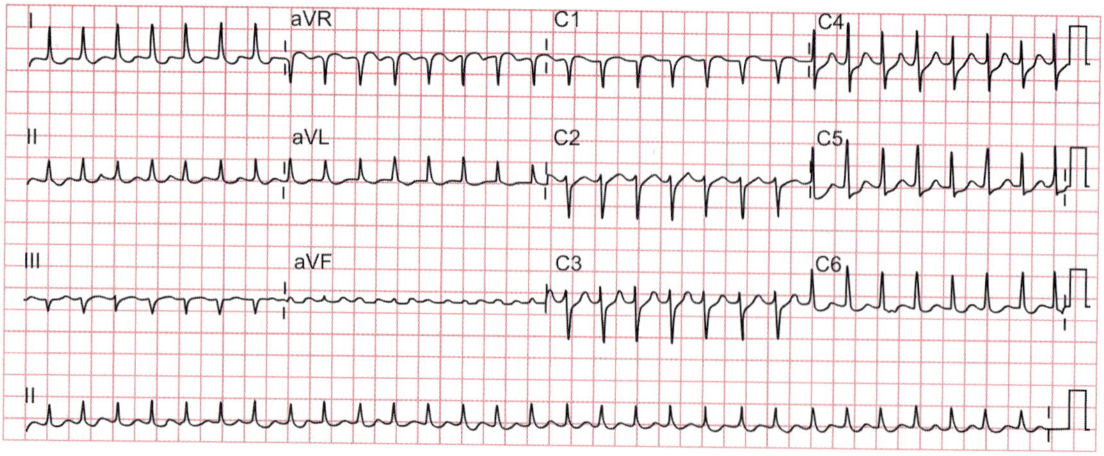

Fig. 3.95: *Twelve-lead electrocardiograph (ECG) showing atrioventricular nodal reentry tachycardia (AVNRT). Retrograde P-waves are not visible in this ECG*

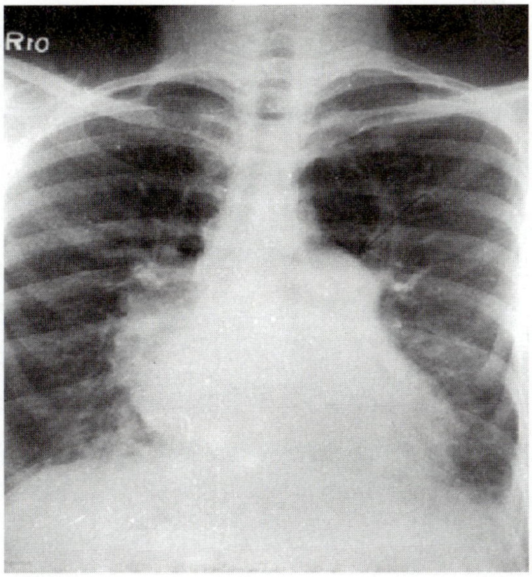

Fig. 3.96: *X-ray chest (PA view) showing cardiomegaly with enlargement of left ventricle with dilated main pulmonary artery along with congested lung fields in left to right shunt*

Phonocardiogram is also an useful aid as there is a close correlation between visual and acoustic events. The severity of lesion can also be assessed by this method besides obtaining graphic record of heart sounds and murmurs.

Echocardiography is being widely used at present and makes use of ultrasonic sounds for the detection of anatomic and physiologic abnormalities. Measurements the dimensions of the ventricles, the outflow tracts, detection of pericardial effusion, congenital and acquired heart dysfunctions are now possible with this technique without risk or injury to the body tissues (Figs 3.97–3.99).

Computed tomography: It is one of the most useful non-invasive techniques employed in the assessment of cardiac functions and its great vessels. In children it is being used in the diagnosis of congenital and acquired cardiac dysfunctions with least discomfort. It also gives most useful information before and after cardiac surgery and medical therapy (Figs 3.100, 3.102, 3.103 and 3.104).

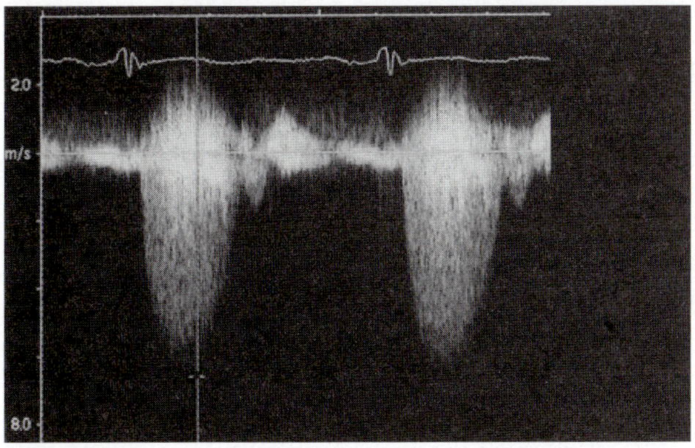

Fig. 3.97: *Continuous-wave Doppler recording across a severely stenosed aortic valve showing an instantaneous pressure gradient by the application of Burnouli equation*

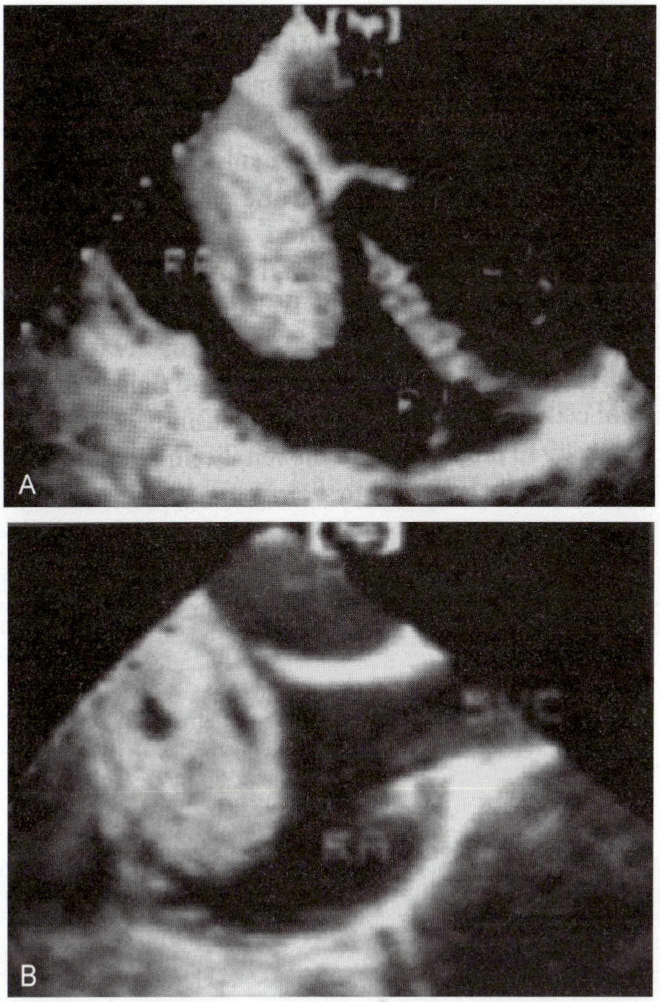

Fig. 3.98: *(A) TEE four chamber view the mass prolapsing across the tricuspid valve during diastole, (B) TEE longitudinal view of the atrial septum and vena cava,showing the mass extending from the IVC-RA junction, and filling the right atrial cavity*

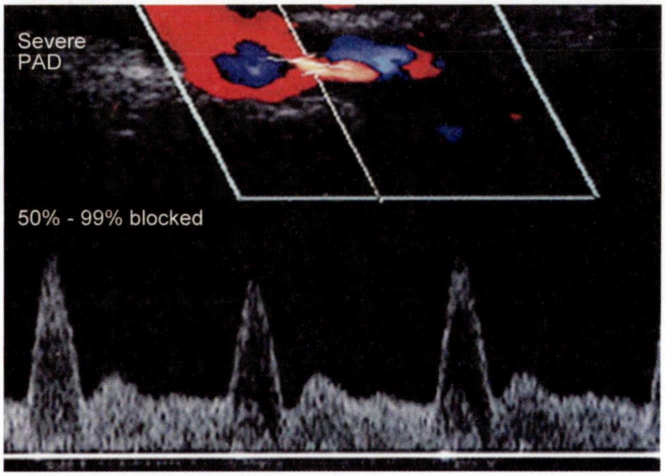

Fig. 3.99: *A duplex ultrasound image of an artery that has been almost completely blocked by peripheral arterial disease (PAD). The blue areas indicate slow blood flow, and not much blood flow is visible beyond the blockage because PAD has nearly closed off the artery*

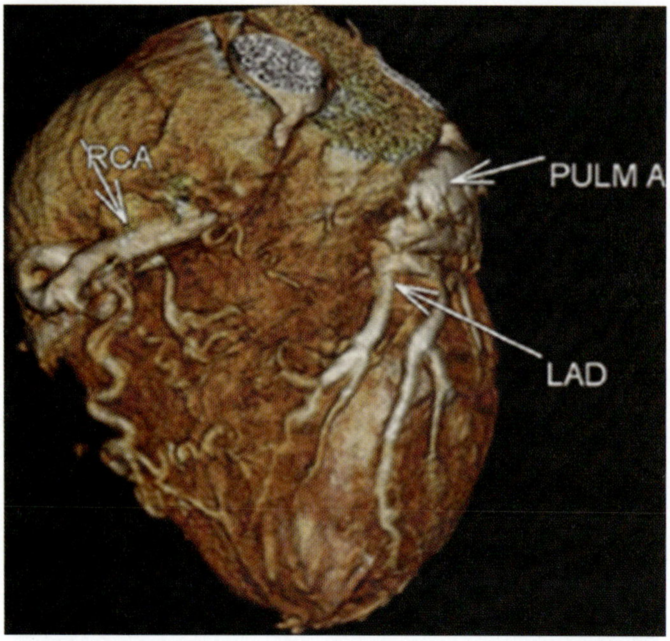

Fig. 3.100: *CT angiography volume rendered image. Right coronary artery (RCA) is dilated and tortious with a large number of collaterals feeding the left coronary system. Left coronary artery (LCA) is emerging from pulmonary artery trunk. PULMA the left anterior descending artery and their diagonal branches are also dilated and tortuous*

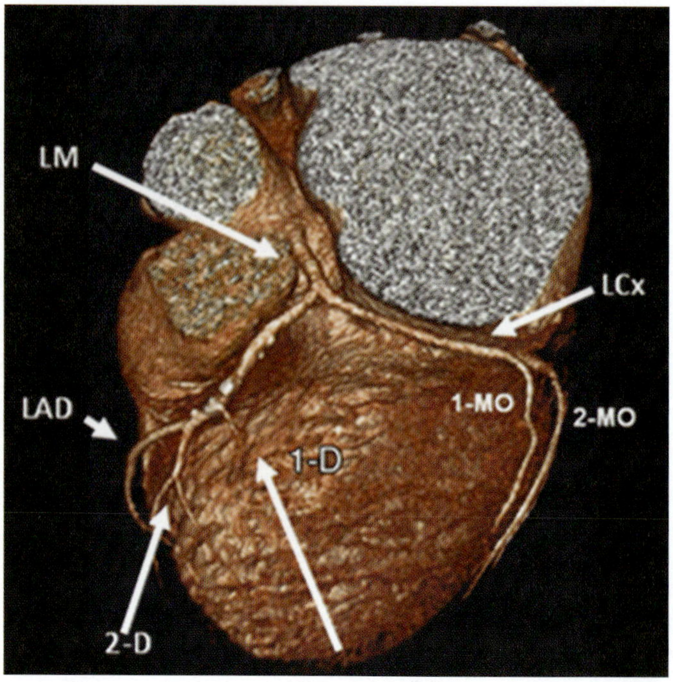

Fig. 3.102: *Coronary CT angiography with (a) volume-rendered CT image (left anterior oblique view and cranial angulation) shows the arteries: left main (LM), left anterior descending (LAD), first diagonal (1-D), second diagnoal (2-D), left circumflex (LCx), and first and second marginal obtuse branches (1-MO, 2MO)*

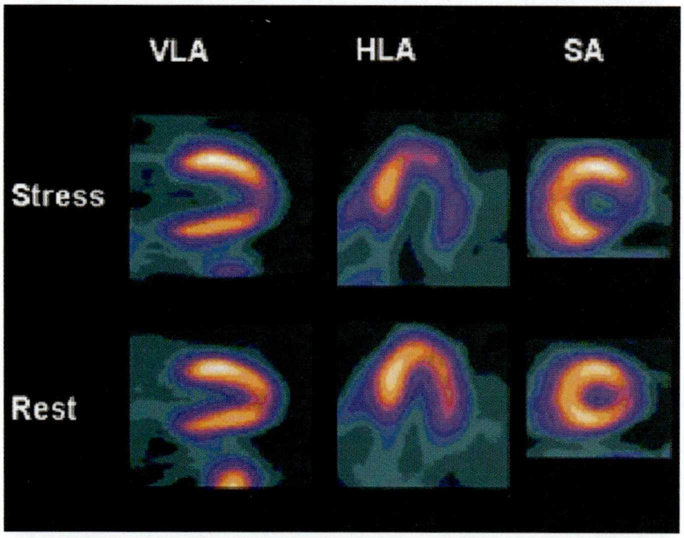

Fig. 3.101: *Stress and rest Rb-82 PET images in a patient with dipyridamole stress-inducible lateral wall and apical ischemia. Notable is the marked LV dilation during stress*

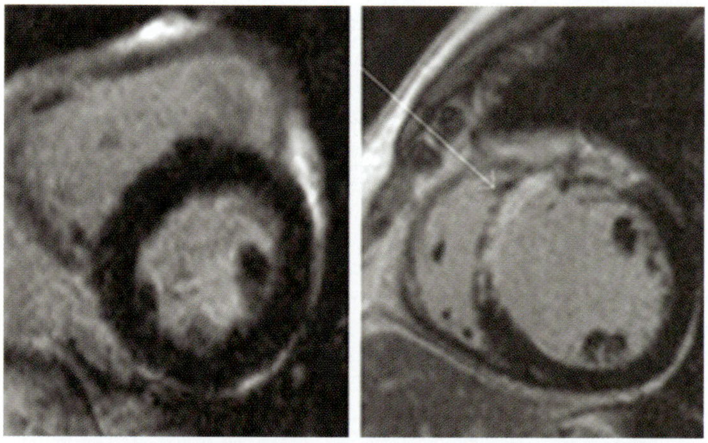

Fig. 3.103: *Cardiac MRI – left: normal heart muscle; right: scarring after a heart attack (arrow)*

Laboratory Tests

Estemation of Hb%, PCV, HIV screening and blood group typing are most essential part of a preoperative workup in both acquired and congenital heart ailments.

Cardiac catheterization aims at defining the anatomical and physiological variation of congenital heart disease and is undertaken only in specialized cardiac centers. It is indicated in infants and children with progressive lesions, complex malformations, severe degrees of cyanosis, severe degrees of refractory heart failure and in those in whom early surgery is contemplated. In competent hands, the technique is low risk procedure and provides data regarding O_2 content in the various chambers, systemic and pulmonary vascular resistance (Fig. 10.5).

Special techniques such as the hydrogen electrode catheter (for very small L-R shunts) and the indicator dilution curves, detection of shunts as well as cardiac outputs, are employed when special indication exists.

Cardiac catheterization is also used for injection of contrast material for angiography and percutaneous

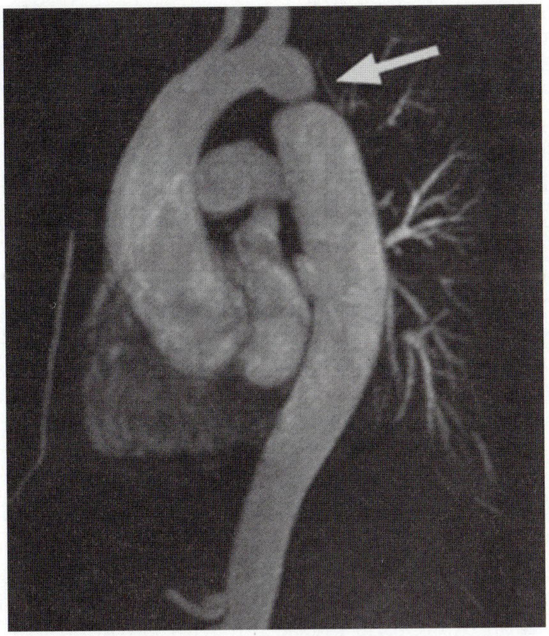

Fig. 3.104: *MR angiography of the thoracic aorta with gadolinium-enhanced 3D gradient-echo imaging in a 17-year-old adolescent with recurrent aortic coarctation (arrow)*

introduction of intracardiac devices in the management of congenital and acquired heart defects.

Angiocardiography: Injection of contrast media into the required chambers or great vessels permits identification of specific anomalies (selective angiocardiography) producing pictures without shadows from other areas of the cardiovascular system. A number of serial X-ray films (6–14/sec and even faster) are taken. Cineangiocardiography is being employed on a large scale in well-equipped centers (Fig. 3.11).

Radioisotopic studies using technetium 99 m is useful for delineating left to right shunts as well as the vessels and location of cardiac chambers (Fig. 3.101).

Cardiac Biomarkers

The use of cardiac biomarkers for the diagnosis and risk stratification of patients in the emergency department (ED) is evolving rapidly. Previously, the role of cardiac enzymes was restricted to the diagnosis of acute myocardial infarction (AMI). The identification of new biomarkers and more sensitive assays has extended the use of biomarkers beyond the diagnosis of cardiac necrosis. As novel biomarkers are identified, emergency physicians should be aware of both the potential clinical usefulness and the limitations of promising biomarkers. Testing should always be guided by a patient's history and physical examination to avoid misusing biomarkers as "screening" tools in critically ill patients. This update focuses on the present and future value of cardiac biomarkers in the care of patients who have suspected cardiac and cardiac-related diseases in the emergency department.

Galectin-3, a biomarker: Galectin-3 is a protein that binds and activates myofibroblasts in damaged heart tissue, which leads to collagen synthesis and subsequently problematic fibrosis. Though the current use case for galectin-3 is simply to get a better sense for the probability of adverse disease outcomes in patients with heart failure, ideally, treatments would be found that work best in patients with high galectin-3 levels. Galectin-3 is a protein that has been shown to play an important role in the development and progression of heart failure in approximately 30% of the patients diagnosed with heart failure. (i) This galectin-3 mediated form of heart failure is associated with progressive fibrosis, or stiffening, in the heart muscle, which impairs the heart's ability to pump. (ii) The role of galectin-3 in heart failure was first established in 2004, and (iii) the clearance of the company's Galectin-3 blood test now for the first time allows physicians to use this product in the evaluation of patients diagnosed with heart failure. "The availability of a galectin-3 test to identify high risk patients with cardiovascular disease and myocardial fibrosis represents another step toward the goal of enabling more efficient targeting of therapeutic approaches to reduce fibrosis in patients with chronic heart failure.

BIBLIOGRAPHY

1. Lee TH, Goldman L: Evaluation of the patient with acute chest pain. N Engl J Med 341:1187, 2000.
2. Ammann P, Sabine M, Kraus M, et al: Characteristics and prognosis of myocardial infarction in patients with normal coronary arteries. Chest 117:333, 2000.
3. Goyal RK: Changing focus on unexplained esophageal chest pain. Ann Intern Med 124:1008, 1996.
4. Hertzer NR, Beven EG, Young JR, et al: Coronary artery disease in peripheral vascular patients: a classification of 1, 000 coronary angiograms and results of surgical management. Ann Surg 199:223, 1984.
5. Diamond GA, Forrester JS: Analysis of probability as an aid in the clinical diagnosis of coronary artery disease. N Engl J Med 300:1350, 1979.
6. Pryor DB, Harrell FE, Lee KL, et al: Estimating the likelihood of significant coronary artery disease. Am J Med 75:771, 1983.
7. Gibbons RJ, Balady GJ, Beasley JW, et al: ACC/AHA guidelines for exercise testing: a report of the American College of Cardiology/American Heart Association Task Force on Practice Guidelines (Committee on Exercise Testing). J Am Coll Cardiol 30:260, 1997.
8. Chou TM, Amidon TM: Evaluating coronary artery disease noninvasively: which test for whom? West J Med 161:173, 1994.
9. Gianrossi R, Detrano R, Mulvihil D, et al: Exercise-induced ST depression in the diagnosis of coronary artery disease: a meta-analysis. Circulation 80:87, 1989.
10. Kwok Y, Kim C, Grady D, et al: Meta-analysis of exercise testing to detect coronary artery disease in women. Am J Cardiol 83:660, 1999.
11. Garber AM, Solomon NA: Cost effectiveness of alternative test strategies for the diagnosis of coronary artery disease. Ann Intern Med 130:719, 1999.
12. Geleijnse ML, Elhendy A, Fioretti PM, et al: Dobutamine stress myocardial perfusion imaging. J Am Coll Cardiol 36:2017, 2000.

13. Gibbons RJ, Chatterjee K, Daley J, et al: ACC/AHA/ACP-ASIM guidelines for the management of patients with chronic stable angina: a report of the American College of Cardiology/American Heart Association Task Force on Practice Guidelines (Committee on the Management of Patients with Chronic Stable Angina). J Am Coll Cardiol 33:2092, 1999.
14. Cheitlin MD, Alpert JS, Armstrong WF, et al: ACC/AHA Guidelines for the clinical application of echocardiography. A report of the American College of Cardiology/American Heart Association Task Force on Practice Guidelines (Committee on Clinical Application of Echocardiography). Developed in collaboration with the American Society of Echocardiography.Circulation 95:1686, 1997.
15. Nissen SE, Grines CL, Gurley JC, et al: Application of a new phased-array ultrasound catheter in the assessment of vascular dimensions. In vivo comparison to cineangiography. Circulation 1990;81(2): 660–6.
16. Hamm CW, Giannitsis E, Katus HA. Cardiac troponin elevations in patients without acute coronary syndrome. Circulation 2002; 106:2871–2.
17. Azzazy HM, Christenson RH. Cardiac markers of acute coronary syndromes: is there a case for point-of-care testing? Clin Biochem 2002;35:13–27.
18. Panteghini M. Role and importance of biochemical markers in clinical cardiology. Eur Heart 1 2004;25:1187–96.
19. Braunwald E, Antman EM, Beasley 1W, et al. ACC/AHA guidelines for the management of patients with unstable angina and non-ST-segment elevation myocardial infarction: executive summary and recommendations: a report of the American College of Cardiology/American Heart Association task force on practice guidelines (committee on the management of patients with unstable angina). Circulation 2000; I 02:1193–209.
20. Laffe AS, Ravkilde 1, Roberts R, et al. It's time for a change to a troponin standard. Circulation 2000;102:1216–20.
21. Laffe AS, Katus H. Acute coronary syndrome biomarkers: the need for more adequate reporting. Circulation 2004;110:104–6.
22. Alpert 1S, Thygesen K, Antman E, et al. Myocardial infarction redefined: a consensus document of The 10int European Society of Cardiology/American College of Cardiology Committee for the redefinition of myocardial infarction. 1 Am Coil CardioI 2000;36:959–69.
23. Wu AH, Apple FS, Gibler WB, et al. National Academy of Clinical Biochemistry Standards of Laboratory Practice: recommendations for the use of cardiac markers in coronary artery diseases. Clin Chern 1999;45:1104–21.
24. Lee-Lewandrowski E, Corboy D, Lewandrowski K, et al. Implementation of a point-of-care satellite laboratory in the emergency department of an academic medical center: impact on test turnaround time and patient emergency department length of stay. Arch Pathol Lab Med 2003; 127:456–60.
25. Wu AH, Smith A, Christenson RH, et al. Evaluation of a point-of-care assay for cardiac markers for patients suspected of acute myocardial infarction. Clin Chim Acta 2004;346: 211–9.
26. Kontos MC, Fritz LM, Anderson FP, et al. Impact of the troponin standard on the prevalence of acute myocardial infarction. Am Heart 12003; 146:446–52.
27. Koukkunen H, Penttila K, Kemppainen A, et al. Differences in the diagnosis of myocardial infarction by troponin T compared with clinical and epidemiologic criteria. Am 1 Cardiol 200 I ;88:727–31.
28. Newby LK. Markers of cardiac ischemia, injury, and inflammation. Prog Cardiovasc Dis 2004;46:404–16.
29. Balk EM, Ioannidis 1P. Salem D. et al. Accuracy of biomarkers to diagnose acute cardiac ischemia in the emergency department: a meta-analysis. Ann Emerg Med 2001;37:478–94.
30. Panteghini M. Acute coronary syndrome: biochemical strategies in the troponin era. Chest 2002; 122:1428–35.
31. Roongsritong C, Warraich I, Bradley C. Common causes of troponin elevations in the absence of acute myocardial infarction: incidence and clinical significance. Chest 2004; 125:1877–84.
32. Cantwell R V, A viles R1, Bjornsson 1, et al. Cardiac amyloid~sis presenting with elevations of cardiac troponin I and angina pectoris. Clin Cardiol 2002;25:33–7.
33. Aviles R1, Wright RS, Aviles 1M, et al. Long-term prognosis of patients with clinical unstable angina pectoris without elevation of creatine kinase but with elevation of cardiac troponin i levels. Am 1 Cardiol 2002;90:875–8.
34. Antman EM, Tanasijevic MJ, Thompson B, et al. Cardiac-specific troponin I levels to predict the risk of mortality in patients with acute coronary syndromes. N Engl J Med 1996; 335:1342–9.
35. Apple FS, Murakami MM, Pearce LA, et al. Predictive value of cardiac troponin I and T for
36. Subsequent death in end-stage renal disease. Circulation 2002; 106:2941–5.
37. Donnino MW, Karriem-Norwood V, Rivers EP, et al. Prevalence of elevated troponin I in
38. End-stage renal disease patients receiving hemodialysis. Acad Emerg Med 2004; II:979–81.
39. A viles RJ, Askari AT, Lindahl B, et al. Troponin T levels in patients with acute coronary syndromes, with or without renal dysfunction. N Engl J Med 2002;346:2047–52.
40. Polanczyk CA, Lee TH, Cook EF, et al. Cardiac troponin I as a predictor of major cardiac events in emergency department patients with acute chest pain. J Am Coli Cardiol 1998;32:8–14.
41. Quiles J, Roy D, Gaze D, et al. Relation of ischemia-modified albumin (IMA) levels following elective angioplasty for stable angina pectoris duration of balloon-induced myocardial ischemia. Am J Cardiol 2003;92:322–4.
42. Sinha MK, Gaze DC, Tippins JR, et al. Ischemia modified albumin is a sensitive marker of myocardial ischemia after percutaneous coronary intervention. Circulation 2003;107: 2403–5.
43. Roy D, Quiles J, Aldama G, et al. Ischemia modified albumin for the assessment of patients presenting to the emergency department with acute chest pain but normal or non-diagnostic 12-lead electrocardiograms and negative cardiac troponin T. Int J Cardiol 2004;97:297–30 I.
44. Libby P. Inflammation in atherosclerosis. Nature 2002;420: 868–74.
45. Smith SC Jr, Anderson JL, Cannon RO III, et al. CDCfAHA workshop on markers of inflammation and cardiovascular disease: application to clinical and public health practice: report from the clinical practice discussion group. Circulation 2004;110:e550—3.

46. Ridker PM, Brown NJ, Vaughan DE, et al. Established and emerging plasma biomarkers in the prediction of first atherothrombotic events. Circulation 2004; 109:IV6–19.
47. Hwang SJ, Ballantyne CM, Sharrett AR, et al. Circulating-adhesion molecules VCAM-I, CAM-I, and E-selectin in carotid atherosclerosis and incident coronary heart disease cases: the Atherosclerosis Risk In Communities (ARIC) study. Circulation 1997;96:4219~25.
48. Blake GJ, Ridker PM. Inflammatory bio-markers and cardiovascular risk prediction. J Intern Med 2002;252:283–94.
49. Ridker PM, Hennekens CH, Roitman-Johnson B, et al. Plasma concentration of soluble intercellular adhesion molecule I and risks of future myocardial infarction in apparently healthy men. Lancet 1998;351:88–92.
50. Ridker PM, Hennekens CH, Buring JE, et al. C-reactive protein and other markers of inflammation in the prediction of cardiovascular disease in women. N Engl J Med 2000;342: 836–43.
51. Ross R. Atherosclerosis-an inflammatory disease. N Engl J Med 1999;340:115–26.

4 Noninvasive Cardiac Imaging

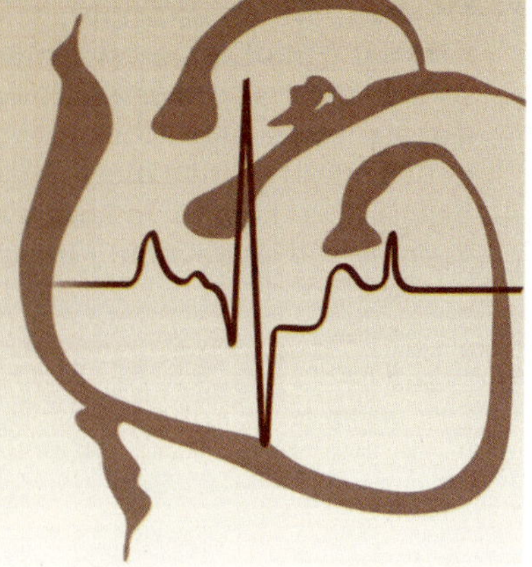

CHEST RADIOGRAPHY

Good quality posteroanterior (PA) and lateral chest X-rays make an important contribution to the cardiac assessment (Fig. 4.3 A, B and 4.4A, B).

1. Cardiac Silhouette

Because the radiodensity of cardiac tissue is similar to that of blood intracardiac structures can rarely be identified unless they are calcified. However, the cardiac silhouette contrasts strongly with the adjacent radiolucent lung fields. permitting accurate appreciation of the heart size. The heart is long and thin in ectomorphic individuals but is more bulky in endomorphic individuals. Nevertheless the maximum transverse measurement should not exceed 50% that of the chest. Cardiac enlargement is caused either by pericardial effusion or by dilatation of the cardiac chambers and great vessels. Myocardial hypertrophy without chamber dihltation rarely causes radiographic cardiac enlargement. The ideal radiograph for assessing the heart and great vessels is the straight, erect, postero-anterior (PA) chest radiograph taken at full inspiration. PA radiographs image true heart size, as opposed to anteroposterior radiographs in which there is variable and indeterminate magnification. As a result of gravity, erect radiographs display small pulmonary vessels in the upper zone and larger ones in the lower; this sign of normality can not be assessed on a supine chest radiograph in which upper and lower zone vessels are equal in size. The high diaphragm and the commonly used short tube-to-film distance supine radiographs also lead to magnification of heart size. In addition, heart size affected by patient rotation. Because the long axis of the heart lies at about 45° to the sagittal plane patient rotation with the right shoulder forward (RAO) enlarges the cardiac image, whereas the reverse rotation (LAO) reduces it. Rotations such as these along the major axis of the body also affect the prominence of various great vessels (aorta and pulmonary arteries), making their evaluation unreliable.

Heart Size

Assessment of heart size is important because apparently enlarged hearts are usually abnormal, though there are exceptions. A small heart is generally not a useful finding.

Transverse cardiac diameter is the horizontal distance between the most rightward and leftward borders. A diameter of 15 cm is regarded as the upper limit of normal. If serial chest radiographs are available, a change in heart size can be assessed; a 1.5 cm difference in diameter is regarded as significant.

Cardiothoracic ratio (CTR): A cardiac diameter of 15 cm in a small individual is likely to be abnormal and, to compensate for body size, the diameter is often expressed as a ratio (transverse cardiac diameter/transverse chest diameter). Conventionally, the transverse chest diameter is measured from the inside rib margin at the widest level of the chest. A CTR of 50% or less is generally considered normal and one of more than 55% is abnormal. The 50–55% range is a 'grey zone' that may or may not be abnormal.

Pericardial effusion: Pericardial disease may manifest as thickening, calcification or effusion. Effusion is a cause of cardiomegaly. Cardiac enlargement caused by pericardial effusion is often nonspecific, but should be suggested by the following finding (Fig. 4.15).

1. Featureless cardiac envelope
2. Rapid increase in heart size (over days)
3. Large heart with normal pulmonary vessels and lungs, particularly if cardiomegaly is a *surprising finding in the clinical context*
4. Large heart with a small, isolated left pleural effusion
5. *Occasionally, the pericardium is manifested as* a line of soft tissue lying between darker mediastinal and epicardial fat, best seen on a lateral chest radio graph over the anterior aspect of the heart, low down behind the

sternum; widening of this line beyond its normal 2 mm width is a specific sign of pericardial fluid or thickening. Rapid accumulation of sufficient pericardial fluid to cause tamponade may not enlarge the cardiac silhouette, because the fibrous pericardium takes time to stretch.

Chamber Size (Figs 4.1–4.3)

Assessment of chamber size and great vessel enlargement requires knowledge of the structures that form the border of the mediastinal silhouette. The chest radiograph is particularly accurate for assessing the left atrium (LA), is less so for the left ventricle (LV) and is poor for the right ventricle (RV) and right atrium (RA). It is fortunate that the chest radiograph allows accurate assessment of the LA because this chamber is commonly affected in adult heart disease and yet is inaccessible to clinical examination.

Left atrium: The signs of LA enlargement include:

1. Increased density in the region of the LA extending to the right of the spine, making the right heart denser than the left (Figs 4.1 and 4.2)
2. A visible right-hand margin to the LA, seen as a curvilinear border, convex inferolaterally through the right heart the distance from the midpoint of this curve to the nearest point of the left main stem bronchus is more than 7.0 cm.
3. Elevation of the distal left main stem bronchus to a horizontal position on the PA chest radiograph, sometimes with widening of the carinal angle beyond the normal 80° on a lateral chest radiograph, the left main stem bronchus is elevated and angled backward, out of alignment with the trachea.
4. A local convexity, where the LA appendage forms the mediastinal border just below the left main stem bronchus, appendage prominence with LA enlargement is unusual other than in chronic rheumatic heart disease (Fig. 4.1).

Left ventricle: With LV enlargement, the LV contour elongates and the cardiac apex is displaced downward and outward. On the lateral radiograph, the inferoposterior aspect of the heart becomes lower and more posterior. LV enlargement may have an additional element of hypertrophy. In pure hypertrophy, however, the LV is commonly not enlarged and a contour change (a more rounded LV border) mayor may not be present. Causes of LV enlargement are, with some exceptions, those of LA enlargement (Figs 4.3–4.5).

Right ventricle: RV enlargement in adult heart disease is often overshadowed and obscured by the enlargement of other chambers. It is seen most convincingly and commonly in congenital heart disease [Fallot's tetralogy and its variants, atrial septal defect (ASD)]. Principal findings area raised cardiac apex with a long, prominent upper contour and a shorter lower contour that turns medially; increased bulk of the anterior heart on lateral view, with the heart contacting the lower half, or more, of the sternum.

Right atrium: Assessment of RA size is too unreliable to be of use but a bulge at the lower right cardiac-border is indicative of RA enlargement.

Pulmonary Vessels

Pulmonary Veins

The principal disorder affecting pulmonary veins is pulmonary venous hypertension (PVH). PVH is a common manifestation of adult heart disease (which is overwhelmingly left-sided). As pulmonary venous pressure rises, radiographic signs tend to occur in a sequence. Exceptions are not uncommon.

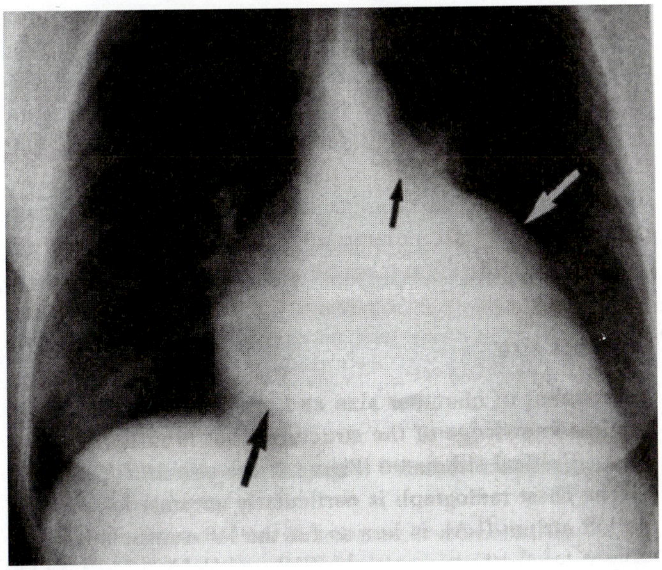

Fig. 4.1: *Left atrial enlargement. There is an area of increased density overlying the right atrium with a curvilinear lower border (large black arrow). The distal left main stem bronchus is elevated (small black arrow) and the left atrial appendage bulges (white arrow)*

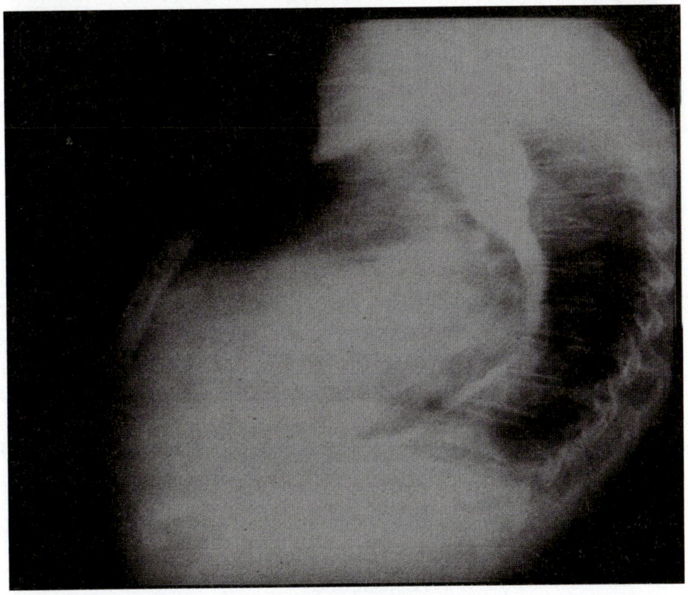

Fig. 4.2: *Indentation of esophagus (arrow) during barium meal study in left atrial enlargement in patient with RHD and moderately severe mitral stenosis*

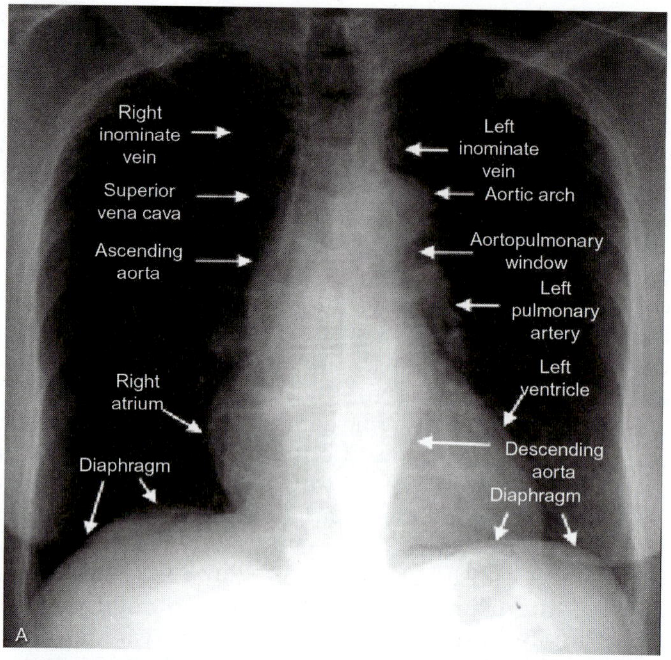

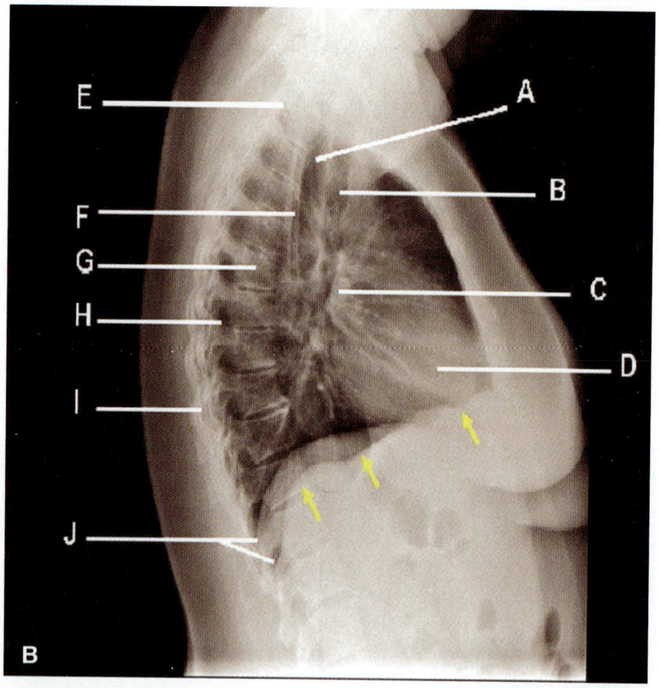

Fig. 4.3: *(A) Photograph of X-ray chest (PA view) showing various anatomical structures of heart and its great vessels (shown written with arrows on skiagram), (B) Structures that should be demonstrated on the left lateral chest radiograph include: esophagus (A), trachea (B), lung hili (C), heart silhouette (D), lung apices (E), scapulae (F), thoracic vertebra (G), thoracic intervertebral foramen (H), superimposed posterior ribs (I), costophrenic angles (J), and diaphragm (yellow arrows)*

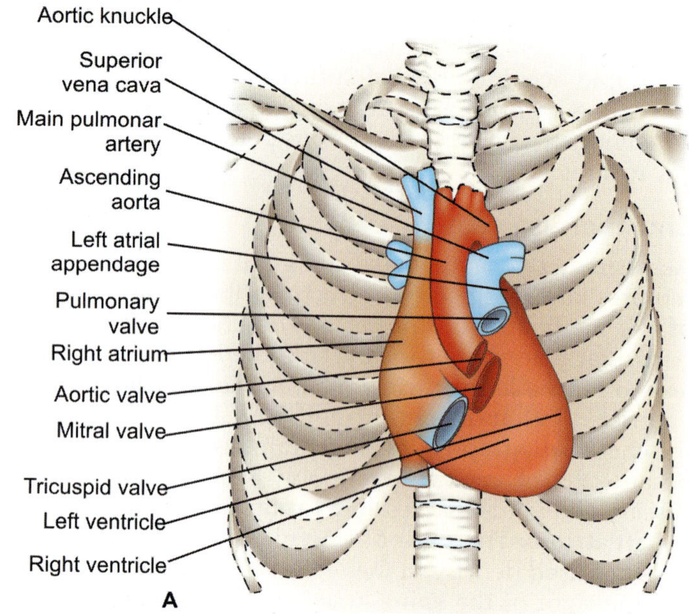

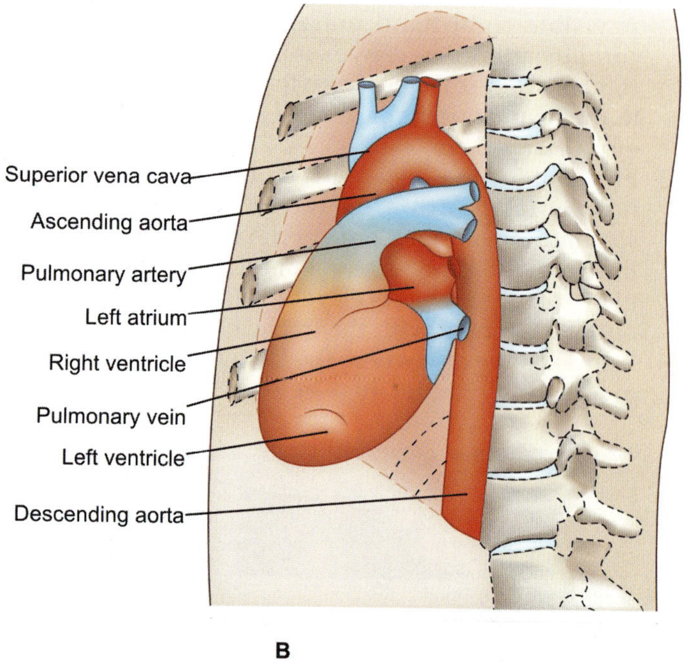

Fig. 4.4: *(A) Line diagram of chest (PA view) showing various anatomical structures of heart and its great vessels (shown written with arrows on diagram, (B) Structures depicted in a left lateral view*

Causes of left atrial enlargement

1. Mitral/aortic valve disease
2. Reduced left ventricular compliance
3. Restrictive or hypertrophic cardiomyopathy
4. Systemic hypertension
5. Congestive cardiomyopathy
6. Ischemic heart disease
7. Shunts (excluding atrial septal defect)
8. Left atrial myxoma.

It is related to the duration and rate of onset of PVH and the use of diuretic therapy. Indeed, modern therapy is so effective that there may be no evidence of PVH in LV disease sufficient to cause cardiac dyspnea.

Redistribution of pulmonary vessel size occurs at LA pressures of 16–22 cm H_2O. On an erect chest radiograph,

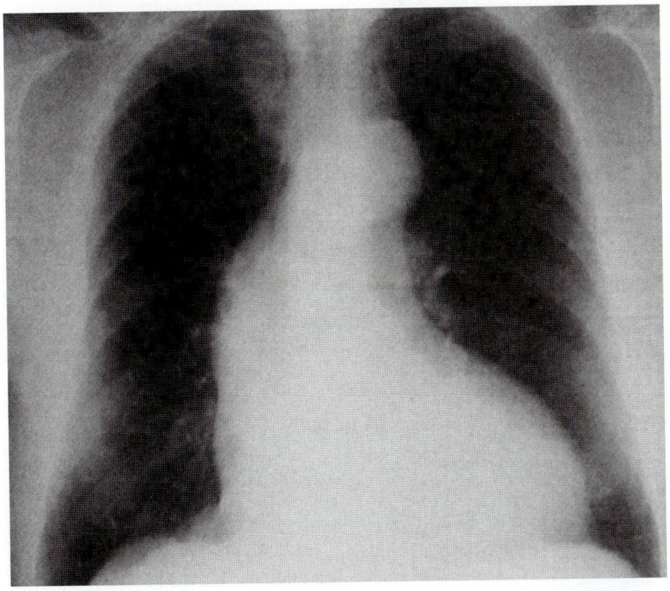

Fig. 4.5: *Left ventricular enlargement-characteristic long, continuous curve to the left ventricular contour with displacement of the apex downward and to the left. The patient has bicuspid valve aortic regurgitation, giving a prominent ascending aorta and a slightly widened arch*

upper zone vessels (arteries and veins) are normally smaller than lower zone vessels of the same generation; the discrepancy in diameter is about 1–3 mm. As pulmonary venous pressure rises, upper zone vessels (arteries and veins) increase in size and ultimately become wider than lower zone vessels. Distension of the upper venous trunk as it crosses the basal artery at the right hilum straightens the normal shallow V-shape of the lateral hilar contour.

Interstitial edema occurs at LA pressures of 22–30 cm H_2O. The lung interstitium is an interconnecting connective tissue framework that has central (perivascular, peribronchial) and peripheral (interlobular, subpleural) components. As tissue fluids accumulate, these normally covert elements become visible (Fig. 4.7).

Causes of pulmonary venous hypertension

1. Aortic valve disease
2. Left ventricular disease
3. Myocardial ischemia
4. Cardiomyopathy
5. Reduced left ventricular compliance (e.g. hypertrophic cardiomyopathy)
6. Mitral valve disease
7. Left atrial myxoma
8. Pulmonary venous obstruction (veno-occlusive disease).

Vessels: Particularly in the perihilar and lower zones, become hazy and ill-defined and airway/walls thicken.

Septal (Kerley) lines appear: B-lines are most commonly seen and are caused by oedema of interlobular septa. They are straight, short (1–2 cm) horizontal lines that touch the parietal pleura and occur most commonly in the region of the costophrenic angles. Their width is usually 1–2 mm but can be up to 5 mm. Septal B-lines can be distinguished from small vessels because they do not branch, they touch the pleura and they are surprisingly dense for their width (Fig. 4.6).

Laminar effusions are caused by fluid in pleural space, giving a vertical band of soft tissue density several millimeters wide against the lateral chest wall in, and just above, the costophrenic angle. Laminar effusions are often accompanied by septal lines, and their size provides a useful guideline for following the progress of heart failure (Fig. 4.6).

Alveolar edema occurs when the LA pressure exceeds 30 mmHg. Alveoli that have become filled with transudate

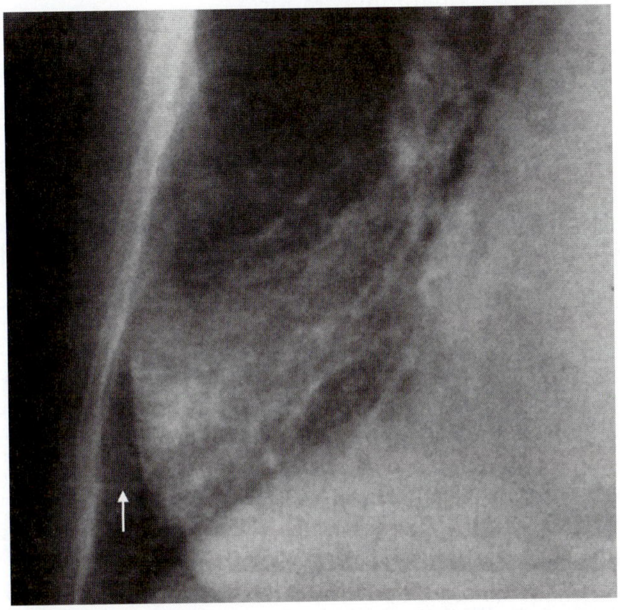

Fig. 4.6: *Septal (Kerley) B-lines linear, nonbranching horizontal lines about 2 mm wide and 1–2 cm long (arrow). When caused by raised pulmonary venous pressure, they are predominantly in the lower zone (arrow)*

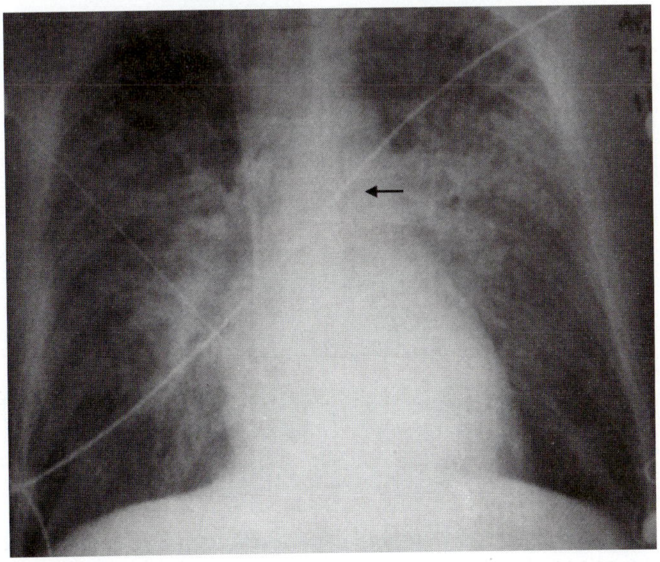

Fig. 4.7: *Cardiogenic alveolar edema. Symmetrical air space opacity with perihilar predominance is one characteristic pattern produced by cardiogenic edema*

become opaque (consolidation). The appearance is characterized by a pulmonary opacity of nondescript shape, with hazy margins. Characteristically, alveolar edema is bilateral with perihilar or lower zone predominance, but occasionally it is unilateral or focal. Unlike infective consolidation, the appearance can change rapidly, particularly under the influence of diuretics.

Pleural effusion is a feature of PVH. It is commonly bilateral or right-sided and may vary in size from small to large. Pleural fluid is sometimes loculated and, when localized in the minor fissure, gives rise to a mass-like opacity that changes size with fluctuations in the degree of heart failure ("phantom tumour").

Main Pulmonary Artery (Fig. 4.8–4.10)

The main pulmonary artery (MPA) forms a border between the aortic knuckle and the left main stem bronchus.

This segment is normally slightly concave, straight or slightly convex. Prominence of the MPA usually implies enlargement. Important causes of MPA prominence. Pulmonary arterial hypertension is characterized by enlargement of both the MPA and the right and left hilar pulmonary arteries. The upper limit of normal diameter for the right pulmonary artery is 16 mm in men and 15 mm in women (measured 1 cm beyond the hilar point; the point at which the outer borders of the superior pulmonary vein and the basal pulmonary artery cross). Distal segmental and smaller vessels may be normal or reduced in size.

Plethora is the term used to describe the pulmonary vascular pattern in which there is a generalized increase in vessel size (arteries and veins). This is associated with loss of the normal size differential between upper and lower zone vessels. Plethora is characteristic of left-to-right shunts and is also seen in venoarterial mixing lesions (e.g. total

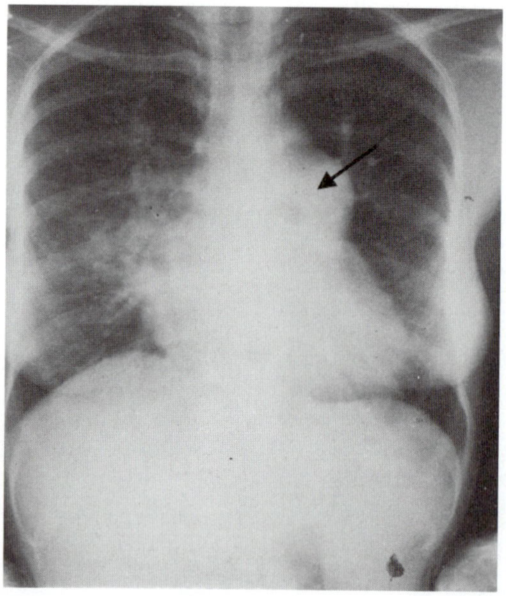

Fig. 4.8: *Pulmonary arterial hypertension in a 16-year-old boy. The principal finding is prominence of the main pulmonary artery (arrow). In addition, the right and left pulmonary arteries an slightly widened*

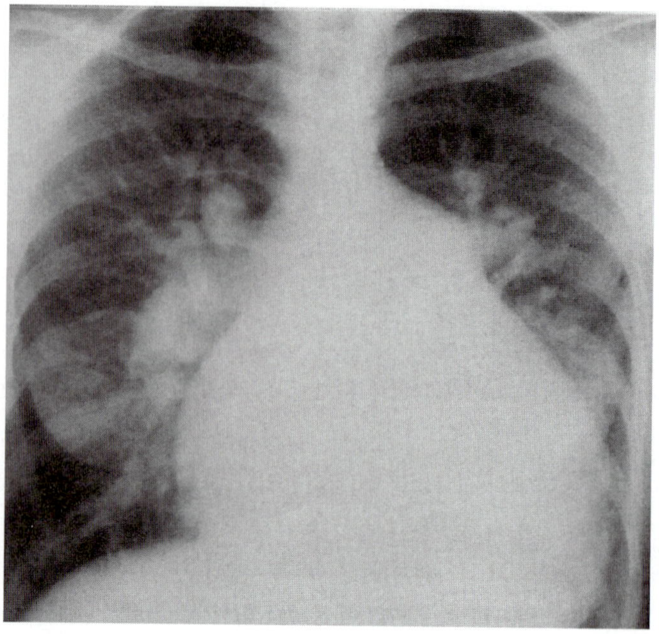

Fig. 4.9: *Secundum atrial septal defect. The main and hilar pulmonary arteries and veins are large. The lungs are plethoric, with general enlargement of segmental and more distal vessels, and loss ofthe upper/lower zone size differential. Other characteristic features are the small (unidentifiable) aortic knuckle and the leftward shift of the heart*

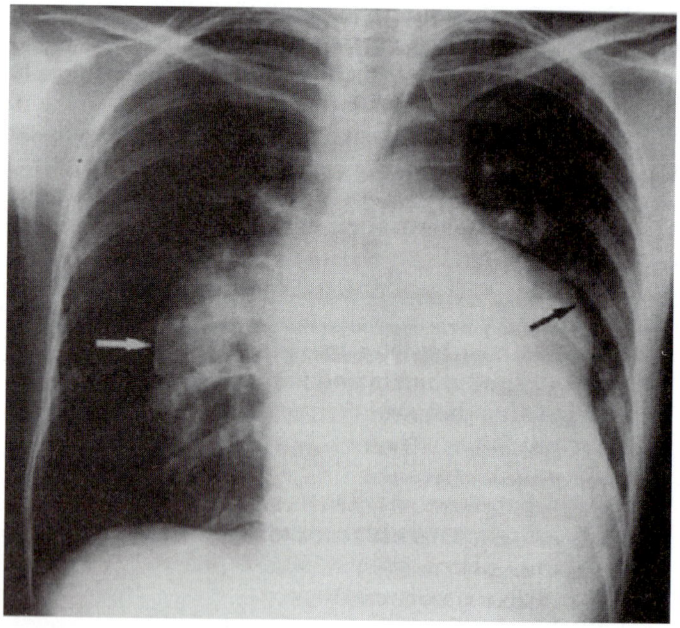

Fig 4.10: *Eisenmenger atrial septal defect. The left-sided bulge (black arrow) is caused by a massively enlarged main pulmonary artery. Enlarged right pulmonary artery and hilar vessels (white arrow)*

anomalous pulmonary venous drainage, truncus arteriosus). Mildly plethoric lungs may be seen in cor pulmonale in chronic obstructive pulmonary disease.

Left-to-right shunts cause enlargement of proximal and distal pulmonary vessels, resulting in plethora. Plethora

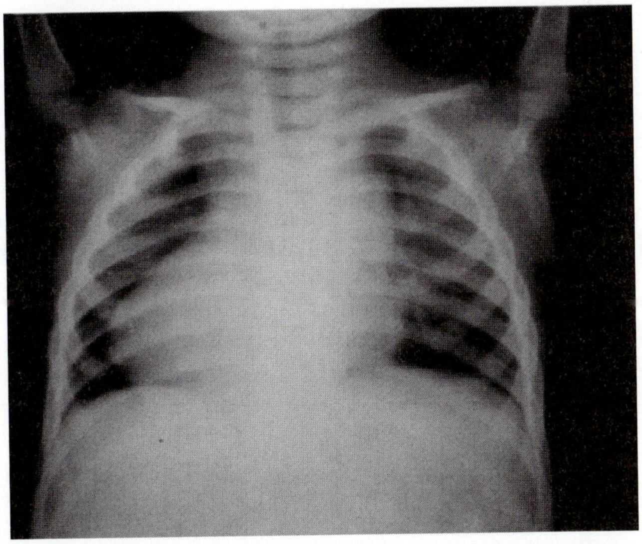

Fig. 4.11: *X-ray chest PA view showing apex of the heart and MPA are located on right side of the heart in a child with dextrocardia*

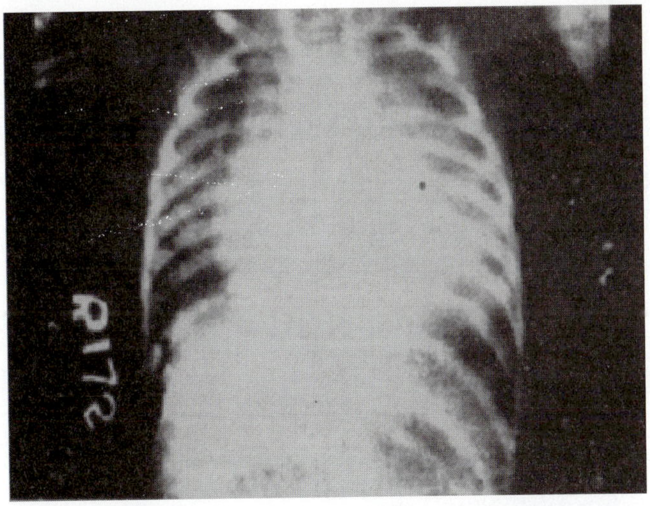

Fig. 4.12: *Gross left ventricular enlargement with pulmonary plethora in a young child with L-R shunt with CCF*

invariably occurs in shunts with a pulmonary flow: systemic flow ratio of more than 2:1, but is often absent in small shunts (<1.5;1).

Causes of a Prominent main Pulmonary Artery

1. Pulmonary Arterial Hypertension
2. **Increased flow:** L-R shunts (Fig. 4.12)
3. Mycotic aneurysm
4. Pulmonary valve stenosis
5. **Displaced by large aortic root.**
6. Mediastinal mass
7. **Corrected transposition of great vessels** (Fig. 4.18)
8. **Secundum atrial septal defect:** The findings are: A large, left-shifted heart, commonly with features of RV dilatation plethoric lungs with large proximal vessels, including the MPA (a small aortic knuckle, a left atrium of normal size) (Fig. 4.12).
9. **Ventricular septal defect (VSD):** Radiological changes generally differ from those of an ASD.
   - The heart and the MPA are less enlarged and may even be normal if the shunt is small.
   - Plethora is also usually less striking than in an ASD and, if the shunt is small, some upper/lower differential in vessel size remains.
   - The left atrium is commonly enlarged.
10. **Patent ductus arteriosus:** As in VSD, heart enlargement and plethora may be slight or even absent in small shunts. The cardiac contour suggests. LV enlargement and mild LA enlargement is usually present. The most important features relate to the aortic arch and the MPA region. This is invariably abnormal, with a large knuckle or with flattening of the angle between the knuckle and the MPA. In adults, the ductus or the adjacent aorta may calcify.

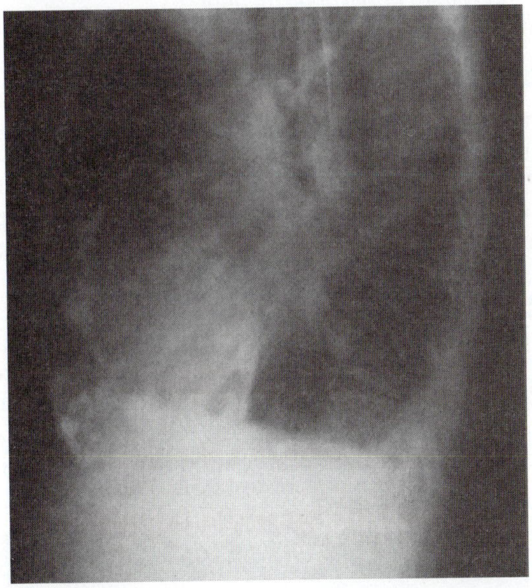

Fig. 4.13: *Pericardial calcification. The calcification here is heavy and craggy with peripheral predominance. Sometimes, it has a more linear configuration. Almost invariably, it is easier to detect in lateral than in frontal views. Pericardial calcification usually follows pericarditis (particularly tuberculous, as in this case) and is commonly associated with constriction*

Causes of Pulmonary Arterial Hypertension

- Pulmonary venous hypertension
- Shunts: Left -to-right
- Eisenmenger's syndrome
- Pulmonary embolism
- Thromboembolism
- Parasites
- Chronic hypoxia
- Diffuse fibrotic lung disease
- Uncommon
- Arteritis
- Drugs/toxins
- Idiopathic.

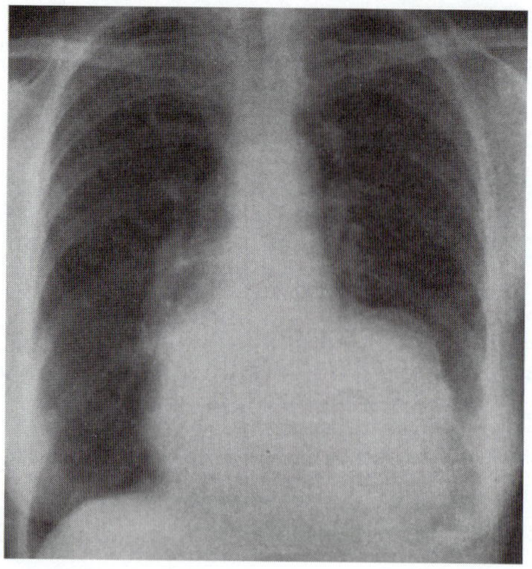

Fig. 4.14: *Left ventricular aneurysm following old myocardial infarction. There is a pronounced bulge to the upper aspect of the left ventricular border. In this patient, the old infarct has also calcified in a thin, curvilinear manner*

Eisenmenger's Syndrome (Fig. 4.10)

In this syndrome there is raised pulmonary vascular resistance, shunt reversal and cyanosis produced by prolonged high flow through pulmonary vessels as the result of a left-to-right shunt. The important radiological difference from non-reversed shunts is that the lungs are no longer plethoric.

Oligemia is a general reduction in pulmonary vessel size. The change is opposite to that in plethora and is caused by low pulmonary blood flow. Oligemia is difficult to assess reliably; it is more commonly associated with congenital heart disease (e.g. Fallot's tetralogy, Fallot variants, occasionally pulmonary valve stenosis) than with adult-acquired disease (e.g. pulmonary embolism, tricuspid valve disease).

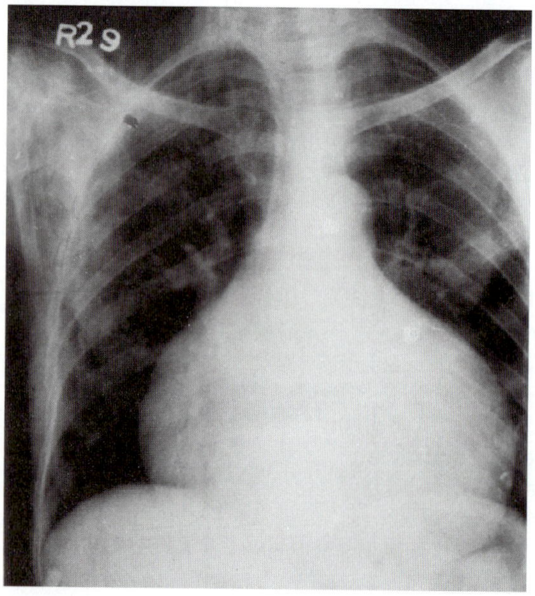

Fig. 4.15: *X-ray chest (PA) view showing global cardiac enlargement with money bag configuration and olegemic lung fields in patient with moderate pericardial effusion*

Aorta

In children and young adults, the ascending aorta is not border-forming on a PA chest radiograph and the lateral margin of the descending aorta is straight. The aorta elongates and "unfolds" outward with age, commonly producing a right-sided convexity to the mediastinum between the superior vena cava and the RA (after 40 years of age) and a lateral bowing of the descending aortic border.

- **Aortic aneurysm:** Aortic disease commonly manifests as an aneurysm, and it may be difficult to distinguish between aneurysm and unfolding aorta. Observations suggesting that a prominent ascending aorta might be the result of aneurysm include:
  1. Age > 40 years
  2. Absent or disproportionately mild prominence of the descending aorta
  3. Abnormally wide aortic arch (more than 40 mm).

There may be radiographic clues to the cause of an aneurysm of the ascending aorta.

Although the width of a prominent descending aorta cannot be assessed on a PA chest radiograph, it can be assessed on a lateral chest radiograph, on which its anterior and posterior borders are often outlined by lung, thus allowing distinction between aneurysm and unfolding.

- **Dissection of the aorta** appears as mediastinal widening. In addition, leakage of blood can cause haziness of the aortic outline, extrapleural opacity andpleural effusion.

Type A dissections involve the ascending aorta with or without distal extension, and are treated surgically.

Type B dissections start at the left subclavian artery and propagate distally into the descending aorta. They are usually treated medically. Previous radiographs may be useful because dissections often occur on the basis of a preexisting aneurysm (e.g. atherosclerosis, Marfan's cystic medial necrosis).

- **Coarctation of the aorta** is a localized congenital narrowing just beyond the left subclavian take-off. It is associated with other congenital anomalies including bicuspid aortic valve. In about 70% of patients the ascending aorta is characteristically most marked in the region of the aortic sinuses; because of this, they cause aortic regurgitation, and may be quite large without distorting the mediastinal envelope.

Coarctation lead to inferior rib-notching (ribs three to eight) and an abnormal configuration of the aortic knuckle region, which may be high, low, flat or double. Heart size is usually normal, possibly with a contour suggesting LV hypertrophy, and occasionally there is mild LA enlargement. Slight prominence of the ascending aorta is common and is caused by hypertension and/or a bicuspid aortic valve.

The main radiographic clues to the cause of an aneurysm of the ascending aorta are:

1. In hypertension, dilatation tends to be mild and generalized, and is often best appreciated in the arch.

2. The ascending aorta and the arch are involved in aortic regurgitation, whereas aortic stenosis affects only the ascending aorta.
3. Syphilis affects the ascending aorta is characterized by thin, continuous, curvilinear marginal calcification that is bestseen on lateral radiographs.
4. Calcification is qualitatively different in atheromatous aneurysms and comprises interrupted, irregular plaques; these aneurysms can affect any segment, but are most common in the descending aorta.
5 Aneurysms in Marfan's syndrome typically affect the ascending aorta are characteristically most marked in the region of aortic sinuses; because of this, they cause aortic regurgitation and may be quite large without distorting the mediastinal envelope.

Calcification (Figs 4.16–4.19)

Both vascular and cardiac lesions may calcify and, if moderate, calcification may be seen on a chest radiograph. The optimal projection may be frontal or, more commonly, lateral.

Causes of cardiovascular calcification

1. *Pericardium* (Old infective, particularly tuberculous, pericarditis
2. *Myocardium:* Old myocardial infarct
3. *Rheumatic heart disease* (left atrium)
4. *Mitral annular calcification*
5. *Endocardium.* Jet lesions
6. *Within chamber*
   - Thrombus
   - Myxoma
7. *Valve*
   - Rheumatic heart disease

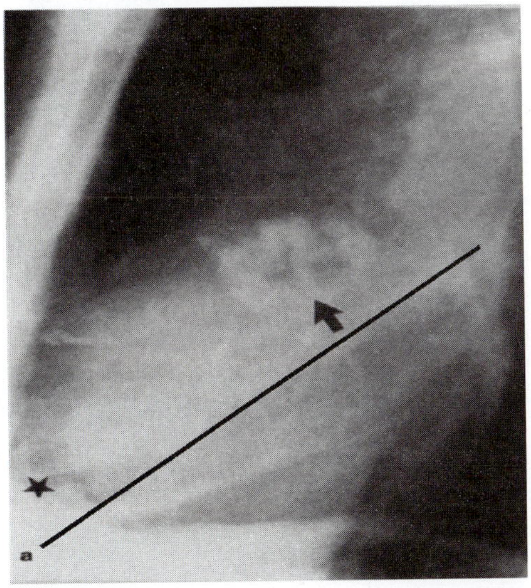

Fig. 4.16: *Calcific, bicuspid aortic stenosis a lateral view the aortic valve is heavily calcified (arrow), indicating severe stenosis, despite which the heart size is normal. The calcification is clear visible and typically lies above an imaginary line joining the costophrenic angle and the lung hilum (both marked with a star The a-like configuration of the calcification is characteristic and clearly outlines the base and free margin of the two cusps*

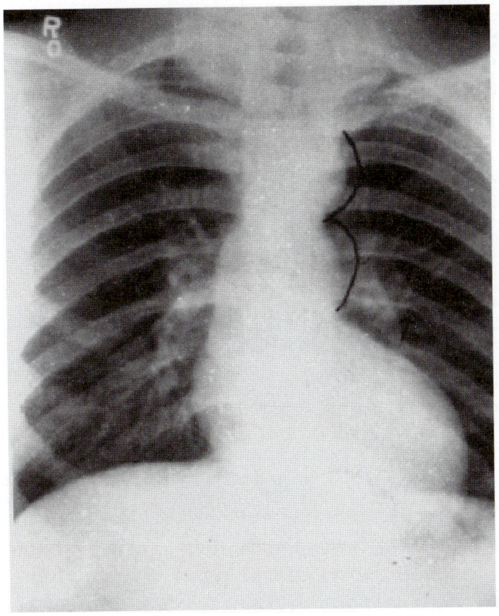

Fig. 4.17: *Chest X-ray PA view showing prominence of left subclavian artery, abcent impression in the region of coarctation and distatal impression of descending aorta giving the configuration of word 3 as shown (arrow) in patient with coarctation of aorta*

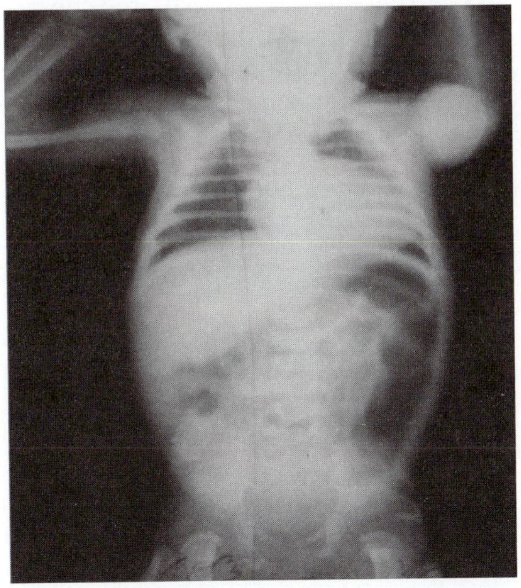

Fig. 4.18: *Chest X-ray PA view showing wider base obliquily placed heart in the chest, abscent pulmonary impression and upward lift of the cardiac apex and egg-shaped configuration of the heart in a child with dextro-transposion of great vessels*

   - Bicuspid/senile aortic valve
   - Aortic homograft
8. *Coronary artery*
   - Atheroma
9. *Pulmonary artery*
   - Pulmonary arterial hypertension
10. *Aorta*
   - Atheroma
   - Aortitis

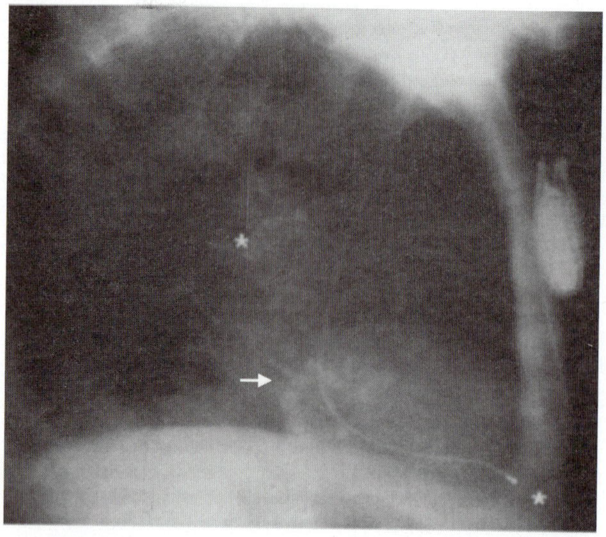

Fig. 4.19: *Mitral annular calcification (arrow) commonly has a C-shaped configuration and lies in the region of the mitral valve (i.e. below a line joining the hilum and the anterior costophrenic angle, both marked with a star). It must not be confused with mitral valve calcification (often an easy distinction based on its configuration). Its presence is associated with systemic emboli and dysrhythmias (note the pacemaker in this patient)*

Ischemic Heart Disease

In acute myocardial infarction (AMI), the chest radiograph enables assessment of hemodynamic disturbance, detects complications and excludes some other causes of chest pain. Hemodynamic disorder is manifested by PVH, which can occur despite a normal heart size.

Complications of Myocardial Infarction

1. Mitral regurgitation is characterized by pulmonary venous hypertension, mild cardiomegaly, and absent or mild LA enlargement.
2. The signs of VSD are similar to those of acute mitral regurgitation, and classic changes of plethora are not usually seen in the acute state.
3. LV aneurysm affects the anterolateral and apical parts of the LV in particular, producing either a large heart with a configuration of LV enlargement or a localized bulge to the LV border (apical or anterolaterally, that occasionally calcifies. Post-MI syndrome (Dressler's syndrome) is a delayed manifestation that gives rise to pericardial and pleural effusions, sometimes with basal lung consolidation (Fig. 4.14).

Valvular Heart Disease

Mitral stenosis has characteristic radiological appearances. There is LA and LA appendage enlargement; the size of the LA correlates poorly with the degree of stenosis. Gross LA enlargement is not seen in pure mitral stenosis and indicates mitral regurgitation or a mixed lesion.

I. *Mitral valve*

- **Mitral valve calcification** is present in long-standing, severe stenosis and is not a feature of mild disease (Fig. 4.19).

A normal heart size is common in uncomplicated disease. There is evidence of PVH. Pulmonary arterial hypertension is evident in long-standing severe disease. At this stage, the heart usually becomes enlarged as the right-sided chambers dilate.

- **Mitral regurgitation:** Radiological findings in mitral regurgitation differ in acute and chronic situations.
  1. **Chronic mitral regurgitation:** The heart is enlarged (with a contour of LV enlargement) and there is LA enlargement, which is often greater than in mitral stenosis. Signs of raised pulmonary venous pressure may be present but are often mild. In the absence of LV disease, heart size correlates with the severity of the mitral regurgitation.
  2. **Acute mitral regurgitation:** The main finding is gross pulmonary edema, often without overall enlargement of either the heart or the LA.

II. *Aortic stenosis*

Aortic stenosis should be suspected if the radiograph shows:

1. Aortic valve calcification with a normal heart size
2. Cardiac contour that suggests left ventricular hypertrophy
3. Prominence of the ascending aorta as a result of post-stenotic dilatation. With decompensation, the heart, including the LA, enlarges and signs of PVH develop.

- **Aortic regurgitation:** The radiological signs of aortic regurgitation are:
  1. A large heart with a contour characteristic of LV dilatation.
  2. Mild LA enlargement (sometimes)
  3. A prominent ascending aorta caused by dilatation

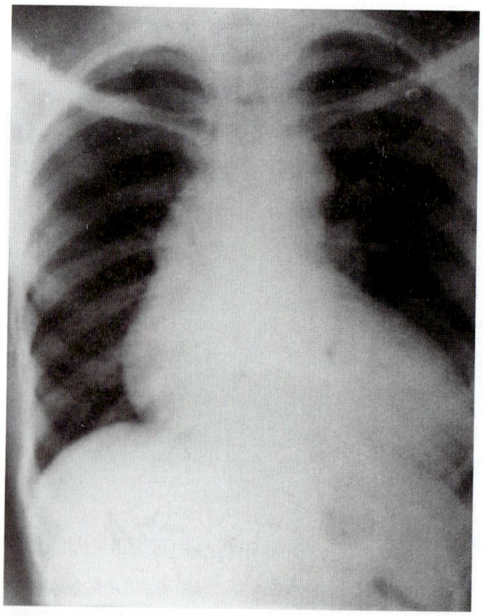

Fig. 4.20: *Chest X-ray PA view showing, absent pulmonary impression,olegemic lung fields, upward lift of the cardiac apex and prominant bulge along the lower right border of the right atrium in an older child with congenital pulmonic stenosis with gross tricuspid regurgitation*

4. A calcified aortic valve (sometimes) PVH may be absent despite marked regurgitation and, when it does develop, it is often late in the course of the disease.

III. *Prosthetic valves* (Fig. 4.21)

A large range of prosthetic valves is available. Apart from homografts, all valves are radiopaque. Radiopaque components in prosthetic valves allow; identification of the type of valve, and usually indicate the direction of flow:

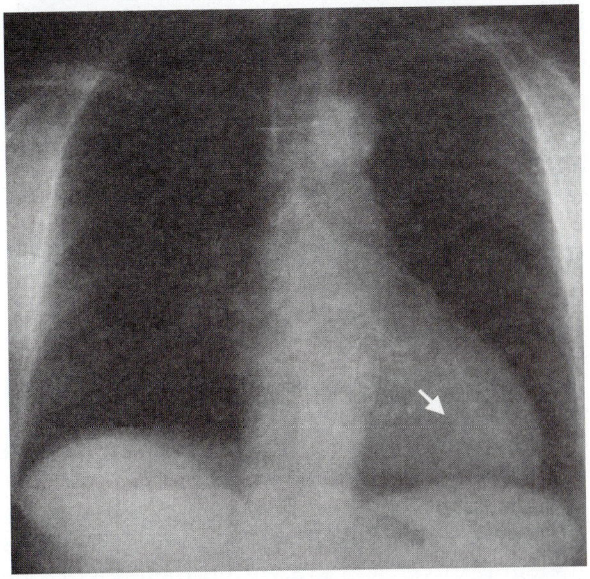

Fig. 4.21: *Porcine (Carpentier-Edward) mitral valve replacement. Flow in such a prosthesis is from the "base" to the tips of the stents and is indicated by the arrow. Flow in this direction could not be aortic but could be tricuspid or mitral. The position of the prosthesis to the left of the spine favors the latter*

1. In hetrografts and caged valves, flow is from the base ring to the strut.
2. In the disk valves, the disc is often radiopaque, and the direction of flow is indicated if the disk is caught in an open position
3. Because most replaced valves in adults are aortic or mitral knowledge of the direction of flow is usually sufficient to identify the valve site
4. Occasionally, the tricuspid valve is replaced. This is oriented, from a flow point of view, like a mitral prosthesis, but it positioned more anteriorly and to the right. Some prosthetic valve abnormalities including struit fracture and bioprosthesis calcification can be detected on a chest radiograph.

2. Medical Devices of the Chest (Figs 4.22–4.26)

Chest devices are encountered on a daily basis by almost all radiologists. A multitude of extrathoracic materials from intravenous catheters to oxygen tubing and electrocardiographic leads, frequently overlie the chest, neck, and abdomen. Chest tubes, central venous catheters, endotracheal tubes, and feeding tubes are very common. Cardiac surgery involves the use of many sophisticated devices and procedures, ranging from valve replacement to repair of complex congenital anomalies. Coronary artery bypass surgery is no longer considered unusual, and in many large medical centers, ventricular assist devices and total artificial hearts are frequently encountered. Breast implants are visible at standard chest radiography, and many ancillary devices not intended for treatment of cardiac or thoracic diseases are visible on chest radiographs. New devices are constantly being introduced, but most of them are variations on a previous theme. Knowing the specific name of a device is not important. It is important to recognize the presence of a device and to have an understanding of

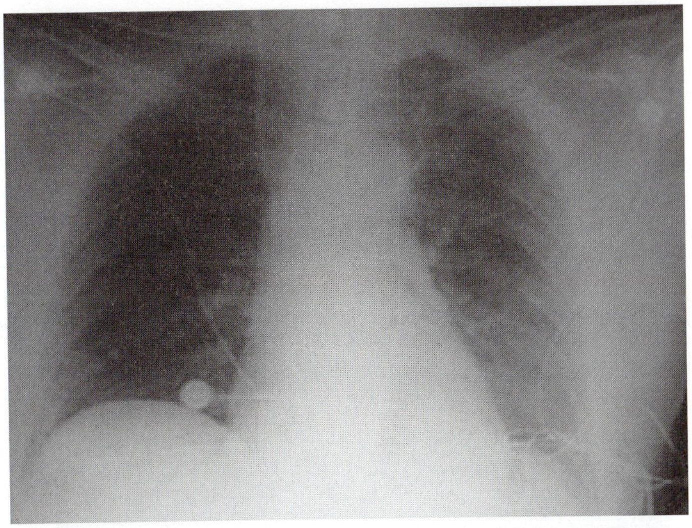

Fig. 4.22: *Typical postoperative cardiac surgery chest radiograph. First postoperative study showing coronary artery bypass graft (CABG) surgery. The image is underexposed and shows a confusing array of apparatus including overlying oxygen tubing, a pulmonary artery catheter, a nasogastric tube, an endotracheal tube, a mediastinal drain, median sternotomy wires, mediastinal clips, electrocardiographic (ECG) leads, and incipient left lower lobe atelectasis and pleural fluid*

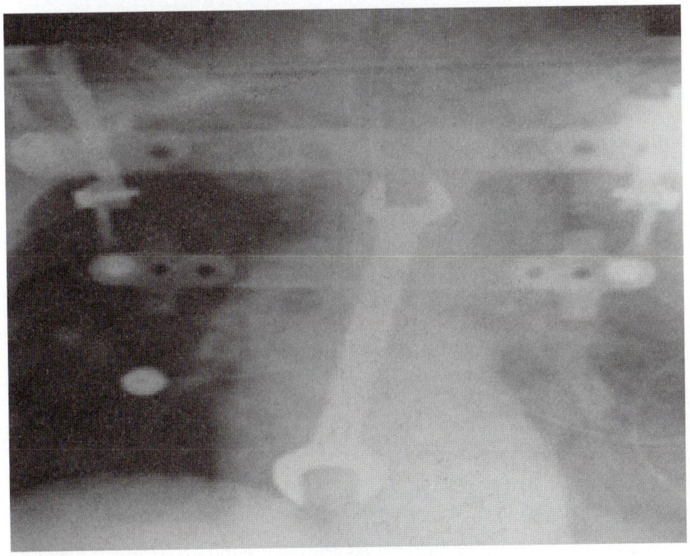

Fig. 4.23: *Chest radiograph shows halo apparatus (with emergency wrench close at hand) for cervical spine stabilization*

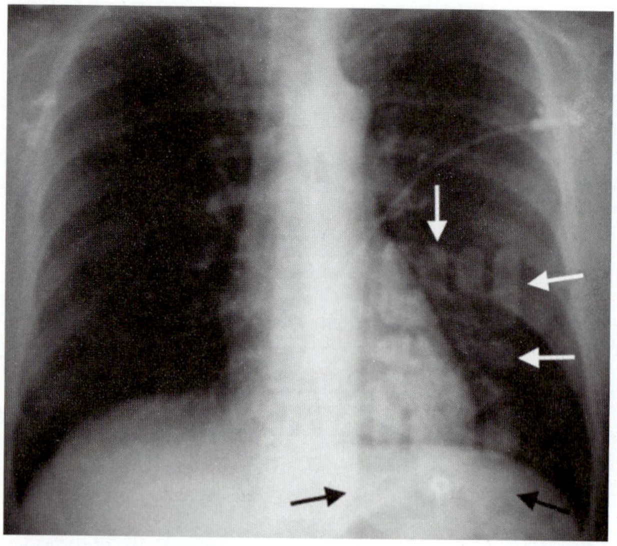

Fig. 4.24: *Chest radiograph reveals an external pacemaker-defibrillator electrode plate overlying the left side of the chest. The rectangular Chinese character-like electrode (white arrows) goes on the patient's back, and the round electrode (black arrows) goes on the patient's front*

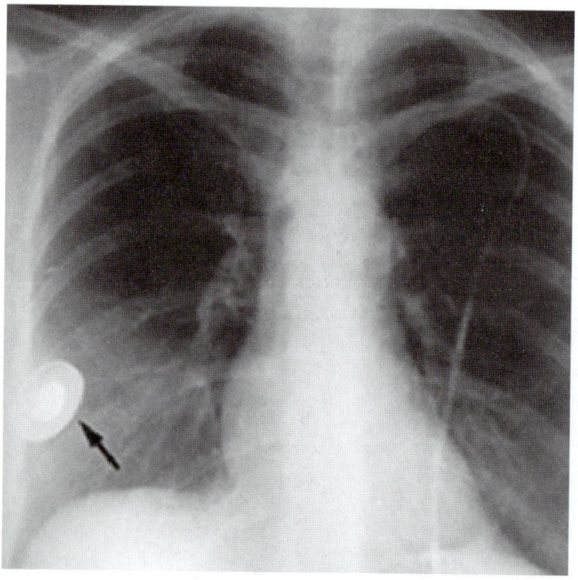

Fig. 4.25: *Frontal view of the chest shows a tissue expander (arrow) for subsequent breast reconstruction*

its function, as well as to recognize the complications associated with its use.

Chest radiography represents a significant percent of the workload of a diagnostic radiology department in a modern general hospital. The proliferation of intensive care units and the advances in the treatment of the very ill have greatly increased the numbers of examinations performed at the patient's bedside. Obtaining a daily chest radiograph is standard practice in most intensive care units, and any change in the patient's condition, or an intervention, can lead to several more studies in a given day. A medical center that has an active cardiothoracic surgery service and a busy trauma center generates large numbers of daily chest

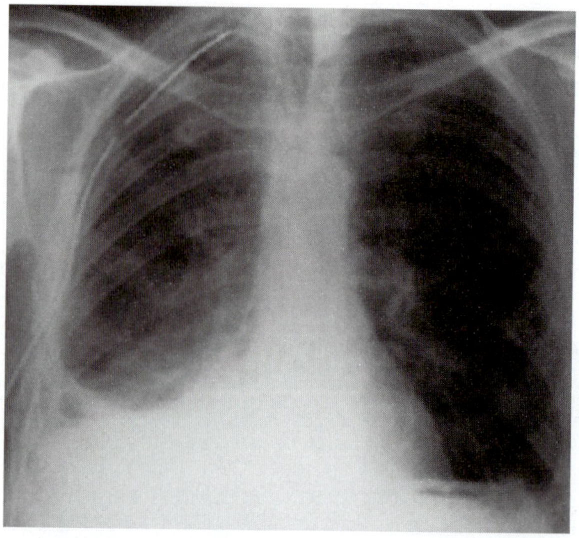

Fig. 5.26: *Frontal view shows a thoracostomy tube in good position for treatment of a pneumothorax but not for an effusion*

radiographs, many of which display a confusing array of medical apparatus used to treat and monitor patients.This article discusses the most common and important devices of the chest to help radiologists recognize their presence, have an understanding of their functions, and recognize the complications associated with their use.

Extrathoracic Devices

Most life-support devices are within the patient's heart, blood vessels, lungs, or pleura. Tubing, clamps, syringes, and other apparatus often lie on or under the patient and are imaged with the chest during the radiographic examination. These objects are usually easy to recognize and of no great importance. Patients may also lie on trauma boards, foam mattresses, or other similar supports that may be visible on radiographs. Ventilator support tubing is almost always visible somewhere on a chest image, as are attachments such as temperature and humidity sensors. ECG electrodes are now so ubiquitous that even healthy newborns rarely escape having them applied. A versatile device commonly used in cardiac patients being transported by helicopter or ambulance is the external pacemaker-defibrillator.

Breast prostheses are usually recognizable on chest radiographs. Sometimes, breast reconstruction following mastectomy may require the gradual preparation of a pocket suitable for the prosthesis; in such cases, a tissue expander is used.

Pleural devices: Thoracostomy (chest) tubes are commonly used for evacuating fluid or air from the pleural space. They vary from 10–40°F in size, depending on the viscosity of the material to be evacuated, and the preferences of the individual physician involved in the treatment of the case. The tube is usually placed antero-superiorly to evacuate a pneumothorax and postero-inferiorly for fluid collections. The normally positioned tube lies on the surface of the expanded lung, between the visceral and the parietal pleurae. Pigtail catheters may be used in place of standard thoracostomy tubes, and they are popular for empyema drainage and for installation of medication for treatment of an empyema. If the thoracostomy tube is not accomplishing its task of adequate fluid drainage or reexpansion of a collapsed lung secondary to a pneumothorax, the tube is probably malpositioned. To accurately assess the position of a tube, both frontal and lateral views of the chest or even chest computed tomographic scans may be needed. A chest tube may enter an interlobar fissure, and, with apposition of the visceral pleura of the two lobes, the end and side holes of the tube may become obstructed and the tube rendered ineffective. Malposition of chest tubes in lung parenchyma or subcutaneous soft tissues sometimes occurs. The proximal port of the chest tube may be in a superficial location outside the pleural cavity, or the tube may become kinked. The tube can also become occluded if its tip lies against the mediastinum (Figs 4.26–4.27).

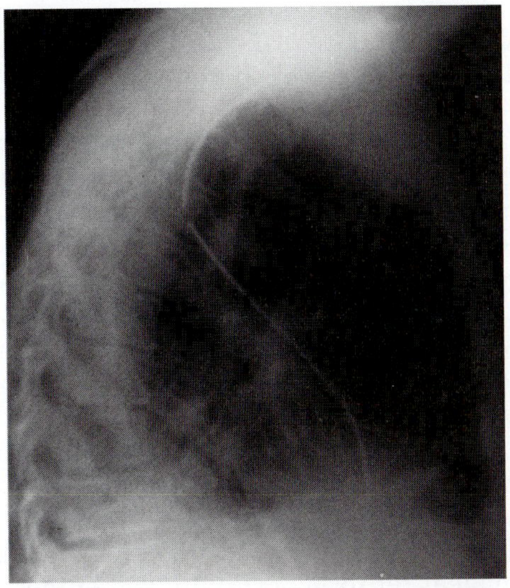

Fig. 4.27: *Lateral view show a thoracostomy tube in good position for treatment of a pneumothorax but not for an effusion*

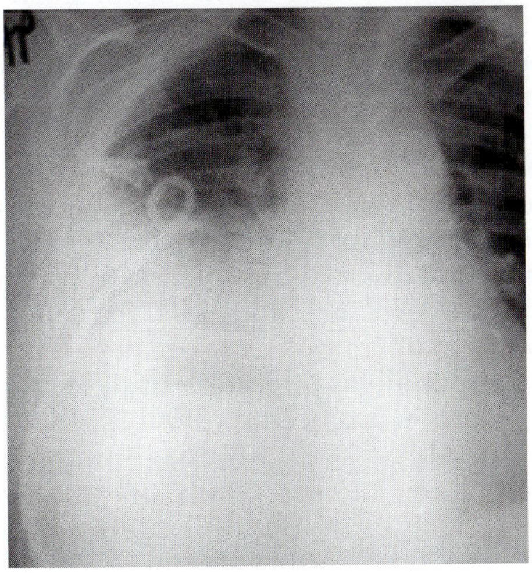

Fig. 4.28: *Frontal view of the chest shows a pigtail catheter that had been inserted under fluoroscopic guidance into a loculated right empyema for instillation of urokinase and fluid drainage*

In the era before antibiotics, a variety of pleural devices were used in the treatment of tuberculosis. These include "ping-pong" ball plombage and wax plombage Their appearance is quite dramatic, and they may occasionally be encountered in an older patient.

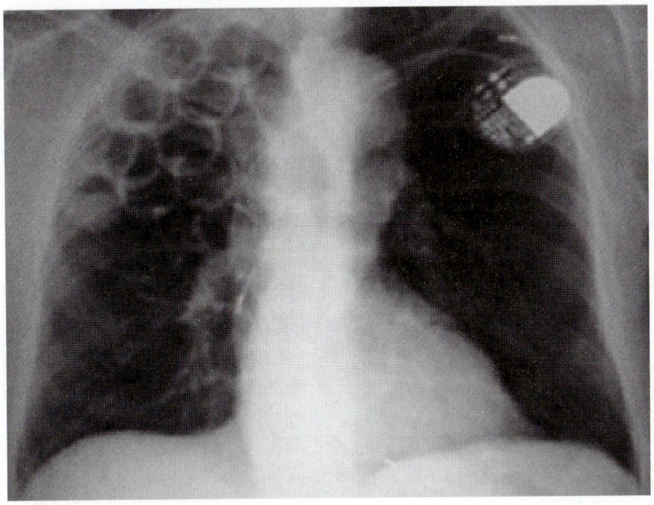

Fig. 4.29: *Frontal view of the chest shows "ping-pong ball plombage" in the right apex, as well as a cardiac pacemaker*

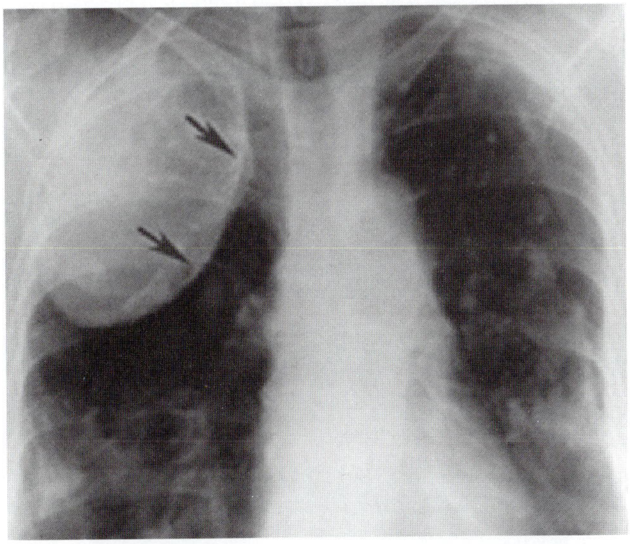

Fig. 4.30: *Frontal view of the chest shows "ping-pong ball plombage" in the right apex, as well as a cardiac pacemaker*

Tracheal and Esophageal Devices (Figs 4.31–4.33)

Endotracheal intubation is a lifesaving procedure, but it can also be life threatening if the tube is incorrectly positioned. In an adult, the tip of the tube should be situated approximately 5 cm above the tracheal carina, so that excursions of 2 cm upward or downward (with neck extension or flexion) can be safely accommodated.

The carina may not be visible on every image, but the aortic "knob" usually is. The carina is just caudad to the aortic arch, so that if the tip of the endotracheal tube is just above the aortic arch, it is in good position, midway

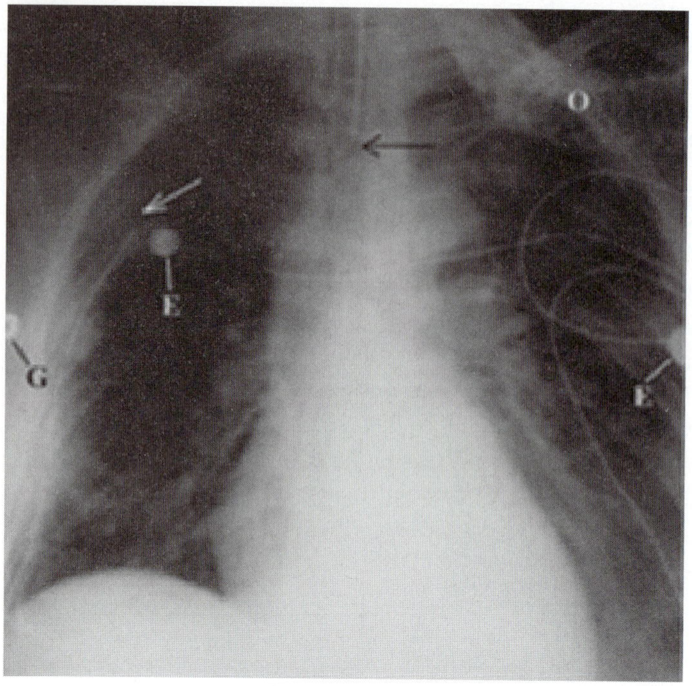

Fig. 4.31: *Chest radiograph shows that the tip of the endotracheal tube (black arrow) is slightly above the aortic arch and well above the carina, in good position. A right chest tube (white arrow), ECG leads (E), a gown snap (G), and oxygen tubing (O) are also visible*

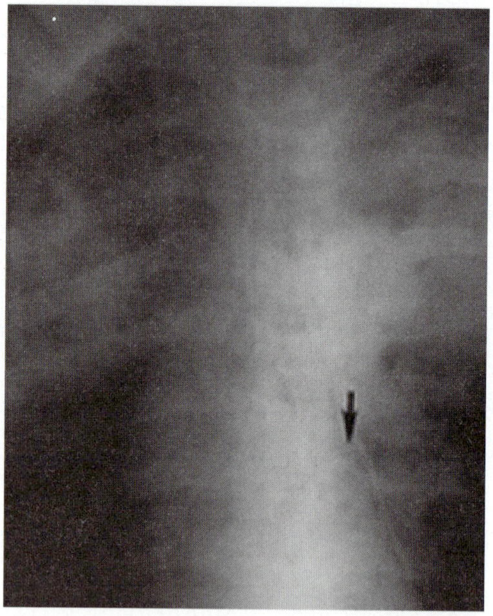

Fig. 4.32: *Frontal view shows a double-lumen endotracheal tube with selective intubation of the left main bronchus (arrow)*

between the vocal cords and the carina. When advanced too far, the endotracheal tube usually enters the right main bronchus, causing various combinations of hyperinflation and atelectasis of the two lungs, depending on the positions of the end and side holes. Besides being placed into the right bronchus, endotracheal tubes can also be inadvertently placed in the esophagus or in the soft tissues of the neck. Sometimes, a double-lumen endotracheal tube is deliberately

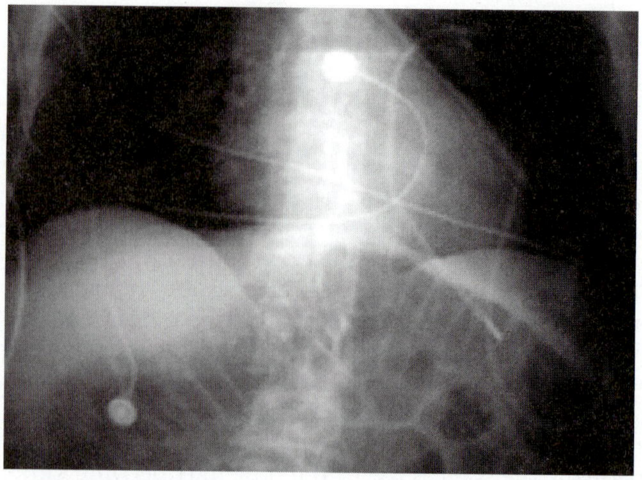

Fig. 4.33: *Frontal view of the chest shows a feeding tube that was inadvertently placed in the patient's airway, perforating the lung and lying in the pleural space*

used for differential ventilation of the two lungs to accommodate differences in compliance between them.

Nasogastric tubes and feeding tubes are frequently visualized passing through the mediastinum on their way to the stomach and intestines. Not infrequently, chest radiographs reveal medical devices in abnormal locations and unexpected foreign bodies.

Esophageal balloons and esophageal stents used to treat benign and malignant esophageal disease may manifest themselves at chest radiography. Balloon dilatation and stent placement in the esophagus are safe, effective procedures for treating esophageal strictures and fistulas, and they provide reasonable palliative relief from malignant esophageal obstruction. Esophageal and gastric balloons are still occasionally used to treat bleeding varices. Probes to measure distal esophageal pH as part of a gastroesophageal reflux workup are sometimes seen and may be confused with a feeding tube if one is not careful or if a proper patient history is not provided. The ideal location for the pH probe is the distal portion of the esophagus, just above the gastroesophageal junction.

Tracheostomy tubes and other tracheal and bronchial apparatus are not infrequently visible on chest radiographs. Tracheoesophageal voice prostheses are not common but may occasionally be seen. Bronchial stents are occasionally seen in patients who have undergone lung transplantation and have developed a stricture at the anastomosis between the native tracheobronchial tree and the transplanted one. These stents may be metallic and easily recognized, or they may be composed of various plastic materials and be hard to recognize, especially if no history of stent placement or lung transplantation has been given. It is wise to look for these stents in all patients who have undergone lung transplantation.

Vascular Devices

Vascular catheters of various types are now routinely used for monitoring hemodynamic function; for performing hemodialysis; and for administering fluids, medications,

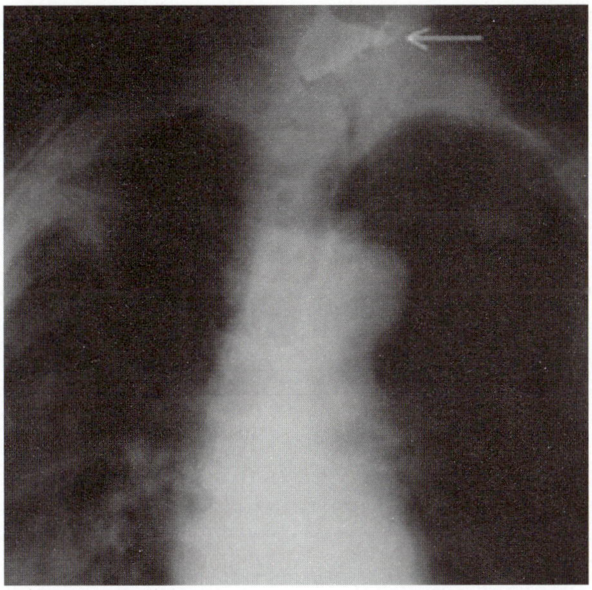

Fig. 4.34: *Chest radiograph of an elderly man with recurrent pneumonia and difficulty swallowing shows a dental appliance (arrow) in the esophagus at the thoracic inlet*

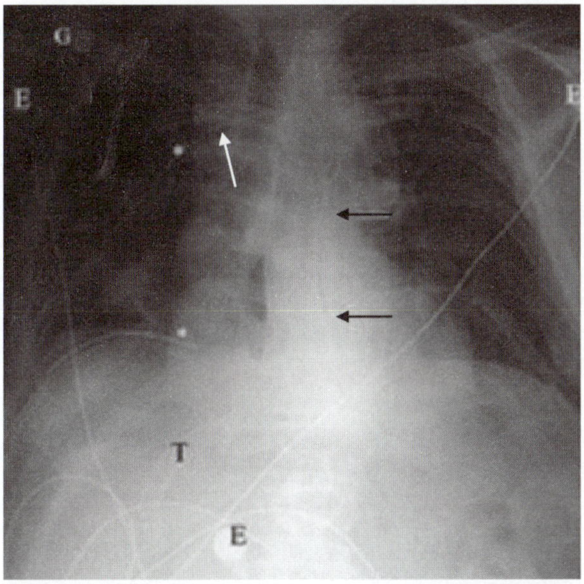

Fig. 4.35: *Frontal view of the chest shows an esophageal stent (black arrows) that was placed to ameliorate the effects of an esophageal malignancy. There are also two chest tubes, a peripherally inserted central catheter (white arrow), ECG leads (E), a gown snap (G), and a transjugular intrahepatic portosystemic shunt (T) in the liver*

and nutrition. Some catheters are designed for short-term use in the postoperative or intensive care unit setting, whereas others are implanted for long-term use, such as those used in cancer patients. Venous devices are usually inserted, either percutaneously or surgically, via the subclavian, internal jugular, or femoral veins. Arterial devices usually are placed through the femoral artery, but sometimes the brachial or axillary route is employed.

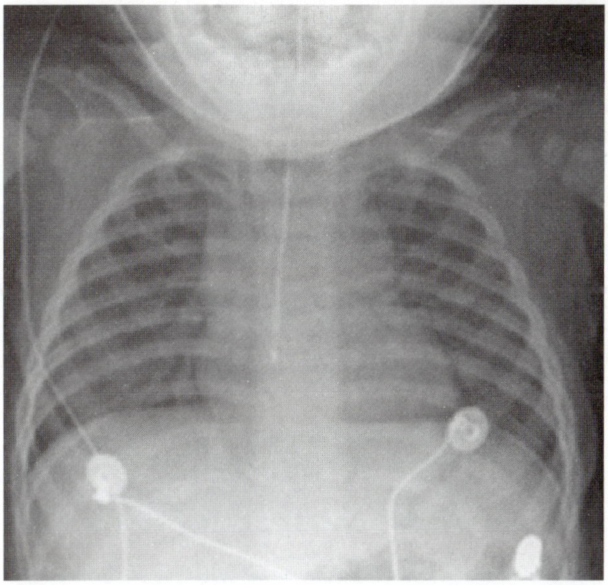

Fig. 4.36: *Frontal chest radiograph of an infant shows a pH probe*

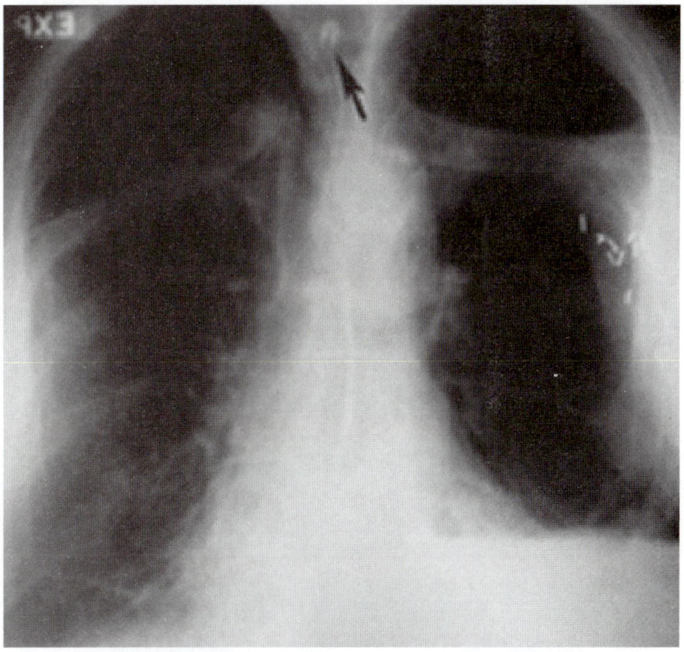

Fig. 4.37: *Frontal chest radiograph demonstrates a tracheoesophageal voice prosthesis (arrow)*

Central venous catheters [also known as central venous pressure (CVP) catheters, central catheters, and central lines] typically have one to three lumens and are constructed out of medical-grade silicone or polyurethane. The nomenclature for central catheters is confusing and inconsistent in daily use. For example, the terms *Hickman, Broviac, Leonard,* and *Hohn* are trademarks of CR Bard, Inc (Miami Lakes, Fla). Cordis sheath is a trademark of the Cordis corporation (Covington, Ga). However, in many medical centers, these names are used generically to represent any central catheter, regardless of its actual construction, manufacturer, or particular use.

Swan-Ganz is a registered trademark of Baxter International (Deerfield, Ill). This name has come to represent any type of multilumen catheter used for measuring hemodynamic pressures and cardiac output. A better term to use is *pulmonary artery catheter*. The Groshong (trademark of CR Bard) catheter is noted for its unusual closed, rounded. Near the tip in the side of the catheter is a three-position valve. The valve is designed to allow fluid to flow in and out through the valve, but it remains closed when it is not in use. This catheter does not require routine clamping or heparin solution to keep open. It does require periodic flushing with 0.9% normal saline.

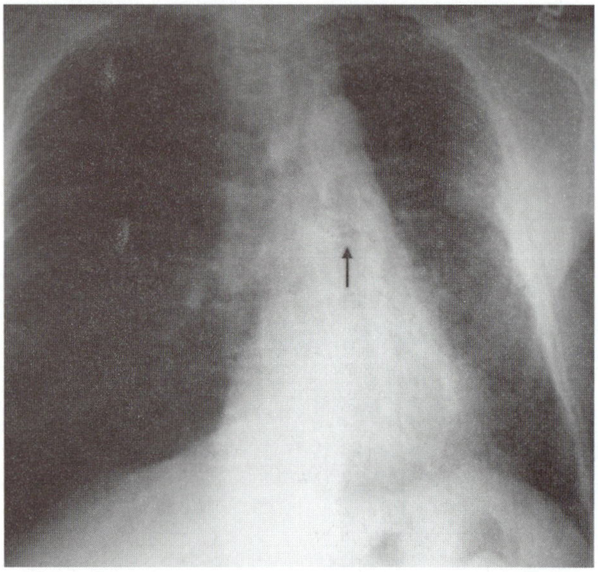

Fig. 4.38: *Frontal view of the chest in a patient with a transplanted left lung reveals a left bronchial stent (arrow) and surgical clips*

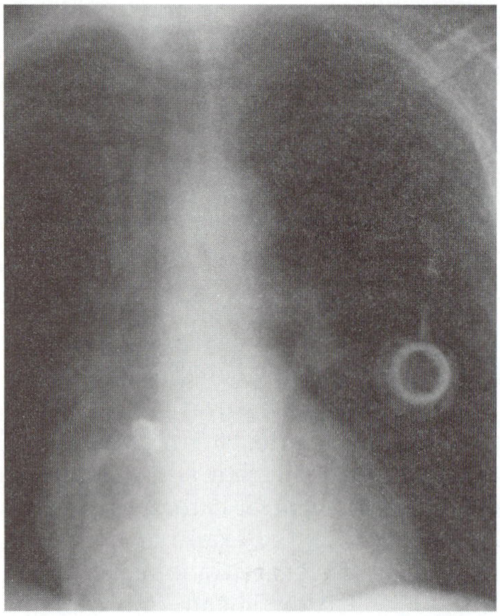

Fig. 4.39: *Portable chest radiograph shows a right subclavian single-lumen central venous catheter and a left subcutaneous port catheter, which enters via the left subclavian vein. Both catheter tips are in the superior vena cava*

There are also a variety of implantable access devices (subcutaneous ports), most commonly represented by the Port-A-Cath (trademark of CR Bard). Such devices are designed for easy, long-term access to the vascular system or peritoneal cavity. Port access is accomplished by percutaneous needle insertion. The port itself typically sits in the infraclavicular fossa, over the upper abdomen, or over the lower ribs. The port is usually connected to a central venous catheter or to an arterial catheter and can be used for instillation of fluids, medications, chemotherapeutic agents, parenteral nutritional solutions, and blood products. It can also be used for withdrawal of blood samples. There are almost as many types of access ports as there are types of standard central venous catheters.

A central venous catheter is ideally positioned in the superior vena cava for the monitoring of pressure or infusion of medication and nutrition. A catheter tip positioned in the right atrium increases the risk of perforation and cardiac arrhythmia. The same holds true for dialysis catheters. However, there is some controversy over the correct position for the tip of a central venous catheter. Some believe the usefulness and longevity of a catheter will be improved if its tip is positioned in the upper portion of the right atrium.

Flow-directed, balloon-tipped catheters (pulmonary artery, Swan-Ganz catheters) are now widely used for monitoring circulatory hemodynamics. Accurate measurement of pulmonary arterial wedge pressure in a supine patient requires the catheter tip to be in the lower lobe (zone 3 of West) so that left atrial pressure, not alveolar pressure, is measured. Over a period of time, pulmonary artery catheters may migrate toward the periphery of the pulmonary bed and become lodged in a small pulmonary artery. Such migration can cause vessel injury by prolonged occlusion or by overdistention of the vessel when the catheter balloon is inflated. Also, pulmonary infarction can

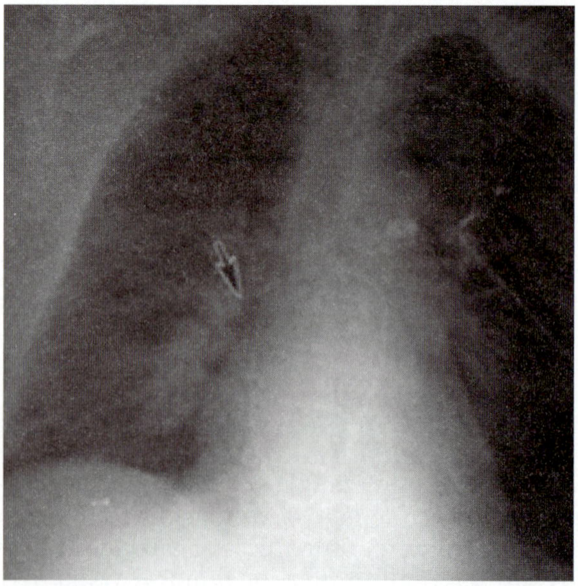

Fig. 4.40: *Frontal chest radiograph shows a right jugular Swan-Ganz catheter with its tip (arrow) in the right lower pulmonary artery*

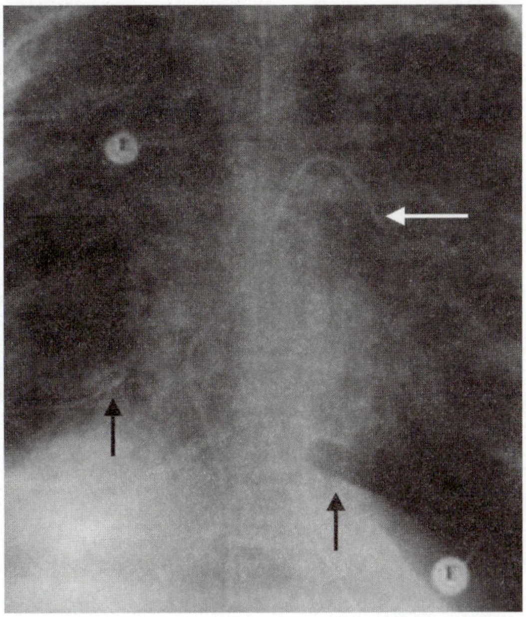

Fig. 4.41: *Frontal chest radiograph shows a Swan-Ganz catheter (white arrow) in the left pulmonary artery via the inferior vena cava. Note also the bilateral chest tubes (black arrows) and ECG leads (E)*

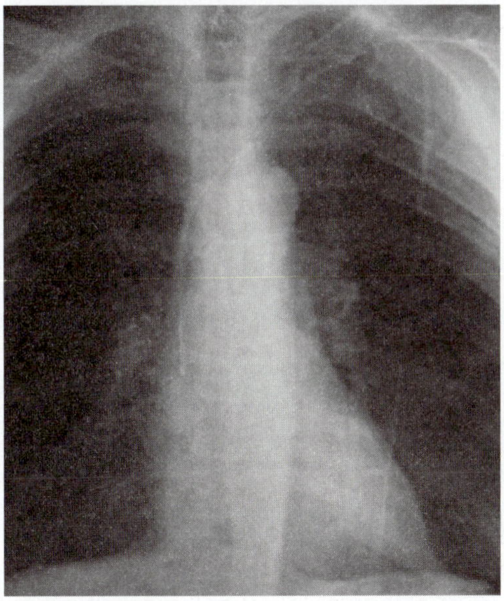

Fig. 4.42: *Frontal view of the chest shows a left subclavian Groshong catheter with its tip in the proximal most portion of the superior vena cava*

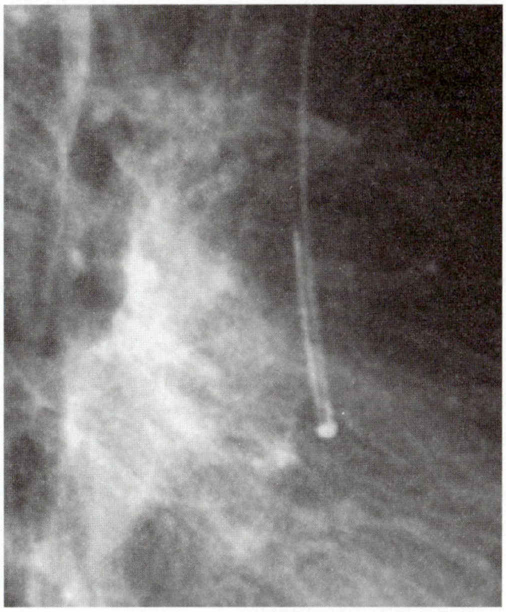

Fig. 4.43: *Frontal view of the chest shows a left subclavian Groshong catheter with its tip in the proximal most portion of the superior vena cava*

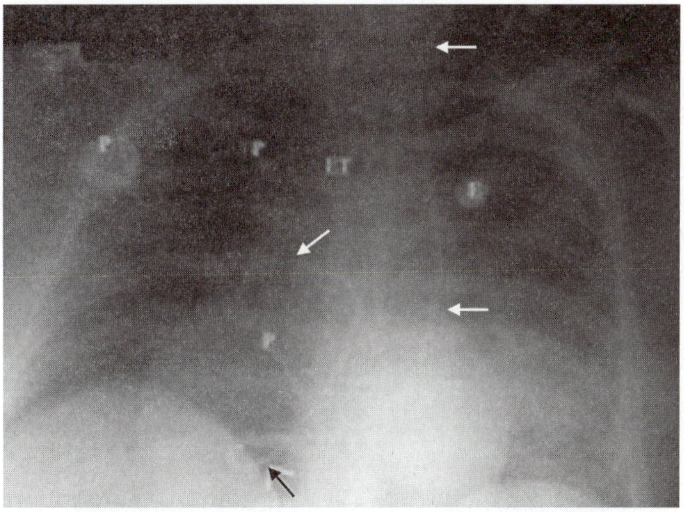

Fig. 4.44: *Frontal view of the chest shows a left jugular Swan-Ganz catheter (arrows), which passes through a persistent left superior vena cava into the coronary sinus, through the right atrium and right ventricle, and into the right pulmonary artery. Also seen are a subcutaneous port (P), an endotracheal tube (ET), an ECG lead (E), and a nasogastric tube (not labeled)*

result from this situation. The period of time during which the balloon remains inflated and wedged should be limited, particularly in patients with pulmonary hypertension. A central location of the catheter tip near the lung hilum helps prevent pulmonary artery perforation and is a good "parking" position for the catheter when it is not being used to measure pulmonary arterial wedge pressure.

The routine use of pulmonary artery catheters has been questioned by some authorities, but they are a common finding on intensive care unit portable chest radiographs. Even though these catheters are widely accepted and widely used, there are no definitive studies demonstrating their benefit.

Complications of catheter insertion vary with the catheters used and the sites employed catheter malposition usually involves the catheter passing into a tributary vessel rather than the one sought. The internal jugular vein, azygous arch, and internal mammary vein are frequent sites of catheter malpositioning. Catheters may take an unusual course or position because of a congenital anomaly. Arterial puncture may lead to an abnormal catheter position with pulsatile flow in the catheter.

Pneumothorax is a common complication of unsuccessful attempts at subclavian or low jugular catheter insertion. Nerve injury is usually a complication of improper puncture technique. Vessel lacerations and perforations can produce hematomas, hemothorax, and infusion of fluid into the mediastinum, thorax, or other inappropriate space. Looping of catheters may lead to knotting. Pinching of catheters and catheter shearing usually occur at the site of entry and suture fixation.

Although central venous catheters inserted into the subclavian vein or into the internal jugular vein represent the standard approach for establishing central venous access, a simpler, potentially less-injurious access to the central venous system is through the use of a peripherally inserted central catheter (PICC). PICC lines are smaller catheters that are peripherally inserted at or slightly proximal to the antecubital fossa, with the tip placed in the superior vena cava. They are often preferred over standard central lines in children.

Cardiac Devices (Figs 4.45–4.51)

Treatment of heart disease has probably fostered more development of sophisticated medical interventions than all the interventions designed for all other organs combined. Coronary artery angioplasty, coronary artery stent placement, CABG surgery, the surgical correction of congenital cardiac defects, and even cardiac transplantation are no longer considered novel, experimental procedures. Cardiac pacemakers, valve prostheses, and artificial hearts are sophisticated biomedical engineering products that have drastically altered the course of many cardiac disorders. Because chest radiography is commonly employed in the assessment of patients with heart disease, recognition of cardiac devices and the problems associated with them is important for all individuals involved in the care of these patients.

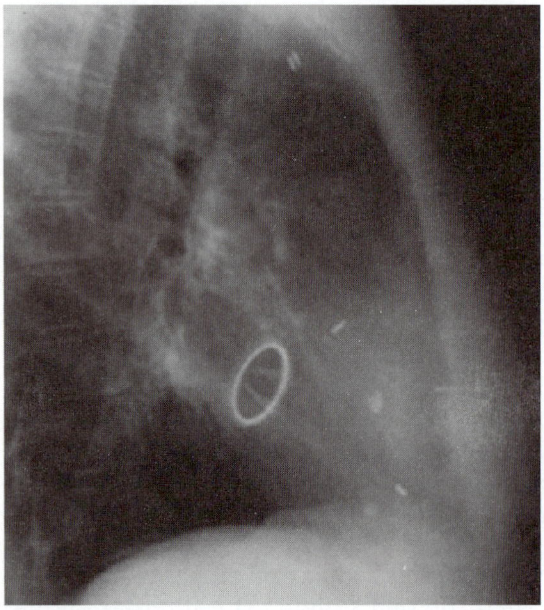

Fig. 4.45: *Mechanical heart valve. Lateral view of the chest shows a Hemex tilting bileaflet mechanical mitral valve prosthesis. Median sternotomy wires and surgical clips are also evident*

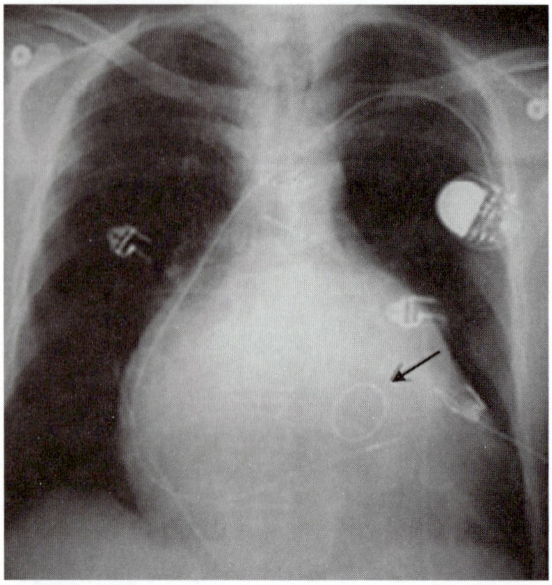

Fig. 4.46: *Biologic heart valve. Frontal view of the chest shows a Hancock porcine mitral valve prosthesis (arrow). A single-lead pacemaker, ECG leads, and median sternotomy wires are also seen*

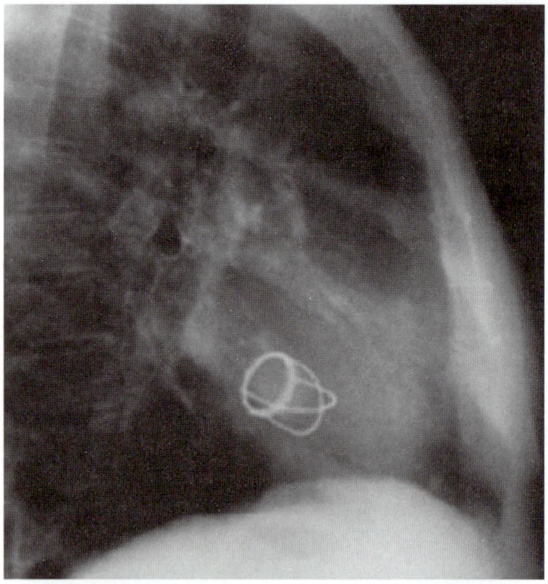

Fig. 4.47: *Mechanical heart valve. Lateral view of the chest shows a Starr-Edwards caged ball mechanical mitral valve prosthesis*

Heart Valves

Heart valve prostheses have been used successfully since the 1960s, and there are two basic types: (1) mechanical and (2) biologic. The number, complexity, and use of prosthetic heart valves have increased dramatically to the point where most radiologists see them on a daily basis in

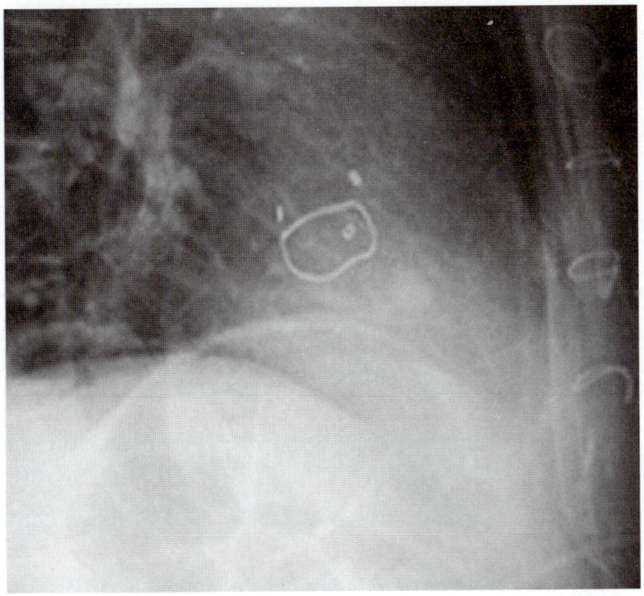

Fig. 4.48: *Biologic heart valve. Collimated lateral view of the chest shows a Medtronic Hancock valve*

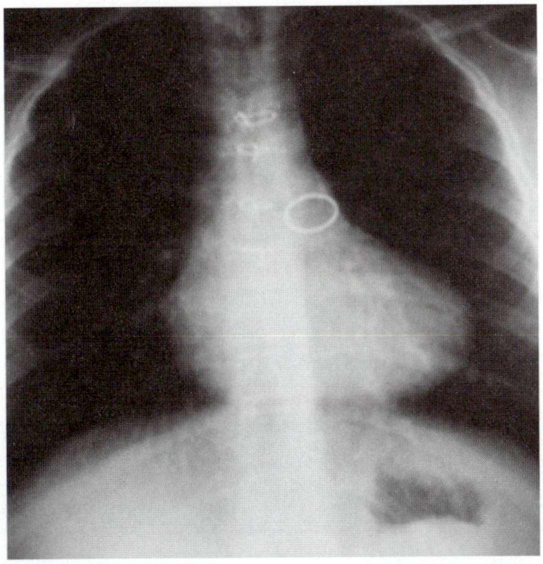

Fig. 4.49: *Biologic heart valve. Frontal view of the chest shows a Hancock porcine valve prosthesis in a Rastelli conduit going from the right ventricle to the pulmonary artery*

their practices. Mechanical valves are composed of metals, polymers, and ceramics. A mechanical valve functions basically as an occluder, moving passively with changes in pressure and flow within the heart. Most require lifelong treatment with anticoagulants. Biologic valves contain tissue from human cadavers (homografts), porcine aortic cusps, or bovine pericardium (xenografts). Biologic valves are less durable than mechanical valves, with some deterioration developing, frequently 5–10 years after placement, but they do not usually require anticoagulant treatment.

There are many types of prosthetic cardiac valves, and it is not possible to discuss them in any detail in this article.

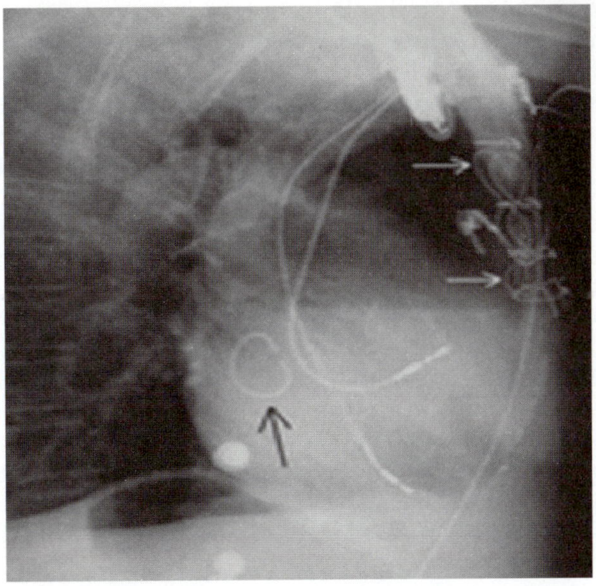

Fig. 4.50: *Lateral view of the chest in patient shows a mitral annuloplasty ring (black arrow) and a dual-lead cardiac pacemaker. Sternal wires, surgical clips, and ECG leads are also present. The sternal wires are used to close a sternal dehiscence. The patient has both horizontal sternal wires and vertical intercostal wires (white arrows)*

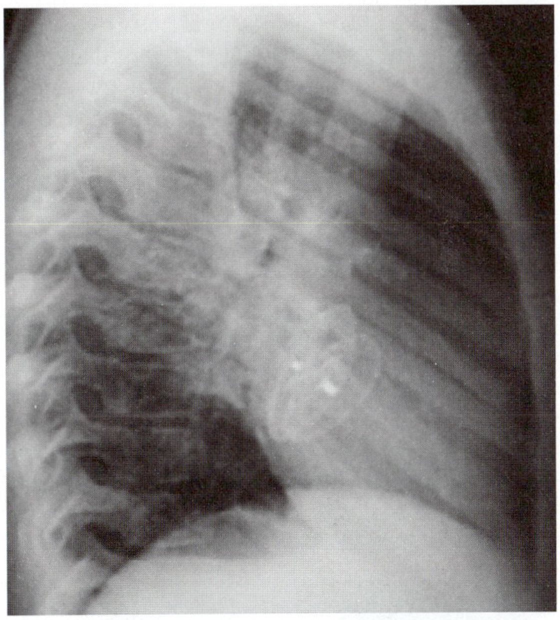

Fig. 4.51: *Lateral view of the chest in a child shows an occlusion basket (umbrella) for treatment of an atrial septal defect*

Some mechanical valves include the Starr-Edwards (Edwards Lifesciences, Irvine, Calif), Bjork-Shiley (Pfizer, New York, NY), Medronic Hall (Medronic, Minneapolis, Minn), St Jude Medical (St Jude Medical, Inc, St Paul, Minn), Sorin Bicarbon (Sorin Biomedica, Italy), and the Carbomedics (Sorin Biomedica). Some bioprosthetic (biologic) heart valves include the Carpentier-Edwards (Edwards Lifesciences), Tissue Med (Aor Tech International PLC, United Kingdom), and the Hancock (Medtronic,

Minneapolis, Minn). It is not important and often impossible to know the specific name of a particular prosthetic heart valve, but it is important to recognize its presence. Because prosthetic heart valves are used in a large variety of congenital and acquired conditions in both adults and children, it is frequently difficult to ascertain which native valve has been replaced by a prosthesis. The heart in such cases may be markedly enlarged, displaced, or altered by cardiac surgery. The mitral and aortic valves are those most commonly replaced, whereas prosthetic tricuspid valves are seen less often. Prosthetic pulmonary valves are rare. There are also various shunts or conduits used as part of a complex cardiac surgical procedure to correct congenital heart disease. These shunts may contain a prosthetic heart valve.

Sometimes, an annuloplasty ring may be used instead of a prosthetic cardiac valve to treat valvular regurgitation. The annuloplasty rings narrow and reshape the heart valve for proper functioning.

There are products designed to close nonphysiologic openings in the heart, such as a patent ductus arteriosus, atrial septal defect, or ventricular septal defect, without the need for open heart surgery. The first of these products was the Rashkind "double umbrella" occlusion device (CR Bard) to close a patent ductus arteriosus. Other devices are the Bard Clamshell Septal Umbrella (CR Bard), the Amplatzer Septal Occluder (AGA Medical Corp, Golden Valley, Minn), and the Sideris device (AGA Medical) to close atrial septal defects, ventricular septal defects, and other intracardiac communications. In general, these devices consist of a basket (umbrella) or filter placed in the defect to occlude it. They are often self-adjusting and lie flat against the atrial or ventricular septum. This flat design helps to create a natural profile (Figs 4.51–4.53).

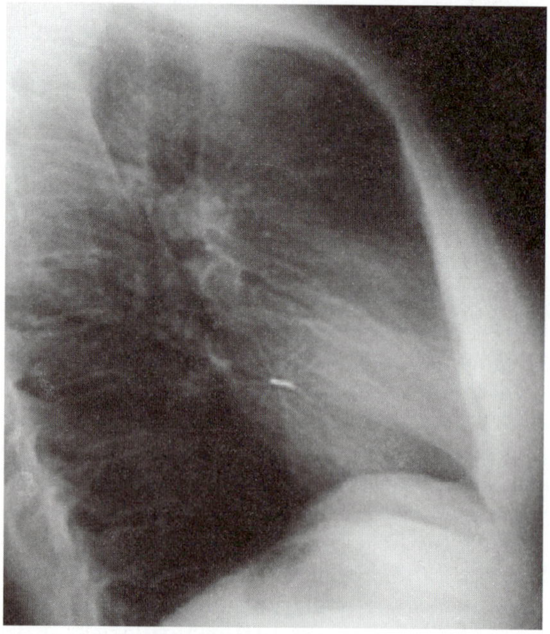

Fig. 4.52: *Lateral view of the chest in an adult with an atrial septal defect shows an occlusion (filter) device*

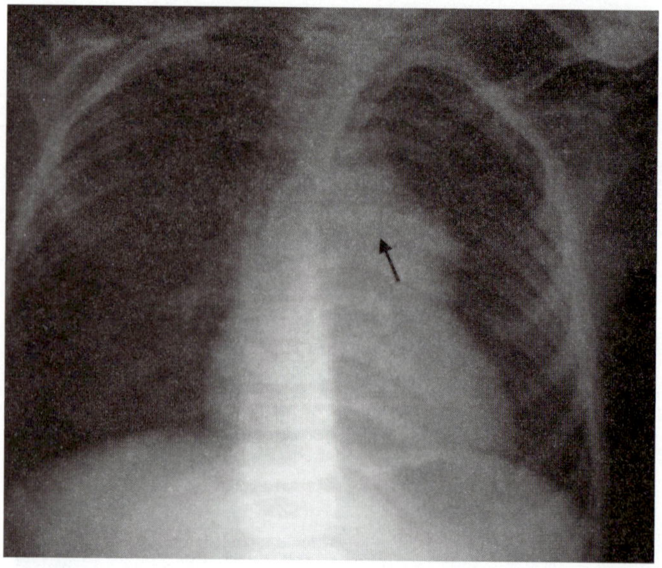

Fig. 4.53: *Frontal view of the chest in a child shows an occlusion filter (arrow) used to close a patent ductus arteriosus*

Cardiac Pacemakers (Figs 4.29–4.30)

Cardiac pacemakers are probably as common as prosthetic cardiac valves and are found in patients of all ages, although they are much more common in older adults being treated for abnormal cardiac rhythms caused by coronary artery disease. Cardiac pacemakers improve cardiac function, reduce the severity of clinical symptoms, and reduce mortality and morbidity (Figs 4.54–4.58).

A cardiac pacemaker is composed of two main elements: (a) a pulse generator and (b) lead wires with electrodes for contact with the endocardium or myocardium. Cardiac pacemakers were first used clinically in the 1960s, with stainless steel electrodes sewn directly onto the myocardium

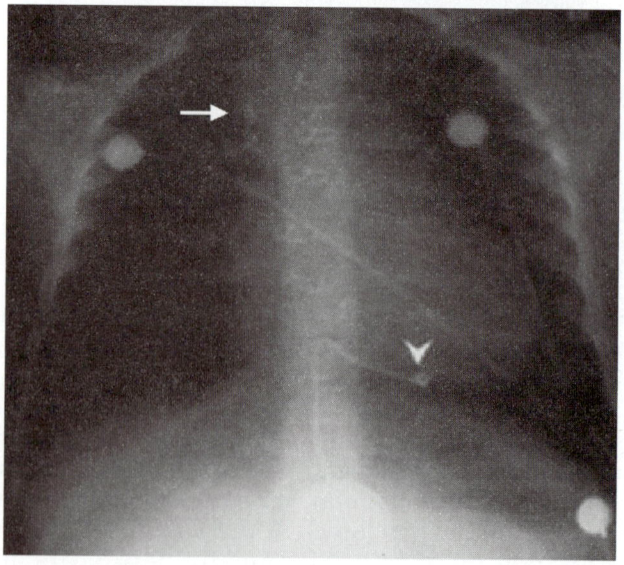

Fig. 4.54: *Frontal view of the chest show a single electrode epicardial "corkscrew" subxiphoid pacemaker. There is also coils (white arrow) occluding a previous right Blalock-Taussig shunt. In addition, ECG leads and sternal wires are evident*

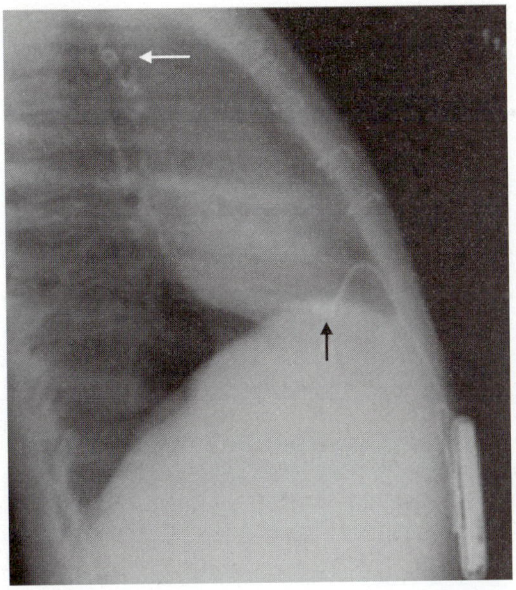

Fig. 5.55: *Lateral view of the chest show a single electrode epicardial "corkscrew" subxiphoid pacemaker (arrow head in a, black arrow). There are also coils (white arrow) occluding a previous right Blalock-Taussig shunt. In addition, ECG leads and sternal wires are evident*

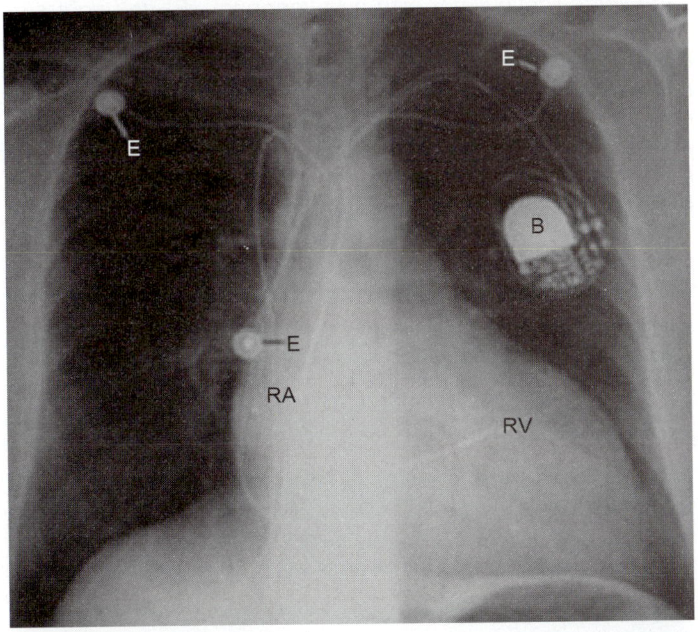

Fig. 4.56: *Frontal view shows an atrioventricular sequential pacemaker with one electrode in the right atrial appendage (RA) and the other at the right ventricular apex (RV). Also shown are ECG leads (E) and the battery-control pack*

and attached to a fixed-rate pulse generator implanted in the subcutaneous tissues of the upper abdomen. Since then, there have been many advances, including small-caliber, fracture-resistant, transvenous leads and programable multichamber atrioventricular pulse generators. The pacemaker generator (battery pack and control unit) is most commonly placed in the infraclavicular area.

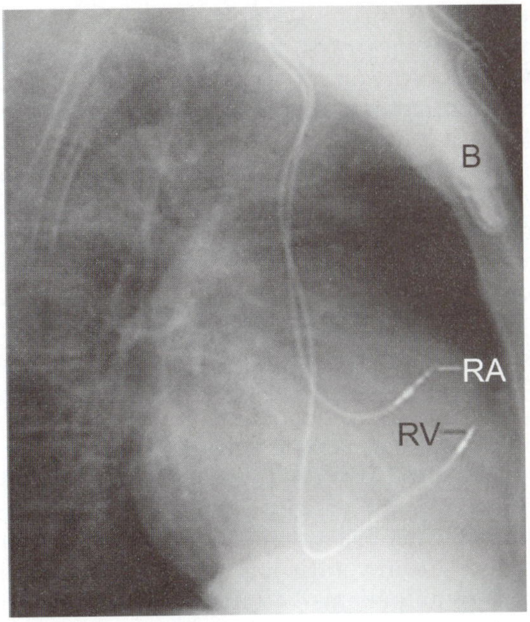

Fig. 4.57: *Lateral view shows an atrioventricular sequential pacemaker with one electrode in the right atrial appendage (RA) and the other at the right ventricular apex (RV). Also shown are ECG leads (E) and the battery-control pack (B) for the pacemaker*

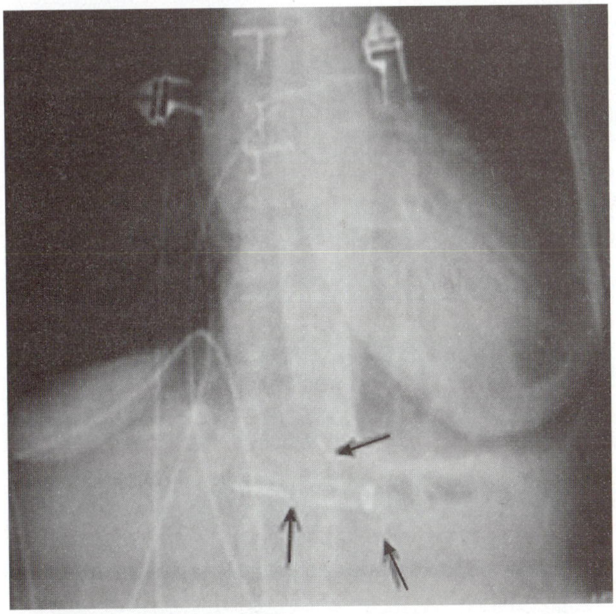

Fig. 4.58: *Collimated frontal view of the chest shows typical epicardial pacing wires (arrows) coiled on the patient's anterior chest wall after heart surgery*

There has been a steady improvement in pacemaker durability and utility. It is now possible for a patient traveling anywhere in the world to phone into his or her physician and have a scheduled periodic evaluation of pacemaker function over the phone. Pacemakers range from simple temporary epicardial electrodes to very complex pacemakers with multiple atrial and ventricular leads. A single-lead intramyocardial pacer electrode may be appropriate in one patient, whereas a right atrial-biventricular synchronous pervenous device is indicated in another. Temporary, easily removable epicardial electrodes are now commonly placed at the time of cardiac surgery for immediate pacemaker access, should the need arise). The leads are simply pulled out through the incision when the patient is discharged from the hospital. Transvenous (pervenous) pacemaker leads are the most commonly used type today and are inserted through the subclavian or jugular vein with use of local anesthesia.

Cardiac resynchronization therapy (CRT) or biventricular pacing is sometimes used to treat severe chronic congestive heart failure. Combined right and left ventricular pacing or left ventricular pacing alone may considerably improve heart function. CRT involves pre-excitation of the left ventricular wall by means of a lead placed in a tributary of the coronary sinus. There is often further benefit to the patient when CRT is combined with an implantable defibrillator, because there is a high risk of sudden death from ventricular tachycardia or ventricular fibrillation in all patients with heart failure. Current CRT usually involves atrial synchronized ventricular pacing to optimize atrioventricular timing with biventricular pacing to promote ventricular synchrony. CRT improves ejection fraction, left ventricular size, and mitral regurgitation.

There are several ways pacemakers can be placed for left ventricular or biventricular pacing. In some cases, left ventricular epicardial leads are used. The leads go directly to the surface of the left ventricle, and they are usually associated with typical pacing electrodes in the right atrial appendage and right ventricular apex. In other cases, the left ventricular pacing electrodes are introduced through the coronary sinus and wedged into a left ventricular cardiac vein. In these instances, the position of the pacing leads may seem unusual, and detailed knowledge of the

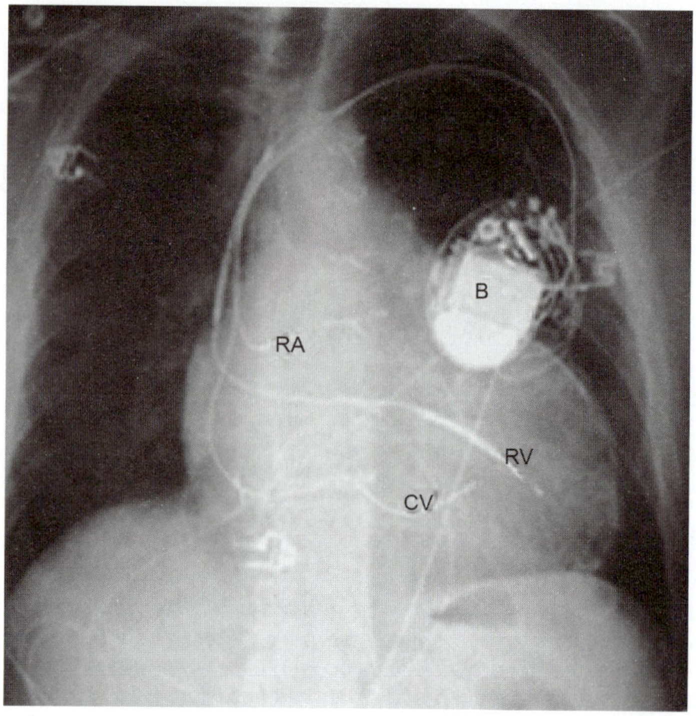

Fig. 4.60: *Frontal view of the chest shows a combination biventricular pacemaker and an automatic implantable cardioverter defibrillator with a battery pack (B) and right atrial (RA), right ventricular (RV), and coronary venous (CV) leads. Note also the left ventricular calcification from a past myocardial infarction. The coronary venous lead is positioned in a vein draining the posterior inferior wall of the left ventricle so that it can stimulate functional myocardial tissue rather than the nonfunctioning tissue represented by the ventricular wall calcification and probable myocardial aneurysm*

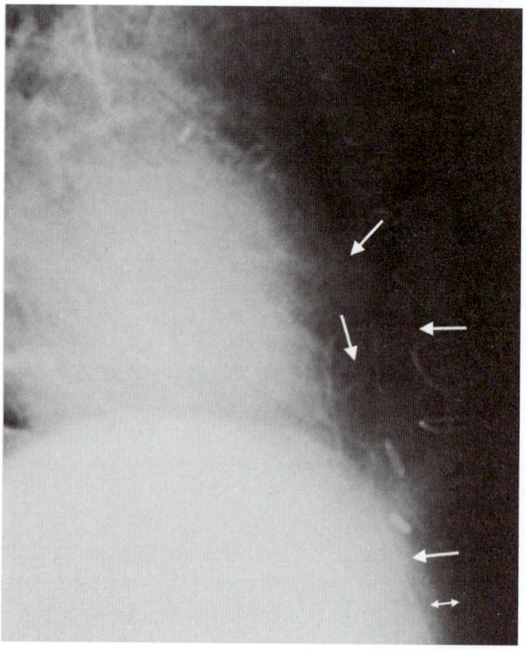

Fig. 4.59: *Collimated lateral view of the chest shows epicardial pacing wires (arrows)*

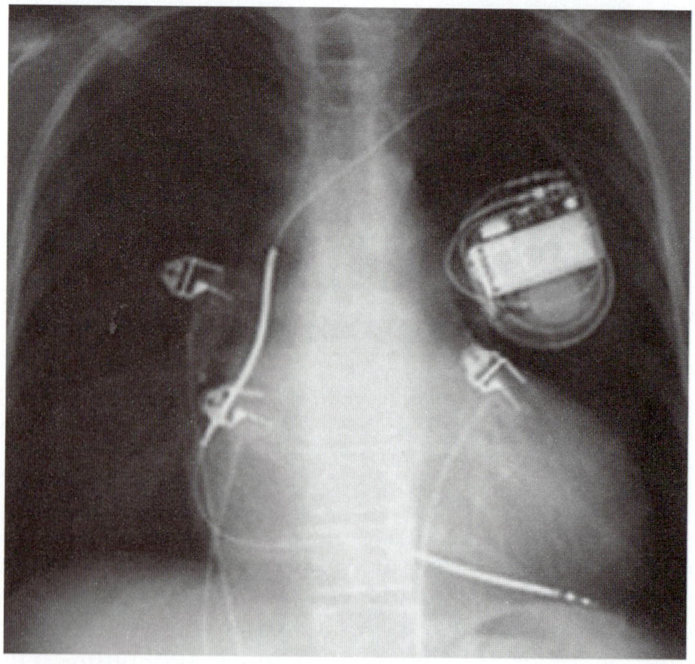

Fig. 4.61: *Frontal view of the chest shows a typical automatic implantable cardioverter defibrillator*

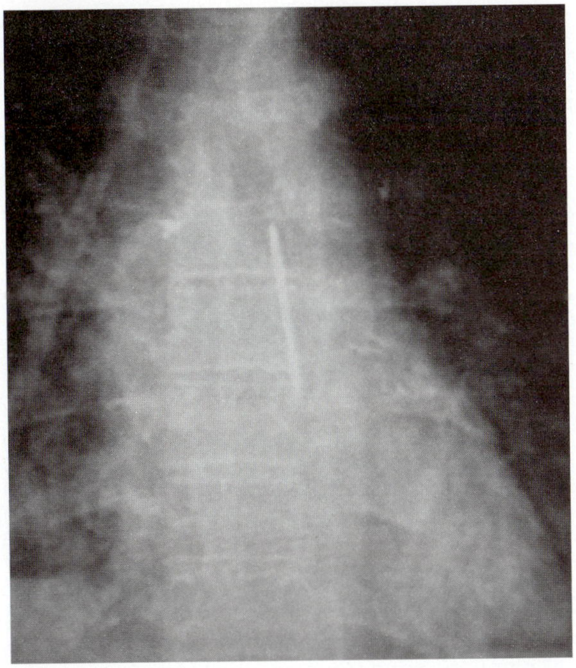

Fig. 4.62: *Frontal view shows a sternal fixation pin or Kirschner wire. This sternal fixation was used for a patient who underwent lung transplantation in which a "clamshell" chest incision was made, resulting in a transverse sectioning of the sternum. In this case, the sternum is best stabilized by a vertical fixation wire or pin. Note also the surgical clips overlying the heart and the root of the aorta*

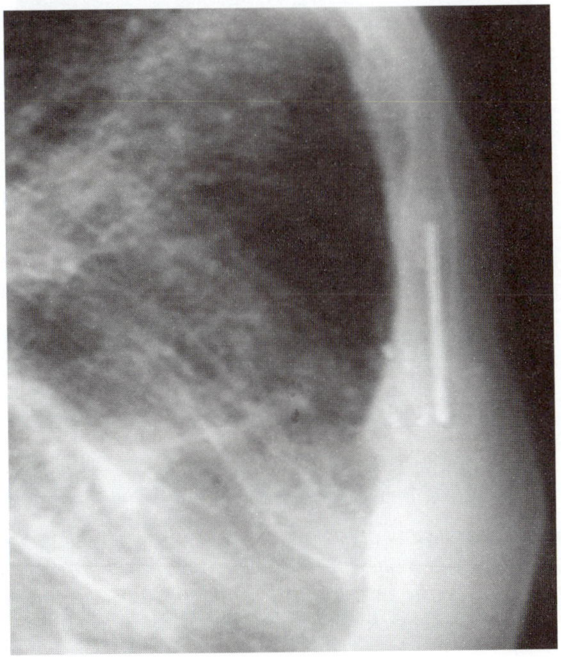

Fig. 4.63: *Lateral view shows a sternal fixation pin or Kirschner wire. This sternal fixation was used for a patient who underwent lung transplantation in which a "clamshell" chest incision was made, resulting in a transverse sectioning of the sternum. In this case, the sternum is best stabilized by a vertical fixation wire or pin. Note also the surgical clips overlying the heart and the root of the aorta*

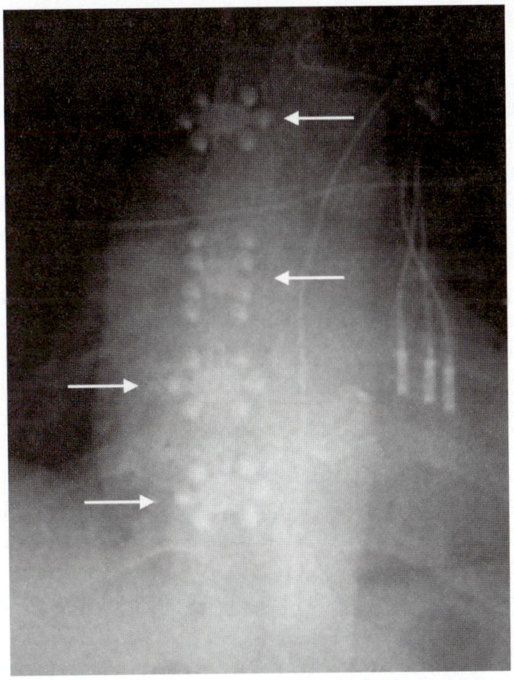

Fig. 4.64: *Collimated view of a cardiac surgery patient shows a synthes maxillofacial sternal fixation system (Synthes, Paoli, Pa) (arrows)*

coronary venous anatomy is necessary for the radiologist and cardiologist to appreciate the location of the leads.

Because there can be such a wide variation in the proper positioning of pacemaker leads, it is often difficult for the average radiologist to know if a pacemaker is properly positioned. Frequent consultation with the cardiologists and cardiac surgeons in one's own medical center is important to gain familiarity with the pacemakers and therapeutic approaches used by the referring physicians. In this way, complications of pacemaker placement are more readily recognized and brought to the attention of the patient's physicians.

Pacemaker lead fracture is now rarely seen because of improvements in the flexibility of the metal alloys used in electrode construction. Even when they are broken, the ends frequently do not separate, so the radiograph does not show the fracture. Electronic testing has largely replaced radiography to investigate cases of suspected lead malfunction. After being in place for several weeks, pacemaker leads become "epithelialized" and firmly attached to the myocardial wall. When a pacemaker is changed, the leads are simply cut for removal of the control pack, and they are left in place because they are adherent to the heart. New leads are then placed with the new pacemaker. If a patient has had his or her pacemaker changed a number of times, there is often a bewildering array of wires about the heart. In this circumstance, it can be impossible to trace the currently functioning pacemaker leads back to the pacemaker battery pack. On rare occasion, a central venous catheter may interfere with a pacemaker lead.

The safety of magnetic resonance (MR) imaging studies for patients with cardiac pacemakers is an important matter and is subject to much discussion. Many radiologists and cardiologists consider MR imaging to be contraindicated for patients with a cardiac pacemaker. This approach is the safest, but it may not always be in the best interest of a patient with a cardiac pacemaker who needs an MR imaging study. There are circumstances in which a patient with a pacemaker may undergo MR imaging, especially if a 0.5-T unit is used. It may also be safe to perform MR imaging with an extremity system for patients with cardiac pacemakers and implantable cardioverter defibrillator systems. It must be emphasized that MR imaging should be performed on patients with a pacemaker or similar device only after the patient has been cleared for the study by his or her physicians. Such a study should be performed in a medical center with experienced staff who are able to monitor the patient before, during, and after the MR imaging study as well as treat any problems that arise from the study. MR imaging is generally safe for patients who have artificial heart valves, who have undergone coronary artery surgery, or who have retained epicardial pacemaker leads after cardiac surgery.

The automatic implantable cardioverter defibrillator (AICD or ICD) is a common cardiac device designed for both patient monitoring and therapy in case of ventricular tachycardia or fibrillation. The early AICD designs consisted of two shocking electrodes, two sensing electrodes, and a generator implanted in the abdominal wall. The new designs are completely different, consisting of various combinations of sensing and shocking electrodes. They are frequently combined with a pacemaker as a bundled system for the patient, treating both the patient's established arrhythmia and also acting as a fail-safe system should ventricular fibrillation or ventricular tachycardia occur.

Coronary Artery Surgery and Stents (Figs 4.65 and 4.66)

Since 1967, when the first aortocoronary saphenous vein bypass graft was performed, direct myocardial revascularization has gained wide acceptance. Revascularization techniques include CABG surgery, coronary artery angioplasty, and coronary artery stent placement. CABG surgery is probably the most common cardiac surgical procedure performed in adults. Until recently, CABG surgery was the primary surgical technique for treating coronary artery disease. Now, it is competing with coronary artery angioplasty and stent placement as well as improved noninterventional medical treatments for coronary artery disease. CABG surgery has been refined over the years and varies from center to center, which is reflected in the variety of devices seen in the postoperative chest radiographs of these patients. Median sternotomy is the usual surgical approach for CABG surgery, and sternal wires the common method of fixation of the two sternal segments vascular clips are used to occlude tributary branches of saphenous vein grafts and anterior intercostal branches of the internal mammary arteries. There may be a few clips or a great many, depending on the number and types of grafts used. Some surgeons place markers on the adventitia of the ascending aorta to indicate the proximal anastomoses of the bypass grafts. These markers, which facilitate subsequent graft angiography, vary considerably from center to center, and even from surgeon to surgeon.

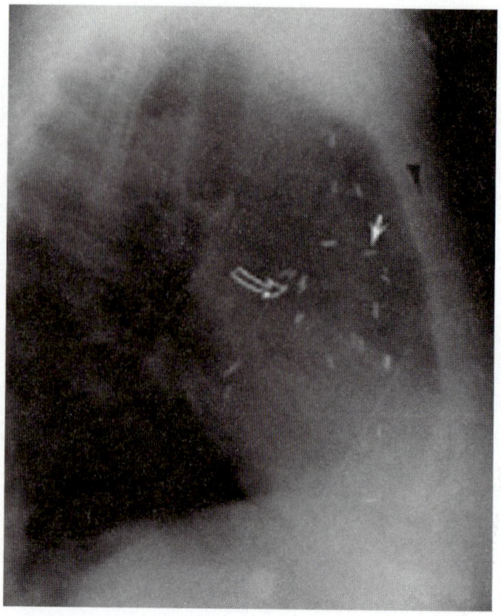

Fig. 4.65: *Lateral view of the chest shows sternal wires (arrowhead), vascular clips of a saphenous vein bypass graft to the right coronary artery (curved arrow), and those of the left internal mammary graft to the left anterior descending coronary artery (straight arrow)*

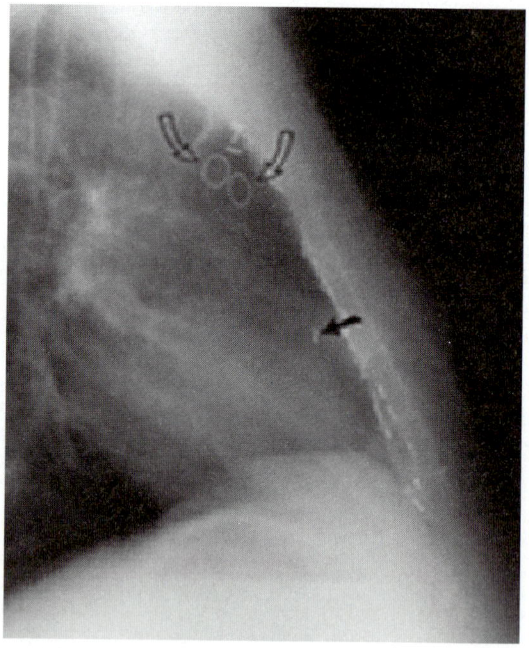

Fig. 4.66: *Lateral view of the chest shows vascular clips of internal mammary artery bypass grafts (solid arrow) and marker rings on the ascending aorta around the ostia of two saphenous vein bypass grafts (open arrows)*

In many cases, CABG surgery has been supplanted by coronary artery angioplasty and stent placement. At present, almost 90% of coronary interventions include stent placement. Coronary artery stent placement was introduced in 1964 by Dotter and Judkins and has been in regular clinical use since the end of the 1980s. The objectives of coronary artery stent placement are to improve on the results of coronary artery balloon angioplasty, to reduce the occurrence of coronary artery restenosis, and to treat an acute or threatened closure of a coronary artery (Fig. 4.67).

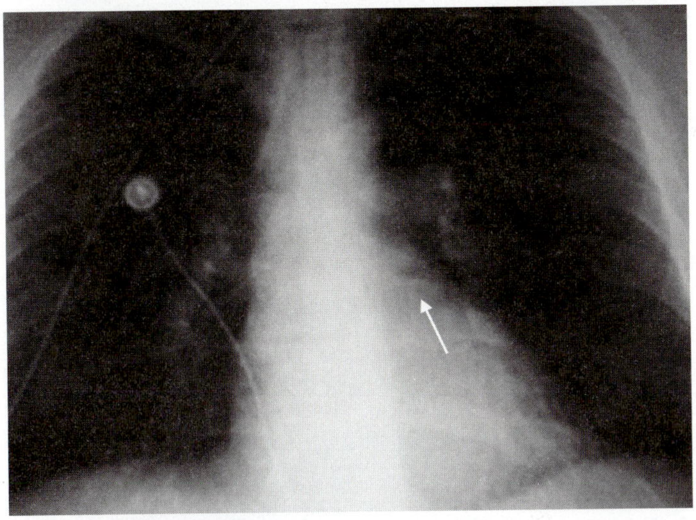

Fig. 4.67: *Frontal view of the chest shows a left anterior descending coronary artery stent (arrow)*

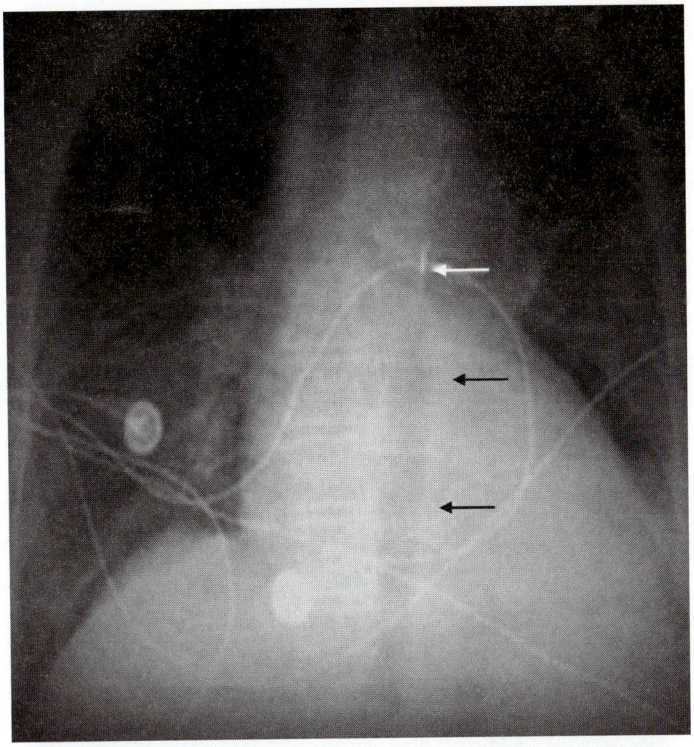

Fig. 4.68: *Frontal view of the chest shows an intraaortic counterpulsation balloon used in a patient with heart failure. The balloon (black arrows) is inflated. Usually, only the balloon tip (white arrow) is visible*

Before 1997, only two coronary artery stents were approved for clinical use in the United States: the Gianturco-Roubin I (Cook, Bloomington, Ind) and the Palmaz-Schatz (Johnson and Johnson, Warren, NJ). By 2002, over 40 stent designs were used in clinical practice. Many more are under investigation, including drug-coated stents. Based on their method of expansion, coronary artery stents are divided into three groups: (1) balloon expandable (most frequently used), (2) self-expandable and (3) thermally expandable. Most stents are composed of 316L stainless steel. Alternative stent designs have also incorporated nitinol, gold, tantalum, and other metals. They must maintain elasticity, radial strength, biocompatibility, and corrosion resistance. At present, the approved coronary artery stents range in size from 2.0 mm to 5.0 mm in diameter and 8.0–38.0 mm in length to accommodate the size of the target vessel. Stents of different designs have variable strut thickness. In addition to improvement in stent design and delivery technologies, further development includes covered stents, biodegradable stents, and drug-delivery stents. Stent selection is determined by a variety of factors, including operator familiarity with the stent, lesion morphology and location, and balloon delivery system characteristics. Complications associated with coronary artery stents are stent thrombosis and restenosis.

Circulatory Assist Devices (Figs 4.68–4.76)

The high mortality from cardiogenic shock continues to spur efforts to develop mechanical support for the circulatory system. It is estimated that 100,000 patients in the United States could benefit from heart transplantation. However, only 2,000 donor hearts are available each year. Most devices currently available provide temporary

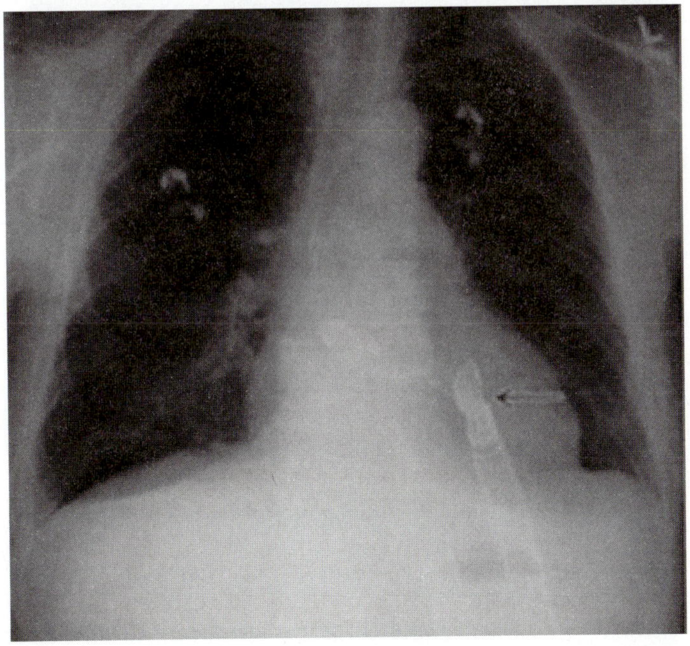

Fig. 4.69: *Frontal views of the chest show a thoratec left VAD (arrow)*

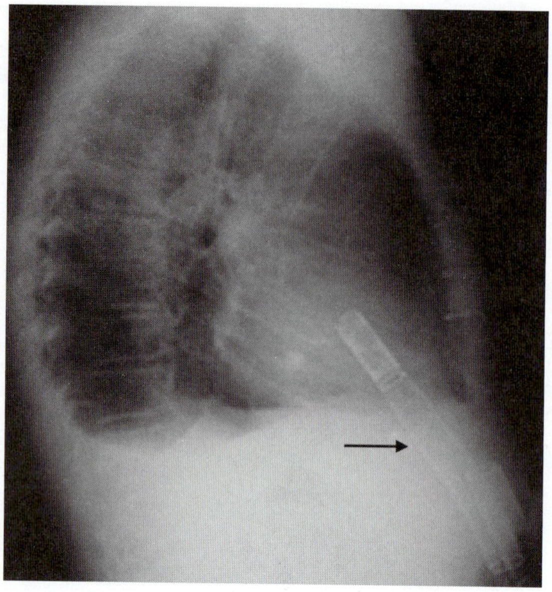

Fig 4.70: *Lateral view of the chest shows a thoratec left VAD (arrow)*

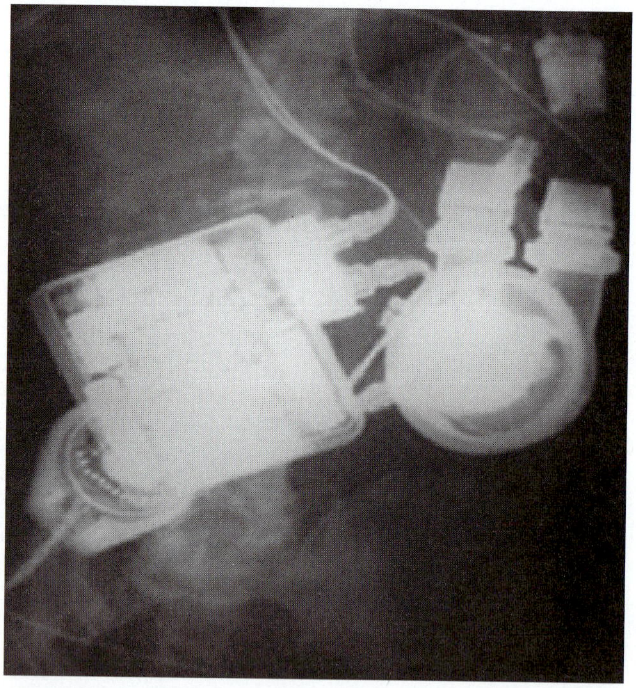

Fig. 4.71: *Abdominal image shows a heart mate VAD1*

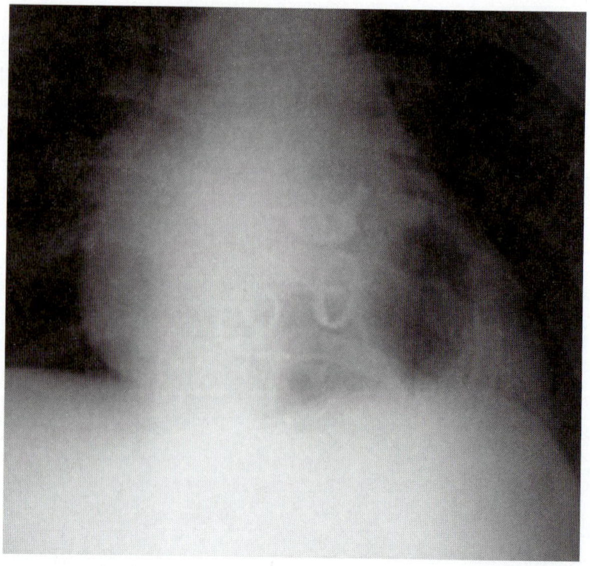

Fig. 4.72: *Abdominal image shows a Novacor VAD*

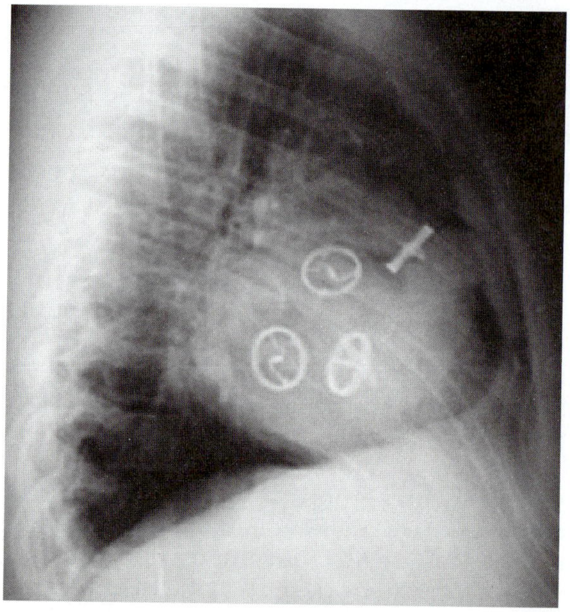

Fig. 4.73: *Cropped frontal view of the chest shows a CardioWest total artificial heart. Note the four prosthetic valves and the two coil, reinforced polyurethane tubes carrying pulses of compressed air to the two artificial ventricles*

assistance until the damaged heart can recover or until a donor heart becomes available for transplantation). Most mechanical support for patients with heart failure consists of devices that assist the heart without replacing it.

Mechanical cardiac assist devices can be divided into three groups: (a) temporary cardiac assist devices, (b) permanent cardiac assist devices, and (c) heart replacement devices. Examples of short-term cardiac assist devices are the intraaotic balloon pump and newer left ventricular assist devices (VADs), such as the Tandem Heart (Cardiac Assist, Inc, Pittsburgh, Pa). The Biventricular System 5000 short-term VAD (ABIOMED, Danvers, Mass), for example, is approved by the US Food and Drug Administration (FDA) for treating post-cardiotomy shock and as a bridge to either heart transplantation or implantation of a long-term device. It consists of two disposable, dual-chamber, extracorporeal blood pumps connected by transcutaneous cannulas to a console. This pump fills passively and ejects actively.

The intraaortic counterpulsation balloon device (also known as IACB, IAB, IABP, IAC, and IACD) is used to support the circulation after cardiac surgery or an acute

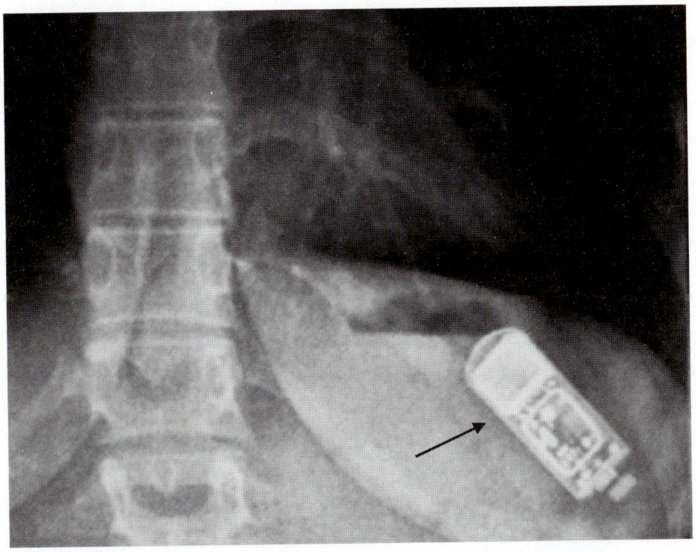

Fig. 4.74: *Collimated frontal view of the chest shows an implantable loop recorder (arrow) in the left breast of a 25-year-old woman with a history of heart palpitations and surgical repair of a tetralogy of Fallot as a young child*

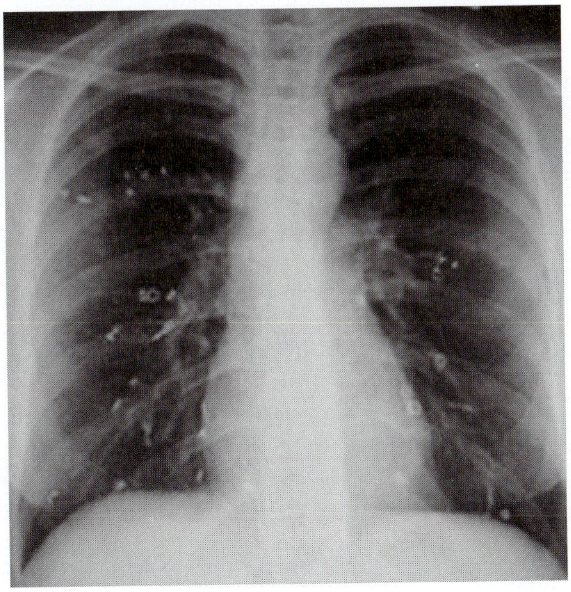

Fig. 4.75: *Frontal view of the chest of a patient with hereditary hemorrhagic telangiectasia (Osler-Weber-Rendu disease) shows numerous coils, which had been used in multiple coil embolizations to treat repeated bouts of significant hemoptysis*

myocardial infarction until the heart recovers adequate function of its own. The device consists of an inflatable balloon approximately 25 cm long mounted on a catheter, which is introduced via a femoral artery. The tip of the catheter is placed just distal to the left subclavian artery in the descending thoracic aorta.The balloon is inflated with gas (carbon dioxide) during ventricular diastole to augment diastolic coronary artery perfusion and to reduce left ventricular afterload. This technique improves cardiac function by both increasing the oxygenation and decreasing the work requirements of the myocardium.

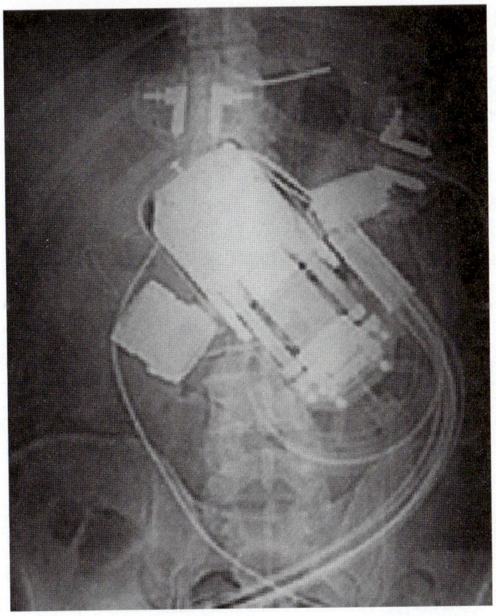

Fig. 4.76: *Abdominal image shows a Novacor VAD*

The mainstays of mechanical support for patients with severe congestive heart failure are VADs. These devices are mechanical pumps used for temporary or permanent blood circulation support. They can be used for a single right or left ventricle or for both ventricles. The left VADs are used in patients with end-stage heart failure, as a bridge to transplantation, but they may also be used as a destination therapy. These devices have been in clinical use since 1984. The Heart Mate (Thoratec Corp, Pleasanton, Calif) became the first left VAD that was FDA-approved as a bridge to transplantation and for treating reversible cardiogenic shock. The newer, vented-electric Heart Mate device is powered by an internal electric motor. This device has been in use since 1991. The Heart Mate blood pump is a flexible polyurethane diaphragm within a titanium shell. The woven Dacron inflow and outflow cannulas each contain a 25 mm caged porcine xenograft valve.

Another left VAD is the Novacor pump (Novacor Corp, Oakland, Calif), which is implanted in the subcutaneous tissue of the left upper abdomen with power lines and sensors exiting via the right lower quadrant to connect with a control console. The pump takes blood through a Dacron conduit from the apex of the left ventricle and pumps it via another Dacron conduit to the aorta. Both the Heart Mate and Novacor devices have a demonstrated durability for periods more than 2 years. Other similar or developing VADs include the Jarvik 2000 left VAD (Jarvik Heart, Inc, New York, NY), the MicroMed DeBackey VAD (MicroMed Technology, Inc, Houston, Tex), the HeartMate II and HeartMate III, the Incor (Berlin Heart, Hamburg, Germany), and the Terumo (Terumo Medical Corp, Somerset, NJ). The risks associated with implantation of a VAD include postoperative hemorrhage, sepsis, thromboembolism, renal failure, technical failure, and neurologic sequelae. It is extremely important to note if any central venous catheter is near the tricuspid prosthetic valve of a VAD or total artificial heart. If a catheter becomes entangled in the valve, it can cause malfunction of the valve, which will in turn stop venous return to the heart, rapidly endangering the patient's life.

The total artificial heart requires removal of the native heart. It serves as a bridge to cardiac transplantation, but occasionally it becomes the patient's permanent circulatory support for the rest of his or her life. The Jarvik 7 was the first attempt at an implantable artificial heart, but the recipient patients were completely hospital bound and suffered major complications. Other artificial hearts include the CardioWest (SynCardia Systems, Inc, Tucson, Ariz) and the AbioCor implantable replacement heart (ABIOMED. The AbioCor, for example, consists of two blood-pumping chambers; the right supplies blood to the lungs, and the left supplies the blood to the rest of the body. It is made of titanium and Angioflex (a proprietary polyether-based polyurethane plastic), and it is powered in part by an internal battery that can be recharged through the intact skin, obviating external power lines. Permanent implantable artificial hearts may be a reality in the not too distant future, but they still suffer the major hurdles of severe infections and thromboembolism, and their use remains very limited.

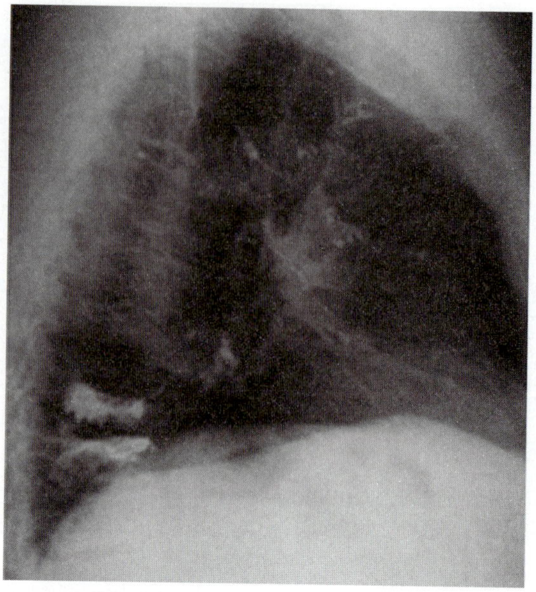

Fig. 4.78: *Lateral views of the chest in a patient who had undergone vertebroplasty. The vertebroplasty material extruded from the vertebrae and entered the spinal venous system with ultimate embolization to the patient's lungs. The patient suffered no known sequelae*

Miscellaneous Devices (Figs 4.77–4.79)

From time to time, other medical devices not commonly found at chest radiography may be seen. These devices include embolization coils, remote telemetry ECG monitoring devices, pericardial drainage catheters, and left atrial catheters. An interesting new device is the insertable (implantable) loop recorder, which is used for prolonged monitoring of the cardiac rhythm. It is a small electronic device implanted in the left pectoral region, and it can provide more than a year of continuous monitoring that may be activated by the patient or automatically activated. It has a variety of uses including monitoring of patients with unexplained syncopal episodes and assessment of patients with atrial fibrillation, ventricular arrhythmias, or conduction disturbances.

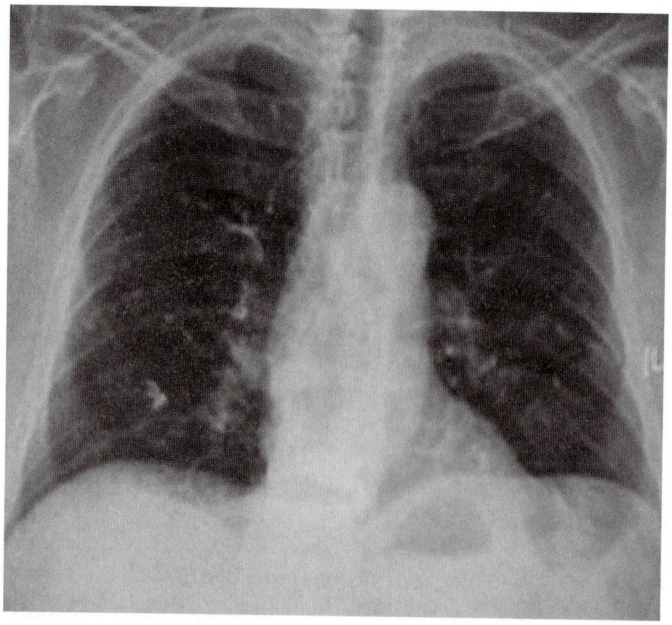

Fig. 4.77: *Frontal views of the chest in a patient who had undergone vertebroplasty. The vertebroplasty material extruded from the vertebrae and entered the spinal venous system with ultimate embolization to the patient's lungs. The patient suffered no known sequelae*

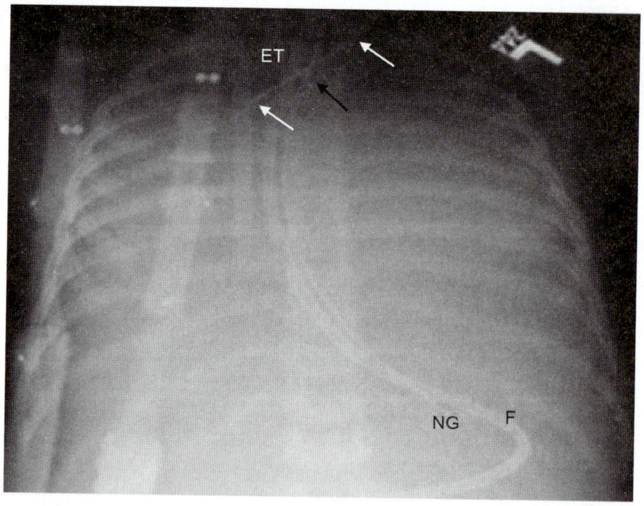

Fig. 4.79: *Portable chest radiograph of a patient undergoing extracorporeal membrane oxygenation shows pulmonary edema in the lungs and the tubing going to the patient's right carotid artery and right jugular vein. Also seen are an endotracheal tube (ET), a right internal jugular vein catheter (black arrow), a left internal jugular vein catheter (white arrows), a nasogastric (NG) tube, and a feeding (F) tube*

Sometimes, unexpected neck, abdomen, and spinal apparatus may be visible at chest radiography. Such objects include tracheostomy tubes; voice prostheses; neck drainage catheters; cervical, thoracic, or lumbar spine fixation apparatus; temperature monitoring catheters in the hypopharynx or esophagus; vagus nerve stimulators; abscess and biliary drainage catheters in the abdomen; umbilical arterial and venous catheters; and transjugular intrahepatic portosystemic shunts (TIPS) in the liver Vertebroplasty is not uncommon, and in some medical centers extracorporeal membrane oxygenation apparatus may be seen in premature infants and other patients with severe heart and lung disease. Most of these devices have nothing to do with the cardiovascular or pulmonary structures in the chest, but they happen to overlie the chest or be visible on chest images, because they lie contiguous to the thorax in the neck, spine, or upper abdomen. Recognizing and evaluating such apparatus is just as important as recognizing and evaluating apparatus primarily designed for the chest.

ECHOCARDIOGRAPHY

Cardiovascular imaging plays an essential role in the practice of cardiology. Two-dimensional (2D) echocardiography is able to visualize the heart directly in real time using ultrasound, providing instantaneous assessment of the myocardium, cardiac chambers, valves, pericardium, and great vessels. Doppler echocardiography measures the velocity of moving red blood cells and has become a noninvasive alternative to cardiac catheterization for assessment of hemodynamics. Transesophageal echocardiography (TEE) provides a unique window for high-resolution imaging of posterior structures of the heart, particularly the left atrium, mitral valve, and aorta (Figs 4.80–4.88).

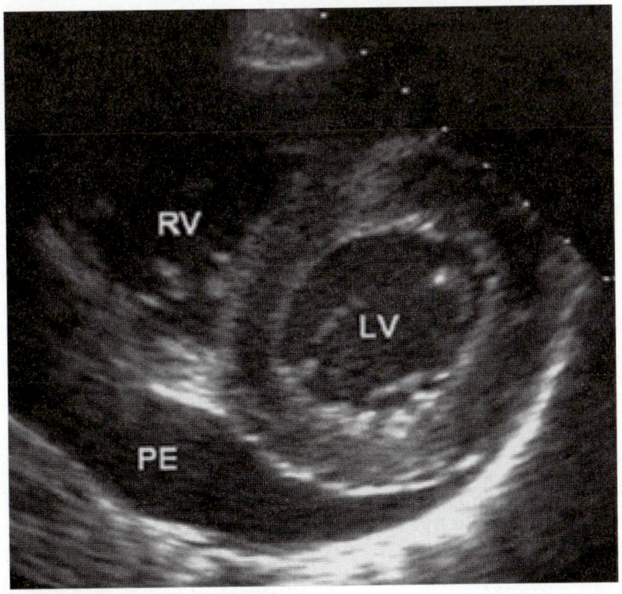

Fig. 4.80: *Pericardial effusion from a parasternal short-axis echocardiographic view. RV indicates right ventricle; LV, left ventricle; PE, pericardial effusion*

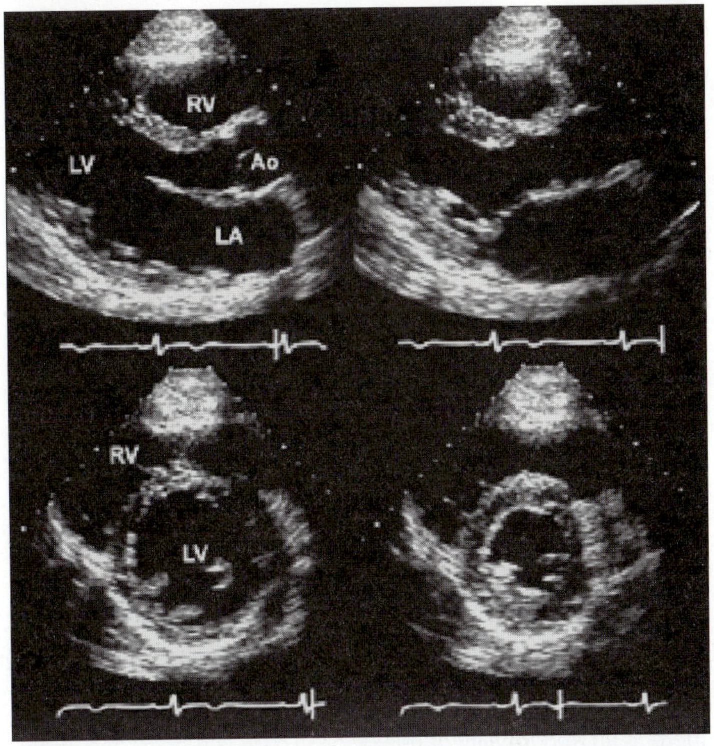

Fig. 4.81: *Two dimensional echocardiographic still-frame images from a normal patient with a normal heart. Upper: parasternal long-axis view during systole and diastole (left) and systole (right). During systole, there is thickening of the myocardium and reduction in the size of the left ventricle (LV). The valve leaflets are thin and open widely. Lower: Parasternal short-axis view during diastole (left) and systole (right) demonstrating a decrease in the left ventricular cavity size during systole as well as an increase in wall thickening. LA, left atrium; RV, right ventricle; Ao, aorta*

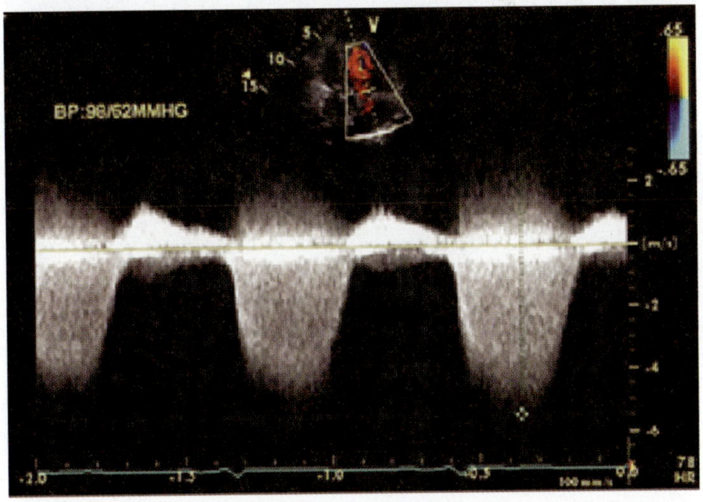

Fig. 4.82: *Continuous-wave Doppler of tricuspid regurgitation in a patient with pulmonary hypertension. There is an increase in the velocity to 5.4 m/s. Using the modified Bernoulli equation, the peak pressure gradient between right ventricle and right atrium during systole is 116 mmHg. Assuming a right atrial pressure of 10 mmHg, the right ventricular systolic pressure is 126 mmHg. In the absence of right ventricular outflow tract obstruction, this indicates there is severe pulmonary hypertension with a pulmonary artery systolic pressure of 126 mmHg*

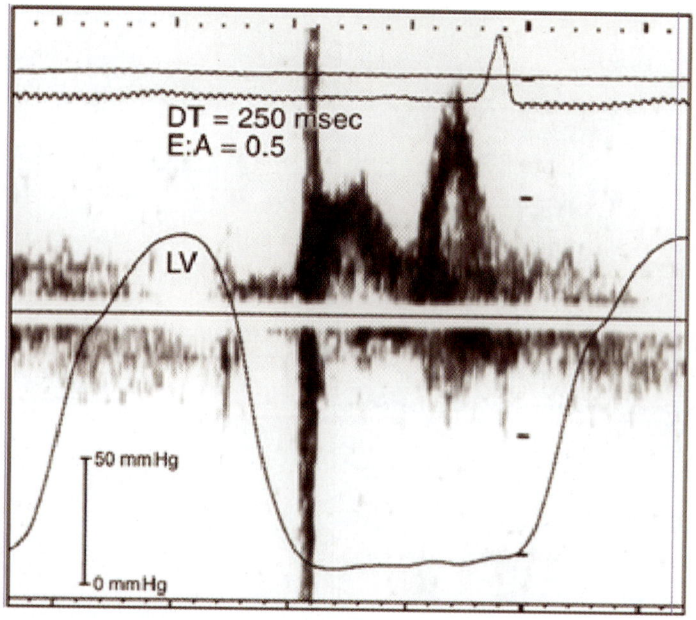

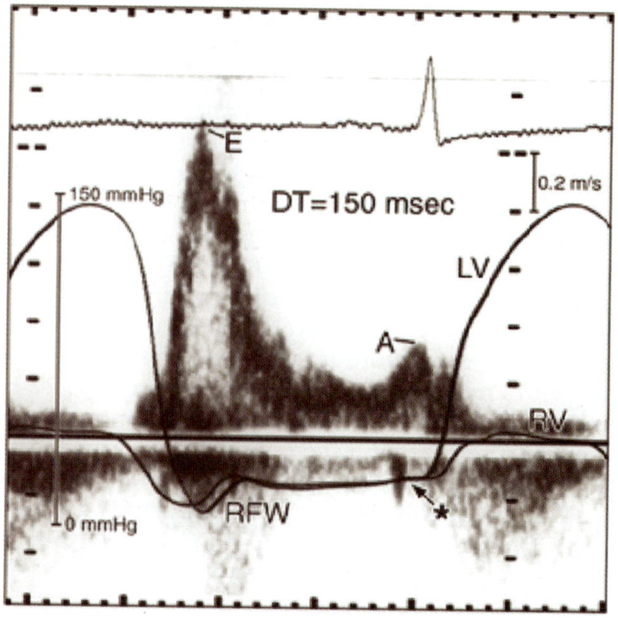

Fig. 4.83: *High-fidelity left ventricular (LV) pressure curves superimposed on a mitral inflow velocity curve obtained by Doppler echocardiography. The ratio of early and late diastolic flows is termed the E:A ratio. The deceleration time (DT) measures the rate of decline of early velocity and reflects the effective operative compliance of the left ventricle. Left: In early stages of diastolic dysfunction, there is an abnormality of relaxation. There is a decrease in the early diastolic filling and an increase with filling at atrial contraction, resulting in a low E:A ratio of 0.5, with deceleration time (DT) of 250 ms. In this instance, the LV diastolic pressure is low at 6 mmHg. Right: as diastolic dysfunction progresses, there is a restriction to filling, in which there is a high early diastolic velocity and low velocity at atrial contraction resulting in a high E:A ratio of 3.0, with DT of 150 ms. In this instance, the LV diastolic pressure is markedly elevated to 34 mmHg*

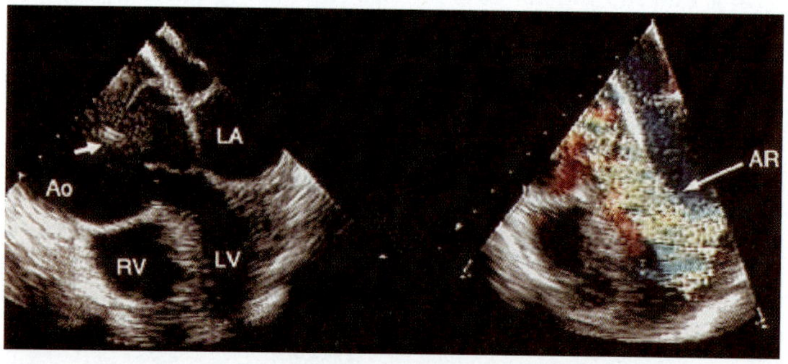

Fig. 4.84: *Transesophageal still-frame echocardiographic view of a patient with a dilated aorta, aortic dissection, and severe aortic regurgitation. The arrow points to the intimal flap that is seen in the dilated ascending aorta. Left: the long-axis apex-down view of the black-and-white two dimensional image in diastole. Right: color-flow imaging that demonstrates a large mosaic jet of aortic regurgitation. Ao, aorta; RV, right ventricle; AR, aortic regurgitation*

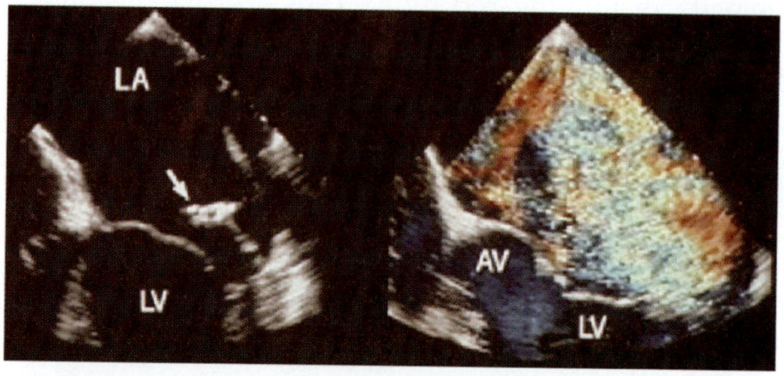

Fig. 4.85: *Left: transesophageal echocardiographic view of a patient with severe mitral regurgitation due to a flail posterior leaflet. The arrow points to the portion of the posterior leaflet that is unsupported and moves into the left atrium during systole. Right: color-flow imaging demonstrating a large mosaic jet of mitral regurgitation during systole. LA, left atrium; LV, left ventricle; AV, aortic valve*

Stress Echocardiography

Stress echocardiography is a universally employed modality in the noninvasive diagnosis and risk stratification of patients with suspected or known CAD. During SE, increased oxygen demand can be achieved through exercise (e.g. on a treadmill or bicycle) or administration of adrenergic α-agonist. In the setting of a significant coronary obstruction, ischemia will manifest as stress-induced wall-motion abnormality. A typical stress examination includes at least the apical four-chamber, apical two-chamber, parasternal long- and short-axis views. Images are obtained at peak stress during pharmacologic and bicycle stress or immediately after cessation of treadmill exercise. The current standard for analysis of SE is visual assessment of wall motion and endocardial systolic thickening. An expert physician assigns a higher score to an increasing severity of wall-motion abnormality (1: normal; 2: hypokinetic;

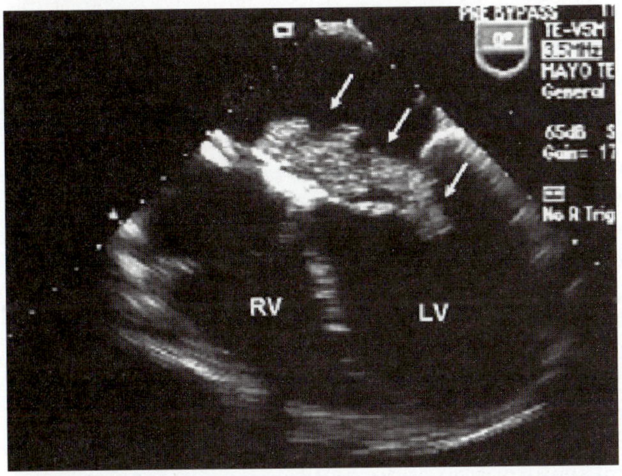

Fig. 4.86: *Transesophageal still-frame echocardiographic images of a patient with a left atrial myxoma. There is a large echo-dense mass in the left atrium, attached to the atrial septum. The mass moves across the mitral valve in diastole. LV, left ventricle; RV, right ventricle*

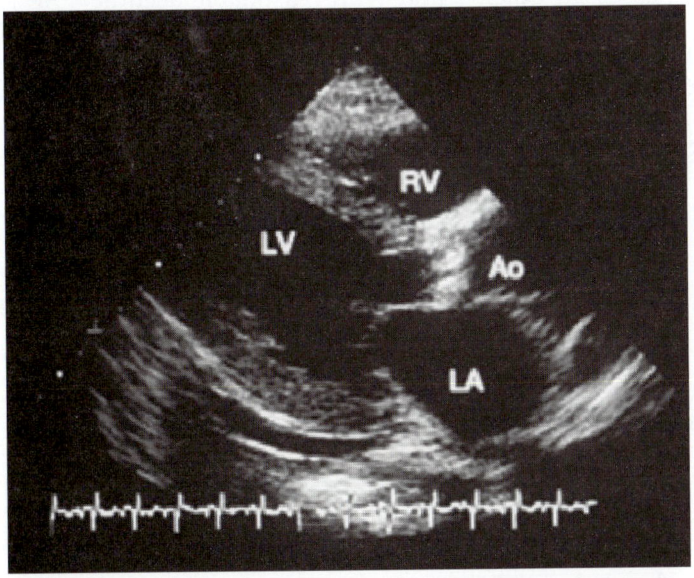

Fig. 4.87: *Two dimensional echocardiographic still-frame images from a patient with aortic stenosis. Parasternal long-axis view shows a heavily calcified aortic valve. RV, right ventricle; LV, left ventricle; AO, aorta; LA, left atrium*

3: akinetic). Regional contractility of the left ventricle (LV) is graded using a 16-segment or, more recently revised, 17-segment American Heart Association model. Myocardial segments are grouped according to their coronary supply (left anterior descending [LAD], right coronary artery [RCA] and left circumflex [LCX]), with the recognition that there is variability in the coronary supply of various segments, including the apical lateral (LAD or LCX territory) and apical inferior (LAD or RCA territory) segments (Fig. 4.88).

Images are obtained at rest, low-dose dobutamine, peak-dose dobutamine and during recovery. There is normal wall

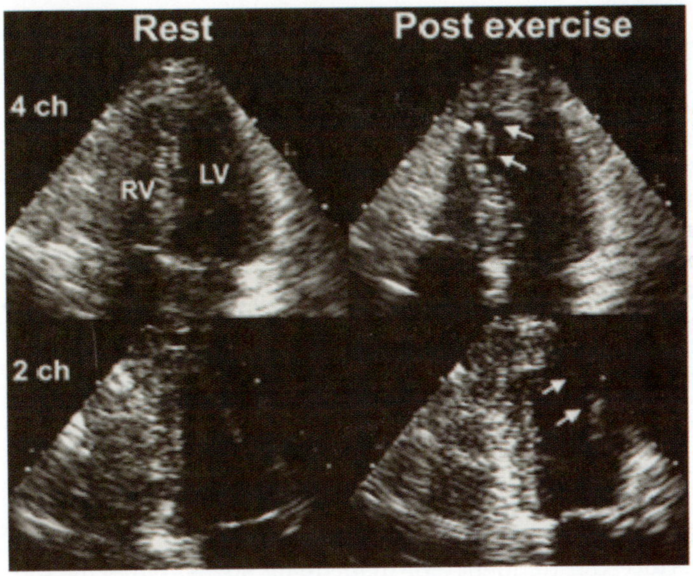

Fig. 4.88: *Systolic still-frame two dimensional echocardiographic images of a patient undergoing a stress echocardiogram. During rest (left), there is contraction of all segments of the myocardium. During exercise (right), there are regional wall motion abnormalities in the anterior and anteroapical segments (arrows). 4 ch, four-chamber view; 2 ch, two-chamber views; LV, left ventricle; RV, right ventricle*

motion at rest, with evidence of extensive wall-motion abnormality involving the septal and lateral walls in addition to left ventricular dilation (white arrows). This is highly suggestive of multivessel coronary disease.

Stress echocardiography can also be successfully performed with vasodilators, mainly high-dose dipyridamole, as the stress agents, with the aid of atropine to increase heart rate and myocardial oxygen demand. In regions supplied by obstructed arteries, improvement of perfusion may not occur with vasodilators, resulting in a reduction in wall motion, relative to wall motion in regions that have improved perfusion with vasodilators. In general, vasodilator stress produces less increase in oxygen demand compared with â-adrenergic stress. Vasodilator SE is less widely employed in the USA than in Europe (Table 4.3).

The diagnostic accuracy of SE, as well as that of all other noninvasive imaging techniques, is generally compared with invasive coronary angiography. This approach has a number of limitations, in part, owing to the variability of an angiographic cutoff for significant disease (usually > 50% diameter stenosis equaling > 70% of area stenosis) in addition to the heterogeneous hemodynamic effect of a stenosis, based on site, length and vessel size.

Data pooled from several studies showed that exercise SE had a weighted mean sensitivity and specificity of 88 and 79%, respectively, for the diagnosis of CAD. The sensitivity of treadmill SE may be reduced if images are not acquired rapidly after treadmill stress, particularly in patients with less-severe disease. The diagnostic accuracy of dobutamine SE is, in general, comparable to that of exercise SE. From a large pool of data, the reported sensitivity and specificity of dobutamine SE is 81 and 80%, respectively.

The high diagnostic accuracy of SE seems to be maintained in specific subject populations, such as women. On the basis of the aggregate data available in studies of nearly 1,000 women with suspected CAD, SE had a mean sensitivity of 81% (89% in women with multivessel disease), a specificity of 86% and overall accuracy of 84% for detecting or excluding significant CAD. However, a number of studies report a relatively higher rate of false-negative SE in women. A potential contributing factor is a greater likelihood of single-vessel coronary disease in this patient population. Women also tend to have a more rapid increase in heart rate with lower dose of dobutamine than men. This leads to more frequent termination of the test at a submaximal dose of dobutamine and less frequent use of atropine.

A number of factors affect the overall diagnostic accuracy of SE. When SE is being performed for diagnostic purposes in a stable patient, withdrawal of medications that would blunt the heart rate response to stress is recommended to reduce the frequency of inadequate stress. Other factors for false-negative studies include the presence of single-vessel disease or failure to detect limited wall-motion abnormalities in patients with suboptimal echocardiographic images. A blunted increase in myocardial oxygen demand owing to lower-wall stress and difficulty in the detection of subtle wall-motion abnormalities may also account for false-negative studies in patients with concentric left ventricular remodeling.

Although some false-positive studies may result from challenges in wall-motion assessment, a significant proportion of false-positive studies are due to myocardial ischemia in the absence of obstruction of epicardial coronary vessels. The presence of microvascular disease and the reduction in capillary density that occurs in patients with left ventricular hypertrophy and cardiomyopathy may account for a higher than expected incidence of stress-induced wall-motion abnormalities in the absence of large epicardial coronary artery obstruction. Coronary vasospasm may be provoked by exercise and, infrequently, by dobutamine. False-positive studies may also result from difficulty in distinguishing ischemic wall-motion abnormalities from those produced by tethering of myocardial segments to less-mobile structures, such as the mitral annulus. Dysynchronous contraction produced by LBBB and right ventricular pacing can be confused with septal wall-motion abnormalities from ischemia.

There are a number of advantages associated with SE. Compared with other noninvasive techniques, it is the most versatile and provides the most ancillary information at the lowest cost. Global and regional left and right ventricular systolic function, valvular disease and hemodynamics can be assessed quickly and with reasonable accuracy. SE is particularly useful in the evaluation of diastolic dysfunction and pulmonary hypertension in patients with dyspnea. The portability of cardiac ultrasound systems permits evaluation of patients in the intensive-care unit and satellite clinics or physician offices.

The primary disadvantage of SE is that a proportion of patients have inadequate or suboptimal images. The

Table 4.1: *Selection of imaging test*

	Echo	*Nuclear*	*CT*[a]	*MRI*[b]
LV size/function	Initial modality of choice Low cost, portable Provides ancillary structural and hemodynamic information	Available from PET imaging	Best resolution Highest cost	Best resolution Highest cost
Valve disease	Initial modality of choice			Visualize valve
Valve motion	Doppler hemodynamics		motion	Delineate abnormal flow
Pericardial disease	Pericardial effusion Doppler hemodynamics		Pericardial thickening	Pericardial thickening
Aortic disease	TEE rapid diagnosis[c] Acute dissection		Image entire aorta Acute aneurysm Aortic dissection	Image entire aorta Aortic aneurysm Chronic dissection
Cardiac masses	TTE–large intracardia masses TEE—smaller intracardiac masses[c]		Extracardiac masses Myocardial masses	Extracardiac masses Myocardial masses

[a]Contrast required.

[b]Relative contraindication: pacemakers, metallic objects, claustrophobic.

[c]When not seen on TTE.

Abbreviations: Echo, echocardiography, PET, positron emission tomography; SPECT, single-photon emission computed tomography, TEE transesophageal echocardiography; TTE, transthoracic echocardiogram.

Table 4.2: *Clinical uses of echocardiography*

Two-dimensional echocardiography Cardia chambers
Chamber size Left ventricular hypertrophy Regional wall motion abnormalities
Valves Morphology and motions
Pericardium
Effusion
Tamponade
Masses Great vessels
Stress echocardiography
Two dimensional
Myocardial is chemia
Viable myocardium Doppler
Valve disease
Doppler echocardiography
Valve stenosis
Gradient Valve area
Valve reguagitation Semi
Intracardiac pressures Volumetric flow Diastolic filling
Intracardiac shorts Transesophageal echocardiography
Aortic disease infective endocarditis
Source of embolism Valve prothesis
Introperative

success of imaging varies from laboratory to laboratory and is, in part, dependent on the sonographer expertise, patient mix and physicians' proficiency and tolerance for technically difficult studies (e.g. obese patients). In approximately 10–20% of examinations, two or more of 16 (or 17) myocardial segments may not be well visualized. Commercial contrast agents can be used to opacify the LV cavity and improve myocardial border detection in patients with suboptimal images with a low incidence of serious complications. Another disadvantage of SE is that visual assessment of wall motion and thickening requires significant expertise and involves some interobserver variability, especially in lower quality images. Interobserver agreement in wall-motion assessment may decline from the above 90% range for high-quality studies to the 70% range for poor-quality studies.

SINGLE-PHOTON EMISSION COMPUTED TOMOGRAPHY (Fig. 4.89)

Single-photon emission computed tomography is a well-validated method commonly used in daily practice in the diagnosis of CAD. A radioactive tracer is injected, followed by imaging of its myocardial distribution using SPECT. Exercise (e.g. treadmill) or pharmacologic (e.g. dobutamine or vasodilators) stress are commonly used. Unless contraindicated, vasodilators (e.g. adenosine, dipyridamole or, more recently, regadenason) are the first choice for pharmacologic stress, since they induce greater levels of hyperemia than α-adrenergic agonists. Adenosine is a direct-acting vasodilator, while dipyridamole inhibits cellular uptake and breakdown of adenosine. Regadenason is a recently introduced selective adenosine A_{2A} receptor agonist that was US-FDA approved in April 2008. It has been developed in an effort to minimize the complications and discomfort from the nonselective activation of A_1, A_{2B} and A_3 receptors. Regadenason produces hyperemia with rapid onset (30 s) and for a longer duration (~2–5 min) than adenosine. These drugs produce coronary vasodilation, resulting in limited hyperemia in regions supplied by arteries with obstructive CAD compared with regions supplied by arteries with no significant disease. Ischemia is induced infrequently with vasodilator administration because there is usually no major increase in myocardial oxygen demand. This heterogeneous perfusion is best detected with a blood flow tracer. Three perfusion tracers are commonly available: thallium (Tl)-201, technetium (Tc)-99m sestamibi, and ^{99m}Tc tetrofosmin. For tracer uptake and retention, all three agents require viable myocytes supplied by adequate perfusion. The agents are injected at peak exercise or during peak vasodilation. Two sets of images are obtained: once after stress and once at rest.

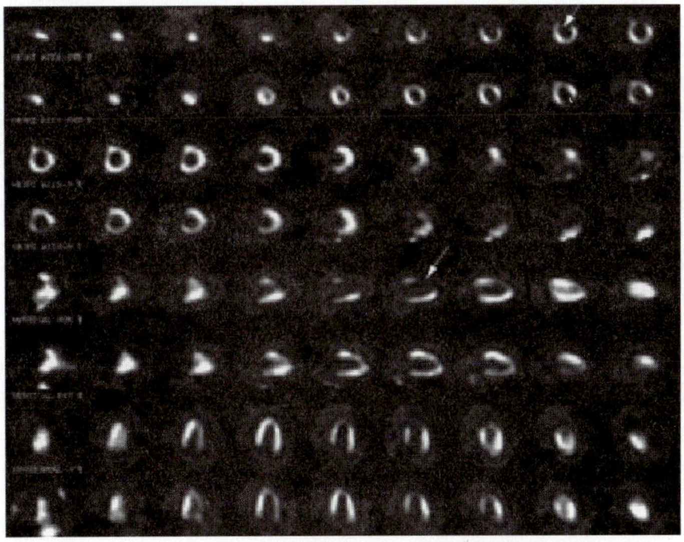

Fig. 4.89: *A reversible defect on adenosine technetium-99m sestamibi single-photon emission computed tomography. A moderate-size, reversible defect is present in the anterior wall, in the short- and vertical long-axis projections, illustrating stress-induced ischemia (white arrows)*

Reconstructed images are displayed in the vertical long-, horizontal long- and short-axis projections. These can be viewed in grayscale or in various color-scale maps, which allow easier grading of severity of defects. Tracer uptake in myocardial segments is normalized to the region with maximal tracer uptake. Assessment is primarily visual and qualitative for routine scan interpretation. Reversible (stress-induced) defects identify viable regions supplied by obstructed vessels, while irreversible (fixed) defects reflect partial or transmurally infarcted myocardium. A standard method is to grade perfusion on a scale of 0–4, with 0 representing normal perfusion and 4 representing no visible tracer uptake. Display of rest and stress images in a single polar plot diagram representing all 17 segments of the LV with automated comparison of tracer uptake values with an established normal gender- and tracer-matched database also permits some degree of quantification of defect size and severity.

POSITRON EMISSION TOMOGRAPHY

Positron emission tomography is another accurate method for assessing myocardial perfusion and metabolism in the evaluation of coronary disease. PET has been used as a research tool for many years, but has not seen extensive clinical application. Similar to SPECT, exercise (e.g. treadmill) or pharmacologic (e.g. dobutamine or vasodilators) stress is used. Pharmacologic stress imaging usually follows resting imaging after the initial activity has been allowed to decay. Three positron-emitting radiotracers are used clinically for cardiac PET imaging: ^{13}N and ^{82}Rb for assessing myocardial perfusion and ^{18}F deoxy-D-glucose (FDG) for evaluating myocardial glucose metabolism and viability assessment. Rb imaging is limited by the high cost of the Rb generator, which, together with the fixed high cost of PET cameras, necessitates two to three reimbursed studies per day to be economically feasible. ^{13}N requires an onsite cyclotron for its production and the current lack of reimbursement limits its clinical use. The short half-lives of ^{82}Rb (75 s) and ^{13}N (10 min) result in low radiation exposure for the patient, and allow other radionuclide imaging studies on the same day. The use of PET in myocardial perfusion imaging is expected to increase in the near future, with the regional distribution of positron-emitting radiotracers and the emergence of relatively low-cost PET systems (Fig. 4.90–4.92).

Positron emission tomography imaging has been combined with computed tomography (CT) for attenuation correction. Hybrid scanners integrating PET and CT account for approximately 80% of new PET units installed. Attenuation-corrected images are displayed in cardiac short-axis, vertical long-axis and horizontal long-axis projections. An experienced reader will visually interpret the myocardial perfusion pattern. Similar to SPECT, a 5-point scoring system (0: normal uptake; 4: absent uptake) and a 17 LV segment model are used to compute a summed stress score, a summed rest score and a summed difference score.

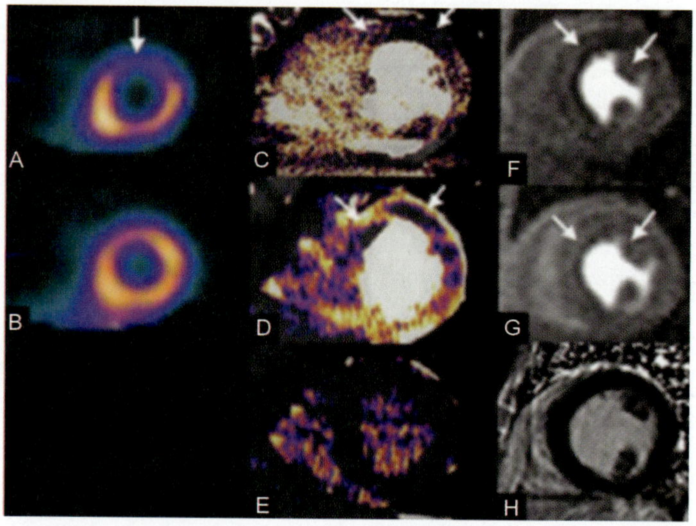

Fig. 4.90: *Contrast-enhanced retrospectively ECG-gated DECT study in a young patient with abnormal SPECT. Short-axis SPECT acquisitions during stress (A) and rest (B) show reversible perfusion defect in the left anterior descending (LAD) artery territory. Corresponding short-axis DECT reconstructions reveal myocardial blood pool defects during both stress (C) and rest (D). DECT images show good agreement with perfusion cardiac MRI during stress (F) and rest (G) delineating a partially reversible subendocardial defect in the LAD territory. Late DECT image acquisition (6 minutes after iodine administration) shows no sign of delayed enhancement (i.e. myocardial infarct; E). Similarly, there also is no evidence of hyperenhancement within the myocardium at delayed-enhancement cardiac MRI [15 minutes after gadolinium (Gd-DTPA) administration]*

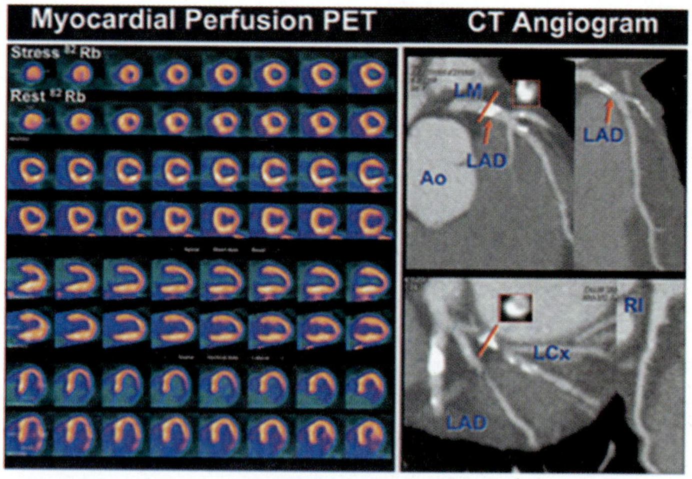

Fig. 4.91: *Showing well correlated myocardial perfusion with PET and CT coronary angiography of an obstructed and calcified left anterior descending artery*

From a large meta-analysis (n = 19 studies), the sensitivity and specificity of PET for the diagnosis of CAD were calculated as 92% (85–98%) and 85% (50–100%), respectively. The same study reported a positive likelihood ratio of 6.2 (CI: 3.3–11.8) and a negative likelihood ratio of 0.11 (CI: 0.08–0.14). On this basis, PET may be an excellent tool at confirming and excluding CAD. This diagnostic

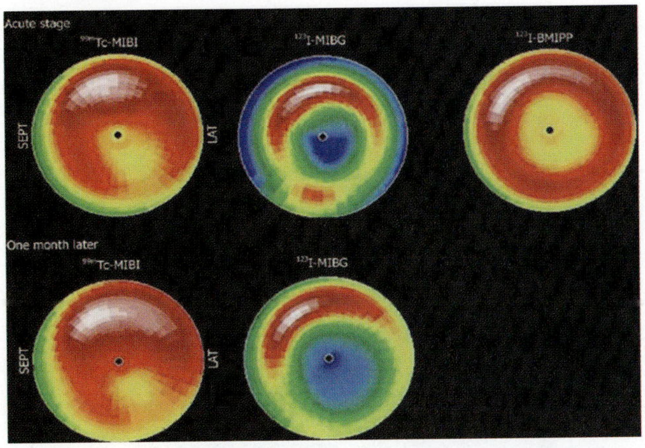

Fig. 4.92: *Scintigraphic features of Takotsubo cardiomyopathy are depicted. Bull's eye maps of 99mTc-sestamibi (MIBI), 123I-MIBG and 123I-methyl-p-iodophenyl-pentadecanoic acid (BMIPP) are shown. Both 123I-MIBG and 123I-BMIPP images show reduced uptake in the apical segment of the myocardium, which are typical features of the disease*

performance seems to be comparable to other functional stress-imaging modalities.

Contrary to SPECT, PET maintains its high diagnostic accuracy in women. Patterson et al. showed that sensitivity and specificity for the detection of CAD in women is equally high to that in men. Bateman and coworkers found that, of women who had undergone both stress SPECT and stress PET, both imaging tests had similar high sensitivity but the specificity of PET was significantly higher than for SPECT.

There are several advantages to PET. When compared with SPECT, image uniformity is probably the most important property of cardiac PET. This is because of its excellent spatial (2–4 mm) and temporal resolution. Bateman et al. found that the PET count exceeded that of SPECT by a factor of 2, despite the shorter imaging time of PET. Attenuation correction is also superior in eliminating attenuation artifacts. This may prove PET to be an attractive alternative to other imaging modalities in selected patients (e.g. obese patients) as an uncertain image finding of a noninvasive test is one of the factors prompting physicians to recommend further diagnostic procedures. In 2748 patients, Patterson et al. found a reduction in the number of uncertain ("probably" normal or abnormal) interpretations from 37% with ^{201}Tl SPECT to 21% with ^{82}Rb PET. PET with FDG has also shown promise in the assessment of atherosclerotic plaque inflammation, a feature that may be of significant clinical importance. Ogawa et al. have shown that macrophages are responsible for the FDG accumulation in vulnerable plaques. Since these plaques are rich with macrophages, FDG imaging was shown to be useful in the detection of vulnerable plaques.

A number of limitations, however, hamper the use of PET for myocardial perfusion assessment in daily practice. It is expensive and not widely available, especially outside of the USA. PET imaging is subject to a number of artifacts related to acquisition techniques, heart drift between rest and stress images, which leads to misregistration, and posterior artifacts due to highly attenuating structures (e.g. the spine). Similar to SPECT, PET has a limited ability in delineating the anatomical extent of disease in patients with multivessel stenosis. Radiation exposure also remains a concern. When combined with CT, a hybrid scan has an estimated radiation dose close to 13mSv.

CARDIAC MRI

Recently, MRI has emerged as a new noninvasive modality for detecting CAD. It uses high-intensity magnetic fields and radiofrequency to generate 3D/tomographic images with high resolution (~0.8 mm) and excellent tissue contrast. The two main imaging techniques employed in CMR are spin echo imaging, which delineates the tissue structures of the heart as bright and the blood pool as dark (black-blood approach), and cine CMR, which produces images in which the blood pool appears as bright and cardiac tissue structure appears dark (bright-blood approach) using gradient echo-based rapid imaging sequences. Cines are typically obtained within single-breath holds using fast schemes. These schemes include fast low-angle shot (FLASH), steady-state with free precession (SSFP), spiral imaging and echo planar imaging (EPI). CMR evaluates the presence of CAD using three very different techniques: evaluation of wall motion and thickening during stress, dynamic first-pass perfusion imaging, which assesses for inducible perfusion defects, and anatomical assessment (coronary MRA), which provides noninvasive visualization of the coronary tree (Figs 4.93–4.97).

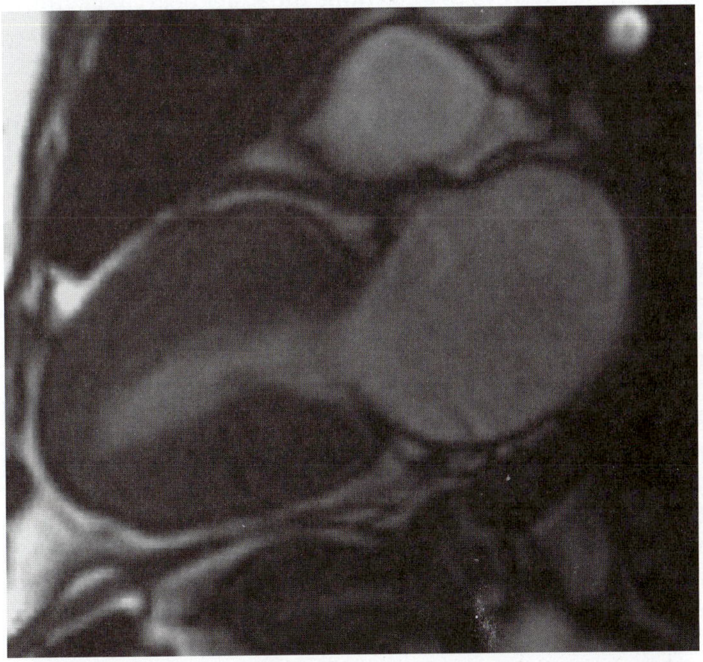

Fig. 4.93: *MRI scan of a patient with hypertrophic cardiomyopathy, showing the severe increase in left ventricular wall thickness. Cardiac MRI is an ideal imaging modality for diagnosing cardiomyopathies*

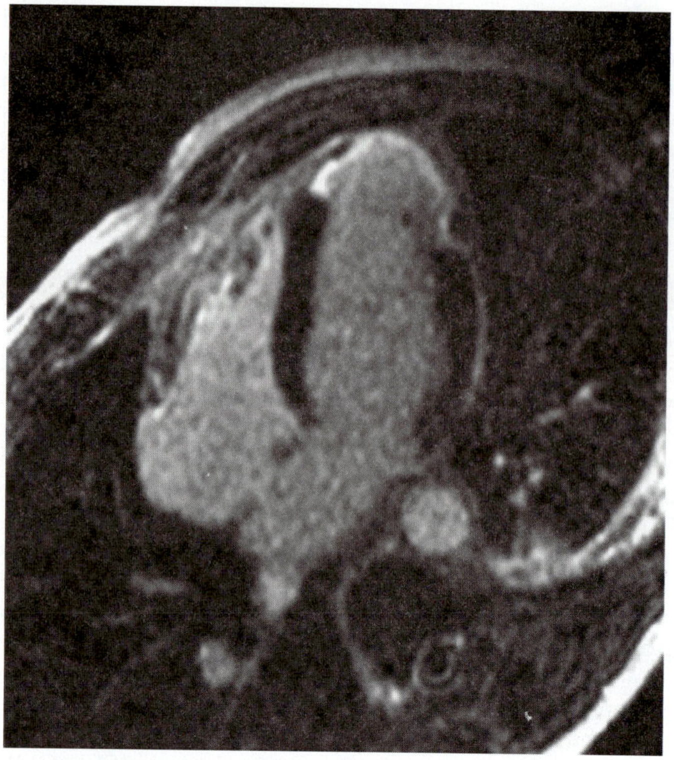

Fig. 4.94: *MRI scan with delayed gadolinium enhancement in a patient with a large anteroapical infarction. The gadolinium (white area) accumulated in the extracellular space in the presence of cell death from myocardial infarction*

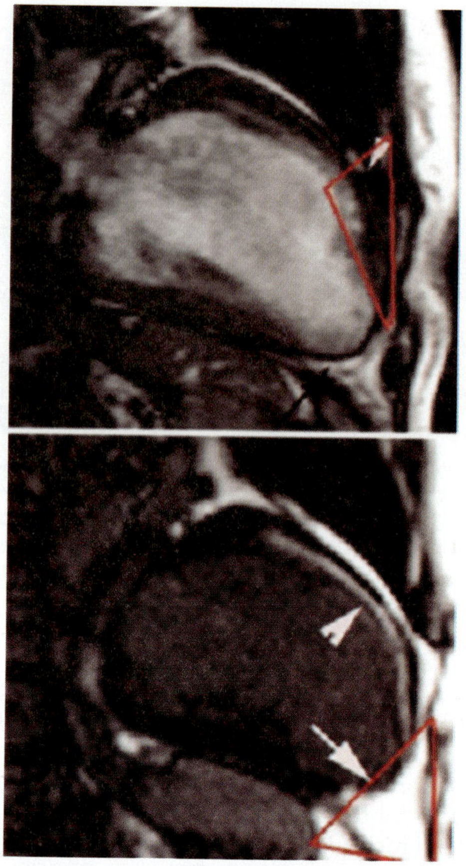

Fig. 4.95: *Cardiac MRI to determine myocardium viability before revascularization. The whole concept of viability on cardiac MRI is based on the fact that all infarcts enhance vividly 10-15 minutes after intravenous contrast administration. Cardiac MRI shows the transmural extent of the infarct very reliably. It tells you that: "white is dead" (all infarcts irrespective of age enhance) In areas of hypokinesia, if there is a rim of "black" or noninfarcted myocardium that is not contracting well, it indicates the presence of hibernating myocardium, which is likely to improve after revascularization of the artery supplying that particular territory. Viability imaging reliably allows identification of areas of hibernation and viable or nonviable myocardium. All infarcts irrespective of age enhance. The percentage involvement of the myocardial wallthickness by an infarct determines viability*

Assessment of wall motion with CMR utilizes dobutamine as the stress agent. Protocols similar to those implemented for dobutamine SE can be used for CMR. After rapid surveys to determine the exact heart axis, three short-axis planes (apical, mid and basal) and four- and two-chamber views are usually acquired. Images can be displayed as continuous cine loops using a quad-screen display for review of a 17-segment LV model. At each level of stress, LV segmental wall motion is assessed as normal, hypokinetic, akinetic or dyskinetic. Inducible ischemia is defined as deterioration of the segmental systolic wall motion within a myocardial segment observed in two orthogonal views.

When compared with invasive coronary angiography, the sensitivity and specificity of stress CMR detection of CAD by wall-motion analysis has been reported to be 83 and 86%, respectively, in a report pooling data from several investigations. Stress MRI evaluation of wall motion has the advantage of providing high-quality images in most subjects, regardless of body habitus. The use of myocardial tagging may also improve the sensitivity of wall-motion analysis. Tagging is a special radiofrequency modulation of the magnetized vector to obtain both line and grid representation of the myocardial segments to help assess regional heterogeneity of systolic segmental contraction.

An alternative approach to detecting obstructive CAD by CMR is based on dynamic first-pass perfusion scanning. Adenosine is the preferred stressor agent. After acquisition of rest cine scans in the standard views (apical, mid and basal short-axis views; four- and two-chamber views), adenosine infusion is started. Within the last minute of the infusion, intravenous gadolinium (typical dose ranging from 0.05 to 0.15 mg/kg/min) is administered, and perfusion scanning is performed during breath holding After a 10–15 min waiting period to allow for equilibration of the contrast agent with the myocardium, an identical rest perfusion scan is repeated. Interpretation of inducible perfusion defects is visually performed. The transmurality of a defect is determined from the single dynamic image showing the maximum extent of regional hypoenhancement. A regional hypoenhancement of at least 25% in any segment not visible on the rest perfusion scan is considered pathological. Alternatively, computer quantification of parameters, such as the signal-intensity upslope or regional contrast transit time, can be used to generate parametric

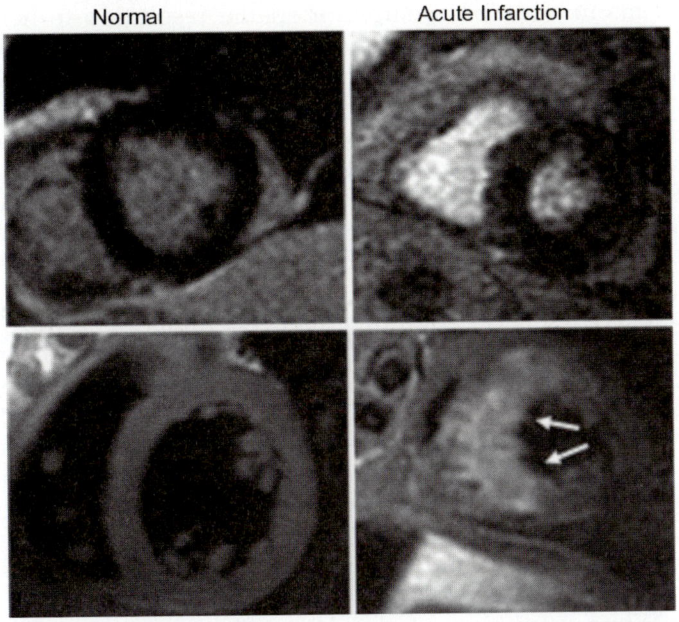

Fig. 4.96: *Left: Normal delayed enhancement and "edema"-sensitive images. Top (left): Delayed enhancement image illustrating normal black myocardium without infarction/fibrosis. Bottom (left): A triple inversion recovery sequence that is T2-weighted demonstrating normal homogenousappearing gray myocardium. Right: A patient postmyocardial infarction and early revascularization without evidence of an infarction and an edematous myocardium in the septum. Top (right): Delayed enhanced with normal black myocardium without infarction or fibrosis. Bottom (right): A triple inversion recovery sequence illustrating edema in the septum without infarction. This is the area of "salvaged" myocardium*

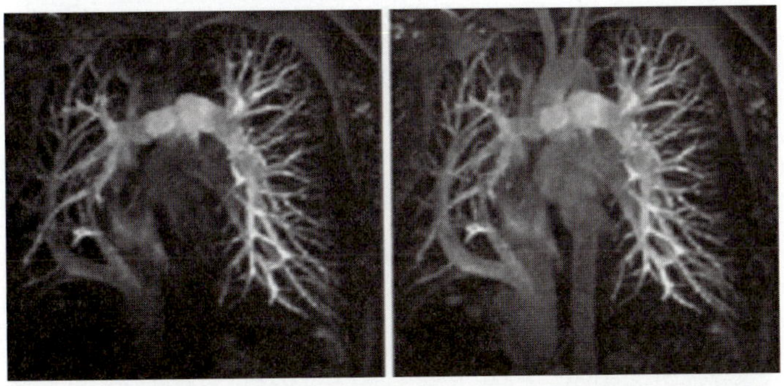

Fig. 4.97: *MRA scan of a patient with partial anomalous pulmonary venous drainage of the right lung into the inferior vena cava (scimitar syndrome). MRA is able to define the abnormal anatomic relationships of cardiac structures and great vessels in patients with congenital heart disease*

relative perfusion maps or measures of relative perfusion index at rest and during stress. A myocardial perfusion reserve index (MPRI) of 1.1 (when the second smallest MPRI is used) has been suggested as a reasonable cut-off value. The reported sensitivity of perfusion imaging averages 91%, with a specificity of 81% using coronary angiography as the gold standard Plein et al. showed that combined assessment of wall motion and perfusion yielded a sensitivity of 96% and a specificity of 83%, which was higher than the values for sensitivity and specificity of each method alone.

To date, few CMR studies have evaluated ischemia provocation in women. The study by Nagel et al. including 208 patients (61 women) revealed no significant differences in sensitivity, specificity and test accuracy of dobutamine CMR when compared with men. CMR maintains its high diagnostic accuracy in patients with single-vessel disease, which may be of particular value to female subsets of the population. CMR may also be well suited to women with chest pain due to microvascular disease and normal coronary arteries, a disease commonly known as syndrome X. Owing to its high resolution, CMR can discriminate between subepicardial and subendocardial flow, which enables the detection of an abnormal subendocardial perfusion index in this syndrome.

The third approach for the detection of CAD by CMR uses anatomical assessment of the coronary tree by angiography. Using the natural T2-weighted signal difference between the blood in the coronary lumen and the surrounding myocardium, coronary artery contrast is generated without exogenous contrast administration. The reconstruction interval is usually performed during mid-diastole, when cardiac motion is the least and coronary flow is the greatest. The duration of data acquisition can vary from 50 to 150 ms per cardiac cycle, with the acquisition extending to several minutes. From pooled data, the sensitivity and specificity of coronary MRA on a patient level were 88 and 56%, respectively.

Cardiac MRI has the advantage of being a highly versatile modality because it provides multiple techniques in one imaging system. It does not involve exposure to radiation. CMR myocardial perfusion has the potential for significant clinical growth given greatly enhanced spatial resolution. The excellent resolution enables the assessment of subendocardial perfusion abnormalities. This may present a significant clinical advantage, since a subendocardial perfusion abnormality is a more sensitive sign of obstructive CAD compared with a transmural perfusion abnormality. The ability to detect subendocardial perfusion abnormalities may also reduce the possibility of false-negative studies owing to balanced multivessel CAD encountered with SPECT and PET imaging. In addition, CMR is well validated for quantifying the volumes, mass and function of the ventricles, and has become the gold standard against which other techniques are measured. Given its 3D nature, CMR does not rely on geometric assumptions, especially in the vertical heart, LV hypertrophy and with regional heterogeneity of CAD. This permits excellent interstudy reproducibility of volume and mass for both the LV and right ventricle. Other clinical applications of CMR include assessment of myocardial infarction and viability by combining delayed enhancement imaging, evaluation of infiltrative or inflammatory disease processes, and study of pericardial and congenital diseases. The disadvantages of CMR include that it is a relatively expensive technology with limited availability. Stress is still largely limited to pharmacologic agents. Exercise is avoided, owing to motion artifacts during imaging.

Monitoring during testing can be suboptimal and ECG tracings and ST-segments can be altered by the strong magnetic field. The entire acquisition and image processing can be time consuming (30 min or more on average). Analysis times may be prolonged when quantitative assessment is performed. CMR cannot be used in patients with severe claustrophobia. It is also absolutely or relatively contraindicated in patients with pacemakers, defibrillators, certain aneurysm clips and other indwelling ferromagnetic materials. Gadolinium administration to patients with moderate-to-severe kidney disease (glomerular filtration rate < 30 mL/min) has been associated with the syndrome of nephrogenic systemic fibrosis, although only rarely. CMR is feasible only in cooperative patients. The need for accurate gating with a stable heart rhythm and the ability to hold breath for long scan-acquisition time are other limitations. More recently, self-gating techniques have been described. These largely rely on cardiac tissue motion and blood flow, which eliminates the need for an external physiologic signal monitoring. Lack of established CMR sequences for first-pass perfusion imaging, standardized protocols for stress testing and analysis are other drawbacks that are being currently addressed.

Coronary MRA also suffers from a number of technical limitations, which continue to hinder its widespread clinical application. Visualization of the entire coronary tree requires several minutes, and multiple beats are needed to reconstruct the coronary arteries. Beat-to-beat variability in the duration of the cardiac cycle and the period of diastasis can produce image blurring. Only proximal and mid LAD and RCA segments can be assessed reliably. Visualization of the LCX is less successful, owing to the close relationship of the accompanying vein and adjacent blood pools of the left atrium and ventricle, in addition to a lower signal related to the greater distance from the receiving coil. The number of uninterpretable segments is still significant, and exclusion of up to 20% of all segments has been reported. In addition, coronary MRA can be affected by motion related to intrinsic cardiac contraction/relaxation and motion attributable to superimposed diaphragm and chest-wall movement during respiration. ECG gating is used to account for the intrinsic cardiac motion, while breath holding is required to reduce artifact from respiratory motion. To overcome some of these limitations, free-breathing navigator coronary MRA has been introduced. This system tracks the patient's diaphragmatic motion and pictures are only obtained when the diaphragm is 3–5 mm within its end expiratory position.

MULTISLICE CARDIAC CT

The first experience with noninvasive coronary arteriography was described in 1995. Since its inception, substantial improvements in temporal and spatial resolution have been made. Mechanically rotating gantries with a rotation time of less than 420 ms are now routinely used. The more recently introduced dual-source MSCTs are able to attain a maximal temporal resolution as low as 83 ms in addition to superior spatial resolution to help improve coronary image quality at faster heart rates.[57] The 64-slice MSCT systems have a spatial resolution of 0.4–0.7 mm. Systems capable of 256 or 320 slices with each gantry rotation are now available. MSCT scanners can be operated in a sequential (step and shoot) or spiral (helical) mode. Data acquisition is triggered by the patient's ECG in sequential mode or, in case of continuous acquisition imaging, the reconstruction is made through retrospective or prospective ECG gating. Imaging is performed within one single breath hold. Most patients undergoing MSCT receive oral or intravenous â-blockers to achieve a heart rate of less than 60–70 bpm to optimize acquisition of gated images during diastolic diastasis. For new dual-source MSCT, acceptable image quality has been obtained at heart rates up to 90 bpm. Sublingual nitroglycerin can also be administered before the scan to achieve adequate coronary vasodilation. The entire procedure can be performed in approximately 30 min with study acquisition requiring less than 10 s (Fig. 4.98–4.101).

When examining arteries, interpreters must review the images on workstations capable of 2D and 3D displays of the commonly available reconstruction formats. These include transaxial 2D image stacks, multiplanar reformation (MPR), maximum intensity projection (MIP), curved multiplanar reformation (cMPR) and volume-rendering technique (VRT) reconstructions. During segmental analysis, a combination of these reconstruction formats can be used, depending on the characteristics of the vessel being examined (e.g. presence of calcification and tortuosity). Each stenosis is interpreted in all three planes (sagittal, coronal and axial) using all postprocessed and axial raw

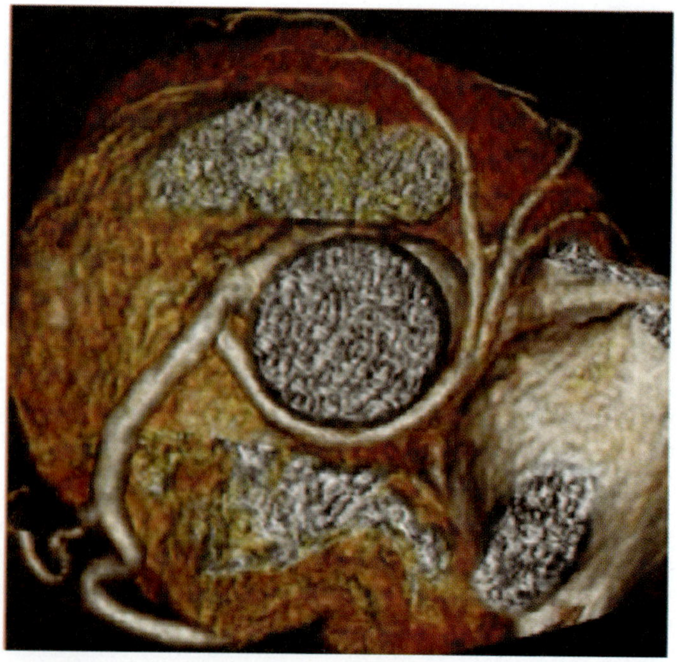

Fig. 4.98: *Three dimensional volume rendered image of a contrast enhanced CT angiogram illustrating an anomalous left coronary artery arising from the right coronary artery and traveling posterior to the aorta*

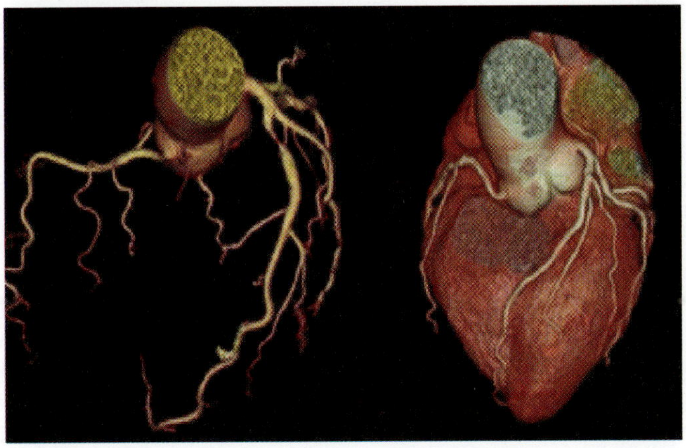

Fig. 4.99: *Three dimensional volume-rendered image of a contrast-enhanced CT angiogram demonstrating a normal left main coronary artery arising from the aorta and its two branches, the left anterior descending artery (left) and the circumflex artery (right) and right coronary artery (left panel)*

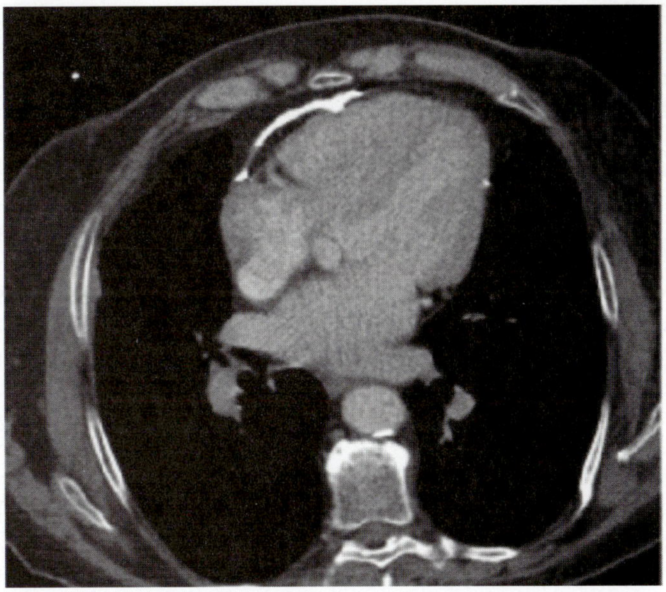

Fig. 4.100: *CT scan showing pericardial calcification, seen as a white linear density anterior to the myocardium*

images. Coronary arteries are scored using the American Heart Association coronary segmentation. The coronary tree should be examined initially for the course and branching of the main coronary vessels. Epicardial coronary arterial luminal stenosis is graded semiquantitatively as minimal (< 30%), mild (30–49%), moderate (50–69%), severe (70–99%) or occluded.

Initial studies with four-slice technology showed encouraging results, with sensitivities and specificities ranging from 66 to 90% and from 71 to 99%, respectively. However, the percentage of segments with nondiagnostic quality was very high (>25%). More recently, MSCT was reported to have high discriminative power to detect significant obstructive CAD with good sensitivity and specificity, which can reach the 90% range. As expected, considerably more segments are now available for evaluation (> 90%). The reported specificity is considered to be on par with other noninvasive imaging modalities (mainly SE and SPECT), whereas the diagnostic sensitivity and negative predictive value (NPV) are higher with MSCT.

For screening purposes, in properly selected patients, MSCT has excellent NPV reaching almost 100%, with a positive predictive value (PPV) of approximately 60%. As a result, a "negative" MSCT excludes high-grade coronary stenosis with very high certainty, as long as image quality is diagnostic and all coronary segments are well seen. This may help identify patients who do not have to undergo an invasive angiography for CAD detection.

The limited available data suggest that MSCT maintains its diagnostic accuracy in women. In a study of 103 consecutive patients (51 men and 52 women) with known or suspected CAD, 64-slice MSCT had high diagnostic accuracy in all patients with no significant differences in accuracy on a segmental or vessel basis.

Multislice cardiac CT may have its greatest value in symptomatic patients with nondiagnostic functional tests or in those with suspected false-positive or -negative functional tests. The use of MSCT in these settings may

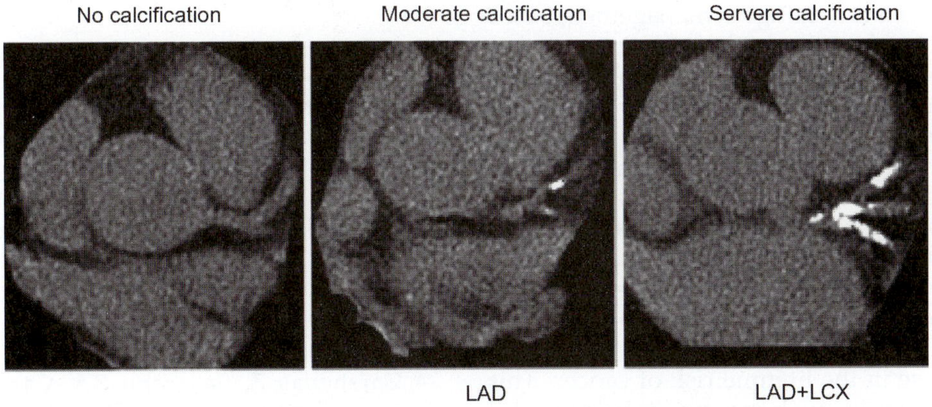

Fig. 4.101: *CT scans of three patients showing the ability to detect coronary calcification. Left: Normal coronary arteries without calcification. Middle: Calcification in the left anterior artery (LAD). Right: Severe calcification in the LAD and circumflex (CX) arteries*

help to avoid overutilization of invasive coronary angiography and exposure to unnecessary procedure-related risks. Another potential role of MSCT is in a specific subgroup of patients with a relative contraindication for physiologic testing. Patients with LBBB may be better served by MSCT for evaluation of suspected CAD. Other imaging modalities may have lower specificity, PPV and higher false-positive results of CAD detection in those with LBBB. The diagnostic accuracy of MSCT for the detection of coronary stenosis was evaluated in 66 patients with LBBB without a history of CAD. The sensitivity and specificity values (97 and 95%, respectively) were similar to those in patients without LBBB. Another potential role of MSCT may include the workup of dilated cardiomyopathy in low- to intermediate-risk CAD patients. A single-center study reported that 64-slice MSCT correctly identified 60 out of 62 patients (97%) without and 28 out of 31 (90%) with ischemic cardiomyopathy. The reported accuracy of MSCT is higher than that reported for SPECT perfusion imaging and SE in distinguishing the cause of dilated cardiomyopathy.

Multislice cardiac CT can also been used for the detection of coronary artery calcification (CAC). Radiologic detection of CAC *in vivo* by fluoroscopy was first described in the late 1950s. The Agaston score is the most widely used and best-established measure of CAC for assessment of the diagnostic and prognostic value of CAC scanning. Use of age-, gender- and race-specific threshold values has improved diagnostic accuracy of CAC scanning. Other measures, such as the volume score and calcium mass, are often reported, and may prove superior to the Agaston score but have been studied less well.

In both men and women presenting with chest pain, CAC detected by CT is highly sensitive for the presence of at least 50% of angiographic stenosis but is only moderately specific—especially in individuals over 60 years of age. The absence of CAC is highly predictive of the absence of CAD. CAC scanning has also been shown to have incremental value in risk stratification above Framingham score and serum biomarkers. Currently, the screening of asymptomatic patients should be limited to clinically selected patients with an intermediate 10-year risk of coronary heart disease (between 10% and 20%), where the result can potentially lead to a change in management based upon reclassification to a lower or higher risk group. Other potential clinical applications of CAC scanning include workup of dilated cardiomyopathy in low-risk patients and emergency department evaluation of chest pain.

A primary disadvantage of MSCT in general is the radiation exposure, estimated to be between 7 and 21 mSv depending on the generation of the MSCT and the use of radiation-reducing algorithms. Supporters of the technique point out that there is little excess radiation exposure compared with diagnostic invasive coronary angiography (>5 mSv). The MSCT radiation dose imparts a small but non-negligible increase in the lifetime risk of cancer. This risk varies markedly and is much greater for women and younger patient Introduction of scanning algorithms using ECG-dependent dose modulation during spiral scan and a reduced tube voltage have been successful in reducing the radiation dose. More importantly, dose reduction does not influence diagnostic image quality The need for iodinated contrast (60–120 mL) makes MSCT relatively contra-indicated in patients at risk for contrast-induced nephropathy or those with a history of allergy to contrast media.

The utility of MSCT is limited in certain patient populations in whom coronary segments cannot be visualized, or in whom the degree of stenosis cannot be assessed. These populations include older subjects or patients with chronic kidney disease with extensive coronary calcification, coronary stents or tortuous coronary arteries. As noted in the assessment by coronary computed tomographic angiography of individuals undergoing invasive coronary angiography (ACCURACY) trial, specificity was reduced in the presence of CAC (86 vs 53% for detection of ≤ 50% stenosis with calcium scores ≥ 400 vs > 400 Agaston units). Dense coronary calcification tends to lead to an overestimation of diameter stenosis. Other patient-related factors that can interfere with the image quality include obesity, tachycardia, irregular heart rhythms or those unable to cooperate or hold their breath for 10–15 s. These create 'stairstep artifacts' due to motion occurring between reconstruction of sequential heartbeats. MSCT also has lower sensitivity for exclusion of distal or branch vessel obstruction in segments less than 1.5 mm in size.

Multislice cardiac CT can be combined with PET and SPECT imaging. This combined approach would noninvasively provide comprehensive information (functional and anatomic) of the presence and physiological significance of the atherosclerotic coronary disease. It is conceivable that patients with known or suspected disease could be studied with sequential stress-rest perfusion imaging and CT angiography, allowing acquisition of superimposed images for the extent of abnormal coronary anatomy, perfusion and wall-motion abnormality. Early studies suggest that this hybrid modality has high sensitivity and specificity, and can add precision and confidence in deciding on the best therapeutic approach, reduce downstream unnecessary testing and be cost effective.

BIBLIOGRAPHY

1. Landay MJ, Mootz AR, Estrera AS. Apparatus seen on chest radiographs after cardiac surgery in adults. Radiology 1990; 174:477–482.
2. Wiener MD, Garay SM, Leitman BS, Wiener DN, Ravin CE. Imaging of the intensive care unit patient. Clin Chest Med 1991; 12:169–198.
3. Henry DA, Jolles H, Berberich JJ, Schmeizer V. The post-cardiac surgery chest radiograph: a clinically integrated approach. J Thorac Imaging 1989; 4:20–41.
4. Zarshenas Z, Sparschu RA. Catheter placement and misplacement. Crit Care Clin 1994; 10:417–436.
5. Trotman-Dickenson B. Radiology in the intensive care unit (part I). J Intensive Care Med 2003; 18:198–210.

6. Trotman-Dickenson B. Radiology in the intensive care unit (part 2). J Intensive Care Med 2003; 18:239–252.
7. Henschke CI, Yankelevitz DF, Wand A, Davis SD, Shiau M. Chest radiography in the ICU. Clin Imaging 1997; 21:90–103.
8. Swensen SJ, Peters SG, LeRoy AJ, Gay PC, Sykes MW, Tastek VF. Radiology in the intensive-care unit. Mayo Clin Proc 1991; 66:396–410.
9. Maffessanti M, Berlot G, Bortolotto P. Chest roentgenology in the intensive care unit: an overview. Eur Radiol 1998; 8:69–78.
10. Therasse E, Oliva VL, Lafontaine E, Perreault P, Giroux M, Soulez G. Balloon dilatation and stent placement for esophageal lesions: indication, methods, and results. RadioGraphics 2003; 23:89–105.
11. Funaki B. Central venous access: a primer for the diagnostic radiologist. AJR Am J Roentgenol 2002; 179:309–318.
12. Vesely TM. Central venous catheter tip position: a continuing controversy. J Vasc Interv Radiol 2003; 14:527–534.
13. Katz JD, Cronau LH, Barash PG, Mandel SD. Pulmonary artery flow-guided catheters in the perioperative period: indications and complications. JAMA 1977; 237:2832–2834.
14. McLoud TC, Putman CE. Radiology of the Swan-Ganz catheter and associated pulmonary complications. Radiology 1975; 116:19–22.
15. Richard C, Warszawski J, Anguel N, et al. Early use of the pulmonary artery catheter and outcomes in patients with shock and acute respiratory distress syndrome: a randomized controlled trial. JAMA 2003; 290:2713–2720.
16. Fowler RA, Cook DJ. The arc of the pulmonary artery catheter. JAMA 2003; 290:2732–2734.
17. Dunbar RD, Mitchell R, Lavine M. Aberrant location of central venous catheters. Lancet 1981; 1:711–715.
18. Henry DA, LeBolt S. Invasive hemodynamic monitoring: radiologist's perspective. RadioGraphics 1986; 6:535–572.
19. Knutstad K, Hager B, Hauser M. Radiologic diagnosis and management of complications related to central venous access. Acta Radiol 2003; 44:508–516.
20. McGee DC, Gould MK. Preventing complications of central venous catheterization. N Engl J Med 2003; 348:1123–1133.
21. Hinke DH, Zandt-Stastny DA, Goodman LR, Quebbeman EJ, Krzywda EA, Andris DA. Pinch off syndrome: a complication of implantable subclavian venous access devices. Radiology 1990; 177:353–356.
22. Hunt R, Hunter TB. Cardiac tamponade and death from perforation of the right atrium by a central venous catheter (letter). AJR Am J Roentgenol 1988; 151:1250.
23. Landay MJ, Estrera AS, Bordlee RP. Cardiac valve reconstruction and replacement: a brief review. RadioGraphics 1992; 12:659–671.
24. Bodner E, Frater R, eds. Replacement cardiac valves New York, NY: McGraw-Hill, 1992.
25. Mandell VS, Nimkin K, Hoffer FA, Bridges ND. Devices for transcatheter closure of intracardiac defects. AJR Am J Roentgenol 1993; 160:179–184.
26. Bejvan SM, Ephron JH, Takasugi JE, Godwin JD, Brady GH. Imaging of cardiac pacemakers. AJR Am J Roentgenol 1997; 169:1371–1379.
27. Cascade PN, Sneider MB, Koelling TM, Knight BP. Radiographic appearance of biventricular pacing for the treatment of heart failure. AJR Am J Roentgenol 2001; 177:1447–1450.
28. Auricchio A, Abraham WT. Cardiac resynchronization therapy: current state of the art: cost versus benefit. Circulation 2004; 109:300–307.

5 Interpretations in Pediatric Electrocardiography

BACKGROUND

- At birth, the right ventricle is larger and thicker than the left ventricle, reflecting the greater physiological stresses placed upon it in utero (i.e. pumping blood through the relatively high-resistance pulmonary circulation).
- This produces an ECG picture reminiscent of right ventricular hypertrophy in the adult: marked rightward axis, dominant R-wave in V1 and T-wave inversions in V1-3 (Tables 5.1 to 5.3).
- Conduction intervals (PR interval, QRS duration) are shorter than adults due to the smaller cardiac size.
- Heart rates are much faster in neonates and infants, decreasing as the child grows older.

Common Findings on the Pediatric ECG

The following electrocardiographic features may be normal in children (Tables 5.3 to 5.5):

- Heart rate >100 beats/min
- Rightward QRS axis > +90°
- T-wave inversions in V1–3 ("juvenile T-wave pattern")
- Dominant R-wave in V1
- RSR pattern in V1
- Marked sinus arrhythmia
- Short PR interval (<120 ms) and QRS duration (<80 ms)
- Slightly peaked P-waves (< 3 mm in height is normal if >6 months)
- Slightly long QTc (>490 ms in infants >6 months)
- Q waves in the inferior and left precordial leads.

This ECG of a healthy 2-year-old boy displays many of the typical features of the pediatric ECG:

- Heart rate of 110 bpm (normal for age).
- Dominant R-waves in V1–3.
- RSR pattern [partial (RBBB) morphology] in V1. Juvenile T-wave pattern (T-wave inversion in V1–V3).

Stepwise Assessment of the ECG

Rhythm (Fig. 5.14)

Sinus: Atrial depolarization starts from the sinoatrial node. This requires:

- P-wave preceding each QRS complex, with a constant PR interval.
- Normal P-wave axis (zero to +90°), i.e. P-wave is upright in leads I and aVF.

Nonsinus: Some atrial rhythms may have P-waves in front of every QRS but with an abnormal P-axis (inverted in lead II).

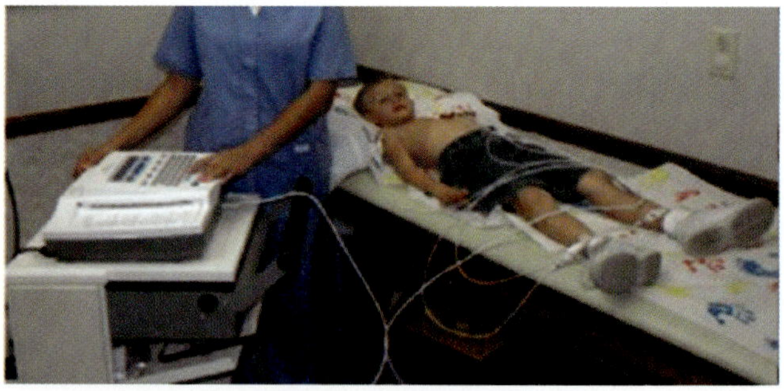

Fig. 5.1: *Electrocardiographic equipment along with precardial leads over the chest prior to obtaining an electrocardiogram ECG*

HEART RATE

Usual paper speed is 25 mm/sec. So, 1 mm (small square) = 0.04 sec, and 5 mm (big square) = 0.2 sec. Calculate atrial and ventricular rates separately if different. Many methods to estimate the rate, for example:

- *For regular rhythms:* 300/number of large squares in between each consecutive R-wave.
- *For very fast rates:* 1,500/number of small squares in between each consecutive R-wave.
- *For irregular rhythms:* Number of complexes on the rhythm strip × 6 (Fig. 5.9).

[Or just use the computer reading]

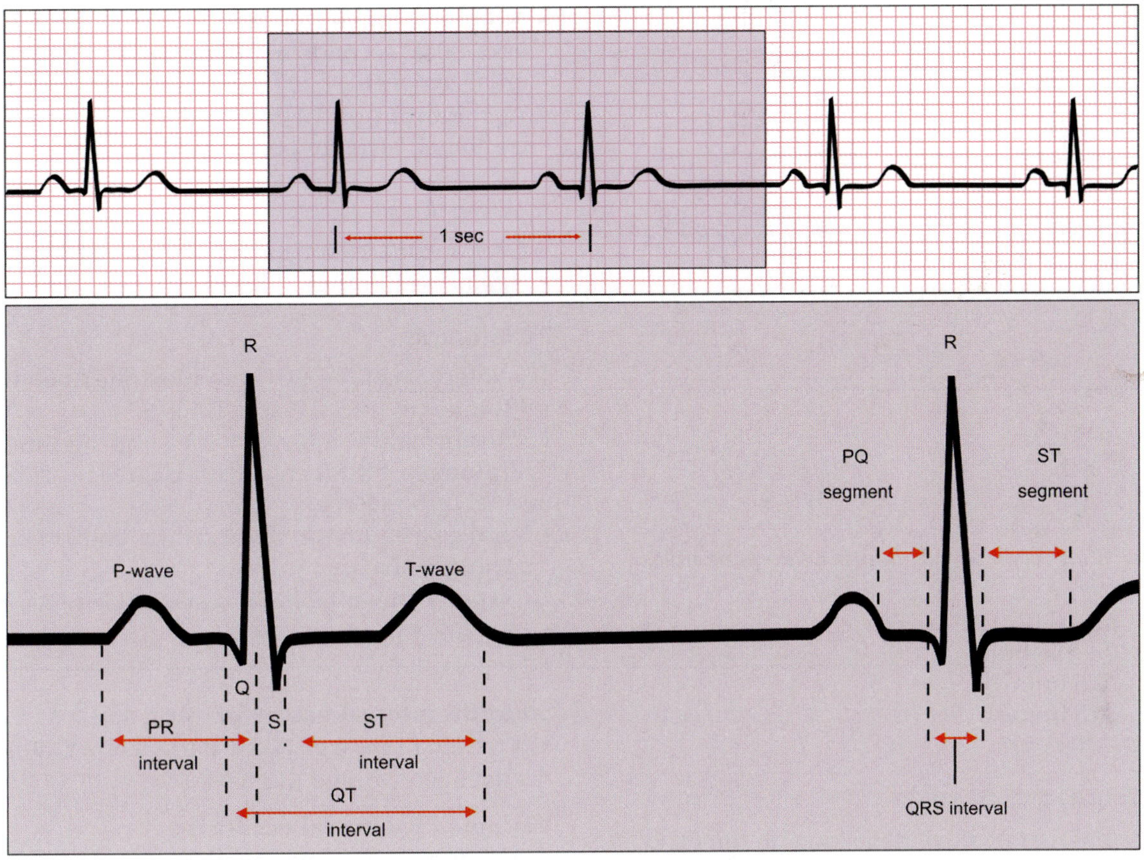

Fig. 5.2: *Diagram showing various waves and intervals above and below the isoelectric line as seen on ECG in a normal individuals*

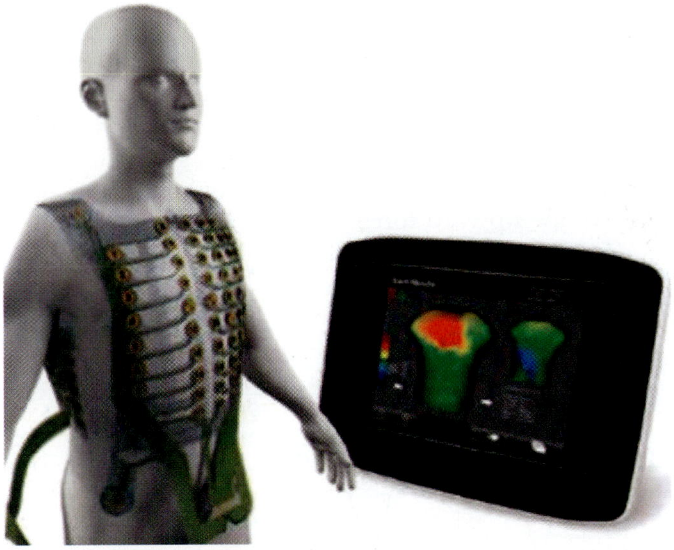

Fig. 5.3: *Heartscape 80-lead 3D ECG system; Heartscape 80-lead 3D ECG System. The concept is not entirely new, as it is the successor to the PRIME ECG system which has the same amount of leads, and has been available since 2003. The Heartscape 3D ECG system aims to give a 360° electrocardiographic view of the heart, to helping in identifying myocardial infarcts without ST-segment elevation on traditional 12-lead ECGs, and in patients with left bundle-branch block. Compared to traditional 12-lead ECG's, the system has shown to be more sensitive while retaining comparable specificity in detecting acute infarcts*

Table 5.1: *Successful use of pediatric electrocardiography*

- Be aware of age-related difference in the indications for performing electrocardiography, the normal ranges for electrocardiographic variables, and the typical abnormalities in infants and children
- Genuine abnormality is unusal if abnormality is suspected, seek a specialist opinion.

Table 5.2: *Indications for pediatric electrocardiography*

• Syncope or seizure	• Electrolyte disturbance
• Exertional symptoms	• Kawasaki disease
• Drug ingestion	• Rheumatic fever
• Tachyarrhythmia	• Myocarditis
• Bradyarrhythmia	• Myocardial contusion
• Cyanotic episodes	• Pericarditis
• Heart failure	• Postcardiac surgery
• Hypothermia	• Congenital heart defects

Table 5.3: *Pediatric electrocardiographic findings that may be normal*

- Heart rate > 100 beats/min
- QRS axis > 90°
- Right precordial T-wave inversion
- Dominant right precordial R-waves
- Short PR and QT intervals
- Short P-wave and short duration of QRS complexes
- Inferior and lateral Q-waves

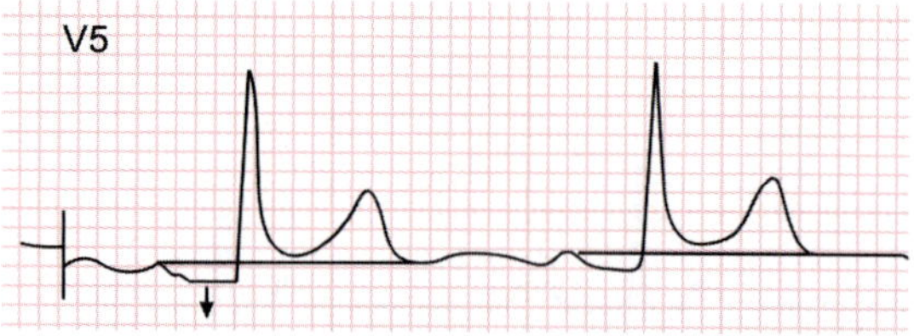

Fig. 5.4: *PR segment depression in V5 due to acute pericarditis*

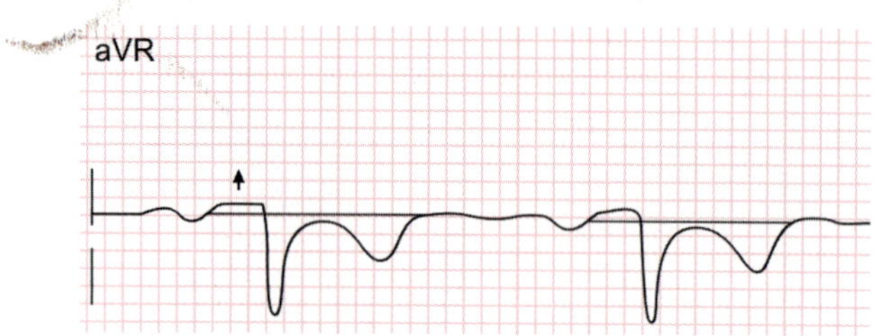

Fig. 5.5: *PR elevation in aVR due to acute pericarditis*

Resting heart rate (HR) varies with age:
- *Newborn:* 110 – 150 bpm
- *2 years:* 85 – 125 bpm
- *4 years:* 75 – 115 bpm
- *6 years+:* 60 – 100 bpm.

P-Wave (Figs 5.10 to 5.31)

The P wave is the first positive deflection on the ECG
- It represents atrial depolarization.

Morphology

- Smooth contour
- Monophasic in lead II (Fig. 5.14)
- Often biphasic in V1 (Fig. 5.20).

Axis

- Normal P-wave axis is between 0° and +75°.

P-Wave Amplitude and Duration

- Normal P-wave amplitude is < 3 mm (tall P-waves = right atrial enlargement) (Figs 5.12 to 5.15).
- Normal P-wave duration is < 0.09 seconds in children and < 0.07 seconds in infants (wide P-waves = left atrial enlargement).
- A combination of tall and wide P-waves occurs in combined atrial hypertophy (Figs 5.10 and 5.11).

P-Wave Axis

- *Over 3 years:* + 60° (range: +20° to +120°)
- *Adult:* + 50° (range: –30° to 105°)

PR Intervals

The intervals of the ECG are illustrated below:
- PR interval (Fig. 5.2 and Table 5.5)
- The normal PR interval varies with age and heart rate

Prolonged PR interval (first degree heart block) may be normal or be seen in:
- Viral or rheumatic myocarditis and other myocardial dysfunctions
- Certain congenital heart disease (Ebsteins, ECD, ASD)
- Digitalis toxicity
- Hyperkalemia

Short PR interval occurs in:
- Preexcitation (e.g. Wolff-Parkinson-White)
- Glycogen storage disease

Variable PR interval occurs in:
- Wandering atrial pacemaker
- Wenckebach (Mobitz type 1) second degree heart block.

QRS Axis

Calculated using the hexaxial reference system that shows the frontal view of the electrical activity of the heart via the six limb leads (Figs 5.5 and 5.8)
- In lead 1, the R-wave represents the leftward force, the S-wave the rightward force.
- In aVF, the R-wave represents the downward force, the S-wave the upward force.

A suggested method of axis calculation: the successive approximation method.

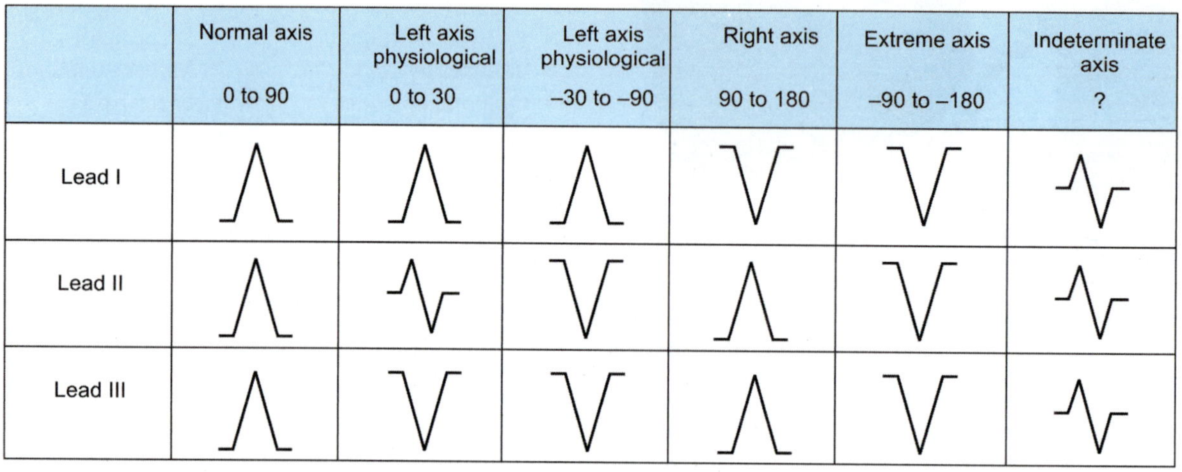

Fig. 5.6: *Determination of axis with the help of leads 11 and 111*

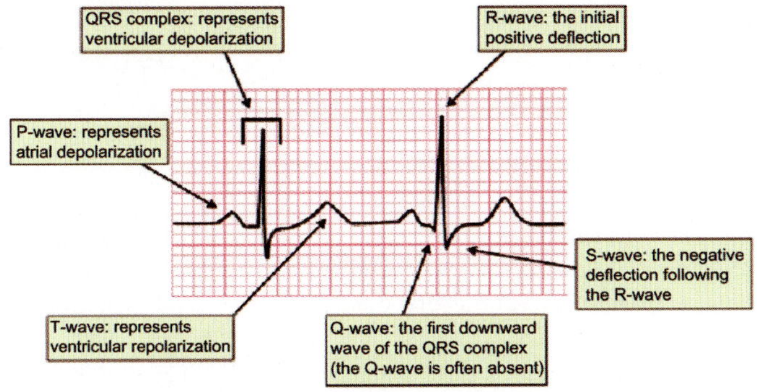

Fig. 5.7: *Graphic representation of genesis of various PQRST-waves as recordede on standard surface ECG*

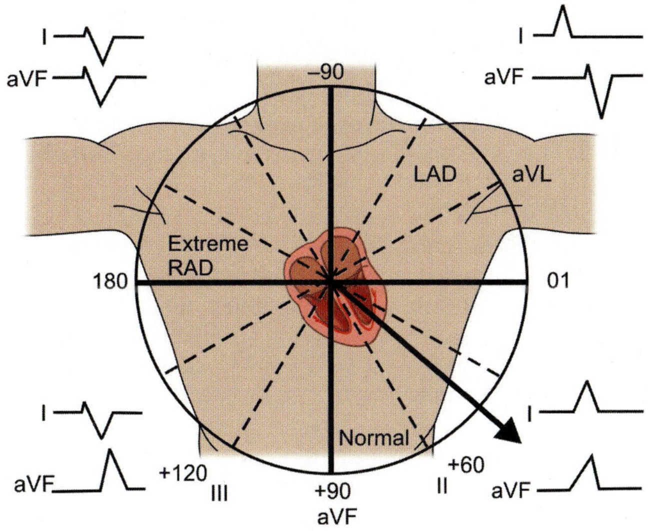

Fig. 5.8: *Graphic representation of axis deviation. ECG representations of each type of axis are shown in each quadrant. Large arrow indicates normal axis*

Normal QRS Axis Varies with Age

- *1 week – 1 month:* + 110° (range: +30° to +180°)
- *1 month – 3 months:* + 70° (range: +10° to +125°)
- *3 months – 3 years:* + 60° (range: +10° to +110°).

Table 5.4: *Normal values of different waves, segments, complexes, intervals, rhythm and conduction abnormalities*

P wave	• Left atrial enlargement: negative portion of the P-wave in lead V1 more than 0.1 mV in depth and more than 0.04 s in duration • Right atrial enlargement: peaked P-wave in leads II and III or V1 more than 0.25 mV in amplitude
QRS complex	• Frontal plane axis deviation: right more than +120° or left –30° to –90° • Increased voltage: amplitude of R or S-wave in in a standard lead more than 2 mV, S-wave in lead V1 or V2 more than 3 mV, or R-wave in lead V5 or V6 more than 3 mV • Abnormal Q-waves more than 0.04s in duration or more than 25% of the height of the ensuing R-wave or QS pattern in two or more leads • Right or left bundle branch-block with QRS duration more than 0.12s • R or R-wave in lead V1 more than 0.5 mV in amplitude and R/S ratio more than 1.
ST-segment T-waves, and QT interval	• ST-segment depression or T-wave flattening or inversion in two or more leads • Prolongation of heart rate corrected QT interval (QTc) more than 0.44s in males and more than 0.46s in females.[c]
Rhythm and conduction abnormalities	• Premature ventricular beats or more severe ventricular arrhythmias • Supraventricular tachycardias, atrial flutter, or atrial fibrillation • Short PR interval (less than 0.12s) with or without "delta" wave • Sinus bradycardia with resting heart rate less than 40 beats/min[a] • First (PR more than 0.21s)[b], second or third degree atrioventricular block.

[a]Increasing less than 100 beats/min during limited exercise test.
[b]Not shortening with hyperventilation or limited exercise test.
[c]A recent study suggests athletes with a QTc > 500 ms should be recommended not to participate in competitive sports.

QRS Duration

QRS duration varies with age: (Fig. 5.8 and Table 5.4)

Prolonged QRS is characteristic of ventricular conduction disturbances:

- Bundle-branch blocks
- Preexcitation conditions (e.g. WPW)
- Intraventricular block
- Ventricular arrhythmias (Fig. 5.19)

QRS Amplitude (Voltages)

High QRS amplitudes are found in:

- Ventricular hypertrophy (Figs 5.33, 5.40 and 5.47)
- Ventricular conduction disturbances, e.g. BBB's, WPW (Figs 5.12 and 5.40)

Low QRS amplitudes are seen in:

- Pericarditis
- Myocarditis
- Hypothyroidism
- Normal newborns.

Ventricular hypertrophy produces changes in one or more of the following areas: the QRS axis, the QRS voltages, the R/S ratio or the T axis.

Table 5.5: *Waves and intervals*

RR interval	The interval between an R-wave and the next R-wave. Normal resting heart rate is between 60 and 100 bpm	0.6–1.2s
P-wave	During normal atrial depolarization, the main electrical vector is directed from the SA node toward the AV node, and spreads from the right atrium to the left atrium. This turns into the P wave on the ECG.	80 ms
PR intervals	The PR interval is measured from the beginning of the P wave to the beginning of the QRS complex. The PR interval reflects the time the electrical impulse takes to travel from the sinus node through the AV node and entering the ventricles. The PR interval is therefore a good estimate of AV node function.	120–200 ms
PR segment	The PR segment connects the P-wave and the QRS complex. This coincides with the electrical conduction from the AV node to the bundle of His to the bundle branches and then to the Purkinje fibers. This electrical activity does not produce a contraction directly and is merely traveling down toward the ventricles and this shows up flat on the ECG. The PR interval is more clinically relevant.	50–120 ms
QRS complex	The QRS complex reflects the rapid depolarization of the right and left ventricles. They have a large muscle mass compared to the atria and so the QRS complex usually has a much larger amplitude than the P-wave.	80–120 ms
J-point	The point at which the QRS complex finishes and the ST segment begins. Used to measure the degree of ST elevation or depression present.	N/A
ST segment	The ST segment connects the QRS complex and the T-wave. The ST segment represents the period when the ventricles are depolarized. It is isoelectric.	80–120 ms
T-wave	The T-wave represents the repolarization (or recovery) of the ventricles. The interval from the beginning of the QRS complex to the apex of the T-wave is referred to as the absolute refractory period. The last half of the T-wave is referred to as the relative refractory period (or vulnerable period).	160 ms
ST interval	The ST interval is measured from the J point to the end of the T-wave.	320 ms
QT interval	The QT interval is measured from the beginning of the QRS complex to the end of the T-wave. A prolonged QT interval is a risk factor for ventricular tachyarrhythmias and sudden death. It varies with heart rate and for clinical relevance requires a correction for this, giving the QTc.	300–430 ms
U-wave	The U-wave is hypothesized to be caused by the repolarization of the interventricular septum. They normally have a low amplitude, and even more often completely absent. They always follow the T-wave and also follow the same direction in amplitude. If they are too prominent we suspect hypokalemia, hypercalcemia or hyperthyroidism usually.	
J-wave	The J-wave elevated J-point or Osborn Wave appears as a late delta wave following the QRS or as a small secondary R-wave. It is considered pathognomonic of hypothermia or hypokalcemia.	

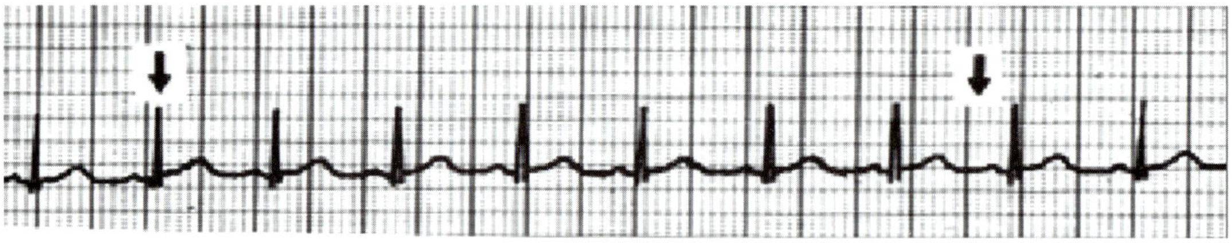

Fig. 5.9: *Showing heart rate of 134 per minute. There are about 6.7 cardiac cycles between the two markers (3.0 seconds) in the top margin of the ECG paper. Therefore, the heart rate is 6.7 × 20 = 134*

Right Ventricular Hypertrophy

Axis: RAD for the patients age (Fig. 5.48).

Voltages:

- Tall R-waves (greater than limits for patient's age) in right-sided leads V4R and V1.
- Deep S-waves (greater than limits for patient's age) in left-sided leads V5 and V6.

R/S ratio: Abnormal R/S ratio in favour of RVH.

- Increased R/S ratio (greater than upper limits for child's age) in V1–2.
- R/S ratio < 1 in V6 (after one month of age).

Left Ventricular Hypertrophy

Axis: LAD for the patients age (marked LAD is rare with LVH) (Figs 5.32 and 5.59).

Voltages:

- Tall R-waves in the left-sided leads V5 and V6 (greater than limits for patient's age).

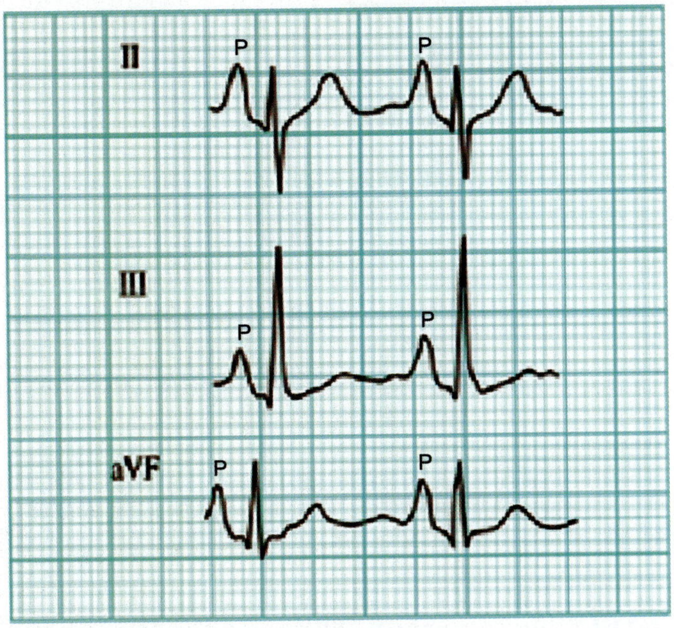

Fig. 5.10: *Large P-waves in leads II, III, and aVF (P pulmonale)*

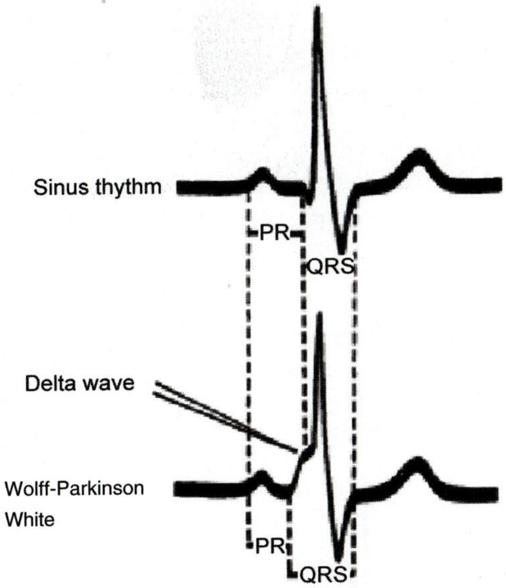

Fig. 5.12: *Normal PQRST morphology and normal intervals (upper panel) and features of WPW syndrome with short PR interval, wide QRS duration, delta wave and normal QRS duration collectively (lower panel)*

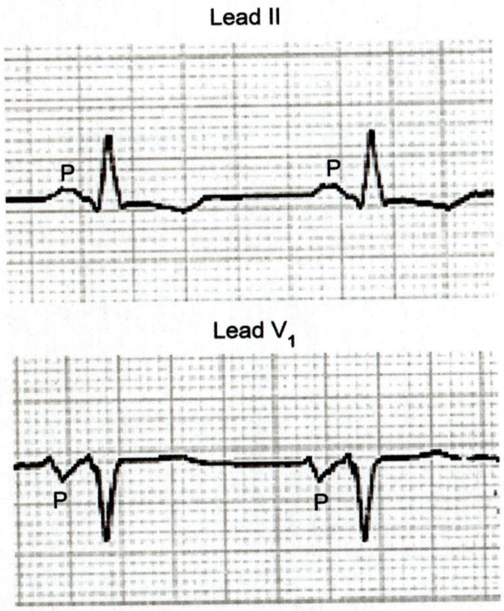

Fig. 5.11: *Left atrial enlargement: in leads II and V1- LAE is best seen in V1 with a prominent negative (posterior) component measuring 1 mm wide and 1 mm deep*

- Deep S-waves in the right-sided leads V4R and V1 (greater than limits for patient's age).
  R/S ratio: Abnormal R/S ratio in favor of LV.
- Decreased R/S ratio in V1-2 (less than upper limits for child's age)
  - Abnormal Q-waves in V5 and V6
  - Inverted T-waves in I and aVL (LV strain pattern)
  - Compare this with the criteria for LVH in adults.

Biventricular Hypertrophy

- Positive voltage criteria for RVH and LVH (with normal QRS duration).
- Positive voltage criteria for RVH or LVH and relatively large voltages for other ventricle.
- Large equiphasic QRS complexes in two or more limb leads and in mid-precordial leads (V2-5).

ST Segment

- The normal ST is isoelectric. Elevation or depression is judged in relation to the TP segment (Fig. 5.39).
- Some ST changes may be normal:

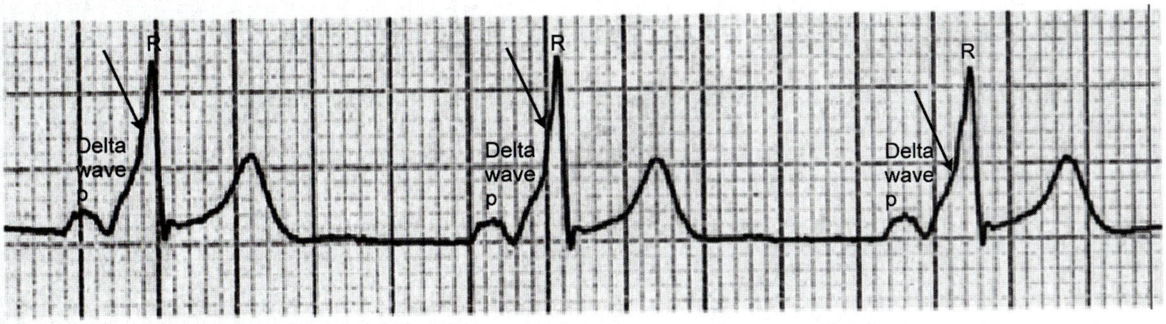

Fig. 5.13: *Short PR (<120 ms), broad QRS and delta waves in WPW syndrome*

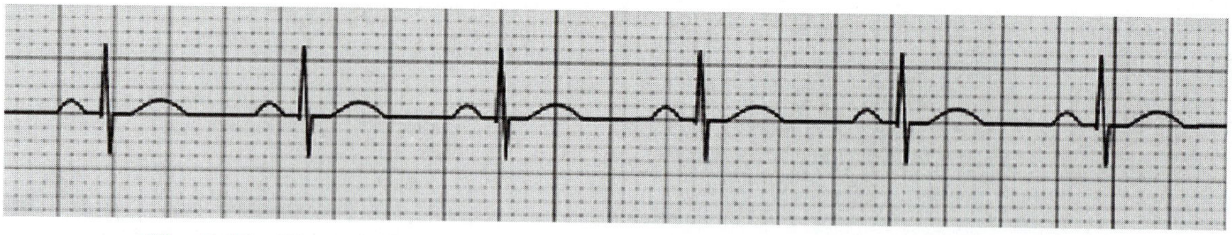

Fig. 5.14: *Sinus rhythm: each narrow complex is preceded by a normal P-wave*

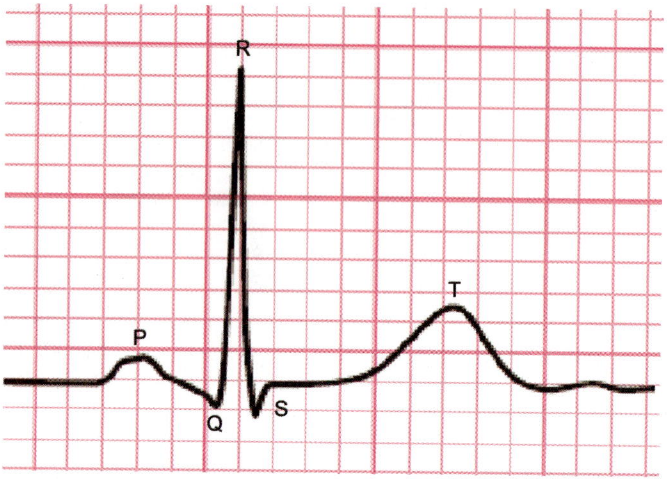

Fig. 5.15: *Normal monophasic P-wave in lead II*

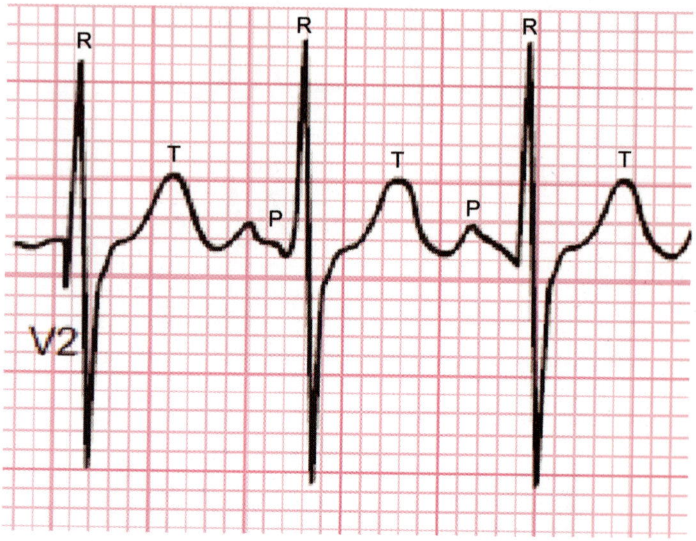

Fig. 5.17: *Peaked P-wave > 1.5 mm in V2*

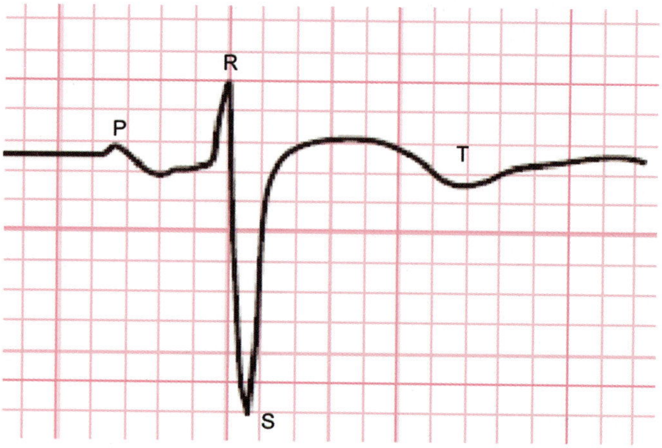

Fig. 5.16: *Normal biphasic P-wave in V1*

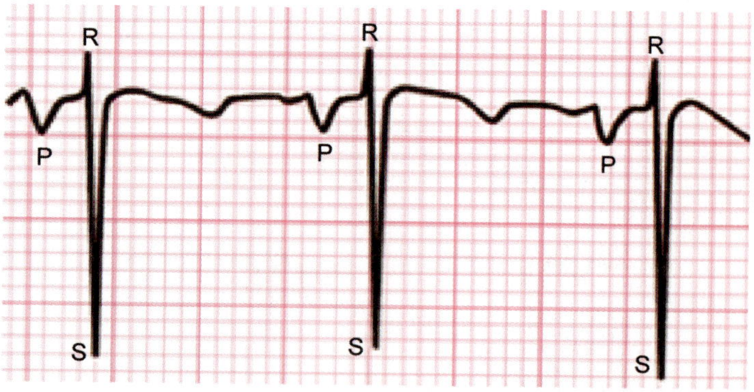

Fig. 5.18: *Biphasic P-waves in V1 with terminal negative portion > 1 mm deep*

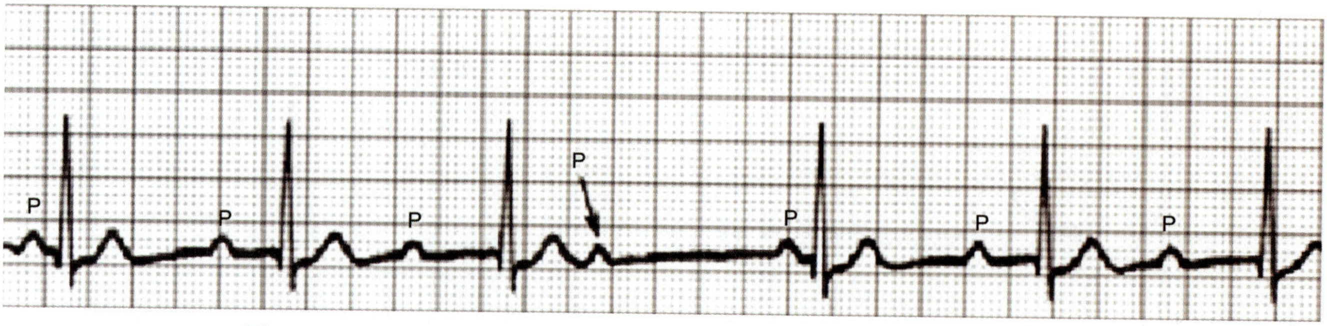

Fig. 5.19: *Progressive lengthening of PR interval till beat is dropped (arrow)*

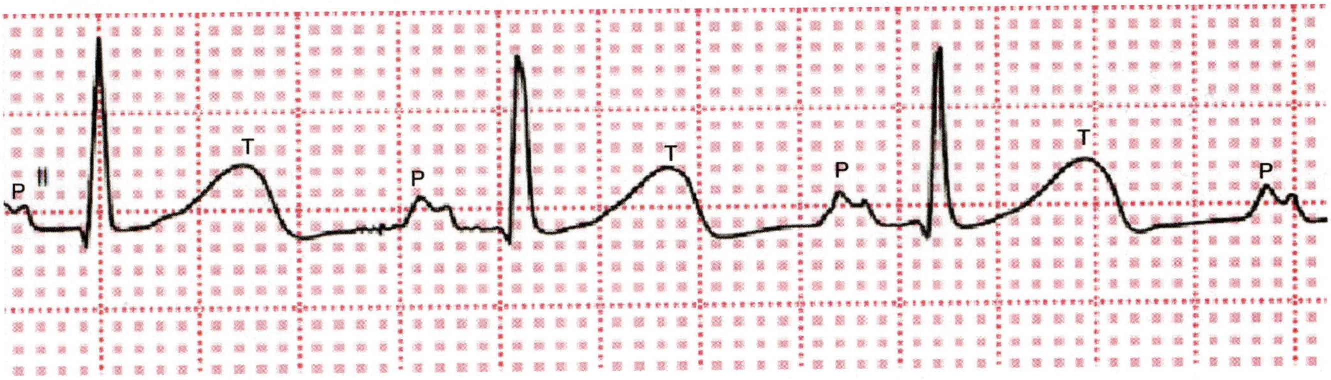

Fig. 5.20: *Bifid P-waves in lead II with > 40 ms between the peaks, total P-wave duration > 110 ms*

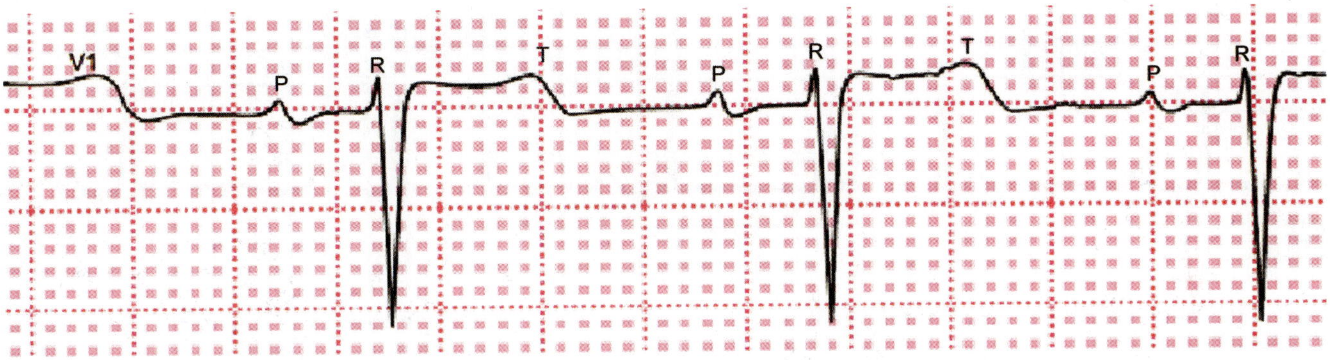

Fig. 5.21: *Biphasic P-waves in V1 with terminal negative portion > 40 ms duration*

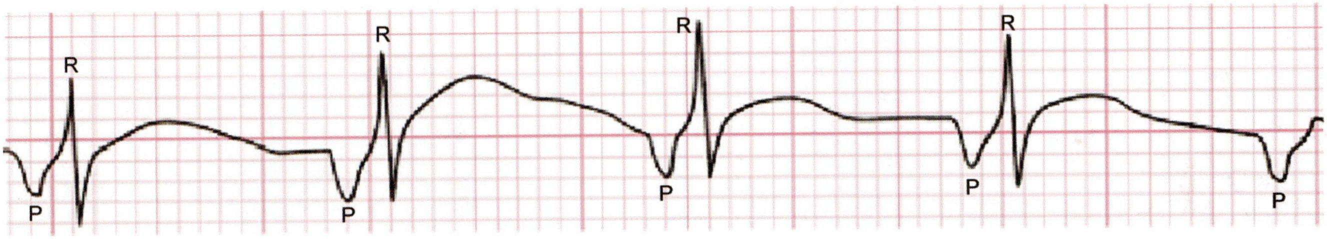

Fig. 5.22: *Accelerated junctional rhythm*

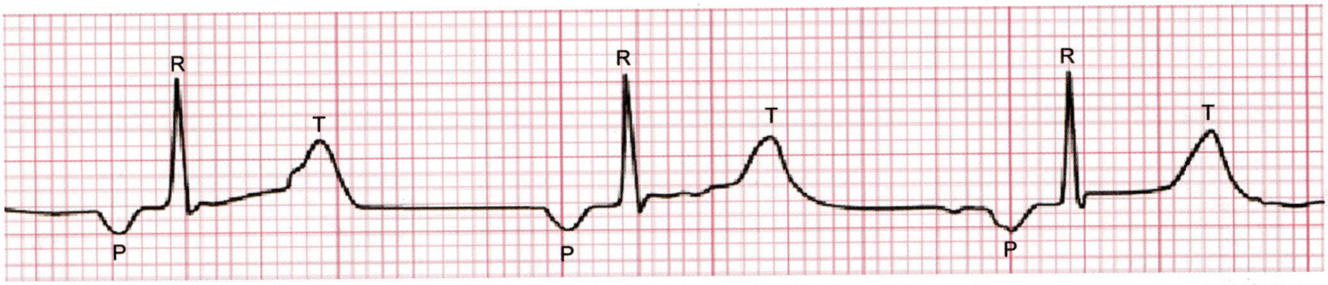

Fig. 5.23: *Accelerated junctional rhythm*

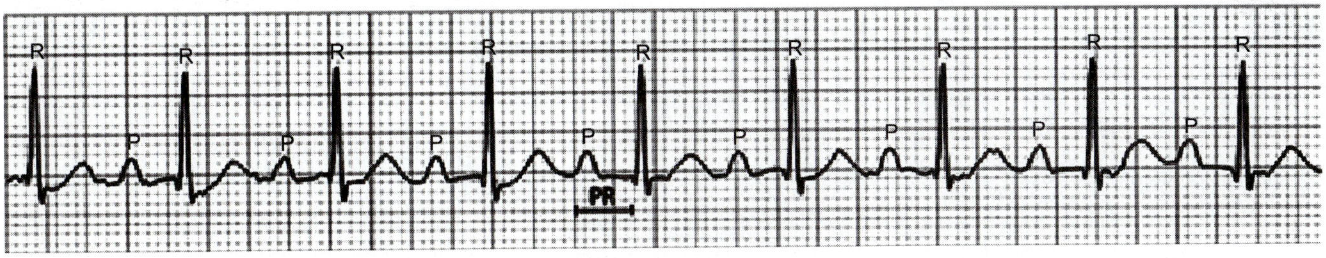

Fig. 5.24: *First degree heart block (PR interval > 200 ms)*

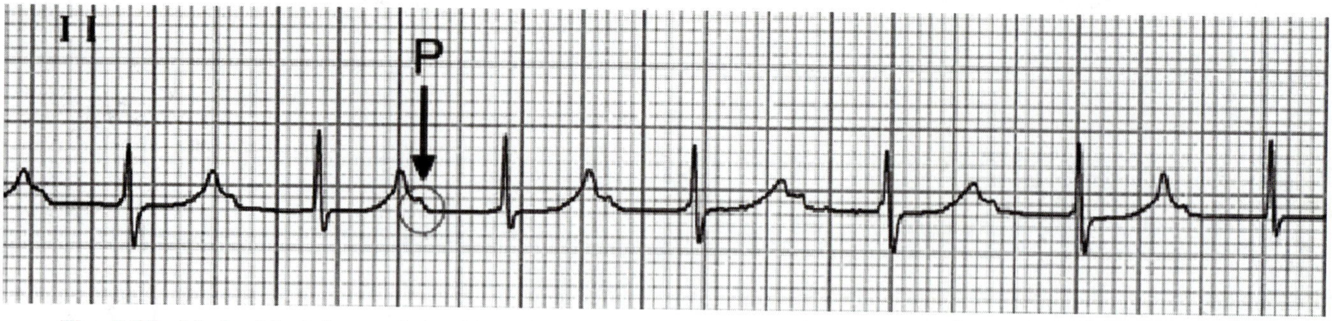

Fig. 5.25: *Marked first degree heart block (PR interval > 300 ms, P-waves are buried in the preceding T-wave)*

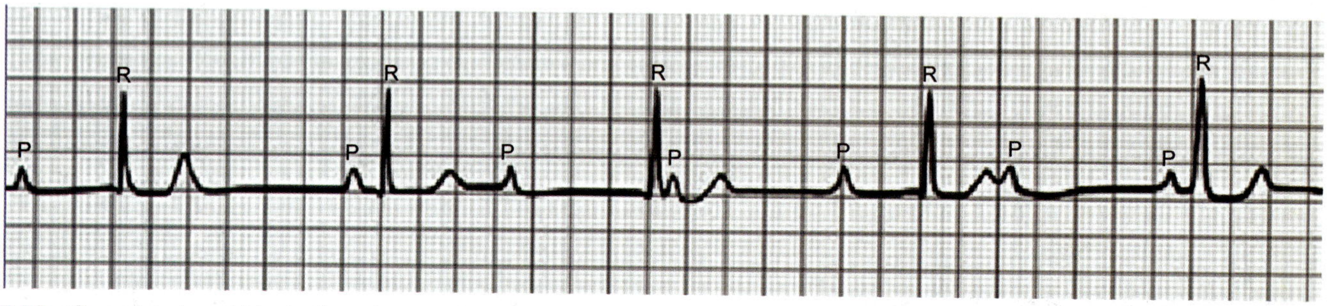

Fig. 5.26: *Complete heart block, there is complete absence of AV conduction—none of the supraventricular impulses are conducted to the ventricles*

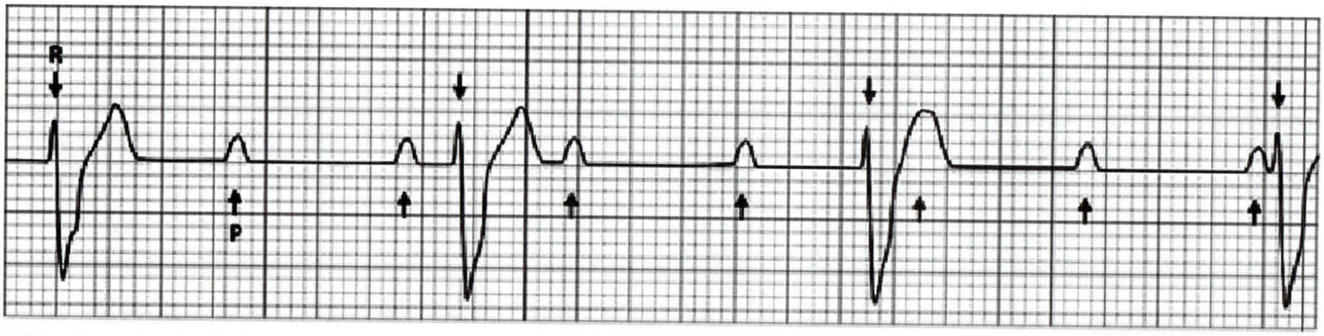

Fig. 5.27: *Complete heart block 3rd degree heart block. The atrial rate is approximately 100 bpm. The ventricular rate is approximately 40 bpm. The two rates are independent; there is no evidence that any of the atrial impulse are conducted to the ventricles*

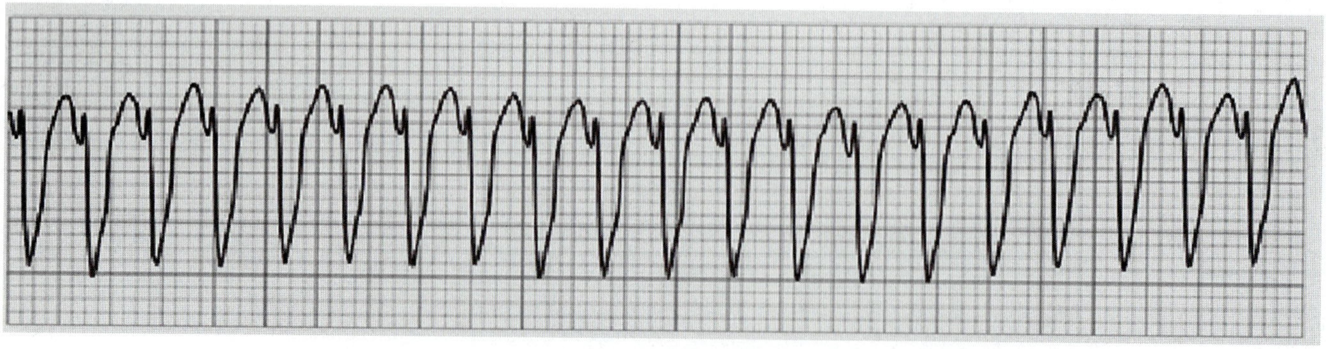

Fig. 5.28: *Ventricular tachycardia: broad QRS complexes with no visible P-waves*

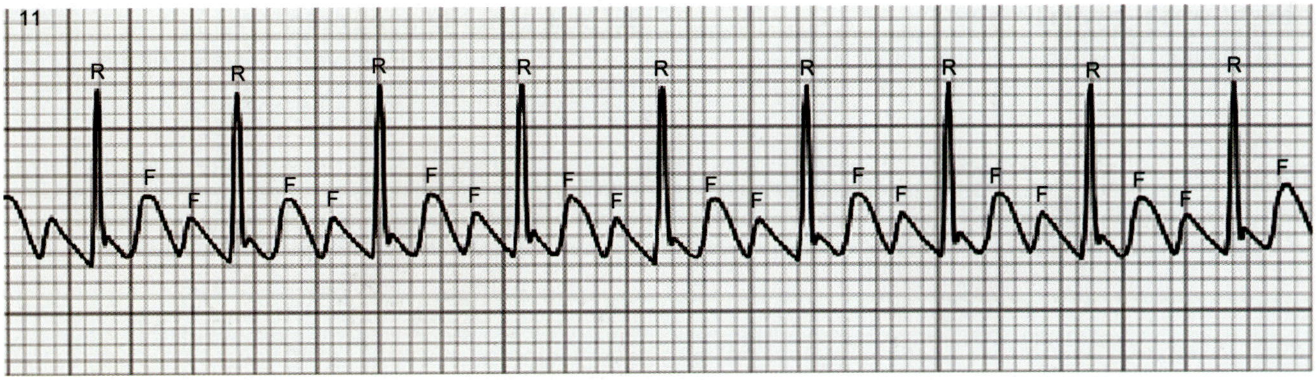

Fig. 5.29: *Atrial flutter: narrow QRS complexes are associated with regular flutter waves*

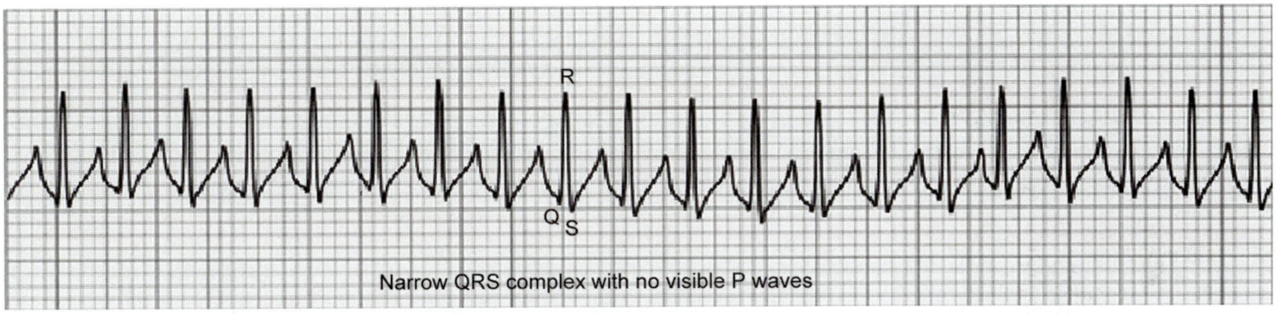

Fig. 5.30: *Junctional tachycardia: narrow QRS complexes with no visible P-waves*

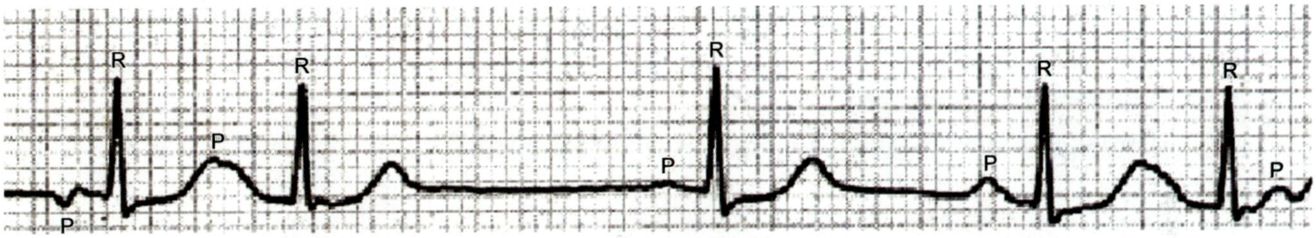

Fig. 5.31: *Multifocal atrial rhythm*

Table 5.6: *Normal values in pediatric electrocardiograms*

Age	*PR interval (ms)*	*QRS duration (ms)*	*R-wave (S-wave) amplitude (mm)*	
			Lead VI	*Lead V6*
Birth	80–160	<75	5–26 (1–23)	0–12 (0–10)
6 months	70–150	<75	3–20 (1–17)	6–22 (0–10)
1 year	70–150	<75	2–20 (1–20)	6–23 (0–7)
5 years	80–160	<80	1–16 (2–22)	8–25 (0–5)
10 years	90–170	<85	1–12 (3–25)	9–26 (0–4)

- Limb lead ST depression or elevation of up to 1–2 mm in the left precordial leads).
- *J-point depression:* The J-point (junction between the QRS and ST segment) is depressed without sustained ST depression, i.e. upsloping ST depression.
- *Early repolarisation in adolescents:* The ST segment is elevated and concave in leads with an upright T-wave. (Fig. 5.39).

Others are Pathological

- A downward slope of the ST followed by a biphasic inverted T.
- A sustained horizontal ST segment depression 0.08 sec or longer.
- A = Upsloping ST depression/J-point depression (normal variant)

1. **Right atrial hypertrophy**
   tall, peaked P-wave in leads I and II

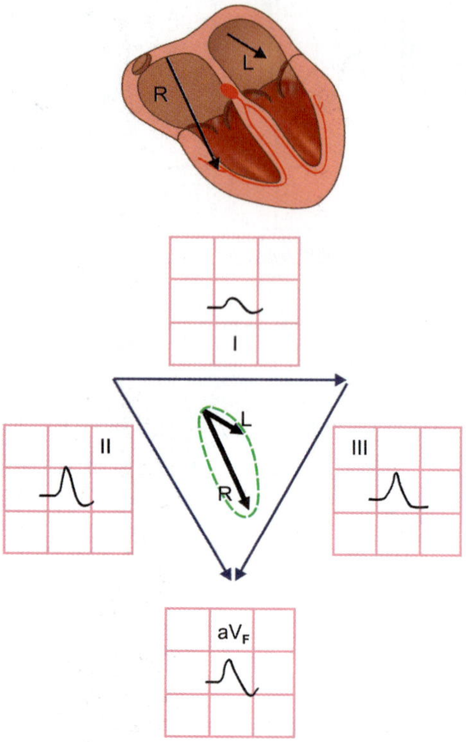

2. **Left atrial hypertrophy**
   Wide, notched P-wave in lead II, diphasic P wave in Vi

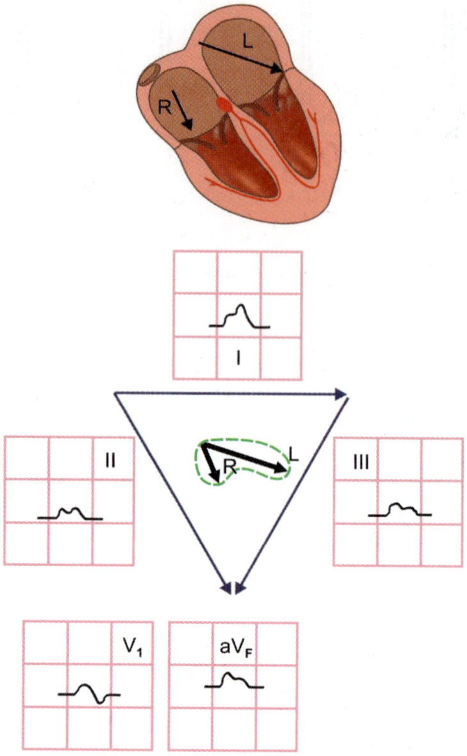

3. **Left ventricular hypertrophy**
   large S-wave in leads V1 and V2, large R-wave in V5 and V6

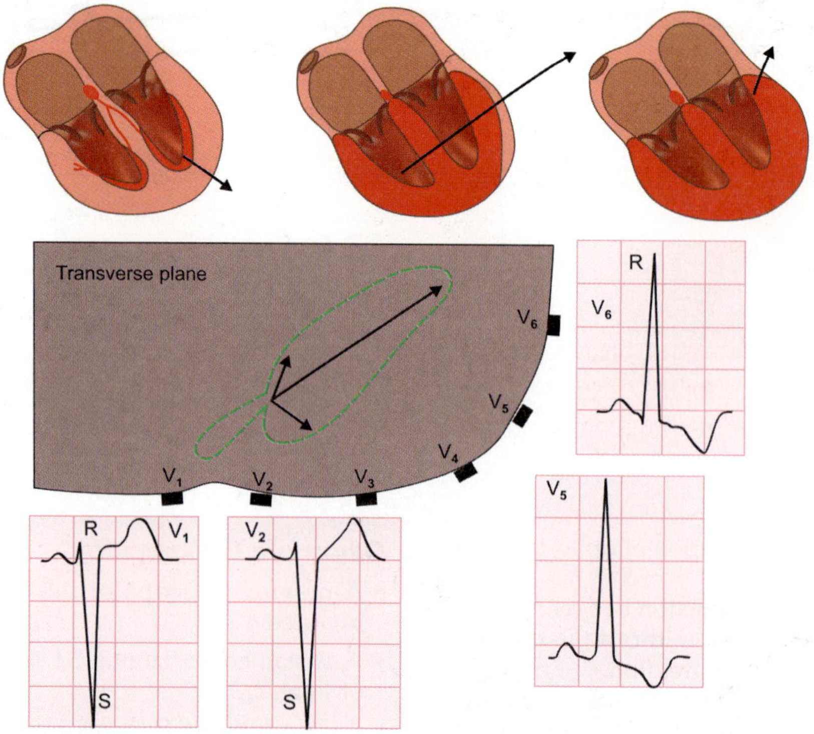

Fig. 5.32: *Illustrations (1–3) showing right atrial, left atrial and left ventricular hypertrophics*

- B = Downsloping ST depression (usually abnormal)
- C = Horizontal ST depression (usually abnormal).

Pathological ST segment changes are commonly associated with T-wave changes and occur in:

- Pericarditis (Figs 5.4 and 5.5).
- Myocardial ischemia or infarction (Figs 5.37, 5.38 and 5.45)
- Severe ventricular hypertrophy (ventricular strain pattern).
- Digitalis effect (Figs 5.51, 5.52 and 5.62).

T-Waves

The precordial T-wave configuration changes over time:

- For the first week of life, T-waves are upright throughout the precordial leads.
- After the first week, the T-waves become inverted in V1–3 (= the "juvenile T-wave pattern")
- This T-wave inversion usually remains until ~ age 8; thereafter the T-waves become upright in V1-3.
- However, the juvenile T-wave pattern can persist into adolescence and early adulthood (= "persistent juvenile T-waves").

Tall, peaked T waves are seen in:

- Hyperkalemia
- LVH (volume overload)
- Benign early repolarization

Flat T-waves are seen in:

- Normal newborns
- Hypothyroidism
- Hypokalemia
- Digitalis
- Pericarditis
- Myocarditis
- Myocardial ischemia.

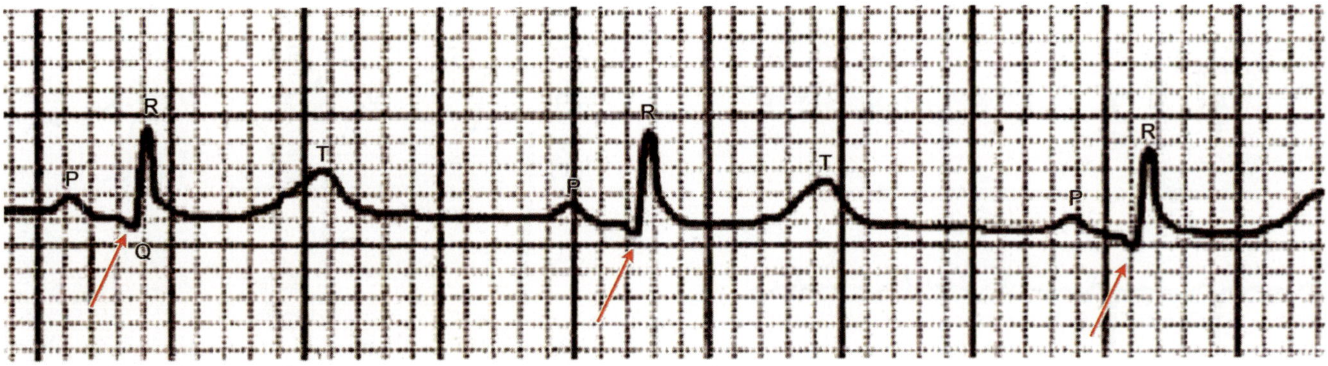

Fig. 5.33: *Normal Q-wave in V6*

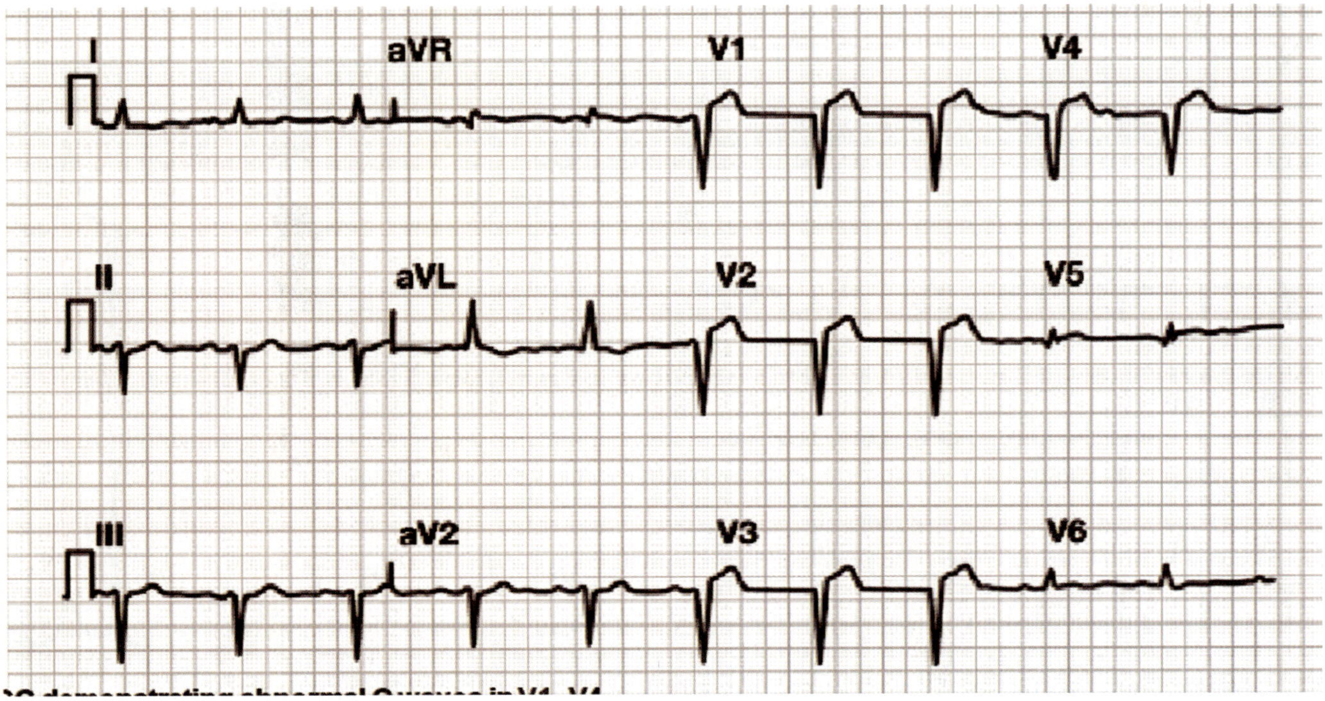

Fig. 5.34: *ECG demonstrating abnormal Q-waves in V1–4*

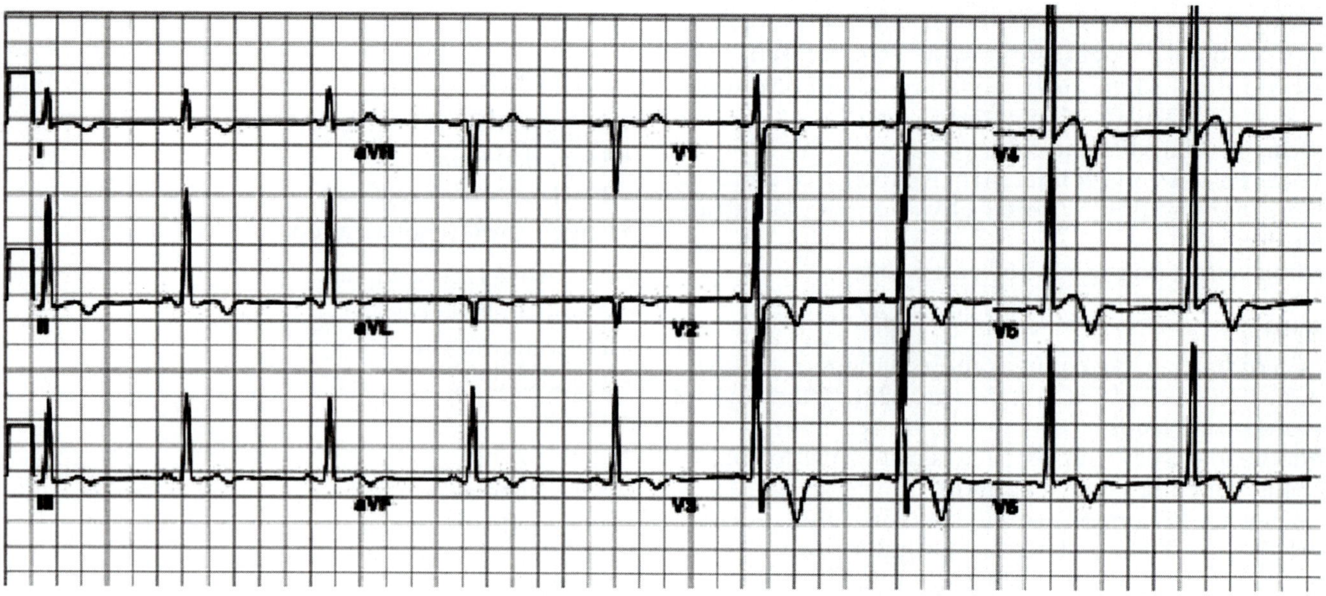

Fig. 5.35: *T-wave inversion in V1-6 due to HOCM*

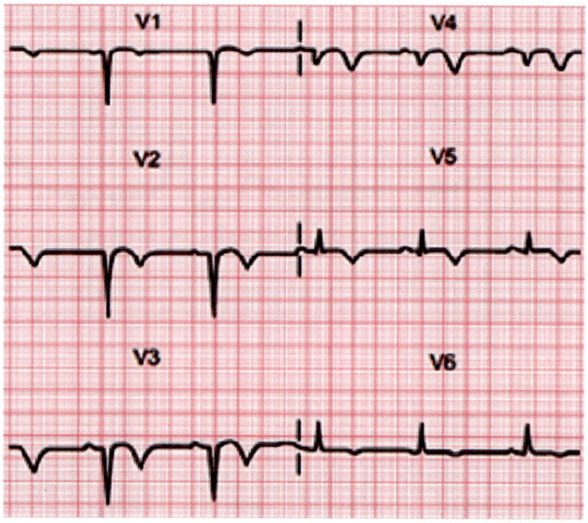

Fig. 5.36: *Anterior Q waves (V1-4) with T-wave inversion due to recent MI*

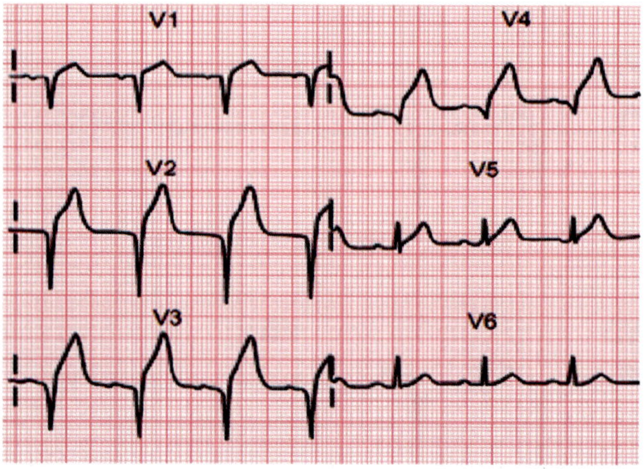

Fig. 5.37: *Anterior Q-waves (V1-4) with ST elevation due to acute MI*

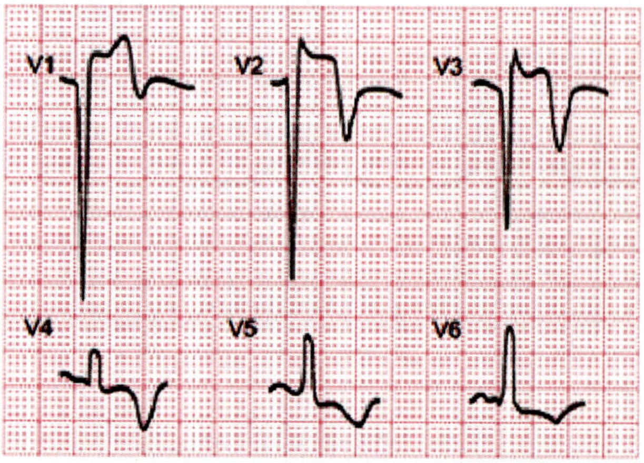

Fig. 5.38: *Persistent ST segment elevation in anterior chest leads in association with left ventricular aneurysm*

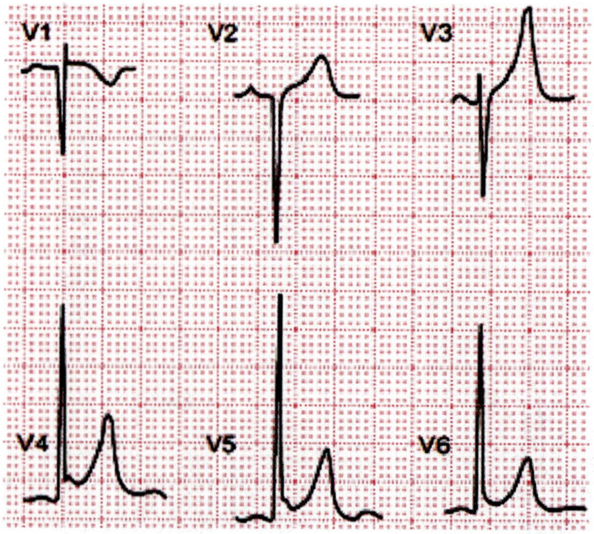

Fig. 5.39: *ST elevation in precordial leads in benign early repolarization*

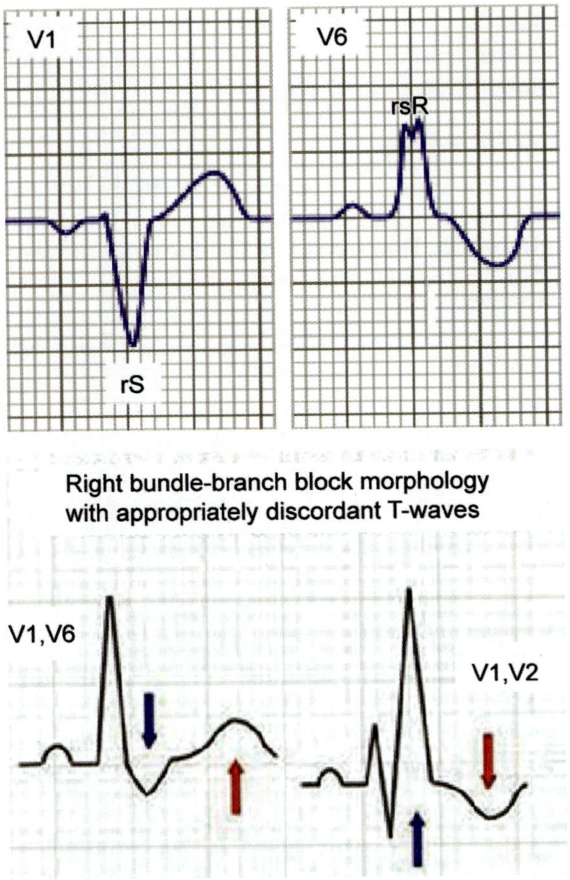

Fig. 5.40: *Right and left in bottom explaining the identification of bundle-branch blocks through QRS duration: If longer than 2–3 square (0.08–0.12 sec), that's bundle-branch block (BBB). RBBB or LBBB? To determine if a block is right BBB versus left BBB, look for the "M" shaped QRS. If you see it in V1 (right chest lead) then it is RBBB, if you see it in V6 (left chest lead), then it is LBBB*

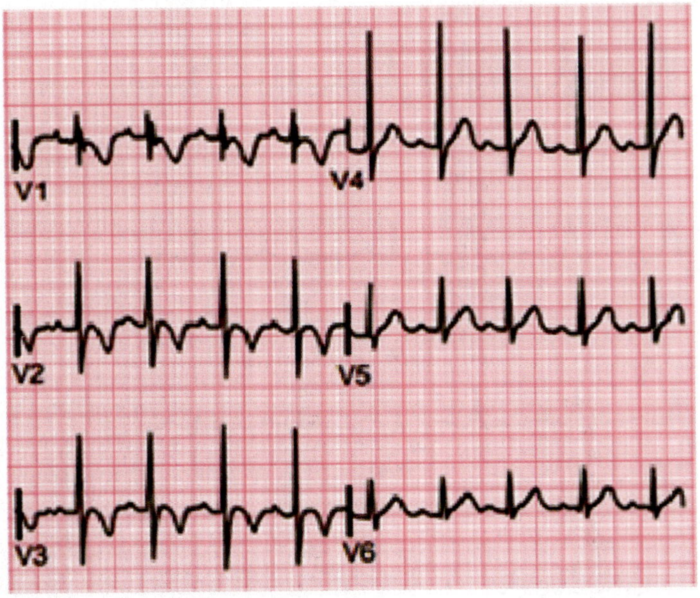

Fig. 5.41: *Normal pattern of T-wave inversions in a 2-year-old boy*

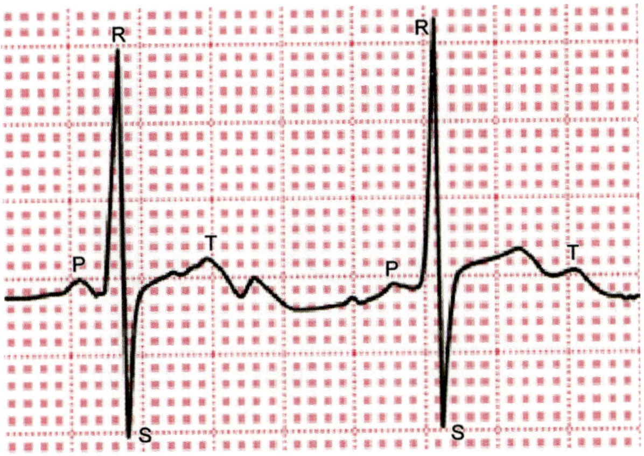

Fig. 5.42: *Biphasic T-waves due to ischemia*

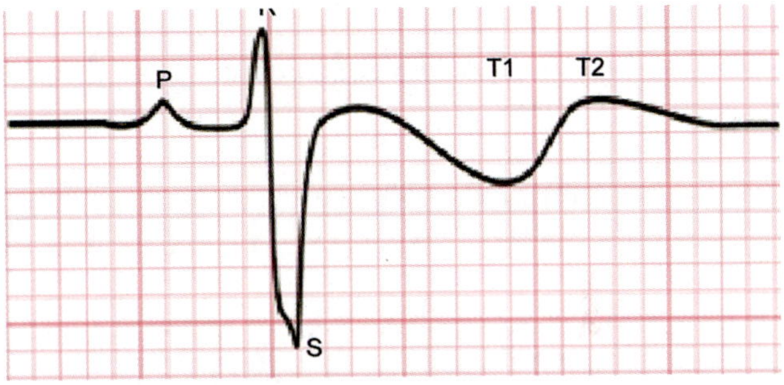

Fig. 5.43: *Biphasic T-waves due to hypokalemia*

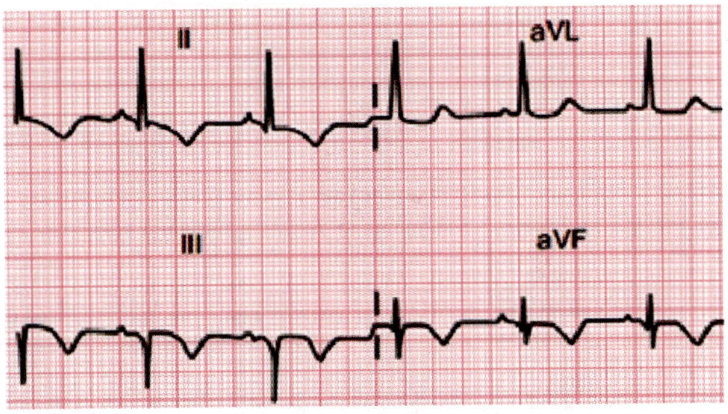

Fig. 5.44: *Inferior T-wave inversion with Q-waves due to prior inferior MI*

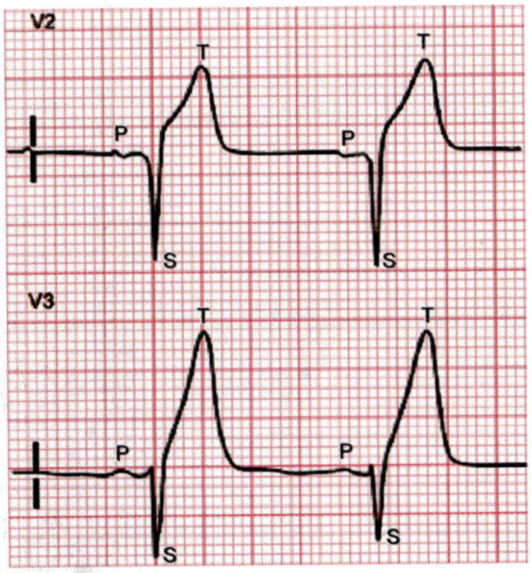

Fig. 5.45: *Hyperacute T-waves due to anterior STEMI*

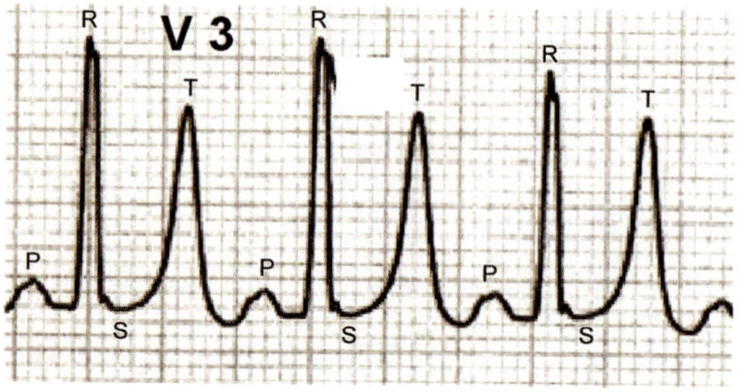

Fig. 5.46: *Showing peaked T-waves due to hyperkalemia*

Large, deeply inverted T-waves are seen with:

- Raised intracranial pressure (e.g. intracranial hemorrhage, traumatic brain injury) (Fig. 5.55).

Abnormal T-waves

- Upright T waves in V1 and V4R in children 3 days to 6 years (provided that T-waves are normal elsewhere, i.e. upright in V6). This is evidence alone of significant RVH. (Figs 5.41, 5.46, 5.60 and 5.61)

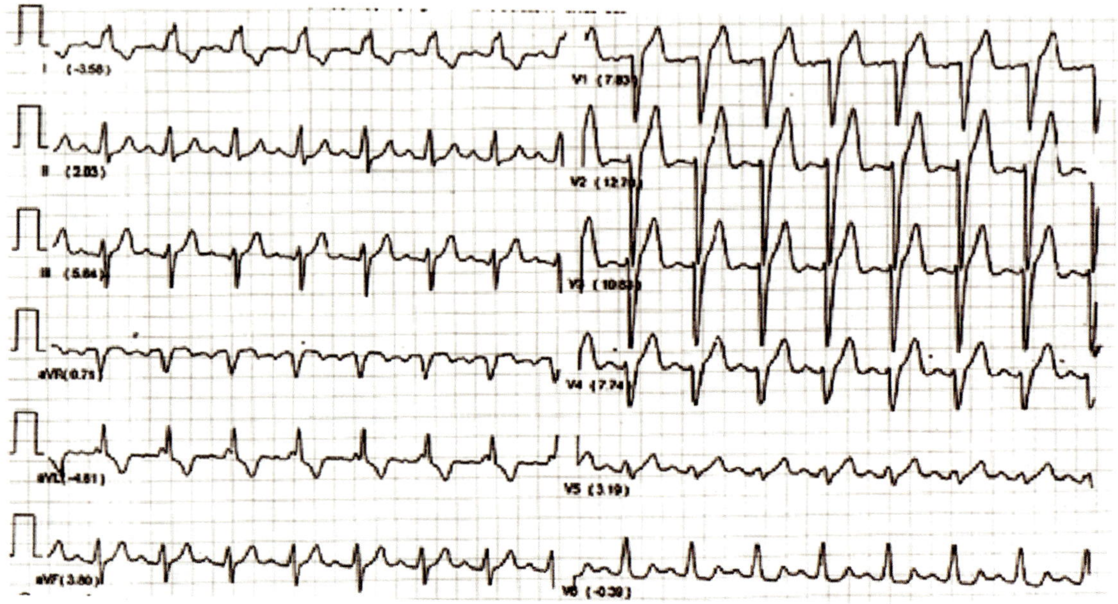

Fig. 5.47: *12 lead ECG showing widened QRS complexes in leads 1 aVL with tall QRS complexes and ST elevation in precordial leads V1-V4 in chronic LBBB as a result of stable coronary artery disease*

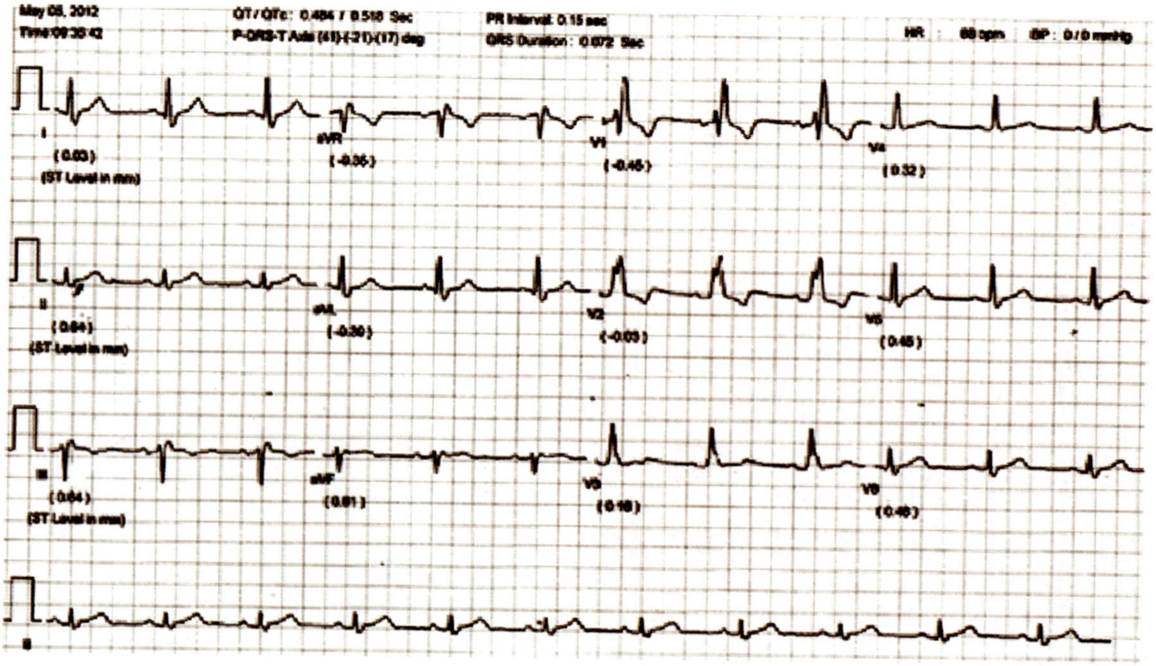

Fig. 5.48: *12 lead ECG showing rSR pattern leads V1-2 with left-axis deviation in right bundle-branch block*

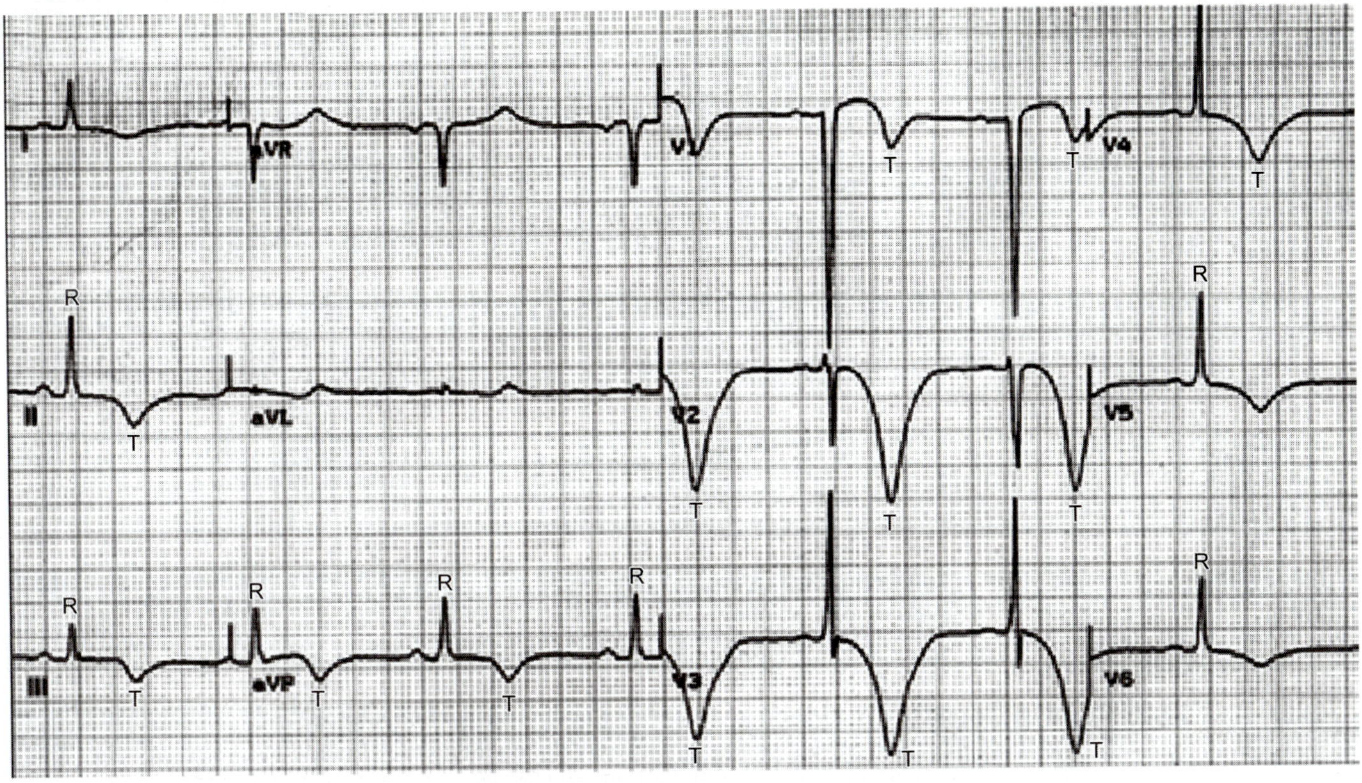

Fig. 5.49: *Long QT with giant negative T-waves*

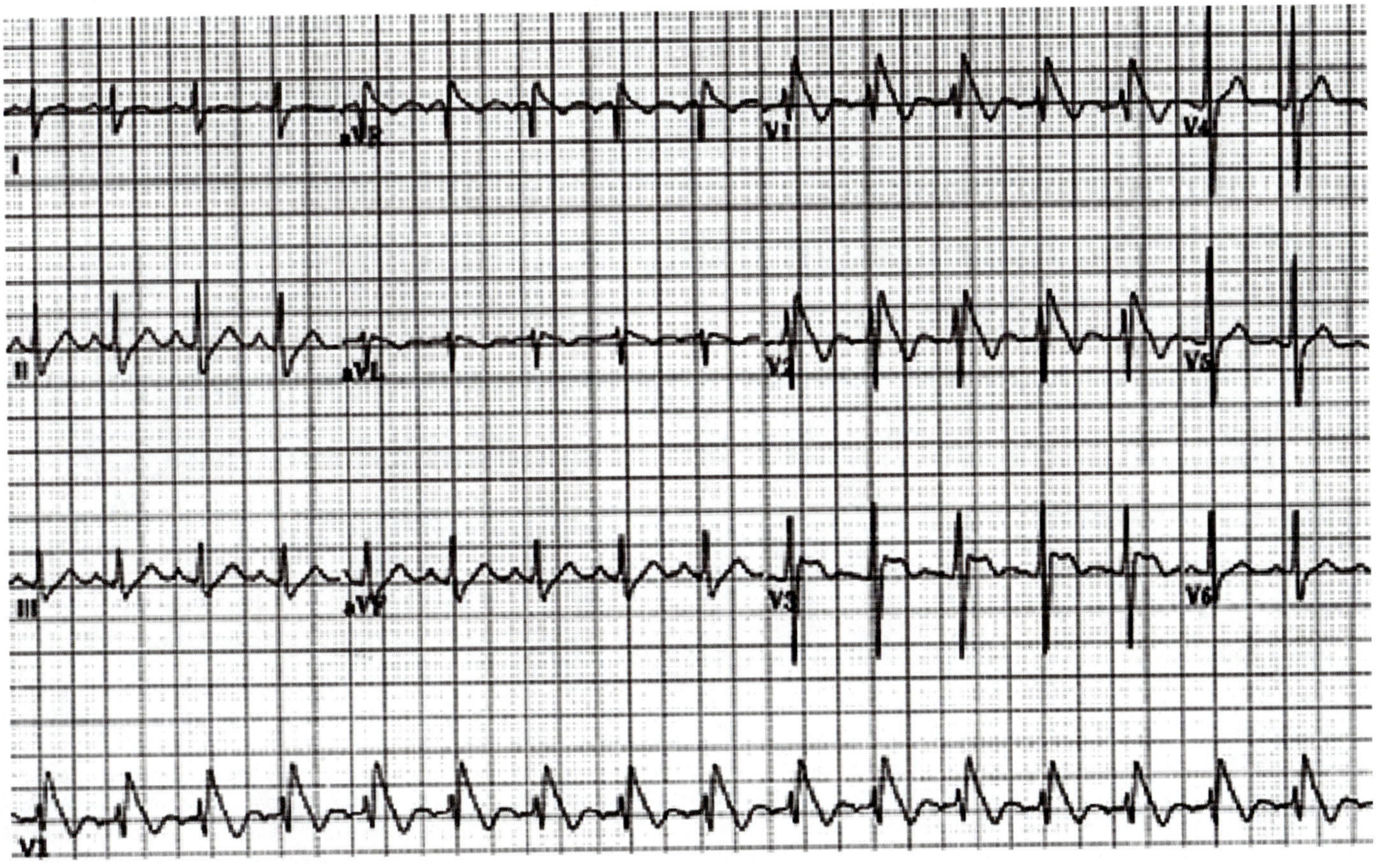

Fig. 5.50: *12 lead ECG showing marked ST elevation in leads V1–3 Brugada syndrome*

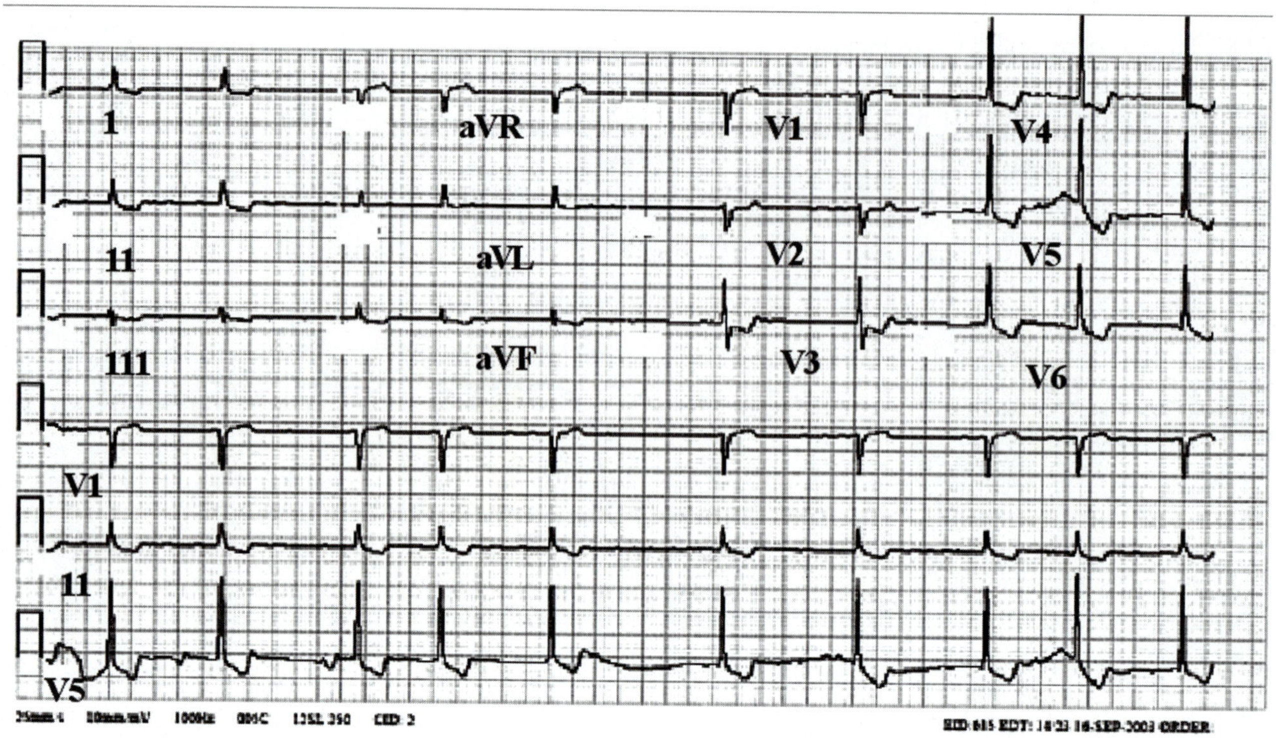

Fig. 5.51: *ECG showing (1) atrial fibrillation with bradycardia, (2) ST segment depression consistent with digoxin effect. The ECG shows a downsloaping ST segment depression in multiple leads that are shaped like the "reverse check mark sign" or a "scooped out" appearance. This pattern is typical of digoxin. This may occur at normal digoxin levels in some people, but becomes more common as the digoxin level increases*

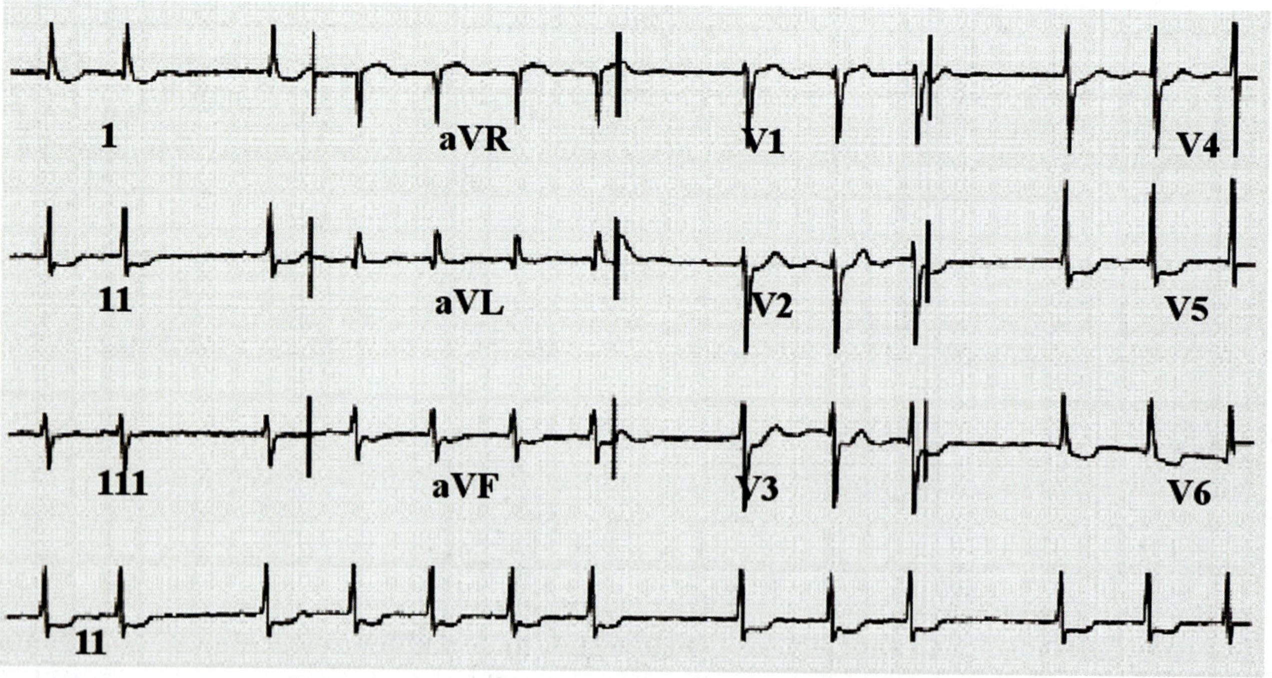

Fig. 5.52: *Top, digitalis effect. Digitalis glycosides characteristically produce shortening of the QT interval with a "scooped" or downsloping ST-T complex (From Goldberger AL: Clinical electrocardiography: a simplified approach. 6th ed. St Louis, CV Mosby, 1999). Bottom, digitalis effect in combination with digitalis toxicity. The underlying rhythm is atrial fibrillation. A "group beating" pattern of QRS complexes with shortening of the R-R intervals is consistent with nonparoxysmal junctional tachycardia with exit (atrioventricular Wenckebach) block. ST segment depression and "scooping" (V6) are consistent with digitalis effect, although ischemia or left ventricular hypertrophy cannot be excluded. Findings are strongly suggestive of digitalis excess; the serum digoxin level wasgreater than 3 ng/mL. Digitalis effect does*

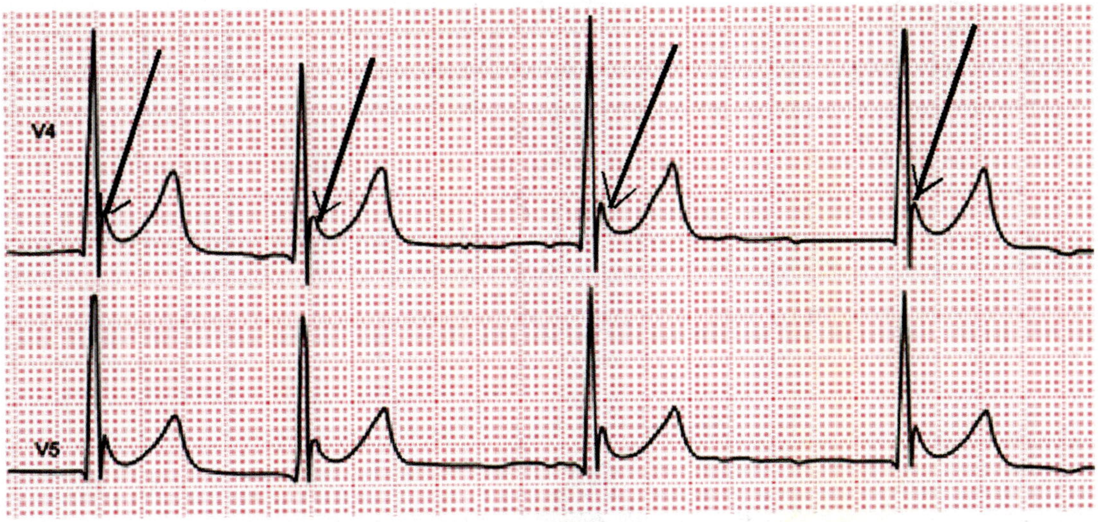

Fig. 5.53: *Osborn (J) waves in moderate hypothermia*

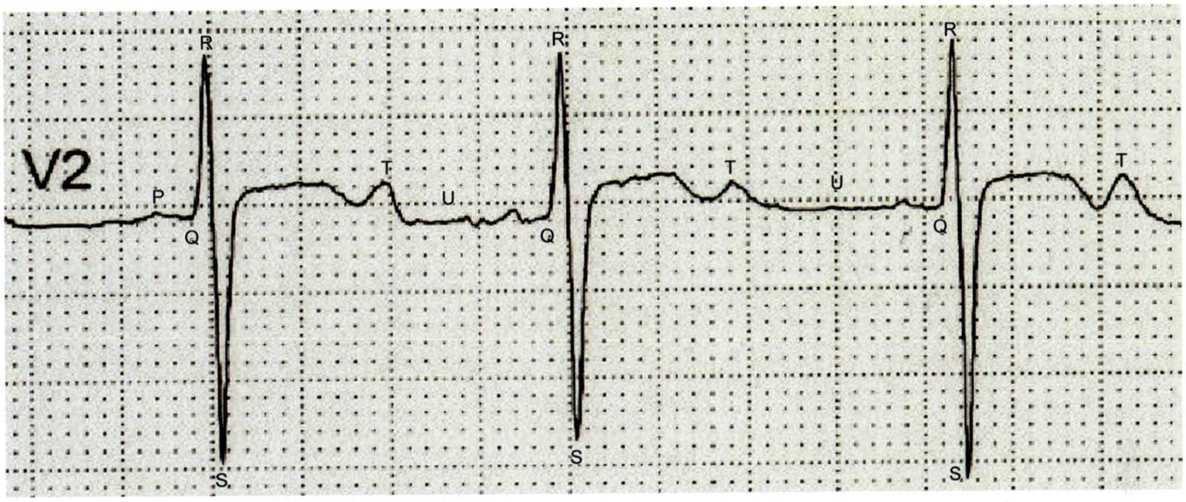

Fig. 5.54: *Prominent U-waves in a patient with a K+ of 1.9*

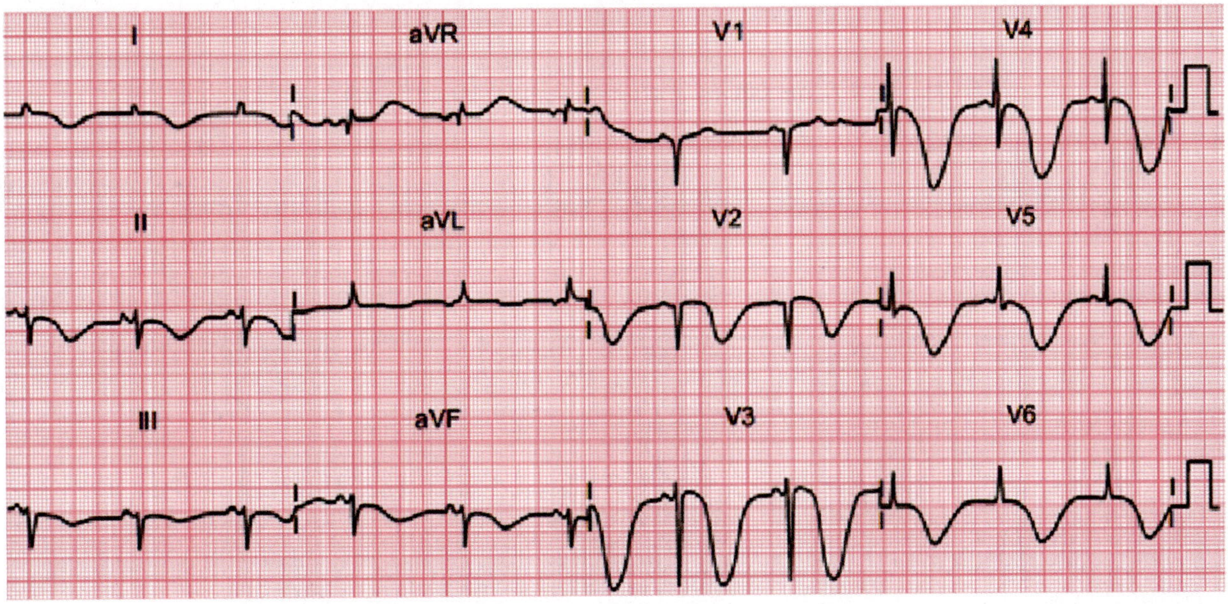

Fig. 5.55: *Prominent U-waves in a patient with a K+ of 1.9*

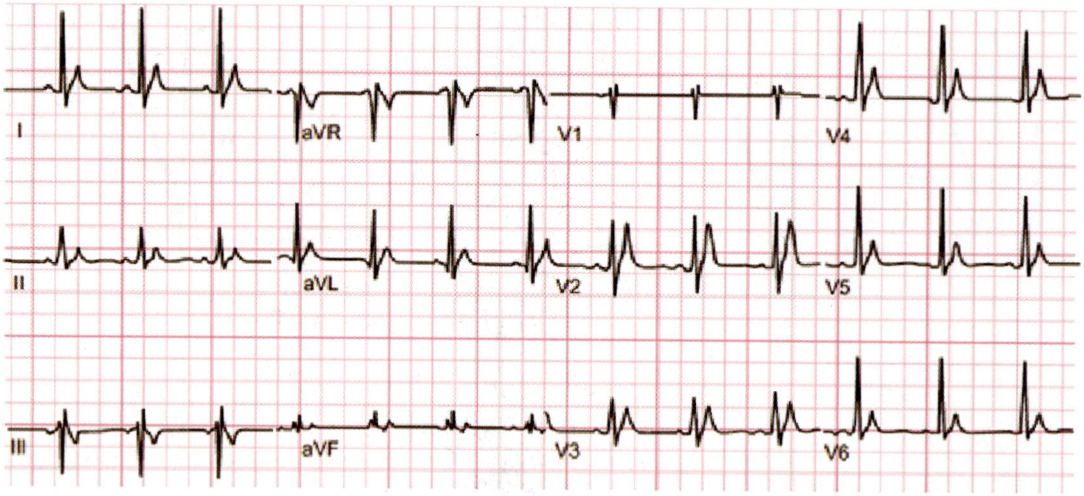

Fig. 5.56: *Very short QTc (280 ms) with tall, peaked T-waves due to congenital short QT syndrome*

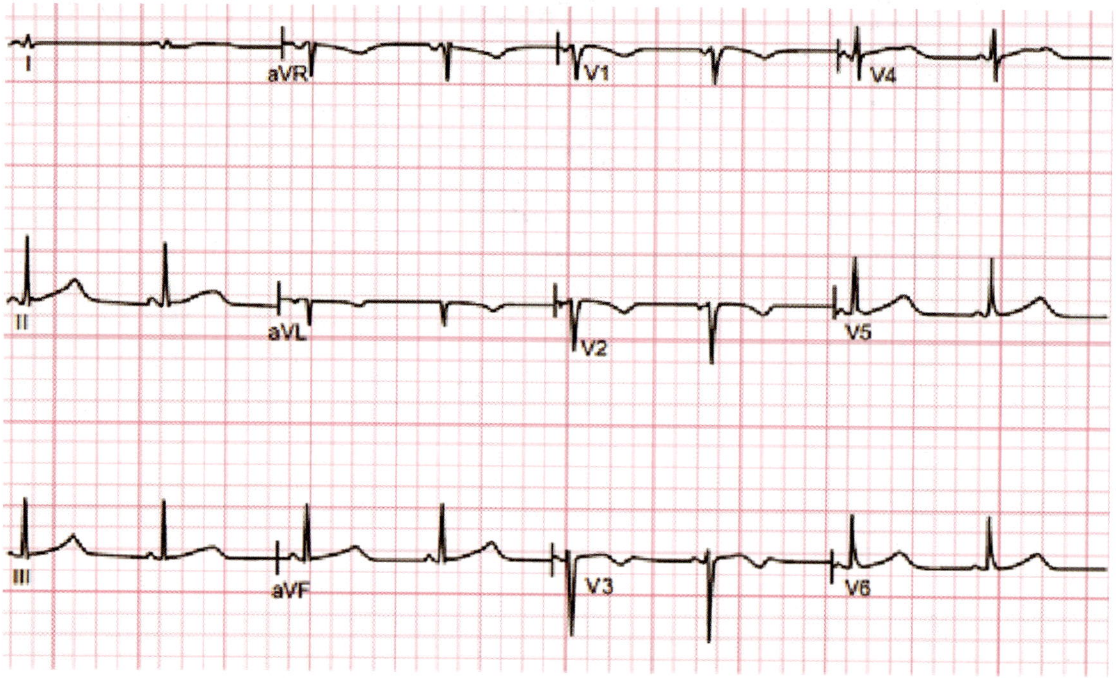

Fig. 5.57: *QTc 550 ms due to congenital long QT syndrome*

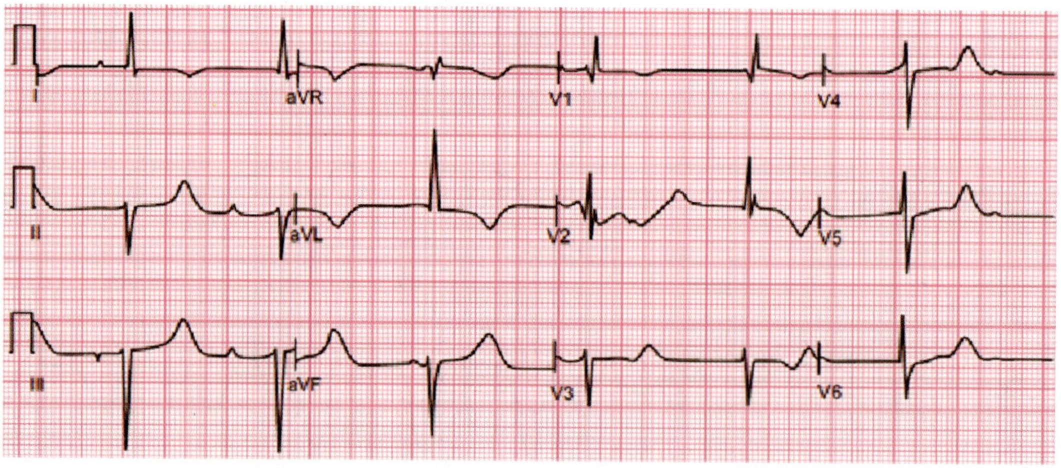

Fig. 5.58: *QTc 620 ms due to severe hypothermia*

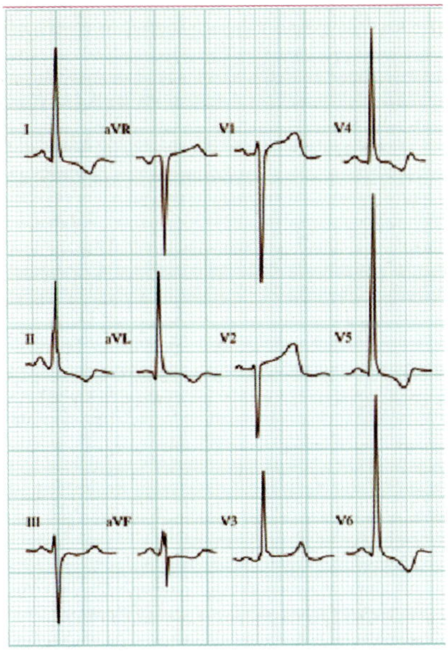

Fig. 5.59: *Left ventricular hypertrophy in patient who presented with ST segment changes in V1 and V2*

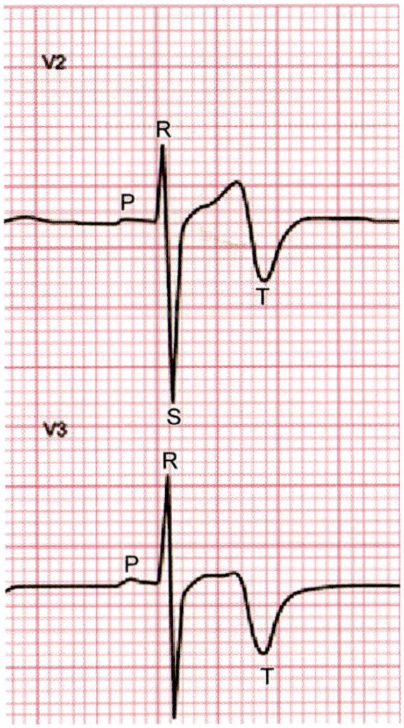

Fig. 5.61: *Showing "Type 2 Wellens" T-waves are biphasic, with the initial deflection positive and the terminal deflection negative*

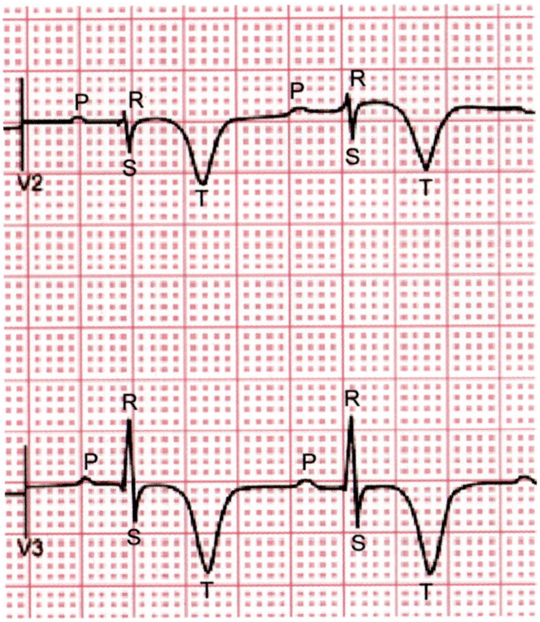

Fig. 5.60: *"Type 1 Wellens" T-waves are deeply and symmetrically inverted*

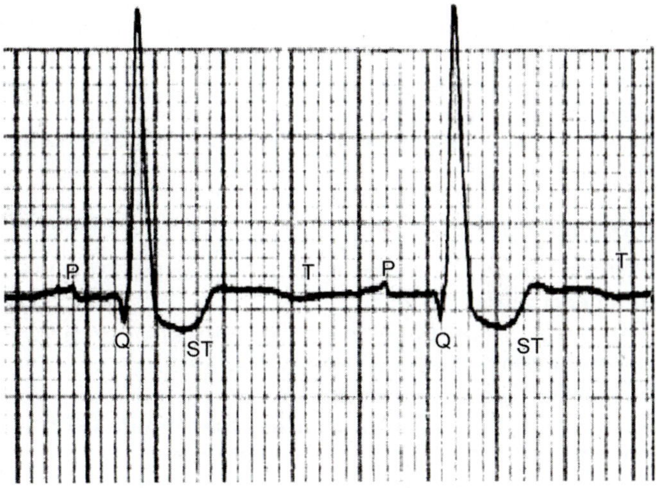

Fig. 5.62: *ECG shows a downsloaping ST segment depression in multiple leads that are shaped like the "reverse check mark sign" or a "scooped out" appearance in digitalis effect*

Q-Waves (Figs 5.33 and 5.34)

Normal Q-Waves

- Narrow (average 0.02 seconds and less than 0.03 seconds).
- Usually less than 5 mm deep in left precordial leads and aVF.
- May be as deep as 8 mm in lead III in children younger than 3 years.

Q-Waves are Abnormal if They

- Appear in the right precordial leads, i.e. V1 (e.g. severe RVH).
- Are absent in the left precordial leads (e.g. LBBB) (Fig. 5.47).
- Are abnormally deep (ventricular hypertrophy of the volume overload type).
- Are abnormally deep and wide (myocardial infarction or fibrosis).

Abnormal Q Waves (Figs 5.36 and 5.37)

- QR pattern in V1 (small Q-wave, tall R-wave) = highly specific for RVH (Fig. 5.48).
- Compare this with the criteria for RVH in adults.

QT Interval (Table 5.7)

- QT interval varies with heart rate
- Bazett's formula is used to correct the QT for HR
- QTc = QT measured/(R-R interval).

Normal QTc

- Infants less than 6 months = < 0.49 seconds.
- Older than 6 months = < 0.44 seconds.

QTc is prolonged in: (Figs 5.49, 5.57 and 5.58)

- Hypokalcemia
- Myocarditis
- Long QT syndromes, e.g. Romano-Ward
- Head injury
- Drugs.

QTc is short in: (Fig. 5.56)

- Hyperkalcemia
- Digitalis effect
- Congenital short QT syndrome.

How to Measure QT?

- The QT interval should be measured in either lead II or V5-6
- Several successive beats should be measured, with the maximum interval taken
- Large U-waves (> 1 mm) that are fused to the T-wave should be included in the measurement
- Smaller U-waves and those that are separate from the T-wave should be excluded
- The maximum slope intercept method is used to define the end of the T-wave.

Corrected QT

- The corrected QT interval (QTc) estimates the QT interval at a heart rate of 60 bpm.
- This allows comparison of QT values over time at different heart rates and improves detection of patients at increased risk of arrhythmias.
  There are multiple formulas used to estimate QTc. It is not clear which formula is the most useful.
- Bazett's formula is the most commonly used due to its simplicity. It over-corrects at heart rates > 100 bpm and under-corrects at heart rates < 60 bpm, but provides an adequate correction for heart rates ranging from 60–100 bpm
- At heart rates outside of the 60–100 bpm range, the Fredericia or Framingham corrections are more accurate and should be used instead.
- If an ECG is fortuitously captured while the patient's heart rate is 60 bpm, the absolute QT interval should be used instead.

There are now multiple i-phone apps that will calculate QTc for you (e.g. MedCalc), and the website MDCalc.com has a quick and easy QTc calculator that is free to use.

Normal QTc Values

- QTc is prolonged if > 440 ms in men or > 460 ms in women (Table 5.7).

Table 5.7: *QTc values for normal and prolonged QT interval after correction with Bazett's formula*

	QTc values by age group and sex (mL)		
	1–15 years	*Adult males*	*Adult females*
Normal	<440	<430	<450
Bordeline	440–460	430–450	450–470
Prolonged (top 1%)	>460	>450	>470

- QTc > 500 is associated with increased risk of torsades de pointes
- QTc is abnormally short if < 350 ms
- A useful rule of thumb is that a normal QT is less than half the preceding RR interval.

Causes of a Prolonged QTc (>440 ms)

- Hypokalemia
- Hypomagnesemia
- Hypocalcemia
- Hypothermia
- Myocardial ischemia
- Postcardiac arrest
- Raised intracranial pressure
- Congenital long QT syndrome (Fig. 5.57)
- Drugs.

Digoxin Effect on ECG

Digoxin produces a relative shortening of the QT interval, along with downward sloping ST-segment depression in the lateral leads ('reverse tick' appearance), widespread T-wave flattening and inversion, and a multitude of arrhythmias (ventricular ectopy, atrial tachycardia with block, sinus bradycardia, regularized AF, any type of AV block) (Figs 5.51, 5.52 and 5.62, 5.63).

Osborn Wave (J-Wave)

- The Osborn wave (J-wave) is a positive deflection at the J-point (negative in aVR and V1) (Fig. 5.53)
- It is usually most prominent in the precordial leads
- Characteristically seen in hypothermia (typically T<30C), but they are not pathognomonic.
- J-waves may be seen in a number of other conditions:
  - Normal variant
  - Hyperkalcemia
  - Medications
  - Neurological insults such as intracranial hypertension, severe head injury and subarachnoid hemorrhage

Typical J-Waves

Hypothermia

The height of the J-wave is roughly proportional to the degree of hypothermia:

Subtle J-waves in mild hypothermia (temperature 32.5°C)

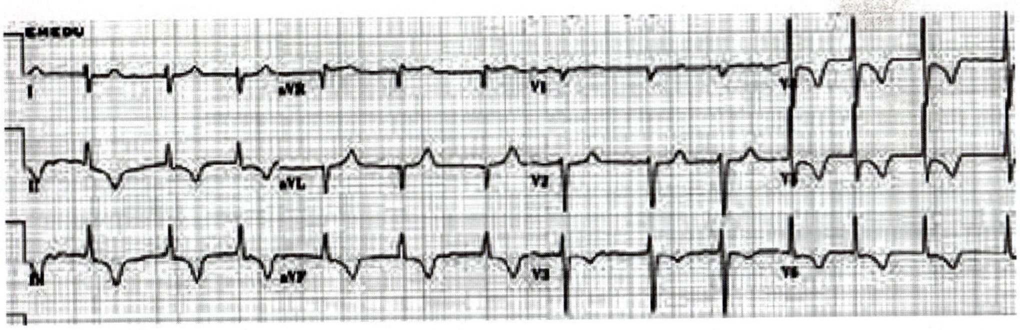

Fig. 5.63: *ECG showing generalised ST depression and T-wave inversion as seen in digitalis toxicity*

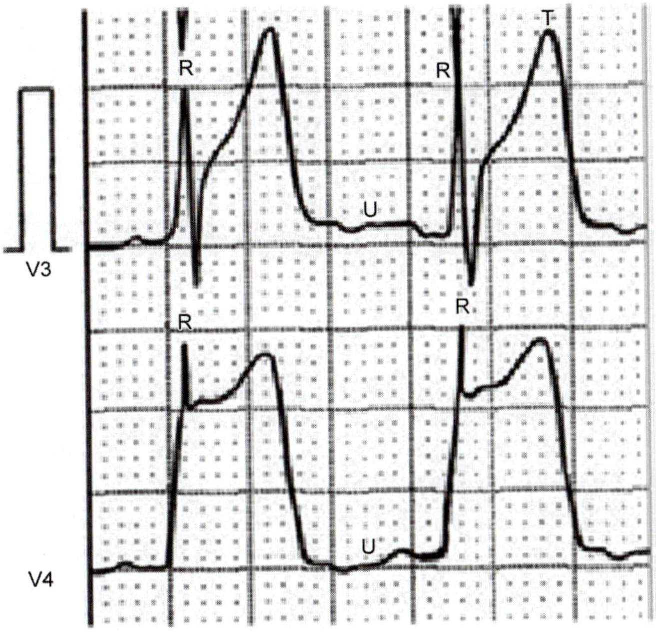

Fig. 5.64: *Inverted U-waves in a patient with Prinzmetal's angina*

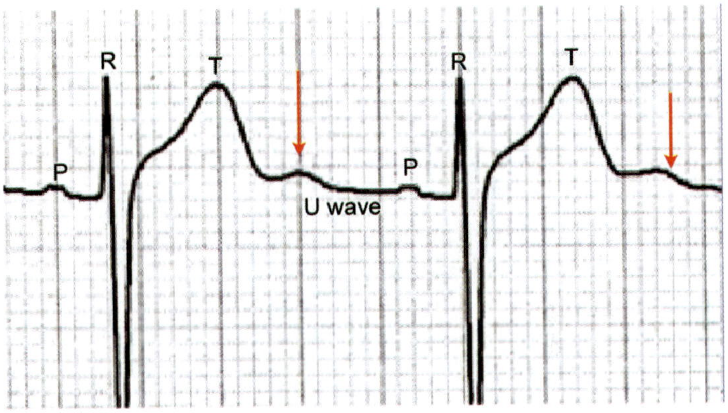

Fig. 5.65: *Normal U-wave*

J-point (Fig. 5.53)

- The J-point is the junction between the termination of the QRS complex and the beginning of the ST segment.

U Waves (Figs 5.54, 5.64 and 5.65)

A U-wave is an extra positive deflection at the end of a T wave. Most common causes:

- Hypokalemia.
- Normal finding at slower heart rates (e.g. sinus bradycardia).
- Normal U-wave in an adolescent

BIBLIOGRAPHY

1. Chan TC, Brady WJ, Harrigan RA, Ornato JP, Rosen P. ECG in Emergency Medicine and Acute Care. Elsevier Mosby 2005.
2. Hampton JR. The ECG Made Easy. 7th edition. London: Churchill Livingstone 2008.
3. Park MK. Pediatric Cardiology for Practitioners. 5th edition. St Louis: Mosby 2007.
4. Surawicz B, Knilans TK. Chou's Electrocardiography in Clinical Practice. 6th Edition. Saunders Elsevier 2008.

6 Cardiovascular Radionuclide Imaging

Radionuclide ventriculography is used to evaluate ventricular function. It is useful for measuring resting and exercise ejection fraction in CAD, valvular heart disease, and congenital heart disease. Some clinicians prefer it for serial assessment of ventricular function in patients taking cardiotoxic cancer chemotherapy (e.g. anthracyclines). However, radionuclide ventriculography has been largely replaced by echocardiography, which is less expensive, does not require radiation exposure, and theoretically can measure ejection fractions as accurately. 99 mTc-labeled RBCs are injected into the ventricles. Left ventricular (LV) and right ventricular (RV) function can be evaluated by first-transit studies (a type of beat-to-beat evaluation) or by gated (ECG-synchronized) blood pool imaging done over several minutes.

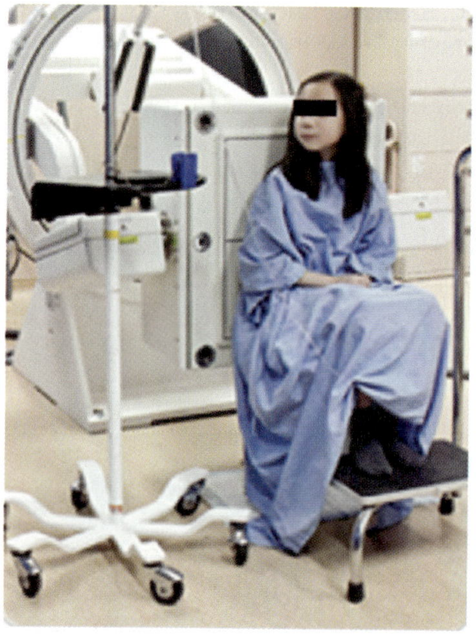

Fig. 6.1: *A young child is being prepared for radionuclide study in a hospital laboratory*

MULTIPLE-GATED ACQUISITION (MUGA)

Either study can be done during rest or after exercise. First-transit studies are rapid and relatively easy, but MUGA provides better images and is more widely used.

In first-transit studies, 8–10 cardiac cycles are imaged as the marker mixes with blood and passes through the central circulation. First-transit studies are ideal for assessing RV function and intracardiac shunts.

In MUGA, imaging is synchronized with the R-wave of the ECG. Multiple images are taken of short, sequential portions of each cardiac cycle for 5–10 min. Computer analysis generates an average blood pool configuration for each portion of the cardiac cycle and synthesizes the configurations into a continuous cinematic loop resembling a beating heart.

MUGA can quantitate numerous indexes of ventricular function, including regional wall motion, ejection fraction (EF); ratio of stroke volume to end-diastolic volume, ejection and filling rates, LV volume, and indexes of relative volume overload (e.g. LV:RV stroke volume ratios). EF is used most commonly.

MUGA during rest has virtually no risk. It is used for serially evaluating RV and LV function in various disorders (e.g. valvular heart disorders); for monitoring patients taking potentially cardiotoxic drugs (e.g. doxorubicin); and for assessing the effects of angioplasty, CABG, thrombolysis, and other procedures in patients with CAD or MI. Arrhythmias are a relative contraindication because there may be few normal cardiac cycles.

LV: MUGA is useful for detecting LV aneurysms; sensitivity and specificity are > 90% for typical anterior or anteroapical true aneurysms. Conventional-gated blood pool imaging shows inferoposterior LV aneurysms less well than it shows anterior and lateral aneurysms; additional views are required. Gated SPECT imaging takes longer (about 20–25 min with a multihead camera) than a single

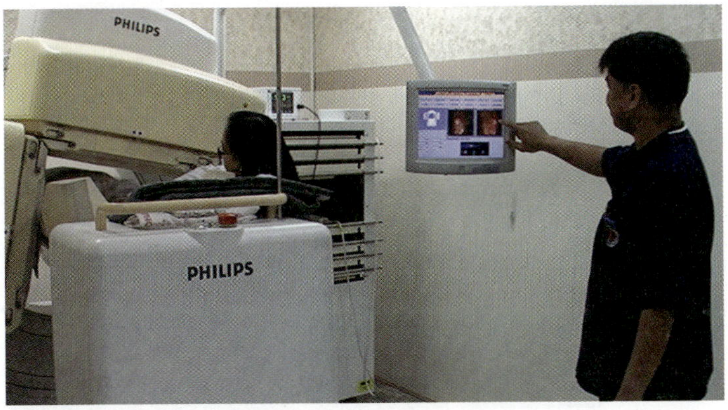

Fig. 6.2: Nuclear medicine set-up with emphasis given to cardiovascular nuclear medicine and radionuclide therapeutic procedures to treat diseases responsive to radioactive materials administered internally. It also provides in vitro procedures and interpretations

planar-gated view (5–10 min) but shows all portions of the ventricles.

RV: MUGA is used to assess RV function in patients who have a lung disorder or an inferior LV infarct that may involve the RV. Normally, RVEF (40–55% with most techniques) is lower than LVEF. RVEF is subnormal in many patients with pulmonary hypertension and in patients with RV infarction or cardiomyopathy affecting the RV. Idiopathic cardiomyopathy is usually characterized by biventricular dysfunction, unlike typical CAD, which usually causes more LV than RV dysfunction.

Valves: MUGA can be used with rest-stress protocols to assess valvular disorders that result in LV volume overload. In aortic regurgitation, a reduction in resting EF or no increase in EF with exercise is a sign of deteriorating cardiac function and may indicate a need for valvular repair. MUGA also can be used to calculate the regurgitant fraction in regurgitation of any valve. Normally, the stroke volume of the two ventricles is equal. However, in patients with left-sided valvular regurgitation, LV stroke volume exceeds that of the RV by an amount proportional to the regurgitant fraction. Thus, if the RV is normal, the regurgitant fraction of the LV can be calculated from the LV:RV stroke volume ratio.

Shunts: With MUGA and commercially available computer programs, size of a congenital shunt can be quantified by the stroke volume ratio or, during the first transit of the marker, by the ratio of abnormal early pulmonary recirculation of radioactivity to total pulmonary radioactivity. Radionuclide stress testing involves injecting a radioactive isotope (typically thallium or cardiolyte) into the patient's vein after which an image of the patient's heart becomes visible with a special camera. The radioactive isotopes are absorbed by the normal heart muscle. Nuclear images are obtained in the resting condition, and again immediately following exercise. The two sets of images are then compared. During exercise, if a blockage in a coronary artery results in diminished blood flow to a part of the cardiac muscle, this region of the heart will appear as a relative "cold spot" on the nuclear scan.

This cold spot is not visible on the images that are taken while the patient is at rest (when coronary flow is adequate). Radionucleide stress testing, while more time-consuming and expensive than a simple ECST, greatly enhances the accuracy in diagnosing CAD.

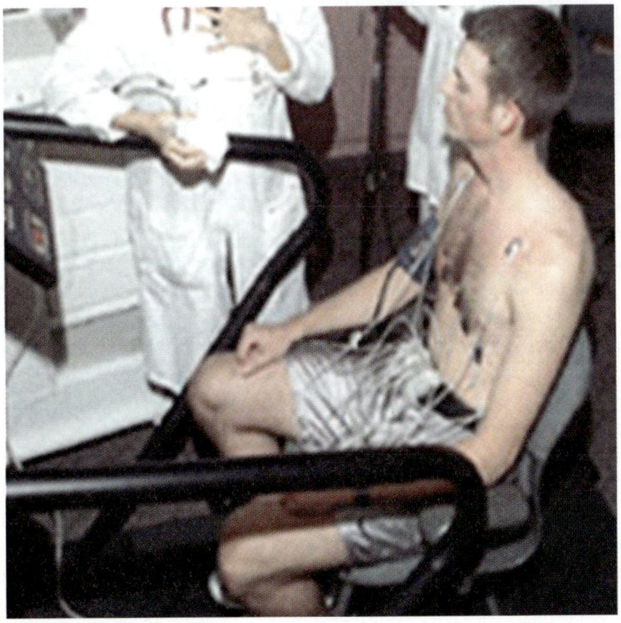

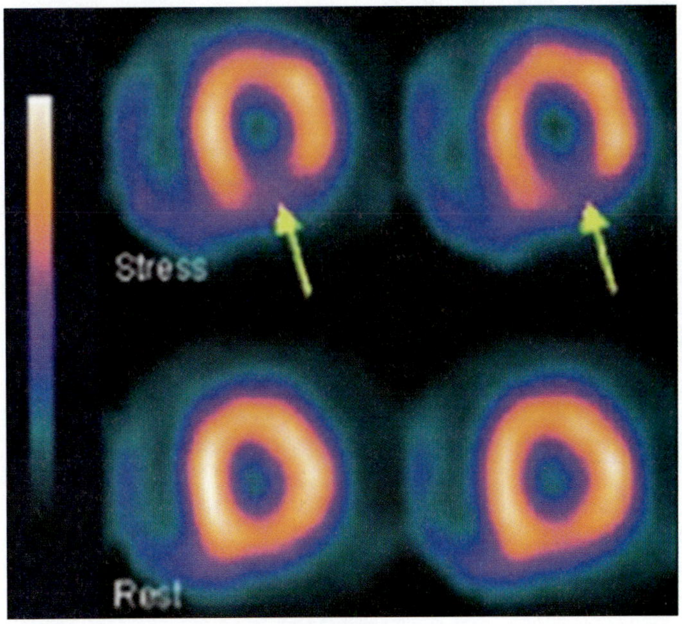

Fig. 6.3: Stress testing and nuclear imaging are often done at the same time, because in combination they are a powerful test to diagnose coronary artery disease. Nuclear heart scans allow your doctor to visualize blood flow to the heart indirectly. During a nuclear heart scan, a safe, radioactive material called a tracer is injected through a vein into your bloodstream. The tracer then travels to your heart. The tracer releases energy, which a special camera outside of your body can detect. The camera uses the energy detected to create pictures of the blood flow to your heart

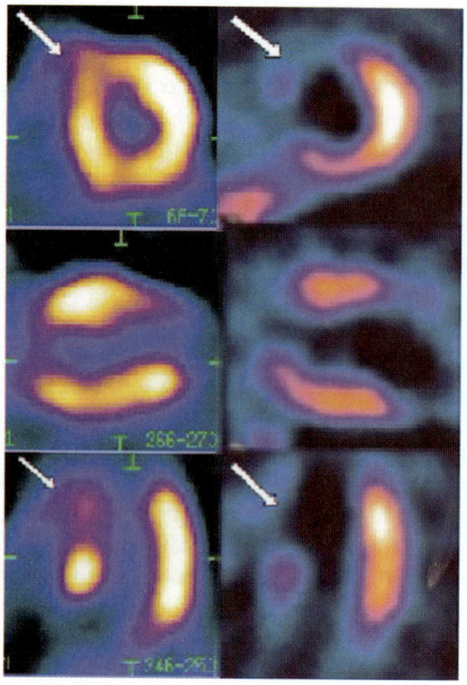

Fig. 6.4: *FDG PET (resting), left, with 99mTc tetrofosmin study in same patient displayed in short axis (A), vertical long axis (B) and horizontal long axis (C). note FDG uptake with corresponding reduction in perfusion in the interventricular septum (arrows) indicating compromised, but viable myocardium. There is no perfusion or viable myocardium at the apex suggesting old infarction*

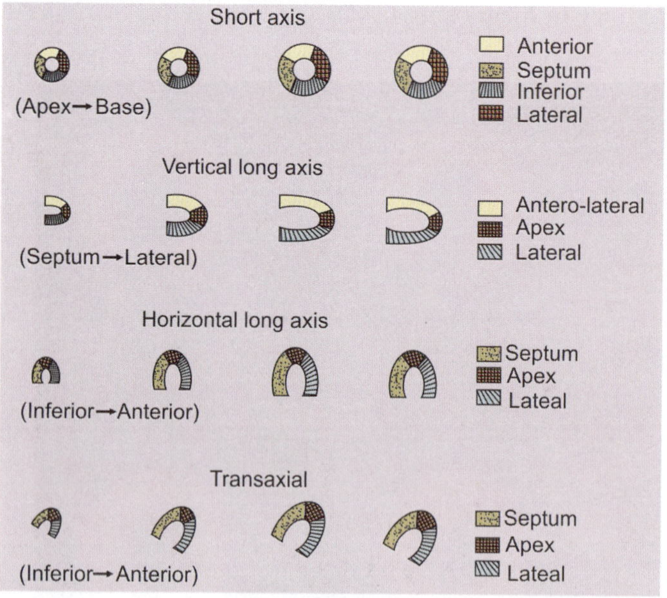

Fig. 6.5: *Diagram showing different myocardial segments in various axis employed in study of nuclear echocardiography*

PRINCIPLES

All radionuelide techniques require the internal administration of a radioisotope; the distribution of radioactivity in the area of interest is then imaged with a gamma camera. Ideally, the isotope should be distributed homogeneously in that part of the cardiovascular system under investigation; thus, isotopes that remain in the intravascular space during imaging are used for radionuclide angiography. In myocardial perfusion scintigraphy, however, isotopes taken up by the myocardium are required. Because of their potential toxicity isotopes with a short half-life are usually used.

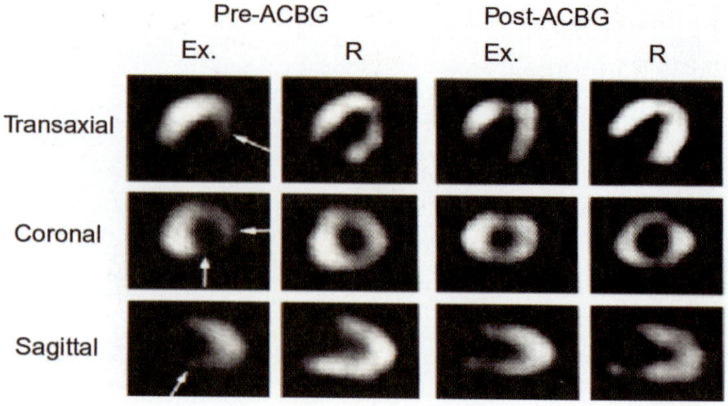

Fig. 6.6: *A young boy with mucocutaneous lymph node syndrome (MCLS) who underwent aortocoronary bypass grafting (ACBG). Stress thallium-20l myocardial imaging using single-photon-emission computed tomography was also performed; on the left side (pre-ACBG), exercise-induced ischemia of the inferolateral segment (arrows) was noted; 5 weeks postoperatively, it disappeared, except for small ischemic areas on the anterior and inferior walls; these results indicated the effectiveness of ACBG*

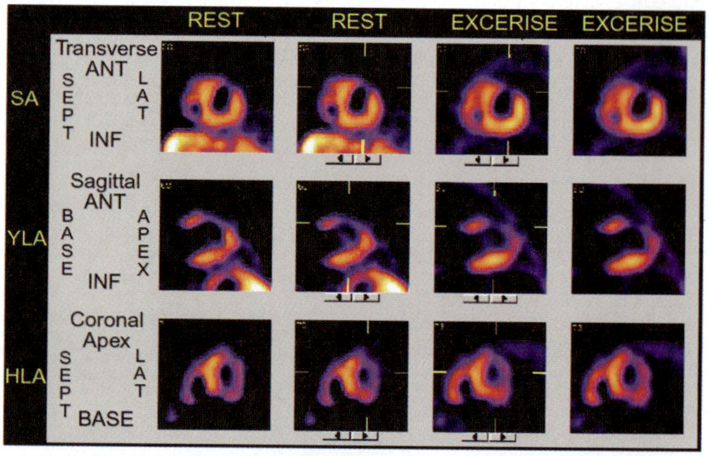

Fig. 6.7: *Eleven days after PTCA, a second rest-exercise myocardial scintigraphy with Tc-99m sestamibi showed a fixed perfusion defect in the anterolateral segment of the left ventricle (shown by thin arrows) with no other significant abnormalities. Ischemia in the apical portion of the anterior wall is no longer seen (thick arrows). (The second study was obtained with different system than the first study). A concomitant echocardiographic study demonstrated left ventricle hypertrophy with an ejection fraction of approximately 61%, hypokinesis of the anterolateral wall and abnormal septal motion*

IMAGING PROTOCOLS

A. Thallium 201

1. **General features:** Stress imaging with thallium 201 involves injection at peak exercise (or with pharmacologic stress) and immediate imaging, followed by redistribution images 3–4 hours after injection.
   a. Because of the long half-life of thallium 201 (i.e. 73 hours), limited amounts are administered. Although a single injection typically is used because of the redistribution phenomenon, a second injection may be given to enhance the filling of reversible defects.
   b. The low energy range of thallium 201 is marginal for imaging with the gamma camera because of scatter and diminished spatial resolution.

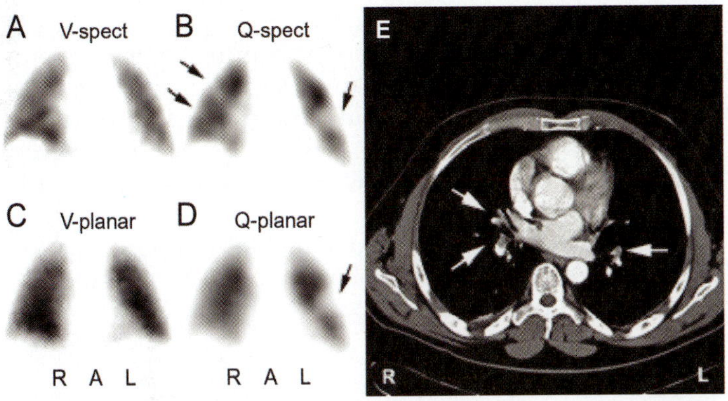

Fig. 6.8: *Patient with multiple embolisms in both lungs: segmental mismatch defect in left lung was detected by both SPECT (A and B) and planar scintigraphy (C and D). Defects are marked by arrows in B and D. However, subsegmental mismatch defects in right lung were only diagnosed by SPECT (B). CT angiography found thrombotic clots in branches of middle lobe artery and both lower lobe arteries (E, arrows). V, ventilation scan; Q, perfusion scan; R, right; A, anterior; L, left*

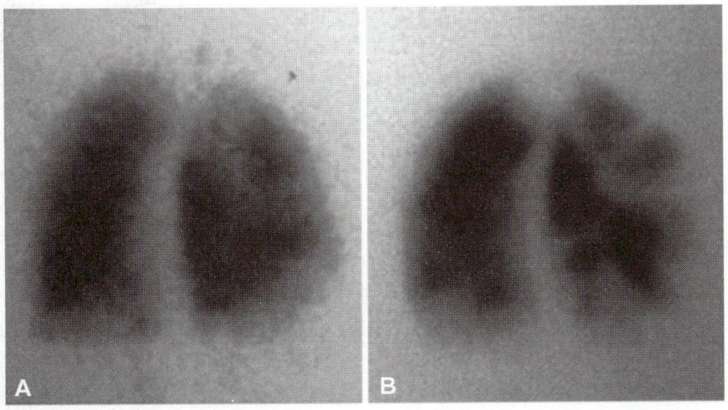

Fig. 6.9: *Ventilation/perfusion lung scintigraphy images of a patient undergoing etiological investigation of pulmonary hypertension and with normal findings on CT angiography of the pulmonary arteries. Right posterior oblique images: ventilation (A) and perfusion (B). Note the normal distribution of ventilation and the multiple, bilateral segmental perfusion defects, predominantly in the right lung. The patient was diagnosed with distal, chronic pulmomary thromboembolism*

2. **Variations from standard protocol:** Exact imaging techniques vary among institutions. Initial thallium 201 doses range from 2 to 3.5 mCi, acquisition times vary from 20 to 40 seconds per image, and the number of images varies from 32 to 64 depending on whether 150° or 360° image acquisition is used.
   a. The use of 360° versus 180° imaging has been the subject of debate. Contrast is better, there is less artifact, and imaging times are shorter with 150° tomography. Slight variations also exist depending on the use of exercise stress testing or pharmacologic stress protocols.
   b. When exercise thallium 201 scintigraphy is performed, the radionuclide (2–3.5 mCi) usually is injected approximately 1 minute before peak exercise to allow time for distribution. Initial images are obtained within 5–10 minutes of injection. Redistribution images are obtained 2.5–4 hours after the initial images.
   c. In some cases, persistent defects that would ordinarily be interpreted as myocardial scar represent viable myocardium.
      i. For this reason, some advocate delayed (late redistribution) imaging 15–24 hours after injection. Some studies indicate that upto 40% of persistent defects exhibit radiotracer uptake after revascularization. Delayed imaging has resulted in further redistribution in as many as 45% of patients.
      ii. Alternative approaches in differentiating viable tissue from scar include rest reinjection of thallium 201, in effect to boost filling in of perfusion defects. As many as 50% of persistent defects have been shown to exhibit improved thallium 201 uptake after rest injection of 1 mCi of thailium 201, suggesting viability.
   d. Minor changes in imaging protocol may be observed with pharmacologic stress testing with adenosine, dipyridamole, or dobutamine.

B. Technetium-99m

The relative lack of redistribution requires two injections of technetium-99m to obtain rest and stress images.

1. Basic protocols

a. Same-day protocol: At peak exercise, 25–30 mCi of technetium-99m is injected. Rest images are obtained first, and stress imaging follows to minimize residual scintigraphic activity caused by the higher-dose stress injection.
   (1) Rest images are obtained with injection of 7–10 mCi of technetium-99m and image acquisition 1–1.5 hours later. Imaging is delayed because of slower liver clearance with rest injection.
   (2) Stress images are obtained approximately 45–60 minutes after injection. Hepatic uptake of technetium-99m occurs within 15–30 minutes of injection, and the tracer is excreted into the gastrointestinal tract through the biliary system.

Appearance of the tracer in the gas trointestinal tract can interfere with imaging of the inferior wall of the left ventricle.

b. The separate-day protocol allows time for decay of activity. Larger doses of technetium-99m can be administered for rest and stress images, and there is minimal interference between the images.
   (1) Between 22 and 30 mCi of technetium-99m is injected for stress and rest imaging, separated by 1–2 days.
   (2) The higher doses possible with the 2-day protocol produce increased count density and better image quality at the cost of inconvenience.

2. Factors that affect image quality: Consumption of a fatty meal can enhance biliary excretion of technetium-99m and improve image quality. Because of possible interference from noncardiac uptake, image processing with technetium 99m relies on normalization to the brightest cardiac pixel.

C. Dual isotope imaging: Use of both thallium 201 and technetium-99m substantially reduces the time required to obtain stress and rest images.
   1. The patient receives thallium 201 at rest (3.5 mCi) and, immediately after rest imaging, undergoes stress. At peak stress, the patient is given an injection of 25 mCi of technetium-99m. Stress images are obtained 15 minutes later.
   2. This technique makes use of the dissimilar energy levels of the two radionuclides to shorten the protocol while still allowing acquisition of ECG-gated images (because of the use of technetium-99m).
   3. The sensitivity (91%) and specificity (75%) of this combination protocol are comparable with the values for conventional technetium-99m SPEC.

STRESS PROTOCOLS

A. Exercise stress testing: Standard exercise testing is frequently complemented with nuclear imaging. The radioisotope is injected at peak exercise, and time is allowed for circulation of the agents (usually at least 1 minute before termination of exercise).

B. For patients who are unable to exercise, pharmacologic testing is used in concert with nuclear imaging. Dipyridamole is an indirect vasodilator that is useful in noninvasive testing because of differences in coronary flow reserve. In the presence of marked coronary stenosis, the distal vessel is maximally dilated and therefore possesses little flow reserve. Dipyridamole substantially enhances coronary flow in normal beds (i.e. normal reserve), although much less so in distributions supplied by a stenotic artery. The resultant disproportionate flow is the basis for heterogenous radiotracer uptake.
   1. **Administration: Dipyridamole** is infused over a 4 minute period (0.142 mg/kg/min). Maximum vasodilatory effect is achieved 4 minutes after completion of the infusion, and the radiotracer is injected at this point. A slight increase in heart rate (10 beats/miri) and decrease in blood pressure (10 mmHg) frequently are observed.
   2. **Side effects:** Headache, nausea, chest pain, hypotension, dizziness, and flushing have been reported. Severe side effects may necessitate reversal of the dipyridamole effect with aminophylline, given as a 50- to 100-mg intravenous bolus.

C. Adenosine is the vasoactive end product of dipyridamole infusion and acts similarly although with a substantially shorter half-life.
   1. **Administration:** Adenosine is infused at 140 µg/kg/min for 6 minutes. The radio tracer is injected after 3 minutes of infusion.
   2. Side effects include chest pain, headache, nausea, flushing, dyspnea and atrioventricular block.

D. Dobutamine
   1. **Administration:** Infusion is begun at 5 µg/kg/min and increased every 3 minutes to a maximum dose of 40 µg/kg/min. The radiotracer is injected at maximum dose (or at 85% of age-predicted maximum heart rate), and the infusion is continued for 2–3 minutes.
   2. Side effects associated with dobutamine include ectopy, headache, flushing, dyspnea, paresthesias, and hypotension.

IMAGE INTERPRETATION

Standard view of normal anatomy: Uptake of radiotracer is homogeneous in persons with normal myocardial perfusion. The predominance of tracer is distributed to the left ventricle; the right ventricle usually appears as a faint, thin structure. Understanding and interpreting these images, however, requires an understanding of standard planar and SPECT views of left ventricular (LV) anatomic features.

CLINICAL APPLICATIONS

Radionuclide Angiography

Radionuclide angiography is used for assessment of ventricular function. Red cells labeled with technetium-99m are allowed to equilibrate in the blood pool and the heart is then imaged under the gamma camera. The waxing and waning of radioactivity within the ventricular chambers during diastole and systole, respectively, permits construction of a dynamic ventriculogram. Left ventricular contractile function can be evaluated quantitatively-by calculation of ejection fraction, or qualitatively-by observation of wall movement. Global Left ventricuiar impairment is characteristic of cardiomyopathy, while regional defects are seen following myocardial infarction. Stress radionuclide angiography using exercise or peripheral cold stimulation (cold pressor test) is used for detection of myocardial ischemia: provocation of reversible regional wall-motion abnormalities is strongly suggestive of coronary artery disease.

Myocardial Perfusion Scintigraphy (Figs 6.10 to 6.13)

Myocardial perfusion scintigraphy is used for diagnosis of coronary artery disease. The investigation requires a standardized exercise stress test with continuous ECG monitoring in order to provoke myocardial ischemia in susceptible subjects. Thallium-201 is used most commonly but the more recently introduced technetium-99m-labeled MIBI (methoxy isobutyl nitrile) provides better image quality. Isotope is injected intravenously at peak exercise and the heart is imaged under a gamma camera. Isotope is distributed homogeneously in normally perfused myocardium.

Ischemic or infarcted areas appearing as scintigraphic defects. If thallium-201 is used, repeat imaging after 2–4 hours' rest permits reassessment of scintigraphic defects, those that disappear (reversible defects) indicating areas of exercise-induced ischemia. Those that persist (fixed defects) indicating infarcted myocardium. If technetium-

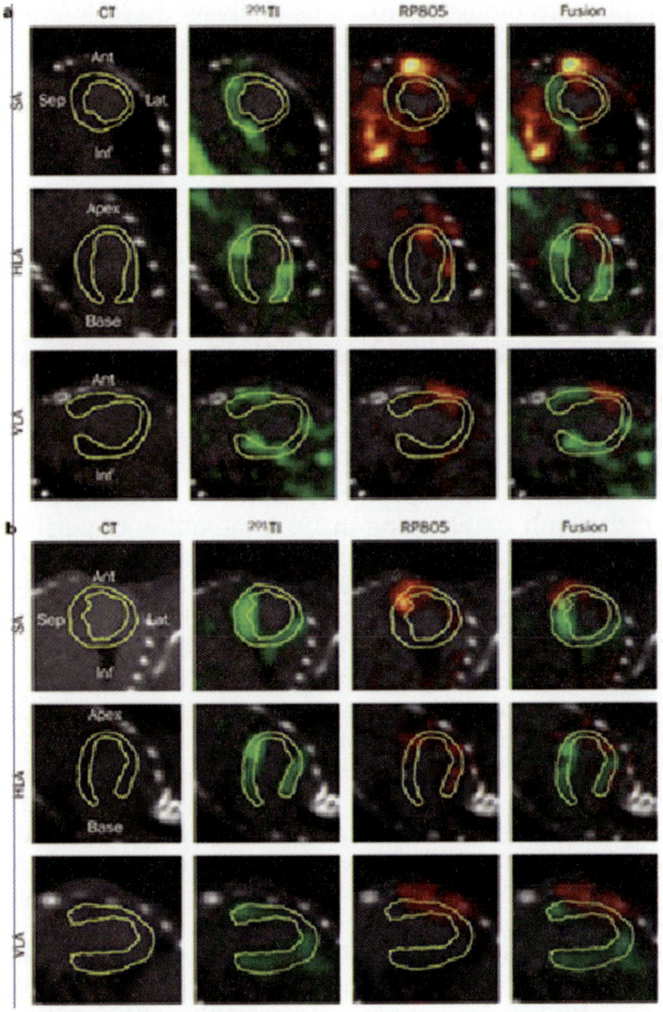

Fig. 6.10: *The contrast agent permitted better definition of the left entricular myocardium (highlighted by yellow line). Representative short-axis (SA), horizontal long-axis (HLA), and vertical long-axis (VLA) images are shown. Focal uptake of 99mTc-RP805 targeted at matrix metalloproteinases is seen within the central infarct and peri-infarct regions, which corresponds to 201Tl perfusion defect*

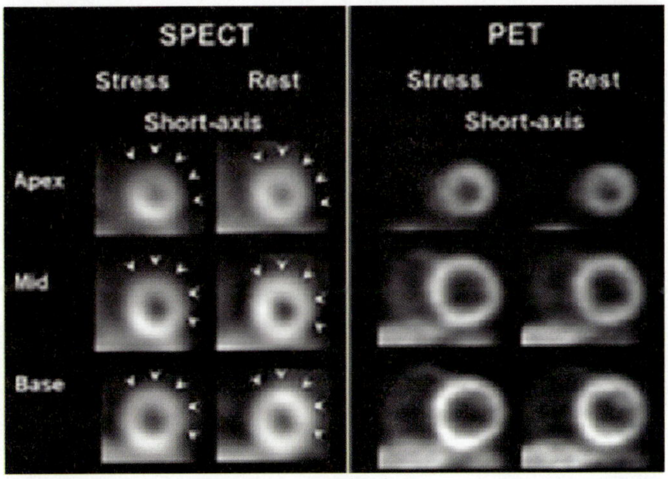

Fig. 6.11: *SPECT and PET images in a 17-year adolescent with atypical chest pain. Images are shown in short-axis views, with stress (left) and rest (right) in each panel. Shifting breast position between the rest and stress SPECT acquisitions produced an apparent reversible apical, anterior, and anterolateral attenuation artifact (arrowheads) resembling ischemia. With PET and its built-in attenuation correction in the same patient, the defect was not present. SPECT, single-photon emission computed tomography; PET, positron emission tomography*

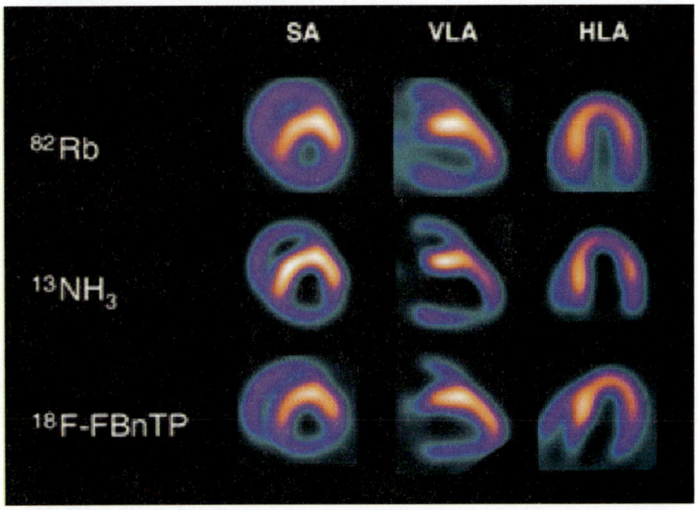

Fig. 6.12: *Showing PET perfusion tracers tomographic positron emission tomography (PET) images of myocardial perfusion after administration of adenosine using three different tracers, the Food and Drug Administration-approved agents 82rubidium (82Rb) (top) and 13N-ammonia (13NH3) (middle), and the novel compound 18F-fluorobenzyl-triphenylphosphonium (18F-FBnTP) (bottom). All images were obtained in a dog model of hemodynamically relevant left circumflex coronary artery stenosis, resulting in reduced perfusion of inferolateral myocardium, as shown by all 3 tracers. Since the canine cardiac anatomy is different from human anatomy, the septum is displayed more superiorly in short-axis (SA) images. HLA, horizontal long axis; VLA, vertical long axis*

99m-labeled MIBI is used resting images for assessment of reversibility require a separate injection of isotope 24 hours after (or before) the exercise images.

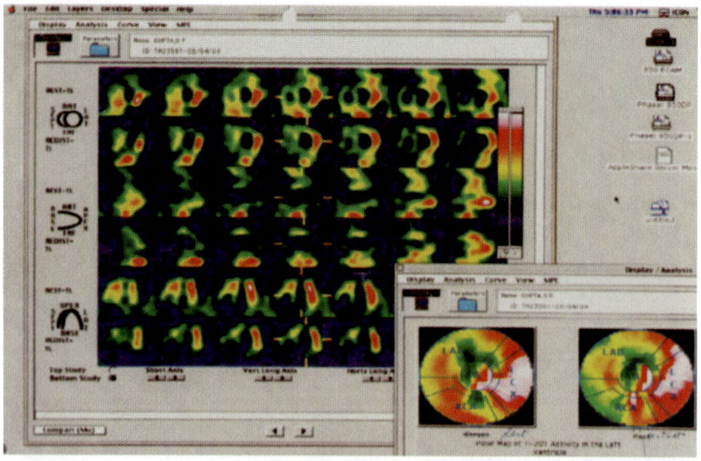

Fig. 6.13: *Photograph featuring rest redistribution SPECT thallium-201 myocardial perfusion scintigraphic study are consistent with myocardial infarction involving septal and anteroapical walls without any evidence of residual hibernation. The patient had echocardiographic LVEF<20% with features of ischemic cardiomyopathy*

Hot-spot Scintigraphy

Hot-spot scintigraphy permits diagnosis of acute myocardial infarction but in practice is rarely used technetium-99m pyrophosphate is taken up by hot-spot scintigraphy. Tectinetium-99m pyrophosphate Is taken up by normal bone and in the normal study.

(a) The ribs are clearly visible. Following myocardial infarction

(b) The isotope has localized in the infarcted area of the left ventricle producing a large "hot spot" which is clearly visible on the scintigram in recently infarcted myocardium, producing a localized "hot spot" of radioactivity on the scintigram. Diagnostic sensitivity is greatest during the first week following infarction.

Pulmonary Scintigraphy (Figs 6.8 and 6.9)

Pulmonary scintigraphy is used for the diagnosis of pulmonary embolism tectinetium-99m-labeled microspheres. injected intravenously, become trapped within the pulmonary capillaries. The normal pulmonary perfusion scintigram shows homogeneous distribution of radioactivity throughout both lung fields. Pulmonary embolism causes regional impairment of pulmonary flow. Which results in a perfusion defect on the scintigram; however, the appearance is nonspecific and occurs in many other pulmonary disorders, particularly chronic obstructive pulmonary disease. Specificity is enhanced by simultaneous ventilation scintigraphy. Inhaled xenon-133 is distributed homogeneously throughout the normal lung and, in pulmonary embolism (unlike other pulmonary disorders) distribution remains homogeneous. Thus a scintigraphic perfusion defect not matched by a ventilation defect is highly specific for pulmonary embolism than one vascular distribution, increased lung thallium uptake, and transient LV dilatation.

Quantitative analysis: The principles of image analysis rely on visual inspection, which is fraught with observer variability.

1. Computer-aided analysis of planar data involves comparison of regional radionuclide activity on stress and rest images; count discordance coincides with reversibility. SPECT data are quantitatively analyzed by means of comparing count densities on short-axis images (displayed as a polar map) with normal count profiles. Although they improve sensitivity, these methods are used in concert with visual analysis.

PET IMAGING

Although evaluated in large part in a visual manner, also possesses great clinical utility with the application of quantitative analysis (similar in principle to that used with SPECT) of coronary flow reserve. On the basis of comparison of baseline blood flow and hyperemia induced by pharmacologic agents, this analysis may have great clinical utility in ascertaining whether a patient needs revascularization and in evaluating the success of revascularization. The administration of adenosine or dipyridamole has demonstrated at least a twofold to threefold increase in coronary blood flow over baseline. Quantitative analysis of coronary flow reserve may prove useful in overcoming the achilles heel of the angiographically present but clinically enigmatic coronary lesion.

CLINICAL APPLICATIONS

Perfusion Analysis

Detection of CAD

a. Sensitivity and specificity: Since the introduction of thallium 201 imaging in 1975, the utility of perfusion agents in the diagnosis of CAD has been well established. Quantitative planar imaging and SPECT demonstrate 90% or greater sensitivity.
   (1) Sensitivity is affected by the number of vessels involved. Single-vessel disease is the most likely to produce a false-negative finding. Multivessel CAD rarely produces a normal perfusion scan result. The specificity of planar imaging is 83%, and that of SPECT is 60–70%.
   (2) In general, radionuclide imaging is best used to evaluate a population at intermediate risk for CAD. The choice of radionuclide agent seemingly has little effect on the accuracy of these techniques.
   (3) The introduction of PET, however, has brought with it advanced diagnostic accuracy, with approximately 10–15% improvement over SPECT. The ability to detect CAD in a noninvasive manner offers numerous additional applications in risk stratification, prognosis, and imaging of acute infarction (Figs 6.12 to 6.14).
b. Causes of false-positive perfusion study results include attenuation defect, technical inadequacies, coronary

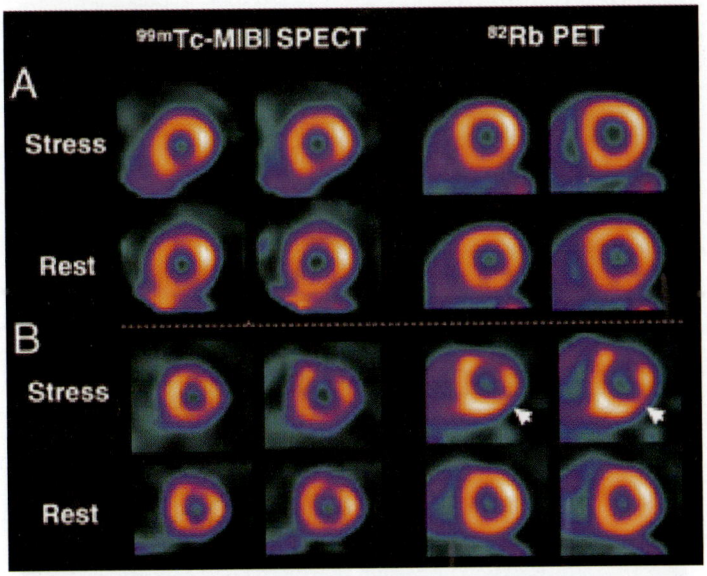

Fig. 6.14: *Comparison of PET and SPECT perfusion imaging shown are matched, representative short-axis slices for single-photon emission-computed tomography (SPECT) (left) and positron emission tomography (PET) (right) in two subjects with suspected coronary artery disease. Panel A illustrates improved specificity with PET. A fixed defect in the inferior wall on SPECT is absent on PET, suggesting the presence of a SPECT attenuation artefact. Panel B illustrates improved sensitivity with PET. Stress-induced perfusion defects in the anterior and inferolateral walls (arrows) are more clearly shown with PET versus SPECT*

vasospasm, anomalous coronary circulation, cardiomyopathy, conduction defects such as left bundle branch block, and recanalization of a thrombosed coronary artery.

c. Causes of false-negative perfusion study results include a submaximal exercise stress test, antiischemic medical therapy, presencse of nonobstructive CAD, collateral or overlap circulation, inaccurate interpretation of perfusion images or angiograms, acquisition of suboptimal images, presence of balanced coronary stenoses, and delay in stress imaging.

Risk stratification: In addition to indicators of higher risk taken from perfusion images, such as increased lung uptake, determinants in the assessment of risk are as follows:

a. Presence of reversible as opposed to fixed defects is associated with greater likelihood of cardiac events at follow-up evaluation. This relation has clinical utility in a number of settings, including risk stratification after MI or in the preoperative setting. In one study involving patients who had MI without complications, patients with single, fixed defects on thallium 201 images had a 6% cardiac event rate, compared with a rate of 51% for those with thallium 201 scans that indicated high risk of such an event.

b. Radionuclide imaging abnormalities have been identified as independent predictors of subsequent infarction or death. In general, the number of abnormal segments identified on nuclear images can be seen as inversely proportional to survival rate. Normal findings on a nuclear perfusion study, however, suggest an excellent prognosis, with a yearly mortality rate less than 1%. The application of such prognostic information to the care of patients preparing for noncardiac operations reflects significantly on the patient's surgical risk and has an established role in preoperative evaluation and clearance. For this population, evidence of ischemia on perfusion images portends higher risk for a perioperative cardiac event.

Myocardial perfusion imaging may aid in diagnosis and risk stratification for patients with acute coronary syndromes.

a. Patients with chest pain of ill-defined origin can be given an injection at rest ofthallium 201 or technetium-99m. In the presence of true ischemia (i.e. without infarction), reversible defects are documented, and insight into regional disiribution of ischemia and extent of myocardium involved is gained. The absence of any perfusion defect with ongoing chest pain makes a diagnosis of angina unlikely.

b. Injection of thallium 201 or technetium-99m within 6 hours of the onset of chest pain in acute infarction allows imaging of non-Q-wave and Q-wave events. As the time from onset of pain to injection increases, perfusion defects tend to normalize, probably as a result of autolysis or administration of thrombolytic therapy.

c. In the setting of thrombolysis, imaging with technetium-99m can provide important information about reperfusion or lack thereof. Injection of technetium-99m before initiation of thrombolysis captures a picture of hypoperfusion, which can, because of the extensive half-life, be imaged at a later time. Subsequent injections reveal the status of perfusion as the period after thrombolysis proceeds (i.e. persistent, large defect that represents failed reperfusion). Such applications in the setting of thrombolysis and in acute coronary syndromes have limited clinical utility because of the logistics of staffing and availability of radiopharmaceuticals.

d. A further application that affects the arena of revascularization and management of ischemic syndromes involves assessment of myocardial viability.

Assessment of ventricular function: In addition to its use in perfusion analysis, radionuclide imaging can establish cardiac performance. Radionuclide-based assessment of ventricular function includes first-pass radionuclide angiocardiography and gated blood pool imaging.

1. First-pass radionuclide angiocardiography involves injection of a radionuclide and analysis as the agent passes through the central circulation.
   a. Technetium-99m-labeled agents typically are administered in bolus form, and scintigraphic data

are recorded for 15–30 seconds after injection. Multicrystal cameras oriented in a straight anterior projection are used for detection of high count rates.

b. This method of ventricular function analysis is more useful in evaluating right ventricular function than is gated blood imaging. In patients with severe LV dysfunction, the radiotracer may be dispersed, and proximal venous access and rapid administration may be necessary.

GATED BLOOD POOL IMAGING OR MULTIGATED ACQUISITION (MUGA)

It relies on ECG gating to correlate multiple individual images of the cardiac blood pool to specific phases of the cardiac cycle.

a. The blood pool is labeled by means of removing a 2- to 3-mL sample of the patient's blood after the intravenous administration of stannous pyrophosphate. The sample is labeled with technetium-99m.
b. A single-crystal gamma camera is used in the LAO, anterior, LLAT, and left posterior oblique projections to obtain serial static images of the cardiac blood pool gated to the R-R interval.
c. Because multiple cardiac cycles are averaged to obtain the final images, this technique is not optimal for evaluating regional wall motion.

ECG-gated perfusion imaging: Perfusion imaging with technetium-99m-labeled tracers produces sufficient count densities on individual images *to* allow ECG gating. The standard injection of 20–30 mCi of technetium-99m. allows evaluation of perfusion and function in a single study. Comparison of this method with two dimensional echocardiography in the evaluation of regional wall motion has shown good correlation between the two. This correlation is not applicable to stress echocardiography, however, because of the time lag from the period of stress to the acquisition of nuclear images. The greatest utility of ECG-gated perfusion imaging may be in elucidating perceived artifacts on perfusion images.

PET in the evaluation of CAD allows blood flow imaging and evaluation of metabolic activity. Positron imaging agents can be considered blood flow tracers and metabolic radiopharmaceuticals.

Blood flow tracers: A number of radiopharmaceuticals exist for the assessment of myocardial blood flow. They can be produced by a cyclotron or generator.

1. Rubidium 82, the most readily used blood flow tracer, can be generated on site without the use of a cyclotron. Much like thallium 201, rubidium 82 is a potassium analogue that is actively transported into myocytes through the Na, K pump. Uptake into myocardium is proportionate to regional blood flow. Approximately 65% of the radiotracer is extracted at first pass. Because of a short half-life (76 seconds), rubidium 82-based imaging protocols can be used to assess myocardial blood flow rapidly (within 1 hour).

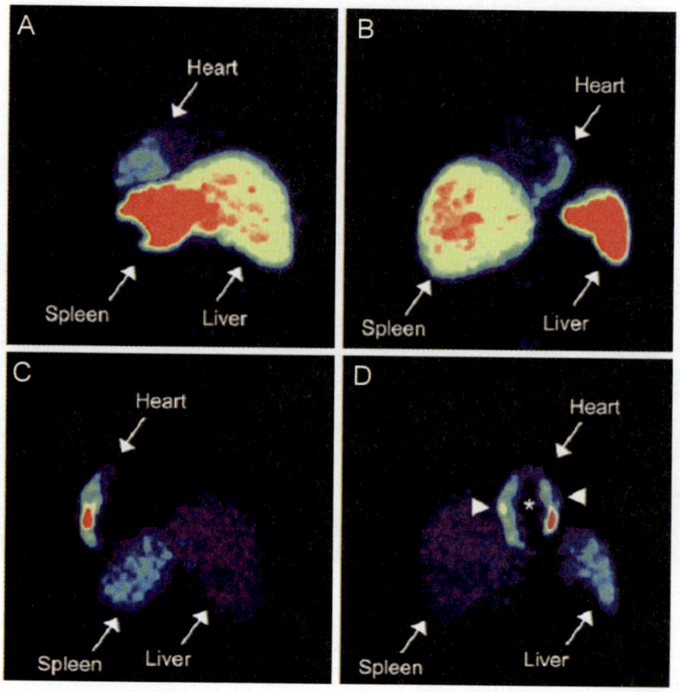

Fig. 6.15: *Evaluation of myocardial homing and biodistribution of 18F-FDG-labeled bone marrow cells after intracoronary delivery in patient after myocardial infarction. (A and B) Representative left posterior oblique (A) and left anterior oblique (B) views at 65 min after injection of 18F-FDG-labeled unselected bone marrow cells into the left circumflex coronary artery. (C and D) Representative left posterior oblique (C) and left anterior oblique (D) views at 70 min after injection of 18F-FDG-labeled CD34-positive subpopulation of bone marrow cells into left anterior descending coronary artery*

2. Copper 62 pyruvaldehyde bis (N-4-methyl-thiosemicarbazone) copper (IT) [(62CU) PTSM] is a blood flow tracer produced by cyclotron. Image quality comparable to that with rubidium 82, but gastro-intestinal activity may interfere with evaluation of specific distributions (inferior wall in particular).

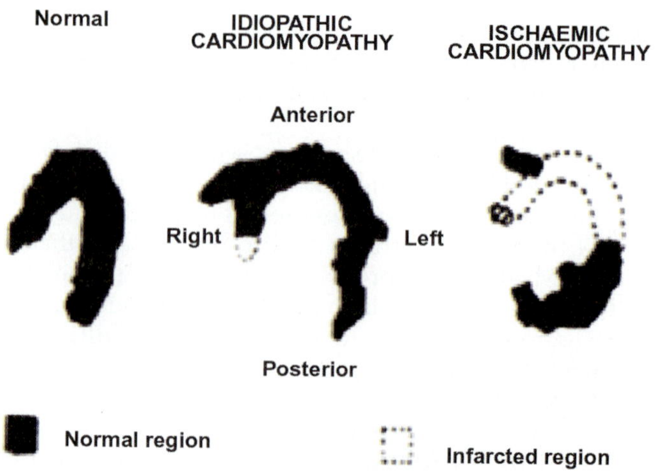

Fig. 6.16: *PET appearance from midventricular levels in idiopathatic and ischemic types of cardiomyopathies*

3. Other cyclotron-produced perfusion agents include nitrogen 13 ammonia and oxygen 15 water. Image quality with oxygen 15 water is poor and requires extensive processing to subtract the blood pool. Nitrogen 13 ammonia image quality is excellent, although the impracticality of cyclotron production is a limiting factor for both agents.

METABOLIC RADIOPHARMACEUTICALS

Metabolic imaging with PET depends on the use of radiolabeled substrates of cardiac metabolism, largely in the form of fluoro-2-deoxyglucose (FDG), carbon 11 palmitate, and carbon 11 acetate.

1. FDG is a glucose analogue used by ischemic myocardium because of a transition to alternative fuel sources in the hypoxic state. Ischemic myocardium diminishes the oxidation of long-chain fatty acids and incorporates glucose as a secondary fuel source. FDG is phosphorylated to FDG-6-phosphate after transport across the cell membrane. FDG imaging therefore reflects myocardial use of exogenous glucose, and FDG is a widely used metabolic radiopharmaceutical.
2. Palmitate is taken up by myocytes, converted to acyl-CoA, and relegated to triglyceride stores or oxidized to produce carbon dioxide. The release of this product of oxidation is reflective of long-chain fatty acid oxidation in myocardium.
3. Acetate is metabolized to carbon dioxide after entering the tricarboxylic acid cycle. Measuring the production of carbon dioxide in this setting correlates with myocardial oxygen consumption.

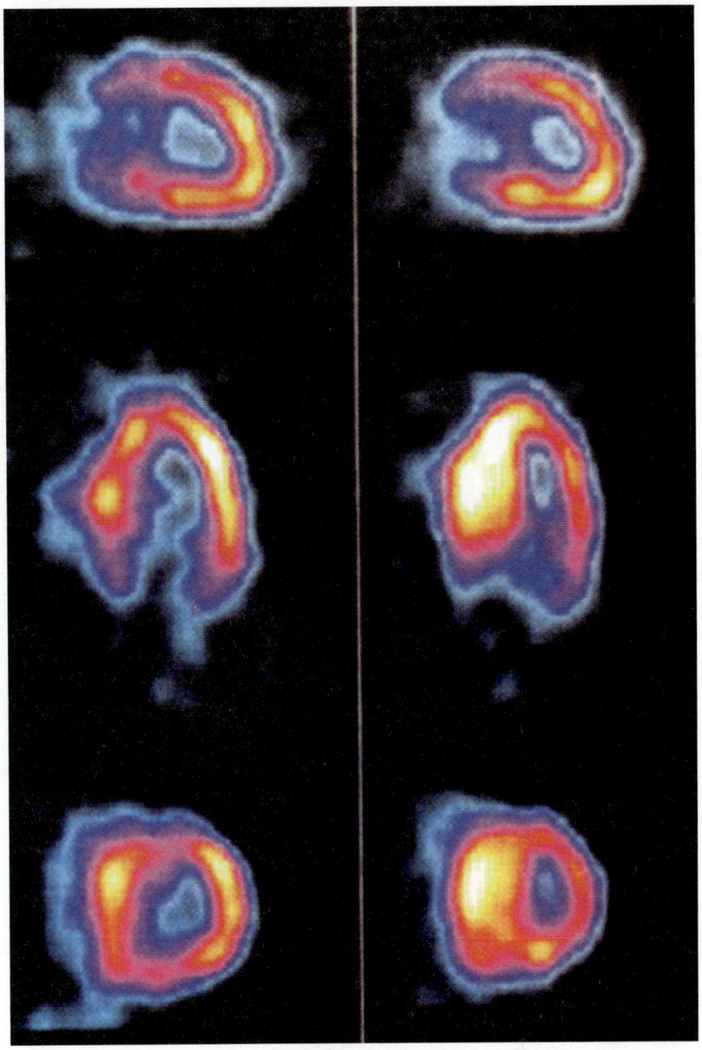

Fig. 6.17: *Significant inducible perfusion abnormality in an asymptomatic patient with HOCM demonstrated by radionuclide myocardial perfusion imaging*

METABOLIC IMAGING WITH SPECT

Metabolic imaging with SPECT cameras allows application of higher-energy photons even when PET is unavailable.

1. FDG has been imaged with SPECT when outfitted with a high-energy collimator. Various fatty-acid radiopharmaceuticals now are available that are SPECT compatible.
2. These techniques allow perfusion, ischemia, and viability assessment with standard SPECT equipment.

Protocols: Image acquisition with PET is similar to that with SPECT in that tomographic images are obtained in short-axis, horizontal long-axis (sagittal), and vertical long-axis (coronal) views. A positron camera consists of an array of crystals arranged in a circle. Unlike in SPECT, the camera remains stationary in PET.

1. The heart is localized with the patient's arms extended above the head. An attenuation scan is performed that allows the density of the surrounding thorax to be subtracted to leave only cardiac count activity. This ability to make allowance for noncardiac interference adds a great deal to the accuracy of PET.
2. After the attenuation scan, the positron radiopharmaceutical is injected, and images are obtained 2–5 minutes later. Up to 21 tomographic images may be acquired concomitantly.
3. Metabolic imaging can be undertaken after flow imaging with the administration of 5–10 mCi of FDG. Tomographic images are typically obtained 30–50 minutes after FDG injection.

Patterns of perfusion and metabolic imaging. Specific patterns of perfusion and metabolic imaging are identifiable. For example, normal flow-normal FDG (match) indicates normal perfusion and normal metabolic activity. Reduced flow-normal or increased FDG (mismatch) demonstrates viability (i.e. hiber-nating myocardium). Reduced flow-reduced FDG identifies scar tissue.

Clinical Applications

1. **Diagnosis of CAD:** Flow imaging with PET is highly sensitive and highly specific for the detection of coronary stenosis, approaching 93% for both.
   a. Certain perfusion agents allow for quantitative analysis of coronary flow reserve (oxygen 15 water)

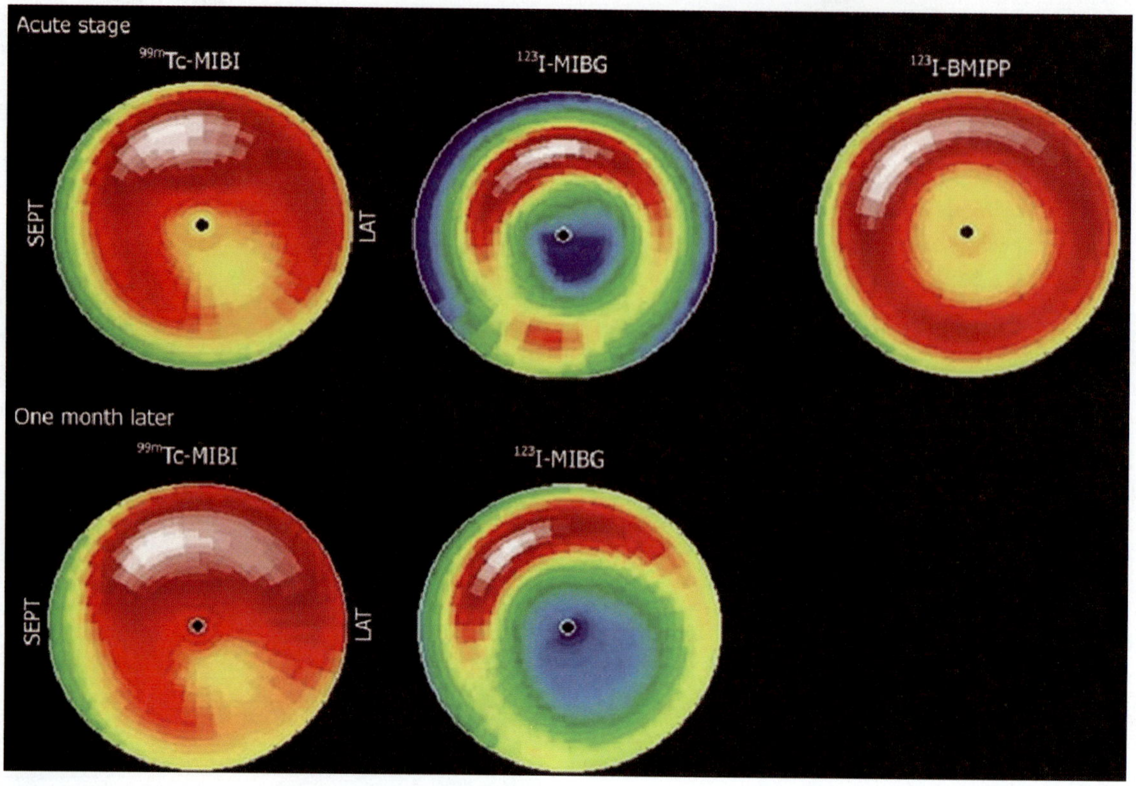

Fig. 6.18: *Scintigraphic features of Takotsubo cardiomyopathy are depicted. Bull's eye maps of 99mTc-sestamibi (MIBI), 123I-MIBG and 123I-methyl-p-iodophenyl-pentadecanoic acid (BMIPP) are shown. Both 123I-MIBG and 123I-BMIPP images show reduced uptake in the apical segment of the myocardium, which are typical features of the disease*

and aid greatly in assessment of the functional significance of a stenotic lesion.

b. Higher-energy photons (511 keY), higher count densities, shorter half-life, and the ability to correct for attenuation place PET substantially ahead of SPECT in the accurate detection of CAD.

2. Assessment of myocardial viability. The use of PET with metabolic radiotracers is the standard for identifying viable myocardium. The presence of a flow-metabolism mismatch, which indicates underperfusion in the presence of metabolically active myocytes, indicates a hibernating myocardium. Revascularization of these zones as identified with PET has been shown to result in improvement in wall motion. This utility of nuclear imaging finds increasing application as the ever-growing population of patients with heart failure and increasingly complex CAD experience demands better methods of viability assessment.

3. What diagnostic questions are addressed by myocardial perfusion imaging (MPI)?

MPI is primarily used in the diagnosis of coronary artery disease (CAD).

Stress perfusion imaging is used to define the severity of physiologic significance of a stenosed vessel already identified by coronary angiography.

MPI is also used for preoperative risk assessment. Dipyridamole perfusion imaging with perfusion tracers is highly predictive of either perioperative or postoperative cardiac-related death or myocardial infarction (MI) in patients with reversible perfusion defects. These reversible perfusion defects are equivalent to ischemic tissue or myocardium at risk of infarction, and therefore the extent and severity is directly related to the risk of a perioperative cardiac event.

MPI has been used to evaluate and define prognosis following acute MI. Areas of fixed defect as well as reversible perfusion abnormalities in vascular distribution other than the original infarct region are risk factors for subsequent myocardial events. Early dipyridamole thallium 201 perfusion imaging following acute myocardial imaging (within 48–96 hours) may be useful for identifying patients at greatest risk for subsequent myocardial nuclear cardiology, Magnetic resonance imaging, and computed tomography.

DIAGNOSIS OF CORONARY ARTERY DISEASE BY RADIONUCLIDE MYOCARDIAL PERFUSION IMAGING

Despite advances in the understanding of the pathophysiology of atherosclerosis and an applaudable reduction in cardiovascular mortality over the past 30 years, coronary artery disease (CAD) remains an important cause of mortality and morbidity in the UK. While primary prevention of CAD is a priority for modern medicine, so too is the need for development of noninvasive techniques for imaging of myocardial ischemia. Radionuclide tests occupy a central position within the cardiac imaging portfolio, and among them myocardial perfusion imaging

(MPI) has an obvious place because it is the only widely available and validated method of assessing myocardial perfusion.

1. Coronary Angiography and Myocardial Perfusion

MPI allows direct assessment of myocardial perfusion and therefore has an important role in the diagnosis of CAD in patients presenting with chest pain. An inducible perfusion abnormality indicates impaired perfusion reserve, which in turn usually corresponds to epicardial coronary obstruction. The site, depth, and extent of the abnormality provide diagnostic and management information. Conversely, a normal stress MPI indicates the absence of coronary obstruction and hence of clinically significant disease. A normal perfusion scan does not exclude non-obstructive CAD, but such disease is unlikely to be related to symptoms or to be prognostically important.

Positron emission tomography (PET) is generally considered the gold standard noninvasive technique for the assessment of myocardial perfusion. Although PET may have better accuracy than MPI, its clinical utility is constrained by high cost and poor availability. Therefore, MPI is the standard clinical technique for assessing myocardial perfusion, while coronary angiography is the technique for assessing epicardial coronary anatomy. Complete accuracy of MPI to predict the findings at angiography is neither expected nornecessary for clinical management, and when MPI is used for the diagnosis of CAD, it is not being used purely to predict the presence of epicardial coronary stenoses. Nevertheless, angiography is the accepted standard for imaging coronary arteries, and functional tests such as MPI are frequently compared with it.

Sensitivity and Specificity of MPI

Many studies have assessed the diagnostic accuracy of MPI for the detection of CAD, but they are of variable size and quality. The highest quality score is 3 (high), when the study involved a clearly defined population, avoided verification bias, and had independent interpretation of MPI and angiography; a quality score of 2 (medium) fulfilled two of these criteria; a score of 1 (low) fulfilled only one criterion. Because of the variation in study size, quality, and design, no attempt was made to provide weighted means of sensitivity and specificity.

In the largest single study of 2,560 patients randomised to one of the three commercial perfusion radiopharmaceuticals, and using mainly adenosine stress (the UK based ROBUST study), overall sensitivity in the subset of patients undergoing angiography was 91% and overall specificity was 87%, with no significant difference between the three tracers. In general, review of the studies showed that the sensitivity of MPI for detecting angiographic CAD was consistently above 70%. Typical sensitivity values were in the region of 85–95% for both thallium-201(Tl-201)6, 8 and technetium-99m sestamibi (sestamibi). There was a significant variation in specificity in low quality studies, ranging from 33–100%, but carefully designed studies have reported specificities of around 75% for exercise Tl-201, and sestamibi and even higher values (up to 94%) with incorporation of ECG-gated data.

For pharmacological stress performed with vasodilators, a number of good quality studies showed a sensitivity 90% for both Tl-201 and sestamibi and a specificity 75%, with some studies reporting values as high as 100%. For dobutamine Tl-201 MPI, the sensitivity was in the region of 90% while the specificity ranged from 70–100%. When it was used in combination with sestamibi, most studies have shown that the sensitivity was above 80%, but the specificity ranged from 64–90%.

Fewer diagnostic studies have been performed using technetium-99m tetrofosmin (tetrofosmin) because of its more recent commercial introduction. For exercise tetrofosmin MPI, the sensitivity and specificity values ranged from 81–96% and 67–91%, respectively.

2. Stress Echocardiography

Stress echocardiography is a well validated technique for diagnosing CAD and identifies wall motion abnormalities in patients with hemodynamically significant coronary stenoses, induced by exercise or pharmacological stress. Stress induced impairment of regional endocardial excursion and of myocardial thickening is a specific marker of myocardial ischemia.

3. Myocardial Contrast Echocardiography and Cardiac Magnetic Resonance Imaging

A small number of studies have directly compared MPI with either myocardial contrast echocardiography (MCE) or cardiac magnetic resonance imaging (CMRI), both of which are novel techniques for the assessment of myocardial perfusion. In a small study of 30 patients who underwent dipyridamole stress testing, Kaul and colleagues found a good agreement (= 0.86) between MPI and MCE for the presence or absence of CAD.

CMRI has also been used for detection of CAD in a similar way to stress echocardiography; in a recent review, this technique has been shown to have a mean sensitivity and specificity of 86% and 84%, respectively, for detecting CAD. In the last few years, direct assessment of myocardial perfusion has become feasible using gadolinium diethylentriaminepenta acid (Gd-DTPA). There have been no studies so far directly comparing the diagnostic accuracies of Gd-DTPA perfusion CMRI and MPI, and the exact role of the former in clinical practice remains to be determined.

When the reference standard for diagnosis (in this case coronary angiography) is not used in all patients, and referral to angiography is more likely when MPI is abnormal, then the findings are affected by post-test referral bias and specificity appears falsely low. Indeed, if only patients with abnormal MPI undergo angiography, the observed sensitivity will be 100% and the specificity 0%. The normalcy rate is therefore a better index for assessing the performance of a test in patients without disease. This is defined as the rate of normal perfusion scans in patients with a low (< 5%) likelihood of CAD based on clinical and exercise ECG features. Studies have consistently reported significantly higher normalcy rates than specificity for MPI in the diagnosis of CAD. The mean normalcy rate for MPI from 12 studies (543 patients) was 88%.

Despite their different physical and imaging characteristics, all three radiotracers have comparable diagnostic accuracies for detecting CAD. As technetium-99m labeled tracers have myocardial uptake curves that plateau at lower levels of hyperemia than Tl-201, it has been suggested that they may not perform well when used with vasodilator stress. However, several studies with sestamibi indicate that the diagnostic accuracy is not compromised when the latter is used with adenosine or dipyridamole. Data from studies with tetrofosmin are less consistent, with some studies reporting good accuracy with vasodilators and others showing it to be less sensitive than Tl-201 or sestamibi for the detection of mild to moderate angiographic disease. Such underestimation has also been reported in some, but not all, studies performed with dobutamine sestamibi MPI.

4. Evaluation in Patients with Extensive CAD

An important function of any noninvasive test for CAD is its ability to identify patients with extensive disease, as their prognosis is particularly poor and thus demands prompt management. It is well documented that patients with three vessel or left main stem disease almost always have an abnormal MPI study and that the sensitivity is higher in patients with multivessel disease compared to those with single vessel disease. However, the perfusion abnormality will not necessarily reflect involvement of more than one vessel; moreover, less than two-thirds of such scans show the typical pattern of multi-vessel disease (Fig. 6.19).

A number of studies have observed a low sensitivity for accurately detecting three vessel disease with visual analysis. Quantitative analysis of the washout rate in the areas of normal Tl-201 uptake was found to improve the sensitivity, which can also be increased by incorporation of the clinical response to treadmill testing. Other scintigraphic features such as transient ischemic dilatation and increased lung uptake of Tl-201 were found by some investigators to be useful predictors of extensive CAD.

5. Left Bundle-Branch Block (LBBB) and other ECG Abnormalities

The non-invasive detection of CAD in patients with resting LBBB poses a particular problem. Although patients with LBBB have a high prevalence of CAD, LBBB also frequently occurs in nonischemic cardiomyopathies. ST segment changes on exercise ECG are nondiagnostic in these patients, and abnormal septal motion associated with the conduction abnormality may reduce the diagnostic accuracy of stress/rest regional wall motion comparisons using radionuclide ventriculography or echocardiography. Even in the presence of angiographically normal coronary arteries, patients with LBBB often have reversible or fixed septal defects on MPI, particularly when combined with exercise or dobutamine stress. The exact mechanism is

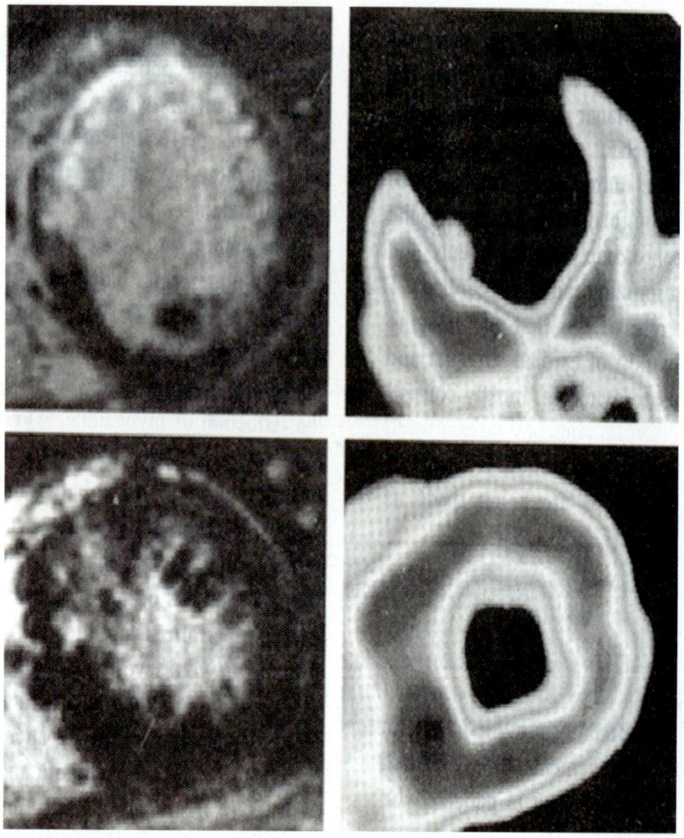

Fig. 6.19: *Midventricular short-axis view of the patient who has AMI (top) and who has HCM (bottom). Left panels demonstrate CMR images, right panels demonstrate anatomic tissue fraction PET images*

unclear but it is possible that a delayed activation of the septum in the presence of LBBB may lead to a reduction in coronary flow and hence tracer delivery to the septum. A high heart rate increases the proportion of diastolic filling that is lost, leading to a further reduction in septal coronary flow and therefore more obvious perfusion defects. When stress is performed with dipyridamole or adenosine alone it is less likely to observe such perfusion abnormalities probably because the effect of vasodilators on the heart rate and septal contraction is less than that of dynamic exercise. It has been shown that specificity with vasodilator stress improves by up to 75% and this is achieved without a reduction in sensitivity. Accordingly, the recently published American College of Cardiology/American Heart Association guidelines for the management of patients with stable angina recommend the use of adenosine or dipyridamole SPECT MPI as the preferred imaging modality for patients with LBBB. The committee does not recommend the use of echocardiography because there is only limited information regarding its clinical utility.

As in LBBB, perfusion abnormalities may be seen in patients with bifascicular block or right ventricular pacemakers even in the absence of epicardial CAD, therefore if a stress test is required, this should be performed with vasodilators. MPI can also be helpful in patients with resting ECG changes (such as those seen in left ventricular hypertrophy (LVH), preexcitation or drug effects) because they can reduce the usefulness of exercise ECG for the detection of CAD.

6. Cardiomyopathies and LVH

Dilated cardiomyopathy (DCM) is often associated with perfusion abnormalities and hence the noninvasive detection of concomitant epicardial coronary stenoses can be difficult. Although a normal scan or a study showing patchy nonreversible defects in a patient with DCM virtually exclude the presence of underlying CAD as the cause of cardiomyopathy, the presence of reversible abnormalities is not always the result of CAD. However, if such abnormalities are found in the distribution of coronary territories, then they are more likely to represent underlying CAD and hence, they can help to differentiate between ischemic and nonischemic aetiology. This distinction is important because it has implications for the patient management (Figs 6.16 and 6.18).

Patients with hypertrophic cardiomyopathy (HCM) often demonstrate an abnormally thickened septum on MPI. However, this technique is of very limited value in the detection of the condition and confirmation of the diagnosis should be performed with echocardiography or CMRI. Perfusion abnormalities are often seen in patients with HCM in the absence of epicardial coronary disease and typically affect the septum. There is evidence that patients with inducible ischemia on MPI demonstrate lactate production during rapid atrial pacing. This supports the view that such abnormalities represent true myocardial ischemia, although this is presumably the result of other mechanisms, such as systolic compression of intramyocardial septal vessels, abnormal coronary flow pattern in the left anterior descending artery, or impaired coronary flow reserve. A negative perfusion scan in HCM, on the other hand, suggests that significant underlying epicardial CAD is unlikely. Inducible ischemia on MPI has been correlated with events (cardiac arrest or syncope) in young patients with HCM, although not in larger unselected populations. At present, the role of MPI in the management of patients with HCM remains undefined.

Inducible perfusion defects can also be seen in patients with more generalised LVH because of abnormalities in the microcirculation which may therefore erode the specificity of MPI for detecting epicardial CAD. The specificity of MPI may be further compromised by changes seen occasionally in the septum and lateral wall in the form of a reversal of lateral wall to septum tracer uptake ratio, which is not caused by CAD. Dobutamine echocardiography does not suffer from these limitations and although some investigators have found it to be equally effective with MPI for detecting underlying CAD more recent data suggest that the former is probably the technique of choice in this clinical setting.

According to Bayes theorem, noninvasive tests are of most value in patients with an intermediate probability of CAD ideally, therefore, such patients should undergo MPI without prior performance of an exercise ECG. Several factors militate against this. The most important is the relative availability of the two techniques, but radiation burden and cost are also relevant. Many centers use a staged approach with the exercise ECG being the initial test followed by MPI if the likelihood of disease is indeterminate after the exercise ECG, or if further information on myocardial perfusion is required to assist management decisions. This strategy has been adopted in recently published guidelines by the British cardiac society/royal college of physicians and European society of cardiology. They also recommend that MPI should be the initial investigation in patients who are unlikely to exercise adequately, in women, and in cases where the exercise ECG is uninterpretable because of resting abnormalities. It is also reasonable to suggest that even patients with a high likelihood of CAD can be considered for MPI before coronary angiography. MPI can assess objectively the extent and severity of myocardial ischemia allowing accurate risk stratification and influencing management decisions.

7. MPI in Asymptomatic Patients

The role of MPI in asymptomatic patients with increased cardiovascular risk profiles is not clearly defined. The existing data suggest that MPI should not be used in screening unselected asymptomatic populations, but it may have a limited role in selected patients considered to be at a high risk for developing CAD. It possesses a high overall diagnostic accuracy for detecting CAD, which increases further with incorporation of ECG-gated data. A normal myocardial perfusion scan makes it extremely unlikely that a patient has hemodynamically significant CAD, whatever the clinical and ECG features are, and therefore invasive investigations can be avoided in such patients.

BIBLIOGRAPHY

1. Go RT, Marwick TH, MacIntyre WJ, et al. A prospective comparison of rubidium-82 PET and thallium-201 SPECT myocardial perfusion imaging utilising a single dipyridamole stress in the diagnosis of coronary artery disease. J Nucl Med 1990;31:1899–905.
2. Stewart R, Schwaiger M, Molina E, et al. Comparison of rubidium-82 positron emission tomography and thallium-201 SPECT imaging for detection of coronary artery disease. Am J Cardiol 1991;67:1303–10.
3. Tamaki N, Yonekura Y, Mukai T, et al. Stress thallium-201 transaxial emission computed tomography: quantitative versus qualitative analysis for evaluation of coronary artery disease. J Am Coll Cardiol 1984;4:1213–21.
4. DePasquale EE, Nody AC, DePuey EG, et al. Quantitative rotational thallium-201 tomography for identifying and localizing coronary artery disease. Circulation 1988;2:316–27.
5. Fintel DJ, Links JM, Brinker JA, et al. Improved diagnostic performance of exercise thallium-201 single photon emission computed tomography over planar imaging in the diagnosis of coronary artery disease: a receiver operating characteristic analysis. J Am Coll Cardiol 1989;13:600–12.

6. Iskandrian AS, Heo J, Kong B, et al. Effect of exercise level on the ability of thallium-201 tomographic imaging in detecting coronary artery disease: analysis of 461 patients. J Am Coll Cardiol 1989;14:1477–86.
7. Maddahi J, Van Train K, Pringent F, et al. Quantitative single photon emission computed thallium-201 tomography for detection and localization of coronary artery disease: optimization and prospective validation of a new technique. J Am Coll Cardiol 1989;14:1689–99.
8. Mahmarian JJ, Boyce TM, Goldberg RK, et al. Quantitative exercise thallium-201 single photon emission computed tomography for the enhanced diagnosis of ischaemic heart disease. J Am Coll Cardiol 1990;15:318–29.
9. Van Train KF, Maddahi J, Berman DS, et al. Quantitative analysis of tomographic stress thallium-201 myocardial scintigrams: a multicenter trial. J Nucl Med 1990;31:1168–79.
10. Coyne EP, Belvedere DA, Vande Streek PR, et al. Thallium-201 scintigraphy after intravenous infusion of adenosine compared with exercise thallium testing in the diagnosis of coronary artery disease. J Am Coll Cardiol 1991;17:1289–94.
11. Quinones MA, Verani MS, Haichin RM, et al. Exercise echocardiography versus Tl-201 single-photon emission computed tomography in evaluation of coronary artery disease. Circulation 1992;85:1026–].
12. Chae SC, Heo J, Iskandrian AS, et al. Identification of extensive coronary artery disease in women by exercise single-photon emission computed tomographic (SPECT) thallium imaging. J Am Coll Cardiol 1993;21:1305–11.
13. Grover-McKay M, Milne N, Atwood E, et al. Comparison of thallium-201 single-photon emission computed tomographic scintigraphy with intravenous dipyridamole and arm exercise. Am Heart J 1994;127:1516–20.
14. Tamaki N, Takahashi N, Kawamoto M, et al. Myocardial tomography using technetium-99m tetrofosmin to evaluate coronary artery disease. J Nucl Med 1994;35:594–600.
15. Ho Y-L, Wu C-C, Huang P-J, et al. Dobutamine stress echocardiography compared with exercise thallium-201 single-photon emission computed tomography in detecting coronary artery disease – effect of exercise level on accuracy. Cardiol 1997;88:379–85.
16. Kiat H, Van Train KF, Maddahi J, et al. Development and prospective application of quantitative 2-day stress-rest Tc-99m methoxy isobutyl isonitrile SPECT for the diagnosis of coronary artery disease. Am Heart J 1990;120:1255–66.
17. Pozzoli MMA, Fioretti P, Salustri A, et al. Exercise echocardiography and technetium-99m MIBI single-photon emission computed tomography in the detection of coronary artery disease. Am J Cardiol 1991;67:350–5.
18. Solot G, Hermans J, Merlo P, et al. Correlation of Tc-99m sestamibi SPECT with coronary angiography in general hospital practice. Nucl Med Commun 1993;14:23–9.
19. Marwick TH, D' Hondt AM, Mairesse GH, et al. Comparative ability of dobutamine and exercise stress in inducing myocardial ischaemia in active patients. Br Heart J 1994;72:31–8.
20. Van Train KF, Garcia EV, Maddahi J, et al. Multicenter trial validation for quantitative analysis of same-day rest-stress technetium-99m-sestamibi myocardial tomograms. J Nucl Med 1994;35:609–18.
21. Heo J, Cave V, Wasserleben V, et al. Planar and tomographic imaging with technetium-99m-labeled tetrofosmin: correlation with thallium-201 and coronary angiography. J Nucl Cardiol 1994;1:317–24.
22. Benoit Th, Vivegnis D, Lahiri A, et al. Tomographic myocardial imaging with technetium-99m tetrofosmin. Eur Heart J 1996;17:635–42 t.echnetium-99m tetrofosmin and thallium-201 single-photon emission computed tomographic imaging for detection of myocardial perfusion defects in patients with coronary artery disease. J Am Coll Cardiol 1998;31:331–7.
23. Francisco DA, Collins SM, Go RT, et al. Tomographic thaalium-201 myocardial perfusion scintigrams after maximal coronary artery vasodilation with intravenous dipyridamole. Circulation 1982;66:370–9.
24. Huikuri HV, Korhonen UR, Airaksinen KEJ, et al. Comparison of dipyridamole-handgrip test and bicycle exercise test for thallium tomographic imaging. Am J Cardiol 1988;61:264–8.
25. Go RT, Marwick TH, MacIntyre WJ, et al. A prospective comparison of rubidium-82 PET and thallium-201 SPECT myocardial perfusion imaging utilizing a single dipyridamole stress in the diagnosis of coronary artery disease. J Nucl Med 1990;31:1899–905.
26. Mendelson MA, Spies SM, Spies WG, et al. Usefulness of single-photon emission computed tomography of thallium-201 uptake after dipyridamole infusion for detection of coronary artery disease. Am J Cardiol 1992;69:1150–5.
27. Cramer M-J, Verzijlbergen JF, Van der Wall EE, et al. Head-to-head comparison between technetium-99m-sestamibi and thallium-201 tomographic imaging for the detection of coronary artery disease using combined dipyridamole-exercise stress. Coron Artery Dis 1994;5:787–91.
28. Ho F-M, Huang P-J, Liau C-S, et al. Dobutamine stress echocardiography compared with dipyridamole thallium-201 single-photon emission computed tomography in detecting coronary artery disease. Eur Heart J 1995;16:570–5.
29. Watanabe K, Sekiya M, Ikeda S, et al. Comparison of adenosine triphosphate and dipyridamole in diagnosis by thallium-201 myocardial scintigraphy. J Nucl Med 1997;38:577–81.
30. Tartagni F, Dondi M, Limonetti P, et al. Dipyridamole technetium-99m 2-methoxy isobutyl isonitrile tomoscintigraphic imaging for identifying diseased coronary vessels: comparison with thallium-201 stress-rest study. J Nucl Med 1991;32:369–76.
31. Miller DD, Younis LT, Chaitman BR, et al. Diagnostic accuracy of dipyridamole technetium-99m-labeled sestamibi myocardial tomography for detection of coronary artery disease. J Nucl Cardiol 1997;4:18–24.
32. Schillaci O, Moroni C, Scopinaro F, et al. Technetium-99m sestamibi myocardial tomography based on dipyridamole echocardiography testing in hypertensive patients with chest pain. Eur J Nucl Med 1997;24:774–8.
33. Soman P, Khattar R, Senior R, et al. Inotropic stress with arbutamine is superior to vasodilator stress with dipyridamole for the detection of reversible ischaemia with Tc-99m sestamibi single-photon emission computed tomography. J Nucl Cardiol 1997;4:364–71.
34. Ogilby JD, Kegel JG, Heo J, et al. Correlation between haemodynamic changes and tomographic sestamibi imaging during dipyridamole-induced coronary hyperaemia. J Am Coll Cardiol 1998;31:75–82.

7 Electrophysiological Study, Catheter Management of Cardiac Arrhythmia and Conduction Blocks

HISTORICAL ASPECTS OF ELECTROPHYSIOLOGY (EP) STUDY

Clinical cardiac electrophysiologic testing has evolved rapidly since 1968, when the technique was first described. In an electrophysiologic study, electrode catheters are positioned within the heart to record electrical activity from the atrium, atrioventricular conduction tissue, and ventricle. Programed stimulation is then performed, which involves pacing of the atrium or ventricle and introducing critically timed premature stimuli during sinus rhythm or paced rhythm. The use of programed stimulation in conjunction with intracardiac recordings in electrophysiologic studies has facilitated the diagnosis of mechanisms of arrhythmia and the assessment of therapy. Electrophysiologic testing is useful in selected patients with sinus node dysfunction, conduction system disorders, supraventricular tachycardia, ventricular tachycardia, or ventricular fibrillation and in survivors of out-of-hospital cardiac arrest and patients with symptomatic but unsubstantiated rhythm disturbances. Therapeutic approaches that can be assessed by electrophysiologic testing include serial drug testing to determine the effectiveness of antiarrhythmic agents, antitachycardia pacing, the implantable defibrillator, transcatheter ablation, and electrophysiologically guided surgical procedures. In this review, the methods of electrophysiologic testing, its clinical applications in diagnosing the various cardiac rhythm disturbances, and its use in assessing various therapeutic modalities (Figs 7.1 to 7.4) have been discussed.

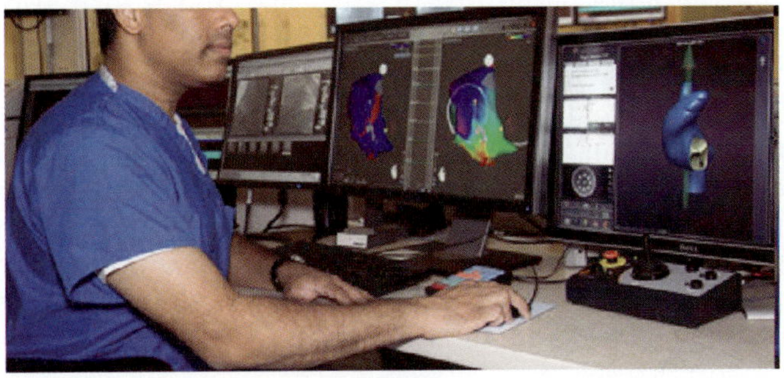

Fig. 7.1: *Electrophysiology laboratory for carrying out EP studies and catheter ablation of various types of drug resistant cardiac arrhythmias*

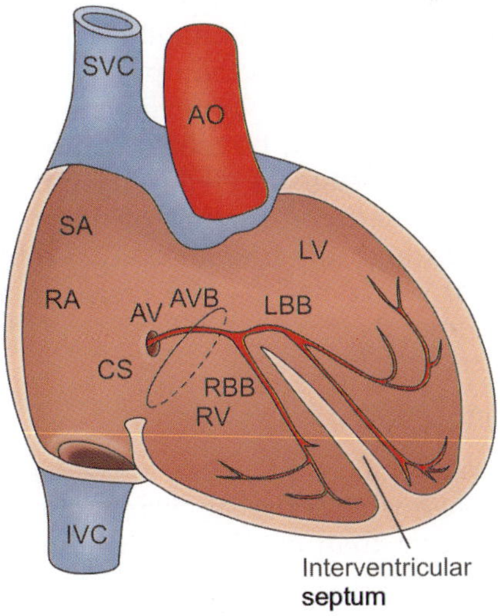

Fig. 7.2: *Anatomical features of bundle of His as a conduction system of the heart close to tricuspid valve*

AN OVERVIEW OF THE PROCEDURE

While ECGs are noninvasive, an EP study is somewhat invasive. The study is performed after giving local anesthesia and conscious sedation (twilight sleep) to keep the patient as comfortable as possible. The procedure involves inserting a catheter-a narrow, flexible tube-attached to electricity monitoring electrodes, into a blood vessel, often through a site in the groin or neck, and winding the catheter wire up into the heart. The journey from entry point to heart muscle is navigated by images created by a fluoroscope, an X-ray-like machine that provides continuous, "live" images of the catheter and heart muscle. Once the catheter reaches the heart, electrodes at its tip gather data and a variety of electrical measurements are made. These data pinpoint the location of the faulty electrical site. During this "electrical mapping", the cardiac arrhythmia specialist, an electrophysiologist, may instigate, through pacing (the use of tiny electrical impulses), some of the very arrhythmic that are the crux of the problem. The events are safe, given the range of experts and resources close at hand and are necessary to ensure the precise location of the problematic tissue.

Once the damaged site or sites are confirmed, the specialist may administer different medications or electrical impulses to determine their ability to halt the arrhythmia and restore normal heart rhythm. Based on this data, as well as information garnered before the study, sometimes the specialist will proceed to place an implantable cardioverter device (ICD) or a pacemaker or will perform radiofrequency ablation. In any case, the information proves useful for diagnosis and treatment.

Throughout the procedure, the patient is sedated but awake and remains still. Patients rarely report pain, more often describing what they feel as discomfort. Some watch the procedure on monitors and occasionally ask questions. The procedure usually takes about 2 hours. The patient remains still for 4–6 hours afterward to ensure the entry point incision begins to heal properly. Once mobile again, patients may feel stiff and achy from lying still for hours.

The Importance of the Flow of Electricity

Each heart has it own normal rhythm brought about by the seamless flow of electrical impulses throughout the organ. This electrical flow begins in the heart's natural "pacemaker" (also know as the sinoatrial node or sinus node) in the upper right heart chamber, the right atrium. The electricity flows through the upper chambers (atria), crosses the bridge between upper and lower chambers (atrioventricular node) and travels to the lower chambers (ventricles). The passage of electricity culminates in a carefully coordinated contraction of heart muscle that pushes blood through the human body. Problems in the precise flow of electricity are the cause of arrhythmia (Figs 7.3 and 7.4).

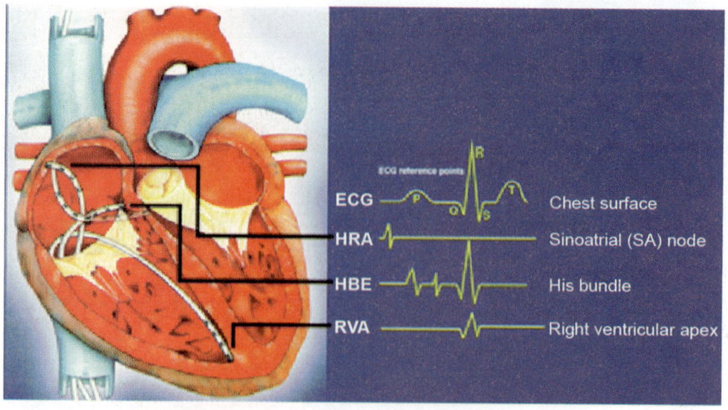

Fig. 7.3: *(Left) diagram shows different intracardiac conduction system from where electrograms are generated (right) shows schematic illustrations of several intracardiac electrograms contrasted with a conventional body-surface electrocardiogram (ECG)*

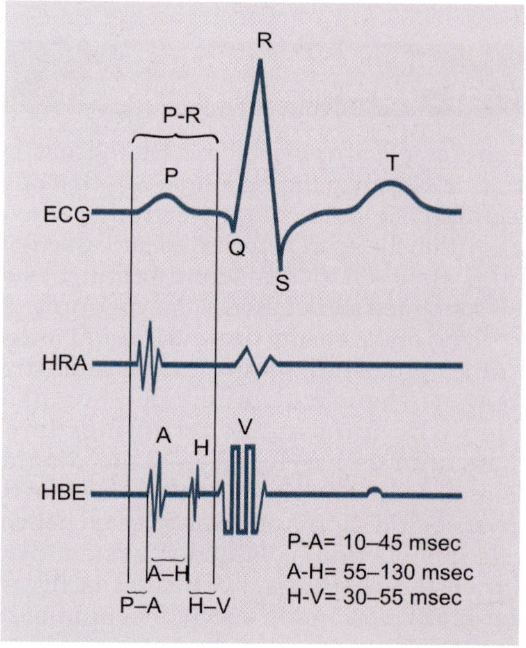

Fig. 7.4: *Intracardiac electrograms. Schematic illustrations of several intracardiac electrograms contrasted with a conventional body-surface electrocardiogram (ECG). HRA, high right atrial electrogram; HBE, His bundle electrogram, in which A = low right atrial activity, H, His bundle activity, and V, ventricular septal activity; also shown are the P-R, P-A, A-H, and H-V intervals*

CLINICAL APPLICATION OF EP STUDY

An electrophysiologic, or EP, study provides information that is key to diagnosing and treating arrhythmia. Although it is more invasive than an electrocardiogram (ECG) or echocardiogram, and involves provoking arrhythmia, the test produces data that makes it possible to:

1. Diagnose the source of arrhythmia symptoms
2. Evaluate the effectiveness of certain medications or procedures in controlling the heart rhythm disorder
3. Predict the risk of a future cardiac event, such as sudden cardiac death
4. Assess the need for an implantable device (a pacemaker or ICD) or treatment procedure (radiofrequency catheter ablation).

Who Performs the Test and Where?

Since potentially dangerous arrhythmia are provoked during an EP study, it is crucial that specialized staff are present to handle all situations. A physician electrophysiologist, with advanced training in the diagnosis and treatment of heart rhythm problems, performs the EP study.

The electrophysiologist leads a team of specially trained healthcare professionals, technicians and nurses, who assist during the procedure. The team performs the EP study in an electrophysiology laboratory, or EP lab, a well-equipped, controlled clinical environment usually located within a hospital or clinic. As a result, the test is quite safe and complications are rare.

Complications in EP Study

The procedure is generally very safe. Possible risks include:

- Arrhythmias
- Bleeding
- Blood clots that lead to embolism
- Cardiac tamponade
- Heart attack
- Infection
- Injury to the vein
- Low blood pressure.

1. TECHNICAL CONSIDERATIONS IN PERFORMANCE OF ELECTROPHYSIOLOGICAL STUDY

I. Before the Procedure

Your physician will explain the procedure to you and offer you the opportunity to ask any questions that you might have about the procedure.

- You will be asked to sign a consent form that gives your permission to do the test. Read the form carefully and ask questions if something is not clear.
- Notify your physician if you are sensitive to or are allergic to any medications, iodine, latex, tape, or anesthetic agents (local and general).
- You will need to fast for a certain period of time prior to the procedure. Your physician will notify you how long to fast, usually overnight.
- If you are pregnant or suspect that you may be pregnant, you should notify your physician.
- Notify your physician if you have any body piercing on your chest and/or abdomen.
- Notify your physician of all medications (prescription and over-the-counter) and herbal supplements that you are taking.
- Notify your physician if you have heart valve disease, as you may need to receive and antibiotic prior to the procedure.
- Notify your physician if you have a history of bleeding disorders or if you are taking any anticoagulant (blood-thinning) medications, aspirin, or other medications that affect blood clotting. It may be necessary for you to stop some of these medications prior to the procedure.
- Your physician may request a blood test prior to the procedure to determine how long it takes your blood to clot. Other blood tests may be done as well.
- Notify your physician if you have a pacemaker.
- If a sedative is given before the procedure, you may need someone to drive your home afterwards.
- The area around the catheter insertion (groin area) may be shaved.
- Based upon your medical condition, your physician may request other specific preparation.

II. During the Procedure (Figs 7.5A and B, 7.6 to 7.9)

An EP study may be performed on an outpatient basis or as part of your stay in a hospital. Procedures may vary depending on your condition and your physician's practices.

Generally, an EP Study Follows This Process

1. You will be asked to remove any jewelry or other objects that may interfere with the procedure.
2. You will be asked to remove clothing and will be given a gown to wear.

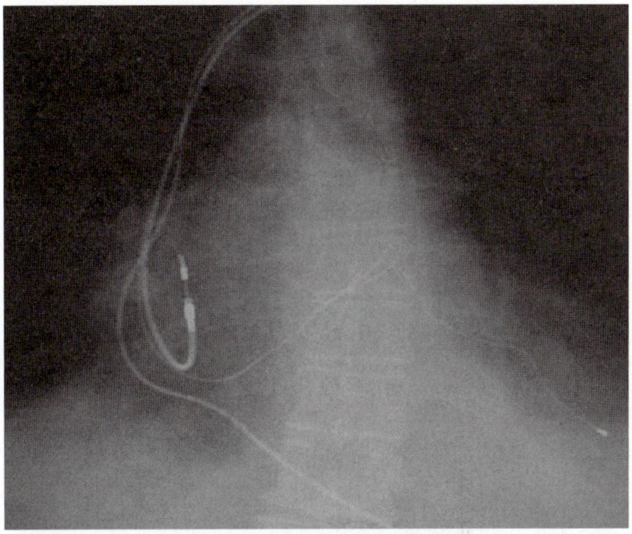

Fig. 7.5A: *X-ray chest AP view showing "granny knot" of left ventricular lead in coronary sinus*

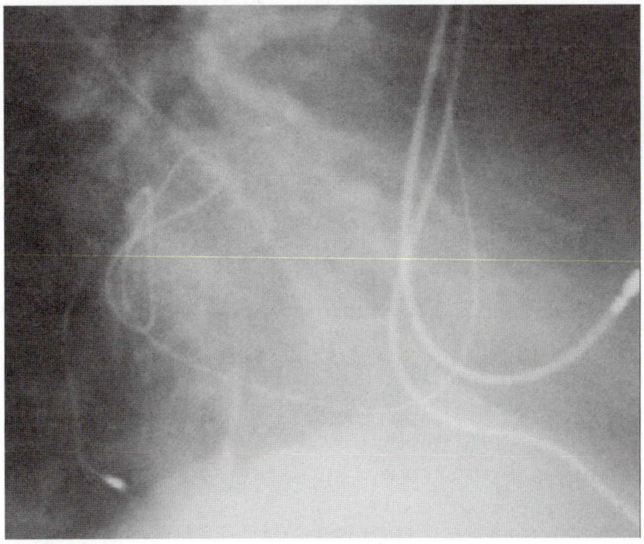

Fig. 7.5B: *X-ray chest lateral view showing "granny knot" of left ventricular lead in coronary sinus*

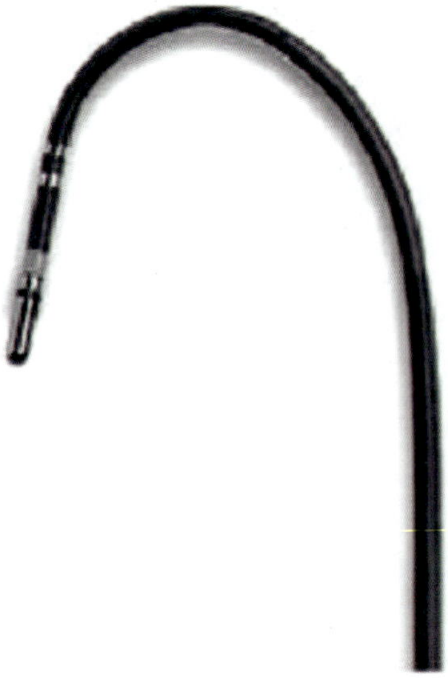

Fig. 7.6: *Image of a typical ablation catheter with a distal tip consisting of electrodes that can measure the electrical activity in the heart as well as deliver radiofrequency, or heat, energy to ablate cardiac arrhythmias*

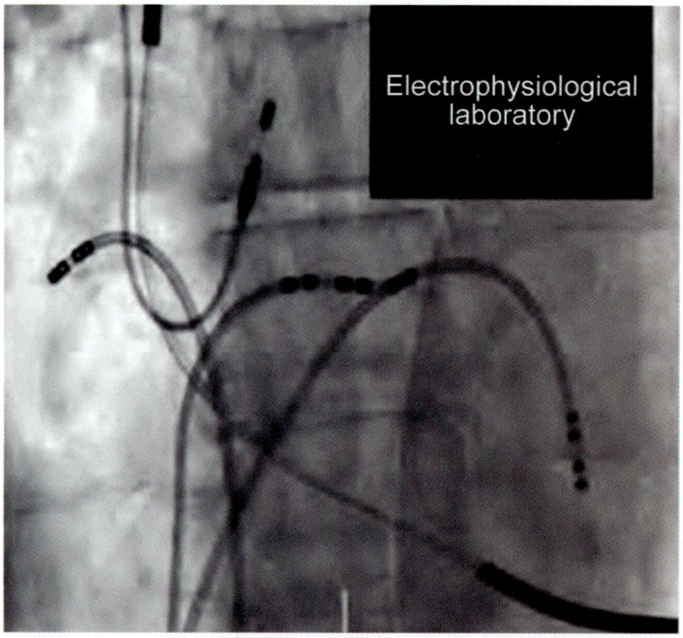

Fig. 7.7: *An X-ray image showing 3 catheters introduced into the heart to record electrical signals and for circuit testing*

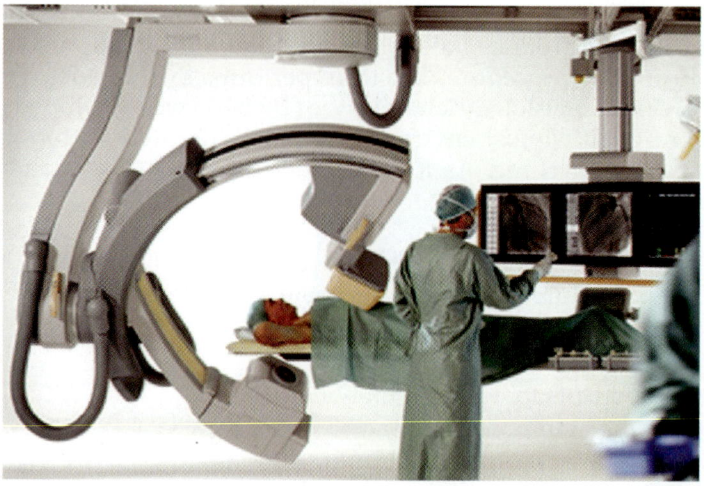

Fig. 7.8: *Cardiac catheterization laboratory. Electrophysiologist is busy in performing electrophysiological study for diagnosis of cardiac arrhythmia*

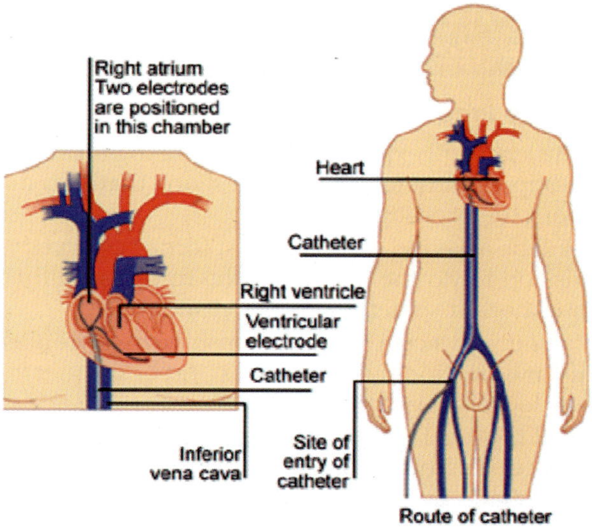

Fig. 7.9: *Routes inserting catheter in intracardiac electrocardiographic study*

3. You will be asked to empty your bladder prior to the procedure.
4. An intravenous (IV) line will be started in your hand or arm prior to the procedure for injection of medication and to administer IV fluids if needed.
5. You will be placed in a supine (on your back) position on the procedure table.
6. You will be connected to an ECG monitor that records the electrical activity of the heart and monitors the heart during the procedure using small, adhesive electrodes. Your vital signs (heart rate, blood pressure, breathing rate, and oxygenation level) will be monitored during the procedure.
7. There may be several monitor screens, showing your vital signs and the images of the catheter being moved through the body into the heart.
8. You will receive a sedative medication in your IV before the procedure to help you relax. However, you will likely remain awake during the procedure.
9. Your pulses below the IV site may be checked and marked with a marker so that the circulation to the limb below the site can be checked after the procedure.
10. A local anesthetic will be injected into the skin at the insertion site. You may feel some stinging at the site for a few seconds after the local anesthetic is injected.
11. Once the local anesthetic has taken effect, a sheath, or introducer, will be inserted into the blood vessel. This is

a plastic tube through which the catheter will be inserted into the blood vessel and advanced into the heart.

12. One or more catheters will be inserted through the sheath into the blood vessel. The physician will advance the catheter through the blood vessel into the right side of the heart. Fluoroscopy (a special type of X-ray that is displayed on a TV monitor), may be used to assist in advancing the catheter to the heart.
13. Once the physician has the catheter(s) placed properly, the electrical testing will begin by sending very small electrical impulses to certain areas within the heart. If a dysrhythmia occurs, you may begin to feel lightheaded or dizzy.

    Medication will be given to you IV to treat the dysrhythmia. Alternatively, a shock will be delivered to stop the dysrhythmia. You will be sedated before this type of shock is given.
14. If a certain area of tissue is found to be causing a dysrhythmia, the physician may perform an ablation to eliminate the tissue. This is done with radiowaves (radiofrequency ablation). The radiowaves are delivered through the catheter to the tissue.
15. If you notice any discomfort or pain, such as chest pain, neck or jaw pain, back pain, arm pain, shortness of breath, or breathing difficulty, let the physician know.
16. Once the procedure has been completed, the catheter(s) will be removed from the insertion site. The physician or an assistant will hold pressure on the insertion site so that the blood can begin to form a clot at the site and stop the bleeding.
17. Once the bleeding has stopped, a bandage will be placed on the site.
18. You will be assisted to slide from the table onto a stretcher so that you can be taken to the recovery area. ***Note:*** If the insertion was in the groin, you will not be allowed to bend your leg for a few hours.

To help you remember to keep your leg straight, the knee of the affected leg may be covered with a sheet and the ends will be tucked under the mattress on both sides of the bed to form a type of loose restraint.

Transseptal Approach Technique in EP Study

Throughout the diagnostic electrophysiological study and transseptal procedure the patients were kept well hydrated with a continuous infusion of normal saline, receiving at least 500 mL before the transseptal procedure. The transseptal procedures were performed using a standard Brockenborough needle and either a Mullins sheath (Bard Inc, Billerica, Massachusetts, USA) or a Swartz sheath and dilator (Daig Corporation, Minnetonka, Minnesota, USA). The needle was connected to a standard catheterization manifold by a short length of flexible tubing, so that contrast could be injected and pressure could be displayed and recorded. Biplane fluoroscopic projections used were (right anterior oblique 45° and left anterior oblique 40°) in all cases, providing en face and longitudinal views of the interatrial septum, respectively. The transseptal sheath/dilator was placed in the superior vena cava and then the dilator/sheath/needle combination was withdrawn inferiorly in the left anterior oblique projection until the tip of the dilator "popped" into the fossa ovalis. Positioning was always checked in the right anterior oblique projection to ensure that the tip of the needle/sheath assembly was pointing directly away from the plane of vision and slightly anterior. A test injection of contrast was delivered through the dilator in the left anterior oblique projection to check for "tenting" of the fossa at the intended puncture site. This was typically just below the level of the his recording catheter in the left anterior oblique 40° projection, and well behind the his catheter electrodes in the right anterior oblique 45°. The needle was then advanced and a second test injection was made following needle advancement to check that the needle had entered the left atrium; left atrial pressure was then recorded. The sheath/dilator were advanced over the needle into the left atrium. Once the dilator was well into the left atrium, the sheath was advanced over the dilator, but the needle remained just inside the dilator to give support for advancement of the long sheath. Once the needle is withdrawn, the tip of the dilator tends to flex. This makes it hazardous to redeploy the needle, since this may result in penetration of the wall of the dilator (Fig. 7.10).

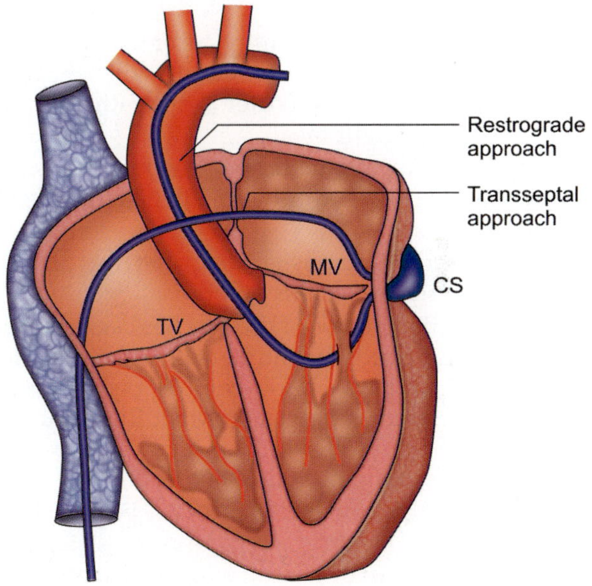

Fig. 7.10: *Illustration showing transseptal and retrograde approaches in EP study*

Patients then received 5,000 units of heparin, with a further 2,500 units being given if left-sided deployment lasted more than 1 hour. If deployment exceeded 90 minutes, activated partial thromboplastin time was estimated. Ablations were performed using 4 mm tipped "Steerocath" or "Blazer-T" thermistor tipped electrodes (EP Technologies, Sunnyvale, California, USA). The ablation catheter was passed through the sheath into the left atrium and positioned on the mitral annulus. Care was always taken to flush the sheath during catheter advancement to avoid entrainment of air. Suitable ablation sites were obtained using conventional criteria. Nine patients remained in the laboratory with transseptal sheath in place for 30 minutes after the procedure (particularly after accessory pathway ablation) for confirmation of success. After successful ablation, transseptal sheaths were withdrawn across the interatrial septum with the ablation catheter tip protruding slightly. This technique was employed to avoid inadvertent displacement of adherent coagulum from the catheter at the sheath tip.

III. After the Procedure

In the Hospital

After the procedure, you may be taken to the recovery room for observation or returned to your hospital room. You will remain flat in bed for a few hours after the procedure. The circulation and sensation of the limb where the catheter was inserted will be monitored. A nurse will monitor your vital signs, the insertion site, and circulation/sensation in the affected leg or arm.

You should immediately inform your nurse if you feel any chest pain or tightness, or any other pain, as well as any feelings of warmth, bleeding, or pain at the insertion site in your leg or arm.

Bed rest may vary from 2–6 hours depending on your specific condition.

In some cases, the sheath or introducer may be left in the insertion site. If so, the period of bed rest will be prolonged until the sheath is removed. After the sheath is removed, you may be given a light meal.

You may be given pain medication for pain or discomfort related to the insertion site or having to lie flat and still for a prolonged period.

You may resume your usual diet after the procedure, unless your physician decides otherwise.

After the specified period of bed rest has been completed, you may get out of bed. The nurse will assist you the first time you get up, and will check your blood pressure while you are lying in bed, sitting, and standing. You should move slowly when getting up from the bed to avoid any dizziness from the long period of bed rest.

When you have completed the recovery period, you may be discharged to your home unless your physician decides otherwise. If this procedure was performed on an outpatient basis, you must have another person drive you home.

IV. Discharge Instructions and Care

Your heart rhythm specialist will discuss specific individualized recommendations in regard to your discharge care. The following are general recommendations:

- Limit heavy lifting or strenuous exertion for 4–5 days after your study
- You may shower after your return home the day of the procedure
- You may remove any dressing or bandages placed at the catheter site after you return home
- You may typically return to work in 1–2 day, as long as it does not involve heavy lifting or strenuous exertion
- Call your physician if your incision site (typically in the groin) appears to swell or become more painful
- It is normal to develop some bruising at the catheter site with a transition to a "black-and-blue appearance" - however, this should not become more painful or lead to increased swelling
- Follow-up with your physician in approximately 1 month for a clinic visit.

At Home

Once at home, you should monitor the insertion site for bleeding, unusual pain, swelling, and abnormal discoloration or temperature change at or near the injection site. A small bruise is normal. If you notice a constant or large amount of blood at the site that cannot be contained with a small dressing, notify your physician.

It will be important to keep the insertion site clean and dry. Your physician will give you specific bathing instructions.

You may be advised not to participate in any strenuous activities. Your physician will instruct you about when you can return to work and resume normal activities.

Post Procedural Information to Your Physician About Your Physical Problems Such As

- Fever and/or chills
- Increased pain, redness, swelling, or bleeding or other drainage from the insertion site
- Coolness, numbness and/or tingling, or other changes in the affected extremity
- Chest pain/pressure, nausea and/or vomiting, profuse sweating, dizziness, and/or fainting

Your physician may give you additional or alternate instructions after the procedure, depending on your particular situation.

MANAGEMENT OF CARDIAC ARRHYTHMIAS WITH CATHETER ABLATION

Radiofrequency catheter ablation (RFCA) has revolutionized treatment for tachyarrhythmias and has become first-line therapy for some tachycardias. Although developed in the 1980s and widely applied in the 1990s, formalized guidelines for its use in clinical practice were not developed until recently.

Different Types of Catheters Employed in Ablation

The design and functionality of catheters is constantly evolving. Most atrial fibrillation ablations today use single point radiofrequency energy catheters, which have a success rate-freedom from atrial fibrillation of about 70%. It's believed that different types of catheters could have higher success rates or fewer complications. Here are the different types of catheters available today for atrial fibrillation catheter ablations:

Single point radiofrequency catheters emit radiofrequency energy from a single point at the catheter tip. To make lesions, electrophysiologists ablate one spot after another, similar to drawing a line by making dots one after the other. If all the dots are not connected, afib could reenter the heart in the unablated space (gap).

Multielectrode radiofrequency catheters have several electrodes, each of which can transmit radiofrequency energy. These catheters can ablate a larger area of tissue than single point radiofrequency energy catheters, which could decrease procedure times. In addition, multielectrode catheters may be better at making contiguous lesions (lesion lines without any gaps) than single point catheters. Finally, these catheters enable the use of bipolar radiofrequency energy, which may reduce certain complications that are seen with unipolar radiofrequency energy. However, there is limited clinical data on multielectrode catheters, which means that complications arising from these procedures may not be fully known or understood.

Contact force sensing radiofrequency catheters. Contact force is one of the variables that affects transmurality. If there is not enough pressure, the lesion may not fully penetrate the tissue, which would allow afib to reenter the heart. If there is too much pressure, complications, such as steam pops, can occur. These catheters tell the electrophysiologist how much pressure is being applied to the catheter and tissue.

Balloon catheters. After the balloon catheter is inserted into the left atrium, the electrophysiologist inflates the balloon at the tip of the catheter. Balloon catheters can ablate a larger area of tissue than single point radiofrequency catheters, which enhances the prospects that lesions will be contiguous (without gaps) and could shorten procedure times. There are balloon catheters using cryothermy, laser energy, and even radiofrequency energy. In general, balloon catheters have difficulty reaching the right pulmonary veins.

Robotic Catheter Navigation for Ablation

Robotic catheter ablation is performed at some centers. Robotic systems could improve navigation of the catheter, keep the catheter in a stable position, and shorten procedure times. In general, robotic catheter ablations have had similar outcomes as traditional (manual) catheter ablation, meaning that the success and complications rates aren't significantly better or worse. Robotic systems are expensive, so not all centers have them (Figs 7.11 to 7.13).

Performing catheter ablation with a single point radiofrequency catheter can be technically challenging, particularly for doctors who have not performed many ablations. In theory, using a robot will simplify the procedure and decrease the expertise needed. However, studies that test this theory have not been performed.

A robotic ablation starts the same way as a traditional catheter ablation. The doctor inserts a catheter into the groin and guides the catheter to the right side of the heart. After making a puncture in the septum, the wall that separates the right and left sides of the heart, the doctor leaves the patient's side and goes to the control system for the robotic system, which is usually located in an adjacent room.

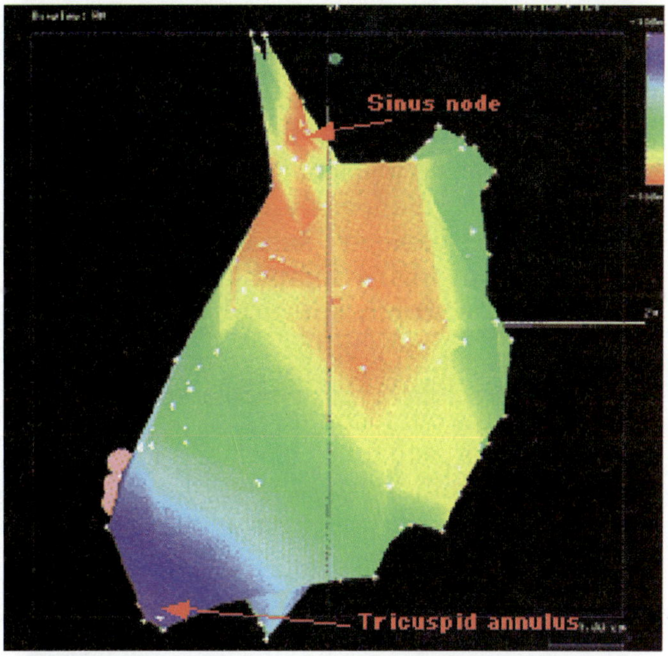

Fig. 7.11: *Activation sequence during sinus rhythm. Electroanatomic mapping of the right atrium with the CARTO system during sinus rhythm shows the earliest activation in the region of the sinus node (red), spreading throughout the atrium. The last part to be activated in the region of the tricupid annulus and coronary sinus so (dark blue/purple). (Reprinted with permission from Cooke, PA, Wilber, DJ pacing CI in Electrophysiol 1998; 21:1802)*

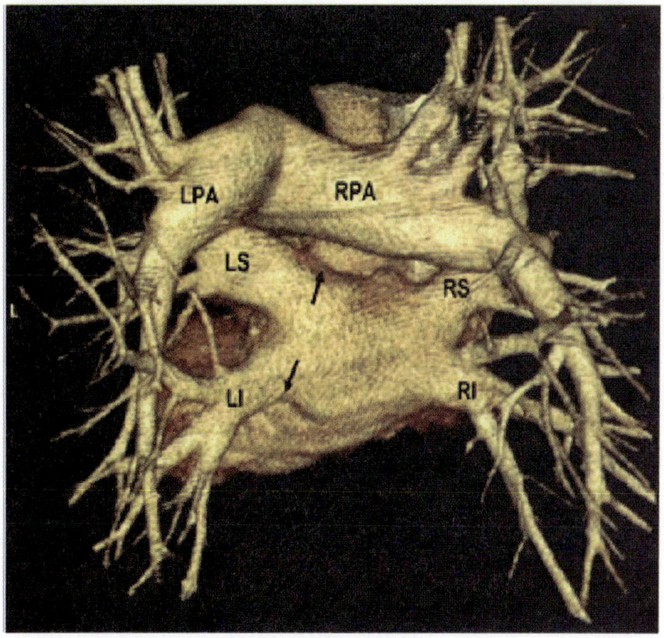

Fig. 7.12: *Multirow spiral computed tomography showing a posterior coronal image of the pulmonary veins in a patient with atrial fibrillation. The right superior (RS) and right inferior (RI) pulmonary veins enter posteriorly into the right atrium. The left superior (LS) and the left inferior (LI) pulmonary veins combine to form an antrum (black arrows) before entering the left atrium. LPA, left pulmonary artery; RPA, right pulmonary artery*

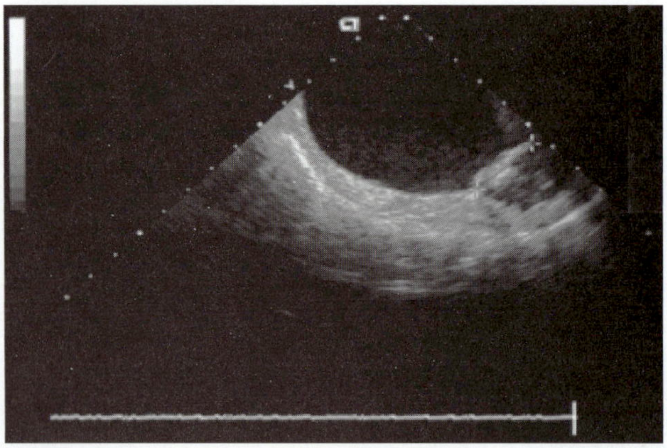

Fig. 7.13: *Intracardiac ultrasound image of the left atrium as obtained from the right atrium. Shown (white pluses) is a left atrial occlusion device positioned into the left atrial appendage. When expanded, this device measured 2.2 cm in diameter*

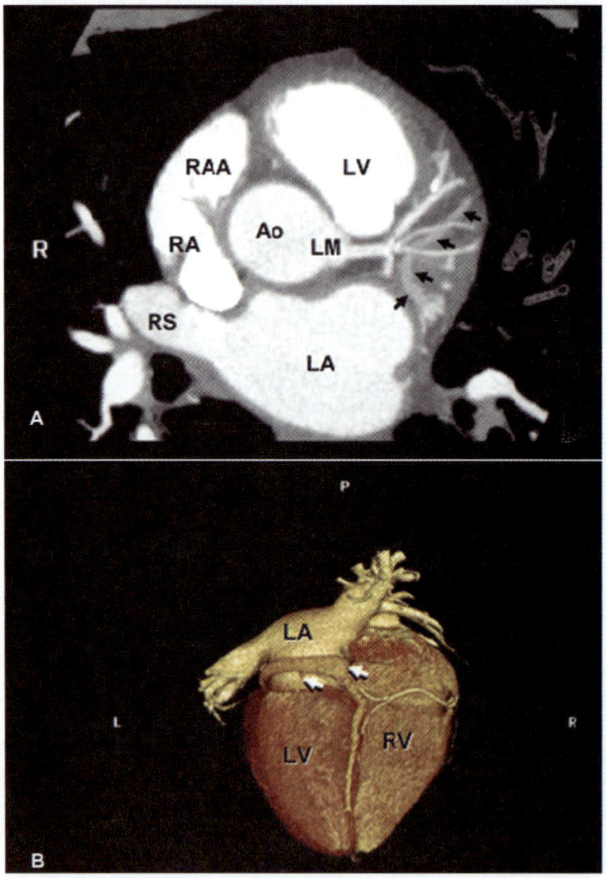

Fig. 7.14: *Helical row, computed tomographic imaging of the distal and proximal venous system of the heart. (A) Oblique view of the heart displaying the greater cardiac vein and its extension into the anterior, interventricular vein (black arrows). (B) Three dimensional, segmented rendering of the heart from a posterior view. Shown are the coronary sinus (white arrow), the middle cardiac vein, a posterior branch of the coronary sinus (black arrow), and the greater cardiac vein extending laterally around the oblique margin of the heart. AO, aortic root; LA, left atrium; LM, left main coronary artery; LV, left ventricle; RA, right atrium; RAA, right atrial appendage; RS, right superior pulmonary vein; RV, right ventricle*

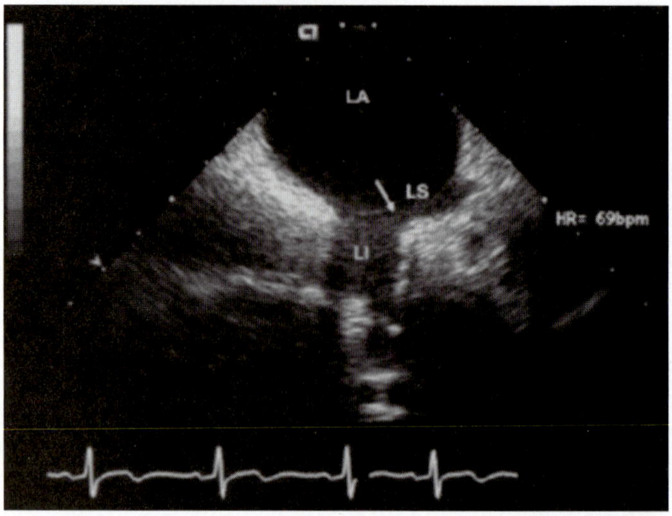

Fig. 7.15: *Intracardiac, phased-array echocardiographic image of the left pulmonary veins. Shown are the left superior (LS) and left inferior (LI) pulmonary veins. This image is obtained with the intracardiac echocardiographic transducer on the right side of the interatrial septum. LA, left atrium*

Leading Robotic Systems Used in Catheter Ablations

Niobe (stereotaxis): Niobe is a magnetic system that only works with the CARTO electroanatomic mapping system and Biosense Webster mapping and ablation catheters. It doesn't look like a robot, but is considered a robotic system. The patient's bed lies between two large magnets, which track the movement in the catheter and send the information to the system. The doctor uses a joystick like those used in video games to change the position of the magnets, which then makes the catheters move. People who have a pacemaker or ICD cannot have a Niobe procedure because these devices would be affected by the magnets.

Sensei (Hansen medical): Sensei has a robotic arm that is attached to the patient's bed. It works with both Ensite NaVx and CARTO as well as standard mapping and ablation catheters. Similar to the Niobe system, the doctor uses a joystick to change the catheter's location. When the doctor moves the joystick in the Sensei system, the robotic arm moves the catheter.

Amigo (Catheter Robotics): Amigo is a less expensive system than Niobe and Sensei and works with a variety of mapping and ablation catheters. It is in a clinical trial in the US.

Artis zeego (Siemens): Artis zeego uses computed tomography (CT) imaging technology to guide navigation, and is also in clinical studies.

CATHETER ABLATION TECHNOLOGY

The goal of any catheter or energy source is to create a transmural lesion while minimizing complications. A transmural lesion-scar tissue that completely penetrates the heart tissue-is key to a successful ablation because it keeps errant electrical signals from being transmitted.

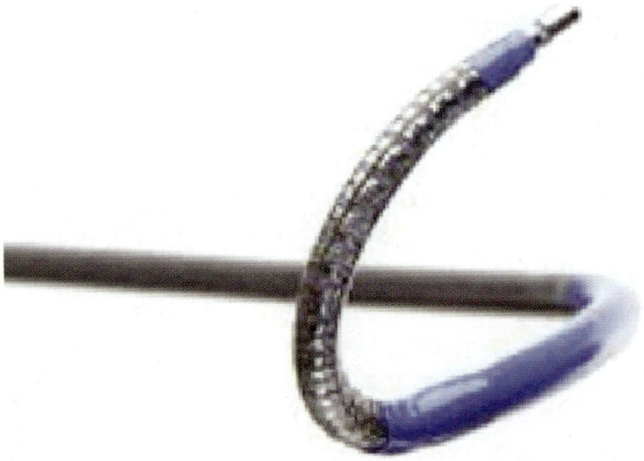

Fig. 7.16: *Hansen medical's robotic catheter control system for EP study*

Making a transmural lesion is as much of an art as it is a science. It depends on the temperature generated by the energy source, how much pressure is applied to the catheter (contact force), and how long the catheter remains in contact with tissue. There are different energy sources that can be used in various types of catheters, and each has advantages and disadvantages, so it is important for patients to understand the different options.

Estech cobra ablation system: The minimally invasive Fusion system uses suction to tug on the target tissue and bring it into probe where RF energy ablates it, isolating the target section from the rest of the blood flowing through the heart and resulting in more predictable lesions. The COBRA fusion ablation system incorporates proprietary Versapolar™ technology—an exclusive innovation that delivers both bipolar and monopolar radiofrequency (RF) energy to the targeted cardiac tissue, enabling transmural lesion formation in thin and thick cardiac tissue. As with all COBRA® ablation systems, the new device is powered by Estech's patented temperature controlled radiofrequency (TCRF) energy which continuously monitors and maintains tissue temperature at target levels throughout the procedure. TCRF avoids the need for multiple applications that other technologies often require and ensures that tissue temperatures remain within a safe and effective range.

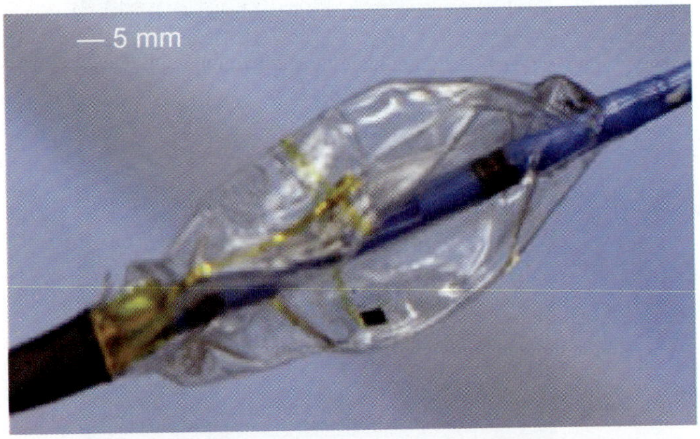

Fig. 7.17: *Flexible electronics with multi-sensing cardiac ablation catheter as an early example that was just announced, an international team of researchers built and tested a balloon ablation catheter capable of measuring intracardiac pressure, EKG, and local temperature around the device tip. All this data can be monitored in real time by the physician during ablation without having to switch devices*

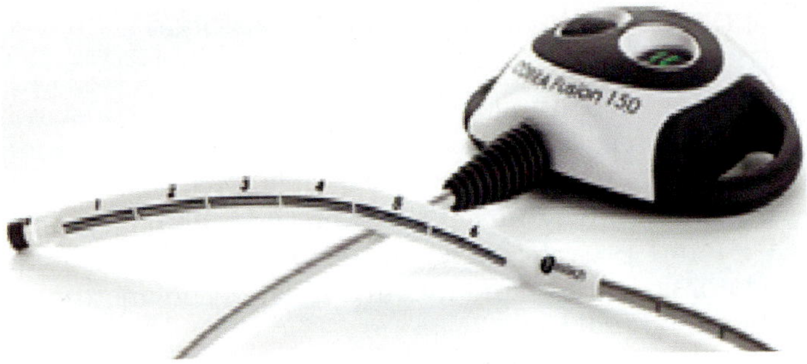

Fig. 7.18: *Estech Cobra ablation system*

Energy Sources

Here are the energy sources being used today in atrial fibrillation catheter ablations:

Radiofrequency (RF) energy is radiowaves that are converted to heat to ablate and create scar tissue. It reliably achieves transmurality and is the most widely used energy source in catheter ablations. In general, high temperatures are needed to make sure that all layers of tissue are ablated. Traditional catheters use unipolar radiofrequency energy, which simply means that the radiofrequency energy is transmitted from a single point at the catheter's tip.

Cryothermy, or cryo energy, is intense cold that is used to form ice crystals within the tissue, causing the cells to die and creating scar tissue. It may be easier to make lesions using cryothermy since the cold temperatures cause tissue to stick to the catheter. In addition, cryoenergy may have fewer major complications. Animal studies have shown cryo energy to have a much lower incidence of thrombus (clot) formation than radiofrequency energy, which suggests that cryothermy could lower the risk of a stroke. Cryo energy can be used in single point catheters or balloon catheters.

Laser energy is light waves that are converted to heat to ablate and create scar tissue. It may be a safer heat-based energy than unipolar radiofrequency energy. With laser energy, the catheter doesn't need to be in direct contact with tissue, which could mean it will have fewer complications than radiofrequency energy. Unlike other energy sources, contact force is not a factor in whether a laser lesion is transmural. In addition, laser energy can be adjusted when ablating tissues of varying thickness, with higher energy applied to thicker tissue and lower energy applied to thinner structures in the heart.

Other energy sources, such as microwave and high intensity focused ultrasound (HIFU), have been studied but these energy sources aren't widely used in catheter ablation. The tools used to assist with catheter ablation are constantly evolving. Here are some of the tools that are commonly used for atrial fibrillation catheter ablations:

Mapping and Navigation Tools for Ablation
(Figs 7.19–7.22)

The tools used to assist with catheter ablation are constantly evolving. Here are some of the tools that are commonly used for atrial fibrillation catheter ablations.

- **CT and MR imaging of the atrium and pulmonary veins:** Provides preablation imaging to help doctors locate anatomic features and identify variations in anatomy of the individual heart.
- **Fluoroscopy X-ray:** Helps doctors guide mapping and ablation catheters in the body by generating 2D (flat) black and white images, but can't show contours in anatomy, such as the "curve" of a pulmonary vein, and also exposes the patient and doctor to radiation.
- **Pulmonary vein venography:** Helps to determine the location of the pulmonary vein ostia, the base of the pulmonary veins, and guide the manipulation of the catheter.
- **Intracardiac echocardiography (ICE):** Provides real-time information about anatomy to facilitate the transseptal puncture (from the right atrium to the left atrium) and to guide catheter ablation.
- **Electroanatomic mapping system:** Reduces fluoroscopy exposure to doctors and patients and allows doctors to visualize structures in 3D and create appropriate lesions, particularly with the incorporation of previously-acquired MR or CT images.
- **Robotic catheter navigation:** Improves navigation precision and may shorten procedures, and includes the stereotaxis' Niobe magnetic navigation system, Hansen Medical's Sensei robot, and Catheter Robotics' Amigo robot.
- **Multielectrode circumferential mapping catheter:** Verifies that the pulmonary veins are electrically isolated.

Electroanatomic Mapping Systems for Ablation

Because of the shortcomings of fluoroscopy, some electrophysiologists use electroanatomic mapping systems like Ensite NaVx (St. Jude Medical) and CARTO (Biosense Webster), which provide colorful 3D images that show variations in a patient's anatomy. These systems may assist doctors in assuring that lesions are contiguous (no gaps) and in reducing complications, such as perforation of the heart or esophagus. In addition, the use of an electroanatomic mapping system may lessen the time that doctors and patients are exposed to radiation. However, the systems are expensive, so they are not available at all facilities.

Using these systems, electrophysiologists create a real time 3D view of the heart by positioning a mapping catheter in the heart. When the doctor moves the catheter in a sweeping motion, the systems track the catheter's location. CARTO and Ensite NaVx use different methods to do this. In a CARTO procedure, the table where the patient lies has an electromagnetic pad that tracks movement of the catheter, whereas in an EnSite NaVx procedure, patches on the patient's skin track the catheter. Both systems use algorithms to translate data on the catheter's location into a 3D image. It usually takes about 20 minutes to complete this process.

Electroanatomic mapping systems are sometimes called multimodality mapping or image integration systems because they can show pictures or data from other sources. For instance, patient CT or MRI scans taken a few days or weeks before the procedure may be loaded onto Ensite NaVx or CARTO and matched with the real-time 3D image

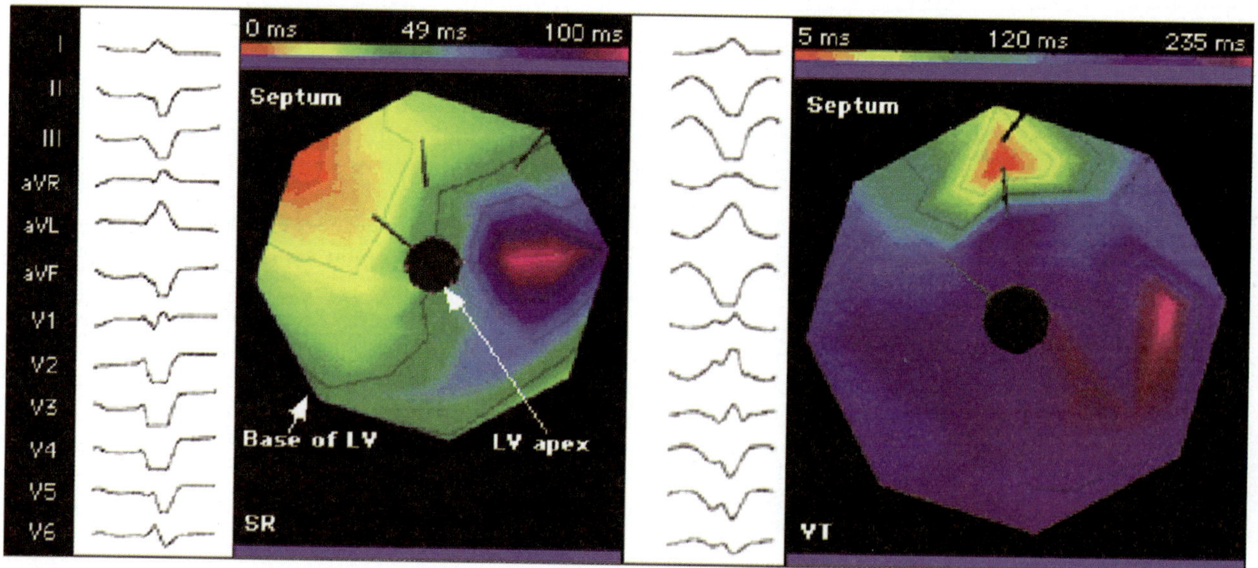

Fig. 7.19: *32-site bipolar mapping of ventricular tachycardia. The outer circle is located near the base of the left ventricle (LV) while the inner circle is positioned within the LV apex. Left panel: mapping during sinus rhythm (SR) shows that the earliest endocardial activation (red) is in the region near the basal septum; activation then spreads rapidly in a radial pattern over the endocarium. The area in purple/pink is activated last. Right panel: during ventricular tachycardia (VT), there is a change in the activation sequence and an increase in the activation time, indicated by the blue/purple color over the majority of the LV endocardium. (Reprinted by permission from Schalij, MJ, van Rugge, P, Siezenga, M, et al., Circulation 1998; 98:2168)*

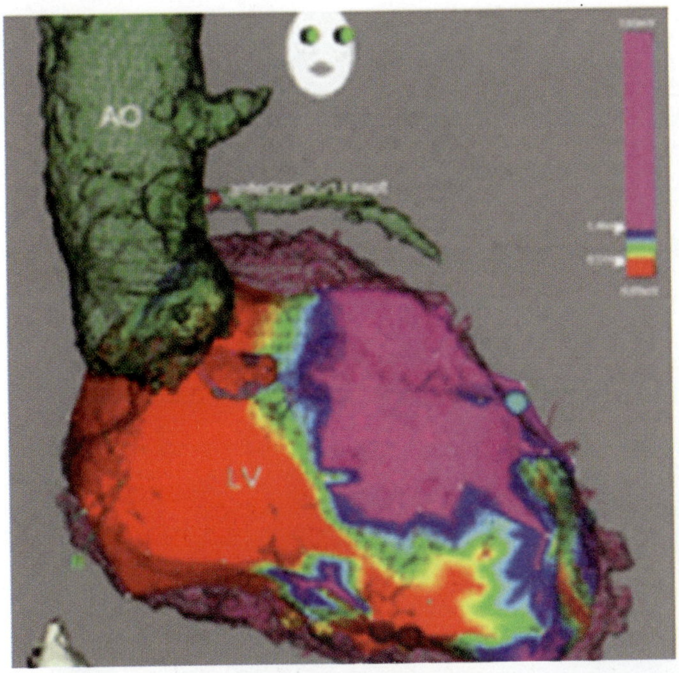

Fig. 7.20: The 3D computed tomographic reconstruction of the left ventricle (LV) displayed as purple wireframe alongwith the 3-D LV endocardial voltage map (Solid collor map). Red areas represented dense scar and purpole area represented normal myocardum; dark-brown points indicate observe sites; AO, aorta

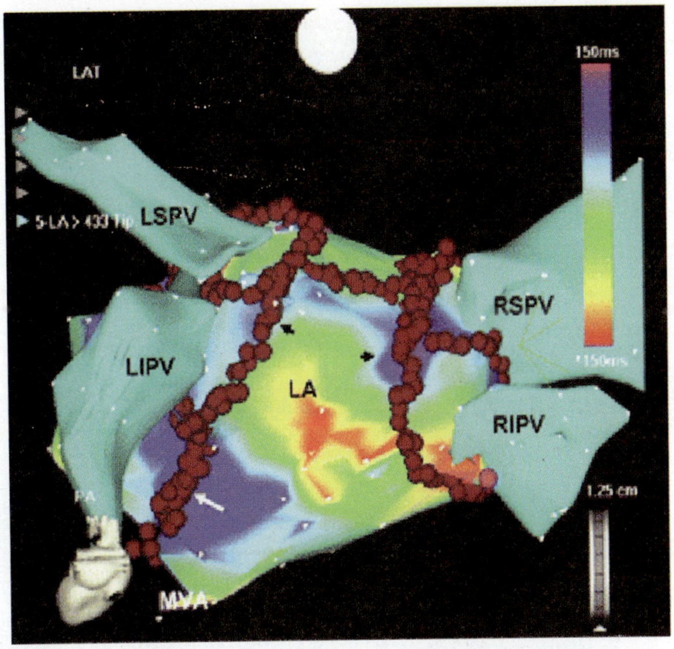

Fig. 7.21: Postablation electroanatomic map showing a wide area circumferential ablation in a patient with persistent atrial fibrillation. Shown are the left superior pulmonary vein (LSPV), left inferior pulmonary vein (LIPV), right superior pulmonary vein (RSPV), and right inferior pulmonary vein (RIPV). Ablative rings circumscribe the left and right pulmonary vein sets. The carinal lines between the veins, a line connecting the right to the left pulmonary vein rings, and an ablative line (white arrow) from the LIPV to the mitral valve annulus (MVA) are also shown. LA, left atrium. (With permission from Packer DL. Catheter ablation for atrial fibrillation: A promising alternative to drug therapy)

of the heart. The doctor does this by moving the catheter slightly, verifying its location in the heart, and taking note of large structures like the pulmonary veins. After several common areas on the two images are identified, the system merges the real-time view and preprocedure scan into one 3D picture. It usually takes about 15 minutes to complete this process, which is called registration. However, the positioning of anatomy can even change within just a week, so if the preprocedure scan doesn't easily correspond with the real-time view of the heart, it can take much longer.

Electroanatomic mapping systems also provide real-time data on electrical activity within the heart, which means that electrophysiologists can see whether conduction block has been achieved. The systems also provide other real-time information, such as atrial pressure and volume, so doctors can easily monitor the patient during the procedure.

CATHETER ABLATION TECHNIQUES

Catheter ablation techniques are constantly evolving. Initial catheter ablations attempted to recreate the lesion set used in the open-chest Cox maze procedure by creating linear ablation lines that interrupted the atrial fibrillation wavelets. However, doctors had difficulty duplicating the Cox maze lesion set during a closed-chest catheter ablation. The procedure had high complication rates and required long fluoroscopy times.

Research in Bordeaux, France, by Michel Haïssaguerre, MD, and colleagues, suggested that electrophysiologists didn't need to duplicate the Cox maze lesion set. Dr Haïssaguerre's group found that over 90% of atrial

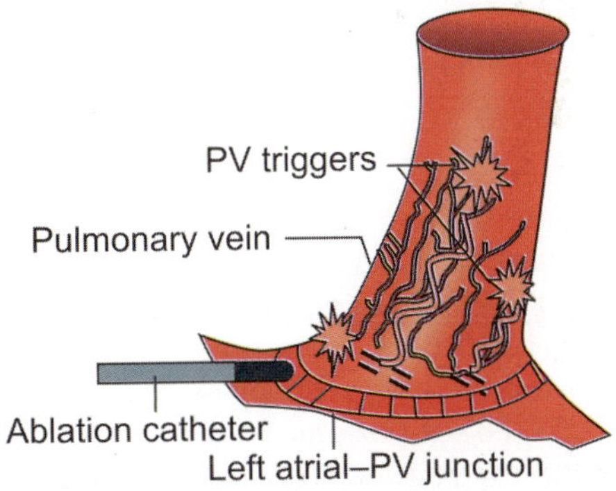

Fig. 7.22: Schema of the left atrial-pulmonary vein ostium. Muscular extensions of the left atrial tissue into the pulmonary veins may serve as the originating foci of premature atrial beats and pulmonary vein atrial tachycardias. It is these foci that lead to the initiation and perpetuation of atrial fibrillation. Catheter ablation at the left atrial-pulmonary vein junction serves to electrically isolate the pulmonary veins, thereby trapping these foci that are now unable to excite the left atrium

fibrillation is triggered (starts) in or near the pulmonary veins. As a result of these findings, a new type of catheter ablation technique, called segmental pulmonary vein isolation or ostial pulmonary vein isolation, was created. Dr Haïssaguerre and his colleagues used radiofrequency

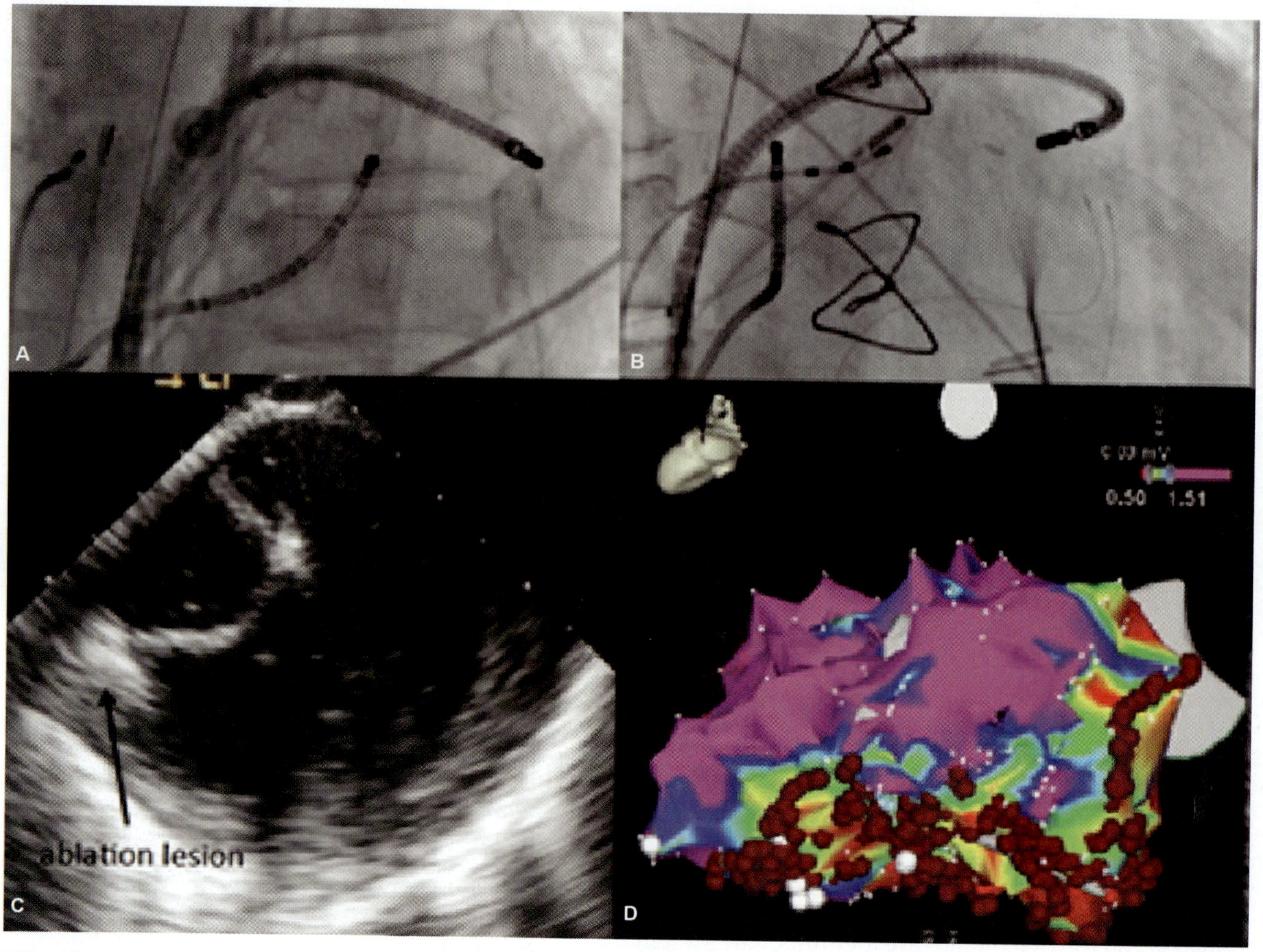

Fig. 7.23: *Mapping and ablation of a basal lateral scar. (A, B) Robotic catheter position in left and right anterior oblique fluoroscopic views, respectively. The mid-lateral wall is being mapped. (C) Intracardiac echocardiographic image showing catheter contact and lesion formation in the left ventricular lateral wall. (D) Three dimensional map of the lateral scar and the ablation lesions created*

energy to ablate the pulmonary vein ostium, the opening to the pulmonary veins. When "isolated", pulmonary veins can no longer be a trigger point for atrial fibrillation. Dr Haïssaguerre and his colleagues were able to terminate atrial fibrillation in, and stop prescribing antiarrhythmic drugs for, 62% (28) of patients in the study.

This pulmonary vein isolation approach continues to be the cornerstone of catheter ablation strategies for the treatment of paroxysmal atrial fibrillation. However, pulmonary vein isolation can mean different things to different doctors. Indeed, it has become a catch-all term to describe any ablation of the pulmonary veins. This can lead to misunderstandings between doctors and patients, and can make a big difference in the rate of freedom from afib after ablation.

Perhaps the most important difference among doctors relates to whether the pulmonary veins are isolated, or just ablated. In order for a procedure to be called a pulmonary vein isolation, the doctor must confirm that the pulmonary veins are "blocked"-in other words, that conduction block was achieved. This is done with a mapping catheter that can determine whether there is any electrical activity around the pulmonary veins. If conduction block isn't confirmed, then the procedure is an ablation, not an isolation. Thus, it is important to ask doctors what type of lesion set will be made and whether they will confirm that conduction is blocked (Figs 7.27 to 7.29).

There have been several updates to the segmental (ostial) pulmonary vein isolation developed by Dr Haïssaguerre and his colleagues. First, it was found that ablating tissue in the ostia (opening) of the pulmonary veins could lead to pulmonary vein stenosis (narrowing), which is a serious complication that can obstruct oxygenated blood from flowing from the lungs into the heart. Second, it has been found that more extensive lesion sets are better at stopping afib. This is probably because the pulmonary veins aren't the only area in the heart that can trigger atrial fibrillation. Over time, afib can create new pathways, called macro re-entry sites, where it can "cycle" in the heart. Macro re-entry sites are different for each patient.

Ablation strategies and techniques continue to evolve, as does the terminology, as doctors learn more about areas

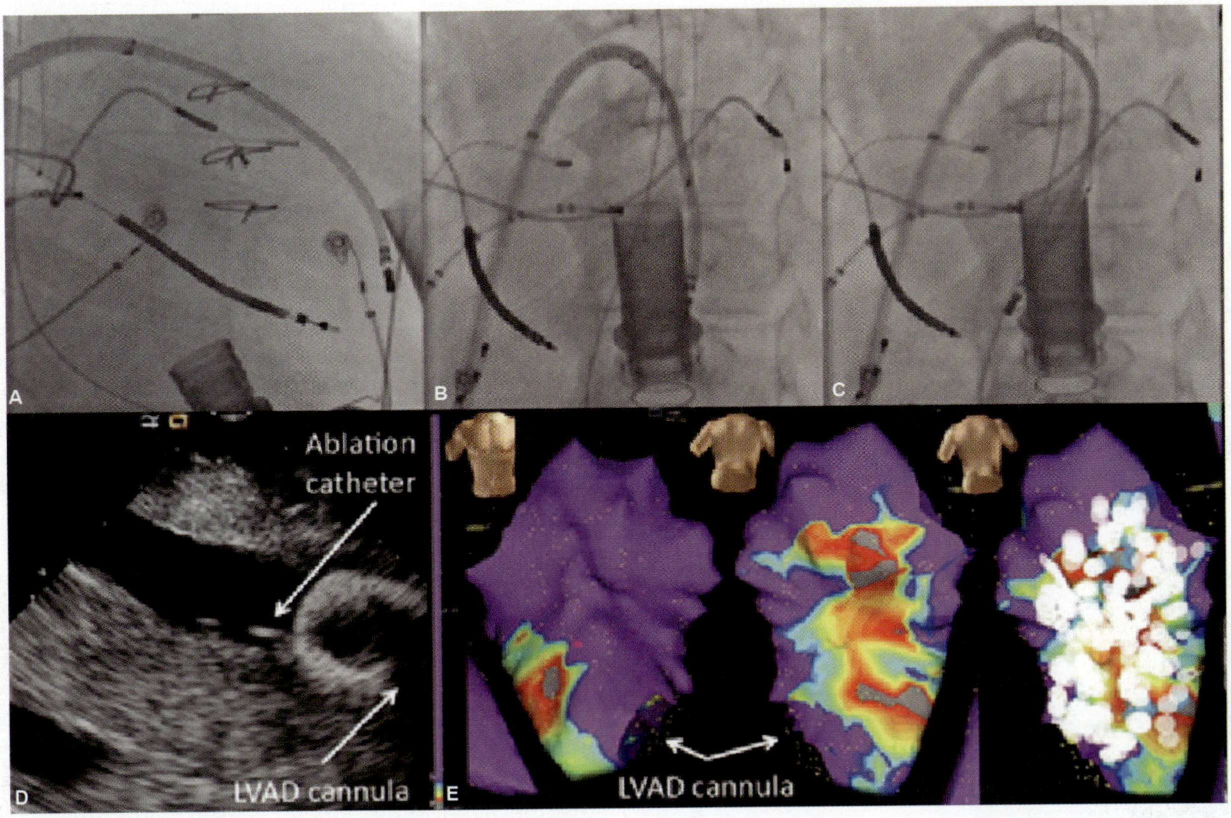

Fig. 7.24: *Mapping and ablation of an inferior wall scar in the presence of a left ventricular assist device (LVAD). (A–C) Robotic catheter position in the right (A) and left (B, C) anterior oblique fluoroscopic views, with the catheter tip around the LVAD inflow cannula. (D) Intracardiac echocardiographic image of the LVAD cannula and the ablation catheter. (E) Three dimensional scar maps and ablation lesions*

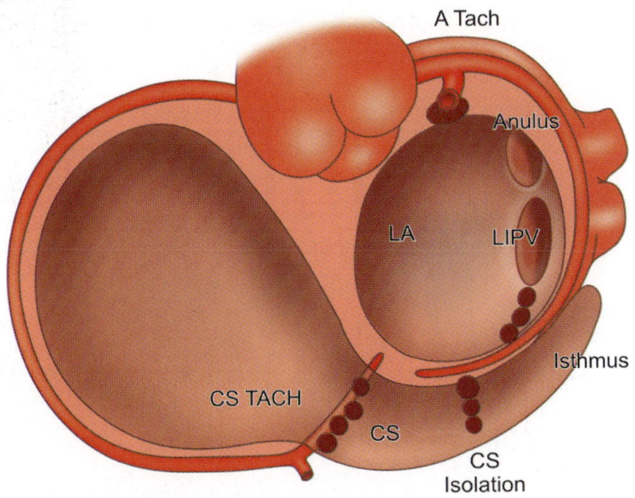

Fig. 7.25: *Diagrammatic representation of ablation sites which may involve injury to the major coronary aterial system. Septal mitral annular tachycardias may result in injury to the proximal circumflex coronary artery, whereas the more distal portions of this artery can be injured during intracardiac or coronary sinus-based ablation*

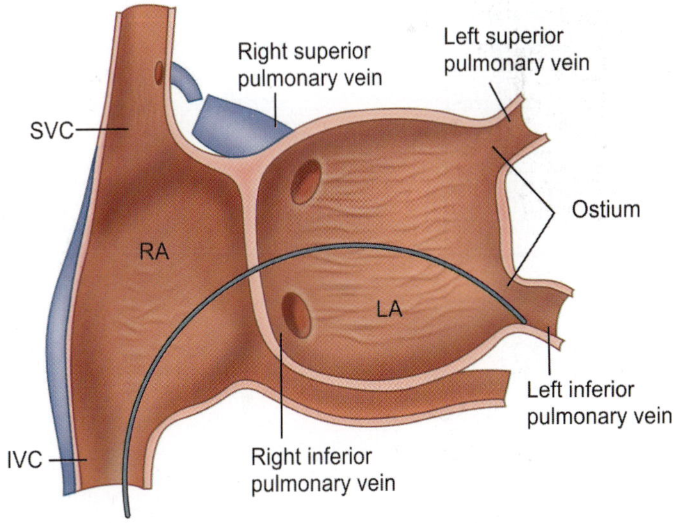

Fig. 7.26: *Targeting the triggers in atrial fibrillation (AF) ablation*

of the heart that could act as a trigger or reentry site. Thus, the term "segmental pulmonary vein isolation" is rarely used today, and instead we refer to the anatomic area that will be ablated or to the technical approach to ablation.

BASIC CATHETER ABLATION TECHNIQUES

Here are the most frequently used basic catheter ablation techniques, shown in order of the fewest to the greatest number of ablation (lesion) lines:

Antrum pulmonary vein ablation: Because of the issues with the ostia, as mentioned above, the antrum (base) of

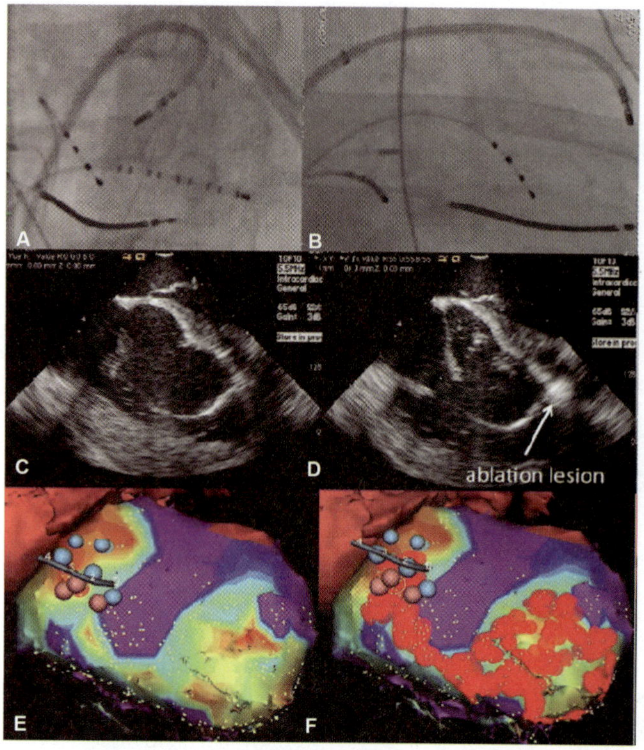

Fig. 7.27: *Mapping and ablation of a septal scar. Stable catheter positioning allowed real-time monitoring of lesion creation on intracardiac echocardiography. (A, B) Robotic catheter position in left and right anterior oblique fluoroscopic views, respectively. The septal aspect of the apex was being mapped. (C, D) Intracardiac echocardiographic images before and 15 seconds after application of radiofrequency. The catheter tip is in the distal septum, where increased echogenicity is seen at the ablation site. (E, F) Three dimensional maps of the large septal and apical scar and the ablation lesions, respectively*

the pulmonary veins became the site of catheter ablations. The antrum includes the posterior (back) wall of the left atrium and extends to the anterior (front) of the right pulmonary veins. In essence, it is a wide perimeter around the pulmonary veins. Antrum pulmonary vein ablation entails lesion lines in this area, but doctors do not confirm conduction block.

Pulmonary vein antrum isolation (PVAI or PVI): Lesion lines are made in the antrum of the pulmonary veins, and doctors confirm that conduction block has been achieved. Some electrophysiologists also make additional lesion lines. These may include the superior vena cava, roof of the atrium, or the septum, the wall that separates the two sides of the heart. You can see these structures in this diagram of the heart. However, the location of the additional lesions varies by doctor. That is, there isn't a standard that requires that all pulmonary vein antrum isolations include a lesion line along the superior vena cava.

Circumferential ablation: Similar to pulmonary vein antrum isolation, circumferential ablation entails lesions encircling the pulmonary veins. Some electrophysiologists also make an ablation line that connects the pulmonary veins on the posterior (back) wall of the left atrium or ablate tissue from the pulmonary veins to the mitral valve. In addition, a mapping catheter is used to identify "potentials", which are areas that could serve as a trigger or macro re-entry site for atrial fibrillation. According to the HRS Consensus statement, there isn't a single endpoint, or goal, for circumferential ablation. Some doctors confirm that conduction block has been achieved, whereas others look for elimination of "potentials" or a reduction in electrical activity in the ablated area.

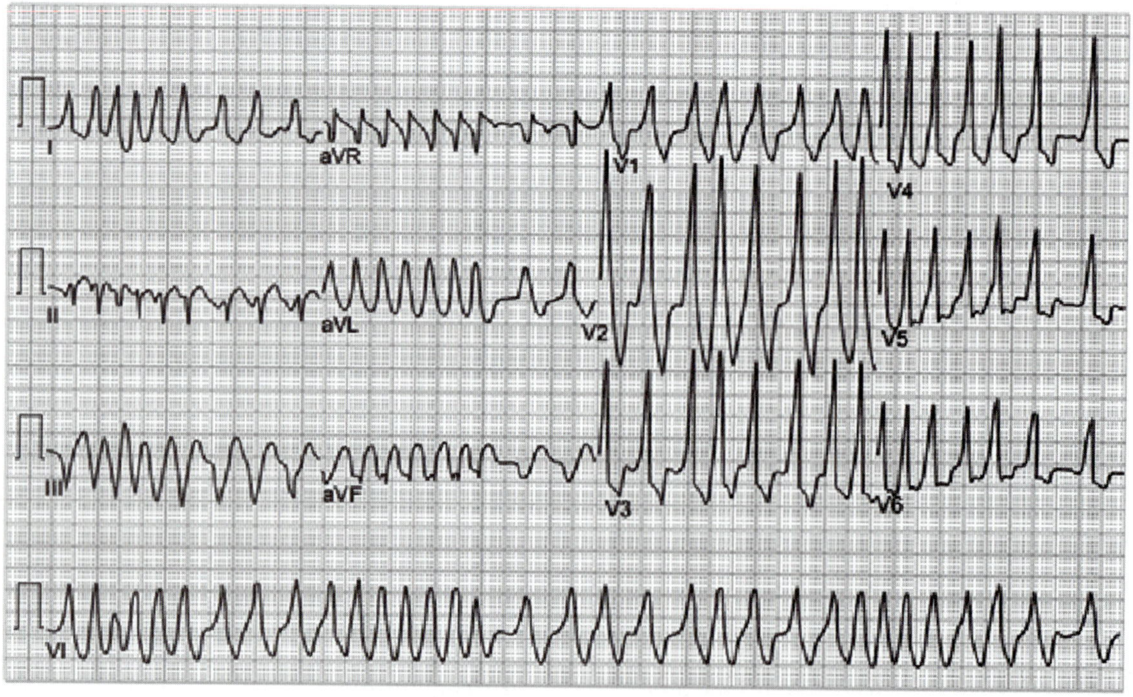

Fig. 7.28: *ECG aberrant conduction*

Advanced Catheter Ablation Techniques

Atrial fibrillation leads to atrial remodeling over time, meaning that afib can change the deeper layers of heart tissue (substrate) or change the way electricity is conducted within the heart. This is also known as substrate modification (Figs 7.23, 7.24 and 7.27).

Advanced catheter ablation techniques, which are primarily used to treat persistent and long-standing persistent afib, target anomalies in the substrate or electrical conduction. However, clinical data is inconclusive, meaning that it is not clear whether these techniques can stop persistent or long-standing persistent afib for the majority of patients.

The most commonly used advanced catheter ablation techniques are (Figs 7.31 to 7.35)

Stepwise ablation: Stepwise ablation is the only ablation strategy with a stated goal of terminating afib. It involves isolation of the pulmonary veins and entails additional lesion lines, which differ by electrophysiologist. It is sometimes called sequential ablation because the additional ablation lines are performed in a specified order. That is, doctors may make a lesion line along the roof of the left atrium, and then pace or use a mapping catheter to determine whether conduction has been stopped. If there continues to be afib activity, the doctor will ablate the next area in the sequence. The lesion lines and sequences vary by doctor. Most electrophysiologists make a lesion on the roof of the left atrium after isolating the pulmonary veins. After this, some doctors will ablate the coronary sinus, the vessel between the left atrium and the left ventricle, whereas others might ablate the mitral isthmus, the area where the mitral valve and the left inferior pulmonary vein meet. There isn't one specific sequence that has proven to have the best results, largely because clinical trials haven't been performed on this.

Complex fractionated atrial electrograms: Ablation of complex fractionated atrial electrograms (CFAE, pronounced cafe) is performed by some electrophysiologists to treat persistent and longstanding persistent afib. A complex fractionated atrial electrogram is a site where there is an unusual electrical pattern, which could be due to the length of the electrical wave (long or short), the frequency of electrical activity (a lot or a little), or the speed of conduction (fast or slow). Complex fractionated atrial electrograms appear to represent macro reentry sites for atrial fibrillation, so ablation of these sites should stop afib, but that hasn't been proven by clinical data. In fact, CFAE ablation has been shown to be less effective in stopping afib than a pulmonary vein antral isolation with additional lesion lines at the roof of the left atrium and along the mitral isthmus. To learn more, see can catheter ablation successfully treat persistent atrial fibrillation, which discusses a session at the Heart rhythm society about ablating persistent afib.

Ganglionated plexi ablation: Another advanced strategy for stopping afib is to ablate the ganglionated plexi (GP), which are "fat pads" in the heart. Nerves that control automatic functions, such as breathing, are located in these ganglionated plexi. These nerves also initiate electrical activity at various places in the heart. It is thought that when one ganglionated plexus is activated, another ganglionated plexus located nearby will also be activated. Some doctors use mapping catheters with high frequency electrodes to

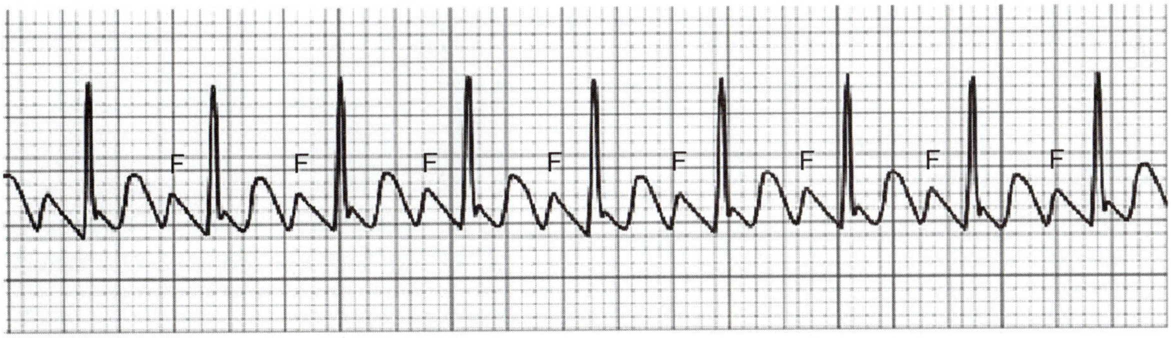

Fig. 7.29: *ECG showing atrial flutter: narrow QRS complexes are associated with regular flutter waves*

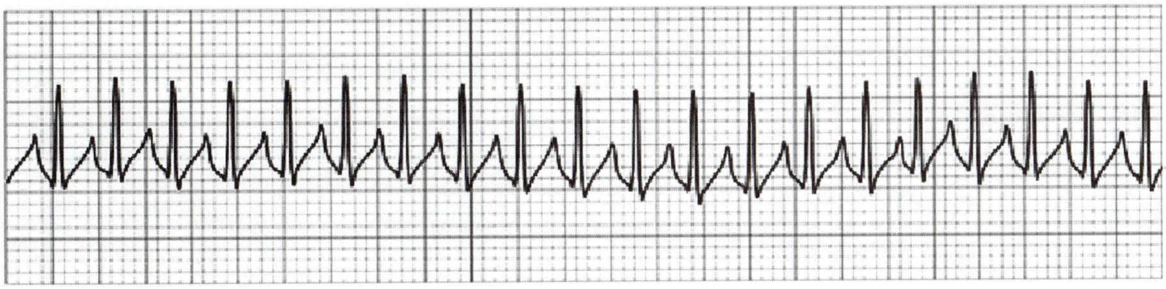

Fig. 7.30: *ECG showing junctional tachycardia, narrow QRS with no visible p-waves*

identify ganglionated plexi, while others simply ablate the four primary ganglionated plexi in the left atrium. Ablation of the ganglionated plexi has not been widely adopted by electrophysiologists, which may be because there is little research data available.

Hybrid ablation: Hybrid ablation is an emerging treatment for patients with more severe forms of atrial fibrillation, typically persistent and long-standing persistent afib. Hybrid ablation is a dual approach in which an electrophysiologist ablates from inside the heart and a cardiac surgeon ablates on the outside of the heart. A hybrid ablation may enhance the prospects that ablation lines fully penetrate all layers of the cardiac tissue, which is crucial to stopping afib. In addition, higher success rates and fewer complications could be possible because each specialty (electrophysiology and cardiac surgery) can ablate areas of the heart that are best suited to their different approaches. See hybrid procedure may offer better outcomes for persistent and long-standing persistent atrial fibrillation for Dr James Edgerton's presentation on hybrid ablations at Boston atrial fibrillation symposium in January 2011. Another dual approach, the convergent procedure, also has surgeons and electrophysiologists collaborate on ablation. The convergent procedure is different from hybrid procedures in that it uses a different entry point and a different device, in this case a unipolar radiofrequency device instead of a bipolar radiofrequency one.

CLINICAL APPLICATIONS OF CATHETER ABLATION

There are three classes of indications for catheter ablation.

1. The first is symptomatic supraventricular tachycardia (SVT) due to atrioventricular nodal reentrant tachycardia (AVNRT), Wolff-Parkinson-White syndrome, unifocal atrial tachycardia, or atrial flutter (especially common right atrial forms). For these conditions, catheter ablation is first-line therapy if that is the patient's preference.
2. The second indication is atrial fibrillation with lifestyle-impairing symptoms and inefficacy or intolerance of at least 1 antiarrhythmic agent. Both left atrial ablation for restoration of sinus rhythm and AV junction ablation for rate control are class I indications, depending on the circumstance.
3. The third indication is symptomatic ventricular tachycardia (VT). Catheter ablation is first-line therapy in idiopathic VT, if that is the patient's preference. In structural heart disease, catheter ablation is generally performed for drug inefficacy or intolerance, or as adjunctive therapy in patients with an implantable cardioverter-defibrillator (ICD) who are experiencing frequent ICD discharges.

Uncommon indications for catheter ablation include the following:

1. Symptomatic drug-refractory (inefficacy or intolerance) idiopathic sinus tachycardia
2. Lifestyle-impairing ectopic beats
3. Symptomatic junctional ectopic tachycardia

RFCA has been applied to most clinical tachycardias, even to polymorphic ventricular tachycardia and ventricular fibrillation in preliminary studies. Success rates are highest in patients with common forms of SVT, namely AVNRT and orthodromic reciprocating tachycardia (ORT).

Ablation in Atrial Fibrillation

The simplest catheter ablation procedure performed in patients with atrial fibrillation is RFCA of the AV junction. AV nodal modification is less therapeutic than AV junction ablation and less commonly performed (Figs 7.50 and 7.51).

Catheter ablation of atrial tissue to cure atrial fibrillation is still evolving. The procedure is technically demanding,

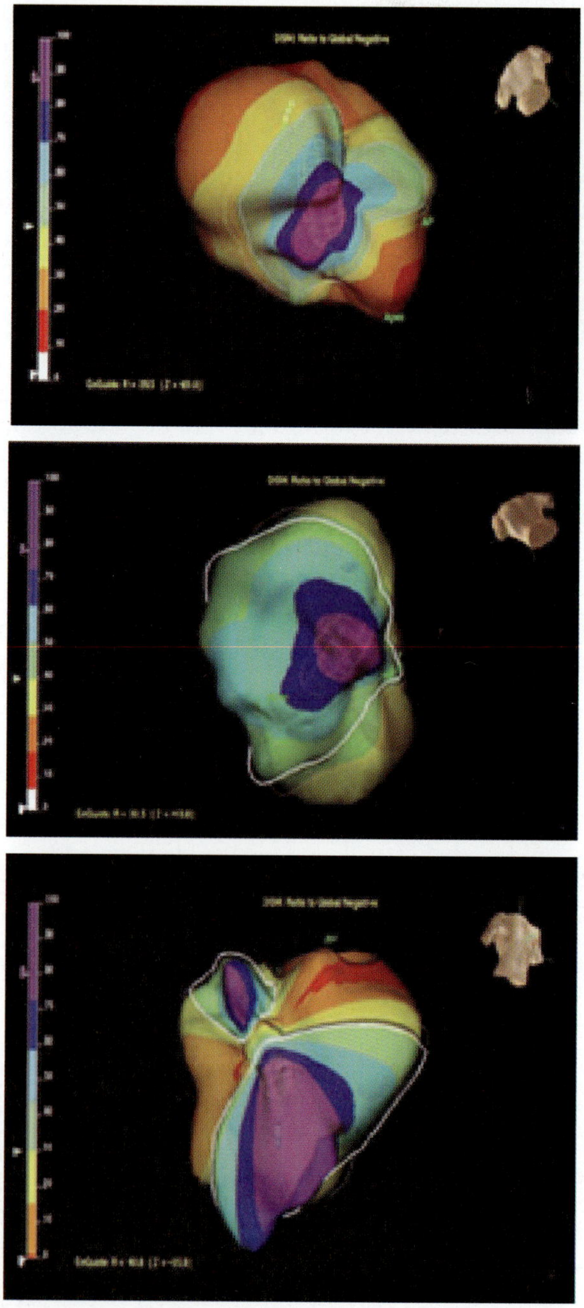

Fig. 7.31: *Upper, middle and bottom show three dimensional views showing large anteroapical scars*

more risky, and less successful than AV junction or AV nodal ablation. Nevertheless, the observation of Haissaguerre and others that pulmonary vein foci can trigger atrial fibrillation has stimulated much additional research, and there is considerable scientific excitement that this common tachyarrhythmia may be amenable to a curative catheter procedure (Table 7.1).

The complete surgical Maze procedure (incisions in both atria +/- transmural radiofrequency lesions) is still the most effective technique for potentially curing atrial fibrillation in all comers, regardless of chronicity or whether structural heart disease is present. The best success rates with left atrial catheter ablation are in patients with paroxysmal atrial fibrillation and hearts that are not too structurally abnormal.

No consensus exists on the optimal left atrial ablation technique or what constitutes a clinically successful procedure. Nevertheless, evidence is accruing that catheter ablation for atrial fibrillation is more effective than

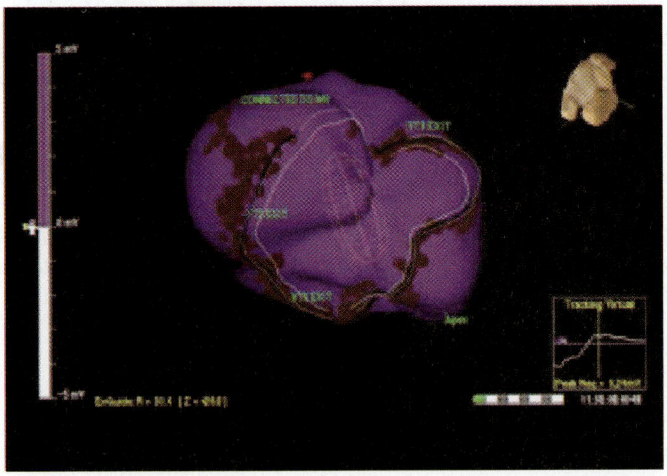

Fig. 7.32: *Three dimensional view of multiple radiofrequency ablations in a line along the border of large anterior scar connecting it to mitral annulus*

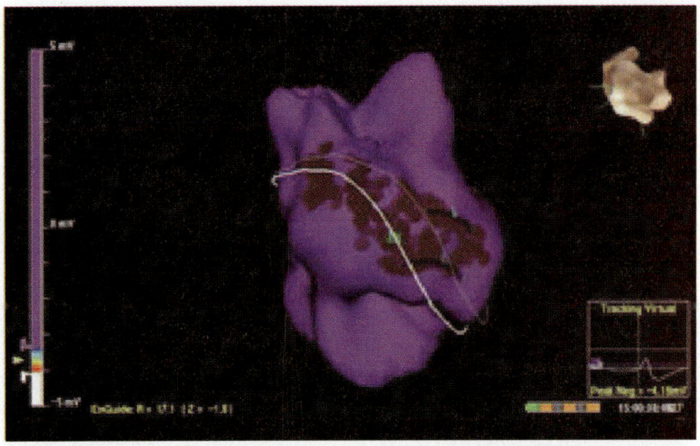

Fig. 7.33: *Three dimensional view of multiple radiofrequency ablations in a line along the border of large posterior scar at the site of VT exit*

Table 7.1: *Characteristics of catheter ablation for selected cardiac arrhythmias*

Arrhythmia	*Ablation location*	*Success rate (%)*	*Complication rate (%)*	*Potential complications*	*Indications*
Atrial tachycardia	Variable, anywhere in right or left atrium	86–100	0–8	Atrioventricular or sinus node dysfunction; cardiac perforation with tamponade; phrenic nerve injury	Incessant tachycardia; symptomatic tachycardia; tachycardia- mediated cardiomyopathy
Atrioventricular nodal reentrant tachycardia	Right atrium, perinodal	96	0.5–1	Atrioventricular nodal block, usually requiring pacemaker implantation	First-line therapy in patients willing and able to undergo catheter ablation
Atrioventricular reciprocating tachycardia	Variable, left or right atrioventricular	Approximately 95	2–4	Complete atrioventricular nodal block; cardiac perforation with tamponade	First-line therapy for symptoms, single or infrequent episodes, or with atrial fibrillation and rapid conduction
Atrial flutter	Right atrium, if common variety of atrial flutter	88–100	2.5–3.5	Cardiac perforation with tamponade; heart block; myocardial infarction; thromboembolic events	First-line therapy for poorly tolerated or recurrent episodes
Atrial fibrillation	Left atrium, pulmonary vein atrial	60–80	6–10	Cardiac perforation with tamponade; phrenic nerve injury; pulmonary vein stenosis; thromboembolic events; vascular complications	Alternative to drug therapy for recurrent atrial fibrillation in symptomatic patients with minimal or no left atrial enlargement

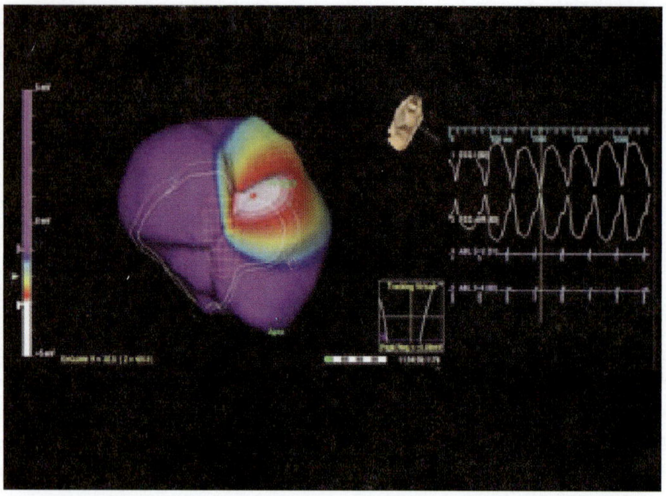

Fig. 7.34: *Three dimensional view showing the exit of ventricular tachycardia from the scar area*

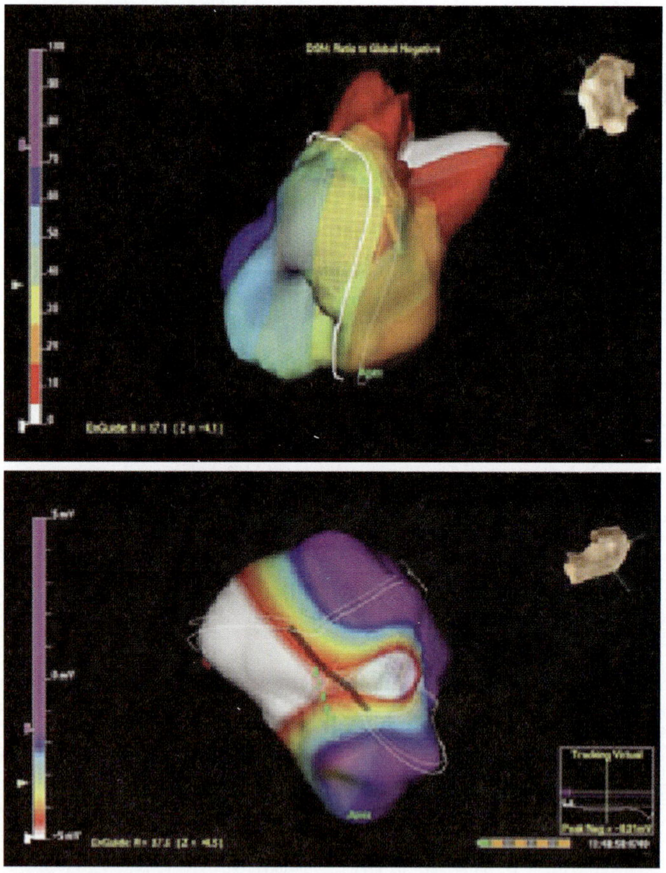

Fig. 7.35: *Upper and bottom show three dimensional views showing large areas of posterior scar*

antiarrhythmic drug therapy, especially in patients who have already failed an antiarrhythmic drug. The 2006 ACC/AHA/ESC guidelines for the management of atrial fibrillation now list catheter ablation as a reasonable strategy for patients with lifestyle impairing symptoms who have failed at least one antiarrhythmic agent.

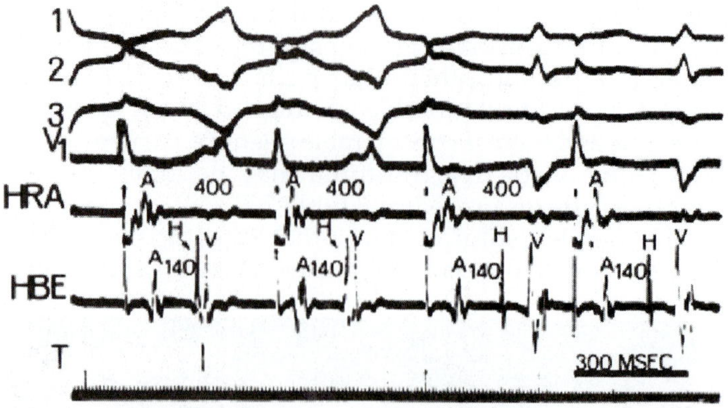

Fig. 7.36: *Graph showing influence of atrial pacing on conduction over an AV bypass tract. In this electrophysiological study, the atria are being paced at a cycle length of 400 msec. First two complexes show marked preexcitation with the antegrade his bundle potential (H) buried in the QRS complex. Constant AH intervals and normal QRS complex results when sudden blockappears during pacing*

ABLATION IN VENTRICULAR TACHYCARDIA

Idiopathic ventricular tachycardia (VT) most commonly arises from the right ventricular outflow tract and less commonly originates in the inferoseptal left ventricle near the apex. These forms of VT are amenable to catheter ablation, although success rates are somewhat lower than those for the common forms of SVT.

For patients with stable VT, the potential benefit of catheter ablation before implantation of an ICD was demonstrated in the ventricular tachycardia ablation in coronary heart disease (VTACHD) study. This prospective, randomized, controlled international trial in 104 patients found that time to recurrence of VT or ventricular fibrillation (VF) was longer in the ablation group (median, 18.6 mo) than in the control group (5.9 mo). At 2 years, estimates for survival free from VT or VF were 47% in the ablation group and 29% in the control group.

CONTRAINDICATION TO RADIOFREQUENCY CATHETER ABLATION

Few absolute contraindication to RFCA exist. Left atrial ablation and ablation for persistent atrial flutter should not be performed in the presence of known atrial thrombus. Similarly, mobile left ventricular thrombus would be a contraindication to left ventricular ablation.

Mechanical prosthetic heart valves are generally not crossed with ablation catheters. Reproductive-aged women should not be exposed to fluoroscopy if any possibility exists that they are pregnant.

Preprocedural considerations in ablation procedure.

Anesthesia for Catheter Ablation

The procedure is typically performed under conscious sedation with intravenous tranquilizers and narcotics. General anesthesia is used in children and selected adults.

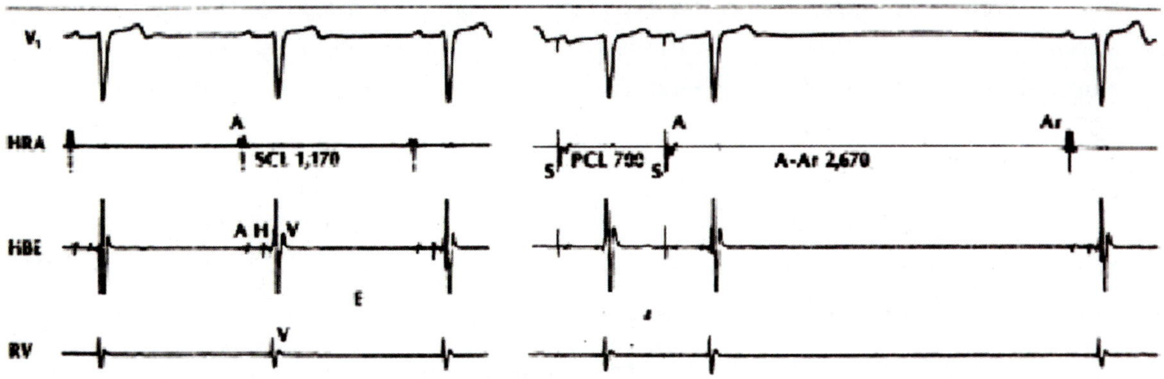

Fig. 7.37: *Graph (upper panel) shows features of sinus bradycardia in sick syndrome (VI). Whereas in HRA there is marked delay in the sinoatrial conduction time (more than 2,670 msecs) with 700 pacing cycle length. His bundle electrogram shows normal HV*

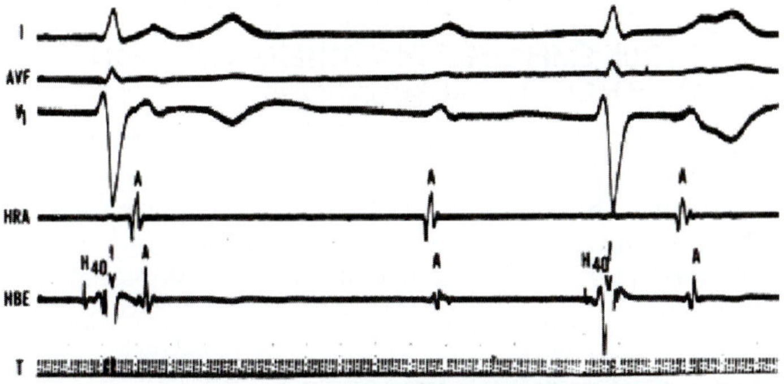

Fig. 7.38: *Graph (upper panel) shows in leads 1 aVF and VI shows morphology of complete heart block in which there is no association of P-wave with QRS compelx and all atrial impulses are unable to conduct due to block at AV junction. His bundle electrogram in this case reveals that each junctional escape QRS complex is preceded by a His bundle deflection (H) with a normal H-V interval (40 msec) in congenital complete heart block*

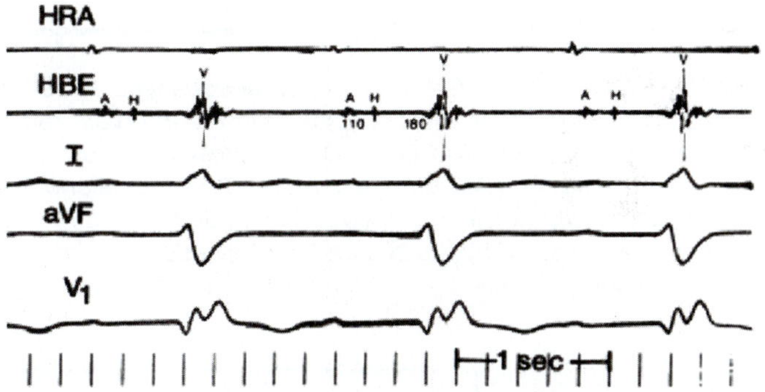

Fig. 7.40: *Spontaneous rhythm with normal features of HBE with normal PA, AH and IIV intervals HRA-high right atrium. HBE = His bundle electrogram I. aVF and Vi are standard and precordial leads, respectively*

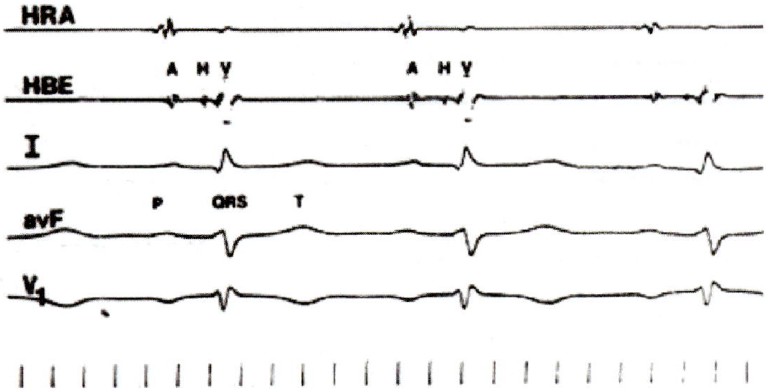

Fig. 7.39: *Graph showing sponlaneous rhythm with normal features of HBE with normal PA, AH and IIV intervals HRA-high right atrium. HBE, His bundle electrogram I. aVF and Vi are standard and precordial leads, respectively*

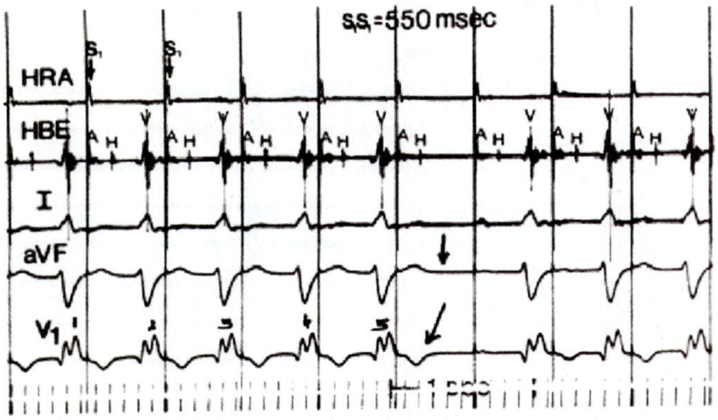

Fig. 7.41: *Graph shows block distal to His bundle during atrial packing Mobitz 11 second degree AV block is seen following 5th beat of atrial pacing at 550 msec (110 beats/min). There is absence of ventricular activity following his deflection in the 5th beat, clearly demonstrating Mobitz II AV block (2nd degree)*

CLINICAL EXAMINATION OF PATIENT PRIOR TO ABLATION

The preprocedural evaluation always includes a thorough history and physical examination, as well as review of electrocardiograms (12-lead, if available) performed during the tachycardia and with the patient in sinus rhythm. At a minimum, preprocedure blood studies typically includes a complete blood cell count and an assessment of renal function and electrolyte levels.

An echocardiogram is frequently obtained to exclude structural heart disease. Other tests that are indicated in

Table 7.2: *Diagnosis of different conduction abnormalities along the His bundle*

	Location	*Character*	*Morphology*
1.	Suprahisian (above HB)	First degree block	Normal QRS or narrow QRS
2.	Intrahisian (inside)	–do–	Widening or split His bundle potentials
3.	Infrahisian (below HB)	–do–	Wide QRS

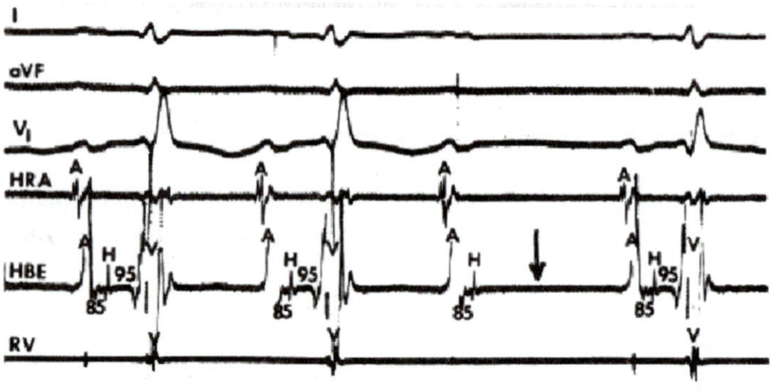

Fig. 7.42: *Graph shows features of spontaneous type 11 second degree infrahisian block. Note that AH and HV intervals remain constant during conducted impulse at 85 msec and 95 msec, respectively. The third AH interval complex, however is suddenly and unexpectedly not followed by a ventricular depolarization. The complex followed by the blocked one revealed no change in the conduction intervals*

specific situations include exercise testing with or without cardiac imaging (especially for exercise-induced tachyarrhythmias), and cardiac catheterization.

The patient should fast overnight before the procedure. Cardiac medications with electrophysiologic effects, such as beta-blockers, calcium channel blockers, digoxin, and class I and III antiarrhythmic drugs, are often tapered and/or discontinued prior to the procedure. Warfarin is typically discontinued for at least a few doses prior to the procedure.

TECHNIQUE EMPLOYED IN CATHETER ABLATION IN DIFFERENT CLINICAL SITUATIONS

Typically, 2–5 electrode catheters are percutaneously inserted via the femoral or internal jugular veins and are positioned within the left heart, right heart, or both. Multiple catheters are needed to induce and map various tachyarrhythmias prior to radiofrequency catheter ablation (RFCA).

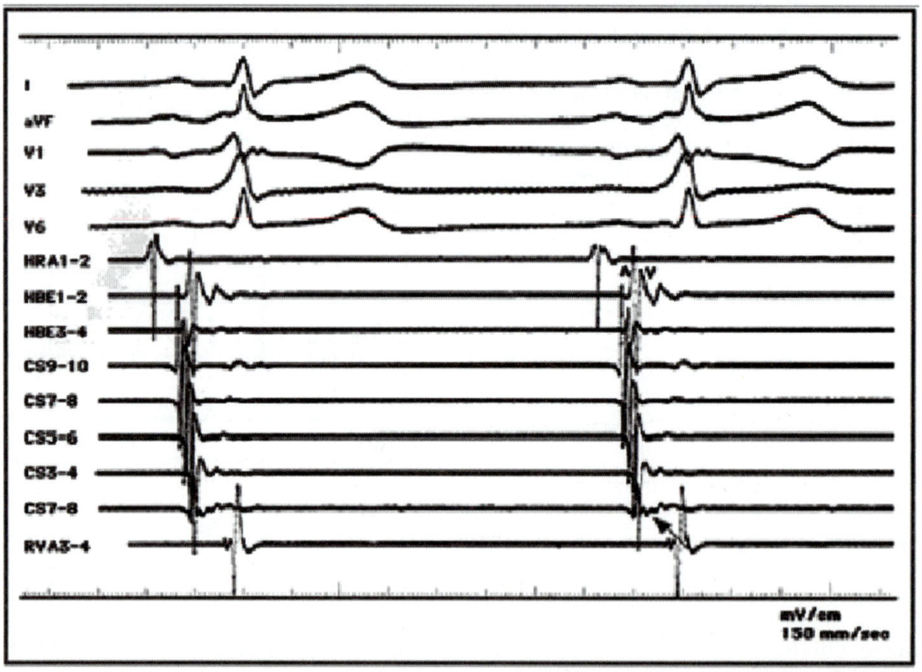

Fig. 7.43: *Electrophysiologic mapping in Wolff-Parkinson-White syndrome. Shown are five surface ECG leads (I, aVF, V1, V3, V6) and intracardiac recording from the high right atrium (HRA), lateral mitral annulus (HBE 1-2 and HBE 3-4), coronary sinus (proximal to distal, CS9-10, CS7-8, CS5-6, CS3-4 and CS1-2), and the right ventricular apex (RVA3-4). During the diagnostaic electrophysiology study, orthodromic atriocventricvular reentrant tachycardia was induced. Recodrings from the CS demonstrated that the earliest site of ventricular activation was at CS7-8, indicating a left lateral location of the accessory pathway (arrow). The mapping catheter (HBE 1-2, 3-4) was advanced through a patent, foramen ovale to the lateral mitral annulus. Activation mapping was used to select the ablation site; during sinus rhythm, the ablation catheter was maneuvered to the site along the mitral annulus which recorded earliest ventricular activity (HBE1-2), i.e. the atrial (A) and ventricular (V) electrograms recorded from the ablation catheter tip were continuous and the local ventricular activity preceded the onset of the delta wave on the surface ECG*

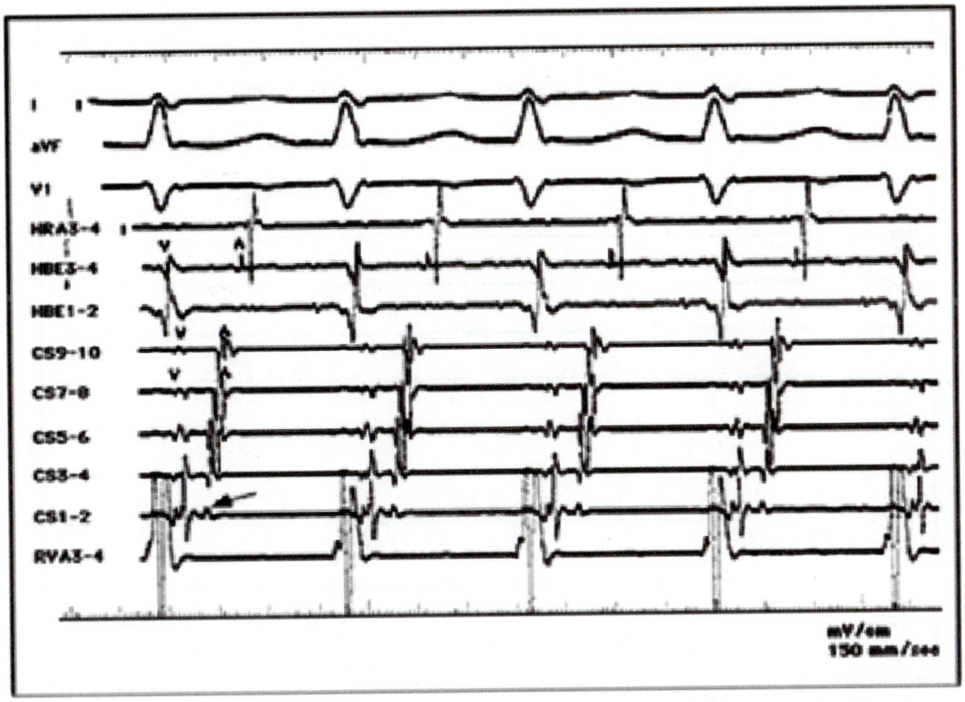

Fig. 7.44: *Orthodromic AV reentrant tachycardia in concealed accessory pathway shown are three surface ECG leads (I, aVF, and VI) and intracardiac recording from the high right atrium (HRA), proximal (HBE3-4) and distal His bundle region (HBE1-2), proximal to distal coronary sinus (CS9-10, CS7-8, CS5-6, CS3-4 and CS1-2), and right ventricular apex (RVA3-4) in a patient with atrioventricular reentrant tachycardia (AVRT). During an orthodromic AVRT, there is retograde atrial (A) activation which occurs after ventricular activation (V); the earliest atrial activation (arrow) is seen in the lateral mitral annulus (CS1-2) due to a concealed left lateral accessory pathway*

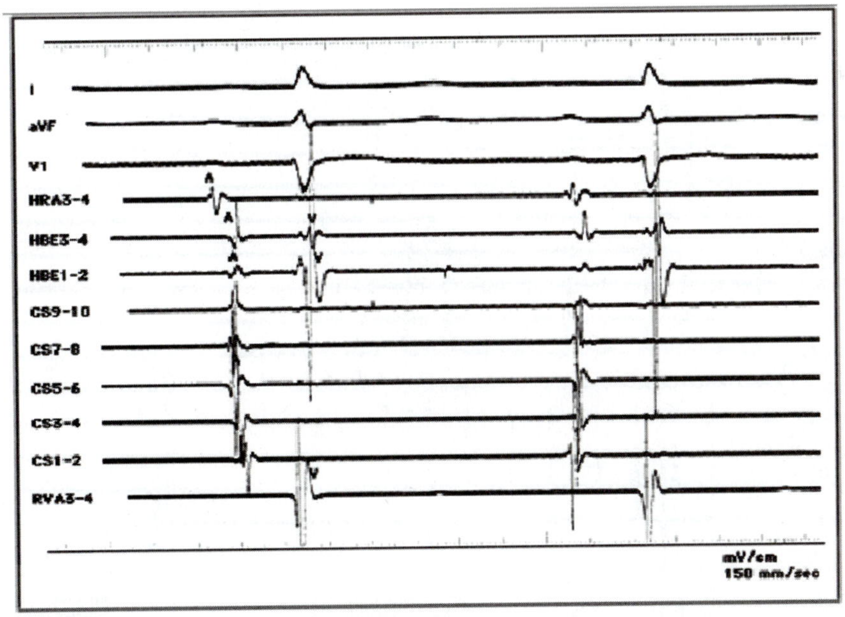

Fig. 7.45: *Identification of slow pathway for ablation of AV nodal reentrant tachycardia. Shown are three surface ECG leads (I, aVF, V1) and intracardiac recordings from the high right atrium (HRA3-4), proximal (HBE3-4) and distal his bundle region (HBE1-2), proximal to distal coronary sinus (CS9-10, CS7-8, CS5-6, CS3-4, and CS1-2), and the right ventricular apex *RVA3-4). The patient had a history of medically refractory sppraventricular arrhythmia and the diagnostic study revealed easily inducible, typical atrioventricular (AV) nodal reentrant tachycardia. The HBE catheter was maneuvered from the His position to the slow pathway region, which is typically inferior and posterior to the His bundle and just anterior to the coronary sinus ostium. This is an ideal site for slow pathway ablation and has a small atrial electrogram (A) and large ventricular electrogram (V), with no evidence of His bundle activity. The tip of the HBE catheter (HBE1-2) records such a signal, and is used for ablation*

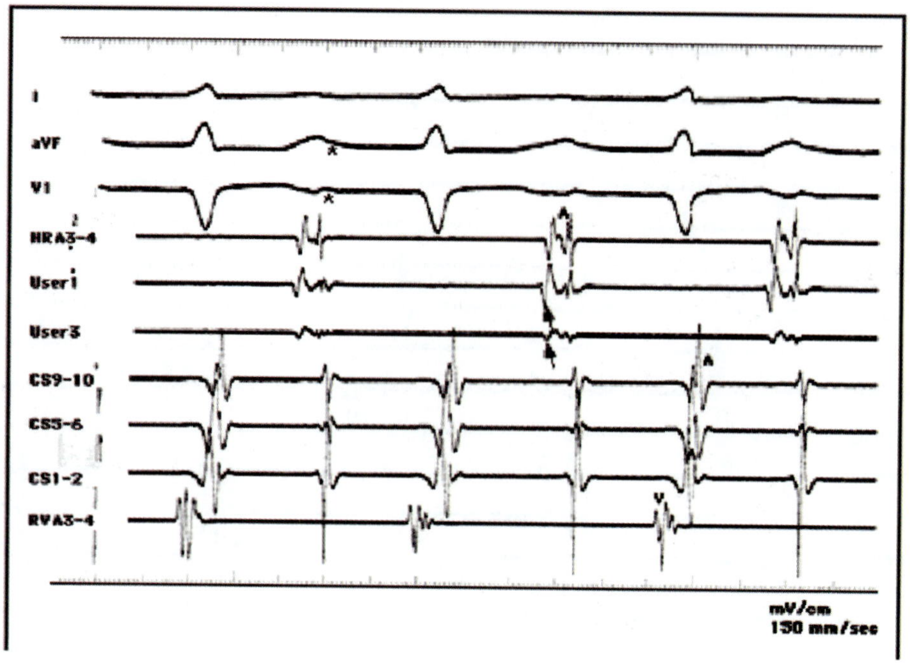

Fig. 7.46: *Electrophysiologic mapping of atrial tachycardia. Three surface ECG leads (I, aVF, VI) and intracardiac recording from the high posterior right atrium (HRA); posterior left atrium (USER1 and USER3); proximal, mid and distal coronary sinus (CS9-10, CS5-6, CS1-2); and right ventricular apex (RVA). The patient had an incessant atrial tachycardia and dilated cardiomyopathy (left ventricular ejection fraction 9%) referred for cardiac transplant evaluation. The P-wave (*) falls at the end of the T-wave on the surface ECG; its onset is difficult to discern. However, the intracardiac electrograms demonstrate obvious atrial (A) and ventricular (V) activity. Activation mapping involves positioning the mapping catheters in the right (HRA) and left atrial (USER) to record earliest electrical activity during the tachycardia. The left atrial catheter records earlier electrical activity (arrow) than the right atrial catheter, but the timing with respect to the surface P-wave is obscured because of the T-wave of the preceding QRS complex*

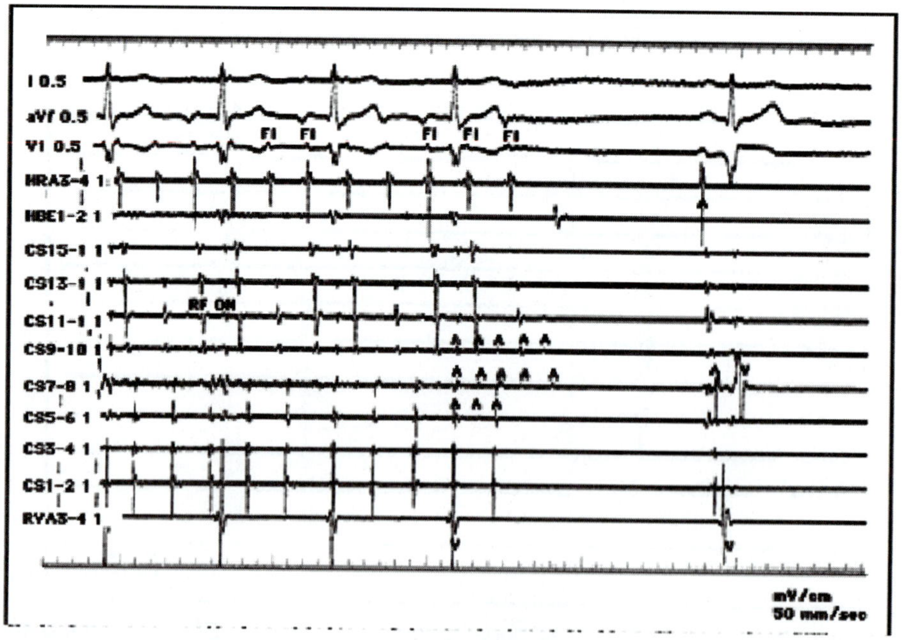

Fig. 7.47: *Radiofrequency catheter ablation of typical atrial flutter. Three surface ECG leads (I, aVF, VI) and intracardiac recordings from the high right atrium (HRA), a mapping catheter in the isthmus between the tricuspid valve and inferior vena cava (TV-IVC) (HBE1-2), eight recordings from a actheter extending from the lateral right atrial wall through the TV-IVC isthmus and into the ostium of the coronary sinus (CS15-1 to CS 1-2), and right ventricular apex (RVA3-4) in a patiene with typical atrial flutter. The tip of the mapping catheter was initially positioned on the tricuspid annulus, and then dragged through the TV-IVC isthmus to the ostium of the iVC during RF application; atrial flutter terminated. Note that the atrial activation (A) blocks between CS7-8 and CS5-6, which on fluoroscopy corresponded to the position of the mapping catheter. F1, flutter waves; V, ventricular electrogram*

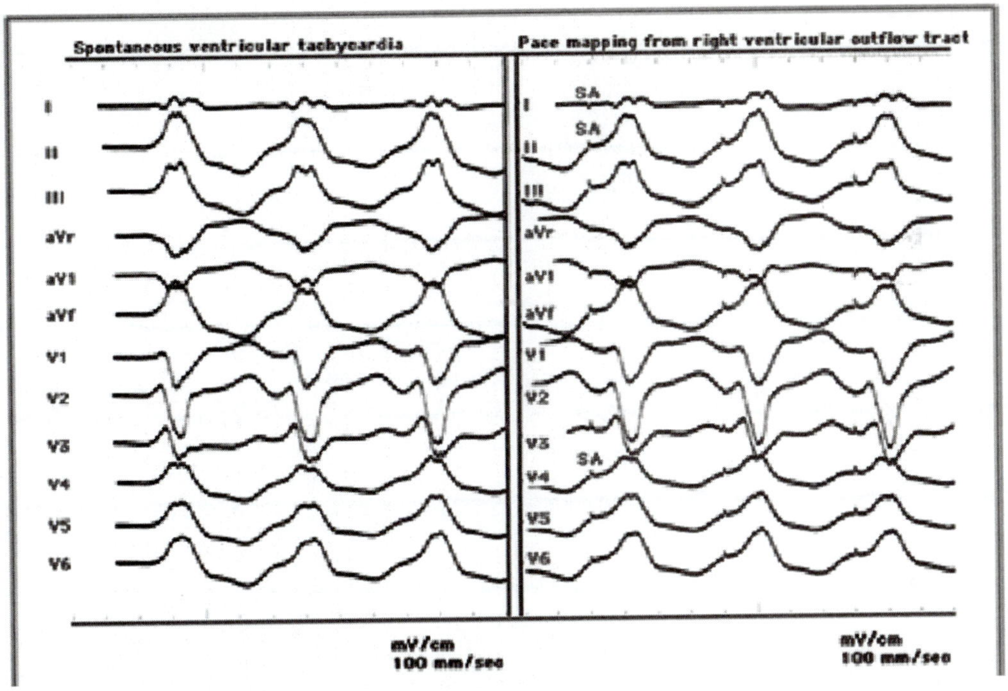

Fig. 7.48: *Pace mapping of an idiopathic RVOT tachycardia. Left panel: 12 lead ECG of spontaneous ventricular tachycardia (VT) in a patient with a structurally normal heart. The VT has a left bundle branch block (LBBB) and an inferior axis morphology, suggesting that the origin is the right ventricular outflow tract (RVOT), Right panel: a mapping catheter has been positioned in the RVOT and pacing is performed from its tip during sinus rhythm. The "pace map" closely approximates the QRS morphology of the spontaneous VT in all 12 leads, suggesting that the mapping catheter is at or near the VT focus, SA, pacing stimulus artifact*

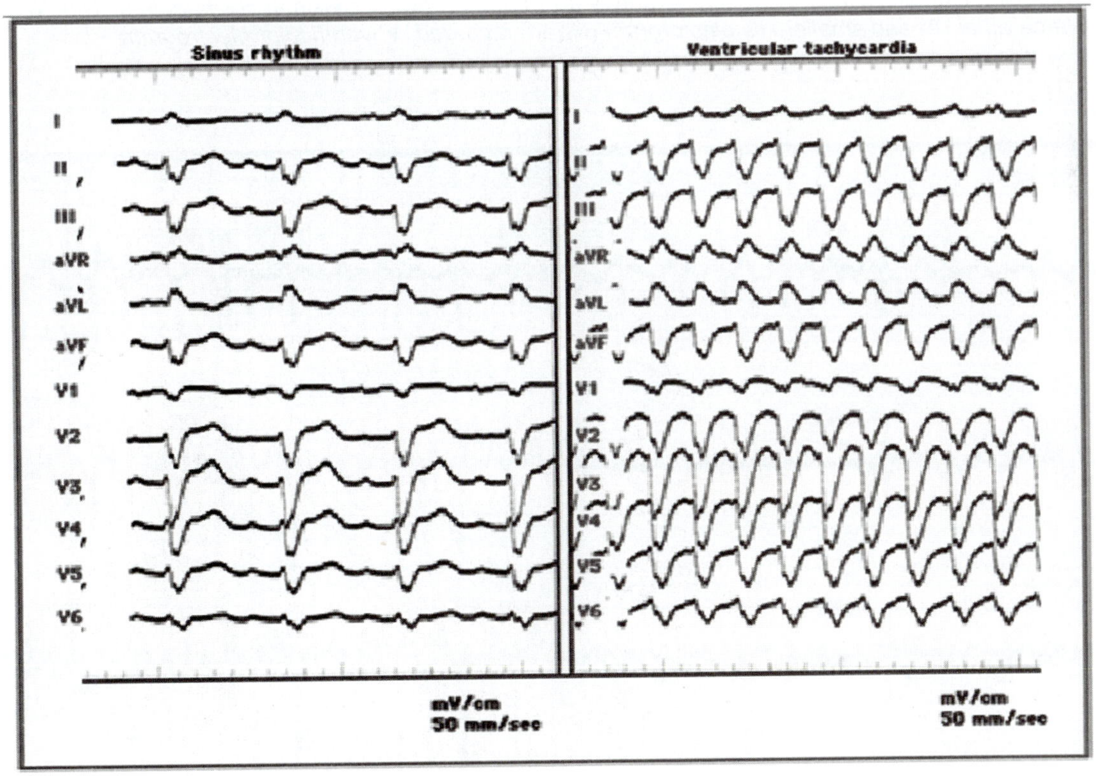

Fig. 7.49: *Bundle branch reentrant ventricular tachcardia. Left panel: 12 lead ECG during sinus rhythm; there is a left bundle type intraventricular conduction delay. Right panel: 12 lead ECG during ventricular 5 tachycardia; there is an remarkable similarity in QRS morphology during VT and sinus rhythm. The HV interval during sinus rhythm was 65 msec, suggesting underlying His-Purkinje conduction disease*

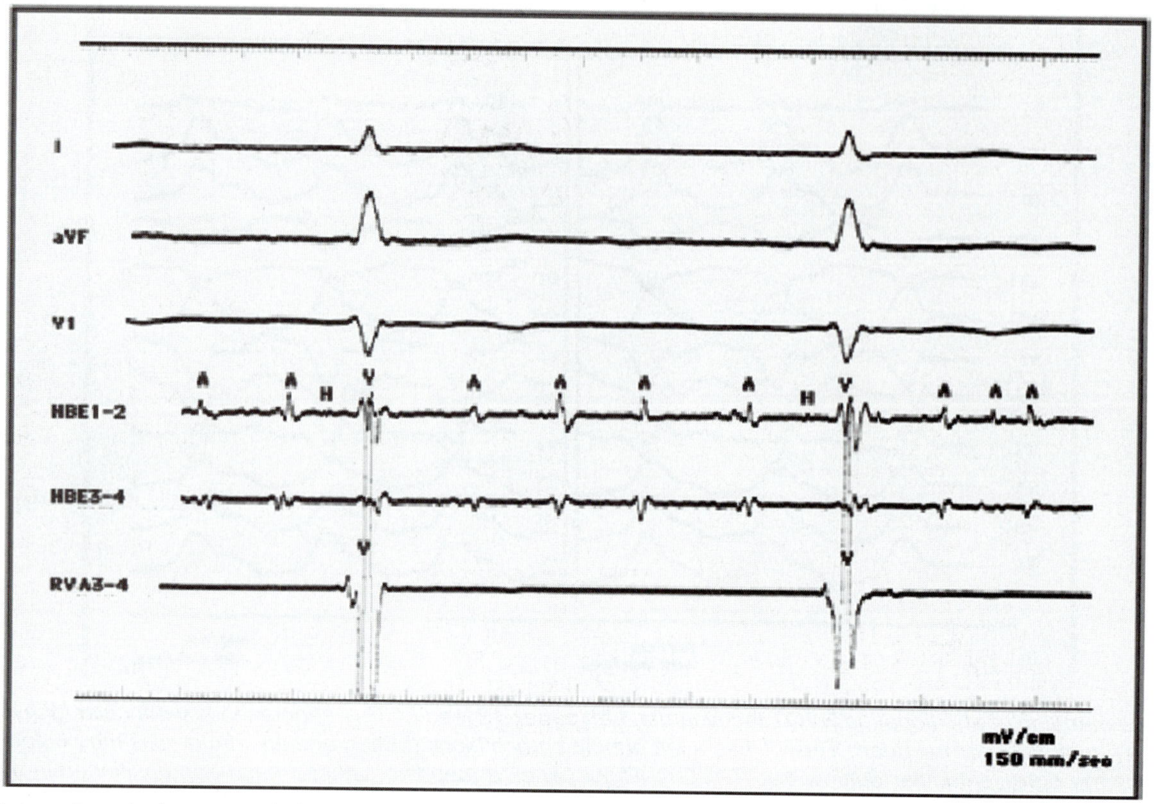

Fig. 7.50: *Intracardiac electrograms during atrial fibrillation. Three surface ECG leads (I, aVF, V1) and ntracardiac recordings from the atrioventricular (AV) junction region (HBE1-2, HBE3-4), and the right ventricular apex (RVA3-4) in a patient with atrial fibrilliation. The patient has extremely symptomatic, medically refractory atrial fibrillation with rapid ventricular rates and recurrent congestive heart failure. The mapping catheter (HBE) has been maneuvered from the area of maximal His bundle activity to a more proximal position, where a large atrial (A) and smaller His electorgram (H) are recorded, V, ventricular electrogram*

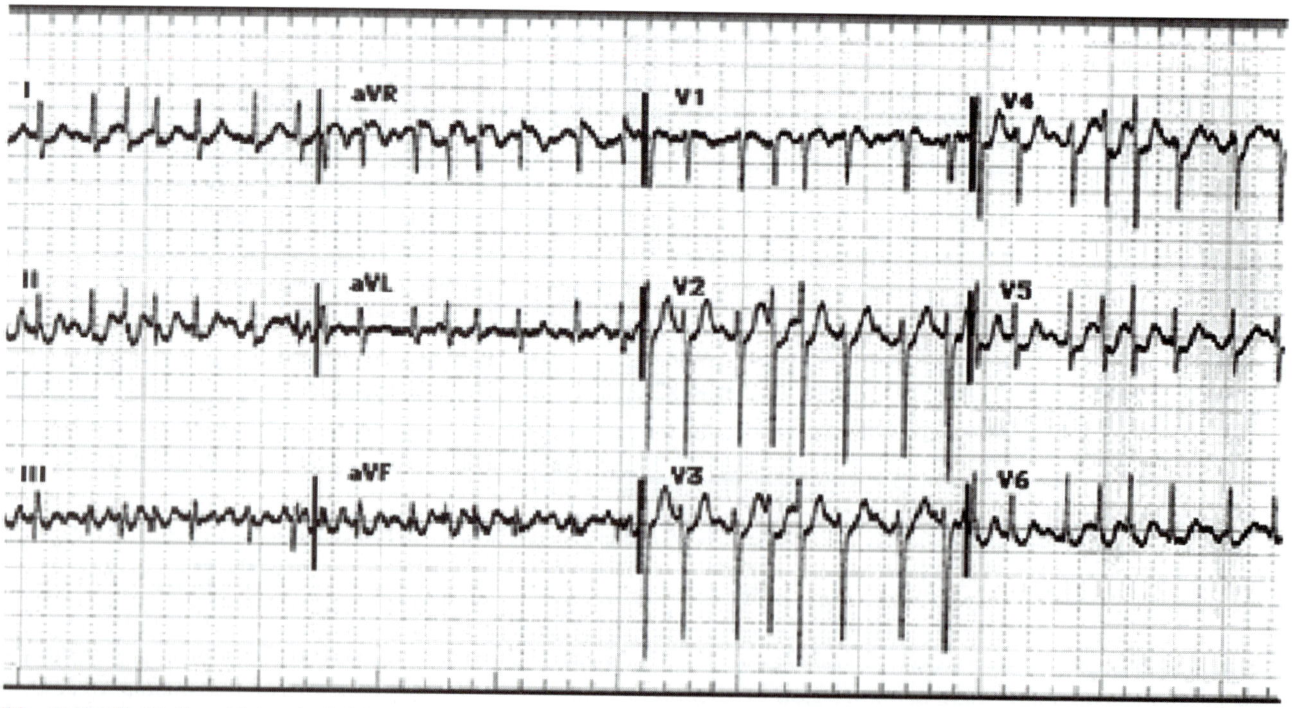

Fig. 7.51: *Atrial fibrillation 12 leads ECG shows an rapid, irregularly irregular rhythm due to paroxsymal atrial fibrillation which was refractory to multiple medications*

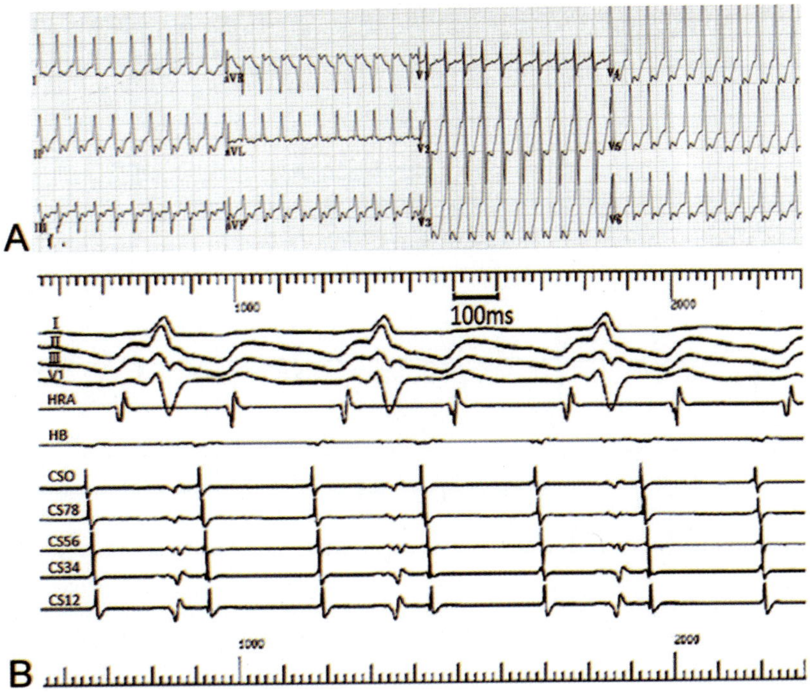

Fig. 7.52: *(A) Electrocardiogram (ECG) showing SVT during the attacks. (B) Intracardiac electrogram showing paroxysmal atrial flutter (2:1) during ablation*

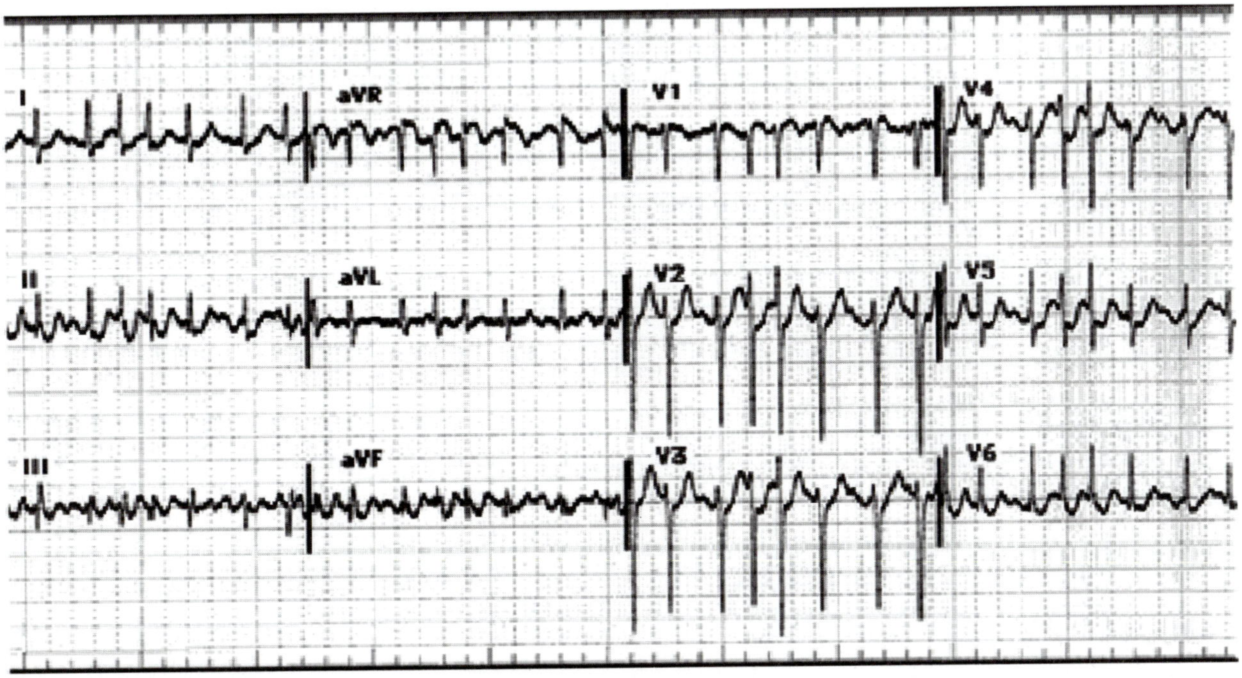

Fig. 7.53: *Bundle branch reentrant ventricular tachycardia. Five surface ECG leads (I, II, aVF, V1, V6) and intracardiac recordings from the His bundle region (HBE2-3, 1-2) the right ventricular apex (RVA3-4), and a mapping catheter (USER1) positioned distal t the His catheter along the RV septum to record a right bundle potential (arrow). The right bundle potential was recorded 30 ms after the His potential (HP). A, atrial electrogram; V, ventricular electrogram*

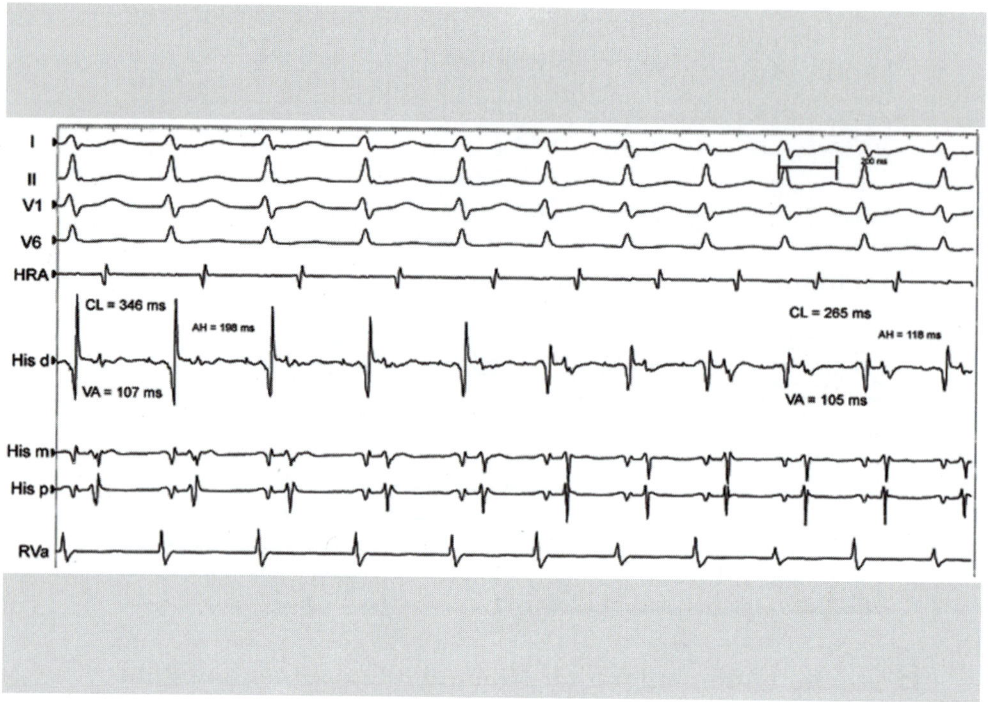

Fig. 7.54: *Narrow complex-tachycardia with 1:1 VA relationship and sudden change in cycle length from 346 to 265 ms. Shown are surface ECG leads I, II, V1 and V6; high right atrial electrogram (HRA); His bundle electrograms - proximal (His p), mid (His m) and distal (His d); right ventricular apex electrogram (RVA)*

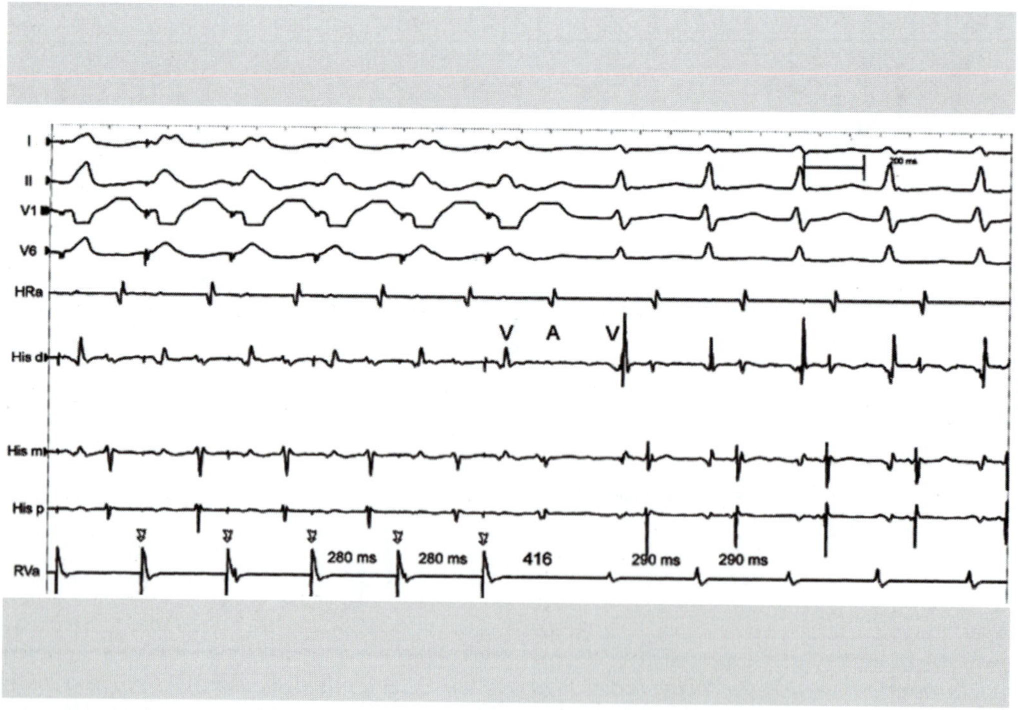

Fig. 7.55: *Tachycardia entrainment from RV apex. When RV pacing was stopped, the response is VAV. The corrected post pacing interval minus tachycardia cycle length is 96 ms (not shown). Arrows represent pacing stimulus*

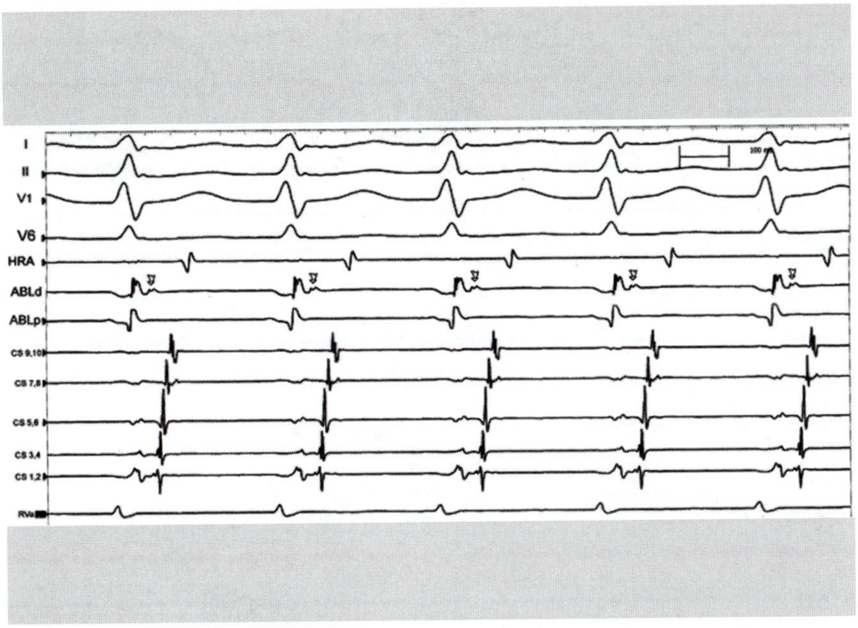

Fig. 7.56: *Narrow complex-tachycardia after CS cannulation. In addition electrograms from proximal (ABLp) and distal (ABLd) ablation catheter and coronary sinus (proximal - 9,10 to distal - 1,2) are shown. The coronary sinus catheter shows eccentric atrial activation pattern. Arrows represent earliest retrograde atrial activation in the ABLd.*

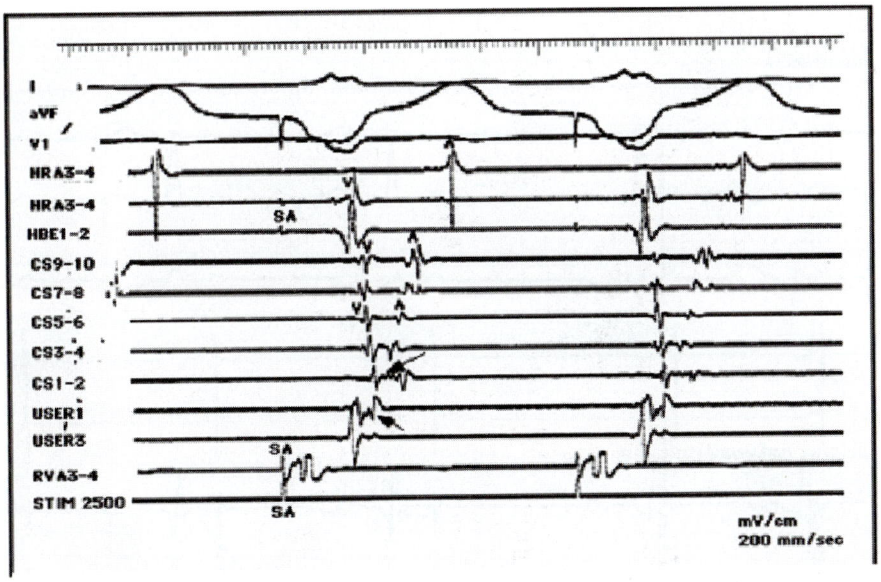

Fig. 7.57: *Electrophysiologic mapping of concealed accessory pathway during ventricular pacing. Shown are three surface ECG leads (I, aVF, and V1) and intracardiac recording from the high right atrium (HRA), proximal (HBE 3-4) and distal His bundle region (HBE1-2), proximal to distal coronary sinus (CS9-10, CS7-8, CS5-6, CS3-4, and CS1-2), right ventricular apex (RVA3-4), from a mapping catheter's distal (USER1) and proximal (USER3) electrode pairs, and a stimulus artifact (SA) channel (STIM). The mapping catheter was advanced through the right femoral artery and retrograde across the aortic valve into the left ventricle. With each ventricular paced beat (V) there is retrograde conduction from the ventricle to atrium (A) via the left free wall accessory pathway. The mapping catheter has been maneuvered to the site along the mitral annulus which records the earliest atrial activity (red arrow); the atrial activity recoreded at the tip electrode of user 1 precedes the earliest atrial activity (black arrow) noted in the coronary sinus (CS1-2) by 25 msec*

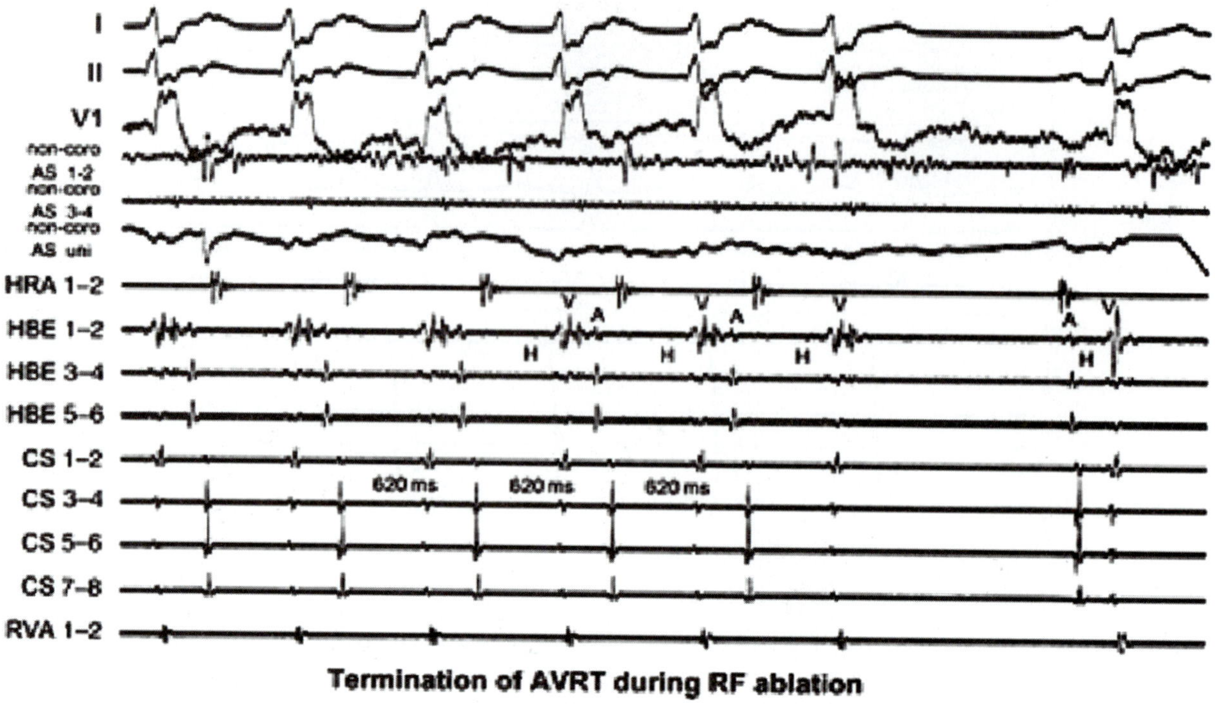

Fig. 7.58: *Tracings are ECG leads I, II, V1, and intracardiac electrograms recorded from a mapping catheter in the noncoronary AS (non-coro AS1-2, non-coro AS3-4, and non-coro AS uni), a catheter in the HRA, a catheter at the region (HBE), a catheter within the CS, and a catheter at the RVA in a patient with an anteroseptal AP during RF ablation in the noncoronary AS. A single RF delivery at this site successfully resulted in tachycardia termination after 15s and ventriculoatrial dissociation*

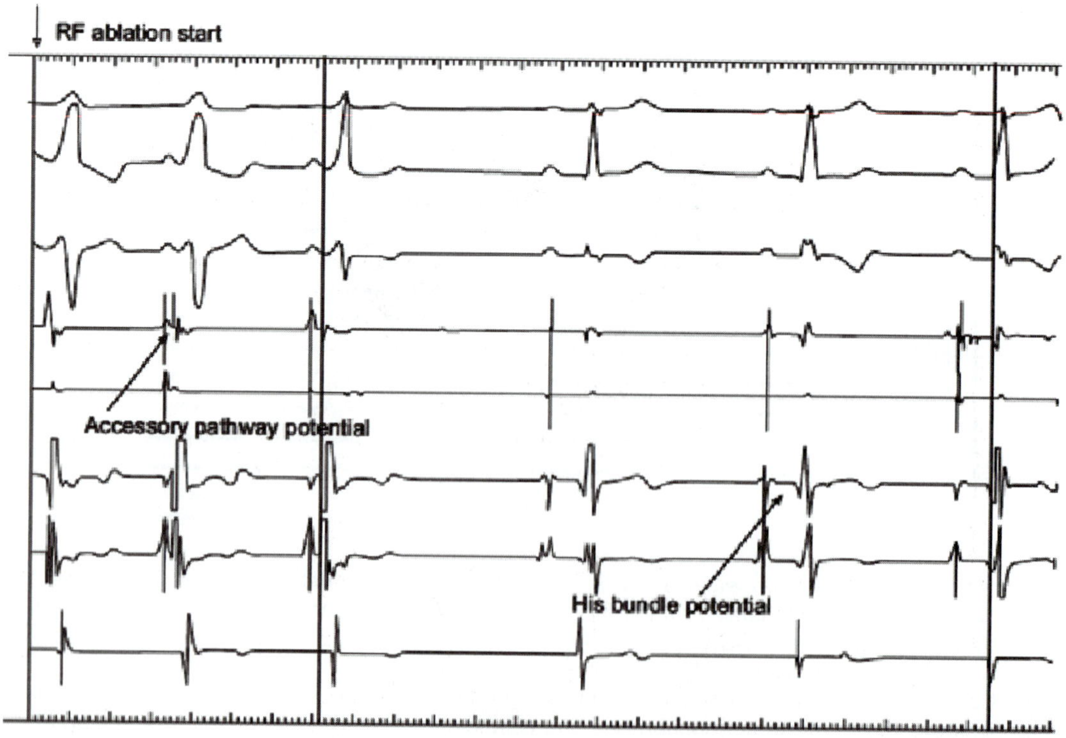

Fig. 7.59: *Accessory pathway potential and local AV fusion at successful RF ablation site with loss of preexcitation and return of normal HV interval*

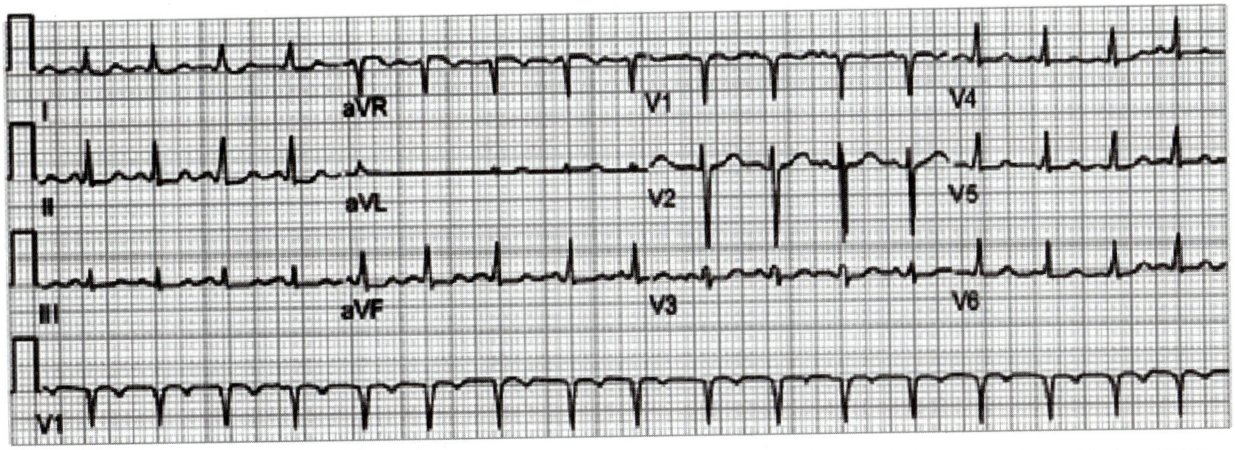

Fig. 7.60: *ECG showing right anteroseptal accessory pathway (AP). A left axis (with a negative delta wave in lead V1) suggests a right lateral AP*

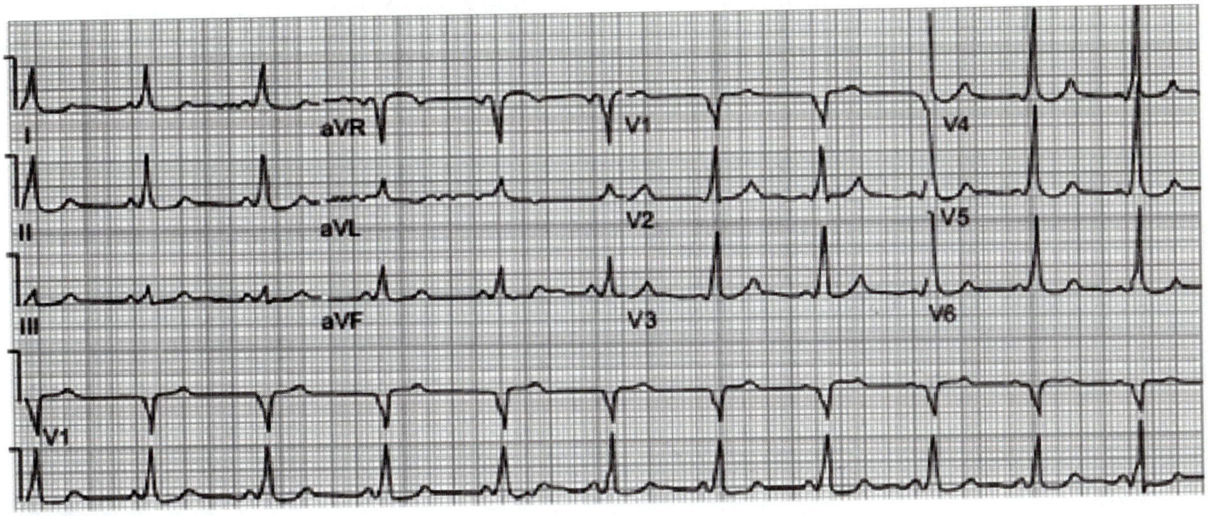

Fig. 7.61: *ECG showing right lateral accessory pathway (AP). If the delta waves in the inferior leads are negative, then it denotes a posteroseptal AP right, or left, depending on the delta wave vector in lead V1 as described above*

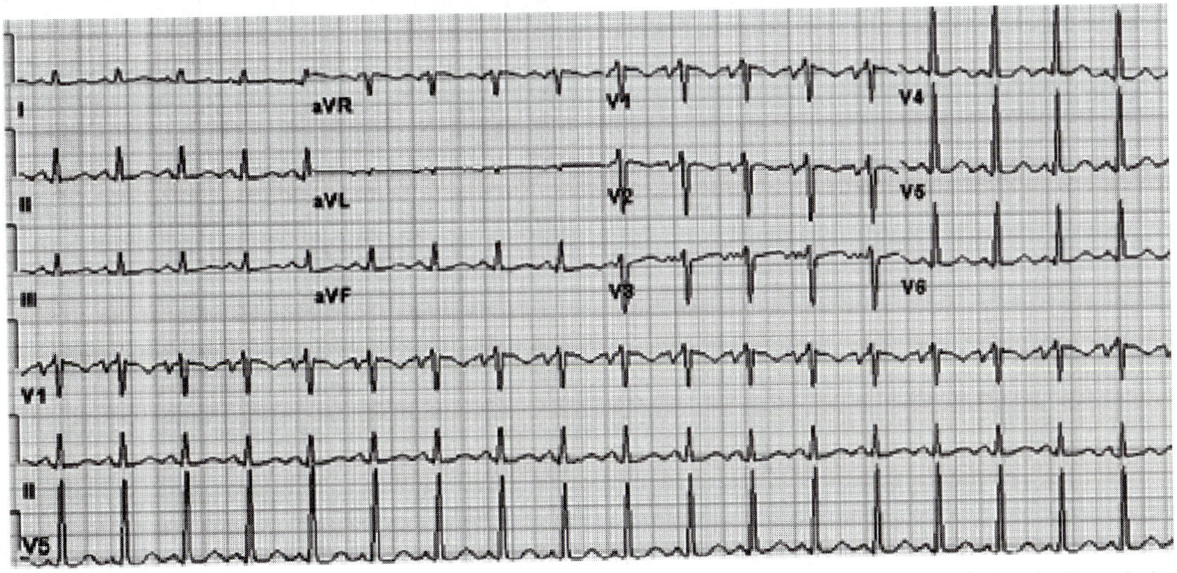

Fig. 7.62: *ECG showing left lateral accessory pathway (AP) showing signs of minimal preexcitation in the inferior leads*

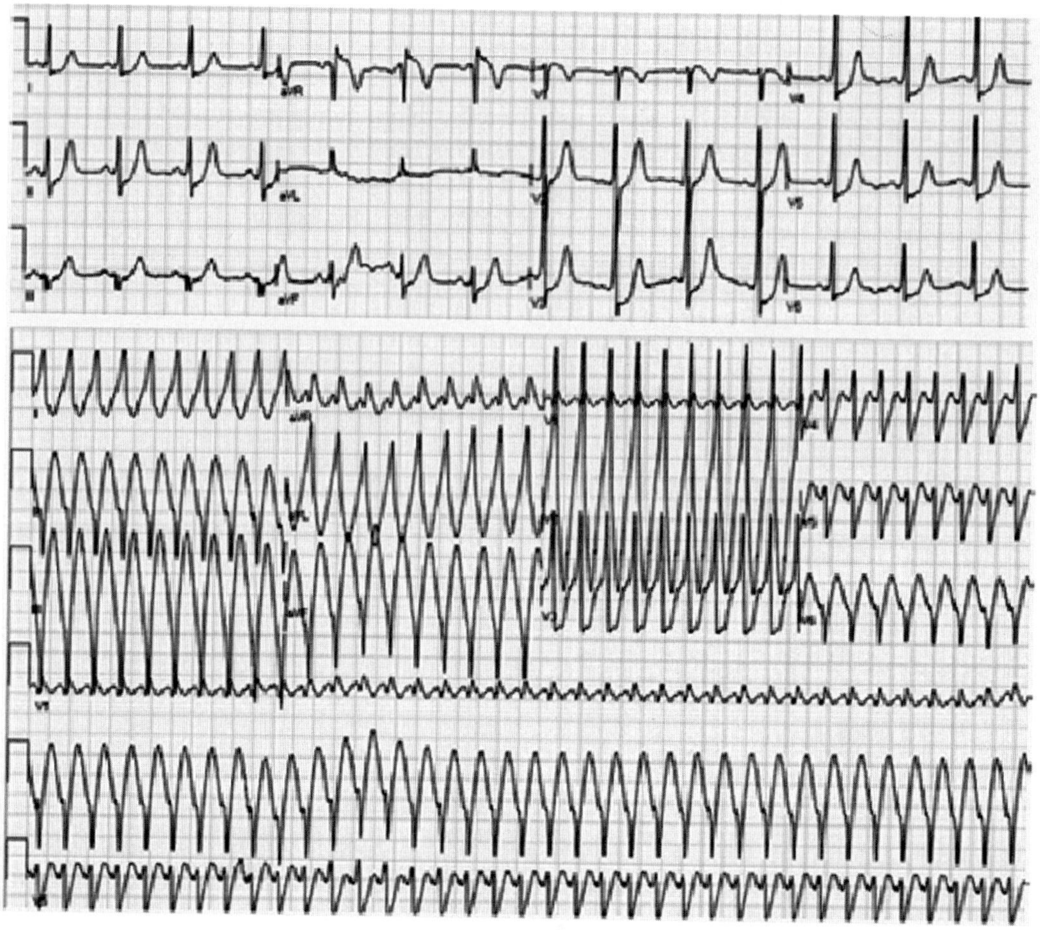

Fig. 7.63: *ECG showing antidromic reciprocating tachycardia in a patient with right posteroseptal accessory pathway (AP)*

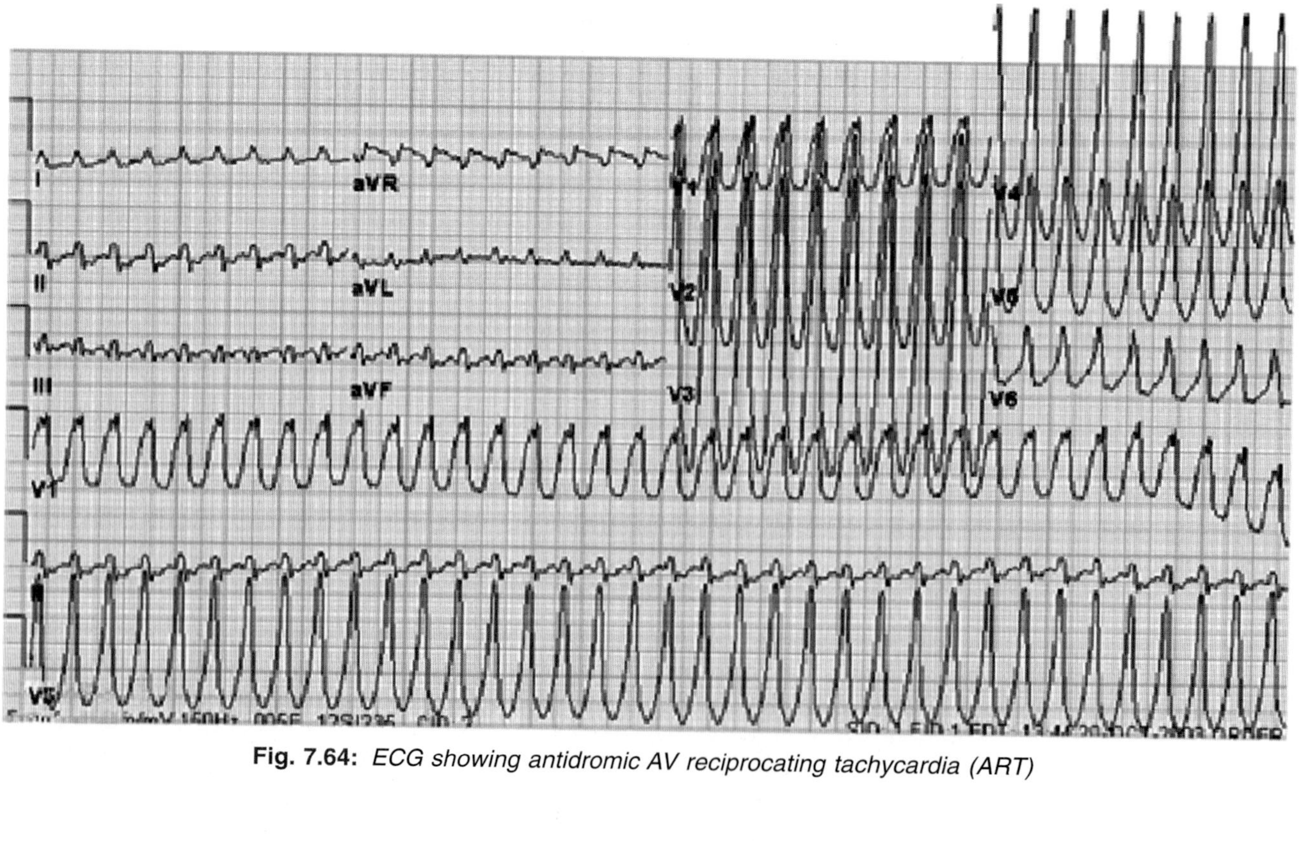

Fig. 7.64: *ECG showing antidromic AV reciprocating tachycardia (ART)*

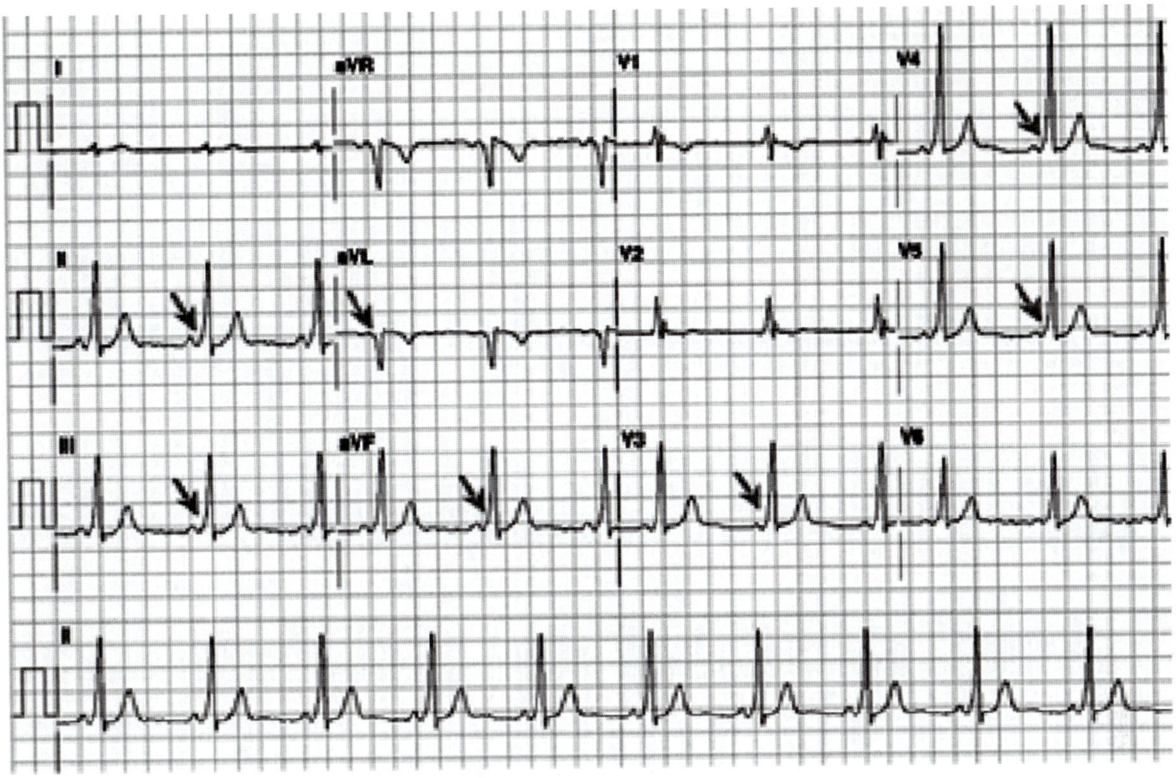

Fig. 7.65: *Resting ECG shows delta waves (red arrows) in the inferior and lateral leads*

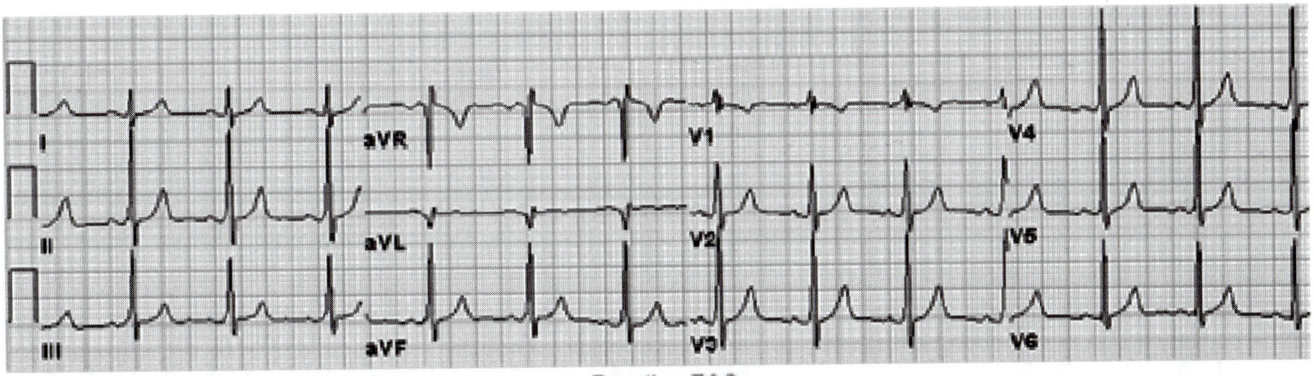

Baseline ECG

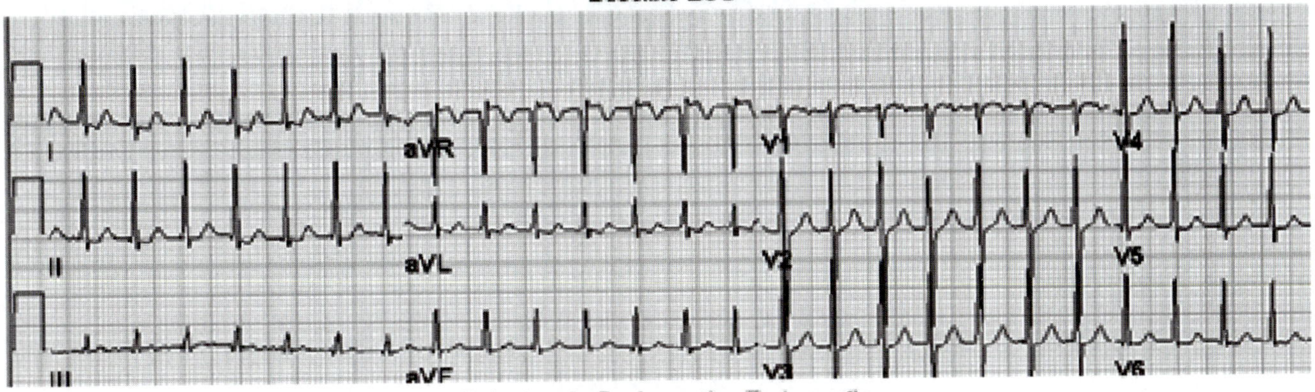

Orthodromic Reciprocating Tachycardia

Fig. 7.66: *Left lateral accessory pathway (AP). It is prudent to recognize that the delta wave vector can only be determined with precision when the ECG shows maximum preexcitation. A right-sided AP with minimal preexcitation but with a posteroseptal location can not be determined with a high probability until ART occurs*

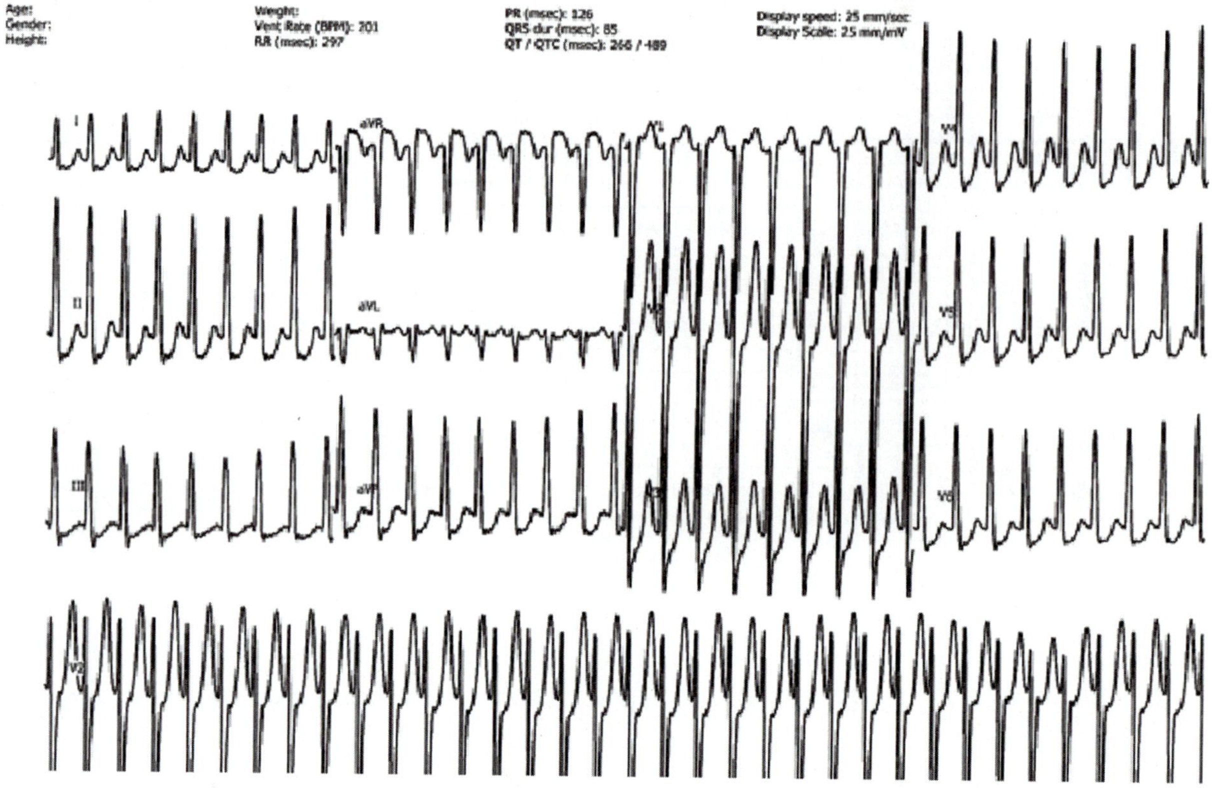

Fig. 7.67: *ECG features of typical atrioventricular nodal reentry tachycardia*

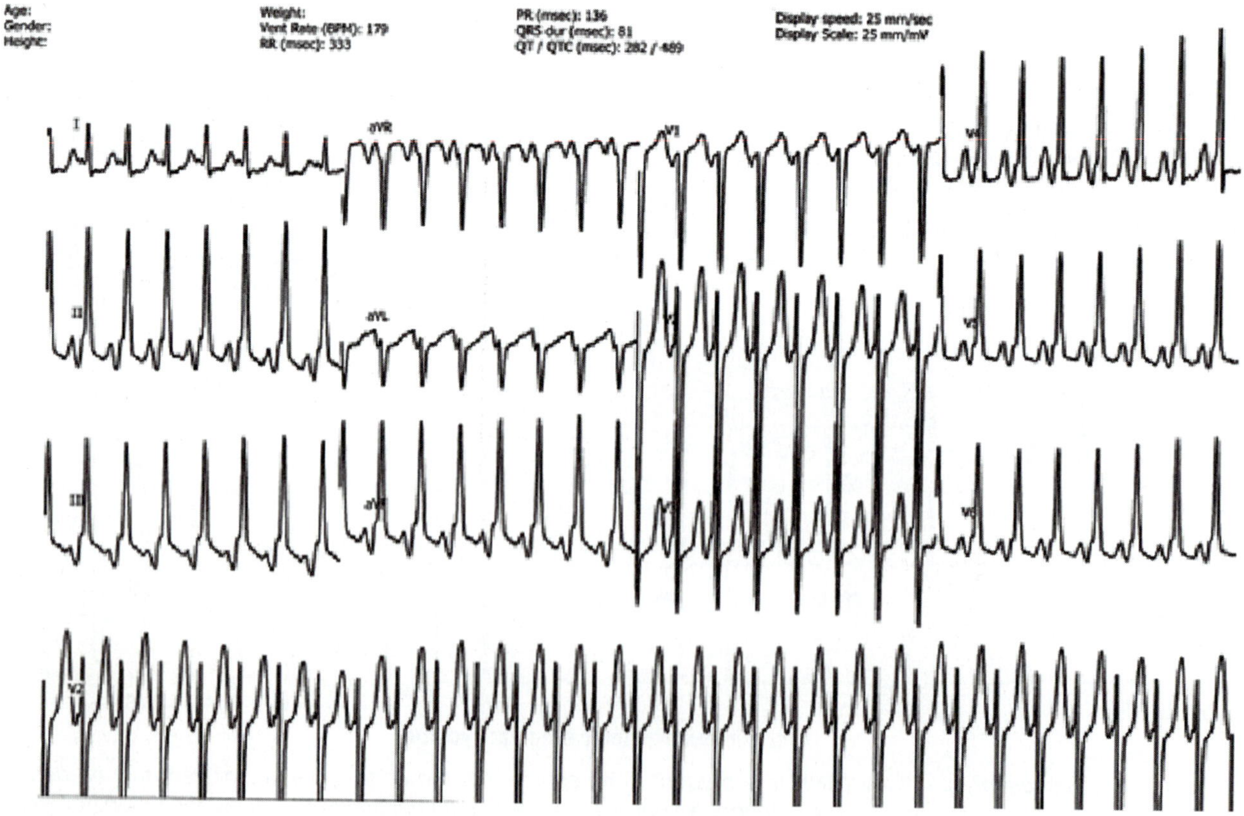

Fig. 7.68: *ECG features of atypical atrioventricular nodal reentry tachycardia*

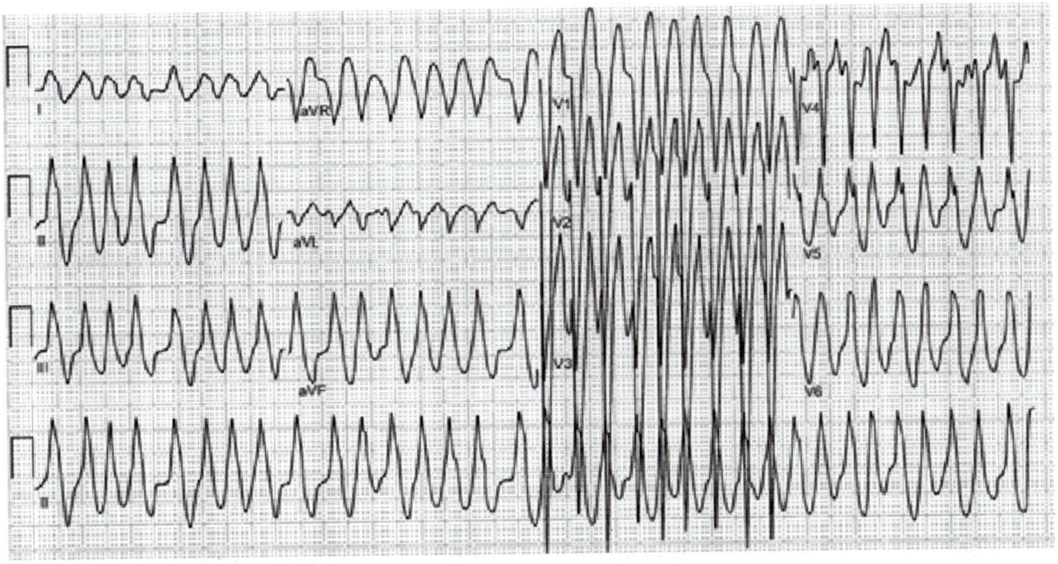

Fig. 7.69: *ECG morphology showing preexcited atrial fibrillation*

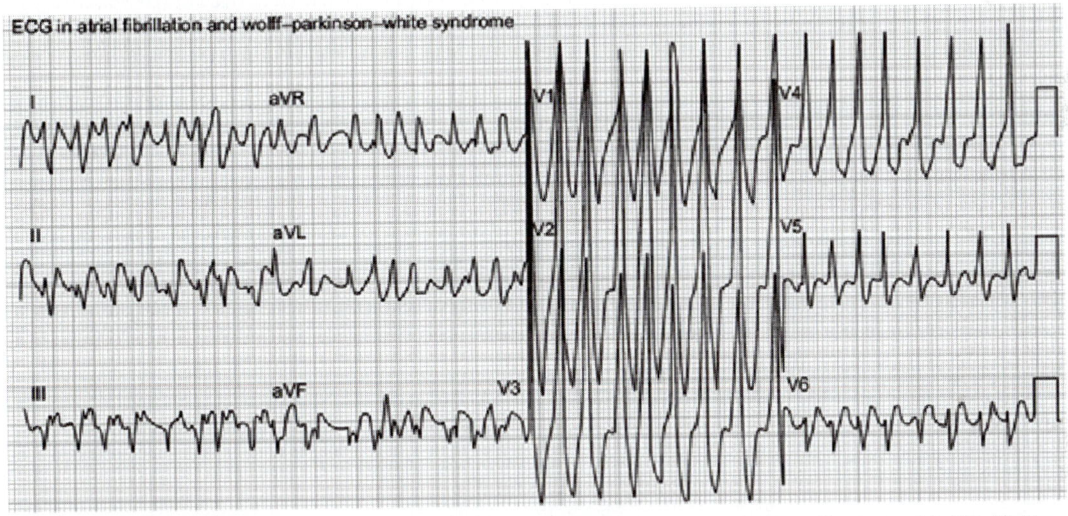

Fig. 7.70: *ECG shows an irregular broad-complex tachycardia. Almost all irregular tachycardias are atrial fibrillation.QRS morphology varies because of the varying contributions of the atrioventricular node and the accessory pathway in atrial fibrillation to activation of the ventricle. This ECG shows preexcited atrial fibrillation. The shortest RR Interval is 200 milliseconds; intervals < 260 milliseconds are associated with a risk of sudden death*

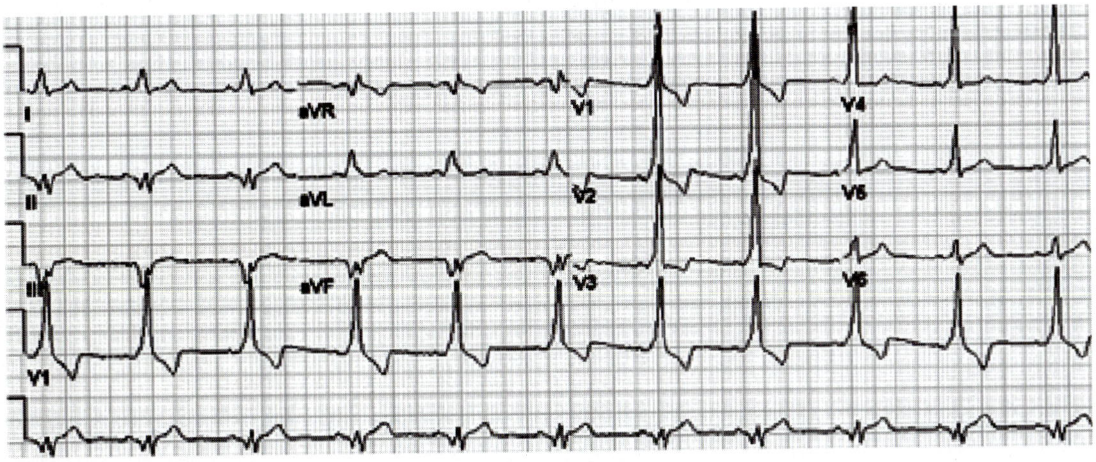

Fig. 7.71: *ECG showing left posteroseptal accessory pathway (AP). A negative delta wave in lead I, aVL and V6 (rightward QRS axis) with a positive delta wave in lead V1 suggests a left lateral pathway*

Cannulation of the coronary sinus is helpful to exclude left-sided accessory pathways or other left-sided tachyarrhythmia substrates.

For left heart catheterization, 1 of 2 approaches may be taken: transseptal catheterization via the interatrial septum or retrograde catheterization across the aortic valve.

Anticoagulation with intravenous heparin is used to reduce the risk of periprocedural thromboembolism.

A. *Atrial Fibrillation*

RFCA of the atrioventricular (AV) junction is the simplest catheter ablation procedure performed in patients with atrial fibrillation. AV nodal modification is less often performed (Figs 7.57, 7.71 and 7.72).

For catheter ablation of atrial tissue for atrial fibrillation, the most commonly used techniques involve ablation of the muscular connections between the pulmonary veins and the left atrium (pulmonary vein isolation), or a wide circumferential ablation around the pulmonary veins. The goal is to electrically isolate foci arising from inside the veins, or adjacent to the pulmonary vein ostia, from the rest of the left atrium.

Electroanatomic map of the posterior left atrium, illustrating the pulmonary veins: right superior pulmonary vein (RSPV), right inferior pulmonary vein (RIPV), left superior pulmonary vein (LSPV), and left inferior pulmonary vein (LIPV). The red circles represent actual discrete radiofrequency applications, predominantly delivered in a circumferential pattern around the pulmonary veins. This ablation strategy can isolate pulmonary vein foci that initiate atrial fibrillation, and/or alter the substrate of the left atrium to inhibit fibrillatory activity due to reentry. Image courtesy of American College of Cardiology Foundation.

B. *Atrioventricular Nodal Reentrant Tachycardia*

In the common form of atrioventricular nodal reentrant tachycardia (AVNRT), the inferior atrionodal input to the atrioventricular (AV) node serves as the anterograde limb (i.e. the slow pathway) of the reentry circuit, and the superior atrionodal input serves as the retrograde limb (i.e. the fast pathway). Typically, AVNRT can be cured by targeting the slow pathway near the inferior tricuspid valve annulus at the level of the coronary sinus os or somewhat higher.

The risk of iatrogenic heart block with ablation in this region is quite low (1–2%). Targeting the slow pathway is safer than targeting the fast pathway, which is located closer to the compact AV node (Figs 7.45 and 7.68).

C. *Orthodromic Reciprocating Tachycardia*

In orthodromic reciprocating tachycardia (ORT) the AV node serves as the anterograde limb and an accessory AV connection (i.e. the accessory pathway) serves as the retrograde limb.

Schema of orthodromic reciprocating tachycardia (ORT). The atrioventricular node serves as the antegrade limb, whereas an accessory pathway (atrioventricular connection) serves as the retrograde limb. For ECG features of ORT, see the image below. Supraventricular tachycardia (SVT) in a patient with orthodromic reciprocating tachycardia (ORT) due to a concealed pathway. Note the retrograde P wave, seen best in lead V2, separated from the QRS complex by an isoelectric baseline (compare to the first ECG above, in which the P-wave is fused to the QRS). This pattern of "short RP tachycardia" (in which the interval between the QRS complex and retrograde P-wave is shorter than the subsequent PR interval and the P-wave is in the first half of the RR interval) suggests an SVT incorporating an accessory pathway (Fig. 7.44).

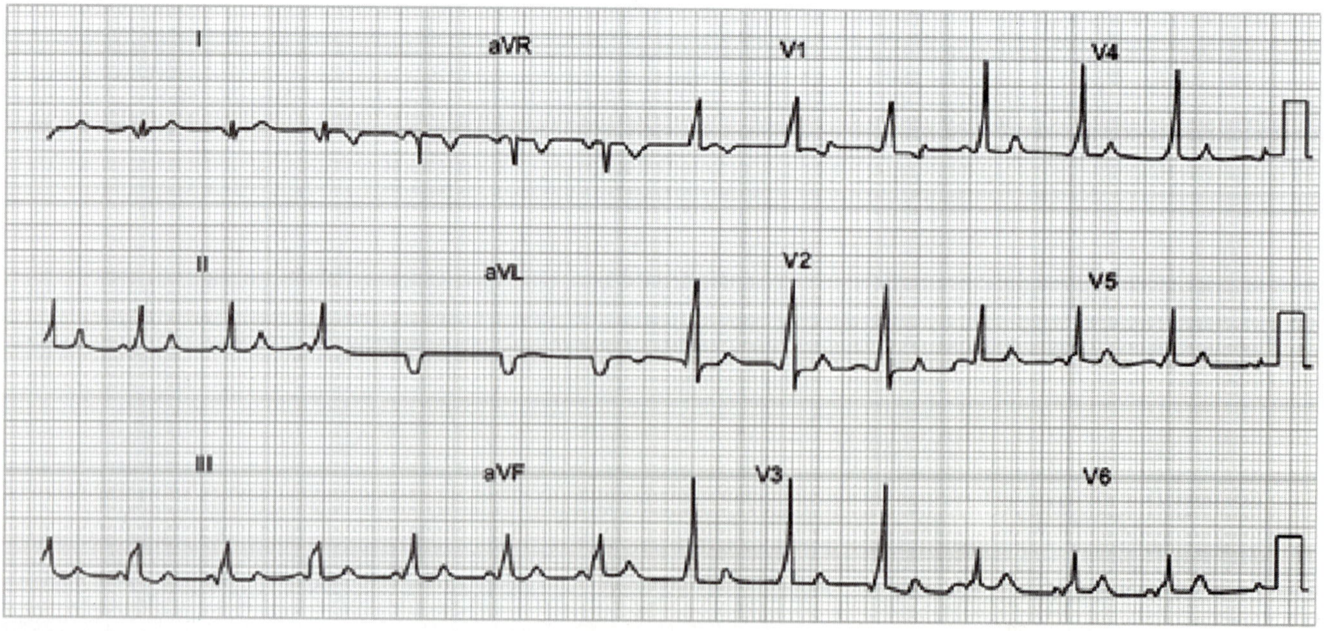

Fig. 7.72: *ECG shows the short PR interval and slurred upstroke of the QRS (delta wave). The QRS is positive in V1 and in the inferior leads; thus, the pathway is left-sided and anterior (free wall)*

Typically, ORT can be cured by targeting the accessory pathway as it crosses the mitral or tricuspid valve annulus.

D. *Unifocal Atrial Tachycardia* (Figs 7.46 and 7.52)

Unifocal atrial tachycardia, which can arise from either atrium, is somewhat more challenging to ablate than the more common forms of generic SVT. For those tachycardias originating from the left atrium, transseptal catheterization via a patent foramen ovale or transseptal puncture is usually required.

E. *Wolff-Parkinson-White Syndrome*

Typically, a transition from ORT to atrial fibrillation can be the cause of rapid preexcited tachycardia in Wolff-Parkinson-White syndrome. Ablation of the accessory pathway cures the syndrome, eliminating ORT and atrial fibrillation in most instances (Figs 7.43, 7.44, 7.56, 7.59, 7.61, 7.65 and 7.67).

F. *Atrial Flutter*

Atrial flutter is most commonly due to a large reentrant circuit in the right atrium, involving an isthmus of tissue between the tricuspid valve annulus and the inferior vena cava. Most commonly, reentry proceeds counterclockwise up the atrial septum and down the lateral wall of the right atrium, inscribing inverted (i.e. "sawtooth") flutter waves in the inferior leads and upright P-waves in V1.

Schema of the common variety of atrial flutter. The reentry circuit is confined to the right atrium and circulates as a counterclockwise macroreentrant circuit proceeding superiorly over the atrial septum and inferiorly over the lateral atrial wall. The wave front circulates through a narrow isthmus of tissue between the tricuspid valve annulus and the inferior vena cava. Linear ablation across this isthmus cures this common form of atrial flutter. For ECG features, see the image below. An example of a typical counterclockwise atrial flutter, the most common form of atrial flutter. The cardinal features are a perfectly regular atrial rhythm with inverted P-waves inferiorly that have a positive overshoot, upright P-waves in V1, and inverted P-waves in V6 (Fig. 7.47).

Clockwise reentry using this same circuit can also occur, giving upright P-waves inferiorly and inverted P-waves in V1. Linear ablation of the cavotricuspid isthmus cures these common forms of atrial flutter.

Nonisthmus-dependent flutters can occur elsewhere in the right atrium as well as in the left atrium. Left atrial flutters are uncommon, may be difficult to ablate, and generally require a three dimensional mapping system to facilitate the procedure.

A three dimensional electroanatomic map of cavotricuspid isthmus flutter. The colors progress from red to purple and represent relative conduction time in the right atrium (early to late). An ablation line (red dots) has been created from the tricuspid annulus to the inferior vena cava. This interrupts the flutter circuit.

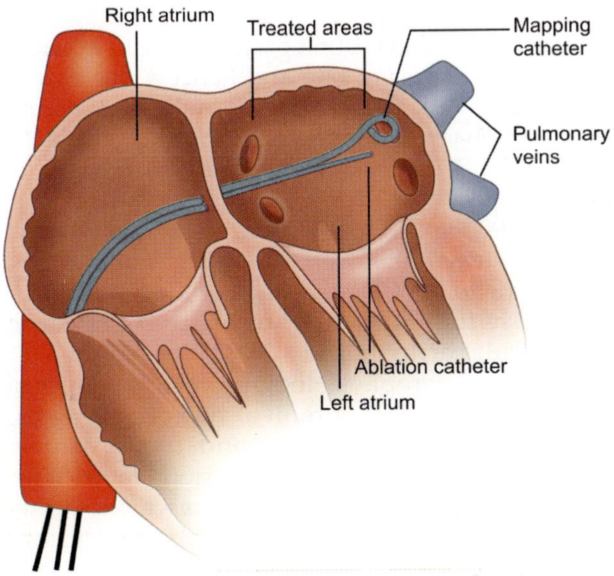

Fig. 7.73: *During catheter ablation of atrial fibrillation, a catheter is passed into the left atrium and is used to cauterize areas surrounding the orifices of the pulmonary veins. The resulting scars prevent conduction of the extra beats arising from the veins, which can trigger atrial fibrillation*

MEASURES TO BE ADOPTED AFTER ABLATION PROCEDURE IN THE FOLLOWING CLINICAL SITUATIONS

Atrial Fibrillation

Radiofrequency catheter ablation (RFCA) of the atrioventricular (AV) junction results in excellent rate control, relieves palpitations, and improves functional capacity; however, patients who undergo this procedure require permanent pacemaker implantation to manage the resulting AV block and require warfarin therapy to prevent stroke because the atrial fibrillation itself is not affected. AV nodal modification is less therapeutic than AV junction ablation and may result in late heart block.

Supraventricular Tachyarrhythmias

The common forms of supraventricular tachycardia (SVT) [e.g. atrioventricular nodal reentrant tachycardia (AVNRT), SVT associated with Wolff-Parkinson-White syndrome] are usually curable with a single procedure; the success rate is typically 90–95%. Cure rates for unifocal atrial tachycardia and common right atrial flutter are somewhat lower but still approach 90%. Recurrent tachyarrhythmias typically occur in the first few months after ablation and may be amenable to cure with a second procedure.

AVNRT is usually amenable to cure with a slow pathway ablation near the inferior atrial septum, where the risk of heart block is 1–2%. In the uncommon circumstances in which ablation near the compact AV node is required (e.g. fast pathway for AVNRT, or an accessory pathway in a para-Hisian location), the risk of heart block may approach 5% or a little higher.

In a number of centers, catheter-based cryoablation is used rather than radiofrequency catheter ablation (RFCA) near the compact AV node to minimize the risk of heart block. With cryoablation, heart block is generally reversible with prompt rewarming. However, cryoablation appears to be slightly less effective than radiofrequency as an energy source, especially for deep accessory pathways.

Success rates for curing atrial fibrillation with RFCA are highest (up to 87% in the 5 randomized trials reported through 2006) for paroxysmal atrial fibrillation in the absence of structural heart disease and lowest (50% or less) with persistent atrial fibrillation in the presence of structural heart disease and left atrial enlargement. Repeat procedures are typically needed in 25% or more of patients.

Success rates have historically been based on patient symptoms and periodic electrocardiographic monitoring. Success rates are lower if intensive ambulatory monitoring to detect asymptomatic atrial fibrillation recurrences is used, such as daily monitoring for a month with an auto-triggering event monitor. Some patients require the use of previously ineffective antiarrhythmic drugs to maintain success.

Ventricular Tachyarrhythmias

Idiopathic ventricular tachycardia (VT) is curable (success rate approximately 80%), assuming it is readily inducible during electrophysiology studies. The most common location for these VTs is the right ventricular outflow tract. Because these VTs are usually not reentrant in nature, a significant percentage are not inducible. Some cannot be ablated because of their deep septal or epicardial location. Some left ventricular VTs originate near a coronary cusp, which may preclude a successful ablation because of concern regarding coronary artery damage. Approximately half the cases of VTs associated with structural heart disease can be palliated by catheter ablation. Extensive scarring in these ventricles may limit the efficacy of the relatively small lesions made by RFCA, and multiple VT circuits may also contribute to this moderate success rate. Some form of three dimensional mapping is helpful for these complex ablations. In practice, many of these patients have ICDs, and catheter ablation is used as adjunctive therapy for frequent device activations.

DIAGNOSTIC PROGRAMED ELECTRICAL STIMULATION

Intracardiac electrogram recordings were measured first in the 1960s, and the methods of diagnostic programed electrical cardiac stimulation were introduced in the 1970s. These procedures are safe when performed under the carefully controlled conditions of the electrophysiology (EP) laboratory. Typically, a number of catheters (wires) are placed in the heart under X-ray fluoroscopic guidance, and electrograms are recorded from various sites, most frequently the high right atrium, His bundle [i.e. atrio-ventricular (AV) junction], coronary sinus, and right ventricle (Figs 7.36–7.42).

In addition to recording the electrograms from these sites, pacing the heart is also possible using an external stimulator. This setup provides the ability to assess the conduction properties of the heart, as well as the ability to induce and terminate cardiac arrhythmias using various pacing protocols. Analysis of the electrogram patterns and the patient's response to pacing interventions and drugs provides an accurate diagnosis of the mechanisms and circuits for most arrhythmias. The introduction of radiofrequency catheter ablation in the 1980s provided the option for therapeutic interventions during the EP study. This has revolutionized the treatment of cardiac arrhythmias and has high success rates, particularly for reentrant supraventricular arrhythmias.

INDICATIONS FOR PROGRAMED ELECTRICAL STIMULATION

- Risk stratification (regarding ventricular arrhythmias) in patients with structural heart disease
- Risk assessment in patients with Wolff-Parkinson-White (WPW) syndrome
- Evaluation of patients with syncope
- Characterization of AV conduction
- Determining the mechanism of supraventricular tachycardia
- Assessment of efficacy of catheter ablation
- Determining the mechanism of a wide QRS complex tachycardia
- Determining the mechanism of ventricular tachycardia
- Determining the impact of pacing on initiation and termination of the tachycardia.

METHODS OF PROGRAMED ELECTRICAL STIMULATION OF THE HEART

Types of pacing protocols are used during EP testing:

- *Burst pacing or continuous pacing:* The atrium or ventricle is paced at a faster fixed rate than the underlying sinus rate, for example, during measurement of sinus node function.
- Decremental pacing is burst pacing but with a continuous increase in the pacing rate and hence a decrease in the cycle length (CL), for example, as in the measurement of the Wenckebach CL or the rate at which the AV node blocks a beat in conduction from the atrium to the ventricle.
- *Extrastimuli:* Typically, 6–8 beats are delivered at a fixed rate (drive train), followed by 1–3 additional premature beats at a shorter CL or faster rate, for example, used particularly for induction of reentrant supraventricular or ventricular arrhythmias.
- A standard electrophysiology protocol involves single premature atrial extra stimuli at two cycle lengths, and from 1 site, single, double, and triple ventricular premature extra stimuli from two right ventricular sites at two cycle lengths. There are various ways to decrement atrial and ventricular premature extrastimuli during fixed rate pacing.
- Occasionally, isoproterenol or other drugs are given to help initiate a tachycardia.
- *Extrastimuli during tachycardias:* Premature atrial or ventricular beats may be introduced during tachycardia to help to differentiate the circuit and mechanism of the

arrhythmia. In addition, accelerating the rate of tachycardia by pacing at a faster rate with a catheter in or near the circuit is possible; this is called entrainment.

- *Pace termination:* Pacing at a faster rate (shorter CL) near the circuit can frequently terminate reentrant tachycardias

Note: A heart rate (HR) of 60 beats per minute (bpm) corresponds to a CL of 1000 milliseconds (1 second); thus, CL (in milliseconds) equals 60,000/HR.

Measurements During Electrophysiology Testing Conduction Intervals

The AH interval is defined as the conduction time from the low right atrium through the AVN to the His bundle. It is measured on the His catheter electrogram. The normal range is 50–150 ms. The AH interval varies tremendously, depending on the patient's autonomic tone (Fig. 7.4).

The HV interval is defined as the time from the His bundle deflection to the earliest ventricular signal, measured in any intracardiac or surface recording. It represents the conduction time through the His Purkinje system and is typically 35–55 milliseconds.

Sinus Node Assessment

The sinus node recovery time is measured by pacing the high right atrium at a rate faster than the sinus rate for up to 1 minute and then measuring the interval from the last paced beat to the first sinus beat. The normal range is less than 1,500 milliseconds. The corrected sinus node recovery time is the difference between the sinus node recovery time and the sinus cycle length; the normal value is <550 ms. Patients with sick sinus syndrome have prolonged sinus node recovery times (Figs 7.36–7.42).

AV Node Assessment

The function of the AV node is to control the rate of impulse conduction from the atria to the ventricles. When the atrial rate increases above a certain rate (typically 150–200 bpm), the AV node initially causes AV block in a Wenckebach pattern and then generates higher degrees of block if the atrial rate increases further, thus controlling the ventricular rate and preserving cardiac output (Fig. 7.45).

- Two measurements of AV nodal function are as follows:
  - Wenckebach CL uses decremental pacing to measure the lowest rate (longest CL) at which a dropped ventricular beat occurs
  - The AV nodal effective refractory period (ERP) is measured by introducing a single extrastimulus (S2) after a drive train of 8 stimuli at a fixed rate (all S1), at which time the S1–S2 interval is decreased until the S2 impulse does not conduct to the ventricle. This is noted on the electrogram where an atrial impulse does not result in a His bundle electrogram and subsequently no ventricular stimulation. This interval defines the AV nodal ERP.

Decremental pacing of the ventricle, as previously described for antegrade (A->V) conduction, assesses retrograde (V->A) conduction.

Extrastimulus pacing in the ventricle, in a method similar to that previously described for the AV node, measures ventricular refractory periods. The ventricular ERP is defined as the longest S1–S2 interval in which S2 fails to capture the ventricle.

His-Purkinje System Assessment

Conduction through the His-Purkinje system and determination of refractory period can provide important information regarding conduction system disease and a need for a permanent pacemaker. The latter is especially important if infra-Hisian block is observed.

Induction of Arrhythmias

Most arrhythmias encountered during EP testing are reentrant in nature and are therefore amenable to induction by the methods of extrastimuli (Fig. 7.44).

A reentrant arrhythmia requires a circuit with different limbs that have different refractory periods. When conduction blocks in one limb, the electrical impulse may travel down the other limb and then return (reenter) via the limb that was blocked. For example, in typical AV nodal reentrant tachycardia (AVNRT), the impulse initially blocks in the fast pathway, conducts antegrade (A->V) over the slow pathway, and is then able to enter retrograde (V->A) over the fast pathway, which has recovered conduction. When the impulse continues to travel around this circuit, a reentrant arrhythmia is generated, yielding a supraventricular tachycardia.

Other examples of reentrant tachycardias are: (1) AV reentrant tachycardia (AVRT), in which antegrade conduction over the AV node and retrograde conduction over a bypass tract occur; (2) atrial flutter, which is a reentrant circuit, usually in the right atrium and (3) scar-related ventricular tachycardia of coronary artery disease, in which the impulse travels through or around the area of scar tissue.

A typical stimulation protocol for induction of reentrant arrhythmias uses a drive train of 8 paced beats (S1 beats) at a fixed CL (e.g. 500 milliseconds) with a premature beat (S2) added to the end of the drive train. The S2 stimulus is brought into atrial or ventricular refractoriness in intervals of 10 milliseconds. When S2 no longer captures, this defines the ERP of the tissue. A second extrastimulus, S3, is then added, with S2 set at a coupling interval 20 milliseconds above the ERP. The S2–S3 interval is also decremented until refractoriness is reached. If no arrhythmia is induced, the pacing sequences may be repeated using a third extrastimulus, i.e. S4.

By convention, drive CLs (S1) of 500 and 400 milliseconds are used in ventricular pacing protocols. Arrhythmias with a reentrant mechanism are most often induced with this method.

Another type of pacing sequence is the continuous (or straight) burst pacing sequence, in which the atrium or ventricle is paced at a fixed rate (S1) for up to 10 seconds. In arrhythmias that have mechanisms other than reentry, this method is more likely to induce such triggered activity In addition, burst pacing at a rate faster than the arrhythmia CL often terminates reentrant arrhythmias.

Termination of Arrhythmias (Figs 7.58 and 7.59)

Programmed stimulation can also be used to terminate reentrant cardiac arrhythmias. In ventricular tachycardia, pacing at a rate faster than the tachycardia rate (overdrive pacing) can capture part of the tissue in the circuit and render it refractory, thus terminating the tachycardia. This is used clinically in the methods of overdrive pacing or antitachycardia pacing used in implantable cardioverter-defibrillator (ICD) devices.

Overdrive pacing in the right atrium can terminate atrial flutter, and either atrial or ventricular pacing can terminate AVNRT and AVRT. Pacing methods are not successful in treatment of atrial or ventricular fibrillation because these arrhythmias comprise multiple small reentrant circuits or breakdown of spiral waves.

COMPLICATIONS AFTER CATHETER ABLATION

Radiation risk in catheter ablation is low, but it may exceed the risk from common radiologic procedures. The average risk for genetic defects has been computed at 1 case per million births. The average risk for fatal malignancies ranges from 0.3–2.3 deaths per 1,000 cases for every 60 minutes of fluoroscopy. Many ablation procedures require less than 60 minutes of fluoroscopy.

Major complications occur in approximately 3% of patients who have ablation procedures including thromboembolism in less than 1% (higher in some atrial fibrillation ablation series) and death in 0.1–0.2% of all procedures. The incidence of cardiac complications varies, based on the site and type of ablation. Cardiac complications include the following:
- High-grade AV block
- Cardiac tamponade (highest in atrial fibrillation ablation, up to 6%)
- Coronary artery spasm/thrombosis
- Pericarditis
- Valve trauma.

Vascular complications, which occur in approximately 2–4% of procedures, include the following:
- Retroperitoneal bleeding
- Hematoma
- Vascular injury
- Transient ischemic attack/stroke
- Hypotension
- Thromboembolism or air embolism.

Pulmonary complications include the following:
- Pulmonary hypertension with and without hemoptysis (secondary to pulmonary vein stenosis)
- Pneumothorax.

Miscellaneous complications include the following:
- Left atrial-esophageal fistula
- Acute pyloric spasm/gastric hypomotility
- Phrenic nerve paralysis
- Radiation or electrically induced skin damage
- Infection at access site
- Inappropriate sinus tachycardia
- Proarrhythmia.

Long-term Monitoring

Some physicians empirically treat patients with 4–12 weeks of aspirin therapy to possibly reduce the risk of thromboembolic sequelae.

Echocardiography is not routinely performed unless a complication may have occurred (e.g. pericardial effusion). Postprocedure electrophysiologic testing is not performed routinely unless recurrent tachyarrhythmias are suspected.

SURGICAL INTERVENTIONS IN THE MANAGEMENT OF CARDIAC ARRHYTHMIAS

Maze Procedure (Surgical Ablation)

The surgical ablation maze procedure, or Cox Maze IV, evolved from the Cox Maze III cut-and-sew procedure. Instead of using incisions, a surgical ablation energy source is used to create a conduction block of scar tissue to stop the errant electrical signals. The surgical ablation version of the maze procedure is much faster than Cox Maze III and is considered very effective.

As an open-chest procedure, it is usually performed on patients needing open-heart surgery for other issues, such as valve replacement or repair or coronary artery bypass (CABG). This is called "concomitant surgery", meaning that it is done along with another procedure. It is performed on either a stopped or a beating heart.

Maze Surgical Ablation (Open Chest)

While this open-chest maze surgery is sometimes done as a standalone procedure on patients with atrial fibrillation only, more often these afib-only cases are handled by the closed chest mini-maze procedure.

Maze Procedure Success Rates

The open-chest maze procedures done by surgical ablation have been found to have similar success rates to Cox Maze III procedures, including those utilizing a variety of surgical ablation energy sources.

Many centers doing this maze surgery also cite freedom from stroke in excess of 99%.

Mini-Maze Procedure Risks

The blood clots and strokes that are occasional complications with catheter ablation are rarely found in the mini-maze procedure as no catheters are involved. And since the surgeon uses a thoracoscope to see the heart directly, there may be less risk of obstructing the pulmonary veins (pulmonary vein stenosis).

However, any procedure dealing with the heart has risks. While we rarely see any of the following, the risks of a mini-maze procedure do include:
- Collapsed lung from deflating the lung in surgery, which is correctable with a chest tube
- Vein inflammation (phlebitis)
- Heart tissue inflammation (pericarditis)
- Blood vessel or heart damage
- Death.

In most studies reviewed, there are minimal complications, though in one study there was one death very early on due to tearing of the left atrial appendage.

Research has also shown that there is some risk of blood clots and a stroke following surgery if the left atrial apendage.

ABNORMAL HEART RHYTHMS AND IMPLANTABLE CARDIOVERTER DEFIBRILLATORS (ICD)

Treatment for abnormal heart rhythms is possible with an ICD, or implantable cardioverter defibrillator. An ICD is an electronic device that constantly monitors your heart rate and rhythm. When it detects a very fast, abnormal heart rhythm, it delivers energy to the heart muscle. This causes the heart to beat in a normal rhythm again.

The ICD has two parts: The lead(s) and a pulse generator. The lead(s) monitor the heart rhythm and deliver energy used for pacing and/or defibrillation (see below for definitions). The generator houses the battery and a tiny computer. Energy is stored in the battery until it is needed. The computer receives information from the leads to determine how well the heart is beating (Figs 7.74–7.76).

Types of ICDs, including

- Single chamber ICD: A lead is attached in the right ventricle. If needed, energy is delivered to the ventricle to help it contract normally.
- Dual chamber ICD: Leads are attached in the right atrium and the right ventricle. Energy is delivered first to the right atrium and then to the right ventricle, helping your heart to beat in a normal sequence.
- Biventricular ICD: Leads are attached in the right atrium, the right ventricle and the left ventricle. This technique helps the heart beat in a more balanced way and is specifically used for patients with heart failure.

Your doctor will determine which type of ICD is best for you.

How Does an ICD Work?

The ICD monitors the heart rhythm, identifies abnormal heart rhythms, and determines the appropriate therapy to

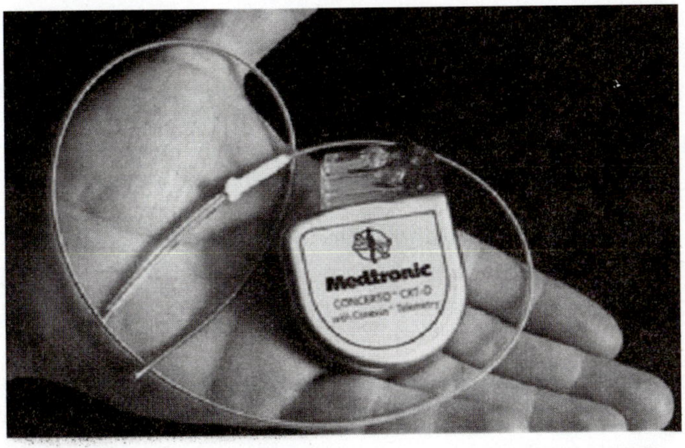

Fig. 7.74: *An implantable cardioverter-defibrillator (ICD)*

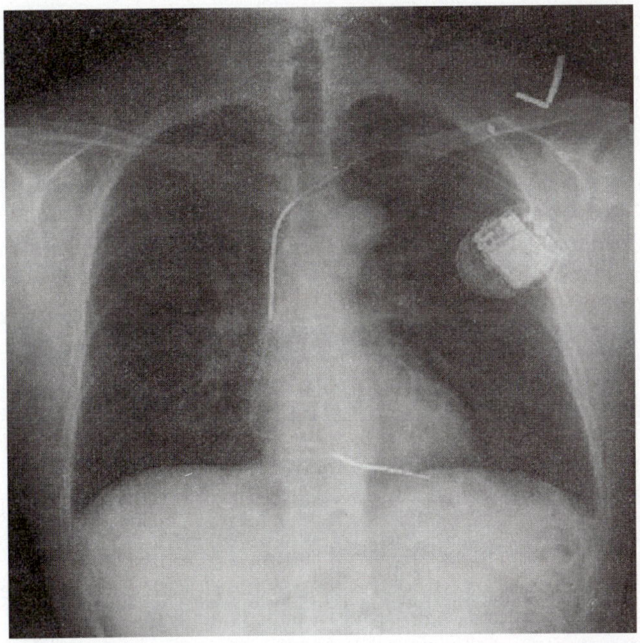

Fig. 7.75: *Chest X-ray showing an implantable cardioverter-defibrillator (ICD), with its battery fixed at left subclavicular region and is connected with a wire placed in the trabecular part of the right ventricular apex*

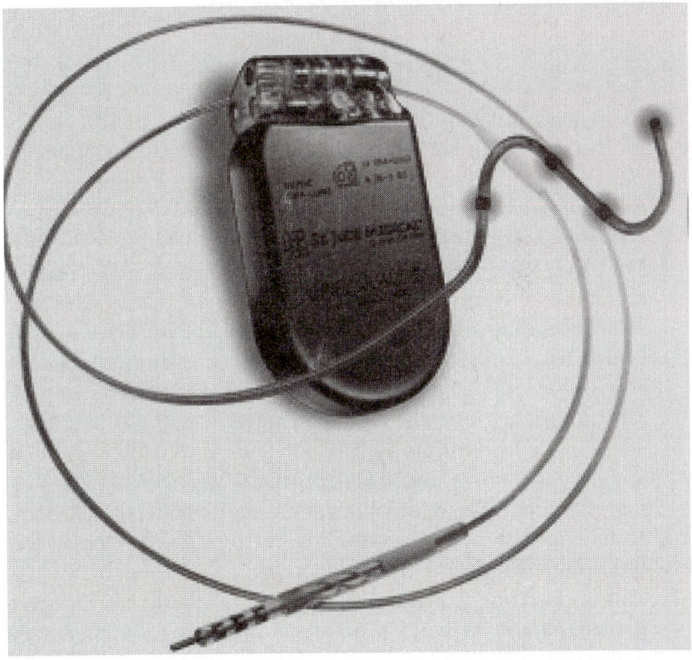

Fig. 7.76: *The ENERGEN cardiac resynchronization therapy defibrillator (CRT-D) and implantable cardioverter defibrillator (ICD) is used to treat heart failure and sudden cardiac death. The system is designed to simplify and reduce the time needed for the implant procedure by combining three separate lead terminals into one integrated connector and reducing the number of connections and set screws needed in the device header. In addition, some patients will receive a remote monitoring system where an at-home communicator will allow physicians to monitor the patient's device, as well as vital signs such as blood pressure and weight, in order to better manage this complex disease*

return your heartbeat to a normal rhythm. Your doctor programs the ICD to include one or all of the following functions:

- *Antitachycardia pacing (ATP):* When the heart beats too fast, a series of small electrical impulses are delivered to the heart muscle to restore a normal heart rate and rhythm.
- *Cardioversion:* A low energy shock is delivered at the same time as your heartbeat to restore a normal heart rhythm.
- *Defibrillation:* When the heart is beating dangerously fast, a high-energy shock is delivered to the heart muscle to restore a normal rhythm.
- *Bradycardia pacing:* When the heart beats too slow, small electrical impulses stimulate the heart muscle to maintain a suitable heart rate.

Who is a Candidate for an ICD?

- People who have had an episode of sudden cardiac arrest or ventricular fibrillation.
- People who have had a heart attack and are at high risk for sudden cardiac arrest.
- People who have hypertrophic cardiomyopathy and are at high risk for sudden arrest.
- People who have had at least one episode of ventricular tachycardia, an abnormal heart rhythm.

BIBLIOGRAPHY

1. Blomström-Lundqvist C, Scheinman MM, Aliot EM, et al., for the European Society of Cardiology Committee, NASPE-Heart Rhythm Society. ACC/AHA/ESC guidelines for the management of patients with supraventricular arrhythmias-executive summary. J Am Coll Cardiol. 2003;42(8):1493–1531.
2. Man KC, Knight B, Tse HF, et al. Radiofrequency catheter ablation of inappropriate sinus tachycardia guided by activation mapping. J Am Coll Cardiol. 2000;35(2):451–457.
3. Walsh EP, Saul JP, Hulse JE, et al. Transcatheter ablation of ectopic atrial tachycardia in young patients using radiofrequency current. Circulation. 1992;86(4):1138–1146.
4. Scheinman M, Calkins H, Gillette P, et al. North American Society of Pacing and Electrophysiology. NASPE policy statement on catheter ablation: personnel, policy, procedures, and therapeutic recommendations. Pacing Clin Electrophysiol. 2003;26(3):789–799.
5. Calkins H, Yong P, Miller JM, et al., for the Atakr Multicenter Investigators Group. Catheter ablation of accessory pathways, atrioventricular nodal reentrant tachycardia, and the atrioventricular junction: final results of a prospective, multicenter clinical trial. Circulation. 1999;99(2):262–270.
6. Scheinman MM. NASPE survey on catheter ablation. Pacing Clin Electrophysiol. 1995;18(8):1474-1478.
7. Langberg JJ, Leon A, Borganelli M, et al. A randomized, prospective comparison of anterior and posterior approaches to radiofrequency catheter ablation of atrioventricular nodal reentry tachycardia. Circulation. 1993;87(5):1551–1556.
8. Calkins H, Langberg J, Sousa J, et al. Radiofrequency catheter ablation of accessory atrioventricular connections in 250 patients. Abbreviated therapeutic approach to Wolff-Parkinson-White syndrome. Circulation. 1992;85(4):1337–1346.
9. Calkins H, Sousa J, el-Atassi R, et al. Diagnosis and cure of the Wolff-Parkinson-White syndrome or paroxysmal supraventricular tachycardias during a single electrophysiologic test. N Engl J Med. 1991;324(23):1612–1618.
10. Jackman WM, Wang XZ, Friday KJ, et al. Catheter ablation of accessory atrioventricular pathways (Wolff-Parkinson-White syndrome) by radio-frequency current. N Engl J Med. 1991;324(23):1605–1611.
11. Kuck KH, Schlüter M, Geiger M, Siebels J, Duckeck W. Radiofrequency current catheter ablation of accessory atrioventricular pathways. Lancet. 1991;337(8757):1557–1561.
12. Lesh MD, Van Hare GF, Scheinman MM, Ports TA, Epstein LA. Comparison of the retrograde and transseptal methods for ablation of left free wall accessory pathways. J Am Coll Cardiol. 1993;22(2):542–549.
13. Hindricks G. The multicentre European radiofrequency survey (MERFS): Complications of radiofrequency catheter ablation of arrhythmias. The Multicentre European Radiofrequency Survey (MERFS) Investigators of The Working Group on Arrhythmias of the European Society of Cardiology. Eur Heart J. 1993;14(12):1644-1653.
14. Chen SA, Chiang CE, Wu TJ, et al. Radiofrequency catheter ablation of common atrial flutter: comparison of electrophysiologically guided focal ablation technique and linear ablation technique. J Am Coll Cardiol. 1996;27(4):860–868.
15. Kottkamp H, Hügl B, Krauss B, et al. Electromagnetic versus fluoroscopic mapping of the inferior isthmus for ablation of typical atrial flutter: A prospective randomized study. Circulation. 2000;102(17):2082–2086.
16. Willems S, Weiss C, Ventura R, et al. Catheter ablation of atrial flutter guided by electroanatomic mapping (CARTO): a randomized comparison to the conventional approach. J Cardiovasc Electrophysiol. 2000;11(11):1223–1230.
17. Tsai CF, Tai CT, Yu WC, et al. Is 8 mm more effective than 4 mm tip electrode catheter for ablation of typical atrial flutter? Circulation. 1999;100(7):768–771.
18. Paydak H, Kall JG, Burke MC, et al. Atrial fibrillation after radiofrequency ablation of type I atrial flutter: time to onset, determinants, and clinical course. Circulation. 1998;98(4):315–322.
19. Pérez FJ, Schubert CM, Parvez B, Pathak V, Ellenbogen KA, Wood MA. Long-term outcomes after catheter ablation of cavotricuspid isthmus dependent atrial flutter: a meta-analysis. Circ Arrhythmia Electrophysiol. 2009;2(4):393–401.
20. Calkins H, Canby R, Weiss R, et al., for the 100W Atakr II Investigator Group. Results of catheter ablation of typical atrial flutter. Am J Cardiol. 2004;94(4):437–442.

8 Stress Testing in Children and Adolescents

Exercise testing has a definite role in pediatrics today. Different methods are presented, and the value of maximal exercise, with determination of oxygen uptake and blood lactate, is stressed (Figs 8.1 and 8.2).

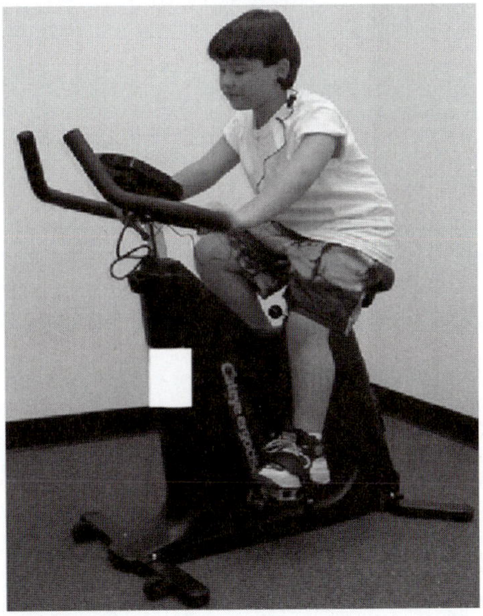

Fig. 8.1: *Pediatric ergometer is suited for exercise stress testing in children*

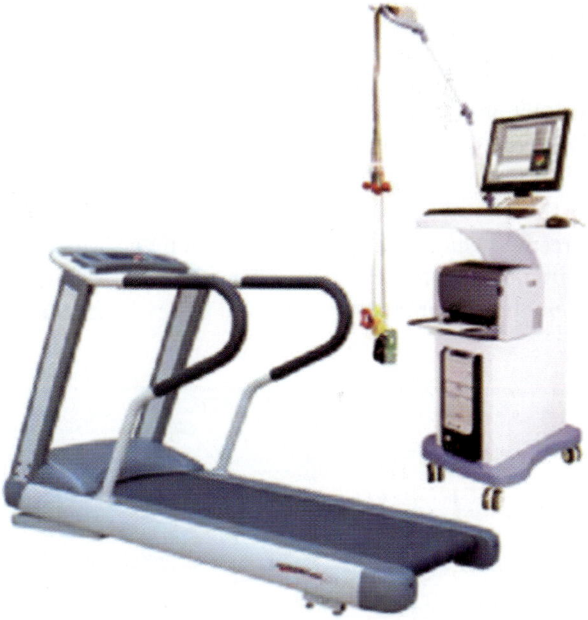

Fig. 8.2: *Morphological features of treadmill machine along with monitor and recording/printing equipment kept over a specially designed trolley*

In children with heart disease, exercise testing, with precordial electrocardiogram, can have both diagnostic and prognostic value. The cardiovascular function, at different intensities of exercise, is evaluated. Serious dysrhythmias may be revealed, hypertension judged, and the effect of drug therapy can be checked by exercise testing. It is an important way for assessing the child's functional capacity, after heart surgery, for deciding whether she or he should take part in physical education and sports activities, and also for choosing a profession. It is also of great psychological value to the parents and the patient himself.

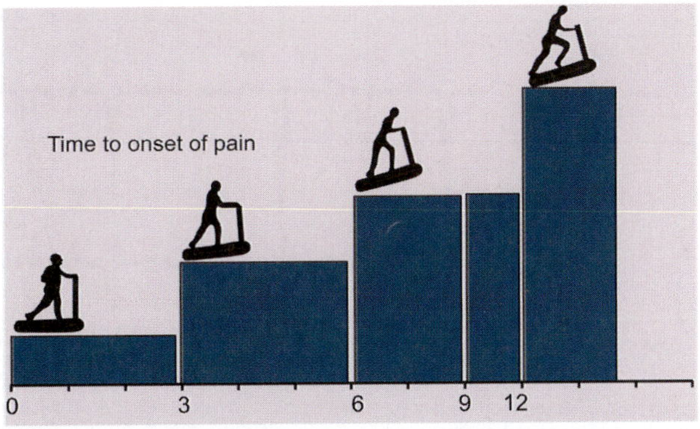

Fig. 8.3: *The various stages and duration of perfonning TMT*

Box 8.1: *Pediatric testing: Exercise testing in children and adolescents*

Class I (Tables 8.1–8.6)

1. Evaluation of exercise capacity in children or adolescents with congenital heart disease, those who have had surgery for congenital heart disease, and children who have acquired valvular or myocardial disease.
2. Evaluation of the rare child with a description of anginal chest pain.
3. Assessment of the response of an artificial pacing system to exertion.
4. Evaluation of exercise-related symptoms in young athletes.

Class IIa

1. Evaluation of the adequacy of the response to medical, surgical, or radiofrequency ablation treatment for children with a tachyarrhythmia that was found during exercise testing before therapy.
2. As an adjunct in assessment of the severity of congenital or acquired valvular lesions, especially aortic valve stenosis.
3. Evaluation of the rhythm during exercise in patients with known or suspected exercise-induced arrhythmia.

Class IIb

1. As a component of the evaluation of children or adolescents who have a family history of unexplained sudden death related to exercise in young persons.
2. Follow-up of cardiac abnormalities with possible late coronary involvement such as Kawasaki disease and systemic lupus erythematosus.
3. Assessment of ventricular rate response and development of ventricular arrhythmia in children and adolescents with congenital complete atrioventricular block.
4. Quantitation of the heart-rate response to exercise in children and adolescents treated with β-blocker therapy to estimate the adequacy of β-blockade.
5. Measurement of response of shortening or prolongation of the corrected QT interval to exercise as an adjunct in the diagnosis of hereditary syndromes of prolongation of the QT interval.
6. Evaluation of blood pressure response and/or arm-to-leg gradient after repair of coarctation of the aorta.
7. Assessment of degree of desaturation with exercise in patients with relatively well-balanced or palliated cyanotic congenital cardiac defects.

Class III

1. Screening before athletic participation by healthy children and adolescents.
2. Routine use of exercise testing for evaluating the usual nonanginal chest pain common in children and adolescents.
3. Evaluation of premature atrial and ventricular contractions in otherwise healthy children and adolescents.

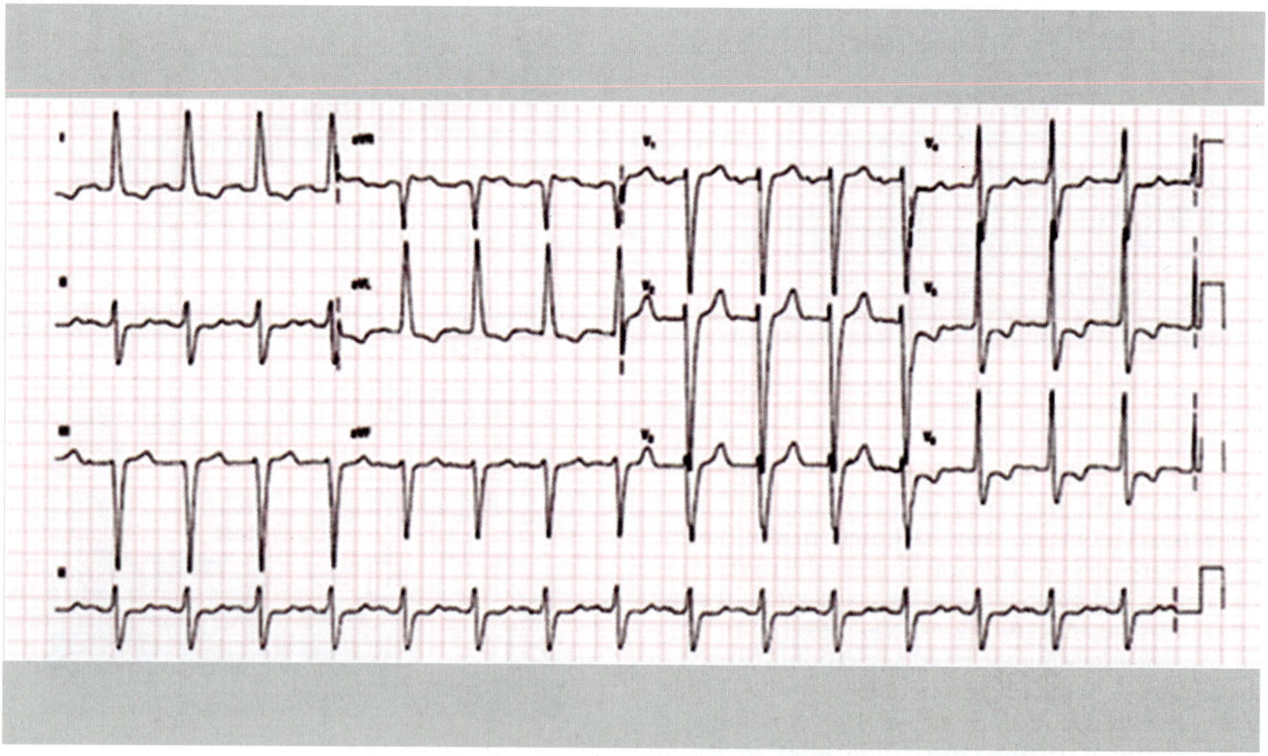

Fig. 8.4A: *ECG showing normal trace*

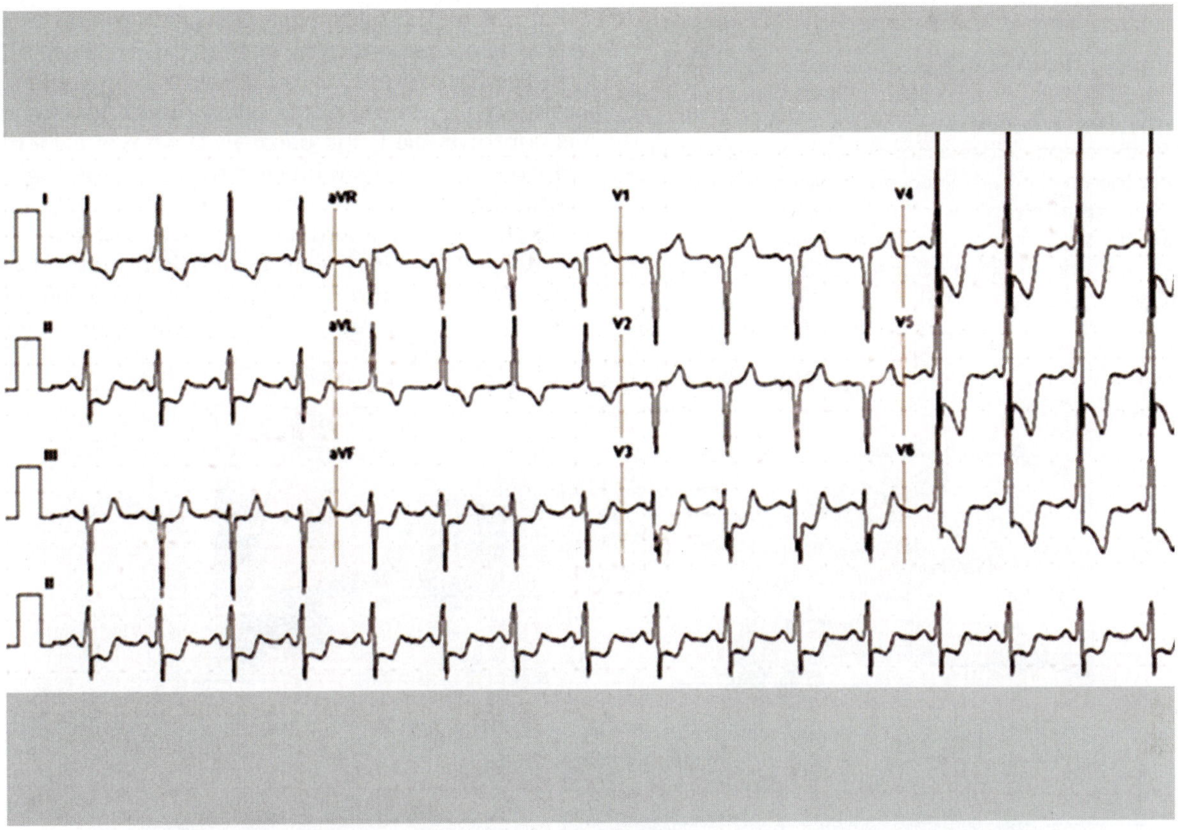

Fig. 8.4B: *Down sloping ST depression of more than 2.0 mm in a stress test*

Table 8.1: *Table exercise protocols for treadmill test*

Routine diagnostic[a]				*Rehabilitation*[b]		
Stage	*Time (Min.)*	*Speed (m.p.h.) %*	*Grade (m.p.h.) %*	*Stage*	*Speed*	*Grade*
I	3	1.7	10	1	1.7	0
2	3	2.5	12	2	2.0	0
3	3	3.4	14	3	2.0	3.75
4	3	4.2	16	4	2.0	3.75
5	3	5.0	18	5	3.0	5.0
6	3	5.5	20	6	3.0	7.5
7	**3**	**6.0**	**22**	7	**3.0**	**10.0**

[a]Exercise for 3 minutes, in each stage, with no rest period in between.
[b]Exercise for 3 minutes, in each stage, followed by resting 1 minute before the next stage.

In children with other chronic diseases, e.g. diabetes, obesity, asthma, neurocirculatory dysfunctions, physical training, together with exercise testing, is for therapy and rehabilitation importance.

Chest pain is the most frequent complaint of ischemic heart disease (IHD). When this symptom is considered as a classical picture of angina, the diagnosis of ischemic heart disease can be made without much difficulty. However, the chest pain may be of atypical variety, location, radiation and factors which aggravate, the discomfort and its response to nitro-glycerin. In this situation, ECG is the most commonly utilized and readily available method of

Table 8.2: *Indications for pediatric stress testing*

1. Evaluate specific signs or symptoms that are induced or aggravated by exercise (Figs 8.26, 8.31 and 8.32)
2. Assess or identify abnormal responses to exercise in children with cardiac, pulmonary, or other organ disorders including the presence of myocardial ischemia and arrhythmias
3. Assess efficacy of specific medical or surgical treatments
4. Assess functional capacity for recreational, athletic, and vocational activities (Fig. 8.34)
5. Evaluate prognosis including both baseline and serial testing measurements
6. Establish baseline data for institution of cardiac, pulmonary, or musculoskeletal rehabilitation

Table 8.3: *Indications for exercise testing in adolescents*

The following are the major indications for exercise stress testing:

1. To aid in the diagnosis of chest pain
2. To evaluate the prognostic severity of coronary heart disease
3. To evaluate therapy of known coronary heart disease
4. To guide rehabilitation following myocardial infarction
5. To evaluate the benefit of surgical procedures
6. To provide a safety check up prior to fitness programme
7. To screen high-risk professionals
8. To assess, in part, the risk factor in asymptomatic persons

diagnosing IHD. The basal ECG may not be that specific as it may be totally normal, even in the presence of significant obstructive atherosclerotic disease of coronary arteries. It is known that only if 80% of the lumen of coronary arteries is compromised, the basal ECG shows ischemic change. However, patients with significant narrowing (50–70%) of coronary arteries may have normal basal ECG, but show ischemic change when subjected to stress. Thus, stress testing of the heart is an established method of detecting the latent or manifest disparity between the demand and the supply of oxygen to the myocardium.

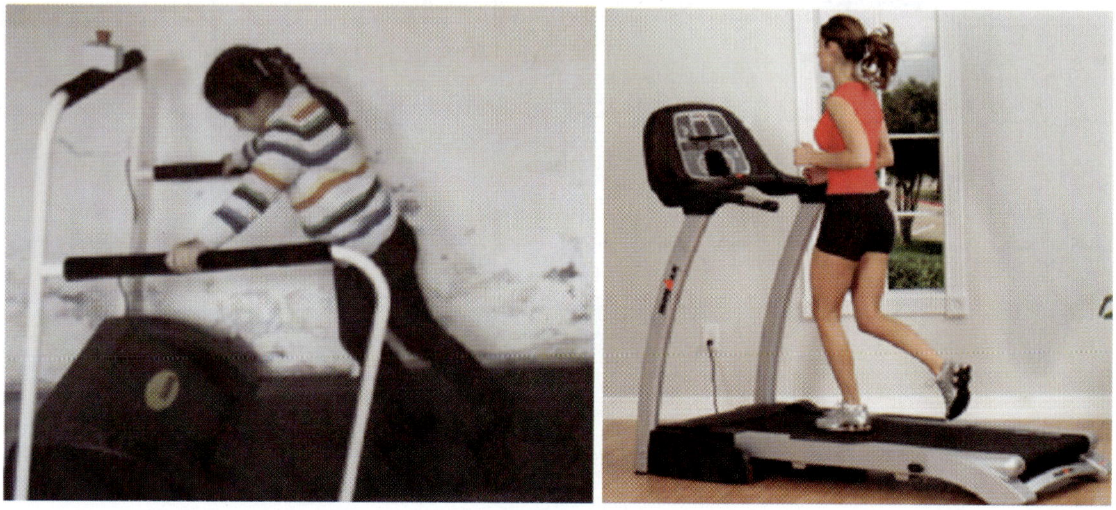

Fig. 8.5: *Left and right panels children are practicing on treadmill prior to undertake exercise stress testing*

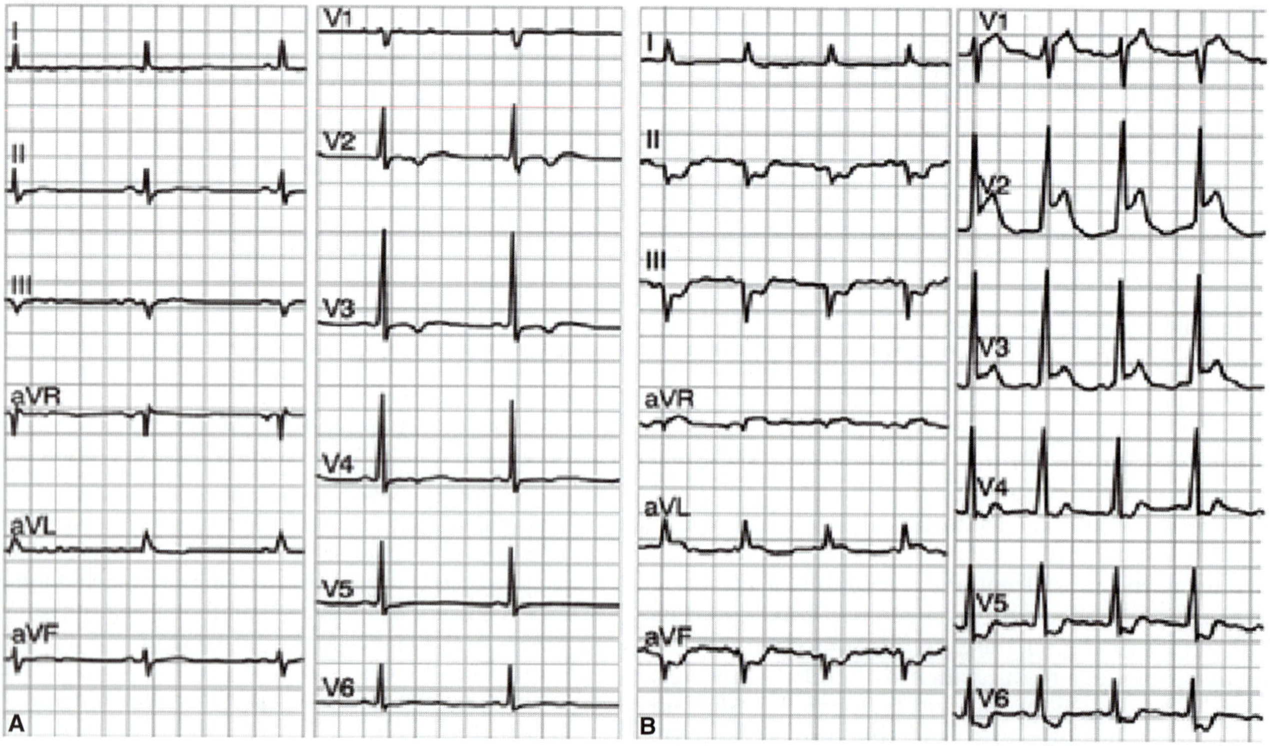

Fig. 8.6: *ECG on admission showing mild T-wave inversion in the precordial leads (A). ECG tracing during exercise stress test at maximal workload demonstrating left-axis deviation and pronounced ST segment elevation in the precordial leads (5 mm in V2) (B)*

TECHNIQUES

The stress testing could be carried out by several methods:

1. *Physical stress testing:*
   (i) Master's two step test
   (ii) Bicycle ergometry
   (iii) Multistage Treadmill test.
2. *Rapid atrial pacing*
3. *Esophageal pill atrial pacing*
4. Exposure to hypoxia.

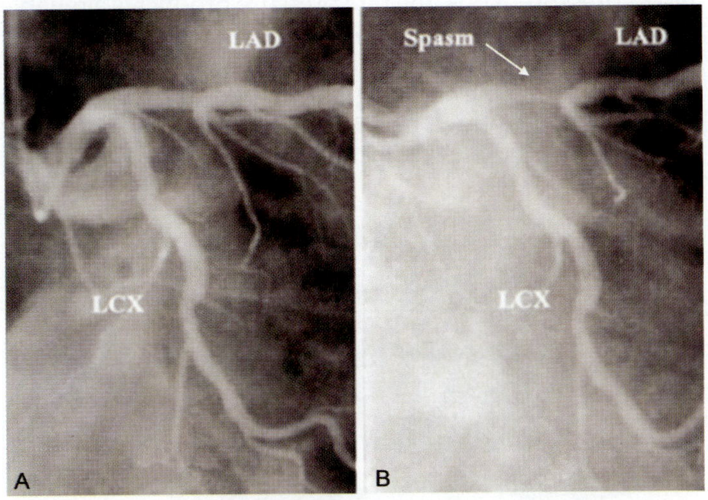

Fig. 8.7: *Angiographic images of the left coronary artery (right anterior oblique) demonstrating a nonsignificantly diseased proximal LAD (A) developing a spontaneous sustained spasm (B)*

Information obtained from noninvasive stress testing:

1. **Physical capacity**
   (i) Symptoms which limit exercise testing
   (ii) Maximum tolerated workload
   (iii) Measured or estimated maximum oxygen uptake.
2. **Hemodynamic adaptation**
   (i) Heart rate response
   (ii) Blood pressure response
   (iii) Ventricular function (any stress-induced decompensation).
3. **Myocardial ischemia:**
   (i) Development of angina during stress test
   (ii) ECG changes (ST-T changes)
   (iii) Thallium scintigraphy.
4. **LV dysfunction**:
   (i) Insufficient (less than 10 mmHg) increase in systolic BP or decrease in systolic BP from the basal level.
   (ii) ECG changes (unchanged or increased R-wave voltage).
   (iii) Blood pool scintigraphy (reduction of ejection fraction).
   (iv) Arrhythmia and conduction defect.
   (v) Development of S3 gallops, MR and other features of papillary muscle dysfunction.

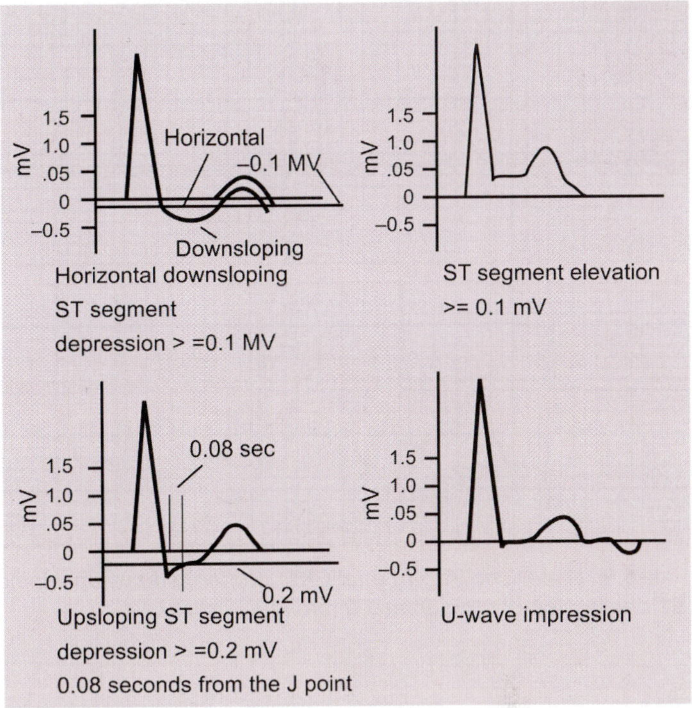

Fig. 8.8: *Clinical significance of ST variations and appearance of U-wave in exercise stress testing*

PHYSIOLOGY OF STRESS TESTING

Like any instrument or machine, human heart and blood vessels can also be subjected to stress testing in order to evaluate the functional reserve. It is known that the disease process may have compromised to a greater extent the cardiac function, yet the circulatory reserves are pumped into action whenever challenged by stress. Therefore, an advanced degree of coronary arterial disease may still exist without obvious myocardial ischemia, owing to remarkable physical flow properties of the fluid. Exercise is, thus, the safest and the most easily available means of stimulating the myocardium to demand maximum or near maximum blood flow, and is the only means of creating such a rigorous demand for oxygen delivery, that even moderate impairment of coronary blood flow capacity becomes obvious. Cardiac output (CO) may rise from 5 to 25 liters per minute during exercise. In spite of vasodilatation, in skeletal muscular bed to accommodate this increased flow, the mean arterial pressure tends to rise; pressure increases of 50% are typical during maximum exercise, along with corresponding increase in contractile force of myocardial fibers, which is a major determinant of myocardial oxygen consumption (MVO_2).

The increase in cardiac output is indicated mainly by increase in heart rate; stroke volume shows only a slight increase. With increasing heart rate, the duration of systolic ejection per beat diminishes, and the normal systolic emptying, in shorter period, is achieved by increased rate of tension development in myocardial fibers. This increases oxygen consumption with each contraction. The heart rate increases proportionately to the workload and enhances

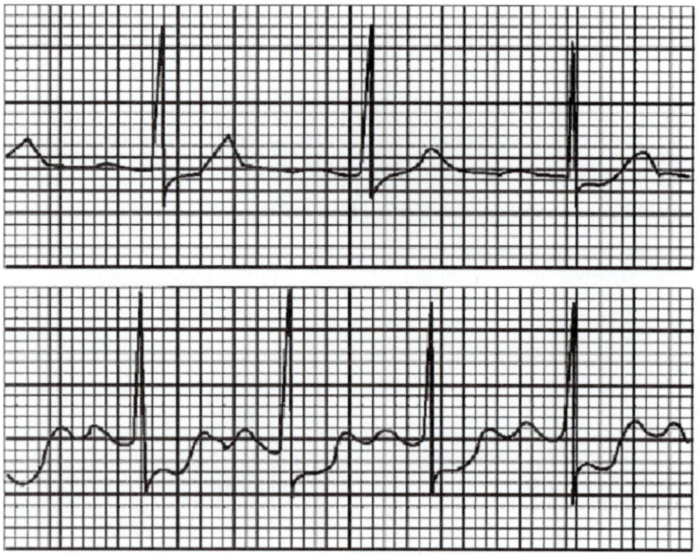

Fig. 8.9: *Upper showing normal EKG. Bottom shows upsloping ST depression of more than 2.0 mm in a stress test*

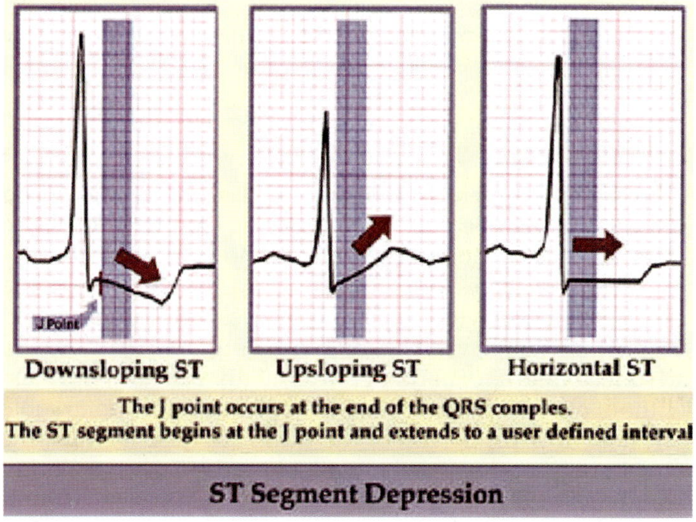

Fig. 8.10: *Left showing downsloping, middle showing upsloping and right showing horizontal ST segment responses during exercise stress testing*

Table 8.4: *Baseline ECG changes that may obscure exercise stress test results*

- ST segment chages (=1 mm) depression or elevation
- Ventricular strain patterns
- Right ventricular hypertrophy
- Left ventricular hypertrophy
- T-wave changes
- Inversion—secondary to strain or old injury
- Conduction abnormalities
- Left bundle-branch block: ST segment and T-wave changes
- Right bundle branch block: ST-segment and T-wave changes (in V1, V2 and V3 leads only)
- Prolonged QT interval

the metabolic requirement for oxygen. At the functional level of aerobic capacity, the heart rate reaches the maximum, which varies inversely with age. MVO_2 which is mainly determined by tension, developed by myofibrils, and the inotropic state is increased greatly by exercise. MVO_2 per minute, a function of heart rate, increases in proportion to the intensity of exercise.

Increase in heart rate accounts for the greatest increase in coronary blood flow, during exercise, in subjects with normal blood pressure. The MVO_2 can be indirectly calculated by the product of the heart rate and the systolic blood pressure. Thus, the rate pressure product is a reliable index of myocardial perfusion requirement in patients with IHD as well as in healthy individuals. It is known that patients with stable angina get chest pain at a reproducible rate-pressure product. In vigorous exercise, the MVO_2 per contraction, increases from $1.2 + 10^3$ mL/100 gm to about

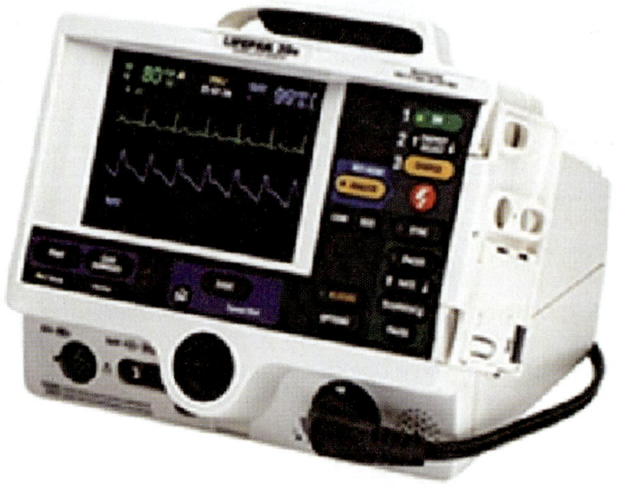

Fig. 8.11: *Viewing features of defibrillator which depicts large and vivid display with three waveforms with ECG and SPO_2 and synchronized cardioversion and AED with biphasic technology*

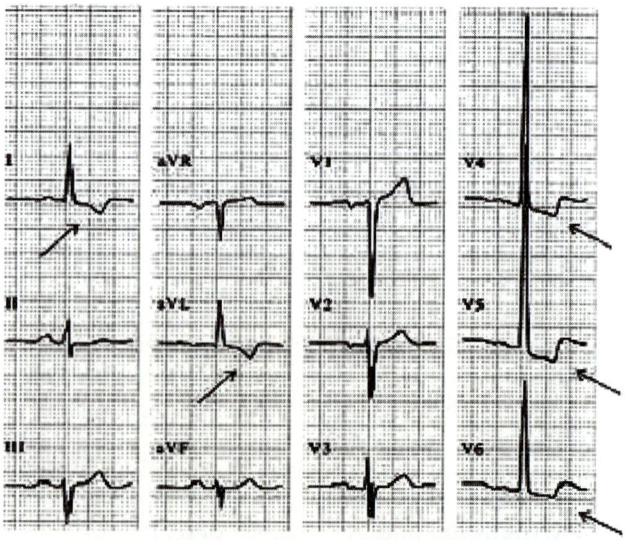

Fig. 8.12: *Showing J-point displacement and ST segment slope in positive exercise test (arrows)*

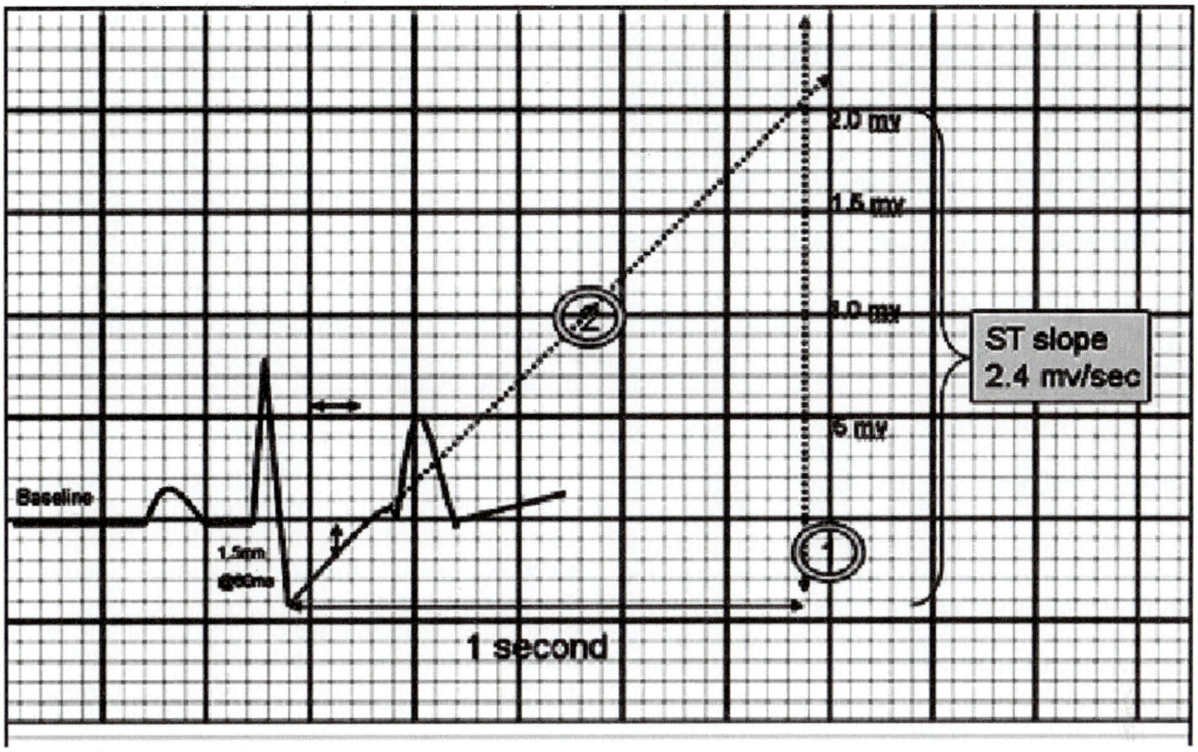

Fig. 8.13: *Rapidly upsloping ST segment: a benign response. Upsloping ST segment with 1.5 mm ST depression at 80 ms after J-point and a upslope reaching 2,4 mv at one second. Line 1 draw a perpendicular line 1 second (5 large squares) after J-point Line 2 connect the ST segment along its inclination to intersect line 1*

1.9 + 10^3 mL/100 gm/per beat. To allow this increased oxygen supply, coronary blood flow (CBF) increases from 60 mL/100 gm, at rest, to about 240 mL/100 gm during vigorous aerobic exercise. This increase in CBF is not possible if there is significant obstructive disease of the main coronary arteries, leading to the development of ischemic areas. Exercise testing is based on the premise that exercise-inducted ischemia is used as diagnostic tool.

There are different types of exercise tests that may be performed, depending on the questions that need to be answered. Exercise tests usually are performed on a stationary bicycle or a treadmill. The equipment is selected and adjusted to meet the individual needs of each patient. During the exercise test, the resistance pedaling or the speed and elevation of the treadmill are gradually increased until the patient can no longer comfortably keep up with the machine. Patients usually exercise for about 10–15 minutes, and are monitored for about 10 minutes before and after exercise.

COMPONENTS OF AN EXERCISE TEST

- ***EKG monitoring:*** All subjects are hooked up to a special exercise-EKG, system to monitor the heart rhythm during exercise and to assess other exercise-related EKG abnormalities that may indicate the presence of a heart problem.
- ***Metabolic measurements:*** By having the patient breathe through a snorkel-like mouthpiece that is connected to a special computer, the air that a patient breathes in and out during exercise can be measured, and a great deal of information can be gathered about response of the heart and lungs to exercise.
- ***Blood pressure measurements:*** Blood pressure cuffs are used to monitor a patient's blood pressure before during and after exercise.
- ***Pulse oximetry:*** A pulse oximeter may be attached to a patient's finger to noninvasively measure his/her oxygen saturation before during and after exercise.
- ***Spirometry:*** Simple measurements of a patient's lung function may be performed before and/or after exercise. These measurements are performed simply by having the subject blow through a special mouthpiece that is connected to a computer. The results are used to identify lung problems that might affect a patient's ability to exercise and to see whether exercise has an adverse effect on a patient's lung function, which may occur in patients with conditions such as exercise-induced asthma.
- ***Echocardiographic measurements:*** Sometimes, it is helpful to perform echocardiographic measurements during, or immediately after, exercise to further assess the effect of exercise on a patient's cardiovascular system.

Myocardial perfusion imaging: Patients who are suspected to have, or are at increased risk for, coronary artery problems may have a special dye injected through an IV before and after exercise. Pictures of the heart may then be obtained to help to determine whether the blood flow to any part of the heart is impaired at rest and/or during exercise.

TECHNIQUE

Double master's test: The patient is asked to climb up and down the 9 inch high, 2 step, ladder during a 3 minutes period. The number of steps are fixed according to the age and sex of the patent. The number of steps, acceptable with patients with severe disease, are considered inadequate in patients with mild to moderate disease as the increase in heart rate is, usually, submaximal. Typical target heart rates, in relation to the age of patients are given in Table. 8.6. The maximum predicted heart rate varies among individuals but is reasonably well-predicted by the formula MPHR (220-age) in years.

Bicycle ergometry: The patient is made to ride a bicycle which can be put to increasing load (resistance), and with succeeding increase in the load, is geared to achieve maximal/submaximal heart rate. The disadvantage of this technique is that some patients, specially females, who never rode a cycle before, feel apprehensive and unstable. There is also increased movement during exercise, causing base line shift of the ECG, leading to erroneous results (Fig. 8.1).

Multistage treadmill test: This is the most frequently used method of exercise testing when the patient is made to walk on a platform. The platform is moved backward using an endless loop of the conveyor belt. The speed of walking (MPH) can be increased by control of the motor as also the elevation of the platform (% of gradient). On the basis of various combinations of the speed of walking, elevation of the platform and the duration of each stage, several protocols have been designed which are given below:

(a) Exercise for 3 minutes, in each stage with no rest period in between.
(b) Exercise for 3 minutes, in each stage, followed by resting 1 minute before the next stage.

Echocardiography Equipment

Accurate interpretation of wall motion abnormalities may be optimized by the use of a high-quality ultrasound system equipped with digital archiving and split- or quad-screen displays. This allows for a side-by-side comparison of resting and stress images. In pediatrics, systems with high frame rates, providing better temporal resolution, are optimal because the heart rate will be quite rapid during administration of stress. Additional equipment should include an ECG system equipped with a stress package enabling display and analysis of ST segment trends, blood pressure monitor, and oximeter. If a pharmacological agent is to be employed for stressing or if contrast agents will be administered, intravenous line equipment is necessary (Figs 8.27, 8.28, 8.29, 8.30 and Table 8.11.

Nuclear Myocardial Blood Flow Imaging

There is an increasing awareness of coronary perfusion abnormalities in children. These occur as a result of congenital coronary abnormalities and acquired coronary disease and as a consequence of corrective surgery for various congenital heart defects. The use of rest and stress nuclear myocardial blood flow imaging has increased significantly in the past decade. Most maximal exercise protocols are acceptable for use with myocardial perfusion imaging (see section on exercise protocols). The only additional equipment requirement during an exercise test is the placement of a peripheral intravenous catheter in a nonexercising extremity. Nuclear myocardial blood flow imaging is frequently combined with pharmacological stress testing. This is especially true for younger patients or when imaging is combined with stress echocardiographic imaging. Specific additional equipment requirements for pharmacological stress testing will be discussed in the protocol section.

Spirometry Equipment (Fig. 8.14)

Spirometry is one of the more commonly performed pulmonary function tests. It provides a flow-volume loop and can assess the degree of airflow obstruction within the airways. Use of spirometry in conjunction with stress tests has become more common. This technique should be performed with the use of equipment and techniques that meet standards such as those developed by the American Thoracic Society. Careful calibration, timing of the study, relationship of medication used at the time of the study, understanding of the correct spirometric technique, and maintaining the equipment are all essential components to achieve meaningful results. Although many of the commercially available spirometry systems provide computer algorithms for determining the acceptability of the patient's technique and interpretation of the study, the individual technician should have sufficient training in identifying the quality of the study and troubleshooting an individual test. Although training courses that are approved by the National Institute for Occupational Safety and Health exist, no approved courses exist for pediatric spirometry. Quality control via consultation with a trained pediatric

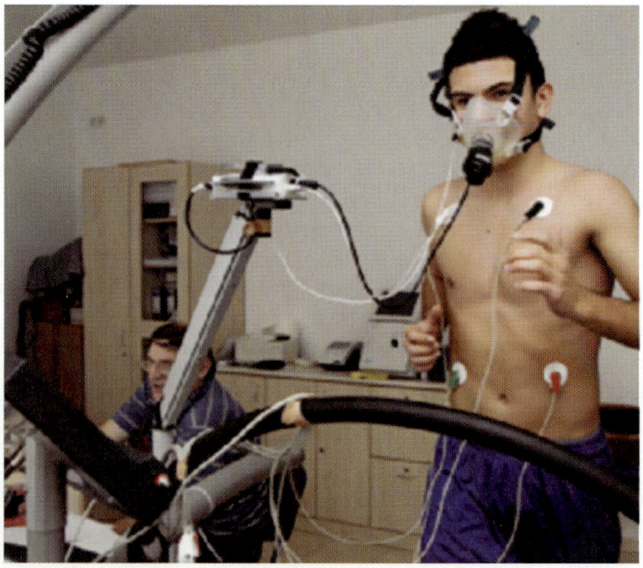

Fig. 8.14: *A adolescent with ASD secondum is performing cardio-pulmonary exercise while sitting on the bycycle ergometer for knowing his degree of cardiac disability*

pulmonary function technician or pediatric pulmonologist should help to optimize the use of spirometry.

Preparation of the Patient

1. The patient is asked to stop all drugs for, at least, 48 hours before the treadmill test. Special care is taken during the withdrawal of beta-blockers as it may cause rebound angina. Hypokalemia (induced by diuretics) and administration of digitalis can cause iatrogenic ST changes, giving false-positive results.
2. Shaving of the entire front of the chest facilitates proper application of electrodes.
3. The patient is asked not to take breakfast tea and coffee, but have a glass of milk 1 hour, before the test.
4. The patient should be accompanied by some near relation.
5. Consent is taken in writing, after explaining the procedure of the test. The patient is familiarized with the setup of the stress laboratory.
6. Skin is rubbed with gauge, soaked in spirit, until it turns red. This removes the superficial most layer of the skin and reduces the electrode-skin interface resistance.
7. Mild erosion of skin with a number 6 spherical dental bur or rubbing with fine sandpaper and scrubbing with acetone a will result in electrodes-skin interface impedance of 1–5 KOhms instead of 10–50 KOhms, present without any kind of skin abrasion.
8. Silver chloride electrodes are the best but stainless steel electrodes are also satisfactory self. Adhesive, disposable electrodes are preferable to reusable electrodes to obtain stable baseline graph without interference.

Lead System

There is no uniform agreement about the number of ECG leads required for optimal exercise electrocardiography. Some investigators have used single bipolar chest lead or a combination of several bipolar chest leads like CMs, CCs' CBs, CSs' CLs', etc. Results may be further improved if 12 or 14 leads are recorded during and after exercise. The positive yield from a single V5-like lead is as low as 60% and may increase to over 90% if 12 conventional leads are recorded. Chaitmen et al. have reported a combination of

it is indicative of more severe IHD as compared to a subject who develops ST change, at peak exercise, or during the recovery phase. The former has very limited coronary reserve and has grave prognosis. Similar significance has

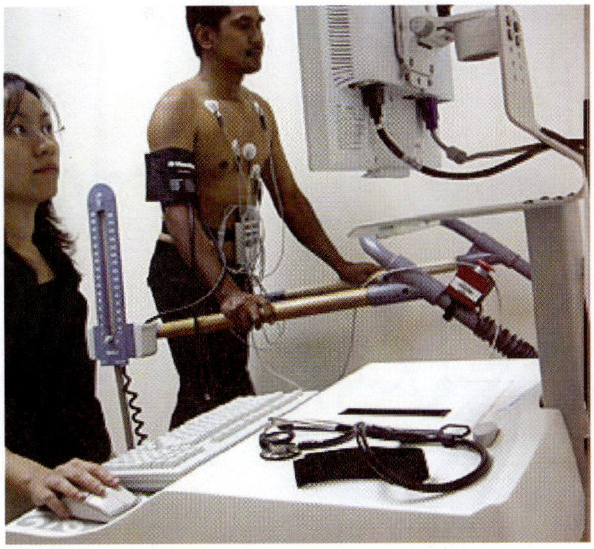

Fig. 8.15: *A subject taking an exercise stress test (front)*

CM5, CC5' CL and V3) leads asan acceptable alternative to the 14 leads system (Fig. 8.15).

Recording Amplifiers

To obtain maximum information from exercise electrocardiography, it is necessary to have records, taken on ECG amplifiers, with an ideal frequency response from DC to 250 Hz, although frequencies up to 100 Hz may also be acceptable. Similarly, an overdamped amplifier may induce artefactual ST changes in an otherwise normal record. Records, obtained on amplifiers, with inadequate frequency response, may be totally misleading.

ST Depression (Figs 8.4B, 8.8, 8.9, 8.10, 8.12, 8.16 and 8.20)

The most important objective evidence of ischemia is the exercise-induced ST segment change. The ST segment is

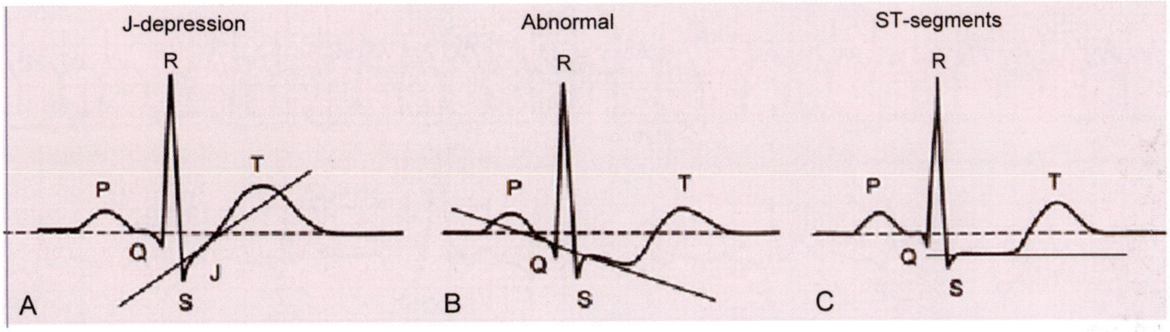

Fig. 8.16: *Showing A, upsloping ST depression/J-point depression (normal variant) B, downsloping ST depression (usually abnormal) C, horizontal ST depression (usually abnormal)*

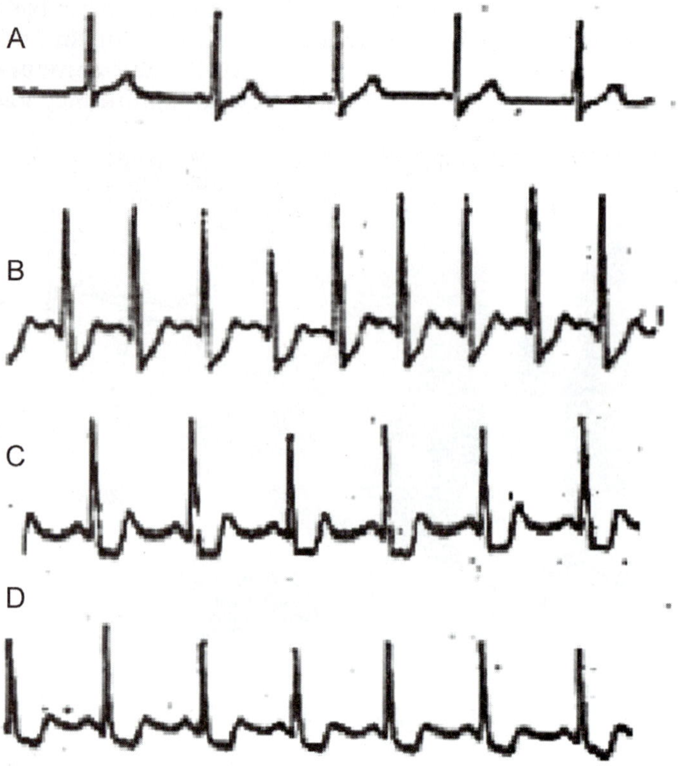

Fig. 8.17: *Typical ischemic response to exercise: (A) Normal or negative response; (B) ST depression of upsloping type 1.5 mm or more 80 msec from J point; (C) Horizontal ST depression of 1 mm or more; (D) Downsloping STdepression. The last two are more pathognomonic of underlying heart disease*

measured at a given interval (60–80 msec) from the J-point, and is compared with the preceding PR segment. Estimation of the ST segment depression, 60 msec from the J point, makes it a more sensitive criterion but considerably less specific (more of false positive). But the ST depression, measured 80 msec from the J-point, is even more important than the degree of its depression. On the basis of time course and configuration, the stress-induced ST segment depression, in symptomatic patients of IHD, has been classified into type lA.

Type IB and type II: By Goldschlarger et al. (1976), using coronary angiographic data, as the evidence of IHD. The type IA response, downsloping ST segment of 1 mm (0.1 mv), during or after the maximal test, and 0.5 mm (0.5 mV), downsloping ST depression, after the submaximal exercise test, is considered to be a positive response for IHD. The type IB response, which is less specific than the type IA, consists of horizontal 1 mm (0.1 mv) and 0.5 mm depression, during the maximal and the submaximal exercises, respectively.

The type II response: An upsloping ST segment depression, is of doubtful significance in the diagnosis of IHD. Many observers consider that slowly upsloping (less than 0.1 mv/sec) ST depression, of 1 mm and/or 1.5 mm, 80 msec from the J-point, may be the only evidence of known IHD, especially when single lead is recorded.

The magnitude of physical work, at which the ECG change appears, is also an important consideration in the interpretation of the ST change. If a subject develops ST segment depression, at nominal work load (stages I and II),

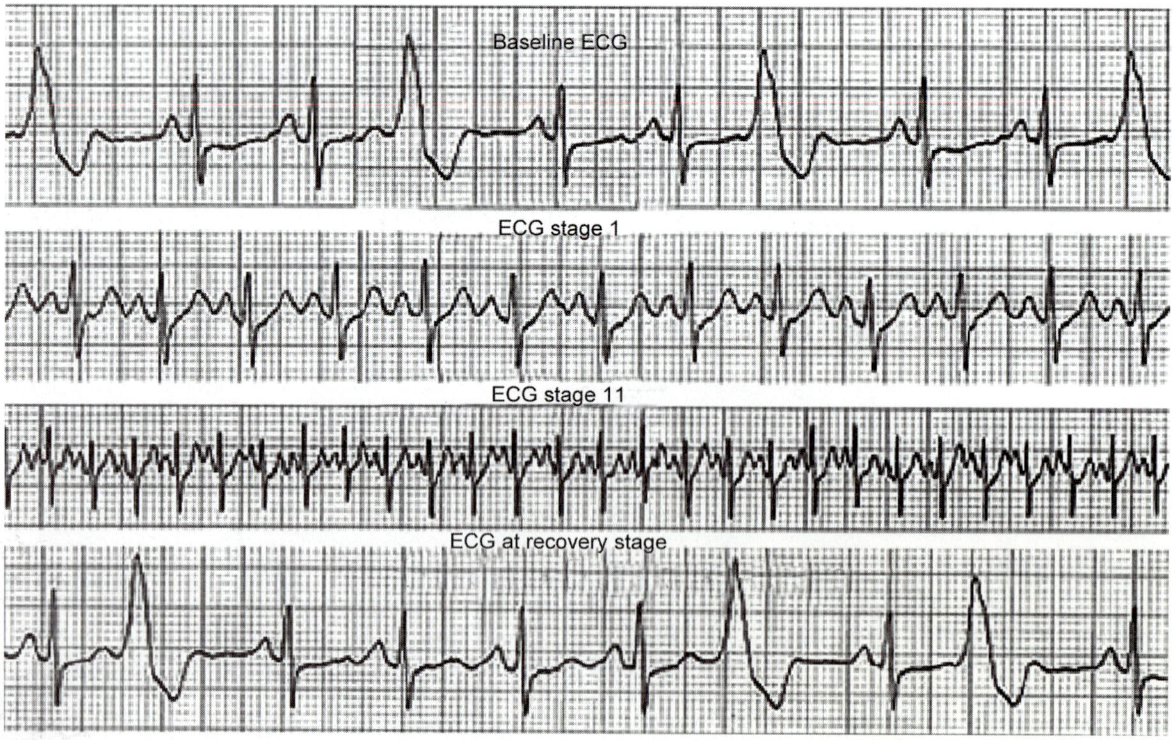

Fig. 8.18: *Exercise stress ECG at different stages as shown on the figure with premature ventricular ectopics both at rest and recovery stages with significant tachycardia during second stage*

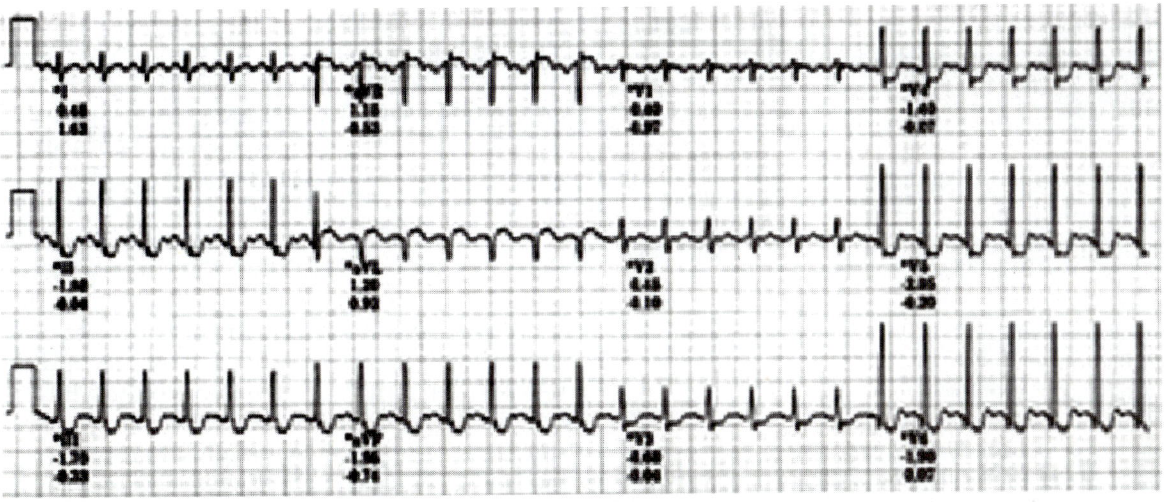

Fig. 8.19: *Peak exercise ECG tracing showing significant horizontal ST depression in inferior and lateral leads*

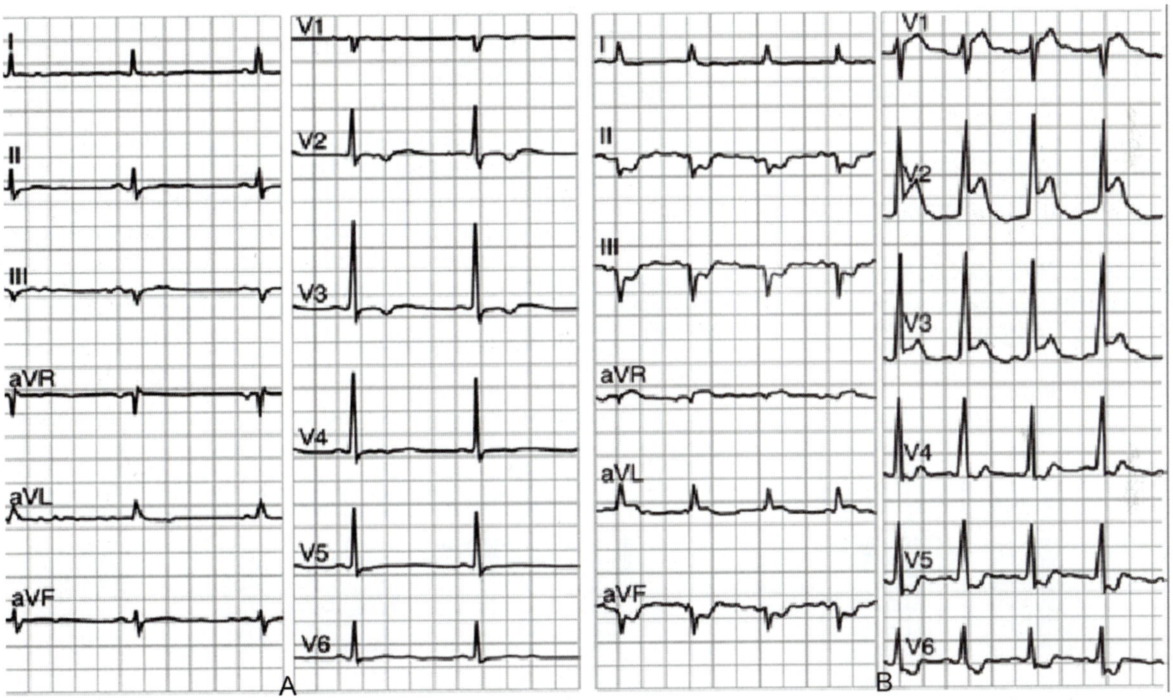

Fig. 8.20: *ECG on admission showing mild T-wave inversion in the precordial leads (A). ECG tracing during exercise stress test at maximal workload demonstrating left-axis deviation and pronounced ST segment elevation in the precordial leads (5 mm in V2) (B)*

been attached to ischemic changes, observed at lower heart rates of 120–130 per minute (less than 70% of predicted maximal heart rate). Persistence of ST depression up to 8 minutes, the after termination of exercise, also suggests advanced coronary artery disease.

Exercise-induced ST Segment Elevation

Paradoxically, one may find ST segment elevation, during stress testing, in 0.5–11.4% of subjects, with suspected IHD. Pathogenesis of ST elevation is different in three clinical patient subsets, as reviewed by Chaitman, et al. (1971). Highest incidence is in patients with old infarction; exercise induced ST elevation, usually, appears in leads with Q-wave, and is more common after anterior wall infarction. It implies underlying akinetic or dyskinetic wall motion. In patients with variant angina, 10–30% patients show exercise-induced ST elevation, which is most likely provoked by arterial spasm. Finally, 0.2–1.7% of symptomatic patients, without infarction or variant angina, who have exercise-induced ST elevation, have fixed high-grade IHD on angiography (Figs 8.21 and 8.34).

ST Integral

ST integral was reported by Scheffield et al. (1968) as an index of myocardial ischemia. They utilized leads V4, V5 and V6 and Frank X, Y and Z leads which were digitized at

Table 8.5: *Relative contraindications to or conditions requiring special consideration for exercise stress testing*

Current medications
Digoxin
- Type I antiarrhythmic agents e.g. quinidine, procainamide (Pronestyl), disopyramide (Norpace)]
- Tricyclic antidepressants
- Vasodilators (nitrates, alpha-adrenergic blockers, alcohol, other antihypertensive agents)
- Beta-adrenergic blockers
- Metabolic abnormalities
- Acid-base disorders
- Thyroid abnormalities
- Abnormal calcium, magnesium or potassium levels
- Vasoregulatory disorders
- Other cardiac conditions
- Mitral valve prolapse syndrome
- Wolff-Parkinson-White syndrome
- Recurrent paroxysmal supraventricular or atrioventricular nodal tachyarrhythmias

Table 8.6: *Criteria of an abnormal exercise test in patients with asymptomatic aortic stenosis*

- Symptoms during exercise: dyspnea, angina, syncope or near syncope
- Fall in blood pressure or < 20 mmHg rise in systolic blood pressure during exercise
- <80% of normal level of exercise tolerance
- >2 mm ST segment depression during exercise (horizontal or downsloping, in comparison to baseline, not attributable to other causes)
- Ventricular arrhythmias

500 samples/sec. They computed the time-voltage integral ST segment, beginning at the QRS, and continuing it until the isoelectric line was crossed or until 80 msec, after the end of QRS. This integral indicates the area of ST segment deviation from the base line. Results with angina yielded a sensitivity of 81% and a specificity of 95%.

R-Wave Changes

Recent reports suggest that the exercise-induced R-wave amplitude change may be a useful index for detecting IHD. Increased sympathetic activity, during stress testing, reduces LV volume in normal subjects and decreases the R-wave amplitude. In patients with IHD, the R-wave amplitude increases or does not change at all, indirectly suggesting impaired LV function during exercise. Exercise-induced R-wave change has been correlated with coronary angiographic data. Patients, with 1 vessel disease, have the lowest incidence of LV dysfunction and poor correlation with the R-wave amplitude change. But patients, with 2 or 3 vessels disease, with LV dysfunction, show the highest frequency of increased or unchanged R-wave amplitude. Bonoris et al. (1978) and Baron et al. (1980) have reported significantly increased sensitivity and specificity of stress testing, using R-wave changes. However, de Caprie et al. (1980) concluded that the R-wave amplitude change improves the sensitivity of the stress test but, concommitently, reduces the specificity. It appears that the usefulness of the stress-induced R-wave amplitude change, as an index of IHD, remains to be determined.

U-Wave Inversion

In a study, involving 248 patients, Gerson et al. (1979) reported exercise induced U-wave inversion in 15% of the

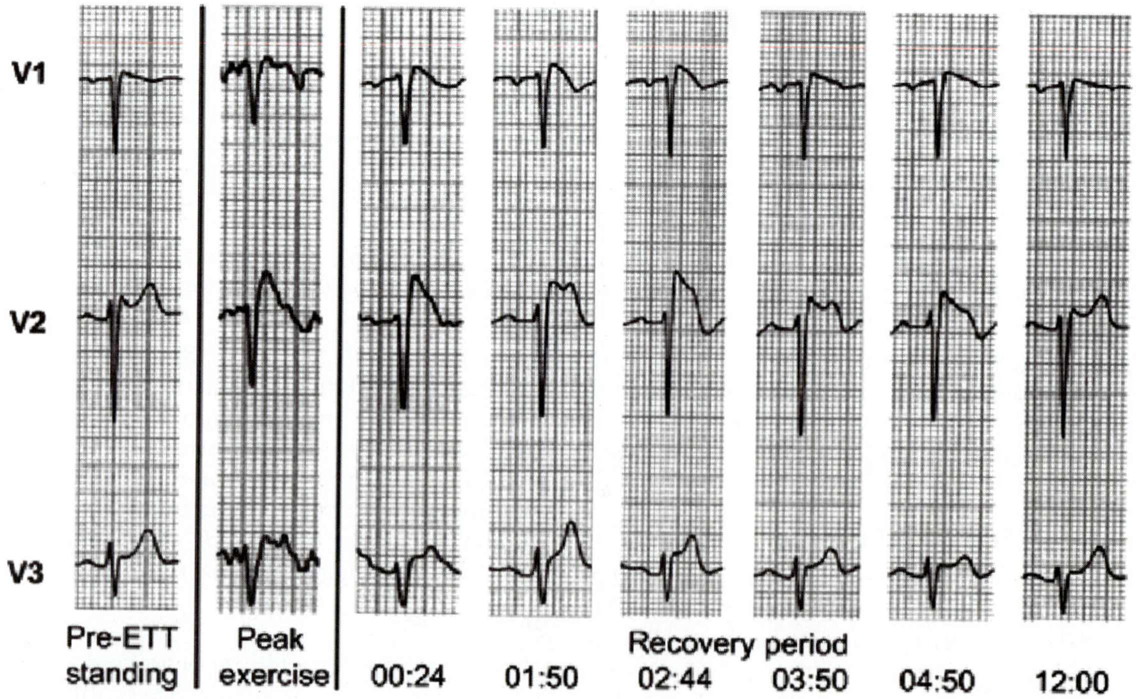

Fig. 8.21: *Persistence of ST segment elevation during the recovery phase of the treadmill exercise stress test*

patients with IHD. Significant disease of the left-anterior descending artery, was present in 92% of these patients. Exercise-induced U-wave inversion was observed in the absence of an abnormal ST segment response in 5% of the patients with IHD. None of the subjects, with normal coronary arteriogram, showed U-wave inversion. Prevalence of exercise-induced U-wave was also low (1.5%), in a large group of asymptomatic, and, presumably, healthy subjects.

Exercise-induced Arrhythmias (Figs 8.22, 8.25, 8.33, 8.36)

Ventricular arrhythmias should not be used as the sole criterion for the diagnosis of IHD. When observed in conjunction with other abnormalities, the combination of abnormalities becomes more specific. Incidence of VPC varies from less than 3%, with heart rate 70–100 per minute, to over 30%, with heart rates higher than 170 per minute. Complex and reproducible arrhythmias, especially at low workload of exercise, occur in patients with IHD, particularly in those who have regional abnormalities of LV contractions and exertional hypotension. Ventricular tachycardia was an indication to terminate exercise in 0.3% of 2,670 healthy men, and 1.7% of 1,650 men with a clinical diagnosis of IHD (Bruce, 1975).

Recently, Mardelli, Morganroth and Drifur (1980) reported markedly increased sensitivity of stress test from 60–95% when occurrence of VPCs with superiorly directed axis was added as a criterion of IHD. All normal subjects had normal QRS axis of exercise-induced VPCs.

Exercise-induced Angina

It is reported that ST segment changes alone were detected in 65% of the patients with IHD. When characteristic anginal pain was also considered a positive finding, the detection rate enhanced to 85%. It is, therefore, inferred that the combination of angina and the ST change was highly predictive of multivessel IHD.

Blood Pressure Response to Exercise

The normal BP response to stress is a progressive rise in the systolic pressure with successive increase in duration and intensity of the exercise. It is not uncommon to find 180–220 mmHg systolic, at peak exercise in normal adults. The diastolic BP shows a minimal fall of 10 mmHg in younger persons but tends to rise in middle-aged and older subjects. On the average systolic BP rises by 8–10 mmHg per minute of treadmill exercise.

Due to obvious reasons, a basal BP of over 160/110 mmHg is considered a contraindication to the stress test. Occasionally, in patients, with established or occult hypertension, BP rise may be disproportionate. Individuals, with normal basal BP, who respond to stress by disproportionately high systolic and diastolic BP rise, are considered latent-hypertensives as their arterial system does not show sufficient fall, in vascular resistance, to allow for increased cardiac output, with exercise. Insufficient rise, less than 10 mmHg, or a fall in systolic BP, is considered an ominous sign and is encountered in 25% of the patients with IHD, 60% of them having three vessel disease.

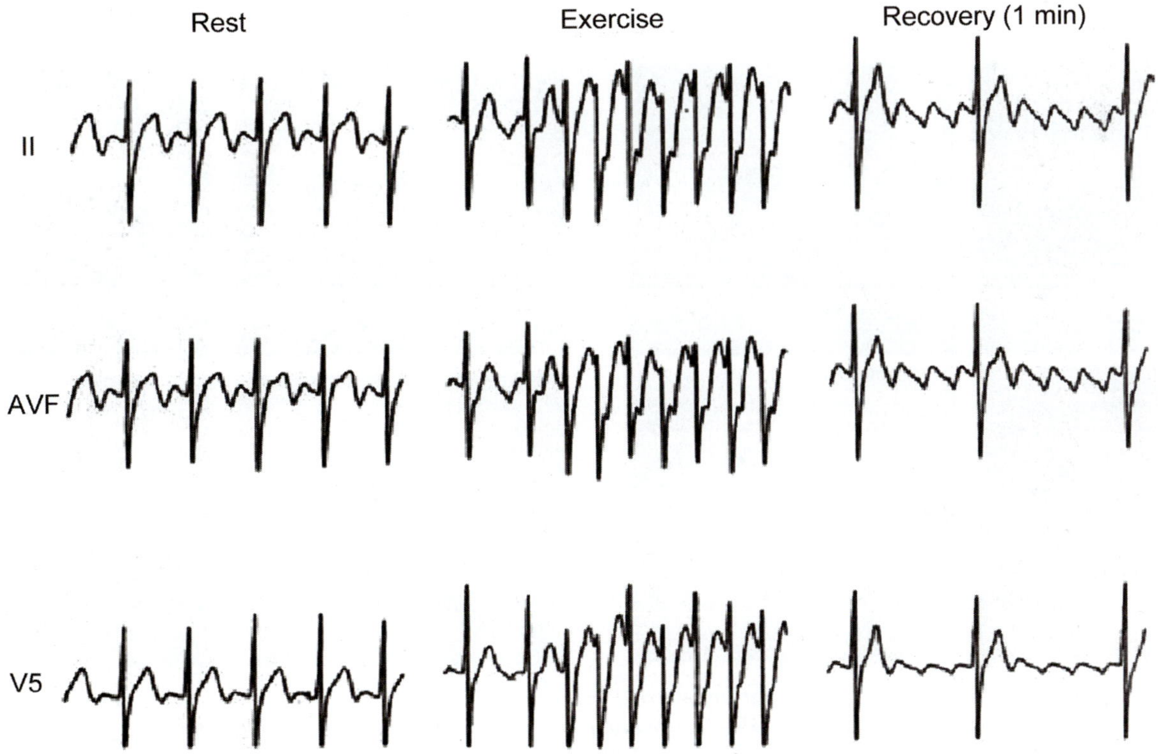

Fig. 8.22: *In a 15-year-old male exercise electrocardiogram shows wide QRS tachycardia during exercise. The recovery ECG shows atrial flutter with variable conduction. The rest ECG probably represents atrial flutter with 2:1 conduction rather than sinus rhythm. Exercise testing helped to establish this atrial arrhythmia*

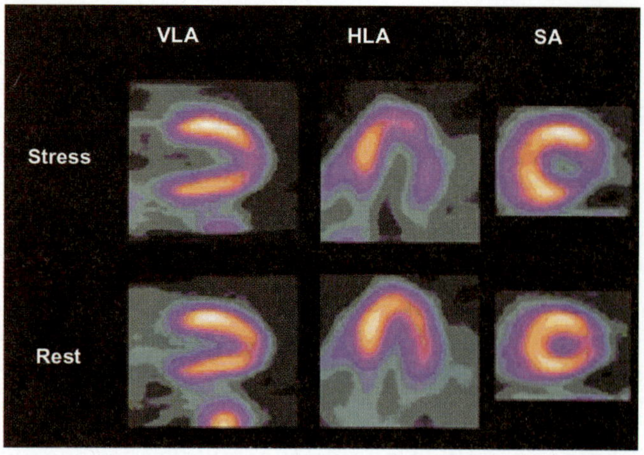

Fig. 8.23: *Stress and rest Rb-82 PET images in a patient with dipyridamole stress-inducible lateral wall and apical ischemia. Notable is the marked LV dilation during stress*

False-Positive Results

1. Healthy women
2. Subjects with labile ST-T changes, during standing or hyperventilation
3. Mitral valve prolapse
4. Pressure overload of the left-ventricle, like aortic stenosis and hypertension
5. Abnormal ventricular activation sequence, like bundle-branch block, pre-excitation syndrome
6. Electrolyte imbalance, especially hypokalemia
7. Digitalis and diuretics
8. Psychotropic drugs; tricyclic and other antidepressant compounds
9. Too rapid exercise without warm up period
10. Asymptomatic adult males.

Precautions required in conducting exercise test

1. Preliminary clinical examination including the record of recent changes in cardiac symptoms.
2. 12-lead ECG.
3. Presence of personnel, trained in cardiopulmonary resuscitation, and the appropriate equipment.
4. Monitoring of systolic blood pressure.
5. Attention to patient's symptoms, gait, and peripheral circulatory changes.
6. Monitoring of electrocardiogram for several minutes after test.
7. Avoidance of heat stress after test.
8. Reliable electrocardiographic electrode and lead system.

Equipment and Supplies for the Management of Complications

1. DC defebrillator with sufficient electrode paste (Fig. 8.11).
2. Airway tube ventilation bag, oxygen and laryngoscope.
3. Intravenous fluid (5% dextrose) with tubing, needles and disposable syringes.
4. Assorted drugs, including lidocaine, quinidine, disopyramide procainamide, diphenylhydantion, propranolol, atropine, isoproterenol, norepinephrine, metaraminol, furosemide, digioxin, dopamine, nitroglycerine.

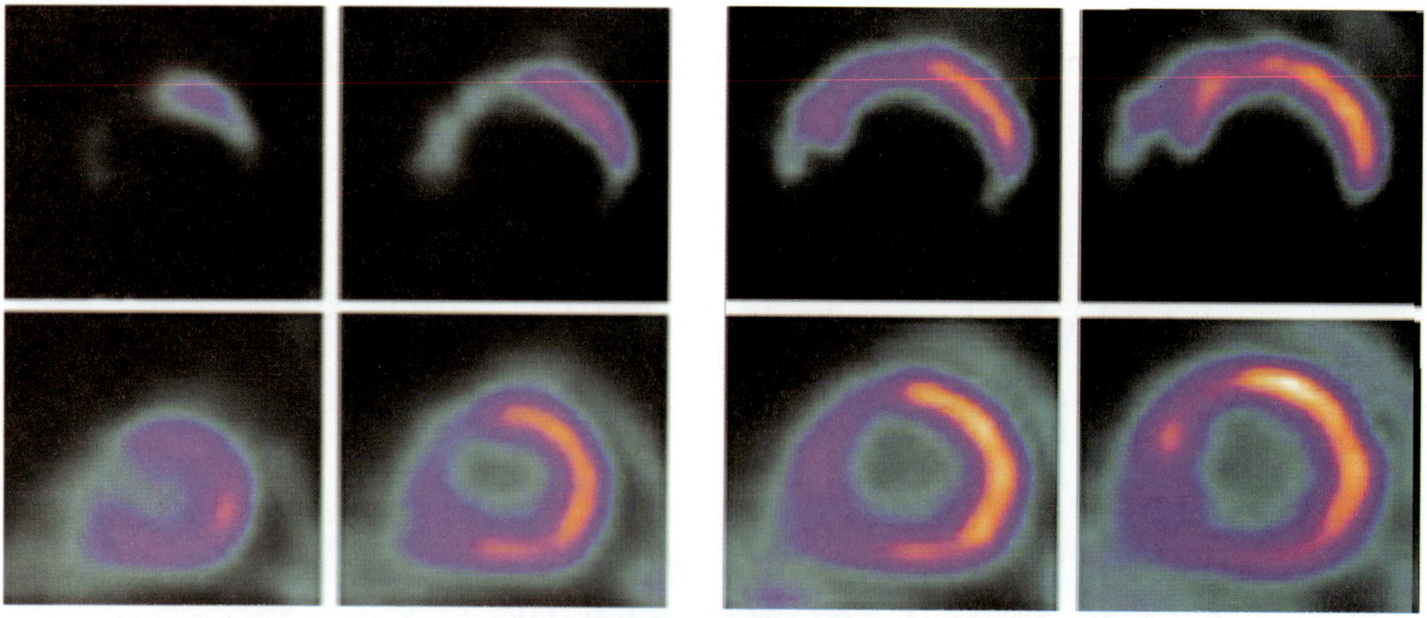

Fig. 8.24: *Resting and dobutamine stress echo for myocardial thinning, contractile reserve and myocardial ischemia integration of resting data and new technologies to predict functional recovery in a patient with severe dysfunction (LVEF 25%). The resting study shows no areas of thinning (1 cm markers in all walls) despite severe LV dysfunction and borderline restrictive filling (deceleration time 150 ms, E/A >2). Dobutamine stress shows basal inferior ischemia and mid-inferior biphasic response. Peak-dose (40 mcg/kg/min) dobutamine response showed hypokinetic septal and lateral walls had deteriorated at peak dose, consistent with extensive ischemia*

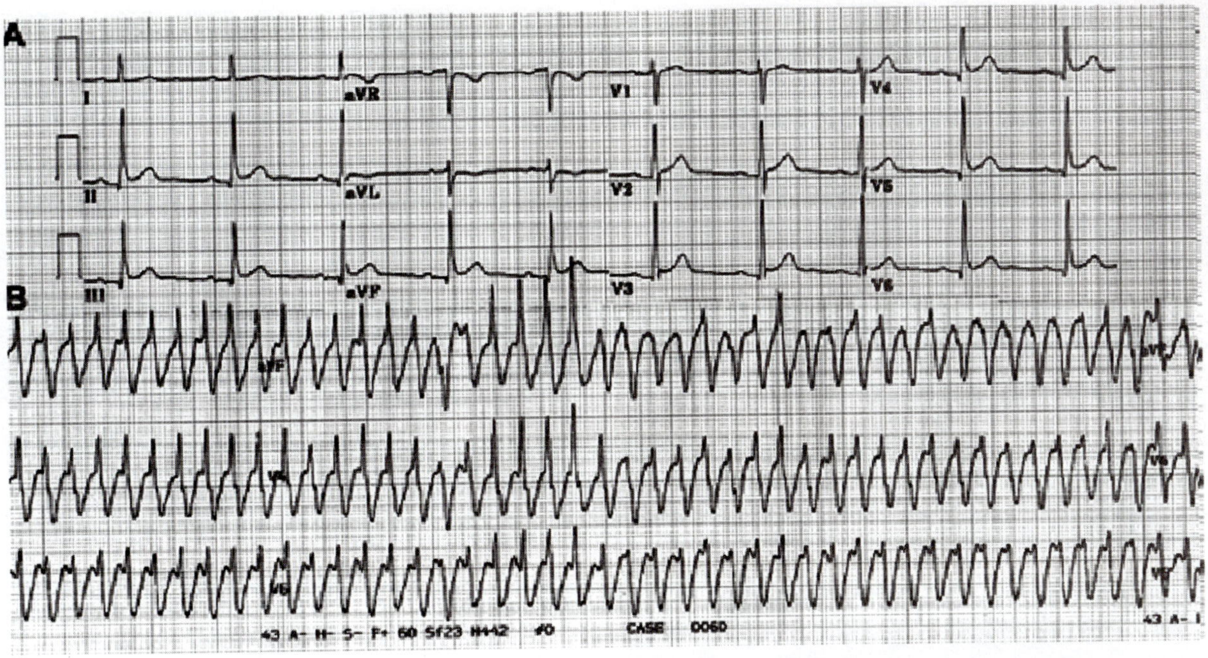

Fig. 8.25: *Note the features of ERPV in the baseline ECG (A) recorded immediately before an exercise stress test (B) that resulted in torsade de pointes*

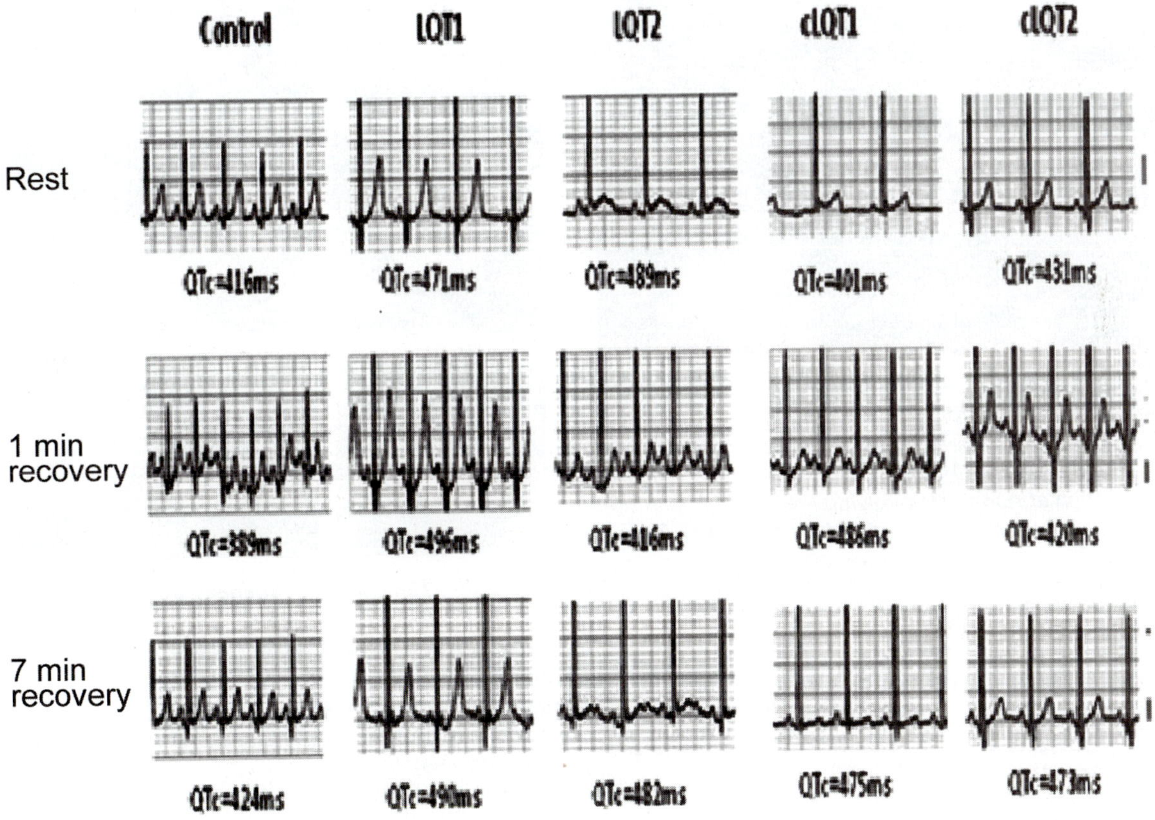

Fig. 8.26: *ECG tracing in patients with long QT syndrome during exercise stress testing. Examples of ECG tracings reflect gene-specific repolarization responses. The control patient had a normal resting heart rate-corrected QT interval (QTc; 416 ms), which shortened in early recovery (389 ms) and returned to near baseline at 7 minutes of recovery (424 ms). The patient with long QT syndrome type 1 (LQT1) had characteristic QTc prolongation at rest (471 ms) that was prolonged further in early recovery (496 ms) and remained prolonged at 7 minutes of recovery (490 ms). The patient with long QT syndrome type 2 (LQT2) also had characteristic QTc prolongation at rest (489 ms) that shortened in early recovery (416 ms) and was prolonged at 7 minutes of recovery (482 ms). Patients with concealed long QT syndrome (cLQT1 and cLQT2) had similar patterns*

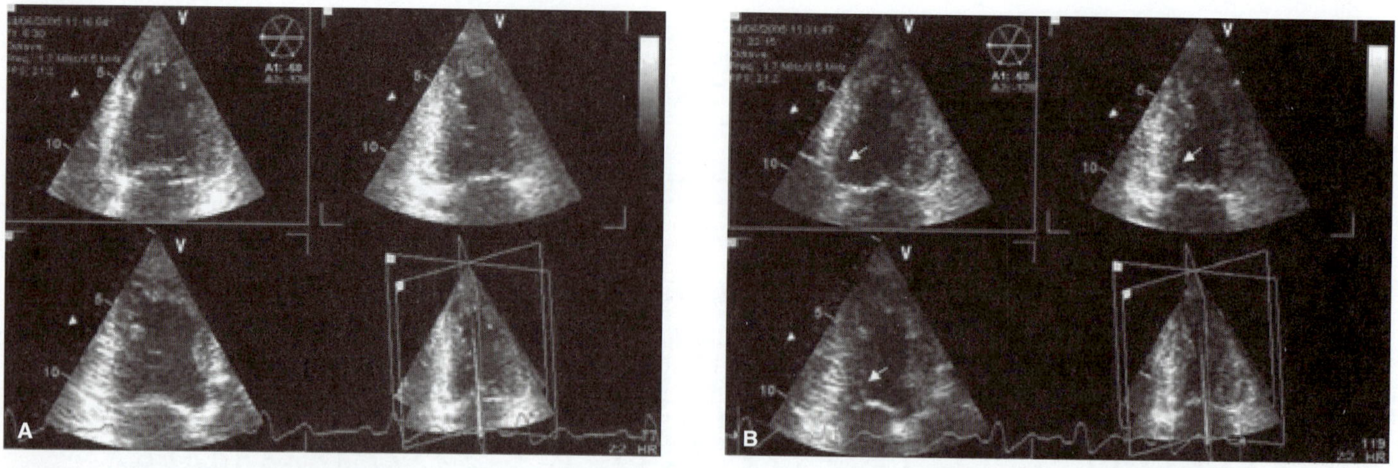

Fig. 8.27: *Assessment of inducible ischemia with RT3P DSE in a 20-year-old patient with CAD. (A) The end-systolic still frame image at baseline showed normal LV systolic wall motion in both apical-4, -2, and -3 chamber views. (B) At peak stress (40 μg/kg/min), the basal segments of the inferior, inferoseptal and the inferolateral walls showed a significant WMA at end-systole (white arrows)*

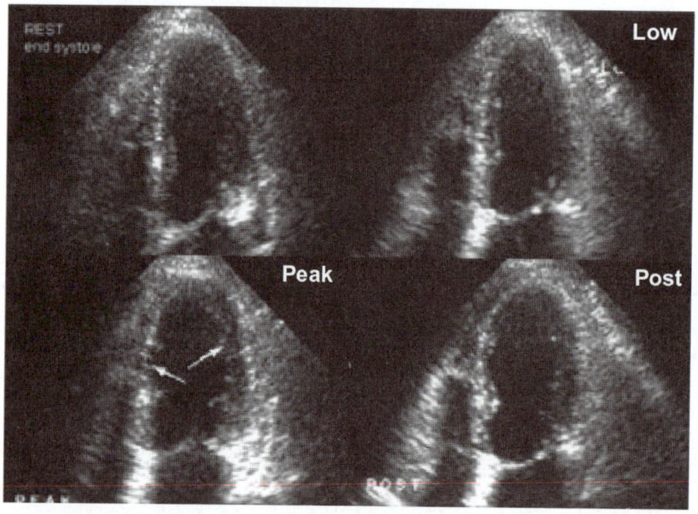

Fig. 8.28: *Example of a stress-induced wall-motion abnormality on dobutamine stress echocardiography. Images are obtained at rest, low-dose dobutamine, peak-dose dobutamine and during recovery. There is normal wall motion at rest, with evidence of extensive wall-motion abnormality involving the septal and lateral walls in addition to left ventricular dilation (white arrows). This is highly suggestive of multivessel coronary disease*

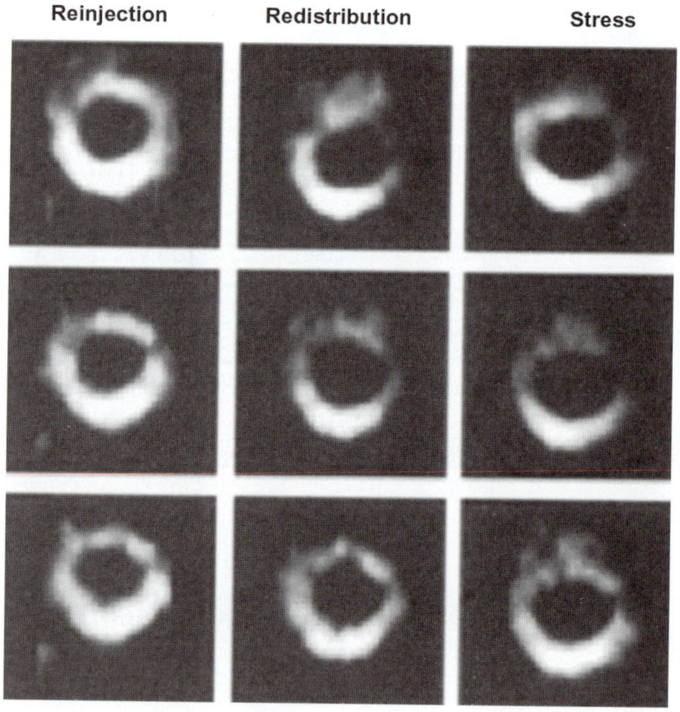

Fig. 8.29: *Thallium-201 imaging for myocardial viability short-axis 201 thallium tomograms during stress, redistribution, and reinjection imaging in a patient with coronary artery disease. There are extensive 201 thallium abnormalities in the anterior and septal regions during stress that persist on redistribution images but improve markedly on reinjection images. (From Dilsizian et al. with permission)*

Complications

Stress testing is considered a very safe, nonivasive, investigation. An analysis of about 2 per 10,000 stress tests, from about 18 centers, reported a mortality of one per 10,000, and a morbidity rate of about 2.4 per 10,000.

Computer Techniques in Stress Testing

Development of ST segment criteria other than few divisions of artefact distortion of ECG, during exercise, and problems of human eye-balling with interobserver and intraobserver interpretation variation have led to the use of computer technology in the analysis of the exercise ECG. By digitizing the ECG signals and sampling them at very fast rate, the ST segment can be very critically analyzed by a process, known as computer averaging.

Recognition of incremental averaging allows critical measurement of the ST segment with much greater precision than is possible with visual measurement of conventionally recorded ECG. One of the greatest advantages of computer averaging is decrease in the

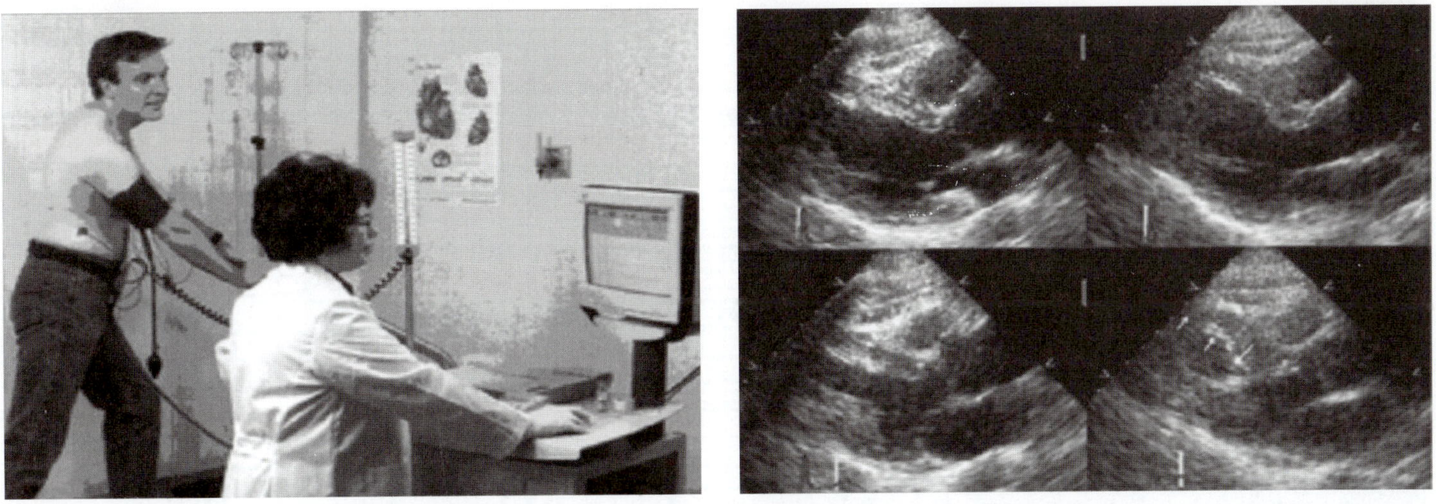

Fig. 8.30: *(Upper) a young person is performing stress echocardiographic study for effort angina. Lower Parasternal long-axis echocardiogram recorded at rest (left) and immediately after exercise (right) in a patient with stenosis of the left anterior descending coronary artery. Diastolic frames are on the top, and systolic frames are on the bottom. At rest, notice the normal contraction of the septum and posterior wall. Immediately after exercise, the proximal septum has normal contractility (downward pointing arrow), and there is dyskinesia of the distal ventricular septum (upward pointing arrows)*

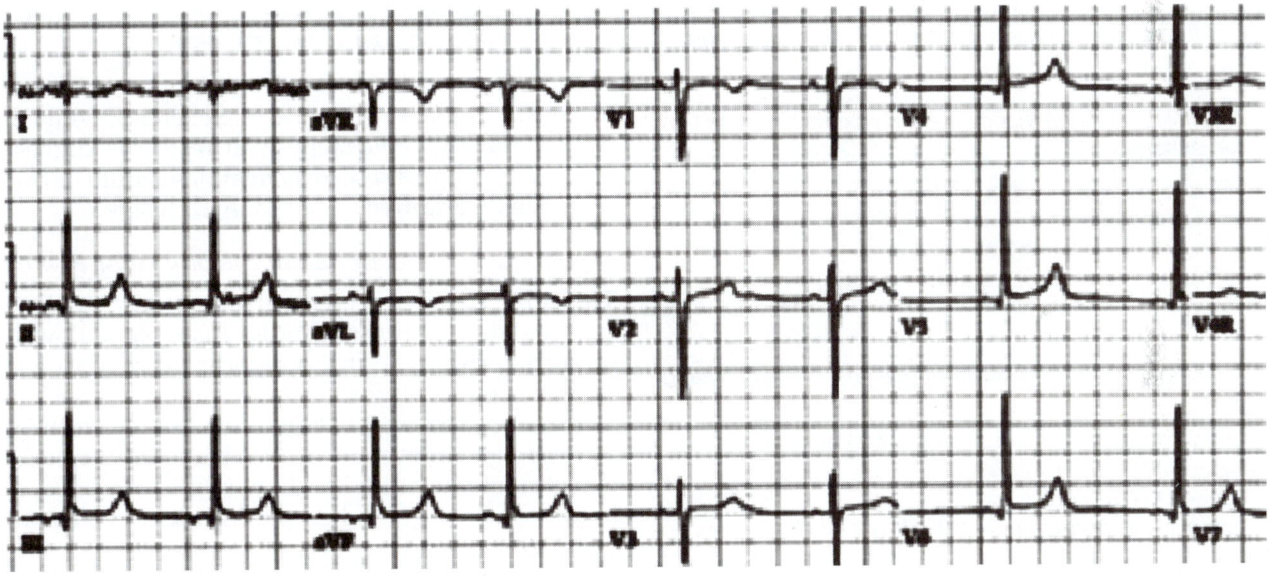

Fig. 8.31: *The QTc prolonged with exercise stress testing in the recovery period to 520 milliseconds, confirming the impression of long QT syndrome (LQTS). She was started on 10 mg of nadolol twice daily and was asked to stop competitive swimming. She was advised to avoid caffeine and stimulants, and not to take medications known to further prolong the QT interval. (A list at www.qtdrugs.org includes azithromycin). Genetic testing confirmed a diagnosis of long QT syndrome, type 1, with a mutation in the KCNQ1 gene. JK will be followed every 6–12 months with exercise stress testing and Holter monitoring and will have medication adjusted as she grows*

amount of distortion, accompanying the stress ECG. In a large series of patients, the sensitivity of computer technique was 76% as compared to 45% by visual analysis.

Prognostic Value of Stress Test

Like any other investigation, the stress test should also be considered as a quantitative risk factor rather than as a simple "disease/no disease" classification. It has been reported that in subjects, with anginal myocardial infarction death, in a 6 years follow-up, who developed ST depression of 2 mm after 7 min of exercise, the incidence of combined events was less than 20% in patients, who developed ischemic change, after 5 minutes of stress; the combined coronary events occurred in 30% of cases, and when ST depression occurred at 3 minutes of exercise, the combined coronary events occurred in 70% of cases. In a prospective seattle heart watch study, it was discovered that the most useful predictors of future development of coronary events

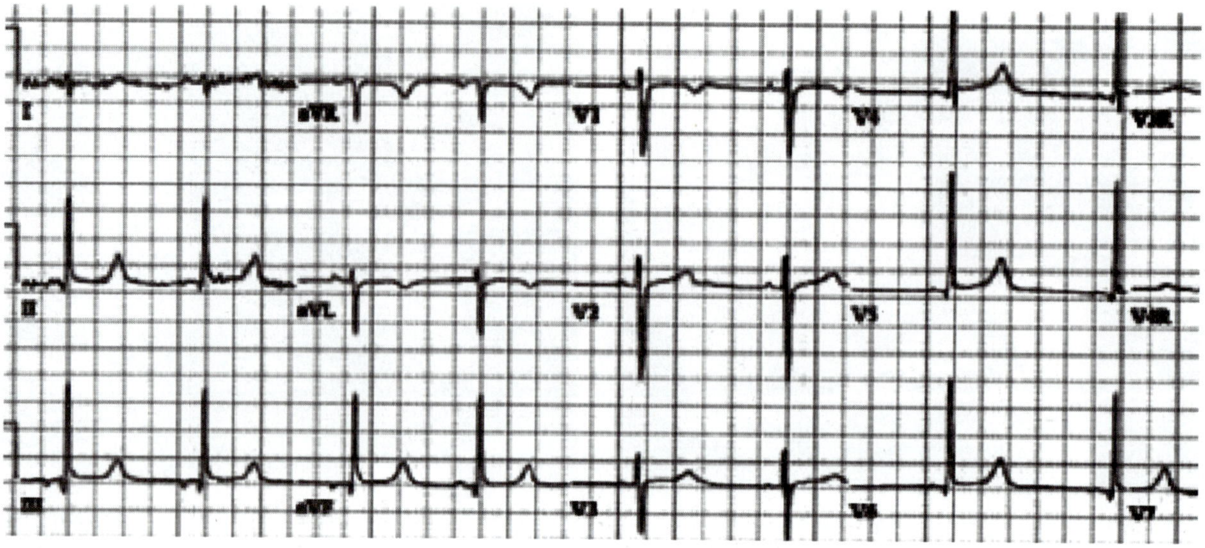

Fig. 8.32: *10-yrs-old child was referred her to a pediatric cardiologist for further evaluation of syncope. She had an electrocardiogram (ECG), showing a prolonged corrected QT interval (QTc) of 490 milliseconds, with abnormal T-wave morphology. The QTc prolonged with exercise stress testing in the recovery period to 520 milliseconds, confirming the impression of long QT syndrome (LQTS). She was started on 10 mg of nadolol twice daily and was asked to stop competitive swimming. She was advised to avoid caffeine and stimulants, and not to take medications known to further prolong the QT interval. (A list at www.qtdrugs.org includes azithromycin). Genetic testing confirmed a diagnosis of long QT syndrome, type 1, with a mutation in the KCNQ1 gene. JK will be followed every 6–12 months with exercise stress testing and Holter monitoring and will have medication adjusted as she grows*

Table 8.7: *Clinical findings that suggest an exercise stress test positive for ischemia*

Exercise-induced hypotension
Exercise-induced angina or anginal equivalents
Appearance of an S3, S4 or heart murmur during exercise

S3 = third heart sound; S4 = fourth heart sound

Table 8.8: *Nonsignificant findings during exercise stress testing*

Fatigue, dyspnea, diaphoresis, flushing
Incremental increase in blood pressure and heart rate
ECG changes
Shortening of QT interval
Functional J-point derpession = 0.2 mV for <0.06 seconds in duration
Peaking of T-wave and P-waves
Shortening of PR interval

ECG = electrocardiogram

are the common occurrence (12%) of horizontal and downslopping ST depression of 1 mV or more, after maximal exercise, and the infrequent occurrence (less than 2%) of chest pain or discomfort, at peak exercise. Without either of the markers, the coronary death rate was 0.5 per 1,000 men at risk per year; with only ST depression it was 4.8%, with only chest pain it was 24%, and with both ST depression and chest pain, it was 53 per 1,000 men at risk per year.

It should be emphasised that stress testing and coronary angiography define two different aspects of coronary circulation. The former delineates the functional adequacy of myocardial blood flow during exercise, while the latter defines the anatomic stenosis at rest. It is suggested that the results of both these investigations should be considered as mutually additive rather than exclusive.

Myocardial Perfusion Scintigraphy after Exercise

Thallium 201 is injected intravenously at the time of maximal stress. In normal individuals, blood flow increases uniformly throughout the myocardium, during exercise, resulting in an uniform distribution of tracer substance. Deficiency or absence of blood flow, caused by hemodynamically significant stenosis, results in tracer-free perfusion defects (cold defects). Thallium scan is repeated, after 3–4 hours of stress test, when the transient perfusion defects get filled up and disappear.

Using thallium 201 scan, patients with IHD (with infarction) revealed abnormal images in 80% cases and, upon comparison with coronary angiography, it revealed the sensitivity of 70, 90 and 73% per single, double, and triple vessel diseases, respectively (Figs 8.23, 8.24 and 8.29).

Contraindication of Stress Test

Absolute

1. Severe cardiac failure
2. Uncontrolled systemic hypertension
3. Recent acute infection
4. Acute pericardities
5. Acute myocarditis
6. Acute thyrotoxicosis
7. Acute myocardial infarction with 10 days of onset
8. Serious dysrhythmia (Figs 8.26 and 8.36).
9. Hepatic and renal failure.

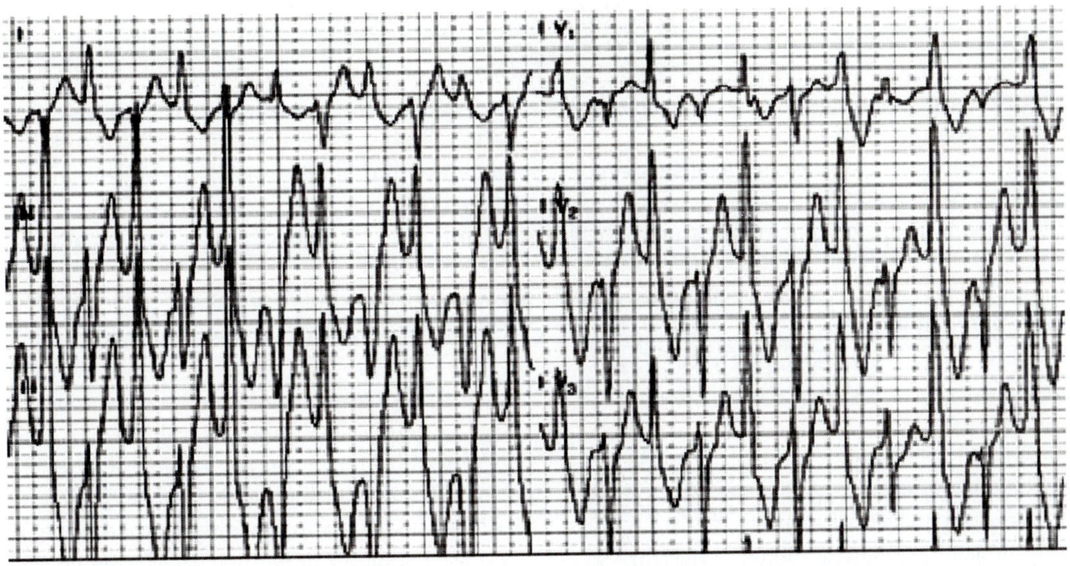

Fig. 8.33: *Bidirectional ventricular tachycardia during exercise stress test in a patient affected by catecholaminergic polymorphic ventricular tachycardia*

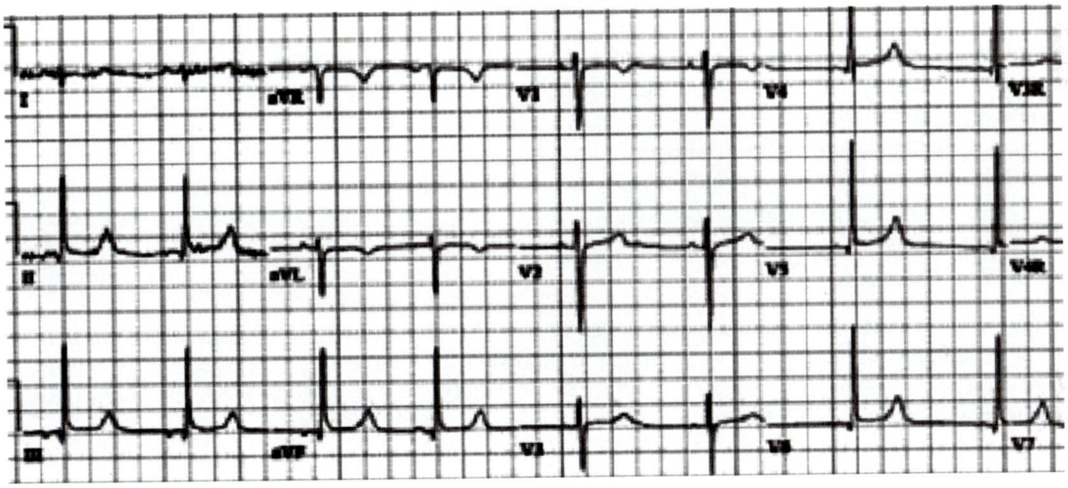

Fig. 8.34: *Exercise in a young athlete. The QTc prolonged with exercise stress testing in the recovery period to 520 milliseconds, confirming the impression of long QT syndrome (LQTS)*

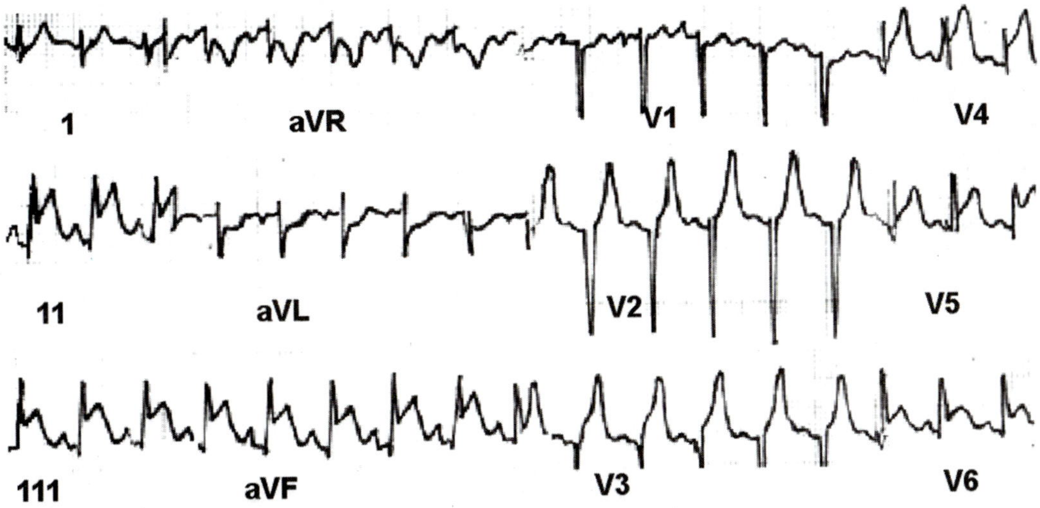

Fig. 8.35: *Post exercise ST elevation in inferiolateral regions*

Table 8.9: *Relative risks for stress testing*

Low risk	*Higher risk*
Symptoms during exercise in an otherwise healthy child who has a normal CVS examination and ECG	Patients with pulmonary hypertension Patient with documented long QT syndrome
Exercise induced bronchospasm studies in the absence of severe resting airways obstruction	Patient with dilated/restrictive cardiomyopathy with CHF or arrhythmia
Asymptomatic ventricular ectopy in patients with structurally normal hearts	Patients with hypertrophic cardiomyopathy who have 1. Symptoms 2. Greater than mild LVOTO 3. Documented arrhythmia.
Patient with unrepaired congenital cardiac lesion who are asymptomatic at rest, including: 1. Left to right shunts (ASD, VSD, PDA, PAPVR) 2. Obstructive right heart lesion without severe resting obstruction (TS, PS ToF) 3. Obstructive left heart lesions without severe resting obstruction (Cor triatriatum, MS, AS, CoA) 4. Regurgitant lesions regardless of severity	Patients with greater than moderate airways obstruction on baseline pulmonary function tests Patient with Marfan syndrome and activity-related chest pain in whom a noncardiac cause of chest pain is suspected Patients suspected to have myocardial ischemia with exertion Routine testing of patients with Marfan syndrome Unexplained syncope with exercise
Routine follow-up of asymptomatic patients at risk for myocardial ischemia, including: 1. Kawasaki disease without giant aneurysms or known coronary stenosis 2. After repair of anomalous LCA 3. After arterial switch procedure	
Routine monitoring in cardiac transplant patients not currently experiencing rejection	
Patients with palliated cardiac lesions withou uncompensated CHF, arrhythmia, or extreme cyanosis	
Patients with a history of hemodynamically stable SVT	
Patients with stable dilated cardiomyopathy without uncompensated CHF or documented arrhythmia	

CVS, cardiovascular system; ASD, atrial septal defect; VSD, ventricular septal defect; PDA, patent ductus arteriosus; PAPVR, partial anomalous pulmonary venous return; TS, tricuspid stenosis; PS, pulmonary stenosis; ToF, tetralogy of Fallot; MS, mitral stenosis; AS, aortic stenosis; CoA, coarctation of aorta; LCA, left coronary artery; SVT, supraventricular tachycardia; CHF, congestive heart failure; and LVOTO, left ventricular outflow trach obstruction.

Relative

1. Severe pulmonary hypertension
2. Known syncope
3. Neurological disease
4. Unstable angina pectoris
5. Outflow tract obstruction of LV, i.e. aortic stenosis
6. Musculoskeletal abnormalities.

Reasons for Terminating the Test

1. Achievement of target heart rate
2. Progressive heart pain
3. ST depression of 6 mm or more
4. Dizziness
5. Severe respiratory difficulty
6. Cardiac arrhythmia (Figs 8.36 and 8.38)
7. Failure for pressure rate product to come up as expected
8. Multifocal ventricular VPCs (Fig. 8.18)
9. Disturbances in impulse transmission
10. Severe symptoms during early part of the test.

What is a MET?

One MET is the energy expenditure per kilogram body weight per minute (kg/min) for an average subject sitting quietly in a chair or at a supine rest. One MET is the approximate equivalent of 3.5 mL of O_2/kg/minute consumption of oxygen by an average individual at rest.

Normal persons can consume 15 METS but according to NYHA, the classification of cardiac disability is

- Class I-II can perform upto 7 METS
- Class II can perform upto 5–6 METS
- Class III can perform upto 3–4 METS only.

Stress Test in Asymptomatic Subjects

This has always been a controversial subject and is dependant upon several factors like as intensity and duration of exercise, age and sex, hereditary and familial background. Recording of the ischemic ST segment depression, in an otherwise asymptomatic subject, is an important clinical finding. Individuals with positive response have four times greater chance of development of coronary events in the next

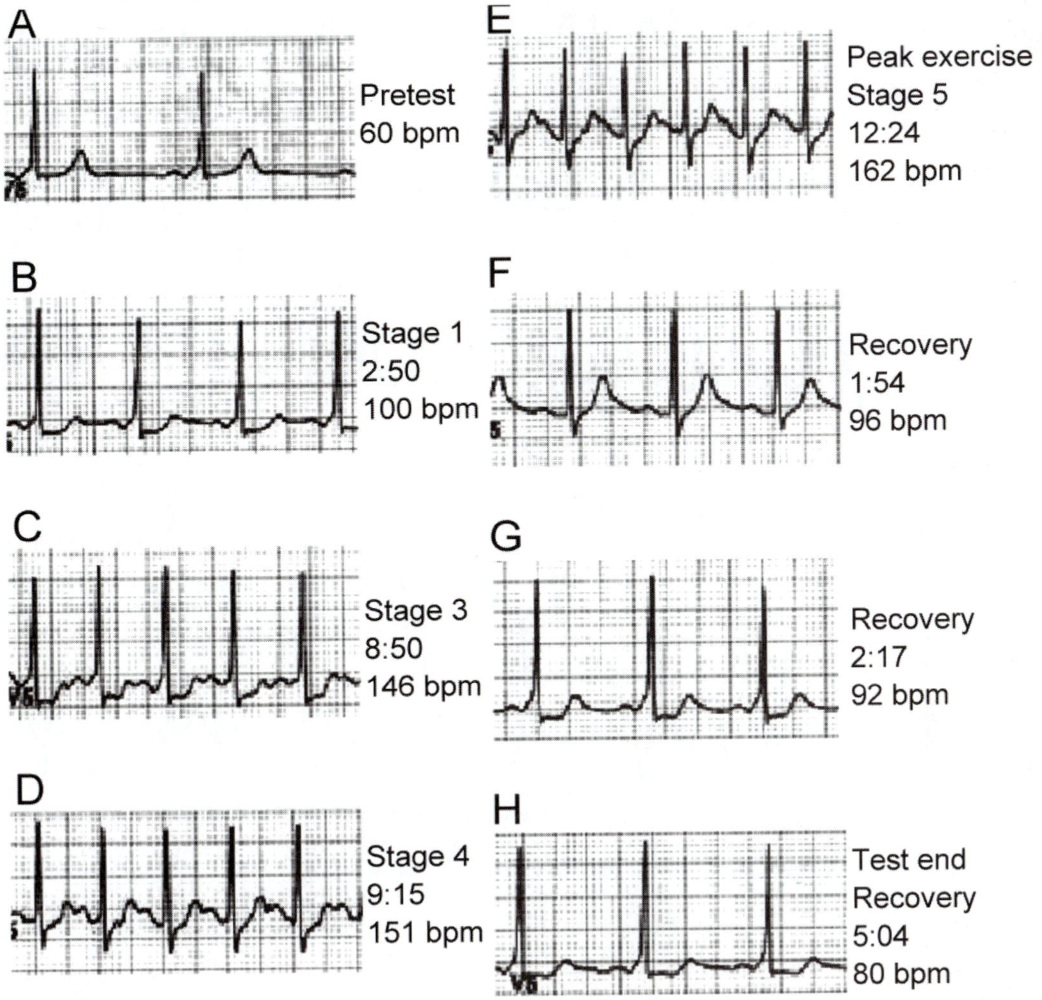

Fig. 8.36: *ECG during testing demonstrated the WPW pattern at baseline, which is consistent with a posteroseptal accessory tract. ST segments were normal at rest (Fig 1, top left, A. An ST-segment depression of 1 mm began at 2 min and 50 s, left top middle; B, reaching a maximum of 2 mm in leads V4 to V6 at 8 min and 50 s (left bottom middle, C. The delta wave suddenly and completely disappeared, and the PR interval lengthened at 9 min and 15 s (left bottom, D. at a heart rate of 151 beats/min with immediate normalization of ST segments extending through maximum exercise (right top, E). In recovery, ST segments remained normal until a heart rate of 90 beats/min occurred, at which time the delta wave reappeared with a recurrence of 1-mm ST-segment depressions (right top middle, F, and right bottom middle, G). At 5 min into recovery, the ECG had returned to baseline (right bottom, H), demonstrating resolution of the ST-segment depression with the normalization of the depolarization abnormality*

8 years as compared to subjects with negative response. Cardiac disability rate was correlated with the magnitude of ST segment depression. The observed mortality was 13 times greater for subjects with ST segment depression in excess of 2.0 mm and five times greater for subjects having ST depression between 1 mm and 2 mm. However. 24-hr Holter monitoring test for the evaluation of ST segment, in such subjects, is gaining better ground. Thallium Stress test and coronary angiography should be advised if the test is strongly positive or if this becomes positive, over a continuous follow up, on long standing negative response (Figs 8.37 and 8.38).

Stress Testing in Old Myocardial Infarction Patients

It is, usually, done about 3–6 weeks after myocardial infarction (MI). It is considered quite a safe guide in rehabilitation and for judging the work capacity of the patient. If, during the course of the test, ventricular irritability or dysfunction occurs, digoxin or some other antiarrhythmic drug is administered. This testing is also useful for the prediction of future coronary events, and the severity of coronary artery disease. In case, the test results are normal, the chances are that there is 0 to 1 inch vessel disease in 62% cases. In old inferior wall MI, a positive test indicates an additional coronary disease in almost 87% of the patients while it is in only 50% patients in anterior myocardial infarction. The incidence of repeated coronary attacks, in the next 2 years, approximates 0–5% over a negative test when compared to the positive test, expected for which it is 30–40%. If the patient has a strongly positive test, it is better to have coronary angiograms done for the management of coronary artery disease.

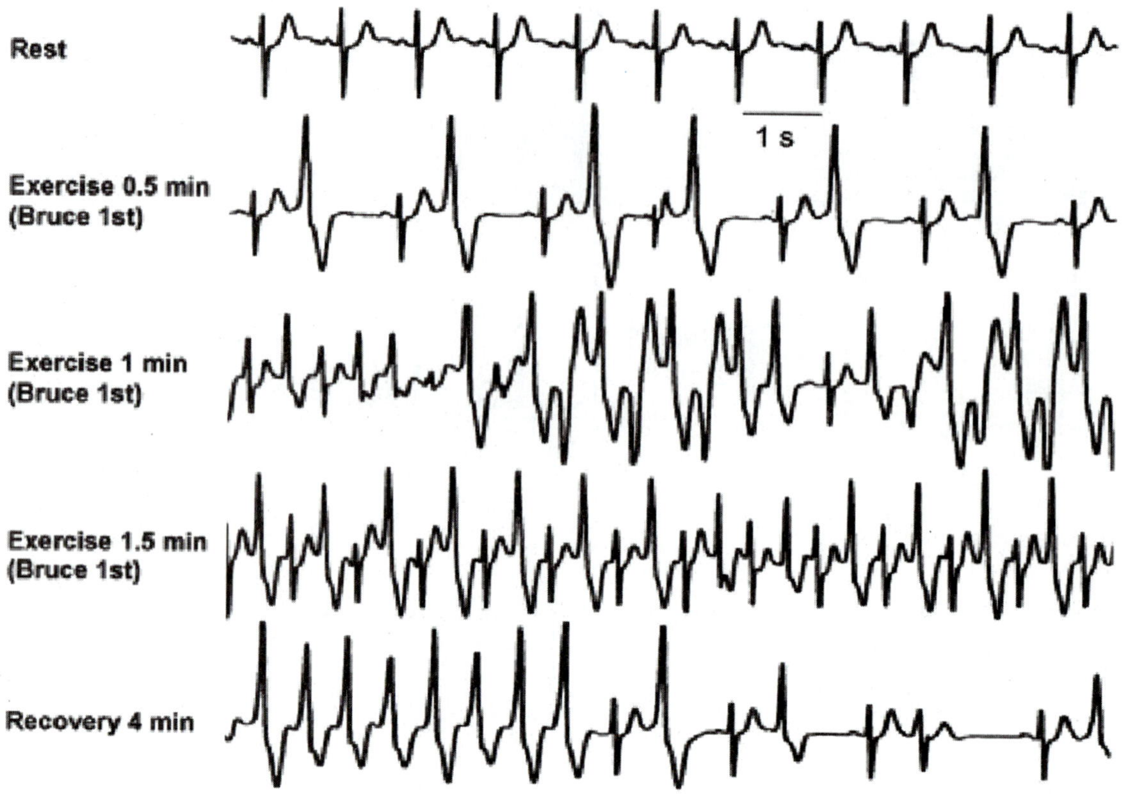

Fig. 8.37: *Exercise stress test in a patient with polymorphic VT and RyR2 mutation. Ventricular arrhythmias are observed with a progressive worsening during exercise. Typical bidirectional VT develops after 1 minute of exercise with a sinus heart rate of approximately 120 beats per minute. Arrhythmias rapidly recede during recovery. (Image from Liu et al. 2008)*

Table 8.10: *Inconclusive, or nondiagnostic, findings on exercise stress testing*

Development of clinically insignificant arrhythmias
Unifocal premature ventricular contractions
Atrial or junctional tachyarrhythmias
Development of blocks
Primary or secondary type I atrioventricular block
Bundle branch blocks
Hemiblocks
Changing atrioventricular conduction
Morphology changes
T-wave flattening
P-wave changes < 0.01 mV
ST depression < 0.10 mV

THE PARAMETERS WHICH INDICATE ABNORMAL TEST

I Electrical:

(a) ST segment depression or elevation of 1 mm at 0.08 sec beyond the J-point.

(b) Downsloping ST segment.

(c) Upsloping ST segment which is, at least, 2 mm depressed at 0.08 see, after the J-point

(d) 25% increase in height of R-wave

(e) Appearance of negative U-waves.

(f) Appearance of multifocal VPCS, VT or VF.

(g) Maximal pressure rate product less than 25×10^3 (25,000). (SBP × heart rate) = < 25,000

For example, a patient having systolic BP of 160 and heart rate of 140 during peak of exercise, then the pressure rate product = 22,400.

II. Symptomatic: Experiencing anginal pain, relieved by nitroglycerine administration.

III. Haemodynamic:

(i) Diminution in systolic BP during exercise.

(ii) Maximum HR of more than 160/minute indicates low risk and, increase in height of R-wave, and fall in BP. When occurring at low work loads (i.e. 4–5 Mets or Bruce stage I) or appearance of progressive fatal arrythmia, are considered signs of strongly positive test.

The various factors which interfere with the ability of interpretation of stress tests are:

1. Left ventricular hypertrophy
2. Left bundle-branch block
3. Baseline ST-T abnormality more than 1 mm
4. Digitalis (with or without baseline ECG abnormality).

Role of exercise ST/HR slope and ST/HR Index in the detection of coronary artery disease

Elamin et al. (1980), Okin et al. (1985) and Finkelhor et al. (1986) have employed the maximum exercise ST/HR slope in the accurate detection of coronary artery disease and for the identification of patients with anatomically and functionally severe coronary obstruction. This method uses linear regression analysis to relate the magnitude of ST

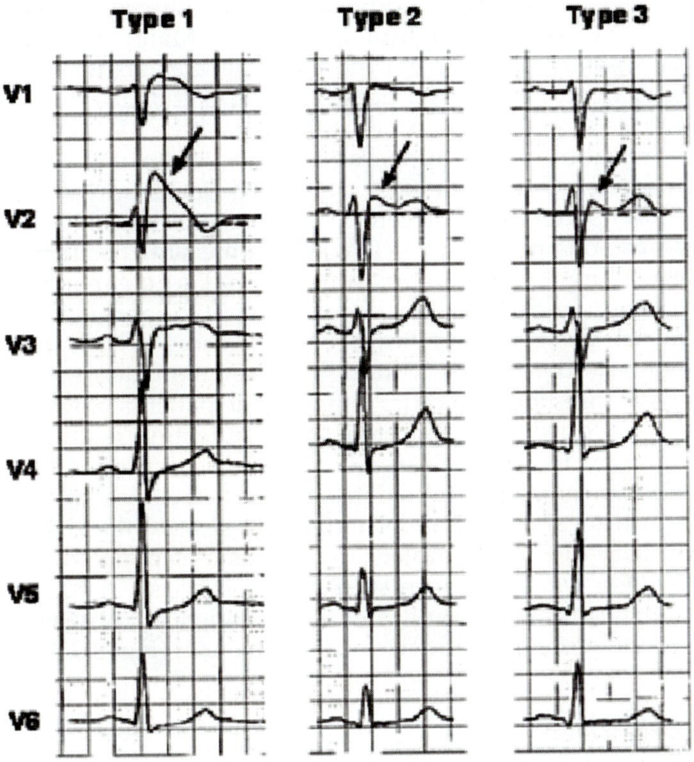

Fig. 8.38: *Three types of ST segment elevation in Brugada syndrome, as shown in the precordial leads on ECG in the same patient at different times. Left panel shows a type 1 ECG pattern with pronounced elevation of the J-point (arrow), a coved-type ST segment, and an inverted T-wave in V1 and V2. The middle panel illustrates a type 2 pattern with a saddleback ST segment elevated by >1 mm. The right panel shows a type 3 pattern in which the ST segment is elevated < 1 mm. According to a consensus report (Antzelevitch, 2005), the type 1 ECG pattern is diagnostic of Brugada syndrome. (Modified from Wilde, 2002)*

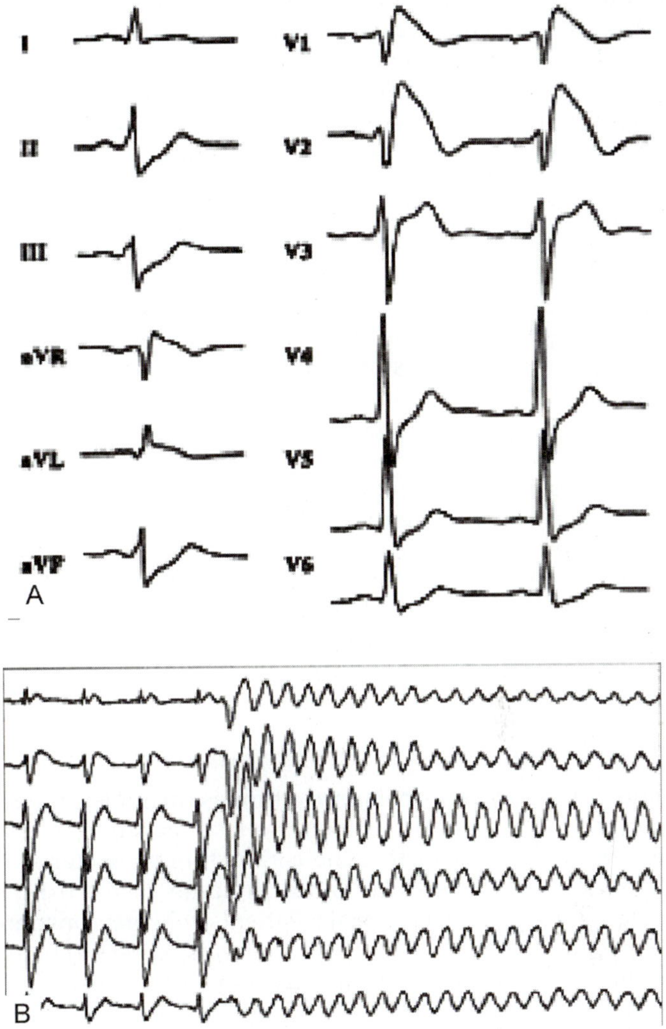

Fig. 8.39: *(A) Typical ECG in Brugada syndrome: atypical right bundle-branch block and ST-segment elevation in right precordial leads in patient who survived episode of cardiac arrest. (B) After exercise stress there is onset of polymorphic ventricular tachycardia with rapid degeneration to ventricular fibrillation in patient with Brugada syndrome*

segment depression to changes in heart rate at higher exercise work loads, thus normalizing the ECG expression of subendocardial ischemia, for estimating exercise-induced augmentation of myocardial oxygen demand. Detrano et al. (1986) have stressed another method, of simpler form, of heart rate adjustment of ST segment depression, which divides the maximum ST segment change, by the total change in heart rate, from rest to peak exercise. It has also been shown to improve the performance of the exercise ECG. This delta ST/HR index tries to show the average rather than the maximal change of ST depression, that occurs with heart rate, over the entire course of exercise, and, often, differs markedly, in magnitude, from the maximum ST/HR slope. Hence, the delta ST/HR index may be a valuable screening method, for the detection of coronary artery disease, and the exclusion of normal subjects, from those suffering from IHD.

Exercise Testing and Autonomic Studies

The manipulation of the autonomic tone, often, provides information regarding the rhythm status that is not always available on a resting electrocardiogram. Enhancement of sympathetic drive during dynamic exercise, permits analysis, not only of the exercise capacity and the hemodynamic response to stress, but also of the sinus node function, intracardiac conduction, and arrhythmias. The most widely employed exercise technique involves the Bruce protocol on an adjustable treadmill, where the belt speed and slope are increased at 3-minute intervals, during which the heart rate, blood pressure, and surface electrocardiograms are recorded. Normal values for exercise tolerance, peak sinus rate, and blood pressure responses are well-established for sex and age.

Exercise testing' can be utilized as a rough indicator of sinus node integrity by comparing the maximal achieved heart rate to the expected normal for age. Some reports suggest a blunted heart rate response to exercise may be observed in patients with the "sick sinus syndrome". The conduction characteristics of the AV node, during sinus tachycardia, can also be used to evaluate low-to-moderate grades of AV blocks. For patients, with known complete heart block, the chronotropic response of their junctional escape rhythm, or the appearance of ventricular ectopy, during exercise, may assist in determining the need for pacemaker insertion.

By far the most common arrhythmic issue, addressed with exercise testing, is ventricular ectopy. Children, who demonstrate ectopy on an electrocardiogram or on Holter monitoring, are, usually, subjected to maximal exercise testing as part of their evaluation. The testing serves two purposes. First, it is, sometimes, helpful to determine whether ectopy is suppressed or aggravated by exercise. In asymptomatic patients, with single premature beats, ectopy, which is suppressed by exercise, is thought to have benign prognosis, although there may be some exceptions to this rule. On the other hand, an increased frequency of premature contractions, at peak exercise, or the new appearance of couplets or ventricular tachycardia, at any stage of testing, may suggest pathology. The second purpose for this testing is to establish a baseline arrhythmia density against which follow-up studies can be compared while the patient is on antiarrhythmic drugs.

Stress Testing in Pre-excitation Syndrome

Generally, supraventricular arrhythmias do not lend them with the WPW syndrome, exercise testing. Often, yields important clues, regarding the conduction characteristics of the accessory pathway, and, in some cases, it may precipitate re-entry tachycardia. Patients, who demonstrate clear delta waves, and short PR intervals, at rest, (i.e. are pre-excited in the anterograde direction), can be exercised to accelerate their atrial rate. A rate may, eventually, be reached, where the capacity of the accessory pathway to conduct anterograde, is exceeded, so that all forward conduction must travel over the AV node, at which point the QRS complex and the PR interval normalize. The rate at which anterograde preexcitation is blocked correlates fairly well with the more accurate measurements of effective refractory periods, for the accessory pathway, obtained from electrophysiologic study. Many accessory pathways are capable of conducting at rates greater than the maximum achieved heart rate. ECG changes during exercise stress testing, such as false-positive ST segment depression and disappearance of the delta wave, are reported in patients with the Wolff-Parkinson-White (WPW) pattern. We present a case of exercise testing in a 53-year-old man with WPW syndrome with ischemic-appearing ECG changes and normal nuclear stress perfusion study findings who was thought to be at clinically low risk for having significant coronary disease. A literature review is discussed. Although ST segment depression typical for ischemia occurs in half of the patients in whom WPW syndrome is reported, exercise testing is still an important tool in their evaluation. Data other than ECG response can be interpreted in the context of clinical history and physical examination findings to stratify the risk of coronary disease. Complete and sudden disappearance of the delta wave has been seen during exercise in 20% of patients with WPW syndrome and can identify those who are at low risk for sudden arrhythmic death (Fig. 8.35).

CONCLUSION

False-positive ST segments are common during exercise testing in WPW syndrome patients, occurring in 49% of cases, regardless of the persistence or absence of the delta wave. Nuclear exercise myocardial perfusion imaging is also associated with a high frequency of false-positive study results. However, exercise testing still is an important diagnostic tool in the evaluation of patients with WPW and should not be categorically avoided. Data such as exercise capacity, symptom reproduction, heart rate, and BP response to exercise, arrhythmia, and prognostic score indexes can be interpreted in the context of the clinical history and physical examination findings to stratify the risk of coronary disease. Nuclear myocardial perfusion imaging findings, when normal, can be reassuring. Conversely, in patients who are thought to be at a higher

Table 8.11: *Stress testing in valve disease: key points*

- Most valvular heart diseases have a dynamic component
- Exercise testing, exercise echocardiography and dobutamine stress echocardiography are the most frequent stress modalities
- Exercise testing is recommended in asymptomatic severe aortic stenosis. A normal exercise test predicts good short term (10 years) outcome
- In symptomatic patients with low gradient aortic stenosis, dobutamine stress echocardiography should be performed to distinguish relative from fixed aortic stenosis. Patients with fixed aortic stenosis, but without contractile reserve by dobutamine stress testing, have a high operative mortality compared with patients with contractile reserve
- In patients with mitral stenosis, the severity of exerciseinduced increases in mean pressure gradient and estimated pulmonary pressures can help in decision making
- Postexercise echocardiography helps to identify patients operated for severe organic mitral regurgitation who are at risk of postoperative left ventricular dysfunction. They are characterised by a larger left ventricular endsystolic volume index and a low contractile reserve
- Ischemic mitral regurgitation is characteristically dynamic. Exerciseinduced changes in effective regurgitant orifice (ERO) area are not predictable by any measurement made at rest
- A large increase in ERO area is associated with a high risk of mortality and of decompensated heart failure

risk for having significant atherosclerosis, a definitive evaluation with coronary angiography should be considered. Finally, the sudden and complete disappearance of the delta wave can be used to identify patients with WPW syndrome who are at low risk for sudden death, and may be a useful noninvasive adjunct to the evaluation of otherwise asymptomatic individuals with structurally normal hearts.

BIBLIOGRAPHY

1. ACP/ACC/AHA. Task Force on Exercise Testing. JACC 1990; 16(5):1061–1065.
2. Ades P A. Grunvald MH. Cardio-pulmonary exercise testing before and after conditioning in older coronary patients, Am. Heart J. 1990, 120:585–589.
3. Ades PAt, Waldmann ML, Gillespie C. A controlled trial of exercise training in older coronary patients. 1. Genontol A Bio. Sci Med. Sci. 1995, 50 A: M7–Mll.
4. Armon Y, Cooper DM, Flores R, Zanconato S. Basstow TJ. Oxygen uptake dynamics during high intensity exercise in children and adults. 1. Apply Physiol., 1991, 70 : 841–848.
5. Becker RC, Alpert JS: Electrocardiographic ST segment depression in coronary heart disease. Am Heart J 1988; 1I5: 862–868.
6. Brouster JP, Douard H, Mora B. Exercise testing in arrhythmias of idiopathic mitral valve prolapse. Eur. Heart 1. 1987; 8 (suppl D):37–42.
7. Bruce RA. Blackmon JR, Jones JW, Strait G. Exercising testing in adult normal subjects and cardiac patients. Pediatrics 1963; 32 (suppl): 742–756.
8. Bruce RA. Fisher ID, Pettinger M, Weiner DA, Chaitman BR. ST segment elevation with exercise: A marker for poor ventricular function and poor prognosis. Circulation 1988; 77: 897–905.
9. Bruce RA, Kusumi F, Hosma D. Maximal oxygen intake and nomographic assessment of functional aerobic impairment in cardiovascular disease. Am Heart J 1973;85: 546–562.
10. Chandrashekhar Y, Anand IS. Can common exercise indices determine peak oxygen consumption. Indian Heart J 1993 ; 45 : 493–495.
11. Chandrashekhar Y, Anand IS. Do haemodynamic indices correlate with maximum exercise capacity and oxygen consumption in chronic congestive failure. Indian Heart J 1992; 44 : 19–22.
12. Cohen-Solal at al. Post-exercise recovery of oxygen consumption in CHF Circulation 1995,91 : 2924–2932. Cohn IN (ed): Quantitative exercise testing/or the cardiac patient: The value of monitoring gas exchanges : Introduction. Circulation 1987; 76 (Suppl. VI : VI-I-VI-2).
13. Dagenais GR, Rouleau JR, Hochart P, Magrina J, Cantin B, Dumesnil JG. Survival with painless strongly positive exercise electrocardiogram. Am J Cardiol 1988; 62:892–895.
14. Damate AN, Galante JG, Smith WM. Haemodynamic response to treadmill exercise in normal subjects. J Appl. Physiol. 1966, 21:959–966.

9 24-Hours Ambulatory Electrocardiography (Holter Monitoring) in Children and Adolescents

Ambulatory electrocardiography (ECG) has become an important tool in the noninvasive assessment of suspected dysrhythmia.

Cardiac dysrhythmias have been reported to occur in 2% of healthy children and in 4% of children with cardiac lesions (Fig. 9.1).

Holter monitoring, the long-term recording of one or two electrocardiographic leads on a portable tape recorder is useful in the diagnosis of dysrhythmias likely to occur but not revealed by routine ECG.

Clinical situations in which Holter monitor recording is indicated include assessment of certain patients following corrective open heart surgery; evaluation of complaints suggestive of episodic tachycardia unexplained syncope; unexplained sudden death in a close family member of young age near-miss sudden infant death syndrome; mitral valve prolapse associated with chest pain, palpitations, or syncope hypertrophic cardiomyopathy; evaluation of antiarrhythmic drug therapy; and evaluation of possible intermittent pacemaker failure.

All ambulatory ECG systems include a recorder, a scanner, and a data analysis system. The battery-powered recorder operates at very slow speed, allowing 24 hours of ECG data to be recorded on a standard cassette tape. It has a built-in timer which is used in conjunction with a patient diary to allow subsequent correlation of symptoms and activities. The scanner is a playback unit that permits rapid review of the tape for documentation of normal and abnormal rhythms. The data analysis system then permits quantitation of dysrhythmias (Fig. 9.2).

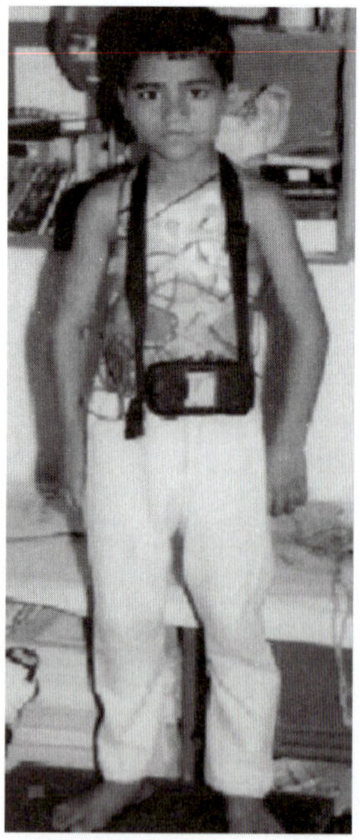

Fig. 9.1: *Photograph showing different leads on the chest along with recorder of Holter-monitoring system in a 12-year-old child with recurrent syncopal attacks and irregular pulse*

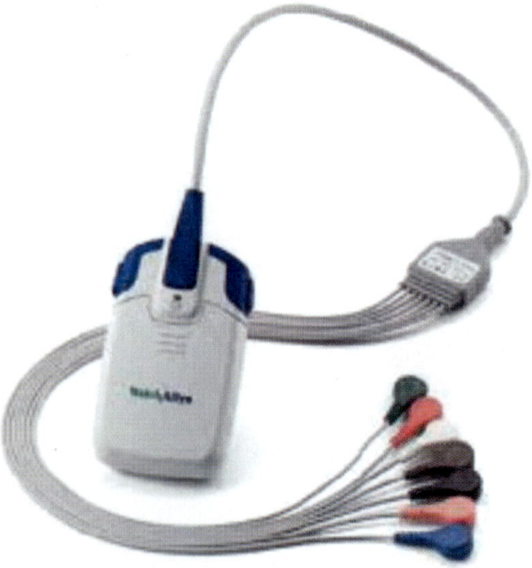

Fig. 9.2: *Holter recorder features*

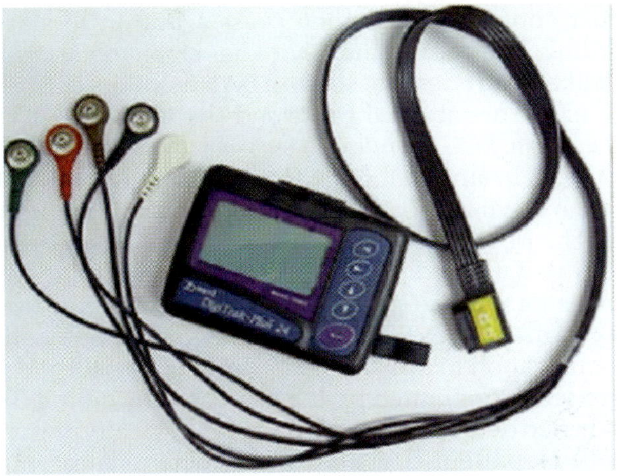

Fig. 9.3: *Showing Holter monitoring system in current use*

Application of ambulatory monitoring techniques for children has been made possible by the reduction in size and weight of the monitoring and recording unit. Many recorders weigh less than 1 lb, allowing easy use in toddlers and infants. Modern Holter systems also continuously record two simultaneous ECG channels for up to 48 hours on a single cassette tape. The two-lead system is especially important in young children for distinguishing artifacts, such as transient lead contact interruption from dysrhythmias.

The usual term of an ambulatory electrocardiogram (EKG or ECG) (Holter monitor recording) means the graphic recording, on magnetic tape, of all cardiac cycles, for periods up to or in excess of 24 hours. The basic knowledge of this technique differs from other methods of intermittent surveillance of the electrocardiogram, in which the recording of only a segment of cardiac electrical activity is allowed for, and, therefore, these other methods cannot be considered to be true. It was for the first time, Holter, in 1949, demonstrated the transmission of electrocardiographic waves by means of radiofrequencies. Later, further developments, by Holter and his colleagues, led to the introduction of the first magnetic tape recording unit.

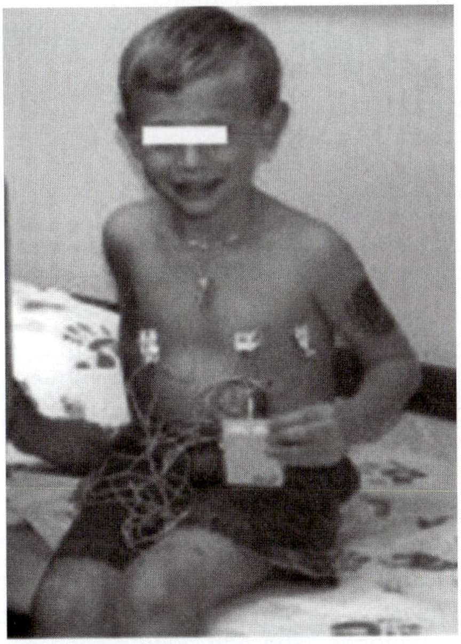

Fig. 9.4: *Photograph showing different leads on the chest along with recorder of Holter-monitoring system in a 6-year-old child with recurrent palpitation*

Subsequently, this method of electrocardiographic recording, over a prolonged period, became the routine technique of choice, in the investigation of ischemic and dysrhythmic heart diseases.

Subsequently, owing to significant advances in electronic component design, the quality and improvement in recordings including multichannel devices, its scope in clinical cardiology has been widened. This technique can be studied in the following modes of application:

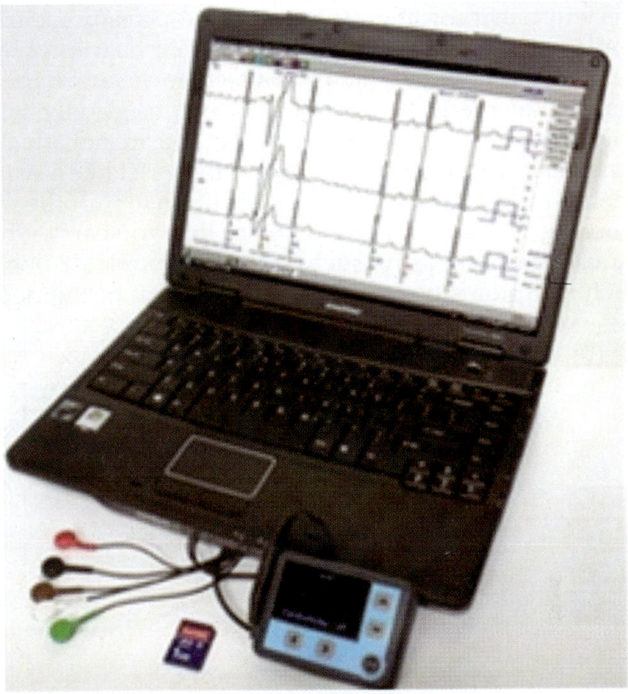

Fig. 9.5: *Holter recording and analyzing system*

RECORDING TECHNIQUES

These are further subgrouped into:

(a) **Method of continuous recording with every beat recorded and available for analysis.**
(b) Event recorders
(c) Microcomputers
(d) Transmitters for online or stored transtelephonic sending of ECG signals during a detected arrhythmia or during symptoms.
(e) **The combination of all the methods (Figs 9.2 to 9.5)**

Many heart problems become noticeable only during activity, such as exercise, eating, sex, stress, bowel movements, or even sleeping. A continuous 24-hour recording is more likely to detect any abnormal heartbeats that occur during these activities. Many people have irregular heartbeats (arrhythmias) from time to time. The importance of irregular heartbeats depends on the type of pattern they produce, how often they occur, how long they last, and whether they occur at the same time you have symptoms. Because arrhythmias can occur off and on, it may be difficult to record an arrhythmia while you are in the doctor's office. There are several different types of ambulatory monitors.

Continuous Recorders (Fig. 9.6)

The most common type is the continuous recorder. It provides a 24–72 hour record of the electrical signals phone to a doctor's office, clinic, or hospital. Two types of intermittent recorders are available:

Loop recorders: A loop recorder constantly records your heart beats. When you have symptoms, you press a button on the monitor to record your heart rhythm. Loop recorders also save a small amount of information about how your heart was beating when you pressed the recording button (presymptom recording). This feature is especially useful for people who lose consciousness when their heart problems occur and can press the button only after they wake up (Fig. 9.8).

Event recorders: This small device is used only when symptoms of the heart problem occur. You are not attached to the machine. One type is worn on the wrist like a watch. When symptoms occur, you press a button to start the EKG recording. The other type is a device that you carry where you can reach it easily, such as in your purse or pocket. When symptoms occur, you press the back of the device against your chest and then press a button to start the recording. The back of the device has small metal disk that work like electrodes. These hand held monitors can be very small (some are about the size and shape of a credit card).

Long-term ECG monitoring system: It has been recently introduced in ambulatory ECG monitoring system that can record and wirelessly transmit heartbeat data for up to 30 days. The device provides immediate online access of all transmitted ECG data. Designed for the diagnosis and management of atrial fibrillation and other cardiac arrhythmias, the TruVue ECG system uses cellular communication to transmit recordings of heartbeat data to secure servers operated by the company. Incoming data is analyzed to detect changes in morphology, rate, or rhythm, as well as patient-triggered alerts when symptoms are experienced. The company employs certified cardiac technicians to validate the findings from the technology. The technicians post real-time reports and notify physicians based on cardiac events or notification criteria.

Risks

There is no risk from ambulatory EKG monitoring. The electrodes placed on your skin detect only the electrical signals from your heart. No electricity is sent through your body, and there is no possibility of receiving an electric

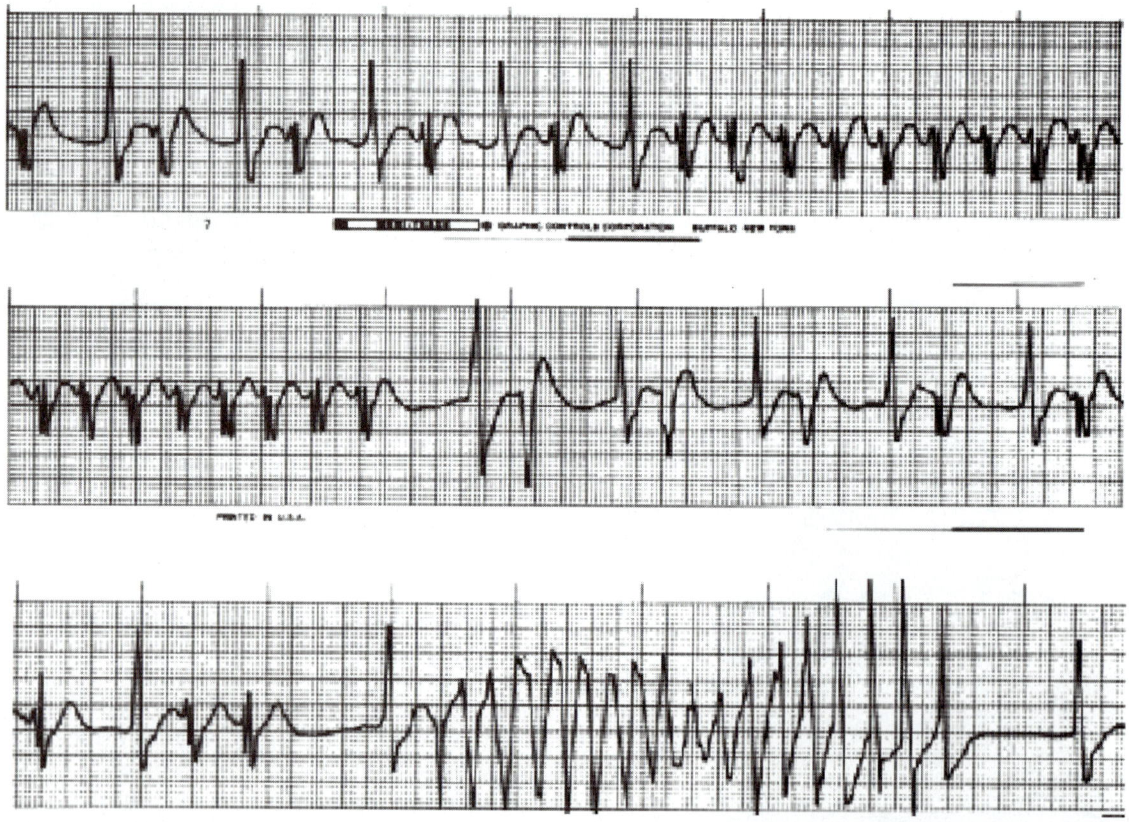

Fig. 9.6: *A continuous rhythm strip from a 14-year-old girl who had undergone repair of tetralogy of Fallot but who had persistently elevated right ventricular pressure due to multiple peripheral pulmonary artery stenoses. She had been placed on quinidine for asymptomatic nonsustained ventricular tachycardia by Holter monitoring. Illustrated is monomorphic ventricular bigeminy, nonsustained monomorphic ventricular tachycardia, and a 4 second episode of polymorphic ventricular tachycardia (torsade de pointes). The latter was a proarrhythmic response to the quinidine*

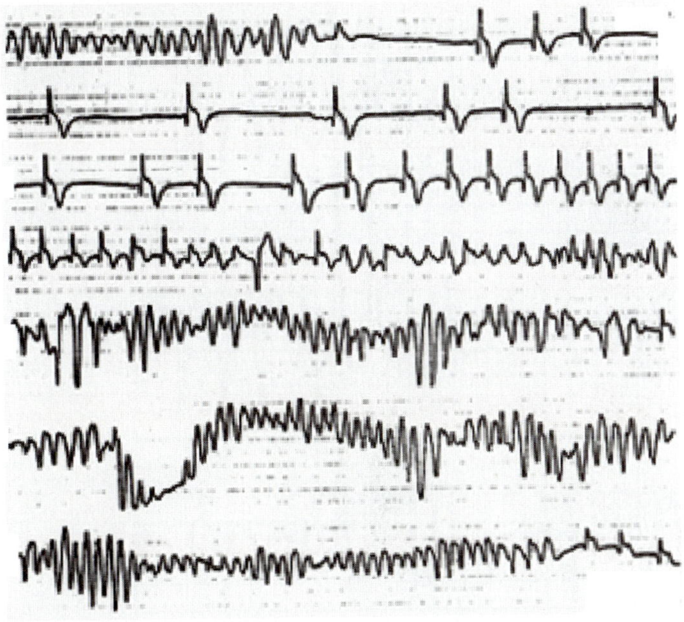

Fig. 9.7: *Showing Holter recording during a syncope showing a polymorphic ventricular tachycardia, ventricular fibrillation with a spontaneous conversion in transient sinoatrial block with postcritical repolarization changes and then a sinus tachycardia, polymorphic ventricular premature beats, and another episode of polymorphic ventricular tachycardia (30 seconds)*

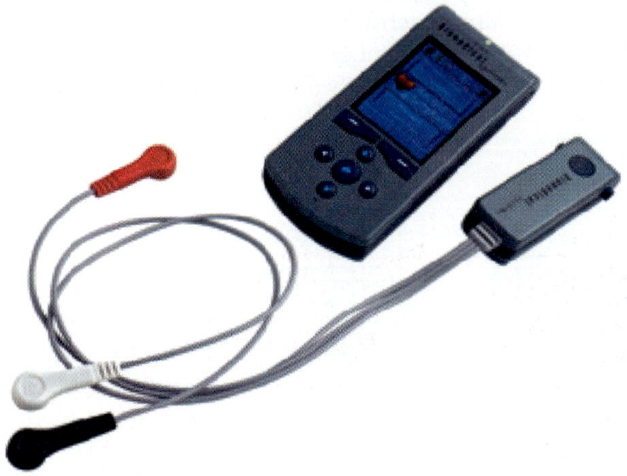

Fig 9.8: *Long-term ECG-monitoring system offers advanced arrhythmia analysis*

shock symptoms that commonly lead to suspicion of arrhythmia are palpitations, syncope, presyncope, or congestive heart failure. The physician must evaluate the patient's overall status, rather than the rhythm disturbance in isolation.

Indications for Holter Monitoring (Figs 9.7–9.12)

- Detection of a suspected rhythm disturbance
- Syncope work-up (Figs 9.7 and 9.11)
- Evaluation after myocardial infarction (MI)
- Evaluation of high-risk cardiac patient
- Risk stratification

Evaluation after cardiac surgery (Fig. 9.20)

- Diagnosis of silent ischemia' (Fig. 9.40)
- Diagnosis of suspected myocardial ischemia
- Evaluation of therapy, i.e. antiarrhythmic drugs, pacemaker function, cardiac ablation.

Evaluation of heart rate variability

The clinical setting has as great a significance as the arrhythmia on choice of work-up and possible risk to the patient. Some arrhythmias are potentially fatal regardless of the clinical setting, whereas others are potentially dangerous because of the clinical setting. The usual tests varies from the less expensive, simpler, noninvasive tests to tests that are more complex and invasive. Certain clinical circumstances, however, necessitate a more complex initial study (e.g. electrophysiology test). In the usual circumstance, Holter monitor and signal-averaged electrocardiogram (SA-EKG) are the first test: i.e. SA-EKG is especially

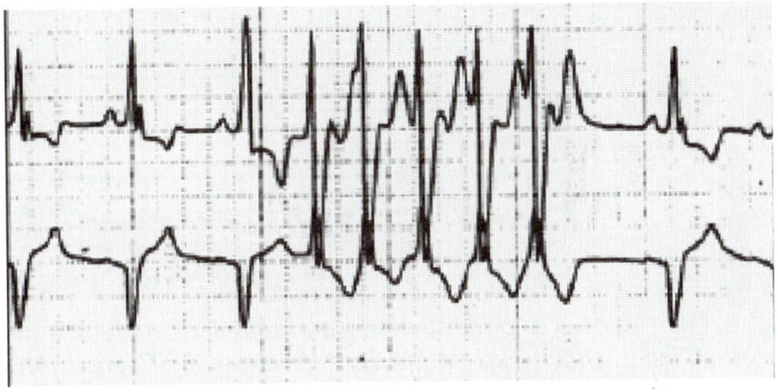

Fig. 9.9: *Two channel Holter recording strip with 5 beats run of ventricular tachycardia*

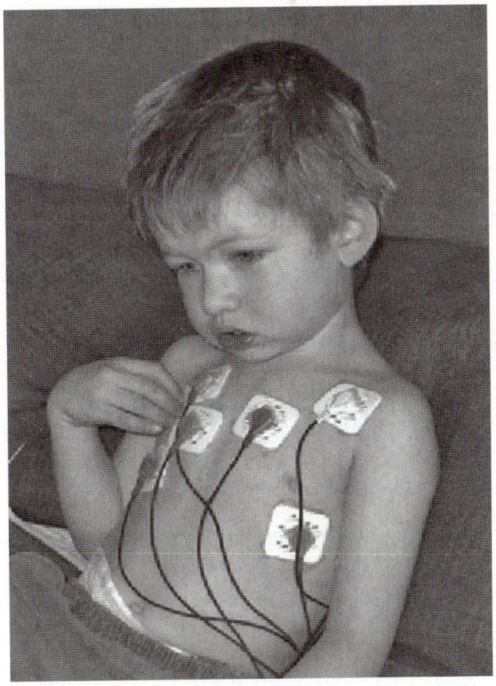

Fig. 9.10: *A 6-year-old boy is investigated for palpitations. Twelve-lead ECG is normal. A 24-hour Holter is reported to detect multiple episodes of nonsustained VT*

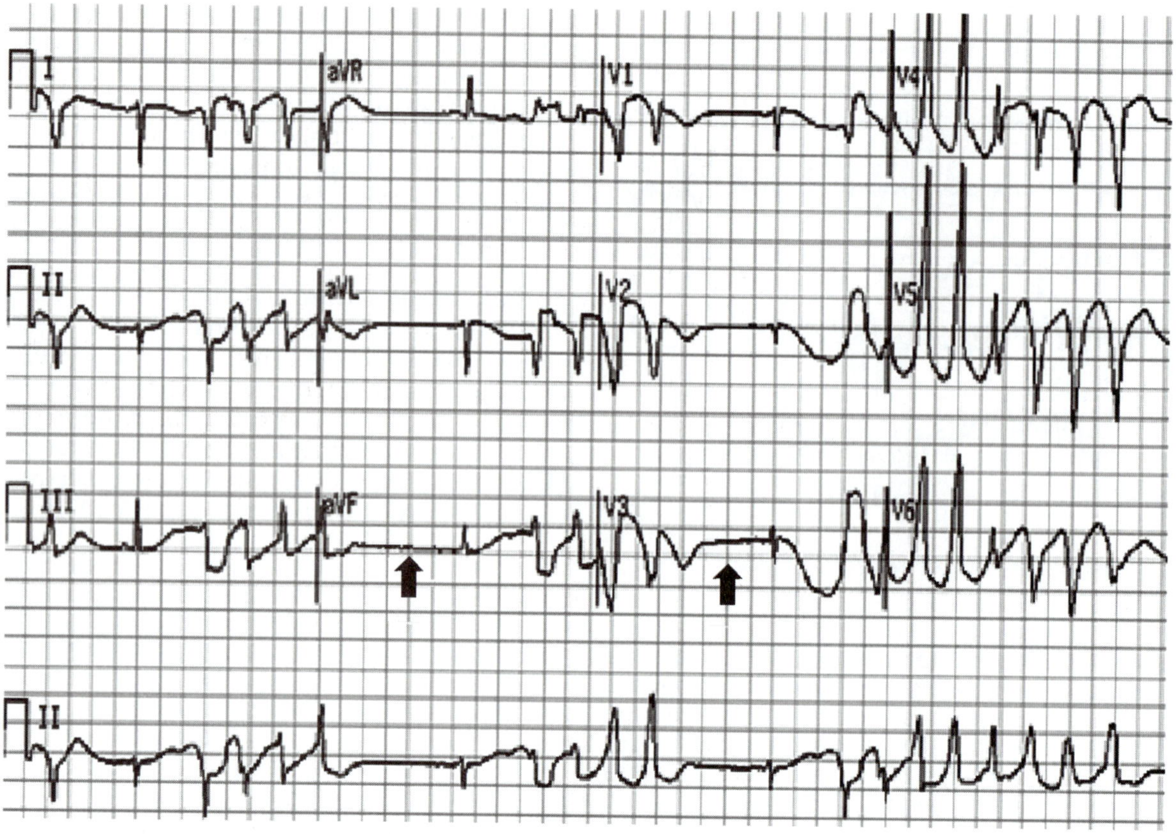

Fig. 9.11: *12 years of patient presented with syncope showed defects in ion channels predispose patients to episodes of torsade de pointes (TdP), which can cause cardiac arrest. TdP is a form of polymorphic ventricular tachycardia that results in a characteristic twisting of the QRS complex around the isoelectric baseline. This arrhythmia is associated with LQTS and can degenerate into more unstable rhythms. In the case of acquired LQTS, a pause usually precedes the onset of TdP. This form of TdP is said to be "pause dependent" (arrows). (Image courtesy of ECG wave-Maven).*

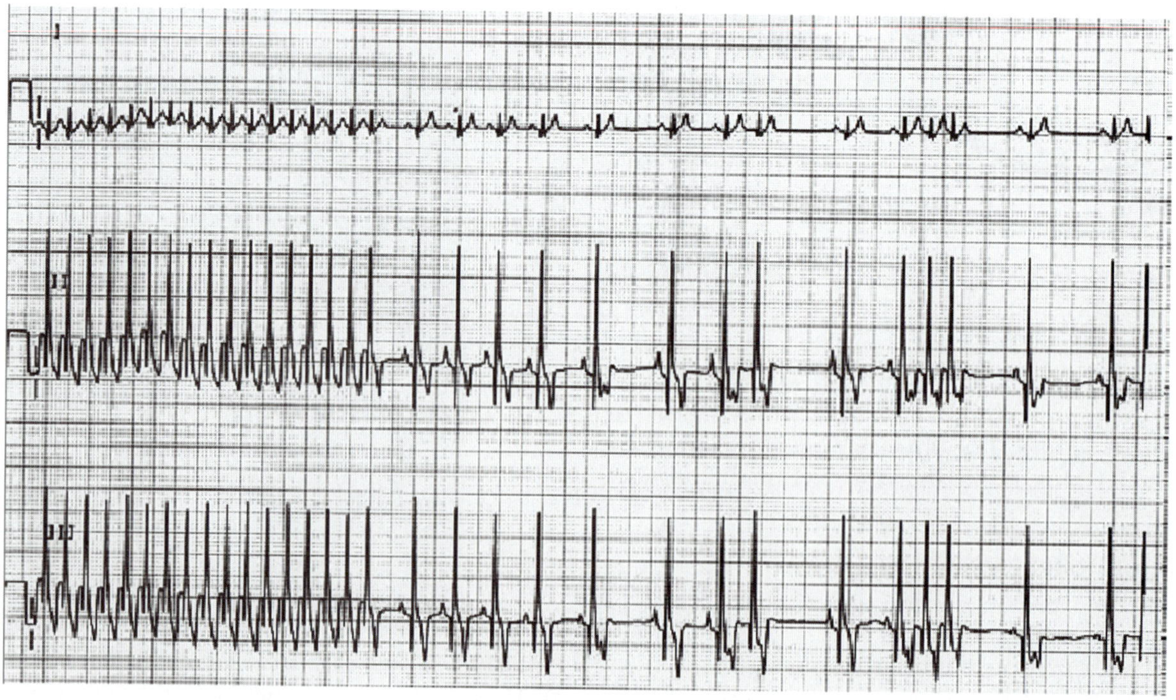

Fig. 9.12: *18-years-old patient presented with syncope showed episodes of supraventricular tachycardia*

appropriate If ventricular arrhythmias are expected: Individualize the type of Holter monitor to the patient, depending on associated symptoms as well as frequency and awareness of arrhythmia. An important consideration in the work-up of rhythm disturbance is underlying heart disease (e.g. valve disease, cardiomyopathy, MI). A resting EKG and echocardiogram may answer any questions and help to categorize the patient as high risk (e.g. low ejection fraction) or low risk (a normal ejection fraction and normal EKG). If the rhythm disturbance is associated with ischemia, an exercise stress test 'may be appropriate'. If the data are positive, or if a diagnosis is not established but symptoms or potentially fatal arrhythmias recur, order an electrophysiology test.

Holter Monitoring and Exercise Tolerance Testing (ETT)

During ETT about one-third of patients with normal hearts develop ventricular ectopy, usually occasional monomorphic pairs or even 3- to 6-beat nonsustained runs. Ectopy may occur in older patients with no coronary artery or other heart disease and is not a predictor of increased mortality or morbidity. Although ETT is more sensitive than a resting, standard 12-lead EKG in detecting ventricular arrhythmias, a Holter monitor is more sensitive than ETT. However, because each may uncover serious arrhythmias that the other does not detect, both tests may be indicated in selected patients, such as those with known or suspected coronary artery disease (CAD).

Positive Holter Results

It is rather uncommon for healthy, young persons to have significant rhythm disturbances; in fact, several arrhythmias are not necessarily abnormal including sinus bradycardias (35–40 beats/minute), sinus arrhythmias (with pauses up to 3 seconds), sinoatrial exit block, Wenckenbach block (second-degree AV block type I), wandering atrial pacemaker, junctional escape complexes, and premature atrial or ventricular contractions. Of concern are frequent and complex atrial and ventricular rhythm disturbances that are less commonly observed in normal subjects including second-degree AV block type II, sinus pauses >3 seconds, and brady- or tachyarrhythmias associated with symptoms. Results of the Holter monitor need to be analyzed with the diary to correlate specific symptoms to the rhythm and rate recorded.

Heart Rate and Rhythm Values in Various Age Groups

Full-term Neonates

Cardiac conduction abnormalities frequent enough to be detected by 12-lead ECG occur in 1% of normal newborns. However, numerous recent studies utilizing 24-hour Holter monitor recordings have now demonstrated that variations in rate and rhythm previously thought to be abnormal in the newborn actually occur quite frequently.

Junctional rhythm was detected in 28% of these infants. Premature ventricular contractions were seen in 4% while another 4% had supraventricular tachycardia.

Premature atrial contractions, the most common dysrhythmia observed in newborns, were seen in 14% of these infants. Sinus pauses were quite frequent, occurring in 72% while 2:1 sinus exit block was seen in 11%.

Southall et al. obtained standard ECGs on 3,383 healthy newborns. Fourteen infants had premature atrial and 11 had premature ventricular contractions. Ventricular tachycardia (200–220 beats/minute) was identified by 24-hour recording in three of eight infants that had demonstrated only premature ventricular contractions on their standard ECGs. Follow-up standard or 24-hour ECGs failed to detect these dysrhythmias after 12 weeks of age. There appears to be a wide range of bradyarrhythmias and tachyarrhythmias in the normal newborn. Indeed, the sinus rate in many neonates can be as low as 75 beats/minute. Ectopy also seems to occur frequently. In the absence of structural heart disease, these dysrhythmias seem to have

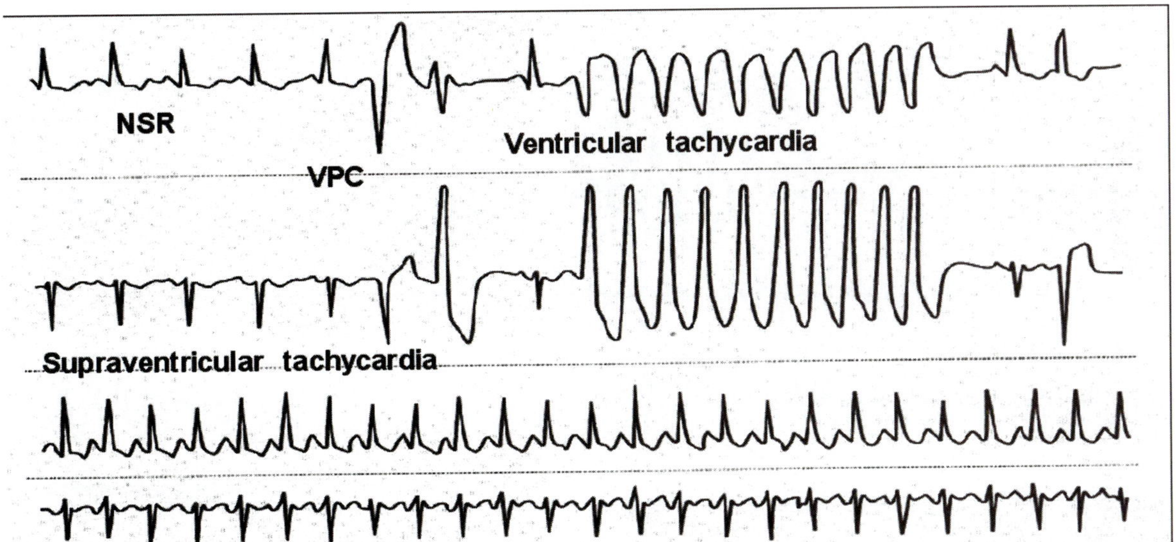

Fig. 9.13: *Holter graph showing ventricular tachycardia in patient with heart failure*

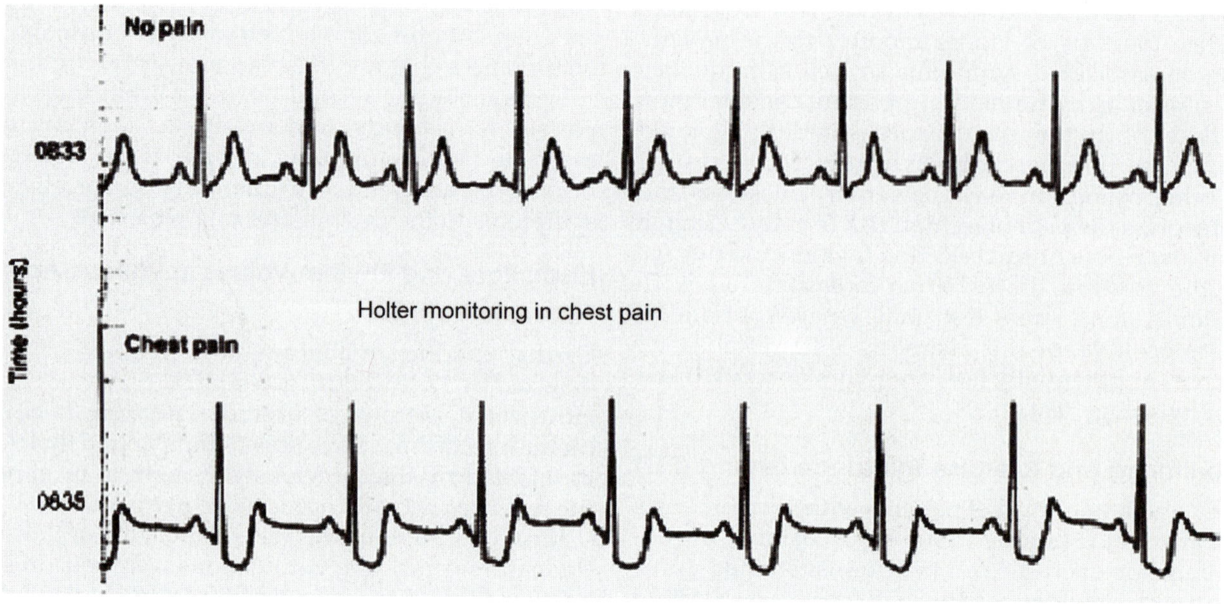

Fig. 9.14: *4.8 Graph (upper panel) normal sinus rhythm at 0833 hours and chest pain with significant ST segment depression at 0855 hours (bottom) on Holter monitor recording of an adolescent patient suffering from silent ischemia*

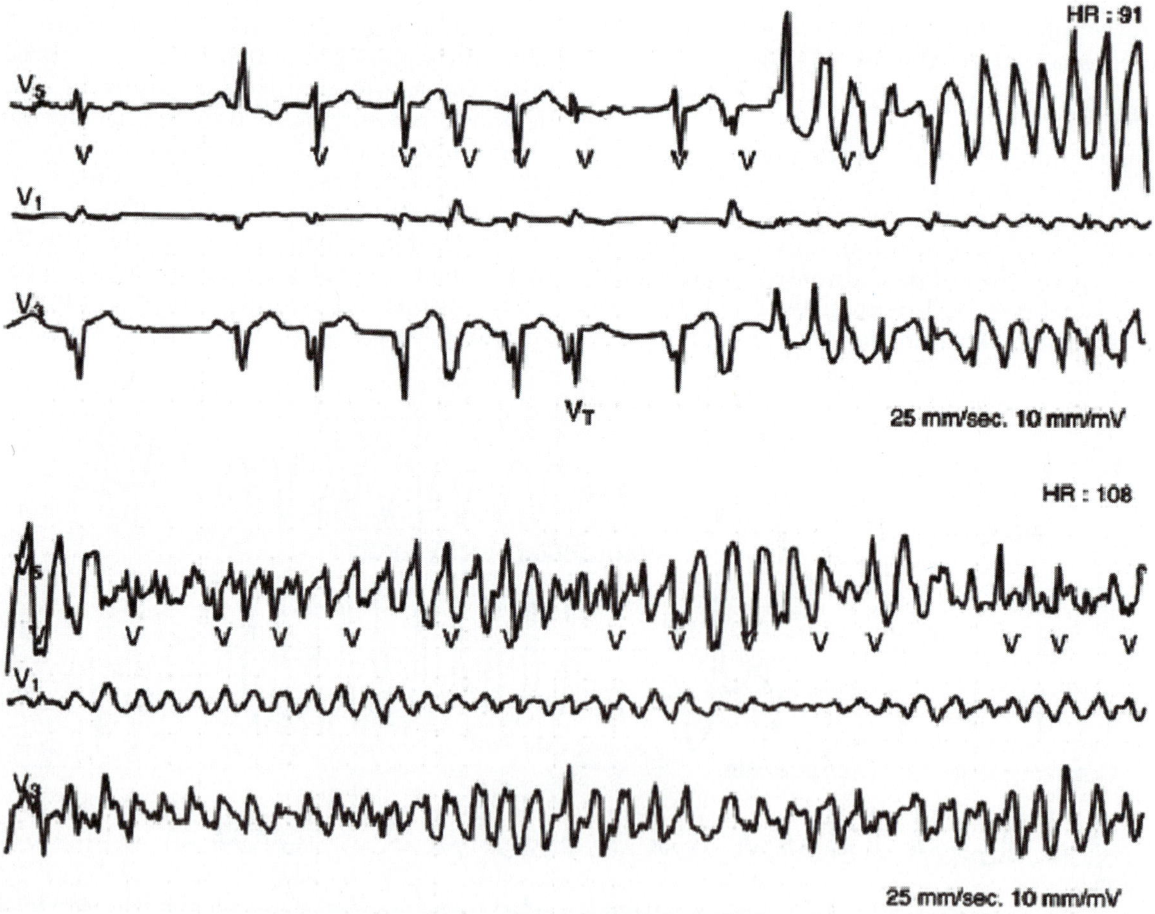

Fig. 9.15: *Holter study shows varying types of cardiac arrhythmia starting from premature ventricular ectopic, sustained VT (two bottom strips) in patient with hypertrophic obstructive cardiomyopathy*

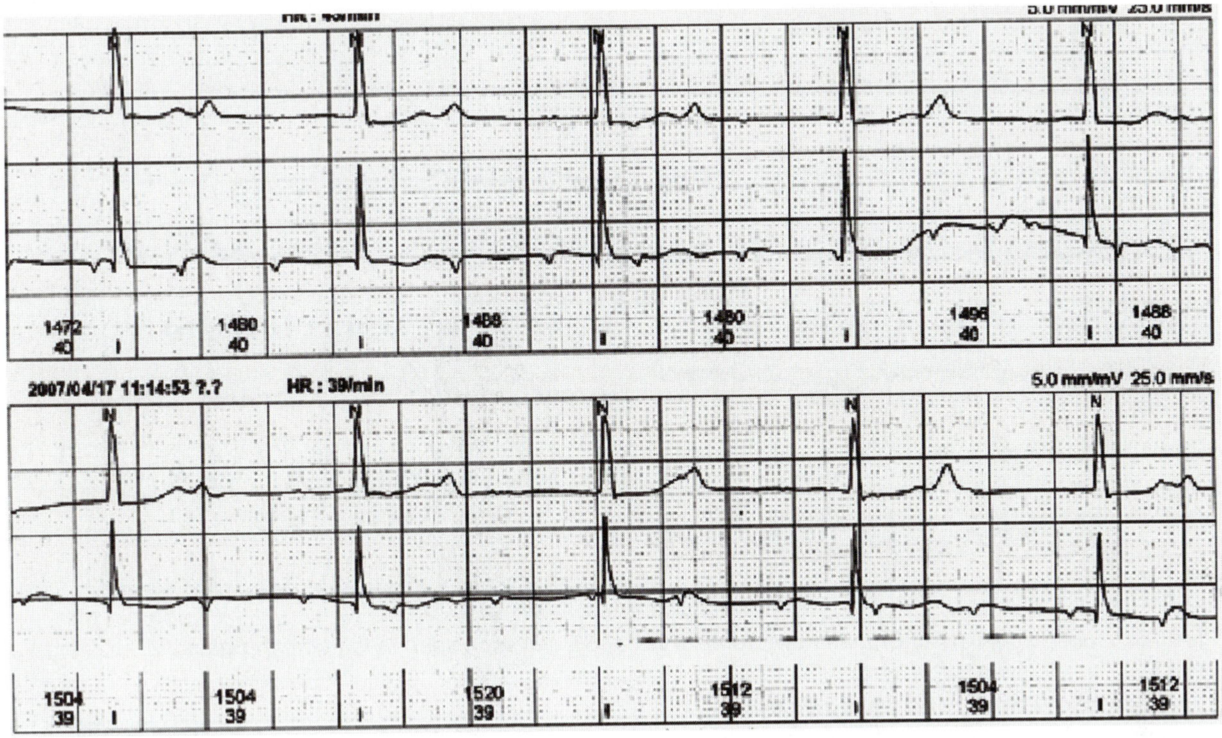

Fig. 9.16: *Holter-recording showing complete heart block in an adolescent who complained of attacks of palpitations and syncope*

a benign prognosis. However, further long-term studies are needed to more fully define the natural history of dysrhythmias in these infants.

Premature and Low-birth-weight Infants

In one Holter study of 100 preterm or low-birth-weight infants, the mean minimum heart rate was 91+: 18 beats/minute. Junctional rhythm was observed in 18% of these babies. Premature atrial contractions occurred in only 2%, and premature ventricular contractions were seen in 6%. In another study of 30 premature infants with birth weight less than 1,500 gm, sinus arrhythmia was seen in 100%. Other dysrhythmias were seen in 90% of these infants including sudden sinus bradycardia of 90 beats/minute or less in 27 babies and sinus arrest of up to 2 seconds' duration in two.

Most of these dysrhythmias were observed with autonomic stimulation.

Marsico et al. obtained Holter recordings in 60 premature infants with a mean gestational age of 33 weeks and a mean birth weight of 1,852 gm. Heart rates ranged from 77 to 211 beats/minute. Sudden sinus pauses not preceded by sinus arrhythmia occurred frequently. Premature atrial contractions occurred in 33% of these infants, while premature ventricular contractions were observed in 17%. There appears to be a high frequency of dysrhythmias in healthy, premature infants. The minimum heart rate in many of these babies can be as low as 73 beats/minute. Sudden sinus bradycardia as well as sinus pauses seem to occur especially frequently. Dysrhythmias, especially bradyarrhythmias, are seen more frequently in the preterm than in the term infant.

Older Children

In a study of 92 healthy 7- to 11-year-old children 24-hour Holter recordings demonstrated that the mean maximum heart rate was 164 :+17 beats/minute, while the mean minimum heart rate was 56 :+ 6 beats/minute. Premature atrial or ventricular contractions occurred in 21%, and the maximum duration of sinus pause was 1.36: + 0.23 seconds.

Scott et al. obtained 48-hour Holter recordings in 131 healthy boys aged 10–13 years. Minimum and maximum awake heart rates were 45–200 beats/minute, respectively, while the same values while sleeping were 30–110 beats/minute. In addition, junctional rhythm was present during sleep in 13% of these children. All had sinus arrhythmia. First-degree atrioventricular block was present in 8.4%,

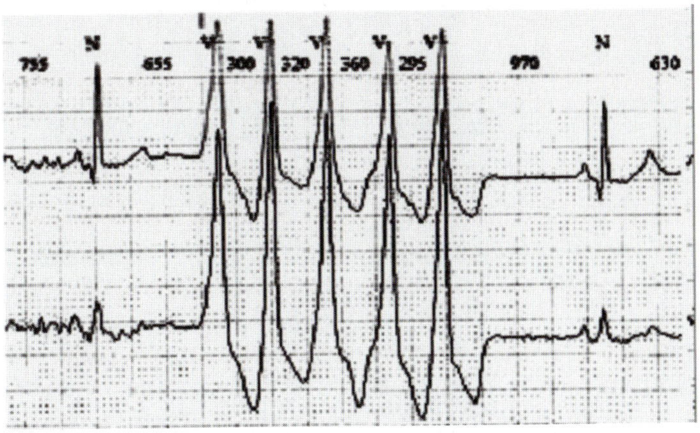

Fig. 9.17: *Holter strip showing nonsustained VT in a young child with recurrent attacks of palpitations and syncope*

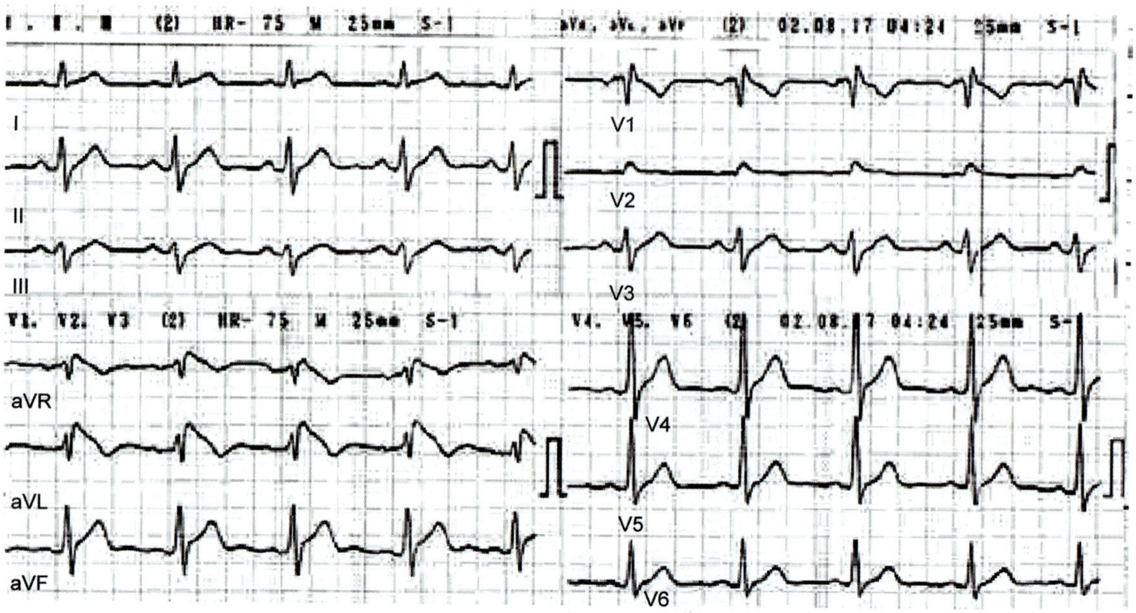

Fig. 9.18: *Holter diagnosis of Brugada syndrome. Typical ST elevation seen in left bottom traces (V1–V2 and V3)*

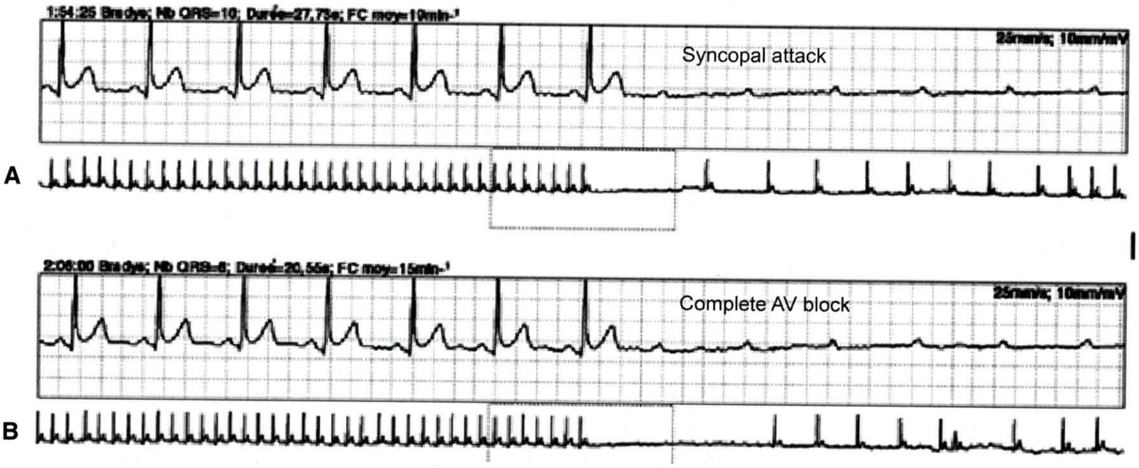

Fig. 9.19: *(A, B) Holter recording of two episodes of spontaneous syncope that occurred a few minutes apart. The two episodes were very similar and were characterized by sudden-onset complete atrioventricular (AV) block without changes in P-P cycle length, which constantly remained 720 ms and long ventricular asystole of 7 and 11 s (top and bottom, compressed traces, respectively)*

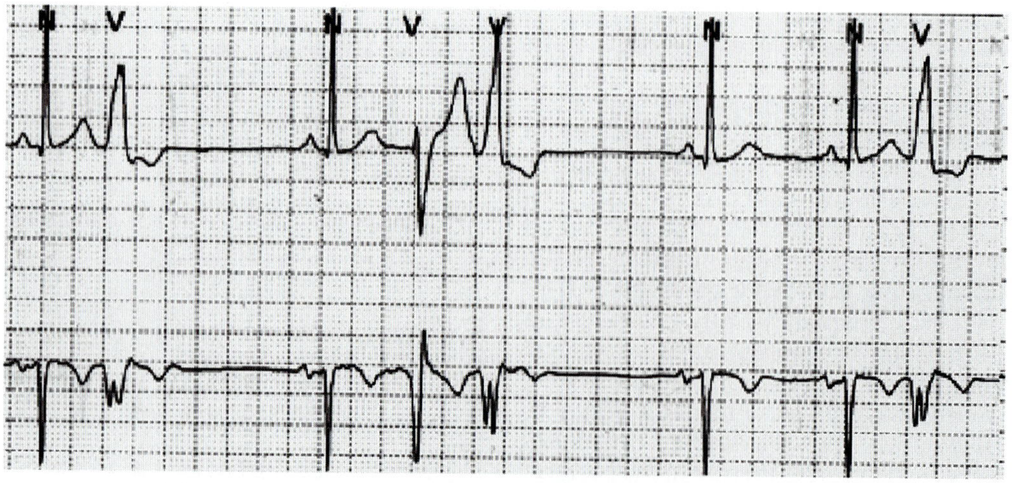

Fig. 9.20: *Polymorphic VPC on Holter after mustard operation*

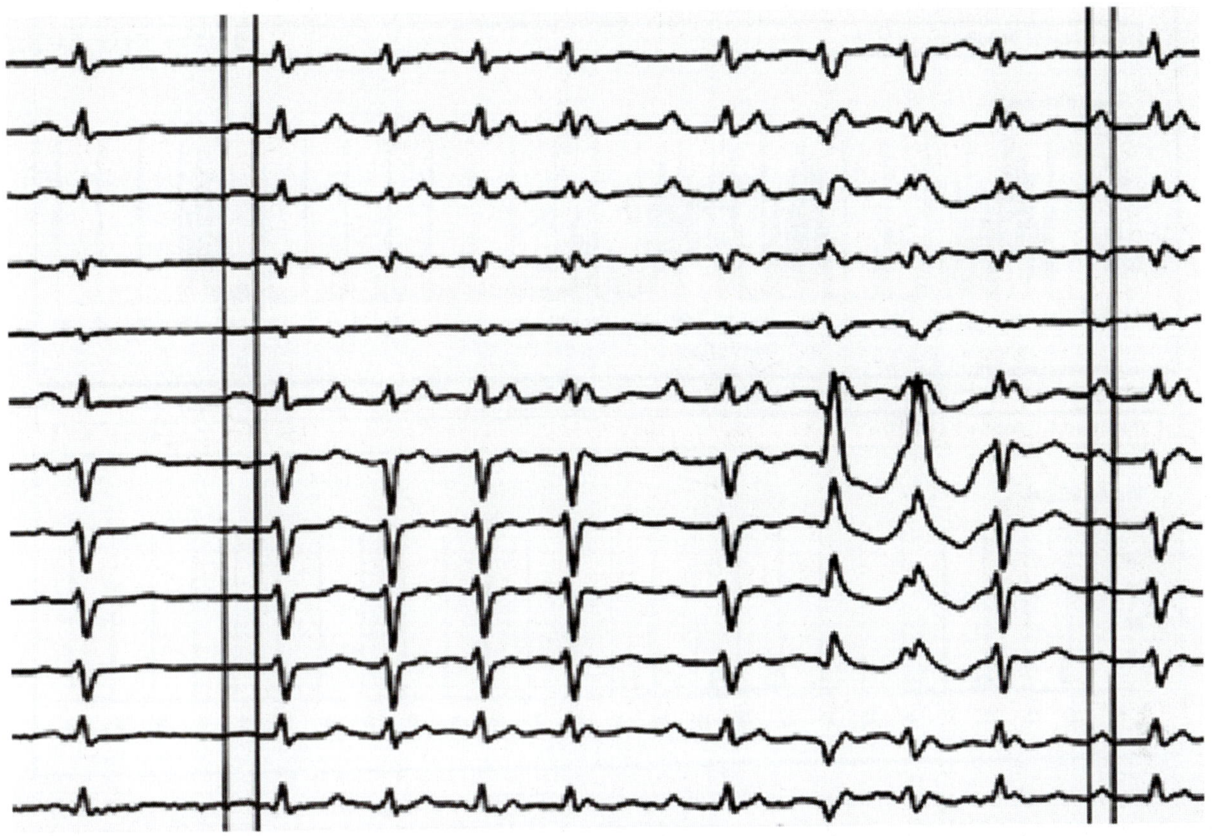

Fig. 9.21: *Holter monitor. Although the electrocardiography of atrial fibrillation is generally straightforward, the onset of arrhythmia (premature atrial contractions or monomorphic atrial tachycardia) should be determined because of the importance of triggers for atrial fibrillation. Such a determination may be done with the help Holter monitoring to guide physicians in counseling patients about atrial fibrillation ablation*

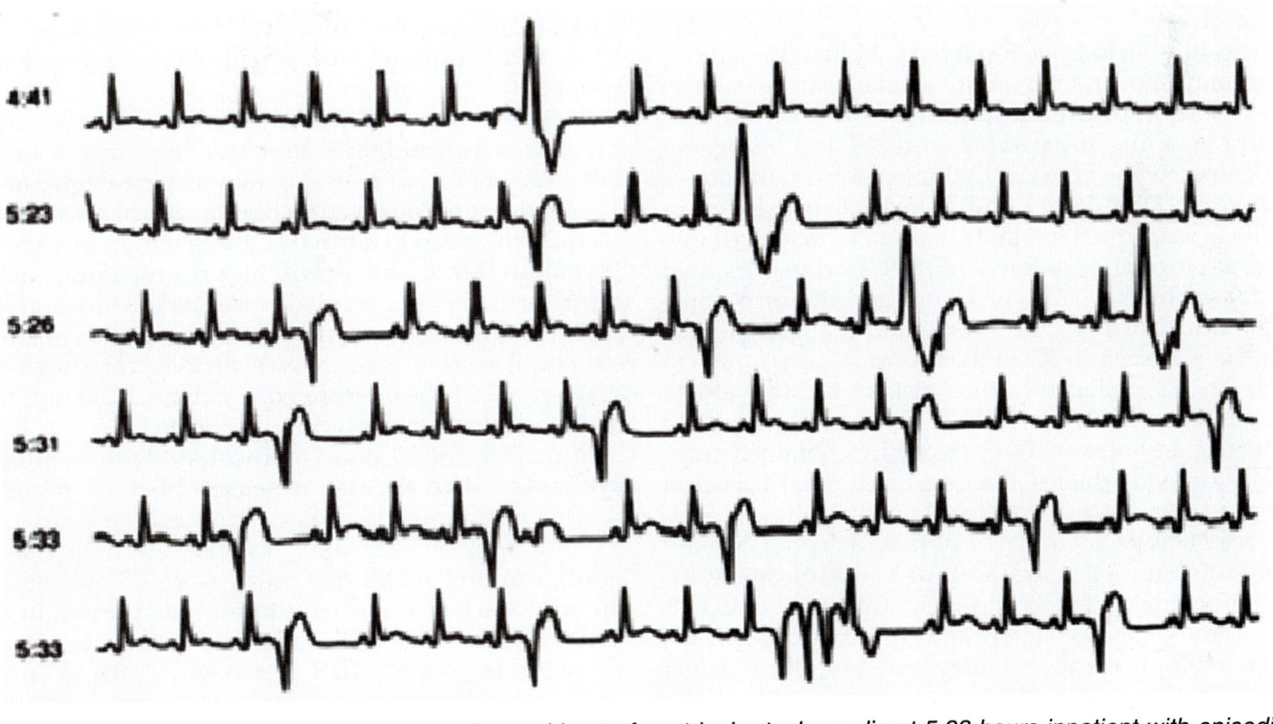

Fig. 9.22: *Holter graph showing ventricular ectopics and bout of ventricular tachycardia at 5.33 hours inpatient with episodic chest pain with palpitation*

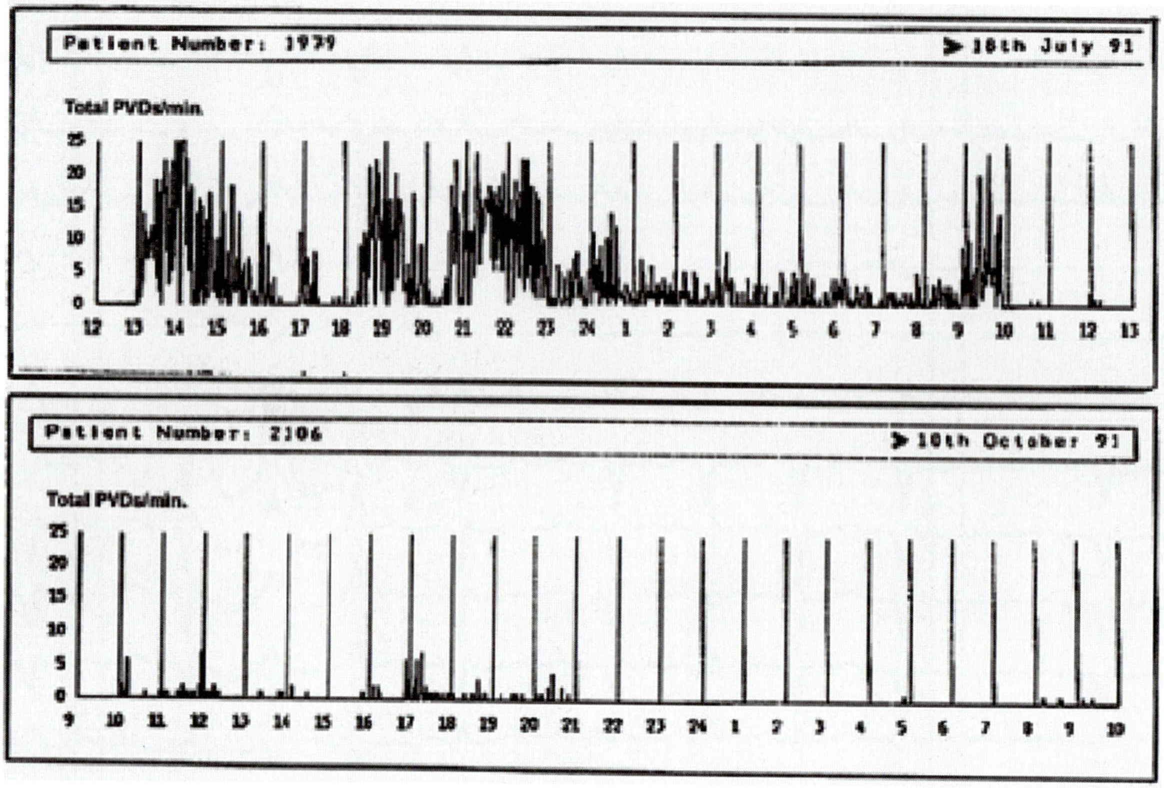

Fig. 9.23: *Arrhythmia trends during 24-hour Holter electrocardiogram (ECG) recordings showing marked reversibility of premature ventricular depolarizations (PVDs) after 3 months of deconditioning in a 18-year-old elite bobsledder. (Top panel) The 24-h ECG performed during peak training shows 3,288 PVDs, distributed relatively homogeneously, with a slight reduction evident during the evening hours. (Bottom panel) marked reduction in ventricular arrhythmias (to 73 PVDs) is evident after 3 months of physical deconditioning. The reduction of ventricular arrhythmia after detraining has occurred throughout the 24-h recording period*

while 10.7% had Wenckebach periodicity. Premature atrial and ventricular contractions were demonstrated in 13 and 26%, respectively.

In 100 healthy 14- to 16-year-old boys, 24-hour recordings revealed minimum and maximum awake heart rates of 45 and 200 beats/minute, respectively. Minimum and maximum sleeping heart rates were 23 and 95 beats/minute, respectively. Sinus arrhythmia was seen in each of these children. First-degree and Wenckebach atrioventricular block were present in 12 and 11%, respectively. Premature ventricular contractions (PVCs) were present in 41% of these children, 75% of whom had uniform while 25% had multiform PVCs. Nonsustained ventricular tachycardia was seen in 3% of these boys.

Frequently, the pediatric cardiologist is asked to evaluate teenage athletes for dysrhythmias. To properly evaluate the results of ambulatory ECG recordings obtained from endurance-trained athletes, the range of normal variation in this group of individuals must be known. Vi-itasalo et al. compared 24-hour recordings obtained from 35 male athletes between 14 years and 16 years of age with recordings obtained from 35 male non-athlete age-matched controls. The athletes had significantly ($p < 0.01$) lower heart rates both while awake and while asleep). In addition, sinus pauses longer than 2.0 seconds occurred in 14% of the athletes but only in 3% of the controls. First-degree atrioventricular block was seen in 23% of the athletes but was only seen in 11 % of the non-athletes. Similarly, atrioventricular Wenckebach was detected in 18% of the athletes but was seen in only 3% of the controls. In contrast, PVCs were observed with equally high frequency in both groups.

Based on these studies, it would seem that normal, asymptomatic children 7–16 years of age can have sleeping heart rates as low as 23 beats/minute. First-degree and type 1 second-degree atrioventricular block are also commonly seen during sleep in normal children within this age range. Premature atrial and ventricular contractions, including multiform PVCs, are also observed in normal young children and adolescents. Of course, if symptoms of structural heart disease are present, these otherwise normal findings should be interpreted as potentially abnormal, and further evaluation should be performed.

In a study of 50 male medical students without any known cardiovascular disease, 24-hour recordings revealed minimum and maximum awake heart rates of 53 and 141 beats/minute, respectively, while sleeping minimum and maximum rates were 43 and 86 beats/minute. Marked sinus arrhythmia was present in 50% of the students, while 28% had sinus pauses longer than 1. 75 seconds and 6% had atrioventricular Wenkebach periodicity. Premature atrial contractions (PACs) were present in 56% although only 2% had more than 100 P ACs/24 hours. Similarly, PVCs were seen in 50% but only

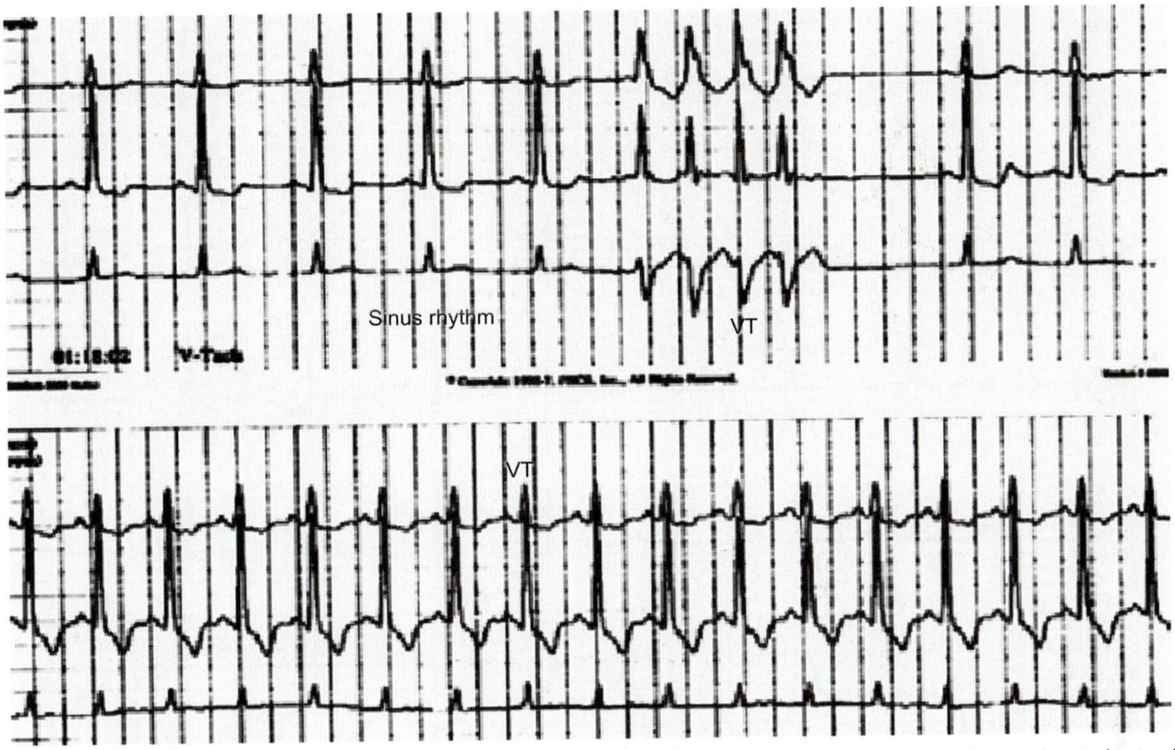

Fig. 9.24: *Holter graph showing ventricular tachycardia at 01;18;02 hours and SVT at 10;24;56 hours in patient with recurrent palpitation*

2% had more than 50 PVCs/24 hours. Thus, although premature atrial and ventricular contractions were seen in this young adult population, bradyarrhythmias were more predominant.

Evaluation of Postoperative Dysrhythmias

Many cardiologists obtain 24-hour recordings on patients following surgical procedures known to predispose to dysrhythmias. The standard 12-lead ECG has been

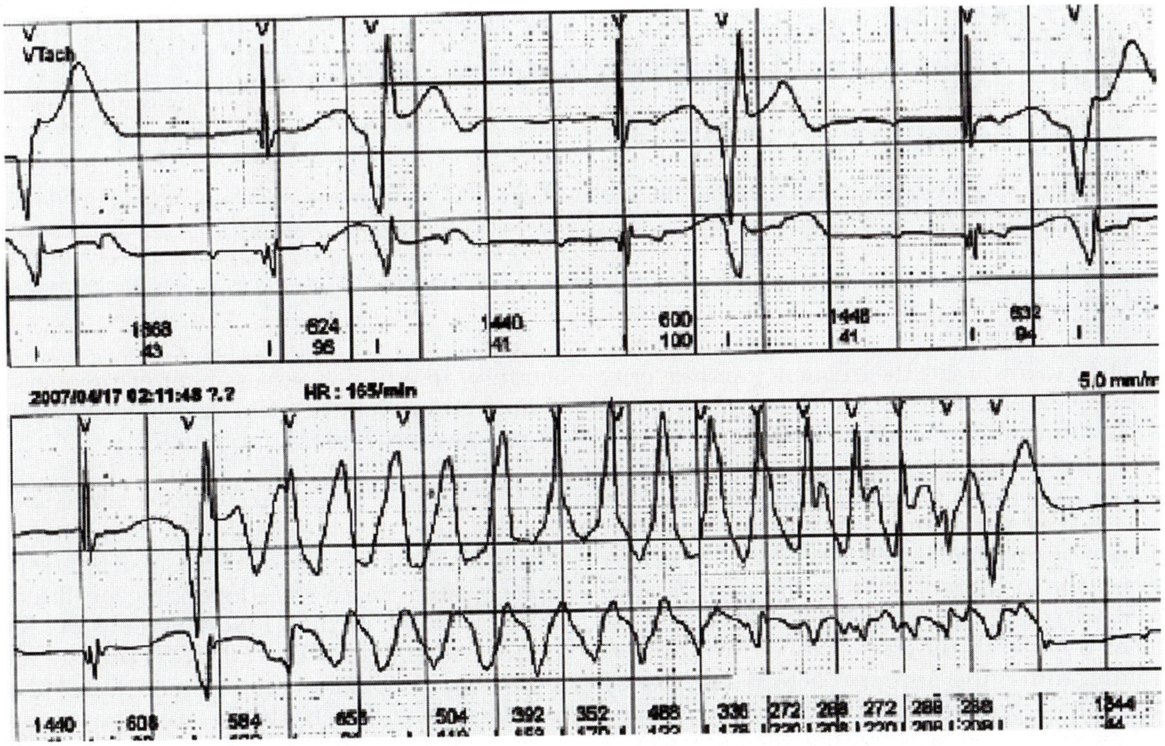

Fig. 9.25: *Holter monitor. Upper strip shows bigeminy pattern, lower strip shows ventricular tachycardia*

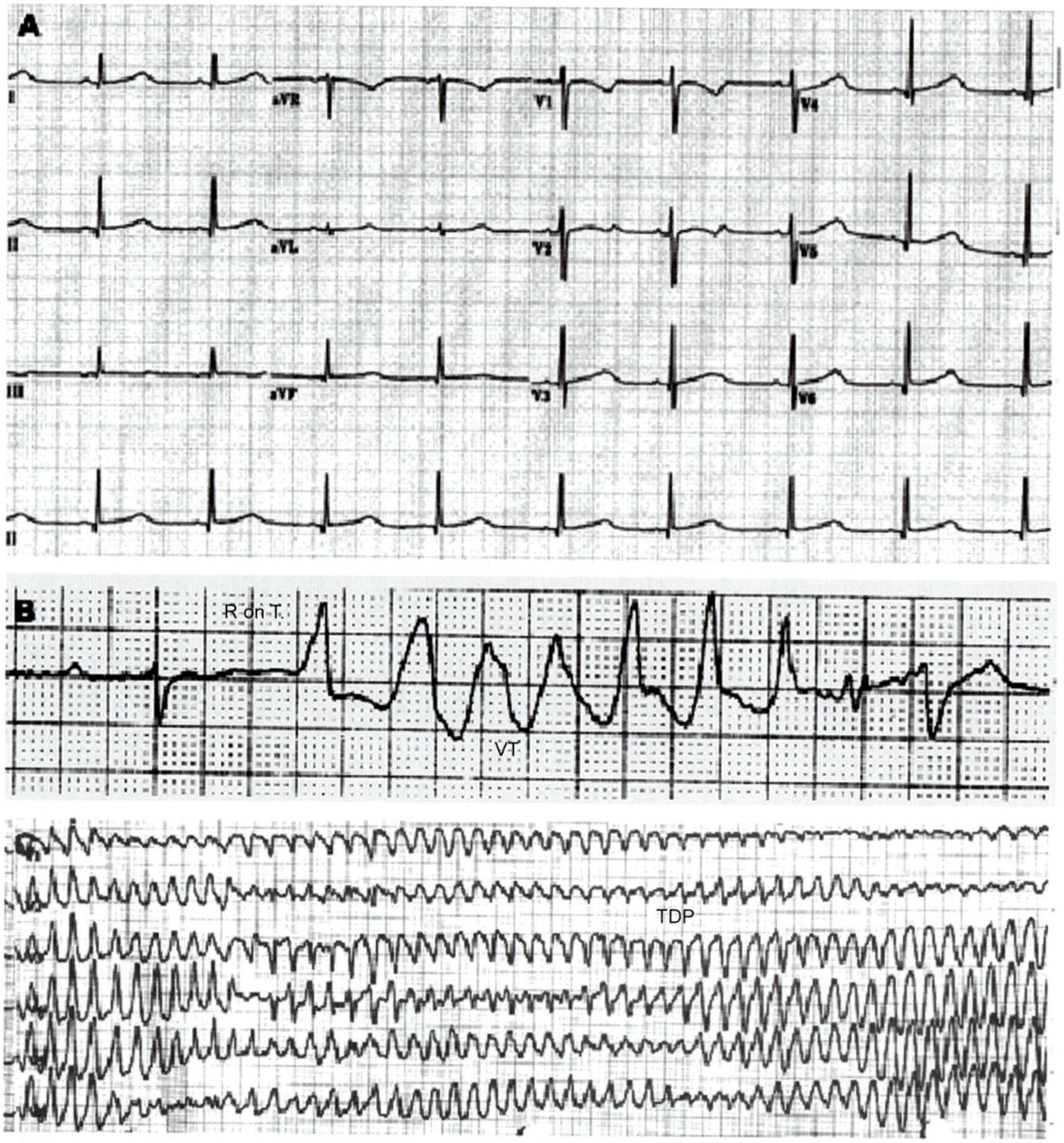

Fig. 9.26: *ECG findings in patient with Long QT syndrome type 2. (A) ECG of an 18-year-adolescent girl with recurrent syncope. As is typical in LQTS, the QTc interval is prolonged at 500 ms. The subtype of LQTS can be predicted from a detailed examination of the T-wave (Zhang et al. 2004). In this case, the biphasic T-waves in V2 and Lead III were consistent with a hERG mutation. (B) Cardiac telemetry recording showed the onset of TdP, with an 'R on T' initiation. (C) Subsequent ECG during syncope, illustrates the characteristic appearance of TdP*

demonstrated to underestimate the frequency and severity of dysrhythmias compared to the Holter monitor. In 65 consecutive children undergoing cardiac surgery with a wide variety of diagnoses, less than 25% of dysrythmias demonstrated by Holter monitor were detected by standard 12-lead ECG. In this same study, 25% of patients had supraventricular dysrhythmias and 39% had ventricular dysrhythmias prior to surgery. Within the first 10 post-operative days, a dramatic increase in both supraventricular and ventricular dysrhythmias was observed. On follow-up 3–12 months following surgery, ectopy frequency decreased but not to preoperative levels. Therefore, the Holter monitor is much more sensitive that the 12-lead ECG for detecting dysrhythmias in patients undergoing cardiac surgery. In addition, assessment of preoperative dysrhythmias is important to evaluate postoperative dysrhythmias in perspective (Figs 9.12, 9.16 to 9.22).

Dysrhythmias Following Mustard Operation

The frequency of dysrhythmias following the Mustard operation for transposition of the great arteries (TGA) varies greatly from 9% to 95% depending on the method used and the length of time following surgery. Southall et al. performed standard 12-lead ECGs prior to and following the Mustard operation and demonstrated that just 1% of patients had dysrhythmias preoperatively and this increased to 4% by 3 months postoperatively. However, 24-hour recordings demonstrated a 53% frequency of

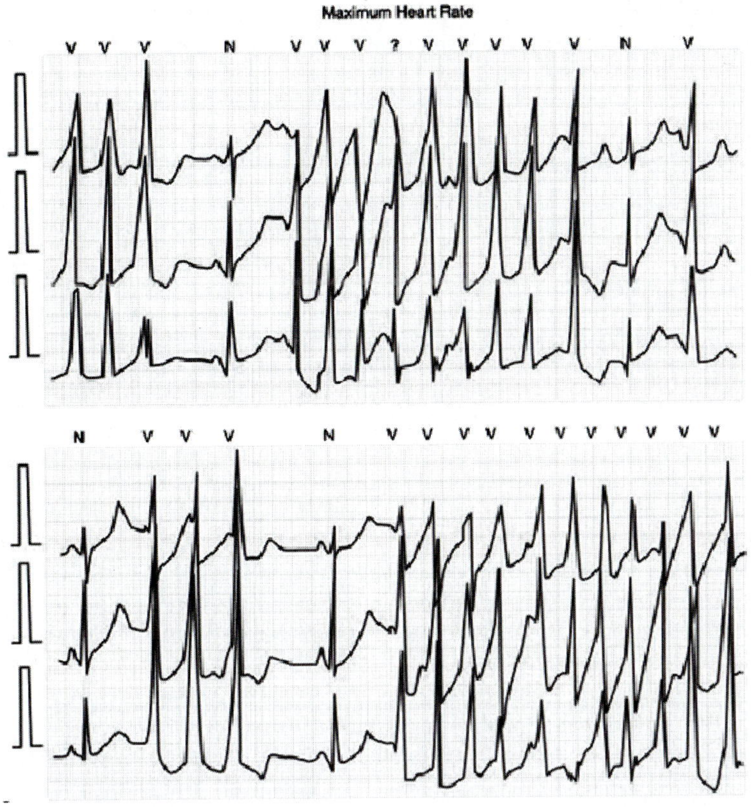

Fig. 9.27: *Torsades de pointes in a patient with long QT syndrome*

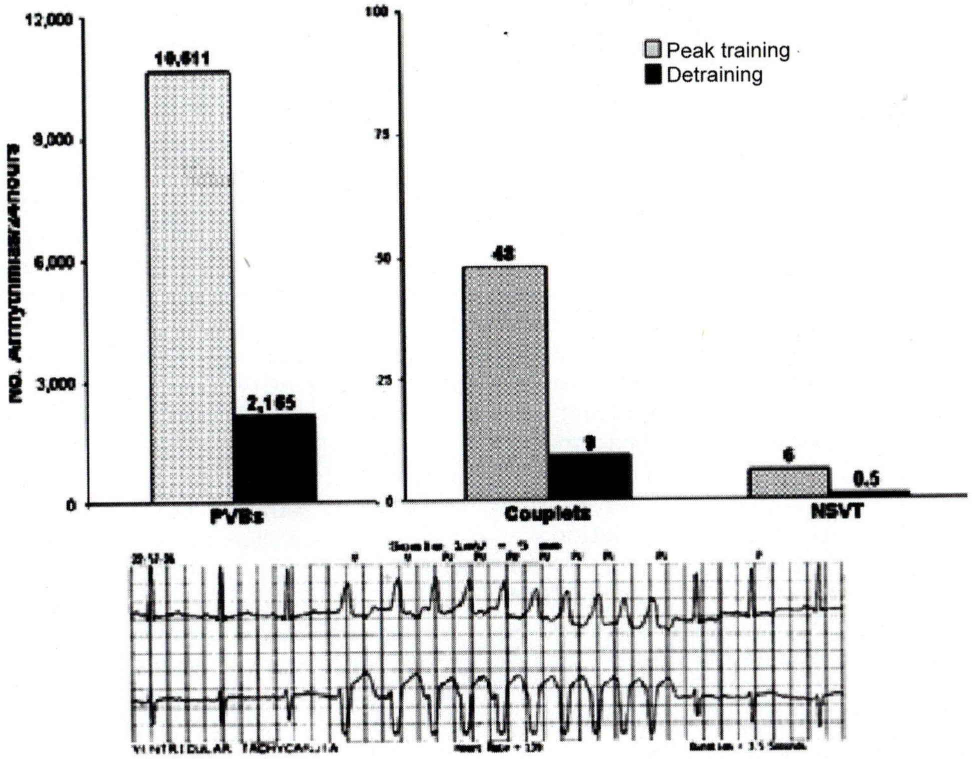

Fig. 9.28: *Ventricular arrhythmias in trained athletes. Top, Frequency of premature ventricular beats (PVBs), ventricular couplets, and bursts of nonsustained ventricular tachycardia (NSVT) recorded during a 24-hour (Holter) ECG at peak training and after a deconditioning period. Bottom, Ambulatory Holter ECG recording from adolescent male basketball player with frequent palpitations showing asymptomatic 10-beat burst of nonsustained ventricular tachycardia*

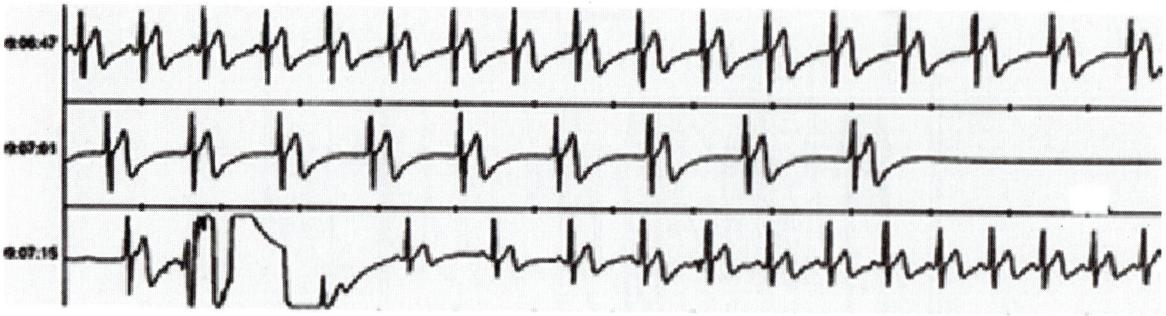

Fig. 9.29: *Utility of implantable loop recorder in the diagnosis of unexplained syncope. Event recorder tracing showing a 4.8 s asystole period in a 13-year-old girl subject. Time is indicated on the right scale. After a few sinus beats, there is a progressive slowing of a junctional rhythm ending into asystole. Recovery of sinus rhythm is evident in the bottom panel*

preoperative and 74% frequency of postoperative dysrhythmias.

In a follow-up study of 95 patients who had Mustard operation for TGA, 52 patients had 12-lead ECGs and 24-hour Holter monitors within the same 24-hour period. Of these 52 patients, 28 had sinus rhythm on ECG and 24 had dysrhythmias. However, by Holter monitor recording only 17 had sinus rhythm while 35 had significant dysrhythmias, including slow junctional rhythm and sinus arrest. Thus, 11 patients had an abnormal 24-hour Holter recording despite a normal 12-lead ECG on the same day. Sick sinus syndrome frequently develops in patients following the Mustard operation for TGA. Since sick sinus syndrome may be progressive, follow-up Holter recordings should be obtained during routine, periodic follow-up in these patients even if they remain asymptomatic. Strict guidelines for permanent pacemaker implantation are not completely agreed upon. However, if syncope or near-syncope is associated with profound bradyarrhythmia on Holter recording, then pacemaker implantation probably should be performed (Fig. 9.20).

Dysrhythmias in Congenital Heart Defects

In 11 children evaluated prior to repair of a secundum atrial septal defect (ASD), six had an abnormal 24-hour Holter recording. Observed abnormalities included sinus arrest with and without junctional escape, second-degree atrioventricular block, premature atrial contractions, paroxysmal atrial flutter, and wandering atrial pacemaker. Of 166 adults evaluated 8–21 years following repair of an ASD, 17% were found to have supraventricular dysrhythmias by Holter recording. Atrial flutter or fibrillation was also detected in 14%.

Dysrhythmias consistent with sick sinus syndrome seem to occur frequently both prior to and following repair of an ASD. Accordingly, symptoms suggesting dysrhythmia in these patients either prior to or following surgery should prompt further investigation, including a 24-hour recording. It is also useful in follow-up of VSD repair (Fig. 9.43).

Dysrhythmias in Tetralogy of Fallot

There is a 3–6% frequency of late sudden death following repair of tetralogy of Fallot (TF). A majority of these patients had PVCs or ventricular tachycardia documented by ECG prior to death. In a study of 207 survivors of repair of TF, 21 had PVCs on their 12-lead ECGs. Of these 21 patients, eight died suddenly a mean of 3.4 years following surgery. Each of these eight patients had a residual right ventricular pressure of 70 mmHg or more. Deanfield et al. noted PVCs on the 12-lead ECG in 15% of 196 patients 1–20 years following repair of TF. However, the 24-hour Holter monitor revealed that 77% had PVCs, including 28% with complex ventricular dysrhythmias (Fig. 9.6).

Although the prognosis of PVCs detected in patients following repair of TF remains uncertain, these patients should have periodic Holter recordings even if they remain asymptomatic. The decisions concerning selection of patients for postoperative electrophysiologic study and antiarrhythmic drug therapy remain controversial.

Sick Sinus Syndrome

Holter monitor recording can provide documentation for the presence of transient dysrhythmias seen in patients with sick sinus syndrome not associated with structural congenital heart disease. Indeed, a diagnosis of sick sinus syndrome cannot be made unless a relationship is established between the presence of dysrhythmias on the ECG and the symptoms such as palpitations, dizziness, or syncope. Conversely, if these symptoms occur without concomitant ECG changes, sick sinus syndrome can be excluded (Fig. 9.32, 9.33 and 9.37).

In a study of 25 children complaining of palpitations, syncope, lightheadedness, or chest pain, three children detected by standard ECG or 24-hour Holter recording in nine patients. Pacemakers were implanted in eight children, two of whom also required antiarrhythmic drug therapy. In a recent study of six children evaluated for unexplained syncope, the Holter monitor detected sinus bradycardia in three patients and supraventricular tachycardia (rate 200 beats/minute) in an additional patient. This latter patient experienced a near-syncopal episode while driving a car at the time that the Holter recorded her dysrhythmia. Pacemakers were implanted in four of these children, one of whom also required antiarrhythmic drug therapy. These studies have demonstrated that sick sinus syndrome can occur in children as an isolated cardiac abnormality. When symptoms suggesting dysrhythmia are associated with inappropriate bradycardia or supraventricular tachycardia, the diagnosis of sick sinus syndrome should be considered. Further investigation, including electrophysiologic study in selected cases, may indicate the need for pacemaker implantation, antiarrhythmic drug therapy, or both.

Sudden Infant Death Syndrome

The possible role of dysrhythmias in sudden infant death syndrome (SIDS) remains controversial. In a large, prospective study of 1,157 preterm infants, Southall et al. obtained 24-hour recordings of breathing, movement, and ECG within 1 week of nursery discharge. Subsequently,

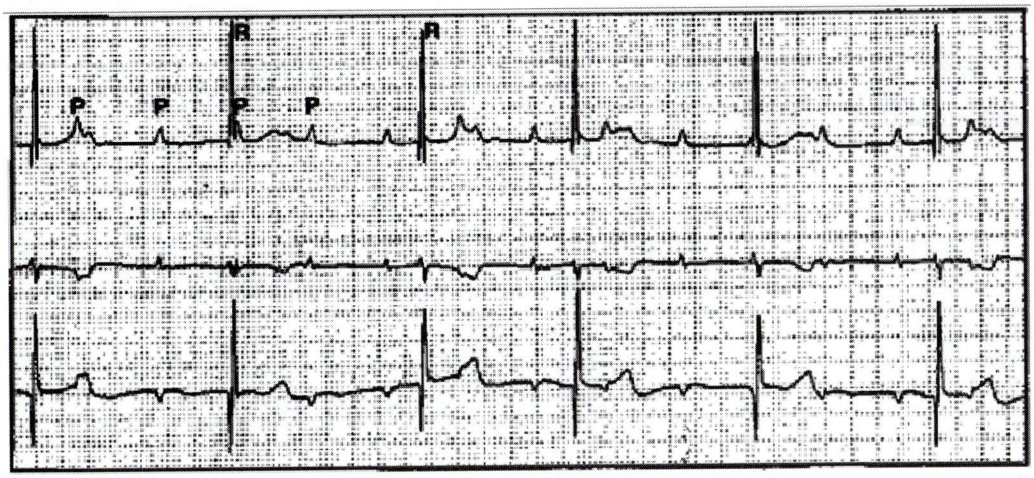

Fig. 9.30: *Ambulatory Holter monitor recording from a patient with congenital complete atrioventricular block. The ventricular rate is 45 beats per minute, and the sinus rate is 108 beats per minute. P = P-wave; R = QRS complex*

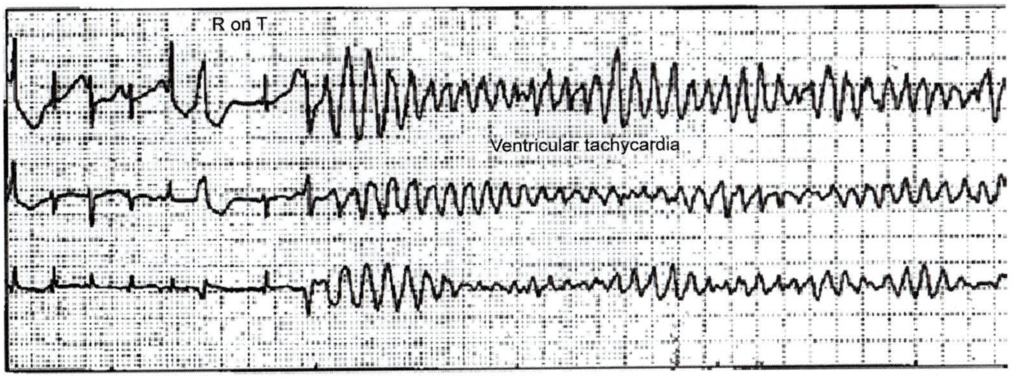

Fig. 9.31: *Ambulatory Holter monitor recording from a patient with long Q-T syndrome. The recording shows sinus rhythm with ventricular premature beats followed by the induction of a polymorphic ventricular tachycardia (torsades de pointes)*

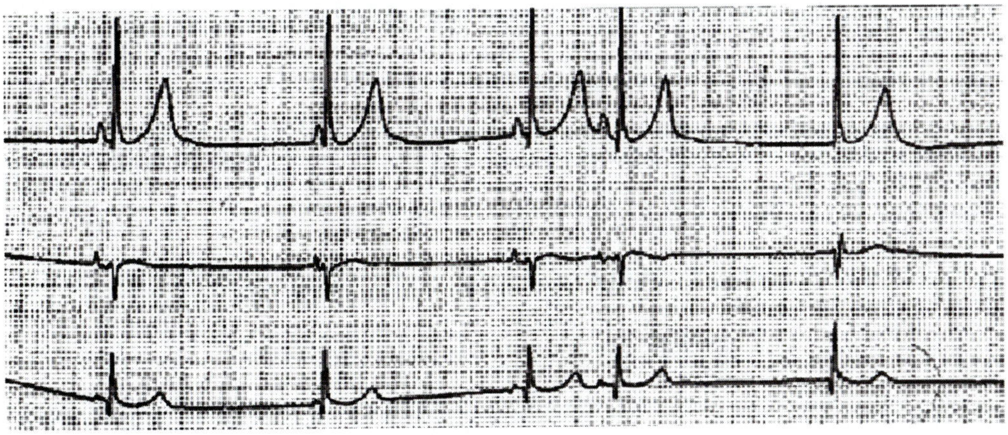

Fig. 9.32: *Ambulatory Holter monitor recording from a postoperative patient with electrocardiographic findings of sinus node dysfunction. The first beat is a conducted sinus beat followed by a sinus pause with a junctional escape beat. The fourth beat is an atrial premature beat followed by sinus arrest with another junctional escape beat*

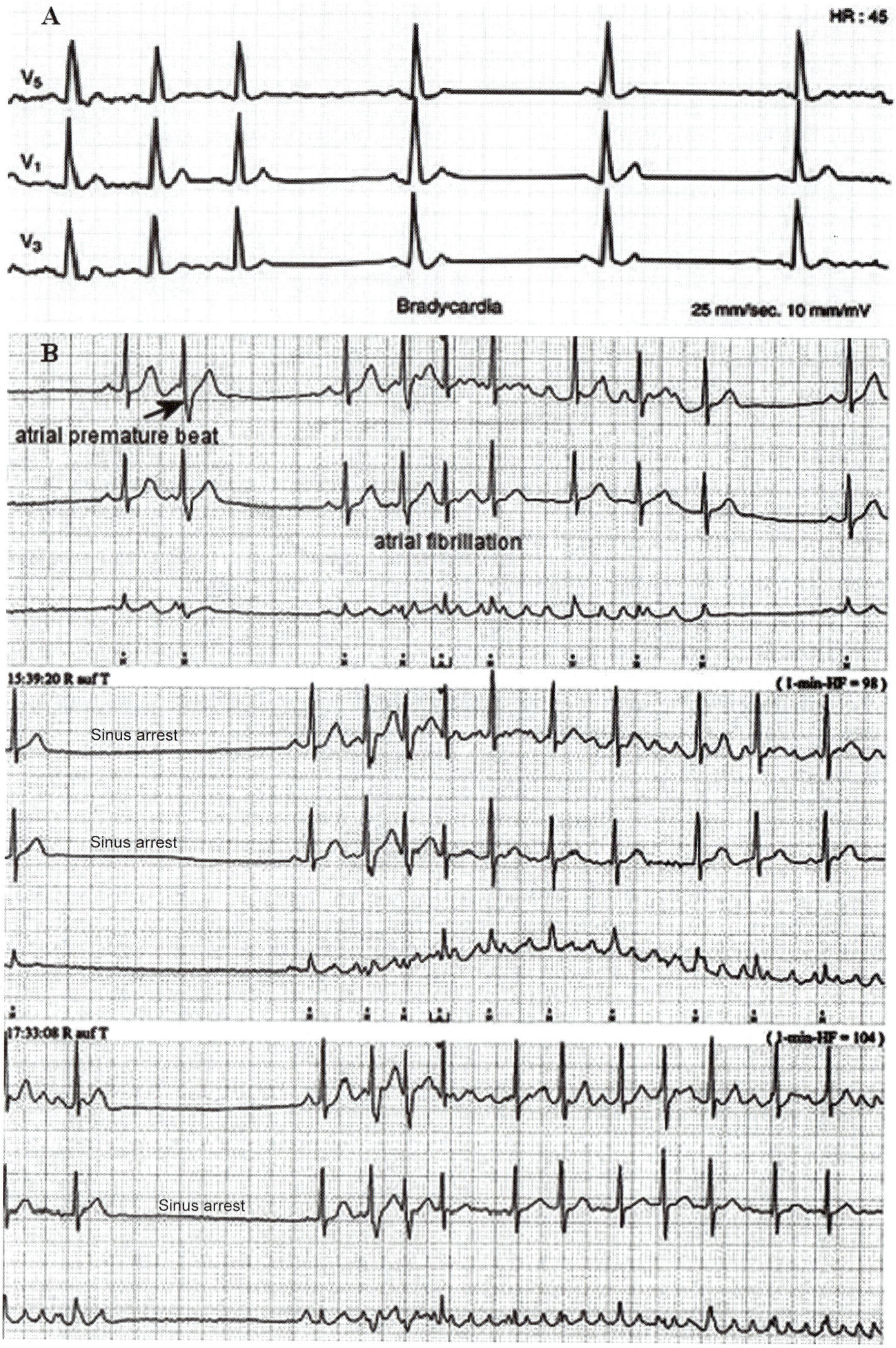

Fig. 9.33: *Examples (A) showing bradyarrhythmia in sick sinus: syndrome (B) shows the irregularity of the QRS complexes with changing rates and the changing P-waves is the diagnosis the sick sinus syndrome, a pattern of atrial malfunction, which can be of the slow or the fast type. The conduction velocity is different from beat to beat and there are blocked beats (arrow)*

five of the infants died of SIDS, but none of these five infants had any dysrhythmias on their recordings. In another prospective study (of full-term infants, only one of 16 infants who subsequently died of SIDS had cardio-respiratory patterns on previously obtained recordings that were outside the normal range when compared to controls. Based on these studies, 24-hour monitoring does not seem to predict infants at risk of sudden death.

Mitral Valve Prolapse (Fig. 9.36)

The Holter monitor is superior to both the standard 12-lead ECG and the exercise test for the detection of dysrhythmias in patients with mitral valve prolapse The myriad of nonspecific symptoms seen in these patients can be correlated with Holter monitor recordings to exclude dysrhythmia as the cause of symptoms in many cases. Complex or frequent PVCs do occur in more than 50% of patients with mitral valve prolapse detected by echocardiography. Supraventricular tachycardia is also seen in 28% of these patients. However, in the Framingham Study, supraventricular and ventricular dysrhythmias were so common in the general population that the difference in frequency of dysrhythmias between mitral valve prolapse subjects and controls did not reach significance.

Hypertrophic Cardiomyopathy (Figs 9.15 and 9.34)

Holter recording has revealed that more than 50% of adults with hypertrophic cardiomyopathy have frequent were found to have a dysrhythmia on Holter monitor at the time of symptoms. Nine others had no evidence of dysrhythmias during symptoms. The remaining 13 had neither symptoms nor dysrhythmias during the Holter study, and thus no conclusions could be drawn concerning the etiology of symptoms.

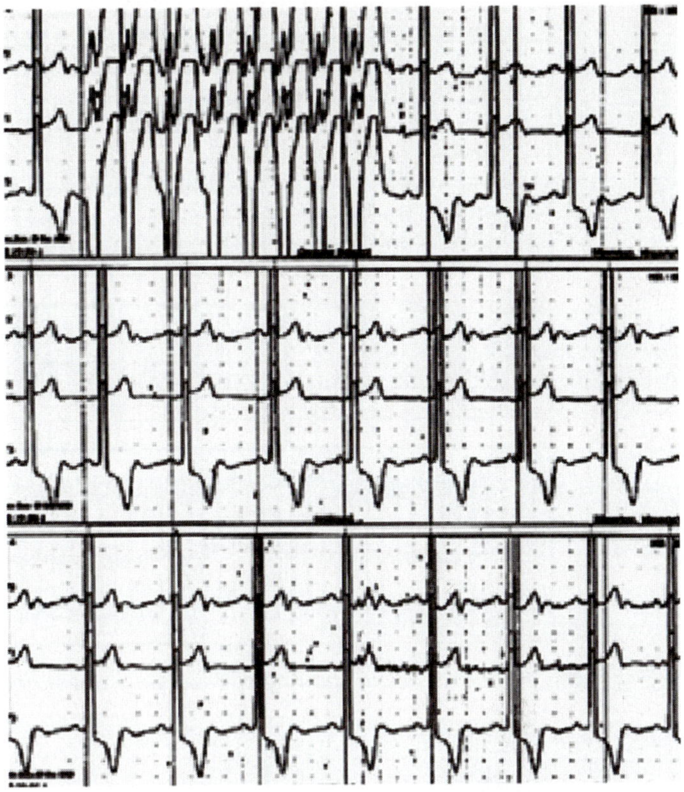

Fig. 9.34: *Holter graph showing giant T-wave inversion and tall R-waves along with ventricular tachycardia at 22.19;50 hours in patient with hypertrophic obstructive cardiomyopathy*

In another study of 11 children presenting with syncope, palpitations, or chest pain, sinus bradycardia was episodes of ventricular tachycardia, supraventricular tachycardia, or other potentially life-threatening dysrhythmias which

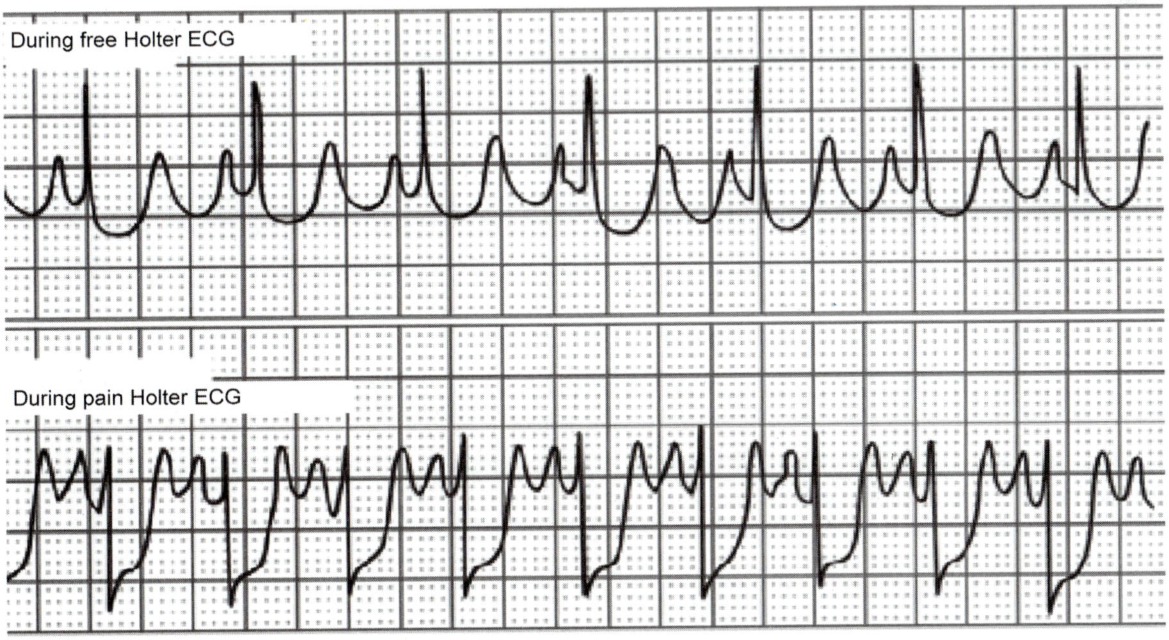

Fig. 9.35: *Holter ECG taken at rest (Upper panel) and marked ST segment depression (Lower panel) during chest pain in patient with unstable angina pectoris*

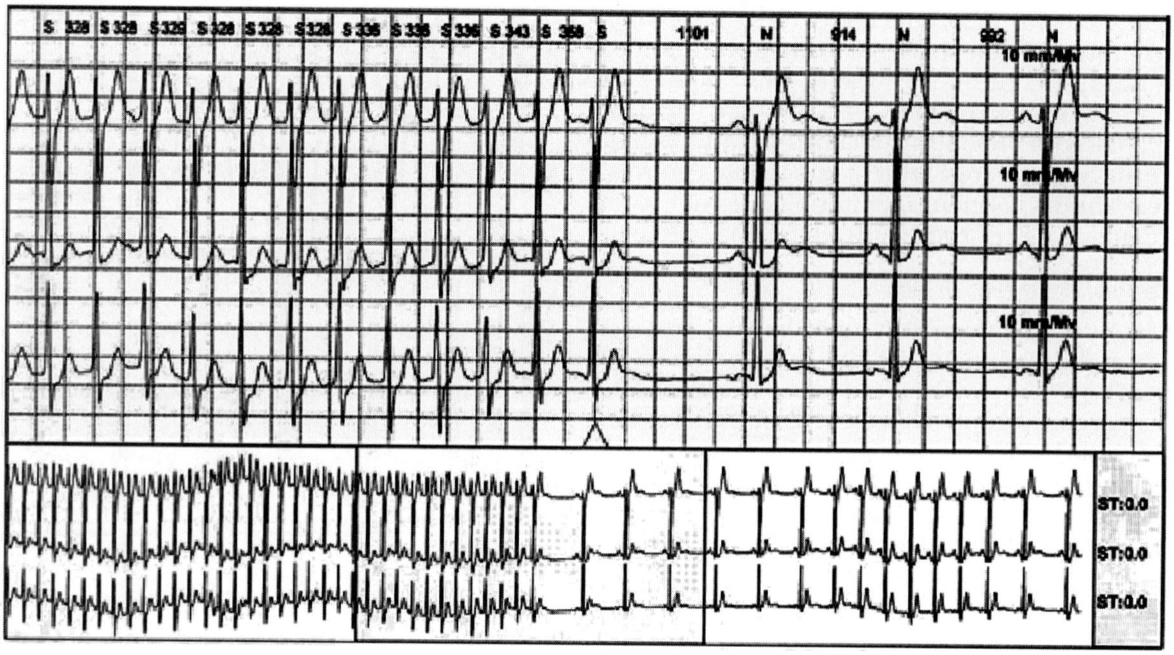

Fig. 9.36: *Holter recording showing spontaneous onset and termination of SVT in a patient with MVP (Mitral valve prolapse)*

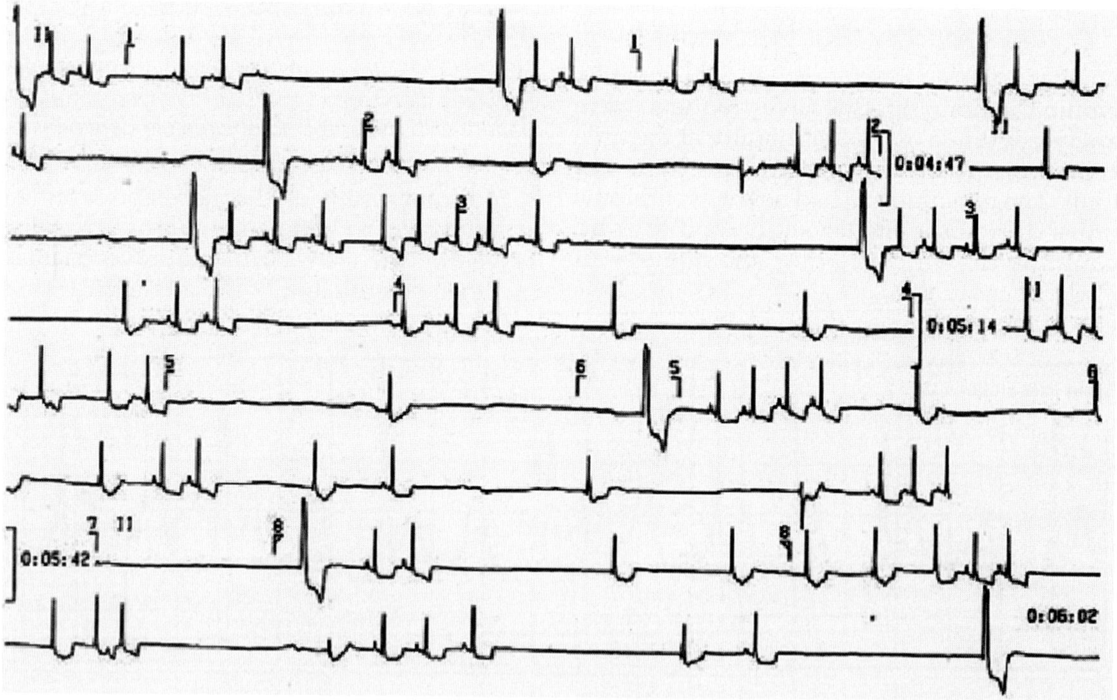

Fig. 9.37: *ECG in sick sinus syndrome: contineous Holter recording shows 1. A slow and irregular atrial rate (impaired sinoatrial activity), severe sinus bradycardia, or long pauses of asystole with no escape beats. 2. Evidence of impaired atrioventricular conduction with 2nd degree heart block. 3. The ventricular rate is very slow and irregular. * Ventricular escape beats are common, though they are often slow to manifest (follow a longer pause than usual). 4. Incomplete 3rd degree heart block. 5. Paroxysms of supraventricular tachycardia alternating with severe sinus bradycardia*

might escape detection by standard ECG. Furthermore, the 24-hour Holter recording has been found to be superior to treadmill exercise testing in revealing these dysrhythmias. In a study of 100 patients, more than 50% had multiform or repetitive ventricular premature depolarizations, including 19% who had ventricular tachycardia. In these latter patients, all episodes of ventricular tachycardia were brief (less than 10 beats/episode) and terminated spontaneously. Nonetheless, 10% of the patients with nonsustained ventricular tachycardia subsequently

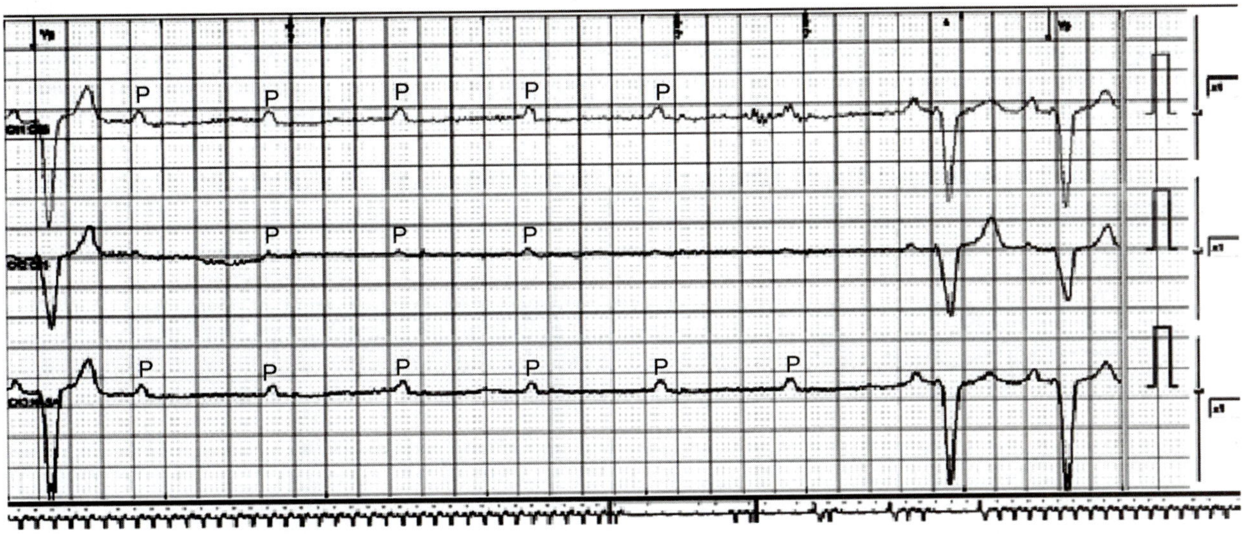

Fig. 9.38: *Holter monitoring showing paced rhythm with a pacemaker malfunction/ventricular standstill (ventricular asystole) approximately (5.6 seconds pause) in a young boy with recurrent palpitation after 2 years of pacemaker implantation*

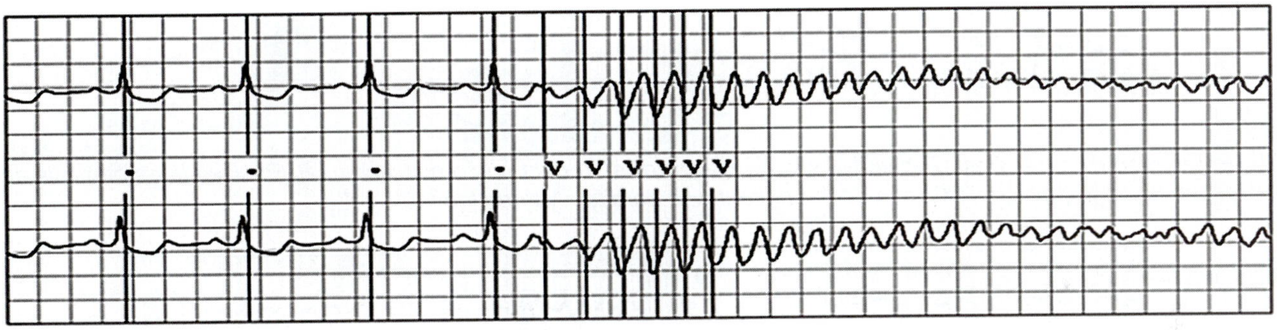

Fig. 9.39: *Holter graph showing ventricular tachycardia degenerating into ventricular fibrillation in sudden death syndrome in an obese adolescent male*

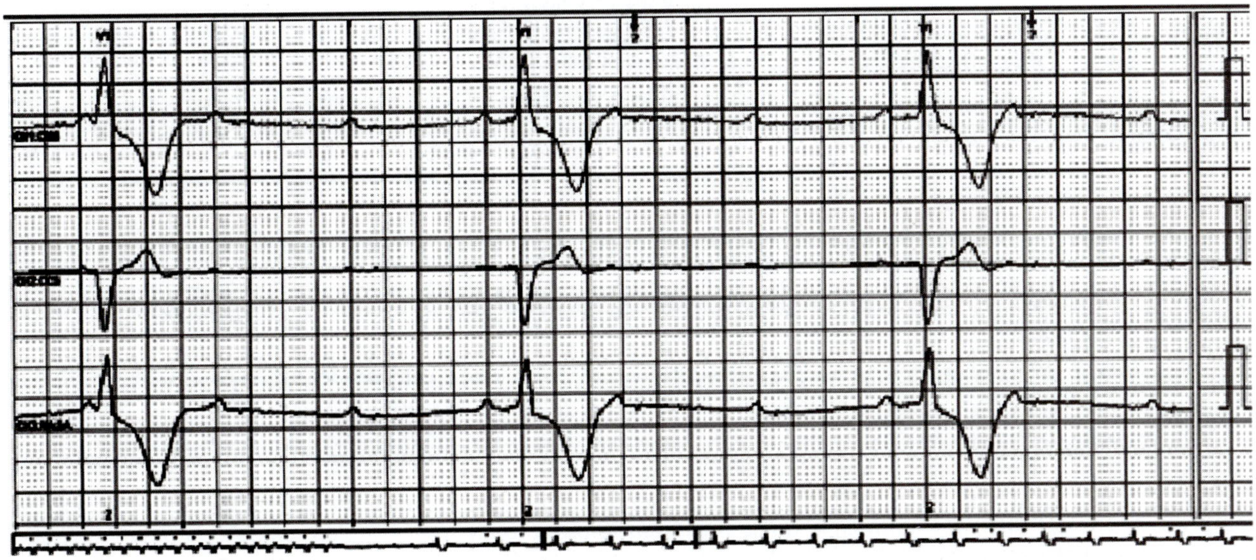

Fig. 9.40: *Holter monitoring shows pacemaker failure to capture ventricular escape rhythm with severe bradycardia (ventricular rate 24 bpm) in 18-years-old girl who had undergone cardiac operation for congenital heart defect 12 years back with permanent pacemaker*

experienced cardiac arrest within 2 months of their Holter studies. These dysrhythmias occurred independently of both symptoms and left ventricular outflow tract gradient.

Drug Efficacy

The Holter monitor is very useful in assessing antiarrhythmic therapy in patients with PVCs, more complex ventricular dysrhythmias, or frequent supraventricular tachycardia. However, it is important to distinguish true drug effect from spontaneous variability in dysrhythmia frequency, and this can be and this can be difficult.

In one study, 22 of 54 patients had at least a 50% reduction in their frequency of PVCs during sleep. In some of these patients, trials of various antiarrhythmic drugs were less

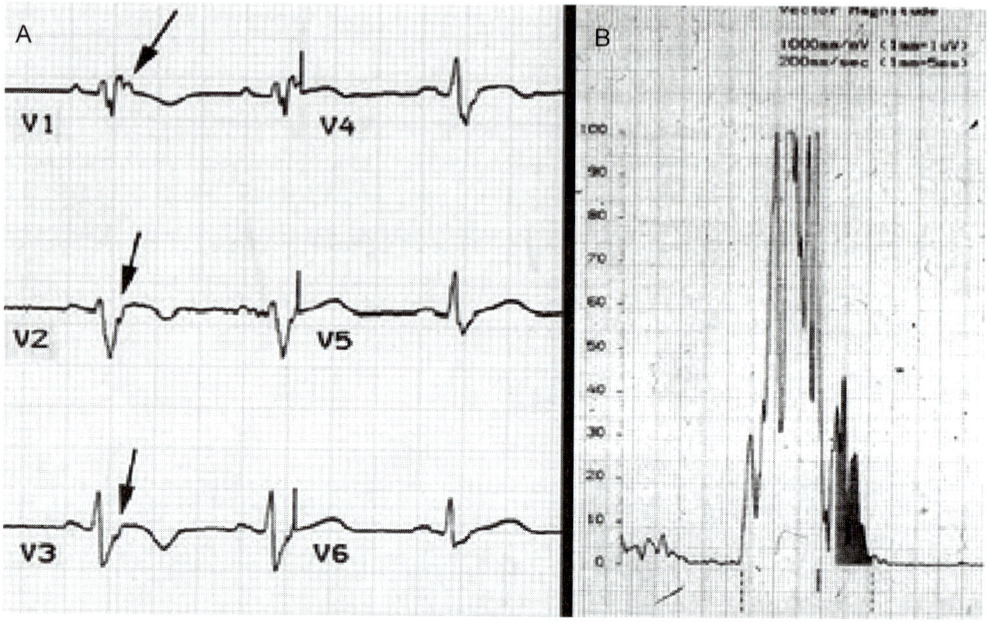

Fig. 9.41: *Holter recording: (A) Postexcitation epsilon wave (arrows) in right precordial leads; (B) Positive late potentials at signal-averaged electrocardiography (SAECG) in a young patient with cardiac dysarrhythmia*

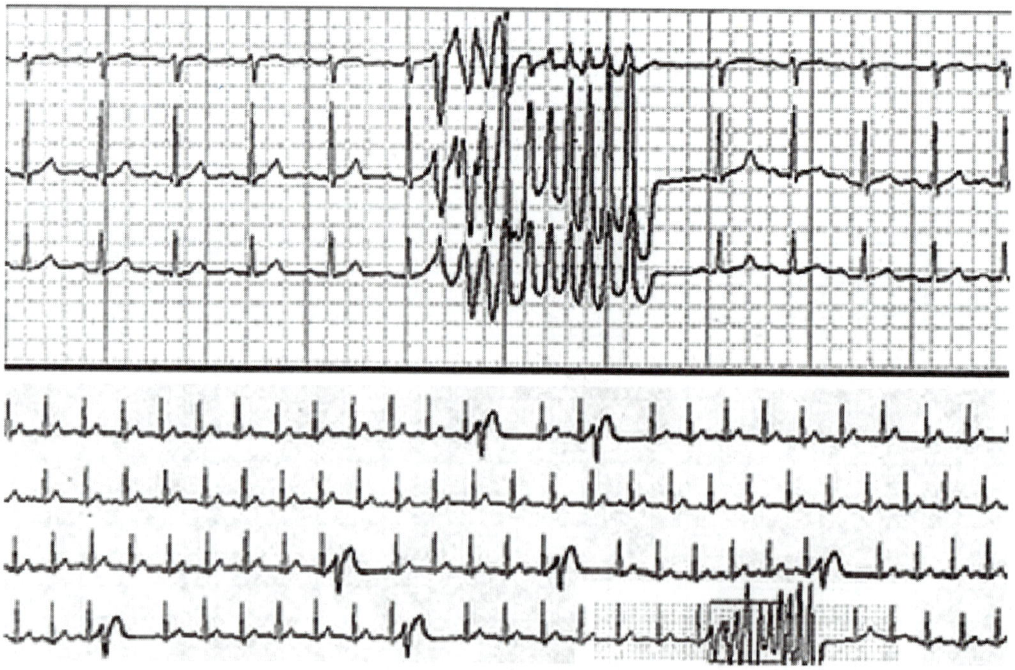

Fig. 9.42: *Holter monitoring shows in upper 3 tracings the onset of rapid polymorphic ventricular tachycardia that occurs near the peak of the T-wave. The QT interval is normal, and this has been referred to as short-coupled torsade de pointes. These patients frequently have premature ventricular contractions that are also short-coupled as noted on the bottom strip (recorded for a more prolonged period). This arrhythmia does not occur frequently enough to evaluate various forms of therapy in a randomized controlled trial, but there are many reports in the literature confirming its lethal nature*

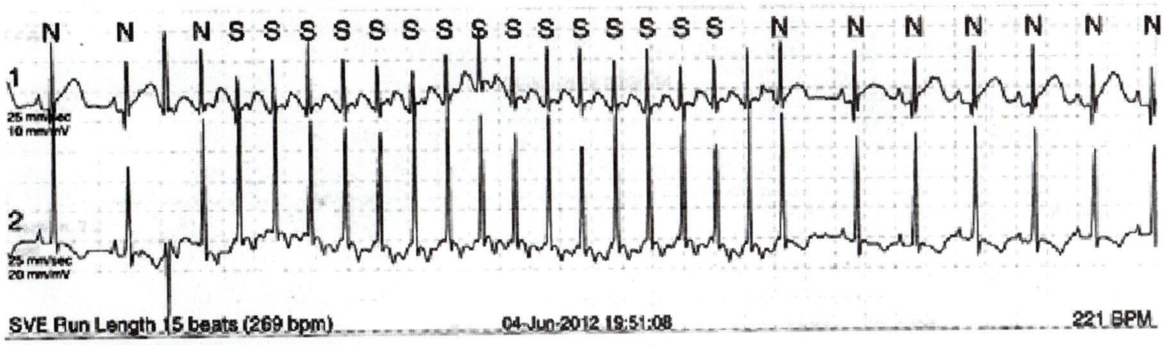

Fig. 9.43: *Holter recording showing spontaneous onset of junctional rhythm (retrograde P-waves) from a 3-month-old patient-after VSD repair*

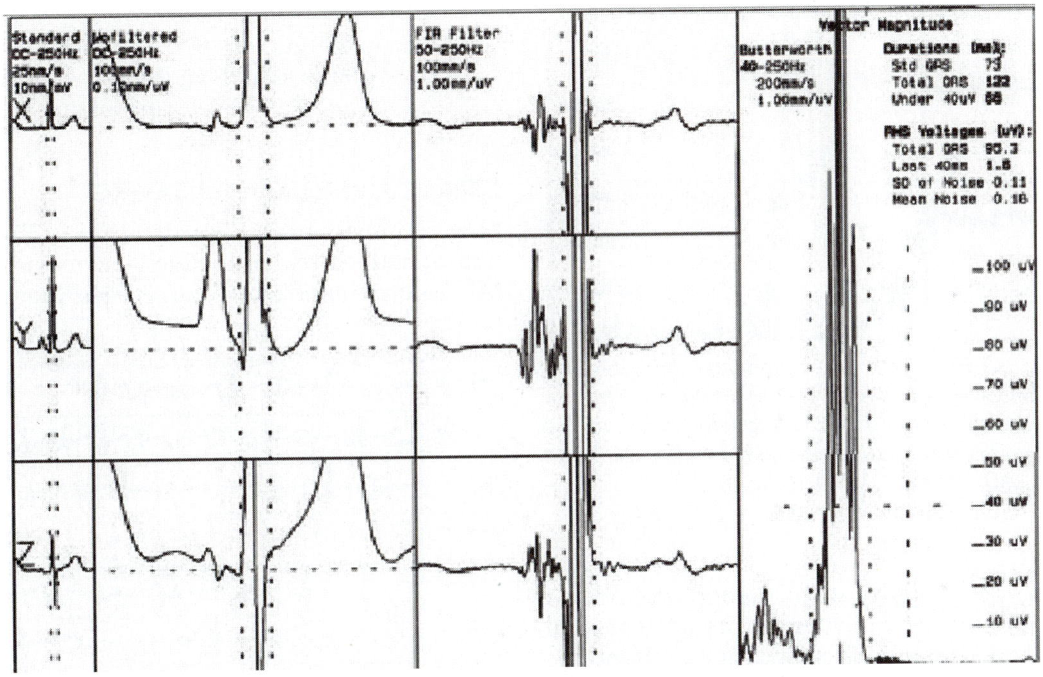

Fig. 9.44: *Ventricular late potentials in patients with mitral valve prolapse reflecting prolapse of mitral leaflet equal to 5.0 mm during systole. SAECG showing ventricular late potentials (fQRS = 122 ms, LAS 40 = 66 ms, RMS 40 = 1.6 μv)*

effective than sleep in reducing the frequency and grade of ventricular dysrhythmias. In an other study of 15 patients with PVCs, it was concluded that an 83% reduction in frequency between two 24-hour Holter monitor recordings was necessary to conclude that a decrease in frequency of PVCs was due to drug intervention rather than to spontaneous biologic variation.

Pacemaker Malfunction (Figs 9.38 and 9.40)

When a thorough pacemaker check fails to detect a suspected pacemaker malfunction, then the 24-hour Holter monitoring is considered for pacemaker evaluation.

Role of Holter Monitors in Angina and Its Pattern of Occurrence (Fig. 9.14)

Holter monitoring has shown that the majority of ischemic episodes that occur during normal daily activities are silent (asymptomatic), and that symptomatic and silent episodes of ST segment depression exhibit a circadian rhythm, with ischemic ST changes more common in the morning. Studies also have shown that nocturnal ST-segment changes are almost always an indicator of two- or three-vessel CAD or left mainstem stenosis.

Role of Holter-Monitoring for Detection of Silent Ischemia

Patients with an "anginal equivalent" and risk factors for CAD (e.g. exertional shortness of breath) are also at high risk for ischemia. Patients with type II diabetes mellitus also have a greater incidence of asymptomatic ischemia as well as silent MIs, and may benefit from Holter evaluation for silent ischemia (Fig. 9.35).

Heart Rate Variability

Holter monitor recordings can be used to assess heart rate variability as a measurement of the standard deviation of

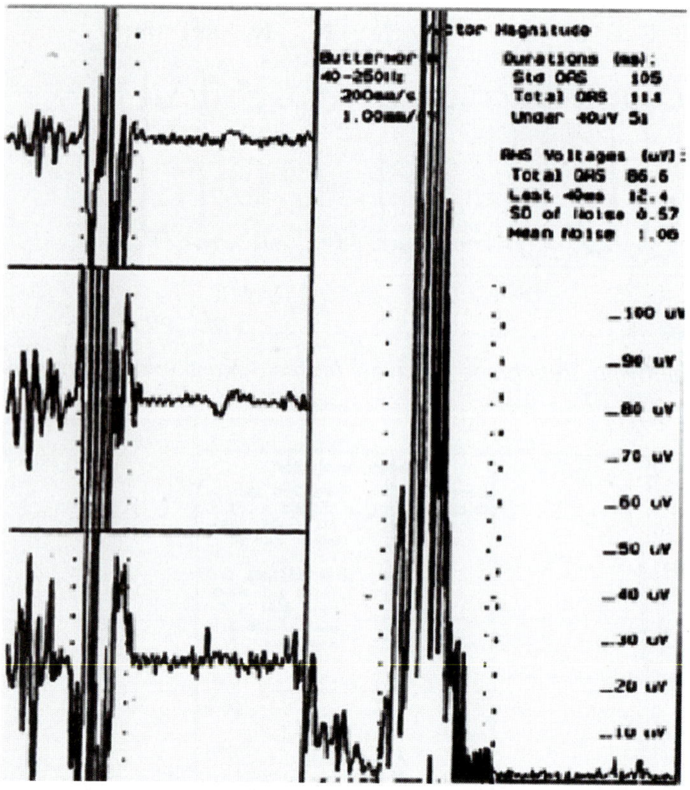

Fig. 4.45: *Positive SA-EKG with late potentials highlighted at the end of the QRS complex between 150 and 190 ms. The low amplitude signals (≤ 25) exceed the voltage for noise at the terminal 40 ms. The QRS duration is normal (114 ms). QRS 114 ms (NL < 120 ms) LAS - 51 ns. RMS 40 12.5 mv*

the sinus rhythm cycle-length (or fluctuation around the mean RR interval). Heart rate variability reflects the parasympathetic and sympathetic balance of the autonomic nervous system and therefore offers insight into the risk for sudden cardiac death.

Recent studies show that analysis of heart rate variability is important in evaluation of postinfarction and diabetic patients. In both groups, decreased heart rate variability is associated with an increased risk of sudden cardiac death. Lower heart rate variability is also recorded with acute MI. Here a predominance of sympathetic activity and reduction in parasympathetic cardiac control result in increased sympathetic activity, which decreases the fibrillation threshold and predisposes to ventricular fibrillation. In addition, anterior wall MI results in a more profound reduction in heart-rate variability than inferior wall infarction.

Signal-averaged Electrocardiography

SA-EKG is a method of recording the EKG in which amplifiers and filters record cardiac signals with amplitudes of only a few microvolts. Electrical potentials corresponding to delayed and fragmental conduction in the ventricle are recorded in microvolts and waveforms continuous with the QRS complex. Three criteria are of importance (Figs 9.28, 9.41, 9.44 and 9.45).

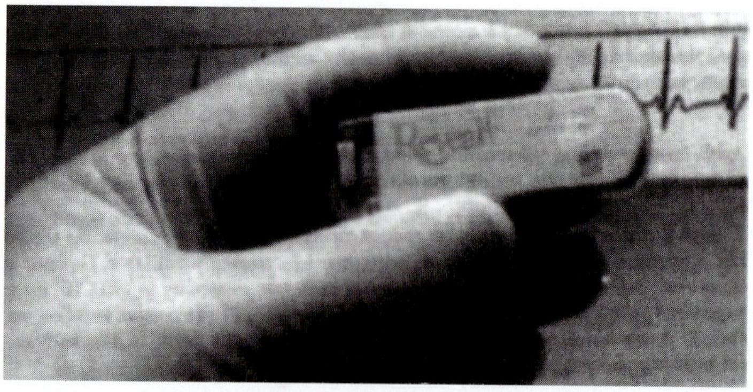

Fig. 9.46: *Showing implantable loop recorder for detecting cardiac arrhythmia*

1. QRS duration
2. Low-voltage signals in the last 40 msec of the QRS
3. Low-frequency waveforms lasting > 30 msec after the terminal QRS complex.

Clinical Applications of SA-EKG

Late potentials have been detected in 73–92% of patients with sustained and inducible ventricular tachycardia after MI. Late potentials also have been identified in patients

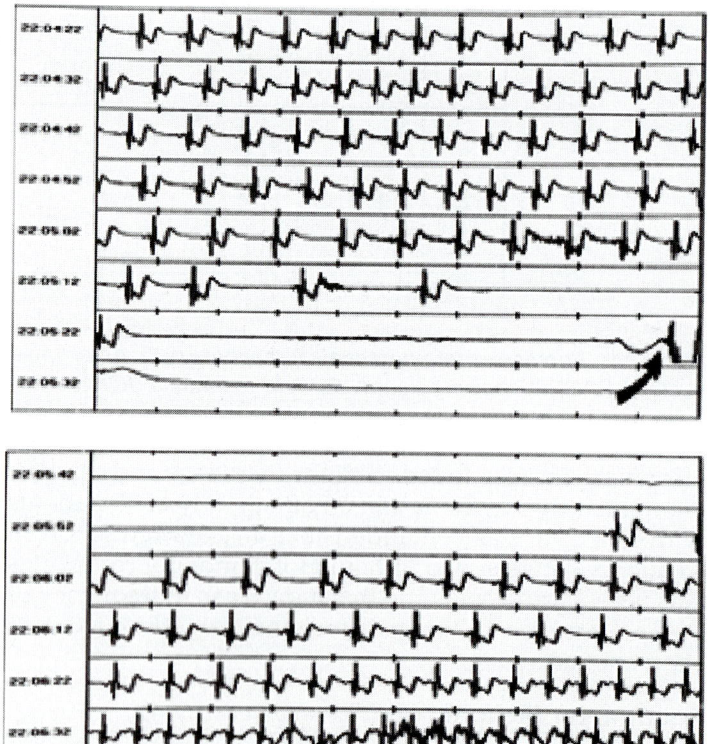

Fig. 9.47: *A rhythm strip from 15-year-old patient with 11 previous episodes of syncope over 7 years before enrollment. Conventional testing did not result in diagnosis. Patient was crossed over to monitoring strategy. Seven months after implantation of loop recorder, patient had recurrent syncope and captured a 43-second pause with a single QRS complex after 4 seconds. There is an impact artifact (arrow) at the point at which patient fell to the floor. The device was removed, and a pacemaker was implanted*

with nonischemic heart disease and ventricular tachycardia, such as those with dilated cardiomyopathy. Early use of thrombolytic agents reduces the prevalence of late potentials after coronary occlusion and therefore the risk of sudden death, ventricular fibrillation, and tachycardia. Late potentials after MI are an independent marker of patients at high risk for ventricular tachycardia. SA-EKG results combined with other noninvasive data (e.g. Holter, ETT, ejection fraction) provide a highly sensitive and highly specific method of identifying patients at risk for ventricular tachycardia or sudden death.

Role of Holter Monitoring in Sudden Cardiac Death in CHF

Though it remains difficult to predict sudden cardiac death in CHF patients, the prediction must be attempted because defibrillation treatment is increasingly available. Galinier et al. looked at time and frequency domain measures of heart rate variability in 190 CHF patients, mean ejection fraction 28%, class II (189 points) and class III or IV (81 points). In follow-up (22 months), 55 deaths had occurred, of which 21 were sudden cardiac death.

In data analysis, depressed heart rate variability was an independent prognostic value (Fig. 9.13).

Role of an Implantable Loop Recorder (ILR) in Cardiac Arrhythmia (Figs 9.29 and 9.47)

An implantable loop recorder (ILR) allows correlation of symptoms and rhythm abnormalities in many patients where these are infrequent or unexpected. The device is small (61 mm × 19 mm; 8 mm thick) and easy to implant with a single chamber lead. It provides up to 14 months of continuous monitoring and has shown a high diagnostic yield (up to 94%). The metronic reveal ILR may reduce cost and inconvenience of repeated testing and hospital visits.

Cardiodefender Smartphone-based ECG, a 21st Century Holter Monitor

Smartphone ECG that can provide continuous readings throughout the day that can help detect arrhythmias that may be hard to spot in an office visit. The system uses a wrist watch-like device to collect data from electrodes and transmit it wirelessly via bluetooth to a smartphone that can then share it with clinicians monitoring the patient. Cardiodefender, that recently won both FDA approval and EU's CE Mark, can activate an alarm to rapidly notify a physician of any particularly unwelcome graph via an email, page, or other electronic means.

- Fully mobile system cardiodefender is the world's first ECG system which delivers hospital based quality ECG and arrhythmia analysis by integrating unique software,

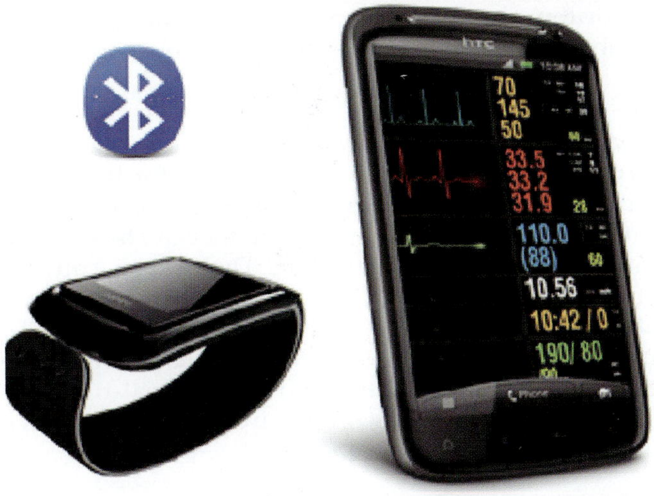

Fig. 9.48: *Showing cardiodefender smartphone-based ECG, a 21st century holter nonitor. Smartphone ECG that can provide continuous readings throughout the day that can help to detect arrhythmias that may be hard to spot in an office visit. The system uses a wrist watch-like device to collect data from electrodes and transmit it wirelessly via bluetooth to a smartphone that can then share it with clinicians monitoring the patient. Cardiodefender, that recently won both FDA approval and EU's CE Mark, can activate an alarm to rapidly notify a physician of any particularly unwelcome graph via an email, page, or other electronic means. Fully mobile system; cardiodefender is the world's first ECG system which delivers hospital based quality ECG and arrhythmia analysis by integrating unique software, algorithms and data compression capabilities which enable a smartphone to perform as a mobile ECG*

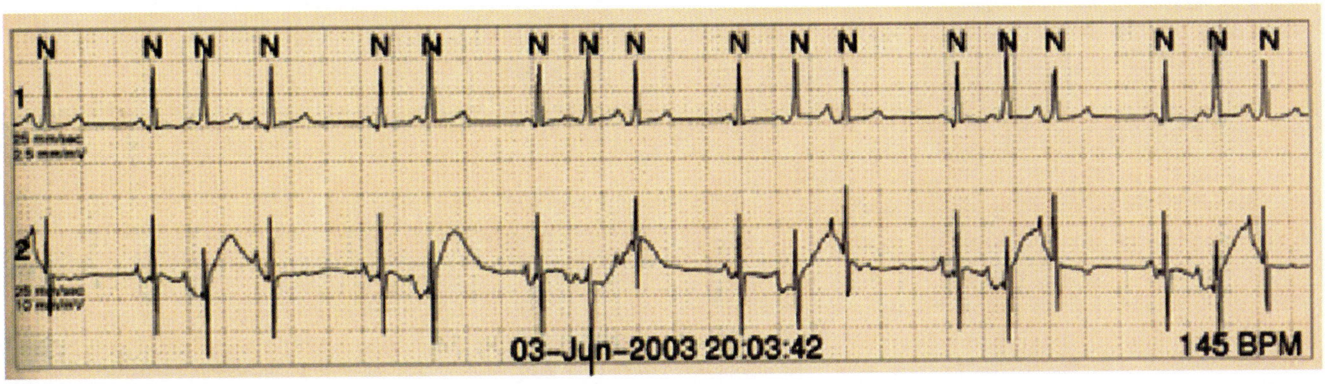

Fig. 9.49: *Holter recording in an infant showing preexcitation and premature atrial beats. Echocardiography showed LV cardiac mass*

algorithms and data compression capabilities which enable a smartphone to perform as a mobile ECG.

Real-time Wireless Holter (Fig. 9.50)

Curvus, a subsidiary of WPR Medical out of Arendal, Norway, has received 510 (K) clearance for its wireless Curvus Arrhythmia Monitoring Device (C-AD), a continuous ECG monitoring system that can be worn 24/7, including during showering. The system can send immediate notifications to clinicians when arrhythmias are detected. The C-AD is a highly differentiated wireless cardiac arrhythmia monitor, which, with its patent-secured design, is able to capture continuous, real-time ECG readings over the broadest spectrum of patient activity with minimal noise artifacts.

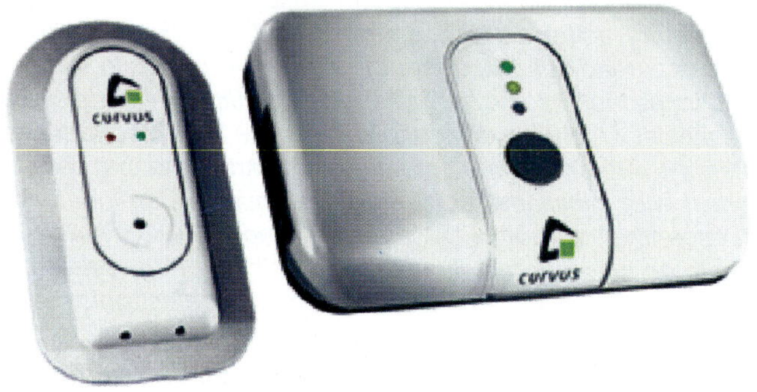

Fig. 9.50: *Real-time wireless Holter*

BIBLIOGRAPHY

1. Cohen TJ, Ibrahim B, Sassower MJ: Revealing data retrieved from an implantable loop recorder. J Invasive Cardiol 12(3): 174–175, 2000.
2. DiMarco JP, Philbrick JT: Use of ambulatory electrocardiographic (Holter) monitoring. Ann Intern Med 113.53–8, 1990.
3. Galinier M, Pathak A, et al: Depressed low-frequency power of heart rate variability as an independent predictor of sudden death in chronic heart failure. Eur Heart J 21(6):475–482, 2000.
4. Kennedy HL: Long-term (Holter) electrocardiogram recordings. In Zipes DP, Jalife J (eds): Cardiac Electrophysiology: From Cell to Bedside. Philadelphia, WB. Saunders, 1990, p 791.
5. Langer A, Freeman MR, Josse RG, et al: Detection of silent myocardial ischemia in diabetes mellitus. Am J Cardiol 67: 1073, 1991.
6. Lazzeri C, La Villa G, et al: 24-hour heart rate variability in patients with vasovagal syncope. Pacing Clin Eleclrophysio 123 (4 Part 1):463–468,2000.
7. Van Ravenswaaij-Arts MA, Kollee AA, Hopman JC, et al: Heart rate variability. Ann Intern Med 118:436–447, 1993.
8. Yeung AC, Barry J, Orav J, et al: Effects of asymptomatic ischemia on long-term prognosis in chronic stable coronary disease. Clin Cardiol. 1992;10:341–356,
9. Crivellaro W, Dassi S, Tinelli M. Raselli G, Cerutti S, Lombardi F, Pagani M. Malliani A. Continuous 24-hour assessment of the neural regulation of systemic arterial pressure and RR variabilities in ambulant subjects. Circulation. 1990;81:537–547.
10. Gohlke C. Gohlke H. Petersen J, Fruh A. Gondolf K. Betz P and Roskmann H: Incidence and prognostic importance of silent ischaemia after PTCA : a prospechigh resolution trend recordings of leads CM5 and CC5 for ST segment analysis. Am J Cardiol 60:796,1987.
11. Josephson MA, Nademanee K. Intarachot V. Lewis H and Singh BN: Abolition of Holter monitor detected silent myocardial ischaemia after percutaneous transluminal coronary angioplasty. J Am Coli Cardiol 10:499,1987.

10 Recognition and Management of Syncope in Children and Adolescents

Syncope in children is most often neurally mediated and usually has a natural history of spontaneous resolution or improvement. Syncope is defined as the temporary loss of consciousness resulting from a reversible disturbance of cerebral function. It is characterized by a loss of consciousness due to a lack of cerebral blood flow, rapid or sudden onset, falling of the patient, if not supported, and transiency of the attack. In children, it is most often benign, but may sometimes herald a more serious, potentially life-threatening cause.

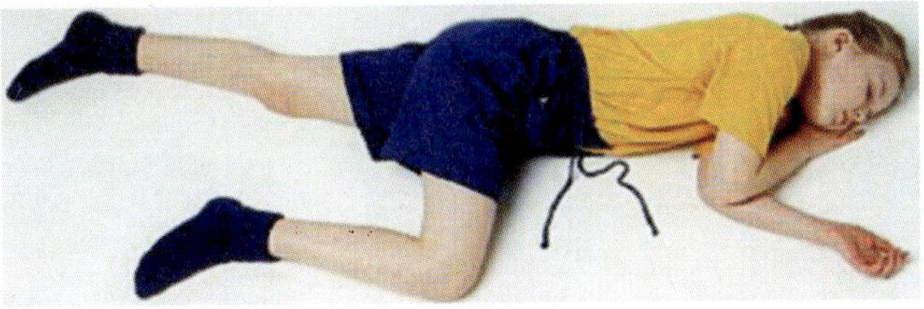

Fig. 10.1: *A young child fells suddenly on the ground with an episode of syncope*

Syncope is a common clinical problem characterized by transient, spontaneously self-terminating loss of consciousness with complete and prompt recovery; the cause is insufficiency of cerebral oxygen/nutrient supply most often due to a transient fall of systemic arterial pressure to levels below those tolerated by cerebrovascular autoregulation. Careful and thorough evaluation of the cause of syncope is warranted in all patients. Determining that certain individuals are at "low mortality risk" is inadequate; syncope, although often benign from a mortality perspective, tends to recur, is

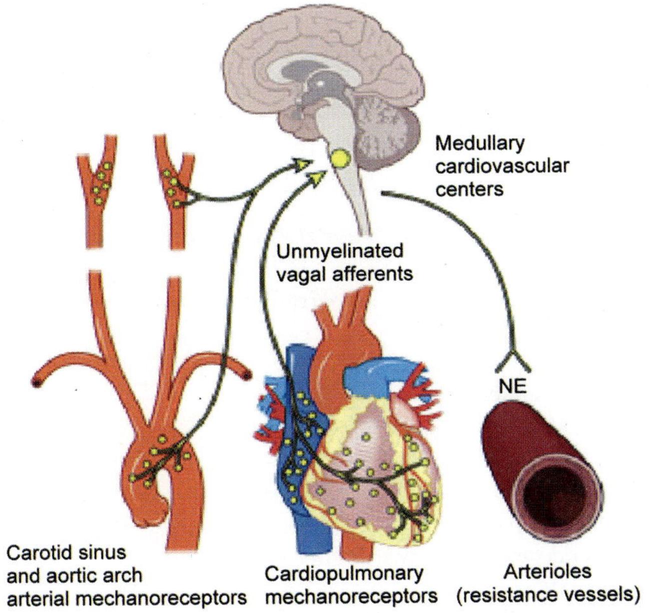

Fig. 10.2: *Diagram showing the importance of autonomous nervus system in the fainting attacks*

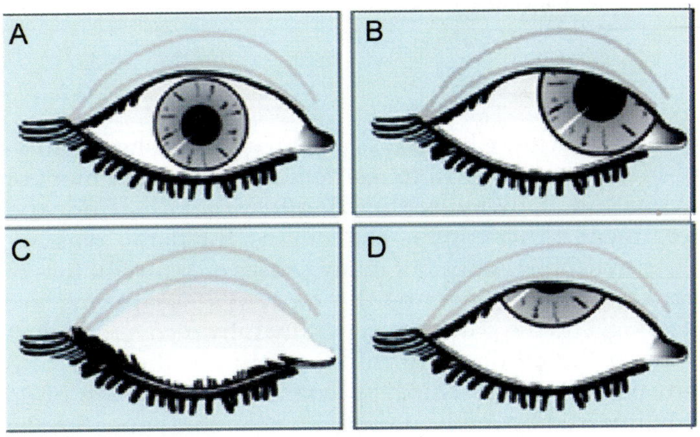

Fig. 10.3: *Eye closure and gaze in various epileptic and nonepileptic seizures. (A) Staring during a temporal lobe seizure; (B) lateral gaze during an extratemporal lobe seizure; (C) closed eyes during a psychogenic; nonepileptic attack, (D) upward gaze during a syncope*

Table 10.1: *Cause of syncope*

Neurally medical (reflex)
• Vasovagal syncope (common faint) – Classical – Nonclassical • Carotid sinus syncope • Situational syncope – Acute hemorrhage – Cough, sneeze – Gastrointestinal stimulation (swallow, defecation, visceral pain) – Micturition (postmicturition) – Postexercise – Postprandial – Others (e.g. brass instrumental playing, weightlifting • Glossopharyngeal neuralgia
Orthostatic hypotension
• Autonomic failure – Primary autonomic failure syndromes (e.g. pure autonomic failure, multiple system atrophy, Parkinson's disease with autonomic failure) – Secondary autonomic failure syndrome (e.g. diabetic neuropathy, amyloid neuropathy) – Drugs and alcohol – Postexercise – Postprandial • Volume depletion – Hemorrhage, diarrhea, Addison's disease
Cardiac arrhythmias as primary cause
• Sinus node dysfunction (including brabycardia/tachycardia syndrome) • Atrioventricular conduction system disease • Paroxysmal supraventricular and ventricular tachycardias • Inherited syndromes (e.g. long QT syndrome, Brugada syndrome) • Implanted device (pacemaker, implantable cardioverter-defibrillator) malfunction • Drug-induced arrhythmias
Structural cardiac or cardiopulmonary disease
• Obstructive cardiac valvular disease • Acute myocardial infraction/ischemia • Obstructive cardiomyopahty • Atrial myxoma • Acute aortic dissection

associated with risk of physical injury, diminishes quality-of-life, and might lead to restriction from employment or avocation. However, the diagnostic evaluation and treatment of syncope is challenging for many reasons. First, syncope is only 1 of many causes of transient loss of consciousness. Second, the patient's symptoms are fleeting, and the patient is generally fully recovered when seen in the clinic; only infrequently are there helpful physical findings. Third, spontaneous events are often unwitnessed by medical professionals; consequently, the medical history of symptom events is usually a "second-hand" or "third-hand" story. Finally, there is often an excessive sense of diagnostic "urgency" that tends to result in a rush to undertake multiple poorly considered "diagnostic" testing procedures; a deliberate approach

Table 10.2: *Cause of nonsyncopal attacks (commonly misdiagnosed as syncope)*

Disorders without any impairment of consciousness
• Falls • Cataplexy • Drop attacks • Psychogenic pseudosyncope • Transient ischemic attacks (TIA) of carotid origin
Disorders with partial or complete loss of consciousness
• Metabolic disorders including hypoglycemia, hypoxia, hyperventilation with hypocapnia • Epilepsy • Intoxicartions • Vertebrobasilar TIA

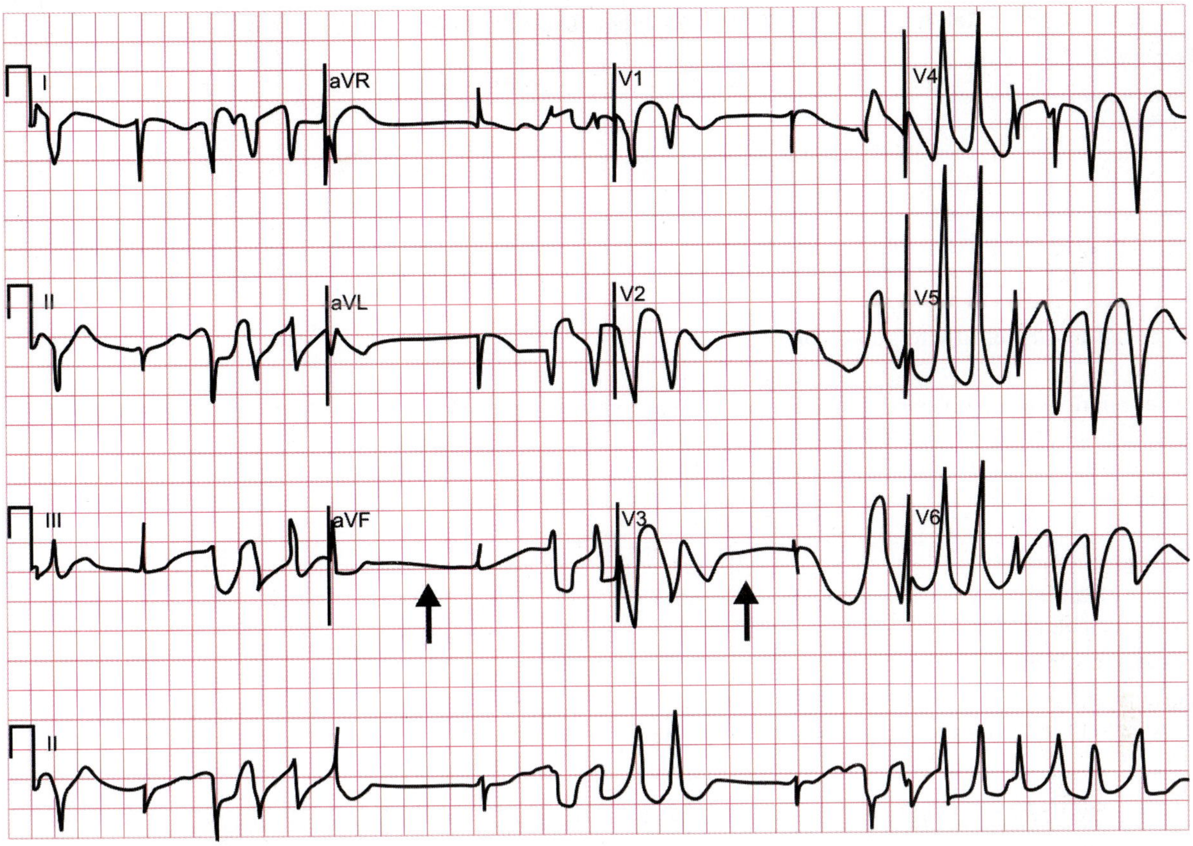

Fig. 10.4: *Eighteen-years-old of patient presented with syncope showed defects in ion channels predispose patients to episodes of torsade de pointes (TdP), which can cause cardiac arrest. TdP is a form of polymorphic ventricular tachycardia that results in a characteristic twisting of the QRS complex around the isoelectric baseline. This arrhythmia is associated with LQTS and can degenerate into more unstable rhythms. In the case of acquired LQTS, a pause usually precedes the onset of TdP. This form of TdP is said to be "pause dependent" (arrows). (Image courtesy of ECG Wave-Maven)*

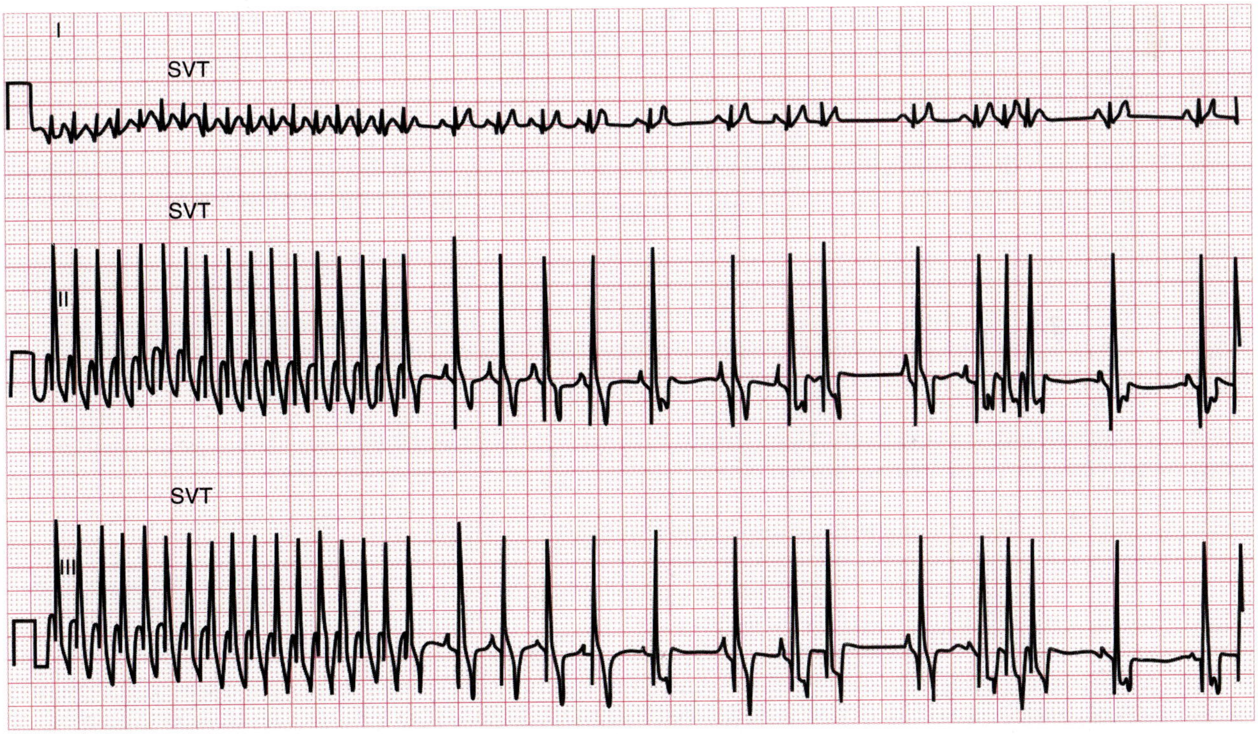

Fig. 10.5: *Holter study in 16-year-old male patient presented with syncope showed episodes of supraventricular tachycardia*

Table 10.3: *Clinical features suggestive of specific causes of syncope*

Neurally-mediated syncope

- Absence of cardiac disease
- Long history of syncope
- After sudden unexpected unpleasant sight, sound, smell or pain
- Prolonged standing or crowded, hot places
- Nausea, vomiting associated with syncope
- During or in the absorptive state after a meal
- With head rotation, pressure or carotid sinus (as in tumors, shabhing, tight collar
- After exertion

Syncope caused by orthostatic hypotension

- After standing up
- Temporal relationship with start of medication leading to hypotension or change of dosage
- Prolonged standing especially in crowded, hot places
- Presence of autonomic neuropathy or parkinsonism

Cardiac syncope

- Presence of severe structural heart disease
- During exertion or supine
- Preceded by palpitation or accompanied by chest pain
- Family history of sudden death

Cerebrovascular syncope

- With arm exercise
- Differences in blood pressure or pulse in the two arms

Table 10.4: *ECG abnormalities suggestive arrhythmic syncope*

- Bifascicular block (defined as either left bundle-branch block or right bundle-branch block combined with left anterior or left posterior fascicular block)
- Other intraventricular conduction abnormalities (QRS duration ≥ 0.12 s)
- Mobitz I second degree atrioventricular (AV) block
- Asymptomatic sinus bradycardia (<50 beats/min) or sinoatrial block
- Pre-excited QRS complexes
- Prolonged QT interval
- Right bundle-branch block pattern with ST elevation in lead V1–V3 (Brugada syndrome)
- Negative T-waves in right precordial leads, epsilon waves and ventricular late potentials suggestive of arrhythmmogenic right ventricular dysplasia
- Q-wave suggesting myocardial infraction

Table 10.5: *Most useful and less useful tests*

	Test	*Suspected diagnosis*
Most useful	Carotid sinus massage	Neurally mediated
	Tilt testing	Neurally mediated
	Echocardiogram	Cardiac
	Holter/external loop monitoring	Cardiac
	Electrophysiological test	Cardiac
	Implantable loop recorder	Neurally mediated and cardiac
Less useful indicated only in selected cases	Electroencephalography	Epilepsy and TIA
	Brain computed tomography	Epilepsy and TIA
	Brain magnetic resonance imaging	Epilepsy and TIA
	Carotid Doppler sonography	Epilepsy and TIA
	Coronary angiography	Cardiac
	Pulmonary computed tomography/scintigraphy	Cardiac
	Chest X-ray	Cardiac
	Abdominal ultrasound examination	Comorbidities

TIA, transient ischemic attack.

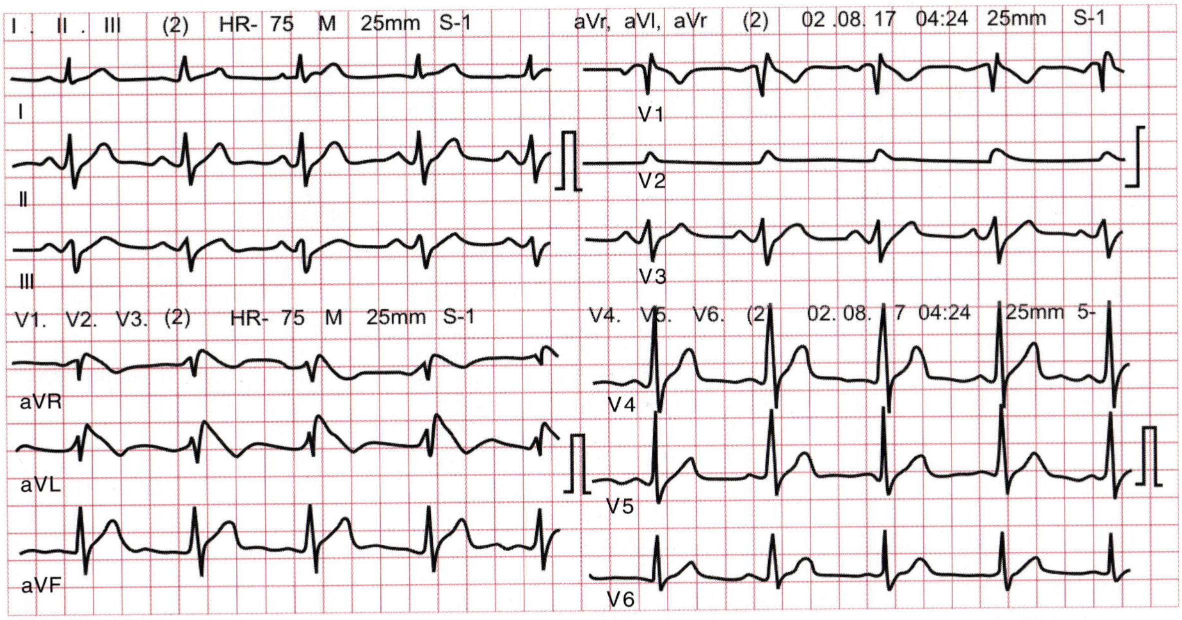

Fig. 10.6: *Holter diagnosis of Brugada syndrome (ST elevation in V1–V3)*

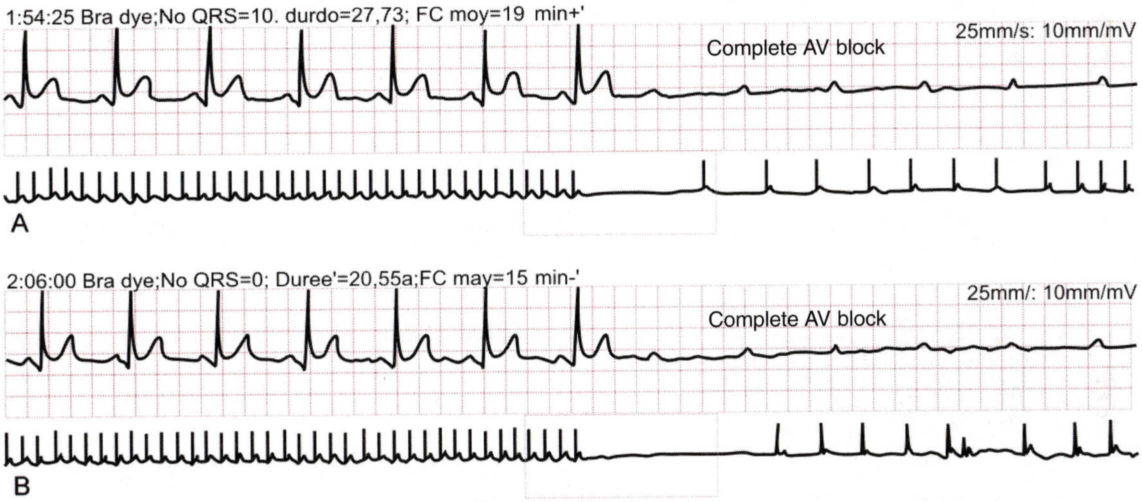

Fig. 10.7: *(A, B) Holter recording of two episodes of spontaneous syncope that occurred a few minutes apart. The two episodes were very similar and were characterized by sudden-onset complete atrioventricular (AV) block without changes in P-P cycle length, which constantly remained 720 ms and long ventricular asystole of 7 and 11 s (top and bottom, compressed traces, respectively).*

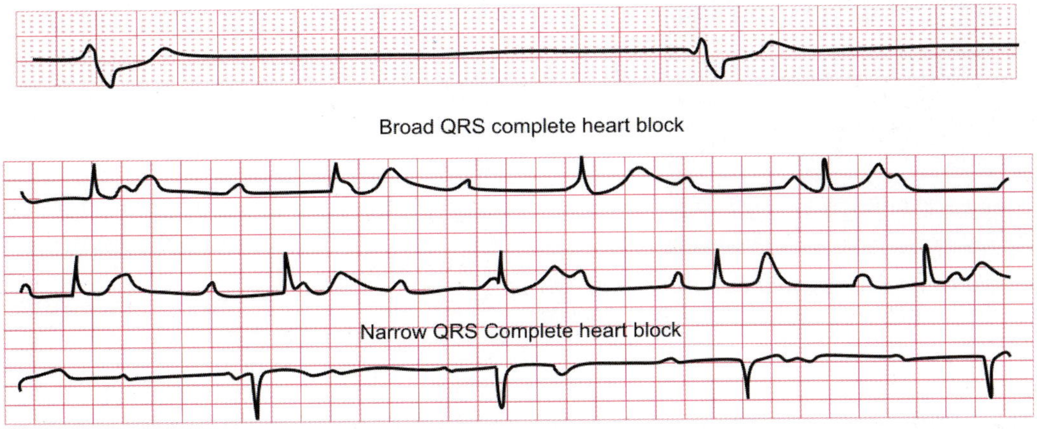

Fig. 10.8: *Holter ECG showing narrow and wide QRS complex in two patients suffering from aquired and congenital complete heart block respectively presening as syncopal attacks*

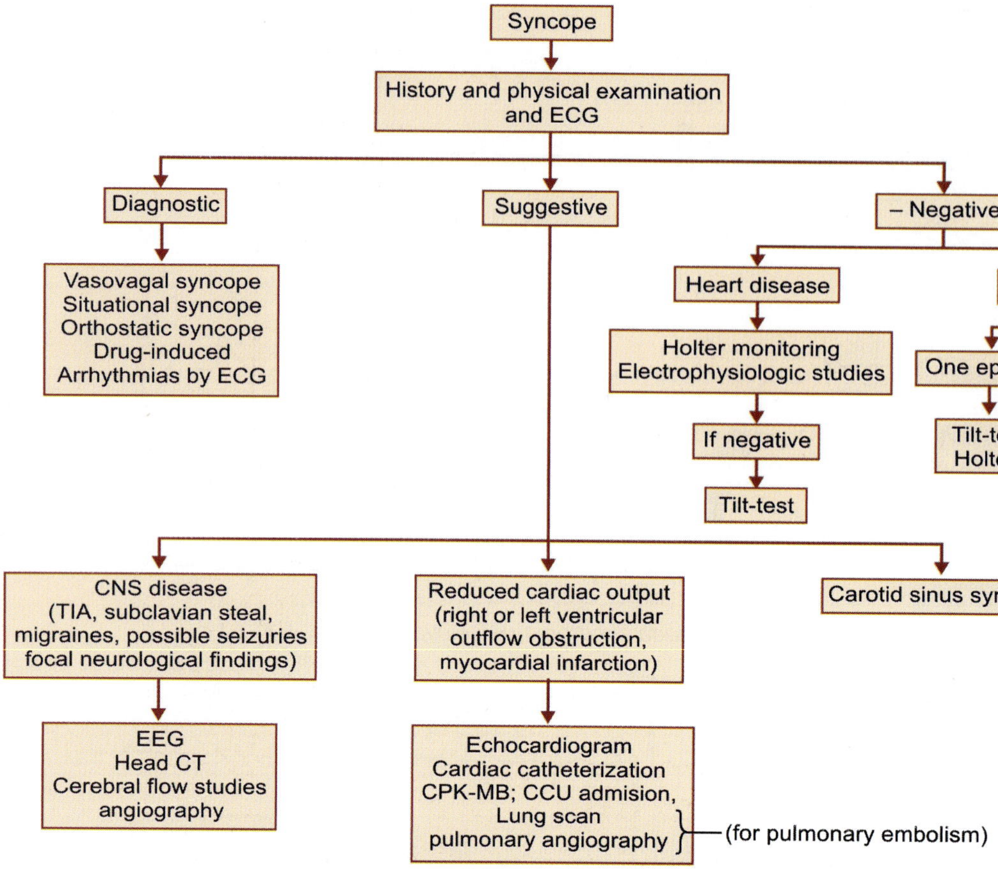

Fig. 10.9: *Schematic algorithm for the evaluation of patients presenting with syncope*

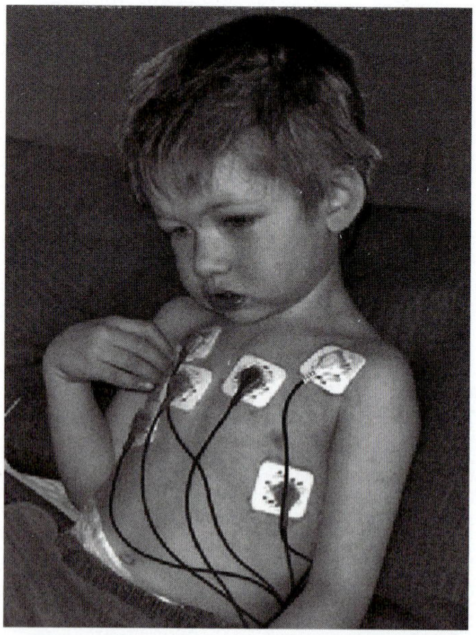

Fig. 10.10: *A 6-year-old boy is investigated for palpitations. 12-lead ECG is normal. A 24-hour Holter is reported to detect multiple episodes of nonsustained VT and amiodarone was started*

based on initial risk stratification is more likely to reap the dual rewards of a correct diagnosis and initiation of effective treatment in a cost-effective manner.

THE FOLLOWING QUESTIONS SHOULD BE ANSWERED

- Was loss of consciousness complete?
- Was loss of consciousness with rapid onset and short duration?
- Was recovery spontaneous, complete, and without sequelae?
- Was postural tone lost?

If the answers to these questions are positive, the episode has a high likelihood of being syncope. If one or more answers are negative, consider other forms of loss of consciousness prior to proceeding with syncope evaluation. The clinician should attempt to gather all information with respect to symptoms preceding the syncope.

Prior faintness, dizziness, or light-headedness occurs in 70% of patients experiencing true syncope. Other symptoms, such as vertigo, weakness, diaphoresis, epigastric discomfort, nausea, blurred or faded vision, pallor, or paresthesias, may also occur in the presyncopal period.

Symptoms of nausea or diaphoresis prior to the event may suggest syncope rather than seizure when the episode was not witnessed, whereas an aura may suggest seizure. Patients with true syncope do not remember actually falling to the ground. Presyncope involves the same symptoms and pathophysiology but terminates prior to loss of consciousness and can occasionally include loss of postural tone.

Table 10.6: *Recommendations: diagnostic criteria with initial evaluation*

Recommendations	*Class*[a]	*Level*[b]
VVS is diagnosed if syncope is precipitated by emotional distress or orthostatic stress and is associated with typical prodrome	I	C
Situational syncope is diagnosed if syncope occurs during or immediately after specific triggers	I	C
Orthostatic syncope is diagnosed when it occurs after standing up and there is documentation of OH	I	C
Arrhythmia-related syncope is diagnosed by ECG when there is: • Presistent sinus bradycardia <40 bpm in awake or repetitive sinoatrial block or sinus pause ≥3S • Mobitz II second or third degree AV block • Alternative left and right BBB • VT or rapid paroxysmal SVT • Nonsustained episodes of polymorphic VT and long or short QT interval • Pacemaker or ICD malfunction with cardiac pauses	I	C
Cardiac ischaemia-related syncope is diagnosed when syncope presents with ECG evidence of acute ischaemia with or without myocardial infarction	I	C
Cardiovascuolar syncope is diagnosed when syncope presents in patients with prolapsing atrial myxoma, severe aortic stenosis, pulmonary hypertension, pulmonary embolus, or acute aortic dissection	I	C

[a]Class of recommendation. [b]Level of evidence.
AV, atrioventricular; BBB, bundle-branch block;
ECG, electrocardiogram
ICD, implantable cardioverter defibrillator
OH, orthostatic hypotension; SVT, supraventricular tachycardia; VVS, vasovagal syncope; VT, ventricular tachycardia.

The duration of symptoms preceding a syncopal episode has been reported to be an average of 2.5 minutes in vasovagal syncope and an average of only 3 seconds in arrhythmia-related cardiac syncope.

Clinicians should specifically inquire as to red flag symptoms, such as exertional onset, chest pain, dyspnea, low back pain, palpitations, severe headache, focal neurologic deficits, diplopia, ataxia, or dysarthria prior to the syncopal event.

Patients should be asked to estimate the duration of their loss of consciousness. Syncope is associated with patient estimates ranging from seconds up to 1 minute in most cases. To discriminate from seizures, patients should also be asked if they remember being confused about their surroundings after the event or whether they have oral trauma, incontinence, or myalgias.

A detailed account of the event must also be obtained from any available witnesses. Witnesses can aid the clinician in differentiating among syncope, altered mental status and seizure.

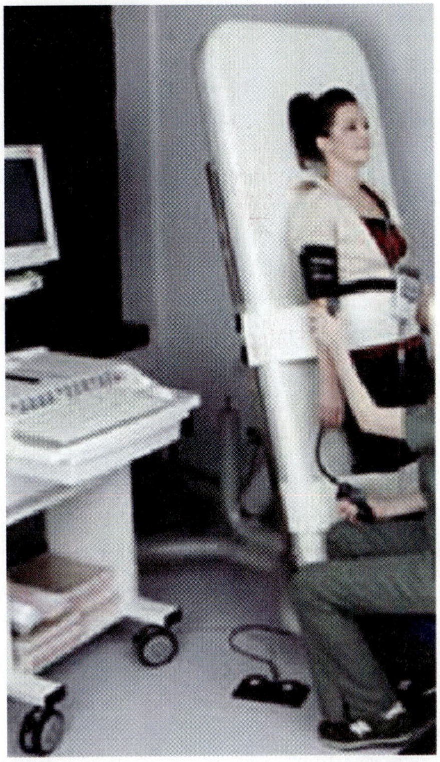

Fig. 10.11: *Showing performance of HUTT test a young lady with syncopal attack*

Convulsive activity, automatisms, or attempts to elicit focality can indicate seizure. Witnesses may be able to estimate the duration of unconsciousness and to assist in ascertaining whether the patient experienced postevent confusion.

Postevent confusion is the most powerful tool for discriminating between syncope and seizure. A postictal phase suggests that a seizure has occurred. Postevent confusion has been described with syncope, but the confusion should not last more than 30 seconds. Seizure like activity can occur with syncope if the patient is held in an upright posture.

A medication history must be obtained in all patients with syncope with special emphasis placed on cardiac and antihypertensive medications. Drugs commonly implicated in syncope include the following:
- Agents that reduce blood pressure (e.g. antihypertensive drugs, diuretics, nitrates)
- Agents that affect cardiac output (e.g. beta-blockers, digitalis, antiarrhythmics)
- Agents that prolong the cardiac output (QT) interval (e.g. tricyclic antidepressants, phenothiazines, quinidine, amiodarone)
- Agents that alter sensorium (including alcohol, cocaine, analgesics with sedative properties)
- Agents that alter serum electrolytes (especially diuretics).

Inquiry must be made into any personal or familial past medical history of cardiac disease. Patients with a history

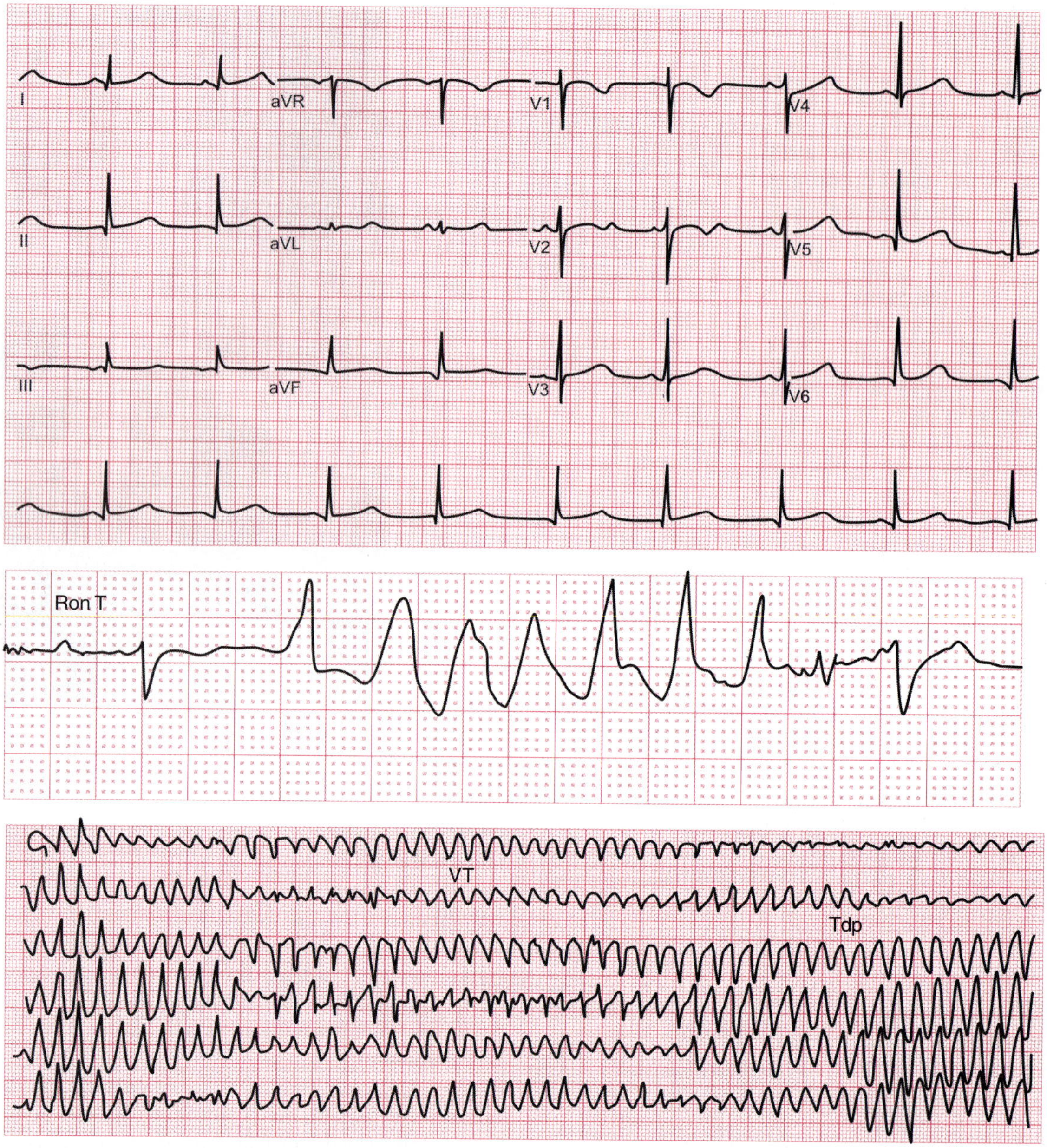

Fig. 10.12: *Holter ECG findings in patient with long QT syndrome type 2. (A) ECG of an 18-year-old woman with recurrent syncope. As is typical in LQTS, the QTc interval is prolonged at 500 ms. The subtype of LQTS can be predicted from a detailed examination of the T-wave (Zhang et al., 2004). In this case, the biphasic T waves in V2 and Lead III were consistent with a hERG mutation. (B) Cardiac telemetry recording showed the onset of TdP, with an 'R on T' initiation. (C) Subsequent ECG, during syncope, illustrates the characteristic appearance of TdP*

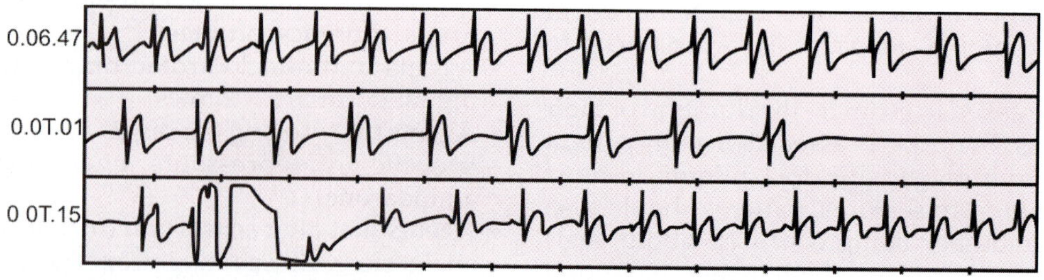

Fig. 10.13: *Utility of implantable loop recorder in the diagnosis of unexplained syncope. Event recorder tracing showing a 4.8 s asystole period in a 13-year-old subject. Time is indicated on the right scale. After a few sinus beats, there is a progressive slowing of a junctional rhythm ending into asystole. Recovery of sinus rhythm is evident in the bottom panel*

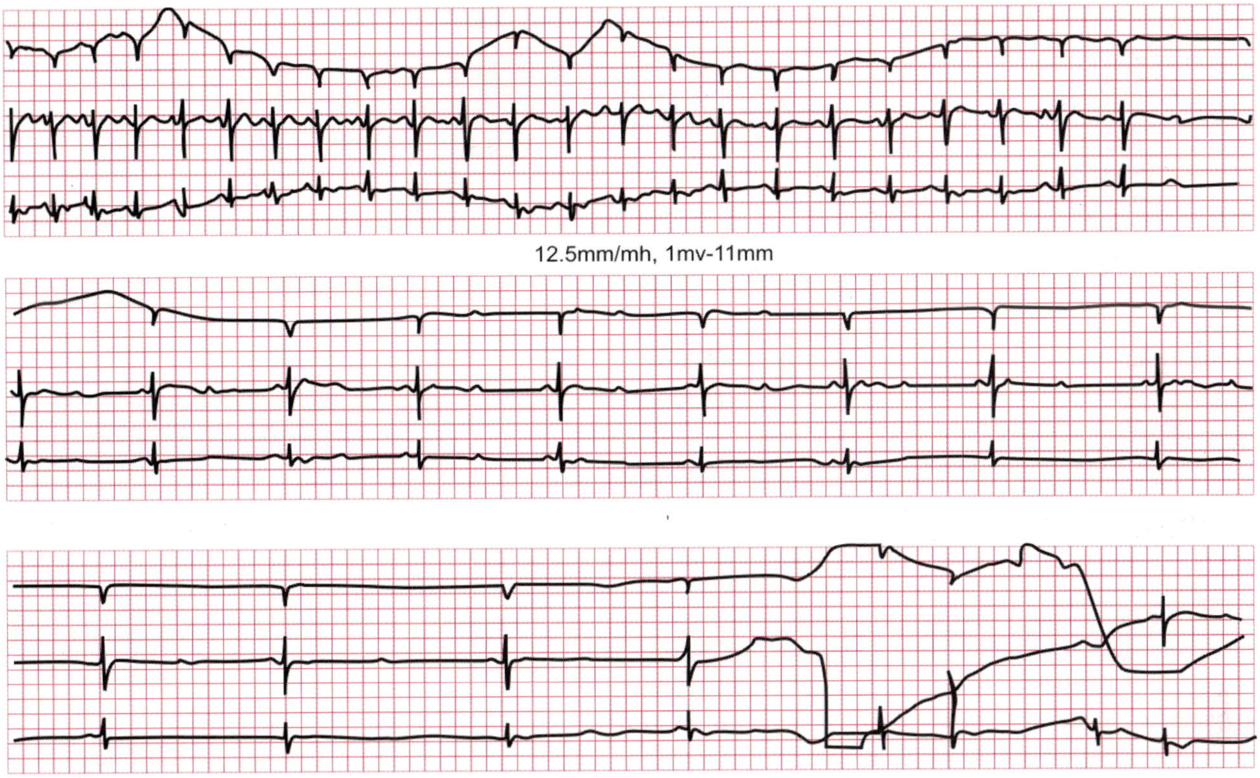

Fig. 10.14: *Electrocardiographic characteristics of atrioventricular block induced by tilt testing. Electrocardiographic Holter recordings at 12.5 mm/s, three consecutive strips. The electrocardiographic tracing begins with sinus rhythm slowing, PR prolongation and then 2:1 atrioventricular block, ending with Mobitz I second-degree atrioventricular block*

Table 10.7: *Recommendations:active standing*

Recommendations	*Class[a]*	*Level[b]*
Indications		
• Manual intermittant determination with sphygmomanometer of BP supine and during active standing for 3 min is indicated as initial evaluation when OH is suspected	I	B
• Continuous beat-to-beat noninvasive pressure measurement may be helpful in cases of doubt	IIb	C
Diagnostic criteria		
• The test is diagnostic when there is symptomatic fall in systolic BP from a baseline value ≥ 20 mmHg or diastolic BP ≥ 10 mmHg, or a decrease in systolic BP to <90 mmHg	I	C
• The test should be considered diagnostic when there is an asymptomatic fall in systolic BP from baseline value ≥ 20 mmHg or diastolic BP ≥ 10 mmHg, or a decrease in systolic BP to < 90 mmHg	IIa	C

[a]class of recommendation. [b]Level of evidence.
BP, blood pressure; OH, orthostatic hypotension.

of myocardial infarction (MI), arrhythmia, structural cardiac defects, cardiomyopathies, or CHF have a uniformly worse prognosis than other patient groups.

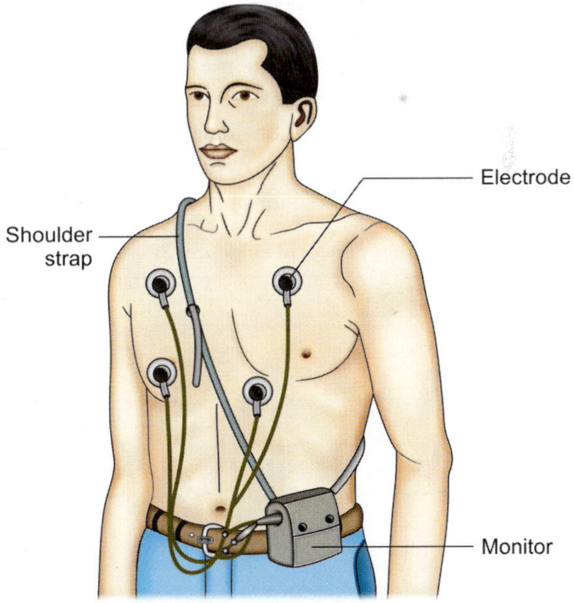

Fig. 10.15: *Diagram showing a 24-hour Holter monitor system which has been attached with leads over the chest of the patient. A monitor is also seen (bottom left) fitted with belt*

Remember to consider the broad differential diagnosis of syncope. Assess whether the patient has a history of seizure disorder, diabetes, stroke (CVA), deep venous thrombosis (DVT), or abdominal aortic aneurysm or if pregnancy is a possibility.

Table 10.8: *Recommendations: tilt testing*

Recommendations	*Class*[a]	*Level*[b]
Methodology		
• Supine pre-tilt phase of at least 5 min, when no venous cannulation, and of at least 20 min, when cannulation is undertaken, is recommended	I	C
• Tilt angle between 60° and 70° is recommended	I	B
• Passive phase of a minimum of 20 min and a maximum of 45 min is recommended	I	B
• For nitroglycerine, a fixed dose of 300–400 µg sublingually administered in the upright position is recommended	I	B
• For isoproterenol, an incremental infusion rate from 1 upto 3 µg/min in order to increase average heart rate by ~20–25% over baseline is recommended	I	B
Indications		
• Tilt testing is indicated in the case of an upexplained single syncopal episode in high-risk setting (e.g. occurrence of, or potential risk of physical injury or with occupational implication, or recurrent episodes in the absence of organic heart disease, or in the presence of organic heart disease, after cardiac causes of syncope have been excluded	I	B
• Tilt testing is indicated when it is of clinical value of demonstrate susceptibility to reflex syncope to the patient	I	C
• Tilt testing should be considered to discriminate between reflex and OH syncope	IIa	C
• Tilt testing may be considered for differentiating syncope with jerking movements from epilepsy	IIb	C
• Tilt testing may be indicated for evaluation patients with recurrent unexplained falls	IIb	C
• Tilt testing may be indicated for evaluation patients with recurrent unexplained falls	IIb	C
• Tilt testing is not recommended for assessment of treatment	III	B
• Isoproterenol tilt testing is contraindicated in patients with ischemic heart disease	III	C
Diagnostic criteria		
• In patients without, structral heart disease the induction of reflex hypotension/bradycardia with reproduction of syncope or progressive OH (with or without symptoms) are diagnostic of reflex syncope and OH, respectively	I	B
• In patients without structural heart disease the induction of reflex hypotension/bradycardia without reproduction of syncope may be diagnostic of reflex syncope	IIa	B
• In patients with structural heart disease, arrhythmia or other cardiovascular cause of syncope should be excluded prior to considering positive tilt test result as diagnostic	IIa	C
• Induction of LOC in absence of hypotension and/or bradycardia should be considered diagnostic of psychogenic pseudosyncope	IIa	C

[a]Class of recommendation. [b]Level of evidence. BP, blood pressure; CSM, carotid sinus massage; HR, heart rate; LOC, loss of consciousness; OH, orthostatic hypotension; TIA, transient ischemic attack; mg, micrograms.

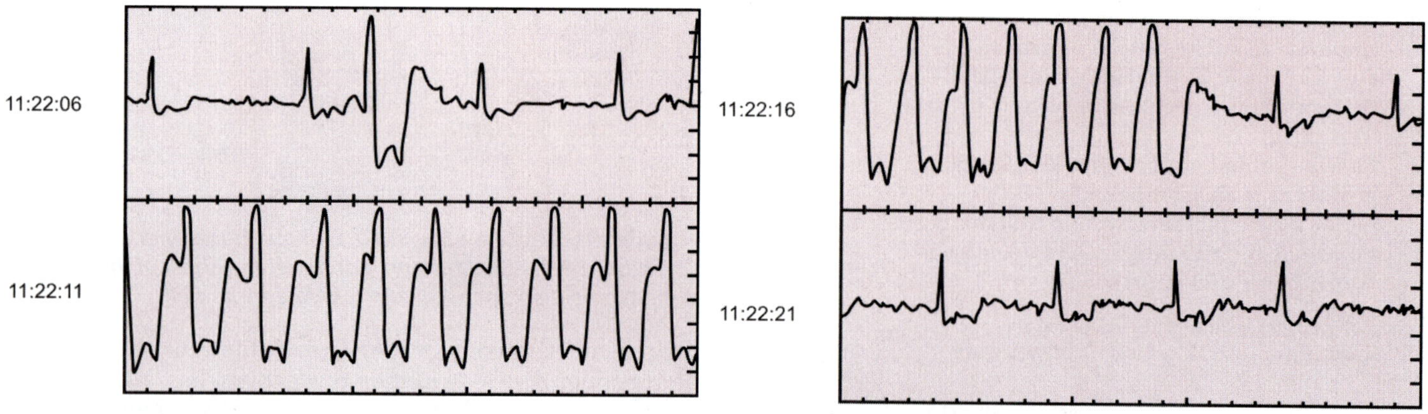

Fig. 10.16: *Utility of implantable loop recorder in the diagnosis of unexplained syncope event recorder tracing showing a bout of wide QRS tachycardia during a syncopal episode*

Causes

Cardiac (cardiopulmonary) syncope may be due to vascular disease, cardiomyopathy, arrhythmia, or valvular dysfunction and predicts a worse short-term and long-term prognosis. Obtaining an initial ECG is mandatory if any of these causes are possible for the differential diagnosis.

Low flow states, such as those associated with advanced cardiomyopathy, CHF, and valvular insufficiency, may result in hypotension and cause transient global cerebral hypoperfusion. Often, these patients are on medications that reduce afterload, which may contribute to the cause of syncope (Figs 10.17 and 10.18).

Ventricular arrhythmias, such as ventricular tachycardia and torsade de pointes, tend to occur in older patients with known cardiac disease. These patients tend to have fewer recurrences and have a more sudden onset with few, if any, presyncopal symptoms. Associated chest pain or dyspnea may be present. This type of syncope is generally unrelated to posture and can occur during lying, sitting, or standing. Often, these arrhythmias are not revealed on the initial ECG but may be captured with prolonged monitoring (Fig. 10.16).

Supraventricular tachyarrhythmias include supraventricular tachycardia and atrial fibrillation with rapid response. These may be associated with palpitations, chest pain, or dyspnea. Patients typically have prodromal symptoms and may have syncope while attempting to stand or walk because of resultant hypotension. These symptoms may spontaneously resolve prior to evaluation but are often noted during initial triage and assessment. Be sure to scrutinize ECG findings for evidence of Wolff-Parkinson-White syndrome, Brugada syndrome, and long QT syndrome.

Bradyarrhythmias include sick sinus syndrome, sinus bradycardia, high-grade atrioventricular blocks, pacemaker malfunction, and adverse medication reactions. Generally, these patients have a history of cardiac problems and are symptomatic. Chest pain, dyspnea, decreased exercise tolerance, and fatigue may all be present. Consider cardiac ischemia and medication side effects as additional causes. Cardiac outflow obstruction may also result in sudden-

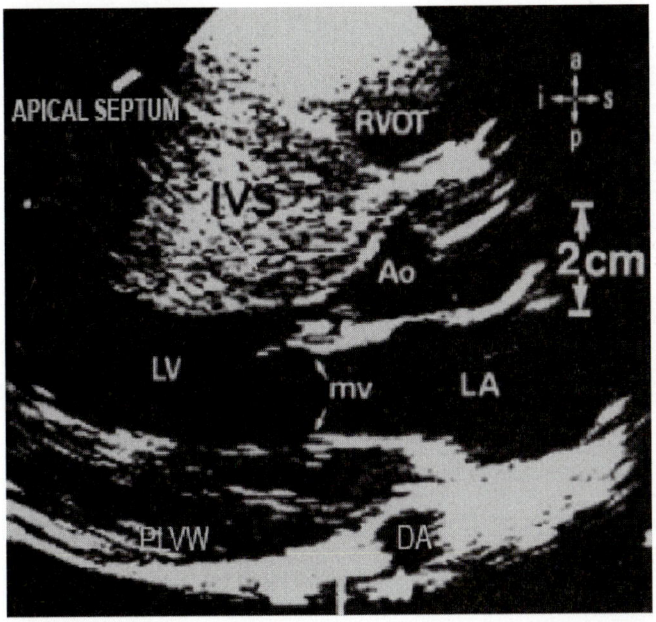

Fig. 10.17: 2-D echocardiogram in long-axis view showing marked hypertrophy of interventricular septum and posterior left ventricular wall ,almost approximating anterior mitral valve leaflet with hypertrophied interventricular septum producing severe left ventricular outflow tract obstruction in patient with hypertrophic cardiomyopathy and presenting as syncopal attack

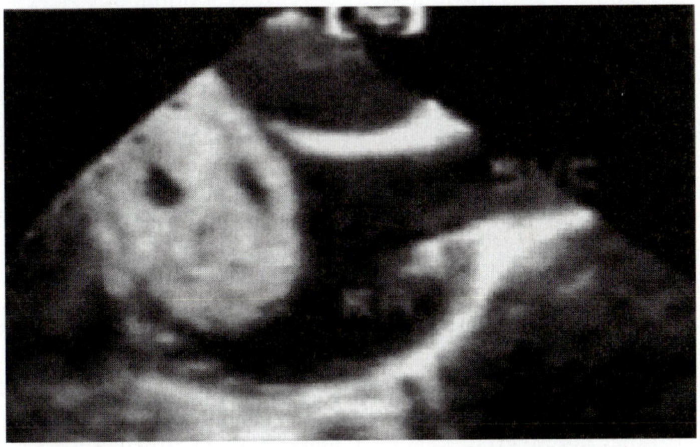

Fig. 10.18: TEE four chamber view the mass prolapsing across the tricuspid valve during diastole in a young patient with arrythmic syncope

Table 10.9: *Classification of vasovagal syncope induced by head-up tilt table testing*

Type	*Classification*
Type 1 mixed	Ventricular rate during syncope 40 bpm or falls to <40 bpm for <10 sec asystole for <3 sec. BP falls prior to heart rate
Type 2A cardioinhibitory	Ventricular rate during syncope <40 bpm for >10 sec or asystole for >3 s. BP falls to <80 mmHg systolic at or after rapid fall in heart rate (as above)
Type 2B cardioinhibitory	Heart rate does not fall more than 10% from its peak at syncope. Fall in BP precipitates syncope.
Type 3 Pure vasodepressor	

Exceptions to this classification include chronotropic incompetence, excessive heart rate rise (>130 bpm) during tilt and where carotid sinus hypersenstivity is demonstrated.

Table 10.10: *Recommendations: electrocardiographic monitoring*

Recommendations	*Class[a]*	*Level[b]*
Indications		
• ECG monitoring is indicated in patients who have clinical or ECG (features suggesting arrhythmic syncope. The duration (and technology) of monitoring should be selected according the risk and the predicted recurrence rate of syncope:	I	B
– Immediated in-hospital monitoring (in bed or telemetric) is indicated in high-risk patients defined in Table 10.11	I	C
– Holter monitoring is indicated in patients who have very frequent syncope or presyncope (≥1 per week)	I	B
– ILR is indicated in:		
o An early phase of evaluation in patients with recurrent syncope of uncertain origin, absence of high risk criteria listed in table 10.11 and a high likelihood of recurrence within battery longevity of the device	I	B
o High risk patients in whom a comprehensive evaluation did not demonstrate a cause of syncope or lead to a specific treatment	I	B
– ILR should be considered to assess the contribution of bradycardia before embarking on cardiac pacing in patients with suspected or certain reflex syncope presenting with frequent or traumatic syncopal episodes	IIa	B
– External loop recorders should be considered in patients who have an intersymptom interval ≤ 4 weeks	IIa	B
Diagnostic criteria		
• ECG monitoring is diagnostic when a correlation between syncope and an arrhythmia (brady-or tachyarrhythmia) is detected	I	B
• In the absence of such correlation, ECG monitoring is diagnostic when periods of Mobitz II or III degree AV block or a ventricular pause > 3s (with the possible exception of young-trained persons, during sleep, medicated patients, or rate-controlled atrial fibrillation), or rapid prolonged paroxysmal SVT or VT are detected. The absence of arrhythmia during syncope excludes arrhythmic syncope	I	C
• The ECG documentation of presyncope without any relevant arrhythmia is not an accurate surrogate for syncope	III	C
• Asymptomatic arrhythmias (other than those listed above) are not accurate surrogate for syncope	III	C
• Sinus bradycardia (in the absence of syncope) is not an accurate surrogate for syncope	III	C

[a]Class of recommendation. [b]Level of evidence. AV, atrioventricular; ECG, electrocardiogram; ILR, implantable loopr recorder; SVT, supraventriculartachyradia; VT, ventricular tachycardia.

Table 10.11: *Recommendations: electrophysiological study*

Recommendations	*Class[a]*	*Level[b]*
Indications		
• In patients with ischemic heart disease EPS is indicated when initial evaluation suggests an arrhythmic cause of syncope unless there is already an established indication for ICD	I	B
• In patients with BBB, EPS should be considered when noninvasive tests have failed to make the diagnosis	IIa	B
• In patients with syncope preceded by sudden and brief palpitations, EPS may be performed when other noninvasive tests have failed to make the diagnosis	IIb	B
• In patients with Brugada syndrome, ARVC and hypertrophic cardiomyopathy an EPS may be performed in selected cases	IIb	C
• EPS is not recommended in patients with normal ECG, no heart disease, and no palpitations	III	B
Diagnostic criteria		
• EPS is diagnostic, and no additional tests are required, in the following cases:		
– Sinus bradycardia and prolonged CSNRT (> 525 ms)	I	B
– BBB and either a baseline HV interval of ≥ 100 ms, or second or third degree His-Purkinje block is demonstrated during incremental atrial pacing, or with pharmacological challenge	I	B
– Induction of sustained monomorphic VT in patients with previous myocardial infarction	I	B
– Induction of rapid SVT which reproduces hypotensive or spontaneous symptoms	I	B
• AV HV interval between 70 ms and 100 ms should be considered diagnostic	IIa	B
• The induction of polymorphic VT or ventricular fibrillation in patients with Brugada syndrome, ARVC and patients resuscitated from cardiac arrest may be considered diagnostic	IIb	B
• The induction of polymorphic VT or ventricular fibrillation in patients with ischemic cardiomyopathy or DCM cannot be considered a diagnostic finding	III	B

[a]Class of recommendation. [b]Level of evidence. ARVC, arrhythmogenic right ventricular cardiomyopathy; BBB, bundle-branch block; CSNRT, corrected sinus node recovery time; DCM, dilated cardiomyopathy; EPS, electrophysiological study; ICD, implantable cardioverter defibrillator; HV, His-ventricle; SVT, supraventricular tachycardia; VT, ventricular tachycardia; MI, myocardial infarction.

onset syncope with little or no prodrome. One critical clue is the exertional nature, and the other is the presence of a cardiac murmur. Young athletes may present with this etiology for syncope. Specific pathology includes aortic stenosis, hypertrophic obstructive cardiomyopathy, mitral stenosis, pulmonary stenosis, pulmonary embolus, left atrial myxoma, and pericardial tamponade.

Syncope can also result from an acute MI, acute aortic dissection, and pulmonary embolus. These conditions can have associated chest pain, neck pain, shoulder pain, dyspnea, epigastric pain, hypotension, alteration of mental status and can result in sudden death.

Reflex (neurally mediated) syncope may be due to vasovagal syncope, which is mediated by emotional distress such as fear or physical pain. Situational syncope describes syncope that occurs with a fixed event such as micturition, deglutition, exercise induced, and carotid sinus syncope. These causes tend to be more benign and do not predict poor outcomes.

Vasovagal syncope is the most common type in young adults but can occur at any age. It usually occurs in a standing position and is precipitated by fear, emotional stress, or pain (e.g. after a needle stick). Autonomic symptoms are predominant. Classically, nausea, diaphoresis, fading or "graying out" of vision, epigastric discomfort, and light-headedness precede syncope by a few minutes. Syncope is thought to occur secondary to efferent vasodepressor reflexes by a number of mechanisms, resulting in decreased peripheral vascular resistance. It is not life threatening and occurs sporadically.

Situational syncope is essentially a reproducible vasovagal syncope with a known precipitant. Micturition, defecation, deglutition, tussive, and carotid sinus syncope are types of situational syncope. These stimuli result in autonomic reflexes with a vasodepressor response, ultimately leading to transient cerebral hypotension. These are not life-threatening but can cause morbidity. The treatment involves avoidance of the precipitant when possible and the initiation of counter maneuvers when anticipated.

Syncope due to orthostatic hypotension can occur through several mechanisms. Pure autonomic failure can be associated with Parkinson's disease or dementia. Secondary autonomic insufficiency can be due to diabetes, uremia, or spinal injury. Drugs such as alcohol cause orthostatic intolerance and medications such as vasodilators and antidepressants block orthostatic reflexes. Volume depletion due to blood loss, vomiting, diarrhea, poor oral intake, and diuretics also cause orthostatic syncope.

Dehydration and decreased intravascular volume contribute to orthostasis.

Orthostatic syncope describes a causative relationship between orthostatic hypotension and syncope. Orthostatic hypotension increases in prevalence with age as a blunted baroreceptor response results in failure of compensatory cardioacceleration. In elderly patients, 45% of these cases are related to medications. Limited evidence suggests that polydipsia may reduce recurrences.

Orthostasis is a common cause of syncope and tends to be recurrent. Bedside orthostatics cannot exclude this as an etiology; if suspected, patients should be referred to a primary care provider for outpatient tilt-table testing.

Dehydration and decreased intravascular volume contribute to orthostasis. Orthostatic syncope describes a causative relationship between orthostatic hypotension and syncope. Orthostatic hypotension increases in prevalence with age as a blunted baroreceptor response results in failure of compensatory cardioacceleration. In elderly patients, 45% of these cases are related to medications. Limited evidence suggests that polydipsia may reduce recurrences. Orthostasis is a common cause of syncope and tends to be recurrent. Bedside orthostatics cannot exclude this as an etiology; if suspected, patients should be referred to a primary care provider for outpatient tilt-table testing.

LABORATORY STUDIES

Currently, no specific testing has sufficient power to be absolutely indicated for evaluation of syncope. Research-based and consensus guideline recommendations are listed below.

Serum Glucose Level

In one study, 2 of 170 patients with syncope tested for serum glucose were found to be hypoglycemic.

Despite this low yield, rapid blood glucose assessment is easy, fast, and may be diagnostic, leading to efficient intervention.

CBC Count

If performed empirically, a CBC count has an exceedingly low yield in syncope. Some risk stratification protocols use a low hematocrit level as a poor prognostic indicator.

A prospective evaluation of syncope found that 4 of 170 patients had signs and symptoms of GI hemorrhage with a confirmatory CBC count. No occult bleeding was diagnosed based on an empiric CBC count in this study.

Table 10.12: *Recommendations: treatment of orthostatic hypotension (OH)*

Recommendations	*Class*[a]	*Level*[b]
• Adequate hydration and salt intake must be maintained	I	C
• Midedrine should be administered as adjuctive therapy if needed	IIa	B
• Fludrocortisone should be administered as adjunctive therapy if needed	IIa	C
• PCMs may be indicated	IIb	C
• Abdominal binders and/or support stocking to reduce venous pooling may be indicated	IIb	C
• Head-up tilt sleeping (<10°) to increase fluid volume may be indicated	IIb	C

[a]Class of recommendation. [b]Level of evidence. PCM, physical counter pressure maneuver.

Table 10.13: *Recommendations: indications for ICD in patients with unexplained syncope and a high risk of SCD*

Clinical situation	*Class[a]*	*Level[b]*	*Comments*
• In patients with ischemic cardiomyopathy with several depressed LVEF or HF, ICD therapy is indicated according to current guidelines for ICD–cardiac resynchronization therapy implantation	I	A	
• In patient with nonischemic cardiomyopathy with several depressed LVEF or HF, ICD therapy is indicated according to current guidelines for ICD–cardiac resynchonization therapy implantation	I	A	
• In hypertrophic cardiomyopathy, ICD therapy should be considered in patients at high risk	IIa	C	In non-high risk, consider ILR
• In right ventricular cardiomyopathy ICD therapy should be considered in patients at high risk	IIa	C	In non-high risk, consider ILR
• In Brugada syndrome ICD therapy should be considered in patients with spontaneous type I ECG	IIa	B	In the absence of spontaneous type I pattern, consider ILR
• In long QT syndrome, ICD therapy, in conjuction with β-blockers, should be considered in patients at risk	IIa	B	In non-high risk, consider ILR
• In patients with ischemic cardiomyopathy without severely depressed LVEF or HF and negative programed electrical stimulation ICD therapy may be considered	IIb	C	Consider ILR to help to define the nature of unexplained syncope
• In patients with nonischemic cardiomyopathy without severely depressed LVEF or HF ICD therapy may be considered	IIb	C	Consider ILR to help to define the nature of unexplained syncope

[a]Class of recommendation. [b]Level of evidence. "HF, heart failure; ECG, electrocardiogram; ICD, implantable cardioverter defibrillator; ILR, implantable loop recorder; LVEF, left ventricular ejection fraction; SCD, sudden cardiac death

Anemia has been shown in several studies to suggest poor short-term outcomes.

Serum Electrolyte Levels with Renal Function

These tests if performed empirically have an exceedingly low yield in syncope. Some risk stratification protocols use electrolyte level abnormalities and renal insufficiency as poor prognostic indicators.

In the study by Martin et al., 134 patients with syncope had electrolytes drawn as part of the routine workup. One patient was unexpectedly found to be hyponatremic secondary to diuretic use.

Serum electrolyte tests are indicated in patients with altered mental status or in patients in whom seizure is being considered.

If arrhythmia is noted, evaluation of electrolytes may be useful.

Cardiac Enzymes

These tests are indicated in patients who give a history of chest pain with syncope, dyspnea with syncope, or exertional syncope; those with multiple cardiac risk factors; and those in whom a cardiac origin is highly suspected.

Total Creatine Kinase (CK)

A rise in CK levels may be associated with prolonged seizure activity or muscle damage secondary to a prolonged period of loss of consciousness.

BNP level >300 pg/mL is a predictor of serious outcomes at 30 days.

Urinalysis/Dipstick

In elderly and debilitated patients, UTI is common, easily diagnosed, and treatable and may precipitate syncope. UTIs may occur in the absence of fever, leukocytosis, and symptoms in this population.

IMAGING STUDIES

Chest Radiography

In elderly patients and in patients who are debilitated, pneumonia is common, easily diagnosed, and treatable and may precipitate syncope. Pneumonia may occur in the absence of fever, leukocytosis, and symptoms in this population.

Evaluation of a select number of etiologies of syncope may be aided by chest radiography. Pneumonia, CHF, lung mass, effusion, and widened mediastinum can all be seen if present and may guide therapy.

Head CT Scanning (Noncontrast)

Head CT scanning is not indicated in a nonfocal patient after a syncopal event. This test has a low diagnostic yield in syncope.

Head CT scanning may be clinically indicated in patients with new neurologic deficits or in patients with head trauma secondary to syncope.

Chest /Abdominal CT Scanning

This imaging study is indicated only in select cases, such as cases in which aortic dissection, ruptured abdominal aortic aneurysm, or pulmonary embolus is suspected.

Table 10.14: *Recommendations: treatment of syncope due to cardiac arrhythmias*

Recommendations	*Class*[a]	*Level*[b]
• Syncope due to cardiac arrhythmias must receive treatment appropriate to the cause	I	B
Cardiac pacing		
• Pacing is indicated in patients with sinus node disease in whom syncope is demonstrated to be due to sinus arrest (symptom—ECG correlation) without a correctable cause	I	C
• Pacing is indicated in sinus node disease patients with syncope and abnormal CSNRT	I	C
• Pacing is indicated in sinus node disease patients with syncope and asymptomatic pauses ≥ 3 s (with the possible exceptions of young-trained persons, during sleep, and in medicated patients)	I	C
• Pacing is indicated in patients with syncope and second Mobitz II, advanced or complete AV block	I	B
• Pacing is indicated in patients with syncope, BBB, and positive EPS	I	B
• Pacing should be considered in patients with unexplained syncope and BBB	IIa	C
• Pacing may be indicated in patients with unexplained syncope and sinus node disease and persistent sinus bradycardia itself asymptomatic	IIb	C
• Pacing is not indicated in patients with unexplained syncope without evidence of any conduction disturbance	III	C
Catheter ablation		
• Catheter ablation is indicated in patients with symptom—arrhythmia ECG correlation in both SVT and VT in the absence of structural heart disease (with the exception of atrial fibrillation)	I	C
• Catheter ablation may be indicated in patients with syncope due to the onset of rapid atrial fibrillation	IIb	C
Antiarrhythmic drug therapy		
• Antiarrhythmic drug therapy including control drugs, is indicated in patients with syncope due to onset of rapid atrial fibrillation	I	C
• Drug therapy should be considered in patient with symptom—arrhythmia ECG correlation in both SVT and VT when catheter ablation cannot be undertaken or has failed.	IIa	C
Implantable cardioverter defibrillator		
• ICD is indicated in patients with documented VT and structural heart disease	I	B
• ICD is indicated when sustained monomorphic VT is induced at EPS in patients with previous myocardial infraction	I	B
• ICD should be considered in patient with documented VT and inherited cardiomyopathies or channelopathies	IIa	B

[a] Class of recommendation. [b] Level of evidence. AV, atrioventricular; BBB, bundle-branch block; CSNRT, corrected sinus node recovery time; ECG, electrocardiogram; EPS, electrophysiological study; ICD, implantable cardioverter defibrillator; SVT, supraventricular tachycardia; VT, ventricular tachycardia; MI, myocardial infraction

Brain MRI /Magnetic Resonance Arteriography (MRA)

These tests may be required in select cases to evaluate vertebrobasilar vasculature and are more appropriately performed on an inpatient basis in consultation with a neurologist or a neurosurgeon.

Ventilation-perfusion (V/Q) Scanning

This test is appropriate for patients in whom pulmonary embolus is suspected.

Echocardiography (Figs 10.17 and 10.18)

In patients with known heart disease, left ventricular function and ejection fraction have been shown to have an accurate predictive correlation with death.

Echocardiography is the test of choice for evaluating suspected mechanical cardiac causes of syncope.

Electrocardiography

Obtain a standard 12-lead ECG in syncope. This is a level A recommendation by 2007 ACEP consensus guidelines for syncope. ECG is used in most every clinical decision rule for risk stratification.

Normal ECG findings are a good prognostic sign.

ECG can be diagnostic for acute MI or myocardial ischemia and can provide objective evidence of preexisting cardiac disease or dysrhythmia such as **Wolff-Parkinson-White syndrome, Brugada syndrome, atrial flutter, or AV blocks (Fig. 10.23).**

Bradycardia, sinus pauses, nonsustained ventricular tachycardia and sustained ventricular tachycardia, and atrioventricular conduction defects occur with increasing frequency with age and are truly diagnostic only when they coincide with symptoms.

Holter Monitor/Loop Event Recorder

This is an outpatient test. In the past, all patients with syncope were monitored for 24 hours in a hospital. Later, loop recorders and signal-averaged event recorders allowed for monitoring over longer time periods, which increased the yield of detecting an arrhythmia.

Recent studies show that age-matched asymptomatic populations have an equivalent number of arrhythmic events recorded by ambulatory monitoring. Loop recorders have a higher diagnostic yield than Holter monitor evaluation with a marginal cost savings (FIgs 10.4 to 10.8).

A study completed through an ECG outpatient registry in Vermont by Gibson and Heitzman involving 1,512 patients referred for syncope, showed that symptomatic arrhythmias were found in just 0.5% of patients. In fact, patients had symptoms without arrhythmias more often than symptoms with arrhythmias, advancing the notion that ambulatory monitoring has a higher negative than positive diagnostic yield (Figs 10.12 to 10.14; 10.19; 10.20 and 10.22).

Head-up Tilt-table Test (Fig. 10.11)

This test is useful for confirming autonomic dysfunction and can generally be safely arranged on an outpatient basis.

The test involves using a tilt table to stand a patient at 70° for 45 minutes. Various modified protocols with concomitant medications, fasting, and maneuvers exist. Normally norepinephrine (NE) levels rise initially and are maintained to hold BP constant.

A positive result occurs when NE levels fatigue with time and a falling BP and pulse rate produce symptoms.

The head-up tilt-table test is less sensitive than electrophysiologic stress testing, and a negative result does not exclude the diagnosis of neurogenic syncope.

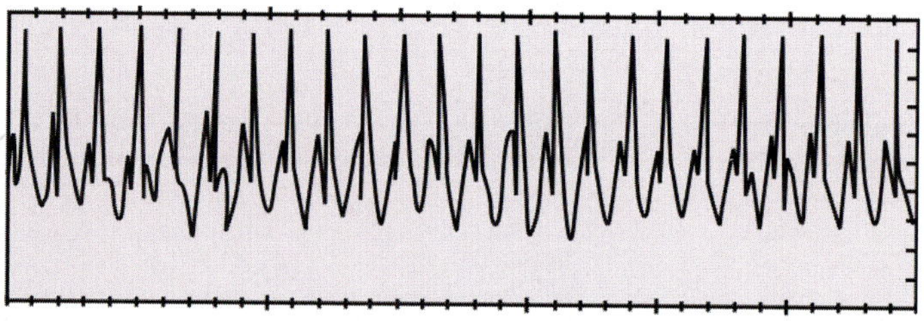

Fig. 10.19: *The single-lead ECG tracing from ILR in patient showing SVT at 214 beats per minute*

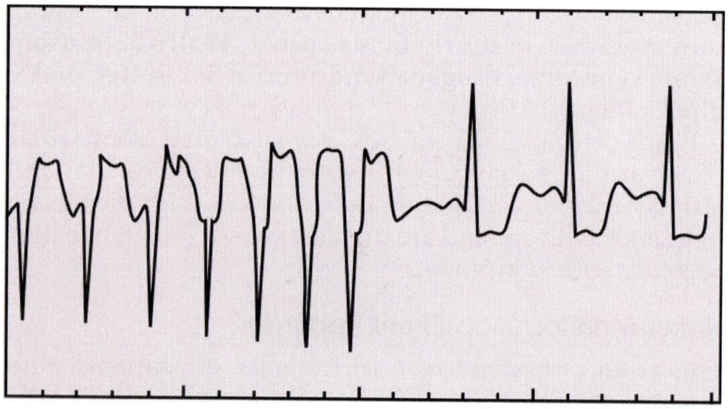

Fig. 10.20: *The single-lead ECG tracing from ILR in patient shows nonsustained VT with abrupt termination, followed by normal sinus rhythm*

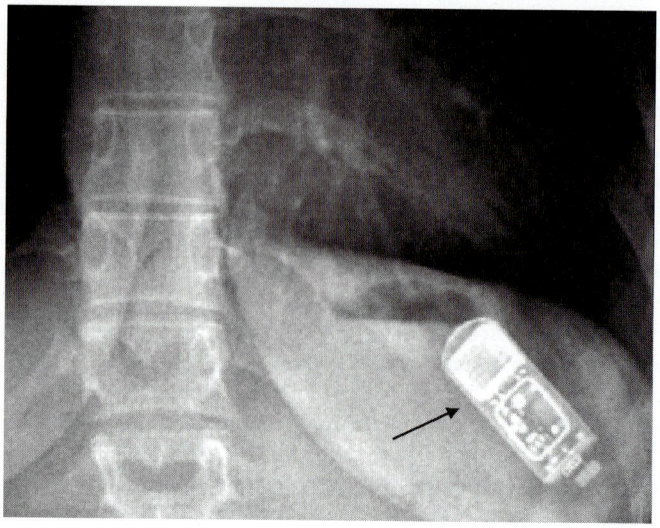

Fig. 10.21: *Collimated frontal view of the chest shows an implantable loop recorder (arrow) in the left breast of a 25-year-old woman with a history of heart palpitations and surgical repair of a tetralogy of Fallot as a young child*

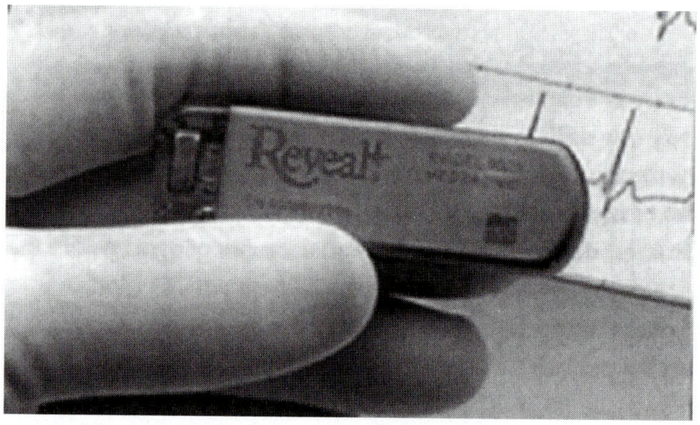

Fig. 10.22: *Showing light weight implantable loop recorder*

Electroencephalography

Electroencephalography (EEG) can be performed at the discretion of a neurologist if seizure is considered a likely alternative diagnosis.

Stress Test

Stress test/electrophysiologic studies (EPS) have a higher diagnostic yield than the Holter monitor and should be obtained for any patient with a suspected arrhythmia as a cause of syncope.

A cardiac stress test is appropriate for patients in whom cardiac syncope is suspected and in whom have risk factors for coronary atherosclerosis. This test can assist with cardiac risk stratification and can guide future therapy.

Procedures

Carotid sinus massage has been used with some success to diagnose carotid sinus syncope.

Patients are placed on a cardiac monitor and beat-to-beat BP monitoring device. Atropine is kept at the bedside.

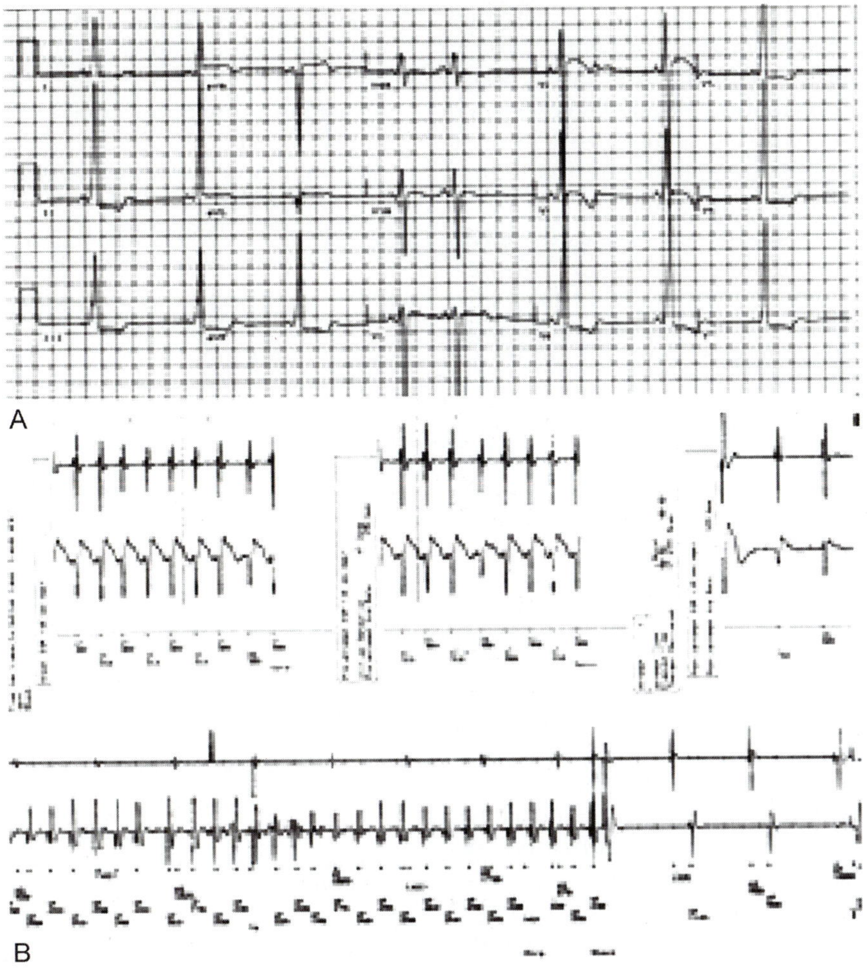

Fig. 10.23: *(A) Shows ECG from a patient with HCM who presented with recurrent syncopal spells, severe left ventricular hypertrophy and Wolff-Parkinson-White pattern. (B) ICD intracardiac electrogram with successful conversion using antitachycardia pacing for VT (top) and an appropriate shock-converting VF (bottom)*

Longitudinal massage lasting 5 seconds is initiated at the point of greatest carotid pulse intensity at the level of the thyroid cartilage on one side at a time.

The maximal response occurs after approximately 18 seconds, and a positive result is one that produces 3 seconds of asystole or syncope. If the result is negative, the process is repeated on the other carotid sinus.

Carotid sinus massage may theoretically precipitate an embolic stroke in persons with preexisting carotid artery disease.

Emergency Department Care

In patients brought to the ED with a presumptive diagnosis of syncope, appropriate initial interventions include intravenous access, oxygen administration, and cardiac monitoring. ECG and rapid blood glucose evaluation should be promptly performed. A study to determine the sensitivity and specificity of the San Francisco syncope rule (SFSR) ECG criteria for determining cardiac outcomes found that when used correctly, the criteria can help to predict which syncope patients are at risk of cardiac outcomes. ECG criteria predicted 36 of 42 patients with cardiac outcomes, with a sensitivity of 86%, a specificity of 70%, and a negative predictive value of 99%.

Syncope may be the manifestation of an acute life-threatening process but is generally not emergent. Clinically ruling out certain processes is important. The treatment choice for syncope depends on the cause or precipitant of the syncope. Patients in whom a cause cannot be ascertained in the ED, especially if they have experienced significant trauma, warrant supportive care and monitoring.

Situational syncope treatment focuses on educating patients about the condition. For example, in carotid sinus syncope, patients should be instructed not to wear tight collars, to use a razor rather than electric shaver, and to maintain good hydration status; they should also be informed of the possibility of pacemaker placement in the future.

Orthostatic syncope treatment also focuses on educating the patient. Inform patients about avoiding postprandial dips in BP, teach them to elevate the head of their bed to prevent rapid BP fluctuations on arising from bed, and emphasize the importance of assuming an upright posture slowly. Additional therapy may include thromboembolic disease (TED) stockings, mineralocorticoids (e.g. fludrocortisone for volume expansion), and other drugs such as midodrine (an alpha1-agonist with vasopressor activity). Patients' medications must be reviewed carefully to eliminate drugs associated with hypotension. Intentional oral fluid consumption is useful in decreasing frequency and severity of symptoms in these patients.

Cardiac arrhythmic syncope is treated with antiarrhythmic drugs or pacemaker placement. Consider cardiologist evaluation or inpatient management since this is more commonly associated with poor outcomes. Trials assessing beta-blockade to prevent syncope have conflicting results, but no clear effect has been demonstrated.

Cardiac mechanical syncope may be treated with beta-blockade to decrease outflow obstruction and myocardial workload. Valvular disease may require surgical correction. This, too, is associated with increased future morbidity and mortality.

KEY POINTS IN DIAGNOSIS AND TREATMENT OF SYNCOPE

- The starting point for evaluation of syncope is the "initial evaluation" that consists of history taking and physical examination, including orthostatic blood pressure measurements and standard electrocardiogram.
- The initial evaluation may lead to certain diagnosis, or suspected diagnosis that needs to be confirmed by appropriate diagnostic tests, or no diagnosis.
- The strategy of evaluation varies according to the severity and frequency of the episodes and the presence or absence of heart disease.
- In general, the absence of suspected or certain heart disease excludes a cardiac cause of syncope. Conversely, the presence of heart disease is a strong predictor of a cardiac cause of syncope and virtually includes all cardiac syncopes, but its specificity is low as about half of patients with heart disease have a non-cardiac cause of syncope.
- Determining the mechanism of syncope is a prerequisite for advising patients with regard to prognosis, and to developing an effective mechanism-specific treatment. Most patients with syncope require only reassurance and education regarding the nature of the disease and the avoidance of triggering events

BIBLIOGRAPHY

1. Chen L, Chen MH, Larson MG, Evans J, Benjamin EJ, Levy D. Risk factors for syncope in a community-based sample (the Framingham Heart Study). Am J Cardiol. May 15 2000;85(10):1189–93.
2. Savage DD, Corwin L, McGee DL, Kannel WB, Wolf PA. Epidemiologic features of isolated syncope: the Framingham Study. Stroke. Jul-Aug 1985;16(4):626–9.
3. Middlekauff HR, Stevenson WG, Stevenson LW, Saxon LA. Syncope in advanced heart failure: high risk of sudden death regardless of origin of syncope. J Am Coll Cardiol. Jan 1993;21(1):110–6.
4. Soteriades ES, Evans JC, Larson MG, et al. Incidence and prognosis of syncope. N Engl J Med. Sep 19 2002;347(12):878–85.
5. Suzuki M, Hori S, Nakamura I, Soejima K, Aikawa N. Long-term survival of Japanese patients transported to an emergency department because of syncope. Ann Emerg Med. Sep 2004;44(3):215–21.
6. Martin TP, Hanusa BH, Kapoor WN. Risk stratification of patients with syncope. Ann Emerg Med. Apr 1997;29(4):459–66.
7. Sarasin FP, Hanusa BH, Perneger T, Louis-Simonet M, Rajeswaran A, Kapoor WN. A risk score to predict arrhythmias in patients with unexplained syncope. Acad Emerg Med. Dec 2003;10(12):1312–7.
8. Quinn JV, Stiell IG, McDermott DA, Sellers KL, Kohn MA, Wells GA. Derivation of the San Francisco Syncope Rule to predict patients with short-term serious outcomes. Ann Emerg Med. Feb 2004;43(2):224–32.
9. Thiruganasambandamoorthy V, Hess EP, Alreesi A, Perry JJ, Wells GA, Stiell IG. External validation of the San Francisco Syncope Rule in the Canadian setting. Ann Emerg Med. May 2010;55(5):464–72.
10. Birnbaum A, Esses D, Bijur P, Wollowitz A, Gallagher EJ. Failure to validate the San Francisco Syncope Rule in an independent emergency department population. Ann Emerg Med. Aug 2008;52(2):151–9.
11. [Best Evidence] Reed MJ, Newby DE, Coull AJ, Prescott RJ, Jacques KG, Gray AJ. The ROSE (risk stratification of syncope in the emergency department) study. J Am Coll Cardiol. Feb 23 2010;55(8):713–21.
12. Costantino G, Perego F, Dipaola F, et al. Short- and long-term prognosis of syncope, risk factors, and role of hospital admission: results from the STePS (Short-Term Prognosis of Syncope) study. J Am Coll Cardiol. Jan 22 2008;51(3):276–83.
13. Andrea U, Attilio DR, Franco G, et al. Early and late outcome of treated patients referred for syncope to emergency department: the EGSYS 2 follow-up study. Eur Heart J. Feb 18 2010.
14. Dipaola F, Costantino G, Perego F, Borella M, Galli A, Cantoni G. San Francisco Syncope Rule, Osservatorio Epidemiologico sulla Sincope nel Lazio risk score, and clinical judgment in the assessment of short-term outcome of syncope. Am J Emerg Med. May 2010;28(4):432–9.
15. Serrano LA, Hess EP, Bellolio MF, et al. Accuracy and quality of clinical decision rules for syncope in the emergency department: a systematic review and meta-analysis. Ann Emerg Med. Oct 2010;56(4):362–373.
16. Pratt JL, Fleisher GR. Syncope in children and adolescents. Pediatr Emerg Care. Jun 1989;5(2):80–2.
17. [Guideline] Huff JS, Decker WW, Quinn JV, et al. Clinical policy: critical issues in the evaluation and management of adult patients presenting to the emergency department with syncope. Ann Emerg Med. Apr 2007;49(4):431–44.
18. Calkins H, Shyr Y, Frumin H, Schork A, Morady F. The value of the clinical history in the differentiation of syncope due to ventricular tachycardia, atrioventricular block, and neurocardiogenic syncope. Am J Med. Apr 1995;98(4):365–73.
19. Moya A, Sutton R, Ammirati F, et al. Guidelines for the diagnosis and management of syncope (version 2009): the

Task Force for the Diagnosis and Management of Syncope of the European Society of Cardiology (ESC). Eur Heart J. Nov 2009;30(21):2631–71.
20. Martin GJ, Adams SL, Martin HG, Mathews J, Zull D, Scanlon PJ. Prospective evaluation of syncope. Ann Emerg Med. Jul 1984;13(7):499–504.
21. Rockx MA, Hoch JS, Klein GJ, et al. Is ambulatory monitoring for "community-acquired" syncope economically attractive? A cost-effectiveness analysis of a randomized trial of external loop recorders versus Holter monitoring. Am Heart J. Nov 2005;150(5):1065.
22. Gibson TC, Heitzman MR. Diagnostic efficacy of 24-hour electrocardiographic monitoring for syncope. Am J Cardiol. Apr 1 1984;53(8):1013–7.
23. Quinn J, McDermott D. Electrocardiogram findings in emergency department patients with syncope. Acad Emerg Med. Jul 2011;18(7):714-8.
24. Shen WK, Decker WW, Smars PA, et a. Syncope Evaluation in the Emergency Department Study (SEEDS): a multidisciplinary approach to syncope management. Circulation. Dec 14 2004;110(24):3636-45.

11 Echocardiography—Overview (Incorporating 2-D, 3-D TTE, TEE, Color Doppler Echocardiography, Tissue and Hormonic Imaging, Strain and Strain Rate Imaging, Point of Care and Virtual Echocardiography in Pediatric Cardiology)

Echocardiography along with its different subtypes such as 2–3 D, color Doppler, TEE and stress systems are established techniques in the diagnosis of both congenital and acquired cardiac defects, myocardial functions, and valvular heart disease. It is also very useful tool in the diagnosis of intracardiac masses, infective endocarditis and coronary artery disease. In pediatric practice besides above said conditions, it is being frequently employed not only in the diagnosis of fetal cardiac malformations but also for the management of cardiac interventions in uterus. An echocardiogram (often called "echo") is a graphic outline of the heart's movement. During this test, high-frequency sound waves, called ultrasound, provide pictures of the heart's valves a and chambers. This allows the technician, called a sonographer, to evaluate the pumping action of the heart. Echo is often combined with Doppler ultrasound and color Doppler to evaluate blood flow across the heart's valves. The echocardiography machine is a powerful computer that images the heart using ultrasound. It reveals cardiac anatomy and physiology, allowing diagnosis of diseases of the myocardium, valves, pericardium and aorta. The functional significance of coronary disease can be determined using stress echocardiography and myocardial perfusion imaging.

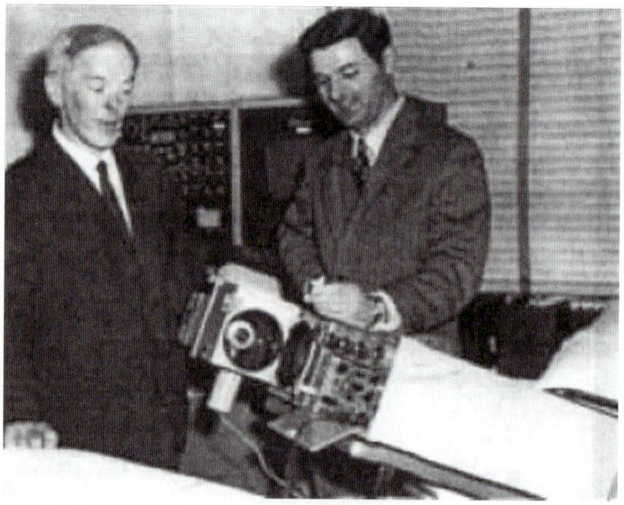

Fig. 11.1: *Photographs of Drs, Elder and Feigenbaum demonstrating their M-mode echocardiographic machine during meeting of cardiac ultrasound Indianpolis in 1968*

The first medical application of ultrasound was started as early as 1950 by Howry, Wild and Keidel. Later on two Swedish scientists, Elder and Hertz in 1954 had the rare honor of visualizing the cardiac structure in motion. This leds to the beginning of M-mode echcardiography by simultaneous recording and displaying the echos on an oscilloscope with respect to time. In 1961, Elder after having modified the existing technique, visualized the various cardiac structures including the heart valves and myocardium. Ultrasound is set at a frequency of more than 20,000 Hz. In the body, frequencies of 1.9–10 MHz are typically used. Most ultrasound entering the body is scattered or absorbed, but some is reflected back to the transducer at interfaces where the acoustic density of tissue changes. The two dimensional echocardiographic image is therefore a map of the acoustic density of the heart. The use of echocardiography as an imaging modality has increased substantially over the past decade. Cardiologists perform most echocardiography studies, with internists being the next most common providers of these studies (15% of all medicare charges submitted for the procedure). The objective of this article is to provide clinicians with a brief review of basic principles and instrumentation of echocardiography.

Neither bone nor air is a good transmission medium for ultrasound waves; accordingly, specific windows (e.g. apical, parasternal, subcostal and suprasternal) are used to image the heart.

PART I. FETAL ECHOCARDIOGRAPHY

Fetal echocardiography is an ultrasound test performed during pregnancy to evaluate the heart of the unborn baby.

Echocardiography assesses the heart's structures and function.

Fetal echocardiography can help to detect fetal heart abnormalities before birth, allowing for faster medical or surgical intervention once the baby is born. This improves the chance of survival after delivery for babies with serious heart defects (Figs 11.2 to 11.4).

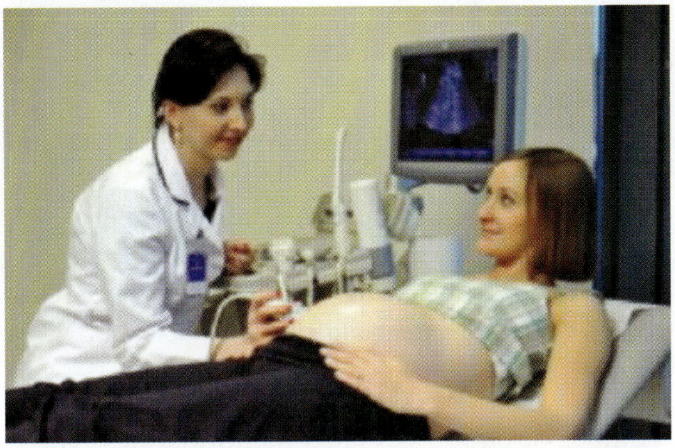

Fig. 11.2: *Doctor is performing fetal echocardiography*

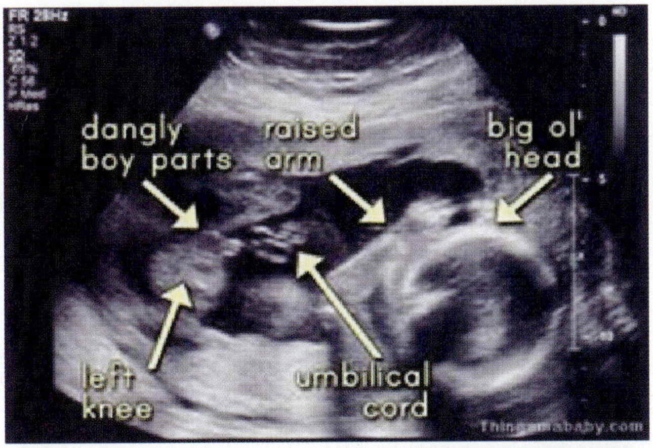

Fig. 11.3: *Abdominal ultrasound showing viable intrauterine 20 weeks old fetus with different parts of the body (labeled)*

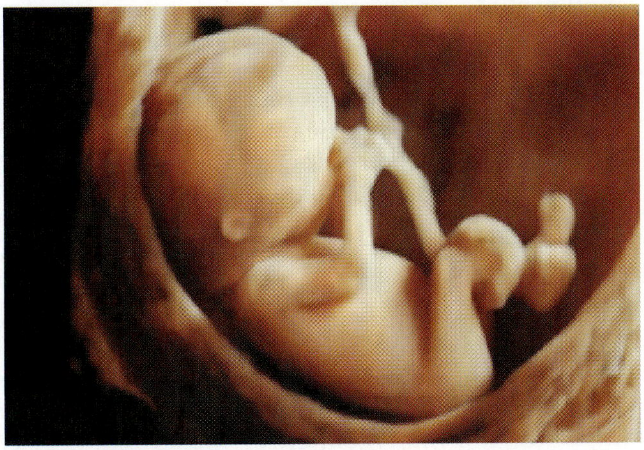

Fig. 11.4: *Abdominal 4D ultrasound showing distinct details of head,ears,umblical cord, upper and lower limbs during 20 weeks of gestation*

Foetal echocardiography (FE) is being increasingly employed to identify the fetal cardiac status during the mid-trimester around the world. It is tending to become the standard of care for optimal health care delivery to the fetus and the mother. Like many other modern techniques, the utility of FE has not been rigorously tested and there are conflicting reports in literature about its precise role? However, FE has provided useful insights into the development of cardiac lesions and fetal physiology.

Clinical Indications

It is not necessary for all pregnancies to receive an echocardiogram. The prenatal ultrasound tests that are done prior to birth can give information about whether the fetal heart has developed with all four chambers. Most unborn babies do not require any further testing. Situations in which a fetal echocardiogram may be necessary include, but are not limited to, the following if a sibling was born with a congenital (present at birth) heart defect a family history of congenital heart disease (such as parents, aunts or uncles or grandparents) a chromosomal or genetic abnormality discovered in the fetus.

1. If a mother has taken certain medications that may cause congenital heart defects, such as anti-seizure medications or prescription acne medications if the mother has abused alcohol or drugs during pregnancy.
2. If a mother has diabetes, phenylketonuria, or a connective tissue disease such as lupus.
3. If the mother has had rubella during pregnancy a routine prenatal ultrasound has discovered possible heart abnormalities.

Early studies from a few centers on selected group of high-risk pregnancies reported a high sensitivity and specificity of FE in the diagnosis of CHD even though the absolute yield was modest. Since it would be impossible for few echocardiographers to screen all pregnancies, it was thought that the obstetrician would evaluate a four-chamber view of the fetal heart for any abnormality during a routine mid-trimester ultrasound scan and pickup important anomalies. However, such an approach has extremely poor sensitivity when applied to the realistic settings. This was clearly demonstrated by Buskens et al. in a recent prospective study of 6,922 routine fetal screening. The fetal four-chamber view examination had a sensitivity of 4.5% (95% CI, 0.6–15%). Various other studies have reported sensitivity ranging from 7–60%. Lesions like tetralogy of fallot, transposition of great vessels or aortic arch interruption could be missed on a four-chamber evaluation by the obstetrician.

Therefore, an extended fetal evaluation by an experienced sonographer might be routinely required to improve upon the case detection as shown by Strumpflen et a1. They reported sensitivity of 85.5% in a study of 3,089 fetal scans. These results are not universal and such expertise is not routinely available even in the developed countries. Further, there are certain other considerations as well.

Fetal Echocardiography in "High-Risk Pregnancies"

The definition of "high risk" pregnancies has not been standardized. It commonly includes history of CHD in the mother or siblings, maternal diabetes mellitus, abnormal results of amniocentesis or obstetric sonography, maternal teratogens, rubella infection, or suspected fetal. Arrhythmias, etc. Maternal age above 35 years, collagen vascular disease in the mother and polyhydramnios were also considered high risk in some studies. It is clear that when an abnormal scan is reported by the obstetrician either due to an abnormal four-chamber view or because of associated anomalies, a detailed foetal echocardiographic study is warranted and the yield is 40–70% under these circumstances. This is not surprising because this group represents a preselected population. The yield in most other so-called 'high risk' pregnancies is not much different from routine pregnancies, conditions like diabetes in the mother (1–2%), previous CHD in the siblings (1–2%) and teratogen exposure (upto 1%) are associated with lower yield of FP. Whether complex CHD occurs any more frequently in the high-risk pregnancies, has not been evaluated. In any case, most CHD lesions occur in pregnancies with no known risk factors (Figs 11.5 and 11.6).

It may be argued that normal fetal scan provides emotional relief to the mother, and is thus justified. This may be true for some cases, but it cannot be generalized. The specter of creating unnecessary anxieties in the mother due to minor abnormalities in the fetus or due to a false positive diagnosis also needs be considered.

Thus, FE is clearly indicated when an abnormal fetal scan is suspected by the obstetrician or the pregnancy has a predisposing high-risk condition that substantially increases the risk of CHD, e.g. trisomy in the fetus, phenylketonuria in the mother (50% chances of CHD), fetal

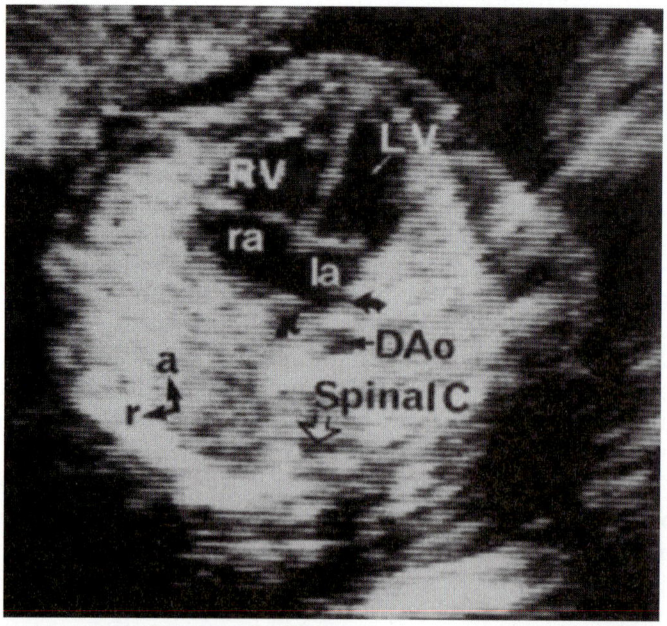

Fig. 11.5: *Fetal echocardiographic graph showing well formed four chambers of the heart with concordant AV valves communicating through their respective chambers*

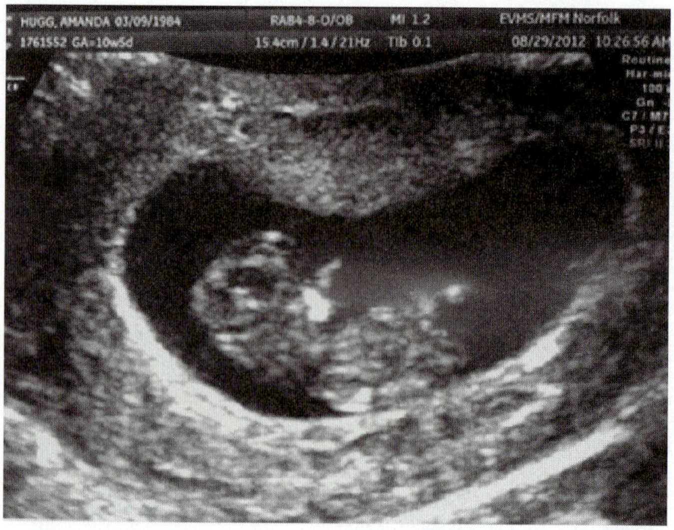

Fig. 11.6: *Abdominal ultrasound showing viable intrauterine 10 weeks old fetus*

arrhythmias or other associated malformations. The yield in many other high-risk pregnancies is low. The distinction between "high-risk" and "low-risk" pregnancies is far from satisfactory. Routine FE, however, neither feasible nor cost-effective, at least for India. Simultaneously, it must be realized that this approach would miss many cases of CHD.

Prognostic Value in Fetal Echocardiography (Figs 11.7 to 11.16)

There are a few other issues that a pediatric cardiologist offering prognosis after FE should take into account.

1. Natural history of CHD lesions diagnosed prenatally may be quite different from that expected for that lesion in the infant, e.g. 75% of tetralogy of fallot diagnosed by FE finally died (including termination of pregnancy) in one series, while most centers report 0–5% mortality though their results may vary from center to centre, after total correction of Fallot's tetralogy in infancy. Similarly, percent of fetuses with complete heart block resulted in still births or early neonatal deaths in another study. The high incidence of chromosomal and extracardiac anomalies in the prenatal group largely accounts for the discrepancy.
   Markers for fetal prognosis on FE are being identified. Fetal hydrops or significant atrioventricular valve regurgitation portends a poor prognosis. Reversal of normal intracardiac flow pattern across foramen ovale, or ductus arteriosus, and certain umbilical vein Doppler flow patterns are also reported to be associated with high fetal mortality.
2. At the same time, diagnosis of CHD should be an indication for karyotype evaluation. High number (30–50%) of abnormal foetal echocardiograms have chromosomal abnormalities and this information may influence the management of the pregnancy, e.g. identifying trisomy would indicate termination of pregnancy due to dismal prognosis, Sometimes, the cardiac lesion may be the only pointer for an abnormal

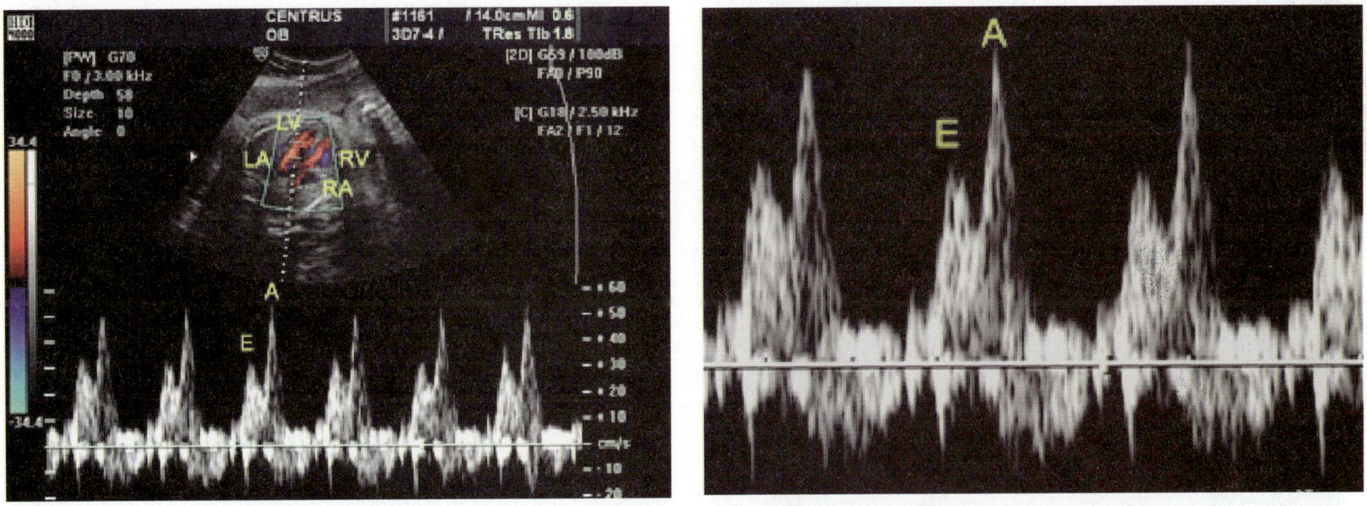

Fig. 11.7: *Low velocity waveform across the tricuspid valve at 28 weeks of gestation (left). (E-wave = early ventricular filling and A-wave = atrial ventricular filling)*

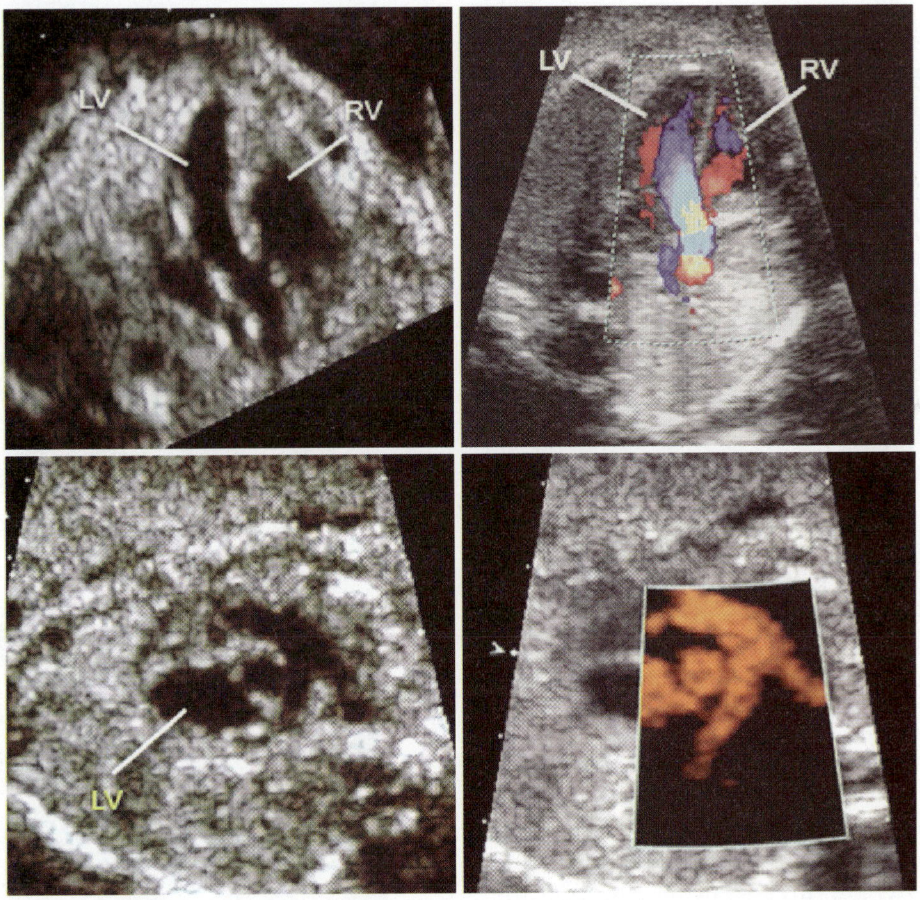

Fig. 11.8: *Five chamber view of the fetal heart with superimposed color Doppler showing the aorta (blue) originating from the left ventricle (top). Short-axis view of the fetal heart with superimposed color Doppler showing the pulmonary artery originating from the right ventricle (bottom)*

karyotype although mostly multiple organ systems are involved.

3. Although cardiac development is complete by 8 weeks of gestation, continuous morphoanatomic alterations occur throughout gestation such that CHD may evolve. FE has clearly thrown new light on this development. Examples of pulmonic stenosis evolving into pulmonary atresia, coarctation worsening later in the gestation and left heart hypoplasia coming on in last trimester with normal mid-trimester echo (probably

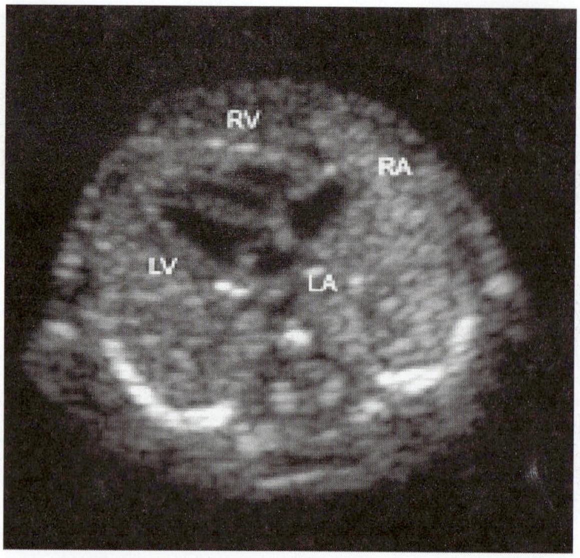

Fig. 11.9: *Fetal echocardiogram showing anatomical orientation of four chambers of the heart*

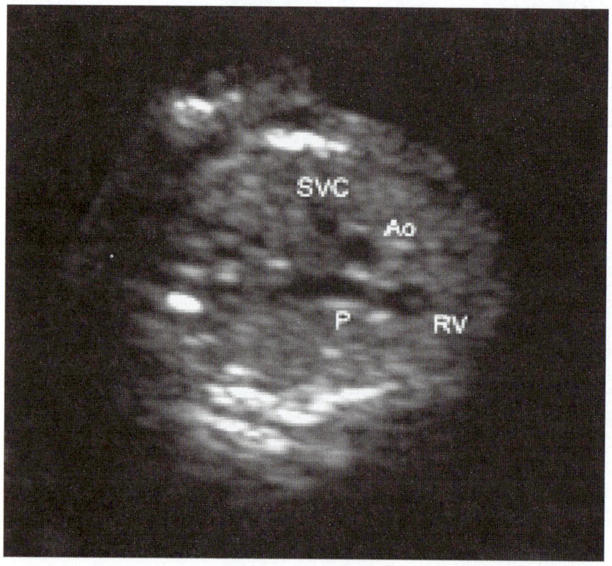

Fig. 11.10: *Fetal echocardiogram showing anatomical orientation superior vena cava (SVC) and pulmonary vein (P)*

due to premature closure of foramen ovale) have been shown. Similarly, complete heart block developing later and cardiac tumors appearing with time are known. Due to peculiarities of fetal circulation, it is difficult to ascertain the severity of valve stenosis although the presence of stenosis is relatively easy to diagnose. Above points may be appreciated while considering the litiginous climate under which FE could be pushed into. Moreover, one may not always be able to have diagnostic images. The quality of fetal echoes is influenced by the duration of pregnancy (best images around 20–22 weeks) and maternal factors like obesity, abdominal scarring, oligohydroaminois, etc. in addition to the operator's experience.

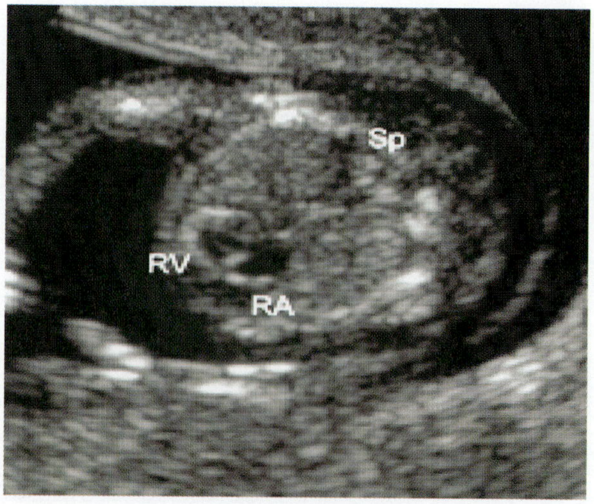

Fig. 11.11: *Fetal echocardiogramin short-axis view showing anatomical two chambers of RA and RV*

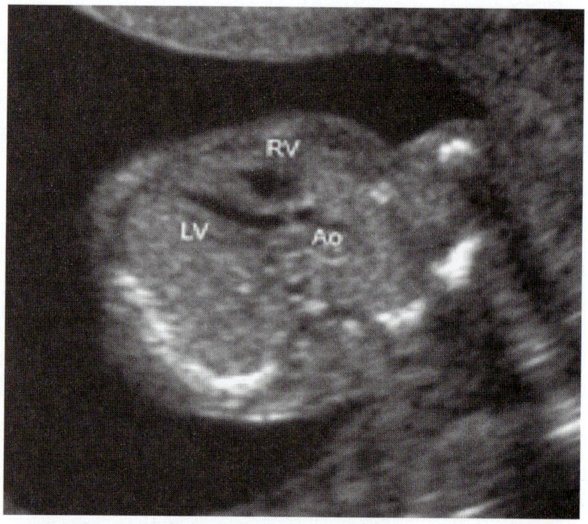

Fig. 11.12: *Fetal echocardiogram showing anatomical orientation aorta (AO)*

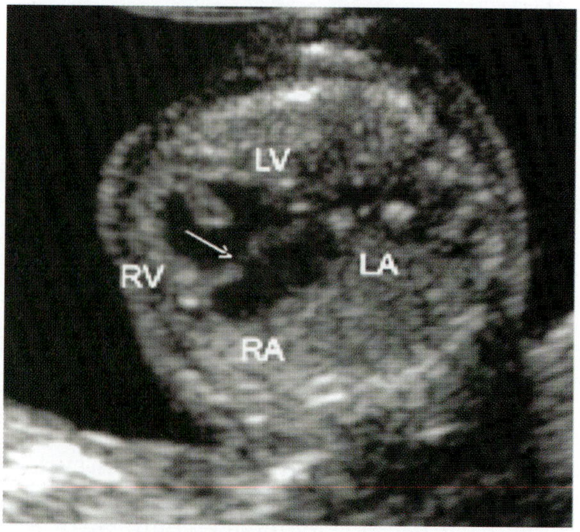

Fig. 11.13: *Fetal echocardiogram showing anatomical location of foramen ovale (arrow) between RA and RV*

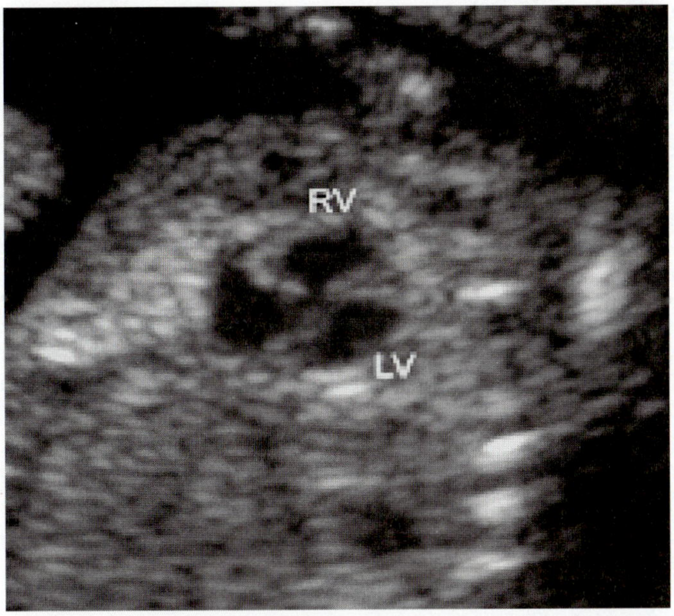

Fig. 11.14: *Fetal echocardiogramin short-axis view showing anatomical two chambers of RV and LV*

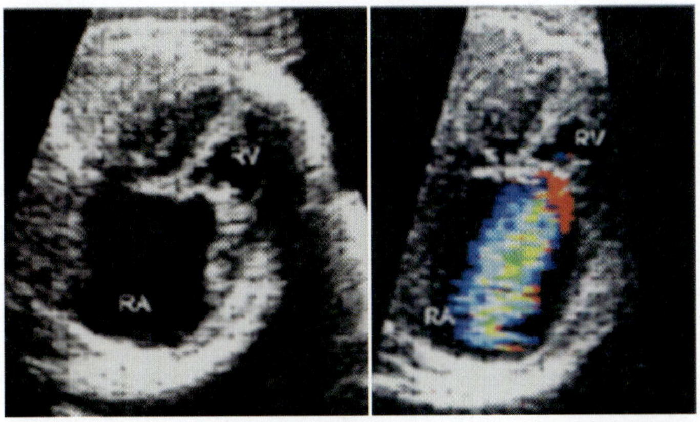

Fig. 11.15: *Fetal echocardiogram showing tricuspid valve dysplasia with severe tricuspid insufficiency and cardiomegaly. Retrograde flow from the right ventricle (RV) to the right atrium (RA) is seen in blue and turbulence is coded by green pixels*

PART II. ECHOCARDIOGRAPHY IN CHILDREN AND ADOLESCENTS

Echocardiography is the most common test used in children to diagnose or rule out heart disease and also to follow children who have already been diagnosed with a heart problem. It can be performed on children of all ages and sizes including fetuses and newborns. Many types of specialized echocardiography services are offered including:

1. Transesophageal echocardiography
2. Intracardiac echocardiography
3. Fetal heart program
4. Three dimensional study
5. Tissue doppler imaging
6. Adult congenital heart disease
7. Cardiac resynchronization evaluation
8. Carotid artery vascular imaging
9. Stress echocardiography
10. Digital echocardiography
11. Tele-echocardiography.

Clinical Application of Echocardiography

Several cardiac conditions may be detected by echocardiography including the following:

1. Heart murmur
2. Chest pain
3. Aneurysm
4. Cardiomyopathy
5. Congenital heart disease
6. Congestive heart failure
7. Pericarditis
8. Valve disease.

What are the different types of echocardiogram?
There are four special types of echocardiography:

M-mode Echocardiography

This is the simplest type of echocardiography, and produces an image that is similar to a tracing rather than an actual picture of heartstructures. M-mode echo is useful for measuring heart structures, suchas the heart's pumping chambers, the size of the heart itself, and the thickness of the heart walls.

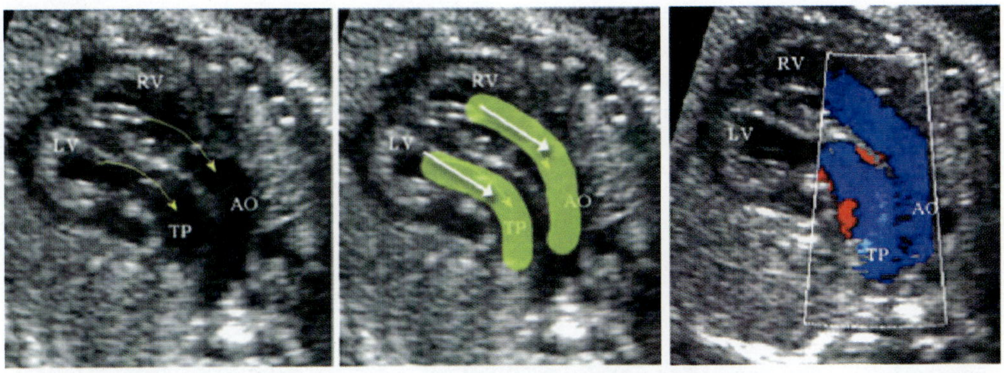

Fig. 11.16: *Fetal echocardiogram showing transposition of the great arteries demonstrating the abnormal connection of the right ventricle (RV) with the aorta (AO) and the left ventricle (LV) with the pulmonary trunk (PT). Both great arteries show a parallel course associated with tricuspid atresia*

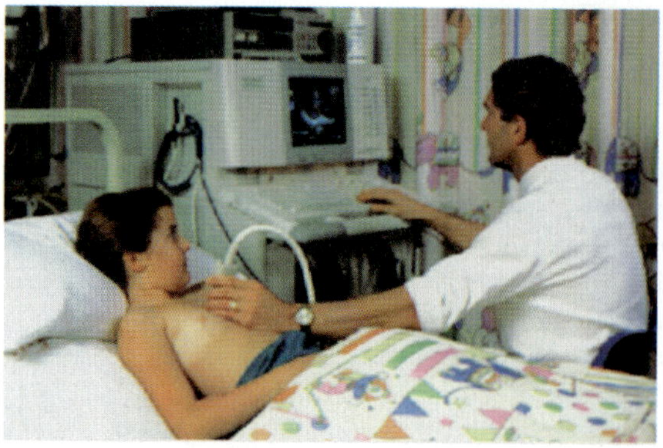

Fig. 11.17: *Echocardiographic evaluation of heart disease in a young child who was admitted into emergency department with cyanosis and heart failure*

Doppler Echocardiography

The Doppler technique is used to measure and assess the flowof blood through the heart's chambers and valves. Also, Doppler can detect abnormal blood flow within the heart, which can indicate such problems as an opening between chambers of the heart, a problem with one or more of the heart's four valves, or a problem with the heart's walls.

Color Doppler

Color Doppler is an enhanced form of Doppler echocardiography. With color Doppler, different colors are used to designate the direction of blood flow. This simplifies the interpretation of the Doppler technique.

2D (two dimensional) Echocardiography

This technique is used to see the actual structures and motion of the heart structures. A 2-D echo view appears cone-shaped on the monitor, and the real-time motion of the heart's structures can be observed.

Electrocardiographic lead placement: The electrocardiogram allows identification of arrhythmias and timing of cardiac events during the echocardiographic examination and is used as a timing marker for digital recording of images. Typically digital "clips" are set to record a predefined number of cardiac cycles (usually one) with timing based on the electrocardiogram. It is important that irregular beats be identified and excluded from analysis. For example, a postectopic beat will falsely increase the two dimensional assessment of ejection fraction and the Doppler assessment of transaortic gradient. In general, any Doppler index requires the average of at least three measurements. For patients in atrial fibrillation, 7–10 beats should be averaged (Table 11.1).

Transducer Selection

The adult echocardiographic examination typically begins with a 2.5- to 3.5-MHz phased array transducer. Transducer frequency is important as at higher frequencies spatial resolution improves but at the expense of reduced depth penetration. Higher frequency (3.0- to 5.0- MHz) transducers may be used in thin or pediatric patients. Therefore, for optimal two dimensional resolution, select the highest frequency transducer that will provide adequate farfield penetration.

Table 11.1: *Standard echocardiographic views in transthoracic echocardiographic examination*

1. **Parasternal long axis (PLAX)** (Fig. 11.19)
   Position transducer in 3rd or 4th intercostal space parasternally (ridge toward right shoulder)
2. **Parasternal short axis (PSAX)** (Figs 11.21 and 11.23)
   Rotate transducer 90° clockwise from PLAX; tilt transducer from superior to inferior (LV apex view, mid-LV view, mitral valve view, aortic valve level, pulmonary valve/main plum artery level)
3. **Apical four-chamber (A4C)** (Fig. 11.20)
   Transducer at apex-ridge toward left (move laterally and inferiorly if necessary to get true apex)
4. **Apical two-chamber (A2C)**
   Rotate transducer: 60–90° anticlockwise tilt posteriorly and rotate clockwise to open out descending aorta
5. **Apical long axis (apical three-chamber)**
   Rotate transducer further 30–45° anticlockwise
6. **Subcostal view:** (Patient supine and legs bent at knees)
   Subxiphoid, midline, tilt anteriorly under sternum with groove toward patients left for four-chamber view
   Color Doppler across interatrial septum to check for PFO or ASD (Fig. 11.22)

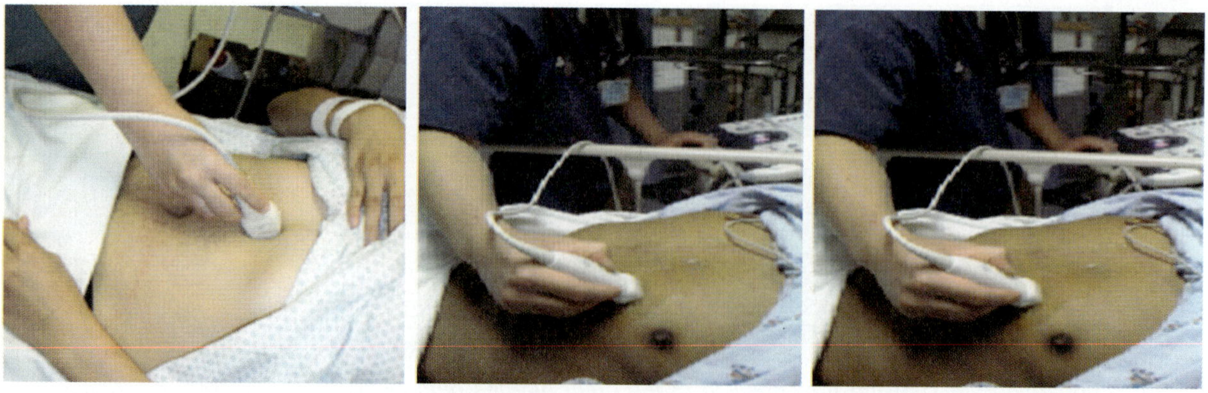

Fig. 11.18: *Transthoacic approach. Top to bottom showing different positions of transducer in obtaining echocardiographic information in emergent situation*

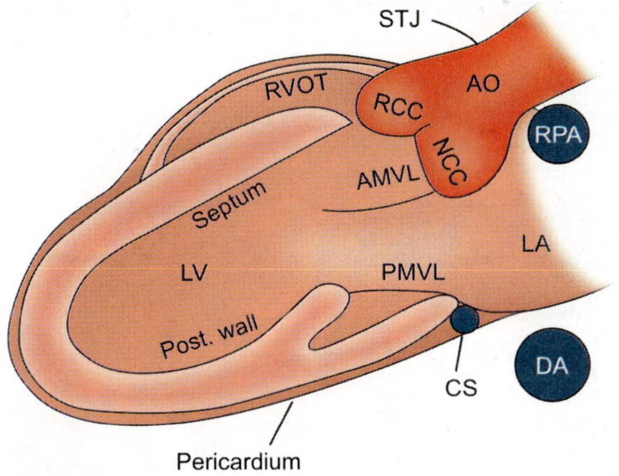

Fig. 11.19: *Schematic diagram of the parasternal long-axis view in diastole. AML, anterior mitral leaflet; Ao, aorta; CS, coronary sinus; DA, descending aorta; LA, left atrium; LV, left ventricle; NCC, noncoronary cusp; PMVL, posterior mitral leaflet; PW, posterior wall; RCC, right coronary cusp; RPA, right pulmonary artery; RVOT, right ventricular outflow tract; STJ, sinotubular junction*

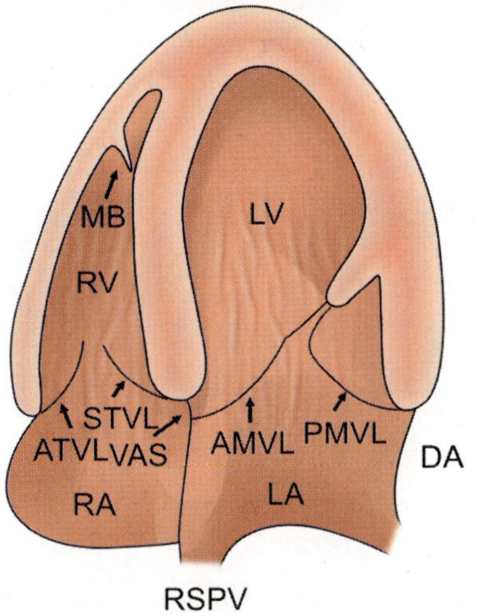

Fig. 11.20: *Schematic diagram of the apical four chamber view. AMVL, anterior mitral leaflet; ATL, anterior tricuspid leaflet; DA, descending aorta; PMVL, posterior mitral leaflet; LA, left atrium; LV, left ventricle; ME, moderator band; RA, right atrium; RUPV, right upper pulmonary vein; RV, right ventricle; STL, septal tricus. pid leaflet*

As regards to transducer frequency for the Doppler examination, lower frequency transducers can record higher velocities. The Pedoff probe is a continuous wave, nonimaging probe (typical frequency 1.8 MHz) used mainly to detect higher velocity profiles and confirm velocities obtained by other imaging methods.

2D Echocardiography Instrument Settings

The following settings can be adjusted in most echocardiography machines (Figs 11.24 and 11.25):

- **Power output:** This adjusts the total ultrasound energy emitted by the transducer
- **Time-gain compensation (TGC):** These controls allow differential adjustment of gain at different image depths; near-field gain can be set at a lower value (since reflected

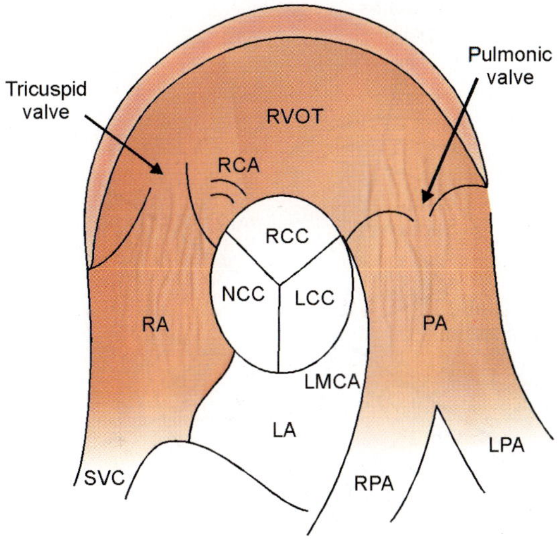

Fig. 11.21: *Schematic diagram of the parastemal short-axis view at the aortic valve level. LA, left atrium; LCC, left coronary cusp; LMT, left main trunk; LPA, left pulmonary artery; NCC, non-coronary cusp; PA, pulmonary artery; PV, pulmonary ventricular; RA, right atrium; RCA, right coronary artery; RCC, right coronary cusp; RPA, right pulmonary artery; RVOT, right ventricular outflow tract; SVC, superior vena cava; TV, tricuspid valve*

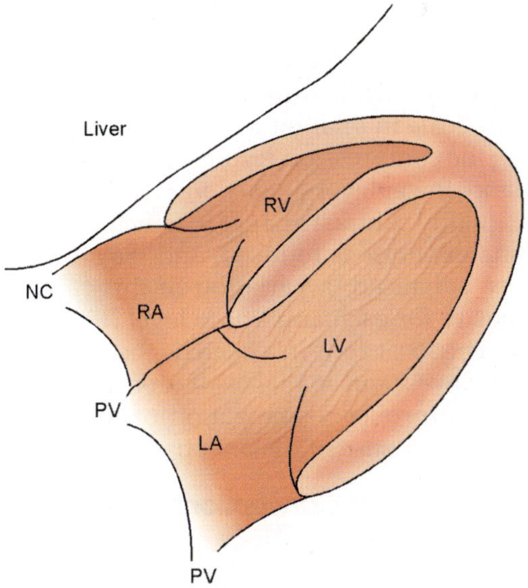

Fig. 11.22: *Schematic diagram of the four chamber view from the subcostal approach. IYC, inferior vena cava; LA, left atrium; LV, left ventricle; RA, right atrium; RV, right ventricle*

signal is strong) with gradual increase at midfield and higher gain in far field; usually, the degree of TGC amplification is displayed beside the echocardiographic image.

- **Depth:** A trade-off exists between depth of image, number of lines per sector (affecting lateral resolution), and number of frames per second (temporal resolution); this control allows the operator to adjust the depth according to body habitus and the structure of interest.
- **Sector width:** This control can be used to increase lateral or temporal resolution by decreasing the number of ultrasound lines in each frame.

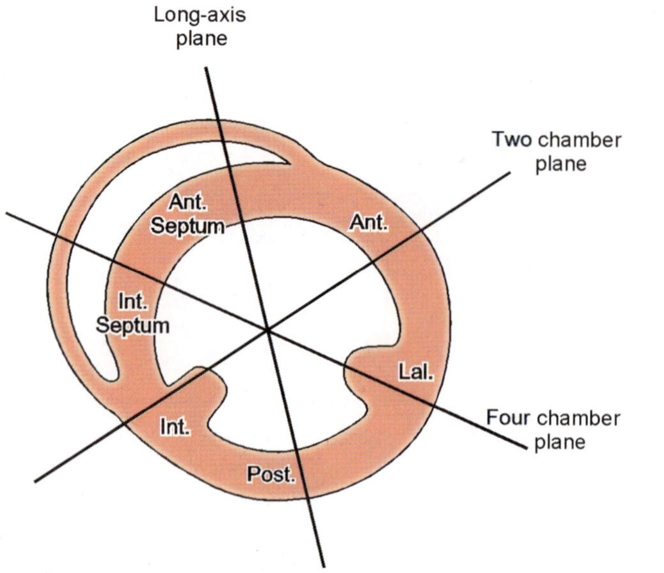

Fig. 11.23: *Schematic diagram of the parasternal short-axis view at the level of papillary muscles. Ant. septum, anterior septum; ant., anterior wall; In. septum, inferior septum; Inf., inferior wall; lat., lateral wall; post., posterior wall*

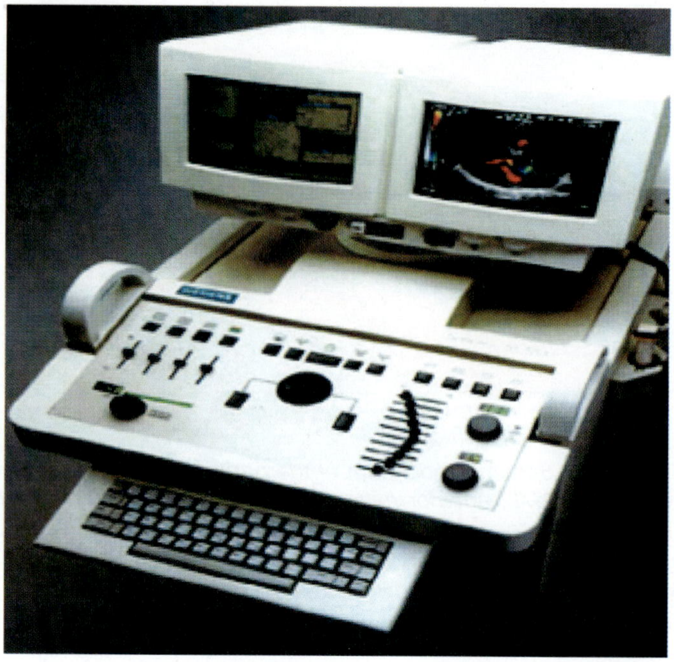

Fig. 11.24: *Showing dedicated color Doppler echocardiographic machine which is being employed for obtaining M-mode, 2D color Doppler scans for investigation of heart patients*

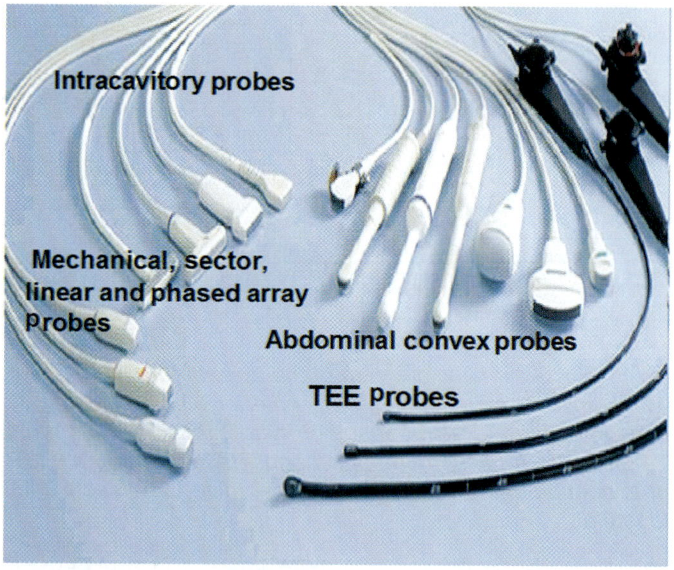

Fig. 11.25: *Showing different types of transthoracic, TEE, intraoperative intravaginal and abdominal probes employed for obtaining echocardiographic/ultrasonographic views*

- **Grayscale/dynamic range (also called compression):** This postprocessing feature allows adjustment of the gray/white scale in relation to received signal intensity; increasing the compression results in a softer picture that may enhance lower level signals, and decreasing it results in higher quality contrast images in which weaker signals are eliminated, noise is reduced, and the strongest echo signals are enhanced; a variation of this function uses color intensity for each amplitude level (Fig. 11.27).
- **Focusing:** The focal zone in a beam is the zone where the beam is narrowest and spatial resolution is therefore best; this feature improves visualization of the structure of interest at the expense of distant structures.

What are the Types of Conventional Echocardiograms? (Fig. 11.24)

There are several types of echocardiograms and your doctor will help to determine which is best for you. The echocardiography functions both as a transmitter or pulsed ultrasound, and receiver of the reflected echos. There are three modes of display of these echoes: A-mode (A = amplitude). B-mode (B = brightness) and M-mode (M = motion).

A-mode displays the reflected echos as vertical spikes on a horizontal baseline. The amplitude of each spike varies with the intensity of each reflected echoe, the baseline being calibrated for distance. Although little used nowadays, it is very useful for adjusting the various echocardiographic controls (Fig. 11.26).

B-mode retains the same horizontal base line, but the reflected echos are displayed as dots rather than spikes. The intensity or brightness of each spot is proportional to the amplitude of the spike. This mode is used for the display of two dimensional echography, and also for the recording of M-mode echocardiograms on strip chart recorders (Fig. 11.26).

M-mode is obtained by electronically tracking the B-mode on an oscilloscope. The B-mode echos are therefore displayed with respect to time and their motion appears as a wavy line; in unidirectional echocardiography, M-mode is a method of presenting the different phases of the cardiac cycle, and of recording and analyzing them. For conveniences, M-mode displayed from left to right on the

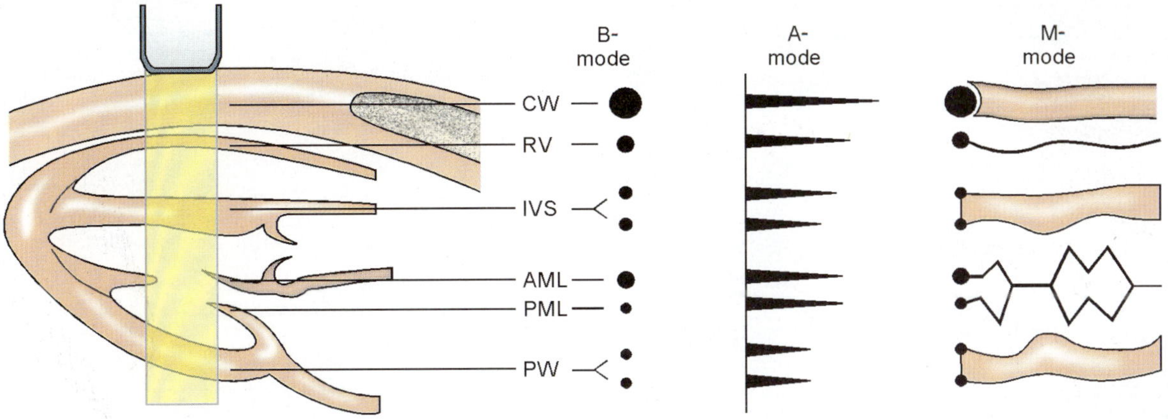

Fig. 11.26: *Illustration shows A-mode, B-mode, and M-mode echocardiograms. The transducer emits an ultrasound beam, which reflects at each anatomic interface. The reflected wavefronts can be represented as dots (B-mode) or spikes (A-mode). The dot brightness and spike magnitude vary with the amplitude of the reflected wave. If the B-mode scan is swept from left to right with time, an M-mode image is produced. AML, anterior mitral leaflet; CW, chest wall; IVS, interventricular septum; PML, posterior mitral leaflet; PW, posterior wall; RV, right ventricle. (Modified with permission from Hagan AD, DeMaria AN. Clinical Applications of Two-Dimensional Echocardiography and Cardiac Doppler. Boston, MA: Little, Brown; 1989)*

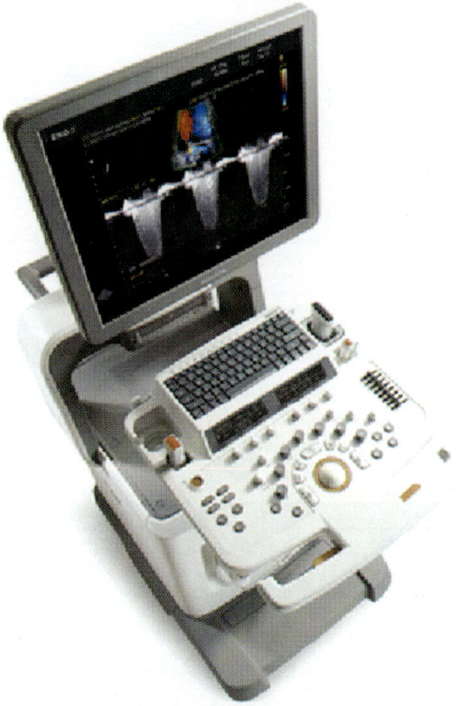

Fig. 11.27: *Showing photograph of a echocardiographic machine which is commonly used in point of care echocardiography*

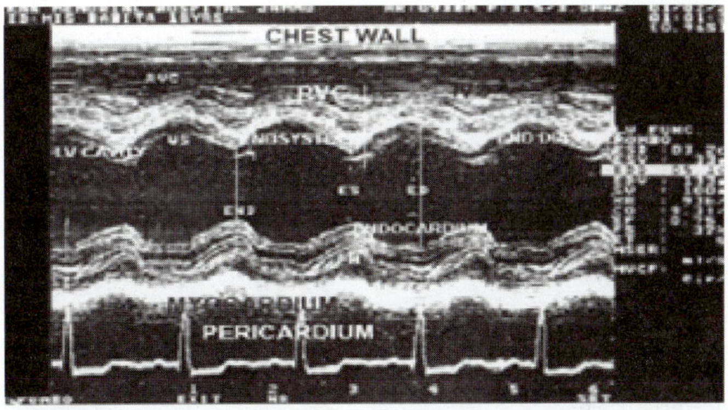

Fig. 11.28: *M-mode echocardiogram showing relationship of different walls and cavities and internal dimensions of LV employed for the calculation of cardiac volumes and hemodynamic functions*

oscilloscope, the top of the screen corresponding to the position of the transducer (Fig. 11.28).

Transthoracic Echocardiogram (B-mode/2D)

This is the standard echocardiogram. It is a painless test similar to X-ray, but without the radiation. The procedure uses the same technology used to evaluate a baby's health before birth. A hand-held device called a transducer is placed on the chest and transmits high frequency sound waves (ultrasound). These sound waves bounce off the heart structures, producing images and sounds that can be used by the doctor to detect heart damage (Figs 11.29 and 11.36).

Transthoracic echocardiography is performed in a darkened room which should be private, temperature controlled and large enough for comfort. The skin of the chest is exposed and electrodes are attached to allow timing of echocardiographic events with the cardiac cycle. The patient then lies semirecumbent on the left side, usually with the left arm behind the neck to enlarge the rib spaces. The echocardiographer sits beside the patient. Ultrasound gel (which must be cold so as not to slip off) acts as a couplant enabling the ultrasound to pass between the probe and the body. Most images are taken from the left of the sternum and around the left breast, but some are obtained in the epigastrium and at the suprasternal notch.

Doppler echocardiography uses similar pulses of ultrasound but analyses them differently. If ultrasound is reflected from blood moving toward the probe, its

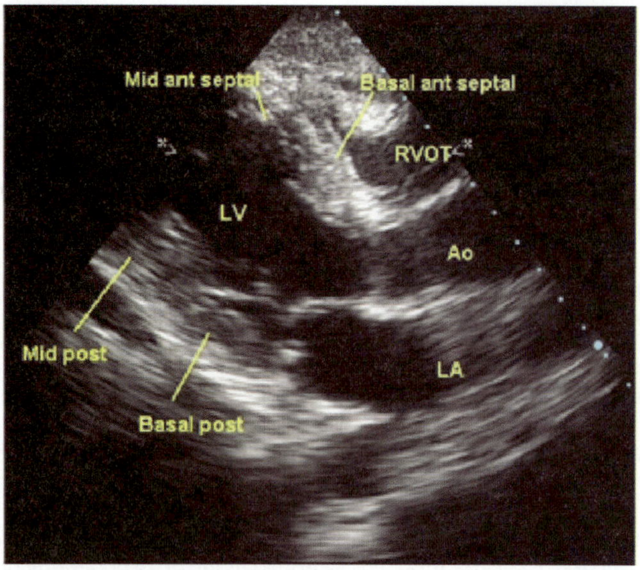

Fig. 11.29: *Segments in parasternal long-axis view are basal anteroseptal and mid-anteroseptal on the septum; and basal posterior and mid-posterior in the posterior wall*

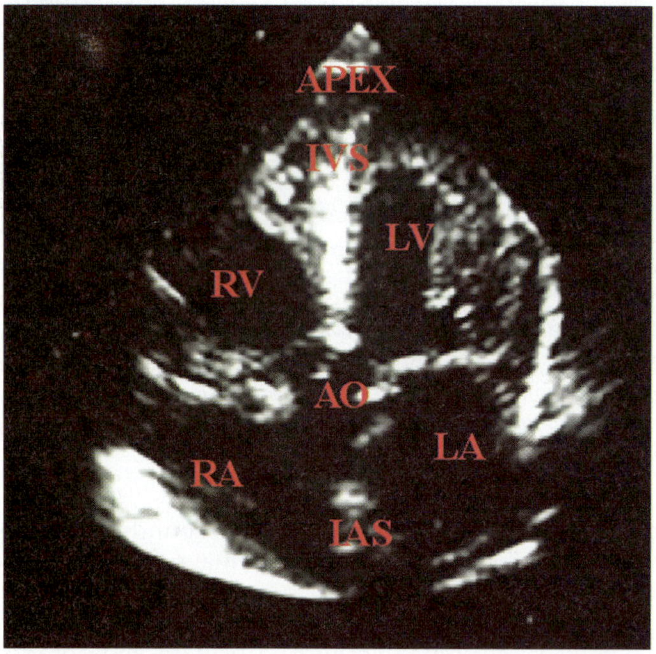

Fig. 11.30: *2D apical four chamber view with superior angulation, the left ventricular outflow tract and proximal aortic root can be seen from the apical view*

wavelength is shortened. Conversely, if the blood is moving away, the wavelength is prolonged. The computer analyzes the change between the transmitted and the returning ultrasound wavelengths and resolves velocities to produce a graph of velocity against time (Fig. 11.34).

Continuous-wave Doppler is the oldest Doppler modality and involves two crystals, one transmitting and the other receiving continuously. This technique is sensitive for short-lived or localized flow abnormalities and can resolve high velocities accurately (Fig. 11.41).

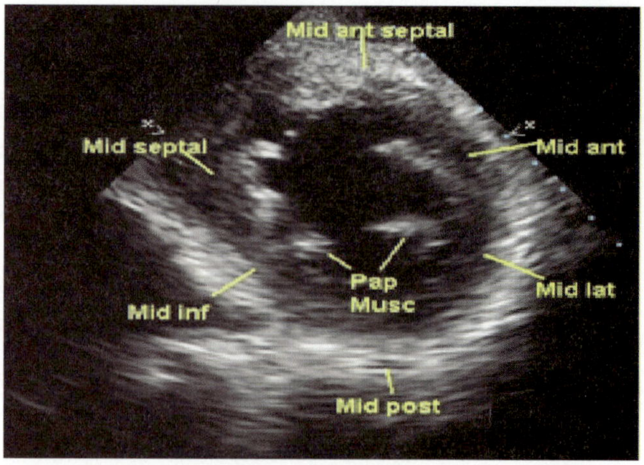

Fig. 11.31: *Short-axis view LV cavity showing different walls of LV*

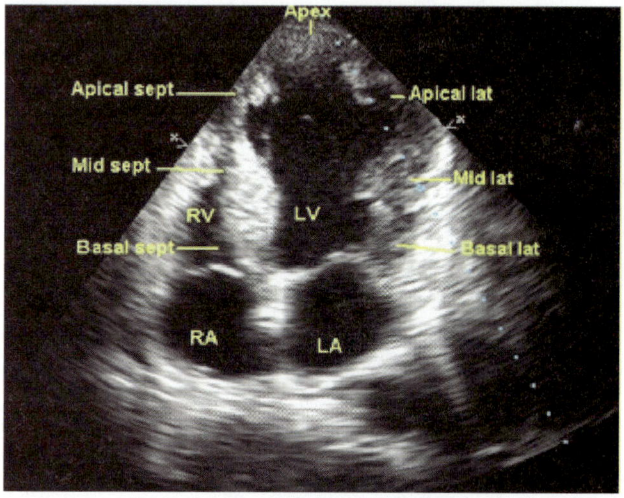

Fig. 11.32: *Apical four chambers view gives information about seven segments: apex, apical lateral, apical- septal, mid-septal, mid-lateral, basal septal and basal lateral*

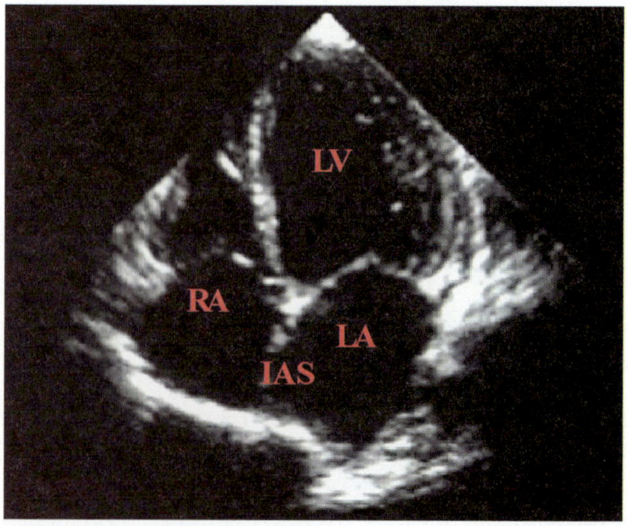

Fig. 11.33: *2D Apical four chamber view. Echocardiographic image of heart during systole. Showing four chambers, IVS, IAS and left and right-sided AV valves (MV and TV)*

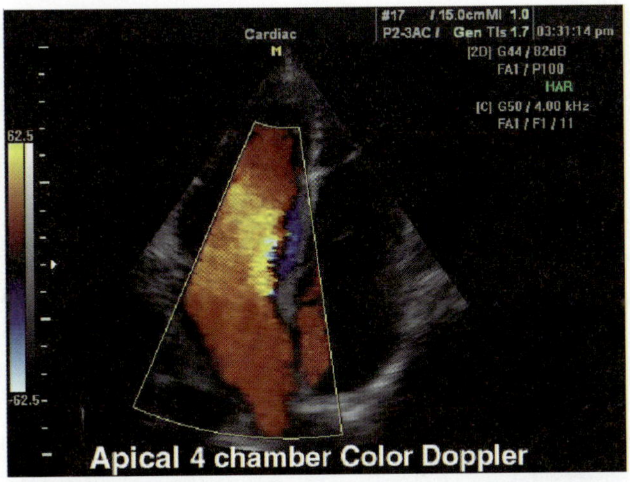

Fig. 11.34: *Apical four chambers, showing color Doppler scan*

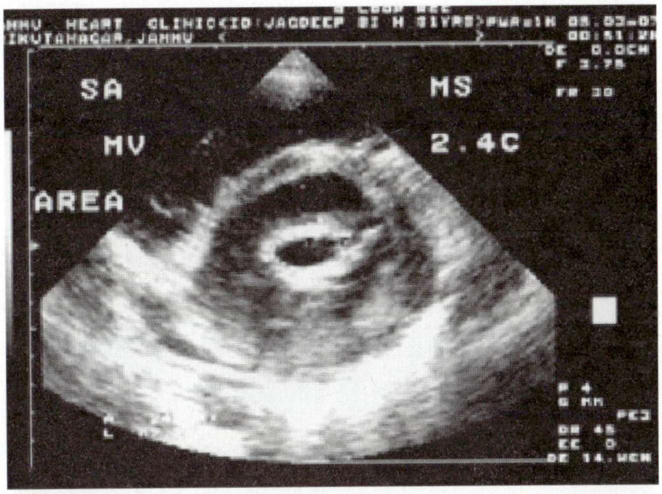

Fig. 11.37: *2D short-axis view of LV showing trace method in the calculation of mitral valve area*

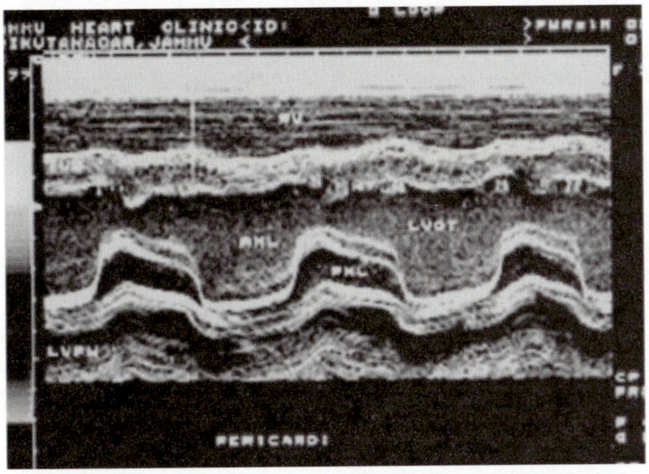

Fig. 11.35: *M-mode echo scan showing thickened both AML and PML with paradoxical movement of PML in patient with moderately severe mitral tenosis*

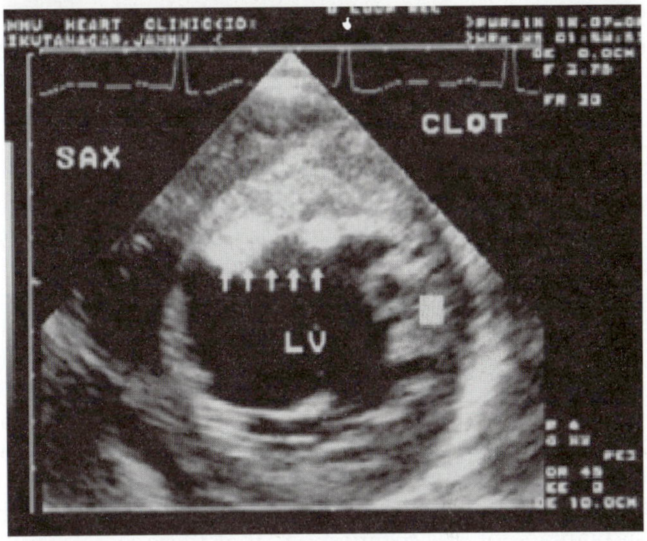

Fig. 11.38: *Apical four chamber view showing apical clot (arrow) in patient with RHD, MS+MR and severe aortic stenosis on digioxin therapy*

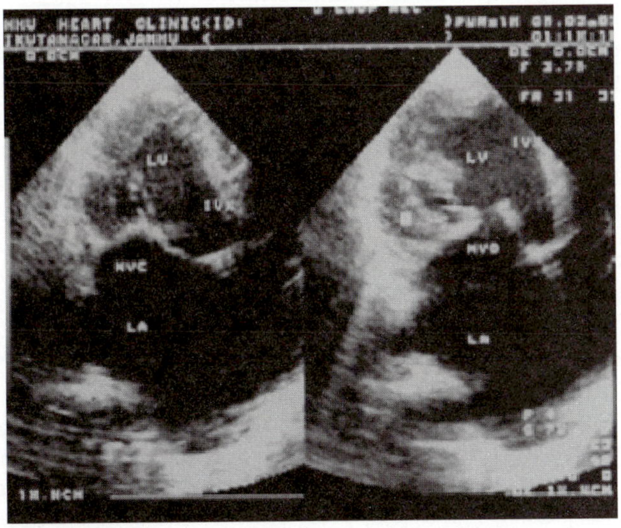

Fig. 11.36: *Apical four chamber view showing closing and opening of thickened mitral valve during systole and diastole respectively with hugely enlarged left atrium in patient with RHD with moderately severe mitral stenosis*

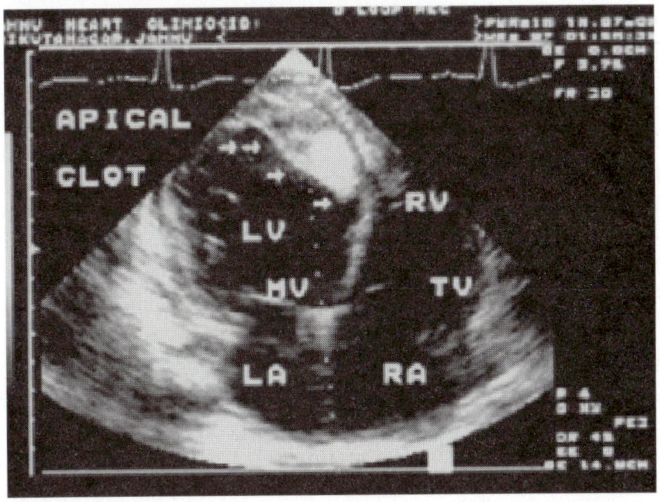

Fig. 11.39: *Subcostal oblique four chamber view showing aneurysm of IAS presenting as a ring like structure in the region of IAS (arrow)*

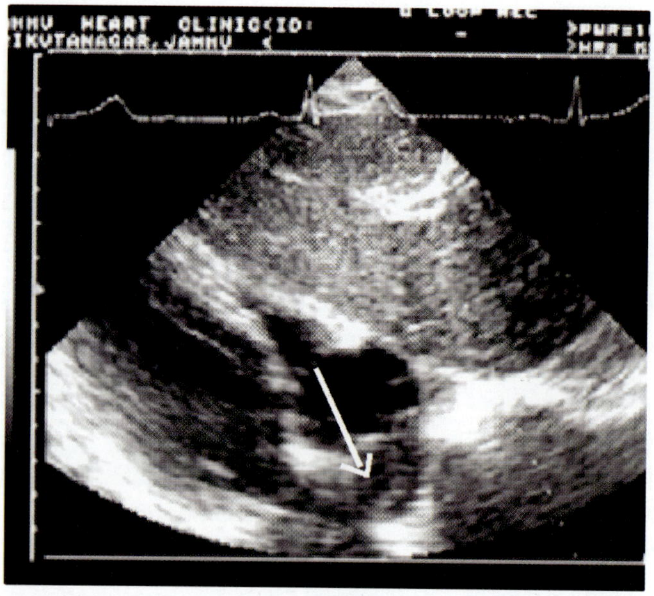

Fig. 11.40: *Subcostal oblique four chamber view showing aneurysm of IAS presenting as a ring like structure in the region of IAS (arrow)*

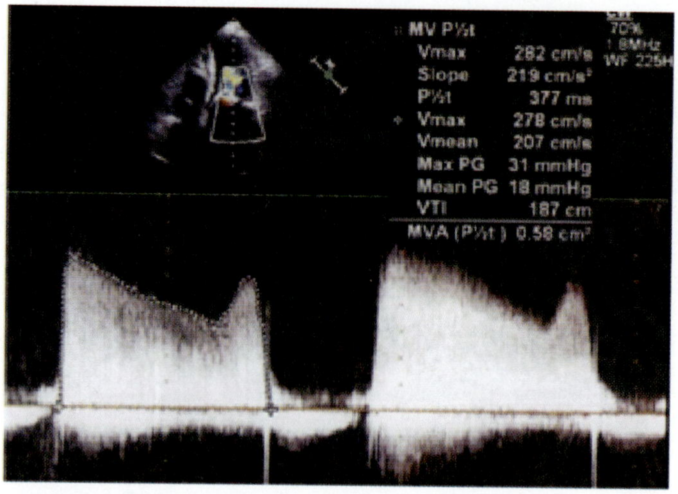

Fig. 11.41: *Mitral gradient by CW Doppler in mitral stenosis demonstrating the maximum gradient (Max PG) of 31 mmHg and mean gradient (Mean PG) of 18 mmHg. The Doppler tracing is obtained by aligning the Doppler cursor along the transmitral jet during diastole in the apical four chamber view. The outline of the tracing is sketched out manually to measure the velocities and gradient, which is calculated by the software package in the echocardiograph. Pressure half time (P1/2t) of the initial slope is calculated as 377 milliseconds. VTI, velocity time intergral; MVA, mitral valve area. Here the mitral valve area calculated by the pressure half time method [MVA(P1/2t)] is 0.58 square cm, indicating critical mitral stenosis. The large left atrium seen in the upper panel is also consistent with severe mitral stenosis. Vmax of 282 cm/s is the peak velocity of the initial peak (E) and the Vmax of 278 cm/s is the peak velocity of the second peak (A). Even though the A-wave is blunted in mitral stenosis in the M-mode echocardiogram, the A of Doppler tracing is not. Slope of 219 cm/s is the slope following the initial E, which is used to estimate mitral valve area. Pressure half time is calculated from the peak velocity and the slope by the software package. The mitral valve area is derived from the pressure half time by dividing 220 by pressure half time. This is because a pressure half time of 220 ms corresponds to a mitral valve area of 1 square cm. Continuous wave Doppler is needed because the velocities are beyond the usual range for pulsed Doppler. If pulsed Doppler is used, the signals will get aliased as the velocity is beyond the Nyquist limit of the pulsed Doppler system*

Doppler Principles

Doppler interrogation traditionally was used to measure velocity of red blood cells, but more recently its use has been expanded to evaluate myocardial motion (tissue Doppler). The Doppler principle states that sound frequency increases as the sound source moves toward the observer and decreases as the source moves away. The change in frequency-pulsed Doppler was introduced to record flow at a relatively focused region within the heart by incorporating a delay between transmission and recording; this allows for the time taken for ultrasound to travel to and from the desired level within the heart. The disadvantage of this technique is that there is a potential sampling error between the transmitted sound and the reflected sound. The Doppler frequency shift relates directly to the velocity component parallel to the ultrasound beam by the Doppler equation.

Therefore, the maximal velocity detected is inversely proportional to the transducer frequency; that is, lower transducer frequencies permit higher velocity detection. The Doppler phenomenon is highly angle dependent. The angle between the ultrasound beam and the blood flow jet of interest should be less than 20°, so that the true flow velocity is underestimated by less than 6%. Adhering to this requirement frequently results in off-axis or unusual two-dimensional images.

Pulsed wave Doppler: In the pulsed wave Doppler mode, a single crystal sends and receives short bursts of ultrasound at a specific pulse repetition frequency (PRF) to a specific location, which are reflected from moving blood cells at this location and received by the same crystal. The maximal velocity that can be measured is limited by the time required to transmit and receive the ultrasound wave. This is called the Nyquist limit (one half of the PRF). The pulsed wave signal appears as a wrap around the baseline for velocities greater than the Nyquist velocity. Hence the peak velocity is limited by the depth of the area of interest and also by the transducer frequency. Pulsed wave Doppler has excellent spatial/depth resolution but has limited capacity to measure high velocities due to the Nyquist limit. It is therefore used primarily to measure low velocity flow (less than 2 m/s), at specific sites in the heart (Fig. 11.42).

Continuous wave Doppler employs two crystals, one sending and the other receiving continuously. The maximal velocity that can be recorded by continuous wave Doppler is not limited by the PRF or the Nyquist phenomenon. Unlike pulsed wave Doppler, continuous wave Doppler measures the maximal velocity along the entire ultrasound beam but does not localize to the precise position where the peak velocity is. However, this is often apparent anatomically or can be deduced using pulsed wave Doppler

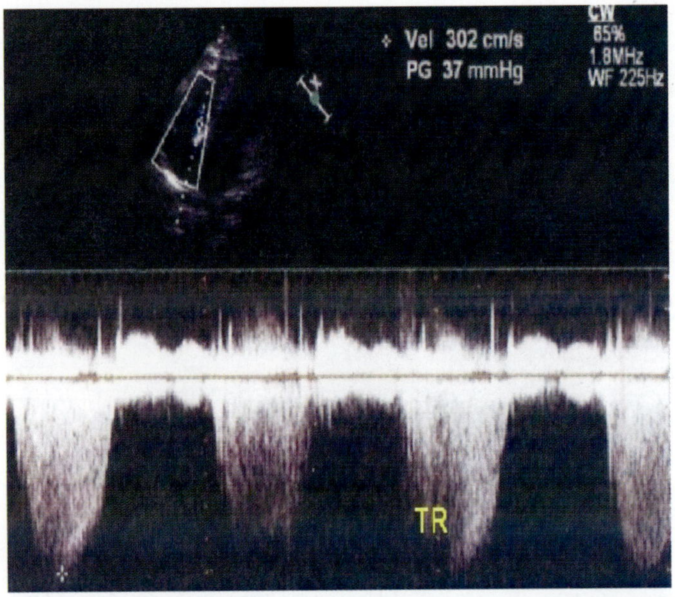

Fig. 11.42: *Continous wave (CW) Doppler interrogation from the apical four chambers view for echocardiography across the tricuspid valve picked up this jet with a velocity of 302 cm/s and a peak gradient (PG) of 37 mmHg. If the right atrial pressure is taken as 10 mmHg (as it is conventionally done), the estimated right ventricular systolic pressure would be 47 mmHg. If the right atrial pressure is elevated as evidenced by a raised jugular venous pressure (JVP), appropriate corrections may be made for the measured JVP. The incomplete envelope in certain cycles is because the heart moves with respect to the Doppler cursor. Changes could also be due to changes in the volume of regurgitation in different phases of respiration. Tricuspid regurgitation increases as the systemic venous return increases in inspiration. Tricuspid regurgitation (TR) is often secondary to right ventricular/pulmonary hypertension as in this case. Sometimes a low pressure TR can occur due to the inherent disease of the tricuspid valve as in carcinoid syndrome or Ebstein's anomaly. In rheumatic heart disease, the mechanism can be a combination of valvular abnormality as well as elevated right ventricular pressures due to pulmonary hypertension secondary to left-sided valvlular lesions. Severe organic tricuspid regurgitation may require tricuspid annuloplasty*

or color flow Doppler. In general, continuous wave Doppler is used to assess high velocity flow and pulsed wave Doppler to measure low velocity flow in specific areas (Fig. 11.43).

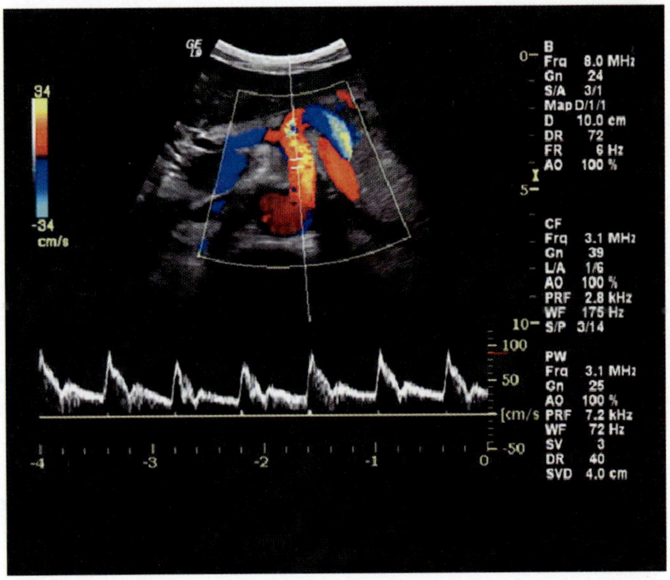

Fig. 11.43: *Celiac trunk using color and pulsed Doppler, CrossX Beam, SRI-HD and matrix technology*

Color Flow Imaging

Color flow mapping is an automated version of pulsed Doppler and is used to screen for flow abnormalities. It calculates mean blood velocity and direction of flow at multiple points down the scan lines. Using color-coding, the velocity information is then superimposed on the image which limits the maximum velocity that can be resolved accurately. While spectral (pulsed wave and continuous wave) Doppler imaging are superior for accurate measurement of specific intracardiac blood flow velocities, the overall pattern of intracardiac flow is best evaluated with color flow imaging. This codes blood velocity as color shades; with red representing flow toward the transducer and blue flow away. Color flow Doppler is based on the principle of pulsed wave Doppler, with multiple sampling volumes at varying depths along a single scan line. A full-color flow map is generated from combining multiple scan lines along the areas of interest. In order to accurately estimate velocity along a given scan line, the instrument compares the Doppler shift changes from several successive pulses (typically eight), and this is known as the **burst length**. Where Doppler shifts are detected, pixels representing those areas are designated a color. The color of the pixel is determined by the mean Doppler shift detected at that site. The maximal number of pulses that can be emitted in 1 second is the PRF, which like pulsed wave Doppler is limited by the depth of the color sector. The number of times per second this entire process can be repeated to provide color information to a specific area equals the **frame rate**. Frame rate and hence color resolution are therefore dependent on the depth of the color sector (dependent on the PRF), the **sector width** (number of scan lines), the burst length, and the density of the scan lines (determined by the machine).

Color flow Doppler has similar limitations to pulsed wave Doppler for velocity determination. When the flow velocity is higher than the Nyquist limit (indicated on the color map), color aliasing occurs (depicted as color reversal).

Factors affecting color Doppler image: Many factors affect spectral Doppler and color flow Doppler, it is therefore important to consider these factors. They can broadly be divided into three groups; machine settings, imaging factors, and hemodynamic factors.

Nyquist limit: At any given depth, for color Doppler imaging the Nyquist or aliasing velocity (which is related to the PRF) can be adjusted. Typically it is set to 50–60 cm/s. The lowest velocity that is displayed on the color map.

The Transthoracic Doppler Examination

1. Doppler (all modalities) is very angle dependent, angle between the ultrasound beam and the blood flow jet of interest should be less than 20°. In order to achieve, this off-axis views are often required.
   PW and CW Doppler
2. Shifting the Doppler baseline up or down can double the maximal velocity detected (still <2 m/s) for PW.
3. Increasing depth, decreases the Nyquist limit, and reduces the maximal velocity that can be measured with PW.
4. Recheck high velocity jets with the Pedoff (CW) probe to confirm peak velocity (include right upper sternal border positions when trying to obtain peak aortic stenosis velocity).
5. Start with high gain setting and reduce until noise and clutter are adequately suppressed.
6. Set wall filter to low to avoid overestimation of low velocities.
7. Decreasing the compress enhances the edges of the spectral envelope, increasing it enhances the various velocities displayed within the Doppler envelope.
8. Initially set "reject" at low (20–40%) to allow the display of a wide range of signals, then increase to remove signals that obscure the image (i.e. to reduce noise).
9. Adjust gate width (1–2 mm for mitral inflow and LVOT, 3–4 mm for pulmonary venous flow, 5–10 for Doppler tissue imaging).

Color Flow Doppler (Figs 11.44–11.49)

1. Narrow the sector and minimize the depth to maximize color resolution (increase frame rate).
2. Spatial resolution is higher axial to the beam than lateral.
3. Higher transducer frequencies result in an increased area of flow disturbance (reduces the Nyquist and increases ability to visualize lower velocities).

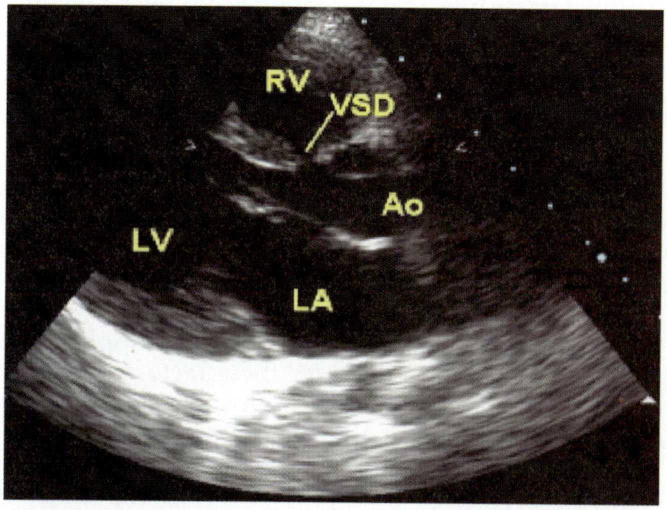

Fig. 11.44: *Ventricular septal defect (subaortic) seen from parasternal long-axis view*

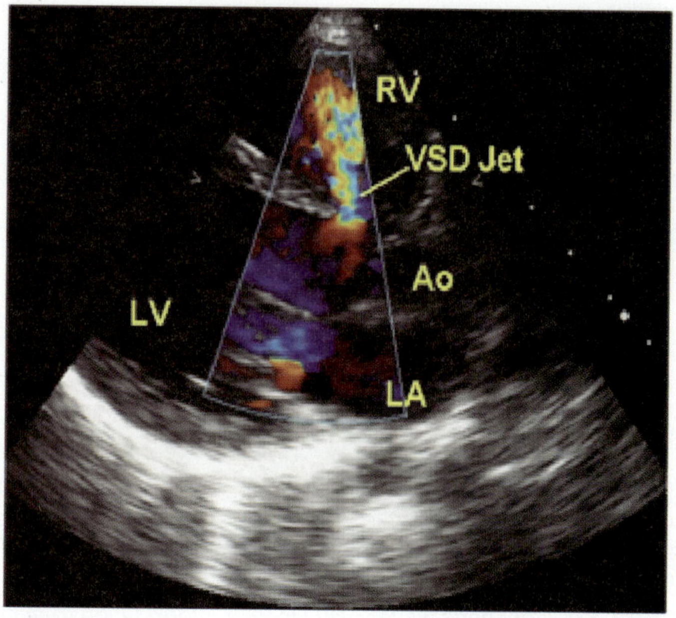

Fig. 11.45: *VSD jet visualized by color flow mapping (color Doppler)*

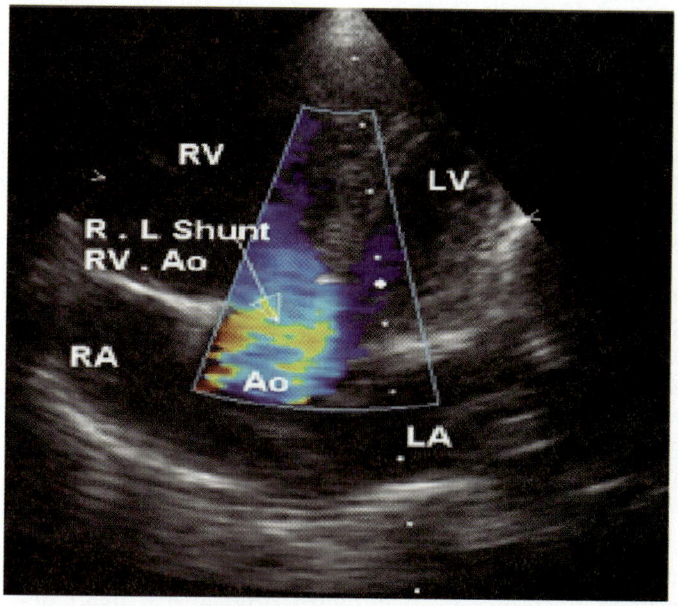

Fig. 11.46: *Apical five chambers view in tetralogy of Fallot with color flow mapping (color Doppler imaging) in systole with right to left shunt across the VSD. Blue stream moving from right ventricle across the VSD to the aorta is clearly visualized in this frame. There is also a blue stream from the left ventricle to the aorta*

4. Adjust color gain until just before noise appears in the color.
5. Minimize wall filters during analysis of PISA/flow convergence, to avoid overestimating low velocities.
6. Decreasing the Nyquist limit increases the size of any regurgitant jet as lower velocities are detected (normally not color coded at higher Nyquist velocities); therefore, set at 50–60 cm/s initially.

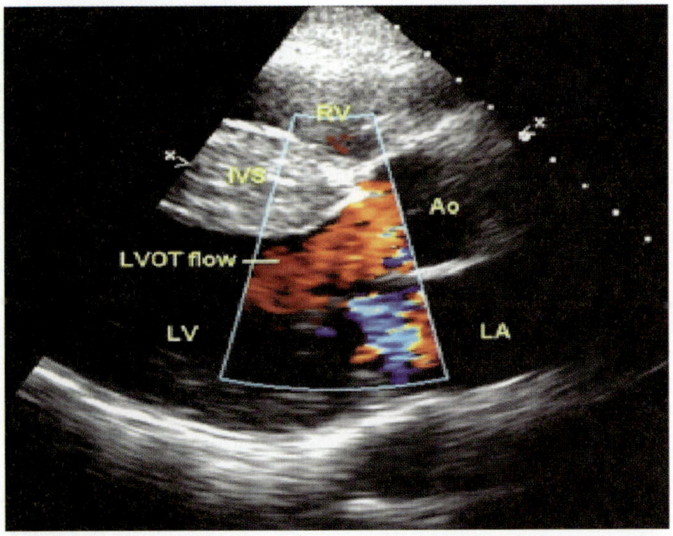

Fig. 11.47: *Color flow mapping (color Doppler imaging) in early systole in hypertrophic cardiomyopathy shows that the flow in the LVOT is not turbulent (red color without any mosaic or variance). This corresponds to the eject phase of the eject-obstruct-leak sequence. The blue color behind the mitral valve is possible a slight back flow during the closing of the mitral valve*

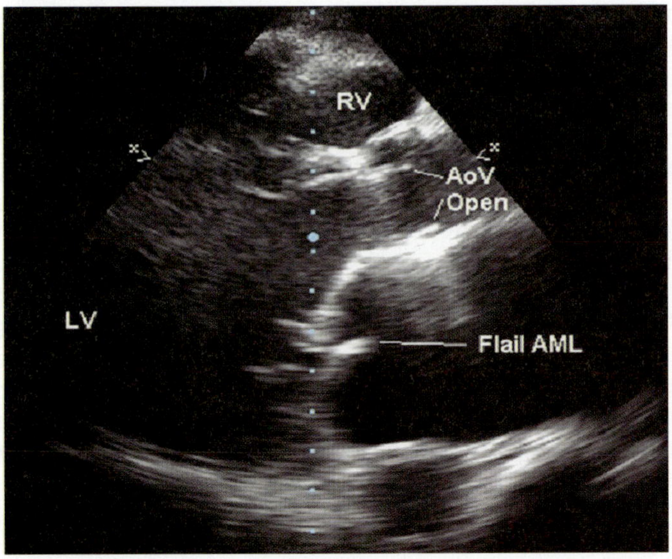

Fig. 11.48: *Flail anterior mitral leaflet with its tip folding back into the left atrium and pointing superiorly. Color Doppler flow mapping showed severe mitral regurgitation with an eccentric jet. The aortic leaflets are widely open (AoV open) and the mitral valve is in closed position, indicating a systolic frame*

Doppler Instrument Settings

The following settings are adjustable on most Doppler instruments:

- **Power output:** This is the electrical energy transmitted to the transducer
- **Filter:** This function eliminates specific frequencies in order to enhance other frequencies that may be of specific interest (e.g. elimination of low frequency Doppler signals due to motion of myocardium and valves in order to yield a cleaner envelope of valvular blood flow)

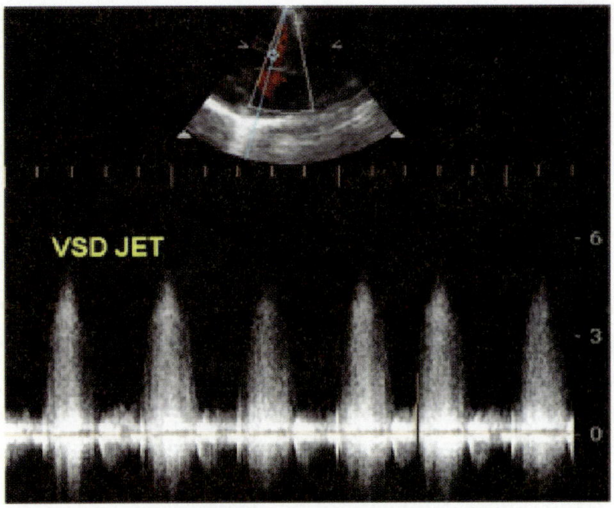

Fig. 11.49: *Continuous wave Doppler interrogation of VSD jet*

- **Baseline shift:** This moves the midline horizontal axis upward or downward to allow displaying of a full-spectrum pulsed wave form.
- **Velocity range:** This expands or compresses the vertical axis scale.
- **Postprocessing options (compression or dynamic range):** This function changes the grayscale in relation to the received signal.
- **Sample volume depth in pulsed Doppler:** This adjusts the depth of the sample volume.
- **Sample volume length in pulsed Doppler:** Typically, a sample volume length of 5 mm is used, but sample volume length can range from 20 mm to 1 mm; a larger sample size can capture weak signals at the risk of displaying more than 1 flow (e.g. a large Doppler sample near the mitral valve may capture both left ventricular outflow and mitral inflow; increasing the sample volume length means increasing the time in which the transducer receives returning Doppler signals spectral Doppler image of mitral valve inflow. Spectral Doppler image of mitral valve inflow.
- **Grayscale/dynamic range (also called compression):** This postprocessing feature allows adjustment the gray/white scale in relation to received signal intensity; for example, decreasing the dynamic range/compress function can improve poor quality images.

Color Doppler Instrument Settings

In addition to depth and sector scan width, instrument settings on color Doppler instruments may include low-pass filter settings, gain, power output, and compression functions. Most instruments provide several choices of the color map used to develop velocity information, which is usually displayed on the echocardiography screen alongside the image. The general recommendation is to adjust color gain until noise appears in the color.

Because color Doppler is a pulsed Doppler technique, aliasing is an important problem. The flow velocity resulting in aliasing (the Nyquist limit) can be adjusted on the machine. Typically, it is adjusted to 50–60 cm/sec. This means that a blood flow velocity equal to 50–60 cm/sec will be properly displayed superimposed on the 2D picture using the correct colors for the blood direction and velocity. On the other hand, the lowest velocity that is displayed on the color map can be calculated from the following equation:

Agents for Contrast Echocardiography

Contrast material is helpful when the endocardial surface of cardiac structures is difficult to visualize. It is also useful in elucidating the presence of intracardiac shunts: it can detect passage of blood from one chamber to another even when the defect itself cannot be clearly seen.

The contrast material used in echocardiography is not nephrotic. The simplest contrast material is agitated saline (saline mixed with some blood drops, exchanged quickly between two syringes across a three way stopcock). Because the bubbles of agitated saline are cleared by the lungs, this material is used to elucidate right heart structures or to rule out right-to-left shunts (i.e. contrast material appearing in the left side of the heart).

Commercially available contrast agents consist of microbubbles of perfluorocarbon gas encased in shells of albumin or synthetic phospholipid. These stable microbubbles reflect ultrasound and opacify intracardiac chambers, resulting in clear delineation of endocardial borders. Contrast agents are utilized in stress echocardiography, where clear visualization of endocardial borders is vital for correct reporting.

Patient Preparation

Anesthesia is generally not necessary for TTE examinations. For most of the echocardiographic examination, the patient should be placed in the left lateral decubitus position, with the left arm extended behind the head. However, for the subcostal view, the patient may be placed in the recumbent position.

Technical Aspects of 2D Echocardiography

Key technical aspects of 2D echocardiography include the transducer type, the shape and size of the ultrasound beam, and the resolution available.

Transducer Type

A detailed description of each different type of transducer is beyond the scope of this brief review. The main element in transducers is the piezoelectric crystal (titanate ceramic or quartz) that both emits and receives ultrasound waves. The frequency of a transducer is related to the nature and thickness of the piezoelectric crystal.

Characteristics of Ultrasound Beam

The shape and size of the ultrasound beam can vary, depending on several factors, including the design of the transducer and the inherent characters of ultrasound waves. Initially, the beam is columnar, but it gradually becomes divergent (less focused), and this divergence results in deterioration of the image quality. The length of the focused beam is directly related to the diameter of the transducer and the ultrasound beam frequency.

The shape of the beam can be altered to have a focal depth (narrowest point) by changing the surface of the piezoelectric crystal to be concave or by adding an acoustic lens. To optimize the picture, the focal length of the beam should be located at the area of imaging interest. Some transducers allow manipulation of the focal zone during the examination.

Axial, Lateral and Elevational Resolution

The ultrasound beam may be thought of as a quadrilateral pyramid with its head at the transducer. It has resolution in 3 dimensions: axial resolution (i.e. resolution along the length of the beam), lateral resolution (i.e. resolution from side to side across the 2D image), and elevational resolution (i.e. resolution across the thickness of the tomographic slice).

Of the three resolutions, axial resolution is the most precise. Accordingly, quantitative measurements are made most reliably by using data derived from a perpendicular alignment of the beam on the structure of interest. To improve axial resolution, a shorter wavelength and a wider bandwidth should be used.

Lateral resolution varies between different depths of the scanned image, being most dependent on beam width or focusing at each depth. With a focused beam at the point of interest, lateral resolution may approach axial resolution; however, with the same image, points at greater depths may be seen in lower resolutions as the beam starts to diverge.

The lack of lateral resolution at greater depths results in blurring of images at far field. This phenomenon is responsible for known echocardiographic artifacts (e.g. a point of calcification at a deep structure may appear as a linear abnormal structure). Other factors that affect lateral resolution include transducer frequency, transducer aperture or footprint, and bandwidth.

Elevational resolution depends on transducer design, beam focusing in the elevational dimension, and transducer frequency. It is the most difficult type of resolution to appreciate, though it can be a source of many artifacts in echocardiography.

In general, echocardiography has a "slice thickness" of 3–10 mm, which may vary with the depth of the image. Accordingly, a strong reflector within the slice (e.g. a calcified structure or prosthetic material) may appear to be within another structure that is being visualized on the image. Examples include a eustachian valve that appears as a linear shadow within the middle of the right atrium and a linear echo in the aortic lumen from an adjacent calcified atheroma that appears as a lumen dissection.

A fourth type of resolution, temporal resolution, is simply resolution across time, which is primarily related to frame rate (expressed in frames/sec).

Image Procession and Production

In 2D echocardiography, the ultrasound beam sweeps across the tomographic plane, emitting bursts of ultrasound wave impulses and receiving the reflected signals from different structures. Accordingly, each ultrasound line in the sector consumes a finite amount of time (which varies with the depth of interest), and each full tomographic scan is composed of many ultrasound lines.

The time needed to acquire a full image is directly related to the width of the sector (i.e. the number of lines) and the depth of the sector (i.e. the length of each line). Moreover, because 2D echocardiography shows real-time images, multiple frames must be acquired every second to yield a real-time display. A trade-off exists between the scan line density and the number of images per second. A high frame rate (> 30 frames/sec) is desirable for accurate display of cardiac movement.

As the ultrasound beam sweeps through the tomographic plane, information is received by the transducer and forwarded for processing. Each ultrasound signal received by the piezoelectric crystal generates an electric signal with an amplitude that is proportional to the acoustic impedance and a timing that is proportional to the distance from the transducer.

The complex process of linking each received signal to a specific point on the sector on the basis of its timing and marking that point with a specific brightness level on the basis of its intensity in comparison to the emitted wave is called image processing. Typically, this process includes signal amplification, time-gain compensation, filtering (to reduce noise), compression, and rectification. Some of these functions (e.g. filtering level or postprocessing) may be manually controlled by the operator to modify the image.

Continuous-wave Doppler Ultrasonography

Continuous-wave Doppler ultrasonography uses two piezoelectric crystals, of which one continuously emits ultrasound and the other continuously receives back-scattered signals. Because, unlike pulsed-wave Doppler, it sends and receives waves continuously, continuous-wave Doppler cannot sample back-scattered waves at any specific point along its pathway. Rather, the returning ultrasound waves represent all ultrasound frequencies reflected by moving bodies in the path of the continuous Doppler beam.

The major advantage of this Doppler modality is that very high velocities can be accurately measured because sampling is continuous. The major disadvantage is that it cannot sample a specific point along its pathway.

Pulsed-wave Doppler Ultrasonography

Pulsed-wave Doppler imaging allows sampling of movement velocity from a specific intracardiac depth (at a specific point of interest, width can be varied by adjusting a sample length function). A pulse of ultrasound is transmitted, and after a specific time interval (determined by the depth of interest), the transducer briefly samples the back-scattered signals. This transmit-wait-receive cycle is repeated at an interval termed the pulse repetition frequency (PRF).

Because the wait time is determined by the depth of interest (i.e. it represents the time needed for the ultrasound signal to travel to and from the point of interest), PRF is depth-dependent. That is, the PRF is high for a nearby point of interest and low for a distant one.

The ability of pulsed-wave Doppler to sample from a specific point is hampered by a phenomenon called signal aliasing. For accurate determination of wavelength, a wave form must be sampled at least twice in each cycle. An analogy may be made with viewing a rotating fan. As long as the fan is rotating at a speed below the eye's natural sampling speed, it appears to be rotating clockwise. However, when the fan accelerates so that is rotating faster than the eye's natural sampling speed, it appears to be rotating counterclockwise.

In pulsed-wave Doppler, signal aliasing results in a wave form that may appear to be moving in the opposite direction to its actual direction (e.g. a signal that should be toward the transducer may appear on the opposite side of the horizontal midline axis).

The Nyquist limit is the maximum frequency shift detectable by pulsed-wave Doppler. Because a wave needs to be sampled at least twice for accurate determination of its wavelength, the Nyquist limit is one-half the PRF.

If the velocity of interest exceeds the Nyquist limit by a small degree, signal aliasing is seen with the signal cutoff at the edge of the display and the top of the waveform appearing on the reverse side of the horizontal midline. If the velocity is much higher than the Nyquist limit, the wave wraps around the whole spectral display, so that determining its original direction may be difficult.

Color Doppler image across mitral valve shows evidColor Doppler image across mitral valve shows evidence of mitral regurgitation; color Doppler scale shown on left indicates Nyquist limit.

Several techniques can be used to mitigate aliasing in pulsed-wave Doppler ultrasonography. If aliasing is minimal, shifting the baseline to allow longer spectrum is the easiest solution. Alternatively, continuous Doppler can be used instead; because this modality continuously emits and receives, aliasing does not occur. Other methods include increasing the PRF for that depth (the greater the depth, the lower the PRF) or using a lower frequency transducer.

Doppler Color Flow Imaging (Figs 11.50 to 11.62)

Doppler color flow imaging is based on the principles of pulsed Doppler echocardiography. However, rather than evaluating one sample volume depth along a single beam, it evaluates multiple sample volumes along multiple sampling lines. Moreover, instead of grayscale spectral analysis, the received backscatters are displayed on a 2D image in a color-coded pattern, with flow toward the transducer shown in red and flow away from the transducer shown in blue (Figs 11.64–11.70).

Because Doppler color flow imaging is a pulsed Doppler modality, aliasing occurs, and velocity above the Nyquist limit would show as bright yellow/white with color reversal.

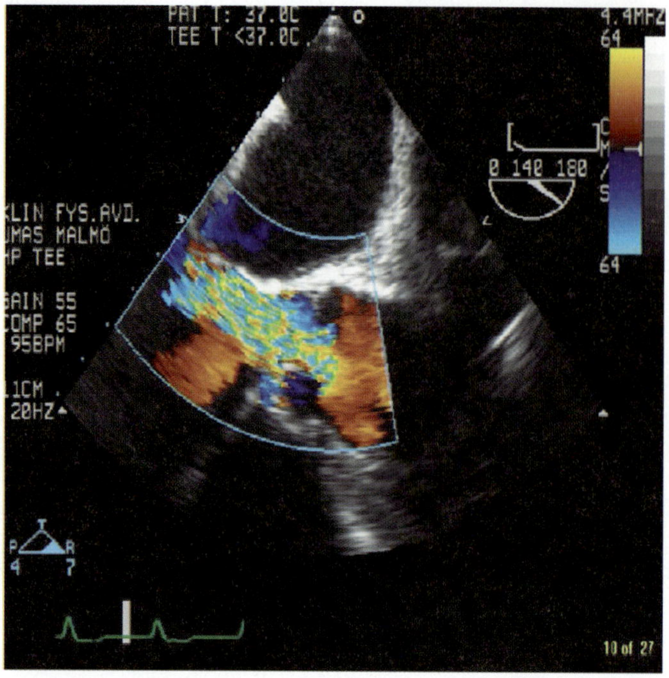

Fig. 11.50: *Transesophageal color-doppler image of severe aortic regurgitation associated with the quadricuspid aortic valve in this case*

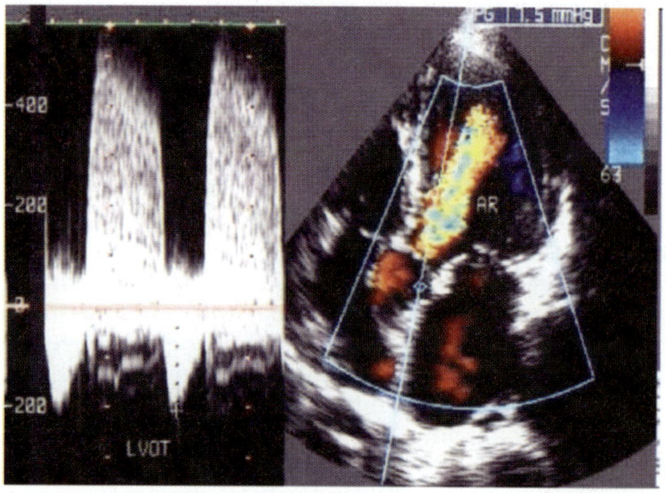

Fig. 11.51: *Doppler echocardiogram showing aortic regurgitation (upward tracing in left panel) and color doppler echocardiogram showing aortic regurgitation (multicolored mosaic jet seen in left ventricle marked AR)*

TRANSESOPHAGEAL ECHOCARDIOGRAPHY

It transesophageal echocardiography is an extremely useful tool in diagnostic cardiology. The proximity of the heart to the esophagus and the use of high frequency transducers allows detailed visualization of cardiac anatomy (Fig. 11.63). Furthermore, Doppler techniques permit evaluation of cardiovascular flow velocities in a safe, semi-invasive manner. Frazim and his associates were the first to perform transesophageal echocardiographic studies by M-mode recordings with certain limitations. In 1981, Souquet, Hanrath and colleagues developed and clinically

Table 11.2: *Indications for transthoracic echocardiography*

Suspected heart failure

1. Symptoms or signs of heart failure, particularly with abnormal ECG or chest radiograph
2. Unexplained hypotension

Pulmonary disease

1. Suspected pulmonary hypertension and evaluation of response to treatment
2. Suspected cor pulmonale

Valve disease

1. Murmur suggesting at least moderate likelihood of organic disease
   - Ejection systolic murmur filling most of systole, or any pansystolic murmur
   - Any diastolic murmur
   - Abnormal second heart sound
   - Wide pulse pressure and displaced apex beat or enlarged cardiac shadow
2. Reevaluation if symptoms change, or severe valve disease even with no symptoms
3. Evidence of endocarditis
4. Known significant valve disease in a pregnant woman
5. Routinely soon after valve replacement, or when symptoms or signs suggest dysfunction, or routinely after 5 years in those with a xenograft

Arrhythmias and syncope

1. Clinical suspicion of structural disease (i.e. ventricular tachycardia and atrial fibrillation) in patient aged <60 years, or abnormal cardiovascular examination.
2. Atrial fibrillation, when decision to start Warfarin will be influenced by left atrial size and left ventricular function.
3. Family history of transmissible disease (i.e. tuberous sclerosis and hypertrophic cardiomyopathy)

Stroke, transient ischemic attack and peripheral emboli

1. Any patient with abrupt occlusion of major peripheral or visceral artery
2. Clinical evidence of relevant structural heart disease (ie mitral stenosis)
3. Clinical suggestion of endocarditis or myxoma (Figs 11.73–11.76)
4. Strong suggestion of cardiac emboli (both peripheral cerebral events)

Chest Pain

1. Suspected aortic dissection
2. Suspicion of postinfarction complication (pansystolic murmur, cardiogenic shock)
3. Postinfarction to access myocardial function, if this will change management (i.e. starting ACE inhibitor)
4. Diagnosis of ischemia if not possible using standard investigations and if echocardiography can be performed soon after pain

Diseases of the aorta

1. Suspected aortic dissection or rupture
2. Widened mediastinum on chest radiography
3. Serial studies, if the ascending aorta is dilated

Screening

1. Family history of genetically transmitted cardiovascular disease (i.e. Marfans syndrome, hypertrophic cardiomyopathy, dilated cardiomyopathy)
2. Before and after potentially cardiotoxic chemotherapy

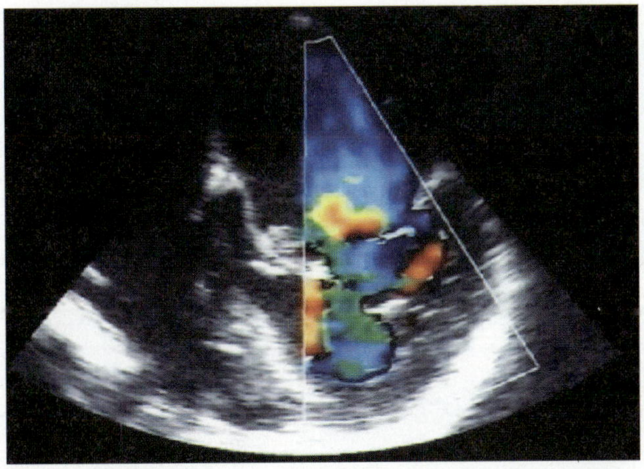

Fig. 11.52: *The transthoracic echocardiogram (TTE) showed left ventricular enlargment, atrial dilatation, moderate/severe mitral regurgitation and moderate aortic regurgitation mitral valve masses were suspected*

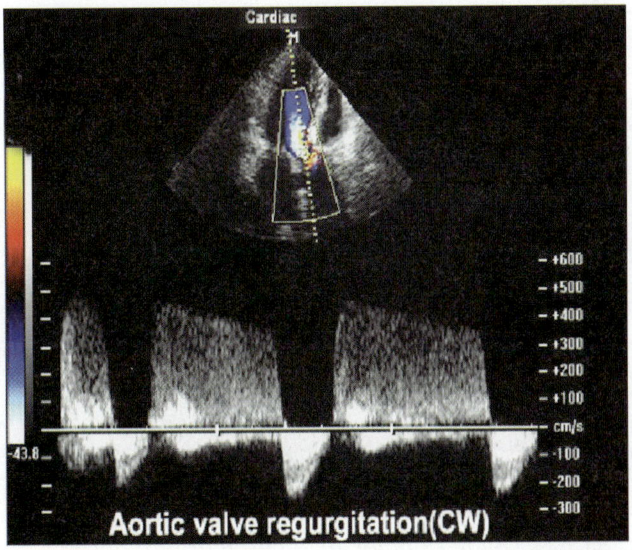

Fig. 11.53: *2D color Doppler image showing severe aortic regurgitation*

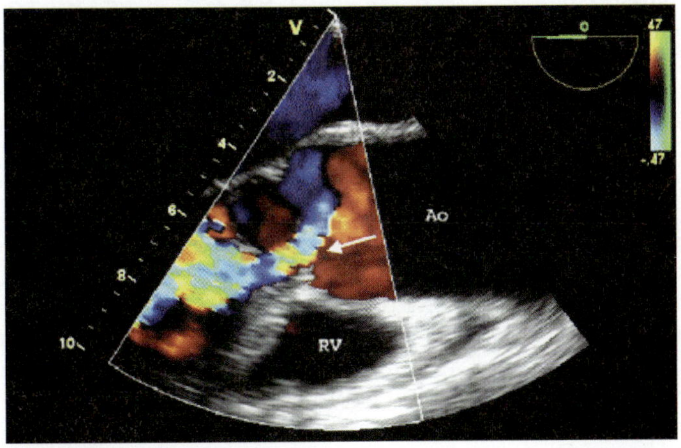

Fig. 11.54: *Transesophageal oblique view using color Doppler, illustrating the eccentric aortic regurgitation (arrow). RV, right ventricle; Ao, aorta*

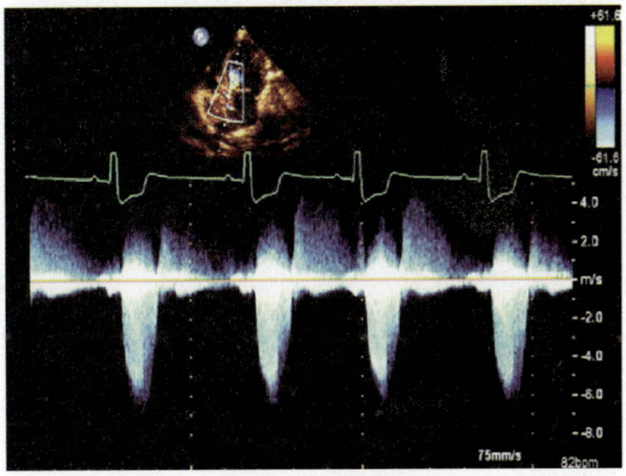

Fig. 11.55: *Left parasternal 2D five chambers apical echocardiographic view from a boxer with severe subaortic stenosis. There is evidence of severe stenosis with a velocity of 6 m/s (144 mmHg) and aortic insufficieny during diastole*

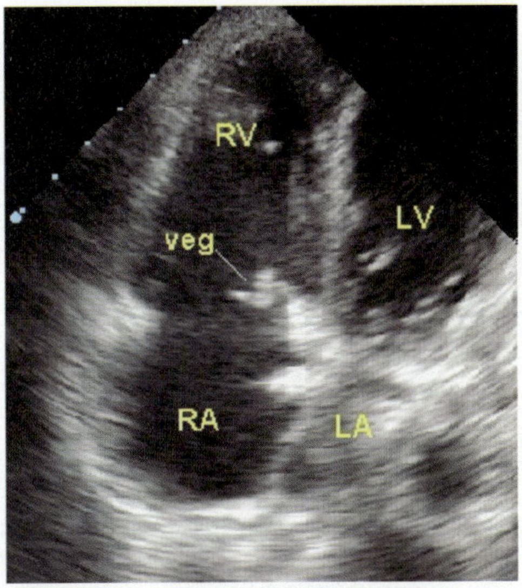

Fig. 11.56: *Vegetation on tricuspid valve*

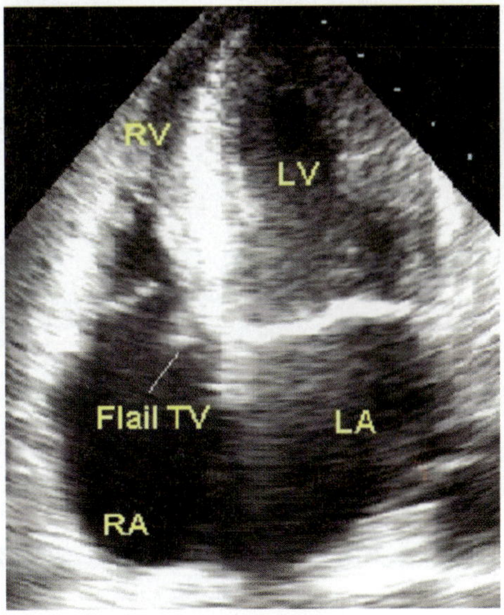

Fig. 11.57: *Flail septal leaflet of tricuspid valve*

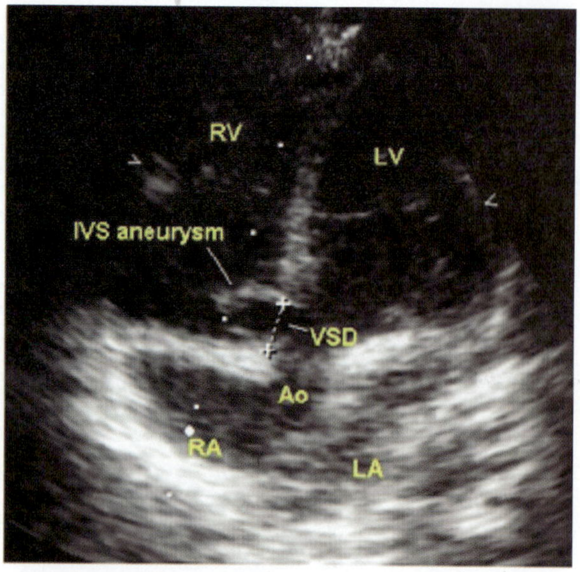

Fig. 11.58: *Perimembraneous ventricular septal defect (VSD)*

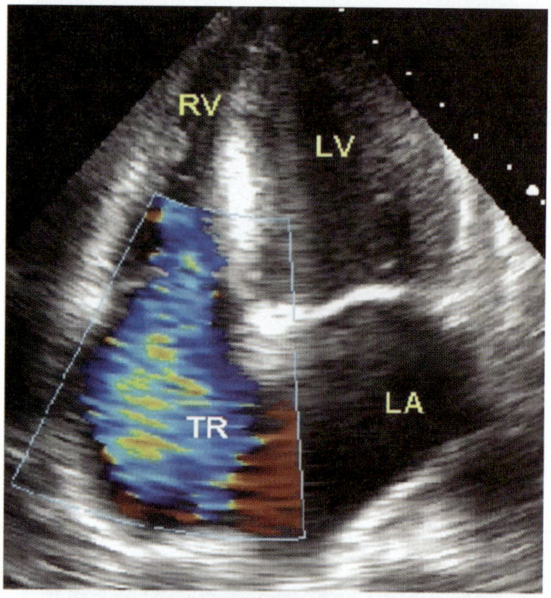

Fig. 11.59: *Tricuspid regurgitation jet*

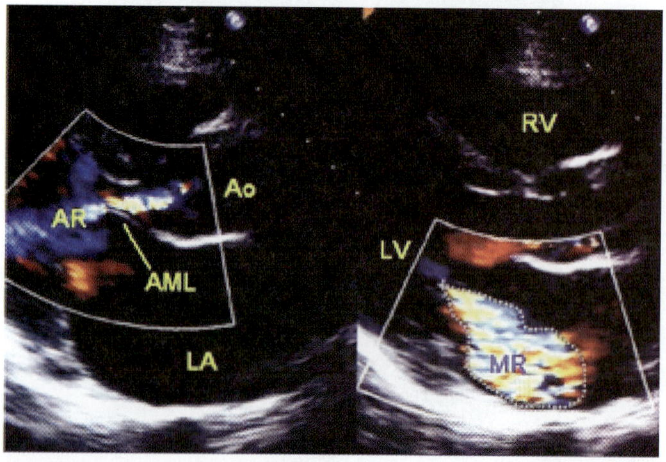

Fig. 11.60: *Color Doppler flow across MV and AOV RHD, MS, MR, AR*

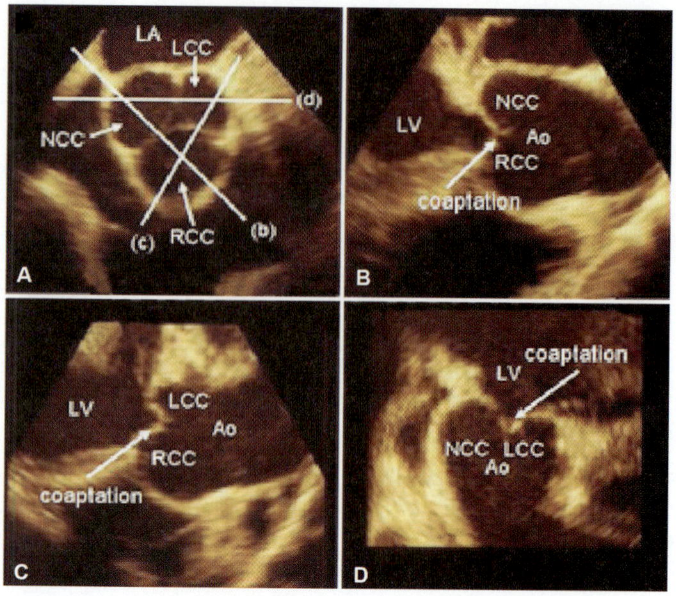

Fig. 11.61: *Aortic valve image on multiple planner reconstruction (MPR) by 3D transesophageal echocardiography*

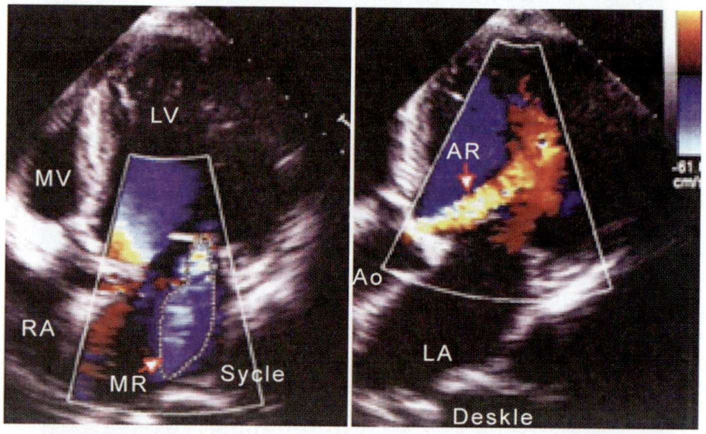

Fig. 11.62: *Color Doppler echocardiogram showing aortic regurgitation (AR) and mitral regurgitation (MR). MR jet is seen in the left atrium (LA) in the systolic frame on the left side of the image, while AR jet is seen in the left ventricle (LV) in the diastolic frame on the right side of the image. RA, right atrium; RV, right ventricle; Ao, aorta. The color bar on the top right corner shows that the Nyquist limit is 61 cm/second. The AR jet shows a good mosaic pattern due to the high velocity and variance in the velocity spectrum. The severity of AR can be assessed by the width of the jet at its origin in relation to the left ventricular outflow tract diameter as well as by the extend of the jet into the left ventricle*

evaluated transesophageal two dimensional phased-array imaging systems, having employed a 2.5 MHz phased-array ultrasound transducers mounted at the tip of an endoscope. However, clinical interest in the technique remained limited as image quality was poor and only morphologic information could be obtained. In 1986 with the introduction of the second generation of single (transverse) plane transesophageal probes which provided the combination of high-resolution imaging centered around 5.0 MHz and color flow mapping that this technique

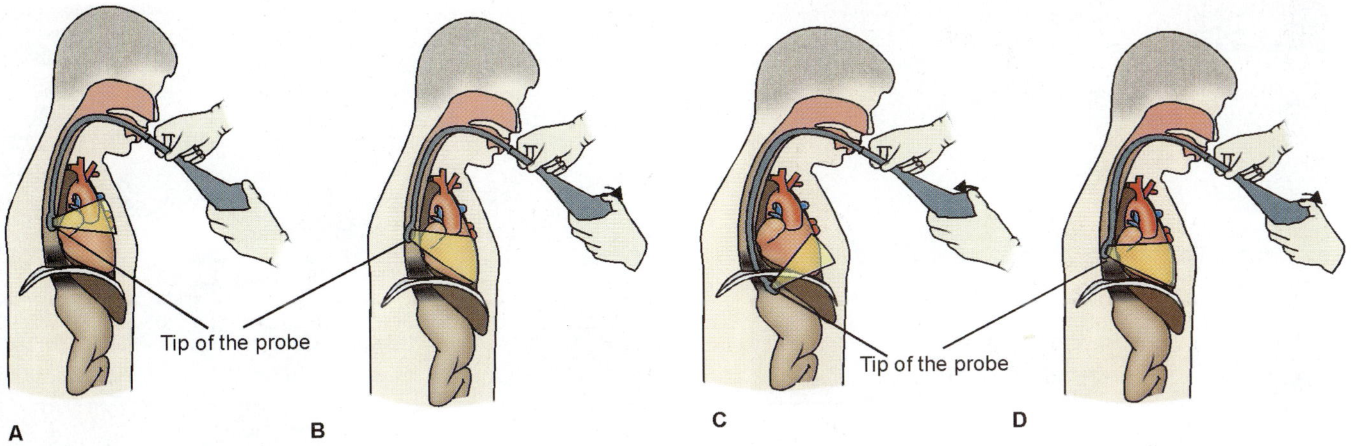

Fig. 11.63: *Diagrammatic reproduction of the three axes around which various cross-sectional views of the heart are obtained in the performance of TEE.(A) Basal short axis (25–30 cm from the incisors). (B) Four chambers longitudinal axis (30–35 cm from incisors). (C) Transgastric short axis (40–45 cm from the incisors) (D) Different maging levels as shown on diagram*

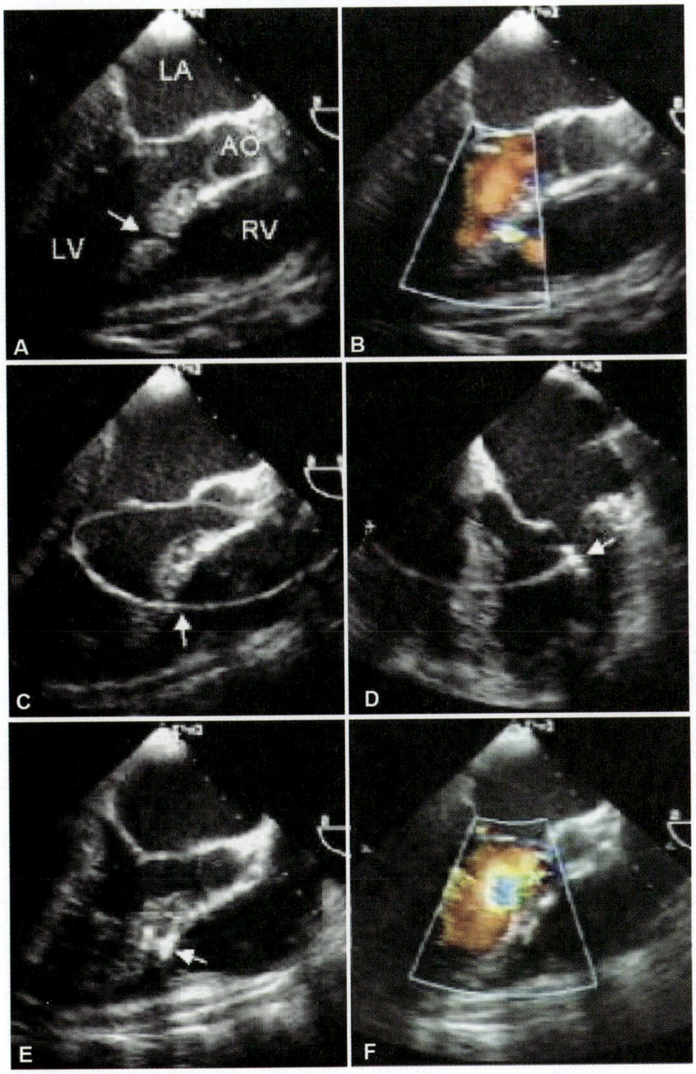

Fig. 11.64: *Severe functional TR and RV enlargement were significantly decreased by TV repair on postoperative 1-year and 5-year follow-up echocardiography (A). Severe TR and RV size were unchanged after PMV alone (B)*

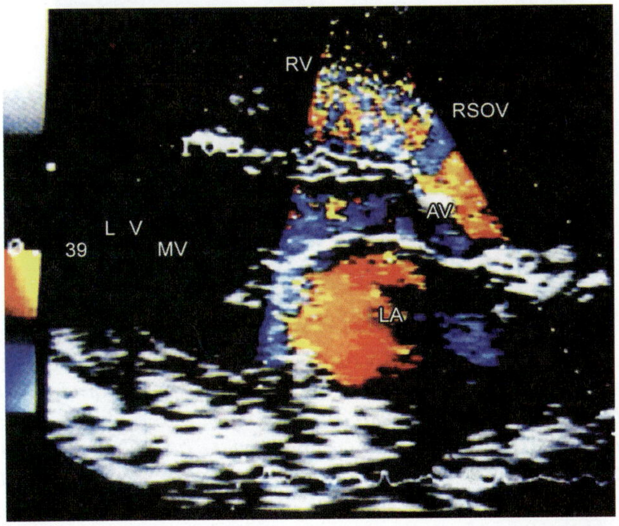

Fig. 11.65: *Color Doppler flow imaging shows the mosaic pattern across the ruptured aneurysm of right sinus of valsalva due to left to right to left shunt*

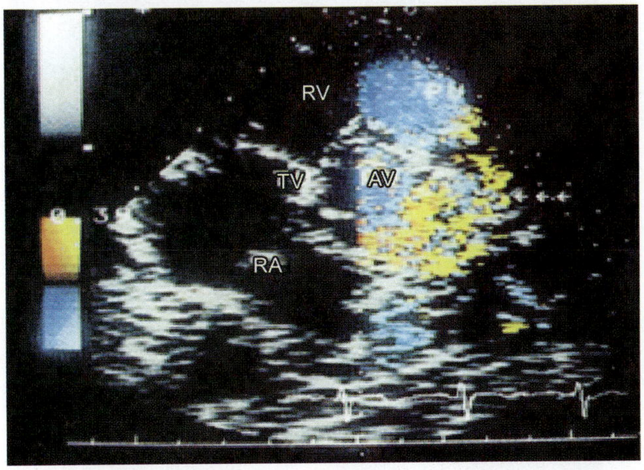

Fig. 11.66: *Color Doppler flow echo scan showing shunt from the aorta into the main pulmonary artery in patient with aorto-pulmonary window*

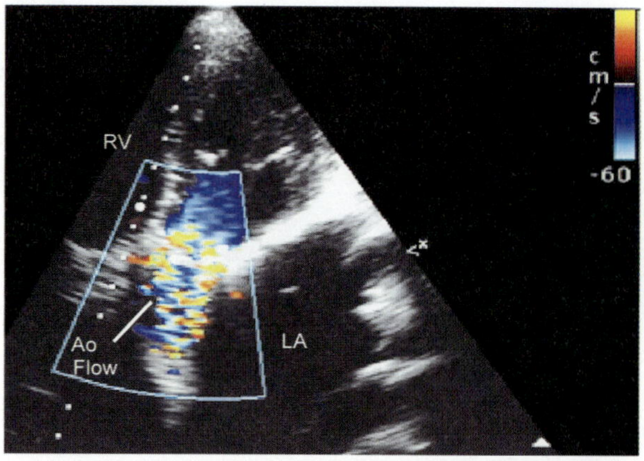

Fig. 11.67: *Turbulent aortic flow in prosthetic aortic valve. Some turbulence can occur even without prosthetic valve dysfunction*

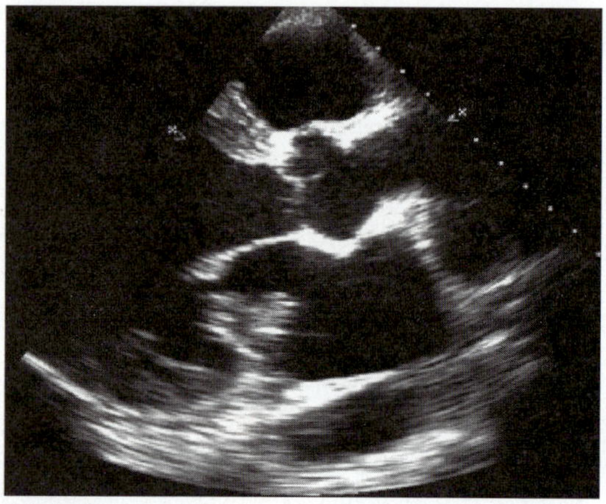

Fig. 11.68: *Left atrial myxoma seen on echocardiogram in parasternal long axis view as a mass prolapsing into the left ventricle in diastole. The site of attachment of the myxoma is not evident in this view. A four chamber view had shown that it is actually attached to the inter atrial septum. Myxoma is the commonest primary cardiac tumor in the adult, and it is usually seen in the left atrium. Right atrial myxomas are rare. Sometimes myxomas can be familial*

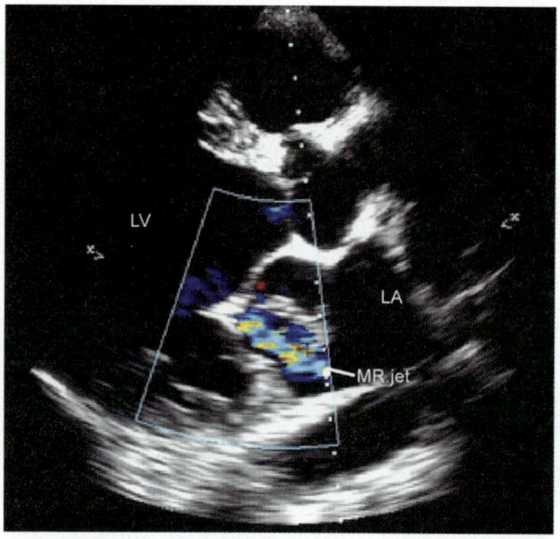

Fig. 11.69: *Mosaic mitral regurgitation jet is seen in the left atrium skirting the myxoma anteriorly and left atrial wall posteriorly*

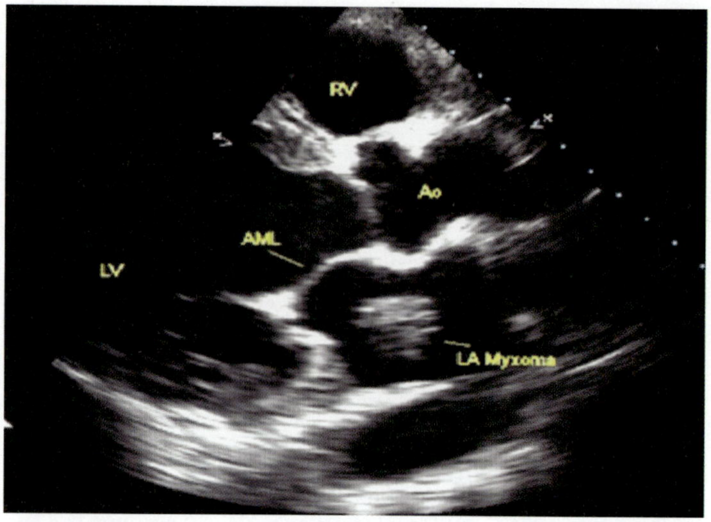

Fig. 11.70: *Left atrial myxoma is a primary cardiac tumor, which is much less common than the secondary cardiac tumors. Echocardiogram demonstrates left atrial myxoma very well*

has become accepted globally as a major new diagnostic technique in the investigation of both congenital and acquired heart ailments and wider number of clinical applications in the field of clinical cardiology. Since then there has been tremendous progress in the development of endosonoscopic probes which has led to the finer views of the normal and altered anatomy of the heart with distinctive objective in the investigation of heart ailments Echocardiographic strain and strain rate imaging is a new technology enabling more reliable and comprehensive assessment of myocardial function. The spectrum of potential clinical applications is very wide due to its ability to differentiate between active and passive movement of myocardial segments, to quantify intraventricular dyssynchrony and to evaluate components of myocardial function, such as longitudinal myocardial shortening, that are not visually assessable. The high sensitivity of both tissue Doppler (TDI) derived and two-dimensional (2D) speckle-tracking derived strain and strain rate data for the early detection of myocardial dysfunction recommend these new noninvasive diagnostic methods for routine clinical use. In addition to early detection of myocardial dysfunction of different etiologies, assessment of myocardial viability, detection of acute allograft rejection after heart transplantation and early detection of patients with transplant coronary artery disease, strain and strain rate measurements are helpful in the selection of different therapies and follow-up evaluations of myocardial function after different medical and surgical treatment. Strain and strain rate data also provide important prognostic information. This Review explains the fundamental concepts of strain and strain rate for both TDI-derived and speckle tracking 2D-strain derived deformation imaging and discusses the clinical applicability with all the major advantages and limitations of these new echocardiographic methods, which recently have become a subject of great interest for clinicians (Figs 11.71, 11.72 and 11.80).

Table 11.3: *Indications of transesophageal echocardiography*

Suspected endocarditis
1. In all cases of prosthetic valve endocarditis
2. Transthoracic study is nondiagnostic.
3. Consider in all cases of native aortic endocarditis
Cerebral infarction, transient ischemic attack, peripheral embolism
1. Patients aged < 50 years with cerebral infarction
2. Patients aged > 50 years without evidence of cerebrovascular disease or other obvious cause in whom the findings of echocardiography will change management (e.g. to start Warfarin if a patent foramen, ovale is found)
Before cardioversion
1. Previous cardioembolic event
2. Anticoagulation contraindicated
3. Atrial fibrillation of <48 hours' duration in the presence of structural heart disease
Prosthetic valve
1. Patient is unwell, even when transthoracic study is normal
2. To improve quantification of mitral regurgitation
3. Suspected endocarditis
Native valve disease
1. To determine feasibility and safety of balloon mitral valvotomy
2. To determine whether cases of mitral regurgitation are repairable
Atrial septal defect
To determine whether percutaneous closure is possible
Aorta
1. To diagnose dissection, intramural hematoma or transection
2. To determine the size of the aorta
Poor transthoracic window
A rare indication

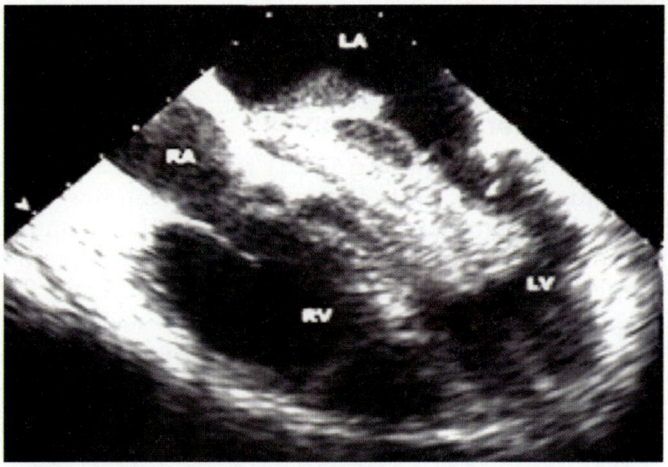

Fig. 11.71: *TEE showing a large mass (M), in the left atrium with attachment to interatrial septum and prolapsing through the mitral valve into the left ventricular cavity in diastole. (M, myxoma).*

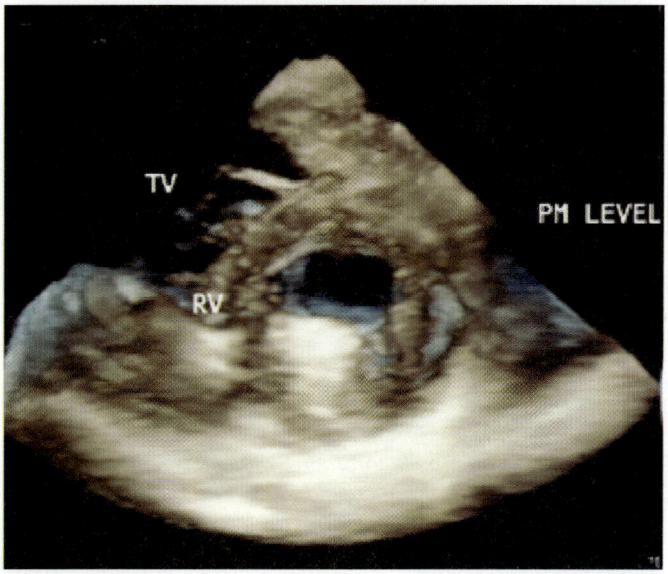

Fig. 11.72: *3D reconstruction of TEE view showing tumor mass occupying most of the right ventricle*

THREE DIMENSIONAL ECHOCARDIOGRAPHY

Whereas computed tomography (CT) and magnetic resonance imaging (MRI) are capable of producing 3D images of cardiac structure by reconstructing slices of images together, 3D echocardiography can acquire 3D images directly. The 3D echocardiography transducer transmits a 3D beam and receives ultrasound waves in a 3D pattern. Effective performance and interpretation of two dimensional (2D) echocardiography requires one to mentally integrate the collected images into a three dimensional (3D) reconstruction of the heart. For example, prolapse of the mitral leaflets may involve the entire leaflet, or only a leaflet portion, requiring the echocardiographer to examine each individual leaflet portion from a series of 2D images and then to mentally "map" the valve to define the location and nature of the abnormality. To do this accurately, one must understand the relationship of each 2D image to one another. Quantification of cardiac structure and function by 2D echocardiography typically requires assumptions about the geometry of the structure being measured so that specific formulae can be accurately used. The shapes of these structures may become altered in various diseases and thus the geometric assumptions about shape become less accurate as do the values calculated from the formulae.

3D echocardiography eliminates the need for cognitive reconstruction of image planes and use of geometric assumptions about shape of structures for cardiac quantitation. This particularly applies to complex shapes such as the right ventricle, an aneurysmal left ventricle (LV), an asymmetrically stenotic or regurgitant valve orifice, eccentric regurgitant jets assessed by color Doppler, valve annulae, and the complex structural relationships observed in congenital heart lesions. 3D echocardiography can be performed from the transthoracic or transesophageal approach. The 3D echocardiographic technique has the potential to decrease the time required for complete image acquisition of the heart. Also, the 3D echocardiogram can be viewed from various projections by rotation of the images resulting in an improved appreciation of the relationships between various cardiac structures (Figs 11.72, 11.79, 11.81 and 11.82).

Tissue Doppler Imaging (TDI)

Tissue Doppler imaging (TDI) is a pulsed Doppler technique that has led to improved understanding of the relation between the hemodynamics of blood flow and the movement of myocardial structures. Tissue motion creates Doppler shifts that are approximately 40 dB higher than Doppler signals from blood flow, whereas tissue velocities rarely exceed 20 cm/sec. Thus, TDI is based on adjusting the pulsed Doppler filter and gain to include low velocity/high amplitude myocardial motion instead of high-velocity/low amplitude blood flow.

In regular Doppler, filtering is increased to eliminate the low velocity signal; in TDI, filtering is decreased to allow detection of low velocity signals. In addition, the Doppler transmit gain is decreased to exclude low amplitude blood signals, mainly allowing high amplitude tissue motion recording.

TDI measurements of tissue strain and strain rate can be used to assess the dynamics of contraction and relaxation. Strain rate is the difference in myocardial velocity between 2 axial points (usually separated by 1 cm) along the path of the ultrasound beam; strain is an integral of strain rate over time. The attractiveness of these measures of ventricular function is their relative load independence (Figs 11.83–11.86).

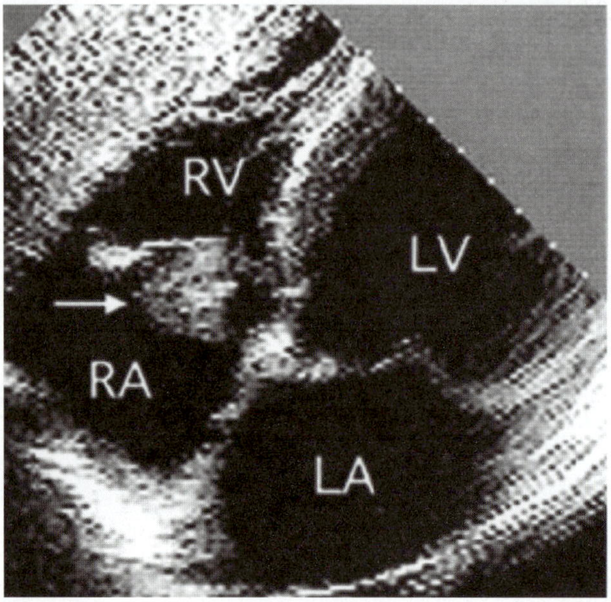

Fig. 11.73: *A large mobile thrombus within the right atrium which is prolapsing through the tricuspid valve into the RV*

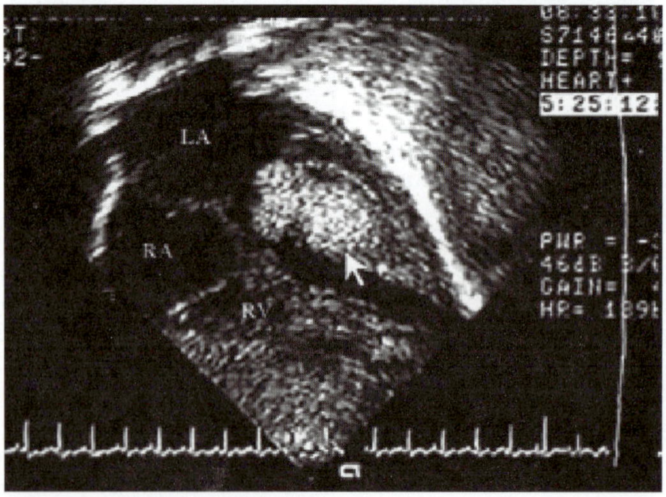

Fig. 11.74: *Echocardiographic subcostal view of a patient with a large mass within the left ventricular cavity invading or connected to the anterior mitral valve leaflet. Mass within the left ventricle fills most of the ventricular cavity. LA, left atrium; RA, right atrium; RV, right ventricle; Arrow, left ventricular mass*

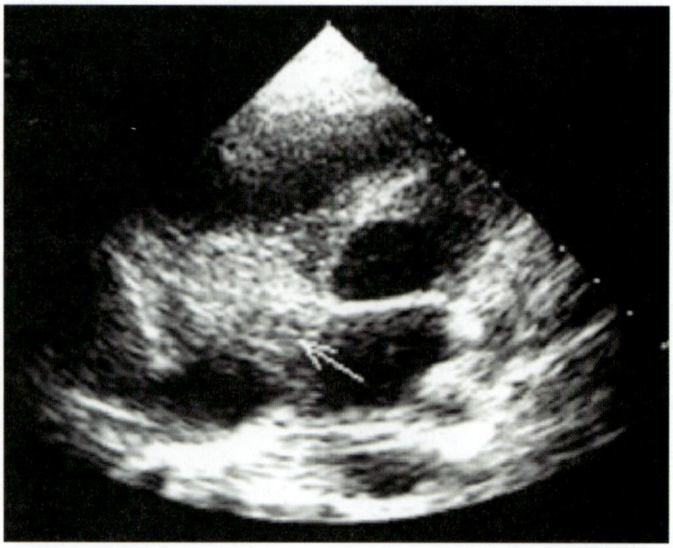

Fig. 11.75: *Echocardiography showing mass lesion over the right atrium after completing chemotherapy*

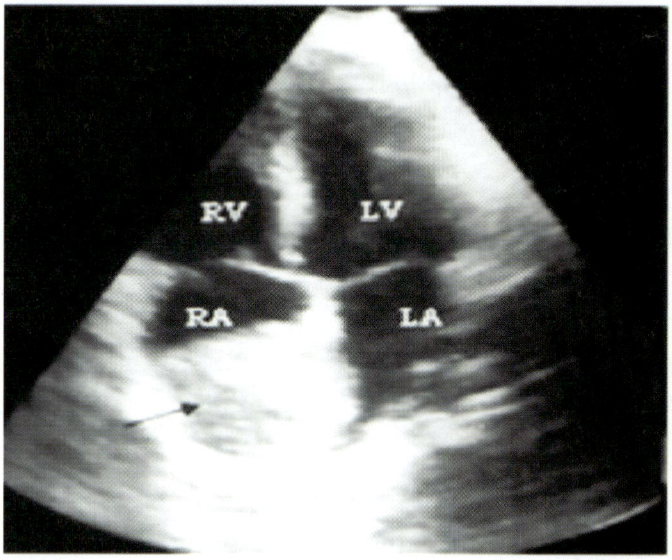

Fig. 11.76: *The transthoracic apical four chamber view below (left panel) illustrates one such situation. The transthoracic echocardiogram shows a mass in the right atrium simulating a right atrial tumor or a thrombus*

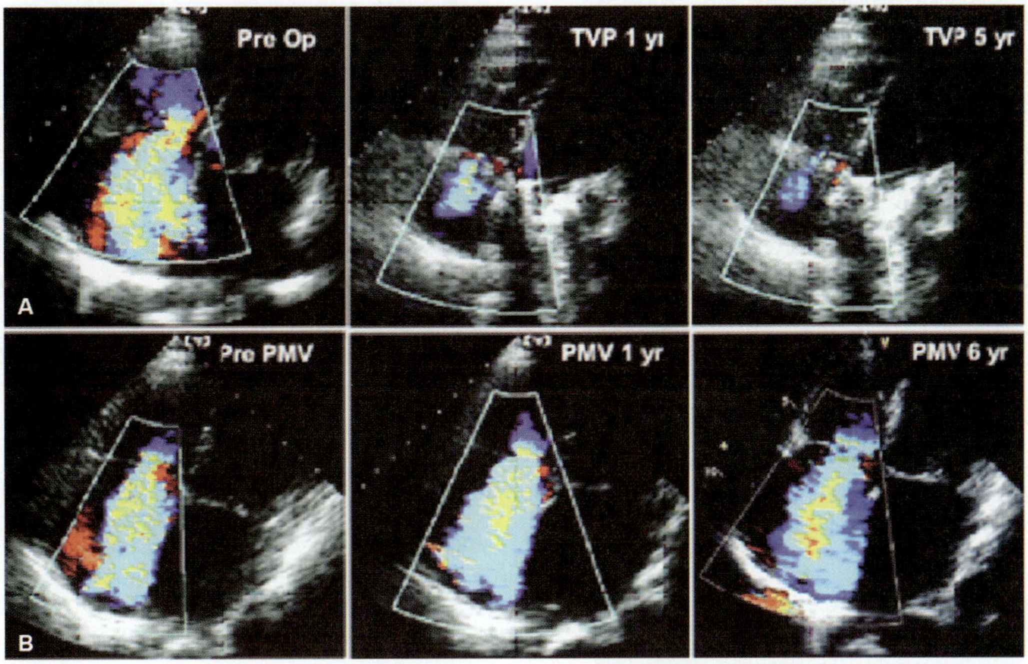

Fig. 11.77: *Transesophageal echocardiographic (TEE) images in a 31.5-year-old, 123.5 kg male patient with a 4.5 mm mid-muscular VSD and a Qp/Qs ratio of 1.5. A and B, Left ventricular long axis view without (A) and with color Doppler (B) showing the muscular VSD (arrow); C, TEE image in the long-axis view demonstrating passage of the delivery sheath from the right to the left ventricle through the VSD. D, TEE image in the four-chamber view during deployment of the LV disk (arrow). (E and F) TEE images without (E) and with color Doppler (F) after a 6 mm Amplatzerâ MVSD device (arrow) has been deployed demonstrating good device position and no residual shunt. AO, aorta; LA, left atrium; LV, left ventricle; RV, right ventricle*

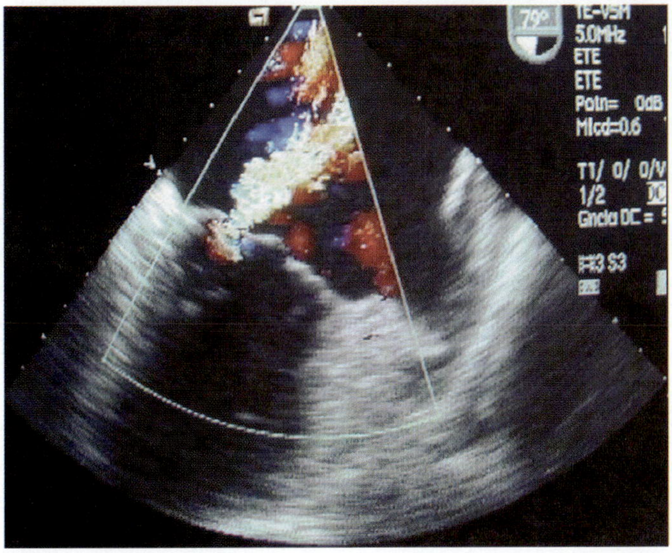

Fig. 11.78: *Transesophageal echocardiogram: 79° projection where a severe mitral regurgitation is visualized. LA indicates left atrium; LV, left ventricle*

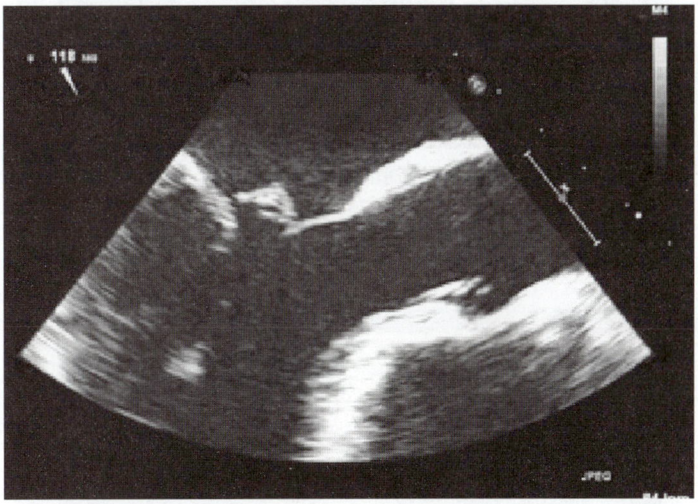

Fig. 11.79: *3D-TEE probe may also be used as a conventional 2D-TEE probe. In this figure, we can see a mitral valve prolaps*

Other TDI-based indices include myocardial performance index, quantification of regional wall motion, and intersegmental delay in peak systolic longitudinal motion between segments. It provides information about movement of cardiac structures. The relation between the dynamics of cardiac structures and the hemodynamics of the blood inside these structures provides information about cardiac diastolic and systolic function. Echocardiography is continuously evolving and constantly being augmented by newer modalities, such as tissue harmonics, speckle tracking, tissue Doppler strain, and tissue characterization.

Dedicated training for competent performance and interpretation of echocardiography is essential. The American College of Cardiology (ACC) and the American Heart Association (AHA) have recommended a set of minimum knowledge and training requirements for the

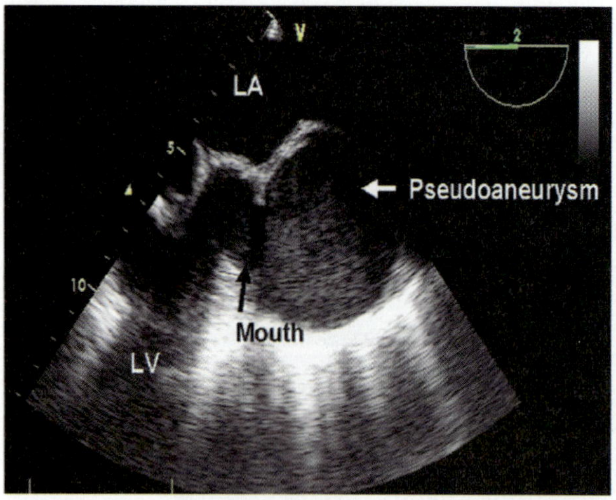

Fig. 11.80: *Transesophageal echocardiography in mid-esophageal short-axis view showing the anatomical relations of pseudoaneurysm*

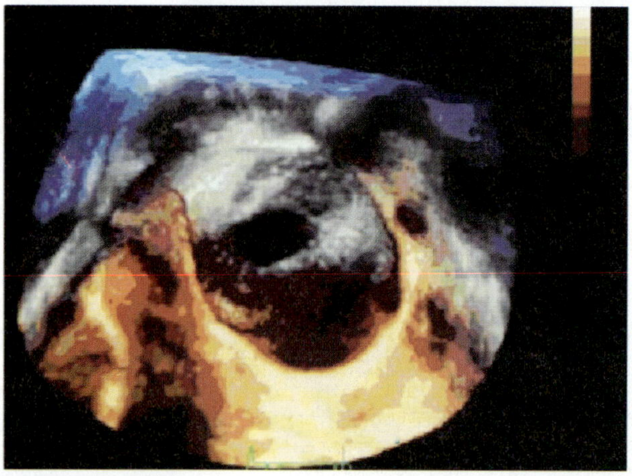

Fig. 11.81: *Ostium secundum atrial septal defect obtained by means of 3D-TEE zoom technique. This view was obtained from the left atrium lateral wall. The septal defect can be see as a black hole in the image*

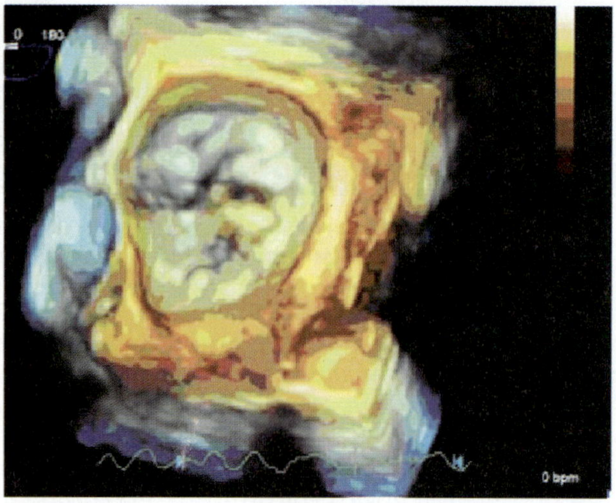

Fig. 11.82: *Mitral valve prolapse evaluation by using 3D-TEE imaging. Mitral valve prolapse evaluation is one of the most common indications for transesophageal 3D echocardiograph*

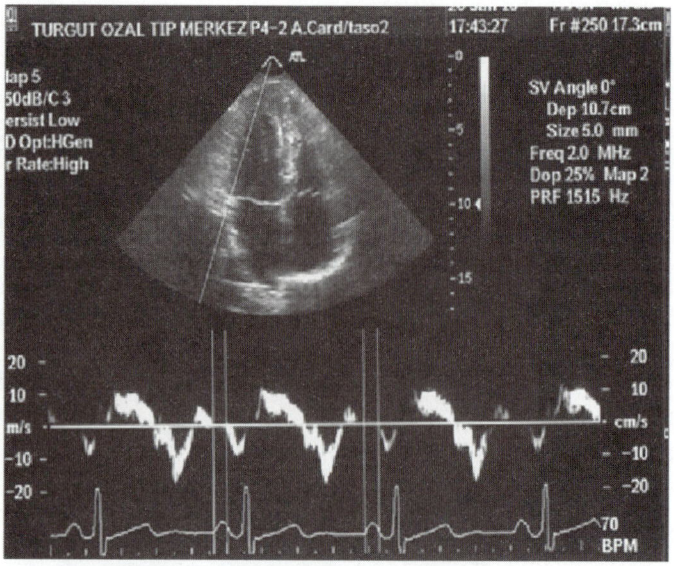

Fig. 11.83: *Measurement of the time interval from onset of the P-wave on surface electrocardiogram to beginning of the A-wave (PA) with tissue Doppler echocardiography*

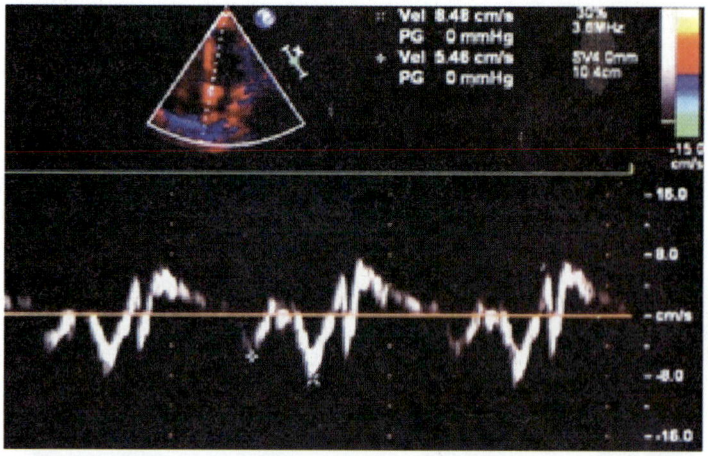

Fig. 11.84: *Tissue Doppler imaging (TDI) measures the velocity of myocardial motion using Doppler principles*

performance and interpretation of echocardiography, including a minimum number of 150 performed and 300 interpreted examinations for level 2 competency in interpreting echocardiography. Similar guidelines have been developed in Canada.

TISSUE HARMONICS IMAGING

Standard ultrasound imaging is based on capturing the reflected ultrasound beam from tissue interfaces, which have the same frequency as the transmitted beam. Tissue harmonics imaging is based on the harmonic frequency energy generated as the ultrasound signal propagates through the tissue. These harmonic frequencies result from the nonlinear effects of the interaction of ultrasound with tissues, resulting in new waveforms of higher frequency that are multiples of the baseline frequency.

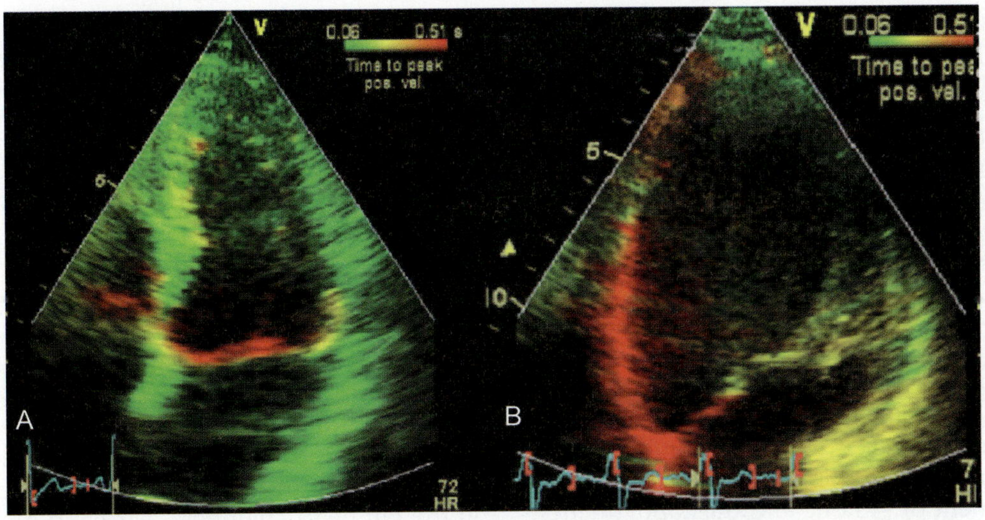

Fig. 11.85: *Tissue synchronization imaging displays color-coded time-to-peak tissue Doppler velocities. The color-coding is green (normal time-to-peak velocity: 20–150 ms), yellow (150–300 ms) and red (300–500 ms) apical four chamber view. (A) TSI in a control patient (only green color coding indicating synchronous contraction). (B) TSI in a patient with LBBB: the basal and mid-septal segments show a delayed time-to-peak velocity (red color)*

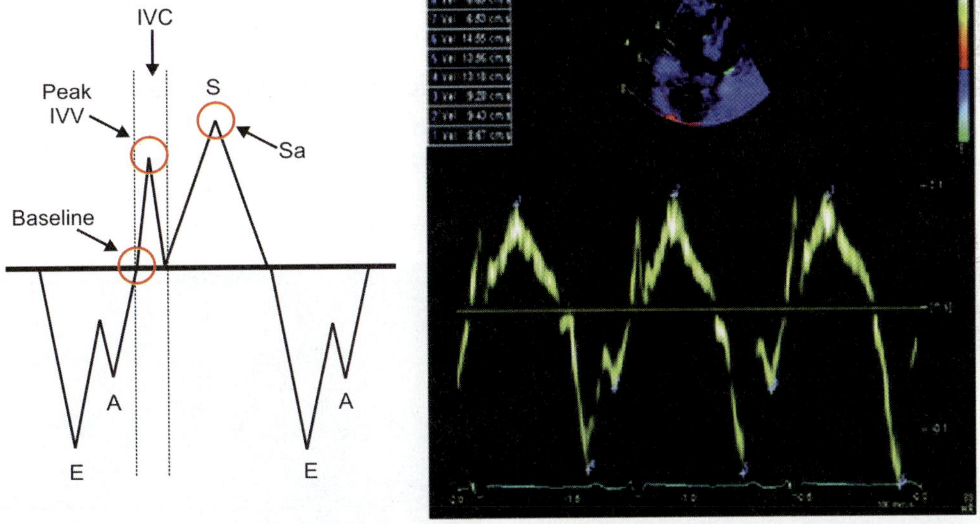

Fig. 11.86: *Normal TDI waveform depicting measured and acquired parameters. E, early diastolic wave; A, late diastolic wave; S, systolic wave; Sa, absolute peak systolic velocity; baseline, onset of isovolumetric contraction; Peak IVV, absolute peak isovolumic velocity; IVC, period of isovolumetric contraction*

Tissue harmonics imaging has two important properties. The first is that the strength of the harmonic signal increases with the depth of propagation; this increased strength can overcome the limitation of traditional ultrasonography in which deeper structures are less well penetrated by ultrasound waves. Thus, harmonic imaging reduces near-field artifacts and improves far-field visualization.

The second property is that stronger fundamental frequencies produce stronger harmonics. Because valves and other planar objects may appear thicker than normal with harmonic imaging, most examiners use both standard and harmonic imaging as needed throughout the examination.

Intracardiac Echocardiography

The first application of ICE was done using mechanical ultrasound systems, which were introduced in the 1980s. These systems provided high resolution imaging, but because of the high frequency of the transducers (20–40 MHz), tissue penetration was only limited and anatomic intracardiac overviews could not be obtained. The subsequent development of lower frequency transducers allowed imaging of intracardiac structures, but these systems were still limited by the low sterability and over-the wire design of the catheters. The clinical use was improved by the development of flexible lower frequency transducers (9 MHz), but depth control of these catheters still was not sufficient to allow visualization of the whole heart from the right side of the heart. In the 1990s, systems modified after transoesophageal echocardiographic probes were introduced. In these systems, depth was improved by the use of lower frequencies (5 MHz). However, the large size of these transducers limited the clinical use. In recent years, the development of steerable phased array ultrasound catheter systems with low frequency newer modes of imaging include tissue characterization and tissue tracking. Tissue characterization is based on quantitation of the back-scattered signals from the myocardium. Tissue tracking (or speckle tracking) involves identification of multiple unique patterns of echocardiographic pixel intensity that are automatically tracked throughout the cardiac cycle. Speckle tracking provides a unique capability for evaluation of myocardial torsion, which can then be used in the assessment of systolic and diastolic functions (Figs 11.87 and 11.88).

Combination of Contrast with Stress Echocardiography

Methods and Interpretation

Contrast echocardiography has an established role for enhancement of the right heart Doppler signals, the detection of intracardiac shunts, and most recently for left ventricular cavity opacification (LVO). The use of intravenously administered microbubbles to traverse the myocardial microcirculation in order to outline myocardial viability and perfusion has been the source of research studies for a number of years. Despite the enthusiasm of investigators, myocardial contrast echocardiography (MCE) has not attained routine clinical use and LV opacification during stress has been less widely adopted than the data would support. The purpose of this review is to facilitate an understanding of the involved imaging technologies that have made this technique more feasible for clinical practice, and to guide its introduction into the practice of the nonexpert user.

I. IMAGING PRINCIPLES

Microbubbles

Two aspects of microbubbles are important—their gas content and the nature of their shell. Recently-approved microbubbles almost universally involve encapsulation of a high molecular weight gas, which improves the persistence of the bubble, optimising the number available in the left heart chambers. Air has a greater propensity to dissolve into solution and although currently unattractive because of loss of gas before arrival on the right side of the heart, better encapsulation may allow its resurgence—the benefit would be more rapid disappearance when the bubble bursts. The nature of the shell or surface modifying agent, which improves stability and prevents dissolution, may become important for new targeted imaging approaches.

Interaction of Microbubbles and Ultrasound

Even when optimal microbubble delivery to the myocardium is achieved with invasive coronary or aortic root injections, detection of reliable myocardial

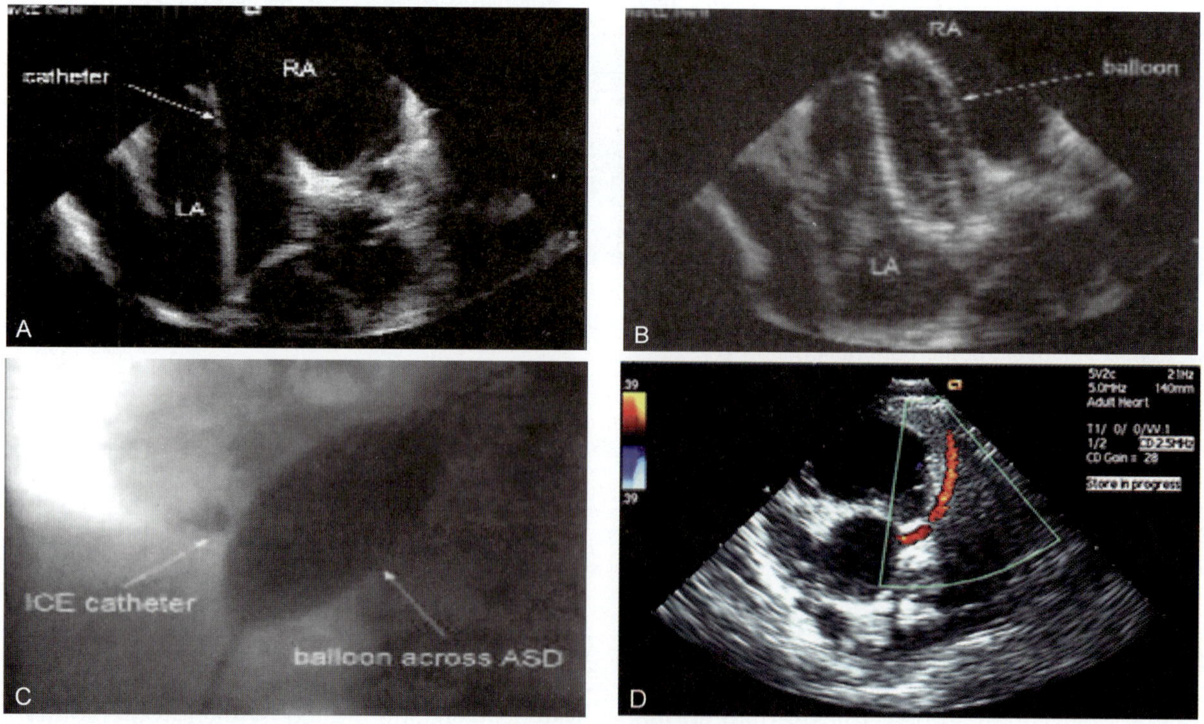

Fig. 11.87: *IC Echocardiograms showing (A) Catheter through the atrial septal defect (ASD) into the left atrium (LA) (B and C) the view from the right atrium (RA) showing balloon sizing of the ASD; (D) Deployment of an atrial septal occluder showing expansion of the LA disk. This was followed by expansion of the RA disk and a good stable position was finally achieved across the ASD*

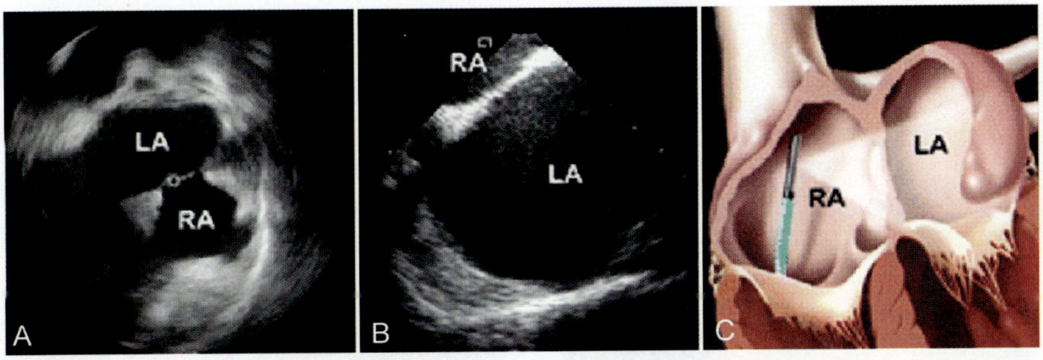

Fig. 11.88: *Comparison of rotational and phased-array ICE (A) Rotational or cross-sectional view of the right atrium (RA), left atrium (LA), and interatrial septum using a rotational intracardiac echocardiography (ICE) catheter. Note that the shaft of the ICE catheter (circular structure) can be seen in the RA, with the tip apposed to the interatrial septum for optimal imaging of the fossa ovalis. (B) Two dimensional view of the interatrial septum using a phased-array ICE catheter. The catheter terminates within the body of the RA. (C) Schematic drawing of a phased-array ICE catheter in the RA in the optimal position to image the interatrial septum. Note that the ultrasound array is facing the septum but is not in apposition to it. (C) Provided by St. Jude Medical and used with permission*

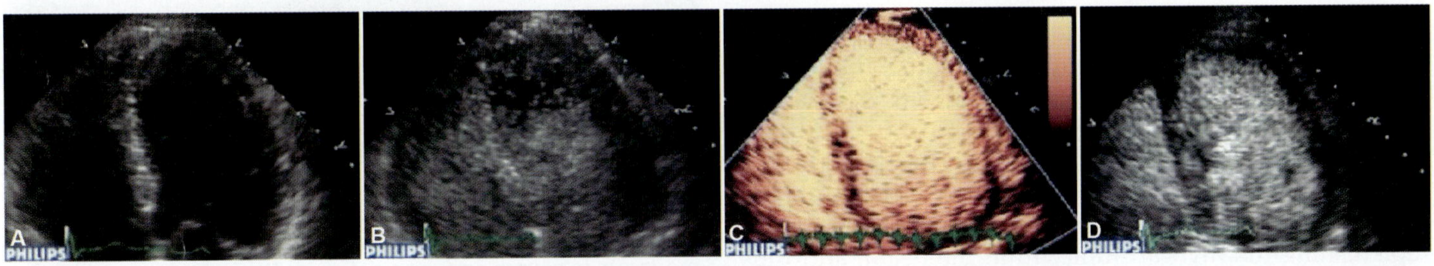

Fig. 11.89: *Importance of machine settings for using contrast for LV opacification. (A) In this example, endocardial border definition is probably adequate with standard tissue harmonic imaging. (B) The use of contrast for LVO with standard diagnostic harmonic imaging machine settings provides worse border definition in the lateral wall, and apical bubble destruction, illustrating the importance of appropriate machine settings. Image (C) shows machine settings for myocardial perfusion imaging – this provides assessment of myocardial perfusion and wall motion, but the frame rate for WMA is 20–25 Hz and thus subtle WMA's could be missed. Therefore, for optimal assessment of WMA image (D) displays specific intermediate MI imaging at high frame rate designed specifically to enhance the endocardial/cavity border. Even in this example, there is some apical swirling despite the focal zone set in the mid LV*

opacification using standard 2D imaging is difficult. Whilst this partly reflects difficulty distinguishing bright, gray scale echo signals from the myocardial tissue from those of microbubbles within the myocardial micro-circulation, the problem is multifactorial and has been overcome by the development of contrast specific imaging modalities, which exploit the unique interaction between the ultrasound field and microbubble to maximize the received contrast backscatter and minimize myocardial tissue backscatter.

Microbubbles oscillate (expand and contract) in the ultrasound field. The pattern and nature of their oscillation, and thus the nature of the backscatter signal, differs, depending on the acoustic power of the transmitted ultrasound field, which is expressed on modern ultrasound machines as the mechanical index (MI). In general echocardiography, the amplitude of returning backscatter depends on the nature of the insonated structure, and is represented by brightness on the formed image. Most backscatter returns at the same frequency as the transmitted ultrasound (fundamental frequency). With very low mechanical index imaging (MI < 0.1), micro bubbles demonstrate linear oscillation, where the contraction and expansion of the microbubble are equal. All returning microbubble backscatter remains within the range of the frequency transmitted by the transducer (the fundamental frequency)—as for surrounding structures.

Low mechanical index imaging (0.1–0.3), generates nonlinear oscillation of the microbubble whereby expansion is greater than contraction. In addition to the usual backscatter of a particular amplitude within the range of the fundamental frequency, the bubbles also produce backscatter of (lesser) amplitude at harmonic frequencies. For example, scatter from a bubble interrogated by a 4 MHz pulse will be composed of 4 MHz and 8 MHz sound. Tissues and surrounding structures do not produce harmonic backscatter when imaged under low power. When exposed to high mechanical index imaging (MI > 0.6, i.e. the MI used for standard imaging) the bubbles oscillate wildly and burst. Upon destruction, microbubbles produce a brief, high amplitude signal, with good resolution, which is rich in harmonic signals, containing backscatter at the second third and fourth harmonics, etc. The bubble dissipates gradually

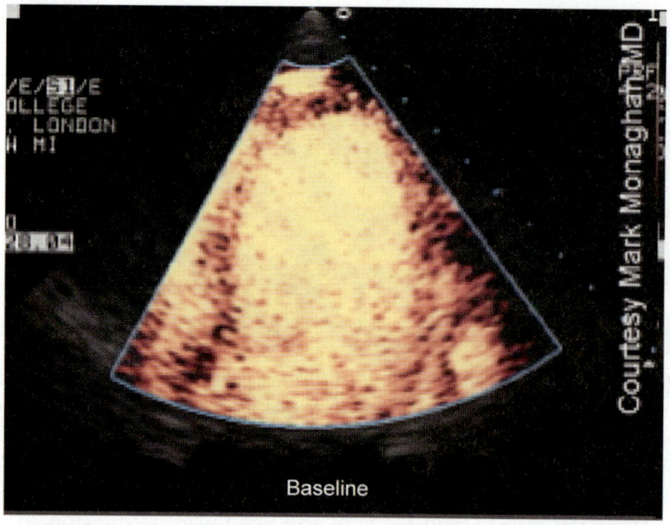

Fig. 11.90: *Low-power scanning shows baseline degree of perfusion, based on presence of microbubbles of contrast agent*

following destruction, depending upon the gas composition of the bubble, with air-based micro-bubbles dissipating much more rapidly. Importantly at high MI, tissues also produce harmonics (Fig. 11.90).

With standard fundamental imaging (high MI), myocardial microbubbles are destroyed continuously, causing apical swirling on LVO images and never replenishing the myocardium within the beam, and thus not returning significant myocardial backscatter. This exacerbates the underlying difficulty of differentiating on gray scale, between tissue backscatter and microbubble backscatter. Changing to standard harmonic imaging (processing only signals returned at the second harmonic of the fundamental frequency) significantly improves LVO, but offers little benefit for myocardial perfusion, with ongoing bubble destruction and suboptimal differentiation between contrast and tissue, because both produce harmonics at high power. Contrast specific imaging modalities, with the aim of enhancing the contrast to tissue backscatter signal ratio (CTR) are required for optimal performance of a myocardial contrast study.

CONTRAST SPECIFIC IMAGING TECHNOLOGY. HIGH POWER TECHNIQUES—INTERMITTENT IMAGING

Triggered Harmonic Imaging (Figs 11.91 and 11.95)

Porter demonstrated that intermittent high power imaging demonstrated significantly better myocardial opacification than continuous imaging, with the best opacification obtained using intermittent harmonic imaging. During intermittent high power imaging, high energy ultrasound is transmitted at specified intermittent intervals, triggered to the ECG (e.g. once every 4 cardiac cycles; 1:4 triggering). The time between destructive pulses allows the micro-bubbles to replenish the myocardium. With each destructive pulse, high amplitude backscatter rich in harmonics is returned to the transducer, enabling static images of myocardial perfusion.

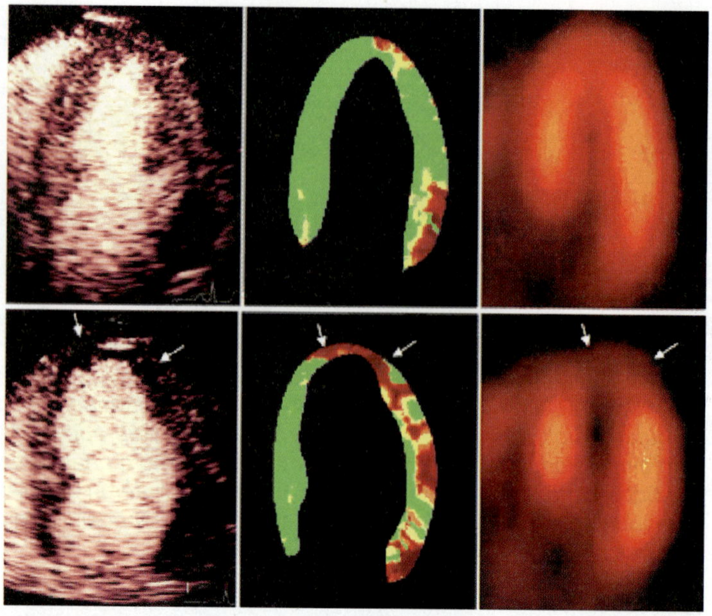

Fig. 11.91: *The upper panels demonstrate a contrast-enhanced apical four-chamber echocardiographic image at rest (left) alongside its corresponding parametric (middle), and single-photon emission computed tomography (SPECT) image (right). The bottom panels demonstrate a contrast-enhanced apical four-chamber echocardiographic image at peak stress (left) alongside its corresponding parametric (middle), and SPECT image (right). The parametric image has been color-coded: red indicates a moderate to severe perfusion deficit; yellow indicates a mild deficit; and green indicates normal perfusion. A stress-induced perfusion defect has developed in the apical segments (arrows), with apical thinning. The basal lateral segment on the parametric image was classified as nonanalyzable, using the goodness-of-fit image*

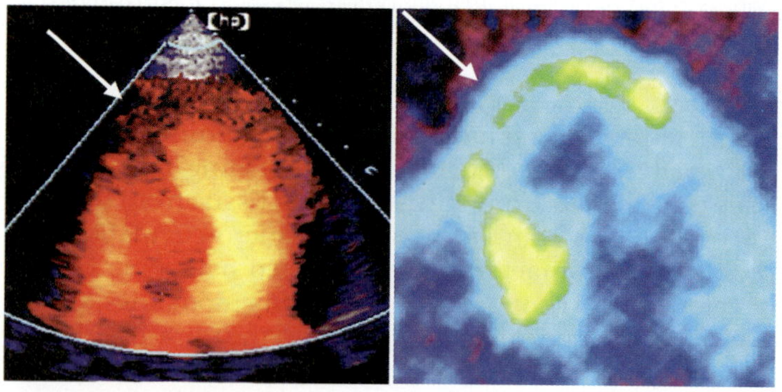

Fig. 11.92: *Assessment of myocardial perfusion abnormalities by intravenous myocardial contrast echocardiography with harmonic power Doppler imaging: comparison with positron emission tomography*

The qualitative assessment of perfusion using intermittent harmonic imaging can be improved by digital subtraction of the myocardial signal, and optimized by color coding techniques to allow better extraction of bubble signals. The first human study validating myocardial perfusion assessment by MCE with SPECT used digital subtraction. However, this approach requires careful superimposition of each frame, and although the analysis

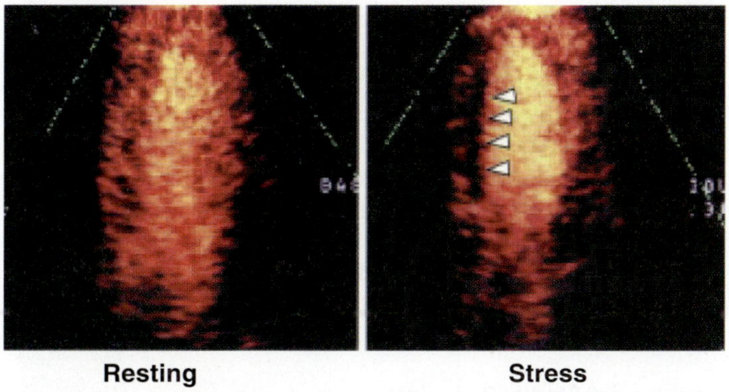

Fig. 11.93: *An example of an inducible inferior myocardial contrast defect (arrows) on pulse inversion Doppler (PID) imaging in the apical two chambers view after intravenous Optison administration in a patient with >50% diameter stenosis in the right coronary artery (RCA). Wall motion was considered normal in this patient both at rest and during stress*

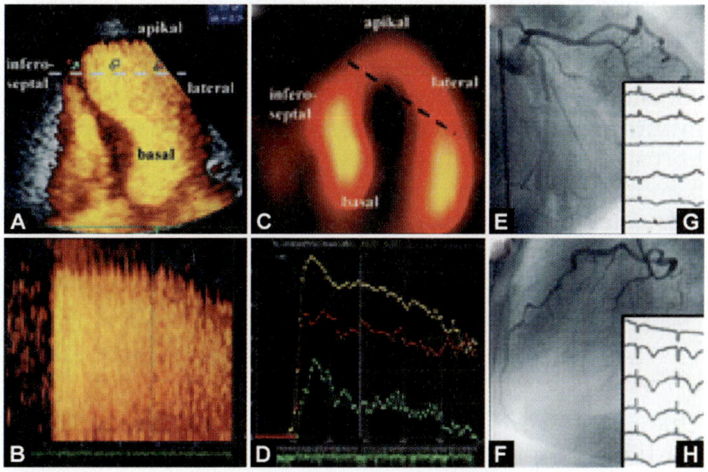

Fig. 11.94: *Power Doppler harmonic imaging measurement of regional myocardial perfusion in a patient with chest pain since 2 days at admission to hospital using intravenous bolus application of Optison®. (A) The color-coded two dimensional image of the apical four-chamber view of a power Doppler harmonic imaging measurement with respective regions of interest put into the left ventricular cavum (yellow), the apical septum (green), and the apical lateral wall (red). In addition, the axis of the colour-M-mode given in (B) is shown. (C) The corresponding scintiscanning of the four chamber view given in (A) documenting hypoperfusion in the apical and mid inferoseptal area as well as the apex. (D) The Doppler intensity kinetics of the regions of interests is given in (A). The Doppler intensity-signals of the septal areas are below the saturation threshold much earlier than those of the lateral wall. Coronary angiography documented normal epicardial arterial vessels (see (E, F)). (G, H). The ECG tracings of the patient*

is becoming more automated, the processing is still performed off-line.

Harmonic Power Doppler

Power Doppler technology is designed to detect motion of blood or tissue, and is used in myocardial contrast echo to overcome the need for off line digital subtraction. As with traditional Doppler, two or more pulses are sent successively along each scan line of the image and the pairs of echo trains are compared for the presence or absence of a frequency shift (indicating movement). However, unlike traditional Doppler, power Doppler ignores the direction and velocity of the moving structure; if a frequency shift is detected, indicating motion of the structure, then color is displayed as an overlay whose saturation is related to the amplitude of the echo which has moved. If no frequency shift (movement) is detected, no color is displayed.

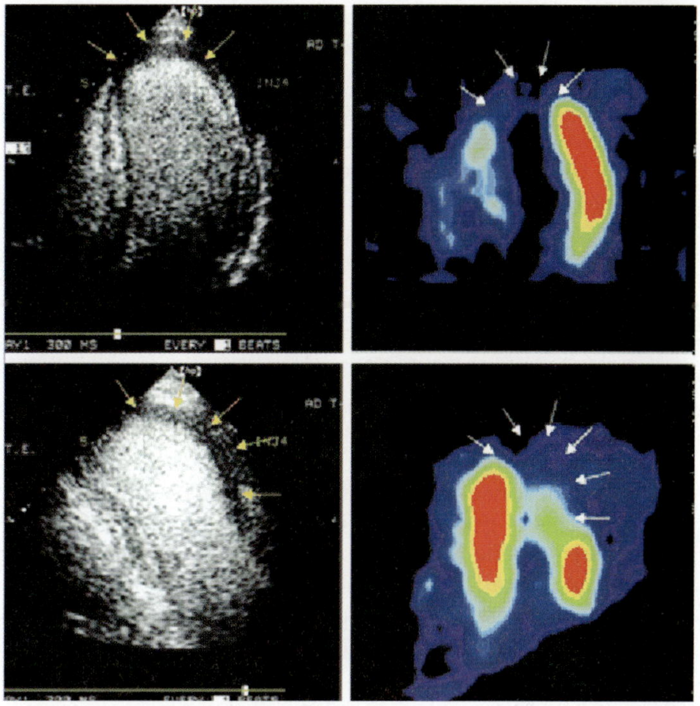

Fig. 11.95: *Representative myocardial contrast echocardiography (MCE) and SPECT images obtained in a patient with anterior myocardial infarction, showing a larger perfusion defect by SPECT than MCE: (top left) apical four chamber MCE; (bottom left) apical two chamber MCE; (top right) apical four chamber SPECT; (bottom right) apical two chamber SPECT. Arrows delineate the area of decreased opacification/tracer uptake. Reprinted from Jucquois et al,14 with permission of BMJ Publishing Group Ltd.*

This method is ideally suited to high mechanical index destructive imaging, as the first pulse destroys the myocardial microbubbles, generating a brief, high amplitude echo rich in harmonics. The second pulse finds that the bubbles have moved, and thus color is overlaid on the echo image over the areas of myocardium that contained microbubbles. In an area with no microbubbles, there is no movement recognized and there is no color overlay applied to that region. Note that the technique is not actually detecting movement of the bubbles in the circulation, but rather their destruction. This technique has been correlated in human subjects with SPECT and has been used extensively in clinical trials (Fig. 11.92 and 11.94).

The most important limitation of this technique is motion artefact from tissue, because tissue motion will be expressed like bubble destruction, potentially showing perfusion when none is present (a false negative). If Doppler frequency is increased, pulse separation is reduced, so tissue movement between pulses can be minimized. However, if the pulses are too close, not all the gas within the bubble will have dissipated before arrival of the next pulse, so the difference between pulses is reduced, possibly leading to false-positive perfusion defects. Air-filled microbubbles are optimal for this technique because of rapid dissipation of the gas, allowing closely spaced pulses.

Pulse Inversion Doppler

Another gray scale high MI technique is pulse-inversion imaging whereby two beam mode pulses are sent in rapid succession into the myocardium. The second pulse sent is a mirror image of the first (i.e. 180° phase shift). The scanner processes the consecutive returning pulses by adding them together. Tissue generates a linear echo, thus the addition of one pulse to the other should cancel out to zero and no signal is generated. Microbubbles produce non-linear echo signals and the summation of returning pulses will not equal zero and a signal will be registered

Ultraharmonic Imaging

With the development of increased bandwidth transducers, another intermittent high MI technique has evolved to improve the contrast to tissue ratio of backscatter. While intermittent harmonic imaging demonstrates myocardial perfusion, it is limited by the presence of tissue signals at the second harmonic. However, bubble destruction causes backscatter at 3rd 4th and subharmonics. At these higher harmonics the tissue signal is negligible, thus processing only backscatter from these further harmonics enables selective enhancement of the contrast signal. Interestingly, current ultraharmonic imaging involves processing signals from between the second and the third harmonic.

The strength of the high MI approaches are their sensitivity for the presence of contrast, because bubble destruction results in the highest amplitude backscatter. The disadvantages are that they lack simultaneous assessment of function, require reliable ECG triggering and image acquisition, and can be both technically challenging and time consuming (of particular importance for stress imaging). While the difficulty maintaining image position with long-triggering intervals has been aided by the use of low MI localization images, respiratory movement is almost inevitable.

Low power techniques—Real-time imaging: In recent years, technologies have been developed which so successfully exploit the nonlinear responses of microbubbles, that even low amplitude microbubble backscatter can be isolated from tissue signals for processing. This allows continuous low power imaging to be performed, with limited bubble destruction, enabling simultaneous assessment of wall motion and perfusion in real-time (although frame-rate is minimized in order to reduce-bubble destruction). Hence, low MI imaging is commonly known as real-time imaging.

The use of low MI has two major benefits:

1. The bubbles undergo stable nonlinear oscillation emitting continuous fundamental and harmonic signals
2. The tissues themselves do not generate harmonic signals at low MI. Like incremental triggered imaging, low MI imaging enables assessment of microbubble replenishment of the myocardium over time after bubble destruction. With low MI imaging, myocardial bubble destruction is achieved by transmission of a series of a high MI pulses ("flashes") after which replenishment can be observed in real-time.

Strain and Strain Rate Imaging

Strain (S) is a measure of tissue deformation, defined as the change in length normalized to the original length, whilst strain rate (SR) measures the rate of deformation Figs 11.6A and B. Strain imaging is derived from TDI and more recently by 2D myocardial speckle-tracking. Unlike TDI measurements, S and SR are not subjected to cardiac tethering Normal ranges for S and SR have been described, and while S is influenced by increasing age, preload and afterload, SR is less load dependent. S and SR can detect subclinical disease in hypertension and diabetes as well as infiltrative myocardial disease, correlates with myocardial fibrosis and has been used to evaluate therapeutic response. S and SR have been used in stress echocardiography. SR correlates with myocardial perfusion during dobutamine stress and is superior to TDI in detecting CAD. S and SR are reduced in ischemia/infarction with augmentation in viable segments (Fig. 11.96).

INTRAVASCULAR ULTRASOUND

This is a form of echocardiography performed during cardiac catheterization. During this procedure, the transducer is threaded into the heart blood vessels via a catheter in the groin. It is often used to provide detailed information about the atherosclerosis (blockage) inside the blood vessels.

Intravascular coronary artery ultrasonography is a unique versatile technique which has already established its place in the diagnosis of coronary atherosclerosis with greater sensitivity. Striking atherosclerotic abnormalities are occasionally evident in patients with totally normal coronary arteries by an angiography. This therefore reveals that a patient should not be absolutely declared atherosclerotic free based exclusively on angiographic report. It being relatively new imaging modality, intravascular ultrasound (IVUS) yields elaborate high resolution pictures of the vessel wall, enabling visualization of atheromas regardless of whether they narrow the lumen. This incremental diagnostic information is proving revolutionary in understanding the pathophysiology of coronary disease, the effects of pharmacological therapy and the effects of interventional devices. Intravascular ultrasound has also been applied to evaluation of angiographically normal coronary arteries following Cardiac transplantation, often revealing occult initial thickening.

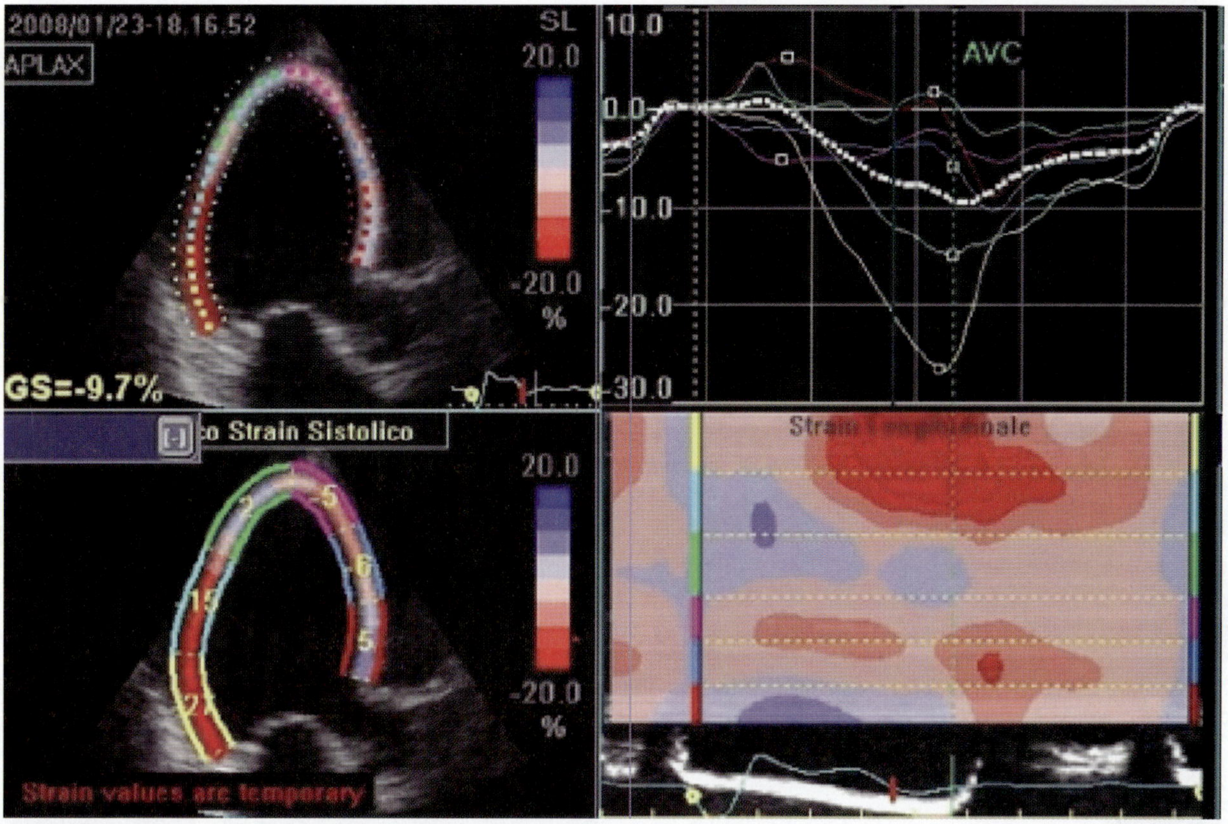

Fig. 11.96: Representation of 2D-strain (speckle tracking) of the left ventricle in the apical long-axis view in a patient with systolic heart failure. The upper right panel depicts the strain curves sampled in each of the analyzed myocardial segments. It is also possible to calculate a global strain index (GS), which in this case is clearly diminished (GS = 9,7%; see upper left panel). The lower left panel shows peak systolic strain for each segment while the lower right panel shows longitudinal strain processed according to a color map of curvilinear anatomical M-mode. From top to bottom: the basal, mid, and apical posterolateral wall, followed by the apical, mid, and basal interventricular anterior septum wall; in red the segments with higher contractility

OPEN-ACCESS ECHOCARDIOGRAPHY

In open-access echocardiography, the general practitioner requests a study and receives a report without the patient being seen by a cardiologist. About 80% of requests are for suspected heart failure or a murmur. Systolic abnormalities are found in about 15% of patients with suspected heart failure who are not yet on treatment.

The role of open-access echocardiography is controversial, and the indications differ from those of hospital-based practice because patients who are ill are not suitable, even if they have an acceptable indication for echocardiography. They should instead undergo echocardiography as part of an emergency or out-patient assessment.

POINT OF CARE ECHOCARDIOGRAPHY

Cardiovascular physical examination (PE), along with patient interview, forms the cornerstone of the evaluation of the patient with suspected heart disease. A broad spectrum of cardiovascular disorders can be detected and graded with bedside inspection, palpation and auscultation. However, the PE skills required to diagnose abnormal cardiovascular findings have been declining. Studies assessing PE abilities have shown significant error and omission rates for physicians at all levels of training. This decline in PE skills has been attributed to the reliance on newer technological methods of diagnosis as well as decreasing availability of time for bedside teaching (Figs 11.97–11.100).

Technological advances over the past two decades have made ultrasound equipment quite portable, with functionality and image quality similar to high-end ultrasound systems used in dedicated imaging laboratories. Echocardiography and vascular laboratories are using these portable ultrasound machines to perform studies on patients who are unable to travel to the imaging laboratory. The same equipment now enables other healthcare providers to perform ultrasound examinations at the point of care (POC), that is, ultrasound examinations performed and interpreted at the bedside in real time. At present, the most commonly used devices for POC ultrasonography include portable, cart-based machines that are smaller and lighter than traditional systems, while offering the same features as larger ultrasound systems. The cart-based machines are often equipped with batteries and have bootup times as short as 15 seconds. Although a wide range of cart-based ultrasound systems is currently available,

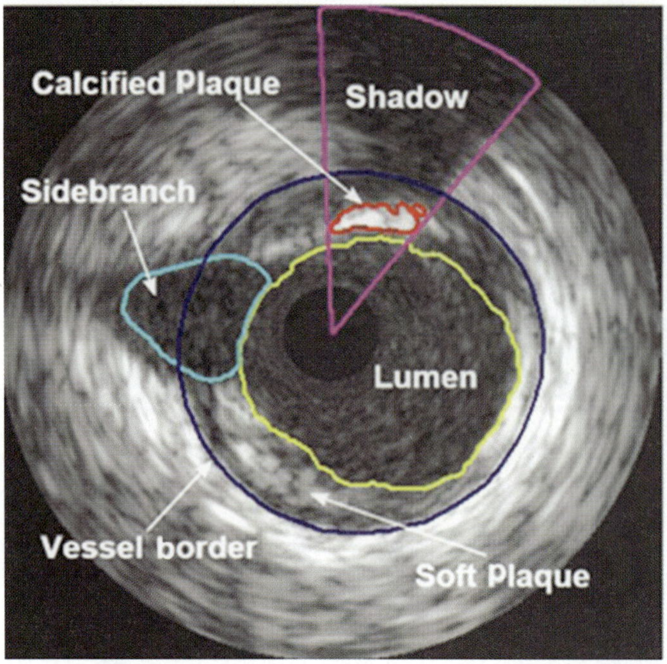

Fig. 11.97: *The intravascular ultrasound cross-section shows an soft and calcified plaques (arrows)*

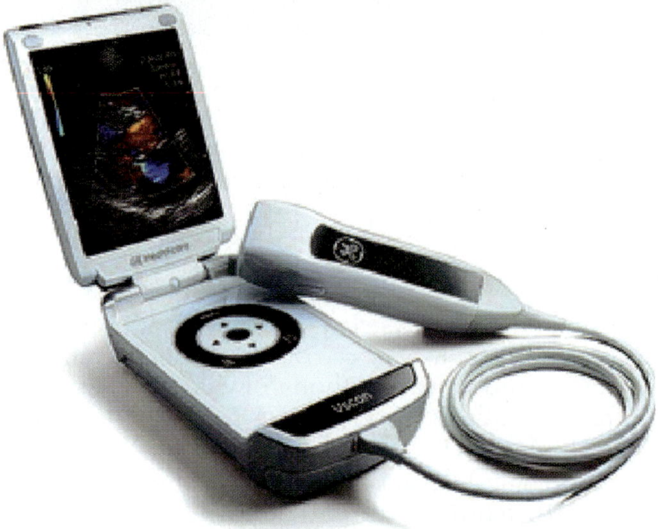

Fig. 11.98: *V scan portable ultrasound device GE healthcare*

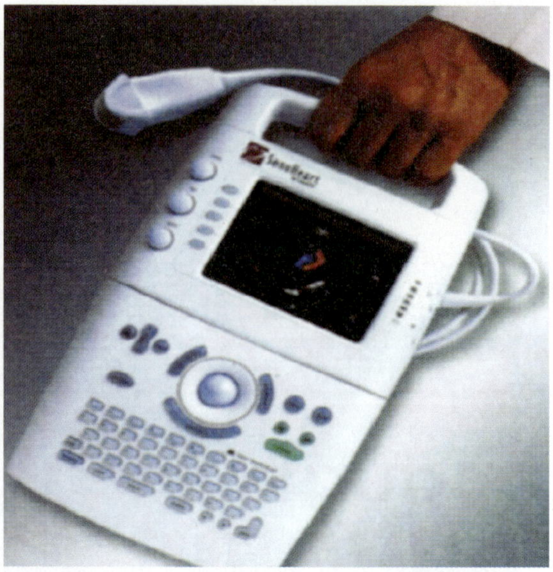

Fig. 11.99: *Showing dedicated mini-hand held color Doppler echocardiographic machine for bedside clinical use*

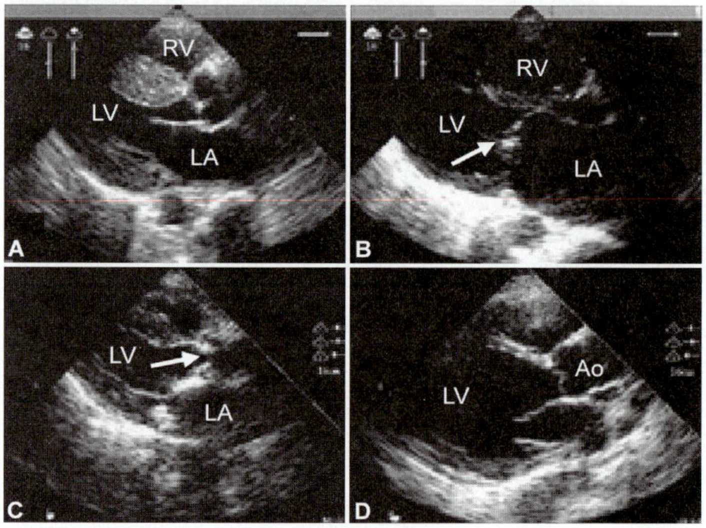

Fig. 11.100: *Examples of still-frames obtained from two-dimensional echocardiographic studies acquired using the miniaturized echocardiographic device. (A) Parasternal long-axis view obtained from a patient with hypertensive heart disease. (B) Parasternal long-axis view obtained from a patient with rheumatic mitral stenosis. (C) Parasternal long-axis view obtained from a patient with severe sclerocalcific aortic valve stenosis and calcification of the mitral valve. (D) Parasternal long-axis view obtained from a patient with a dilated cardiomyopathy. Ao = aorta; LA, left atrium; LV, left ventricle; RV, right ventricle*

these systems have demonstrated adequate image quality to answer focused POC questions, even in patients with obesity or chronic obstructive pulmonary disease.

More recently, pocket-size ultrasound devices have been developed by various vendors. These devices have sizes approaching those of smart phones and are equipped with a battery and a single transducer. Although these devices currently do not have advanced features such as spectral or tissue doppler, they allow for gray-scale imaging (B-mode) and color-flow Doppler and are capable of recording both still images and video clips. These attributes, along with their low cost, allow providers to use these devices like a stethoscope of the future and arguably places them in a disruptive technology category. In a recent study comparing the accuracy of a pocket-size ultrasound device with high-end ultrasound systems in 349 patients, concordance with respect to regional wall motion, ejections fraction, and left ventricular (LV) dimensions was very good between the systems, and no relevant findings were missed. Whether pocket-size systems provide sufficient high-quality images to answer focused clinical questions in difficult-to-image patients warrants further investigation.

The usefulness of these handheld devices is currently being assessed in clinical studies and has evoked a lively discussion regarding the benefits and potential perils of POC echocardiography performed by nonexperts and raised concerns regarding training, documentation, and reimbursement.

Current Role of Point-of-Care Echocardiography

Although diagnostic ultrasound has been used in medical practice for more than five decades, it has only been used by US clinicians at the patients' bedside during the past 15 years. In this short period of time, POC ultrasonography has become an indispensable diagnostic tool for clinicians from various specialties in the assessment and management of patients in the acute care setting and is used to examine almost all organs of the body, including heart, lungs, intraabdominal organs, and blood vessels. For example, multiple studies have demonstrated that clinician-performed ultrasound is reliable in detecting free intraperitoneal fluid in trauma patients and has thus replaced diagnostic peritoneal lavage at many trauma centers. In central line placement, ultrasound guidance confers a significantly lower complication rate and is rapidly becoming standard of care. The latter is one of the reasons why portable ultrasound systems are now available throughout many hospitals.

POC echocardiography has been proven equally beneficial, in the detection of pericardial effusions or the determination of cardiac activity in patients with pulseless electrical activity. In parallel with the improvement of image quality and provider skills, more advanced assessments, including global LV function, right ventricular dilatation, and inferior vena cava diameter have been adopted. Furthermore, European critical care physicians and cardiologists expanded on the sonographic assessment of the chest beyond the detection of pleural effusions and identified the usefulness of ultrasound artifacts in the assessment of pneumothoraces and extravascular lung water (pulmonary edema). Pulmonary ultrasonography as an adjunct to echocardiography is gaining increasing interest among US clinicians and is the focus of ongoing research efforts (Figs 11.101, 11.102 and 11.103).

In many European and other countries, acquisition and interpretation of sonographic images is exclusively performed by physicians. In these countries, the main differentiation between comprehensive and POC ultrasonography is usually based on the question whether the physician performing and interpreting the study is directly involved in the care of the patient who is being imaged or functions on a consultative basis. In these countries, clinicians from various specialties commonly perform their own ultrasound studies, for example, obstetricians (fetal ultrasonography) and cardiologists (echocardiography). In the United States, however, ultrasound studies are typically performed by sonographers and interpreted by physicians.

Although the use of POC echocardiography allows for more rapid and less costly sonographic imaging, it has led to a more distinct differentiation between comprehensive and POC ultrasonography. It has also resulted in controversial debates on who should (and should not) be permitted to perform sonographic examinations, what the training requirements and credentialing process should be, and whether POC imaging should be reimbursed.

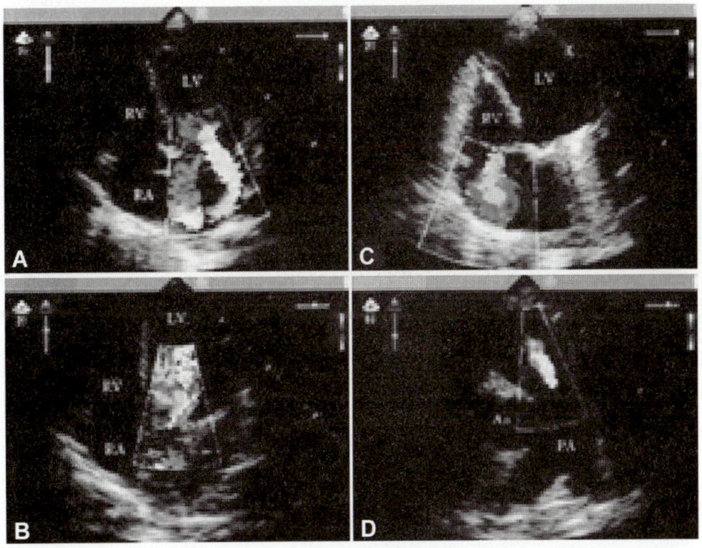

Fig. 11.101: *Examples of color Doppler still-frames acquired using the miniaturized echocardiographic device. (A) Apical four chamber view depicting moderately severe mitral regurgitation. (B) Apical four chamber view depicting moderate tricuspid regurgitation. (C) Apical four-chamber view depicting moderately severe aortic insufficiency. (D) Parasternal short-axis view depicting pulmonic insufficiency. Ao, aorta; LV, left ventricle; PA, pulmonary artery; RA, right atrium; RV, right ventricle*

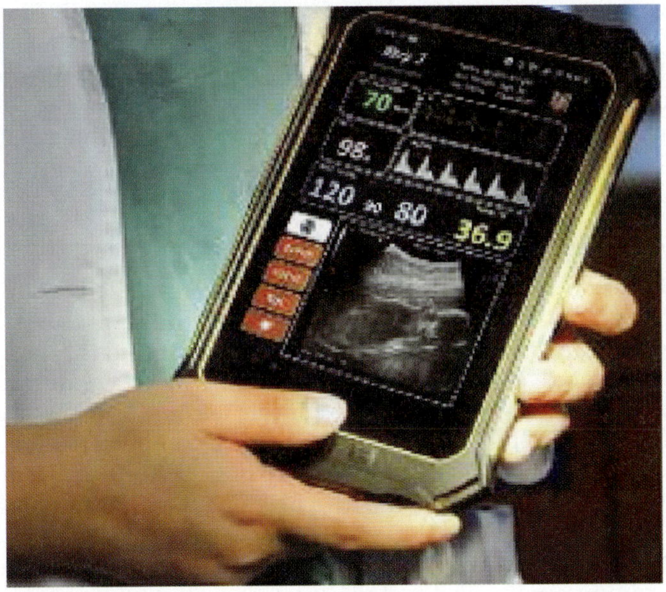

Fig. 11.102: *Pocket ultrasound used for point of care assessment of heart health*

VIRTUAL ECHOCARDIOGRAPHY

Evaluation of intracardiac anatomy from multiple two-dimensional echocardiographic images requires a mental

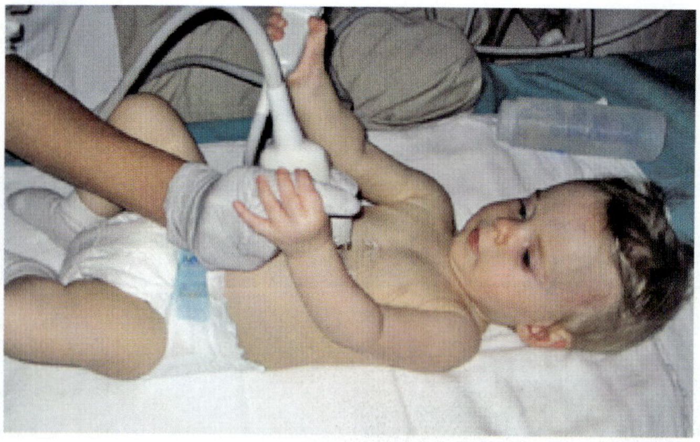

Fig. 11.103: *A young child is being investigated with point-of-care echocardiography, who had systolic murmur since birth*

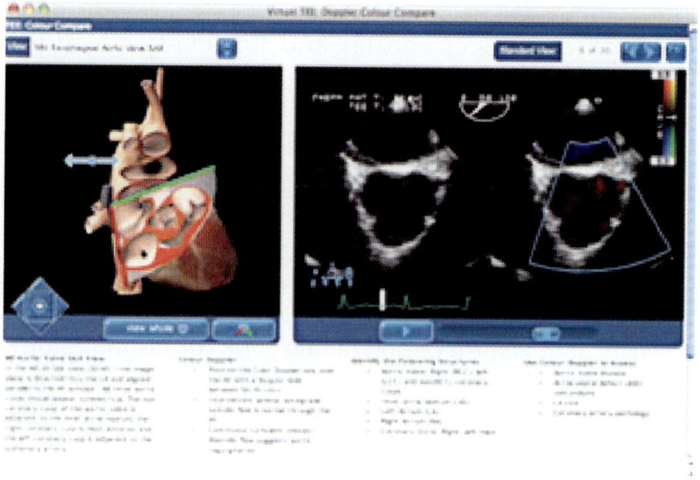

Fig. 11.104: *Showing frozen photograph of 3D virtual echocardiography*

conceptualisation process that is complicated by cardiac dynamics. Currently, real-time 3D echocardiographic images of the heart do no longer demand this difficult and individually variable conceptualisation processes, by offering an equivocal presentation of cardiac anatomy throughout the cardiac cycle. However, the full 3D potential of these imaging modalities cannot be appreciated, since the 3D data are presented on a flat 2D screen. Virtual dynamic systems, known as virtual reality, can assist with the interpretation of 3D data of the heart in space and makes it possible to "dive" into the 3D model of the heart. This study is an attempt in the technological process of the future to evaluate whether virtual reality is feasible for 3D echocardiography and if 3D echocardiographic images in a virtual reality can advance to a clinically useful tool (Figs 11.104 and 11.105).

Methods

Data sets from normal subjects and from patients with mitral valve disease, referred for a diagnostic echocardiogram, were selected with the aim of gathering a representative series of mitral valve pathological conditions with sufficient image quality. For this feasibility study, we selected 3D data sets of clinical conditions which have advantage of 3D perspective: (1) two patients with a normal mitral valve, (2) a patient with a mitral valve prolaps of the P2 segment of the posterior leaflet, (3) a patient with mitral valve stenosis, (4) a patient with hypertrophic obstructive cardiomyopathy and systolic anterior motion of the mitral valve, and (5) a patient with an atrioventricular septal defect (AVSD) where there is a commissure present between the superior and inferior bridging leaflets. Ten observers (5 cardiologist, 3 cardiologist-in-training and 2 cardiothoracic surgeons), who were blinded for the type of mitral valve morphology, were instructed to assess mitral valve anatomy/pathology and function.

Three Dimensional Echocardiographic Data Acquisition

The 3D data sets were acquired with the Philips Sonos 7500 echo system (Philips Medical Systems, Andover, MA, USA) equipped with a 3D data acquisition software package. Real-time 3D echocardiographic (RT-3DE) acquisition was done with ECG gating and in an end-expiratory breath-hold, lasting 6–8 seconds (depending on the heart rate). The 3D image data was stored on CD-ROM in DICOM 3.0 format and transferred to the computer (SGI Onyx4 Ultimate Vision, Silicon Graphics, Inc., Mountain View, CA, USA) driving the I-space.

Visualisation in a Virtual Reality Environment

The BARCO (Barco N.V., Kortrijk, Belgium) I-space installed at the ErasmusMC, is a so-called four-walled CAVE(tm)-like virtual reality system In the I-space researchers are surrounded by computer-generated stereo images, which are projected by four high quality DLP-projectors on three walls and the floor of a small "room". The virtual reality system has a resolution of 1280 by 1024 pixels per projector. This is comparable to or greater than the resolution of the CRT monitors and LCD flat panels used in ultrasound systems and with workstations. The CAVORE (Cave Volume Renderer) volume rendering application is used to investigate 3D ultrasound images during the cardiac cycle. In the I-space, this result in an animated "hologram" of the dataset being visualized, floating in space in front of the viewers. The viewers wear a pair of lightweight glasses with polarizing lenses that allows seeing the hologram with depth. Interaction with this "hologram" is by means of a virtual pointer and makes it possible to assess the interior of the heart, or on a monitor (CRT or LCD).

TRANSMITRAL FLOW PROPAGATION VELOCITY (VP)

Echocardiographic Doppler assessment of left ventricular (LV) filling is the mainstay of our evaluation of myocardial diastolic function (DF) and dysfunction (DD). Due to its insight into LV filling, pulse wave Doppler (PWD) has been termed as the "clinician's Rosetta stone" for simplifying our understanding of this complex process. An understanding and appreciation of DF has introduced

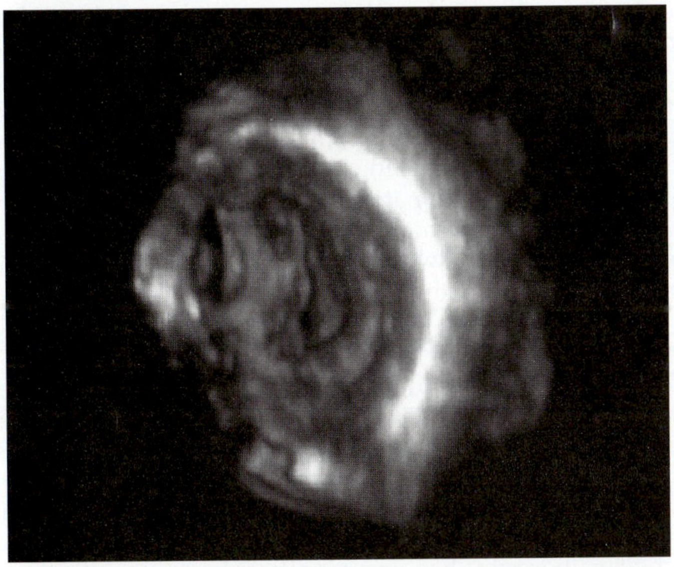

Fig. 11.105: *A 3D hologram of a patient with an atrioventricular septal defect is seen from a ventricular view. The arrow points out the commissure between the superior (SBL) and inferior bridging leaflets (IBL) view obtained from virtual echocardiography. (RV = right ventricle)*

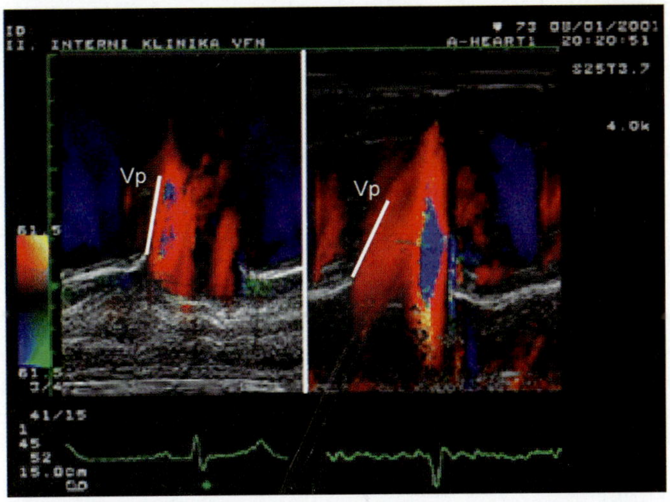

Fig. 11.106: *Representative examples of color M-mode recordings with the method of measuring Vp as the slope of the first aliasing velocity during early filling (yellow or white line). The subject with normal LV diastolic function (left) and the patient with abnormal LV diastolic function (right). Vp, flow propagation velocity*

clinicians to a new paradigm of a comprehensive ventricular assessment", i.e. systolic as well as diastolic function. Traditional means of left ventricular (LV) DF assessment, i.e. PWD of the transmitral inflow (E, A waves and deceleration time) and the pulmonary venous inflow (S, D and atrial reversal waves) are highly load dependent and require significant postacquisition manipulation for accurate diagnosis. Also, due to the unique history of DD (impaired relaxation to pseudo-normal to restrictive pattern), the clinicians are sometimes required to do "unmasking preload reduction maneuvers" to correctly identify the type of diastolic abnormality. Because of the aforementioned reasons, these parameters have limited application in the operating room (Fig. 11.106).

Transmitral flow propagation velocity (Vp) is a recently described parameter of the assessment of the rapid filling phase (active relaxation component) of the diastole. It is obtained by a combination of color-flow Doppler and m-mode interrogation of the mitral inflow during diastole. The concept of Vp is based on the principle of the development of progressive negative intraventricular pressure gradients (suction force) during the active relaxation phase. The presence of a negative intraventricular pressure gradient has been validated in experimental studies to correlate with the invasively measured time constant (Tau) of relaxation, i.e. –dP/dT. Clinically, the vortex and slope of flow of blood from left atrium to LV is determined by this "suction force", which in turn depends upon the diastolic properties (active relaxation) of the left ventricle. The clinical application of Vp as a measure of DD was first described by Brun and Takatsuji et al. and was later validated by Garcia et al. by simultaneous Doppler and cardiac catheterization studies. Initially the slope between flow and no flow in the LV was used to describe the filling pattern, but the slope of the "first aliasing velocity" obtained by adjustment of Nyquist limit to 30–40 cm/sec generated more reproducible results. A value of Vp of < 0.45 m/sec was identified as diagnostic of "impaired relaxation"

Technical Steps to Obtain Vp with Transesophageal Echo (TEE) Include

1. A mid-esophageal four-chamber (00) or long-axis (1200) view for an absolute parallel alignment of Doppler.
2. Placement color-flow box on the LV cavity.
3. Activation of M-mode of the color-flow pattern.
4. Adjustment of the Nyquist limit to obtain a clear wave front of propagation.
5. Tracing the slope of the "first aliasing velocity" from the opening of the mitral valve for 4 cm into the LV cavity.

Vp in not entirely load independent, and there is recent evidence that it displays some age related changes in the same pattern as the traditional transmitral PWD, i.e. there is a degree of "pseudo-normalization". Furthermore, Vp assesses only the "active relaxation" part of the diastole, and is not a measure of the "compliance" of the LV, i.e. change in pressure with volume, which is determined during the atrial contraction phase. The main advantages of Vp are that it is easily and quickly obtained, has been validated, relatively load independent, and does not require postacquisition manipulation for further diagnosis. It has also been utilized in the operating room for assessment of DD and found to be more reliable and reproducible than the traditional PWD methods. A ratio of transmitral E wave and Vp (E/Vp) has also been shown to predict a range of left ventricular end-diastolic pressures.

An abnormal Vp identifies the presence or absence of DD, but cannot be used to assign a severity grade at this stage with decreasing value. Further studies will be needed to achieve this goal. However, Vp is a very practical parameter to assess perioperative relaxation abnormalities and improve our understanding of LV function..

Digital Echocardiography

Echocardiographic images were initially stored on videotapes; however, digital imaging is now the state of the art in echocardiography and is endorsed by the American Society of Echocardiography (ASE). Advantages of digital echocardiography include more efficient reading, easy comparison between studies, and higher image quality. However, two important challenges faced digital echocardiography: managing the size of the electronic files stored and standardizing the storage format to enable interoperability between laboratories (Figs 11.107 and 11.108).

Typical echocardiography cine loops consists of 480 rows and 640 columns, with 24 bits used to represent the color of each pixel. The typical frame rate is 30 Hz. Multiplying these numbers together yields an enormous storage requirement: 221,184,000 bits/sec, or more than 16 gigabytes of storage for a 10 minute study. To accommodate these storage requirements, a combined strategy of clinical compression (storage of only a single cardiac cycle or a few cycles for a given view) and digital compression is required.

To facilitate interoperability between laboratories, the Digital Imaging and Communications in Medicine (DICOM) image formatting standard was adopted as the standard for echocardiographic imaging. DICOM is simply a set of rules to specify how images and other data should be exchanged between compliant pieces of equipment. An in-depth review of the DICOM standard for echocardiography is available elsewhere

Contraindications of Echocardiography

Echocardiography has no contraindications. It should be kept in mind, however, that this modality may yield only limited information in patients at the extremes of adult body weight, because a thick chest wall (in markedly obese patients) or overcrowded ribs (in severely underweight patients) may limit the penetration of ultrasound waves.

Complications in Echocardiography

Theoretically, ultrasonographic waves have a thermal effect (i.e. increased tissue temperature) and cavitation effects (i.e. small gas-filled bodies created or vibrated by the ultrasonographic beam). In practice, however, current diagnostic ultrasonography systems have minimal thermal or cavitation effects. No evidence has suggested that echocardiography has any significant adverse effects at current ultrasonographic output levels. The use of a contrast agent to enhance intraventricular viewing has several relative and absolute contraindications. In October 2008, the US Food and Drug Administration (US-FDA) mandated the addition of a black box warning to echocardiography contrast agents that listed new contraindications for the use of these agents (other than allergy to the contrast agent). These new contraindications, which remain the subject of considerable debate, include the following:

1. Clinical instability or recent worsening of congestive heart failure
2. Acute coronary syndromes
3. Respiratory failure, severe emphysema, or pulmonary embolism

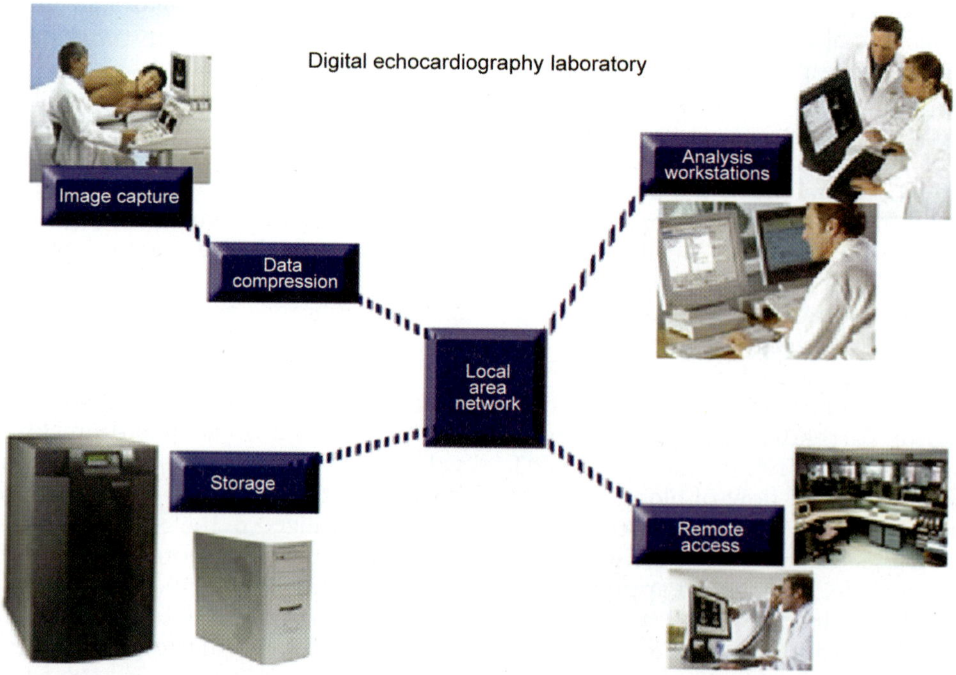

Fig. 11.107: *Diagrammatic representation of working of digital echocardiography*

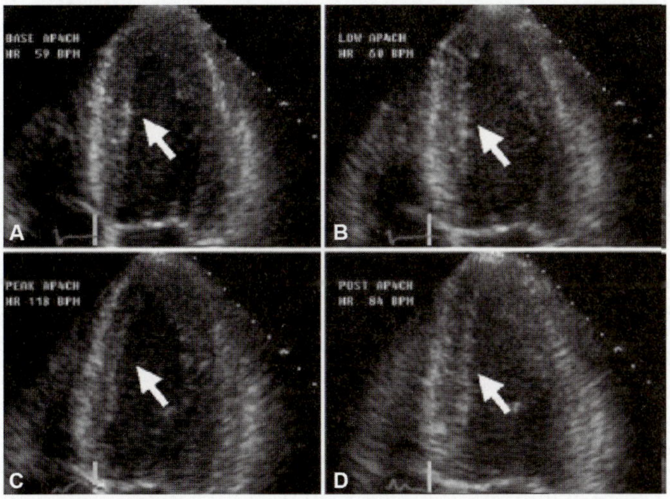

Fig. 11.108: *Digital laboratory. Example of a stress induced wall motion abnormality on dobutamine echocardiography. Panels A, B, C, and D are obtained during rest, low dose (10 g/kg/min) and high dose dobutamine (40 g/kg/min), and recovery. In the septal region (white arrow), normal wall motion is present at rest and during low dose dobutamine infusion, whereas dyskinesia is induced at high dose dobutamine*

4. Serious ventricular arrhythmia or significant QT-interval prolongatio
5. Right-to-left, bidirectional, or transient right-to-left ardiac shunts.

BIBLIOGRAPHY

1. Pearlman AS, Ryan T, Picard MH, Douglas PS. Evolving trends in the use of echocardiography: a study of Medicare beneficiaries. J Am Coll Cardiol. Jun 12 2007;49(23):2283–91.
2. Ryan T, Armstrong WF, Khandheria BK. Task force 4: training in echocardiography endorsed by the American Society of Echocardiography. J Am Coll Cardiol. Jan 22 2008;51(3):361–7.
3. Burwash IG, Basmadjian A, Bewick D, Choy JB, Cujec B, Jassal DS, et al. 2010 Canadian Cardiovascular Society/ Canadian Society of Echocardiography Guidelines for Training and Maintenance of Competency in Adult Echocardiography. Can J Cardiol. Jul 26 2011
4. Otto C. Textbook of clinical echocardiography. 2nd ed. Philadelphia, Pa: WB Saunders Co; 2000.
5. Cheitlin MD, Armstrong WF, Aurigemma GP, Beller GA, Bierman FZ, Davis JL. ACC/AHA/ASE 2003 Guideline Update for the Clinical Application of Echocardiography: summary article. A report of the American College of Cardiology/American Heart Association Task Force on Practice Guidelines (ACC/AHA/ASE Committee to Update the 1997 Guidelines for the Clinical Application of Echocardiography). J Am Soc Echocardiogr. Oct 2003;16(10): 1091–110.
6. Douglas PS, Garcia MJ, Haines DE, Lai WW, Manning WJ, Patel AR, et al. ACCF/ASE/AHA/ASNC/HFSA/HRS/ SCAI/SCCM/SCCT/SCMR 2011 Appropriate Use Criteria for Echocardiography. A Report of the American College of Cardiology Foundation Appropriate Use Criteria Task Force, American Society of Echocardiography, American Heart Association, American Society of Nuclear Cardiology, Heart Failure Society of America, Heart Rhythm Society, Society for Cardiovascular Angiography and Interventions, Society of Critical Care Medicine, Society of Cardiovascular Computed Tomography, and Society for Cardiovascular Magnetic Resonance Endorsed by the American College of Chest Physicians. J Am Coll Cardiol. Mar 1 2011;57(9):1126–66.
7. Nash P, Lin S, Armstrong G. Transthoracic echocardiography. In: Griffin B, Topol EJ. Manual of cardiovascular medicine. 2nd ed. Philadelphia, Pa: Lippincott Williams and Wilkins; 2004:780–815.
8. Feigenbaum H. Echocardiography. In: Braunwald E. Heart Disease: a Textbook of Cardiovascular Medicine. 5th ed. Philadelphia, Pa: WB Saunders; 1997:53–97.
9. Pellerin D, Sharma R, Elliott P, Veyrat C. Tissue Doppler, strain, and strain rate echocardiography for the assessment of left and right systolic ventricular function. Heart. Nov 2003;89 Suppl 3:iii9–17.
10. Marwick TH. Measurement of strain and strain rate by echocardiography: ready for prime time?. J Am Coll Cardiol. Apr 4 2006;47(7):1313–27.
11. Kirkpatrick JN, Vannan MA, Narula J, Lang RM. Echocardiography in heart failure: applications, utility, and new horizons. J Am Coll Cardiol. Jul 31 2007;50(5):381–96.
12. Weyman AE. The year in echocardiography. J Am Coll Cardiol. Apr 28 2009;53(17):1558–67.
13. Thomas JD, Adams DB, Devries S, Ehler D, Greenberg N, Garcia M, et al. Guidelines and recommendations for digital echocardiography. J Am Soc Echocardiogr. Mar 2005; 18(3):287–97.
14. Thomas JD. The DICOM Image Formatting Standard: what it means for echocardiographers. J Am Soc Echocardiogr. May-Jun 1995;8(3):319–27.
15.Mulvagh SL, Rakowski H, Vannan MA, Abdelmoneim SS, Becher H, Bierig SM. American Society of Echocardiography Consensus Statement on the Clinical Applications of Ultrasonic Contrast Agents in Echocardiography. J Am Soc Echocardiogr. Nov 2008;21(11):1179–201; quiz 1281.
16. Pandian N.G, Ramasamy S, Martin P, Banerjee A; Ultrasound stecthoscopy as an extension of clinical examination during hospital patient rounds. J Am Soc Echocardiogr. 13 2000:486
17. Johnson J.E, Carpenter J.L; Medical house staff performance in physical examination. Arch Intern Med. 146 1986:937–941.
18. Roldan C.A, Shively B.K, Crawford M.H; Value of the cardiovascular physical examination for detecting valvular heart disease in asymptomatic subjects. Am J Cardiol. 77 1996:1327–1331.
19. Rahko P.S; Prevalence of regurgitant murmurs in patients with valvular regurgitation detected by Doppler echocardiography. Ann Intern Med. 111 1989:466–472.
20 St. Clair E.W, Oddone EZ, Waugh R.A, Corey G.R, Feussner J.R; Assessing housestaff diagnostic skills using a cardiology patient simulator. Ann Intern Med. 117 1992:751–756.
21 Mangione S, Nieman LZ; Cardiac auscultatory skills of internal medicine and family practice trainees. JAMA. 278 1997:717–722.
22. Grayburn PA, Smith MD, Handshoe R, Friedman B.J, DeMaria A.N; Detection of aortic insufficiency by standard

echocardiography, pulsed Doppler echocardiography and auscultation. Ann Intern Med. 104 1986:599–605.

23. Attenhofer Jost C.H, Turina J, Mayer K; Echocardiography in the evaluation of systolic murmurs of unknown cause. Am J Med. 108 2000:614–620.
24. Rispler S, Rinkevich D, Markiewicz W, Reisner S.A; Missed diagnosis of severe symptomatic aortic stenosis. Am J Cardiol. 76 1995:728–730.
25. Badgett R.G, Lucey C.R, Mulrow C.D; Can the clinical examination diagnose left-sided heart failure in adults?. JAMA. 277 1997:1712–1719.
26. Bruining N, Roelandt JR, Grunst G, Berlage T, Waldinger J, Mumm B: Three-Dimensional Echocardiography: The Gateway to Virtual Reality! Echocardiography 1999, 16:417–423.
27. Bruining N, Lancee C, Roelandt JR, Bom N: Three-dimensional echocardiography paves the way toward virtual reality. Ultrasound Med Biol 2000, 26:1065–1074.
28. Agati L: Three-dimensional echocardiography: the virtual reality in cardiology – luxury or useful technique? Eur Heart J 1996, 17:487–489.
29. Gallagher AG, Cates CU: Virtual reality training for the operating room and cardiac catheterisation laboratory. Lancet 2004, 364:1538–1540.
30. Salustri A, Roelandt JR: Three-dimensional echocardiography: where we are, where we are going. Ital Heart J 2000, 1:26–32.
31. Yambe T, Yoshizawa M, Tabayashi K, Takeda H, Nitta S: Virtual percutaneous transluminal coronary angioplasty system for an educational support system. Artif Organs 1998, 22:710–713.
32. Klein LW: Computerized patient simulation to train the next generation of interventional cardiologists: can virtual reality take the place of real life? Catheter Cardiovasc Interv 2000, 51:528.
33. Issenberg SB, Gordon MS, Gordon DL, Safford RE, Hart IR: Simulation and new learning technologies. Med Teach 2001, 23:16–23.
34. Koning AHJ: Applications of Volume Rendering in the CAVE.
35. Simulation and Visualization on the Grid: Parallel-datorcentrum, seventh annual Conference, Stockholm 1999.
36. Nishimura RA, Tajik AJ. Evaluation of diastolic filling of left ventricle in health and disease: Doppler echocardiography is the clinician's Rosetta Stone. J Am Coll Cardiol 1997; 30:8–18.
37. Brun P, Tribouilloy C, Duval AM, et al. Left ventricular flow propagation during early filling is related to wall relaxation: a color M-mode Doppler analysis. J Am Coll Cardiol 1992; 20:420–32.
38. Takatsuji H, Mikami T, Urasawa K, et al. A new approach for evaluation of left ventricular diastolic function: spatial and temporal analysis of left ventricular filling flow propagation by color M-mode Doppler echocardiography. J Am Coll Cardiol 1996; 27:365–71.
39. Garcia MJ, Thomas JD, Klein AL. New Doppler echocardiographic applications for the study of diastolic function. J Am Coll Cardiol 1998; 32:865–75.
40. Khouri SJ, Maly GT, Suh DD, Walsh TE. A practical approach to the echocardiographic evaluation of diastolic function. J Am Soc Echocardiogr 2004; 17:290–7.
41. Mahmood F, Matyal R, Subramaniam B, et al. Transmitral flow propagation velocity and assessment of diastolic function during abdominal aortic aneurysm repair. J Cardiothorac Vasc Anesth 2007; 21:486–91.
42. Garcia MJ, Ares MA, Asher C, Rodriguez L, Vandervoort P, Thomas JD. An index of early left ventricular filling that combined with pulsed Doppler peak E velocity may estimate capillary wedge pressure. J Am Coll Cardiol. 1997;29(2):448–54.

12 Interventional Cardiac Catheterization

Cardiac catheterizations are performed on people of all ages, from the fetus to the adult with congenital heart disease. Sedation varies from local anesthesia only to general anesthesia depending on the type of procedure (Figs 12.1 and 12.13).

The procedures are done in the cardiac catheterization lab, which looks like a small operating room. The role of the cardiac catheterization laboratory has changed perceptibly in the past few years. In the 1940s and 1950s, the laboratory was used as a research tool to understand the physiology of the normal circulation and the alterations in patients with heart disease. By the 1960s and 1970s, the physiology was understood, but further advances in the surgeon's ability to correct cardiac abnormalities required better evaluation of the anatomy. Although physiologic data was still collected and frequently was important, the major component of study in the catheterization laboratory was devoted to angiography. In the 1980s, the remarkable

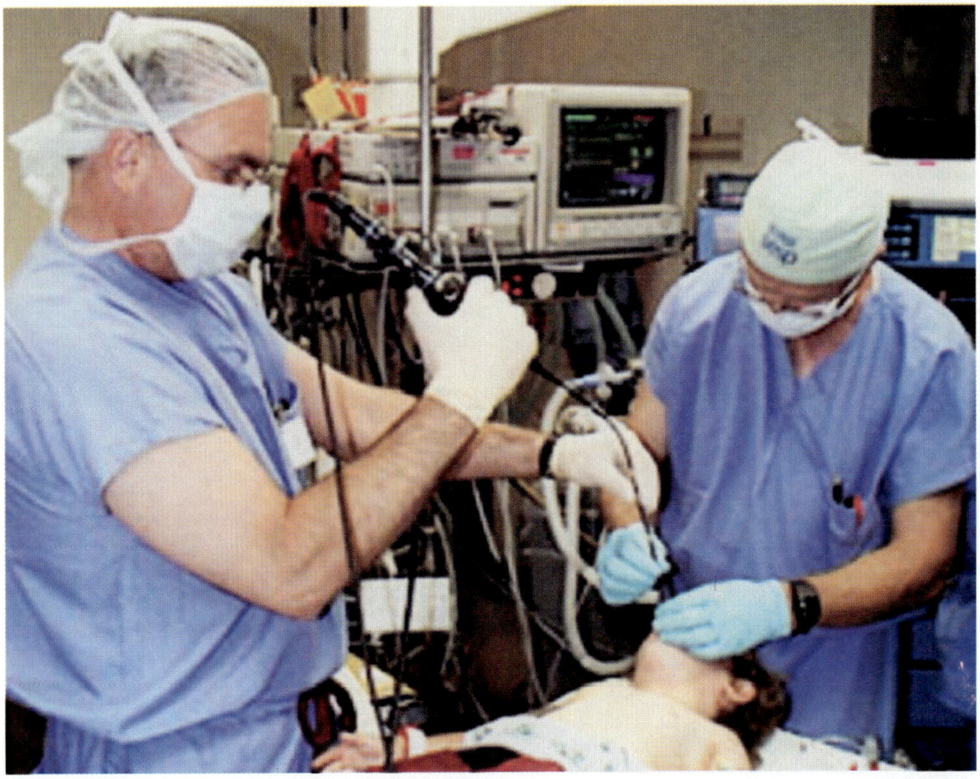

Fig. 12.1: *Doctors are busy in inducing anesthesia to a child in a cardiac catheterization laboratory prior to conducting a interventional procedure*

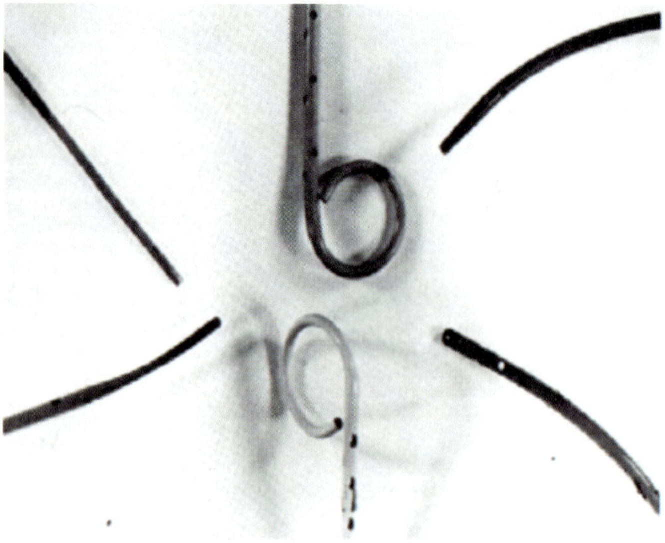

Fig. 12.2: *Examples of injection catheters in current use. Beginning at top and proceeding clockwise: pigtail, 8.2F (Cook); Gensini, 7F; NIH, 8F; pigtail, 8F (Cordis); Lehman ventriculography, 8F; Sones, 7.5F tapering to 5.5F*

advances in imaging by 2D echocardiography and to some extent by magnetic resonance imaging (MRI) have diminished the importance of angiography. Fortunately, interventional techniques have become available so that the catheterization laboratory has retained the excitement of four decades ago, when Cournand and Richards were the first to investigate the fascinating abnormalities of congenital heart disease. Cardiac catheterization is a procedure in which a thin flexible tube (catheter) is passed into the heart and its surrounding blood vessels (Figs 12.1 to 12.3 and 12.5–12.6).

INDICATIONS OF DIAGNOSTIC CATHETERIZATION

Cardiac catheterization and angiography have transformed the care of children with CHD and have greatly increased the safety and efficacy of surgery for CHD. As a result of advances in noninvasive imaging diagnostic catheterization is no longer indicated in the routine preoperative evaluation of most congenital defects, such as ventricular septal defects (VSDs), atrial septal defects (ASDs), atrioventricular canal, tetralogy of Fallot, double-outlet right ventricle (RV), coarctation of the aorta, hypoplastic left heart syndrome (HLHS), and other complex CHD. Details of anatomy, including situs, venous, and arterial connections; septal integrity; severity of valvular stenosis or insufficiency; size of pulmonary arteries; coronary artery origins; and aortic arch anatomy are easily established with echocardiography to the degree of certainty required for surgical intervention. Assessment of patient hemodynamics and, when necessary, assessment of anatomy by angiography should be

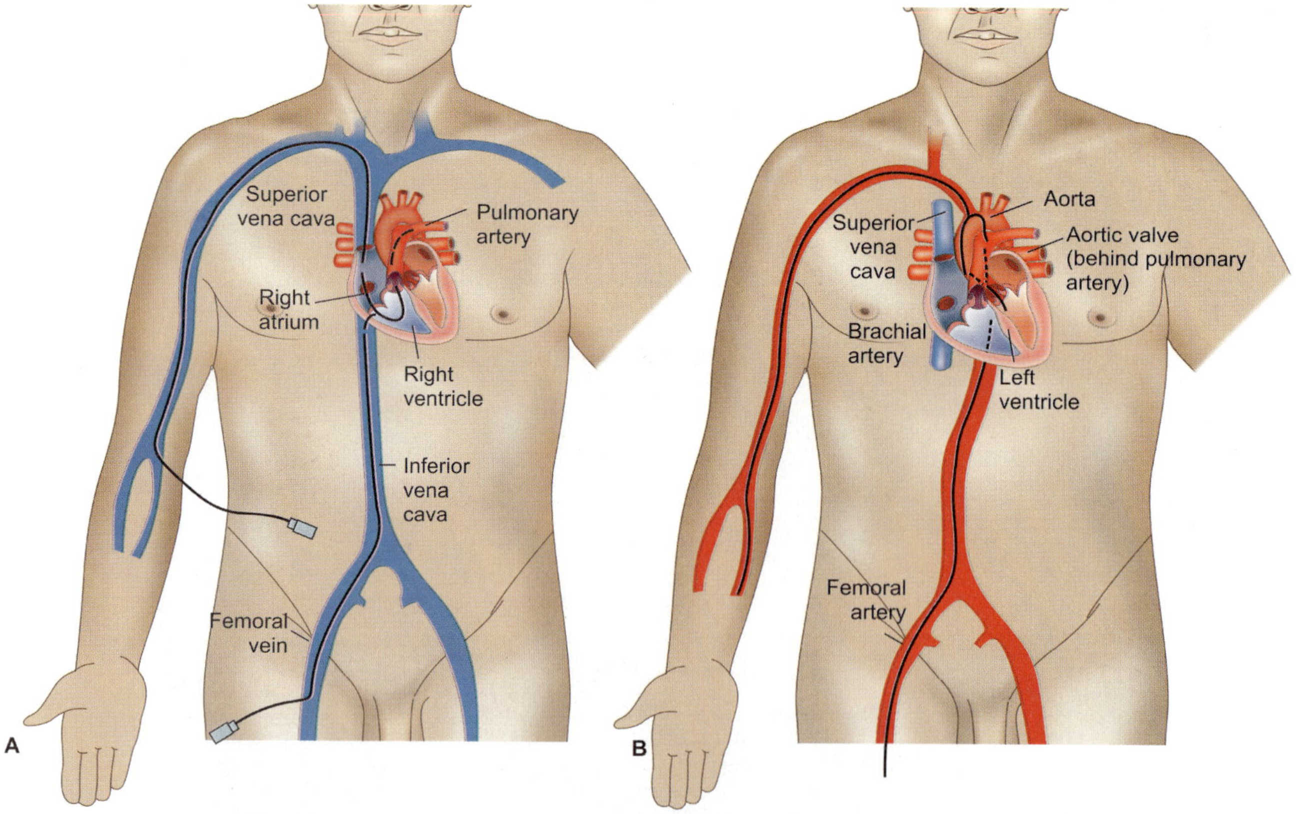

Fig. 12.3: *(A) Right-sided heart catheterization. The catheter is inserted into the femoral vein and advanced through the inferior vena cava (or, if into an antecubital or basilic vein, through the superior vena cava), right atrium, and right ventricle and into the pulmonary artery. (B) Left-sided heart catheterization. The catheter is inserted into the femoral artery or the antecubital artery. The catheter is passed through the ascending aorta, through the aortic valve, and into the left ventricle*

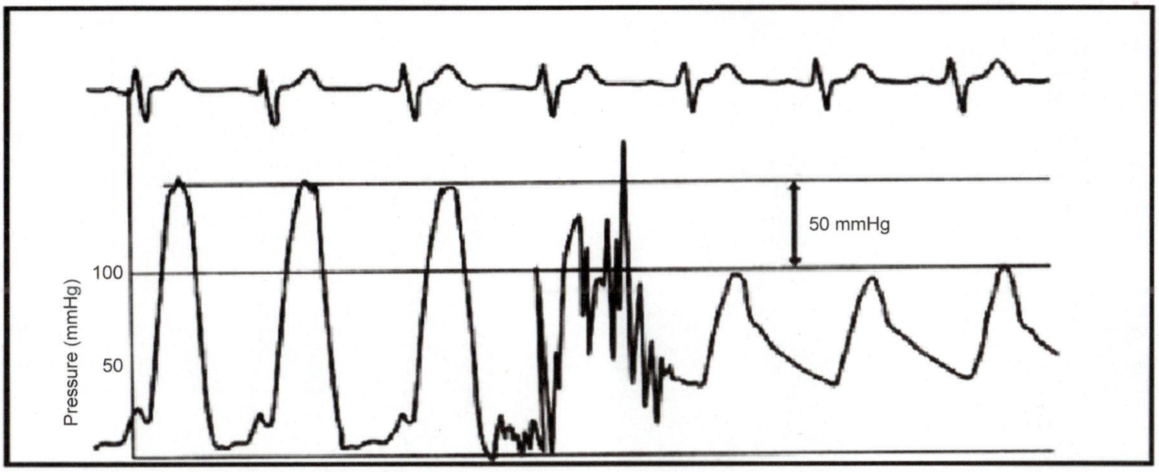

Fig. 12.4: *Pull back across the aortic valve showing a peak to peak gradient of 50 mmHg in patient with valvular aortic stenosis*

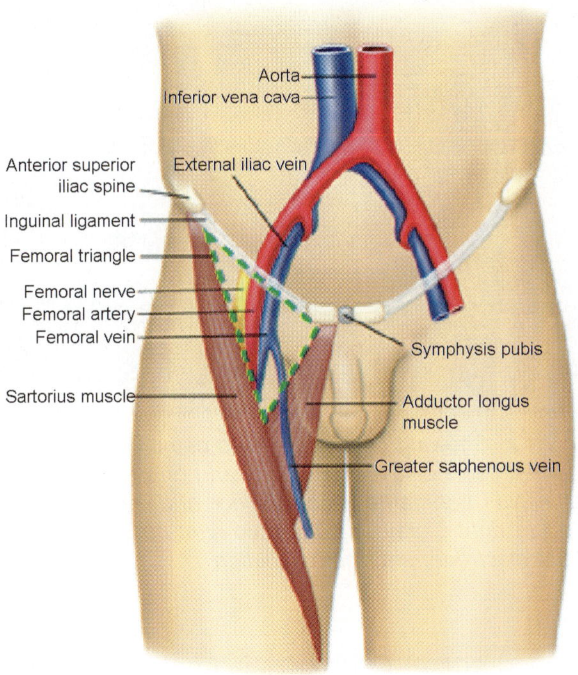

Fig. 12.5: *Anatomy of the common femoral artery. The common femoral artery is the terminal branch of the external iliac artery, and provides the main arterial supply to the lower limb. The common femoral artery enters the femoral triangle deep to the midpoint of the inguinal ligament, posterior to the deep fascia, and overlying the head of the femur bone. These features facilitate arterial puncture, but necessitate deep pressure for compression hemostasis. At this point, the artery has a diameter of 7–10 mm and lies within the femoral sheath close to the common femoral vein and the femoral nerve and its branches*

accomplished before international catheterization to confirm congenital or acquired heart disease in infants and children (Figs 12.4, 12.7 and 12.10).

The availability of adequate noninvasive imaging is not uniform at all centers. At centers where MRI and CT imaging for congenital diagnosis are not state-of-the-art and where echocardiography does not provide sufficient detail,

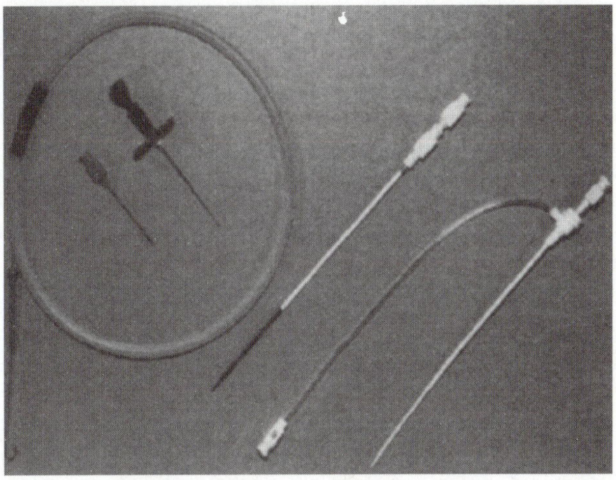

Fig. 12.6: *Showing equipment used for percutaneous catheterization 0.35-inch teflon wire with a 3 mm curve at the end with two percutaneous introducer needles; right, two sheaths, one with a side arm*

diagnostic catheterization is indicated. However, diagnostic catheterization should not be considered routine for diagnosis of congenital defects, and the performance of complete right- and left-sided heart studies may subject patients to unnecessary risk and exposure to radiation. All diagnostic catheterization may lead to the necessity for an interventional procedure. As a consequence, the capability to proceed with the interventional procedure should be a requirement of the individual and institution that will perform the diagnostic portion of the catheterization. Individual centers must assess their abilities as they relate to this ability when determining which catheterization cases they might perform.

It is not the purpose of the present statement to provide a comprehensive list of all indications for diagnostic catheterization; however, there are certain broad categories in which the need for diagnostic catheterization is well established in current practice. In most instances, these indications have been developed empirically, and there are no prospective studies, controlled or otherwise, that prove

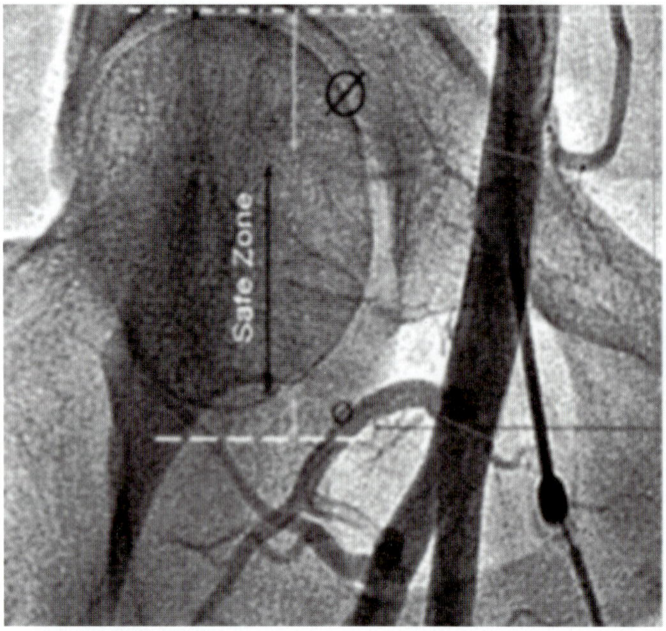

Fig. 12.7: *Femoral angiogram performed in the 30° RAO angulation. Arteriotomy at the center of the femoral head between the inferior border of the inferior epigastric artery and common femoral artery bifurcation is considered "safe". Arteriotomy above these landmarks has been linked with increased risk of retroperitoneal bleeding, and below these landmarks increases the risk of local vessel complications*

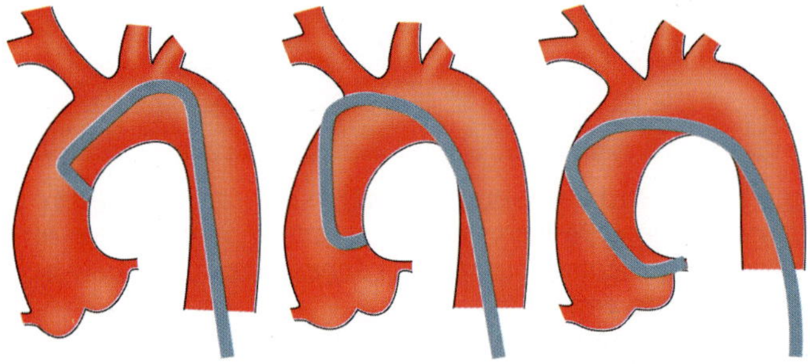

Fig. 12.8: *Selective catheterizationof the left coronary artery by the Judkins technique. In LAO position, the catheter is rotated so that it appears unfolded and enface; it is then slowly advanced until it engages the left coronary orifice. A size 4 (4-cm curve) catheter is adequate for most patients, but with moderate or severe aortic dilatation, a size 5 or 6 catheter may be required*

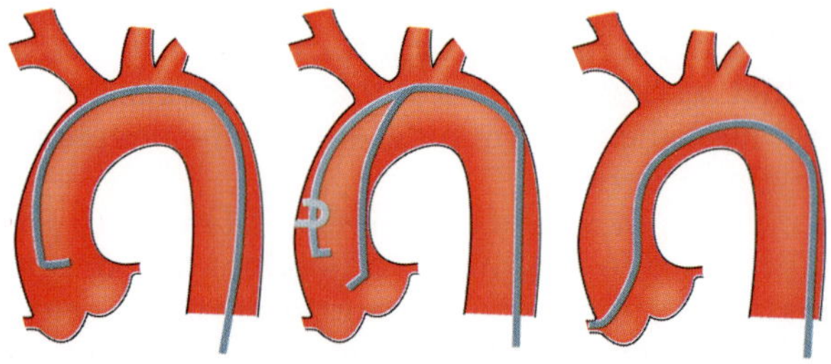

Fig. 12.9: *Diagrammatic representation of selective catheterization of the right coronary artery by the Judkins technique (LAO projection)*

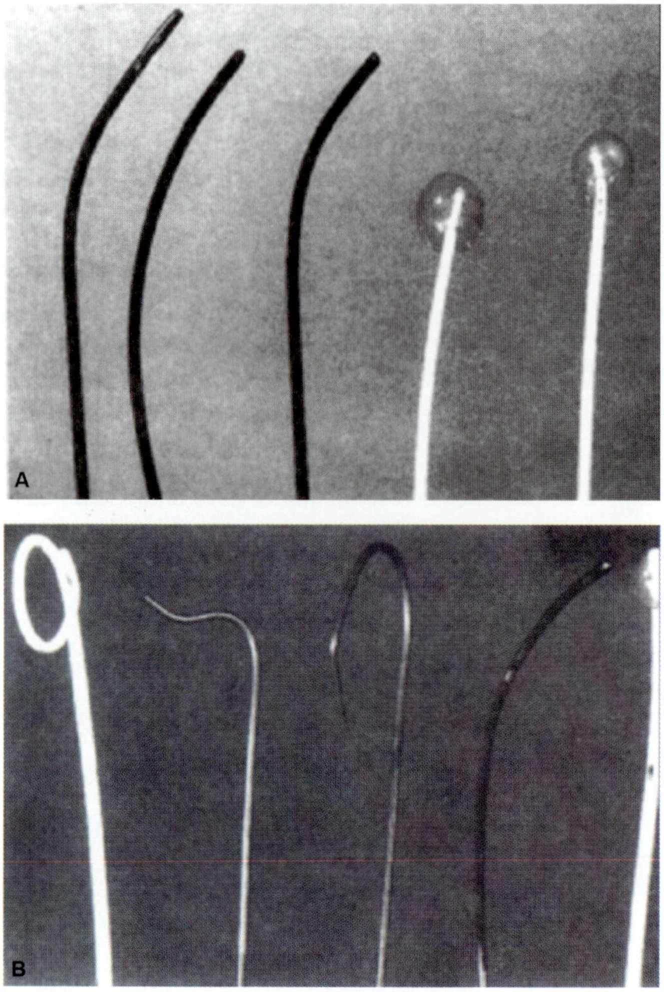

Fig. 12.10: *Showing commonly used catheters for the study of congenital heart disease in infants and children (A) left to right Gensini, NIH, Lehman-end hole balloon and angiographic balloon (B) left to right pigtail angiographic right coronary. Sidewinder, multiple electrode, and thermodilution*

the superiority of catheterization over other diagnostic modalities. Therefore, most indications are supported by patient series, retrospective case reviews, or opinion of authorities. Diagnostic catheterization is or may be indicated in the circumstances outlined in the following section.

Cardiac catheterization should be used in any circumstance in which the anatomy of a child with CHD is inadequately defined by noninvasive means. Although many congenital cardiac lesions are diagnosed and referred directly to surgery on the basis of noninvasive studies, there are some occasions, particularly in very complex lesions, on which more specific details about the anatomy or hemodynamics are necessary. The diagnostic cardiac catheterization remains the "final authority" for this definitive anatomic and hemodynamic information for many of the very complex lesions. Some circumstances that suggest the need for diagnostic catheterization include the following:

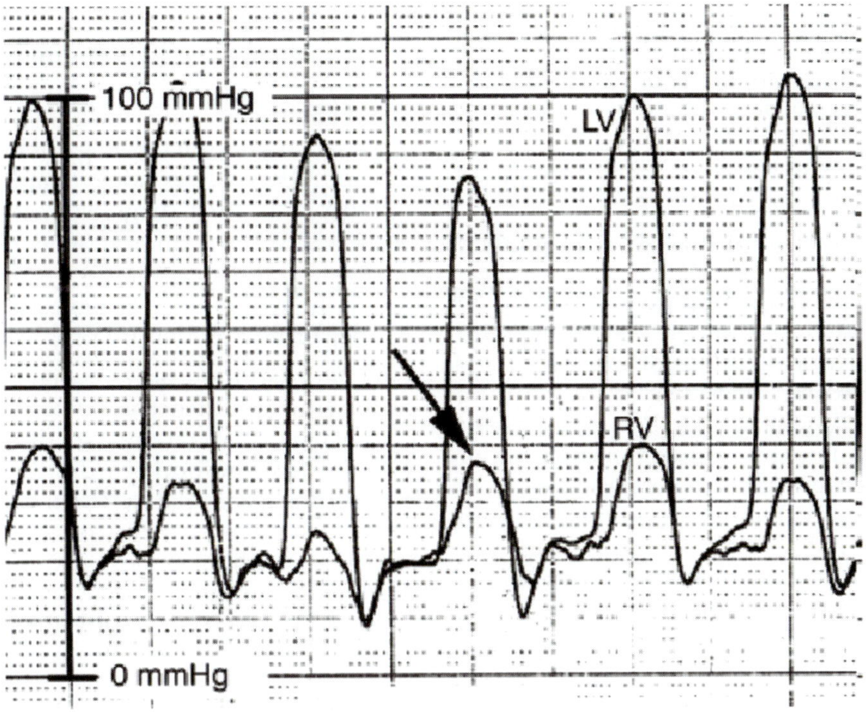

Fig. 12.11: *Pressures in the left (LV) and right ventricle (RV) of a patient with constrictive pericarditis. During peak inspiration (arrow), there is a decrease in LV pressure and a concomitant increase in RV pressure, indicating discordance of ventricular pressures*

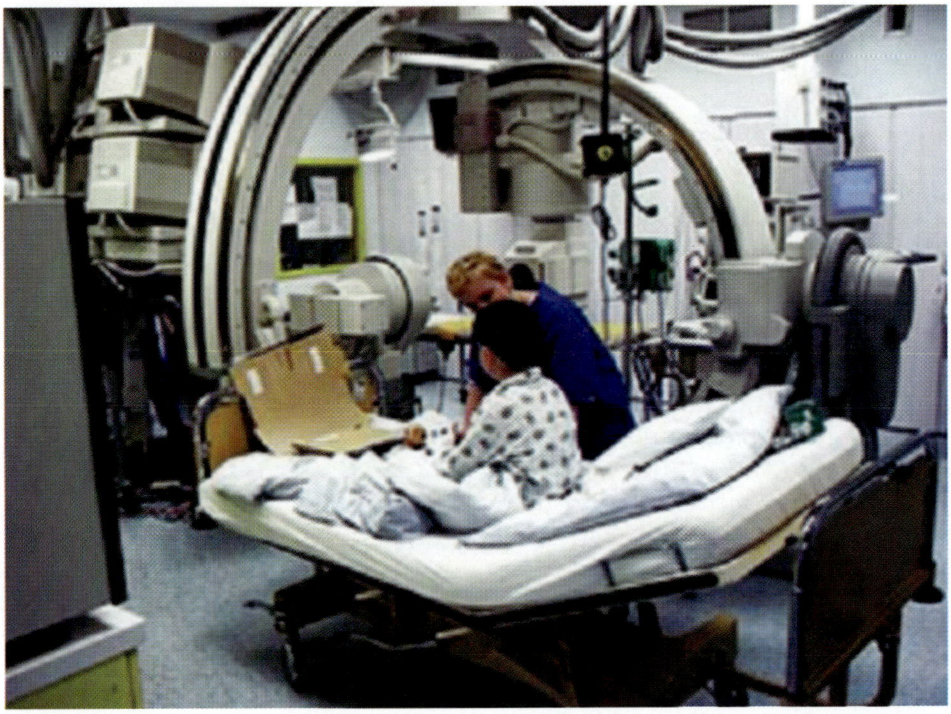

Fig. 12.12: *Child is sitting comfortabily on the bed and nurse is explaining him the reason why this procedure was essential for his future health care*

1. High-flow or low-flow physiology associated with semilunar valve stenosis can lead to inaccurate gradients determined by noninvasive Doppler assessment. Combined aortic stenosis (AS) and insufficiency and pulmonary stenosis and insufficiency, especially with multiple levels of obstruction of both the systemic and pulmonary circulation, can be confusing when examined on the basis of echocardiographic studies alone. A diagnostic catheterization is necessary to determine true peak-to-peak gradient

measurements, which still represent the standard by which the need for both surgical and catheter interventions is determined in some conditions. In many cases, noninvasive determination of pressure gradients is sufficient to proceed with surgical intervention; however, catheterization may be required to resolve conflicting noninvasive data.

2. Low-flow lesions for which calculation of pulmonary arteriolar resistance can be misleading may be best studied by combining angiographic assessment of pulmonary artery anatomy and transit time with pulmonary artery pressures. Details of anatomy alone without corresponding pressure data can be misleading. This is often the case in the assessment of patients after cavopulmonary anastomosis and after Fontan completion. Diagnostic catheterization is useful in these patients in the evaluation for proceeding with completion of Fontan, revision of Fontan, or transplantation. In addition, assessment of a fenestrated Fontan with trial occlusion is useful in patients with excessive cyanosis and in making the decision to proceed with closing the fenestration. The ability to proceed with closure of fenestrations is required. Similar to the above category of patients, the postoperative patient who is not following an anticipated clinical course merits strong consideration for cardiac catheterization.

There are many potential problems that can occur after surgery for congenital defects for which diagnostic catheterization is indicated because of the inability of noninvasive tests to provide the diagnosis. As noted above, the diagnostic procedure may become an interventional procedure, and cardiologists performing these studies should be prepared to proceed with intervention. Examples of some but certainly not all of the more common indications in this setting are provided below:

1. In situations in which excessive desaturation occurs after a systemic-to-pulmonary artery shunt has been created, catheterization is useful to exclude branch pulmonary artery stenosis and shunt stenosis or occlusion. Such a situation may arise if the patient is too unstable to tolerate an MRI or MRI/magnetic resonance angiography (MRA), which can readily show pulmonary artery stenosis and shunt occlusion.
2. If excessive systemic desaturation is present after cavopulmonary anastomosis, catheterization is indicated to exclude venovenous, venoatrial, or pulmonary arteriovenous malformations. The ability to proceed with venous collateral occlusion is a requirement in this setting. State-of-the-art MRA and CT angiography may help to detect and define the presence of these lesions.
3. If an excessive residual left-to-right shunt is suspected after closure of a VSD that included atrioventricular canal repair, catheterization is indicated to calculate shunt size and severity.
4. If the presence of excessive aortopulmonary collateral flow is suspected, diagnostic catheterization should be performed. The ability to proceed to occlusion of the offending systemic-to-pulmonary collateral arteries is required.
5. When there is suspected RV outflow tract obstruction after surgery for tetralogy of Fallot or double-outlet RV and MRI is either not available or the patient is unable to tolerate MRI, diagnostic catheterization is indicated.
6. If there is an unexplained need for extracorporeal membrane oxygenator support or failure to wean without obvious reasons, catheterization should be performed to identify problems and direct care.

In the past, the utility of diagnostic catheterization for providing a definitive diagnosis in the setting of unexplained heart failure with diminished systolic function was limited. Endomyocardial biopsy with routine light microscopic examination is useful when positive findings of myocarditis are found, but in most cases, light microscopic findings of myocarditis or specific criteria by light and electron microscopy that suggest a specific diagnosis of cardiomyopathy are absent. The Dallas criteria for myocarditis are rarely met. MRI with assessment of myocardial edema and delayed enhancement is useful in this situation but does not provide a definitive diagnosis. Although there may be situations in which the clinical condition of the patient precludes catheterization, catheterization with biopsy should be considered whenever possible, and if performed, appropriate samples of myocardium should be obtained for histological diagnosis and viral polymerase chain reaction. In addition, in some instances, examination of biopsy material for abnormalities in contractile proteins and for other molecular abnormalities may enable a definitive diagnosis of cardiomyopathy. The latter should occur in the setting of a comprehensive evaluation of potential heritable causes of cardiomyopathy. Cardiac catheterization continues to play an important role in the assessment of pulmonary hypertension and its responsiveness to medical therapy. This may be the case in patients with CHD in whom an accurate assessment of pulmonary resistance is needed to make surgical and medical decisions. In addition, catheterization to assess resistance is essential in the management of patients with pulmonary vascular disease to assess response to pharmacological agents. Laboratories that perform catheterization to assess reactivity of the pulmonary vascular bed must have the capability to deliver inhaled nitric oxide or other pulmonary vasodilators.

A preoperative evaluation of pulmonary resistance is commonly performed in patients undergoing a staged Fontan approach to single-ventricle palliation. Some authorities do not recommend catheterization in this setting, but for most, catheterization to assess patients with single-ventricle physiology before stage 2 and 3 palliation remains common practice. However, the presence of elevated pulmonary arteriolar resistance, unsuspected pulmonary venous obstruction, and elevation of ventricular filling pressures all impact the outcome of second- and third-stage Fontan palliation. Catheterization in this setting is justified on this basis until prospective studies demonstrate the safety of its omission from preoperative assessment of these patients.

In specific cases, such as patients with pulmonary valve atresia, the pulmonary arterial supply of the lungs may be complex. Catheterization in patients with pulmonary atresia–VSD or pulmonary atresia and complex ventricular anatomy is directed toward determining details of the aortopulmonary collateral supply to the lungs and the size of the true pulmonary arteries. Accurate characterization of dual supply by collaterals and true pulmonary arteries versus single supply by collaterals is important in planning the surgical approach to be used. The ability to perform selective catheterization of collaterals, balloon occlusion angiography, and pulmonary venous wedge angiography is essential. Noninvasive imaging such as MRI/MRA may be helpful in delineating these vessels.

Likewise, the coronary artery anatomy in patients with pulmonary valve atresia and an intact ventricular septum can influence the success of the intervention (catheter-based or surgical) and patient survival. Although the presence of RV-to-coronary artery fistulae in patients with pulmonary atresia and severe RV hypoplasia can be recognized with echocardiography, an RV-dependent coronary circulation cannot. The exclusion of RV dependence of the coronary circulation is essential before procedures are performed to decompress the RV and establish RV-to-pulmonary artery continuity either through a transcatheter or surgical approach. Catheterization for this indication requires the ability to perform RV angiography in the hypoplastic RV, aortic angiography, and in some instances selective coronary angiography.

Diagnostic catheterization is indicated in the evaluation of patients for listing for cardiac transplantation in most instances, both in patients with congenital heart defects and in those with cardiomyopathy. Catheterization is indicated for endomyocardial biopsy, determination of filling pressures, and assessment of pulmonary resistance. Many patients are clinically compromised, and catheterization may need to be delayed or omitted. Catheterization is part of a multimodality evaluation and should be used in combination with echocardiography, MRI, and multislice CT. Likewise, situations may exist in which prior catheterization data suffice for transplantation listing (e.g. the postoperative patient being listed who had a preoperative catheterization).

Graft vasculopathy in cardiac transplant patients is a reflection of chronic rejection and occurs eventually in most patients. Graft vasculopathy is less common in children, although with time, most will develop some degree of coronary disease. Coronary angiography is performed routinely in the assessment of heart transplant patients to monitor for graft vasculopathy. It is well recognized that coronary angiography is an insensitive method for the detection of graft vasculopathy; it is usually only positive in the setting of moderate to severe disease. Intravascular ultrasound, however, is highly sensitive in detecting vasculopathy even in its earliest stages. Although intravascular ultrasound is established as the definitive procedure in adults, its use in children has been limited. Several reports have demonstrated that intravascular ultrasound can be performed safely in children >6 years of age. The addition of intravascular ultrasound to surveillance in pediatric heart transplantation programs has been limited by inexperience and lack of training and, in part, because of the size of the catheters and sheaths that are required. Yet, intravascular ultrasound should be used increasingly as part of the routine annual or semiannual evaluation of pediatric heart transplant recipients, especially given the progressive nature of coronary disease, the potential for sudden death or need for retransplantation, and increasing evidence that changing or augmenting immunotherapy may slow the process of intimal proliferation in the early stages of graft vasculopathy.

Despite promising new diagnostic methods, such as surveillance that includes biomarkers (brain natriuretic peptide), catheterization with endomyocardial biopsy is the mainstay of rejection identification. Endomyocardial biopsy does not diagnose rejection in all cases of unexplained deterioration in graft function but remains the "gold standard". Samples obtained at catheterization should be studied for both cellular and antibody-mediated rejection. Criteria for the diagnosis of both are well developed at this time, including the International Society for Heart and Lung Transplantation revised criteria for cellular rejection and newly published criteria for diagnosis of humoral rejection. Diagnosis of antibody-mediated rejection by biopsy requires both light microscopic findings and fluorescent microscopy for recognition of deposition of complement fragments C4D and C3D.

Recommendations for Diagnostic Catheterization

Class I

1. It is recommended that hemodynamic and anatomic data be obtained (via angiography when necessary) at the time of a planned interventional cardiac catheterization *(Level of Evidence: A)*.
2. It is recommended that cardiac catheterization be used to assess pulmonary resistance and irreversibility of pulmonary hypertension in patients with CHD or primary pulmonary hypertension when accurate assessment of pulmonary resistance is needed to make surgical and medical decisions (Level *of Evidence: B)*.
3. Cardiac catheterization is indicated in patients with complex pulmonary atresia for the detailed characterization of lung segmental pulmonary vascular supply, especially when noninvasive imaging methods incompletely define pulmonary artery anatomy *(Level of Evidence: B)*.
4. Cardiac catheterization is indicated in determination of coronary circulation in pulmonary atresia with intact septum (Level *of Evidence: B)*.
5. Cardiac catheterization is indicated in patients being assessed for cardiac transplantation unless the patient's risk for catheterization outweighs the potential benefit *(Level of Evidence: C)*.

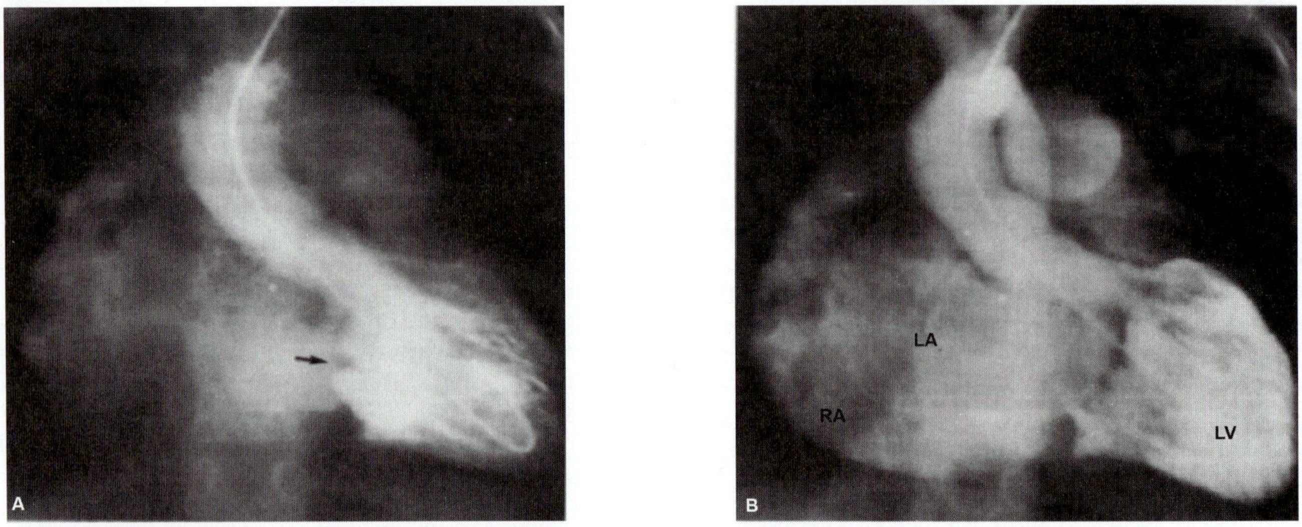

Fig. 12.13: *Left ventriculogram, frontal view. (A) Systole. The right border of the left ventricle is scalloped. The lucent niche (arrow) indicates a cleft in the anterior mitral valve leaflet. The valve is regurgitant, and contrast material refluxes in the left atrium. (B) Diastole. The upper segment of the anterior mitral valve leaflet has swung into the outflow portion of the left ventricle producing an apparent narrowing (arrow). This has been termed the "gooseneck" deformity. Contrast material has refluxed from the left ventricle (LV) into the left atrium (LA) and across the ostium primum defect into the right atrium (RA). Antegrade flow from the righ atrium has filled the right ventricle and pulmonary artery in patient with endocardial cushion defect*

6. Cardiac catheterization is recommended for surveillance of graft vasculopathy after cardiac transplantation *(Level of Evidence: B).*

Class IIa

1. It is reasonable to perform a cardiac catheterization to determine pulmonary pressure/resistance and transpulmonary gradient in palliated single-ventricle patients before a staged Fontan procedure *(Level of Evidence: B).*
2. Cardiac catheterization is reasonable in any CHD patient in whom complete diagnosis cannot be obtained by noninvasive testing or in whom such testing yields incomplete information *(Level of Evidence: C).*
3. Cardiac catheterization is reasonable for the assessment of cardiomyopathy or myocarditis *(Level of Evidence: B).*
4. Cardiac catheterization is reasonable for the assessment of coronary circulation in some cases of Kawasaki disease in which coronary involvement is suspected or requires further delineation or in the assessment of suspected congenital coronary artery anomalies *(Level of Evidence: B).*
5. Cardiac catheterization is reasonable to perform for the assessment of anatomy and hemodynamics in postoperative cardiac patients when the early postoperative course is unexpectedly complicated and noninvasive imaging techniques (e.g. MRA, CT angiography) fail to yield a clear explanation *(Level of Evidence: C).*

Cardiac Catheterization Procedure

Cardiac catheterization is a procedure in which a thin flexible tube (catheter) is passed into the heart and its surrounding blood vessels. Cardiac catheterizations can be used in two ways:

1. **Diagnostic,** to gather information (Figs 12.14–12.25)
2. **Interventional**, for treatment.

Through a tiny incision in the arm, neck, or groin, the catheter is inserted into a blood vessel (artery or vein) and directed into the heart by real-time X-ray imaging, or fluoroscopy. The catheters are used for blood sampling, pressure measurements, dye injection (angiogram), and to repair specific areas of the heart and the surrounding blood vessels.

The length of hospital stay varies according to the type of cardiac catheterization procedure. Many catheterizations are performed on an outpatient basis.

Therapeutic or interventional catheterizations include balloon atrial septostomies, balloon angioplasties, valvuloplasties, and device and stent implantations. Cardiac catheterizations can repair the heart without open-chest surgery in many heart conditions.

Indications

Catheterization has been a routine part of treatment of patients with congenital heart disease for the past 30 years. Initially it was used as a diagnostic modality. More recently (since the early 1980s) "interventional" catheterization has become increasingly important and more common. "Interventional" catheterization includes performance of a corrective or therapeutic procedure during the catheterization either complementing surgical therapy or treating a congenital or acquired defect without surgery.

The majority of cardiac catheterizations performed in children are now performed solely for correction or treatment of a defect, or include an interventional procedure during a diagnostic catheterization.

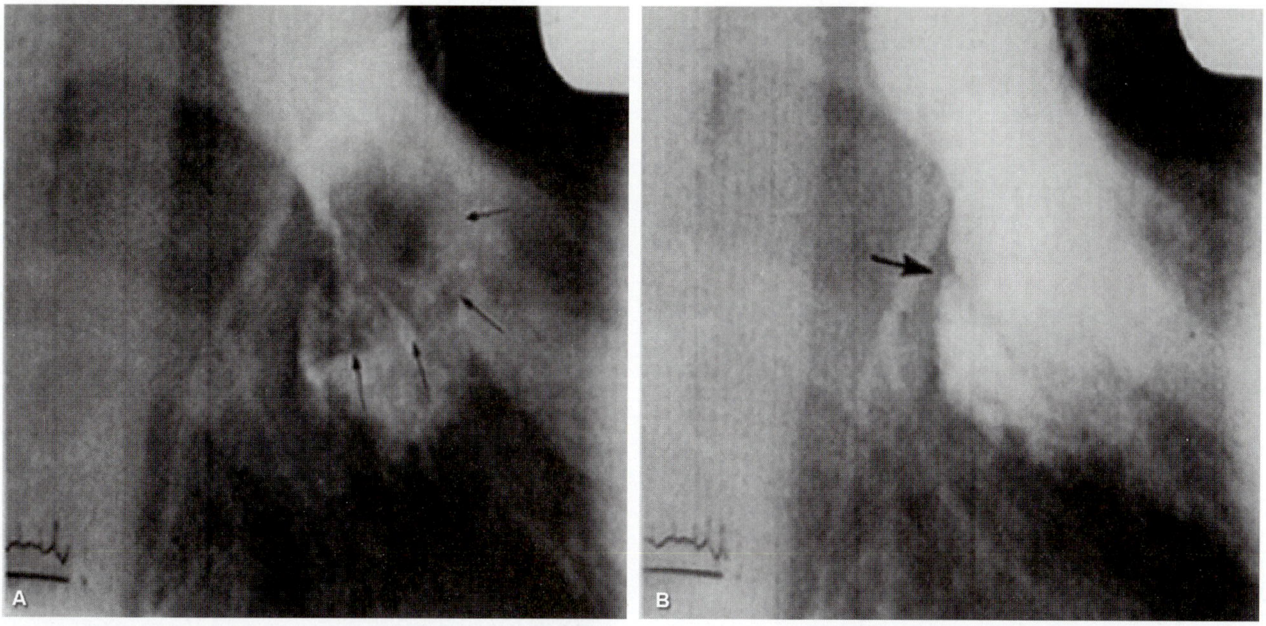

Fig. 12.14: *Left ventricular angiogram, right anterior oblique view. (A) Diastole: the mitral valve cannot open completely and forms a dome (arrows) that bulges into the left ventricle during atrial contraction. The leaflets are outlined by contrast material within the left ventricle and radiolucent blood in the atrium. (B) Systole: the mitral valve (arrow) is closed. The wide excursion of the leaflets between the two phases of the cardiac cycle indicates that they are pliable in patient with mitral stenosis*

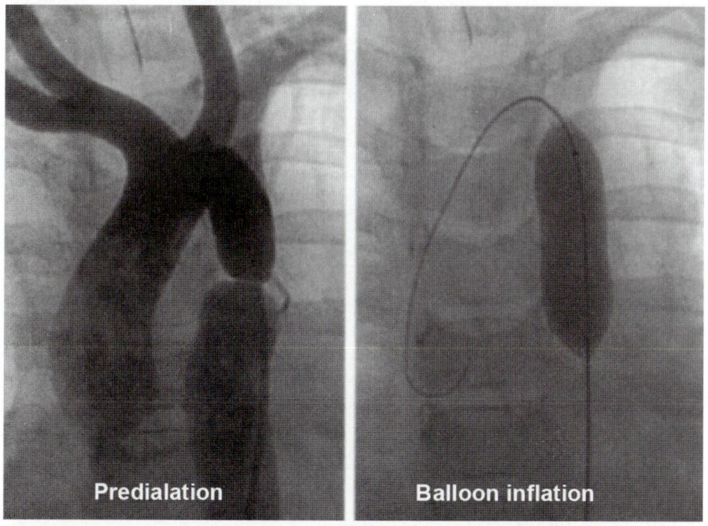

Fig. 12.15: *(Left) Balloon angioplasty has emerged as an alternative to surgery for selected patients with native and recurrent (or residual) coarctation of the aorta (Right) shows complete opening of the aortic lumen after ballon inflation*

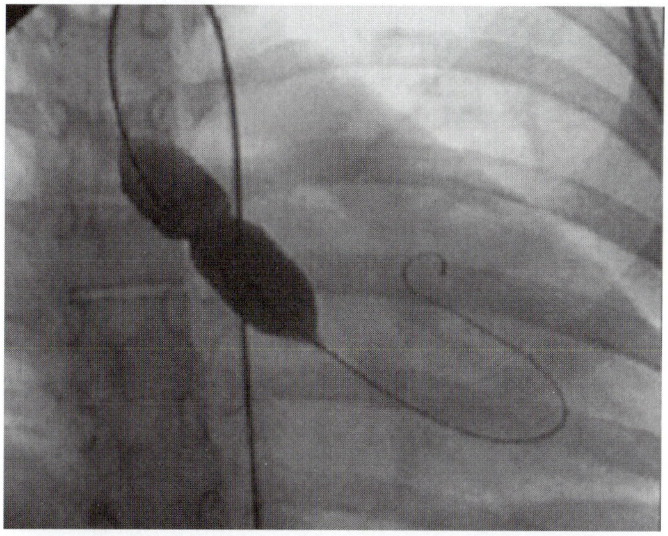

Fig. 12.16: *Percutaneous aortic balloon valvuloplasty. The valvuloplasty balloon is inserted across the aortic valve over a stiff wire into the left ventricle. The fluid-filled balloon is inflated for a few seconds to dilate the stenotic valve*

When cardiac defects are diagnosed and meet criteria for intervention (these criteria vary over time and from defect to defect) the treatment plan must be defined. This plan may include diagnostic or therapeutic (interventional) catheterization. What follows is a summary of the congenital and acquired heart defects that currently can be treated via interventional catheterization.

- Native defects treated via catheterization
- Valvar pulmonary stenosis (PS) (Fig. 12.32)
- Valvar aortic stenosis (AS) (Figs 12.34–12.35; and 12.49)
- Pulmonary artery stenosis
- Coarctation of the aorta (Fig. 12.31)
- Patent ductus arteriosus (PDA)
- Atrial septal defect (ASD)
- Patent foramen ovale (PFO)
- Ventricular septal defect (VSD)
- Arteriovenous fistulae
- Coronary artery fistulae

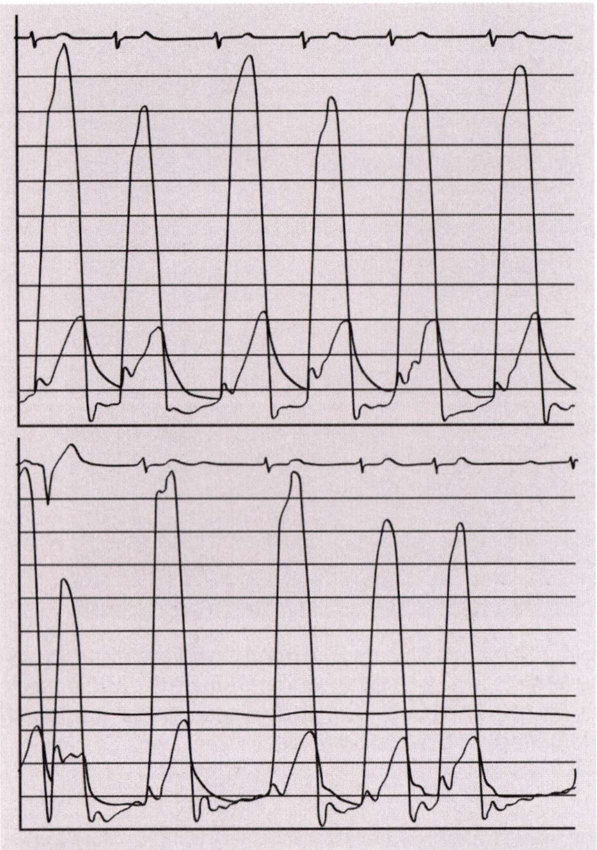

Fig. 12.17: *Left atrial and ventricular pressure measurements and the change in the transvalvular mitral gradient after mitral valvuplasty*

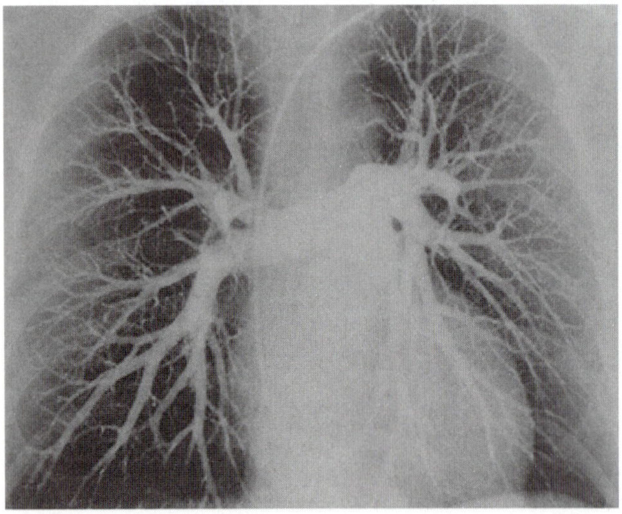

Fig. 12.18: *Pulmonary angiography. Angiograms are created by injecting an iodine solution into the bloodstream. Iodine was chosen because it is a high atomic weight material which differentially attenuates X-rays but is nonetheless well tolerated by the body (it is mostly excreted in the urine). When a catheter is threaded into the pulmonary artery and an iodinated solution ejected from its tip, the pulmonary arteries are quickly first opacified showing a relatively vertically oriented branching pattern, originating at the hilum. Normal arteries progressively reduce in diameter after multiple branches*

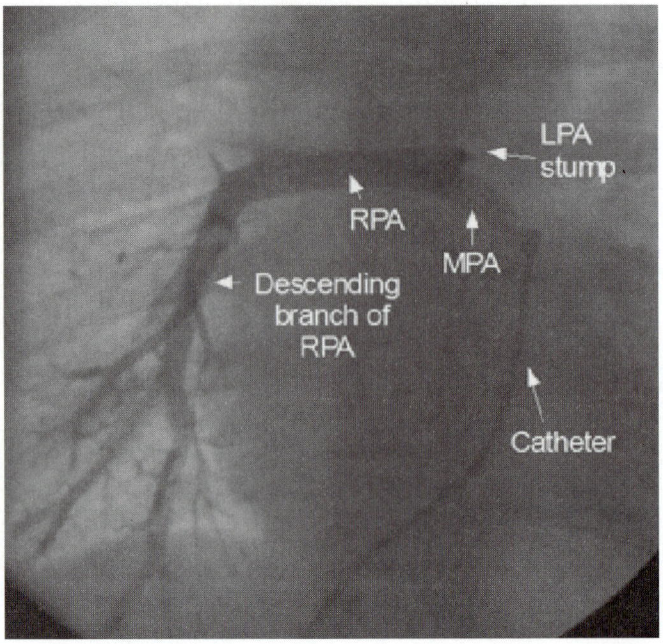

Fig. 12.19: *Pulmonary angiography shows hypoplastic right pulmonary artery and atretic left pulmonary artery*

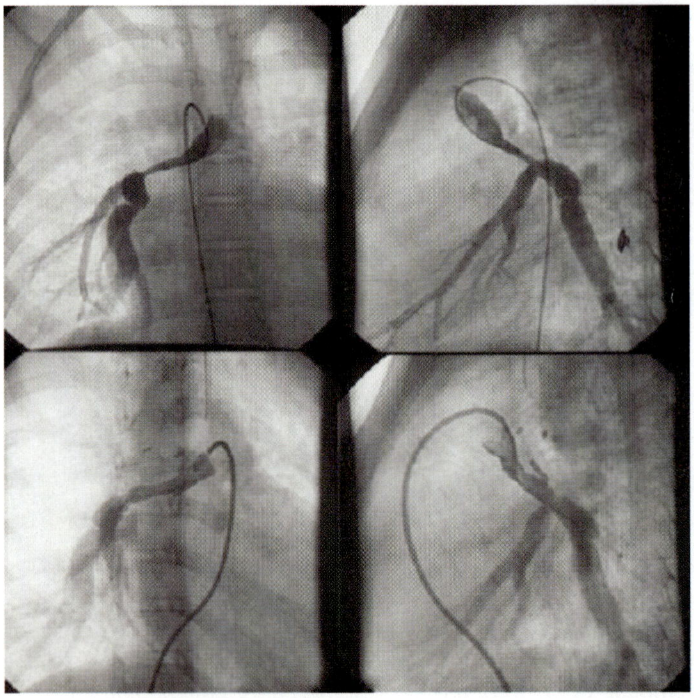

Fig. 12.20: *Right pulmonary artery angiogram demonstrating significant long segment stenosis (A). The stenosis extends fairly distally into the hilum, best appreciated in the lateral projection (B). Initial angiography was performed with a catheter advanced retrograde through the central shunt. (C, D). Following balloon angioplasty, there is marked improvement in the stenosis. Note the catheter is now accessing the shunt in a prograde fashion from the right ventricle to the ascending aorta and through the central shunt. By accessing the pulmonary artery from a venous approach to perform balloon angioplasty, it was possible to avoid placement of a large sheath in the femoral artery*

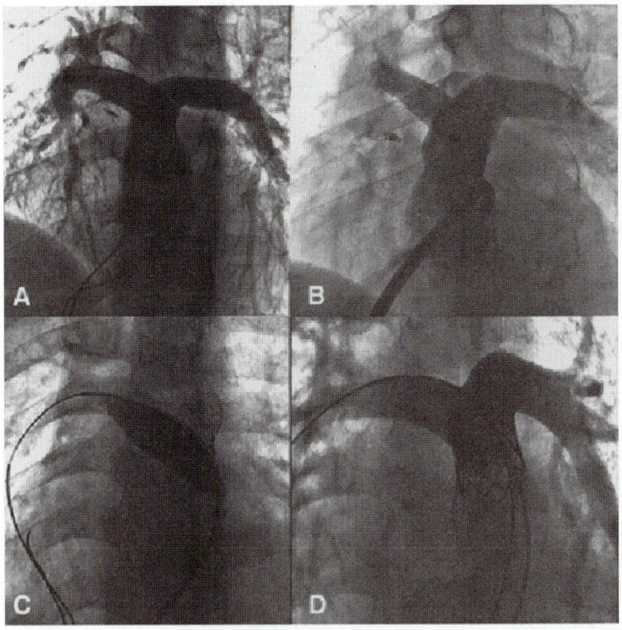

Fig. 12.21: *Cineangiogram still frames demonstrate the jailing technique in patient 1. (A) Angiogram on four-chamber view shows the anatomy of the right ventricular outflow tract (RVOT) and pulmonary artery (PA) tree. (B) RV angiogram after placement of open-cell, bare metal stents shows symmetrical perfusion of the 2 PAs and incomplete apposition of the stents to the RVOT. (C) Angiogram shows opening of the cells at the level of the jailed PA before melody insertion. (D) Final angiogram shows reduction of pulmonary regurgitation with a small amount of paraprosthetic leak*

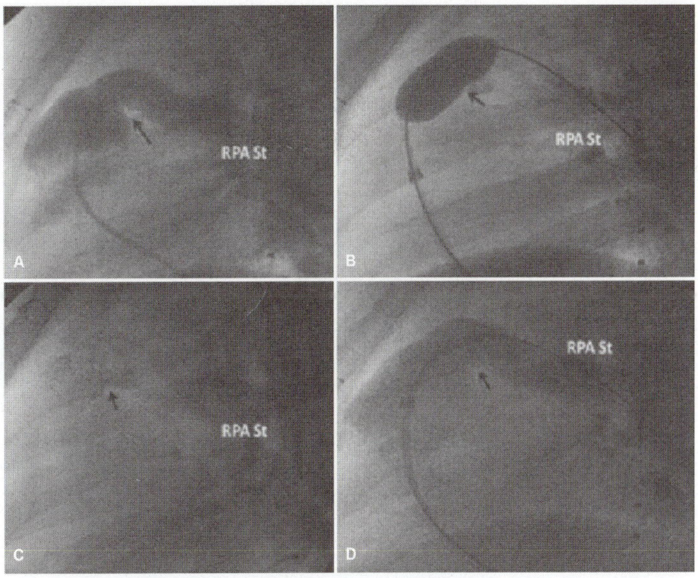

Fig. 12.22: *Superior vena caval (SVC) cineangiographic frame (A) in lateral view demonstrating narrowed SVC in a child who had previously undergone surgical repair of sinus venous atrial septal defect and partial anomalous pulmonary venous connection. Following deployment of the stent (B), the SVC constriction is completely relieved (C). Pressure gradient was abolished and facial edema improved (D)*

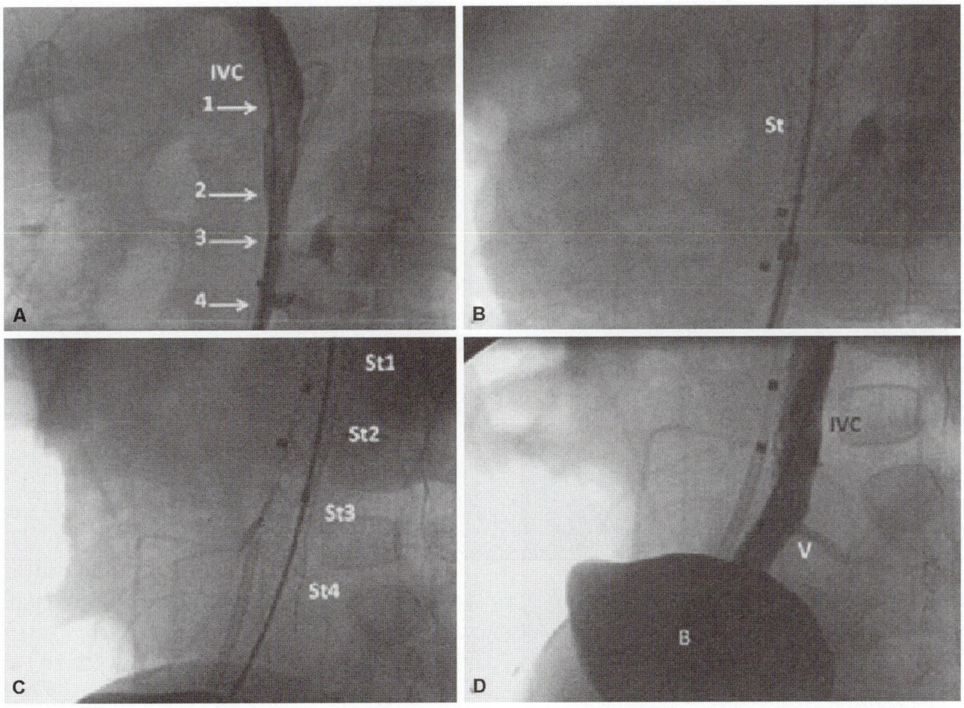

Fig. 12.23: *Inferior vena caval (IVC) cineangiographic frame (A) in lateral view demonstrating narrowed IVC. The narrowing starts at arrow 1, tappers down up to the arrow 2 and remains narrow thru' arrows 3 and 4 and beyond. Cineradiographic frames after implantation the first stent (B) and additional stents (St2 thru' St4) (C) clearly show the stents. Cineangiographic frame (D) shows wide-open stents in the IVC. B, bladder filled with contrast. Faint retrograde filling of a vein (V) suggests that veins emptying into the stented IVC are not obstructed*

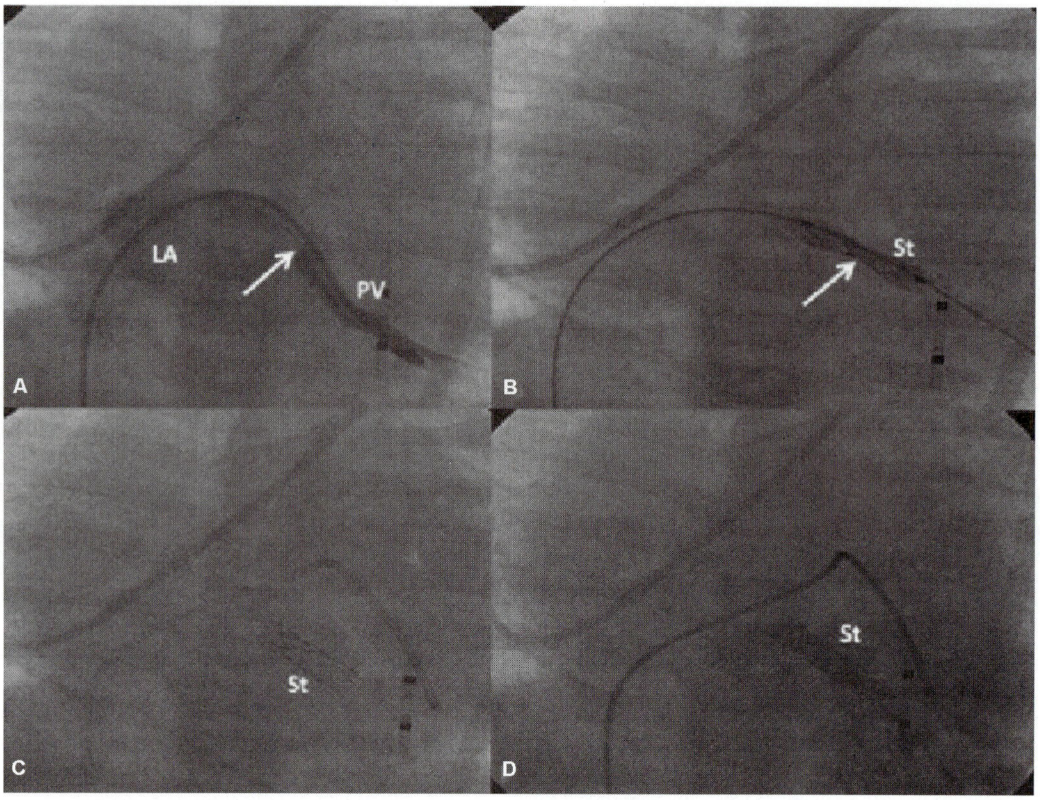

Fig. 12.24: *Selected frame from pulmonary vein (PV) cineangiogram demonstrating narrow jet of contrast (arrow) suggestive of severely stenotic PV (A). During implantation of stent, waist of the balloon/stent (St) assembly (arrow) is seen (B); this waist disappeared with further inflation of the balloon (C). Levophase of left pulmonary artery cineangiogram filling of the stent with contrast is seen in D. LA, left atrium*

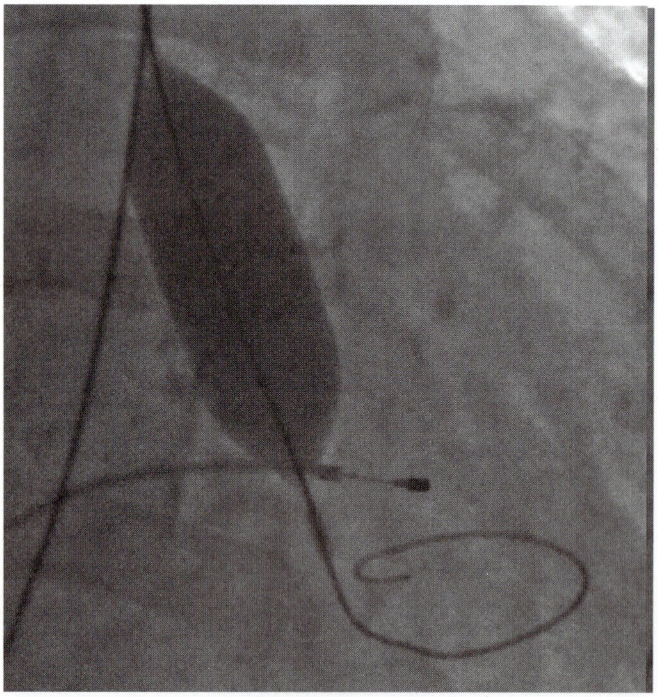

Fig. 12.25: *Balloon aortic valvuloplasty (BAV) via the retrograde approach. After correctly positioning across the stenotic valve the balloon is inflated with dilute contrast material. Note the temporary pacing wire in the right ventricle and the pigtail shaping of the left ventricular wire*

- Wolff-Parkinson white (WPW) or other accessory electrical connections that can cause SVT
- Acquired/postoperative defects treated via catheterization
- Residual/recurrent pulmonary stenosis
- Residual/recurrent valvar aortic stenosis
- Residual/recurrent coarctation of the aorta
- Residual ventricular septal defect
- Fontan fenestration (surgically created defect for right to left shunt) (Fig. 12.62)
- Systemic venous obstruction.

GENERAL METHODS OF INTERVENTION

Balloon Valvuloplasty

Balloon valvuloplasty was the first reported in pediatrics in the early 1980s. Patients who have isolated valvar aortic (AS) or pulmonary stenosis (PS) will likely be appropriate candidates for balloon valvuloplasty. Patients may present at birth with "critical" aortic or pulmonary stenosis requiring immediate ICU care and prostaglandin administration, or may present as a child outside of the newborn period.

The general technique involves placement of a balloon catheter across the affected valve. The pulmonary and aortic valves are most commonly affected although rheumatic mitral stenosis is also treated this way in countries with

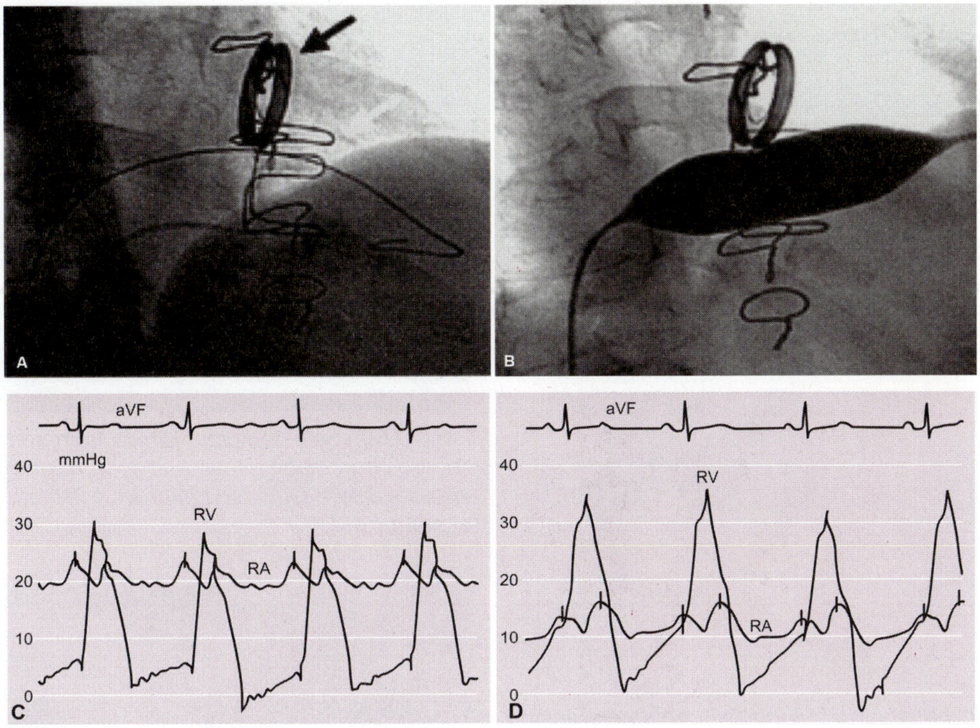

Fig. 12.26: *(A) Fluoroscopic image in the right anterior oblique/cranial view demonstrates the guide wire that was passed through the center of the stenotic bioprosthetic valve (Movie II). Mechanical mitral valve (black arrow) and bioprosthetic tricuspid valve (yellow arrow) are shown. (B) Balloon valvuloplasty was performed with the use of a balloon with a maximum diameter of 25 × 40 mm and an inflation pressure of 16 atm (Movie III). (C) Before the procedure, the mean right atrial pressure was 21 mmHg and the right ventricular end-diastolic pressure was 5 mmHg. The mean diastolic gradient across the tricuspid valve was 13 mmHg. (D) After the procedure, the mean right atrial pressure was 12 mmHg and the right ventricular end-diastolic pressure was 10 mmHg. The mean diastolic gradient across the tricuspid valve was improved to 6 mmHg*

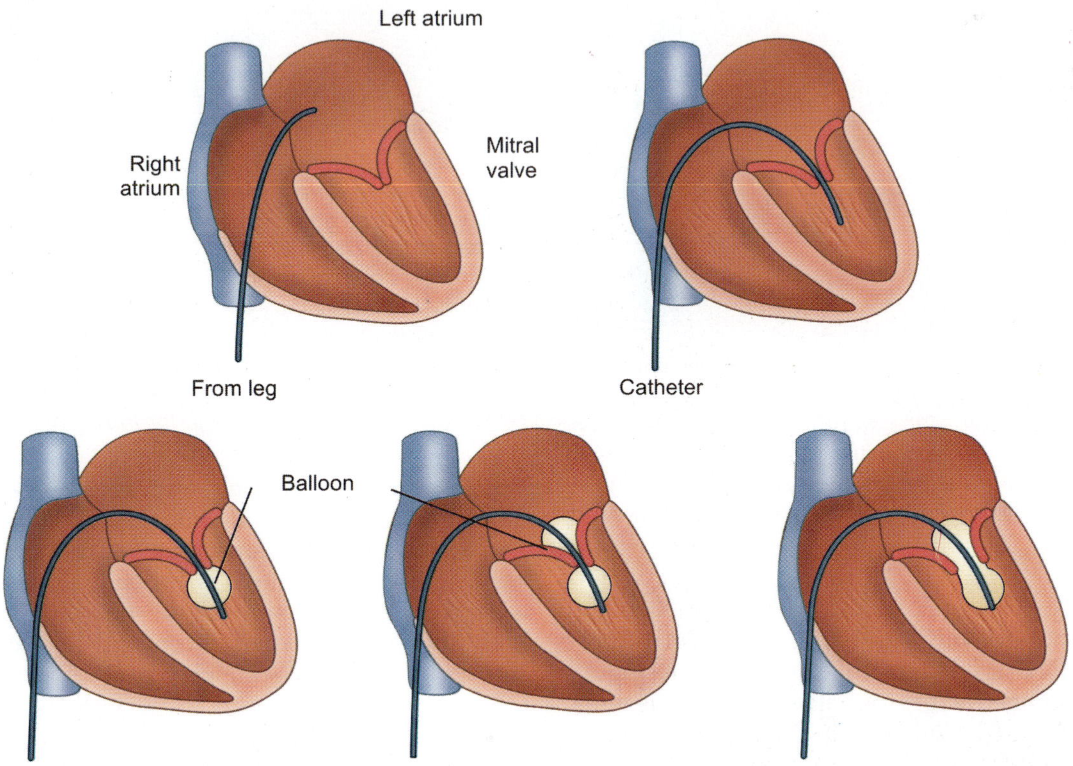

Fig. 12.27: *Diagram showing transcatheter balloon management of mitral valve*

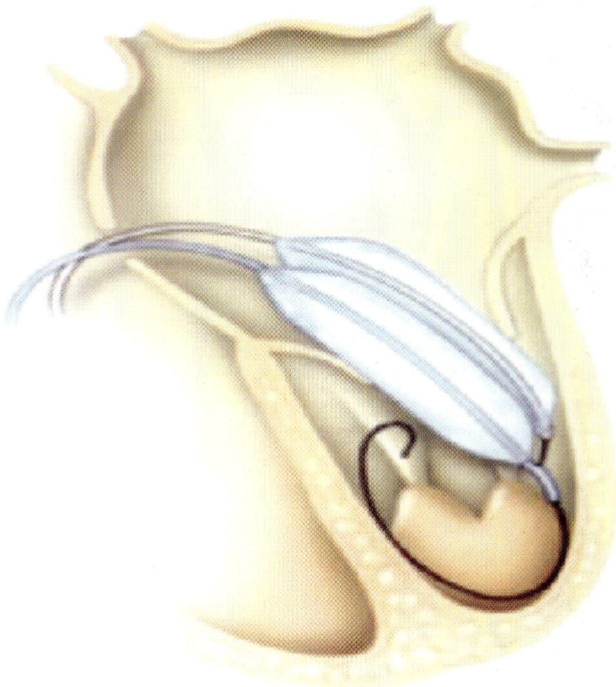

Fig. 12.28: *Showing balloon valvuloplasty catheter crossing across punctured foramen ovale to dilate the stenosed mitral valve*

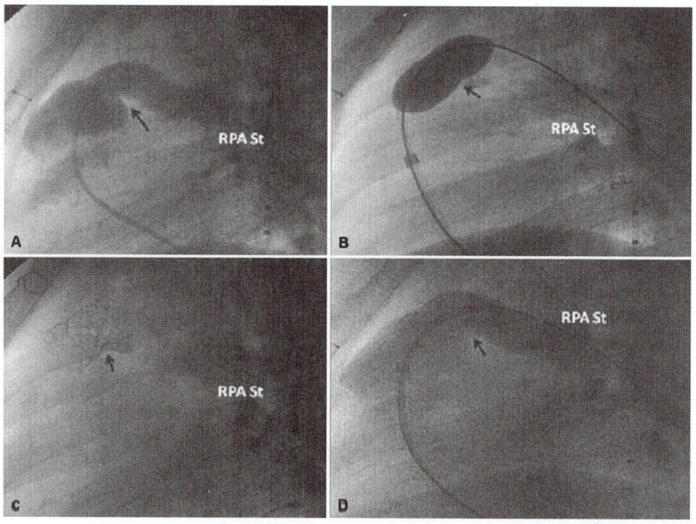

Fig. 12.29: *Selected frames from lateral view of a right ventricular outflow tract cineangiogram (A) demonstrating narrowed outflow tract (arrow). The position of the stent mounted balloon during stent implantation with residual waist (arrow) is shown in (B). Following the removal of the balloon, the stent (C) is seen with residual indentation (arrow). Follow-up angiogram (D) shows wide open stent*

endemic rheumatic fever. The balloons are introduced through the femoral artery, femoral vein, or internal jugular vein and are positioned across the valves using guide wires. The balloon is inflated, deflated, and then removed. The hemodynamic and angiographic evaluation is then repeated and the need for further therapy is assessed.

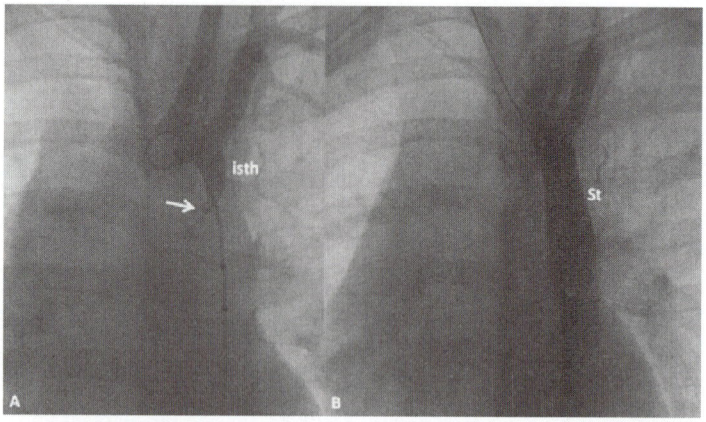

Fig. 12.30: *Selected cine frames from aortogram demonstrating severe coarctation (white arrow) with isthmic hypoplasia (isth) in an adolescent (A) which improved (B) following the deployment of stent (St)*

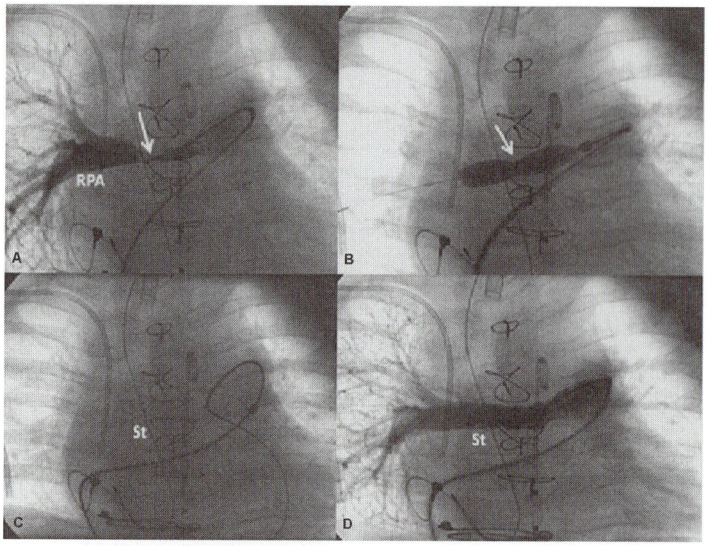

Fig. 12.31: *Selected cineangiographic frames from pulmonary artery cineangiogram demonstrating severe narrowing (solid arrow in A) in the right pulmonary artery (RPA). During implantation of the stent (B) a waist of the balloon was seen (solid arrow in B) which was completely abolished following further inflation of the balloon. Following the removal of the balloon, the stent (St) is seen and is widely open (C). Follow-up angiogram shows wide open St in the RPA (D). Multiple radio-opaque structures such as catheters, sternal wires, pacemaker wires and endo-tracheal tube are seen and are not germane for the stent implantation result*

The results are excellent with about 90% success rate for pulmonary stenosis and about 80–85% immediate success for aortic stenosis. Conscious sedation is used for most while general anesthesia is applied in critically ill or high-risk patients. Outside of the neonatal period balloon valvuloplasty is usually accomplished as an outpatient procedure and is associated with rapid recovery.

Balloon Angioplasty

Balloon angioplasty can be used to treat native or recurrent coarctation of the aorta, native or postoperative peripheral

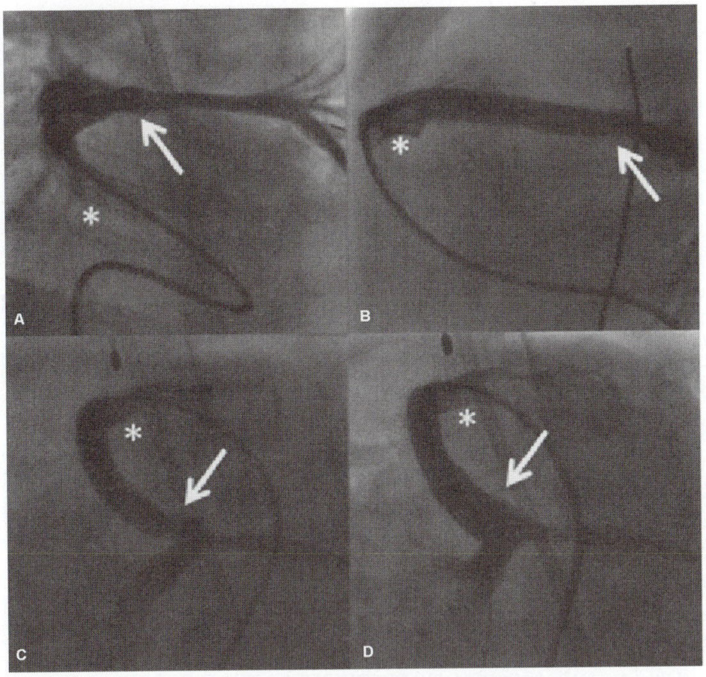

Fig. 12.32: *Angiographic example of distal RV-PA conduit stenosis (arrow) using various camera angulations after proximal conduit stent placement (asterisk). Left anterior oblique cranial (A) and lateral (B) angulations might allow for underestimation of distal conduit stenosis, which was better profiled using left anterior oblique caudal angulation, before (C) and after intervention (D)*

pulmonary artery stenosis, or more rarely acquired systemic venous obstruction [i.e. superior vena cava obstruction following extracorporeal membrane oxygenation (ECMO) therapy.

The general technique is similar to valvuloplasty and involves placement of a balloon catheter across the narrow portion of the affected blood vessel. The balloons are introduced through the femoral artery, femoral vein, or internal jugular vein and are positioned across the narrowed vessel using guide wires. The balloon is inflated, deflated, and then removed. The hemodynamic and angiographic evaluation is then repeated and the need for further therapy is assessed.

The rate of success for recurrent or residual obstructions is the highest, although the long-term success rates in native lesions can be quite variable. Even when a long-term cure is not achieved during the catheterization, the procedure can benefit the patient greatly by allowing definitive therapy (either surgical or transcatheter) to be delayed until the patient has grown significantly or is more medically stable.

Intravascular Stent Placement

Stents are tubular, metallic, balloon expandable devices that can be delivered using techniques similar to balloon angioplasty, however, the stent remains within the vascular space providing a more rigid framework to expand the affected vessel. The stents used in pediatrics are designed

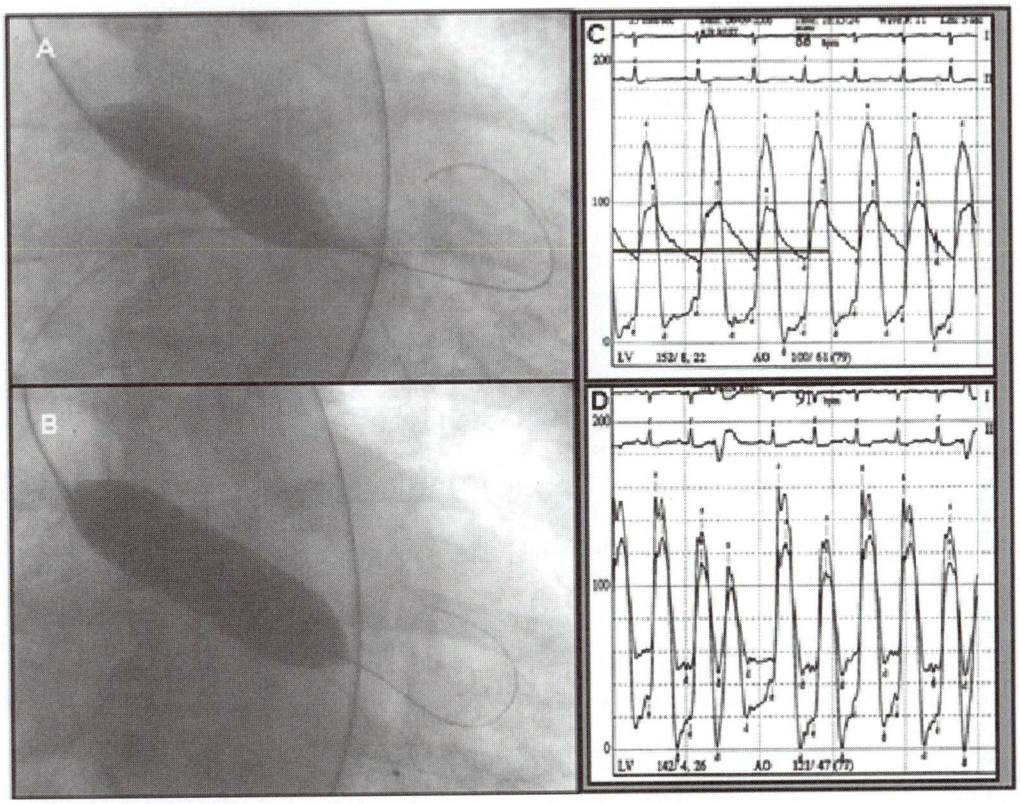

Fig. 12.33: *(A) Shows preinflated balloon catheter across aortic valve (B). Shows fully inflated aoretic valve. Aortic and left ventricular traces pre- (C) and post-(D) valvuloplasty. The mean aortic pressure gradient has reduced significantly from 50 mmHg to 25 mmHg*

for use in the bile ducts and peripheral arteries of adults and are similar to but larger than the stents used to treat adult coronary artery disease.

When used in conjunction with balloon angioplasty to treat peripheral pulmonary artery stenosis, coarctation of the aorta and rarely systemic venous obstruction stent use has been associated with improved short-term and long-term rates of success compared to balloon angioplasty alone. Stent use in pediatrics has less follow-up data than balloon valvuloplasty and the true long-term results have yet to be defined, however the short and midterm results would suggest that stent placement is an important and successful adjunct to current therapy. Balloon angioplasty and stent placement have been uniquely useful in treating stenoses, such as distal branch pulmonary artery stenosis, not approachable by surgical techniques.

Most patients with newly placed or dilated stents will spend a single night in the hospital for close monitoring and empiric anticoagulation.

Embolization Coil Placement

Stainless steel or platinum coils (most dacron covered) can be used to occlude a variety of unwanted blood vessels or structures. PDAs, coronary artery fistulae, pulmonary arteriovenous fistulae, and a variety of undesirable collateral blood vessels that are usually found in patients with complex heart disease, can all be effectively treated using coils or one of the many modified coils available on the market.

The technique involves identification and measurement by angiography of the structure to be closed or occluded. A catheter, usually quite small in caliber (4–5 french), is then threaded into the structure and the coil is then delivered through the catheter. The size of the structure to be occluded determines the choice of coils, which are available in multiple loop diameters and lengths. The angiograms and hemodynamics are then repeated and the need for further intervention is assessed.

When used in stable patients during an uncomplicated catheterization, the procedure is usually performed as an outpatient.

Septal Occluder Placement (Figs 12.52, 12.63 and 12.64)

Atrial septal defects (ASD), patent foramen ovale (PFO), and ventricular septal defects (VSD) can all be closed non-surgically using trans-catheter techniques. The FDA approved the Amplatzer Septal Occluder in November 2001 for closure of uncomplicated ASDs. The CardioSEAL device as well as the Amplatzer PFO device have a limited approval from the FDA under humanitarian device exemption (HDE) guidelines to close PFOs. The CardioSEAL device also has HDE approval to close muscular VSDs or residual VSDs. The anatomy of the ASD or VSD determine whether the patient is good candidate for transcatheter closure. Some ASDs will still require surgical closure and surgery remains an option for all patients with an uncomplicated ASD.

The techniques used are similar to above but generally involve larger introducing sheaths and catheters. This limits the use of these devices to patients out of the newborn age range and usually greater than 3 years of age. Transesophageal echocardiography is utilized to continuously guide device placement, and for this reason most cases are completed with general anesthesia. After placement of a septal occluder, an overnight inpatient stay is currently required to allow assessment of the device position and effectiveness by echocardiography the morning following the procedure.

Radiofrequency Catheter Ablation (Figs 12.46–12.49)

Patients with reciprocating supraventricular tachycardia (most common form of SVT) or with WPW are candidates a transcatheter curative procedure. Catheters tipped with electrodes are introduced through the femoral veins and are used to identify the unwanted accessory connections that cause SVT. Once identified these "pathways" can be eliminated using radiofrequency energy (heat) applied through the same types of catheters used to identify the short circuits (accessory pathways).

This procedure has a greater than 90% success rate and is nearly always curative when used in patients with accessory pathway mediated SVT. The procedure is done as an outpatient and is accompanied by a rapid recovery.

DIAGNOSTIC CATHETERIZATION

Catheters introduced into the heart or great vessels are used both for the delivery of radiographic contrast medium (angiography) and for the measurement of pressure within the chambers of the heart and cardiac output.

Cardiac Angiography

Four diagnostic investigations account for the majority of angiographic procedures:

1. Aortic root angiography (Figs 12.40 and 12.41)
2. Left ventricular angiography (Fig. 12.14)
3. Coronary arteriography (Fig. 12.51)
4. Pulmonary arteriography (Fig. 12.19 and 12.20)

For coronary arteriography, relatively small volumes of contrast (5–8 mL) injected manually are used but, for other angiographic procedures much larger amounts up to 50 mL), introduced by power injection, are required. Digital subtraction techniques permit reductions in contrast volume but have. At present, only a limited role in cardiovascular angiographic diagnosis. Until recently images have been recorded on high-speed cine film or video, to provide a dynamic record of ventricular wall movement, blood flow and intravascular anatomy. The current generation of angiographic laboratories, however, utilize digital technology and provide better quality images which maybe electronically stored.

Aortic Root Angiography (Figs 12.40 and 12.41)

Contrast injection into the aortic root demonstrates the vascular anatomy in suspected aneurysm or dissection, and also permits evaluation of aortic valve function. The normal aortic valve prevents diastolic backflow of contrast, but in aortic regurgitation variable opacification of the left ventricle occurs, depending on the severity of the valve lesion.

Left Ventricular Angiography (Fig. 12.14)

Contrast injection into the left ventricle defines ventricular anatomy and wall motion, and also permits evaluation of mitral valve function. Dilatation of the ventricle and contractile dysfunction occurs in left ventricular failure. Exaggerated contractile function with systolic obliteration of the cavity occurs in hypertrophic cardiomyopathy. Filling defects within the ventricular lumen may indicate thrombus or, less commonly, neoplasm. The normal mitral valve prevents systolic backflow of contrast into the left atrium, but in mitral regurgitation variable atrial opacification occurs, depending on the severity of the valve lesion.

Pulmonary Arteriography (Figs 12.19 and 12.20)

Injection of contrast medium into the main pulmonary artery pacifies the arterial branches throughout both lung fields. The normal flow distribution is homogeneous lung fields. Vascular occlusions with regional perfusion defects usually indicate pulmonary thromboembolism (particularly when intraluminal filling defects are present) but may also occurs in advanced emphysema.

TYPES OF INTERVENTIONAL CATHETERIZATION

Interventional catheterization represents one of the most exciting fields in the treatment of cardiovascular disease and has found important application in both paediatric and adult practice, often extending the role of the cardiologist into areas that were once exclusively surgical. The earliest example was the insertion of electrode-tipped catheters into the heart for pacing patients with bradyarrhythmias. Pacing technology has now reached a high level of sophistication and the interventional management of arrhythmias has expanded to include treatment of resistant tachyarrhythmias by overdrive pacing and, more recently, by the electrical ablation of conduction tissue with catheters placed strategically within the heart. Balloon angioplasty is a cath eter technique used widely for the treatment of coronary artery disease, particularly when medical treatment fails to control symptoms. Intracoronary stents mounted on balloon catheters are also widely used for maintaining patency after angioplasty Balloon valvuloplasty is finding increasing application in the treatment of mitral stenosis, and in paediatric practice is the treatment of choice for congenital pulmonary stenosis. The insertion of obstructors for closure of patent ductus arteriosus using specially adapted catheters represents a recent advance that is reducing the requirement for surgery in young children while in neonates with transposition of the great arteries emergency balloon atrial septostomy is potentially life-saving.

Balloon Dilation

(Figs 12.23, 12.26, 12.28, 12.29, 12.34 and 12.35)

A catheter with a balloon on the tip is passed into the heart, where it is inflated to open up a narrowed area or widen an existing hole. A balloon atrial septostomy is a technique used to enlarge a hole between the right atrium and the left atrium. It is often used to manage patients with transposition of the great arteries. The larger hole improves oxygenation of the blood. This is also known as the Rashkind procedure.

Procedure in Balloon Atrial Septostomy

A balloon atrial septostomy is performed with a special catheter that has a balloon attached to its tip. The catheter is introduced into the body through a blood vessel in the groin or belly button. Once the catheter is advanced into the left atrium of the heart, the balloon tip is inflated and pulled into the right atrium of the heart. This results in the small hole between the left and the right atrium being enlarged. The balloon is deflated and the catheter is

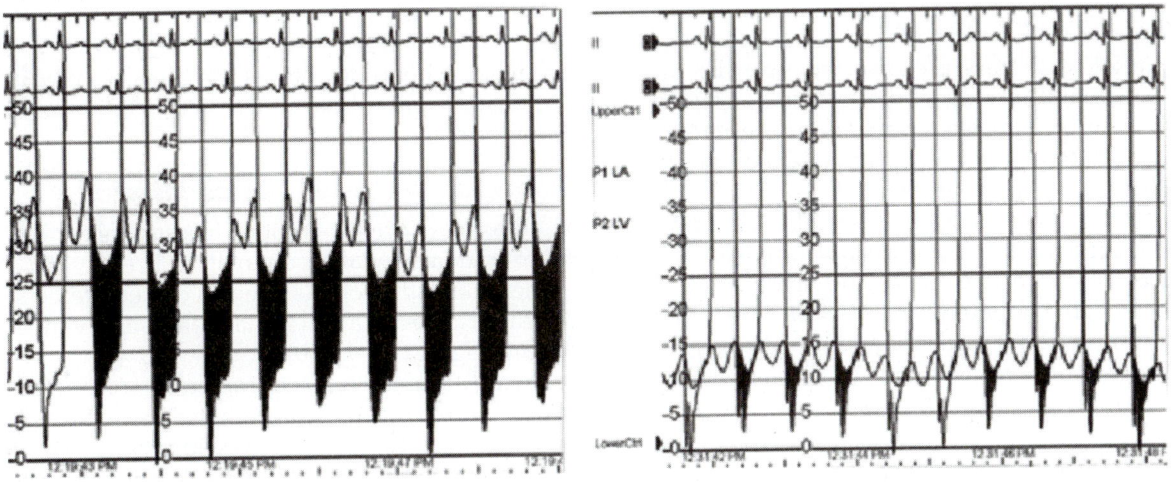

Fig. 12.34: *Hemodynamic tracing of pre- (A) and postdilatation (B) of the mitral valve. It shows considerable reduction in pressure gradient across stenosed mitral valve after successful dilatation*

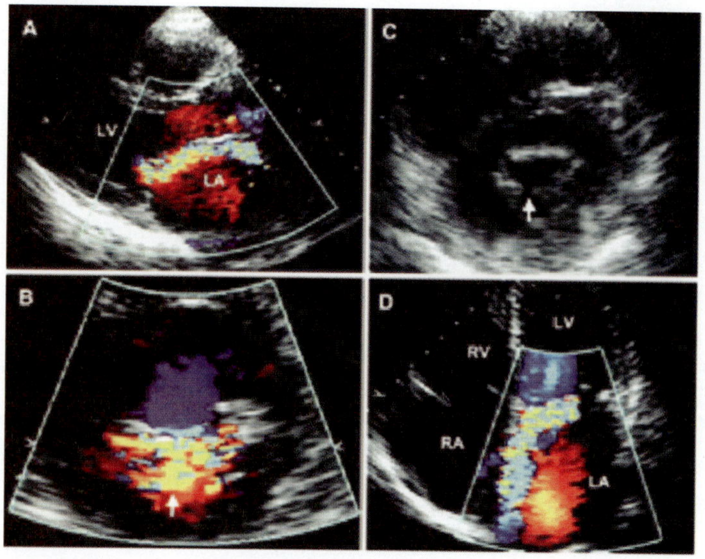

Fig. 12.35: *An illustrative case of development of significant MR as a result of isolated leaflet laceration or tear after PMV. Parasternal long-axis (A) and apical (D) views show an eccentric MR jet. A parasternal short axis view shows a new echocardiographic dropout (C) at the mid portion of the posterior mitral leaflet with proximal flow convergence (B), which suggests a leaflet tear (arrow). LA indicates left atrium; LV, left ventricle; RA, right atrium; RV, right ventricle.*

removed from the body. The entry site on the groin, which is less than 5 mm, is covered with a bandage (Figs 12.27 to 12.29).

Balloon Angioplasty

When any part of the heart's circulation becomes narrowed (as in pulmonary stenosis), balloon angioplasty, which is also known as balloon dilation, can help to open up the narrowed area and improve blood flow. It can also be done to improve the narrowing that occurs with other arteries such as the aorta (coarctation of the aorta) or veins (pulmonary veins or the systemic veins such as the superior vena cava or inferior vena cava).

Balloon Angioplasty Procedure

Thin tubes called catheters are inserted into the blood vessels in the groin at the top of the leg (sometimes both legs). X-ray pictures and measurements of the narrowed area are usually taken. A catheter with a balloon on its tip is threaded through the first catheter to this narrowed area. Once the balloon reaches the right place, it is blown up to open up the narrowed area. The balloon forces the narrowed area open and stretches the artery wall. The balloon is deflated, the catheters are taken out, and the entry site on the leg is covered with a bandage. Sometimes, a stent (a wire mesh tube) is inserted to help keep the newly opened area patent (Fig. 12.50–12.51).

Balloon Valvuloplasty

A balloon valvuloplasty is a procedure done to open a heart valve that is abnormally obstructed. Heart valves are like gates that control the flow of blood between the upper and the lower chambers of the heart, as well as the flow out of the heart. If the opening of a valve is narrow, it is called stenotic valve.

Procedure in Balloon Valvuloplasty (Fig. 12.26)

A catheter is inserted into a blood vessel at the top of the leg and moved through the vessel to the narrowed valve. X-ray pictures are taken of this area. A special catheter with a balloon at the tip is then threaded across the narrowed (stenotic) valve. After the catheter has reached the valve, the balloon is blown up, which opens the valve. The catheters are then taken out and the entry sites at the top of the leg are covered with a bandage.

POTENTIAL COMPLICATIONS

Pulmonary Valve Dilations

Sometimes the valve becomes leaky after a balloon valvuloplasty. This condition, called valve incompetence, is usually mild and occurs after surgical valvuloplasty as well. Most pulmonary valves (80%) are narrowed because parts of the valve are stuck together, but they respond well to dilation. Some valves, however, do not improve enough with the procedure and may need surgery. For example, a so-called dysplastic valve, with leaflets that may not be so stuck together, does not always improve with dilation, although the procedure is often tried before surgery is considered (Figs 12.30 and 12.32).

Aortic valve dilations: The goal of aortic valvuloplasty is to make the narrowing wide enough so that sufficient blood can flow through to reduce the pressure to safe levels without causing a significant leak. Then surgery can be avoided. In a small percentage of cases, the valve becomes very leaky, even when the right-sized balloon is used. If this occurs, your child may need surgery to repair the valve (Figs 12.16, 12.31, 13.34 and 12.35).

Closure Device Insertion

Closure Device

A catheter with a little device on the tip is inserted into the heart to fill a hole in the heart.

For some heart defects, a little device can be inserted into the heart to fill a hole in the heart. In some cases, this is enough to correct the problem.

Procedure in Closure Device Insertion

The closure procedure is done in a special cardiac procedure room with a special medicine that keeps your child asleep (general anesthetic). It's used to correct defects like patent ductus arteriosus, atrial septal defect, and ventricular septal defect (Figs 12.55–12.60).

Once your child is asleep, an echocardiogram taken from the esophagus or stomach tube; a transesophageal echocardiogram is done to measure the size of the hole and to help place the device. If the echocardiogram shows that the hole is too big to close with the device, your child will be awakened and sent to the recovery room.

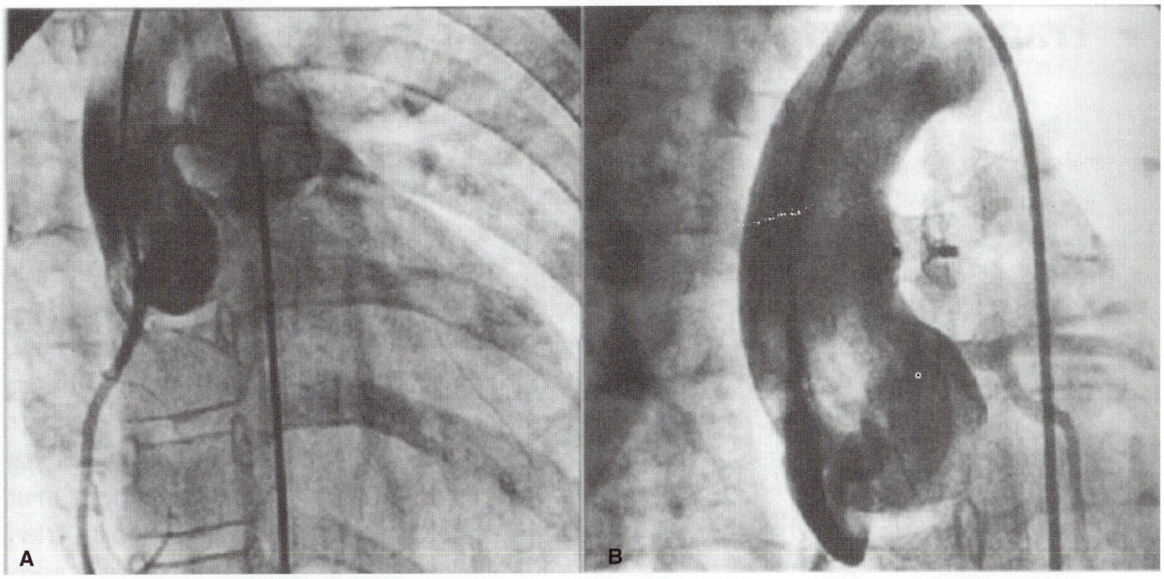

Fig. 12.36: *(A) Angiogram in ascending aorta depicting aortopulmonary window as a communication between ascending aorta and pulmonary trunk. (B) After successful implantation of Amplatzer occluder in aortopulmonary window showing complete closure of the defect*

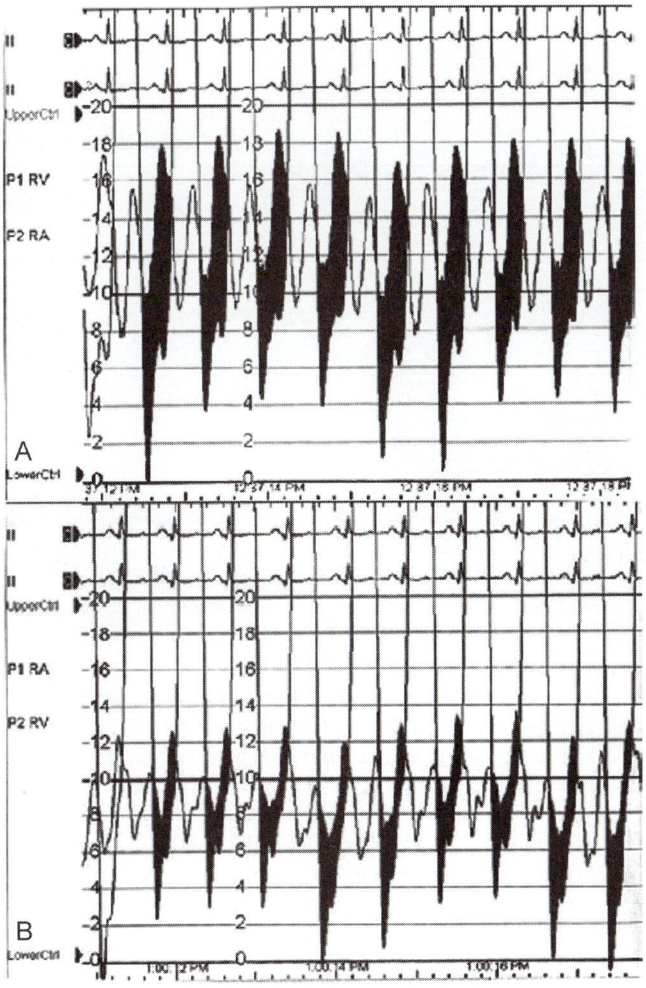

Fig. 12.37: *Hemodynamic in TV stenosis . (A) Shows increased pressure gradient across stenosed tricuspid valve. (B) Shows considerable reduction of gradient after tricuspid valvoplasty*

If the hole is small enough and in the right position, thin tubes called catheters will be inserted through the blood vessels in the groin at the top of the leg (sometimes both legs are used). The catheter is moved up the blood vessel into the heart and into the affected area of the heart. The closure device is inserted through one catheter, while the other is used to help to measure the hole. After the device is in place, the catheters are taken out and the entry sites are covered with a bandage. An echocardiogram might be done to check the placement of the device.

What does the Closure Device Look Like and How does It Work?

There are a number of different kinds of closure devices. For example, one looks like two-opened umbrellas. Its arms stay closed until it reaches the right position in the hole. It is then opened up like an umbrella. The device has spring arms that hold it in the proper place and prevent blood from flowing through the hole. When it comes to repairing a PDA, you may hear this device referred to as a PDA coil.

If the device doesn't fit properly after it is opened, it may be taken out and a second attempt made to close the hole. If the device cannot be taken out, which is rare, surgery will be necessary. A more common complication is a small leak through the closure device. Usually, this disappears with time. In this case, a second device may be placed over the first to stop the leak completely (Fig. 12.52).

Stentoplasty

A stent is a small metal tube made of metal alloy. When part of a major blood vessel or conduit becomes narrowed, it is called stenotic. The stent helps to widen the narrowed passage by supporting the walls of the blood vessel or conduit to keep it open (Figs 12.70 and 12.71).

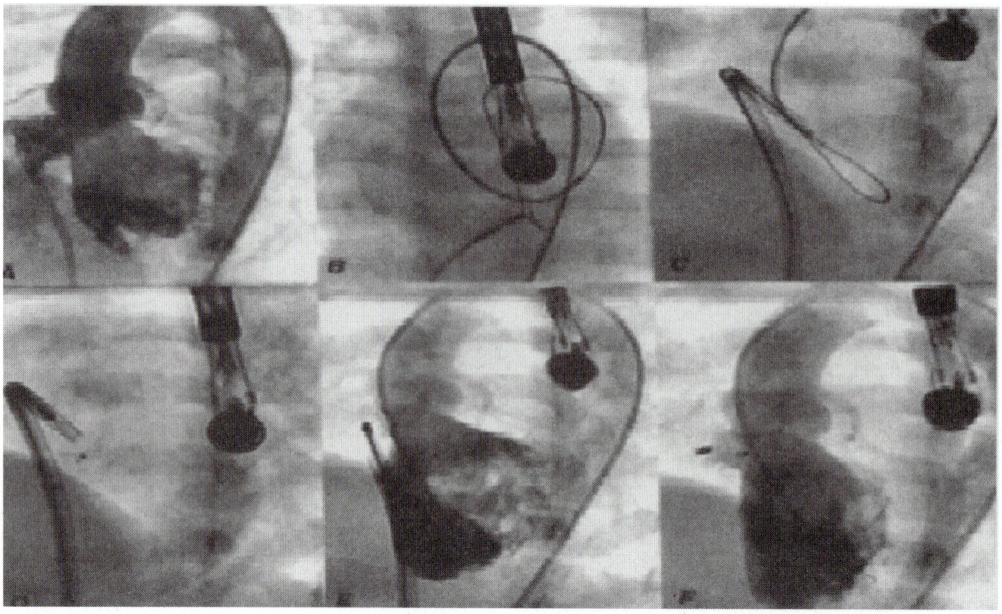

Fig. 12.38: *Different steps in closure of perimembranous ventricular septal defect with asymmtrical amplatzer membranous VSD occluder*

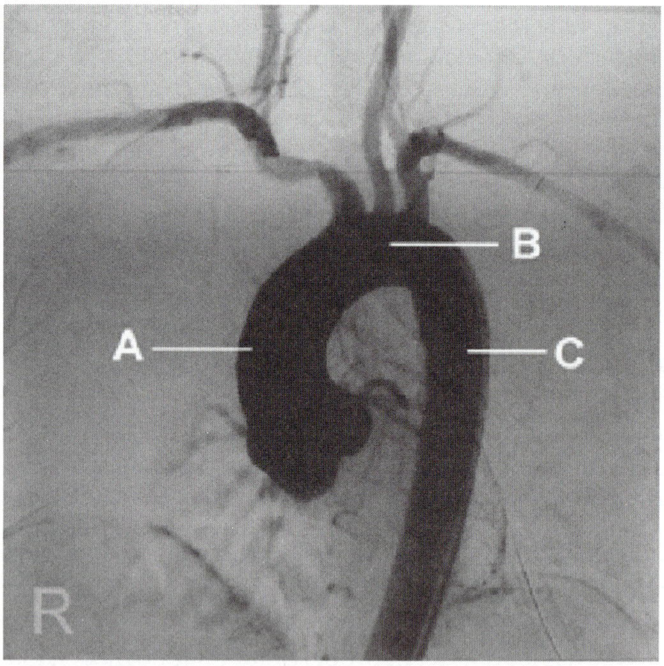

Fig. 12.39: *Showing ascending thoracic aorta (A), the aortic arch, which is the curved continuation of the ascending part (B), and the descending thoracic aorta (C), after aortic root angiography*

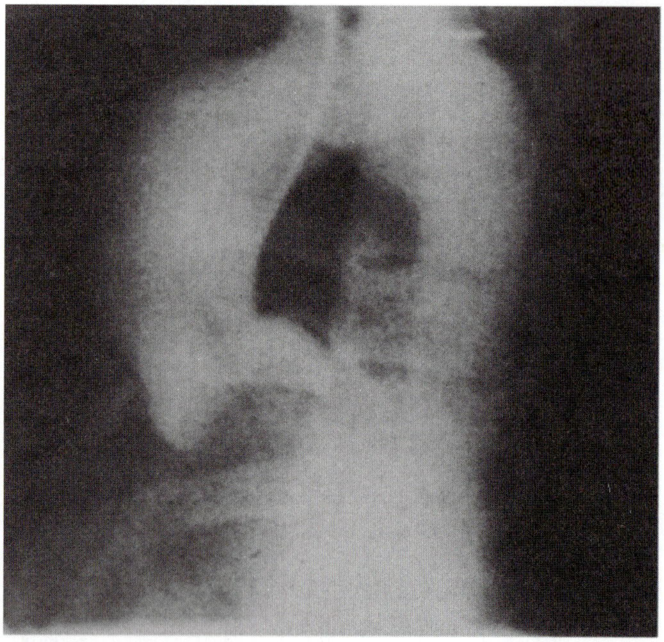

Fig. 12.40: *Aortic stenosis, 45° LAO cine projection. Catheter positioned clear of the aortic valve. Systolic frame shows doming of the valve cusps with negative jet of blood (the Prussian helmet sign). Note also the poststenotic dilatation of the ascending aorta*

Procedure in Stent Insertion

The stent is inserted in a special cardiac procedure room under a general anesthetic that keeps your child asleep. Once your child is asleep, a thin plastic tube called a catheter is inserted into the blood vessel in the groin at the top of one leg or both legs. Pictures are taken of the narrowed vessel using a type of X-ray called fluoroscopy. The special catheter with the balloon and stent is placed across the narrowed blood vessel or conduit. The balloon is inflated, forcing the narrowing open, expanding the stent, where it remains permanently to keep the vessel open. The catheter is then removed and the entry site at the top of the leg is covered with a bandage.

Potential Complications of Stentoplasty

The stent may be misplaced and a second stent needed, although this rarely occurs. If a stent is in an unsafe position,

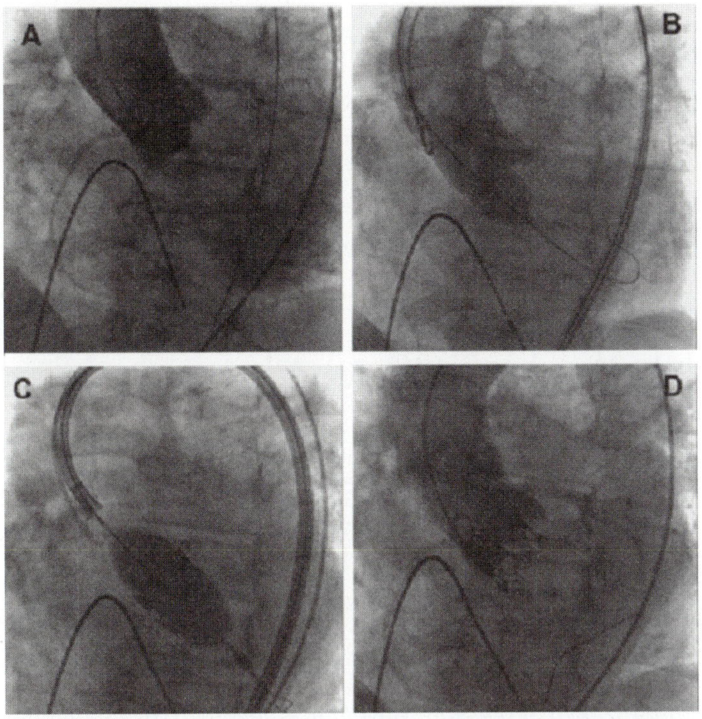

Fig. 12.41: *Percutaneous transcatheter aortic valve implantation by right transfemoral approach. (A) Baseline aortic angiography. (B) 23 mm balloon aortic valvuloplasty. (C) Implantation of the 26 mm Edwards Sapien XT valve across the aortic valve during rapid pacing. (D) At final aortic angiography, only a mild paravalvular leak was present*

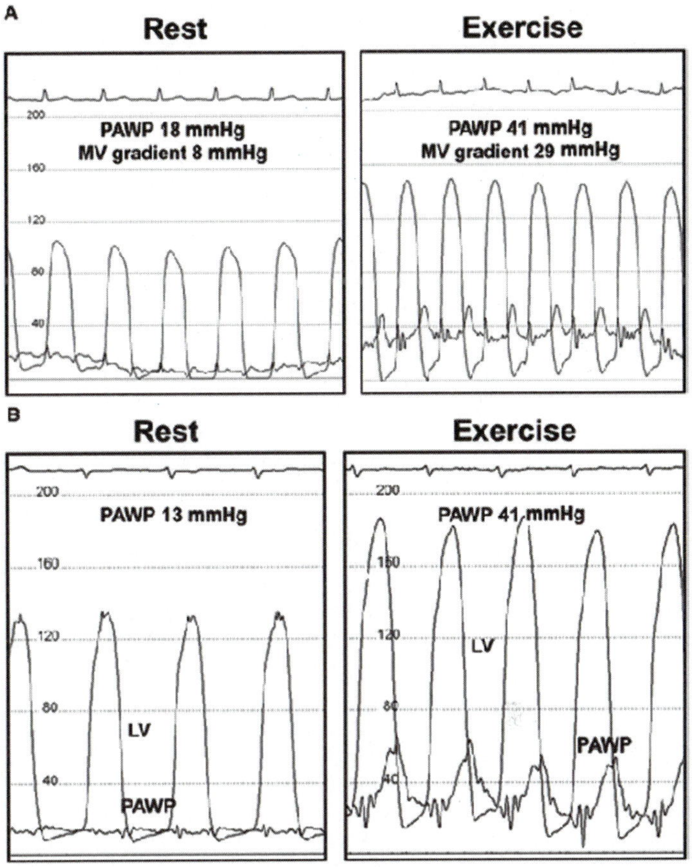

Fig. 12.42: *Exercise is frequently helpful in the cardiac catheterization laboratory to determine the cause of dyspnea in patients who do not have marked abnormalities of pressures in the resting state. (A) In this patient with mitral stenosis, the mean resting gradient was only 8 mmHg and the pulmonary artery wedge pressure (PAWP) was only 18 mmHg. This patient had significant symptoms out of proportion to the resting hemodynamics. With supine bicycle exercise, the mean gradient rose to 29 mmHg and the pulmonary artery wedge pressure rose to 41 mmHg, indicating that the mitral stenosis was hemodynamically significant and causing the severe symptoms. (B) This patient had no significant valve disease, normal left ventricular (LV) systolic function, but significant dyspnea on exertion. In the resting state, the pulmonary artery wedge pressure was only 13 mmHg. However, at a low level of supine bicycle exercise, there was a marked increase in pulmonary artery wedge pressure to 41 mmHg with a large V wave. There was not significant mitral regurgitation by simultaneous echocardiography, indicating that these symptoms were due to noncompliance of the left atrium and left ventricle. MV indicates mitral valve*

it will be removed, usually during catheterization. Surgery may be necessary in a few cases (Figs 12.72 and 12.73).

The opening may need to be enlarged later, usually because it could not be fully widened during the initial procedure. Less often, tissue grows into the interior of the stent, causing it to become narrowed again. Rarely, a clot may form on the stent. It can be dissolved using medicine.

Radiofrequency (Catheter) Ablation

Radiofrequency ablation is a non-surgical treatment for children with certain types of rapid heart beats. It involves using energy—like the kind of energy that makes your radio work (a low-voltage, high-frequency alternating current)—to correct the problem. This energy is given through a thin tube (catheter) placed in the heart.

To "ablate" something means to get rid of it. This approach is often suggested if drugs are unable to control an arrhythmia, and the arrhythmia is considered to be life-threatening. Ablation can, in some cases, completely eliminate an arrhythmia, but in others the success may not be complete and so the arrhythmia could recur.

Procedure in Radiofrequency Ablation

(Figs 12.53 and 12.54)

Radiofrequency ablation is done in a special cardiac procedure room under a general anesthetic. The catheters used in the test are inserted through blood vessels at the top of the leg (groin) or in the arm. The location of the catheters is watched throughout the procedure.

Electrical signals sent by the heart travel through the catheters and give the cardiologist information about the heart's electrical system and where the electrical system is not working properly. This is called an electrophysiology study. The kind of cardiologist who performs this procedure is an electrophysiologist. Cardiologist uses the catheters to find out the exact place of disturbance. Once the area that is causing your child's heart to beat fast is found, the cardiologist uses the energy to get rid of this area, so the rapid heart rate does not happen any more.

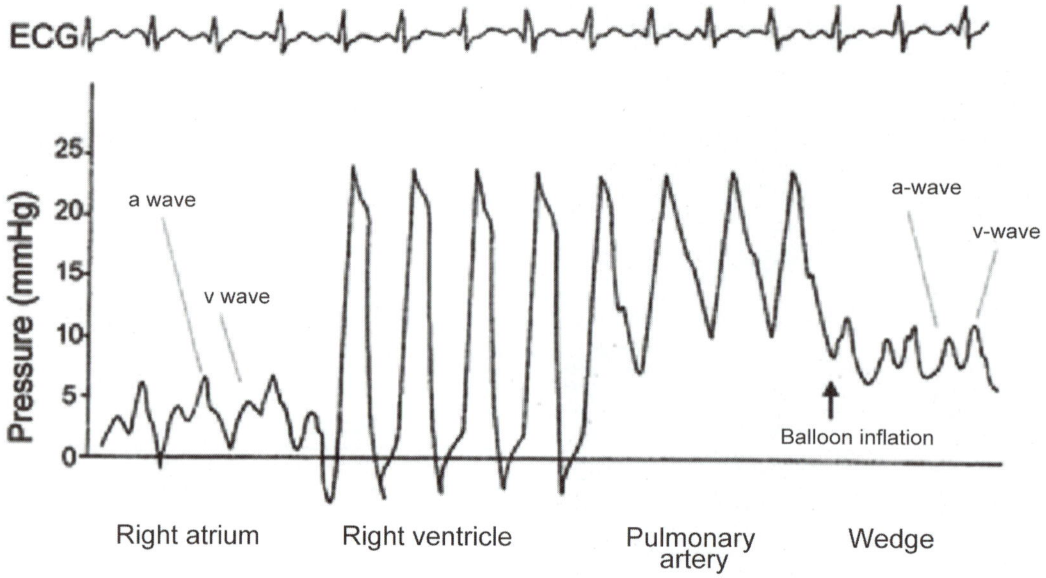

Fig. 12.43: *Representative recording of pressures as a balloon flotation catheter is inserted through a central vein into the right side of the heart into the pulmonary artery. The first recorded waveform is a right atrial tracing with characteristic a- and v-waves (note that the a-wave is usually larger than the v-wave in the right atrium and, conversely, in the left atrium or wedge, below). In the right ventricle, note that end-diastolic pressure is zero. In the pulmonary artery, a normal pressure waveform is recorded. (Note that the pressure in the pulmonary artery decreases during diastole as opposed to the increase in the diastolic pressure in the right ventricle; this difference in pressure contour helps to distinguish catheter position during placement, because the actual values for systolic and diastolic pressures can be virtually identical). The catheter is then advanced to the wedge position with the balloon inflated. The wedge pressure tracing shows a- and v-waves transmitted from the left atrium. The wedge tracing is not always this clear, but it should not be overly damped. The pressures shown here are in the range of normal*

Duration of procedure in cardiac catheterization

The procedure lasts 3–6 hours. Your child will go to the recovery room for about 2 hours after the procedure before going back to the ward.

Intracardiac Pressure Measurement

(Tables 12.1 and 12.2)

Cardiac catheterization for measurement of blood flow and pressure within the heart and great vessels is widely used both for diagnostic purposes and to guide treatment. The fluid-filled catheter is attached to a pressure transducer which converts the pressure waves into electrical signals. For measurement of right-sided pressures, the catheter is directed by the venous route into the right atrium and then advanced through the right ventricle into pulmonary artery. For measurement of left-sided pressures, the catheter is directed by the arterial route into the ascending aorta. Since retrograde guidance of catheter through left atrium is technically difficult, hence left atrial pressure is usually measured indirectly using the pulmonary artery wedge pressure (Figs 12.11 and 12.18).

The pulmonary artery wedge pressure is obtained during the right heart catheterization by advancing the catheter distally into the pulmonary arterial tree until the tip wedges in a small branch. Alternatively, a catheter with a preterminal balloon (Swan-Ganz catheter) may be used. Inflation of the balloon in the pulmonary artery causes the catheter tip to be carried with blood flow into a more distal branch which becomes occluded by the balloon. Regardless

Table 12.1: *Normal resting values for pressures in the heart and great vessels*

Site	*Systolic pressure (mmHg)*	*Diastolic pressure (mmHg)*	*Mean pressure (mmHg)*
• Right atrium	a ≤ ? v ≤ 5	x ≤ 3 y ≤ 3	< 5
• Right ventricle	≤ 25	End-pressure before a ≤ 3 End-pressure on a ≤ 7	Not applicable
• Pulmonary artery	≤ 25	≤ 15	≤ 18
• Left atrium (direct or indirect pulmonary capillary wedge	a ≤ 12 v ≤ 10	x ≤ 7 y ≤ 7	≤ 10
• Left ventricle	120	End-pressure ≤ 7 End-pressure on a ≤ 12	Not applicable

Table 12.2: *Oxygen saturation within the heart and great vessels*

Region	Normal sat. (%)	Sinus venosus defect (%)	Atrial septal defect (%)	Ventricular septal defect (%)	PDA (%)
Superior vena cava	75	85	75	75	75
Right atrium	75	85	85	75	75
Inferior vena cava	75	75	75	75	75
Right ventricle	75	85	85	85	75
Pulmonary artery	75	85	85	85	85
Left ventricle	95	95	95	95	

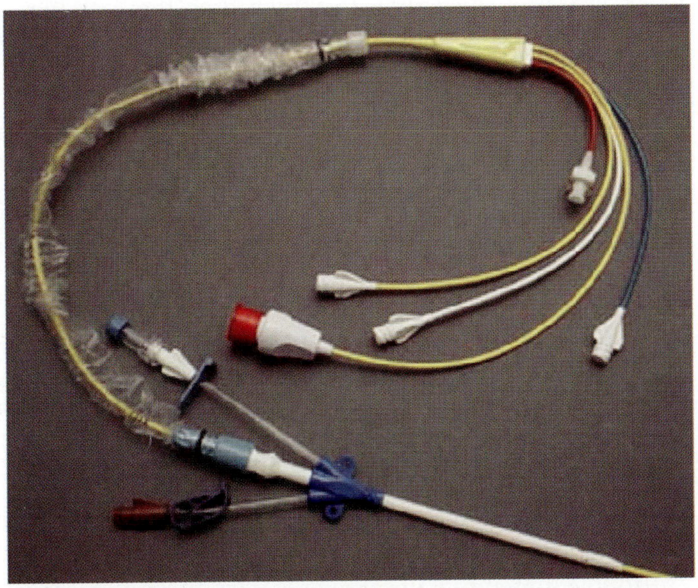

Fig. 12.44: *Multi-hub pulmonary artery catheter: This long catheter has 4 separate hubs on one end. The large hub is the themistor connector, and is used for thermodilution to assess cardiac output (more on that later). There is the distal lumen hub, which connects to a distal outlet on the tip of the catheter, and a proximal hub, which connects to a more proximal hub on the catheter. The fourth hub is a balloon inflation valve which is used to inflate a small balloon on the end of the catheter in order to attain pulmonary capillary wedge pressure (more on that later as well!) If you look closely, the length of the catheter has markings every 10 cm along its length to help the operator determine the position of the catheter within the vasculature and heart*

of which method is used. The wedge pressure recorded at the catheter tip is a more-or-less accurate measure of the left atrial pressure transmitted retrogradely through the pulmonary veins and capillaries.

Hemodynamic Evaluation of Valvular Stenosis

In the normal heart, there is no pressure gradient across an open valve. Such a gradient usually indicates valvular stenosis and, as stenosis worsens, the pressure is increased it. Provides therefore a useful index of the severity of stenosis. However, it must be recognized that the pressure gradient is itself influenced by the flow through the valve.

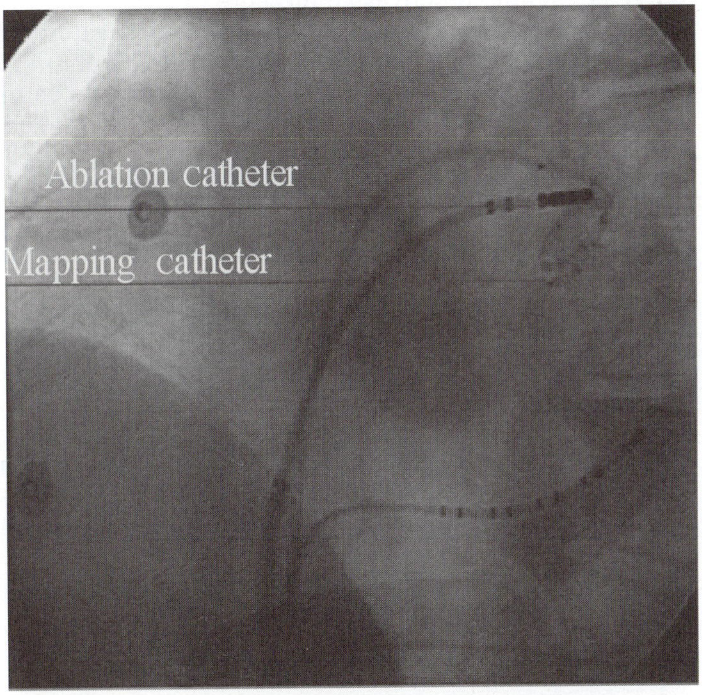

Fig. 12.45: *Fluoroscopic image of the circular mapping catheter and the ablation catheter during segmental pulmonary vein isolation, showing the anteroposterior view*

This applies particularly to the aortic valve because flow velocity is normally high (Figs 12.27 to 12.29).

Hemodynamic Evaluation of Intracardiac Shunts

Left-to-right intracardiac shunts through atrial or ventricular septal defects introduce 'arterialized' blood into the right side of the heart. This results in an abrupt increase or 'step-up' in the oxygen saturation of venous blood at the level of the shunt, which can be detected by right heart catheterization. Thus, by drawing serial blood samples for oxygen saturation from the pulmonary artery, right ventricle, right atrium and vena cava, the shunt may be localized to the site at which the step-up in oxygen saturation occurs. The magnitude of the step-up is related to the size of the shunt but precise quantification of the shunt requires measurement of pulmonary and systemic blood flow. The extent to which the pulmonary systemic flow ratio exceeds 1 is a measure of the size of the shunt (Fig. 12.44).

Measurement of Cardiac Output (Fig. 12.45)

Cardiac output is usually measured by application of the Fick principle. A Swan-Ganz catheter with a right atrial portal and a terminal thermistor is positioned in the pulmonary artery. A known volume of cold saline (usually 10 mL) is injected into the right atrium and the temperature reduction in the pulmonary artery is recorded at the thermistor. The contour of the cooling curve is dependent upon cardiac output, which is calculated by measurement of the area under the curve using a bedside computer. A relatively simple noninvasive measure of cardiac output can be obtained by Doppler echocardiography using the 'area-length' method. Thus, the length of the column of blood ejected by the left ventricle during a single beat is obtained by multiplying the Doppler aortic flow velocity (cm/second) by the ejection time (seconds). The length of the column of blood is then multiplied by the echocardiograpic cross sectional area of the aorta to yield stroke volume (mL/beat). Cardiac output is the product of stroke volume and heart rate.

Coronary Arteriography

Coronary arteriography is the only reliable technique for diagnostic imaging of the coronary arteries, it requires selective injection of contrast into the left and right coronary arteries and multiple views in different projections are necessary for a complete study. Intraluminal filling defects or occlusions indicate coronary artery disease, which is nearly always caused by atherosclerosis (Fig. 12.51).

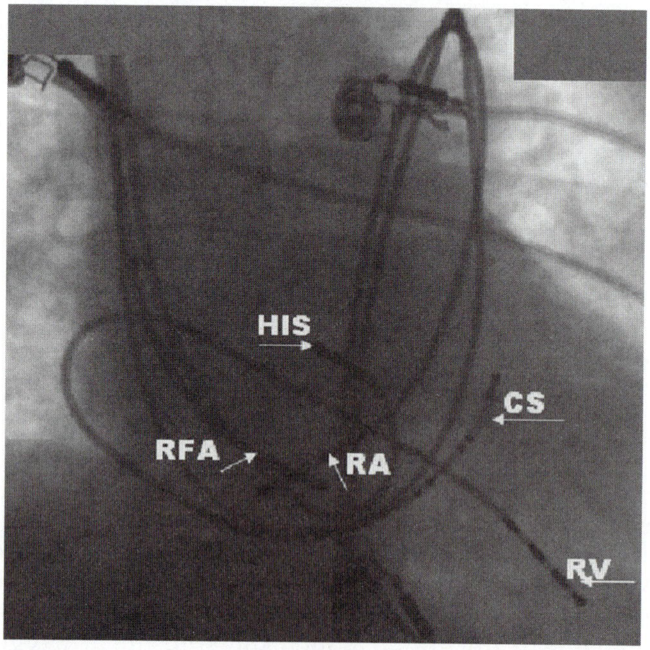

Fig. 12.46: *Fluoroscopy in the RAO view shows recording and ablation catheter positions. CS, coronary sinus catheter, HIS, HIS bundle catheter; RA, right atrial catheter; RV, right ventricle catheter; RFA, radiofrequency ablation catheter*

Crossing the Aortic Valve

1. ***Normal aortic valve:*** The pigtail catheter is most commonly used to cross native aortic valves. Tissue valves can also be crossed, but crossing mechanical valves (e.g. St. Jude, Bjork-Shiley, Medtronic-Hall) risks catheter entrapment and is best avoided. The catheter should be made to loop above the aortic valve. Pulling back very slowly, the catheter should give, and can then be rapidly advanced into the left ventricle during systole. Having the patient take a deep breath and hold it while the pigtail catheter is being unlooped can facilitate the passage of the catheter into the left ventricle. Sometimes, the guidewire itself may be useful in crossing the valve, in which case the catheter is simply advanced over the guidewire into the left ventricle. A single operator can cross the aortic valve without assistance, but if two operators are present, one can move the catheter and change its orientation while the other moves the wire back and forth. The pressure in the left ventricle is recorded continuously; the catheter is pulled back into the aorta in a single motion to determine the aortic pressure, and the pullback pressure gradient can be calculated.
2. ***Aortic stenosis:*** In more severe cases of aortic stenosis, difficulty may be encountered in passing any catheter across the aortic valve. In this circumstance, a 0.038 inch straight-tipped wire can be used to cross the valve. If this method is elected, some operators recommend a 5,000-U bolus of heparin. The timer should be started, and no more than 3–4 minutes should be allowed per attempt at crossing. Between each attempt the wire should be withdrawn and wiped, blood aspirated and a double lumen pigtail catheter is introduced to measure the left ventricular and aortic pressures simultaneously.

Left Ventriculography (Fig. 12.14)

1. **Setting up the view:** The pigtail catheter (commonly the angled version) is positioned in the midcavity of the left ventricle. The pigtail should look like a "6" in the RAO projection. If the pigtail twists with each beat, this indicates it is caught in the mitral valve apparatus and needs to be repositioned. The monitor should be observed for ectopy. Once a stable rhythm is present, ventriculography can proceed. First, the left ventricular end-diastolic pressure (LVEDP) should be measured on a 40 scale. In patients with an elevated LVEDP (greater than 25 mmHg), a left ventriculogram is generally contraindicated. If the decision to proceed with the left ventriculogram is made, sublingual nitroglycerin should first be given to lower the LVEDP. With more moderate degrees of left ventricular dysfunction, nonionic dye, which is less of a myocardial depressant, can be used. Digital subtraction can be used instead of cinefluoroscopy to obtain the left ventriculogram. This allows a smaller amount of contrast to be used. With digital subtraction, the view must be carefully centered because panning is not possible. The left ventriculogram is best avoided in

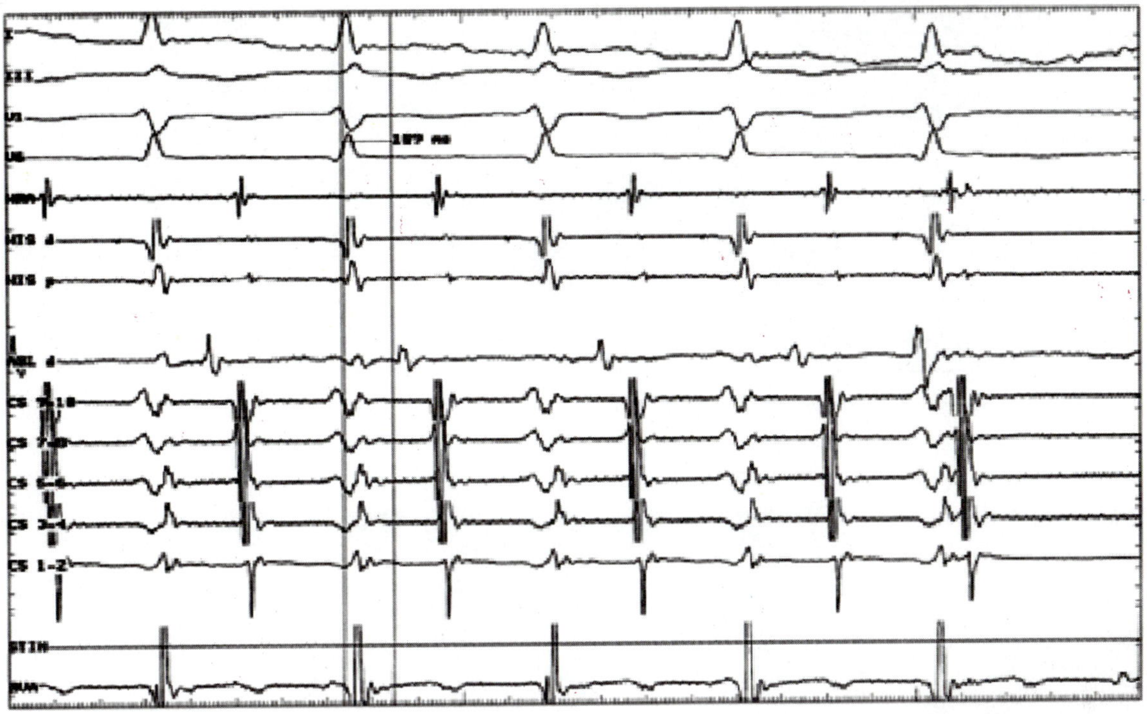

Fig. 12.47: *Surface leads and intracardiac electrograms during radiofrequency catheter ablation of the accessory pathway are shown. Application of energy led to termination of arrhythmia. The VA interval at successful ablation site is 109 msec. Recording speed: 100 mm/sec.*

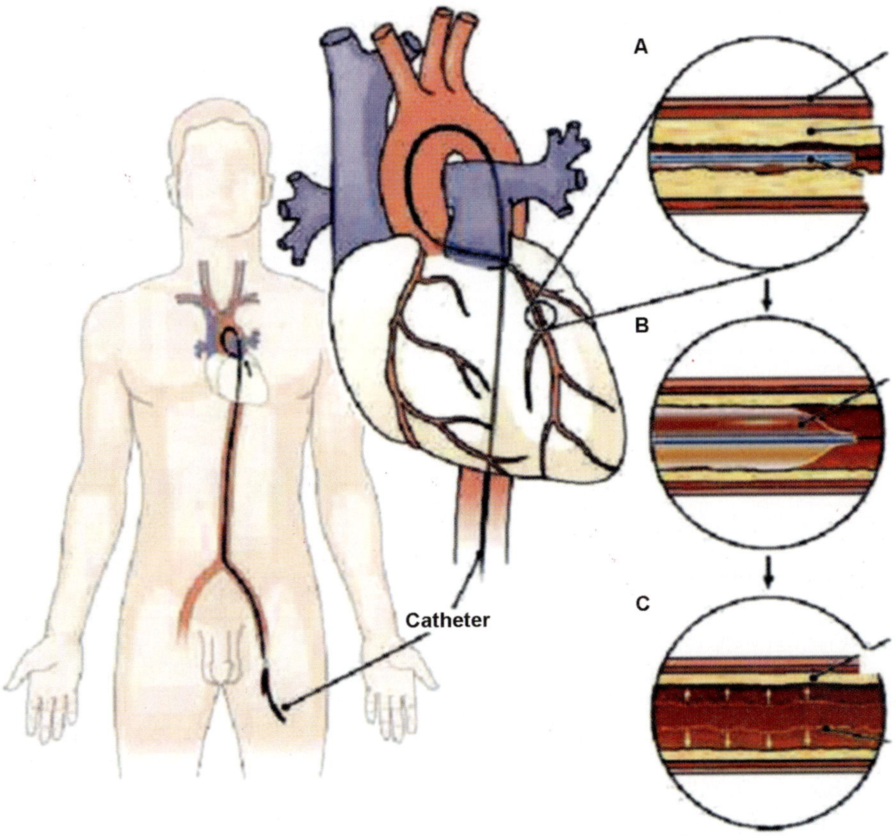

Fig. 12.48: *Illustration explains the intravascular path taken by balloon catheter to reach upto the obstructed coronary artery and finally dilated to its near normal lumen*

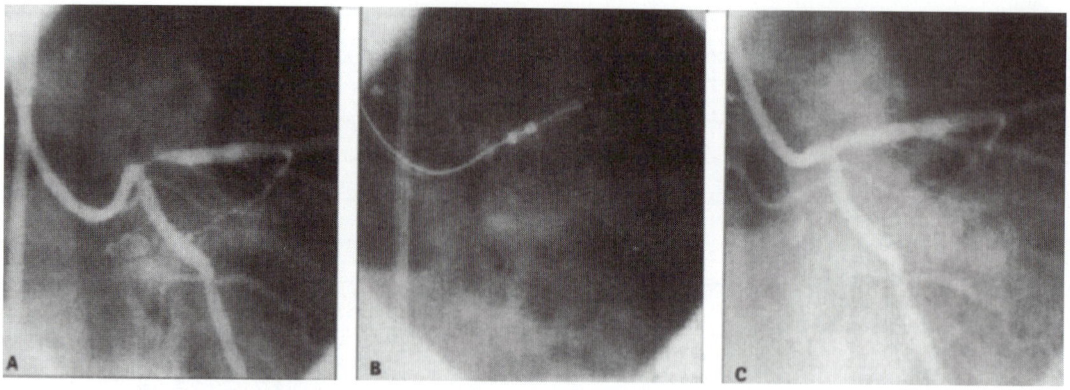

Fig. 12.49: *(A) Coronary angiography showing obstruction of LCx. (B) Stent in position with balloon (C) showing restoration of blood flow*

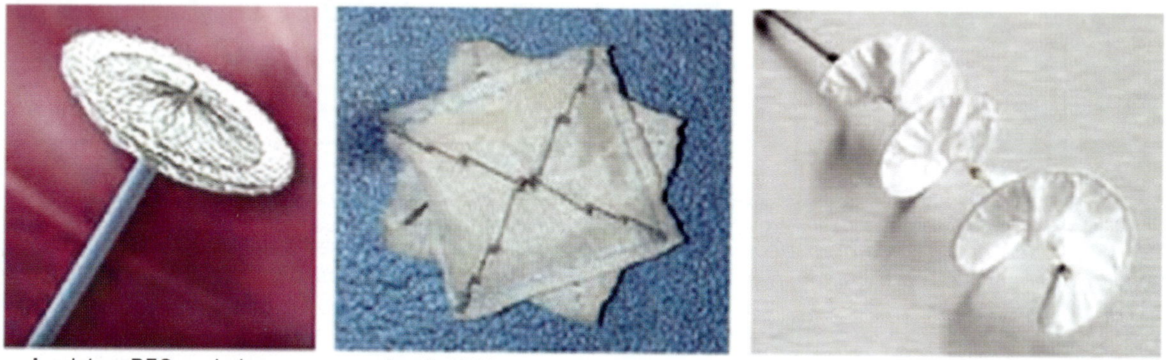

Amplatzer PFO occluder CardioSEAL septal occluder Gore helix Septal occluder

Fig. 12.50: *Different types of closure devices for management of congenital heart defects*

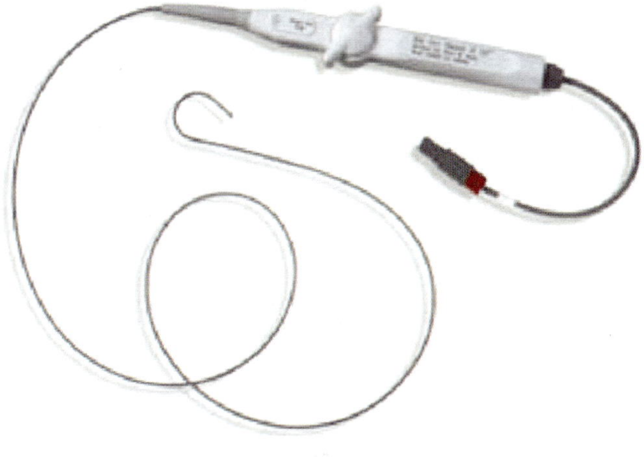

Fig. 12.51: *Radiofrequency ablation catheter*

patients with critical aortic stenosis, significant left main artery disease, or severe left ventricle dysfunction.

2. *Views:* The 30° RAO view is used to look at overall left ventricular function. In particular, the anterior, apical, and inferior walls can be assessed. Some operators routinely pan to the LIMA to assess its patency in a patient who might require CABG. The RAO view is also useful to assess mitral leaflet prolapse and MR. The LAO cranial view can also be used to assess MR,

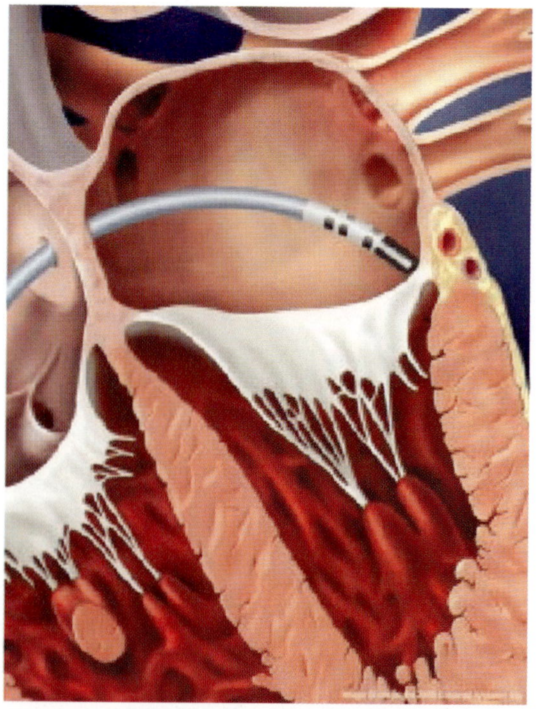

Fig. 12.52: *Radiofrequency ablation catheter close to one of the pulmonary veins after entering left atrium through foramen ovale*

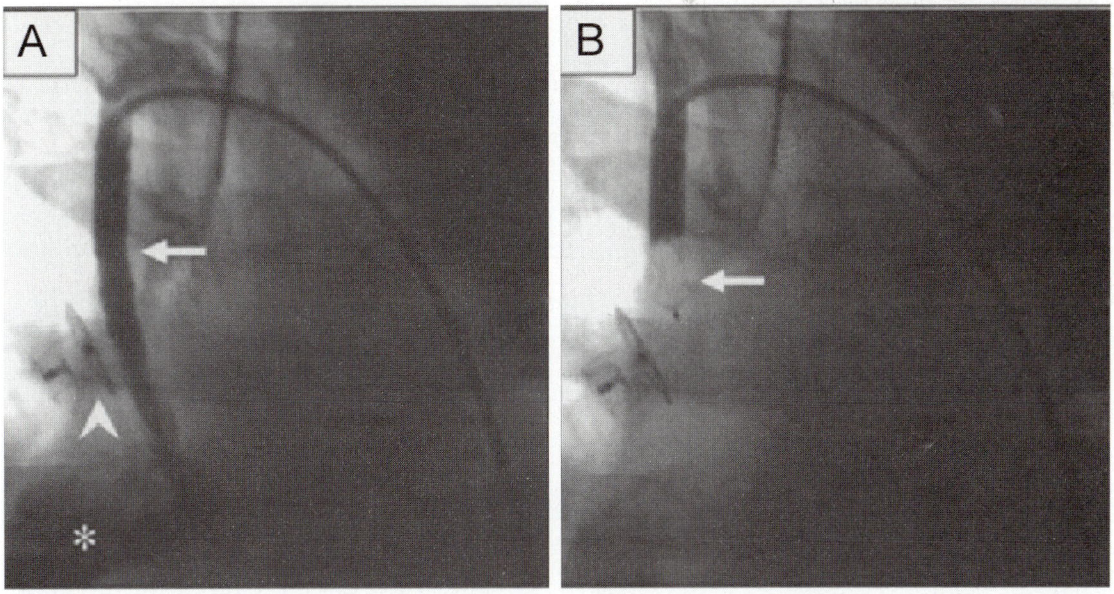

Fig. 12.53: *Occlusion of RSPA with AVP (patient 3). (A) permeable RSPA (arrow), right pulmonary artery (asterisk); ADO occluding fistula between innominate and right superior pulmonary veins (arrowhead). (B) AVP (arrow) occluding RSPA. ADO, amplatzer duct-occluder; AVP, amplatzer vascular plug; RSPA, right systemic-pulmonary anastomosis*

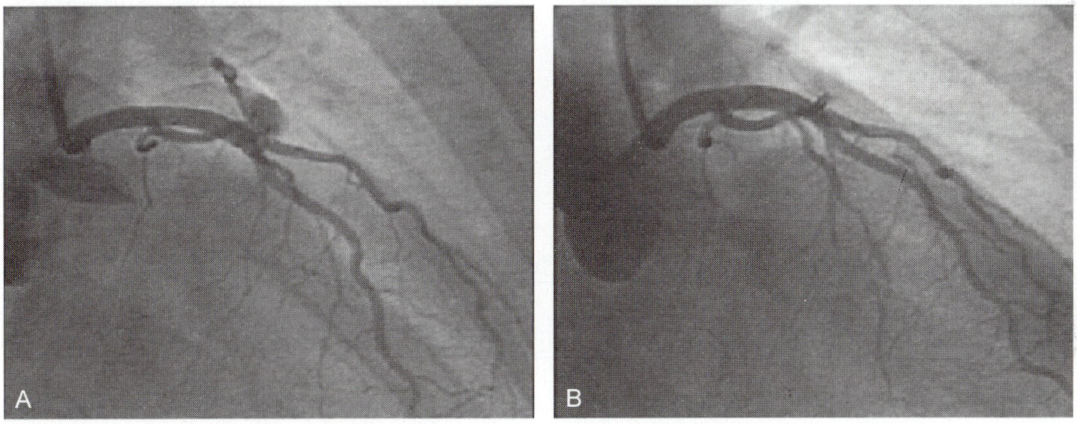

Fig. 12.54: *Coronary fistula between anterior descending artery and origin of pulmonary artery. Oblique right anterior projection before (A) and after (B) closure with coils*

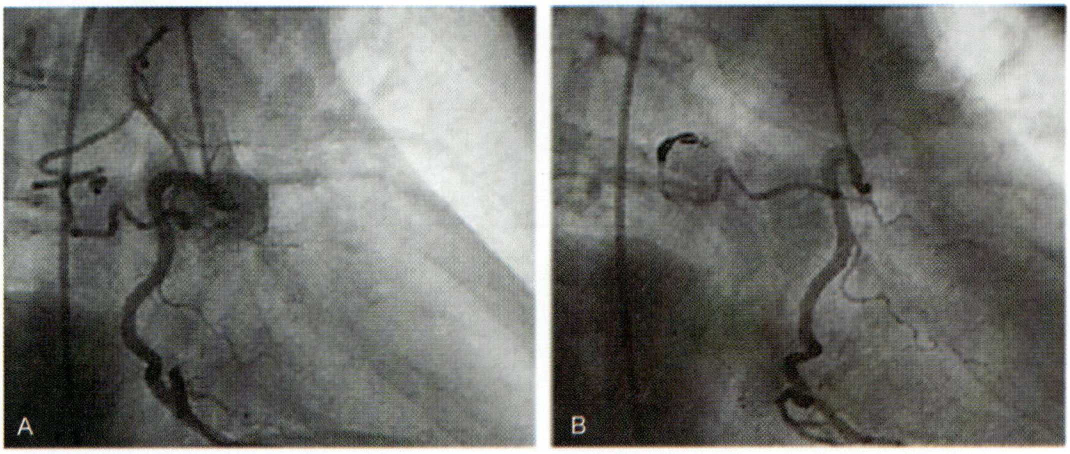

Fig. 12.55: *Fistula from right coronary artery to posterior segment of left lung. Images in oblique anterior right projection before (A) and after (B) closure with coils*

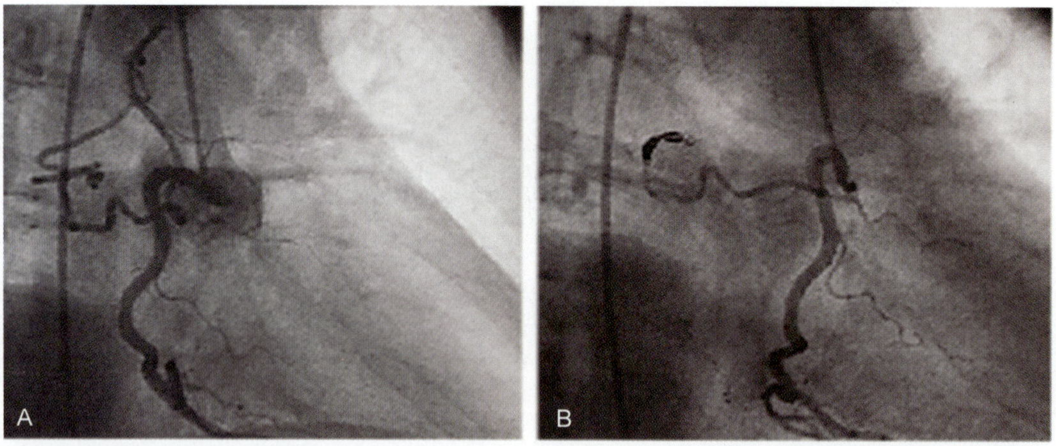

Fig. 12.56: *Fistula from right coronary artery to posterior segment of left lung. Images in oblique anterior right projection before (A) and after (B) closure with coils*

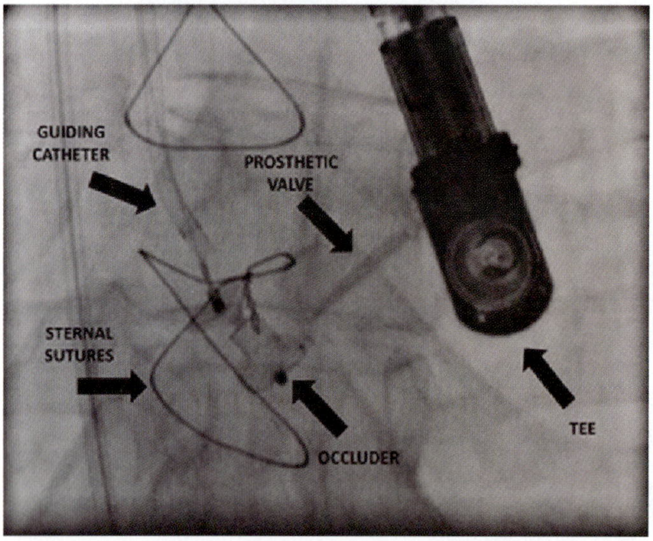

Fig. 12.57: *Aortic valve mechanical prosthesis paravalvular leak closed with AVP III*

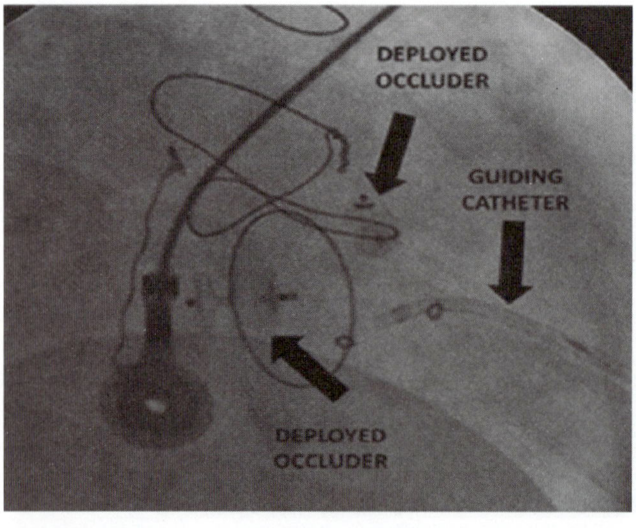

Fig. 12.58: *A mitral valve paravalvular leak closed with two AVP II occluders using the transapical approach*

and it avoids the overlap of the aorta with the left atrium that occurs in the RAO view. MR can be graded on a scale of *1 to 4:*

i. Represents trace MR, with mild left atrial opacification that clears with one beat.
ii. Represents a mild to moderate degree of opacification, though less than the left ventricle.
iii. Represents moderate to severe opacification of the left atrium equal to the left ventricle.
iv. Represents complete opacification of the left atrium greater than the left ventricle.

Panning toward the left atrium may be needed if MR is present. The catheter itself can cause MR if it is caught in the mitral valve apparatus or if it induces premature ventricular contractions. The correlation between angiographic and echocardiographic MR is excellent. The 60° LAO projection allows evaluation of the septum and the posterior and lateral walls. Ventricular septal defects are best identified in the LAO projection with slight cranial angulation. If biplane imaging capability exists, RAO and LAO views of the left ventricle can be obtained simultaneously.

3. ***Settings:*** For a ventriculogram, the flow injector can be set at a rate of 10–15 cm^3/s for a total volume of about 35–50 cm^3, with a rate rise of 0.4 (to minimize ectopy and to keep the catheter from moving abruptly) and a pressure of 600. The exact settings will vary depending on the size of the heart and the need to limit contrast.

Aortography: Aortography is usually performed in the LAO position, with the catheter about 2 cm above the aortic leaflets. Compared to a ventriculogram, a larger volume of contrast is needed to opacify the aorta. The flow injector is set to a higher total volume than for the left ventriculogram, usually about 60 cm^3 at 20–25 cm^3/s. No rate rise is necessary (other than to keep smaller catheters from moving), and a pressure limit of 600 is used. Aortic insufficiency can be identified with a grading system similar to that for MR:

1. Represents trace aortic insufficiency that clears from the left ventricle with each beat

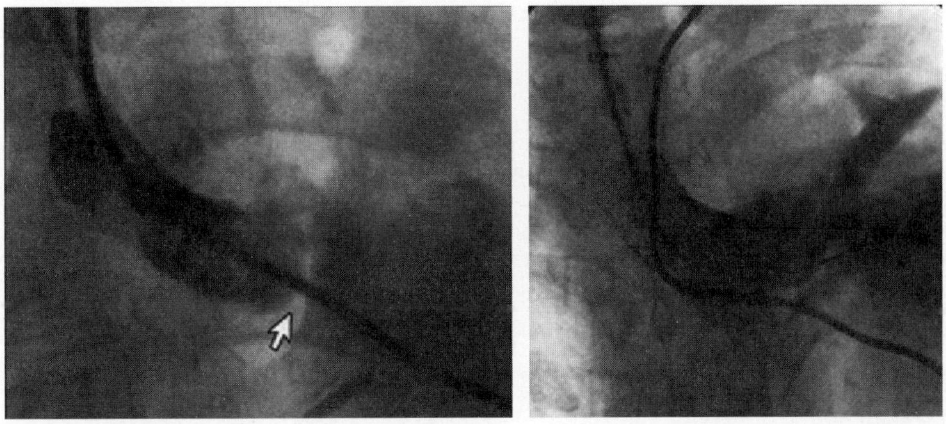

Fig. 12.59: *Complete superior vena cava occlusion in a 16-year-old patient with mustard operation and pacing lead in situ, who presented with near syncopal episodes and exercise intolerance. The obstruction (left, arrow) was relieved after placement of 3 Palmaz stents (right). A new pacing system was inserted a few days later*

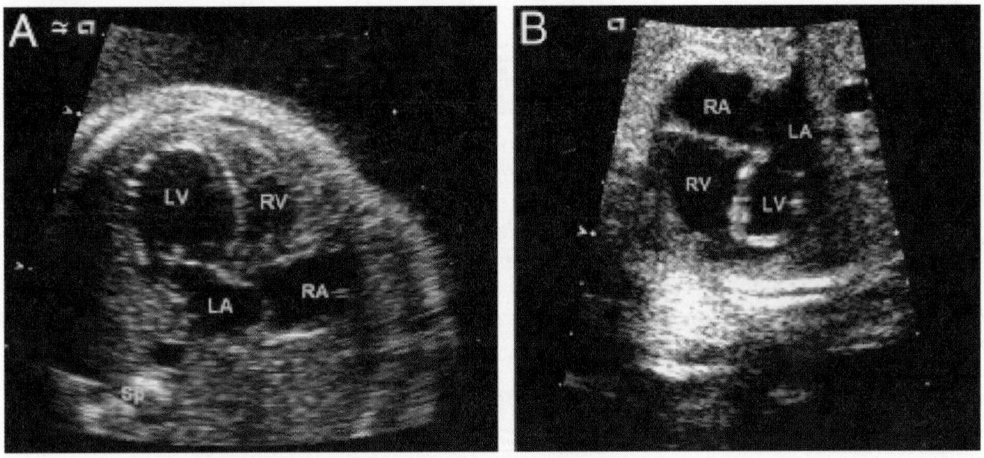

Fig. 12.60: *Fetal echocardiograms (A) Four chamber view of a fetal echocardiogram at 20 weeks' gestation demonstrates a dilated left ventricle with echo bright endocardium suggestive of endocardial fibroelastosis. The position of the atrial septum suggests abnormal left atrial to right atrial shunting in utero. (B) Four chambers view of a fetal echocardiogram in the same fetus imaged at 33 weeks' gestation demonstrates that the left ventricle has become hypoplastic. The echo bright endocardium is even more evident. LA, left atrium; LV, left ventricle; RA, right atrium; RV, right ventricle; Sp, spine*

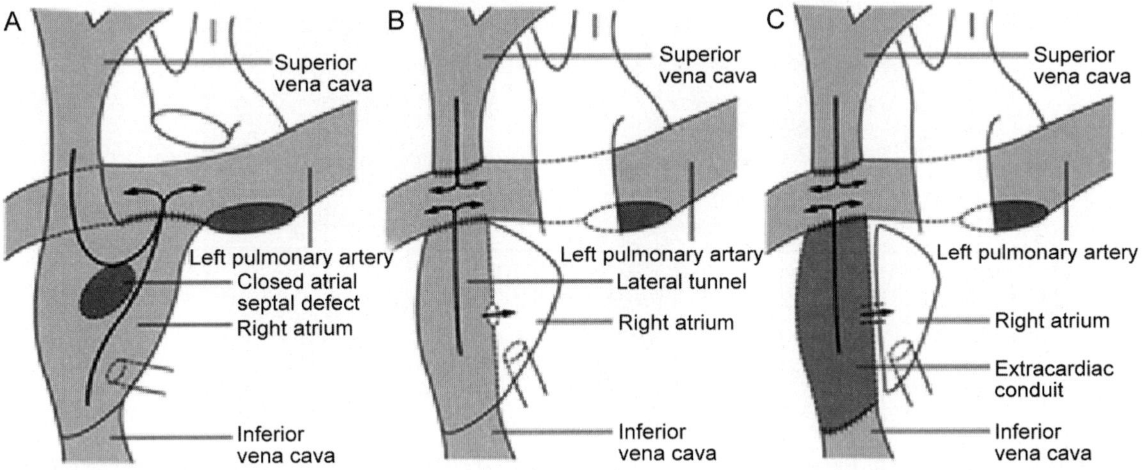

Fig. 12.61: *Fontan surgical techniques the original atriopulmonary fontan (A) has been replaced with the lateral tunnel (B) and extracardiac conduit (C) Fontan*

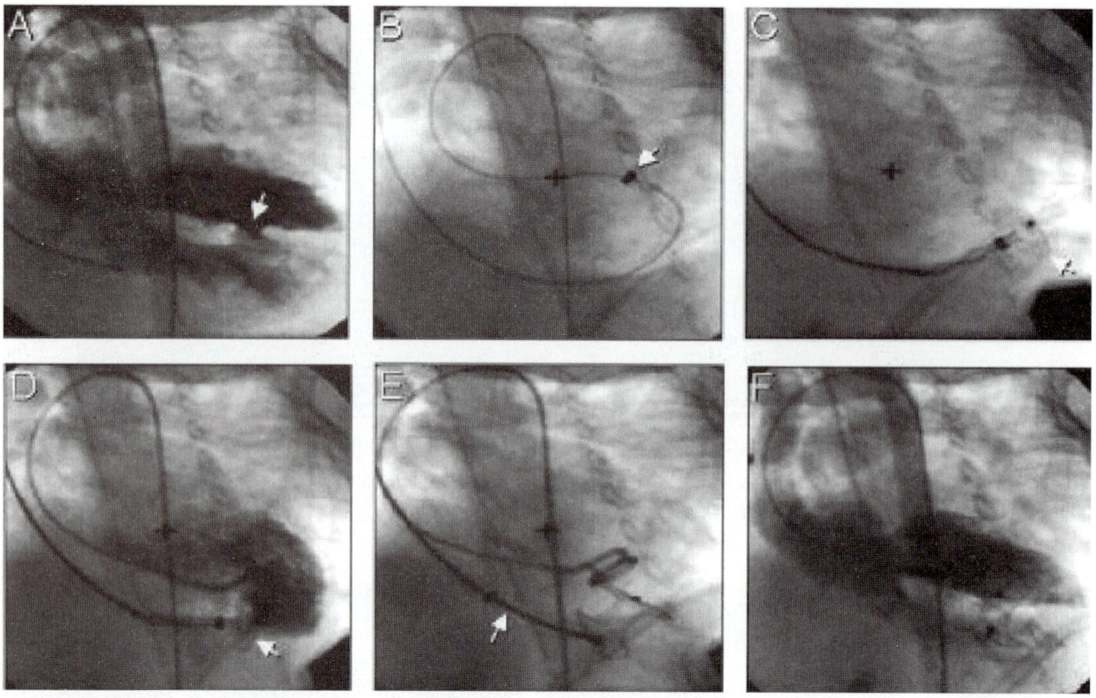

Fig. 12.62: *Angiogram in a 9-month old, 8.4-kg child during transcatheter closure of muscular VSD using an Amplatzerâ muscular VSD occluder. (A) Left ventricle (LV) angiogram in the four-chamber view demonstrating a 7.2 mm mid-muscular VSD (arrow). (B) Cine image demonstrating a 7 Fr Cook sheath (arrow) from the right internal jugular vein through the VSD with an exchange guide wire forming an arteriovenous loop from the jugular vein out the femoral artery. (C) Cine-image demonstrating passage of the device (arrow) out the distal part of the sheath while pulling the wire from the jugular vein. The LV disk is deployed (arrow) in the LV, note there is a pigtail in the LV for angiography. (D) An angiogram in the LV while the LV disk (arrow) was positioned in place. (E) Cine image releasing the device from the cable (arrow). (F) An angiogram in the left ventricle after the device has been released revealing good device position and no, residual shunt*

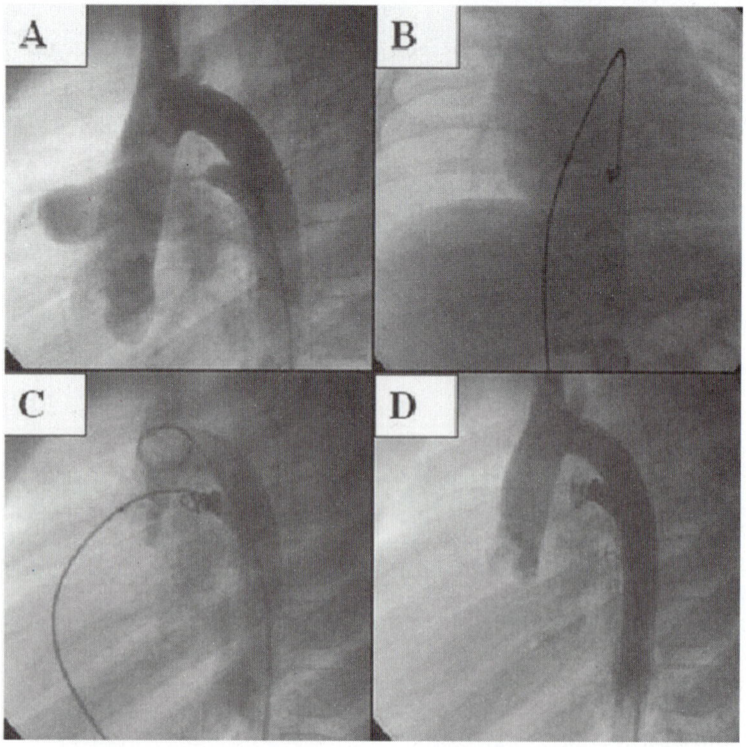

Fig. 12.63: *Angiographic sequence of the implantation of the Nit-Occlud device in patent ductus arteriosus. (A) Lateral arteriography showing the ductal morphology. (B) and (C) Presenting and positioning of the device. (D) Implanted device, with no immediate residual shunt*

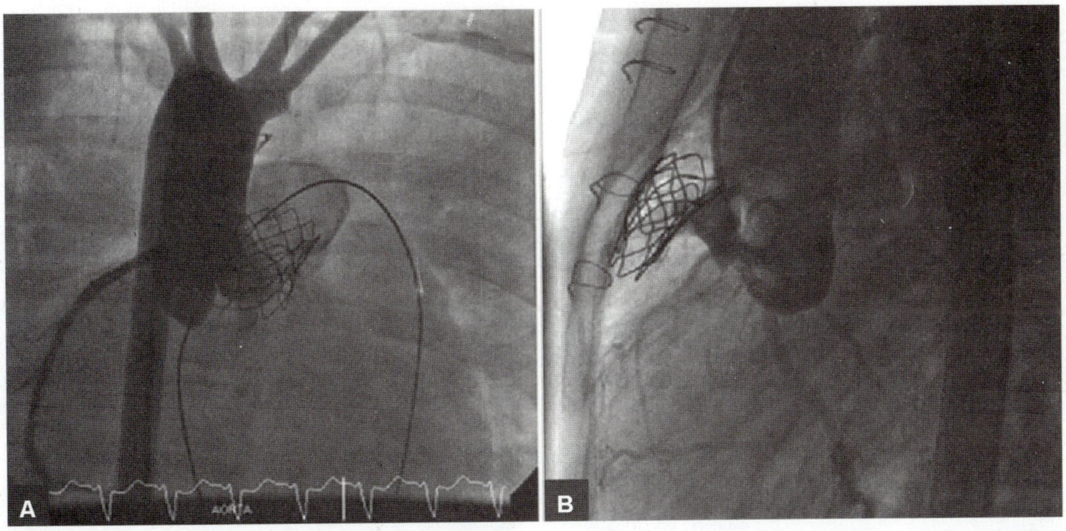

Fig. 12.64: *(A) Left coronary artery occlusion after melody stent implantation. (B) Massage flow was reestablished after external cardiac*

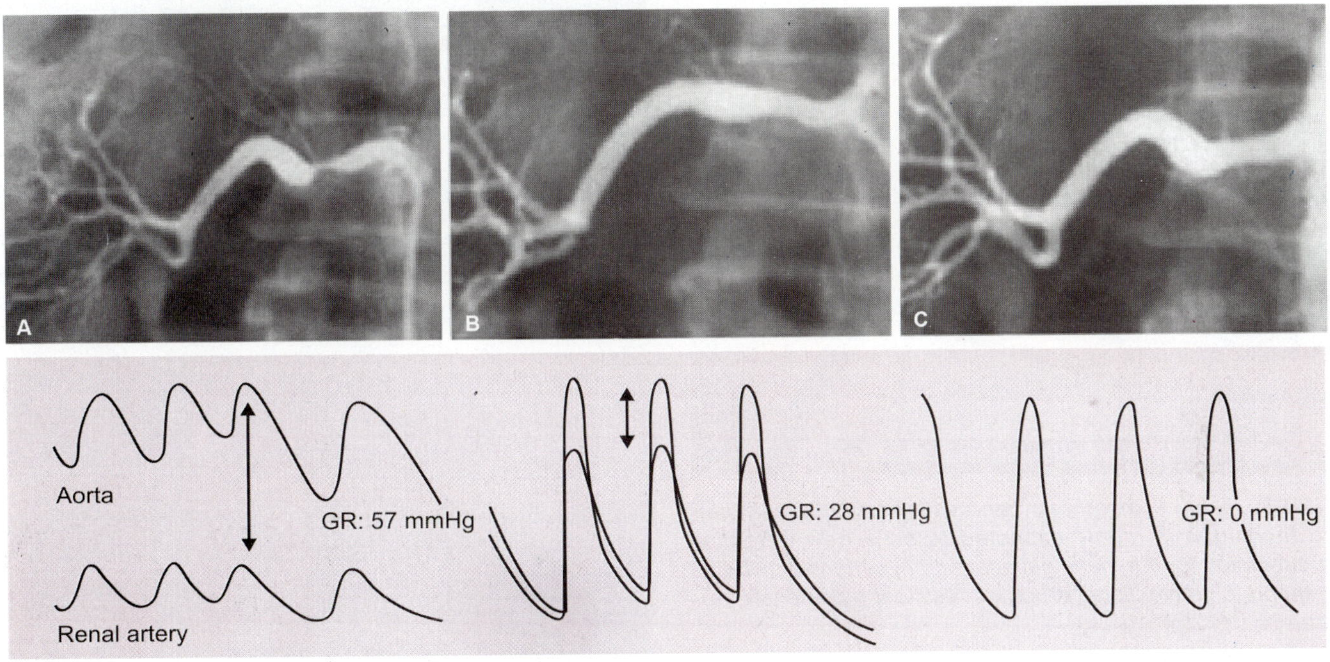

Fig. 12.65: *Treatment of renal artery stenosis with balloon angioplasty and stenting. (A) Angiogram showing substantial narrowing of the renal artery and a systolic pressure gradient of 57 mmHg. (B) After balloon angioplasty, the angiographic stenosis is improved with a residual translesional gradient of 28 mmHg. (C) Following stent placement, minor angiographic improvement is evident, but the hemodynamic gradient has completely resolved*

2. Represents mild left ventricular opacification that takes more than one beat to clear;
3. Represents moderate left ventricular opacification equal to the aortic root; and
4. Represents complete opacification of the left ventricle greater than the aortic root. Diseases of the aorta such as aneurysms or dissection can also be identified. An aortogram can also aid in nonselective visualization of anomalous coronary arteries or grafts that are difficult to engage. However, the absence of filling of a bypass graft on an aortogram does not exclude its presence. The aorta must be well and heavily opacified to ensure that grafts are seen.

Renal Angiography (Figs 12.67–12.69)

An aortogram can be performed with the pigtail catheter placed in the descending aorta slightly above the level of the origins of the renal arteries (L1 vertebral body) to rule out renal artery stenosis. A JR 4 catheter can be used to obtain selective renal arteriograms by turning the tip of the catheter so that it points to either the left or right in the posteroanterior view. The catheter is then pulled gradually

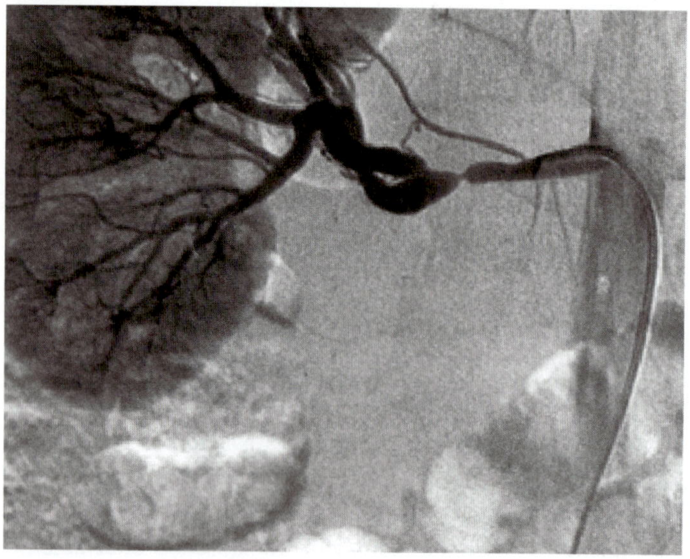

Fig. 12.66: *Selective renal angiography in patient with renal artery stenosis due to fibromuscular dysplasia*

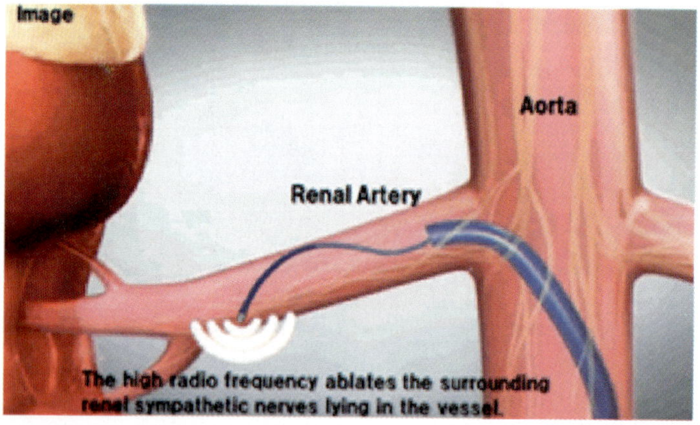

Fig. 12.67: *Renal sympathetic denervation using a catheter-based technique is highly expected to be a new, effective treatment option for the many patients with hypertension who do not respond to conventional drugs, or resistant hypertension*

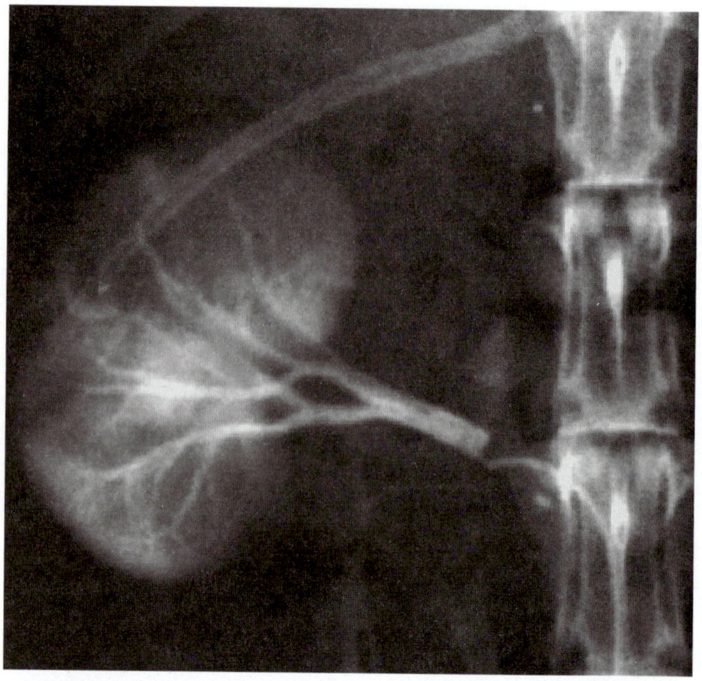

Fig. 12.68: *Renal sympathetic nerve ablation for refractory hypertension*

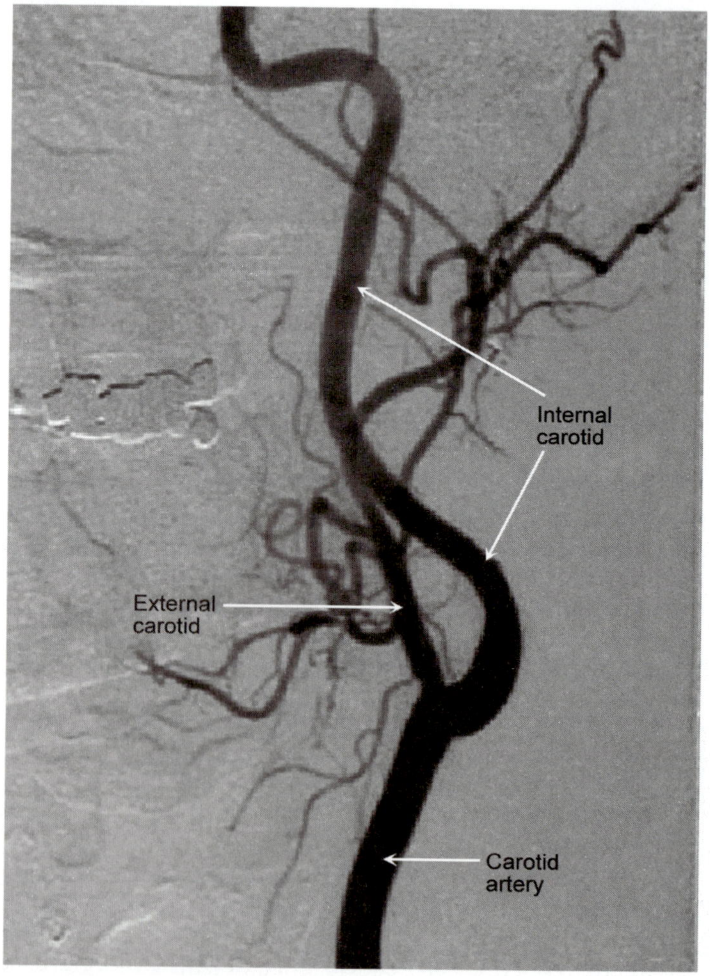

Fig. 12.69: *Normal carotid angiogram*

back when it is in the vicinity of the renal artery ostia until it engages. Digital acquisition should be used.

Carotid angiography is sometimes necessary to confirm the degree of carotid artery stenosis seen on a noninvasive study. A variety of catheters (the Headhunter and Newton series) can be used to selectively cannulate the common carotid artery. These catheters are advanced to the aortic arch over a guidewire and pulled back to engage the artery of interest. A Newton 5 can be used to engage the right common carotid artery and Newton 2, with its smaller curve, can be used to engage the left common carotid artery. There is a 0.5–1% risk of stroke with this procedure. Digital acquisition and use of nonionic contrast are mandatory (Figs 12.70 and 12.71).

Provocative testing: In patients in whom coronary artery spasm is suspected, intravenous methylergonovine can be given to provoke spasm. Once significant angiographic

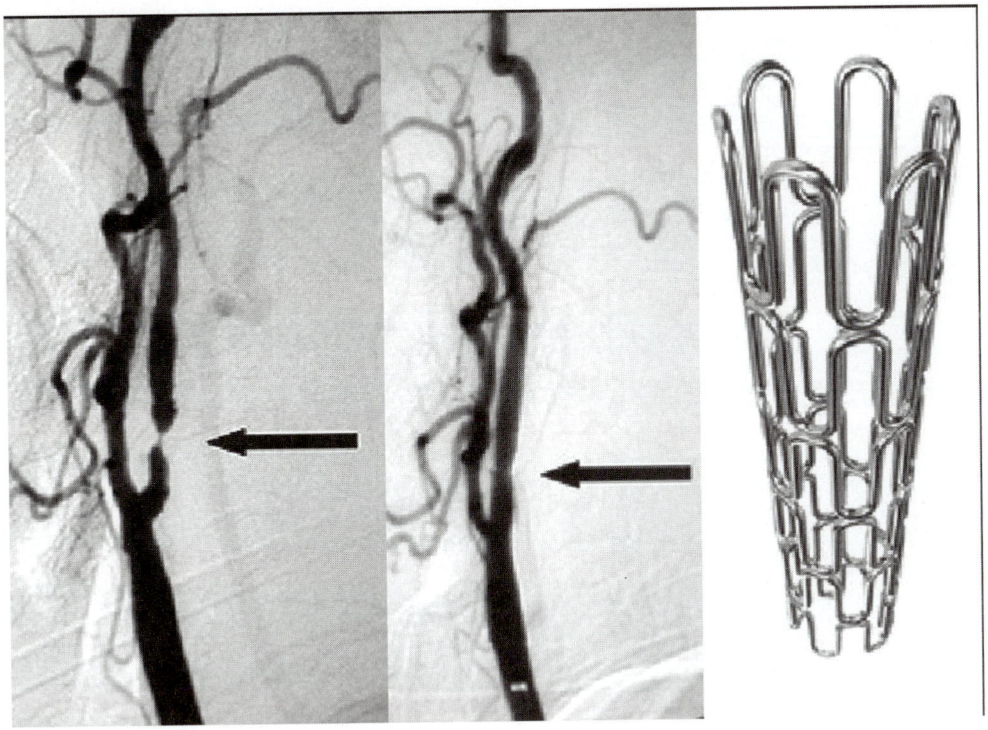

Fig. 12.70: (Left) Angiogram showing carotid stenosis and (middle) the reopening of the carotid artery after angioplasty and stent placement. (Right) Photograph of actual stent used

stenosis has been ruled out, 0.05 mg of intravenous methylergonovine is administered. If the patient develops his or her typical chest pain or ST elevation on electrocardiographic monitoring, the coronary arteries are catheterized immediately.

The electrocardiographic changes can help to determine which coronary artery to cannulate first. If there are no electrocardiographic changes or chest pain, the right coronary (which is statistically more likely to have spasm) and then the left coronary should be recatheterized 5 minutes after the methylergonovine has been administered. A positive response consists of a focal area of spasm that is relieved by intracoronary nitroglycerin (a usual dose of 100–200 µg). Diffuse spasm can be physiologic, and is also managed with nitroglycerin and verapamil. Since the half-life of methylergonovine is longer than that of sublingual nitroglycerin, it is important to realize that spasm can recur after a dose of nitroglycerin. If the initial dose of methylergonovine does not provoke a response, an additional dose of 0.2 mg can be given a few minutes after the first. Alternatively, some operators prefer giving a single dose of 0.2 mg.

Postcatheterization Care

A. ***Sheath removal:*** The sheath is removed once the procedure is complete. Adequate local anesthesia should be reinjected if the previously given dose has lost its efficacy. After the sheath is removed, hemostasis is generally obtained with direct manual pressure of the fingertips over the pulse, without sterile gauze to obscure the view. Pressure is held for approximately 20 minutes (about 3 minutes for each French size) until there is no bleeding. To shorten the time of manual pressure, a new device called the Syvek 'patch (Marine Polymer technologies) is available. This is paper-based and is made up of algae. It is supposed to accelerate the process of hemostasis when used on the skin over the arteriotomy site while holding manual pressure. Another, similar device is the Chito Seal (Abbott), which is a patch that can be applied to stop bleeding from femoral arteriotomy sites. Manual pressure is held for about 10 minutes when using this patch. In patients who have coagulopathy, poorly controlled hypertension, or aortic regurgitation with a wide pulse pressure, a longer duration of pressure is necessary. Care must be taken to intermittently allow adequate blood flow to the distal extremity. It is therefore best if one can directly visualize the extremity to assess its color. If both arterial and venous sheaths are present, it is best to remove the venous sheath first and obtain hemostasis before removing the arterial sheath. In patients with severe aortic stenosis or significant left main coronary artery disease, laboratory personnel should be prepared to rapidly manage a vagal episode, which can be life-threatening in these situations. Adequate administration of anesthesia before removal of the sheath decreases the chance of a vagal reaction.

Bed rest is generally required for 6 hours after a femoral sheath is removed, though some operators require 1 hour for each French size. In fact, 2.5 hours is a

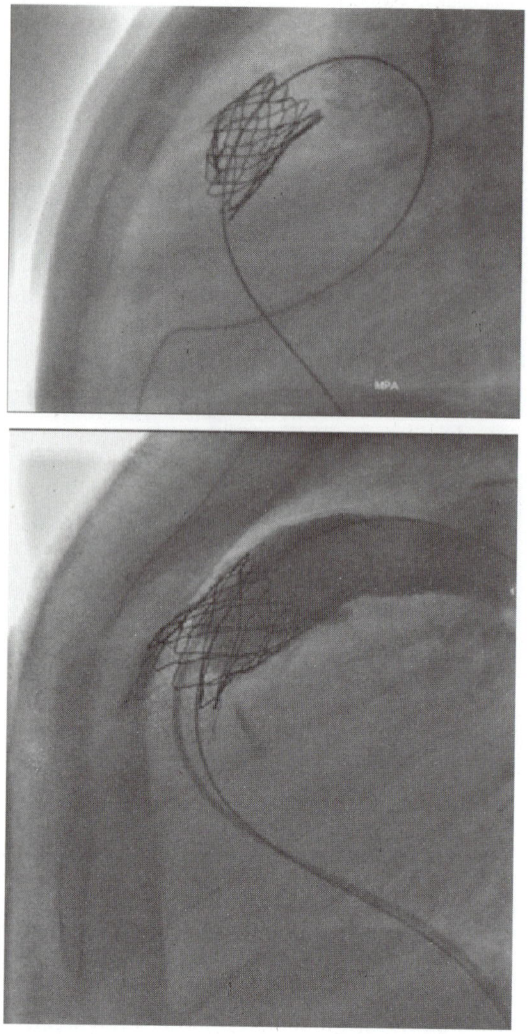

Fig. 12.71: *(Upper) Fracture of the stent due to compression by RVOT muscle bundles. (Lower) Shows use of multiple bare metal stents to relieve long segment stenosis and provide a landing zone for the melody valve*

sufficient period of bed rest for 5F sheaths. Two hours of keeping the arm straight is necessary after a brachial or radial procedure.

During the postprocedure observation period it is necessary to monitor heart rate, temperature, blood pressure, urine output, distal pulses, and the access site (for pain, bleeding, or hematoma).

The use of sandbags placed over the groin site is discouraged. Before discharge it is best to have the patient ambulate under observation. Specific discharge instructions should include the possibility of late access-site bleeding and the need to hold pressure and call for emergency help. Intravenous fluids are often given after a cardiac catheterization. The osmotic load of the contrast dye can cause a large diuresis. Intravenous fluids (e.g. normal saline at 100 cm^3/hour for several hours) can prevent volume depletion. Care should be used in patients with a history of congestive heart failure, in whom liberal intravenous fluids could contribute to pulmonary edema.

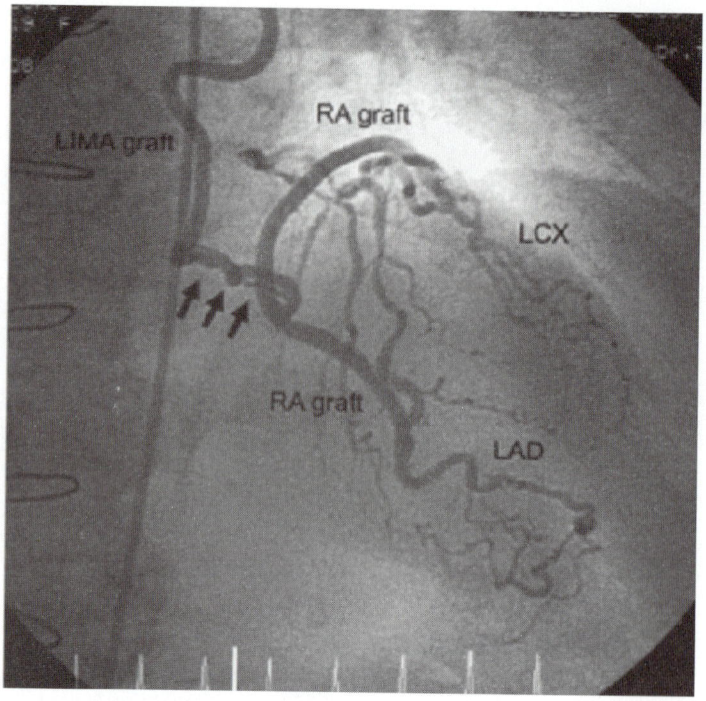

Fig. 12.72: *Cardiac catheterization performed 2 years after the coronary artery bypass grafting surgery showed a spiral dissection of left internal mammary artery (LIMA) graft. RA indicates radial artery*

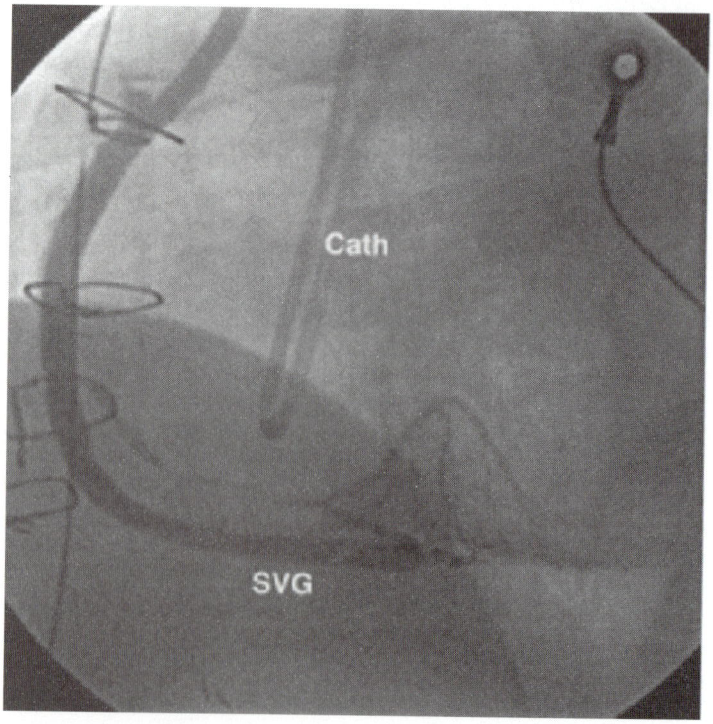

Fig. 12.73: *Severe native coronary artery spasm of the posterior descending artery. Saphenous vein graft (SVG) bypass to*

B. ***Compression/closure devices:*** The use of femoral artery closure devices offers the advantages of improved patient comfort, potentially lower complication rates,

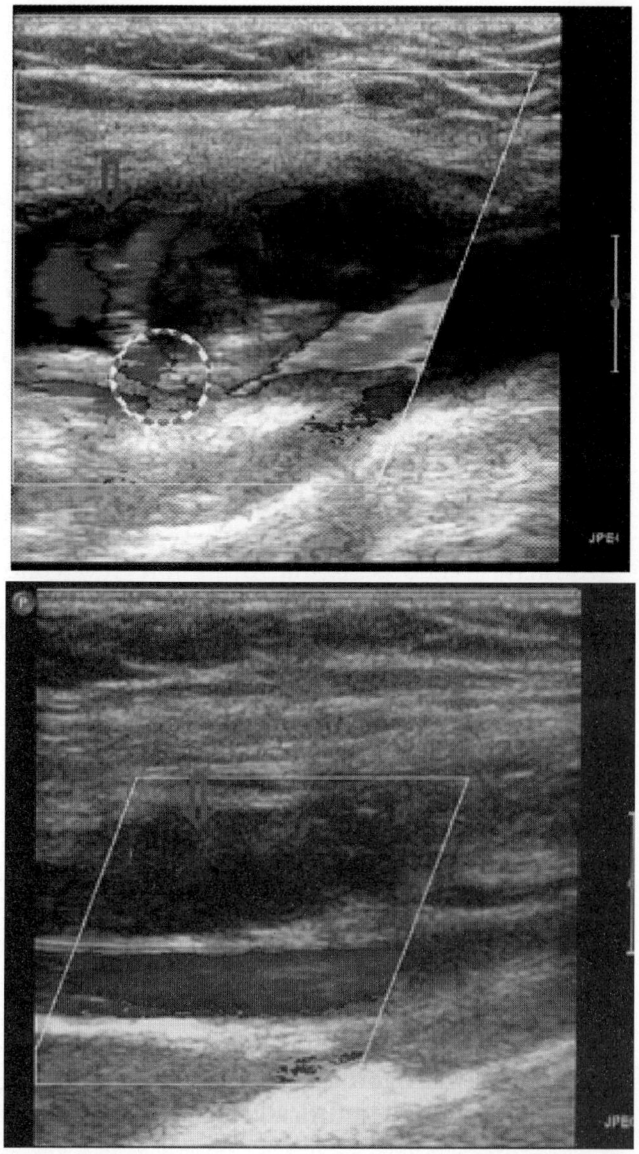

Fig. 12.74: *Upper panel echocardiographic scan of femoral artery showing pseudoaneurysm pre-compression (arrow). Broken circle revealing "neck" of the pseudoaneurysm following a complication of cardiac catheterization. Lower panel showing closure of aneurysmal cavity (arrow) after compression therapy*

early sheath removal, early hospital discharge, and in some patients anticoagulation may be continued without interruption. The currently available products include compression devices such as the FemoStop (RADI Medical Systems) and the C clamp, biosealants (Duett, vascular solutions), collagen plugs (Vasoseal; Datascope), vascular sandwiches (Angioseal; Daig), and percutaneous sutures (Perclose, Prostar, Techstar; Abbott).

Complications of Catheterization in General

A. *Death:* There is a 0.1% risk of death from left heart catheterization (LHC). This risk is substantially higher in patients undergoing urgent catheterization for acute coronary syndromes. In addition, patients with left main coronary artery disease, severe aortic stenosis, or severe left ventricular dysfunction are known to be patient subgroups with a particularly increased risk. Advanced age increases the risk of death.

B. *Myocardial infarction:* There is a 0.05% risk of MI from LHC. Myocardial infarction can result from coronary dissection, disruption of a preexisting atheromatous plaque, a large air embolus, or a thrombus. Patients with acute coronary syndromes have a higher risk of MI.

C. *Stroke:* Stroke occurs in 0.05% of catheterizations. There is a risk of stroke from an inadvertent air embolus or thrombus. Presence of aortic atheroma is a risk factor for embolic complications. Dislodgment of atheromatous debris in the aorta can lead to a stroke. This risk can be minimized by use of 260-cm exchange wires for catheter changes in patients with known severe aortic disease.

D. *Coronary artery dissection:* Engagement of the coronary arteries can rarely cause dissection. It is most often due to injection of contrast through a catheter that is not coaxial to the coronary artery, causing rupture of a preexisting plaque, or placement of the catheter too deeply into the coronary artery (so-called deep throating). Particular caution should be used with Amplatz catheters. In cases of left main coronary artery dissection, a stent can be placed emergently and the patient can be placed on peripheral cardiopulmonary support until the surgical team can be mobilized.

E. *Coronary artery spasm:* Engagement of the coronary arteries, in particular the RCA, can. cause spasm. This is best treated with withdrawal of the catheter. Subsequent reengagement and administration of intracoronary nitroglycerin (100–200 μg) may also be necessary for more rapid resolution of spasm (Fig. 12.74).

F. *Renal failure:* Contrast dye can precipitate renal failure in any patient, although certain patients (those with elevated creatinine, diabetes, proteinuria or dehydration) are at higher risk. Adequate prehydration with normal saline can reduce this risk. In some cases (especially in diabetics with renal insufficiency and those with renal artery stenosis), patients may need to be admitted to the hospital for hydration with 0.45% saline for several hours before the left heart catheterization (LHC) to minimize risk of contrast-induced nephrotoxicity. The best way to minimize contrast-induced renal failure is limiting the amount of dye used. Using less than 30 cm^3 of contrast dye dramatically reduces the incidence of renal failure in even the highest-risk patients. Biplane cineangiography can maximize the amount of information obtained with each view.

G. *Emergency coronary artery bypass graft:* There is a risk of needing emergency CABG as a complication of the catheterization (e.g. dissection of the left main coronary artery). There is also the possibility of identification of critical disease, such as severe left main coronary artery disease, that may prompt emergency CABG as the most expedient treatment.

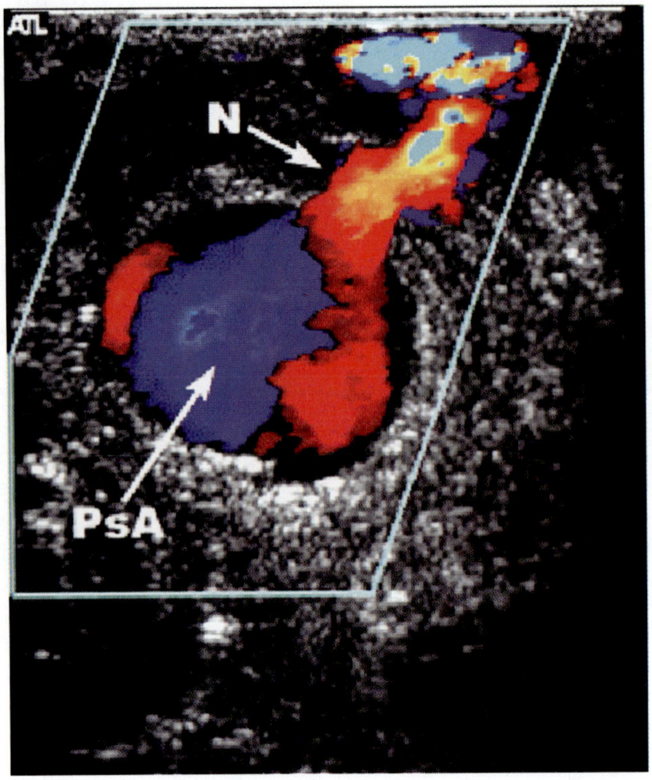

Fig. 12.75: *Color Doppler US image of the pseudoaneurysm clearly depicts the pseudoaneurysmal neck (N) and the yin-yang (red-blue) Doppler US appearance of the pseudoaneurysmal sac (PsA)*

H. ***Arrhythmias:*** A risk of ventricular fibrillation (0.5%) exists with catheterization. This rhythm is treated with electrical defibrillation. In particular, over injection of contrast into the RCA can cause ventricular fibrillation. Contrast dye (less so nonionic dye) can cause transient bradycardia, best dealt with by having the patient cough and by minimizing the amount of dye injected with each angiographic procedure.

I. ***Heart failure:*** The osmotic load of contrast dye can put a patient with diminished cardiac or renal function into overt pulmonary edema. In patients with severe cardiac or renal disease, injection of contrast should be limited and use of nonionic, low-osmolar dye should be considered.

J. ***Vagal reaction:*** If a patient develops hypotension and/or bradycardia, a vagal reaction should be considered. It is common to see this when local anesthetic is being administered or when the sheath is being removed. Atropine 1 mg IV should be available and given in these situations. Adeqpate anesthesia can help to prevent such reactions. In a patient with severe aortic stenosis or left main coronary artery disease, a vagal reaction can lead to death. Levophed (about 10 μg) should always available and used immediately in such cases of hypotension.

K. **Vascular** (Fig. 12.75 to 12.77)

1. ***Femoral:*** Pseudoaneurysms, arteriovenous fistulas, arterial thrombosis, and peripheral emboli are possible vascular complications. Careful technique can minimize these events. In particular, paying attention to puncture location and obtaining adequate hemostasis after sheath removal are the best ways to decrease vascular complications. For example, the smaller sheaths (5F) are preferred in patients with significant peripheral vascular disease. Frequent aspiration and discarding of blood from the arterial sheath, followed by gentle flushing, is useful (Fig. 12.78).

If an attempted cannulation is unsuccessful but an arterial puncture has been made, the needle should be withdrawn and adequate manual pressure held (about 5 minutes). If an venous puncture has been made inadvertently, the needle should be removed and pressure held (for about 3 minutes). Proceeding directly to arterial puncture without removing the needle and holding pressure increases the chance of arteriovenous fistula formation. If a venous puncture is planned, it should be made lower than the arterial puncture site. Bruits should be auscultated both before and after the procedure. A new bruit may indicate a vascular complication. Ultrasound is an essential part of the management of groin complications. If there is a large pseudo aneurysm present, surgery may be required after a trial of ultrasound-guided compression. Small pseudoaneurysms (less than 2 cm) tend to close spontaneously but should be followed by serial ultrasound examinations. An arteriovenous fistula that does not close spontaneously in 2–4 weeks may require surgical repair.

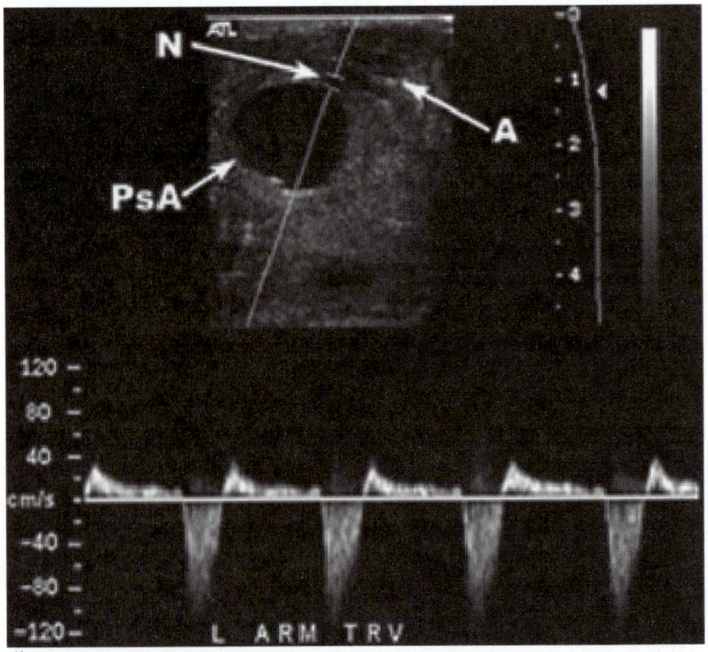

Fig. 12.76: *Duplex Doppler US image depicts a pseudoaneurysm (PsA) with bidirectional flow within the neck (N). The donor artery supplying the pseudoaneurysm can also be seen (A)*

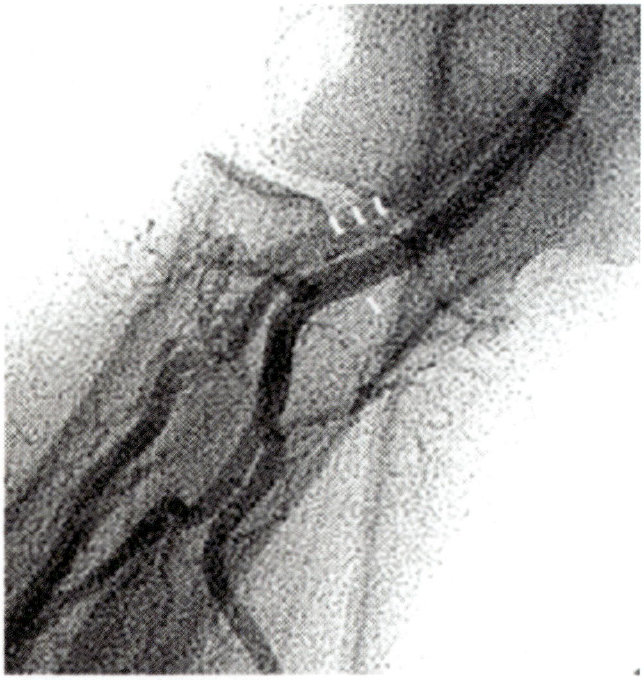

Fig. 12.77: *Arteriovenous fistula as a complication of a radial perforation (angiography at 6 months). The trajectory of the vein is marked by arrows*

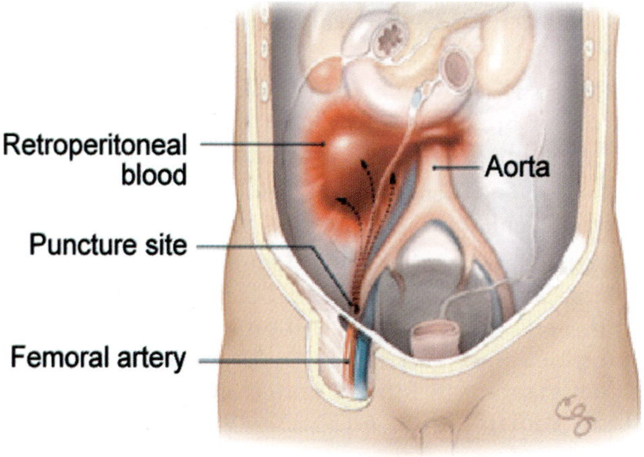

Fig. 12.78: *Retroperitoneal bleeding from the femoral artery*

2. ***Brachial/radial:*** When using an upper extremity approach, blood pressure should first be checked in both arms. If there is a difference between arms, peripheral vascular disease should be suspected and the side with the higher blood pressure should be used. For a radial approach, **an Allen test** must be performed to assess the patency of collateral ulnar circulation. The rate of vascular complications such as thrombosis is higher with the upper extremity approach than with the femoral approach.

L. ***Bleeding:*** Access site bleeding can be significant. If there is a great deal of oozing around the sheath, it can be exchanged for a sheath one French size larger. Adequate manual pressure is usually sufficient to stop bleeding after sheath removal. It is typical practice to

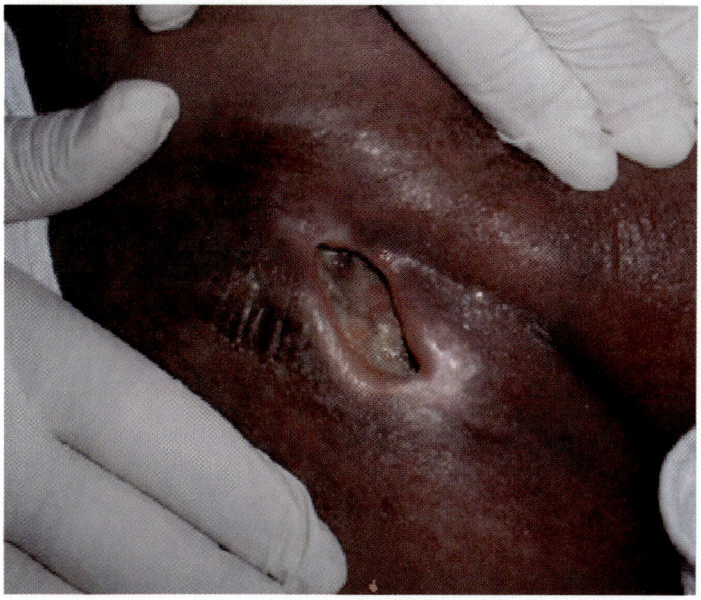

Fig. 12.79: *Deep ulcerative wound in the femoral artery puncture site (Note the presence of an ulcerative purulent area in which cutaneous and subcutaneous tissues are destructed and surrounded by a hyperemic area)*

check the activated clotting time on patients who had been on heparin prior to the procedure and only proceed with sheath removal if the clotting time is below 160. Some institutions use protamine (1 mg/100 U heparin) to reverse heparinization, but this exposes the patient to the potential for allergic reactions to protamine (namely, hypotension). Even more concerning is retroperitoneal bleeding. If a patient complains of severe back pain after a catheterization, this should be considered. An unexpected drop in hemoglobin after a catheterization should also raise this possibility. Obese patients, in particular, can have a major bleed without obvious external signs. The test to diagnose a retroperitoneal bleed is a noncontrast computed tomography scan (Fig. 12.78).

M. ***Infection:*** There is a risk of infection, as with any invasive procedure. This risk can be minimized with proper attention to sterile technique. There is usually no need for prophylactic antibiotics. However, some operators do give antibiotics after use of a percutaneous vascular suture device in patients who are at elevated risk for infection, such as obese or diabetic patients. Endocarditis prophylaxis for patients with valvular heart disease or prosthetic valves is unnecessary (Fig. 12.80).

N. ***Neuropathy:*** There is a slight risk of damage to the femoral nerve from inadvertent puncture. Femoral hematoma (or retroperitoneal bleeding) can also cause compression of the femoral nerve. Function usually improves with time, but complete recovery can take several months.

O. ***Allergy:*** As discussed above, contrast dye can cause adverse reactions, ranging from hives to anaphylaxis. Severe anaphylactoid reactions to contrast dye occur in about 0.1% of cases. Local anesthetic can also cause problems due to specific allergies to the amide or ester component, or to the preservative. A variety of agents are available. Procaine (an ester agent), lidocaine (an amide agent), and bupivacaine (a preservative-free amide agent) are alternative agents.

BIBLIOGRAPHY

1. Grossman W (ed): Cardiac Catheterization and Angiography, ed 3. Philadelphia, Lea & Febiger, 1986, p 5.
2. Lock JE,' Keane JF, Fellows KE: Diag-nostic and I nterventional Catheterization in Congenital Heart Disease. Boston, Mar-tinus Nijhoff, 1987, p 3.
3. Graham TP, Gessner IH: Recommendation for use of laboratory studies for pediatric patients with suspected or proven heart disease: a statement of the Committee on Congenital Cardiac Defects of the Council on Cardiovascular Disease of the Young of the American Heart Association. Dallas, American Heart Association, 1986.
4. Lauer RM: Guidelines for pediatric cardiology diagnostic and treatment centers. Pediatrics 62:258–261, 1978.
5. Friesinger GC, Adams DF, Bourassa MG, et al.: Optimal resources for examination of the heart and lungs: cardiac catheterization and radiographic facilities. Circulation 68:893A–903A, 1983.
6. Rudolph AM: Congenital Diseases of the Heart. Chicago, Year Book, 1974, p 62.
7. Graham TPJr, Atwood GF, Werner B: Use of Droperidol-Fentanyl sedation for cardiac catheterization in children. Am Heart J 87:287–293, 1974.
8. Faithfull NS, Haider R: Ketamine for cardiac catheterization: an evaluation of its use in children. Anaesthesia 26:318–323, 1971.
9. Filston HC, Grant JP: A safer system for percutaneous subclavian venous catheterization in newborn infants. J Pediatr Surg 14:564–570, 1979.
10. Lock JE, Keane JF, Fellows KE: Diagnostic and Interventional Catheterization in Congenital Heart Disease. Boston, Mar-tinus Nijhoff, 1987, p 15.
11. Freed MD, Keane JF: Cardiac output by thermodilution in infants and children. J Pediatr 92:39–42, 1978.
12. Freed MD, Miettinen OS, Nadas AS: Oximetric detection of intracardiac left-to-right shunts. Br Heart J 42:690–694, 1979.
13. Nihill MR, McNamara DG, Vick RL: The effects of increased viscosity on pulmonary vascular resistance. Am Heart J 92:65–72, 1976.
14. Gorlin R, Gorlin SG: Hydraulic formula for calculation of the area of the stenotic mitral valve, other valves, and central circulatory shunts. Am Heart J 41:1–29, 1951.
15. Hakki A, Iskandria AS, Bemis CE, Kim-biris D, Mintz GS, Segal BL, Brice C: A simplified formula for the calculation of stenotic cardiac valve areas. Circulation 63:1050–1055, 1981.
16. Dillon TR, Janos GG, Meyer RA, Benzing G, Kaplan S: Vasodilator therapy for congestive heart failure. J Pediatr 96:623–629, 1980.
17. Landmark K, Sire S, Mavlow E, Amlie JP, Nitter-Hauge S: Haemodynamic effects of nifedipine and propranolol in patients with hypertrophic obstructive cardiomyopathy. Br Heart J 48:19–26, 1982.
18. VogelJHK, Grover RF, Jamieson G, Blount SG: Long-term physiologic observations in patients with ventricular septal defect and increased pulmonary vascular resistance. Adv Cardiolll: 108–122, 1974.
19. Lock JE, Einzing S, Bass JL, Moller JH: The pulmonary vascular response to oxygen and its influence on operative results in children with ventricular septal defect. Pediatr Cardiol 3:41–46, 1982.
20. Beekman RH, Rocchini AP, Rosenthal A: Cardiovascular effects of breathing 95 percent oxygen in children with congenital heart disease. Am J Cardiol 52:106–111, 1983.
21. Cumming GR: Hemodynamics of supine bicycle exercise in "normal" children. Am Heart J 93:617–622, 1977.
22. Lock JE, Einzig S, Moller JH: Hemodynamic responses to exercise in normal children. Am J Cardiol 41:1278–1284, 1978.
23. Cohn HE, Freed MD, Hellenbrand WF, Fyler DC: Complications and mortality associated with cardiac catheterization in infants under one year: a prospective study. Pediatr Cardiol 6:123–131, 1985.

13 Invasive and Noninvasive Coronary Angiography

Anomalies and disease processes of the coronary arteries in children are uncommon. However, with the recent advances in cardiac surgical techniques, many of these lesions are amenable to surgery that requires accurate anatomic delineation by angiography. Ascending aortography is the angiographic procedure commonly used to image the coronary arterial anatomy in children. In some instances, this procedure fails to show the extent or nature of the pathologic process. In some cases, selective coronary arteriography is essential for successful management. Nonselective opacification of the coronary arteries is often adequate for practical purposes in children, especially for studying the coronary circulation before operating congenital heart disease. However, selective coronary angiography is essential to demonstrate some abnormalities of distribution poorly visualized by the nonselective method and especially in cases of coronary anomalies or

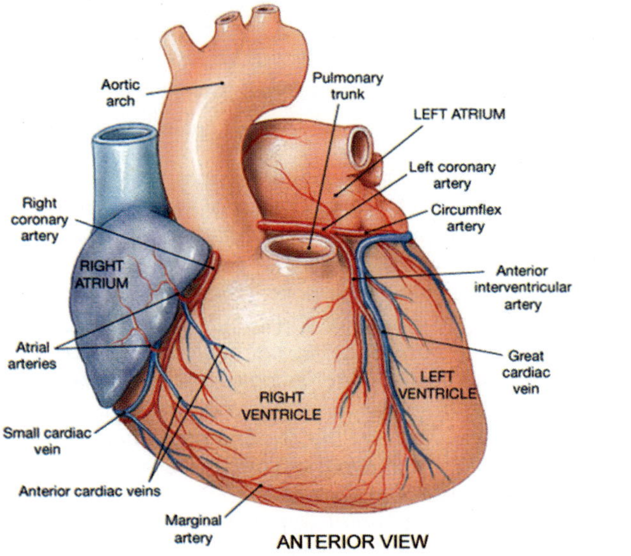

Fig. 13.1: *Main coronary arteries involved in the pathophysiology of angina pectoris*

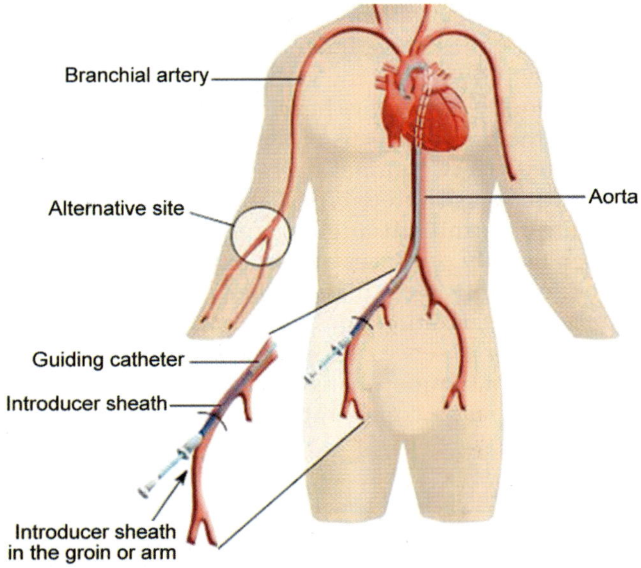

Fig. 13.2: *Different catheter routes of cardiac catheterization including coronary angiography*

acquired coronary disease before procedures of reimplantation of revascularization. The indications must be carefully considered and the technique particularly adapted using pediatric catheters and trained personnel skilled in retrograde arterial catheterization in children.

A coronary catheterization is a minimally invasive procedure to access the coronary circulation and blood filled chambers of the heart using a catheter. It is performed for both diagnostic and interventional (treatment) purposes.

Coronary catheterization is one of the several cardiology diagnostic tests and procedures. Specifically, coronary catheterization is a visually interpreted test performed to recognize occlusion, stenosis, restenosis, thrombosis or aneurysmal enlargement of the coronary artery lumens; heart chamber size; heart muscle contraction performance; and some aspects of heart valve function. Important internal

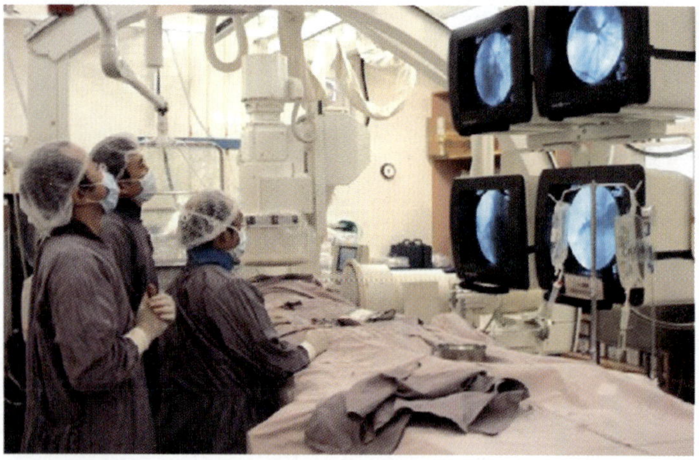

Fig . 13.3: *Catheterization laboratory and busy medical personel in preparing patient for heart catheterization*

heart and lung blood pressures, not measurable from outside the body, can be accurately measured during the test. The relevant problems that the test deals with most commonly occur as a result of advanced atherosclerosis—atheroma activity within the wall of the coronary arteries. Less frequently, valvular, heart muscle, or arrhythmia issues are the primary focus of the test.

Coronary artery luminal narrowing reduces the flow reserve for oxygenated blood to the heart, typically producing intermittent angina. Very advanced luminal occlusion usually produces a heart attack. However, it has been increasingly recognized, since the late 1980s, that coronary catheterization does not allow the recognition of the presence or absence of coronary atherosclerosis itself, only significant luminal changes which have occurred as a result of end stage complications of the atherosclerotic process.

Historical Background

The technique of angiography was first developed in 1927 by the Portuguese Physician Egas Moniz at the University of Lisbon to provide contrasted X-ray in order to diagnose nervous diseases, such as tumors, coronary heart disease and arteriovenous malformations. He is recognized as one of the pioneers in this field (Figs 13.1 and 13.2).

Coronary catheterization was further explored in 1929 when the German physician Werner Forssmann inserted a plastic tube in his cubital vein and guided it to the right chamber of the heart. He took an X-ray to prove his success and published it on November 5 1929 with the title "Über die Sondierung des rechten Herzens" (About probing of the right heart). The coronarography of the left heart was introduced in 1953 with the report by a Portuguese group, published in Cardiologia, International Archives of Cardiology volume 22, pages 45–61, by E Coelho et al. entitled "Arteriografia das coronárias no homem vivo/ L'artériograpie des coronaires chez l'homme vivant" (arteriography of the coronaries in the living man). They were the first to nonselectively inject radiocontrast in the coronary arteries.

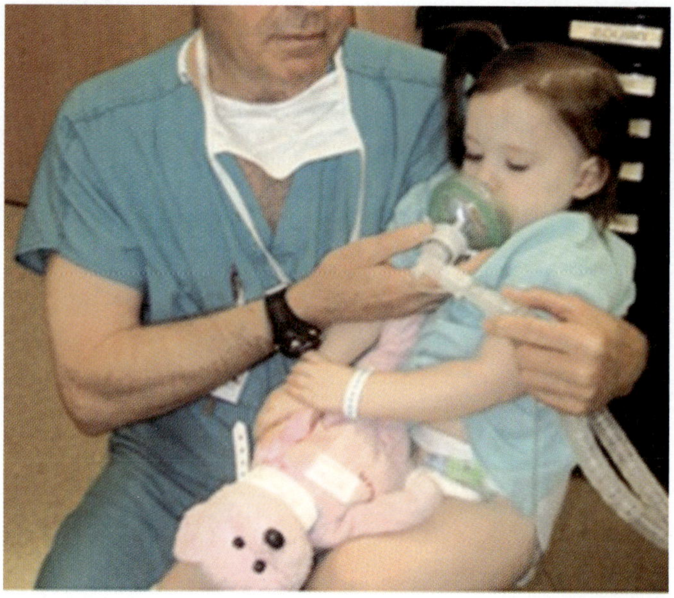

Fig. 13.4: *Child in the lap of anesthesiologist for sedation prior for interventional catheterization*

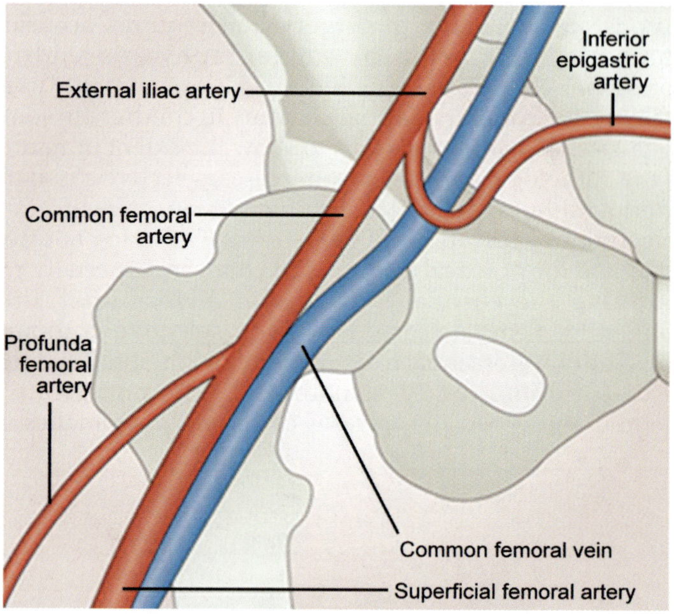

Fig. 13.5: *Anatomy of the common femoral artery. The common femoral artery is the terminal branch of the external iliac artery, and provides the main arterial supply to the lower limb. The common femoral artery enters the femoral triangle deep to the midpoint of the inguinal ligament, posterior to the deep fascia, and overlying the head of the femur bone. These features facilitate arterial puncture, but necessitate deep pressure for compression hemostasis. At this point, the artery has adiameter of 7–10 mm and lies within the femoral sheath close to the common femoral vein and the femoral nerve and its branches. Just proximal to the inguinal ligament, the external iliac artery gives off the clinically important inferior epigastric artery which courses superomedially and anastomoses with distal end of the internal mammary artery. Inferior to the neck of the femur, the common femoral artery divides into the profunda femoris and superficial artery end branches*

In 1960 F Mason Sones, a pediatric cardiologist at the Cleveland Clinic, accidentally injected radiocontrast in a coronary artery instead of the left ventricle. Although the patient had a reversible cardiac arrest, Sones and Shirey developed the procedure further, and are credited with the discovery (Connolly 2002); they published a series of 1,000 patents in 1966 (Proudfit et al.) (Fig. 13.2).

Since the late 1970s, building on the pioneering work of Charles Dotter in 1964 and especially Andreas Gruentzig starting in 1977, coronary catheterization has been extended to therapeutic uses:

1. The performance of less invasive physical treatment for angina and some of the complications of severe atherosclerosis
2. Treating heart attacks before complete damage has occurred
3. Research for better understanding of the pathology of coronary artery disease and atherosclerosis.

In the early 1960s, cardiac catheterization frequently took several hours and involved significant complications for as many as 2–3% of patients. With multiple incremental improvements over time, simple coronary catheterization examinations are now commonly done more rapidly and with significantly improved outcomes.

Death, myocardial infarction, stroke, serious ventricular arrhythmia, and major vascular complications each occur in less than 1% of patients undergoing catheterization. However, though the imaging portion of the examination is often brief because of setup and safety issues the patient is often in the laboratory for 20–45 minutes. Any of multiple technical difficulties while not endangering the patient (indeed added to protect the patient's interests) can significantly increase the examination time.

Equipment Required for the Procedure

Coronary catheterization is performed in a cardiac catheterization laboratory, usually located within a hospital. With current designs, the patient must lie relatively flat on a narrow, minimally padded, radiolucent (transparent to X-ray) table. The X-ray source and imaging camera equipment are on opposite sides of the patient's chest and freely move, under motorized control, around the patient's chest so images can be taken quickly from multiple angles. More advanced equipment, termed a bi-plane catheterization laboratory, uses two sets of X-ray source and imaging cameras, each free to move independently, which allows two sets of images to be taken with each injection of radiocontrast agent.

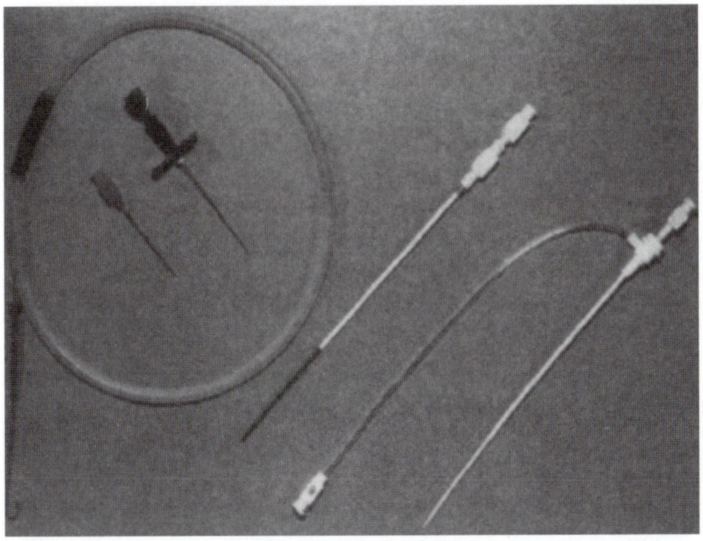

Fig. 13.6: *Equipment used for percutaneous catheterization 0.35-inch. Teflon wire with a 3 mm curve at the end with two percutaneous introducer needles two sheaths, one with a side arm (right)*

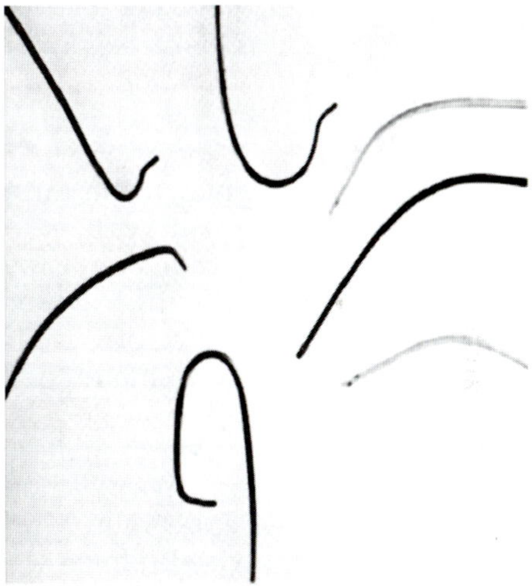

Fig. 13.7: *Different types of catheters in greater use for selective right and left coronary angiography*

Explanation of Test to the Patient

The patient being examined or treated is usually awake during coronary catheterization, ideally with only local anesthesia such as lidocaine and minimal general sedation, throughout the procedure. Performing the procedure with the patient awake is safer as the patient can immediately report any discomfort or problems and thereby facilitate rapid correction of any undesirable events. Medical monitors fail to give a comprehensive view of the patient's immediate well-being; how the patient feels is often a most reliable indicator of procedural safety.

Diagnostic Techniques (Figs 13.2 to 13.7)

During coronary catheterization (often referred to as a **cath** by physicians), blood pressures are recorded and X-ray motion picture shadow-grams of the blood inside the coronary arteries are recorded. In order to create the X-ray pictures, a physician guides a small tube-like device called a catheter, typically ≈ 2.0 mm (6-French) in diameter through the large arteries of the body until the tip is just within the opening of one of the coronary arteries. By design, the catheter is smaller than the lumen of the artery it is placed in; internal/intraarterial blood pressures are monitored through the catheter to verify that the catheter does not block blood flow.

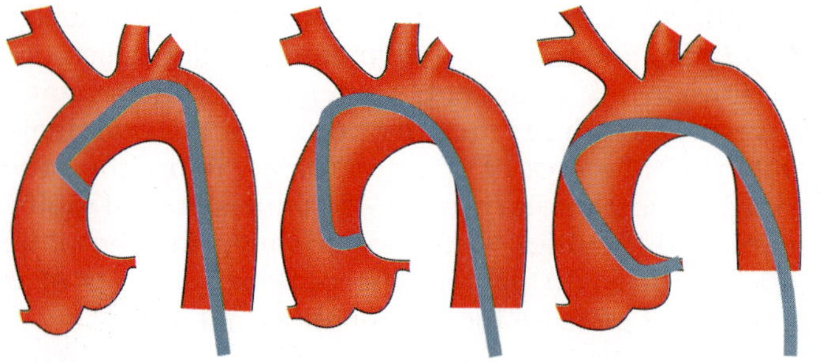

Fig. 13.8: *Selective catheterization of the left coronary artery by the Judkins technique. In LAO position, the catheter is rotated so that it appears unfolded and enface; it is then slowly advanced until it engages the left coronary orifice. A size 4 (4 cm curve) catheter is adequate for most patients, but with moderate or severe aortic dilatation, a size 5 or 6 catheter may be required*

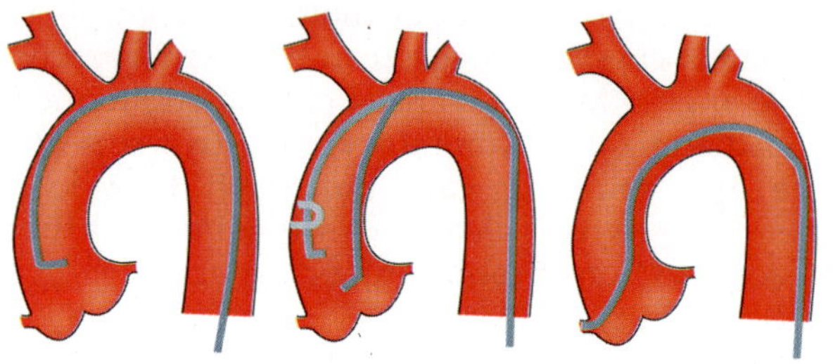

Fig. 13.9: *Diagrammatic representation of selective catheterization of the right coronary artery by the Judkins technique (LAO projection)*

The catheter is itself designed to be radiodense for visibility and it allows a clear, watery, blood compatible radiocontrast agent, commonly called an X-ray dye, to be selectively injected and mixed with the blood flowing within the artery. Typically, 3–8 cc of the radiocontrast agent is injected for each image to make the blood flow visible for about 3–5 seconds as the radiocontrast agent is rapidly washed away into the coronary capillaries and then coronary veins. Without the X-ray dye injection, the blood and surrounding heart tissues appear, on X-ray, as only a mildly-shape-changing, otherwise uniform water density mass; no details of the blood and internal organ structure are discernible. The radiocontrast within the blood allows visualization of the blood flow within the arteries or heart chambers, depending on where it is injected.

If atheroma, or clots, are protruding into the lumen, producing narrowing, the narrowing may be seen instead as increased haziness within the X-ray shadow images of the blood/dye column within that portion of the artery; this is as compared to adjacent, presumed healthier, less stenotic areas. See the single frame illustration of an coronary angiogram image on the angioplasty page.

For guidance regarding catheter positions during the examination, the physician mostly relies on detailed knowledge of internal anatomy, guidewire and catheter behavior and intermittently, briefly uses fluoroscopy and a low X-ray dose to visualize when needed. This is done without saving recordings of these brief looks. When the physician is ready to record diagnostic views, which are saved and can be more carefully scrutinized later, he activates the equipment to apply a significantly higher X-ray dose, termed cine, in order to create better quality motion picture images, having sharper radiodensity contrast, typically at 30 frames per second. The physician controls both the contrast injection, fluoroscopy and cine application timing so as to minimize the total amount of radiocontrast injected and times the X-ray to the injection so as to minimize the total amount of X-ray used. Doses of radiocontrast agents and X-ray exposure times are routinely recorded in an effort to maximize safety.

Though not the focus of the test, calcification within the artery walls, located in the outer edges of atheroma within the artery walls, is sometimes recognizable on fluoroscopy (without contrast injection) as radiodense halo rings partially encircling, and separated from the blood filled lumen by the interceding radiolucent atheroma tissue and endothelial lining. Calcification, even though usually present, is usually only visible when quite advanced and calcified sections of the artery wall happen to be viewed on end tangentially through multiple rings of calcification, so as to create enough radiodensity to be visible on fluoroscopy.

Therapeutic Procedures

By changing the diagnostic catheter to a guiding catheter, physicians can also pass a variety of instruments through the catheter and into the artery to a lesion site. The most commonly used are 0.014-inch-diameter (0.36 mm) guide wires and the balloon dilation catheters (Figs 13.8 and 13.9).

By injecting radiocontrast agent through a tiny passage extending down the balloon catheter and into the balloon, the balloon is progressively expanded. The hydraulic pressures are chosen and applied by the physician, according to how the balloon within the stenosis responds. The radiocontrast filled balloon is watched under fluoroscopy (it typically assumes a "dog bone" shape imposed on the outside of the balloon by the stenosis as the balloon is expanded), as it opens. As much hydraulic brute force is applied as judged needed and visualized to be effective to make the stenosis of the artery lumen visibly enlarge (Fig. 13.10).

Typical normal coronary artery pressures are in the <200 mmHg range (27 kPa). The hydraulic pressures applied within the balloon may extend to as high as 19,000 mmHg (2,500 kPa). Prevention of over-enlargement is achieved by choosing balloons manufactured out of high tensile strength clear plastic membranes. The balloon is initially folded around the catheter, near the tip, to create a small cross-sectional profile to facilitate passage though luminal stenotic areas and designed to inflate to a specific pre-designed diameter. If over inflated, the balloon material simply tears and allows the inflating radiocontrast agent to simply escape into the blood.

Additionally, several other devices can be advanced into the artery via a guiding catheter. These include laser catheters, stent catheters, intravascular vetrasound (IVUS) catheters, Doppler catheter, pressure or temperature measurement catheter and various clot and grinding or removal devices. Most of these devices have turned out to be niche devices, only useful in a small percentage of situations or for research.

Stents, which are specially manufactured expandable stainless steel mesh tubes, mounted on a balloon catheter, are the most commonly used device beyond the balloon catheter. When the stent/balloon device positioned within the stenosis, the balloon is inflated which, in turn, expands the stent and the artery. The balloon is removed and the stent remains in place, supporting the inner artery walls in the more open, dilated position.

Advances in Catheter Based Interventions

Interventional procedures have been plagued by restenosis due to the formation of endothelial tissue overgrowth at the lesion site. Restenosis is the body's response to the injury of the vessel wall from angioplasty and to the stent as a foreign body. As assessed in clinical trials during the late 1980 and 1990s, using only balloon angioplasty (POBA, plain old balloon angioplasty), up to 50% of patients suffered significant restenosis but that percentage has dropped to the single to lower two digits range with the introduction of drug-eluting stents. Sirolimus, paclitaxel and everolimus are the three drugs used in coatings which are currently FDA approved in the United States. As opposed to bare metal, drug eluting stents are covered with a medicine that is slowly dispersed with the goal of suppressing the restenosis reaction. The key to the success of drug coating has been (a) choosing effective agents, (b) developing ways of adequately binding the drugs to the stainless surface of the stent struts (the coating must stay bound despite marked handling and stent deformation stresses) and (c) developing coating controlled release mechanisms that release the drug slowly over about 30 days. One of the newest innovations in coronary stents is the development of a dissolving stent. Abbott laboratories has used a dissolvable material, polylactic acid, that will completely absorb within 2 years of being implanted.

Even with the advent of new noninvasive imaging modalities such as cardiac CT and MRI, coronary angiography remains the gold standard for detecting clinically significant coronary atherosclerotic disease. The technique was first performed by Dr Mason Sones at the Cleveland Clinic in 1958. And still involves the same basic premise, using a series of specially designed catheters to deliver X-ray contrast medium to image the luminal integrity of the coronary epicardial bed. Additionally, through both arterial and venous access, each chamber of the heart can be hemodynamically assessed. Typically, a complete left heart catheterization involves not only coronary angiography, but also some measure of the ventricular filling pressures and cardiac hemodynamics.

Indications

It is estimated that cardiac catheterization will be performed nearly 3 million times/year by 2010. While the overall risk for major complications is relatively low (<2%), it is not negligible. Therefore, patient selection and appropriateness of procedure is vital.

Contraindications

There are no absolute contraindications to cardiac catheterization. Relative contraindications include:

Risk

The overall risk of major complications with left heart catheterization is 1–2%. An include death, bleeding, vascular complications, myocadial infarction (MI), CVA , and contrast reaction. Factors increasing patient risk include age, left main trunk (LMT) or three vessel coronary disease, decompensated heart failure, severe aortic stenosis, diabetes, renal failure and prior CVA.

TECHNIQUE

Vascular Access

Common Femoral Arterial Access is the most common arterial access for performing left heart catheterization. The original catheterization procedure was performed via brachial access. This site is still commonly used in patients with lower extremity peripheral access issues. Arm access also facilitates internal mammary access, especially in patients with tortuous innominant or subclavian arteries. Radial artery access is also used commonly in some practice settings. Before radial access is performed, competence of the radial artery arch should be assessed with the Allen Test. Use of pulse oximetry can facilitate interpretation of the test (Figs 13.2 and 13.5).

Anatomic landmarks are used to identify the correct site of arterial puncture. For the femoral artery access, the femoral head provides the best visible landmark. Arterial puncture at this site remains below the inguinal ligament, is generally above the bifurcation of the superfical femoral and deep femoral arteries, and allows for hemostasis. It is recommended that this site should be observed under floroscopy in any patient prior to access. In obese patients, the inguinal skin crease is generally too low.

After the administration of subcutaneous anesthetic, an 18G Cook needle is used to puncture the the front wall of the artery. This technique is known as the modified Seldinger technique and prevents posterior arterial bleeding or venous communication from the puncture. Complications from arterial access include arterial dissection, artrioventricular (AV) fistula formation, retroperitoneal hemmorhage, and pseudoanuerysm formation (Fig. 13.11).

Once access is obtained, the Cook needle is steadied while the artery is accessed with a wire through the lumen of the Cook needle. The Cook needle is then removed and a sheath is inserted into the artery. Under floroscopy, catheters are then introduced using an 0.35 J-tipped guide wire into the aortic root. The catheters are then attached to a three way manifold. Manifold used allows for continuous pressure monitoring, saline flush instillation, and contrast administration through the catheter tip.

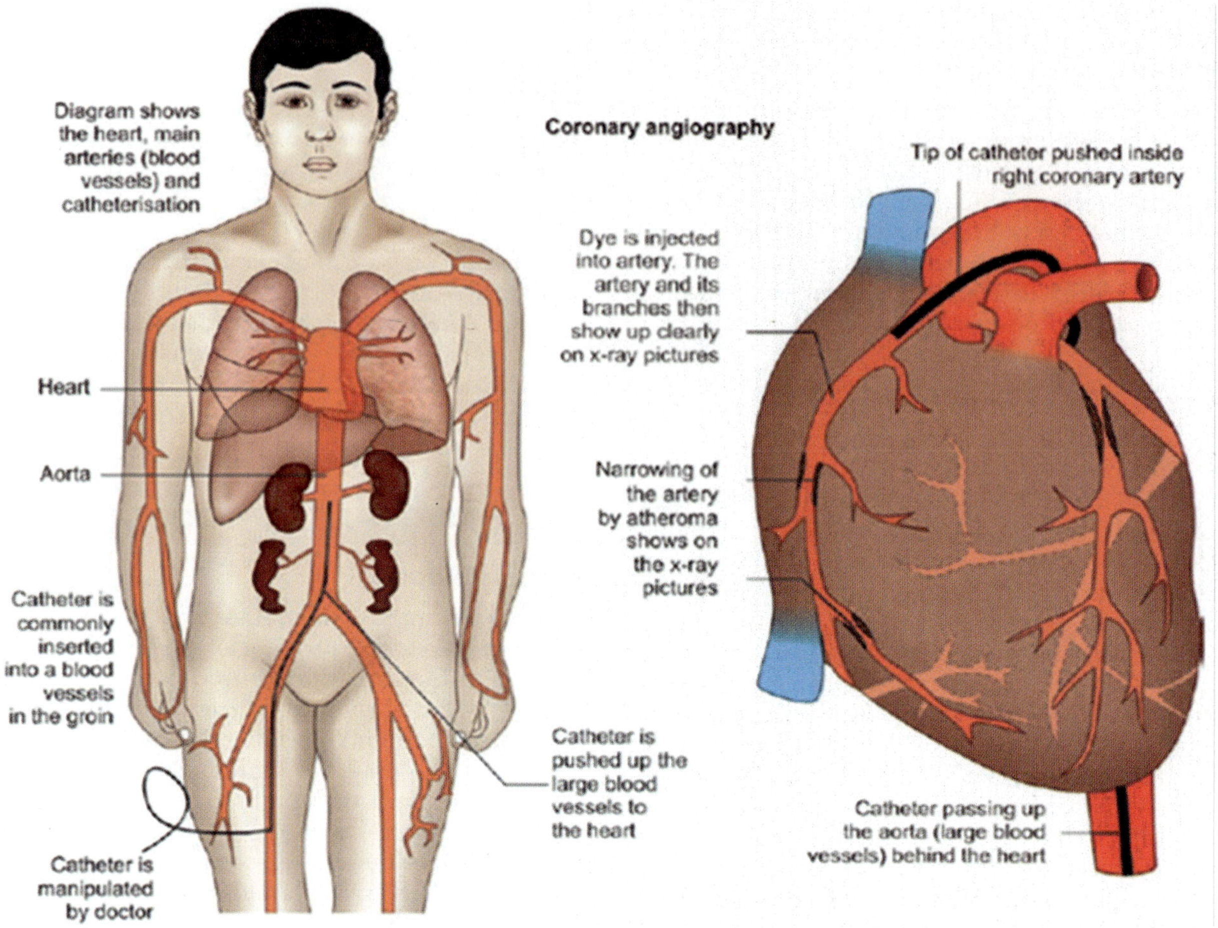

Fig. 13.10: *Diagrammatic representation of procedure in coronary angiogram*

BASICS OF CORONARY ANATOMY

The trileaflet aortic valve gives rise to 3 cusp or sinuses in the aortic root. The left coronary and right coronary cusp give rise to their respective coronary arteries while the noncoronary cusp which arises from the posterior root usually does not give rise to a coronary artery (Figs 13.15 and 13.16).

The major epicardial vessels supplying the myocardium are the left main coronary artery that divides into the Left anterior Descending artery and left circumflex artery, and the right coronary artery. These arteries lie on the epicardial surface and supply smaller branch vessels that eventually give rise to the microvascular network supplying the myocardium.

Coronary dominance is based on the vessel that gives rise to the posterior descending artery (PDA) which travels in the posterior interventricular groove and supplies the Atrio-ventricular node (AV node). This vessel, which can be recognized by the presence of septal perforating branches arises from the RCA in 80% of the population and the LCx in 10% of the population. Co-dominance of the arterial circulation is found in 10% of the population where the posterior interventricular artery is formed by both the RCA and LCx.

The left main coronary artery or LMT originates from the left coronary cusp and bifurcates to give rise to the LAD and LCx coronary arteries. Occasionally, a third branch vessel, the ramus intermedius (RI) arises from the LMT. The LMT varies in length in many patients and in a small number of patients, the two major branch vessels arise from separate origins.

The LAD coronary artery LAD provides blood supply to the anterior wall of the left ventricle. As it courses through

Table 13.1: *ACC/AHA classifications of class I, II and III. These classes summarize the indications for coronary angiography*

Class I: Conditions for which there is evidence and/or general agreement that this procedure is useful and effective.
Class II: Conditions for which there is conflicting evidence and/or a divergence of opinion about the usefulness/efficacy of performing the procedure.
Class IIa: Weight of evidence/opinion is in favor of usefulness/efficacy.
Class IIb: Usefulness/efficacy is less well established by evidence/opinion.
Class III: Conditions for which there is evidence and/or general agreement that the procedure is not useful/effective and in some cases may be harmful.

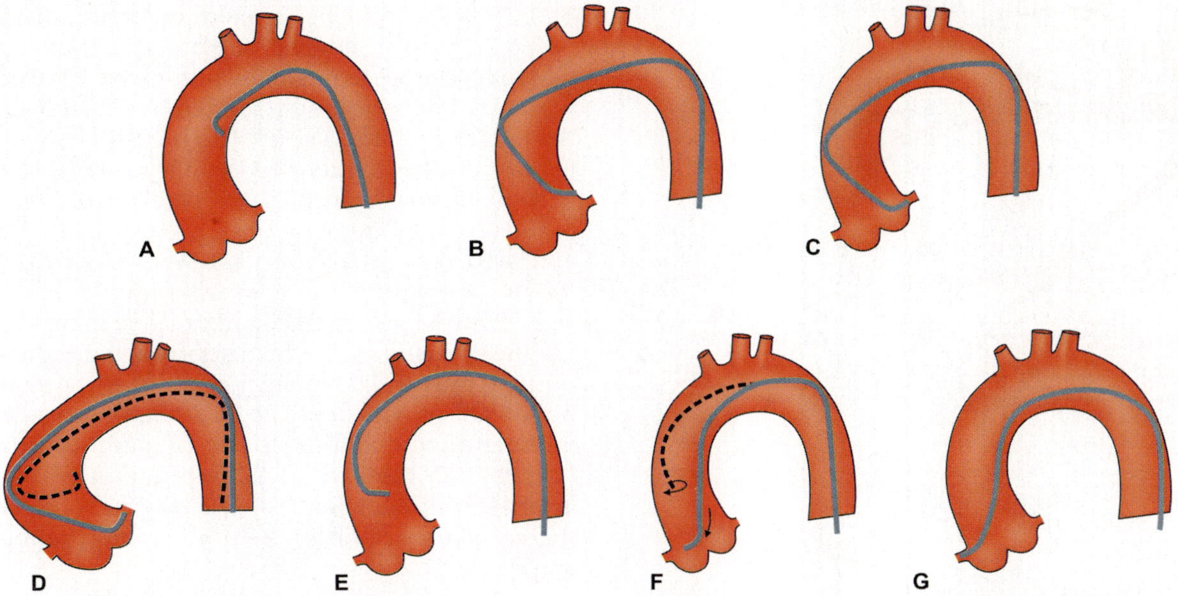

Fig. 13.11: *Left and right judkins catheters Constructed from polyethylene or polyurethane with a fine wire braid within the wall to allow advancement and directional control and to prevent kinking. The left Judkins catheter: This catheter is preshaped to allow entry into the left coronary ostium from the femoral approach with minimal catheter manipulation. A preformed left Judkins catheter can also be used from the left brachial or radial artery, but a catheter with 0.5 cm less curvature than required for the femoral approach is generally better suited for coronary cannulation. The right Judkins catheter: this catheter is shaped to permit entry into the right coronary artery (RCA) with a small amount of rotational catheter manipulation from any vascular approach.*

(A) When Judkins left catheter is applied via a right upper limb approach, the catheter sometimes does not engage coaxially. The distal tip may injure the top of the left main trunk. (B) With Judkins left, the catheter easily loses engagement when the device is pushed into a tight lesion. (C) Ikari left fits the awkward angle at the brachiocephalic artery (black arrow). The angle induces the catheter to attach on the other side of the aorta against the left coronary ostium (triangle). In Judkins, the attachment is limited to a small point of contact (triangle, A) but with Ikari catheter the contact area is much wider (triangle, C). This generates a coaxial engagement and good back-up support (C). (D) When the Judkins right catheter is applied via the right upper limb, the catheter usually does not attach on the other side of the aorta. (E) The catheter easily loses engagement when the device is pushed into a tight lesion. (F) However, the Ikari right catheter fits the angle at the brachiocephalic artery (black arrow). The catheter attaches on the other side of the aorta (triangle). This generates a coaxial engagement and good back-up support

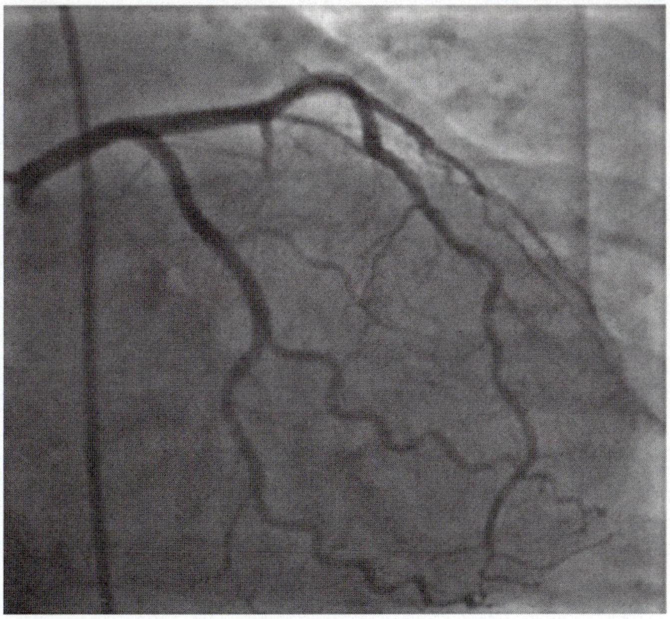

Fig.13.12A: *Right anterior oblique coronary angiographic view with caudal angulation demonstrating normal left anterior descending and circumflex coronary arteries*

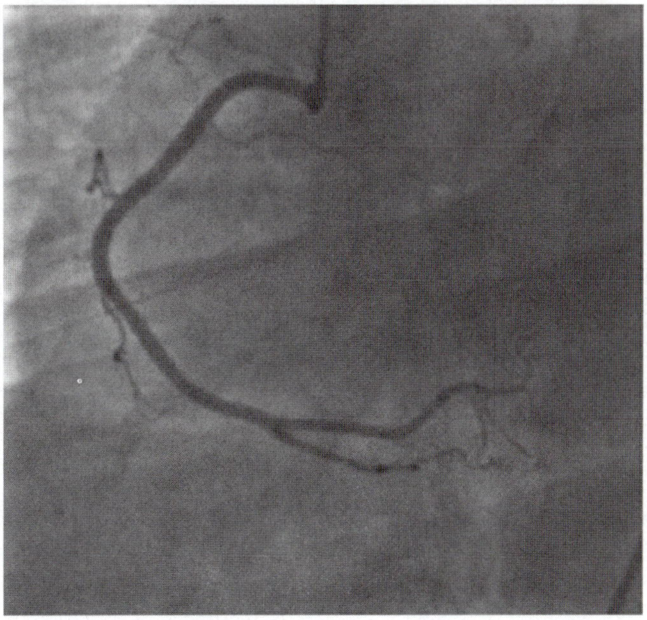

Fig. 13.12B: *Left anterior oblique coronary angiographic view showing normal right coronary artery*

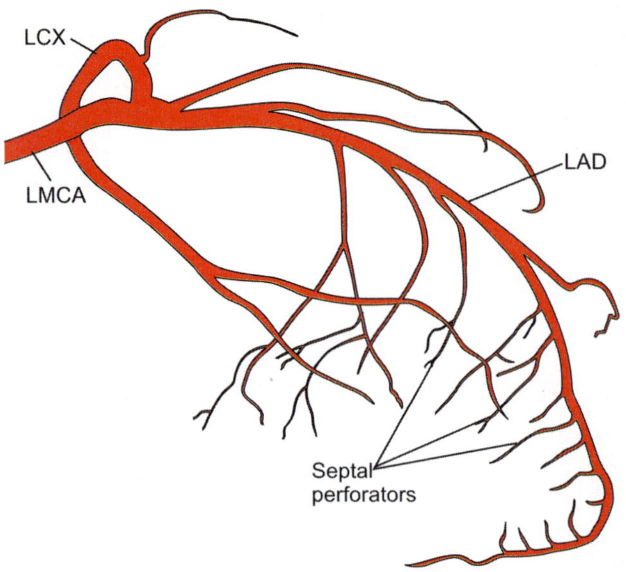

Fig. 13.13: *Right anterior oblique cranial view of left coronary artery. LMCA, left main coronary artery; LCx, left circumflex coronary artery; LAD, left anterior descending artery.*

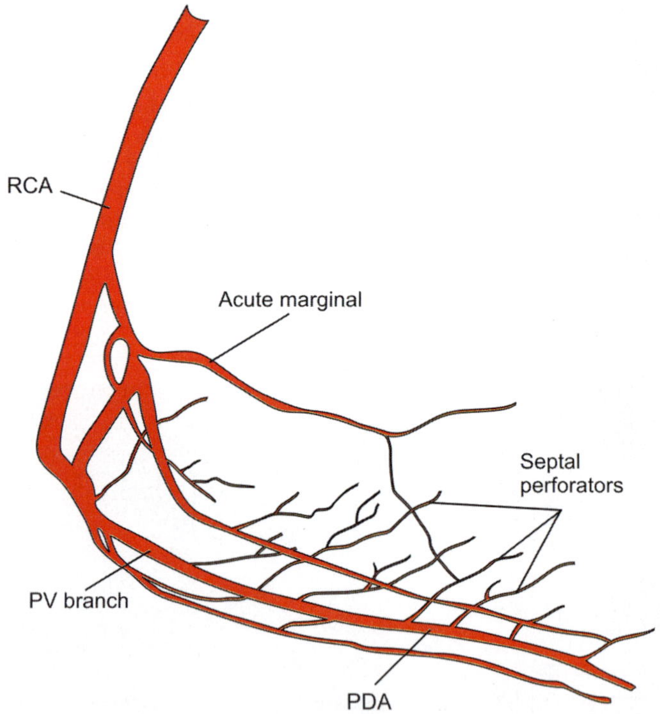

Fig. 13.14: *Right anterior oblique view of right coronary artery. RCA, right coronary artery; PV branch, posteroventricular branch; PDA, polsterior descending artery.*

the anterior intraventricular groove it provides multiple septal branches to the interventricular septum and diagonal branches to the anterior lateral wall. The LAD then courses to the ventricular apex and in some patients wraps around the apex to supply a small amount of the posterior apex.

The LCx coronary artery courses around the lateral or left AV groove and gives rise to multiple marginal or lateral branches. The branches are termed obtuse marginal (OM) or lateral branches depending on institutional preference. OM branches are sequentially numbered (OM1, OM2 etc...) while lateral branches are termed based on the segment of the lateral wall they supply (high lateral, lateral, posterior lateral). As the LCx courses the AV groove it also gives rise to several atrial branches, and occasionally the sino-atrial branch (40% of the population).

The RCA arises from the right coronary cusp. This vessel follows the right AV groove and provides branches to the right ventricle. The most proximal branches of the RCA are the conus-branch which supplies the right ventricular outflow tract and a branch that supplies the sinoatrial (SA) node (60% of patients). The RCA then courses through the interventricular and gives rise to marginal branches and branches to the atrium. Manipulation of the coronary arteries in threedimensions via spacial reconstructions of the coronary arteries is helpful in interpreting coronary angiographic images.

STANDARD ANGIOGRAPHIC VIEWS

For the beginner angiographer, the anatomic landmarks formed by the spine, catheter and diaphragm provide information to discern which tomographic view from which the image is obtained. In the left anterior oblique (LAO) view, the catheter and spine are seen on the right side of the image while in the right anterior oblique (RAO) they are found on the right. posterior anterior (PA) imaging places these landmarks in the center of the image. Cranial angulation can usually be distinguished from caudal angulation by the presence of the diaphragm. For cranial imaging, the patient should be asked to inspire to remove the diaphragmatic shadow from the image.

CATHETERS

Catheter selection for a routine left heart catheterization is generally straight forward.

Most often, Judkins catheter types are most routinely used. For engagement of the left main coronary artery, A Judkins left size 4 (JL4) catheter generally will generally engaged the left coronary artery in most patients with relative ease. Increasing catheter size (JL5) for tall patients or patients with dilated aorta or decreasing size (JL 3.5) in small patients is sometimes required. Engagement of the LMT is usually most straightforward in the LAO projection. For extremely dilated roots or anomalous arteries, other catheters such as Amplatz catheters can be used. For the right coronary artery, a Judkins right size 4 (JR4) is most often used. The right coronary artery is engaged in the LAO projection. Usually, slow clockwise rotation of the JR4 in the aortic root will engage the ostium of the RCA. Specialized catheters are available to engage anomalous origins of coronary arteries and saphenous and internal mammary artery bypass grafts (Figs 13.7 to 13.9).

Once the artery is engaged is is important to examine the pressure wave form. Normally, the waveform should mimic aortic root pressure. Dampening or ventricularization of the pressure waveform may indicate over engagement of the catheter or significant vessel stenosis. Extreme care should be taken before instillation of contrast medium without normal pressure waveforms.

LEFT CORONARY ARTERY (Figs 13.12A, 13.12B and 13.24)

The Left main coronary artery gives rise to the left anterior descending artery and the LCx coronary artery. Complete visualization of these arteries and their branches requires care and rigor to ensure complete anatomical documentation. Often bifurcations and vessel foreshortening and overlap cause errors in stenosis estimation. There are no steadfast rules in which tomographic views are most useful. Generally, for circumflex and proximal epicardial visualization the caudal views are most useful. For LAD and LAD/diagonal bifurcation visualization the cranial views are most useful. Overall, if there is not a significant limitation on contrast utilization, standard "around the world" angiography using a selection of the following angiographic views will document left coronary anatomy (Figs 13.17–13.21).

RIGHT CORONARY ARTERY (Figs 13.13 and 13.14)

The Right coronary artery is engaged in the LAO position.

Initial angiographic imaging of the RCA in this view (LAO 30) gives the best view of significant ostial and proximal RCA disease.

The mid-RCA is best visualized in the straight RAO 30 position (Fig. 13.23).

The bifurcation of the distal RCA and rPDA is best seen in the PA 0 Cran 30 view with a small breath in.

ACC and AHA Update Guidelines for Coronary Angiography

The American College of Cardiology (ACC) and the American Heart Association (AHA) have updated their guidelines for coronary angiography. The executive summary and recommendations are published in the May 4, 1999, issue of circulation. The entire guidelines are published in the May 1999 issue of the Journal of the ACC.

The ACC/AHA coronary angiography guidelines represent an update of the 1987 guidelines. In addition to reviewing the previous guidelines, the 12-member ACC/AHA Committee on Coronary Angiography also conducted a search of the pertinent literature for the previous 10 years. The weight of evidence in support of each recommendation was then ranked into three categories: (A) the presence of multiple randomized clinical trials; (B) the presence of a single randomized trial or nonrandomized studies and (C) expert consensus.

The recommendations are also classified on the basis of conditions for which coronary angiography has demonstrated usefulness/efficacy. The definitions of these categories are as follows:

The following is an excerpt of the recommendations for coronary angiography in the evaluation of patients with known or suspected coronary artery disease who are asymptomatic or have stable angina:

Class I

1. Canadian Cardiovascular Society (CCS) class III and class IV angina on medical treatment. (Level of evidence: B)
2. High-risk criteria on noninvasive testing regardless of angina severity. (Level of evidence: A)
3. Patients who have been successfully resuscitated from sudden cardiac death or have sustained (more than 30 seconds) monomorphic ventricular tachycardia or nonsustained (less than 30 seconds) polymorphic ventricular tachycardia. (Level of evidence: B)

Class IIa

1. CCS class III or IV angina, which improves to class I or II with medical therapy. (Level of evidence: C)
2. Serial noninvasive testing with identical testing protocols, at the same level of medical therapy, showing progressively worsening abnormalities. (Level of evidence: C)
3. Patients with angina and suspected coronary disease who, because of disability, illness or physical challenge, cannot be adequately risk-stratified by other means. (Level of evidence: C)
4. CCS class I or II angina with intolerance to adequate medical therapy or with failure to respond, or patients who have recurrence of symptoms during adequate medical therapy. (Level of evidence: C)
5. Individuals whose occupation involves the safety of others (e.g., pilots, bus drivers) who have abnormal but not high-risk stress test results or multiple clinical features that suggest high risk. (Level of evidence: C)

Class IIb

1. CCS Class I or II angina with demonstrable ischemia but no high-risk criteria on noninvasive testing. (Level of evidence: C)
2. An asymptomatic man or postmenopausal woman without known coronary heart disease with two or more major clinical risk factors and abnormal but not high-risk criteria on noninvasive testing (performed for indications stated in the ACC/AHA noninvasive testing guidelines). (Level of evidence: C)
3. Asymptomatic patients with prior MI with normal resting left ventricular function and ischemia on noninvasive testing but without high-risk criteria. (Level of evidence: C)
4. Periodic evaluation after cardiac transplantation. (Level of evidence: C)
5. Candidate for liver, lung or renal transplant 40 years of age or older as part of the evaluation for transplantation. (Level of evidence: C)

Class III

1. Angina in patients who prefer to avoid revascularization even though it might be appropriate. (Level of evidence: C)
2. Angina in patients who are not candidates for coronary revascularization or in whom revascularization is not likely to improve the quality or duration of life. (Level of evidence: C)

3. As a screening test for coronary artery disease in asymptomatic patients. (Level of evidence: C)
4. After coronary artery bypass grafting or angioplasty when there is no evidence of ischemia on noninvasive testing, unless there is informed consent for research purposes. (Level of evidence: C)
5. Coronary calcification on fluoroscopy, electron-beam CT or other screening tests without criteria listed above. (Level of evidence: C)

CORONARY ANGIOGRAPHY FOR SPECIFIC REASONS

A. Known or Suspected Coronary Artery Disease (CAD)

Coronary atherosclerosis is a slowly progressive process that can be clinically inapparent for long periods of time. Coronary disease often becomes clinically evident because of the occurrence of symptoms, such as angina or those associated with MI. Patients with known CAD are those in whom the disease has been documented by either angiography or MI (i.e. using WHO criteria). "Suspected coronary disease" means that a patient's symptoms or other clinical characteristics suggest a high likelihood for significant CAD and its related adverse outcomes but that evidence of CAD has not yet been documented as defined above (Figs 13.26–13.38).

Patients may develop symptoms at one point in time but may become asymptomatic thereafter as the result of a change in the disease or as the result of therapy. For instance, many patients are asymptomatic after an uncomplicated MI, as are patients with mild angina, who can be rendered asymptomatic by medications. The severity of clinical presentations and the degree of provokable ischemia on noninvasive testing are the principal factors used in determining the appropriateness of coronary angiography. Although the extent of coronary disease defined by coronary angiography does predict outcome, use of coronary angiography as a "screening tool" in unselected populations is neither prudent nor cost-effective. The same can be stated regarding the routine use of exercise testing, radionuclide imaging and stress echocardiography in unselected patients. With only a few exceptions, coronary angiography is not clearly indicated in asymptomatic patients with either known or suspected CAD, unless noninvasive testing (performed as recommended in the ACC/AHA noninvasive guidelines), reveals findings that suggest a high risk for adverse outcome. Coronary angiography is also frequently done during evaluation for

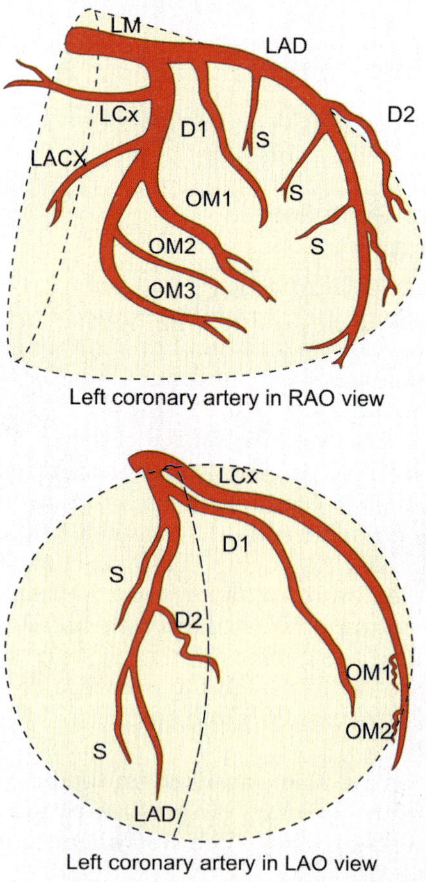

Fig. 13.15: *Diagram showing various branches of left and right major coronary arteries. LM, left main; SN, sinus node branch; D, diagnol ; S,septal branches; LAD, left anterior descending; OM , obtuse marginal; RV, right ventricular branch; AC, atrial circumflex; M, marginal. PDA, posterior descending artery; AVNA,atrioventricular nodal artery; LCX ,left circumflex artery; SANA, sinoatrial nodal artery.*

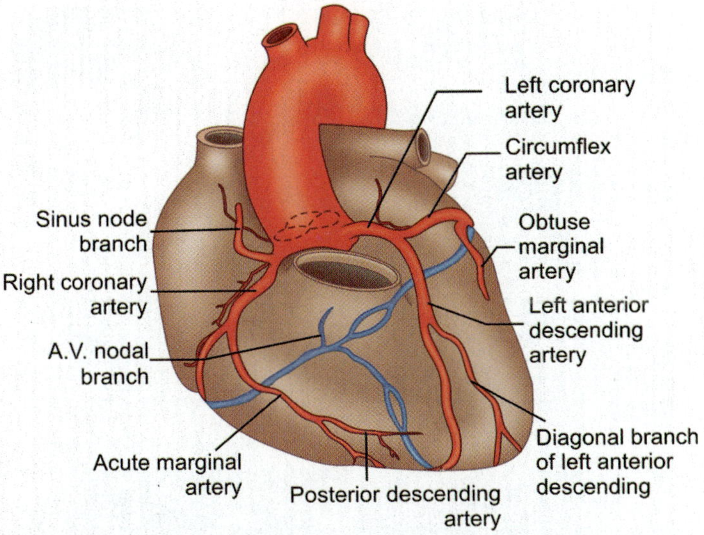

Fig. 13.16: *Blood supply of the heart through coronary arterial system and tries to explain as to how the coronary arteries originate from the ascending aorta to supply the heart with oxygenated blood. The demand for fresh, oxygenated blood is substantial for the heart. Like brain cells, the cells that work collectively to form the structure of the heart will not live for very long (respirate anaerobically) without oxygen*

other cardiac conditions, such as valvular heart disease, congestive heart failure, or assessment of congenital heart disease. In this setting, angiography may be performed in asymptomatic patients. The details of indications for coronary angiography in specific conditions are described below.

B. Recommendations for Use of Coronary Angiography in Patients With Congestive Heart Failure

Class I

1. Congestive heart failure due to systolic dysfunction with angina or with regional wall motion abnormalities and/ or scintigraphic evidence of reversible myocardial ischemia when revascularization is being considered. *(Level of Evidence: B)*
2. Before cardiac transplantation. *(Level of Evidence: C)*
3. Congestive heart failure secondary to postinfarction ventricular aneurysm or other mechanical complications of MI. *(Level of Evidence: C)*

Class IIa

1. Systolic dysfunction with unexplained cause despite noninvasive testing. *(Level of Evidence: C)*
2. Normal systolic function, but episodic heart failure raises suspicion of ischemically mediated left ventricular dysfunction. *(Level of Evidence: C)*

Class III

Congestive heart failure with previous coronary angiograms showing normal coronary arteries, with no new evidence to suggest ischemic heart disease. *(Level of Evidence: C)*

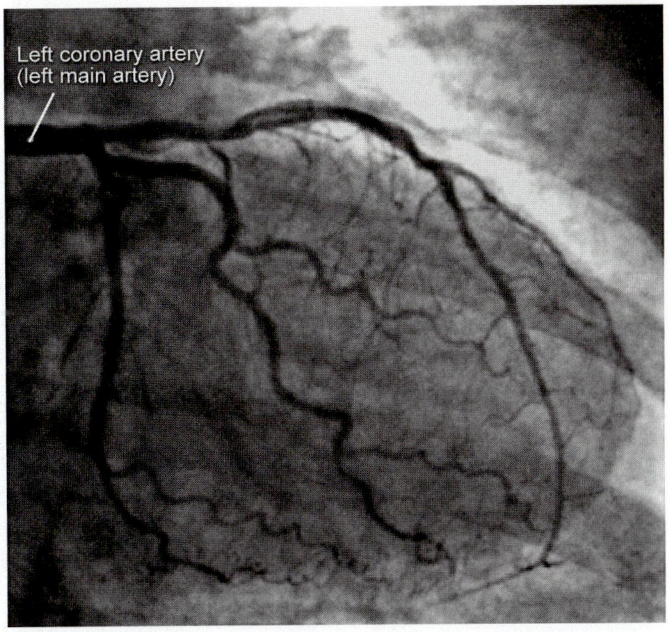

Fig. 13.17: *Left coronary angiography showing left main coronary artery*

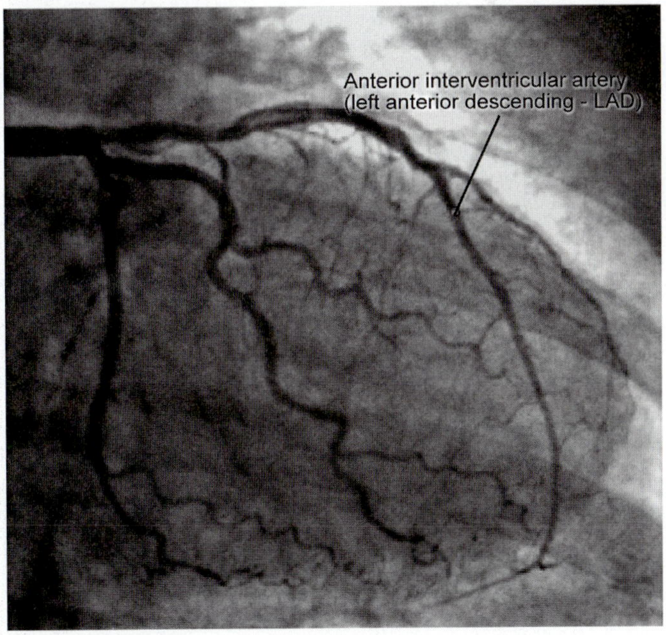

Fig. 13.18: *Left coronary angiography showing left anterior descending artery*

C. Other Conditions

1. *Aortic Dissection*

The need for coronary angiography before surgical treatment for aortic dissection remains controversial because there are no large trials to support its use. In young patients with dissection due to Marfan syndrome or in dissection in peripartum females, coronary angiography is unnecessary unless there is suspicion that the dissection has affected one or both coronary ostia. In older patients, in whom dissection is usually related to hypertension,

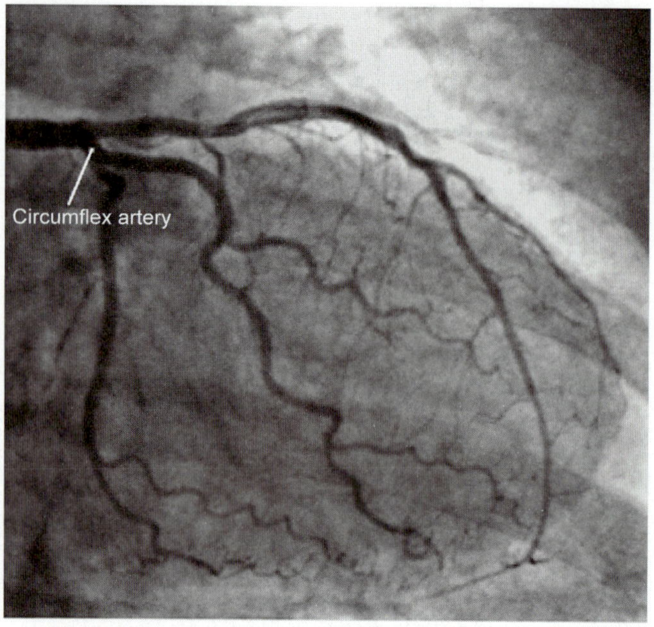

Fig. 13.19: *Left coronary angiography showing circumflex artery*

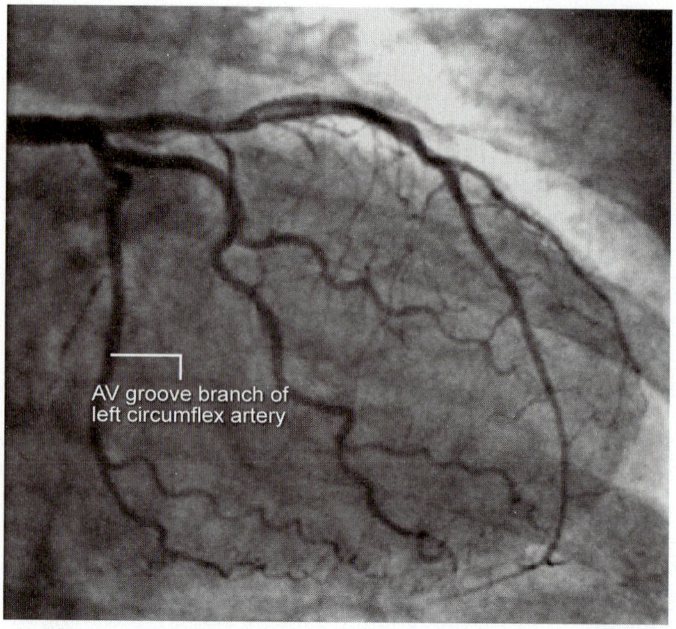

Fig. 13.21: *Left coronary angiography showing AV groove branch of left coronary artery*

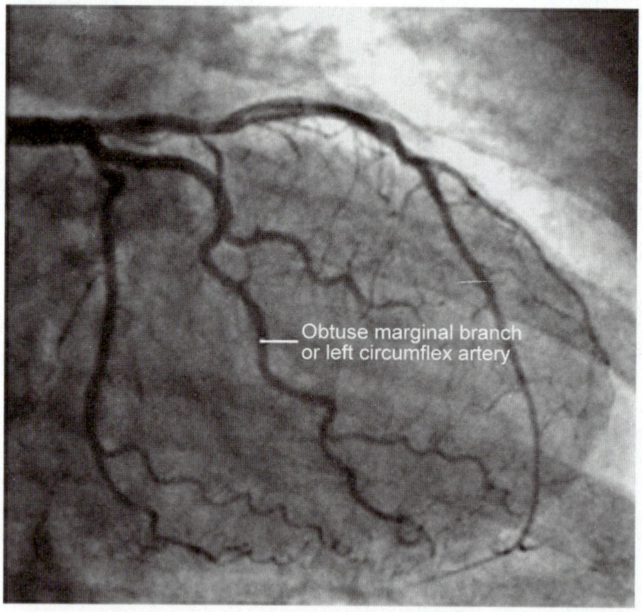

Fig. 13.20: *Left coronary angiography showing obtuse marginal branch of left coronary artery*

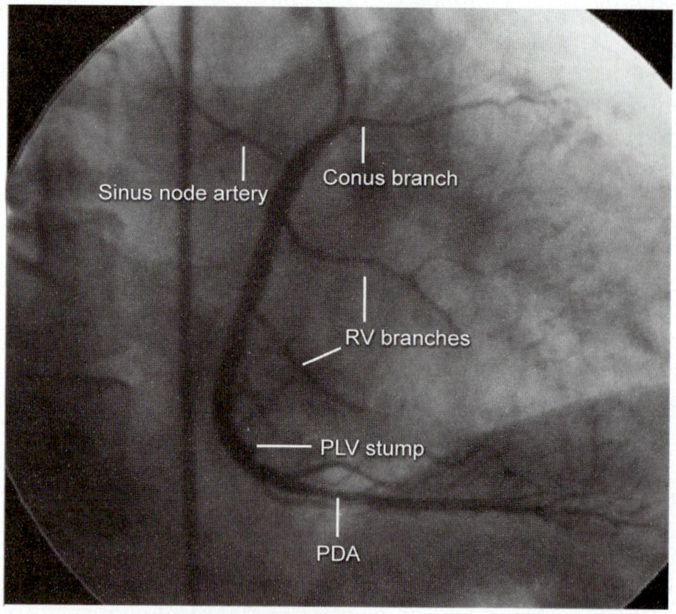

Fig. 13.22: *Angiogram: showing branches of the right coronary artery as indicated on the skiagram*

coronary angiography is often necessary, especially if patients are suspected of having coronary disease because of a history of angina or objective evidence of myocardial ischemia. In patients who have no history of coronary disease, the indications for coronary angiography are much less certain. Because of the high incidence of coronary disease in older patients with dissection, some studies have advocated routine coronary angiography, whereas others have found increased mortality when angiography is performed.

2. *Arteritis*

Some patients with inflammatory processes affecting the aorta, such as Takayasu arteritis, may have coronary artery involvement requiring coronary artery revascularization. In such patients, coronary angiography is required before the surgical procedure. Kawasaki disease can result in coronary artery aneurysm and coronary artery stenosis producing myocardial ischemia or silent occlusion and may require coronary angiographic assessment.

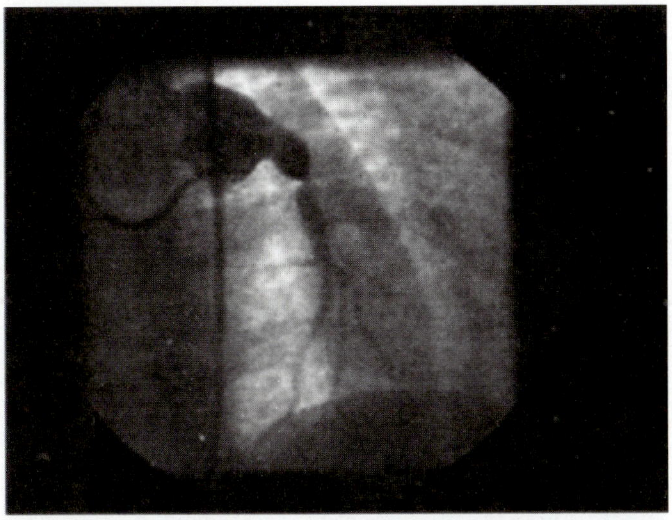

Fig. 13.23: *Coronary angiography showing aneurysm of left main coronary artery and 90% ostial left anterior descending artery*

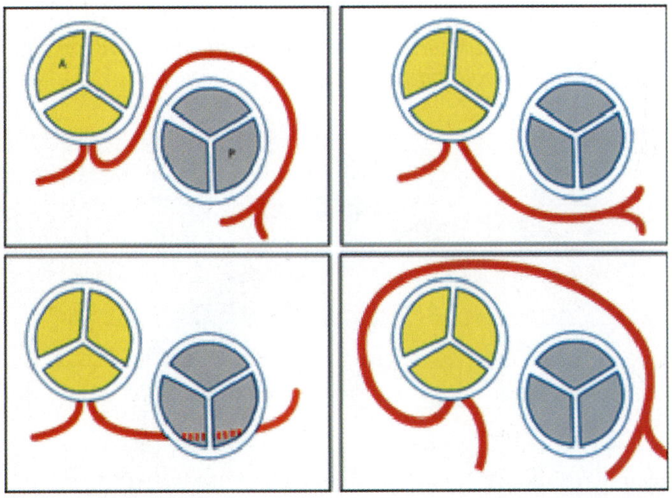

Fig. 13.24: *Origin of the left main coronary artery (LMCA) from the right sinus of valsalva. Top left: the LMCA passes between the aorta and pulmonary trunk, posteriorly and adjacent to the pulmonary trunk. Top right: the LMCA passes anteriorly over the right ventricular outflow tract. Bottom left: the LMCA may course along the crista supraventricularis intramyocardially or subendocardially, surfacing in the proximal interventricular sulcus. Bottom right: the LMCA may rise to the right of the right coronary artery and pass posteriorly to the aortic root*

3. *Hypertrophic Cardiomyopathy*

Significant CAD due to atherosclerosis is found in 25% of patients aged >45 years with hypertrophic cardiomyopathy. Because symptoms due to CAD and hypertrophic cardiomyopathy are similar, patients with ischemic symptoms not well controlled with medical therapy may require coronary angiography to resolve the cause of chest pain. Coronary angiography also is indicated in patients with chest discomfort and hypertrophic cardiomyopathy in whom a surgical procedure is planned to correct outflow tract obstruction.

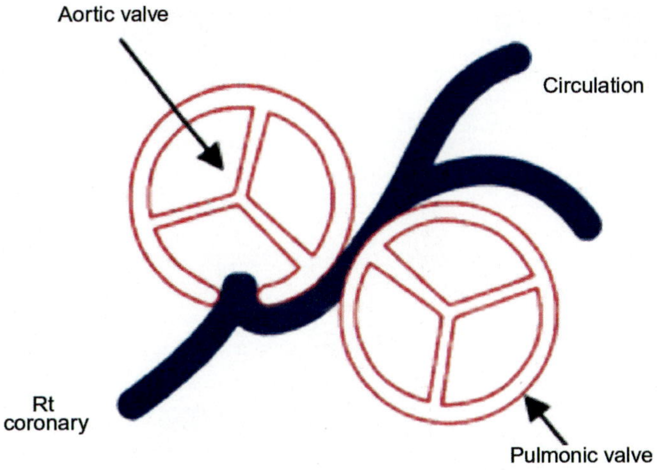

Fig. 13.25: *Coronary artery compression*

4. *Chest Trauma*

Patients who have an acute MI shortly after blunt or penetrating chest trauma may have atherosclerotic CAD, but coronary artery obstruction or damage has been reported in the absence of coronary atherosclerosis. Furthermore, myocardial contusion may simulate acute MI. Infrequently, coronary angiography is indicated in the management of such patients.

5. *Miscellaneous Conditions* (Figs 13.39–13.45)

Preoperative coronary angiography may be indicated in patients undergoing cardiac operations such as

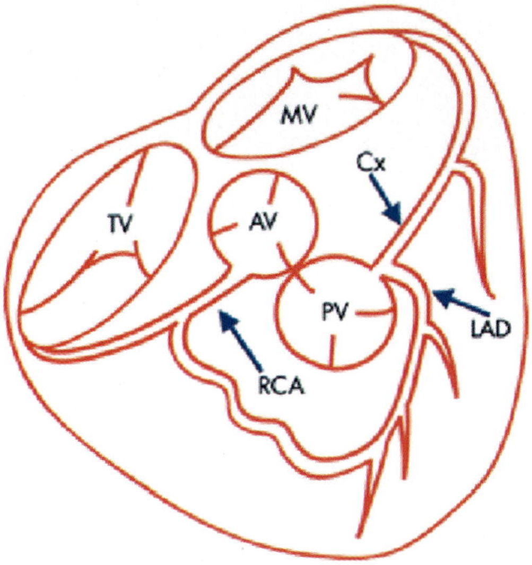

Fig. 13.26: *Anomalous origin of the left coronary artery from the pulmonary artery (ALCAPA). AV, aortic valve; Cx, circumflex coronary artery; LAD, left anterior descending coronary artery; MV, mitral valve; PV, pulmonic valve; RCA, right coronary artery; TV, tricuspid valve.*

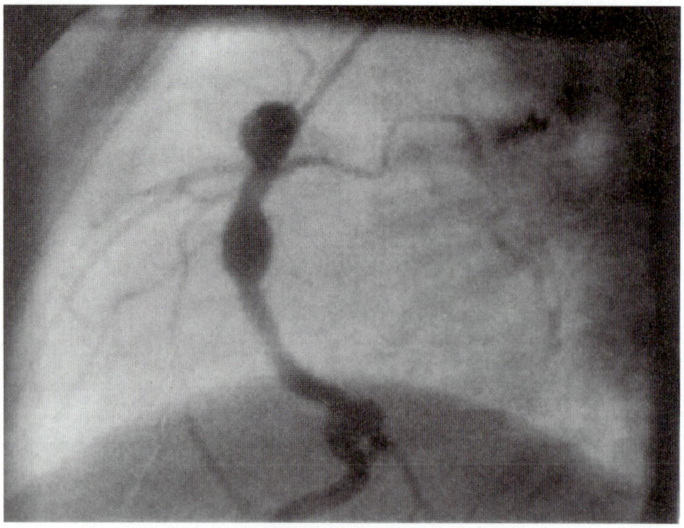

Fig. 13.27: *Aneurysm and stenosis affecting right coronary artery and obliterated left anterior descending*

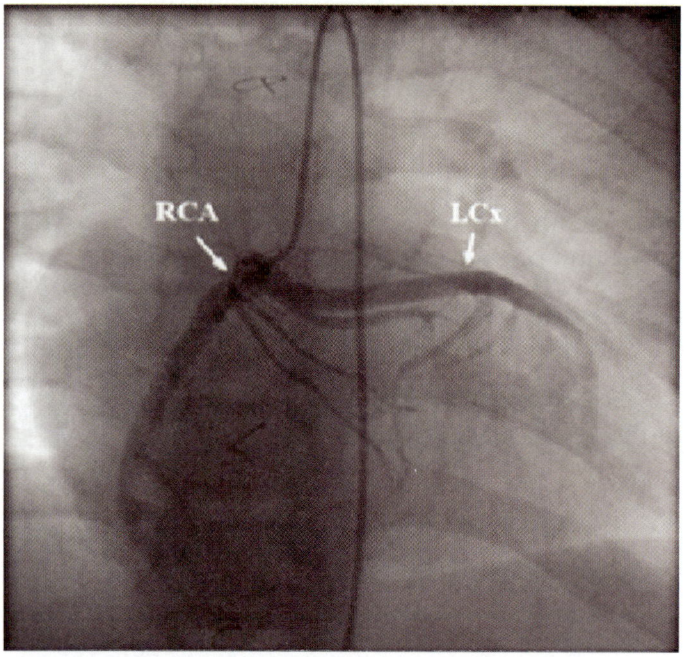

Fig. 13.28: *Selective right coronary angiography, early phase, the left circumflex artery (LCx) originating from the right coronary artery (RCA)*

pericardiectomy or removal of chronic pulmonary emboli if they have 1 risk factor for coronary disease, especially advanced age. Because of the concern about transplanting a donor heart affected by coronary disease, many advocate coronary angiography before transplantation, at least for those donors with a significant likelihood of CAD.

PHARMACOLOGIC ASSESSMENT OF CORONARY SPASM

a. Coronary Artery Spasm

Epicardial coronary arteries exhibit vasoactivity similar to that of many systemic arteries of a similar caliber. The

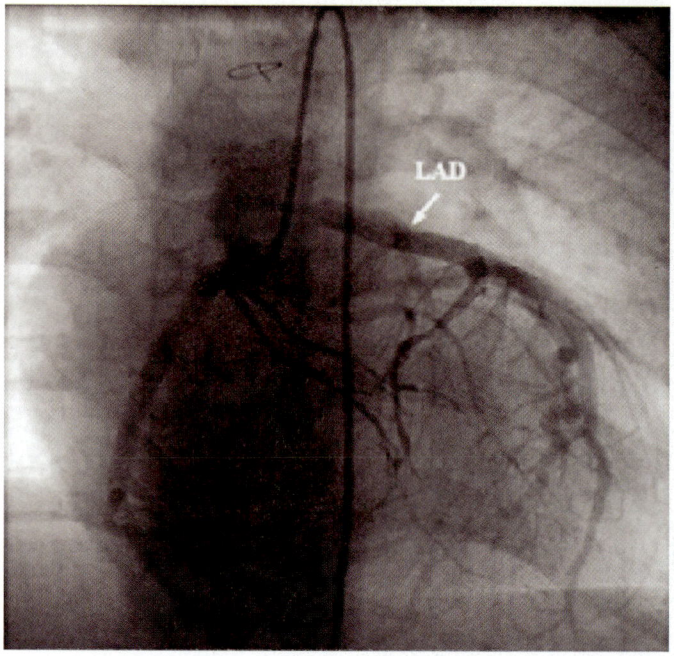

Fig. 13.29: *Late phase of contrast injection to the right coronary artery demonstrated retrograde filling of the left anterior descending coronary artery (LAD) via intramyocardial collaterals and shunting to pulmonary artery*

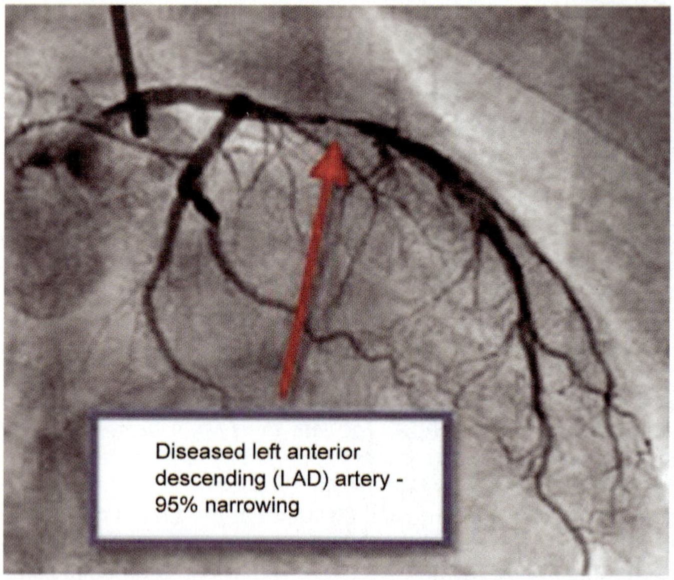

Fig. 13.30: *Selective right coronary angiography, showing 95% narrowing of left anterior descending coronary artery*

presence of atherosclerotic plaque is associated with endothelial dysfunction, which can increase or decrease segmental responses to endogenous and exogenous vasoactive substances. Thus, patients with coronary atherosclerosis may have spontaneous increases in coronary vasomotor tone, resulting in myocardial ischemia. These regional coronary vasospastic events can cause ischemia associated with a variety of ST and T-wave changes. Tobacco and cocaine abuse are important risk factors for the provocation of vasospasm. Provocative

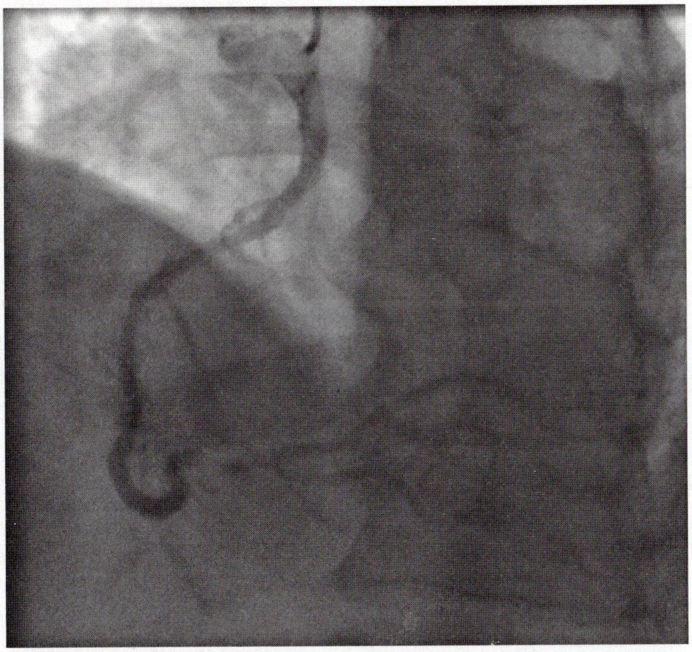

Fig. 13.31: *Nonselective injection into the ascending aorta revealed the abbrant high take-off of the RCA from the aorta. Nonslective injection revealed 90% stenosis with calcification as the distal portion of the RCA*

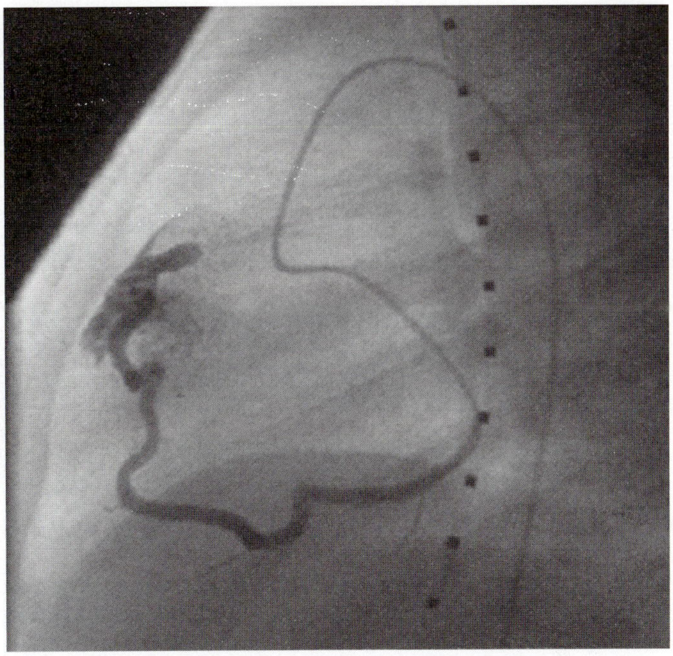

Fig. 13.33: *Coronary angiogram during interventional catheterization in a patient with coronary artery fistula*

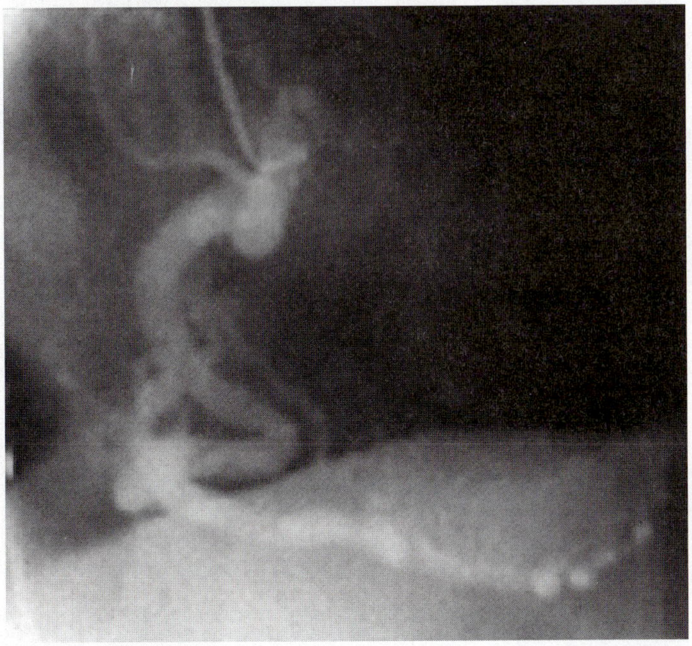

Fig. 13.32: *Dilated right coronary artery associated with ALCAPA*

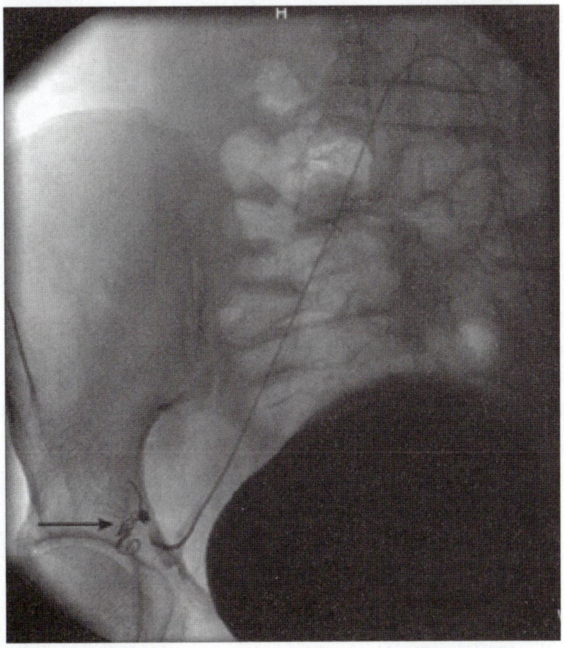

Fig. 13.34: *Treatment of bleeding point by coil embolization (arrow)*

testing with either methylergonovine or acetylcholine often demonstrates the presence of coronary spasm. Although vasomotion can result in as much as a 20% change in lumen diameter, coronary spasm is considered to be present when a reduction in lumen caliber of >50% occurs during a provocative test and reversal is achieved with intracoronary nitroglycerin.

Prinzmetal variant angina is a clinical syndrome occurring in a small percentage of patients without angiographic evidence of significant stenosis or normal angiograms in whom ischemia is caused by severe spasm of an epicardial coronary artery. Variant angina, as described by Prinzmetal in 1959 is an unusual syndrome characterized by ischemic myocardial pain that usually occurs at rest, with accompanying ECG ST-segment elevation. Basal coronary artery vasoreactivity and tone are increased in variant angina. Studies using ^{123}I metaiodobenzylguanidine (^{123}I MIBG) SPECT demonstrate

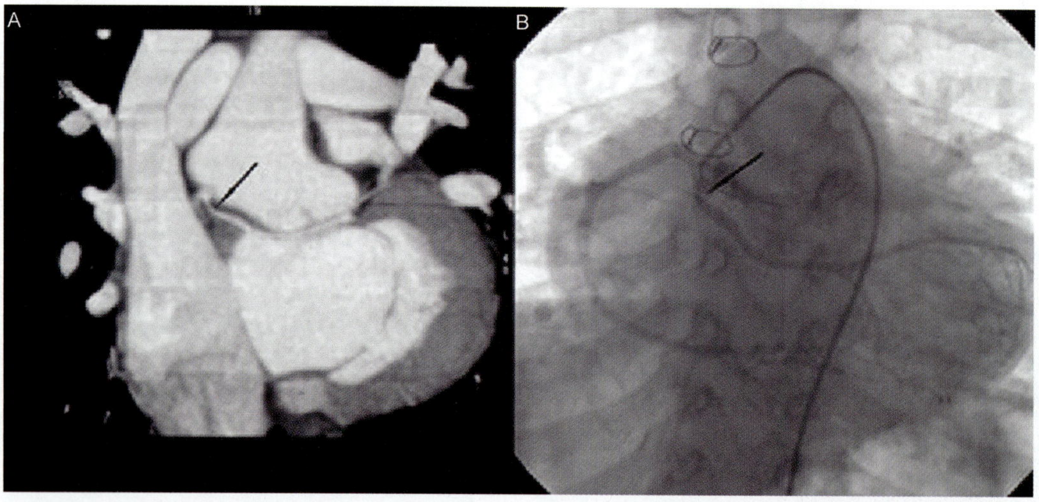

Fig.13.35: *Stretching of the circumflex artery oblique multiplanar reconstruction (A) showing the origin of the right coronary artery in a child presenting with a Yacoub type D coronary distribution. The left circumflex artery arises from the right neosinus and follows a long retroaortic course with substrantial stretching of its proximal segment (arrow). A neosinus had been surgically created to treat a stenosis of the right ostium. (B) Corresponding invasive angiogram: selective catheterization of the right neosinus, showing the right coronary artery and the stenosis (arrow) of the proximal segment of the retroaortic circumflex artery*

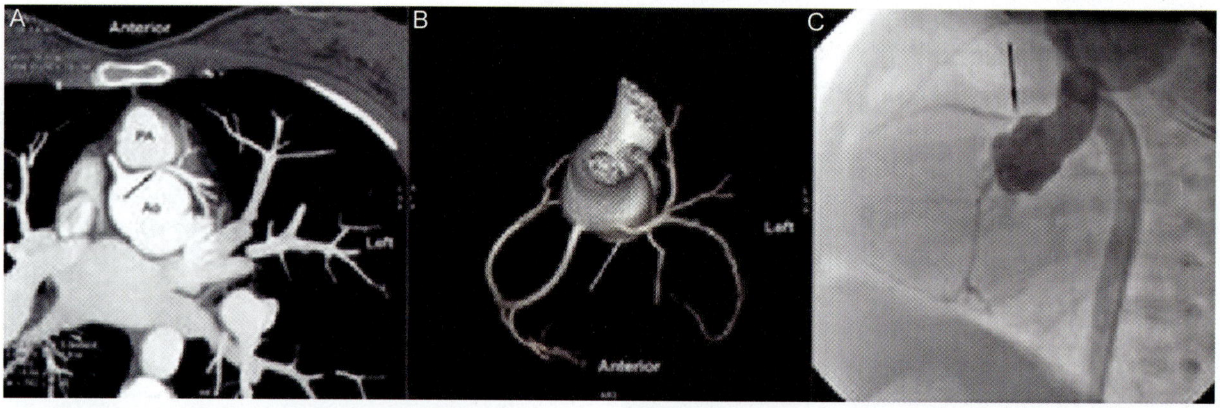

Fig. 13.36: *Ostial stenosis of the left main coronary artery axial cross-section (A) and three dimensional reconstructed image in anterosuperior orientation (B) showing a tight stenosis (arrow) at the ostium of the left coronary artery. Please note that the left ostium is reimplanted at an anterior 12 o'clock position so that it is localized between the great arteries. (C) Corresponding invasive aortography showing the tight stenosis of the left coronary artery ostium*

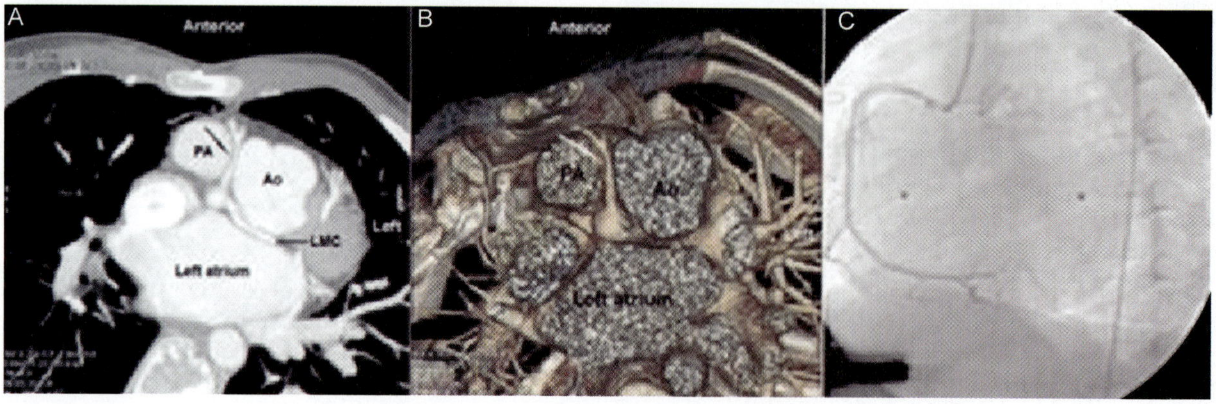

Fig. 13.37: *Mild compression of the right coronary artery axial cross-section (maximum intensity projection) (A) and three dimensional reconstruction (B) showing a single coronary ostium from which both the right and left coronary arteries arise. There is mild compression of a long segment of the right coronary artery between the great arteries. The left coronary artery has a retroaortic loop with no stretching or compression. (C) Selective invasive angiogram of the right coronary artery: the proximal segment was classified as normal*

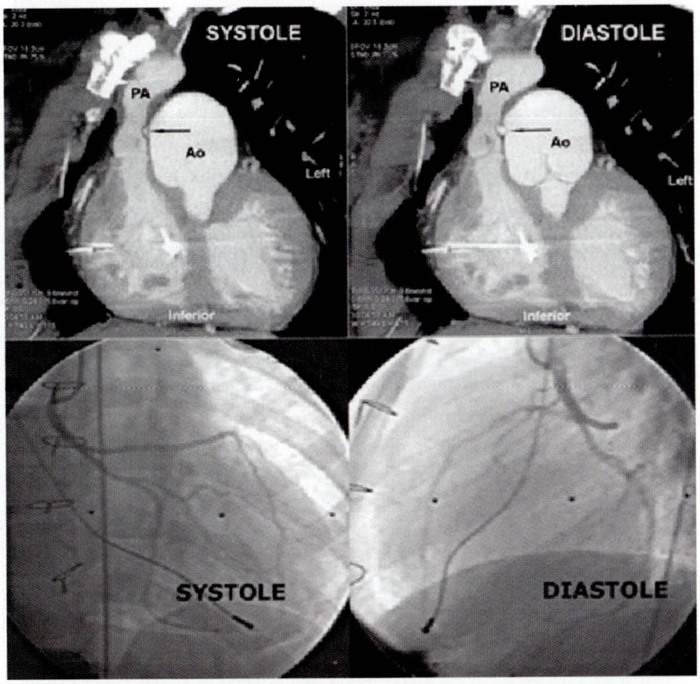

Fig. 13.38: *Systolic compression of the left coronary artery (top) Sagittal oblique cross-section on CT. Note the banana-shape of the left coronary artery (arrow) caused by systolic compression between the anterior pulmonary artery and the posterior aorta (left panel). During diastole, caliber and shape of the coronary artery are normal (right panel). (Bottom) Corresponding invasive angiogram: the systolic compression of the proximal segment of the left coronary artery appears nonsignificant*

regional myocardial sympathetic dysinnervation in patients with variant angina. Tobacco and cocaine may cause episodes of variant angina, the latter because it blocks presynaptic uptake of norepinephrine and dopamine, thereby facilitating alpha-adrenergically mediated vasospasm. Cardiac arrhythmias including ventricular tachycardia and fibrillation, heart block, acute infarction and sudden death, may occur in association with variant angina. Studies using ^{123}I BMIPP, a branched fatty acid, have demonstrated myocardial injury in association with some episodes of variant angina.

b. Provocative Testing for Spasm

Of the tests available to demonstrate coronary spasm, provocation by ergonovine maleate, methylergonovine maleate, acetylcholine or hyperventilation are the most useful. Ergonovine maleate for injection is no longer available, and the availability of methylergonovine is limited. The intravenous administration of incremental doses of methylergonovine starting at 0.05 mg to a maximum of 0.40 mg is both sensitive and specific, and there is an inverse relationship between the dose required to provoke spasm in the laboratory and the frequency of spontaneous episodes experienced by the patient. To ensure a valid test, nitrates and calcium antagonists must be withdrawn for 48 hours before testing. Women are more sensitive than men to methylergonovine.

The intracoronary route of administration of methylergonovine for provocation of spasm is safe, sensitive and specific. This route is preferable in hypertensive patients and affords the opportunity to evaluate the left and right coronary circulations separately. Small dosing increments of 5–10 µg are used with a total dose not to exceed 50 µg.

Absolute contraindications to methylergonovine include pregnancy, severe hypertension, severe left ventricular dysfunction, moderate to severe aortic stenosis and high-grade left main coronary stenosis. Relative contra-indications include uncontrolled or unstable angina, uncontrolled ventricular arrhythmia, recent MI and advanced coronary disease.

Alternatively, intracoronary acetylcholine can be used as a provocative test for spasm, and its effectiveness is comparable to methylergonovine. Acetylcholine is infused over 1 min into a coronary artery in incremental doses of

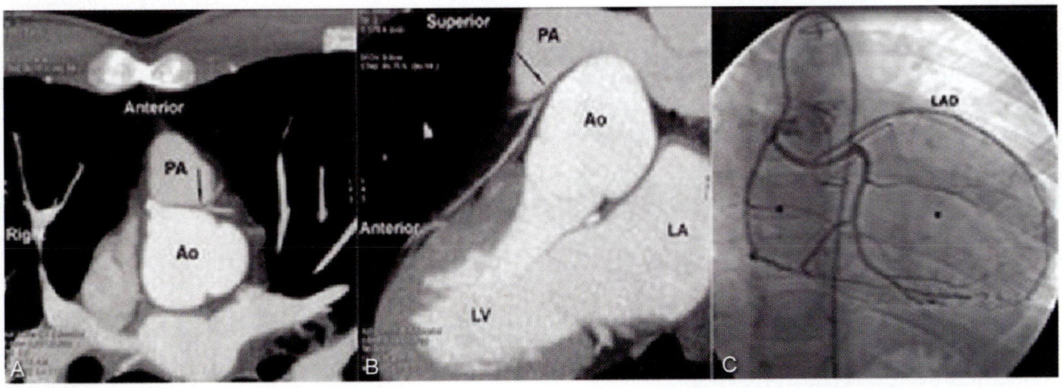

Fig. 13.39: *Left main coronary artery with a course between aorta and pulmonary artery axial (A) and sagittal oblique (B) cross-section through the origin of the left coronary artery. The left coronary artery displays a tight stenosis (arrow) and follows a course between the aorta and pulmonary artery. (C) Corresponding invasive angiogram: selective catheterization of the left coronary ostium was not achieved. Selective right coronary angiography shows a dominant right coronary artery giving rise to a circumflex artery retrogradely filling the left anterior descending artery. Ao, aorta; LA, left atrium; LAD, left anterior descending coronary artery; LV, left ventricle; PA, pulmonary artery.*

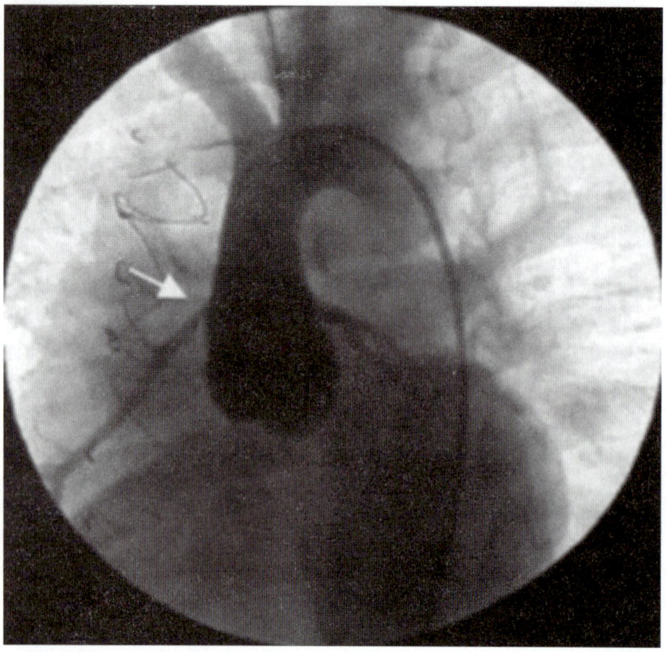

Fig. 13.40: *Late assessment after the arterial switch operation for transposition of the great arteries, coronary angiogram shows lumen reduction at the origin of the right coronary artery*

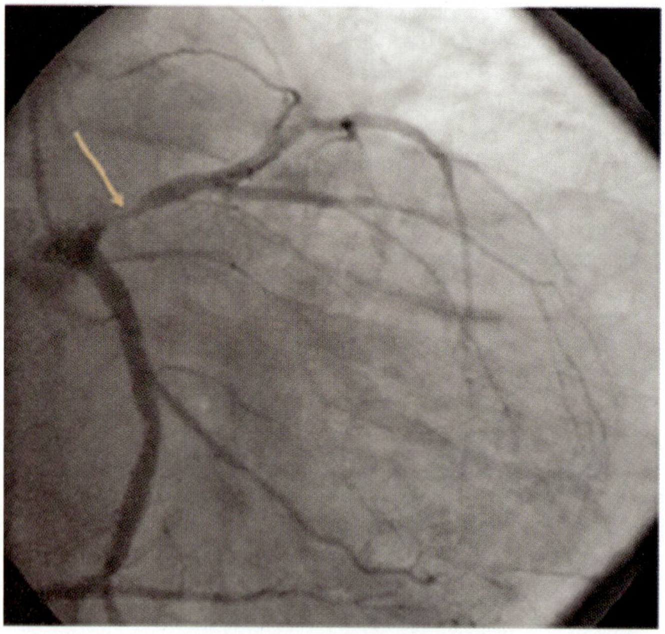

Fig. 13.41: *Caudal view in selective coronary angiogram showing subtotal paraosteal occlusion of LAD*

10, 25, 50 µg and 100 µg. Doses should be separated by 5-min intervals. The same procedural safeguards must be used with acetylcholine and methylergonovine.

In patients with 1 episode of variant angina per day, the hyperventilation provocative test is nearly as effective as methylergonovine in causing vasospasm. In patients with less frequent attacks, hyperventilation is less sensitive. The test requires a patient to hyperventilate vigorously at 30 respirations per minute for 5 min. With this degree of

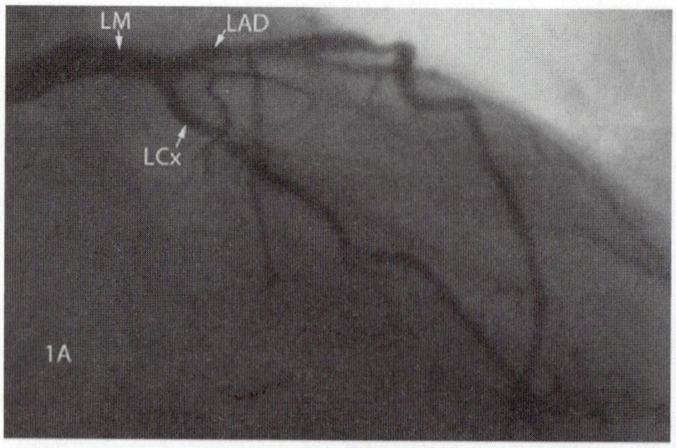

Fig. 13.42A: *The origin of left circumflex artery from left main coronary artery. LCx, left circumflex artery; LAD, left anterior descending artery; LM, left main*

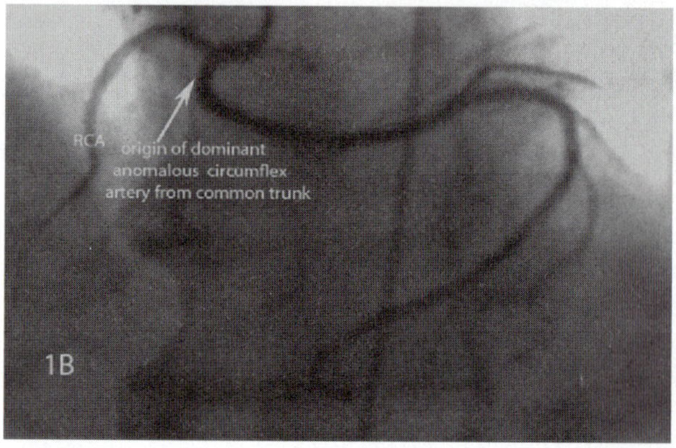

Fig. 13.42B: *The origin of dominant anomalous circumflex artery from a common trunk originating from the right coronary cusp. RCA, right coronary artery*

hyperventilation, arterial pH will increase to 7.60 and pCO_2 will decrease to 20 mmHg. Variant angina if provoked, will occur during hyperventilation and will subside more rapidly than after methylergonovine infusion. The cold presser test can also provoke coronary spasm but is less reliable than pharmacologic techniques.

In patients with ST-segment elevation during episodes of chest pain and a normal coronary angiogram, provocative tests are usually not necessary because ample clinical evidence is present to confirm the diagnosis of coronary spasm.

Recommendations for Intracoronary Doppler Ultrasound

Class I

None.

Class IIa

Assessment of the physiological effects of intermediate coronary stenoses (30–70% luminal narrowing) in patients with anginal symptoms. Doppler velocimetry may also be useful as an alternative to performing a noninvasive functional study to determine whether an intervention is

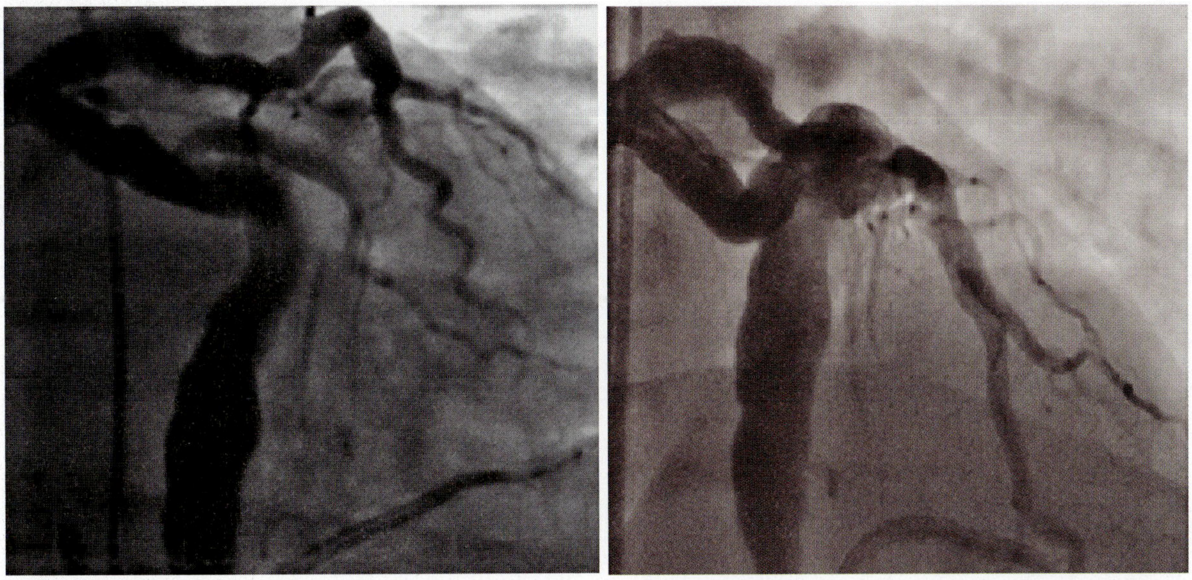

Fig. 13.43: *Heart catheterization images showing severe diffuse coronary artery ectasia with left circumflex dominant circulation in a patient with adult Kawasaki's disease*

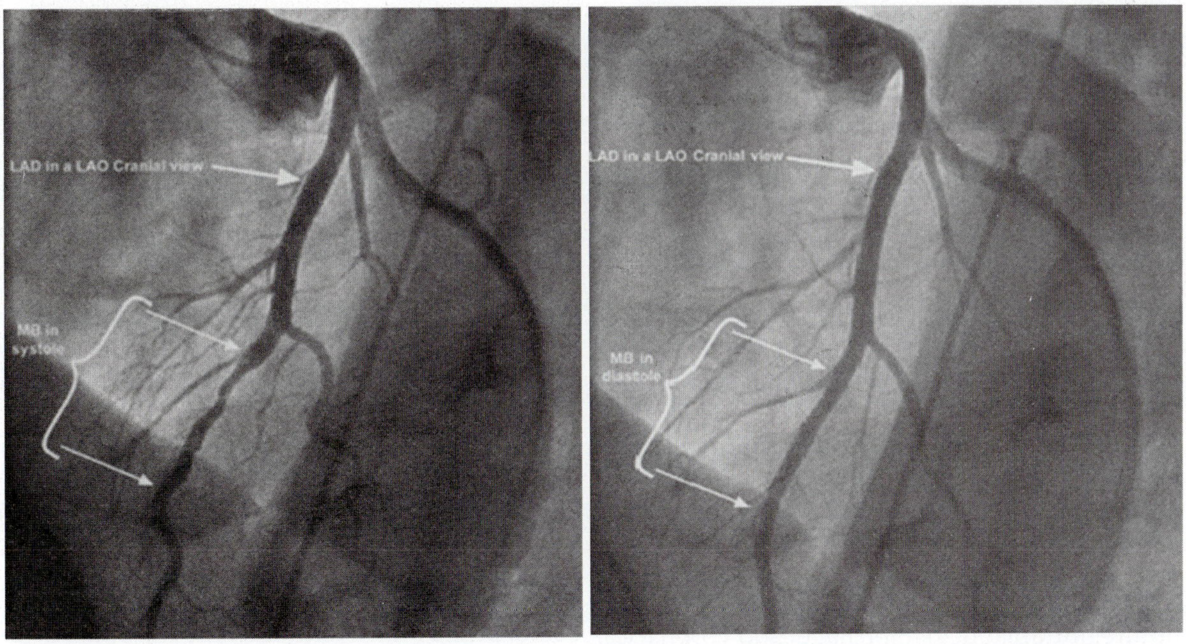

Fig. 13.44: *(A) Selective angiography showing coronary constriction (terminal part of LAD) during systole and normal lumen during diastole (B) in a patient who presented with angina pectoris, HT and nonspecific ECG alterations in anterolateral leads and finally found to have muscular banding of LAD*

warranted for intermediate lesions (or when the functional study is ambiguous). *(Level of Evidence: C)*

Class IIb

1. Evaluation of the success of percutaneous coronary revascularization in restoring flow reserve and to predict the risk of restenosis. *(Level of Evidence: C)*
2. After cardiac transplantation, diagnosis of impaired CFR in patients with anginal symptoms but no apparent angiographic culprit lesion. *(Level of Evidence: C)*
3. Assessment of the severity of coronary flow abnormalities in patients with anginal symptoms and a positive noninvasive functional study but no apparent angiographic lesion. *(Level of Evidence: C)*

Class III

Routine assessment of the severity of angiographic disease in patients with a positive noninvasive functional study.

(Level of Evidence: C).

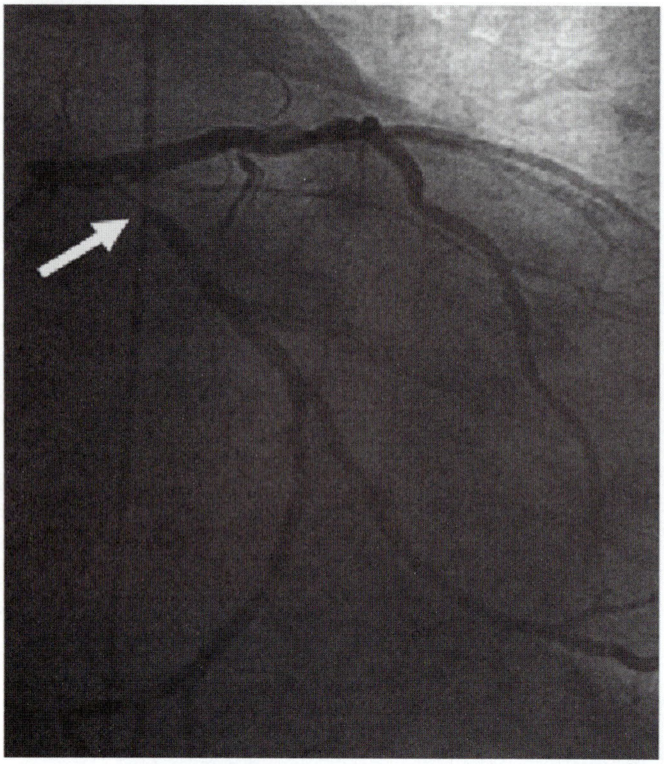

Fig. 13.45: *Invasive coronary angiogram in a patient demonstrates moderate lesion in the proximal left circumflex coronary artery (arrow) which was hemodynamically significant (FFR, 0.67)*

CORONARY ANGIOSCOPY IN THE EVALUATION OF CORONARY ARTERY DISEASE

CORONARY ANGIOSCOPY

Coronary angioscopy uses visible light conducted through fiberoptic filaments to provide direct visual assessment of the surface characteristics and intraluminal morphology in vivo. The images appear in color on a television monitor, which enables examination of the hue of the target lesion and associated plaques. Although difficult to use, angioscopy allows the differentiation of platelet-rich from fibrin-rich thrombus, and it may provide evidence of atheroma rupture, intraplaque hemorrhage, and coronary dissection. Accordingly, this diagnostic imaging modality yields information on the pathogenesis of acute coronary syndromes.

1. Angioscopy Equipment and Technique

All angioscopes require a blood-free field for clear visualization of the arterial wall. This is obtained by inflating a proximal balloon to temporarily occlude blood flow, followed by continuous saline irrigation, which requires a second catheter lumen. Two additional lumens are required for the optical fibers, one for visualization and another to serve as a light source. Videotape recording allows for more detailed offline analysis. A commonly used device is a 120-cm-long 4.5 monorail catheter with an imaging bundle containing 3,000 fibers that permits a viewing arc of 55° and a depth-of-field of 0.5 mm. A video camera displays the images in real time on a color monitor, while videotape recording allows for more detailed offline analysis (Fig. 13.3).

2. Angioscopy of Unstable Coronary Syndromes

Small-scale studies of fiberoptic angioscopy demonstrate differences in the intraluminal appearance of stable versus unstable coronary lesions. An intraoperative study of 32 patients showed distinctive intimal abnormalities in all 10 patients with unstable angina: four patients had "complex plaque" and seven had overt intraluminal thrombus. Neither complex plaques nor thrombi were observed by angioscopy in any patient with stable coronary disease. These findings were later confirmed by percutaneous angioscopy. In 16 patients with unstable angina, 50% had thrombus and 14% had overt dissection. Neither thrombus nor dissection was seen in any of the four patients with stable angina.

In addition to identifying the presence of thrombus, angioscopy can differentiate platelet-rich from fibrin-rich thrombi. Mizuno et al performed angioscopy in 15 patients with unstable angina and 16 patients with acute MI. Angioscopy identified intraluminal thrombus in 29 of 31 patients. However, the typical thrombus in patients with unstable angina was grayish-white in color, suggesting the predominance of platelets, whereas in patients with acute MI, angioscopy identified a preponderance of red thrombi, suggesting an erythrocyte and fibrin-rich clot. Angioscopy can distinguish other surface features of coronary atheromata. Stable plaques are recognized by their elevated contour, smooth configuration, and yellowish-white color. In a study of 199 patients, those with predominantly yellow plaques were found to have higher low-density lipoprotein (LDL) cholesterol and apolipoprotein B levels.

3. Angioscopy during Interventions

Assessment of lesions before or after coronary intervention represents the most commonly reported application of coronary angioscopy. Angioscopy after balloon angioplasty demonstrates that dissections and thrombus are present in almost all cases. However, no prospective data exist that demonstrate a different outcome for patients on the basis of angioscopic findings. The preprocedural identification of thrombus may also prove useful in selecting candidates for coronary stenting and for the use of any of the new antiplatelet agents. Although the value of angioscopy in identifying thrombus is well established, no data exist to suggest that angioscopy can reduce stent-related complications.

4. Limitations of Coronary Angioscopy

Despite recent technical advances, angioscopy is still limited to the proximal and mid portions of relatively straight, large epicardial coronary arteries. Furthermore, the rapid development of ischemia during balloon inflation limits the time of examination. For successful imaging, lesions need to be located 20 mm distal to the balloon site,

Table 13.2: *Relative contraindications to coronary angiography*

- Acute renal failure
- Chronic renal failure secondary to diabetes
- Active gastrointestinal bleeding
- Unexplained fever which may be due to infection
- Untreated active infection
- Acute stroke
- Severe anemia
- Severe uncontrolled hypertension
- Severe symptomatic electrolyte imbalance
- Severe lack of cooperation by patient due to psychological or severe systemic illness
- Severe concomitant illness that drastically shortens life expectancy or increases risk of therapeutic interventions
- Refusal of patient to consider definitive therapy such as PTCA, CABG, or valve replacement
- Digitalis intoxication
- Documented anaphylactoid reaction to angiographic contrast media
- Severe peripheral vascular disease limiting vascular access
- Decompensated congestive heart failure or acute pulmonary edema
- Severe coagulopathy
- Aortic valve endocarditis

PTCA, percutaneous transluminal coronary angioplasty; CABG, coronary artery bypass graft.

which makes it impossible to visualize ostial or very proximal lesions. Angioscopy shows only the surface characteristics of plaques and cannot discern the underlying atheroma morphology. Accordingly, it remains unproved whether visualization of surface anatomy alone warrants the time, expense and risk of angioscopy. In addition, occlusion of coronary flow may produce important imaging artifacts. A recently published study of the European Working Group on Coronary Angioscopy demonstrated that the identification of red thrombus and dissection has relatively close interobserver agreement. However, other angioscopic diagnoses have wide interobserver variability.

5. Recommendations for Coronary Angioscopy

Class I

None.

Class II

None.

Class III

Coronary angioscopy should be considered a research tool for which there are no established clinical indications.

FRACTIONAL FLOW RESERVE OF CORONARY ARTERY

FRACTIONAL FLOW RESERVE (FFR)

The measurement of pressure gradients across coronary stenoses was the earliest method used to assess the adequacy of coronary angioplasty. However, because of the size of the catheter and changes in technology, angiographic and now ultrasonic assessments are more commonly used. Recently, small catheters and guidewires have been developed to more accurately measure pressure gradients across stenoses before and after interventional procedures. Pijls and colleagues demonstrated that just as with CFR measurements by Doppler ultrasound, FFR is useful in assessing the severity of a coronary stenosis. The ratio of the mean pressure distal to a coronary stenosis to that proximal to the stenosis, usually measured through the guiding catheter after maximal vasodilation induced by adenosine or papaverine, can assess the severity of the stenosis. When this ratio falls below 75%, there is an 88% sensitivity and an 84% specificity for an abnormal exercise test. Similar correlations have been made with PET and CFR measured by Doppler ultrasound. The technique is easier to use than Doppler ultrasound. Although it is still in development and validation, it appears likely to be a useful tool in the future to assess coronary stenoses (Fig. 13.47).

What is fractional flow reserve?

Myocardial FFR is a new index of the functional severity of a coronary stenosis that is calculated from pressure measurements made during coronary arteriography. This new approach enables an "on the spot" diagnosis as to what extent a given stenosis (coronary blockage) contributes to reversible myocardial ischemia and the decision whether revascularization of the stenosis is warranted.

How does FFR work?

- FFR closely relates distal coronary pressure to myocardial blood flow during maximum arteriolar vasodilatation.
- The functional state of a patient with a coronary artery stenosis is determined by the maximum blood flow that can reach the heart muscle. As soon as maximum achievable blood flow, at a given level of exercise, is no longer sufficient to match oxygen demand, myocardial ischemia and angina will occur.

How are FFR measurements performed?

- FFR can be measured during a routine cardiac catheterization (Figs 13.46, 13.48 and 13.52)
- The stenosis is crossed with an 0.014" pressure guidewire for recording the trans-stenotic pressure, and administering a maximum hyperemic stimulus. (intracoronary adenosine—12–20 µg or intravenous adenosine—140 µg/kg/min infused into the femoral vein).

What do the FFR values mean?

FFR value < 0.75 discriminates functionally significant lesions.

- FFR > 0.75 means the blockage is not severe enough to limit blood flow to the heart.
- FFR < 0.75 means that the blockage is severe enough to limit blood flow to the heart and should be opened if possible.

What are the benefits of FFR?

- FFR is a specific index for the epicardial stenosis and therefore better indicates to what degree a patient can be helped by revascularization.
- FFR has a normal value of 1.0 in every patient and every coronary artery.
- FFR is independent of changes in heart rate, blood pressure, and contractility.
- FFR takes into account the contribution of the collateral flow.
- FFR can be applied in multivessel disease and for serial lesions within one vessel.

How are FFR measurements performed?

- FFR can be measured during a routine cardiac catheterization.
- The stenosis is crossed with an 0.014" pressure guidewire for recording the trans-stenotic pressure, and administering a maximum hyperemic stimulus. (intracoronary adenosine—12–20 µg or intravenous adenosine—140 µg/kg/min infused into the femoral vein).

When is FFR used?

- FFR is used as a diagnostic tool to determine whether a particular coronary stenosis, found at angiography, is responsible for reversible ischaemia (and consequently should be dilated or bypassed if medical treatment fails).
- Specifically in respect to intermediate stenosis.
- Identification of the culprit lesion in case of multivessel disease.
- Justification to perform (or avoid) angioplasty in a patient without documented evidence of ischemia at non-invasive testing.

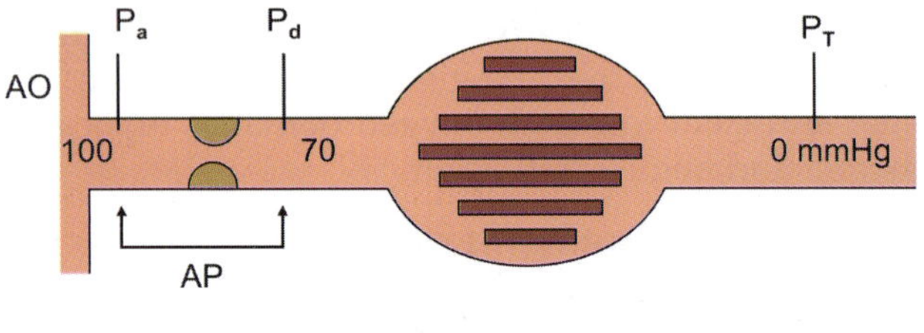

Fig. 13.46: *Simplified illustration of a coronary artery and the dependent myocardial bed. If that system is studied under conditions of maximum arteriolar vasodilatation, myocardial resistance will be minimal and equal to R min. Under such circumstances the flow limiting effect of the epicardial stenosis is maximal, as is the pressure drop across the lesion, expressed as the ratio of driving pressure to resistance, maximum attainable blood flow through the myocardium equals the ratio of the perfusion pressure across the myocardium (distal coronary pressure minus central venous pressure) and the resistance R min. If there is no epicardial stenosis, the perfusion pressure across the myocardium equals Pa Pv where Pa is mean aortic pressure and Pv is central venous pressure. In the presence of a coronary stenosis, the perfusion pressure across the myocardium has decreased to Pd Pv, where Pd represents hyperaemic coronary pressure distal to the stenosis*

- To indicate the exact location of a lesion in case of overprojection and other situations where the angiographic image is unclear.
- Coronary intervention.
- A high value of FFR after regular balloon angioplasty is associated with a favorable long term outcome.
- Coronary stenting.
- Evaluation of optimum stent deployment.

Noninvasive Coronary Multidetector CT Angiography

Preoperative evaluation of patients scheduled to undergo noncoronary cardiovascular surgery includes the use of invasive coronary angiography (ICA) to rule out the coexistence of significant CAD. Despite the absence of apparent clinical symptoms of angina, prevalence of significant CAD in this population has been reported to be between 8% and 41% . The relevance of this finding lies in the observation that revascularization in these patients in addition to the procedure of noncoronary cardiovascular surgery reduces the occurrence of perioperative and postoperative adverse major clinical events (Figs 13.53–13.70).

Multidetector coronary CT angiography of the coronary arteries is nowadays a reliable technique to rule out significant CAD, with a proved high negative predictive value, particularly in patients with low or intermediate pretest probability of disease. Thus, the technique has been applied in the preoperative screening of noncoronary cardiovascular surgery although initial reports are limited to patients with valvular heart disease, in regular sinus rhythm. In the largest study to date, patients with atrial fibrillation also were included. All these studies, however, consist basically of a comparison between ICA and coronary CT angiography without testing the actual value of coronary CT angiography in terms of avoiding routine ICA in these patients.

The findings of the various studies can be summarized as follows: first, preoperative routine ICA can be safely avoided in a considerable number of patients scheduled to undergo noncoronary cardiovascular surgery by use of coronary CT angiography; second, the presence of a controlled atrial fibrillation does not preclude performing diagnostic coronary CT angiographic examination; third, an Agatston score of coronary calcification higher than 579 significantly increases the likelihood of a subsequent nondiagnostic coronary CT angiography. The performance of ICA as a screening preoperative test before major noncoronary cardiovascular surgery in patients at risk for CAD is recommended. The rationale for this approach lies in the proved adverse prognosis after surgery in patients with undetected CAD and in the reduction in terms of mortality observed when coronary revascularization is performed simultaneously with noncoronary cardio-vascular surgery. Although noninvasive tests for inducible ischemia could represent an alternative to ICA, its usefulness is limited in practice because of a proved suboptimal predictive value of postoperative complications in these patients. As an invasive procedure, ICA is costly

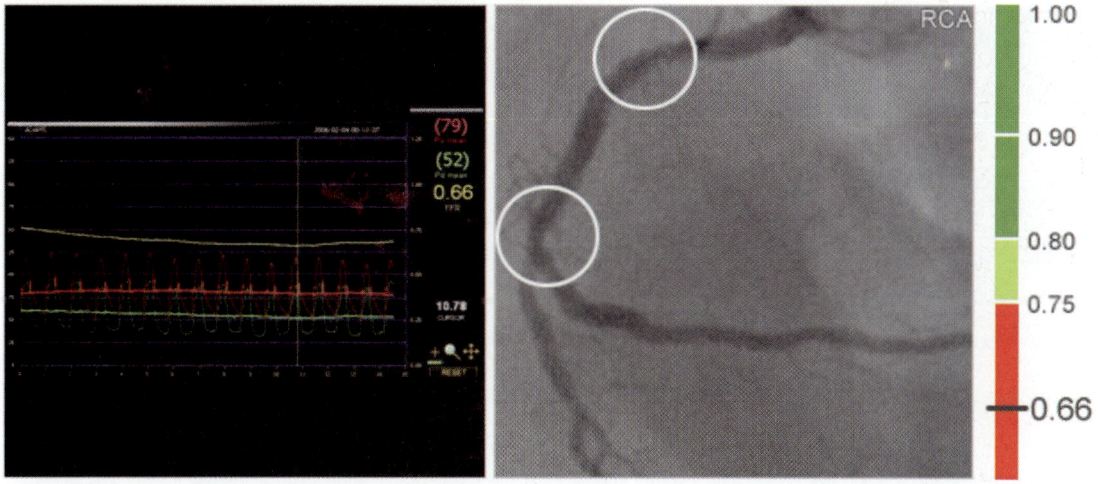

Fig. 13.47: *The FFR in the RCA was well below 0.75. The most proximal stenosis was stented first and a new FFR measurement was performed. A continued low FFR prompted stenting of the distal lesion as well*

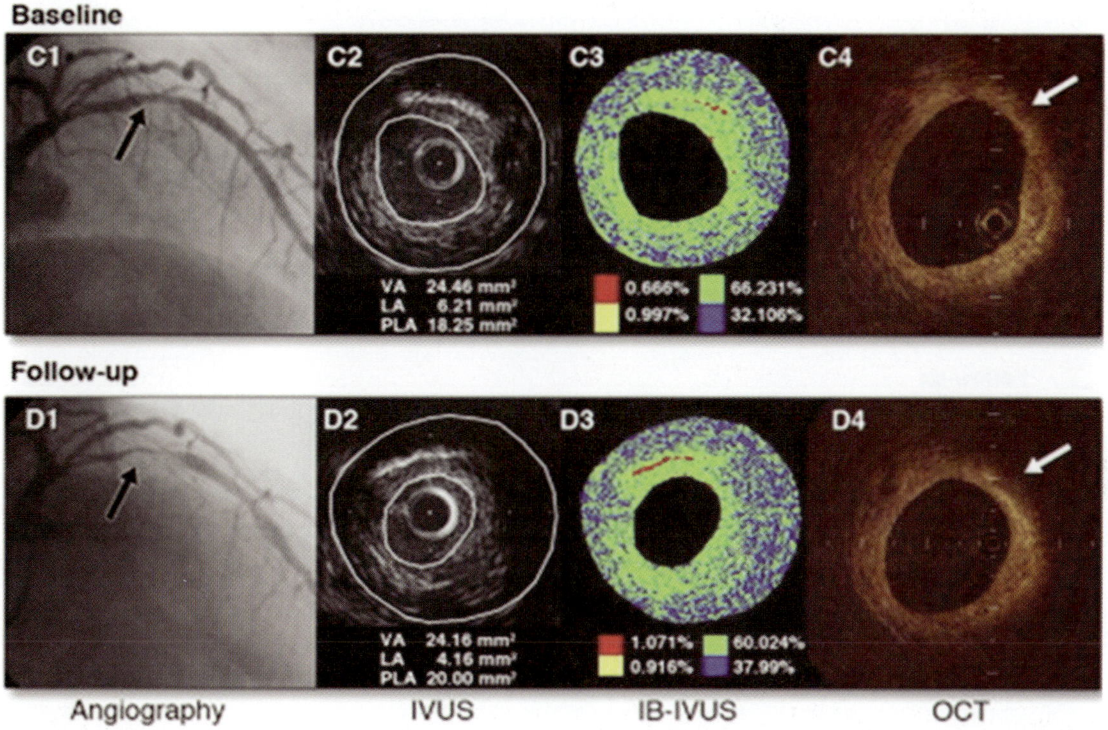

Fig. 13.48: *Coronary angiographic, grayscale IVUS, IB-IVUS, and OCT at baseline and follow-up for the dietary groupwhilst significant progression was observed by angiography during follow-up (C1 and C2), plaque volume index (e.g., plaque area in this slice) increased from 18.2 to 20.0 mm² by grayscale IVUS during follow-up (C2 and D2). Lipid(blue) volume index increased from 32.1% to 37.9%, whereas fibrous (green) volume index decreased from 66.2% to 60.0% by IB-IVUS (C3 and D3). OCT revealed that the fibrous cap thickness of 110 µm did not change during follow-up (arrows in C4 and D4)*

and carries a small but definite risk of complications (1.5%) and even a certain mortality risk (0.15%), and these numbers are higher when the population involved has an increased associated comorbidity, as is the case in those patients scheduled to undergo noncoronary cardiovascular surgery. Furthermore, most of these patients will have normal results at ICA examination; the prevalence of significant CAD in these patients has been reported to range between 10% and 20% because coronary CT angiography has recently emerged as a valuable noninvasive tool for the diagnosis of CAD in symptomatic patients with low to intermediate pretest risk, it seems appropriate to apply the technique to rule out CAD in patients scheduled to undergo noncoronary cardiovascular surgery. Some previous studies have shown a good correlation between coronary CT angiographic and ICA results in selected groups of patients submitted to undergo noncoronary cardiovascular surgery. Of note, in our study, patients did not undergo

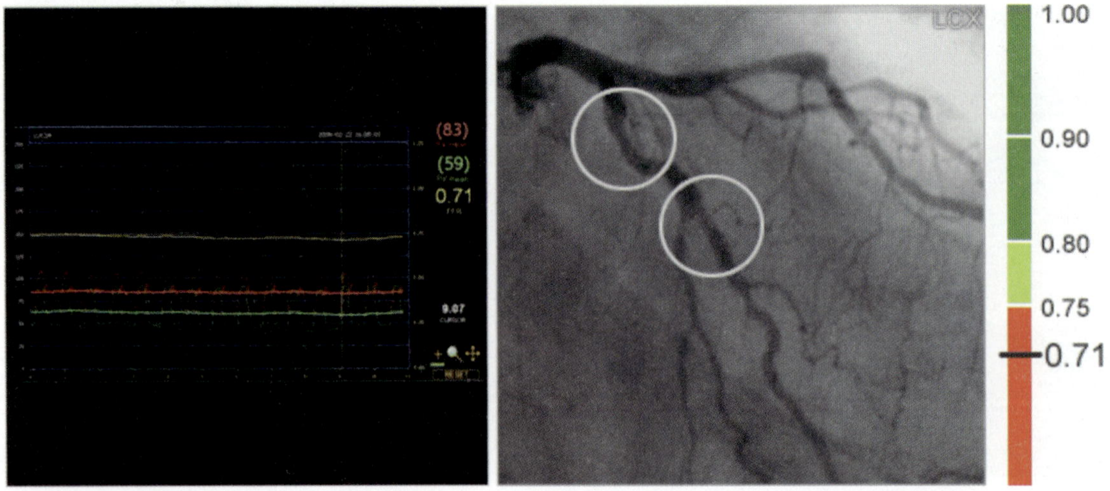

Fig. 13.49: *The FFR in the LCX was below 0.75 and a pressure pullback recording showed both lesions to be significant. Two stents were placed satisfactorily as confirmed by FFR >0.90*

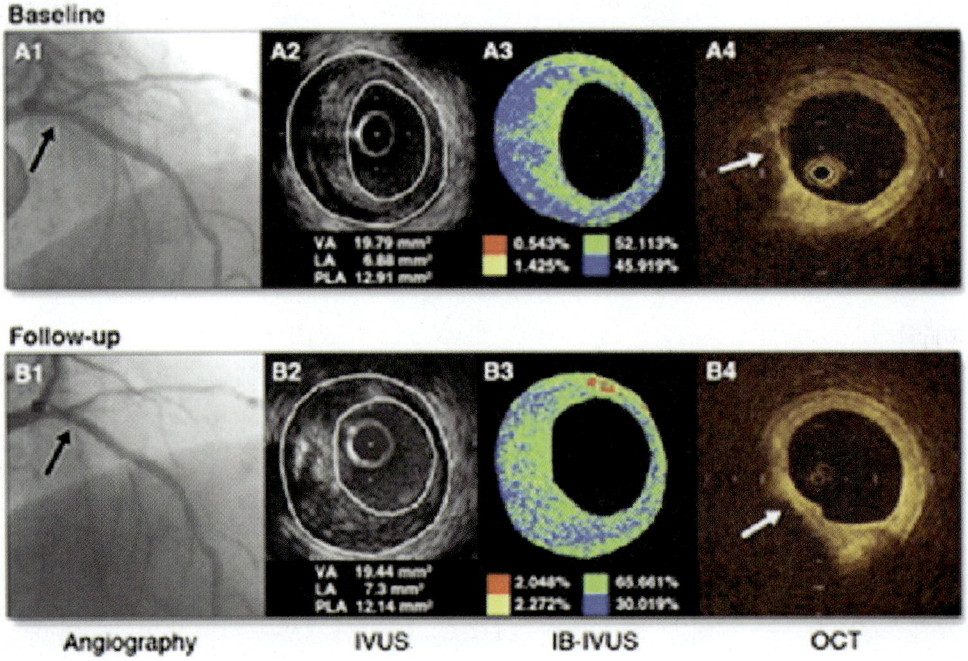

Fig. 13.50: *Coronary angiographic, Grayscale IVUS, IB-IVUS, and OCT at baseline and follow-up for the pitavastatin groupwhile no significant difference was found between baseline and follow-up angiography (A1, B1), plaque volume index (i.e., plaque area in this slice) decreased from 12.9 mm² to 12.1 mm² by grayscale IVUS during follow-up (A2 and B2). Lipid (blue) volume index decreased from 45.9% to 30.0%, while fibrous (green) volume index increased from 52.1% to 65.6% by IB-IVUS (A3 and B3). OCT revealed that the fibrous cap thickness increased from 80 μm to 220 μm during follow-up (arrows in A4 and B4). IB-IVUS, integrated backscatter-intravascular ultrasound; IVUS, intravascular ultrasound; LA, lumen area; OCT, optical coherence tomography; PLA, plaque area; VA, vessel area*

preoperative ICA if deemed to be free of significant CAD after diagnostic coronary CT angiographic examination. Most important, none of these patients had peri- or postoperative complications potentially because of CAD, thus proving the safety of this approach. ICA was performed, in addition to coronary CT angiography, in a total of 40 patients. In those with nondiagnostic coronary CT angiographic studies, ICA results showed a relatively low (5 of 25) prevalence of significant CAD. In most of those patients catheterized because of apparently significant CAD at coronary CT angiography (11 of 15), severity of CAD was confirmed. This is in agreement with the reported suboptimal positive predictive value of coronary CT angiography for defining significant coronary artery lesions

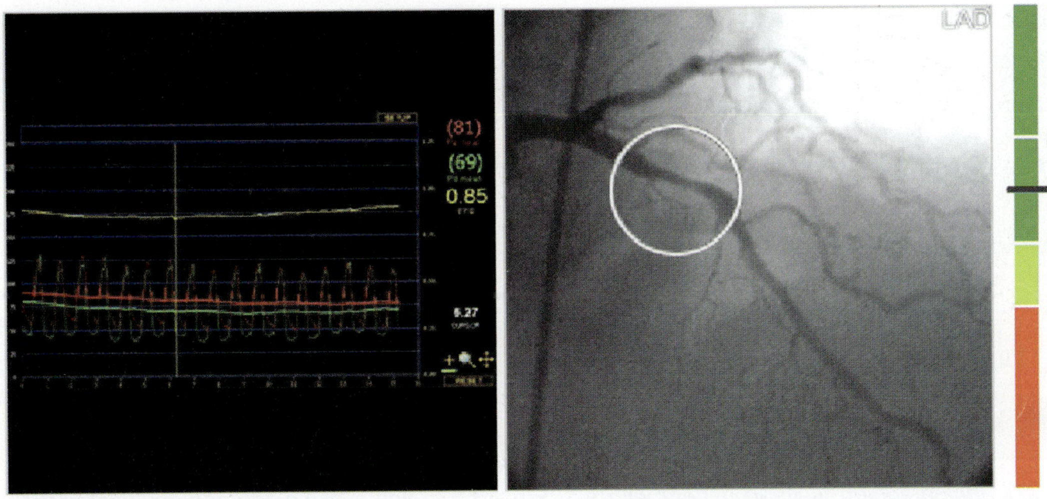

Fig. 13.51: *Angiography showed three-diseased vessels. FFR helped to identify which lesions required treatment. A pressure pullback in the long disease segment of the LAD revealed that there was no significant reduction in flow in this vessel (FFR >0.75)*

In practice, however, this is not a major limitation in the setting of noninvasive preoperative screening for CAD, where it is more relevant to avoid underdiagnosis of CAD rather than overdiagnosis. The consequence will be that a small proportion of patients without significant CAD will still be referred to undergo ICA.

Most important, preoperative coronary CT angiography provides additional information about the thoracic aorta and other mediastinal structures, which is relevant for the cardiac surgeon's choice of cannulation and cross-clamping sites.

The consecutive recruitment of subjects without exclusions due to atrial fibrillation, which was present in nearly half of our population, is also important. Atrial fibrillation has been traditionally considered a relative contraindication to coronary CT angiographic examination. However, when the mean heart rate is appropriately controlled by means of medical therapy, the deleterious effect of an irregular heart rhythm on the quality of the images is notably minimized. The availability of systems for editing ECG synchronization improves the retrospective reconstruction in cases of arrhythmia. This is proved by the results of our study, which showed a similar proportion

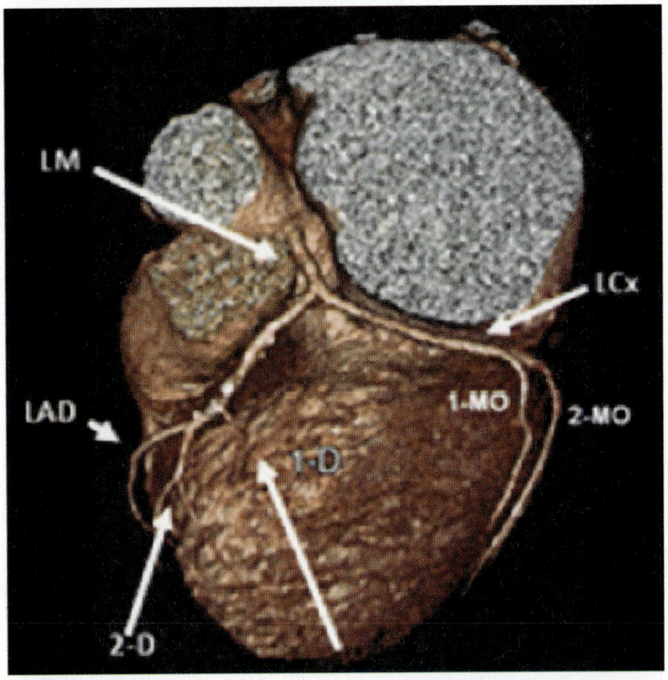

Fig. 13.53: *Coronary CT angiographic results in patient with a dilated left atrium and atrial fibrillation with mean heart rate of 73 beats per minute at coronary CT angiographic acquisition. Volume-rendered CT image (left anterior oblique view with cranial angulation) shows the arteries: left main (LM), left anterior descending (LAD), first diagonal (1D), second diagonal (2D), left circumflex (LCx), and first and second marginal obtuse branches (1-MO, 2-MO)*

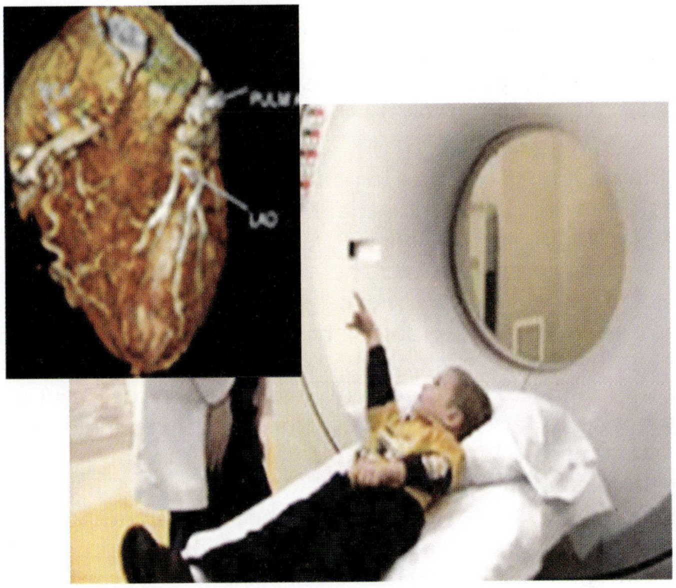

Fig. 13.52: *Photograph of a CT scan machine. Noninvasive coronary multidetector CT angiography in patients with tortous coronary arteries in young child with recurrent chest pain*

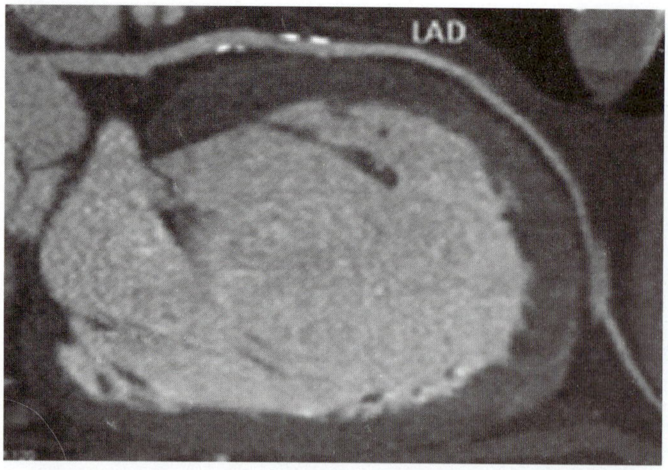

Fig. 13.54: *Coronary CT angiographic results in patient with a dilated left atrium and atrial fibrillation with mean heart rate of 73 beats per minute at coronary CT angiographic acquisition. Curved multiplanar reconstruction of left anterior descending coronary*

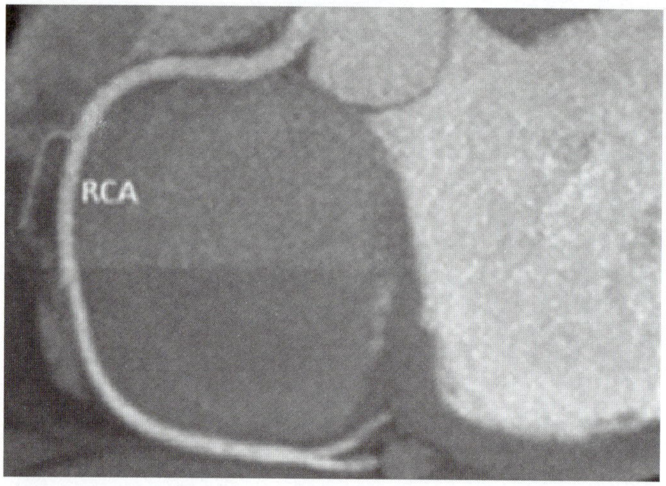

Fig. 13.55: *Coronary CT angiographic results in patient with a dilated left atrium and atrial fibrillation with mean heart rate of 73 beats per minute at coronary CT angiographic acquisition. Maximum intensity projection of right coronary artery*

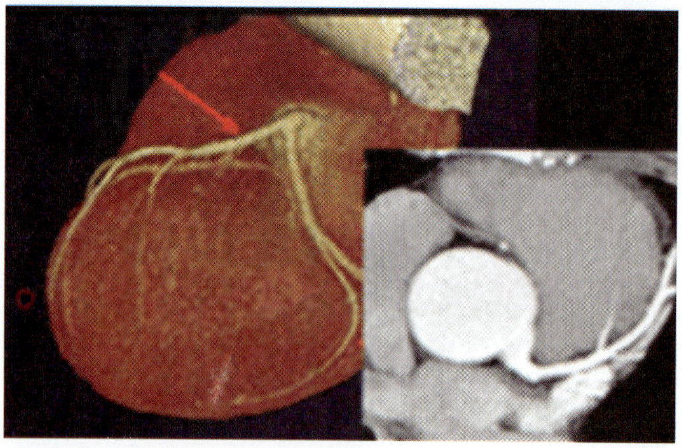

Fig. 13.56: *Noninvasive coronary multidetector CT angiographic images of diagnostic categories. Normal left anterior descending coronary artery (arrow)*

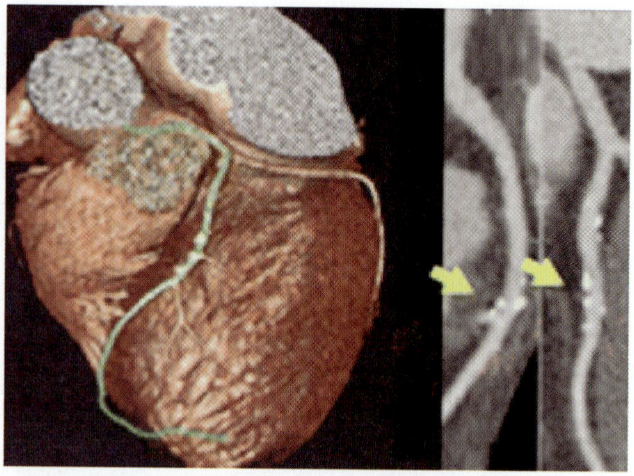

Fig. 13.57: *Noninvasive coronary multidetector CT angiographic images of diagnostic categories. Left anterior descending coronary artery with nonsignificant stenosis (arrows)*

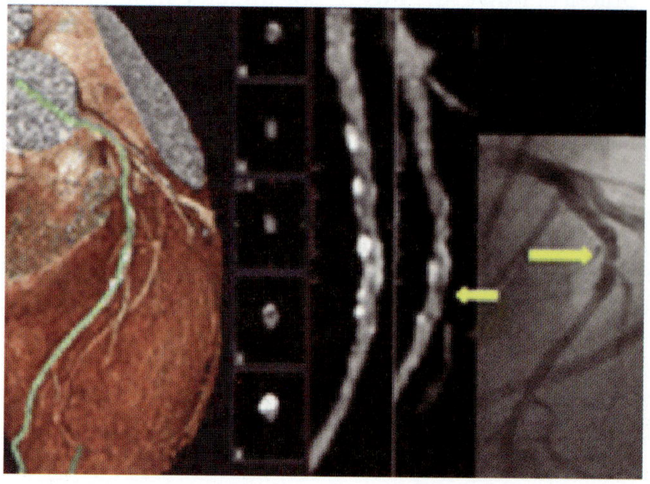

Fig. 13.58: *Noninvasive coronary multidetector CT angiographic images of diagnostic categories. Coronary CT angiogram is nondiagnostic because of severe calcification and shows significant stenosis (arrows) on ICA image (far right)*

of nondiagnostic studies in patients with sinus rhythm and in those with controlled atrial fibrillation.

Nondiagnostic coronary CT angiography accounted for 19% of patients studied. The amount of coronary artery calcium, quantified by means of the Agatston score, was the determinant for a diagnostic study, with a cutoff of 579 being the best predictor. In view of these data, it could be questionable to proceed with noninvasive coronary CT angiography after coronary calcium scanning yielded an Agatston score higher than this value. For example, a rise in the Agatston score from 579 to 1,000 or 1,500 increases twofold and sixfold, respectively, the risk of nondiagnostic coronary CT angiography. As with any other procedure that involves CT, radiation associated with coronary CT angiography is an issue of concern. In particular, the estimated doses of radiation in our study proved to be significantly higher than those reported for diagnostic ICA.

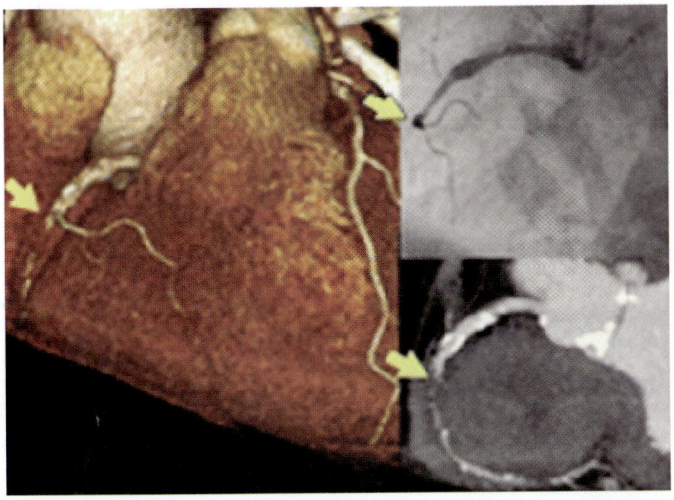

Fig. 13.59: *Noninvasive coronary multidetector CT angiographic images of diagnostic categories. Right coronary artery with a significant stenosis; a total occlusion of the midpart of the right coronary artery (arrows). Top right: ICA image*

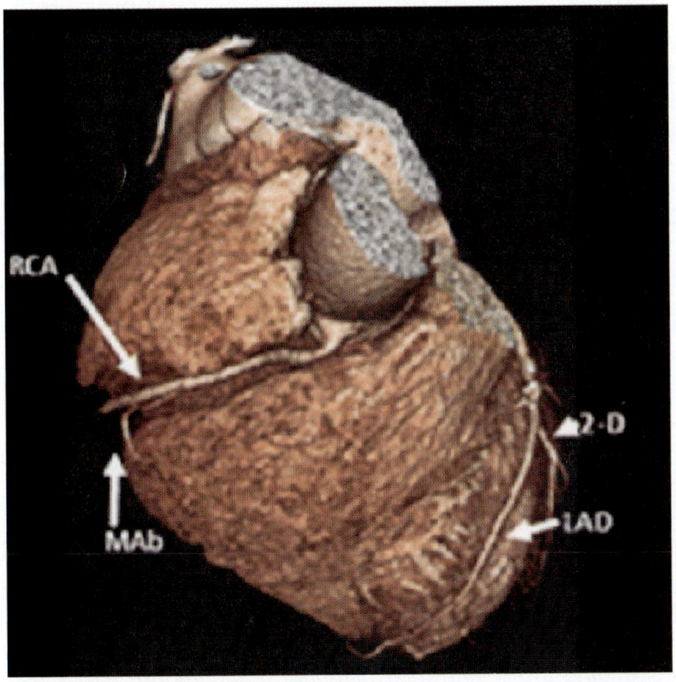

Fig. 13.60: *Coronary CT angiographic results in patient with a dilated left atrium and atrial fibrillation with mean heart rate of 73 beats per minute at coronary CT angiographic acquisition. Volume-rendered CT image (right anterior oblique view with cranial angulation) shows the arteries: right coronary artery (RCA), marginal acute branch (MAb), left anterior descending (LAD), and second diagonal (2D).*

Strategies to limit radiation dose include reduction of tube current or voltage, which is not always feasible in patients with large body mass, and the use of prospective X-ray tube current modulation, which cannot be used in patients with atrial fibrillation, which is a frequent occurrence in this clinical setting. The new generation of CT systems

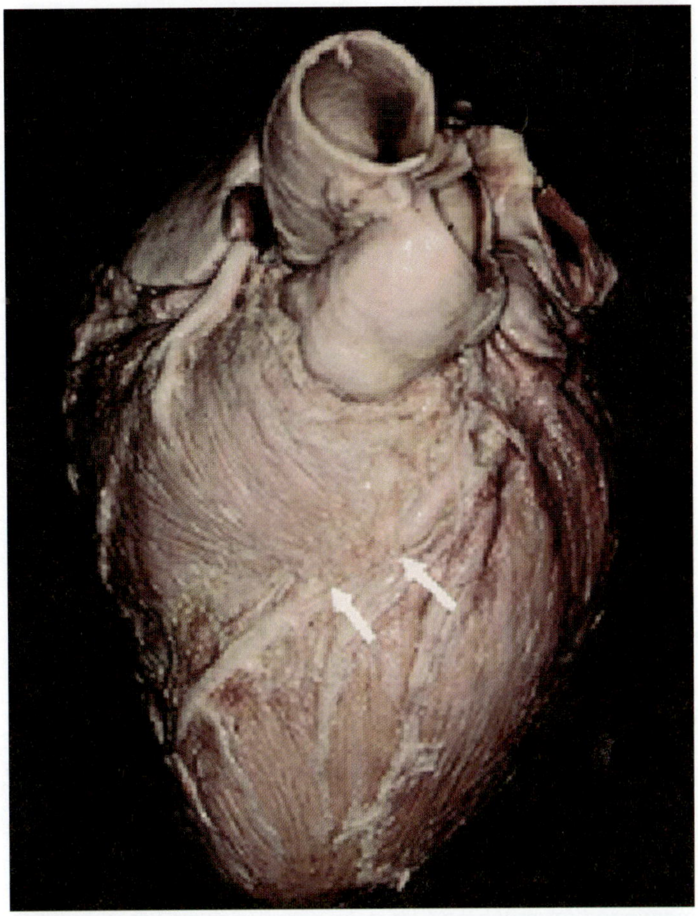

Fig. 13.61: *MB in the LAD of an autopsied heart. The epicardial adipose tissues were manually removed after fixation with formaldehyde. The two arrows indicate the entrance and exit of the MB, respectively*

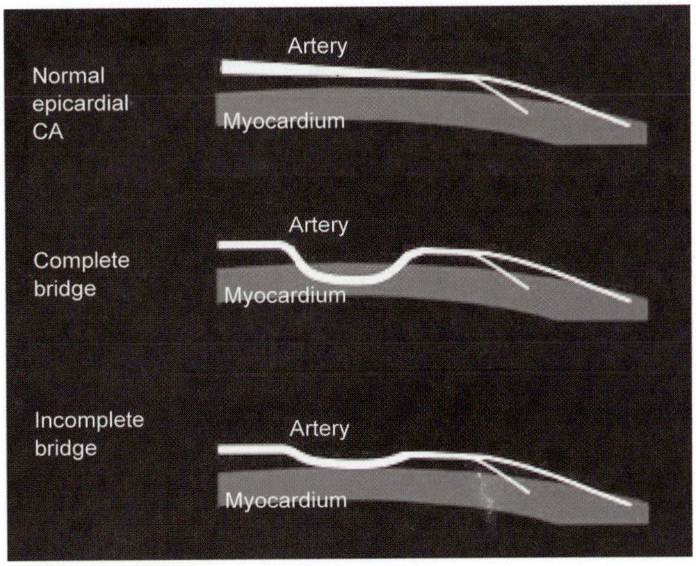

Fig. 13.62: *(Top) normal epicardial artery (middle) shows complete bridging of the artery (bottom) shows incomplete bridging of the epicardial artery*

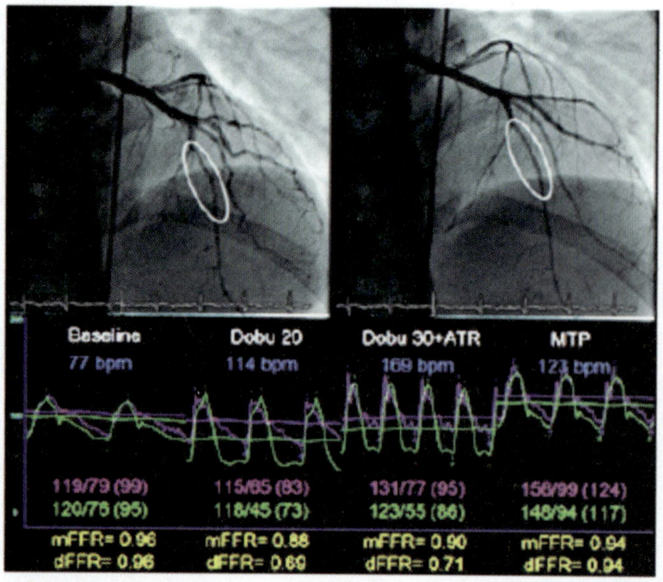

Fig. 13.63: *Midsystolic image of the left coronary artery in anteroposterior view, with 20° of cranial inclination. Just distal to a septal branch, myocardial bridging and "milking" is observed in the left anterior descending artery (encircled in white). Right, End-diastolic view in the same incidence. The segment just distal to the septal branch is smooth and free of atherosclerotic disease. The lower insert of the figure depicts the pressure tracings and their respective values in mmHg at the level of the aorta (in purple) and in the left anterior descending artery distal to the segment with systolic compression (in green). The ratio of distal pressure to aortic pressure (FFR) is depicted in yellow. Values are mentioned for mean and diastolic pressures (mFFR and dFFR, respectively). The distal measurements were obtained using a 0.014-inch pressure wire, after induction of maximum hyperemia with an intracoronary bolus of adenosine. Left to right: Measurements in baseline condition, during intravenous infusion of dobutamine at 20 µg/kg/min, during intravenous infusion of dobutamine at 30 µg/kg/min and administration of 1 mg of atropine, and finally after intravenous administration of 10 mg of metoprolol. The respective heart rates (bpm) are mentioned in blue. At a dose of 20 µg /kg / min of dobutamine, systolic pressure overshoots distally to the dynamic lesion with a diastolic pressure gradient <0.75. At the highest dose of dobutamine and after administration of atropine, an important diastolic pressure gradient is seen (55/77=0.71), indicating impaired myocardial perfusion by the myocardial bridge. This gradient disappeared almost instantly after the intravenous administration of metoprolol, despite a higher heart rate than that during the intravenous infusion of dobutamine*

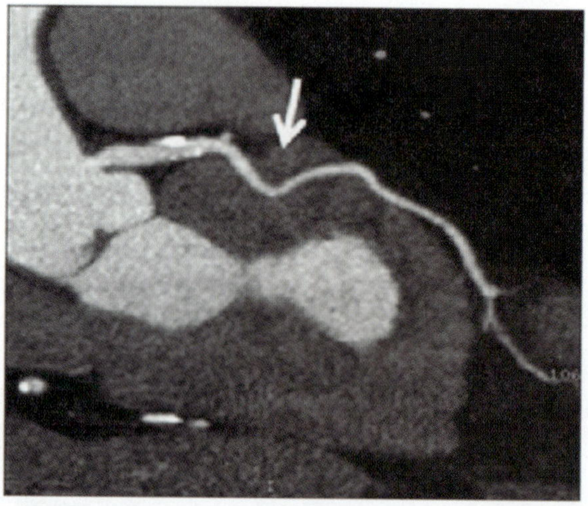

Fig. 13.64: *An adolescent with suspected coronary artery disease. Curved MPR shows long segment of myocardial bridging of mid LAD*

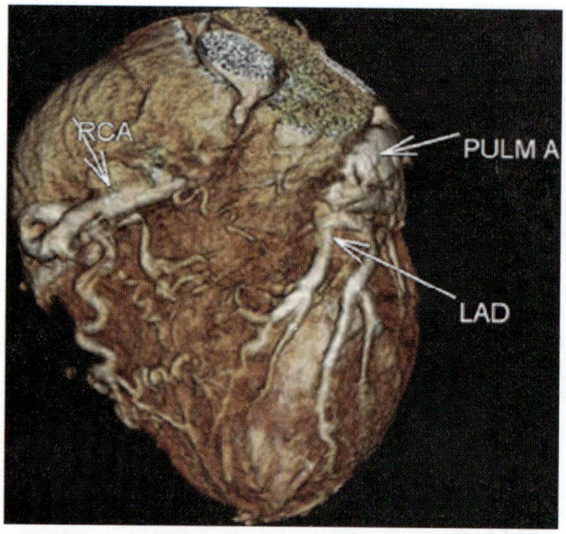

Fig. 13.65: *CT angiography volume rendered image. Right coronary artery is dilated and tortious with a large number of collaterals feeding the left coronary system. Left coronary artery is emerging from pulmonary artery trunk. The left anterior descending artery and their diagonal branches are also dilated and tortuous*

already available, which are based on a single heart beat volume acquisition, will greatly overcome this limitation by means of an important reduction of radiation.

A potential limitation of the study was that its results cannot be extrapolated to other populations of patients usually submitted to preoperative ICA, as those scheduled to undergo major vascular surgery, in whom the presumably higher prevalence of significant CAD would probably lead to a lower number of avoided ICA studies. A further study particularly addressing this issue is warranted.

In conclusion, in patients scheduled to undergo noncoronary cardiovascular surgery, including those with controlled atrial fibrillation, the presence or absence of CAD can be reliably assessed preoperatively by using coronary CT angiography in a majority of cases. Preoperative ICA was safely avoided in those patients without significant CAD. A proportion of nondiagnostic coronary CT angiographic studies still remained, mainly because of severe coronary calcification, and a high Agatston score was the only predictor of an adequate coronary CT angiographic examination.

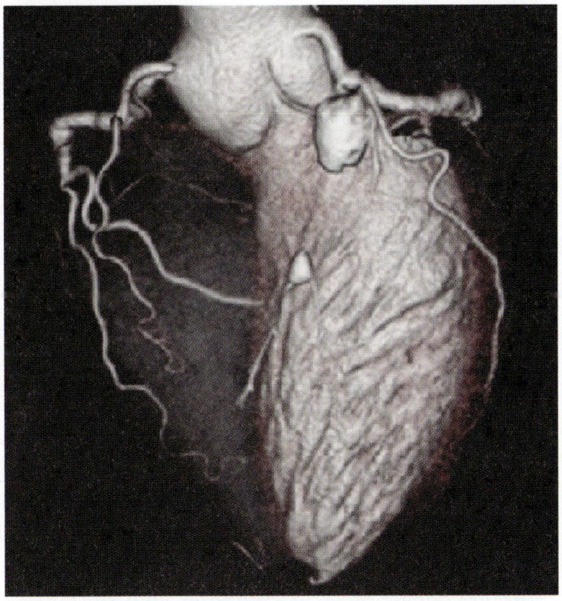

Fig. 13.66: *20-year-adolescent with Kawasaki disease. VR image show partly calcified thrombosed saccular aneurysm in proximal LAD. He has another fusiform aneurysm in the right coronary artery*

Advances in Knowledge of CT Angiography

- In patients scheduled to undergo noncoronary cardiovascular surgery, coronary CT angiograms are of diagnostic image quality in 81% of cases.
- The presence of atrial fibrillation is not a limitation for performing diagnostic coronary CT angiography, provided that the ventricular heart rate is adequately controlled to less than 70 beats per minute.
- The presence of severe coronary artery calcification is the only independent predictor of nondiagnostic coronary CT angiography; an Agatston score cutoff of about 600 shows the best predictive accuracy for performing diagnostic coronary CT angiography.
- Preoperative ICA can be safely omitted in patients without significant CAD (defined as >50% stenosis) by using coronary CT angiography.

Implications for Patient Care

- Coronary CT angiography is a useful preoperative test for safely avoiding ICA in most of the patients scheduled to undergo noncoronary cardiovascular surgery.
- Coronary CT angiography provides additional anatomic information on extracoronary structures that may be relevant in relation to the surgical procedure.

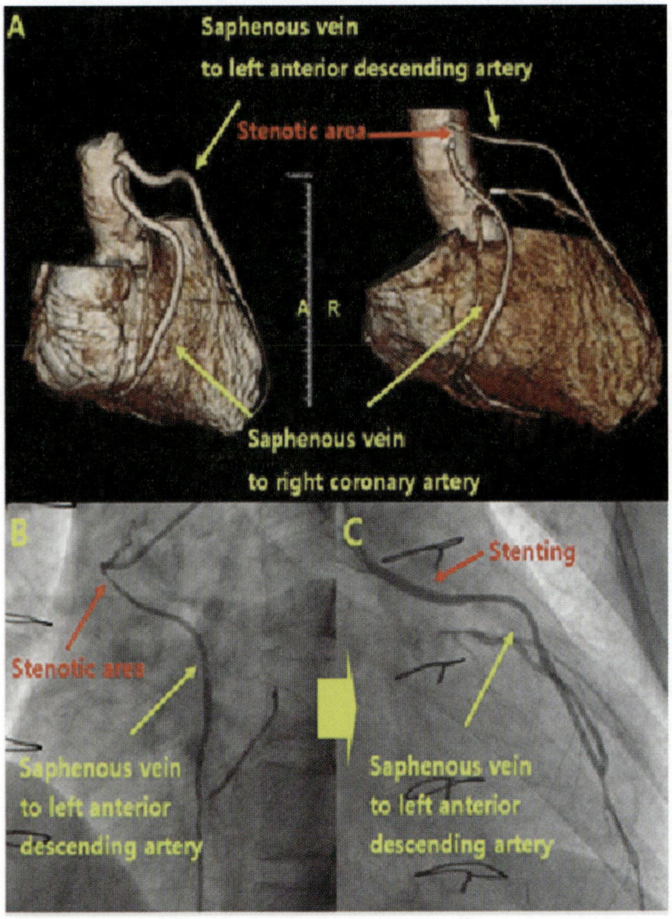

Fig. 13.67: *Chronic occlusion of left saphenous vein graft (SVG). (A, left panel) Immediate after CABG surgery, three dimensional volume-rendered image showed that left SVG was patent with its anastomsis to the mid-portion of LAD artery. There was a patent right SVG, which was attached to the distal-portion of right coronary artery (RCA). (A, right panel) At 8 months after CABG surgery, three dimensional volume-rendered image showed severe stenosis at proximal-portion of SVG, which was attached to the mid-portion of LAD artery. Right saphenous vein graft (SVG) was still patent despite the graft had diffuse mild narrowing from proximal anastomosis site to distal anastomosis site. (B) Invasive coronary angiography showed the proximal-portion of left saphenous vein graft (SVG) was severely occluded. (C) Percutaneous coronary intervention was performed successfully. Note that the findings of invasive coronary angiography is similar to those of three dimensional volume-rendered images of 64-MDCT*

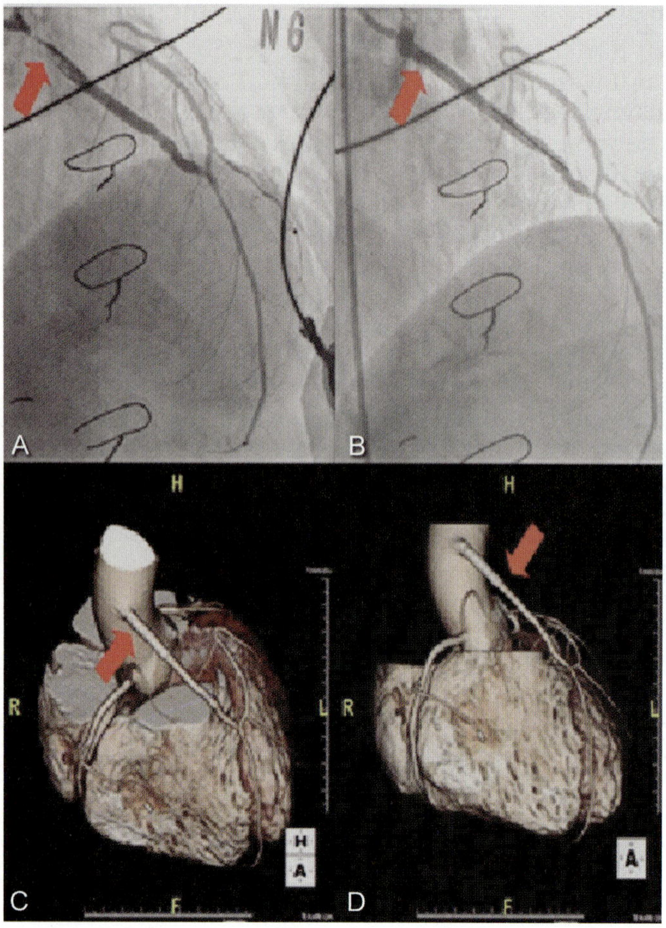

Fig. 13.68: *Acute occlusion of saphenous vein graft (SVG). (A) Invasive coronary angiography showed the proximal-portion of SVG was severely occluded with thrombi. (B) After successful percutaneous coronary intervention (PCI), invasive coronary angiography showed the proximal-portion of SVG with stenting was patent. (C, D) At 6-month follow-up, three-dimensional volume-rendered image showed the proximal-portion of SVG with stenting was still patent. Note that the findings of invasive coronary angiography is similar to those of three dimensional volume-rendered images of 64-MDCT. The figures also demonstrate that 64-MDCT has a useful role to follow-up of patients who have undergone percutaneous intervention for bypass graft stenosis and occlusion*

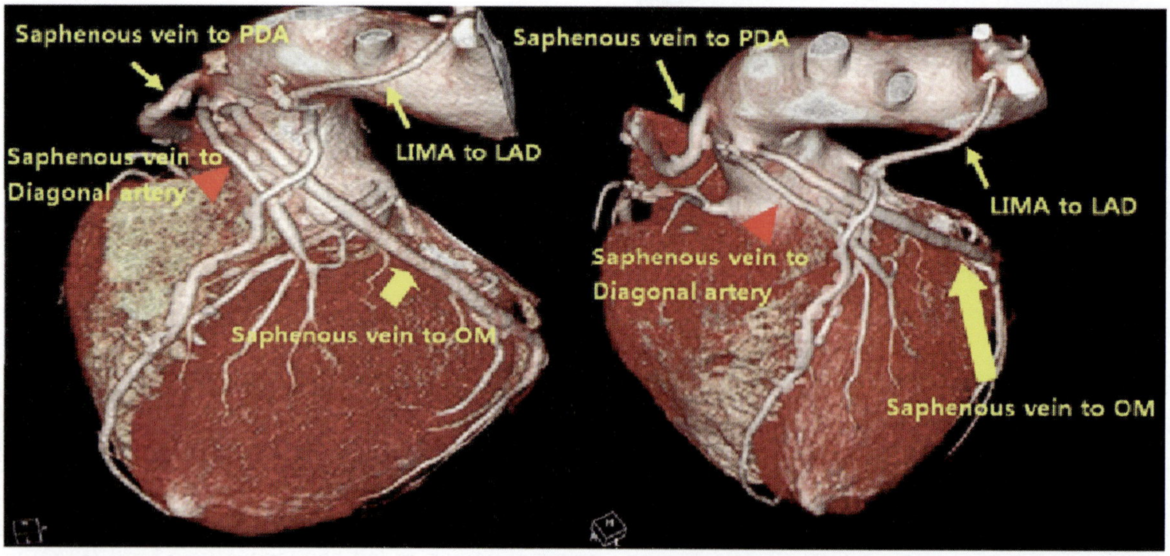

Fig. 13.69: *Left internal mammary artery (IMA) graft. Three dimensional volume-rendered images show the left IMA graft from its origin at the left subclavian artery to its anastomosis with the left anterior descending (LAD) artery. There is also a right saphenous vein graft (SVG) sutured to the anterior aorta with its anastomosis with the posterior descending artery (PDA). The left SVG are attached to diagonal artery and the obtuse marginal (OM) artery*

BIBLIOGRAPHY

1. Ross J Jr, Brandenburg RO, Dinsmore RE, et al. ACC/AHA Guidelines for coronary angiography. A report of the American College of Cardiology/American Heart Association Task Force on Assessment of Diagnostic and Therapeutic Cardiovascular Procedures (Subcommittee on Coronary Angiography). *J Am Coll Cardiol*. 1987;10:935–9502.
2. Selker HP, Zalenski RJ, Antman EM, et al. An evaluation of technologies for identifying acute cardiac ischemia in the emergency department: executive summary of a National Heart Attack Alert Program Working Group Report. *Ann Emerg Med*. 1997;29:1–12.
3. Pepine CJ, Allen HD, Bashore TM, et al. ACC/AHA guidelines for cardiac catheterization and cardiac catheterization laboratories: American College of Cardiology/American Heart Association Ad Hoc Task Force on Cardiac Catheterization. *J Am Coll Cardiol*. 1991;18:1149–1182
4. Marcus ML, Schelbert HR, Skorton DJ, et al. Cardiac Imaging: A Companion to Braunwald's Heart Disease. Philadelphia, Pa: WB Saunders; 1991.
5. Grossman WB, Baim DS. Cardiac Catheterization, Angiography and Intervention. Philadelphia, Pa: Lea & Febiger; 1991.
6. National Heart, Lung, and Blood Institute Coronary Artery Surgery Study. A multicenter comparison of the effects of randomized medical and surgical treatment of mildly symptomatic patients with coronary artery disease and a registry of consecutive patients undergoing coronary angiography. *Circulation*. 1981;63:I-1–I-81 Monograph 79.
7. The BARI Protocol. Protocol for the Bypass Angioplasty Revascularization Investigation. *Circulation*. 1991;84:V-1–V-27.
8. Ringqvist I, Fisher LD, Mock M, et al. Prognostic value of angiographic indices of coronary artery disease from the Coronary Artery Surgery Study (CASS). *J Clin Invest*. 1983;71:1854–1866.
9. Califf RM, Phillips HR III, Hindman MC, et al. Prognostic value of a coronary artery jeopardy score. *J Am Coll Cardiol*. 1985;5:1055–1063.
10. Gensini GG. Coronary Angiography. Mount Kisco, NY: Futura Publishing; 1996.
11. Emond M, Mock MB, Davis KB, et al. Long-term survival of medically treated patients in the Coronary Artery Surgery Study (CASS) Registry. *Circulation*. 1994;90:2645–2657.
12. Hanley PC, Vlietstra RE, Fisher LD, Smith HC. Indications for coronary angiography: changes in laboratory practice over a decade. *Mayo Clin Proc*. 1986;61:248–253.
13. Noto TJ Jr, Johnson LW, Krone R, et al. Cardiac catheterization 1990: a report of the Registry of the Society for Cardiac Angiography and Interventions (SCA&I). *Cathet Cardiovasc Diagn*. 1991;24:75–83.
14. Johnson LW, Lozner EC, Johnson S, et al. Coronary arteriography 1984–1987: a report of the Registry of the Society for Cardiac Angiography and Interventions, I: results and complications. *Cathet Cardiovasc Diagn*. 1989;17:5–10.
15. Laskey W, Boyle J, Johnson LW. Multivariable model for prediction of risk of significant complication during diagnostic cardiac catheterization: the Registry Committee of the Society for Cardiac Angiography and Interventions. *Cathet Cardiovasc Diagn*. 1993;30:185–190.
16. Guidelines for professional staff privileges in the cardiac catheterization laboratory: Laboratory Performance Standards Committee. *Cathet Cardiovasc Diagn*. 1990;21:203–204.
17. Ritchie JL, Phillips KA, Luft HS. Coronary angioplasty: statewide experience in California. *Circulation*. 1993;88:2735–2743.
18. Kimmel SE, Berlin JA, Laskey WK. The relationship between coronary angioplasty procedure volume and major complications. *JAMA*. 1995;274:1137–1142.
19. Hirshfeld JW Jr, Ellis SG, Faxon DP. Recommendations for the assessment and maintenance of proficiency in coronary interventional procedures: statement of the American College of Cardiology. *J Am Coll Cardiol*. 1998;31:722–743.
20. Solomon R, Werner C, Mann D, D'Elia J, Silva P. Effects of saline, mannitol, and furosemide to prevent acute decreases in renal function induced by radiocontrast agents. *N Engl J Med*. 1994;331:1416–1420.
21. Taliercio CP, Vlietstra RE, Fisher LD, Burnett JC. Risks for renal dysfunction with cardiac angiography. *Ann Intern Med*. 1986;104:501–50422.
22. Parfrey PS, Griffiths SM, Barrett BJ, et al. Contrast material-induced renal failure in patients with diabetes mellitus, renal insufficiency, or both: a prospective controlled study. *N Engl J Med*. 1989;320:143–149.
23. Schwab SJ, Hlatky MA, Pieper KS, et al. Contrast nephrotoxicity: a randomized controlled trial of a nonionic and an ionic radiographic contrast agent. *N Engl J Med*. 1989;320:149–153.
24. Deray G, Jacobs C. Radiocontrast nephrotoxicity: a review. *Invest Radiol*. 1995;30:221–225.
25. Matthai WH Jr, Kussmaul WG III, Krol J, Goin JE, Schwartz JS, Hirshfeld JW Jr. A comparison of low- with high-osmolality contrast agents in cardiac angiography: identification of criteria for selective use. *Circulation*. 1994;89:291–301.
26. Bettmann MA. Safety and efficacy of iodinated contrast agents. *Invest Radiol*. 1994;29:S33–S36.
27. Mikkonen R, Kontkanen T, Kivisaari L. Acute and late adverse reactions to low-osmolal contrast media. *Acta Radiol*. 1995;36:72–76.
28. Rudnick MR, Goldfarb S, Wexler L, et al. Nephrotoxicity of ionic and nonionic contrast media in 1,196 patients: a randomized trial. The Iohexol Cooperative Study. *Kidney Int*. 1995;47:254–261.
29. Tommaso CL. Contrast-induced nephrotoxicity in patients undergoing cardiac catheterization. *Cathet Cardiovasc Diagn*. 1994;31:316–321.
30. Greenberger PA, Patterson R, Tapio CM. Prophylaxis against repeated radiocontrast media reactions in 857 cases: adverse experience with cimetidine and safety of beta-adrenergic antagonists. *Arch Intern Med*. 1985;145:2197–2200.
31. Greenberger PA, Patterson R. Adverse reactions to radiocontrast media. *Prog Cardiovasc Dis*. 1988;31:239–248.
32. Wittbrodt ET, Spinler SA. Prevention of anaphylactoid reactions in high-risk patients receiving radiographic contrast media. *Ann Pharmacother*. 1994;28:236–241.
33. Myers GE, Bloom FL. Cimetidine (Tagamet) combined with steroids and H1 antihistamines for the prevention of serious radiographic contrast material reactions. *Cathet Cardiovasc Diagn*. 1981;7:65–69.

34. Lasser EC, Berry CC, Talner LB, et al. Pretreatment with corticosteroids to alleviate reactions to intravenous contrast material. *N Engl J Med*. 1987;317:845–849.
35. Graves EJ. National hospital discharge survey: annual summary, 1993. *Vital Health Stat 13*. 1995;:1–63.
36. American Heart Association. Heart and Stroke Facts: 1996 Statistical Supplement. Dallas, TX: American Heart Association; 1996. p. 22.
37. Medicare claims data. Provided by the Physician Payment Review Commission; 1996.
38. Spertus JA, Weiss NS, Every NR, Weaver WD. The influence of clinical risk factors on the use of angiography and revascularization after acute myocardial infarction: Myocardial Infarction Triage and Intervention Project Investigators. *Arch Intern Med*. 1995;155:2309–2316.
39. Bates DW, Bernstein SJ. Coronary Angiography in Acute Myocardial Infarction: A Review of the Literature Regarding Efficacy and Risks. Boston, MA: Harvard Medical School, Department of Health Care Policy; 1995.
40. Pashos CL, Newhouse JP, McNeil BJ. Temporal changes in the care and outcomes of elderly patients with acute myocardial infarction, 1987 through 1990. *JAMA*. 1993;270:1832–1836.
41. Every NR, Larson EB, Litwin PE, et al. The association between on-site cardiac catheterization facilities and the use of coronary angiography after acute myocardial infarction: Myocardial Infarction Triage and Intervention Project Investigators. *N Engl J Med*. 1993;329:546–551.
42. Blustein J. High-technology cardiac procedures: the impact of service availability on service use in New York State. *JAMA*. 1993;270:344–349.
43. DiSalvo TT, Paul SD, Lloyd-Jones D, et al. Care of acute myocardial infarction by noninvasive and invasive cardiologists: procedure use, cost and outcome. *J Am Coll Cardiol*. 1996;27:262–269.
44. Pilote L, Califf RM, Sapp S, et al. Regional variation across the United States in the management of acute myocardial infarction: GUSTO-1 Investigators. Global Utilization of Streptokinase and Tissue Plasminogen Activator for Occluded Coronary Arteries. *N Engl J Med*. 1995;333:565–572.
45. Guadagnoli E, Hauptman PJ, Ayanian JZ, Pashos CL, McNeil BJ, Cleary PD. Variation in the use of cardiac procedures after acute myocardial infarction. *N Engl J Med*. 1995;333:573–578.
46. Selby JV, Fireman BH, Lundstrom RJ, et al. Variation among hospitals in coronary-angiography practices and outcomes after myocardial infarction in a large health maintenance organization. *N Engl J Med*. 1996;335:1888–1896.
47. Mark DB, Naylor CD, Hlatky MA, et al. Use of medical resources and quality of life after acute myocardial infarction in Canada and the United States. *N Engl J Med*. 1994;331:1130–1135.
48. Rouleau JL, Moye LA, Pfeffer MA, et al. A comparison of management patterns after acute myocardial infarction in Canada and the United States: the SAVE investigators. *N Engl J Med*. 1993;328:779–784.
49. Tu JV, Pashos CL, Naylor CD, et al. Use of cardiac procedures and outcomes in elderly patients with myocardial infarction in the United States and Canada. *N Engl J Med*. 1997;336:1500–1505.
50. Leape LL, Park RE, Solomon DH, Chassin MR, Kosecoff J, Brook RH. Does inappropriate use explain small-area variations in the use of health care services? *JAMA*. 1990;263:669–672.
51. Bonow RO, Carabello BA, Chatterjee K, et al. ACC/AHA 2006 guidelines for the management of patients with valvular heart disease: a report of the American College of Cardiology/American Heart Association Task Force on Practice Guidelines (Writing Committee to Revise the 1998 Guidelines for the Management of Patients With Valvular Heart Disease) developed in collaboration with the Society of Cardiovascular Anesthesiologists endorsed by the Society for Cardiovascular Angiography and Interventions and the Society of Thoracic Surgeons. J Am Coll Cardiol 2006;48:e1-e148.
52. Vahanian A, Baumgartner H, Bax J, et al. Guidelines on the management of valvular heart disease: The Task Force on the Management of Valvular Heart Disease of the European Society of Cardiology. Eur Heart J 2007;28(2):230–268.
53. Salas-Lara VM, Rangel-Abundis A, Solorio-Meza S, Albarrán-López H. Assessment of a predictive index for coronary artery disease in patients with rheumatic valvular disease. Cir Cir 2005;73(2):85–89.
54. Potter DD, Sundt TM 3rd., Zehr KJ, et al. Operative risk of reoperative aortic valve replacement. J Thorac Cardiovasc Surg 2005;129(1):94–103.
55. Czer LS, Gray RJ, Stewart ME, De Robertis M, Chaux A, Matloff JM. Reduction in sudden late death by concomitant revascularization with aortic valve replacement. J Thorac Cardiovasc Surg 1988;95(3):390–401.
56. Meijboom WB, van Mieghem CA, Mollet NR, et al. 64-slice computed tomography coronary angiography in patients with high, intermediate, or low pretest probability of significant coronary artery disease. J Am Coll Cardiol 2007;50(15):1469–1475.
57. Budoff MJ, Dowe D, Jollis JG, et al. Diagnostic performance of 64-multidetector row coronary computed tomographic angiography for evaluation of coronary artery stenosis in individuals without known coronary artery disease: results from the prospective multicenter ACCURACY (Assessment by Coronary Computed Tomographic Angiography of Individuals Undergoing Invasive Coronary Angiography) trial. J Am Coll Cardiol 2008;52(21):1724–1732.
58. Meijboom WB, Mollet NR, Van Mieghem CA, et al. Pre-operative computed tomography coronary angiography to detect significant coronary artery disease in patients referred for cardiac valve surgery. J Am Coll Cardiol 2006;48(8):1658–1665.
59. Russo V, Gostoli V, Lovato L, et al. Clinical value of multidetector CT coronary angiography as a preoperative screening test before non-coronary cardiac surgery. Heart 2007;93(12):1591–1598.
60. Bettencourt N, Rocha J, Carvalho M, et al. Multislice computed tomography in the exclusion of coronary artery disease in patients with presurgical valve disease. Circ Cardiovasc Imaging 2009;2(4):306–313.

14 Congenital Heart Diseases in Children

THE SEQUENTIAL SEGMENTAL APPROACH IN CHD

This newer nomenclature approach has remarkably simplified the classification of congenital heart disease (CHD). It is based on following the blood flow into the heart (systemic venous and pulmonary venous) through the heart (the atrioventricular valves and ventricles) and then out the great vessels (semilunar valves and great vessels). This nomenclature system is extraordinarily helpful to those conducting echocardiographic examinations as it forms a systematic guide for verification that all the pertinent chambers and valves and their relationships have been documented. The system is dependent on a few words that are very important in describing the various lesions:

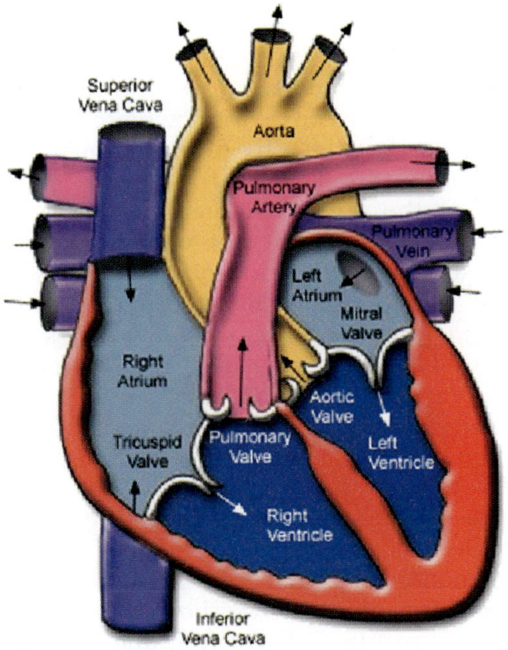

Fig. 14.1: *Diagram showing concodant placement of both atria, ventricles and their ventriculoarterial connections and normally connected four pulmonary veins incoming from both the lungs. Both interventricular and interatrial septa are positioned in their anatomical place in the heart. Similarily, great vessels and coronary blood circulation are found to be normal. The knowledge of normal structures of the heart is as important as the study of abnormally developed structures of the heart*

Connection: It refers to the sequence of anatomic structures. Normally, the right atrium is connected to the right ventricle by means of the tricuspid valve. The right ventricle is then connected to the pulmonary artery by means of the pulmonic valve. Therefore, there are atrioventricular connections and ventriculo-great arterial connections (Fig. 14.1).

Concordance: It describes the relationship between the various chambers, valves, and great vessels. In the normal heart, all the connections and relationships in the anatomic sequence are concordant (Fig. 14.2).

Discordance: It describes abnormal relationships between the various chambers and the great vessels. For example, when the right atrium leads into the morphologic left ventricle and the left atrium into the morphologic right ventricle, the atrioventricular relationships are discordant. Likewise, the atrioventricular relationships may be concordant (normal) but the ventriculo-great arterial relationships may be discordant where the aorta rises from the right ventricle and the pulmonary artery from the left ventricle. Known formerly as transposition of the great vessels, these abnormal relationships would now be termed ventriculo-great arterial discordance.

Absent or imperforate connections: Valves normally form the connections between chambers. There are atrioventricular connections that lead from the right atrium to right ventricle or left atrium to vessels. When connections are not present, the term absent connection is used. Thus, when the tricuspid valve is absent, an absent right atrioventricular

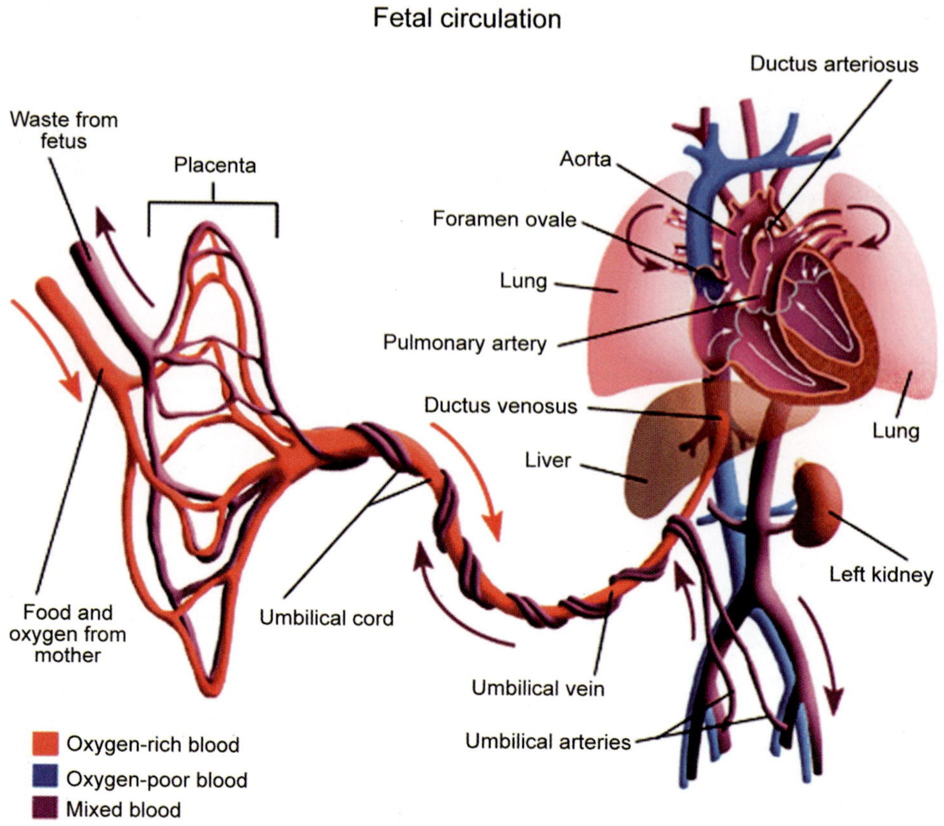

Fig. 14.2: *Placental and fetal heart circulation*

connection may not be totally absent, only severely malformed and does not allow blood to pass antegradely. In this setting, the term imperforate connection may be used.

Commitment: It further describes possible abnormalities of flow through valves into ventricles and great vessels. For example, in a patient with tetralogy of Fallot, the atria, atrioventricular valves, and ventricles are positioned normally, and concordant. Since the aorta overrides a ventricular septal defect, the aorta is doubly committed to both ventricles. Likewise, in cases where there is only one ventricle (univentricular heart), both atrioventricular valves are usually doubly committed to the single ventricle.

Ambiguous: It is used when precise identification of a ventricle or other structure cannot be made. For example, in a univentricular heart with a doubly committed atrioventricular connection it may not be possible to always identify clearly whether it is the right or left ventricle. Thus, the single ventricle would be ambiguous.

Inlet: It refers to anomalies of the structures and flow into the ventricle.

Outlet: It refers to anomalies of the structures and flow out of the ventricles into the great vessels.

The system assumes that flow through the heart is normal and begins with properly identifying the atria, and their position in the chest. In a normal individual there are two atria, each with venous inflow. One must identify the inferior and superior vena cava inflows into the right atrium and, where possible, identify four pulmonary veins into the left atrium.

Following the normal sequence of flow, one then identifies the atrioventricular valves and ventricles. Normally, there are two atrioventricular valves, tricuspid and mitral. The tricuspid valve is committed to the right ventricle and the mitral valve to the left ventricle. Normally, both the atrial and the ventricular septa are intact.

Again following the normal sequence of flow, blood should emerge out of the ventricles into the great vessels. The pulmonary artery, taking flow to the lungs, is normally committed to the right ventricle while the aorta, taking blood to the systemic circuit, is normally committed to the left ventricle.

The pulmonary artery emerges from the right ventricle and passes anterior to the aorta. The pulmonary artery then bifurcates and is differentiated from the aorta that forms an arch, giving off vessels to the head and neck. The pulmonary artery and aorta "criss-cross" as they arise from their respective ventricles.

Given these normal sequences and relationships the terms previously mentioned are used to describe abnormal hearts. Chambers, valves, or vessels may be absent (atretic) or small (hypoplastic). Relationships between chambers and valves may be concordant (normal) or discordant. In addition, chambers or valves may be doubly committed or normally committed.

Atrial situs: In the complex myriad of possible anomalies, some of the most difficult to determine are those involving abnormalities of atrial situs. Mention of atrial situs is made only to point out that any complex malposition of the atria may occur.

Four possible atrial arrangements are encountered in CHD: the normal arrangement of the right atrium and left atrium (***situs solitus***), the direct opposite to the normal where the right atrium is on the left and the left atrium on the right (***situs inversus***), bilateral right atria (right atrial isomerism associated with the asplenia syndrome) or bilateral left atria (left atrial isomerism associated with the polysplenia syndrome). For the purposes of this volume, we shall assume atrial situs to be normal in all patients.

It is easiest to begin with disorders where chambers and valves are in the normal, or relatively normal position. Such disorders comprise those of atrial and/or ventricular septal defects and those disorders where chambers and valves are absent or small, causing obstruction. As a consequence, these types of defects will be divided into those when shunting (abnormal blood flow between the left and the right circulations), obstruction, or regurgitation are predominant.

When Shunting is Predominant

In the structurally normal heart, right and left sides are divided and are without communication. Shunting refers to those flow anomalies where there is an abnormal communication, such as an atrial or ventricular septal defect, that allows abnormal flow between the right and the left sides. Since right-sided pressures are normally lower than those on the left side, when such defects are encountered abnormal flow is usually left-to-right and increased flow into the lungs results. Normally, the lungs can accommodate the increased flow without significant symptoms if the degree of shunting is small or moderate. When significant shunting is present and exceeds the ability of the lungs to accept the increase, the lungs are literally flooded and symptoms of cardiac failure ensue. Where no failure is clinically evident, such shunting, over time, may result in reactive changes in the pulmonary vasculature where normally low pressures then rise within the right heart and exceed those on the left side. Depending on the clinical situation, such changes may be permanent and cause right-to-left shunting (Eisenmenger's syndrome). Without early recognition and correction, these simple problems may result in permanent, inoperative damage to the lungs. In addition, any communication between right and left sides of the heart may allow for the possibility of venous emboli entering the arterial circuit.

Role of Specialist in Congenital Heart Diseases

Initial assessment of patients with known or suspected CHD (Fig. 14.3).

Surgical and nonsurgical interventions, e.g. transcatheter closure ASD.

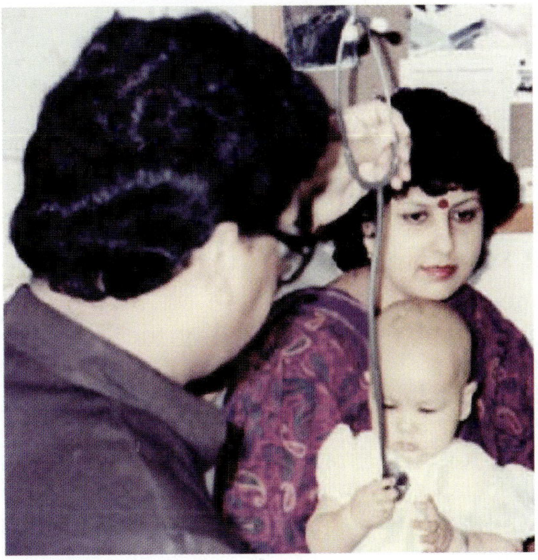

Fig. 14.3: *The best position for a child under examination is the lap of the mother and tool of examination should be made familiar prior to further examination*

Continuing care of patients with moderate and complex CHD.

Advice and ongoing support for noncardiac surgery and pregnancy. Training new specialists and evidence based clinical decision making. Provide feedback of late results to refine early treatment.

Pediatric to Adult Care Transition

A smooth transition from the pediatric to the adult CHD, specialist is essential. This should be tailored to the individual patient with in-built flexibility. Transfer to the adult unit should occur at around 18 years of age. Patient education about the diagnosis and specific health behavior including contraception/pregnancy planning. should be included. Patient passports which include detailed diagrams of the individual cardiac defect and relevant information on topics such as exercise and need for antibiotic prophylaxis should be prepared for each patient.

No patient with CHD should reach adulthood without a clear management plan.

Treat adult CHD with respect. Many problems or errors arise. Percutaneous transcatheter interventions for CHD from arrogance or ignorance. The patients may often know more about their condition and its management than the "emergency" medical team he/she consult; therefore be patient and listen. Patients are often accompanied by a parents even well into late teens/second or third decade. They can prove a great source of information and help; keep them on your side.

ASSESSMENT OF PATIENTS WITH CHD

History

- Family history of CHD.
- Exposure to teratogens toxins during pregnancy.
- CHD suspected during pregnancy or at birth (ask the mother).

- History of prolonged childhood illnesses.
- Prior interventions.
- Any previous hospitalizations for catheter or surgical-based interventions.
- Names of previous paediatric cardiologists and surgeons as well as unit in which surgery, if any, was performed.
- Dental hygiene.

Current Symptoms

- Shortness of breath on exertion?
- Ability to climb stairs, hills, walk on the flat, and distance covered?
- Breathless on lying down?
- Chest pain?
- Precipitating/relieving factors?
- Any associated symptoms?
- Syncopal episodes?
- Palpitations?
- Onset, duration.
- Associated presyncope/chest pain?
- Ask patient to tap out rate and rhythm of palpitations.
- Assess ability index.

General Inspection (Figs 14.4 to 14.7)

- Chart the patient's height, weight, and blood pressure against standard reference charts.
- Does the patient have an obvious syndrome?
- Down's syndrome (one-third associated with CHD, especially atrioventricualr septal defect)?
- William's syndrome (supravalvular aortic and pulmonary stenosis)?
- Noonan's syndrome (dysplastic pulmonary valvular stenosis, hypertrophic cardiomyopathy)?
- Turner's syndrome (coarctation of the aorta/aortic valve stenosis)? Is the patient anaemic or jaundiced?
- Are there any features to suggest infective endocarditis?

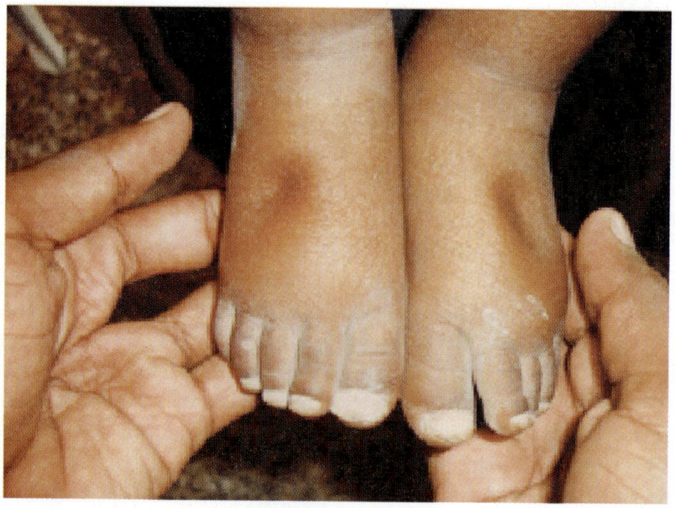

Fig. 14.5: *Pitting edema feet ina child with heart failure*

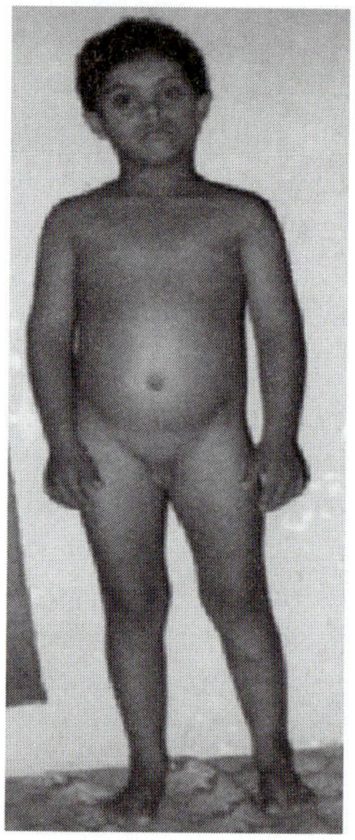

Fig. 14.6: *Physical features of mongolism associated with VSD*

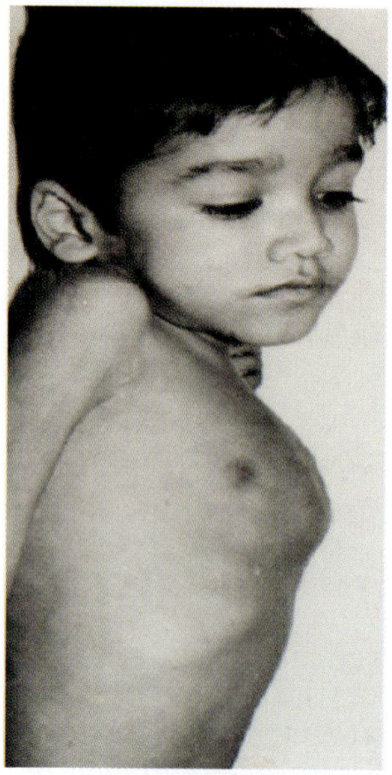

Fig. 14.4: *Pigeon-shaped chest deformity in a child with VSD*

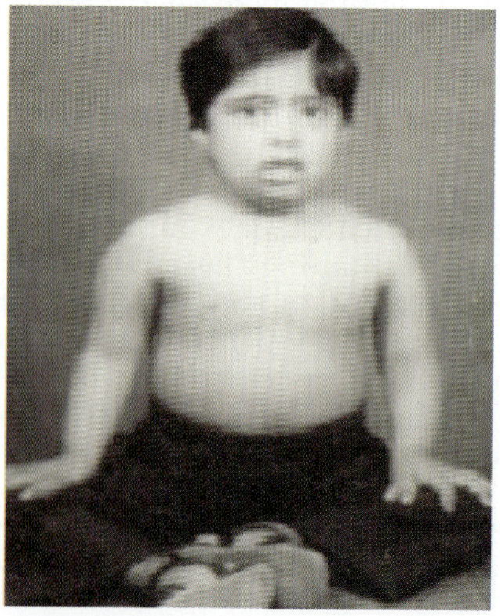

Fig. 14.7: *Stunted growth, polydactylism and chest deformity in a child with endocardial cushion defect*

- Is there evidence of poor oral hygiene with dental caries or infected gums?
- Any tattoos or body piercing?

Inspection of cyanosis or clubbing? (Fig. 14.8)

Oxygen saturation should always be measured by pulse oximetry. Central cyanosis is an indication of arterial saturation and is noted when more than 5 g/dL of reduced hemoglobin is circulating. Thus, it is dependent in part on the total hemoglobin concentration and may be missing in a patient with significant desaturation but who is anemic. Differential cyanosis implies flow of deoxygenated blood from the pulmonary trunk into the aorta distal to the left subclavian artery, e.g. nonrestrictive patent arterial duct with pulmonary vascular disease and right to left shunt.

Previous operation scars?

Lift patient's arms and look for evidence of thoracotomy scars. Is the apex beat displaced or even to the right chest? Assess co-morbidity, e.g. scoliosis and respiratory dysfunction related to prior lateral thoracotomy.

Jugular Venous Pulse (Fig. 14.9)

This can give information about conduction effects and arrhythmias, waveform and pressure. Increased resistance to atrial filling results in an exaggerated "a" wave which may occur in isolated severe pulmonary stenosis or in tricuspid atresia. Episodic "cannon" waves occur in cases of heart block when the atrium contracts against a closed tricuspid valve. A prominent "v" wave is characteristic of tricuspid regurgitation.

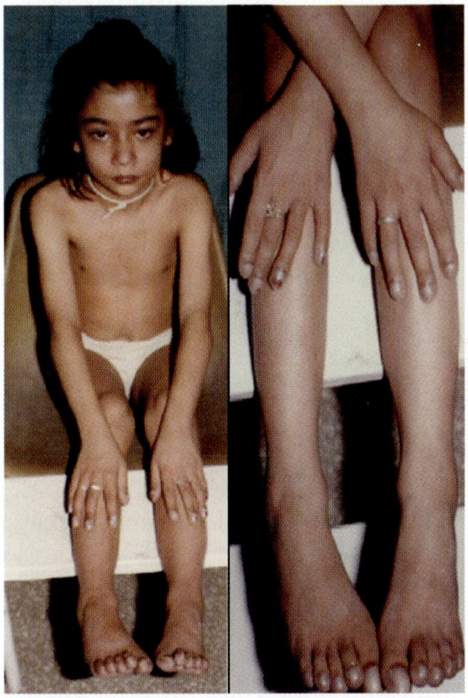

Fig. 14.8: *Central cyanosis and digital clubbing in a child with fallots tetratology who had h/o recurrent cyanotic spells*

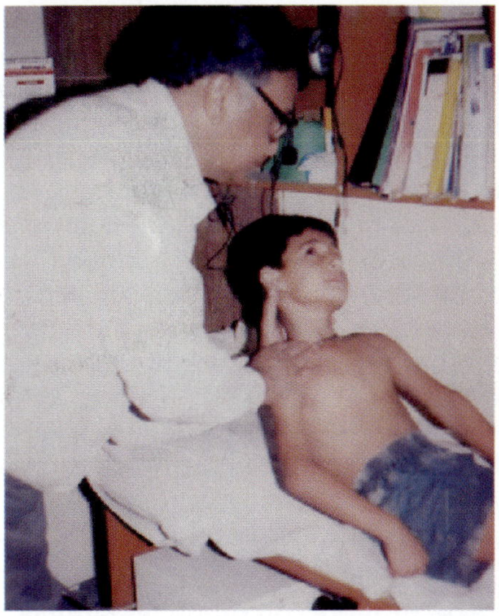

Fig. 14.9: *Demonstrating the RA pressure in relation to anatomical position of both RA, RV and internal jugular vein to the body positioned at 45°*

Systematic Approach to Auscultation of CHD Patient

Innocent versus pathological murmur: How should a clinician distinguish between innocent murmurs and pathological murmurs, and what factors should be evaluated? If the primary care physician is unsure whether the murmur is innocent, then referral to a pediatric cardiologist is the next step. Murmurs are common findings in infants and children. Most murmurs in infants and children originate through normal flow patterns with no structural or anatomic abnormalities of the heart or vessels and are referred to as "innocent", "physiological", or "normal" murmurs. "Innocent" is the preferred term because it strongly conveys that nothing is abnormal, as opposed to the older term "functional", which is not always understood clearly by parents and patients as being "normal". Although murmurs may be heard in virtually anyone, they are most commonly heard in children. Virtually all children will have a murmur sometime while they are growing up. Conversely, murmurs may be created by abnormal flow patterns in the heart and vessels resulting from congenital heart abnormalities, valve disease, or other acquired conditions. In evaluating, the infant or child with a murmur, the clinician must make a complete assessment of the cardiovascular system—not just listen to the murmurs—because there are some serious cardiovascular abnormalities that may have no murmurs. Looking for clues of heart disease, the clinician must obtain a focused history from the patient's parents. For infants, this history will include birth history, feeding patterns, breathing difficulties, color changes, growth pattern, and activity levels. Changes in feeding patterns, particularly a progressively longer time to complete the feeding, may be an early sign of congestive heart failure. For children, parents should be asked about activity capacity: can the child keep up with peers while playing vigorously? Have there been complaints of shortness of breath, palpitations, or chest pain? Chest pain is a common complaint, but a cardiac cause is found in less than 1% of children complaining of chest pain. Syncope occurs in about 15% of children before they reach 21 years of age, and it is most often not the result of primary heart problems; however, the practitioner will want to know whether syncope has occurred and under what circumstances so cardiac causes can be excluded. Although not commonly associated with cardiac disease in childhood, syncope and chest pain may be manifestations of serious cardiac conditions such as aortic stenosis or hypertrophic cardiomyopathy, which are common causes of sudden unexpected death in childhood. If these symptoms are present, particularly if they are related to exercise or there is a positive family history of hypertrophic cardiomyopathy, then they should be evaluated carefully.

Obtaining a thorough family medical history is extremely important in assessing a child because congenital heart defects occur more commonly in families in which a first-degree relative has been born with a heart defect. In addition, hypertrophic cardiomyopathy, a primary muscle disorder of the heart, is an inherited autosomal dominant condition that may result in sudden unexpected death, especially during or after vigorous exercise, in young people. Obtaining a history of this condition or of sudden unexplained death in young people with first-degree relatives who have a heart defect entails a search for hypertrophic cardiomyopathy which may be silent.

Physical examination of a child includes an assessment of general appearance, color, respiratory effort, and vital signs, including heart rate, respiratory rate, and blood pressure. The vital signs should be evaluated by comparing them with age-established norms. The neck should be evaluated for prominence of vessels and abnormal pulsation and listened to for bruits. The chest should be auscultated for abnormal breath sounds. The pulses in the arms and legs should be checked. If the pulses are not equal, then coarctation of the aorta may be present and extremity blood pressures should be obtained. Examination of the heart begins with observation and palpation of the chest for abnormal impulses and thrills. Auscultation begins with listening for the normal sounds of the valves closing and for S1 and S2. It is important not to focus on murmurs initially. Atrial septal defect accounts for about one-third of the congenital defects first detected in adulthood. This is because the characteristic murmur, a pulmonary flow murmur, also is one of the most common childhood innocent murmurs. The key to diagnosis is appreciating the wide fixedly split-second heart sound resulting from right volume overload. This will not be easily appreciated if the clinician focuses on murmurs before defining the heart sounds. Gallop sounds also may be present, signaling difficulty in keeping up with the demands placed on the heart. Conversely, isolated S3 gallop sounds may be heard in healthy adolescents.

When murmurs are heard, they should be defined by the following characteristics (Fig.14.10):

- Timing—when during the cardiac cycle they occur.

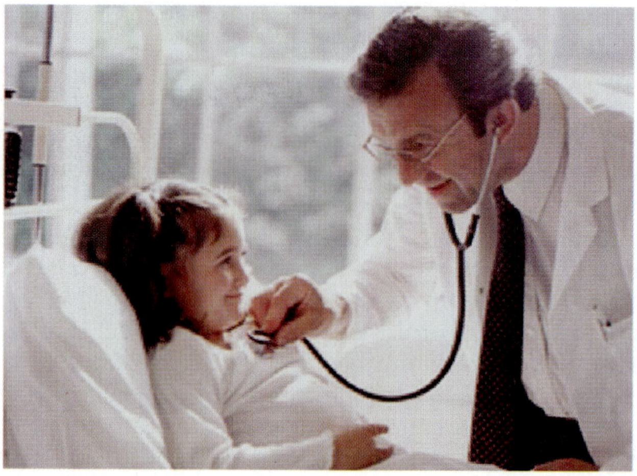

Fig. 14.10: *A young child is being examined by the pediatric cardiologist for heart murmur*

- Location—where in the heart they may originate, keeping in mind that vibrations are transmitted in both directions along a column of blood.
- Quality or pitch—how they sound, which is important in differentiating normal flow murmurs from abnormal
- Intensity or loudness—not necessarily defining the severity, but changes in intensity may help to determine the type of murmur being heard.
- Ejection or nonejection clicks—presence or absence.

Innocent murmurs are murmurs produced by normal flow. Changing the flow should therefore change the intensity of the murmur. Characteristically, maneuvers that decrease the flow of blood returning to the heart through the venous system will decrease the intensity of flow murmurs, suggesting that the murmur is flow related or innocent. Changing the child's position from supine to sitting, then to standing, and finally to squatting during the examination will change the flow and is useful in helping to define innocent murmurs. The child may be asked to push out the abdomen or bear down to perform a valsalva maneuver, which reduces venous blood flow to the heart and the intensity of innocent murmurs. An examiner can coax even a young toddler into doing this by placing a hand on the child's abdomen and asking the child to push it out.

The following are the classic types of innocent or flow murmurs:

Still's murmurs: These murmurs are low-pitched sounds heard at the lower left sternal area. They are musical or have a relatively pure tone in quality or may be squeaky. These most commonly occur between age 3 and adolescence. Because they are low pitched, they are heard best with the bell of the stethoscope. They are related to flow, and they can change with position alteration and then can decrease or disappear with the valsalva maneuver. No clicks are present.

Pulmonary flow murmurs: These are high-pitched, harsher murmurs heard at the upper left sternal border. Because they are high pitched, they are heard best with the diaphragm of the stethoscope. They are flow dependent and also will change with position alteration and decrease or disappear with the valsalva maneuver. These murmurs originate from the right ventricular outflow tract and radiate along the pulmonary arteries and thus may be well heard in the back and axilla bilaterally. They are differentiated from pulmonic stenosis by their quality and from valvular pulmonic stenosis by the absence of an ejection click. Pulmonary flow murmurs can occur at any age, but they are common particularly in adolescents or in children with pectus excavatum. They are prominent in high-flow situations, such as when a child has a fever or is anemic, because flow increases in these situations. In infants, these sounds may be most prominent in the back or axilla because turbulence occurs when the blood flows from the larger main pulmonary artery to the smaller, less well-developed distal pulmonary arteries. In fetal life, the main pulmonary artery transports about 90% of the blood to the ductus arteriosus and only about 10% to the distal pulmonary arteries. The main pulmonary artery is thus large, whereas the distal pulmonary arteries are relatively smaller and come off at more acute angles than they do later as the child's chest grows. An analogy from nature would be the noise that is created as a large stream narrows into smaller streams. This innocent murmur has been termed "benign peripheral pulmonary stenosis of the newborn" to differentiate it from true anatomic obstructions to distal pulmonary arteries that occur in pathological conditions such as congenital rubella syndrome.

Systemic flow murmurs (supraclavicular systemic bruits). These are harsh high-pitched murmurs caused by normal blood flow into the aorta and into the head and neck vessels and are heard best high up in the chest and above the clavicles. They are also heard best with the diaphragm of the stethoscope. No ejection click is associated with these murmurs. They are transmitted to the arch vessels and are heard when listening over the carotid arteries of the neck. It has been said that because of these sounds "all children have carotid bruits"; however, the sounds differ in quality from true carotid bruits and are not associated with aortic outflow pathology.

Venous hums: These are low-pitched continuous murmurs made by blood returning from the great veins to the heart. They are heard best with the bell of the stethoscope. By changing the position of the patient's head or by pressing in the area of the major neck veins, the flow may be changed and these murmurs will change or disappear. Having the child look down or to the side while listening will often make these murmurs or sounds disappear. They are differentiated from the murmurs of patent ductus arteriosus in that they are louder in diastole, when maximal flow occurs in the venous system, and are often heard bilaterally. Venous hums are sensitive to posture and head and neck position, whereas the murmur of patent ductus is not. Although an ECG is usually part of the evaluation and may be helpful, further testing is not needed in the overwhelming majority of infants and children to distinguish between normal or pathological hearts. It has been shown that a competent pediatric cardiologist can determine with a high degree of certainty whether there is heart disease. Because of the characteristics of the sounds and the maneuvers that can be used to facilitate identifying them as flow-related phenomenon, these murmurs can be correctly identified without further testing. After concluding that the murmur or murmurs (a child may have more than one kind) are innocent, the practitioner should explain the findings to the parents and child. The practitioner should emphasize during the discussion that murmurs simply mean sounds or noises and that in and of themselves they are not synonymous with abnormalities of the heart. The clinician should stress that although a large percentage of infants and children have murmurs, less than 1% are born with the congenital heart defects that are the most common cause of heart disease in children. Parents should not be promised that their children will outgrow these murmurs because this is not necessarily true; adults can have innocent murmurs as well. Assurances should be given that because the heart is normal, whether or not the murmur disappears or changes is of no consequence. In addition, because flow changes the murmur, with growth and the changing configuration of chest and heart dynamics, murmurs may change, disappear, and reappear at various times—further evidence that the murmurs are indeed flow related and innocent.

1. ***Listen to the heart sounds*** (Fig. 14.10).

   First heart sound (S1): The first heart sound is usually heard as a single sound but since mitral closure is loudest, it is best heard at the apex. A loud first heart sound may be heard in mitral stenosis or sometimes with an atrial septal defect. Soft first heart sounds are a feature of poor myocardial contractility or a long PR interval.

   Second heart sound (S2): Fixed splitting in the presence of a significant atrial septal defect and is best appreciated in the high or mid left sternal border.

Accentuated in the presence of pulmonary hypertension. Widely split following repair of tetralogy of Fallot, the second heart sound is reflecting the right bundle branch block, characteristic of the postoperative electrocardiogram.

2. ***Check for systolic/diastolic murmurs*** (Draw an imaginary line between the nipples).

Murmurs loudest above nipple line: Ejection systolic in type. Arise from the right or left ventricular outflow tract.

If associated with a carotid or suprasternal thrill, usually from the left ventricular outflow tract. If an ejection click is heard, the murmur is valvular in origin.

Ejection click of aortic valve stenosis is best heard at the apex. Ejection systolic murmur best heard in the interscapular region and associated with a left thoracotomy may indicate turbulence across a prior coarctation repair.

Murmurs loudest below nipple line: Pan-systolic and arise from mitral/tricuspid regurgitation or from a ventricular septal defect.

A 'to and fro' murmur best heard at the upper left sternal edge following cardiac surgery usually results from combined right ventricular outflow tract obstruction and pulmonary regurgitation.

The mid-systolic click and systolic murmur of mitral valve prolapse is best heard with the patient standing up.

A continuous murmur arises from an arterial duct. systemic to pulmonary shunt or arteriovenous fistulas.

Measure height, weight. blood pressure, and oxygen saturation in all patients. 12 lead ECG is essential at every visit.

Electrocardiogram (Fig. 14.11)

Rate and rhythm: Consider atrial flutter with variable block if constant rate of 120 or 150/minute-easily confused with 'sinus rhythm'. Atrial tachycardias are especially common after all forms of atrial surgery, e.g. intra-atrial repair for transposition of the great arteries.

Look for signs of chamber enlargement-atrial or ventricular hypertrophy.

Assess presence/absence of bundle-branch block. Measure duration of QRS in all postoperative tetralogy of Fallot patients: QRS duration >180 ms associated with higher risk of arrhythmias, right heart dilatation and late sudden death.

If tachycardia suspected, record 12 leads ECG during administration of intravenous adenosine.

Role of Exercise Testing

- Assess heart rate and blood pressure response to exercise (blunted response in important aortic valve stenosis).
- Compare upper and lower limb BP following coarctation repair.
- Monitor oxygen saturation by pulse oximetry to improve risk stratification in cyanosed patients.
- Also, improves counseling and planning for pregnancy.
- Formal cardiopulmonary exercise testing reserved for decision making retiming of surgical or catheter-based intervention.
- Can help distinguish limitation due to lack of aerobic fitness and assess maximal effort.

Chest X-ray

Cheap and invaluable investigation in CHD.

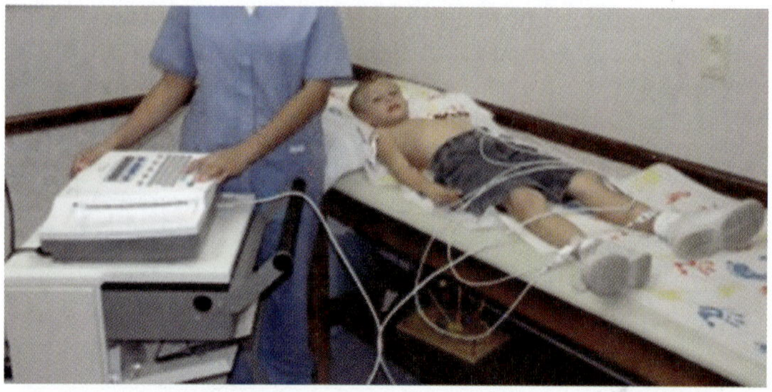

Fig. 14.11: *Electrocardiographic equipment along with precardial leads over the chest prior to obtaining an electrocardiogram*

Identify right-left orientation to assess cardiac and visceral positions. Assessment of the bronchial branching permits diagnosis of isomeric cardiac defects, e.g. symmetric morphologic right bronchi characteristic of right atrial isomerism (usually associated with complex CHD-common right atrial a common atrioventricular orifice, a great artery arising form one ventricular chamber and total anomalous pulmonary venous connection).

Identify situs inversus (mirror image anatomy with liver on the left and stomach bubble on the right with cardiac apex in right chest). Consider Kartagener syndrome. Discordance between position of the apex and visceral situs usually associated with CHD.

Record cardiothoracic ratio in the notes. Look for rib notching related to collateral blood supply in severe coarctation of the aorta. Assess pulmonary vasculature.

Chest X-ray assessment of Pulmonary Vasculature in CHD Patients (Fig. 14.12)

- Increased vascularity
- Left to right shunt atrial septal defect (ASD), ventricular septal defect (VSD)
- Pulmonary edema
- Obstructed pulmonary venous drainage
- Decreased vascularity
- Right ventricular outflow obstruction, e.g. isolated severe pulmonary stenosis, following tetralogy repair
- Pulmonary hypertension
- Unilateral increased pulmonary vascular markings
- Consider ipsilateral systemic to pulmonary arterial shunt
- Over-perfused major arterial pulmonary collateral artery
- Obstructed pulmonary venous drainage, e.g. following Mustard-Senning intra-atrial repair for transposition of the great arteries.

Imging in Congenital Heart Disease Echocardiography (Figs 14.13 to 1.15)

Most useful investigation in CHD but only when directed by detailed history taking and clinical examination.

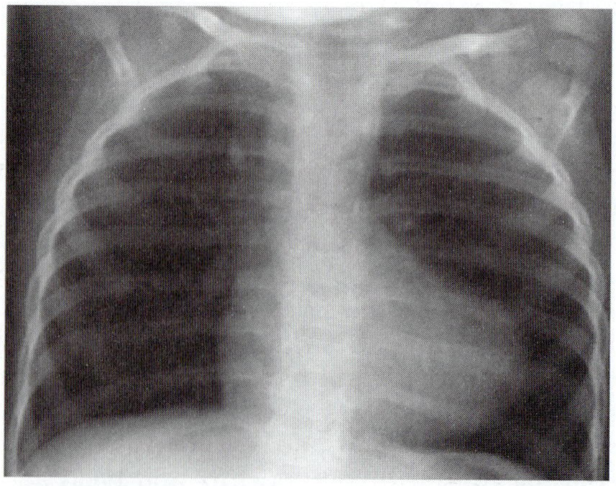

Fig. 14.12: *Frontal chest radiograph of pediatric patient with tetralogy of Fallot (TOF) shows characteristic boot-shaped heart with hyperlucent lungs, diminished central hilar pulmonary vessels, and an upturned cardiac apex. Main pulmonary artery segment is flat to concave, and right aortic arch is seen*

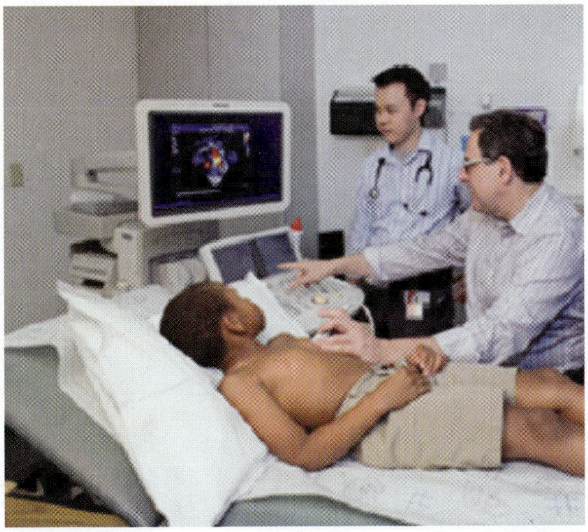

Fig. 14.13: *Tansthoracic echocardiography is applied for assessment of congenital heart defect*

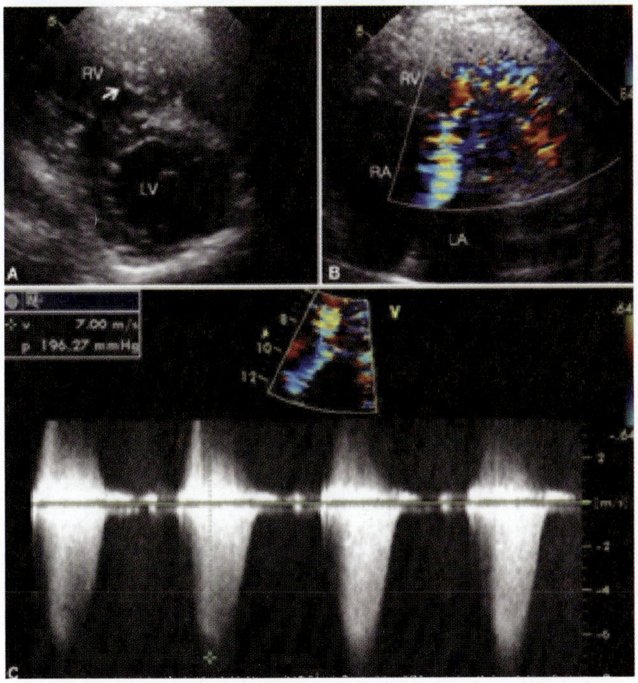

Fig. 14.14: *Double-chambered right ventricle demonstrated by transthrorasic echocardiography. (A) Two dimensional echocardiography showing a stenotic mid-right ventricle with an anomalous muscle bundle (arrow). (B) Turbulent Doppler color flow with mosaic pattern. (C) Continuous-wave Doppler showing tricuspid regurgitation between the right atrium and the right ventricle and indicating the flow acceleration and pressure gradient. RV, right ventricle; LV, left ventricle; RA, right atrium*

This should be performed by an experienced examiner with detailed knowledge of all aspects of CHD.

There is no substitute for sequential data and a protocol for regular, standardized analysis is required.

Imaging in adults may be limited by poor echogenic windows.

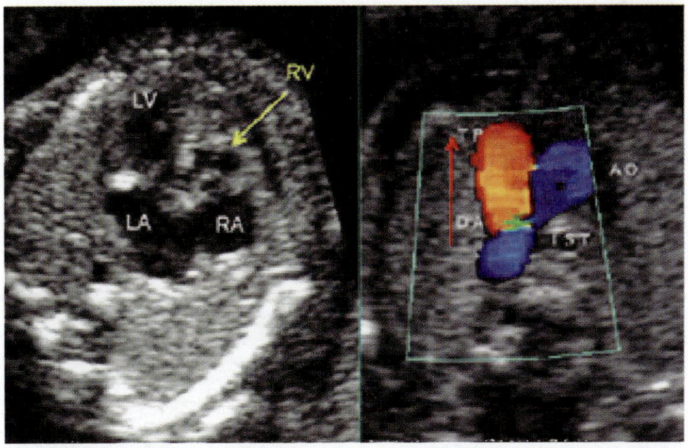

Fig. 14.15: *Echocardiography showing hypoplastic right ventricle (arrow) in a fetus with pulmonary atresia and intact ventricular septum (a). Color doppler of the four chamber view with asymmetric flow between the left heart and the right heart. Pulmonary valve atresia can be diagnosed using color Doppler by visualizing the great vessels-aorta (Ao) and pulmonary trunk (TP)-in the upper thorax and demonstrating the retrograde flow from the descending aorta across the ductus arteriosus toward the pulmonary valve*

Magnetic Resonance Imaging (Figs 14.16)

Ideal for the assessment of extra-cardiac pulmonary arterial and venous trees. Accurate quantification of valvular regurgitation, e.g. assessment of pulmonary regurgitation and right ventricular function following repair of tetralogy of Fallot. Its utility is limited by scarcity of expert radiologists in the field of CHD.

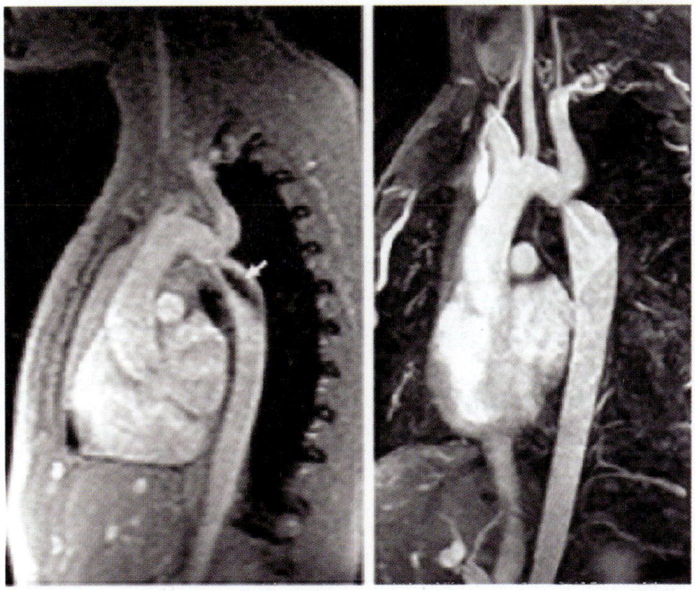

Fig. 14.16: *Axial MR image shows marked stenosis of the main pulmonary artery (MPA) and the origin of the right pulmonary artery (RPA). The descending left pulmonary artery (LPA) is large and isolated. Ao, aorta. Surgery involved unifocalization of the nonconfluent pulmonary arteries and repair of the tetralogy of*

Computerized Axial Tomography (Figs 14.17 to 14.19)

It is very useful in identification of different types of cardiac defects particularily congenital coronary anomalies.

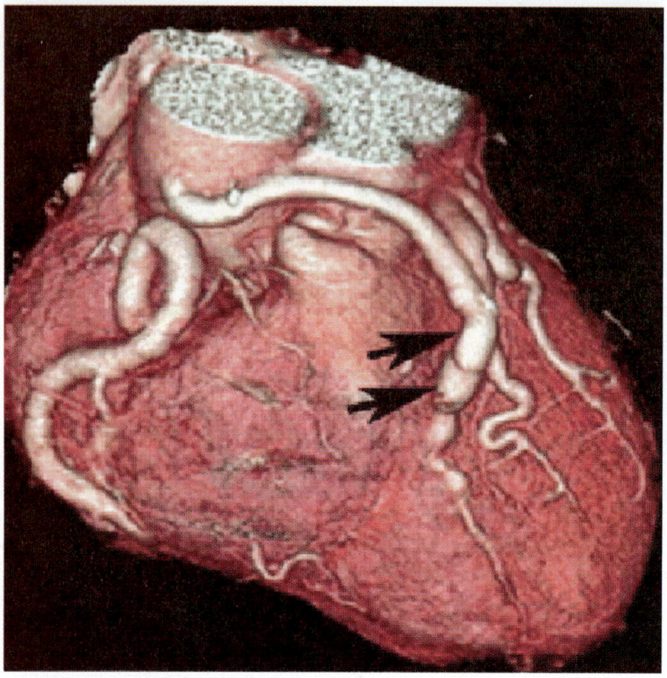

Fig. 14.17: *CABG placement with ligation in an adolescent with ALCAPA syndrome. Volume-rendered CT image shows a venous graft extending from the aorta to the mid-LAD artery with focal atherosclerotic dilatation but no narrowing (arrows). Volume-rendered CT image shows a second graft extending from the aorta to the first marginal artery; this graft is occluded (arrows)*

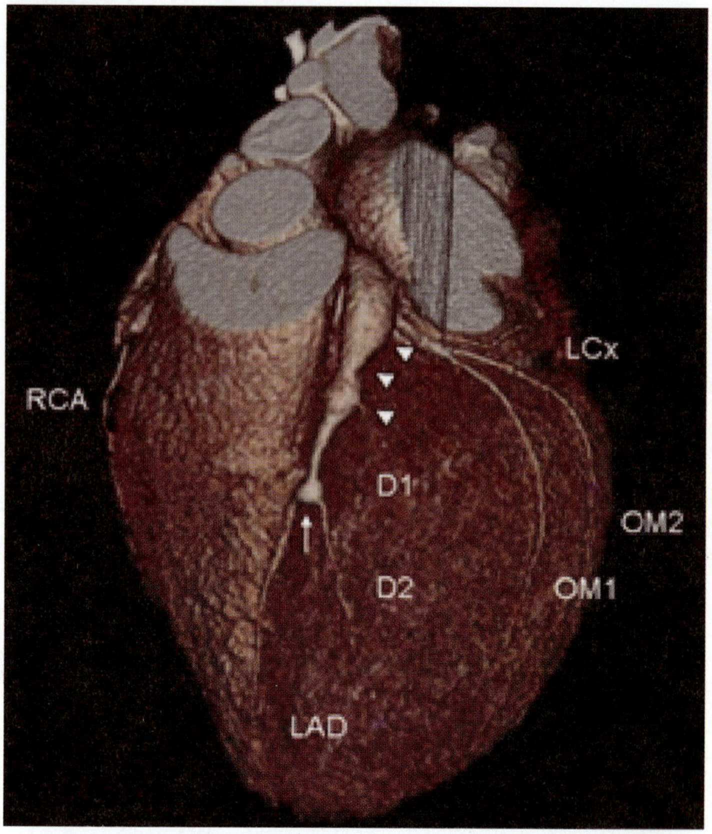

Fig. 14.18: *Kawasaki's disease: multiple fusiform aneurysms throughout the LAD (white arrowheads) with one arising at the origin of the second diagonal branch*

Table 14.1: *Example of gene products and associated features*

	MYH6	*GATA4*	*NKX2–5*	*TBX5*	*TBX1*
Locus	14q11.2–q13	8p23.1–p22	5q34	12q24.1	22q11.2
Syndrome				Holt-Oram	DiGeorge
Atrial septal defects	✓	✓	✓	✓	
Ventricular septal defects		✓	✓	✓	
Electrical conduction abnormalities			✓	✓	
Outflow abnormalities					✓
Noncardiac manifestation*				Upper limb abnormalities	Small or absence thymus small or absence parathyroids facial abnormalities

*The notch signaling pathway, a regulatory mechanism for cell growth and differentiation, plays broad roles in several aspects of cardiac development.

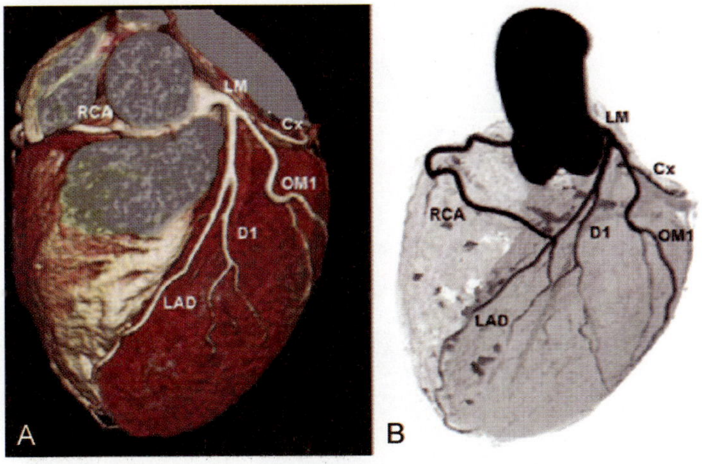

Fig. 14.19: *Coronary CT angiogram with prospective ECG-triggering in an adolescent with atypical chest pain. (A) 3D volume rendering. (B) Angiography-like rendering. Normal coronary arteries are observed. The study allows reliably ruling out coronary artery disease using minimal radiation dose (<3.5 mSv). LM, left main; LAD, left anterior descending coronary artery; D1, first diagonal branch; Cx, circumflex coronary artery; OM1, first obtuse marginal branch; RCA, right coronary arter.*

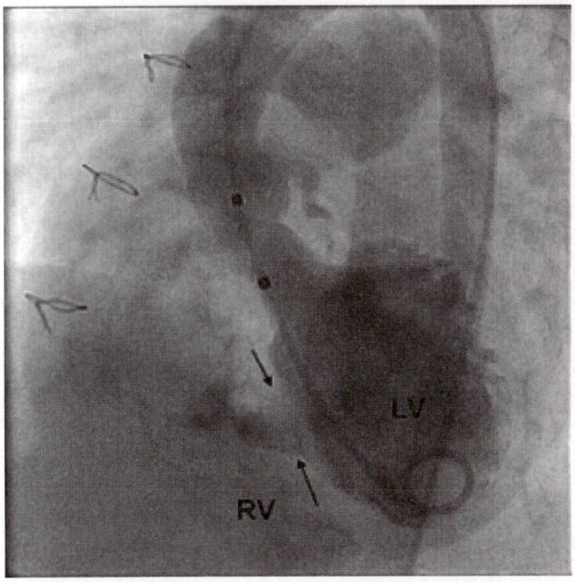

Fig. 14.20: *Angiographic imaging of the muscular VSD. LV angiography performed with LAO and cranial imaging profiles the muscular ventricular septum well and delineates the muscular VSD (arrows). LV, left ventricle; RV, right ventricle*

Cardiac Catheterization (Fig. 14.20)

This still has its place in quantifying shunts and obtaining accurate hemodynamic data. Increasingly this is carried out to facilitate percutaneous transcatheter procedures such as occlusion of atrial septal defects. With an ageing population, many patients with CHD need to undergo coronary angiography as combined surgical procedures may be required.

Genetic Testing (Table 14.1)

The notch signaling pathway, a regulatory mechanism for cell growth and differentiation plays broad roles in several aspects of cardiac development (Table 14.1).

SEPTAL DEFECTS

ATRIAL SEPTAL DEFECTS

An ASD is an opening in the interatrial septum between the right and the left atria. These include (Fig. 14.21):
- Secundum atrial septal defect
- Septum primum defect
- Atrioventricular defect
- Sinus venosus defect.

Etiology

ASD are virtually all congenital, except for the rare defects that result either from marked enlargement of the left atrium (which opens a functionally closed fossa ovalis) or from the passage of large catheters across an intact septum at the time of balloon mitral valvuloplasty.

Pathology (Figs 14.21 and 14.22)

There are three major types of congenital atrial septal defects:
1. ***Ostium secundum***, the most common type, in which the septum secundum does not form in region of the fossa ovalis.
2. ***Ostium primum***, in which the septum primum does not fuse to the endocardial cushion and which is frequently associated with defects of one or both atrioventricular valves.
3. ***Sinus venosus defect***, in which there is a defect In the septum superior to the fossa ovalis and which is often associated with anomalous pulmonary venous return.

Occasionally, the foramen ovale is probe-patent but does not permit the shunting of blood unless the septum is stretched and/or the pressure in one atrium is markedly elevated.

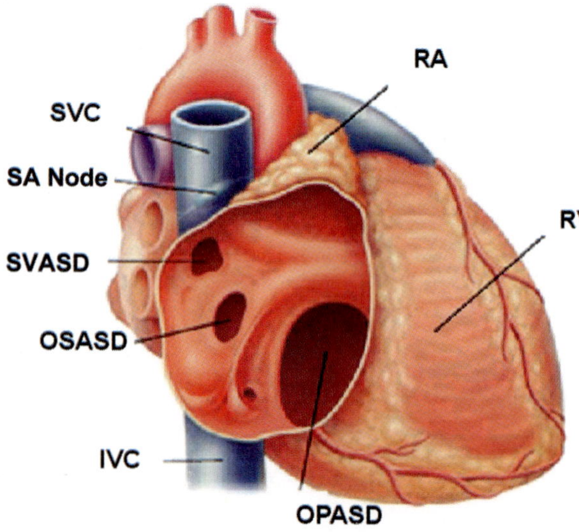

Fig. 14.21: *Anatomy of atrial septal defects (ASDs). OPASD, ostium primum ASD; OSASD, ostium secundum ASD; SVASD, sinus venosus ASD.*

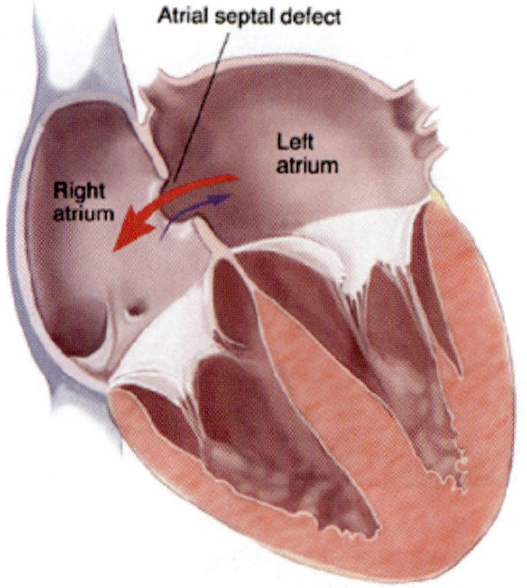

Fig. 14.22: *Diagram showing atrial septal defect (ASD). There are two atria in the heart; one on the right and one on the left. The right atrium carries deoxygenated blood and the left atrium carries oxygenated blood. An ASD is when there is a hole between these two atria, resulting in a mixing of oxygenated and deoxygenated blood*

Clinical Manifestations

History

Many persons with ostium secundum defects or Sinus venosus defects have no symptoms although others may have increased fatigability and dyspnea on exertion, and occasionally palpitations. With the development of severe pulmonary vascular disease, which occurs in about 5–10% after the age of 20, there is often a worsening dyspnea and fatigue, the developmenr of a right-to-left shunt with cyanosis, possibly hemoptysis, and, rarely, a paradoxical embolus or brain abscess. Patients with ostium primum defects frequently have symptoms of severe mitral regurgitation from early childhood and tend to develop severe pulmonary vascular disease (Eisenmenger's syndrome) at an earlier age.

Physical Examination

The condition occurs more often in females. The patients are usually thin and gracile in habitus. Cyanosis is not apparent. There is frequently a right ventricular lift or heave along the left sternal edge; and the pulmonary artery may be palpable in the second left intercostal space. Patients with a secundum type defect may have congenital defects of the bones of the arms and hand (Holt-Oram syndrome). Patients with Eisenmenger's syndrome may have cyanosis. Signs of left ventricular hypertrophy may occur with a primum defect.

Auscultation

The first heart sound is usually split with a loud tricuspid component.

Wide, fixed splitting of the second heart sound (S2) in both the supine and standing positions is usually present.

The delay of the pulmonic component of the second heart sound (P2) is due to prolonged right ventricular ejection and a "hangout", or delay of closure, of the pulmonary valve due to the very distensible pulmonary vasculature.

There is usually a mid-systolic, crescendo-decrescendo murmur that is heard maximally at the left second or third intercostal space and that is produced by the increased flow across pulmonary valve. Occasionally, patients with a large left-to-right shunt have a diastolic flow rumble and opening snap of the tricuspid valve, both best heard along the lower left sternal border. Patients with severe pulmonary hypertension may develop the murmurs of tricuspid regurgitation or pulmonary regurgitation. Persons with ostium primum (or "endocardial cushion") defects usually also have murmurs of mitral, and occasionally tricuspid, regurgitation.

Diagnostic Tests

Chest X-ray (Fig. 14.23)

The chest roentgenogram usually shows moderate cardiomegaly with dilatation of the right ventricle, right atrium, and pulmonary arteries in association with increased pulmonary blood flow. The aortic arch appears small. In neonates, the heart size may be normal and the pulmonary flow may appear normal. Older patients with severe pulmonary vascular disease may have diminished peripheral vascular markings ("pruned-tree" appearance). Patients with ostium primum defects and mitral regurgitation may have left ventricular enlargement.

Electrocardiogram

The electrocardiogram usually shows normal sinus rhythm, although atrial arrhythmias are common. The PR interval

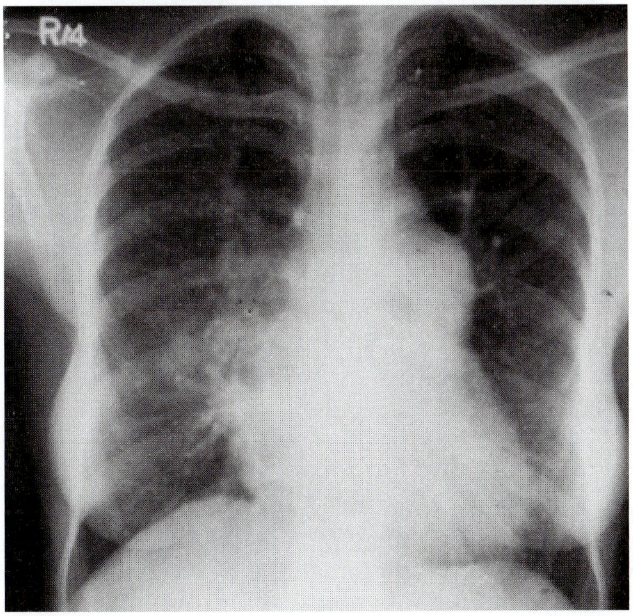

Fig. 14.23: *Photograph of X-ray chest PA view showing moderate cardiomegaly with dilatation of right ventricle, right atrium and pulmonary arteries in association with increased pulmonary blood flow in ASD secundum type*

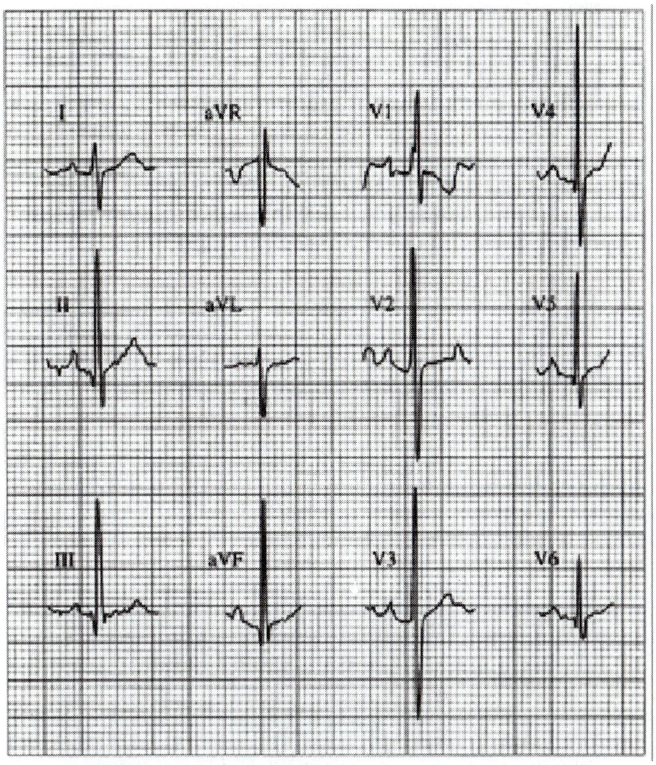

Fig. 14.24: *ECG trace in secundum atrial septal defect: note the right axis deviation and dominant R wave in lead VI*

is prolonged in about 20%. A right ventricular conduction defect is very characteristic of ostium secundum defects. This is usually manifest by the presence in lead VI of one of the following types of QRS complexes: RsR', rSr', or rsR'. The P axis tends to be horizontal or superior in patients with a sinus venosus defect. The QRS complex in a patient with an ostium primum defect characteristically shows right bundle-branch block and left-axis deviation (Fig. 14.24).

Diagnostic: Evaluation

Echocardiogram (Figs 14.25 to 14.30)

The echocardiogram of an ostium secundum defect demonstrates dilatation of a hyperdynamic right ventricle, right atrium, and pulmonary artery with paradoxic motion of the ventricular septum. Occasionally, the atrial defect may be seen. About one-third of secundum defects have evidence of mitral valve prolapse.

Doppler echocardiography can demonstrate flow across the atrial septum. Patients with primum defects may have left ventricular dilatation, defects of the mitral or tricuspid valves, and demonstrable defects of "the atrial and upper ventricular septa". There may be evidence of pulmonary artery hypertension from decreased motion of the pulmonary valve leaflets during atrial systole.

Cardiac Catheterization

Cardiac catheterization remains the procedure of choice for the diagnosis of ASD and shows the following: an abnormal step-up of oxygen saturation occurs in the right atrium

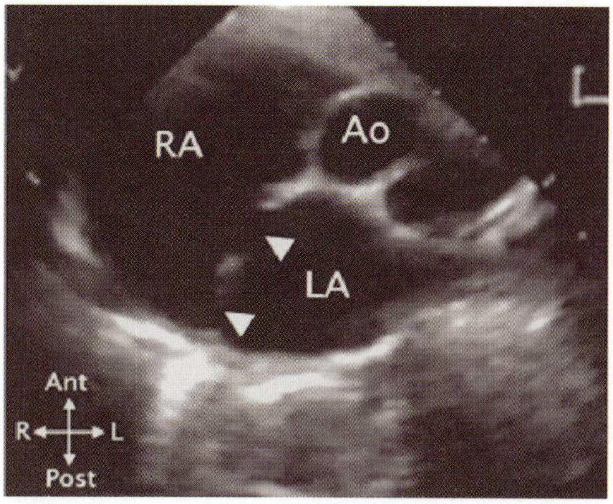

Fig. 14.25: *An echocardiogram in right sternal border view in a patient with multiple ASD2 (arrow heads). Ao, aorta; LA, left atrium; RA, right atrium*

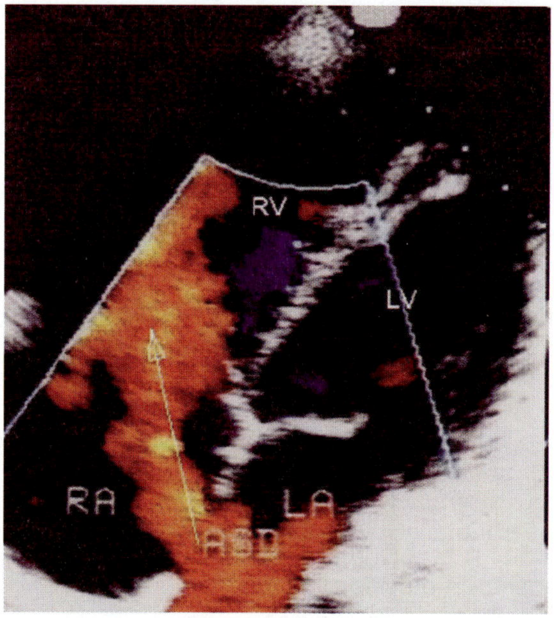

Fig. 14.26: *ASD color Doppler flow mapping showing the red colored flow across the atrial septum from left atrium (LA) to the right atrium (RA). The flow is red colored because it is toward the echotransducer in this view. RV, right ventricle; LV, left ventricle. The flow reversal (blue colour and jet moving from RA to LA) can occur when there is severe pulmonary hypertension. Reverse flow across the ASD (right to left) can also be seen in total anomalous pulmonary venous connection*

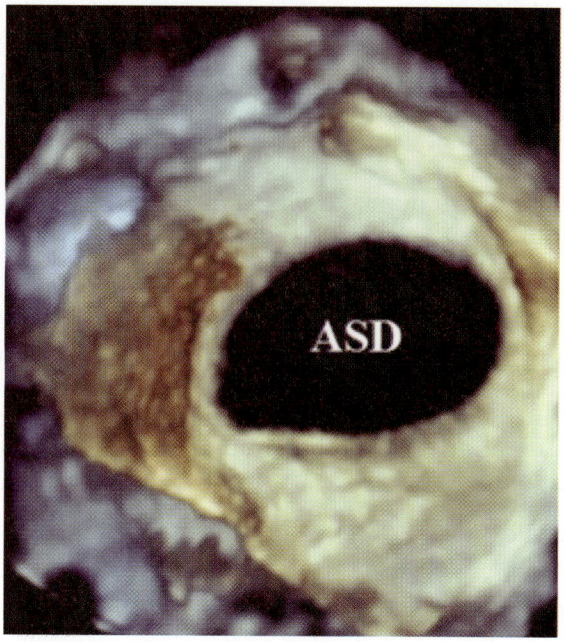

Fig. 14.27: *3D echocardiographic image of an atrial septal defect (ASD)*

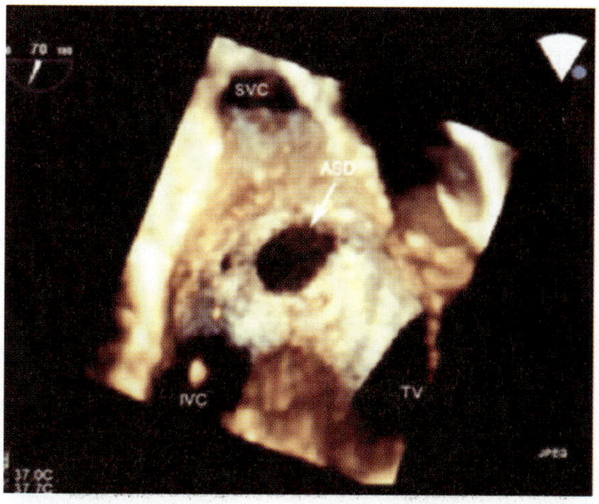

Fig. 14.28: *Three dimensional echocardiogram of a secundum atrial septal defect (ASD; arrow). This is a right atrial en-face view that shows the size, shape, and position of the defect in relation to the right atrial septal surface. SVC, superior vena cava; IVC, inferior vena cava; TV, tricuspid valve*

Cineangiography may demonstrate a "goose" neck of left ventricle in patient with primum defect.

Differential Diagnosis

The differential diagnosis includes anomalous pulmonary venous return with intact atrial septum, mitral stenosis, mitral regurgitation, and Eisenmenger's syndrome. The latter, which occurs as a late complication of ASD, can also result from ventricular septal defect or patent ductus arteriosus.

Natural History and Prognosis

Many secundum ASDs probably close spontaneously in the first year of life. Many patients remain asymptomatic or only minimally symptomatic until the age of 30 or 40, and some never develop symptoms. The major determinants of survival are the amount of left-to-right shunt and the development of pulmonary vascular disease. Death from ASD is usually the result of pulmonary hypertension (which occurs in about one-quarter of patients

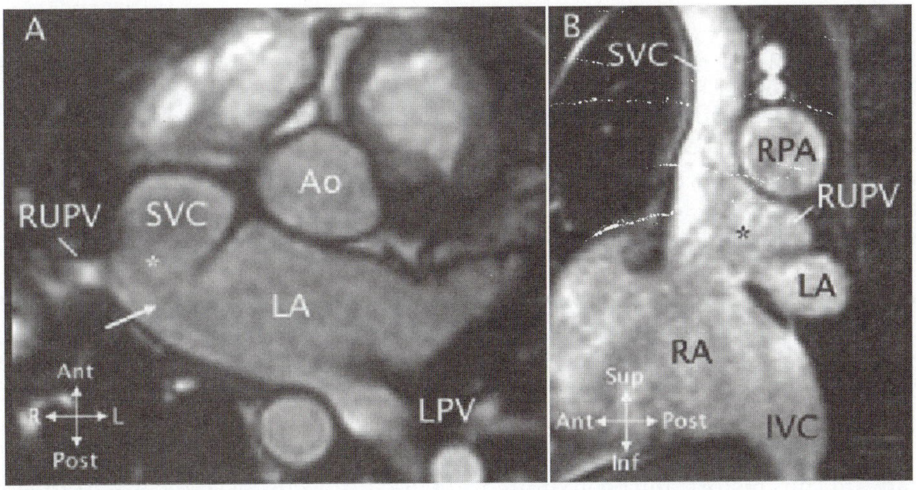

Fig. 14.29: *(A) A MRI 3D SSFP axial view showing a superior vena cava (SVC) type of SVD (*). The right upper pulmonary vein (RUPV) drains to the SVC-right atrial junction near the SVD. The orifice of the RUPV into the left atrium (LA) (white arrow) is the interatrial communication. (B) Sagittal projection of the same data set shows the defect (*) between the SVC - RA junction and the RUPV. Ao, aorta; IVC, inferior vena cava; LPV, left pulmonary vein; RPA, right pulmonary artery. (Reprinted from Valente et al. with permission)*

over the age of 40 but in only about 10% under the age of 40), congestive heart failure (CHF), or pulmonary artery thrombosis. Patients with ostium primum defects with A V valve regurgitation often develop congestive heart failure and severe pulmonary hypertension at a much younger age. Bacterial endocarditis is rare in the secundum or sinus venosus types, but patients with ostium primum defects are vulnerable to the disease.

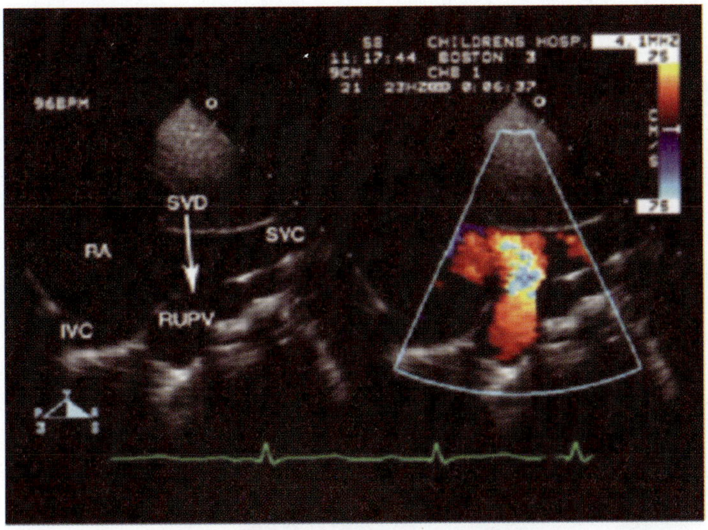

Fig. 14.30: *Superior sinus venosus defect. High right parasternal border long-axis echocardiogram view in this patient with superior sinus venosus defect (SVD) demonstrates the absence of tissue ("unroofing") defect between the right upper pulmonary vein (RUPV) and the distal superior vena cava (SVC). Color Doppler flow demonstrates left-to-right flow from the RUPV to the SVC/ RA, with mild flow acceleration across the defect. IVC, inferior vena cava; RA, right atrium*

Medical Care

Medical therapy is of no benefit in children with asymptomatic atrial septal defects (ASDs). With the exception of ostium secundum types, ASDs are structural defects that do not spontaneously close. Surgical closure is ultimately required for most ASDs, other than ostium secundum ASDs. Occasionally, small primum ASDs may not require closure, but due to their association with mitral valve abnormalities, they may be closed at the time of mitral valve repair, if such a repair is indicated. An ostium secundum atrial septal defect that measures 6 mm in diameter or smaller in the patient's first year of life is likely to spontaneously close; however, such closure is substantially slower than that of a typical small, muscular ventricular septal defect.

Infants who are severely affected with an ASD and who develop CHF may be treated as any other child with CHF from a left-to-right shunt. This treatment, which includes diuretics, afterload reduction, and less commonly, digoxin, is covered in other articles. As noted previously, it is of particular importance to rule out other etiologies of symptoms in these infants, especially those with secundum ASDs due to the typical paucity of symptoms associated with this lesion in infancy and early childhood.

Arrhythmias associated with ASD are similarly uncommon in childhood become increasingly common with age. In fact, the development of atrial fibrillation may trigger CHF in adults with ASD who are younger than 40 years. Arrhythmias may result from atrial distention, and these individuals may require antiarrhythmic therapy until the ASD is repaired. Some children with an ASD present with recurrent respiratory tract infections, which may be poorly tolerated. If immunologically normal, these children are not at a higher risk for infection in general, but the chronically increased pulmonary bloodflow, when combined with the inflammatory changes associated with lower respiratory tract infections, can lead to prolonged symptoms and altered cardiopulmonary interactions.

Bacterial endocarditis prophylaxis is not necessary for the typical patient with an isolated ASD, regardless of the type of ASD. Prophylaxis is recommended prior to surgical repair if the ASD is part of complex cyanotic congenital heart disease (CCHD). Endocarditis prophylaxis is recommended for 6 months following either surgical or percutaneous repair of ASDs and, in some instances, may be recommended for longer in patients with residual mitral valve abnormalities after surgical repair of primum ASDs. For more information see Antibiotic Prophylactic Regimens for Endocarditis.

Surgical Care

Definitive therapy for an ASD has historically been limited to surgical closure. However, with the advent of transcatheter techniques, many children undergo successful treatment in the cardiac catheterization laboratory. The most common surgical approach to the defect is primary repair with suture closure or with patch repair [generally with glutaraldehyde treated autologous pericardium or fabric made of polyester fiber (Dacron)]. Not all children with an ASD are candidates for surgery, which is only indicated for those children with clinically significant left-to-right shunting. In general, a pulmonary-to-systemic flow ratio of 1.5:1 or more is considered the principal indication for surgical repair. Shunting less than this in children with small defects and in those with existing pulmonary hypertension may be observed. Because cardiac catheterization is rarely necessary, echocardiographic evidence of right atrial and right ventricular enlargement is usually considered evidence of a clinically significant left-to-right shunt and an indication for surgical closure of the ASD. Surgery is ideally performed in children aged 2–4 years and has a very low mortality rate. However, surgery may be performed earlier than this if the child has evidence of CHF.

Newer, minimally invasive surgical techniques have been developed. These improve cosmetic appearances and decrease hospital stays. These techniques are ideally suited for simple closure of a secundum atrial septal defect. The surgical mortality rate is low in patients with uncomplicated ASD. In an experienced pediatric center, the mortality rate should be less than 1%. Postoperative morbidity in individuals with ASD is almost exclusively due to accumulation of pericardial fluid (postpericardiotomy syndrome), which occurs in approximately one-third of patients. On occasion, tamponade occurs and requires pericardiocentesis. Pericardial effusion should be suspected in any pediatric patient who undergoes postsurgical repair of an ASD and who presents with chest pain, fever, shortness of breath, or general malaise. In young children, symptoms may be nonspecific and include irritability and decreased appetite (Figs 14.31 and 14.32).

Transcatheter approaches to ASD closure are well accepted in the pediatric population. Secundum ASD are currently the only subtype of ASD that are amenable to this approach. Such techniques require individuals with considerable expertise in the field of interventional pediatric cardiology and cooperation between the interventionalist and the noninvasive imaging specialists.

Benefits of the transcatheter approach include its minimal invasiveness, the lack of median sternotomy, the avoidance of cardiopulmonary bypass, and the relatively quick recovery time. Potential drawbacks and concerns include residual shunting around the device, embolization during placement requiring surgical intervention, lack of

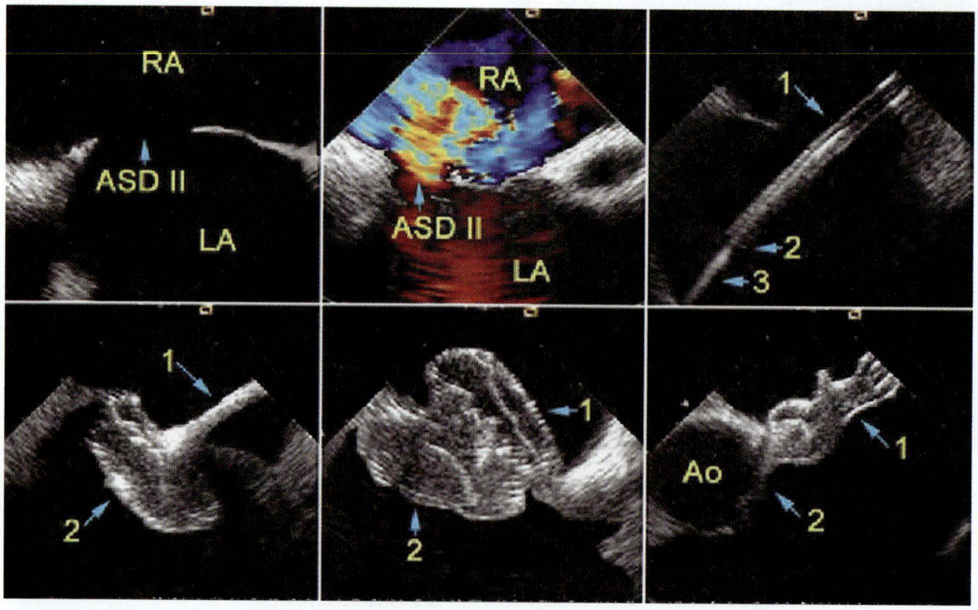

Fig. 14.31: *Guidance of ASD device closure by intracardiac echocardiography. Ao, aorta; ASD, atrial septal defect; LA, left atrium; RA, right atrium; 1c, long access sheath; 2c, end of access sheath in the left atrium; 3c, guidewire; 1d and 2d, delivery cable with the left-sided countercluder opened; 1e and 2e, implanted device still connected to the delivery cable; 1f and 2f, device in its final position*

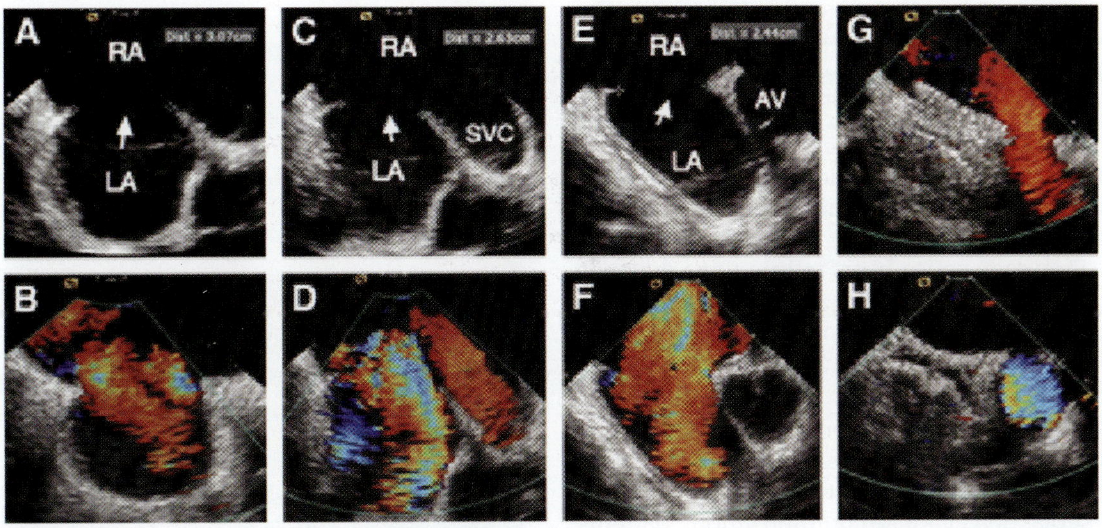

Fig. 14.32: *Intracardiac echocardiographic images during transcatheter closure of a large secundum ASD in a 12.5-year-old male child (A, B) Images in septal view without (A) and with (B) color Doppler, demonstrating the presence of a large defect (arrow) measuring 31 mm. (C, D) Images in long-axis (caval) view without (C) and with (D) color Doppler, demonstrating the large defect (arrow) measuring 26 mm. (E, F) Images in short-axis view without (E) and with (F) color Doppler, demonstrating the large defect (arrow) measuring 24 mm. (G, H) Images after a 34 mm device was implanted in caval (G) and short-axis (H) view, demonstrating good device position and no residual shunt. ASD, atrial septal defect; AV, aortic valve; LA, left atrium; RA, right atrium; SVC, superior vena cava*

adequate septal rims to properly seat the device and the need for specific technical expertise and equipment. Long-term safety concerns are noted because device placement in smaller children is still relatively new. Long-term follow-up studies will provide further information. Overall however, the medium- to long-term outcomes of ASD closure, either surgically or percutaneously, appear very good.

Consultations

Diagnosis of an ASD in a newborn or an older child should prompt consultation with a pediatric cardiologist. Almost all newborns have a small left-to-right shunt at the foramen ovale, as detected during echocardiography in the neonatal period. In the absence of a murmur or other signs of a true ASD on subsequent well-child care visits, consultation with a cardiologist is probably not necessary, although review of the initial echocardiogram report is prudent to verify the description of the defect.

Activity

Children with ASD generally have no restrictions on their activity. Children with compensated CHF with an ASD are candidates for surgical or catheter-based intervention and should be able to resume normal activity after the defect is corrected.

Further Outpatient Care

Provide routine medical care with special attention to signs of CHF or increased pulmonary vascular resistance (PVR). Most patients with an ASD are asymptomatic and require only routine well-child care until they undergo elective surgical repair or transcatheter device placement for their defects.

Most children with uncomplicated ASD are followed up by their primary care provider and receive follow-up with a pediatric cardiologist every year or every other year. Children who require medical intervention or who have other comorbidities are seen by a cardiologist more frequently than this.

ATRIOVENTRICULAR SEPTAL DEFECT

Atrioventricular canal defect; endocardial cushion defect; persistent ostium primum.

Atrioventricular (AV) septal defect consists of primum type ASD with AV valve malformation, with or without a VSD. These defects result from maldevelopment of the endocardial cushions. Defects may be asymptomatic if small. If large, they may cause heart failure with dyspnea with feeding, poor growth, tachypnea, diaphoresis or arrhythmias. Heart murmurs are common. Diagnosis is by echocardiography. Treatment is surgical repair for all but the smallest defects (Fig. 14.33).

AV septal defect accounts for about 5% of congenital heart anomalies. The defect may be complete or partial; 30% of patients with the complete form have Down syndrome. AV septal defect is also common among patients with asplenia or polysplenia (heterotaxy) syndromes.

Complete AV septal defect: Congenital cardiovascular Anomalies: Atrioventricular septal defect (complete form) consists of a large ostium primum ASD in the anteroinferior aspect of the septum, an inlet VSD, and a common AV valve orifice. A left-to-right shunt occurs at the atrial and ventricular levels; AV valve regurgitation may be significant, sometimes causing a direct left ventricle-to-right atrial shunt. These abnormalities result in enlargement of all four cardiac chambers. Hemodynamic findings are similar to those of a large VSD. Over time, the increase in pulmonary blood flow, pulmonary artery pressure, and pulmonary vascular resistance may lead to reversal of shunt direction with cyanosis and Eisenmenger's syndrome (see Congenital Cardiovascular Anomalies: Eisenmenger's Syndrome). Partial AV septal defect: A partial defect consists of an ostium primum ASD, partitioning of the common AV valve into 2 separate AV orifices, and a cleft in the mitral valve (left AV orifice). The ventricular septum is intact, or there may be a small VSD. Hemodynamic abnormalities are similar to those of ostium secundum ASD with the additional finding of variable degrees of mitral regurgitation (Figs 14.34 and 14.35).

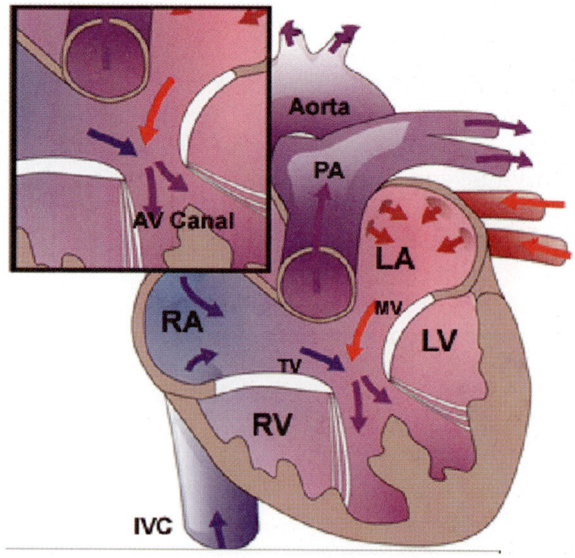

Fig. 14.33: *Disturbed anatomy and circulation in atrioventicular septal defect*

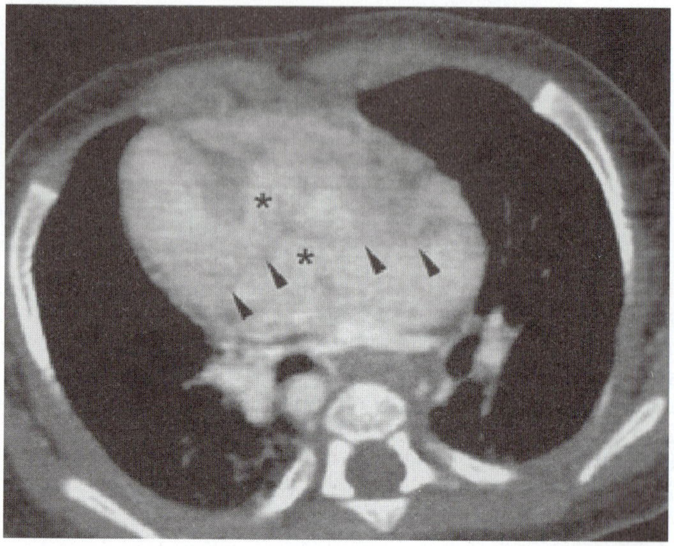

Fig. 14.34: *Atrioventricular septal defect. CT scan shows an atrioventricular septal defect (arrows) and a free-floating common atrioventricular valve with a bridging leaflet (arrow heads) that involves the adjacent atrial and ventricular septa as well as the atrioventricular septum. Dextrocardia and a right descending aorta are also noted*

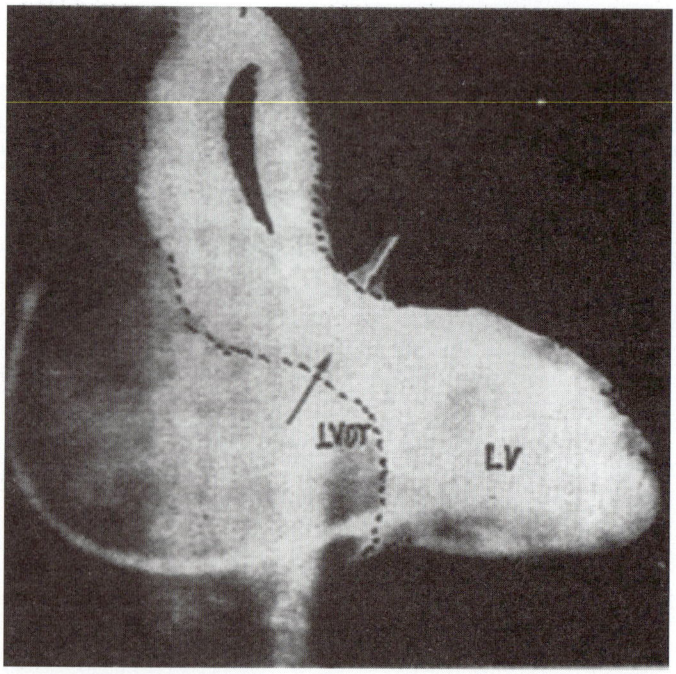

Fig. 14.35: *Cine-angiocardiography showing goose neck deformity of LVOT in patient with septum primum defect*

Symptoms and Signs

Complete AV septal defect with a large left-to-right shunt causes signs of heart failure (HF)—e.g. tachypnea, dyspnea with feeding, poor weight gain, diaphoresis) by age 4–6 week. Pulmonary vascular obstructive disease (Eisenmenger's syndrome) is usually a late complication but may occur earlier, especially in children with Down syndrome.

Partial AV septal defects are asymptomatic during childhood if mitral regurgitation is mild or absent. However, symptoms (e.g. exercise intolerance, fatigue, palpitations) may develop during adolescence or early adulthood. Infants with moderate or severe mitral regurgitation often have signs of HF.

Physical examination in children with complete AV septal defects shows an active precordium due to volume and pressure overload of the right ventricle; a single, loud 2nd heart sound (S2) due to pulmonary hypertension; a grade 3 to 4 of 6 systolic murmur; and sometimes a diastolic murmur at the apex and low left sternal border. Most children with a partial defect have wide splitting of the S2 and a midsystolic (e.g. ejection systolic) murmur audible at the upper left sternal border. A mid-diastolic rumble may be present at the lower left sternal border when the atrial shunt is large. A cleft in the left AV valve results in a blowing apical systolic murmur of mitral regurgitation. Thus, cardiac findings in children with the partial form are the same as those described for secundum ASD; if mitral regurgitation coexists, there will also be a high-pitched holosystolic murmur at the apex.

Diagnosis

Diagnosis is suggested by clinical examination, supported by chest X-ray and ECG, and established by two dimensional echocardiography with color flow and Doppler studies (Fig. 14.34).

Chest X-ray: Chest X-ray shows cardiomegaly with right atrial enlargement, biventricular enlargement, a prominent main pulmonary artery segment, and increased pulmonary vascular markings.

Electrocardiography (ECG) (Figs 14.36 and 14.37)

ECG shows a superiorly directed QRS axis (e.g. left-axis deviation or northwest axis), frequent 1st-degree AV block, left or right ventricular hypertrophy or both, and occasional right atrial enlargement and right bundle-branch block.

Echocardiography: Two dimensional echocardiography with color flow and Doppler studies establishes the diagnosis and can provide important anatomic and hemodynamic information. Cardiac catheterization is not usually necessary unless hemodynamics must be further characterized before surgical repair (Figs 14.38 to 14.48).

Cardiac catheterization and cineangiography: It is done rarely as most of the information can be obtained with 2-D color doppler and transesopageal echocardiography (Fig. 14.35).

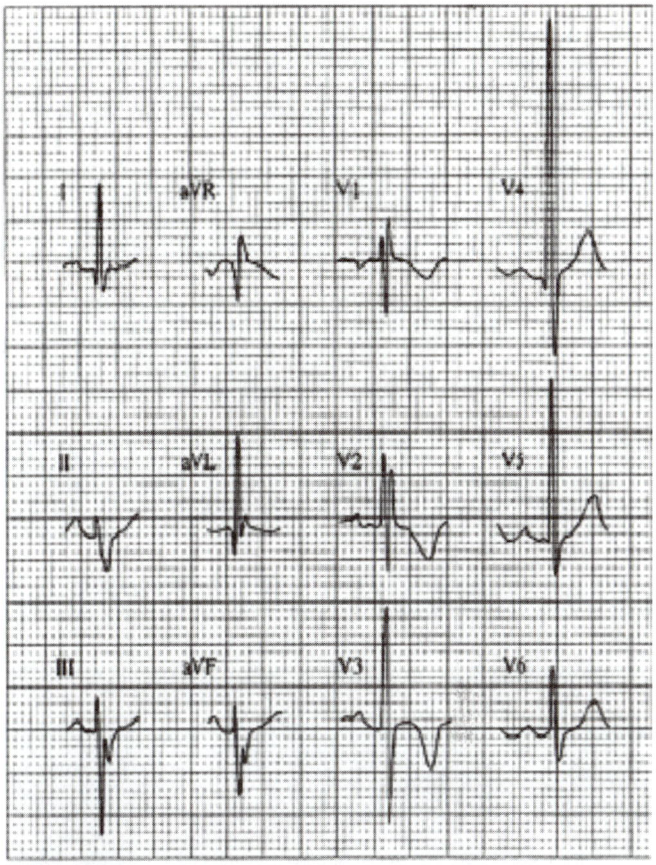

Fig. 14.36: *ECG trace in primum atrial septal defect: note the left-axis deviation (superior axis)*

Surgical Interventions

Treatment for a complete atrioventricular septal defect is surgical.

Single-stage complete repair is currently preferred, but occasional cases of refractory CHF in a low-birth-weight infant may be palliated with the placement of a pulmonary artery band.

Some patients with complete atrioventricular septal defect have additional muscular VSDs. Banding of the pulmonary artery may alleviate their CHF for 6–12 months, during which time the VSDs may spontaneously close and thus simplify eventual complete repair.

The surgical mortality rate should be low. In a published review of surgical outcomes of 363 patients with atrioventricular septal defects who were treated between 1982 and 1995, the early mortality rate was 10.3%, and the 10-year survival rate was 83%.

The Pediatric Heart Network Investigators recently published a multicenter observational study on the contemporary results after repair of complete atrioventricular septal defect. In this series of 120 children, in-hospital and 6-month mortality rates were 2.5% and 4%, respectively. The incidence of residual septal defects and the degree of left atrioventricular valve regurgitation was independent of repair type, presence of trisomy 21, and

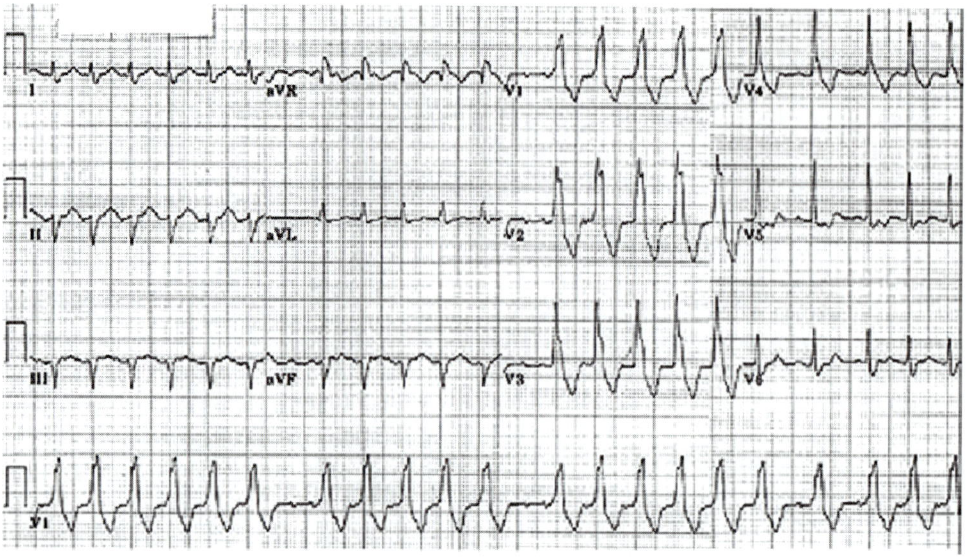

Fig. 14.37: *ECG trace showing RBBB with left posterior fascicular block, QRS duration = 0.12 s. (2) A secondary R wave in V1. (3) Mean QRS axis is more positive than +90° in a patient with congenital endocardial cushion defect*

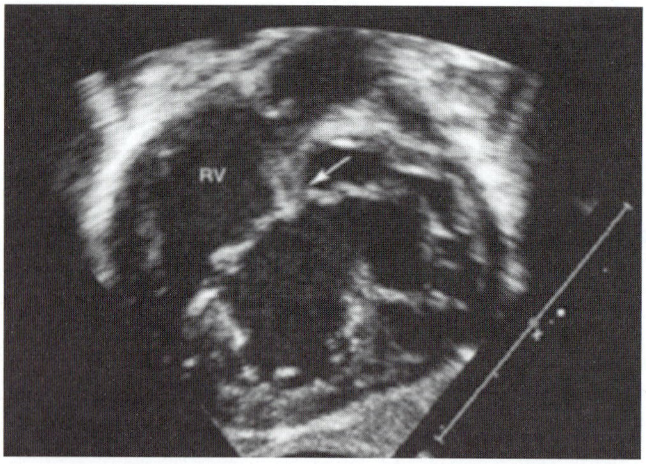

Fig. 14.38: *En-face echocardiogram view of complete common atrioventricular canal, Rastelli type A. En-face imaging from subxiphoid view shows the multiple leaflets of the common atrioventricular valve; note the attachment of the superior bridging leaflet to the ventricular septum (arrow). RV, right ventricle*

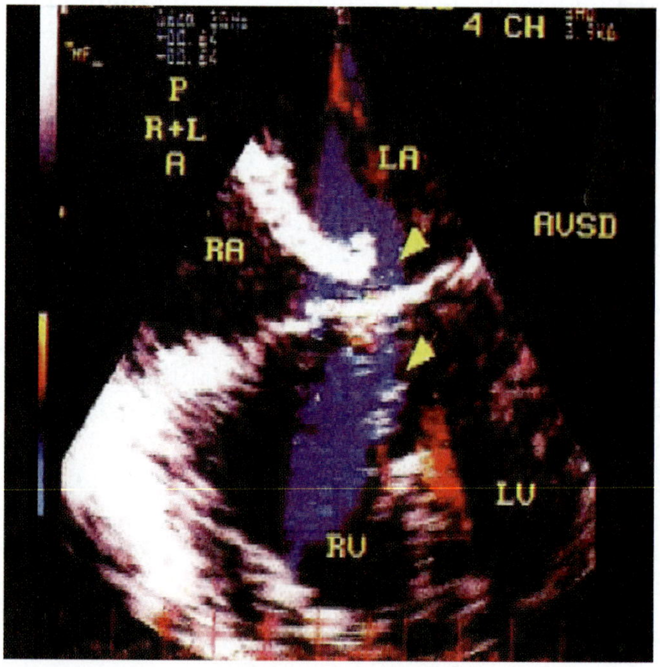

Fig. 14.39: *TEE four chamber view showing atrioventricular defect with blue colored tricuspid regurgitation as a part of AV canal defect*

age of operation although younger age of operation was associated with a longer hospital stay.

Another study, also from the Pediatric Heart Network Investigators, assessed the influence of atrial VSD subtype on outcomes after repair. Preoperatively, transitional patients showed the highest prevalence of moderate or severe left atrioventricular valve regurgitation (LAVVR). In data obtained 1 and 6 months post AVSD repair, the results noted that complete atrial VSD and canal-type VSD patients showed the highest prevalence of trisomy 21 and were younger, had lower weight-for-age z scores, and had more associated cardiac defects. Annuloplasty was similar among all subtypes while complete atrial VSD showed a longer duration of ventilation and hospitalization. At 6 months, weight-for-age z scores improved and improvement was similar in all subtypes.

A pulmonary artery band, placed on the main pulmonary artery by means of a small lateral or anterior thoracotomy incision, obviates cardiopulmonary bypass in a premature neonate or small infant. However, it has the risks of distorting the origins of the branch pulmonary arteries if it migrates and of complicating the eventual definitive surgery if it erodes through the media and intima. Pulmonary artery banding is best used, when deemed necessary, for only a few months in a patient who then undergo complete intracardiac repair and pulmonary artery band takedown.

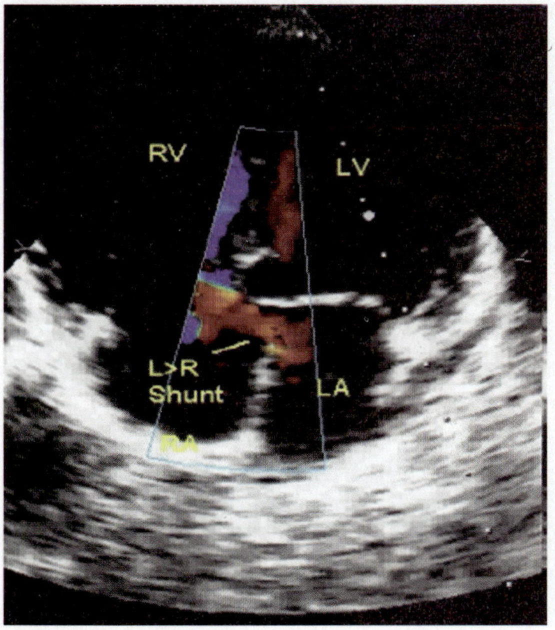

Fig. 14.40: *Color Doppler echocardiogram showing left to right shunt in ostium primum ASD*

A major aspect of atrioventricular septal defect repair involves creating a competent mitral valve. A pericardial patch can be used for this augmentation and for tricuspid valve repair. Repair is occasionally done with two patches: (1) a pericardial patch for the atrial septal defect and (2) a polytetrafluoroethylene patch for the VSD, with routine

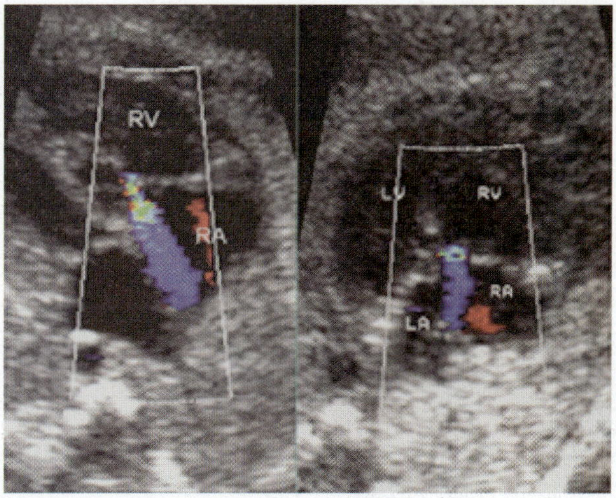

Fig. 14.41: *Fetal color Doppler ultrasonography demonstrating tricuspid regurgitation (blue color) in atroventricular septal defect*

closure of the mitral valve cleft. The two-patch technique with routine cleft closure and atrial septal incision may lower the incidence of residual mitral regurgitation.

Ten Harkel et al reported intermediate follow-up results in patients who underwent surgical repair of atrioventricular septal defects. During a mean follow-up of 66 months, 19% had severe mitral valve regurgitation, and 9% required reoperation. Of note, 13% of patients with severe mitral valve regurgitation in the immediate postoperative period had significantly improved mitral

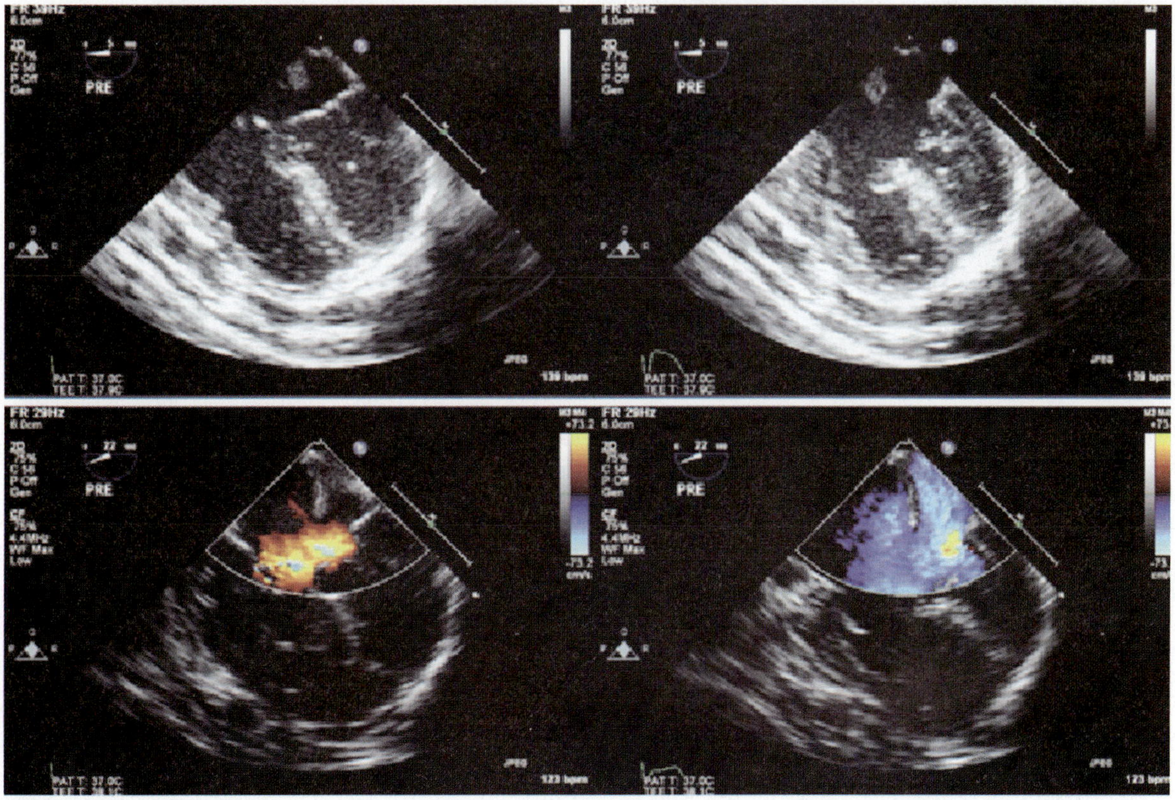

Fig. 14.42: *Color Doppler echocardiography demonstrating in atroventricular septtal defect before repair*

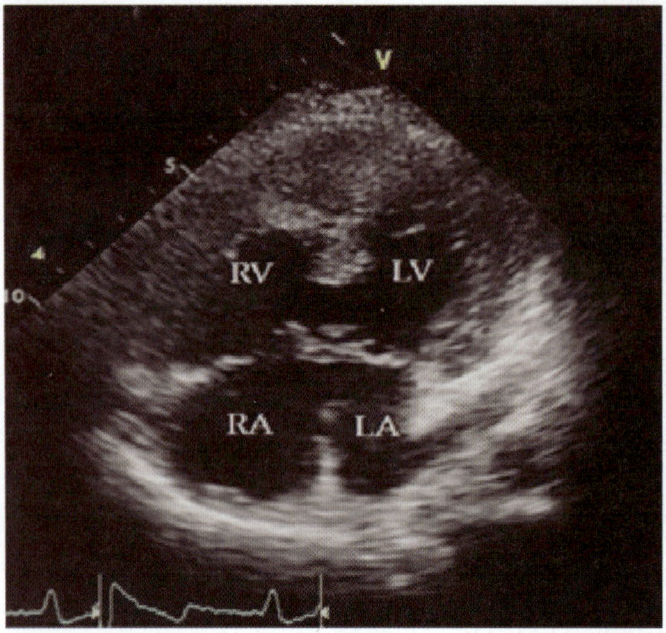

Fig. 14.43: *Apical four chamber image of an inlet ventricular septal defect and an ostium primum atrial septal defect (complete AV canal defect). The ventricular septal defect (VSD) is situated more inferiorly than the typical position of a perimembranous VSD*

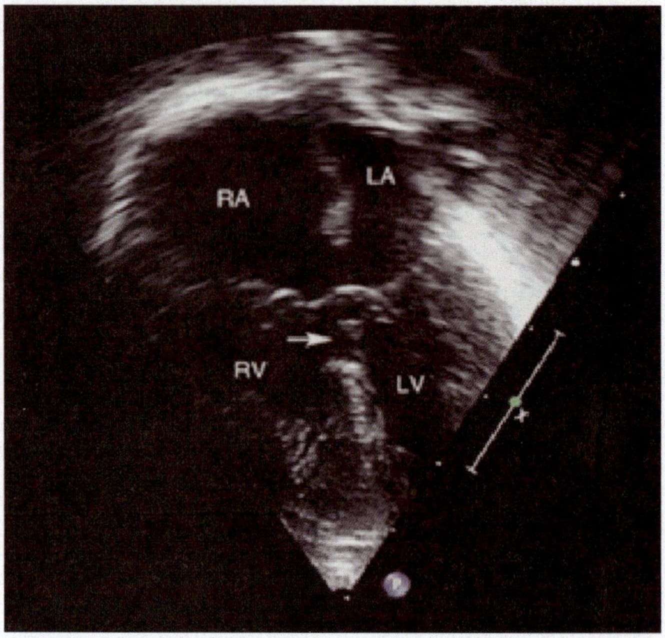

Fig. 14.44: *Apical four chamber echocardiogram view of complete common atrioventricular canal, Rastelli type A. Note the large deficiency of both atrial and ventricular septa as well as the single common atrioventricular valve. The arrow points to the attachment of the superior bridging leaflet to the ventricular septal crest. LA, left atrium; LV, left ventricle; RA, right atrium; RV, right ventricle*

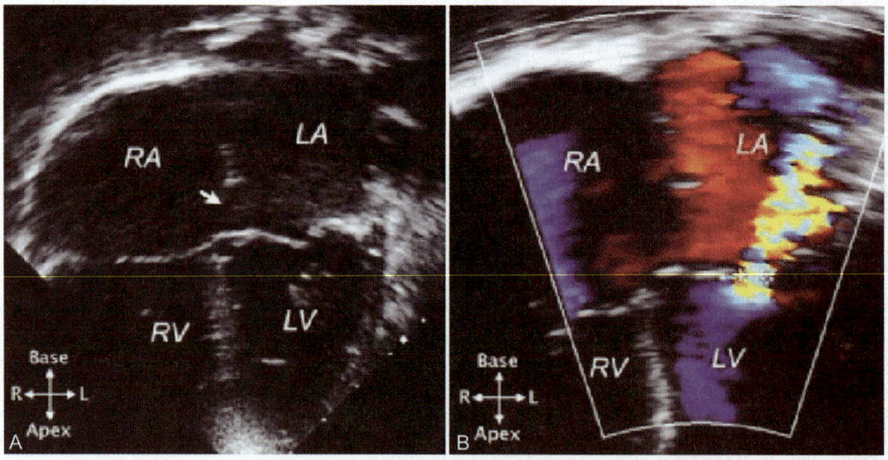

Fig. 14.45A and B: *(A) An echocardiogram in apical four chamber view in a patient with ASD1 (arrow). The defect is just above the closure plane of the AV valves. (B) Color Doppler examination in the same view showing mitral regurgitation (++), most likely through the cleft in the anterior mitral leaflet. LA, left atrium; LV, left ventricle; RA, right atrium; RV, right ventricle. (Reprinted from Valente et al. with permission)*

valve function. For this reason, the authors cautioned against reoperation in the early postoperative period unless it is absolutely necessary.

Additional aspects of complete repair of common atrioventricular canal may include relief of associated left ventricular outflow tract (LVOT) obstruction, patent ductus arteriosus (PDA) ligation, removal of a previously placed pulmonary artery band, repair of stenosis of a pulmonary arterial branch, or relief of aortic arch obstruction. Recent data suggest that children with atrioventricular septal defects and Down syndrome have a prognosis better than that of children with the same cardiac lesion but not Down syndrome.

Residual atrioventricular valve insufficiency or stenosis is a major determinant of long-term outcome.

Total circular annuloplasty is a simple procedure to help reduce atrioventricular valve regurgitation although most patients with severe atrioventricular valve insufficiency or stenosis require more complex mitral valvuloplasty techniques. The need for mitral valve replacement is not

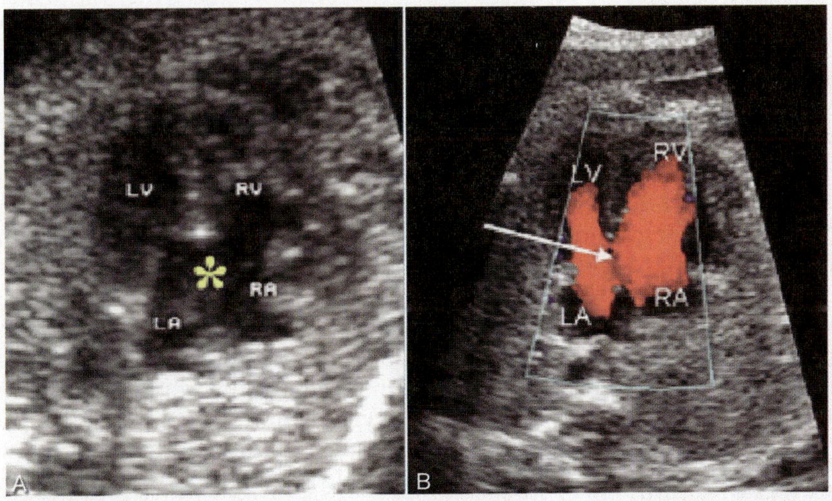

Fig. 14.46A and B: *Four chamber view in a fetus with Down syndrome demonstrating a complete atrioventricular septal defect (AV canal). The defect (*) can be recognized during diastole when the valves are patent but is better assessed using color Doppler, which demonstrates the interatrial and interventricular connection during diastole (H-shape).*

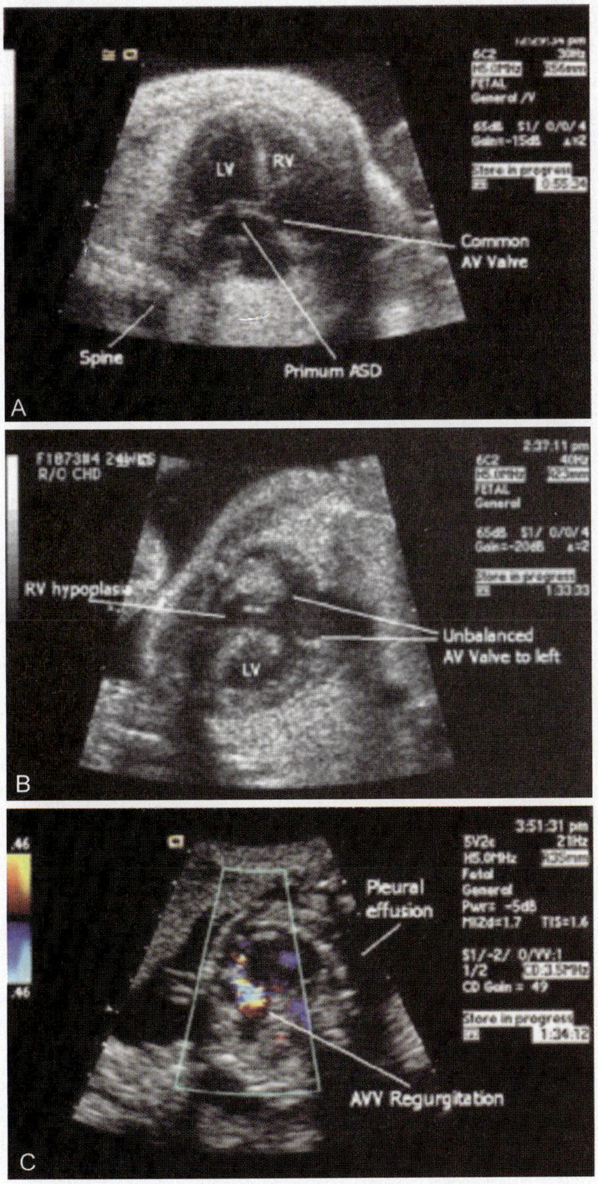

Fig 14.47: *(A) Two dimensional fetal echocardiographic image of a four chamber view of the heart demonstrating a balanced complete common atrioventricular canal defect with a large primum atrial septal defect (ASD) and a common atrioventricular (AV) valve. RV, right ventricle; LV, left ventricle. (B) Four chamber view of the heart demonstrating an unbalanced complete common atrioventricular canal defect to the left with associated right ventricular (RV) hypoplasia. (C) Four chamber view of the heart with color Doppler demonstrating common atrioventricular valve (AVV) regurgitation. The canal defect is severely unbalanced with common atrium and pleural effusions indicating hydrops fetalis. This fetus also had complete heart block*

rare over the course of long-term follow-up but is ideally delayed until an adult-size prosthetic valve can be implanted.

Atrioventricular septal defect may be associated with other surgical conditions including subaortic stenosis, coarctation of the aorta, tetralogy of Fallot (TOF), and total anomalous pulmonary venous return. Each associated lesion may complicate complete repair and make it difficult to achieve a good hemodynamic result. In addition, these defects may add potential risk over follow-up (e.g. recoarctation after coarctation of the aorta repair or pulmonary insufficiency after repair of TOF).

Surgically induced atrioventricular block is a known complication of atrioventricular septal defect repair. Permanent pacing is required if atrioventricular conduction does not return postoperatively.

For complex cardiac lesions involving an unbalanced atrioventricular septal defect, total cavopulmonary connection, otherwise known as a Fontan operation, may be indicated.

In the presence of TOF, an aortic monocusp is used to compensate for deficient right atrioventricular valve tissue. Right-dominant, unbalanced biventricular repair can be successfully completed in patients with mild LV hypoplasia. However, careful preoperative evaluation of the adequacy of the LV to support the systemic circulation is imperative.

De Oliveira et al reported their experience with two-ventricular repair of patients with unbalanced atrioventricular septal defect and small right ventricles (RVs). Patients with a small RV had a high mortality rate, with an 87% 10-year survival, compared with a 100% survival rate in surgical patients with balanced atrioventricular septal defect. Although a median sternotomy is the usual surgical approach, the thoracotomy approach was safely used for common atrioventricular canal repair in some centers.

Medical Management

In heart failure medical therapy with diuretics, digoxin and ACE inhibitors should be started before surgery.

Complete AV septal defect should be repaired by age 2–4 months, because most infants have HF and failure to thrive. However, even if infants are growing well without significant symptoms, repair should be done before 6 mo to prevent development of pulmonary vascular disease, especially in infants with Down syndrome. In patients with two adequately sized ventricles and no additional defects, the large central defect (combination of the primum ASD and inlet VSD) is closed and the common AV valve is reconstructed into two separate valves. For a single-stage complete repair, mortality rate was 5–10% in older series but more recently was as low as 3–4%. Surgical complications include complete heart block (3%) and mitral regurgitation. Pulmonary artery banding is no longer recommended unless associated abnormalities make complete repair in a small infant high risk. For asymptomatic patients with a partial defect, elective surgery is done at age 1–3 years. Surgical mortality rate should be very low.

For patients with large shunts and HF, diuretics, digoxin, and ACE inhibitors are indicated before surgery.

Endocarditis prophylaxis is not needed preoperatively and is required only for the first 6 months after repair or if there is a residual defect adjacent to a surgical patch.

VENTRICULAR SEPTAL DEFECT

Definition, Classification and Pathophysiology

A VSD is a communication
1. Superior to the crista supraventricularis
2. Inferior to the crista supraventricularis
3. Below the septal tricuspid leaflet
4. There may be multiple muscular defects.

The majority of defects are para membranous. The small VSD (less than 0.5 cm^2/m^2) usually produces no hemodynamic changes but may predispose to endocarditis. The moderate VSD (0.5–1.0 cm^2/m^2) results in mild to moderate pulmonary hypertension and moderate elevation of right ventncular pressure. The large VSD (greater than 1.0 cm^2/m^2) results in no resistance to flow, is similar to a common ventricle, and may result in heart failure in early infancy while the survivors usually develop pulmonary hypertension. Aortic regurgitation may result from prolapse of an aortic leaflet into the VSD (Figs 14.48 and 14.49).

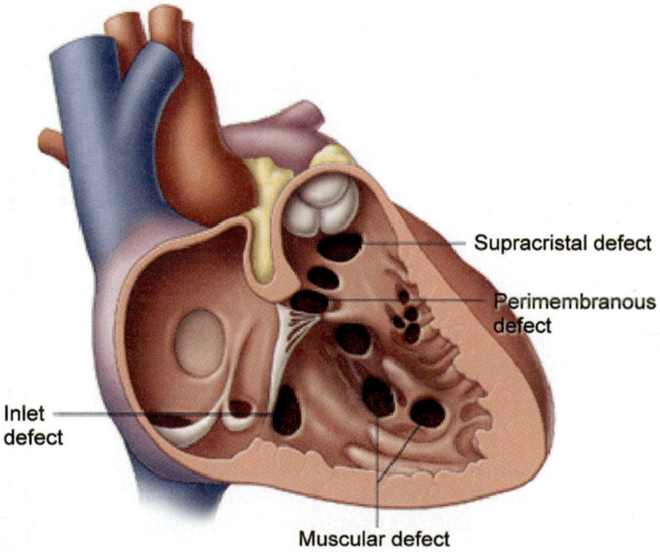

Fig. 14.49: *Depicts the inlet, muscular, perimembranous, and supracristal types of ventricular septal defect*

Clinical Manifestations

History

A small VSD is usually asymptomatic. A moderate to large VSD can be associated with fatigue or effort intolerance. Patients may not seek medical help unless complications (right ventricular outflow tract obstruction, aortic regurgitation, endocarditis, or Eisenmenger's reaction) develop, and most of these are identified on routine physical examination.

Physical Examination

The VSD is usually recognized by a harsh holosystolic murmur localized at the left sternal border which may be associated with a thrill. Moderate to large defects may be associated with a diastolic rumble at the cardiac apex. A few patients will have a murmur of aortic regurgitation due to a poorly supported aortic valve. The murmur may disappear if the VSD closes spontaneously.

The murmur of the VSD may decrease if right ventricular outflow obstruction or pulmonary hypertension develops, decreasing the left-to-right shunt.

If advanced pulmonary vascular disease develops (i.e. Eisenmenger's syndrome), cyanosis, clubbing, and the signs of pulmonary hypertension and right ventricular hypertrophy appear.

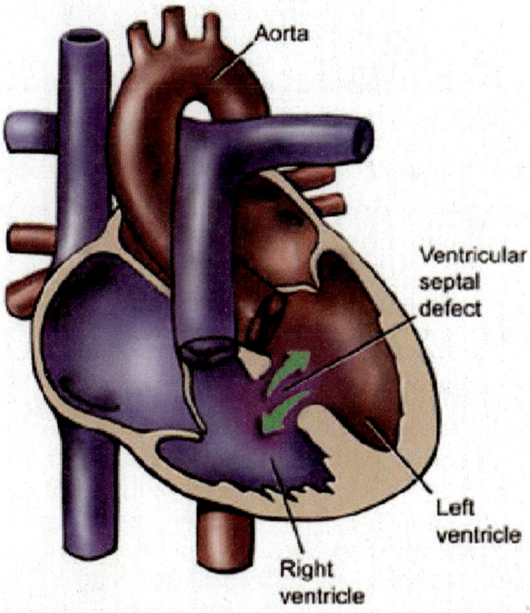

Fig. 14.48: *Common type of interventricular septal defect*

Diagnostic Tests

Chest X-ray (Fig. 14.50)

The chest film is usually normal in the presence of a small VSD. A large VSD is associated with increased pulmonary

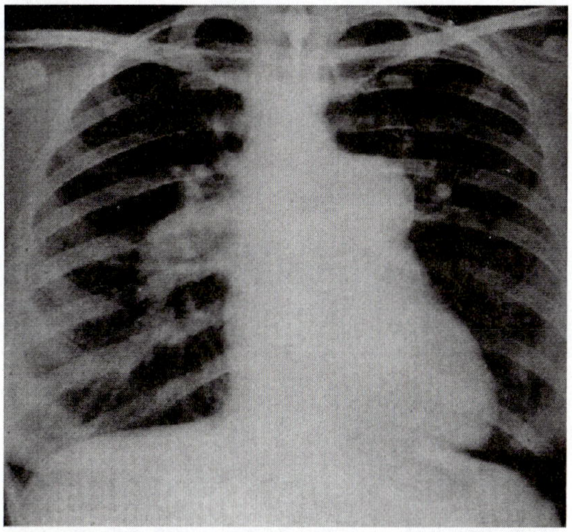

Fig. 14.50: *Photograph of X-ray chest PA view showing prominant pulmonary conus, dilated right pulmonary artery and diffuse congestion in the lungs with boderline cardiomegaly in patient with moderate L-R shunt of VSD*

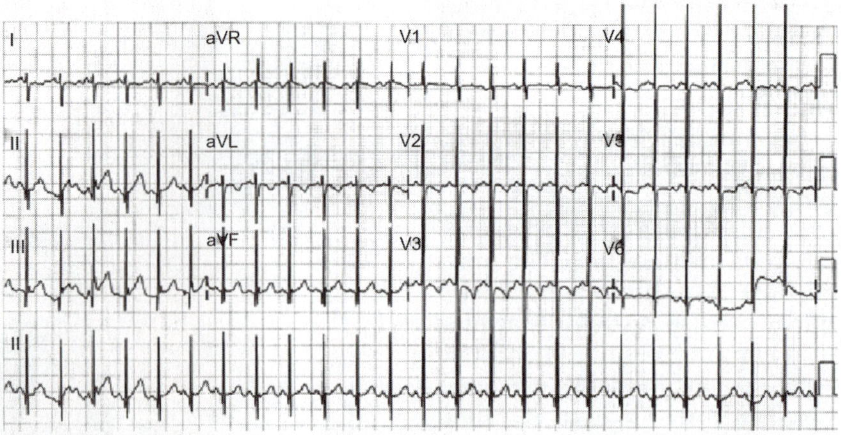

Fig. 14.51: *ECG trace in VSD showing. Katz-Wachtel sign having tall diphasic RS complexes at least 50 mm in height in lead V2, V3 or V4 with mid-precordial leads. The sign has been described in ventricular septal defect with biventricular hypertrophy in children. It can be seen with isolated ventricular septal defect as well as in complex ventricular septal defect*

flow until pulmonary vascular obstructive disease develops after which cephalization of flow develops with dilated proximal and "pruned" peripheral pulmonary arteries. The left atrium and ventricle may be enlarged.

Electrocardiogram (Fig. 14.51)

The ECG is normal in patients with a small VSD. With a large VSD, left atrial abnormality and left ventricular hypertrophy may develop. The development of evidence of combined ventricular hypertrophy or right-axis deviation suggests the presence of pulmonary hypertension or pulmonary outflow tract obstruction.

Differential Diagnosis

A VSD must be differentiated from ASD, patent ductus arteriosus and pulmonary stenosis.

Echocardiogram (Figs 14.52 to 14.59)

The echocardiogram may be useful in evaluating left atrial and left ventricular dilatation. It may visualize the site and size of the VSD, particularly with larger defects, and it may aid in ruling out other congenital heart defects.

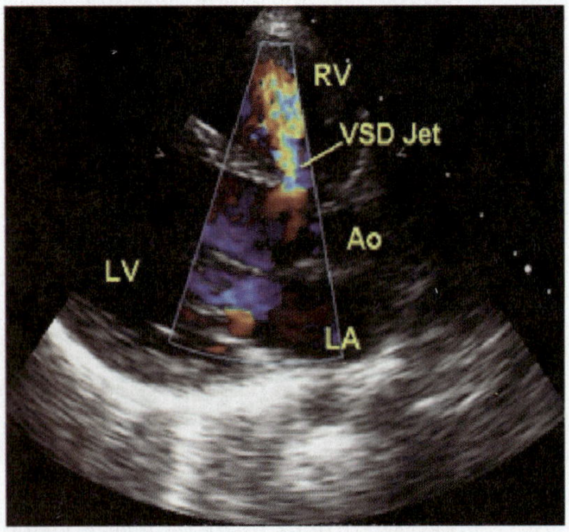

Fig. 14.52: *VSD jet visualized by color flow mapping (color Doppler)*

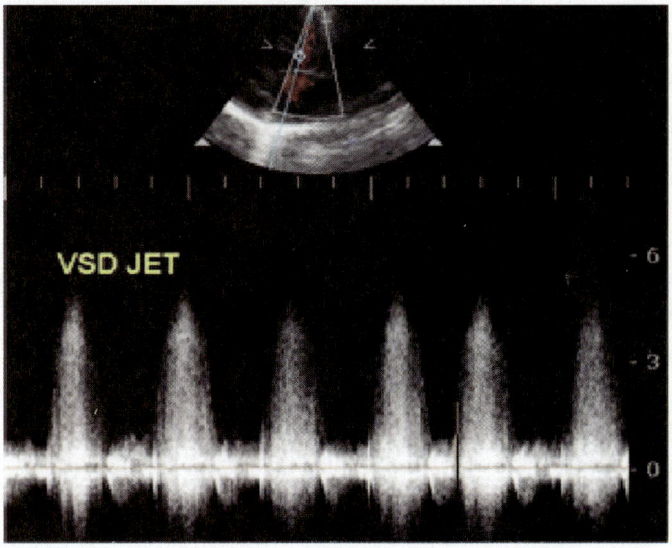

Fig. 14.53: *Continuous wave Doppler showing VSD jet*

Cardiac Catheterization (Figs 14.55 and 14.56)

Cardiac catheterization is useful to confirm the presence and magnitude and direction of shunting. Ventriculography confirms the precise location.

In addition, catheterization is essential to establish the state of pulmonary vascular resistance.

Natural History and Prognosis

A small VSD poses little risk other than the possibility of endocarditis. Small defects may close, usually in childhood. The large VSD usually causes heart failure in infancy, but may not cause heart failure in patients reaching older ages. The prognosis of the patient with irreversible pulmonary obstructive disease is poor. Complications of VSD include aortic regurgitation, endocarditis, and pneumonia, and with large defects, right ventricular outflow tract

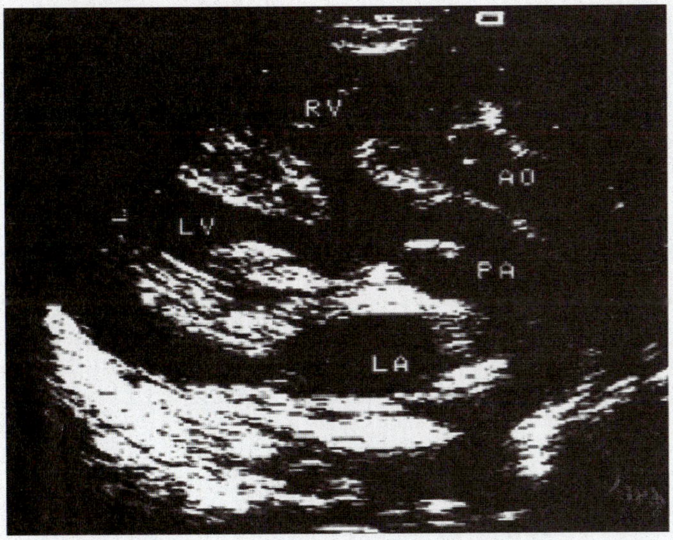

Fig. 14.54: *Two dimensional LAX view showing subaortic VSD (asterex)*

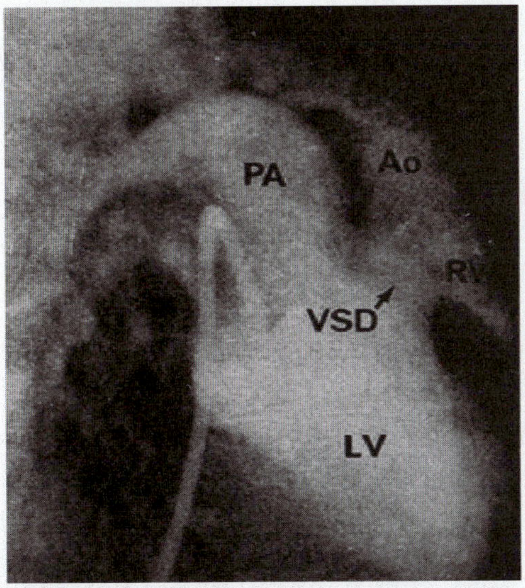

Fig. 14.55: *Cineangiography showing supracristal ventricular septal defect (arrow)*

obstruction, pulmonary hypertension, and eventually irreversible pulmonary vascular obstructive disease.

Management Approach

Children with small VSDs are asymptomatic and have an excellent long-term prognosis. Neither medical therapy nor surgical therapy is indicated. Prophylactic antibiotic prophylaxis against endocarditis is no longer indicated. For more information, see Antibiotic Prophylactic Regimens for Endocarditis. Maintenance of good oral hygiene is of paramount importance in reducing the risk of endocarditis.

In children with moderate or large VSDs, a trial of medical therapy is indicated to manage symptomatic CHF because many VSDs may become smaller with time.

Uncontrolled CHF with growth failure and recurrent respiratory infection is an indication for surgical repair.

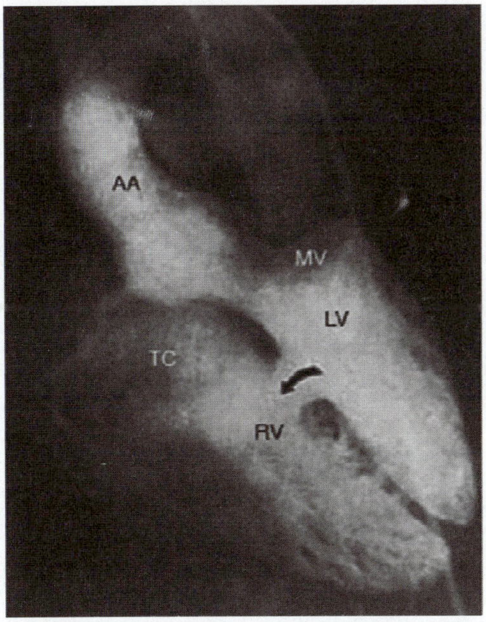

Fig. 14.56: *Multiple trabecular ventricular septal defects (VSDs). Retrograde left ventriculogram, four-chamber projection, profiles the mitral and tricuspid valves, and the midtrabecular VSD (arrow). Additional VSDs closer to the apex are more anterior in location and are not profiled in this projection. AA, ascending aorta; LV, left ventricle; MV, mitral valve; RV, right ventricle; TV, tricuspid valve. (Reproduced with permission from Lock JE, Keane JF, Perry SB).*

Neither the age nor the size of the patient is prohibitive in considering surgery. Large, asymptomatic defects associated with elevated pulmonary artery (PA) pressure are often repaired when infants are younger than 1 year, typically around age 6 years. Surgical repair is indicated in older asymptomatic children with a normal pulmonary pressure if the pulmonary-to-systemic flow ratio (Qp:Qs) is greater than 2:1.

Prolapse of an aortic valve cusp is an indication for surgery even if the VSD is small. Early repair may prevent progression of the aortic insufficiency.

Elevated pulmonary resistance may be maintained in some patients despite therapy directed at the VSD and may, in fact, represent a primary disease of the pulmonary vessels.

Medical Management of Symptomatic CHF

Therapies used to manage symptomatic CHF in children with moderate or large VSDs may include the following:

- Increased caloric density of feedings to ensure adequate weight gain. Occasionally, oral feeds must be supplemented with tube feeds because a baby in CHF may be unable to consume adequate calories for appropriate weight gain.
- Diuretics (e.g. furosemide) to relieve pulmonary congestion—furosemide is usually given in a dosage of 1–3 mg/kg/d divided in two or three doses; long-term furosemide treatment results in hypercalcemia and renal damage and electrolyte disturbances

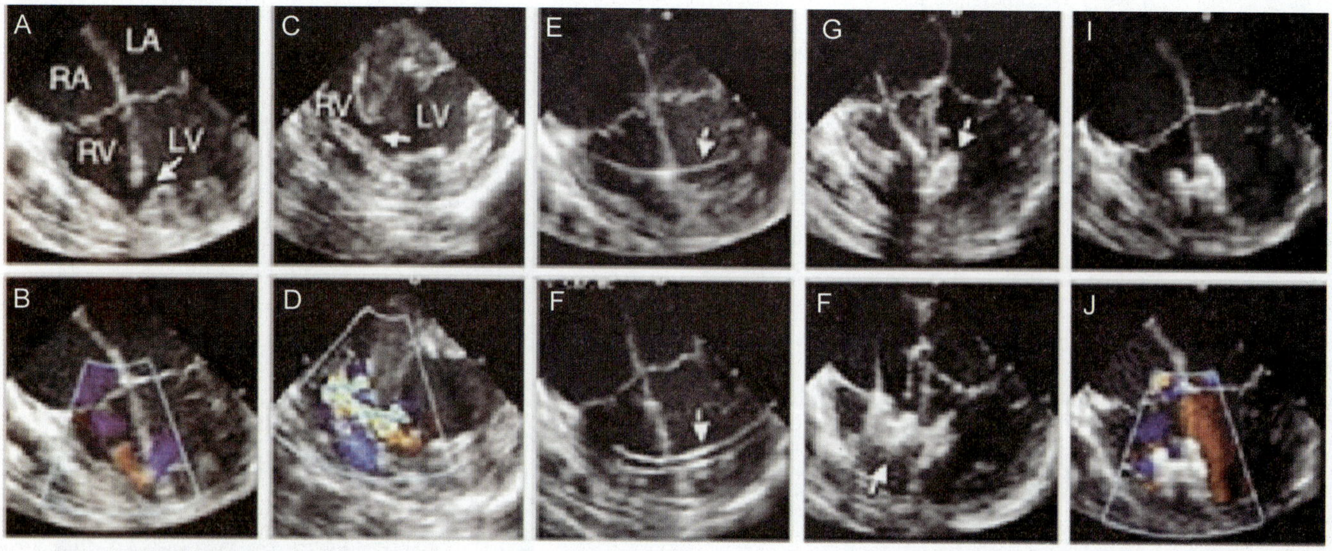

Fig. 14.57: *Transesophageal echocardiographic (TEE) images of muscular ventricular septal defect closure with an Amplatzer muscular VSD device. (A) Apical four chamber view of a muscular VSD; (B) Color Doppler flow across the VSD; (C) The muscular VSD in the short-axis view; (D) Color Doppler flow across the muscular VSD in the short-axis view; (E) Wire across the VSD; (F) Sheath across the VSD; (G) The left ventricular disc is deployed in the left ventricle; (H) The right ventricular disc is deployed in the right ventricle; (I) The device is released from the delivery cable; (J) There is no residual shunt across the VSD by color Doppler. RA, Right atrium; RV, Right ventricle; LA, left atrium; LV, left ventricle*

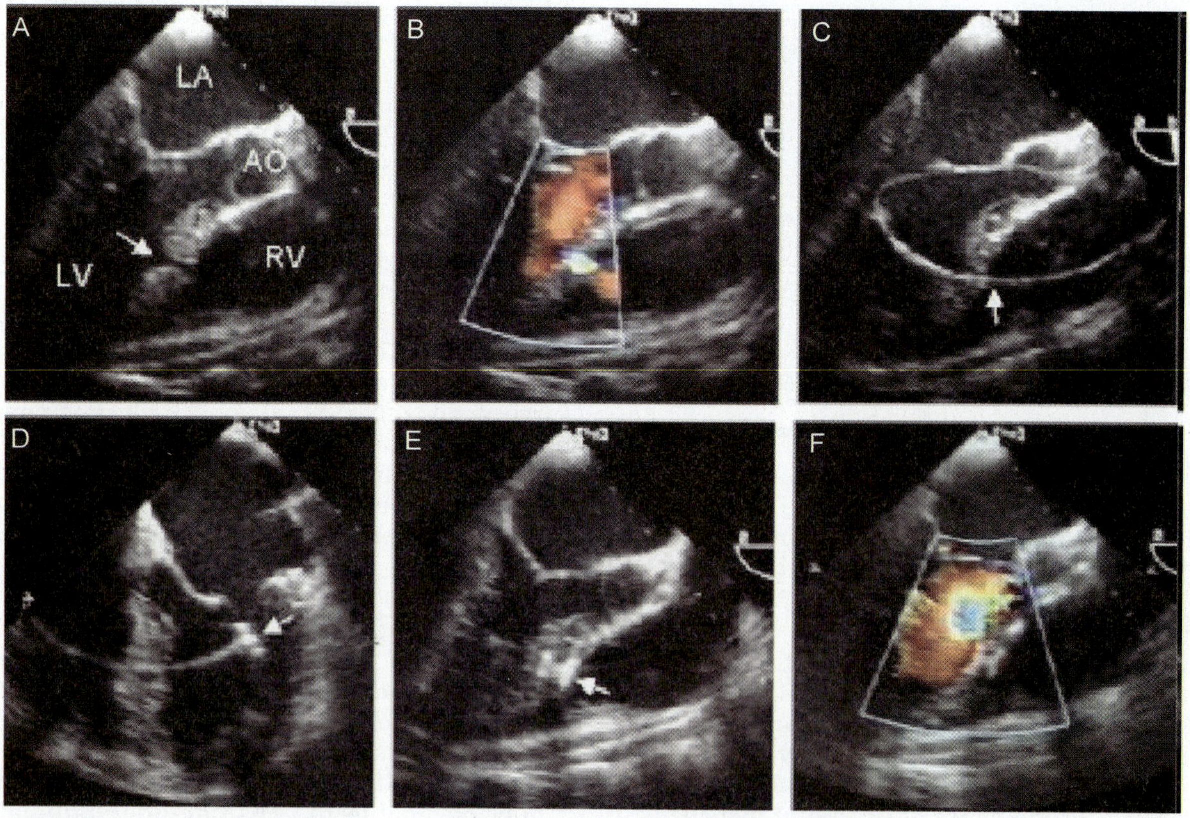

Fig. 14.58: *TEE images in a 15-year-old male patient with a 4.5-mm mid-muscular VSD and a Qp/Qs ratio of 1.5. (A and B) Left ventricular long axis view without (A) and with color Doppler (B) showing the muscular VSD (arrow); C, TEE image in the long-axis view demonstrating passage of the delivery sheath from the right to the left ventricle through the VSD. D, TEE image in the four chamber view during deployment of the LV disk (arrow). E and F, TEE images without (E) and with color Doppler (F) after a 6-mm Amplatzer MVSD device (arrow) has been deployed demonstrating good device position and no residual shunt. AO, aorta, LA, left atrium; LV, left ventricle; RV, right ventricle*

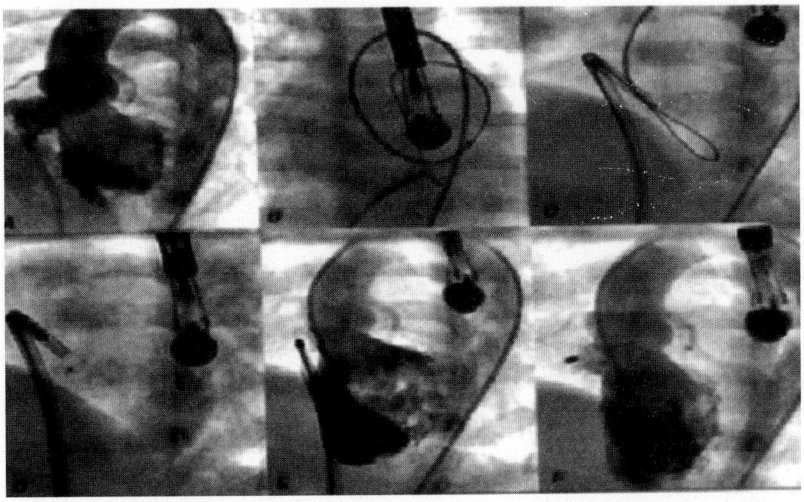

Fig. 14.59: *Different steps in closure of perimembranous ventricular septal defect with asymmtrical amplatzer membranous VSD occluder*

- Angiotensin-converting enzyme (ACE) inhibitors (e.g. captopril and enalapril): These medications reduce both the systemic and pulmonary pressures (the latter to a greater degree), thereby reducing the left-to-right shunt
- Digoxin (5–10 μg/kg/day): This may be indicated if diuresis and afterload reduction do not relieve adequately symptoms.

Intracardiac Repair of Defect

The first operation described for the treatment of a VSD was a palliative one and involved placing a restrictive band across the main PA. This approach was proposed because pulmonary vascular disease as a result of unimpeded flow to the lungs was recognized as a dreaded complication of a VSD. The procedure was popular for about 2 decades because it was associated with low mortality and morbidity.

Surgical Closure

At present, direct surgical repair using cardiopulmonary bypass is the preferred surgical therapy in most centers. PA banding, part of a 2-stage procedure, is largely reserved for critically ill infants with multiple VSDs or for those with associated anomalies. Most perimembranous and inlet VSDs are repaired via a transatrial surgical approach. Defects in the outlet septum are approached through the pulmonary valve. Multiple muscular defects, especially near the apex, pose a difficult problem. Initial pulmonary banding or LV approach through an apical left ventriculotomy and closing the defect with a single patch are the standard techniques.

Short-term results of video-assisted cardioscopy for intraventricular repair of VSD have led to its wide adoption as a means of reducing surgical trauma. Short-term results are excellent.

Transcatheter therapy remains an experimental approach. A hybrid operation is a joint procedure involving the interventional cardiologist and the cardiac surgeon, who concomitantly optimize surgical management of complex CHD. This approach may be used for multiple VSDs where the perimembranous VSD is repaired surgically and the muscular VSDs are closed with a transcatheter device.

Transcatheter Closure (Figs 14.57 to 14.59)

Muscular VSDs have been closed with transcatheter devices for the past 15 years. Perimembranous VSDs though relatively common, can be difficult to close percutaneously. With previous devices (e.g. Rashkind or button devices), attempts to close the VSDs have been unsuccessful, because of the proximity of the defects to the aortic valve and potential aortic valve damage.

The Amplatzer membranous VSD occluder (AGA Medical Corporation; Golden Valley, Minnesota) has undergone phase I trials in the United States. This device is an asymmetric, self-expandable, double-disk unit. Current recommendations are to use this device in older patients who weigh more than 8 kg and who have a subaortic rim of more than 2 mm.

Most procedures are performed with the patient under general anesthesia and with echocardiographic guidance. Reported complications have included aortic and tricuspid regurgitation, device embolization, complete heart block, transient left bundle-branch block (LBBB), hemolysis, small residual shunts and perforation.

In a phase I study, Fu et al reported three adverse events of complete heart block, perihepatic bleeding, and rupture of tricuspid valve chordae tendineae. In a previous article, they reported two cases of transient heart block that responded to high-dose steroids. Subsequent studies found that the Amplatzer membranous VSD occluder resulted in excellent closure rates but had an unacceptably high rate of complete heart block.

Complications

A murmur of a residual VSD is not infrequent. Selective use of intraoperative transesophageal echocardiography

(TEE) to assess closure may be useful. Decisions regarding reoperation are based on symptoms, left heart size, pulmonary pressure, and degree of shunting.

Right bundle branch-block (RBBB) is common and may be caused by ventriculotomy or direct injury to the right bundle itself. Complete heart block can rarely occur and is associated with late mortality. LV dysfunction may occur after left ventriculotomy to close a muscular VSD. Ventricular arrhythmia can be a late problem.

Activity Restriction

Lifestyle changes (i.e. exercise before and after surgery or catheterization) may not be required.

A restrictive VSD with a functional normal heart imposes no exercise limitation. Although patients can safely participate in competitive sports without restriction, adults in this category are uncommon. An important exception is the adult whose moderately restrictive perimembranous VSD decreased in size or closed spontaneously in infancy. However, two dimensional (2D) echocardiography with Doppler interrogation and color flow imaging should be performed to determine whether the defect closed by means of formation of a septal aneurysm.

Unrestricted exercise after surgical closure of a moderate-to-large VSD is permitted if the following criteria are met:

Acceptable Postoperative PA Pressure

Absence of clinically significant disturbances in ventricular rhythm during maximal exercise stress testing and during 24-hour ambulatory electrocardiography 2D echocardiographic evidence of an intact ventricular septum with normalization of LV and left atrial (LA) size and LV function 12-lead scalar ECG revealing little or no evidence of LV volume overload or RV pressure overload.

Long-term Monitoring

After intracardiac repair of a VSD, long-term follow-up is necessary. Even patients with small VSDs require indefinite follow-up. Patients with perimembranous VSDs who have undergone aneurysmal closure have a high incidence of LV-to-RA shunting and a 6% incidence of subaortic ridge, as shown in a large Chinese study. With increasing age, the incidence of aortic leaflet prolapse and aortic insufficiency increases in children with the doubly committed and perimembranous type of VSD.

PATENT DUCTUS ARTERIOSUS

Definition

PDA is an abnormal persistence of the normal fetal connection (ductus arteriosus) between the aorta and the pulmonary artery.

Etiology

The cause of the failure of the ductal wall (medial muscle layer) to constrict in response to PO_2 in the newborn infant's first hours of birth is unknown. Normally, the ductus undergoes complete closure by 2–3 weeks although closure is frequently delayed In premature infants (Figs 14.60 to 14.62).

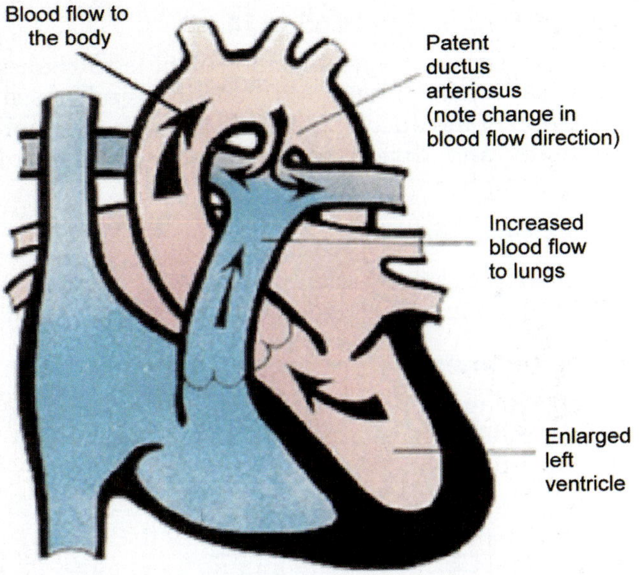

Fig. 14.60: *Anatomical place of PDA in relation to surrounding structures*

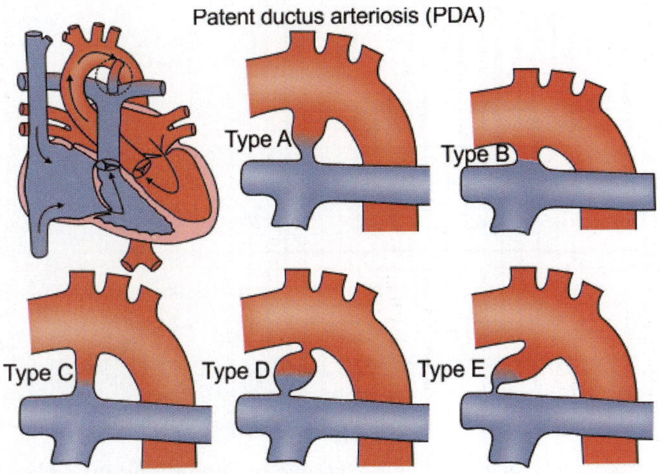

Fig. 14.61: *Anatomy of different types of PDA in relation to surrounding structures*

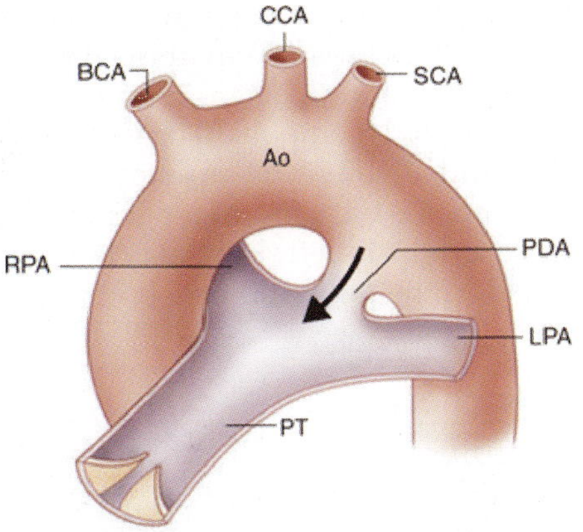

Fig. 14.62: *The anatomy of a patent ductus arteriosus is shown. Note the relation between the position of the ductus, the left subclavian artery, and the pulmonary artery bifurcation. Ao, aorta; BCA, brachiocephalic; CCA, common carotid artery; L, left; PDA, patent ductus arteriosus; PT, pulmonary trunk; RPA, right pulmonary artery; SCA, subclavian artery*

Pathology

There is persistence of the fetal vessel connecting the aorta and the pulmonary artery. Patients with a large ductus may develop severe pulmonary vascular disease.

Clinical Manifestations

History

Females predominate over males by about 3:1. Patients who are born prematurely, who are born at high altitude, or whose mother had rubella during the first trimester of pregnancy are more likely to have a patent ductus. The predominant symptom is breathlessness from pulmonary congestion and CHF. This can become apparent at 1–3 months of age with the normal regression of fetal vascular resistance.

Symptoms of failure may decrease with the redevelopment of increased pulmonary vascular resistance. Later, many patients have no symptoms while others have only minimal fatigue and breathlessness on exertion, even while insidiously developing increased pulmonary vascular disease with Eisenmenger's syndrome and a reversal of the shunt through the ductus. Patients with severe pulmonary vascular disease may develop hemoptysis, extreme fatigue and dyspnea.

Physical Examination

The arterial pulse tends to have an increased pulse pressure. Characteristically, there is a continuous "machinery" murmur that is loudest toward the end of systole and continues through the aortic component of the second heart sound. It is usually loudest in the second and third left intercostal space adjacent to the sternum.

It may be associated with a palpable thrill and a widely split or paradoxically split second heart sound. Some patients may have only a systolic component to the murmur. The apex impulse is usually displaced laterally and is sustained. A diastolic rumble may be heard at the apex. Patients with pulmonary hypertension may have a palpable right ventricular heave along the left sternal border, a loud pulmonic component of a closely split second heart sound, and a diastolic murmur of pulmonary regurgitation. Patients with Eisenmenger's syndrome who have developed a right-to-left shunt may have cyanosis that is more marked in the left hand and both feet than in the right hand.

Differential Diagnoses

- Acute pericarditis
- Aortopulmonary septal defect
- Coarctation of the aorta
- Coronary artery fistula
- Pediatric acute respiratory distress syndrome
- Pediatric sinus of valsalva aneurysm
- Pediatric tachycardia
- Pediatric tetralogy of fallot with absent pulmonary valve
- Pulmonic valvular stenosis
- Sickle cell anemia.

Diagnostic Tests

Chest X-ray (Fig. 14.64)

The chest film may be normal with a small shunt, but with a sizable shunt, there is evidence of enlargement of the aorta, left ventricle, left atrium, and pulmonary artery in association with evidence of increased pulmonary blood flow. Patients with severe pulmonary vascular disease and Eisenmenger's syndrome have a "pruned-tree" appearance of the smaller, peripheral pulmonary arteries.

Electrocardiogram (Fig. 14.63)

The rhythm is usually normal, as is the mean QRS axis. A small percentage (10–20%) of patients have a prolonged PR interval. Almost all patients with a sizable shunt have evidence of left ventricular hypertrophy, and those with significant pulmonary hypertension may have combined ventricular hypertrophy.

Differential Diagnosis

The differential diagnosis includes the normal venous hum, VSD with aortic regurgitation, aorto-pulmonary window, coronary AV fistula, peripheral pulmonary artery stenosis, and anomalous origin of the left coronary artery from the pulmonary artery (LCAPA).

Laboratory Evaluation

Echocardiogram (Figs 14.65 to 14.67)

The echocardiogram shows dilatation of the left atrium and ventricle, a hyperdynamic left ventricle, and possibly visualization of the ductus. It may be possible to establish the patency and direction of shunting by Doppler echocardiography.

Computerized Axial Tomography

It is considered as an exellent noninvasive technique in the diagnosis of many CHDs (Figs 14.68 and 14.69).

Medical Treatment

Prophylaxis against infective endocarditis is very important. Indomethacin (lndocin) may induce closure of a patent ductus in infants.

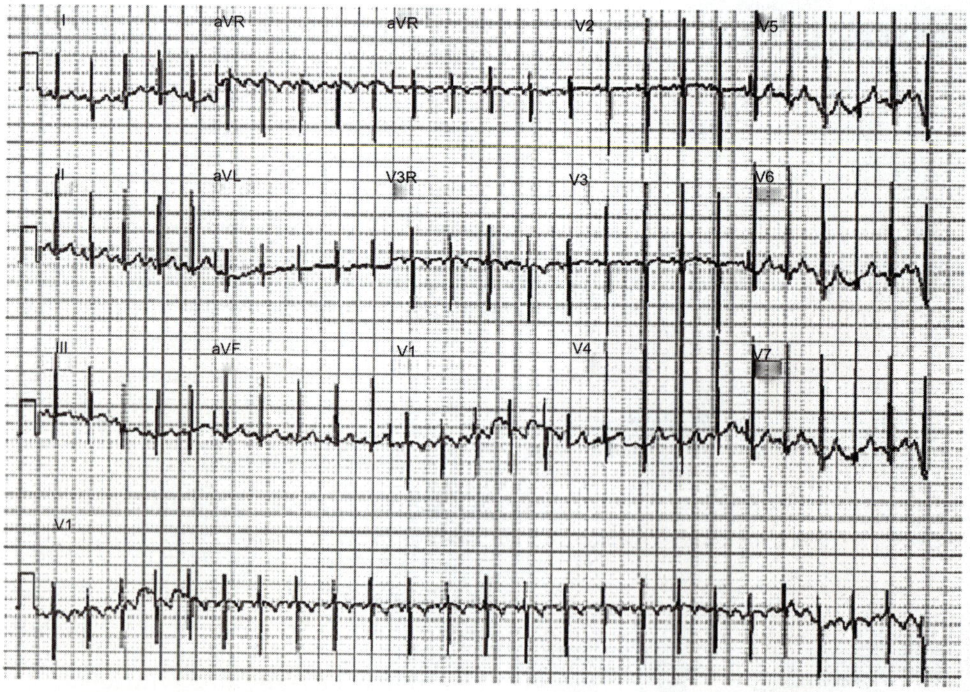

Fig. 14.63: *ECG trace in a 3-month-old infant with large (5 mm) PDA associated with one-half systemic pulmonary artery pressure and left-sided volume overload. The tracing shows left atrial enlargement (biphasic P wave V1) and left ventricular hypertrophy (27 mm R wave V6)*

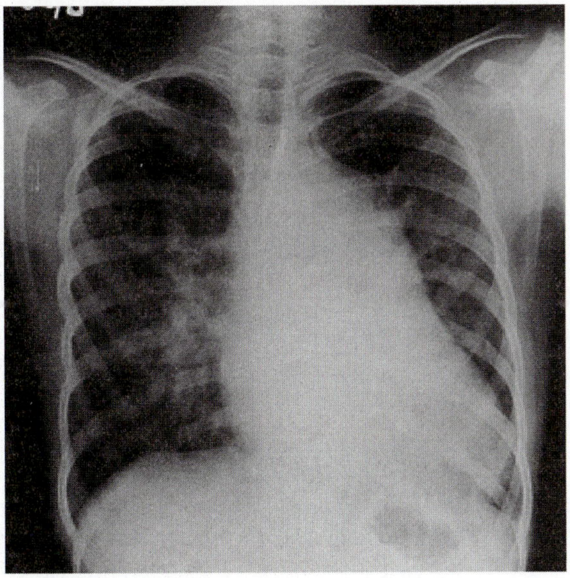

Fig. 14.64: *Patent ductus arteriosus. PA view of the chest shows cardiomegaly with enlargement of the left ventricle and left atrium, dilatation of the main pulmonary artery segment, prominence of the central pulmonary arteries, and overall diffuse increase in pulmonary vascularity. The right ventricle may also show enlargement when pulmonary hypertension is present*

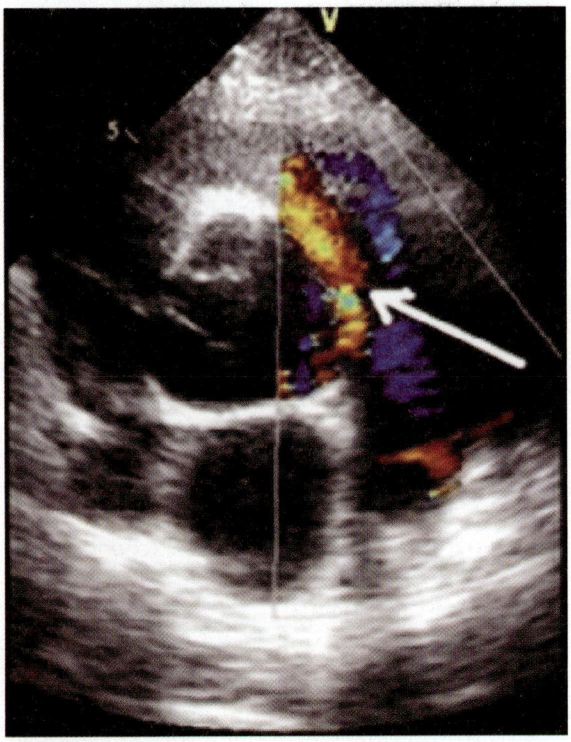

Fig. 14.65: *Transthoracic echocardiography image showing the patent ductus arteriosus (arrow)*

Digitalis and diuretics are useful for the treatment of CHF.

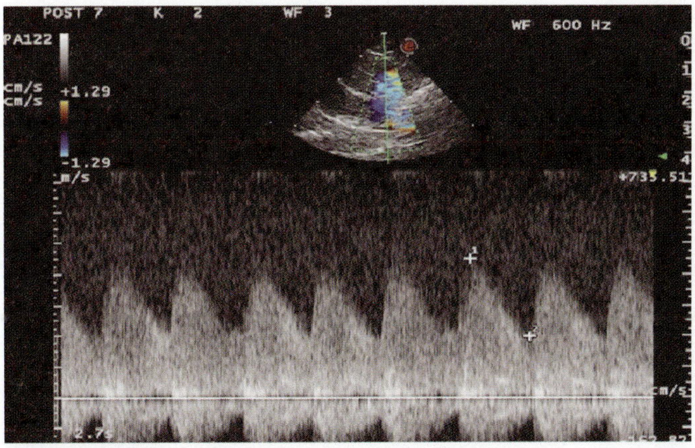

Fig. 14.66: *Patent ductus arteriosus. Color Doppler echo scan (upper) shows contineous blood flow through PDA both during systole and diastole (bottom)*

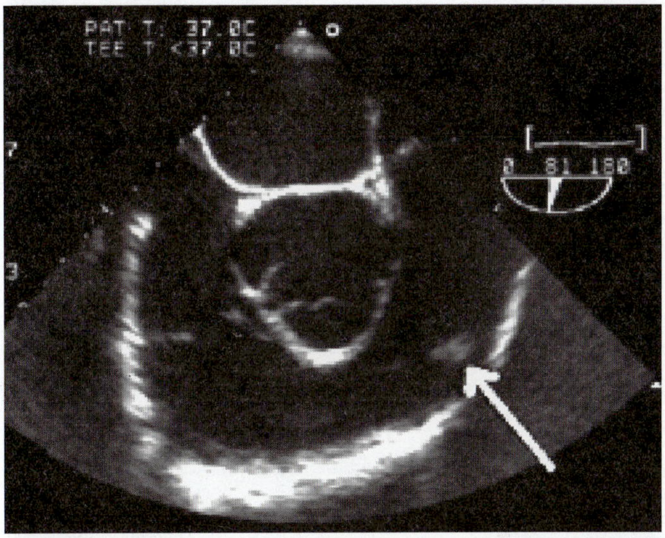

Fig. 14.67: *Transesophageal echocardiography image showing vegetation in main pulmonary artery (arrow)*

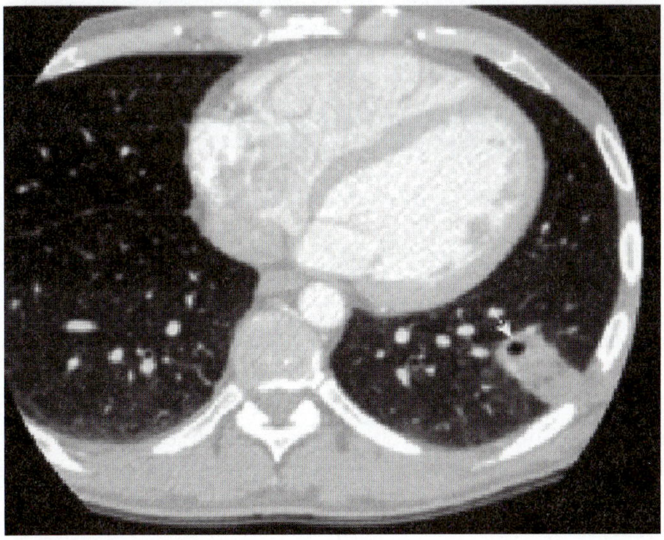

Fig. 14.68: *Lung abscess in PDA. CT scan of the chest demonstrating the area of air space shadowing with a cavity (arrow) in the apical segment of left lower lobe*

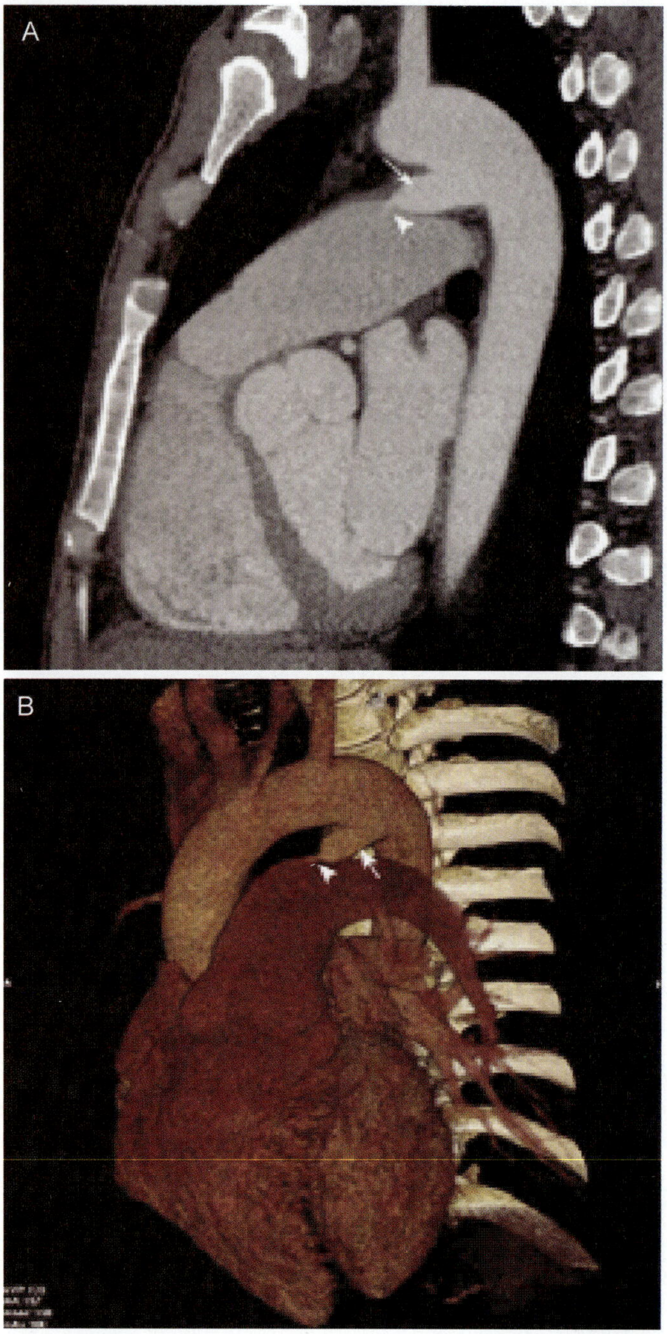

Figs 14.69A and B: *ECG-gated CT scan: sagittal oblique multiplanar reconstruction (A) and 3D reconstruction (B) showing the PDA (arrow) with the narrow end towards the main pulmonary artery*

Cardiac Catheterization and Percutaneous Implantation of Occluder Devices (Fig. 14.70)

The use of the percutaneous route to close the PDA is becoming more common. Transcatheter occlusion is an effective alternative to surgical intervention and is becoming the treatment of choice for most cases of PDA in children and adults.

Most patients with an isolated PDA can have successful treatment by catheterization after the first few months of life.

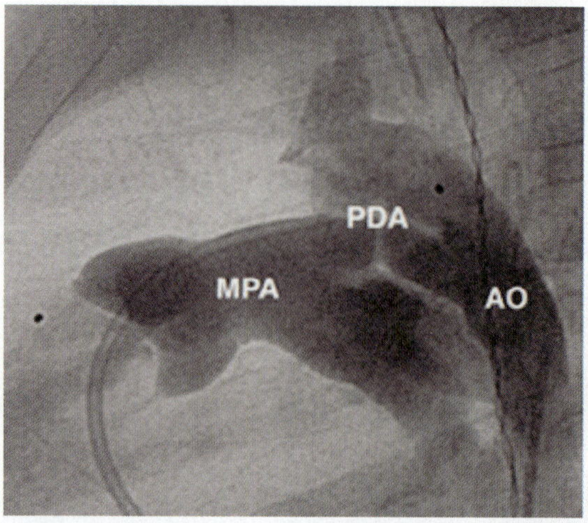

Fig. 14.70: *Patent ductus arteriosus angiogram. Lateral angiogram demonstrating a large tubular type duct (type C) with aortic (AO) to pulmonary flow (MPA). The catheter can be seen entering the MPA from the right ventricle, a second pigtail catheter is positioned in the descending aorta from which contrast is delivered*

After the first birthday, the most common treatment for a PDA is occlusion at cardiac catheterization. In fact, as catheterization techniques advance, the ability to close defects in smaller infants has also been reported with high levels of success. Over the last 4 decades, many techniques and devices have been used for PDA occlusion although definitive closure rates do not approach those of surgery. Contraindications to catheter-based closure involve the size of the patient.

Gianturco Spring Occluding Coils

Introduced in 1992, Gianturco spring occluding coils have been the most common device used for PDA occlusion for many years. The coils are delivered to the PDA via venous or arterial systems: 1–5 coils are placed in the ductus. In experienced hands with proper patient selection, this has become a procedure associated with high success and low morbidity. This method has been reported to be 75–100% effective but is limited to ductus that are only 4–5 mm in diameter. Coil occlusion is best suited to close a PDA with a minimal internal diameter of less than 2.5 mm. Fue et al showed that very high closure rates could be obtained in ducts less than 3 mm using coils, but that success significantly dropped when the ducts exceeded 3 mm.

Amplatzer Duct Occluder

More recently, the Amplatzer device has expanded the ability to close PDA at cardiac catheterization. This device is more reliable and easier to implant in a large PDA than spring occluding coils. The major disadvantage of the design is that the aortic part of the device can protrude into the descending aorta and partly obstruct the lumen, especially in infants. However, the Amplatzer duct occluder II (ADO II), a nitinol flexible mesh with a symmetrical design to provide high conformability, has been approved in Europe for treatment of all types of PDA.

Rashkind Ductus Occlusion Device

The Rashkind ductus occlusion device consists of a 2-umbrella system delivered to the ductus in either the transvenous pathway or transarterial pathway. This therapy has a reported occlusion rate of 83%. Although used internationally, it is not approved for use in the United States (Figs 14.71 to 14.73).

Postcatheterization Risks

Typically, complete occlusion is achieved at catheterization. Occasionally, a tiny residual left-to-right shunt remains at the end of the procedure, which closes by thrombus formation over the following days or weeks. Left-to-right shunt rarely persists through a partially occluded PDA. Usually, the magnitude of the shunt is significantly smaller than before occlusion. Due to concerns about the long-term risk of endocarditis, this residual defect should be closed. Often, this can be accomplished with a second catheter procedure. Rare reports describe association of a persistently patent ductus after occlusion attempts with hemolysis or endocarditis.

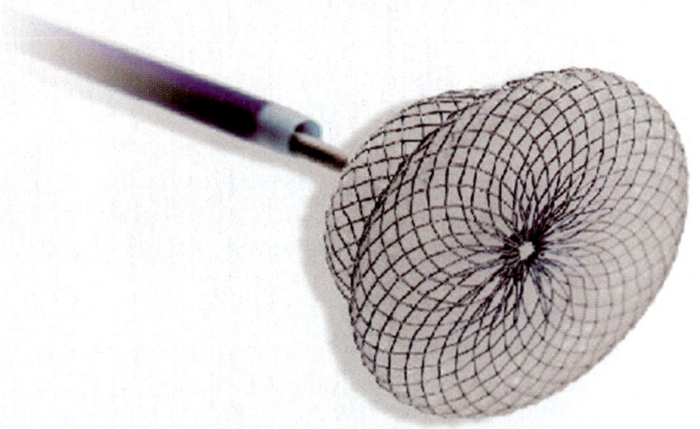

Fig. 14.71: *Structure of PDA amplatzer duct occluder*

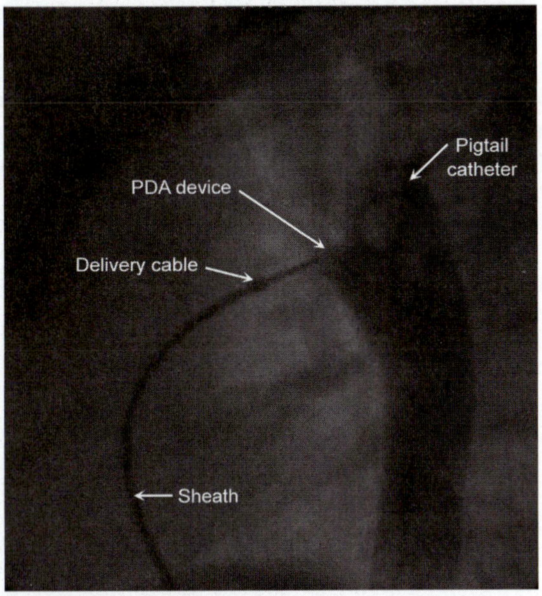

Fig. 14.72: *Implantation of patent ductus arteriosus occlusion device during cardiac catheterization*

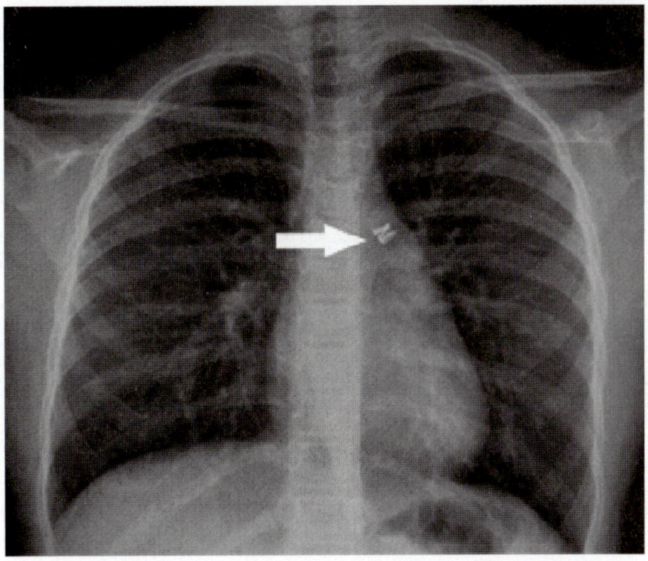

Fig. 14.73: *X-ray chest PA view showing coil embolization in treatment of PDA*

Procedural risks of PDA occlusion by catheter are few and largely influenced by the experience of the physician performing the procedure. These risks include embolization of the device being used to occlude the PDA, blood vessel injury, access site bleeding, infection, and stroke, among others. In the case of device embolization, the device can usually be retrieved by transcatheter techniques, and a second device can be successfully placed in the PDA.

Surgical Ligation

Surgical ligation or surgical ligation and division remain the standard treatment of large PDA that require treatment in infancy (see the following image). This is a particularly successful, low-risk procedure in the hands of an experienced pediatric cardiovascular surgeon. This is true even in the smallest premature babies.

Indications

With rare exceptions, the presence of a PDA is an indication for surgical closure. Clearly, attention must be paid to the existence of other congenital heart lesions that impair pulmonary blood flow. In these patients, all attempts should be made to preserve ductal flow until a more permanent palliative shunt can be constructed or definitive repair can be undertaken. Very small premature infants still require surgical closure.

In the infant, repair may be urgent for the symptomatic patient with evidence of cardiac or respiratory failure not adequately controlled with medications, or it may be delayed in the patient who is asymptomatic or well controlled on medical therapy.

Postoperative results are best if the PDA is closed while the patient is younger than 3 years. An increased incidence of elevated PVR and pulmonary hypertension occurs if the lesion closed in those older than 3 years.

Indications for surgical treatment include the following:
1. Failure of indomethacin treatment
2. Contraindications to medical therapy (e.g. thrombocytopenia, renal insufficiency)
3. Signs and symptoms of CHF
4. PDA found in an older infant
5. Infants found to have an asymptomatic PDA after the neonatal period should undergo surgical ligation preferably before the age of 1 year to prevent future complications of a PDA
6. Ductal closure is indicated for cardiovascular compromise (i.e. pulmonary complications) and for reduction of the risk of infective endocarditis (subacute bacterial endocarditis).

Contraindications

The primary contraindication to repair is severe pulmonary vascular disease. If transient intraoperative occlusion of the PDA does not decrease elevated pulmonary arterial pressures with a subsequent increase in aortic pressure, then the closure must be undertaken carefully and may be contraindicated. Closure of the ductus does not reverse preexisting pulmonary vascular disease.

A subset of associated cardiac anomalies—so-called ductal-dependent lesions—depend on flow through the PDA to maintain systemic blood flow. Premature closure of the ductus without concurrent repair of the following defects is contraindicated and may be fatal:
- Aortic valve atresia
- Mitral valve atresia with hypoplastic left ventricle
- Pulmonary artery hypoplasia
- Pulmonary atresia
- Severe coarctation of the aorta
- Tricuspid atresia
- Transposition of the great arteries
- Other contraindications to surgical closure include concurrent uncontrolled sepsis and an inability of the patient to tolerate general anesthesia.

Medical vs Surgical Therapy

Although indomethacin therapy is preferred in most intensive care units (ICUs) as the first-line approach to effect PDA closure, the benefits of this approach over surgical ligation are not obvious. In most studies that attempt to evaluate differences in the outcomes for indomethacin therapy and surgical closure, results are similar. A cochrane review failed to demonstrate that the net harm-to-benefit ratio favored either surgical ligation or medical therapy. Observational studies suggest that surgical ligation is associated with higher likelihood of chronic lung disease, retinopathy of prematurity, and neurosensory impairment. These data may be questionable, because surgical ligation is not available in every nursery, whereas medical therapy is widely available.

Post-treatment Management

Typically, hospitalization following treatment for PDA is minimal. Patients who have catheter closure of PDA are usually sent home on the day of the procedure. Even patients who have standard surgery with a thoracotomy rarely are hospitalized for longer than 2 or 3 days.

The appropriate care and length of hospitalization of premature neonates with a PDA are primarily determined based on abnormalities of other organ systems. However, babies who have effective closure of PDA appear to have shorter hospital stays than babies whose PDA remains a problem.

Complications

Complications of untreated PDA include bacterial endocarditis, late CHF, and the development of pulmonary vascular obstructive disease. PDA can complicate other circulatory or ventilatory abnormalities, such as the following:
- Aortic rupture
- Eisenmenger physiology
- Left heart failure
- Myocardial ischemia
- Necrotizing enterocolitis
- Pulmonary hypertension
- Right heart hypertrophy and failure.

Prostaglandin E1 (PGE1) should be used to maintain patency of the ductus arteriosus once it is established that a ductal dependent lesion exists. However, PGE is a pulmonary vasodilator and could cause exacerbation of CHF by means of increasing pulmonary blood flow.

Long-term Monitoring

Parents of children with this lesion should be aware that PDA does not have any significant inheritance pattern.

Once the PDA is closed, no special limitations or care is necessary. No exercise restriction is required in the absence of pulmonary hypertension.

Most physicians recommend antibiotic prophylaxis at times of risk of bacteremia for 6–12 months following closure, whether by catheter or surgery. Specific recommendations for prophylactic antibiotics can be found in any current infectious disease or antibiotic reference, or refer to the American Heart Association recommendations. Although rare reports exist of recanalization and recurrence of a left-to-right shunt after PDA ligation, the risk is extremely low. If a PDA has been closed by interventional radiologic techniques, obtaining follow-up echocardiograms echocardiography 2–3 weeks after the procedure until complete closure is confirmed is wise.

Natural History and Prognosis

Spontaneous closure is unlikely after 2 years of age. Over 90% maintain a left-to-right shunt and less than 10% develop Eisenmenger's syndrome with a reversal of the shunt. The life-expectancy is one-half normal after 17 years, of age if the PDA is uncorrected.

The risk of infective endocarditis is very high, especially after the first decade of life. The causes of death if the PDA is uncorrected are CHF, infective endocarditis, Eisenmenger's syndrome, and, rarely, dissection of the ductus.

AORTOPULMONARY SEPTAL DEFECT (APSD)

Aortopulmonary Window

Aortopulmonary septal defect (APSD), an uncommon congenital cardiac defect, is a deficiency in the septum between the aorta and the pulmonary artery, resulting in a communication between the two. This defect is present as an isolated lesion in about one-half of patients and in conjunction with another defect or more complex heart disease in the other half of patients.

Developmentally, the defect results from incomplete separation of the common tube of the truncus arteriosus and the aorticopulmonary trunk. During early embryonic development, the aorta and pulmonary arteries separate by growth of a spiral septum dividing the common trunk into the aorta and the pulmonary artery. The spiral septum is created by fusion of a truncal septum growing cephalad from the semilunar valves and the aorticopulmonary spiral septum growing caudally from the pulmonary bifurcation. Incomplete development of these septa results in aortopulmonary septal defect (Figs 14.74 and 14.75).

van Mierop subdivided aortopulmonary septal defect into three subtypes. The first subtype is believed to result from nonfusion between the aorticopulmonary septum above and the truncal septum below, resulting in a small-to-moderate defect midway between the semilunar valves and the pulmonary bifurcation. The second type is also believed to arise from a failure of fusion of the aorticopulmonary septum above and the truncal septum below; however, this failure of fusion results in a large, nonrestrictive defect without a continuous posterior border, in which the defect describes more than one spiral turn. The third type is absence of the aorticopulmonary septum; the defect is large and without a posterior border, and the right pulmonary artery may arise directly from the aorta.

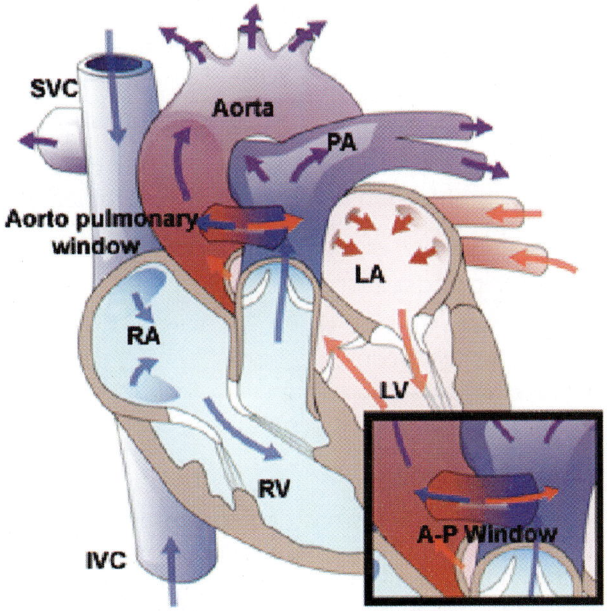

Fig. 14.74: *Demonstrating anatomy and circulation in aortopulmonary window*

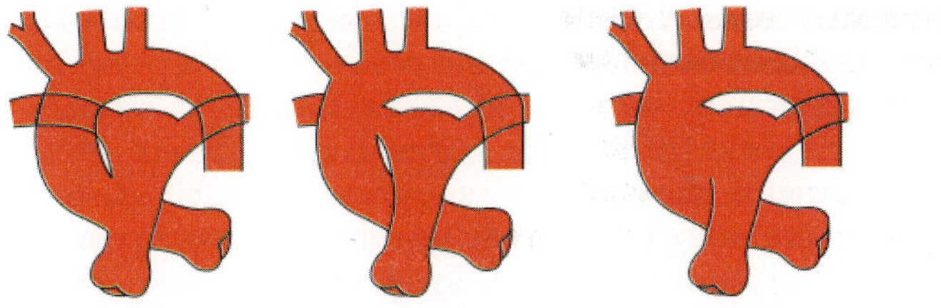

Fig. 14.75: *Mori classification of aortopulmonary window. Type I or proximal communication occurs near the semilunar valves. Type II or distal communication involves the pulmonary bifurcation at the level of the right pulmonary artery. In type III, there is a wide communication between the aorta and pulmonary artery owing to total absence of the aortopulmonary septum*

Although this classification system may correlate with the various embryologic origins of aortopulmonary septal defect itself, it does not account for other anomalies encountered with aortopulmonary septal defect.

Patent ductus arteriosus (PDA) is encountered in almost three fourths of patients with aortopulmonary septal defect. An interrupted aortic arch type A or severe coarctation is present in 10–15% of patients with aortopulmonary septal defect. Discontinuity of the aorta in interrupted aortic arch type A occurs distal to the left subclavian artery, as in a severe form of aortic coarctation. This is quite different developmentally from interrupted aortic arch type B, in which discontinuity occurs between the left carotid artery and the left subclavian arteries. Interrupted aortic arch type B is frequently associated with DiGeorge/velocardiofacial/22q-chromosome arm deletion, unlike interrupted aortic arch type A. When interrupted aortic arch occurs without a ventricular septal defect (VSD), an aortopulmonary septal defect is usually present.

Tetralogy of Fallot and anomalous coronary from pulmonary artery are each present in about 5% of cases. Other reported anomalies associated with aortopulmonary septal defect include VSD, aortic atresia, transposition of the great arteries double aortic arch, and other more complex heart diseases.

Aortopulmonary septal defect has been described in other mammals including dogs, cats and horses.

History

The clinical presentation of aortopulmonary septal defect (APSD) depends on the size of the defect, pulmonary vascular resistance (PVR), and associated anomalies. In a large defect with falling PVR, aortopulmonary septal defect presents with typical signs and symptoms of congestive heart failure (CHF) indistinguishable from those of a large ventricular septal defect (VSD) or ductus arteriosus.

Symptoms usually emerge between the second and eighth weeks of life. Caregivers typically report signs of CHF as tachypnea and diaphoresis (especially with feeds), poor feeding, and usually poor growth. If aortopulmonary septal defect is associated with interrupted aortic arch or severe coarctation, the infant may present with signs and symptoms of shock in newborn period as the ductus arteriosus closes. In less common scenarios (about 10% of patients), the defect is small and restrictive and presents as an asymptomatic murmur in the first weeks to months of life. In presence of a large, nonrestrictive defect, PVR in some patients may not fall significantly, CHF does not develop, and the patients may be relatively asymptomatic. Because pulmonary and systemic resistances are comparable, some right-to-left shunting and mild cyanosis may be present yet not clinically apparent. Unfortunately, despite lack of symptoms, irreversible pulmonary vascular obstructive disease (PVOD) typically develops with time. At this stage, fatigue, exercise intolerance, and cyanosis may appear.

Children with persistently elevated PVR are most difficult to identify clinically, and many years pass before diagnosis with serious heart disease.

Physical Examination

If a large, nonrestrictive defect with low PVR is present, then physical examination findings are indistinguishable from those of a large patent ductus arteriosus (PDA). These findings include tachypnea, tachycardia, and increased work of breathing.

Continuous run-off into the pulmonary circuit during diastole, in combination with an elevated stoke volume, causes a wide pulse pressure with bounding pulses.

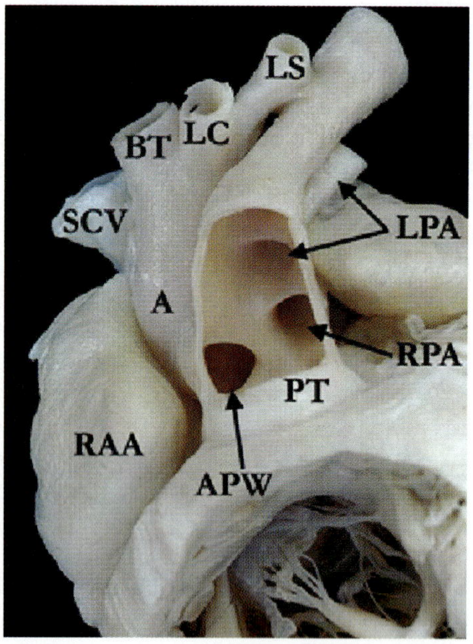

Fig. 14.76: *The pulmonary trunk has been resected anteriorly to show the aortopulmonary window (APW). The defect is seen in the right lateral wall of the pulmonary trunk with the right coronary orifice (RCO) just inferior to the defect. There is a separate aortic valve not shown in this image. The right pulmonary artery (RPA) origin is just superior and to the left of the aorto-pulmonary window (APW). The left pulmonary artery origin is distal and not shown in this image. The aortic arch is interrupted distal to the left subclavian artery (LS) and the arterial duct is widely patent. SCV, superior caval vein, RAA, right atrial appendage;LAA, left atrial appendage; BC, brachiocephalic trunk; LC, left common carotid; DA, descending aorta; PV, pulmonary valve*

Palpation reveals a hyperdynamic precordial impulse from increased volume load on the left ventricle.

Auscultation reveals a loud and single second heart sound with a continuous murmur at the left upper sternal border. Often, a gallop rhythm and an apical diastolic rumble from increased volume load are present.

Hepatic congestion and hepatomegaly develop in proportion to the degree of heart failure.

Failure to thrive is concomitant with the degree of heart failure.

In situations in which PVR fails to fall significantly after birth, findings may be subtler.

The second heart sound is single, yet no murmur or only a soft systolic murmur may be observed. Pulses are not bounding; little diastolic run-off is noted.

Subtle cyanosis may be present from a small amount of right-to-left shunt when pulmonary and systemic resistances are comparable. With irreversible pulmonary vascular changes and Eisenmenger syndrome, cyanosis may become more prominent. Cyanosis will be present if other cyanotic lesions are present (e.g. transposition of the great vessels, tetralogy of Fallot).

A continuous murmur may be the only physical finding if the defect is small and restrictive.

Etiology

Aortopulmonary septal defect is likely caused by multifactorial genetic etiologies. No clear inheritance pattern is noted in most patients. Although this defect appears to have clinical similarities with truncus arteriosus and interrupted aortic arch type B, aortopulmonary septal defect is not associated with the 22q-/DiGeorge syndrome as are the other malformations. Note that the aortic arch interruption commonly associated with aortopulmonary septal defect occurs as type A rather than type B.

Rarely, aortopulmonary septal defect has been described in children affected by other syndromes, including vertebral, anorectal, cardiac, tracheoesophageal, renal, and limb (VACTERL) association, with one case report of an infant with terminal 2q deletion.

One small case series described 3 unrelated children with iris hypoplasia and aortopulmonary septal defect. The hypothesized association between the two problems is an error in neural crest development.

Differential Diagnoses

- Coronary artery anomalies
- Patent ductus arteriosus
- Truncus arteriosus
- Ventricular septal defect, general concepts.

Laboratory Studies

Preoperatively in patients with an aortopulmonary septal defect (APSD), obtain a CBC count, cross match, and urinalysis. If the infant has been on diuretics and digoxin preoperatively, checking electrolyte and digoxin levels is prudent. Infants with congestive heart failure (CHF) are at risk for potassium depletion from diuretics and may be at

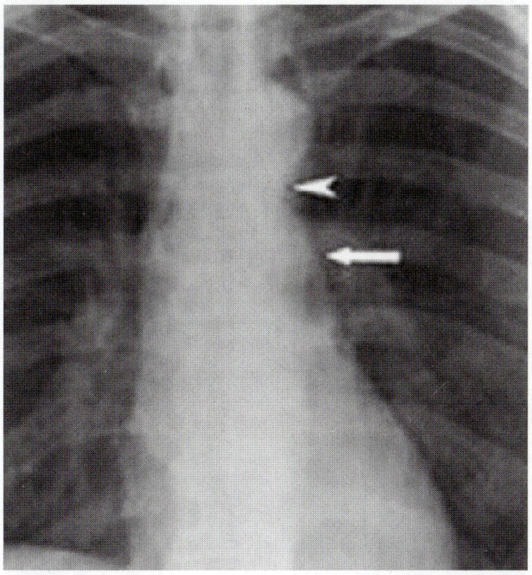

Fig. 14.77: *AP window reflection. On a posteroanterior chest radiograph, the AP window reflection (arrowhead) extends from the aortic knob to the left pulmonary artery and has a normal concave appearance. The aortic-pulmonary reflection (arrow) is a more anterior line and extends from the aortic arch to the level of the left main bronchus*

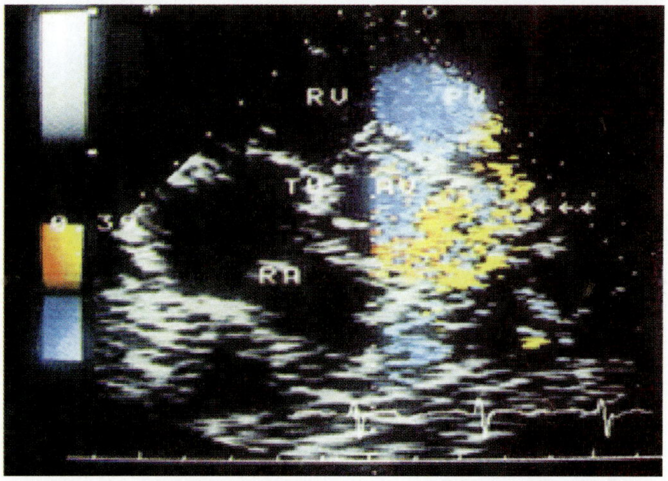

Fig. 14.78: *Color Doppler flow echoscan showing shunt from the aorta into the main pulmonary artery in patient with aorto-pulmonary window*

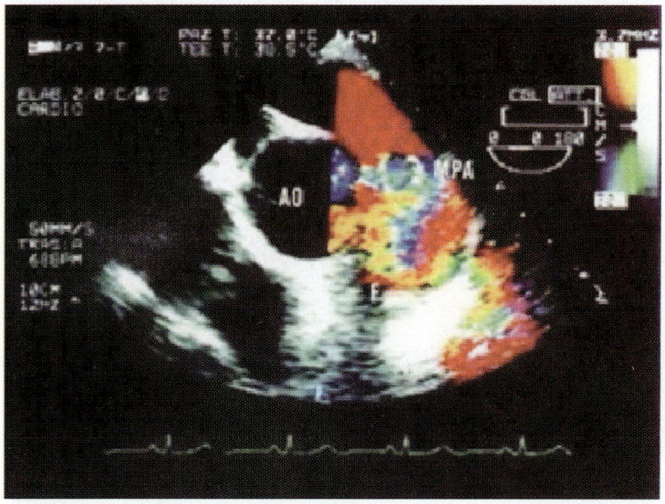

Fig. 14.79: *Color Doppler flow echoscan showing mosaic pattern of flow from main pulmonary artery to aorta in patient with aorto-pulmonary window*

risk for digoxin toxicity from routine dosing during decreased renal perfusion. The combination of a volume-loaded circulation with potassium depletion and an elevated serum digoxin level may be a risk factor for ventricular fibrillation at the time of sternotomy.

Chest radiography: Radiography typically reveals cardiomegaly with increased pulmonary blood flow. Pulmonary congestion is proportional to the degree of CHF.

Electrocardiography

ECG typically reveals biventricular hypertrophy or right ventricular hypertrophy. Electrical evidence for left atrial enlargement may present.

Echocardiography

In infants and children, this test (if performed by experienced personnel and reviewed by a skilled pediatric echocardiographer) should reveal the defect and associated abnormalities in virtually all cases.

Doppler color flow mapping shows retrograde flow in the transverse arch during diastole. By contrast, in an infant with a large left-sided patent ductus arteriosus (PDA) and a left aortic arch, diastolic flow in the arch is antegrade. For patients with poor echocardiographic windows, transesophageal echocardiography or cardiac MRI may be an option (Figs 14.78 to 14.80).

When an aortopulmonary septal defect is found, the echocardiographer should be especially careful to look for other abnormalities, which are present in 50% of cases of aortopulmonary septal defect. In addition to identifying the aortopulmonary septal defect, the ventricular septum, origins of the pulmonary arteries, aortic arch, presence of a PDA, and origins of the coronary arteries should be carefully scrutinized.

In addition, three dimensional echocardiography has been used to help to characterize an aortopulmonary septal defect.

Computerized axial tomography and MRI: These noninvasive techniques are not only helpful in the preoperative assessment cardiac anatomy of the congenital heart defects but also useful in their postoperative follow up (Figs 14.81 to 14.83).

Cardiac Catheterization (CC)

Cardiac catheterization should not be required if anatomy has been well defined by noninvasive means and if the clinical and noninvasive data are both consistent with low pulmonary vascular resistance (PVR). If questions or

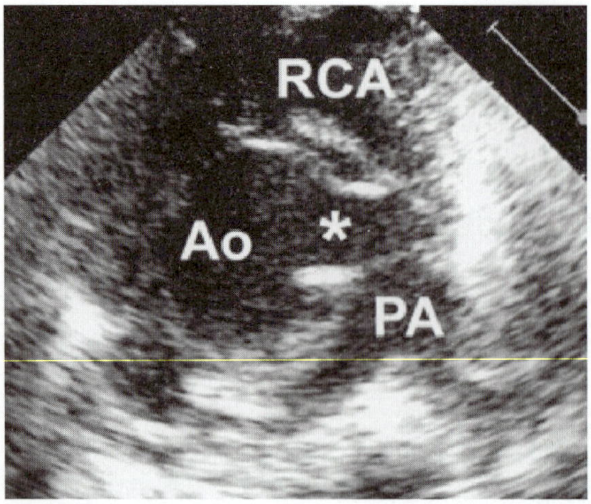

Fig. 14.80: *Preoperative echocardiography of patient shows the anomalous right coronary artery (RCA) originates from the pulmonary artery (PA). (Ao = aorta, * = aorto-pulmonary window.)*

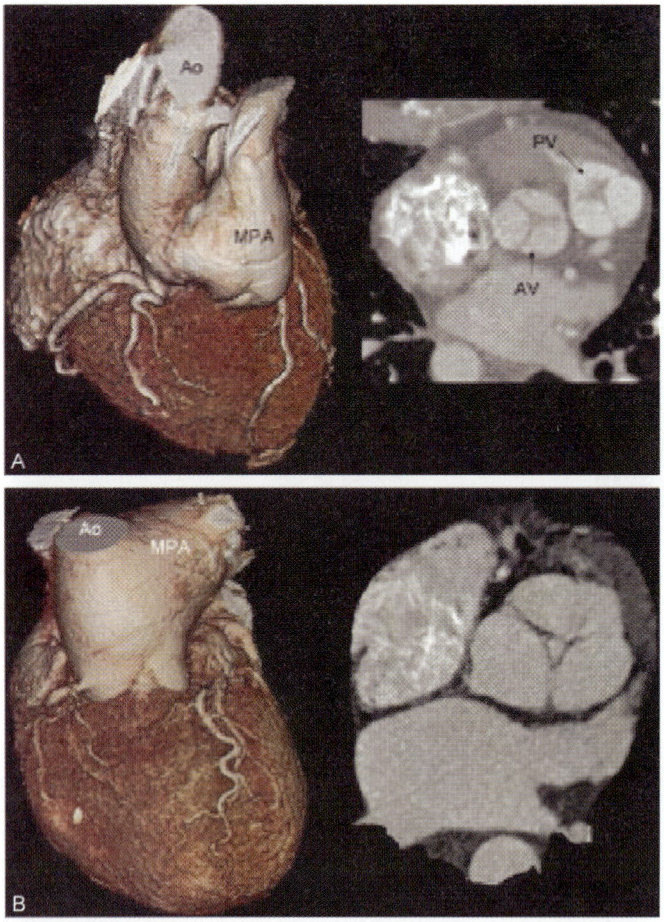

Fig. 14.81: *(A) Aorto-pulmonary window. Note presence of normal aortic and pulmonary valves (in contrast to B). (B) Truncus arteriosus: a single truncal valve comprising of components of both aortic and pulmonary valves*

additional incompletely characterized defects are noted, careful hemodynamic and angiographic assessment may be helpful (Fig. 14.84).

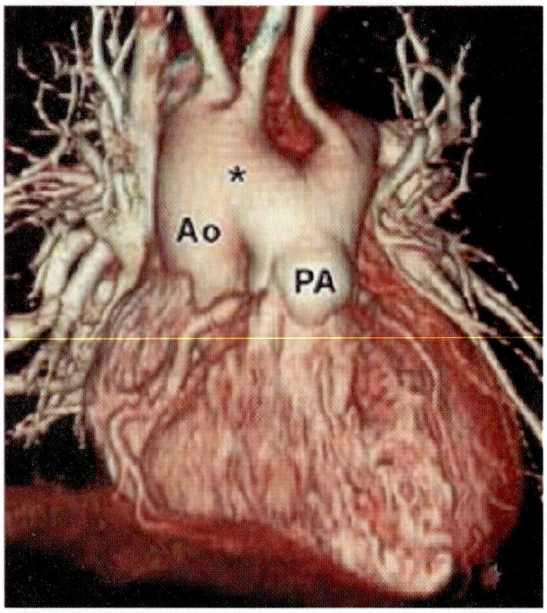

Fig. 14.82: *Anatomic positions of aortopulmonary window on CT angiography*

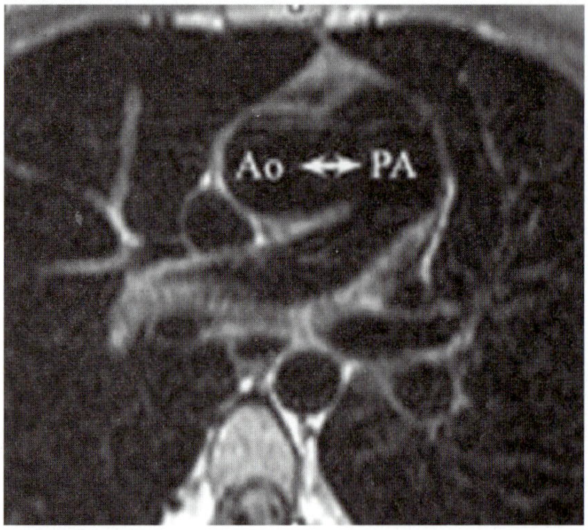

Fig. 14.83: *Anatomic position of aortopulmonary window on MRI angiography (arrow)*

Beyond infancy, CC may be required to exclude irreversible pulmonary vascular obstructive disease (PVOD) before performing surgical repair. In older children with a diagnosis of a nonrestrictive aortopulmonary window, CC is advisable to establish pulmonary vascular reactivity before performing surgical repair. In the rare instance of a small restrictive defect, catheter therapy with device occlusion of the defect may be an option.

Medical Treatment

Medical palliation of aortopulmonary septal defect (APSD) may be performed for several days to weeks to allow elective surgical scheduling. Because an aortopulmonary window does not spontaneously close, surgical repair is necessary to prevent the development of pulmonary vascular obstructive disease (PVOD). Meanwhile, digoxin

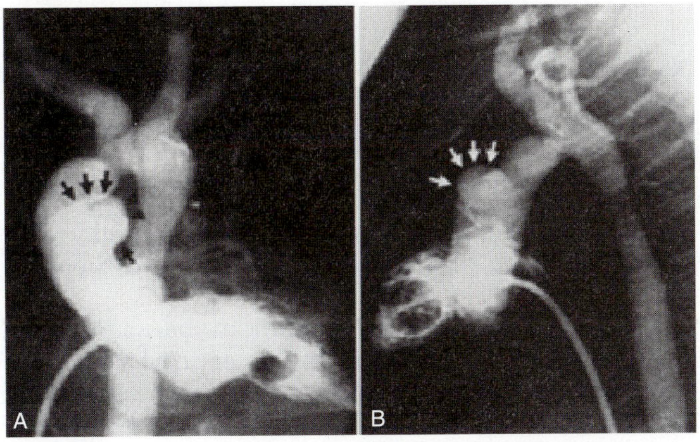

Fig. 14.84: *Anteroposterior (A) and lateral (B) aortograms made after repair demonstrating aortic sac (arrows), new aortopulmonary septum (arrow heads) without any residual leaks at the site of the aortopulmonary window, and a large anastomosis between the ascending and descending aorta. The distal portion of the ascending aorta is pulled backward and somewhat twisted because of the direct anastomosis; however, there is no evident stenosis at the site of cannulation*

and diuretics may provide some symptomatic benefit before surgical repair.

In rare instances (e.g. active sepsis), postponing surgery may be desired. In this situation, provide medical therapy (i.e. digoxin, inotropic drugs, diuretics) for a brief time in anticipation of surgery.

The effect of vasodilator agents [e.g. angiotensin-converting enzyme (ACE) inhibitors, phosphodiesterase inhibitors, nitrates] is uncertain because these drugs all affect pulmonary resistance in addition to systemic resistance. Intubation and positive pressure ventilation with permissive hypercarbia and limiting inspired oxygen concentration to 21% may help limit pulmonary blood flow in infants with torrential pulmonary flow requiring medical palliation. Consider using lower inspired oxygen concentrations (15–19%) to elevate pulmonary vascular resistance (PVR) in more extreme cases. Sedation and muscle relaxants may prove necessary to limit spontaneous ventilation.

Previous common practice consisted of medically treating a small infant with congestive heart failure (CHF) with the expectation that he or she would grow and become a "better" surgical candidate. This approach is seldom successful because caloric demands of an infant with CHF typically exceed the amount of nutrition delivered by even the most aggressive means.

Case reports and small case series report closure of small aortopulmonary septal defects in the cardiac catheterization (CC) laboratory. The Rashkind double umbrella device, the Amplatzer duct occluder, the Amplatzer septal occluder, muscular ventricular septal defect (VSD) occluder, and perimembranous VSD occluder have all been used to close small (type I) defects. The limiting factor to catheter closure of these defects is the anatomy. Only relatively small defects with circumferential tissue rims are amenable to transcatheter device closure, limiting this therapeutic option to a relatively small number of patients. Digitalis and diuretics may be used to palliate this condition for a short time before surgical repair.

Surgical Intervention

Various surgical techniques allow correction of this lesion. Most centers use techniques that involve cardiopulmonary bypass (Figs 14.85 and 14.86).

The aorta and pulmonary artery may be divided, and the defects in the walls may be closed primarily or with patch material. Alternatively, the aorta or pulmonary artery may be opened and the defect patched using autologous, homologous, xenograft, or synthetic material. Two larger case series have reported that transaortic repair is associated with a more favorable outcome and has less risk of causing late pulmonary artery stenosis.

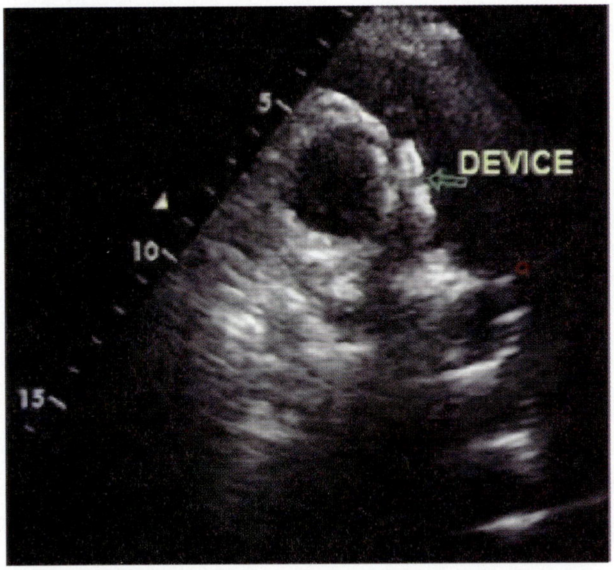

Fig. 14.85: *Anatomic position of aortopulmonary window on echo with closure of the defect with device (arrow)*

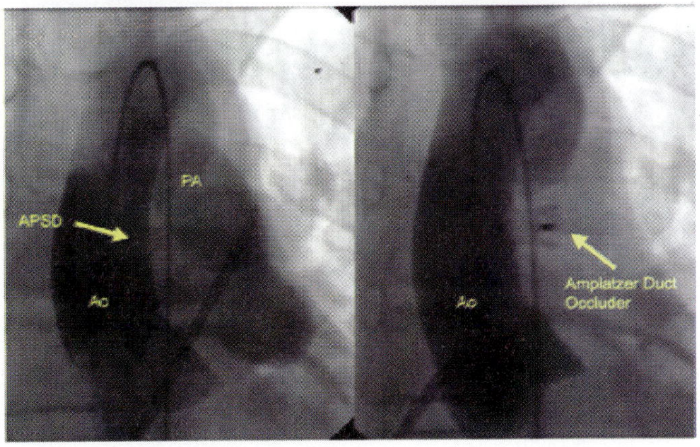

Fig. 14.86: *Angiogram of a small-to-moderate aortopulmonary septal defect in a 4-year-old child. Complete occlusion of the aortopulmonary septal defect with an Amplatzer duct occluder. Ao, ascending aorta; PA, pulmonary artery*

Other defects may be addressed at the same operation; however, in rare instances, a staged approach may be undertaken. Specific techniques for unique anatomy must be individualized.

Postoperatively, evidence of a good surgical repair should be confirmed. Residual anatomic problems may be anticipated from preoperative anatomy and include, but not be limited to, pulmonary artery stenosis or distortion, residual left-to-right shunt at the aortopulmonary septal defect site, and ascending aortic obstruction or distortion. Postoperative data should be consistent with a complete repair.

If a pulmonary artery catheter was left in place, it should indicate low pulmonary artery pressure and pulmonary artery oxygen saturation less than 80%.

An elevated pulmonary artery pressure may indicate pulmonary artery vasoreactivity or a persistent left-to-right shunt. Pulmonary artery saturation and left atrial pressure should differentiate the two conditions. If concerns persist, transthoracic or transesophageal echocardiography may be informative. Rarely, cardiac catheterization (CC) may be needed to detect residual abnormalities.

Apart from anatomic concerns, an older infant or child with elevated preoperative PVR is at risk for postoperative pulmonary hypertension that may require aggressive management. Inhaled nitric oxide may be useful in the management of postoperative pulmonary hypertension by acting as a selective pulmonary arteriolar vasodilator. Other drugs such as sildenafil or calcium channel blockers may provide ongoing pulmonary vasodilatation.

OBSTRUCTIVE CARDIAC ANOMALIES

AORTIC VALVULAR STENOSIS

Abnormalities of the left ventricular outflow tract are common congenital cardiac disorders. In particular, as much as 2% of the population have congenitally bicuspid aortic valves. A bicuspid aortic valve may present as an incidental finding on physical examination or echocardiography done for other reasons; as significant aortic stenosis (AS) or AR; or when it results in infective endocarditis (Fig. 14.87).

Pathophysiology

A stenotic bicuspid aortic valve will produce pressure overload of the LV, which leads to LVH and eventually to heart failure, angina pectoris, or sudden death from tachyarrhythmias. Similarly, the patient with an incompetent bicuspid aortic valve will exhibit LV dilatation, initially with normal systolic function; the condition will later progress to heart failure.

Physical Examination

On physical examination, the cardinal sign of a bicuspid aortic valve is an early systolic ejection click. If no significant hemodynamic abnormality is present, either no murmur or a soft ejection murmur may be heard; a very mild murmur of AR is not uncommon, even with hemodynamically insignificant bicuspid aortic valves. Moreover, significant AS or AR will produce findings similar to those in patients with other disorders that cause these lesions.

Laboratory Tests

Electrocardiography: The ECG will be normal unless hemodynamically significant stenosis or regurgitation is present, in which case it will show LVH (Fig. 14.88).

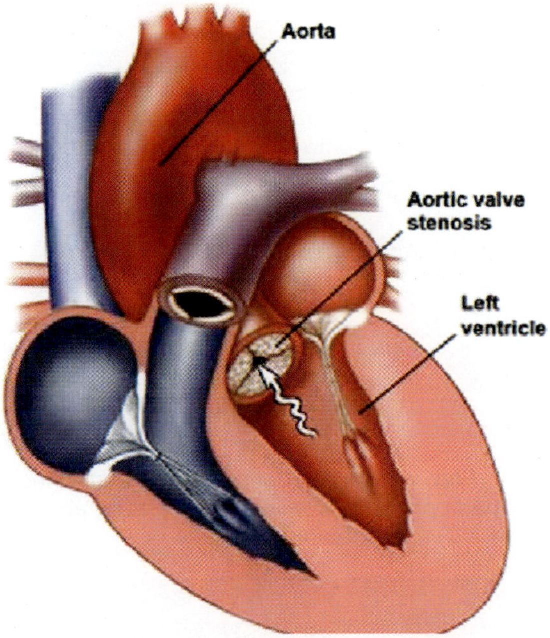

Fig. 14.87: *Anatomical features of valvular aortic stenosis (AS)*

Chest Radiography (Fig. 14.89)

Findings in patients with hemodynamically significant bicuspid aortic valves are similar to those in patients with AS and AR from other etiologies. These may include LV dilatation in AR or in AS progressing to heart failure; the latter will also produce pulmonary congestion.

Echocardiography: Both the presence of a bicuspid aortic valve and its hemodynamic significance can be determined by echocardiography.

Serial studies are useful in following the progression of the lesion (Figs 14.90 to 14.95).

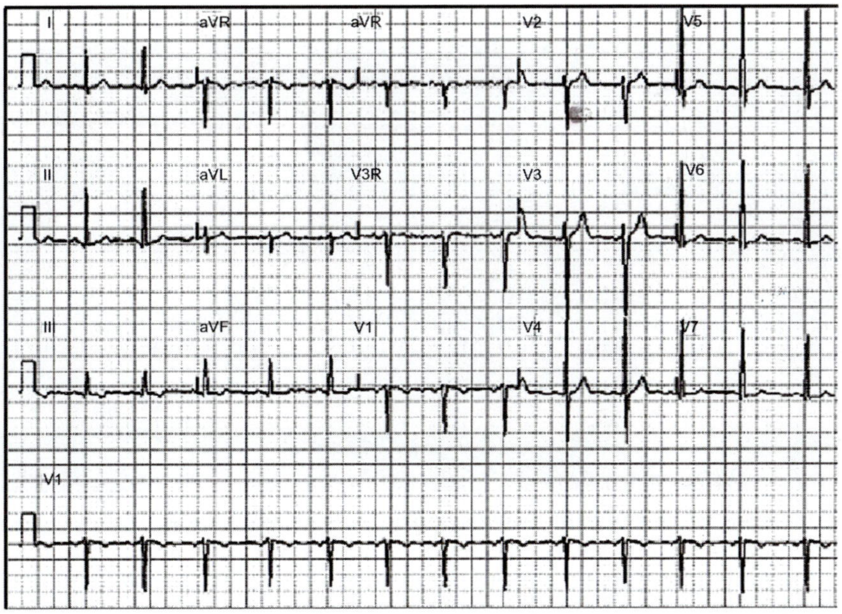

Fig. 14.88: *Aortic stenosis: electrocardiogram obtained in a 16-year-old adolescent with severe valvular aortic stenosis. The tracing shows nonspecific T wave changes in inferior leads III and aVF, and left ventricular hypertrophy (24 mm R wave V5, >98 % for age)*

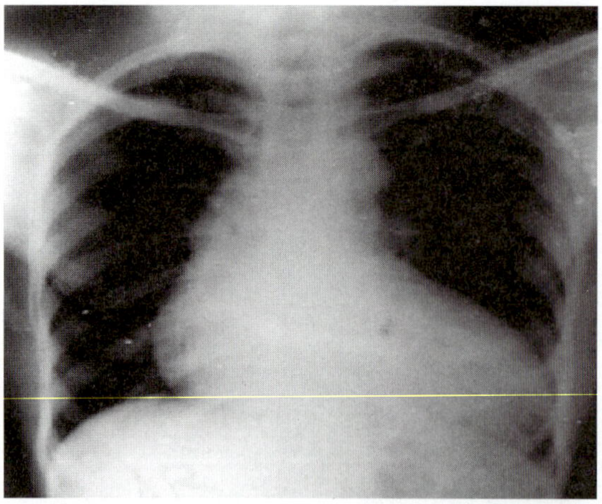

Fig. 14.89: *Photugraph X-ray chest PA view showing LV type cardiac hypertrophy with prominanat ascending aorta in patient with congenital valvular aortic stenosis*

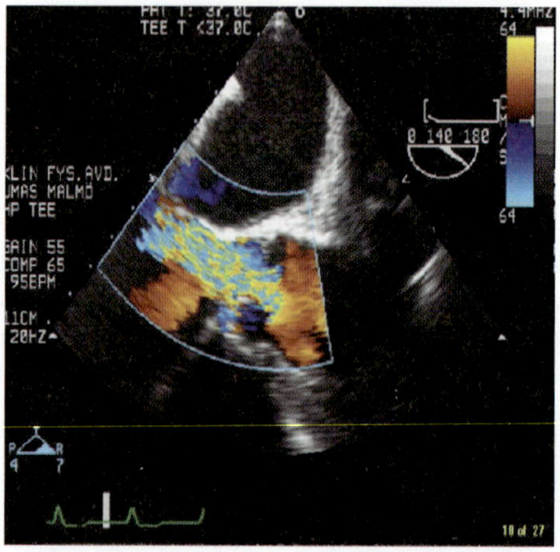

Fig. 14.91: *Transoesophageal color-Doppler image of severe aortic regurgitation associated with the quadricuspid aortic valve in this case*

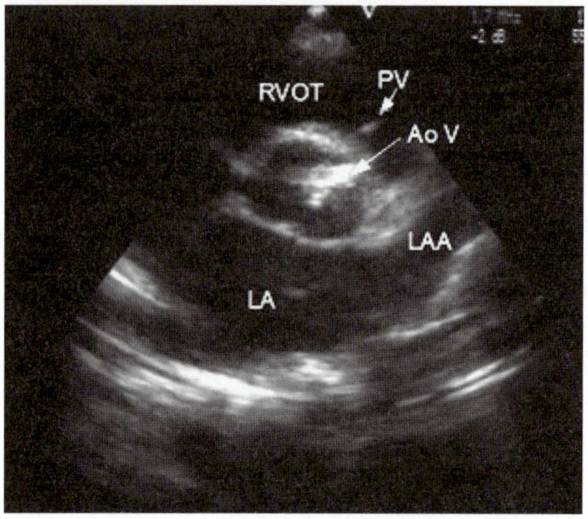

Fig. 14.90: *Parasternal short axis view—valve closed showing markedly thickened valves in valvular aortic stenosis*

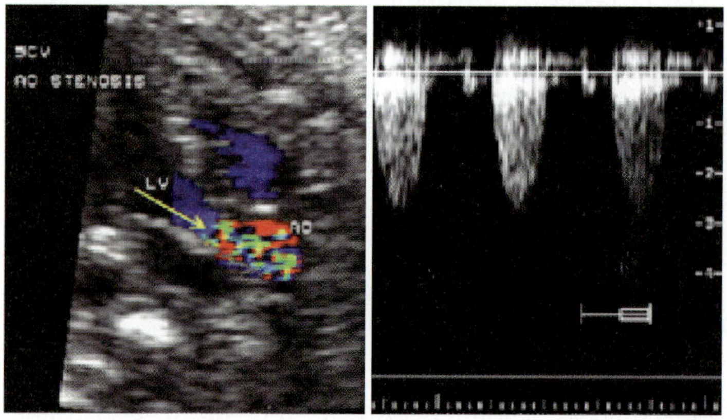

Fig. 14.92: *Fetal ultrasonography in a aortic stenosis with turbulent flow (green pixels), as seen in the five chamber view. Continuous wave Doppler allows a quantification of the stenosis*

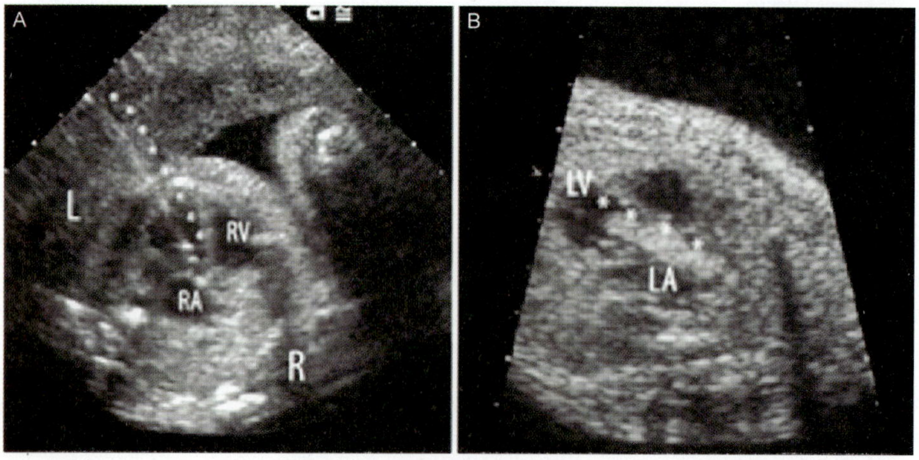

Fig. 14.93: *Fetal catheter intervention for severe aortic valve stenosis at 25 weeks. (A) After positioning of the fetus to ensure the left ventricular apex was oriented toward the maternal abdominal wall, a needle was used to puncture through the maternal abdomen, uterus, fetal chest and fetal left ventricular apex (*course of the needle). A wire was then passed through the needle into the left ventricular outflow tract and through the aortic valve. (B) A coronary balloon catheter was subsequently guided over the wire through the aortic valve and expanded to dilate the valve (*course of balloon). LA, left atrium; RA, right atrium; LV, left ventricle; RV, right ventricle; L, left; R, right*

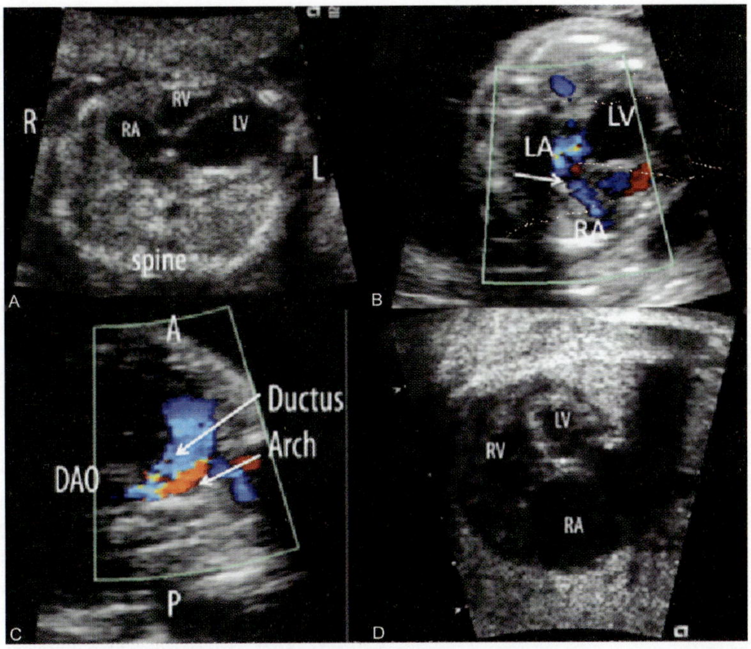

Fig. 14.94: *Images from a 21 week fetus with critical aortic stenosis. (A) At this stage in addition to a thickened and hypoplastic aortic valve, the left ventricle (LV) was found to be severely dilated and akinetic. There was (B) left to right atrial flow and (C) retrograde aortic arch flow in keeping with high left heart filling pressures and severely reduced left ventricular output (D), respectively. With redistribution of blood flow to the right heart and decreased filling of the left ventricle, there was progressive left heart hypoplasia such that by 35 weeks the fetus had findings consistent with hypoplastic left heart syndrome. LA, left atrium; RV, right ventricle; RA, right atrium; L, left; R, right; DAo, descending aorta*

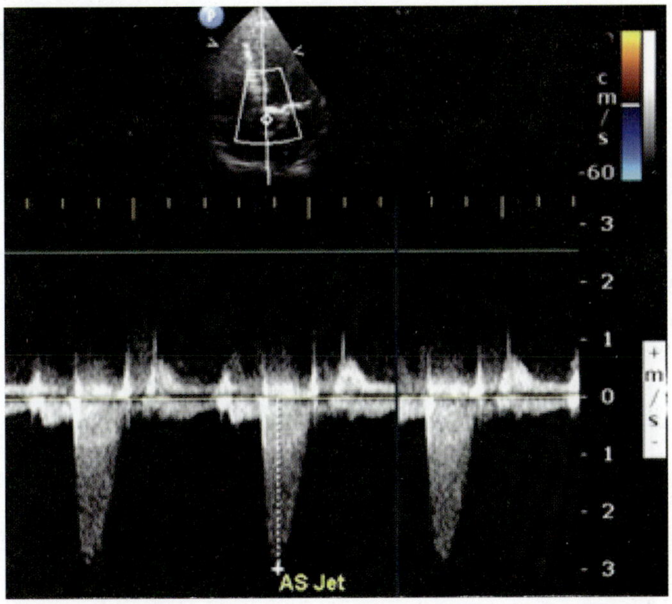

Fig. 14. 95: *Color flow-guided evaluation of aortic stenosis jet from apical five chamber view with continuous wave Doppler interrogation*

Cadiac catheterization and angiography: It is very helpful in hemodynamic evaluation and percutaneous implantation of aortic valve and balloon aortic valvoplasty. It can also be useful in delineating coronary anatomy during aortic valve replacement (Figs 14.96 to 14.99).

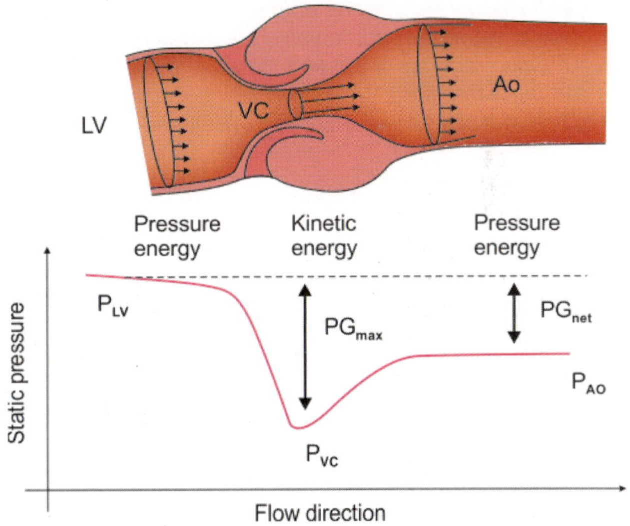

Fig. 14.96: *Pressure recovery distal to the AV. High static pressure in the left ventricle (LV) is converted to kinetic energy, maximal at the vena contracta (VC). In the ascending aorta (Ao), kinetic energy can be either lost as thermal energy or recovered as pressure energy. Pressure recovery is more prominent when the ascending aorta is not dilated. The maximal pressure gradient (PGmax) is the difference in static pressures between the left ventricle (PLV) and the vena contracta (PVC), and correlates with the Doppler gradient. The net pressure gradient (PGnet) is the difference in static pressures between the left ventricle and the ascending aorta (PAo) after pressure recovery has occurred, and correlates with the catheterization gradient. AV, aortic valve*

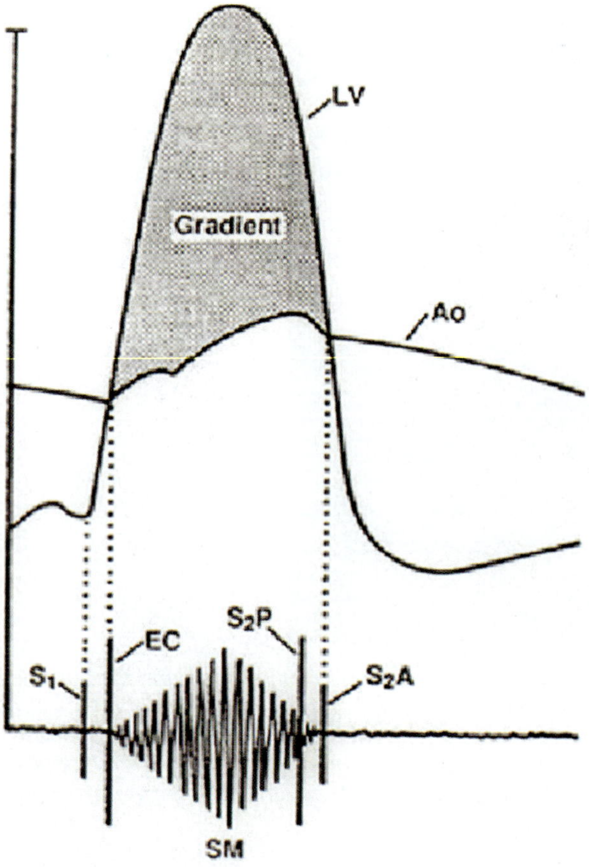

Fig. 14.97: *The diagram represents the pressure relationship in a patient with significant aortic valve stenosis. The narrowing of the aortic valve requires a marked increase in systolic pressure within the left ventricle (LV) to drive blood through the stenotic valve orifice with classical ejection click (EC) and systolic murmur (SM)*

Management

Surgical or balloon valvuloplasty (in younger patients) should be considered in a patient with AS who has heart failure, syncope or chest discomfort. A variety of surgical procedures are available including direct repair of the valve; replacement with a bioprosthesis or mechanical prosthesis; replacement of the valve and proximal aortic root with a cadaver homograft; and the Ross procedure, in which the abnormal bicuspid valve is removed surgically and replaced with the patient's native pulmonic valve, which in turn is replaced with a cadaver homograft. The Ross procedure eliminates the need for a prosthetic valve in the aortic position. Postoperative management focuses on assessment for recurrent stenosis or progressive AR (Figs 14.100 and 14.101).

BICUSPID AORTIC VALVE

A bicuspid aortic valve (BAV) is most commonly a congenital condition of the aortic valve where two of the aortic valvular leaflets fuse during development resulting in a valve that is bicuspid instead of the normal tricuspid configuration. Normally, the only cardiac valve that is bicuspid is the mitral valve (bicuspid valve) which is situated between the left atrium and the left ventricle. Cardiac valves play a crucial role in ensuring the unidirectional flow of blood from the atrium to the ventricles, or the ventricle to the aorta or pulmonary trunk.

Incidence/Prevalence

Bicuspid aortic valves are the most common cardiac valvular anomaly, occurring in 1–2% of the general population. It is twice as common in males as in females.

Bicuspid aortic valve is an inheritable condition, with a demonstrated association with Notch 1. Both familial clustering and isolated valve defects have been documented. The incidence of bicuspid aortic valve can be as high as 10% in families affected with the valve problem. Recent studies suggest that BAV is an autosomal dominant condition with incomplete penetrance. Other congenital heart defects are associated with bicuspid aortic valve at various frequencies including coarctation of the aorta.

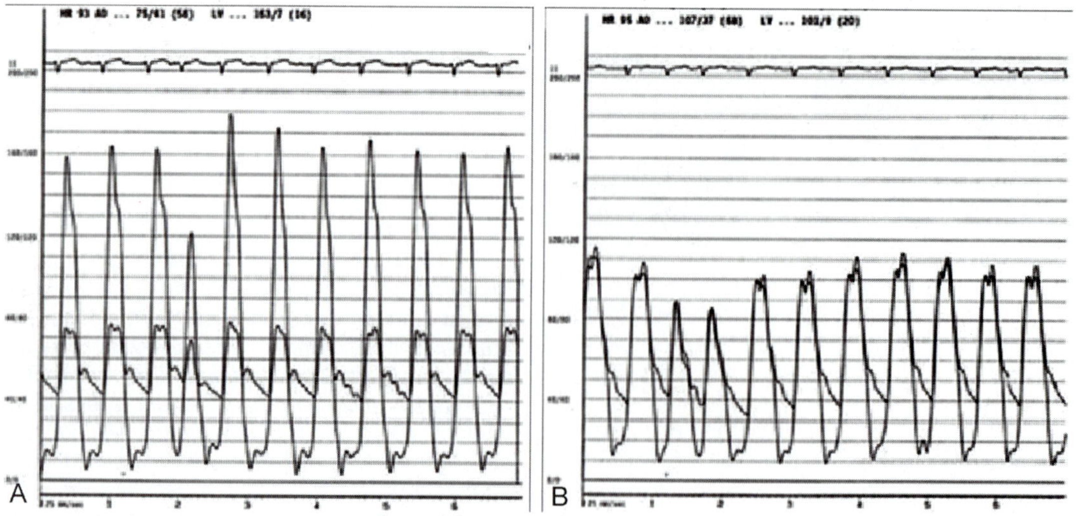

Fig. 14.98: *Intraventricular and intraaortic pressure gradients before (A) and after (B) aortic valve implantation*

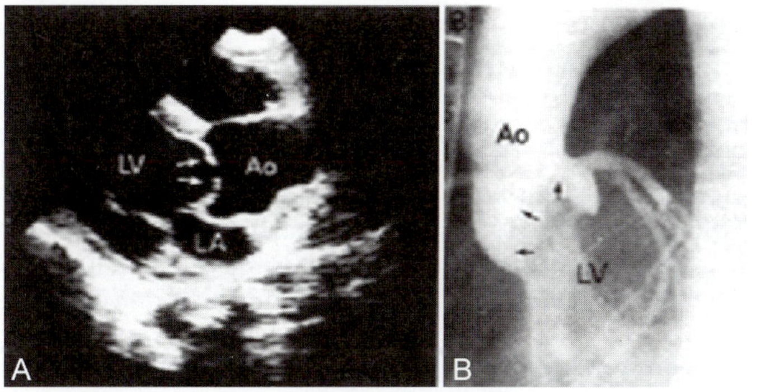

Fig. 14.99: *(A) 2D echocardiographic study with the transducer in the long-axis parasternal position demonstrating leaflet doming and thickening. (B) Aortogram from the same patient showing doming of the aortic valve leaflets. The negative shadow in the proximal aortic root (Ao) is caused by a jet of nonopacified blood from the left ventricle (LV) as it exits through the stenotic aortic valve*

Types of Bicuspid Aortic Valves

Bicuspid aortic valves may assume three different types of configuration (Figs 14.102A and B):

1. "Real" bicuspid valves with two symmetric leaflets
2. A tricuspid architecture with a fusion of two leaflets
3. A tricuspid architecture with a fusion of three leaflets.

Clinical Manifestations

In many cases, a bicuspid aortic valve will cause no problems. However, BAV may become calcified later in life, which may lead to varying degrees of severity of aortic stenosis that will manifest as murmurs. If the leaflets do not close correctly, aortic regurgitation can occur. If these become severe enough, they may require heart surgery. People with BAV may become tired more easily than those with normal valvular function and have difficulty maintaining stamina for cardio-intensive activities due to poor heart performance. The heart is put under more stress in order to either pump more blood through a stenotic valve or attempt to circulate regurgitation blood through a leaking valve.

Laboratory Studies

In the case of a child with bicuspid aortic valve and family history of hypercholesterolemia or early coronary artery disease, baseline cholesterol levels may be helpful in recommending dietary modification. Total and high-density lipoprotein (HDL) cholesterol or fasting lipid panel should be measured in children older than 3 years. Elevated low-density lipoprotein (LDL) cholesterol may accelerate sclerosis of the bicuspid aortic valve (Figs 14.104A and B).

Imaging Studies

Chest radiography may reveal mild prominence of the ascending aorta in the posteroanterior projection along the superior right heart border. Left ventricular enlargement implies progressive aortic valve insufficiency. Chest radiography is generally not helpful as a screening tool for bicuspid aortic valve (Figs 14.104A and B).

Echocardiography (Figs 14.104 to 14.109)

Two-dimensional echocardiography provides accurate confirmation of a bicuspid aortic valve. Two dimensional echocardiogram of typical bicuspid aortic valve in diastole and systole. Valve margins are thin and pliable and open widely, creating the fishmouth appearance. Imaging can show the bicuspid aortic valve in multiple planes. Most important information is obtained from the parasternal long-axis and short-axis views.

The long-axis view reveals the typical systolic doming due to limited valve opening. An approximation of valve orifice diameter can be obtained at peak systole. This view is also important for sizing the sinus of valsalva, sinotubular junction and ascending aorta. Parasternal long-axis echocardiogram showing doming of a bicuspid aortic valve. The short-axis view is used to examine commissures, leaflet morphology, mobility, and the presence or absence of a low raphe. The diameter or area of the valve opening is

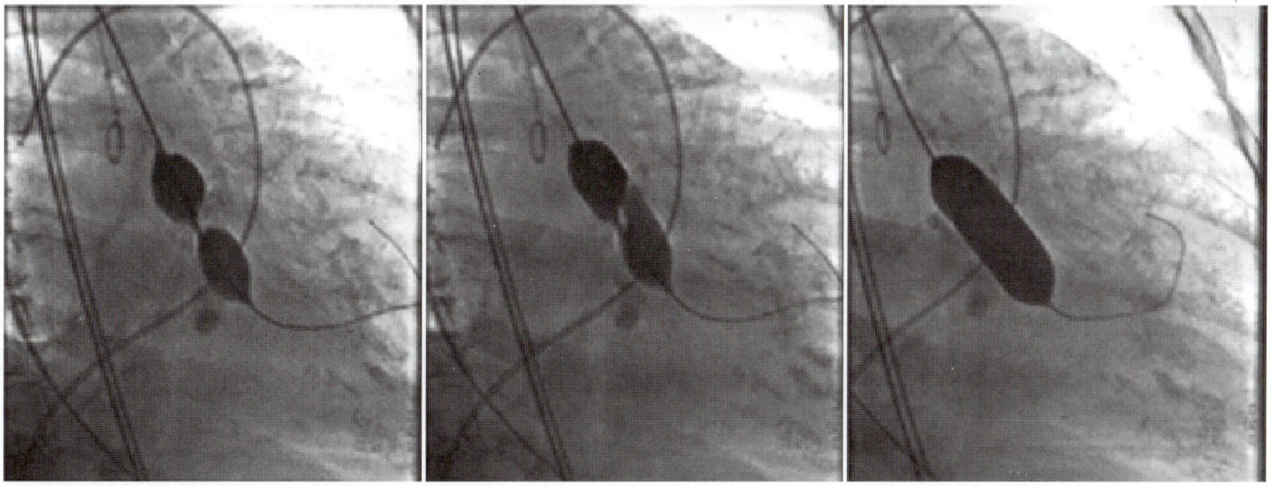

Fig. 14.100: *(A) Shows full waist after balloon position at aortic valve level. (B) Showed less waist in a partially opened valve and Complete disappreance of the waist after the valve has been fully dilated (right)*

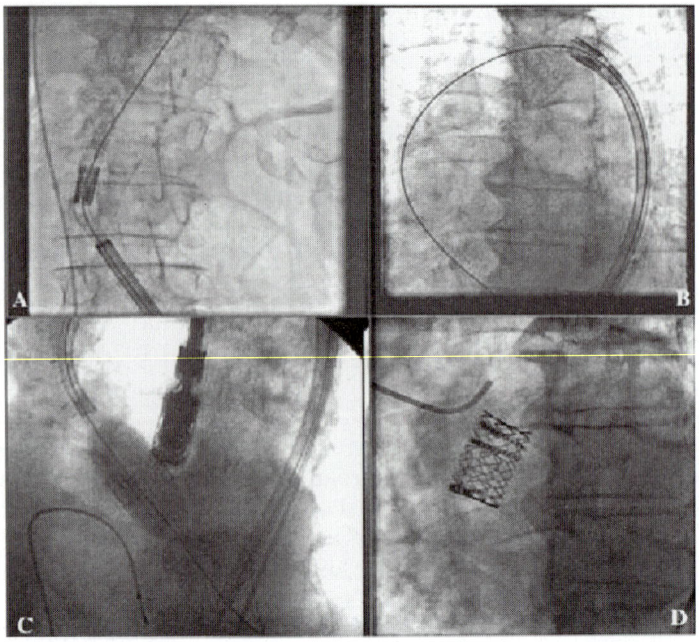

Fig. 14.101: *Percutaneous implantation of aortic prosthetic valve in aortic valvular stenosis. Angiographic sequence of device implantation in the aortic valve. (A) Catheter introduction through the femoral artery. (B) Catheter deflection in the aortic arch. (C) Prosthesis inflation. (D) Angiographic outcome*

generally overestimated in this view because the true orifice usually lies above this plane. The bicuspid valve typically looks like a fish's mouth on opening. Parasternal short-axis echocardiographic view in diastole, showing bicuspid aortic valve with nearly equal cusp size and right-left orientation of the commissure. Note the two color signals showing minimal aortic insufficiency.

Doppler measurements of peak and mean systolic velocities and gradients can be recorded from the apical five-chamber, the suprasternal, or the high right parasternal views. Doppler signal should be lined up as closely as possible and parallel to the jet to provide accurate estimates of flow velocities. Estimates of flow velocity from the apical view can sometimes be improved by moving the transducer more medially toward the sternum.

Parasternal long-axis and short-axis views can also be used for color Doppler studies, which evaluate for aortic insufficiency. The severity of aortic valve insufficiency can be assessed by several methods. One of the simplest and most reliable is to measure the insufficiency jet diameter at the aortic valve annulus and compare this diameter to the annulus diameter.

False-positive diagnosis of bicuspid aortic valve may arise from incomplete demonstration of all three valve closure lines. The typical normal (trileaflet) aortic valve shows a rotated Mercedes sign on closure. The bicuspid valve may not be recognized if a high raphe is observed with valve closure.

Angiography

The bicuspid aortic valve is viewed best in the anteroposterior 30° right anterior oblique (RAO) projection. Injection is into the left ventricle and also into the aortic root.

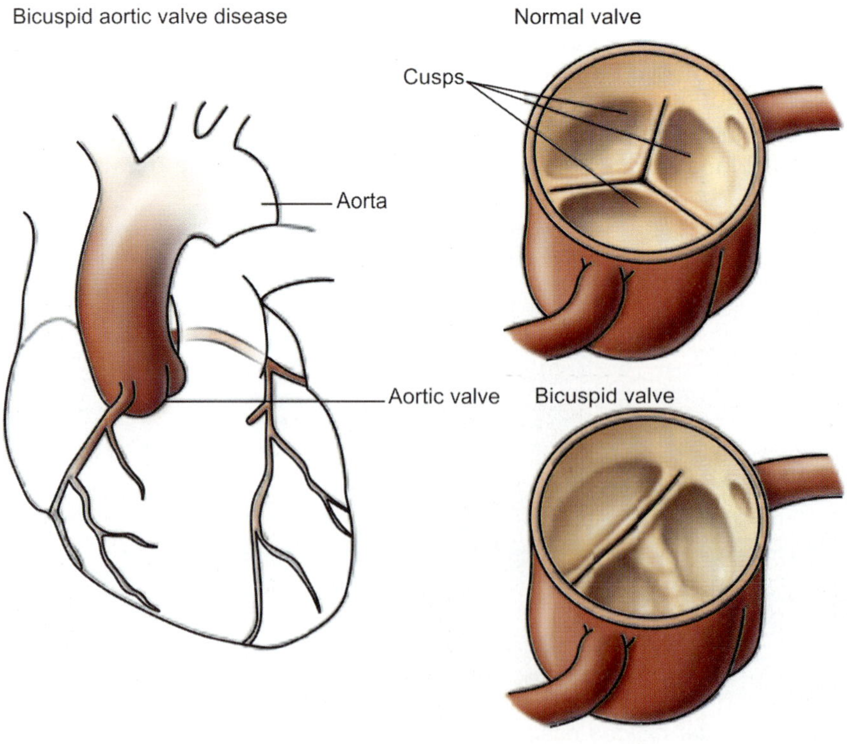

Fig. 14.102: *Normal tricuspid aortic valve (top) and bicuspid valve (bottom) in adult*

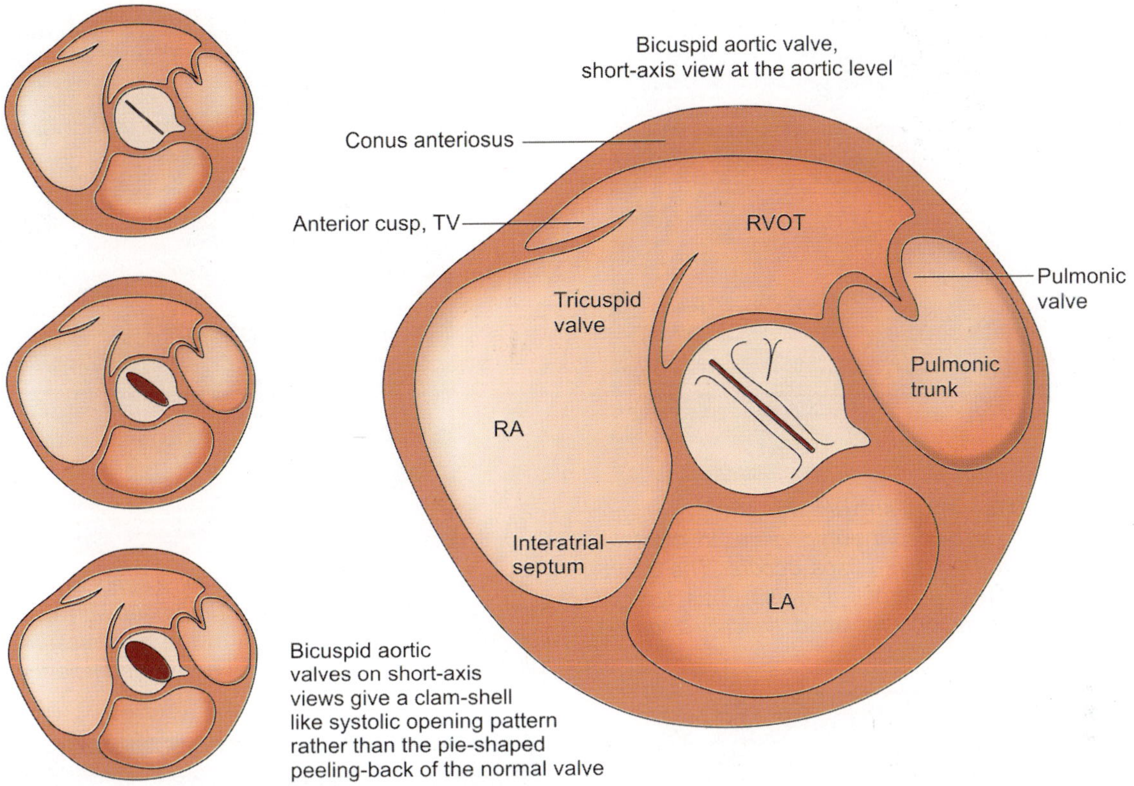

Fig. 14.103: *Anatomy of bicuspid aortic valve*

Electrocardiography

ECG findings are generally normal for an isolated bicuspid aortic valve without stenosis or insufficiency.

Progression of stenosis or insufficiency leads to left atrial enlargement and left ventricular hypertrophy.

Testing in Family Members

Two dimensional echocardiography is recommended as a screening tool for the offspring and first-degree relatives (especially males) of patients identified as having a bicuspid aortic valve because a high recurrence rate (as much as 12–17%) has been shown in several families.

Angiography is not the primary diagnostic method to diagnose a bicuspid aortic valve.

Typical finding is systolic doming of the valve margins due to incomplete opening.

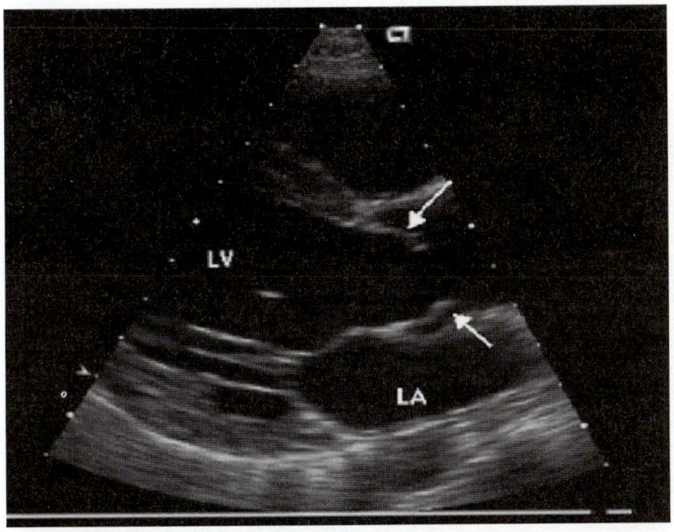

Fig. 14.104A: *Parasternal long-axis echocardiogram showing doming of a bicuspid aortic valve*

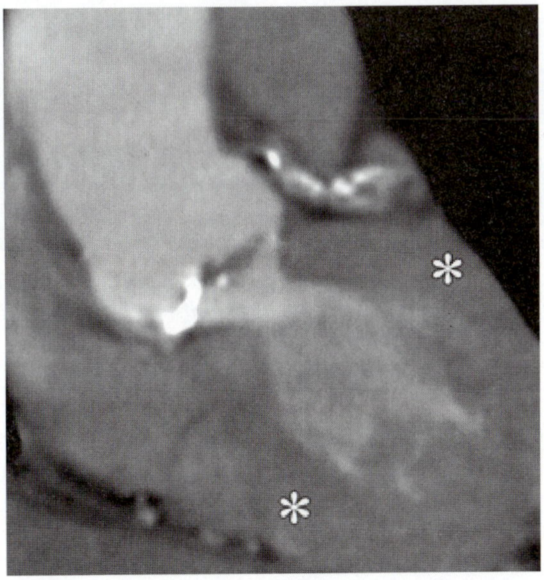

Fig. 14.104B: *Oblique MIP reformatted images show thickening and coarse calcification of the cusps of the aortic valve. Secondary findings include marked left ventricular hypertrophy (*)*

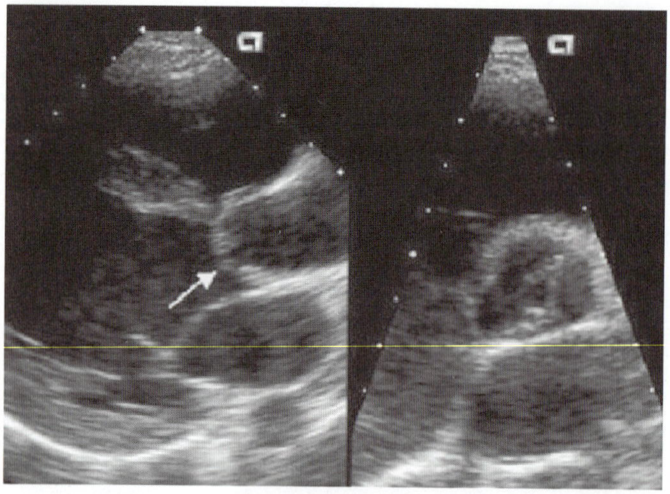

Fig. 14.105: *Long-axis and short-axis transthoracic echocardiograms showing a bicuspid aortic valve. In diastole, hammocking (prolapse) of the valve cusps occurs. The short-axis view shows the irregular sclerotic margins. This type of bicuspid valve is the most commonly replaced, typically because of insufficiency*

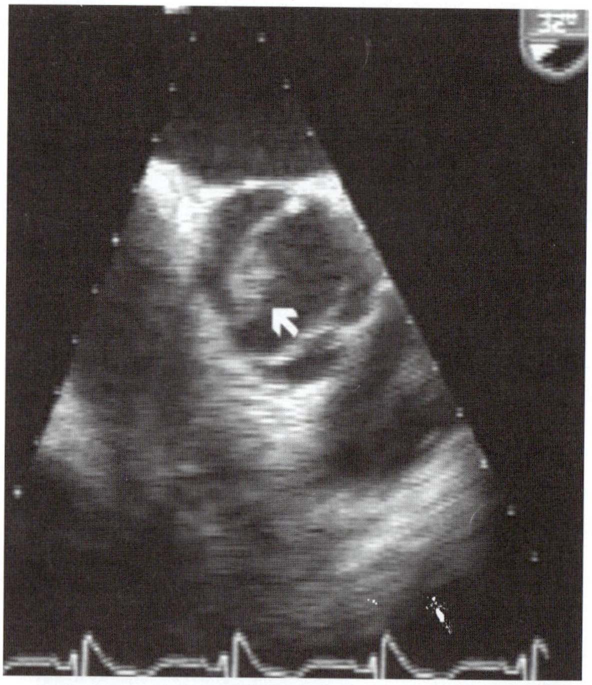

Fig. 14.106: *Basilar oblique transesophageal image showing congenitally bicuspid aortic valve with vegetation (due to Streptococcus viridans endocarditis)*

Aortic insufficiency can be looked for on the aortic root injection.

MRI: It is generally not helpful for the diagnosis of bicuspid aortic valve alone but may be helpful for complete assessment of the thoracic aorta, particularly in cases of coarctation, Turner syndrome, or Williams syndrome (Figs 14.110 and 14.111).

Transesophageal echocardiography: It may be necessary to define valve commissures and vegetations in adolescents

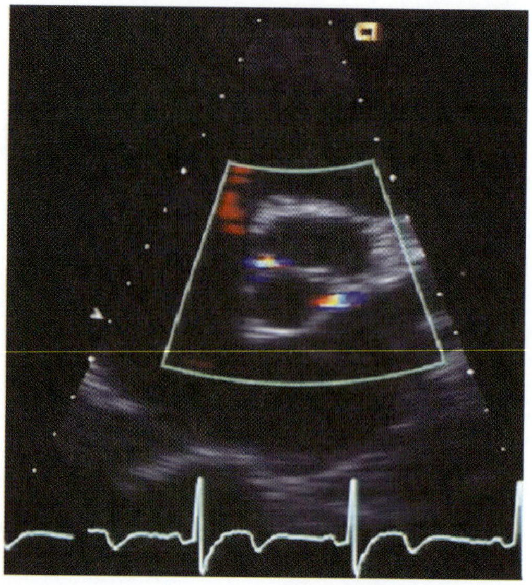

Fig. 14.107: *Parasternal short-axis echocardiographic view in diastole, showing bicuspid aortic valve with nearly equal cusp size and right-left orientation of the commissure. Note the two color signals showing minimal aortic insufficiency*

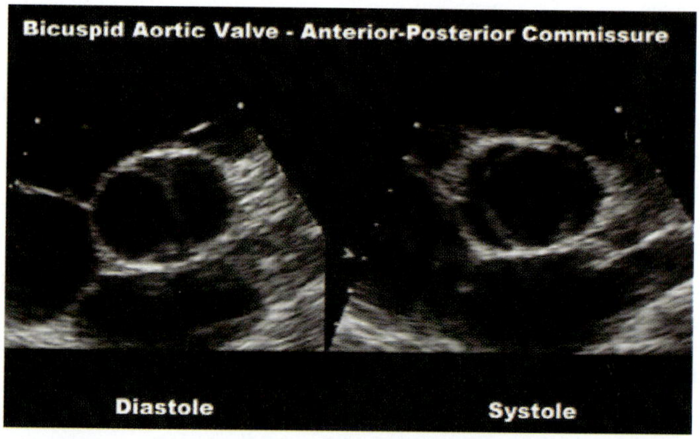

Fig. 14.108: *Two dimensional echocardiogram of typical bicuspid aortic valve in diastole and systole. Valve margins are thin and pliable and open widely, creating the fish-mouth appearance*

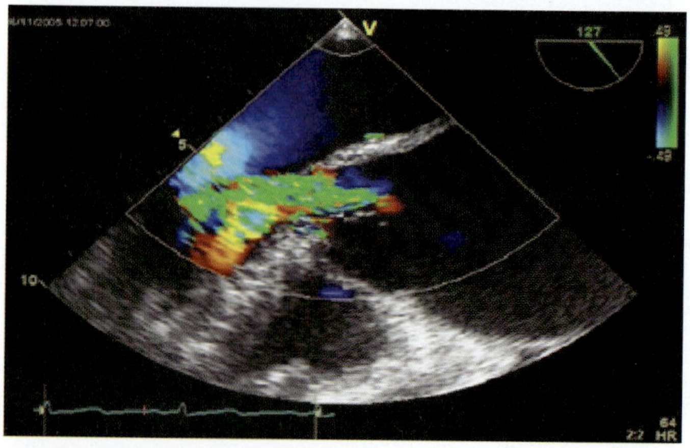

Fig. 14.109: *TEE scan showing color Doppler echoscan in bicuspid aortic stenosis with AR*

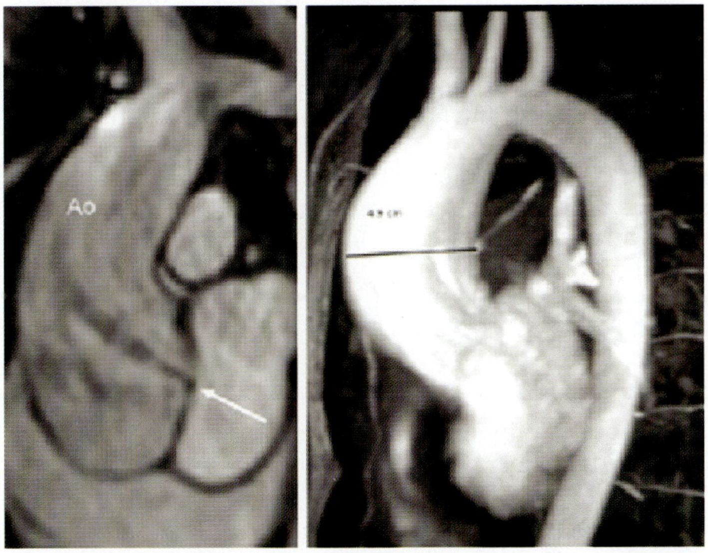

Fig. 14.110: *Patients with bicuspid aortic valves often have enlargement of the ascending aorta, regardless of valve function as shown here in both cine imaging (left) and MR angiography (right). Enlargement may be found at any level of the ascending aorta, and CMR can help define and follow diameter over time, to guide decisions about potential aortoplasty. CMR is preferred over computed tomography for this purpose in younger patients needing serial study. Ao, aorta*

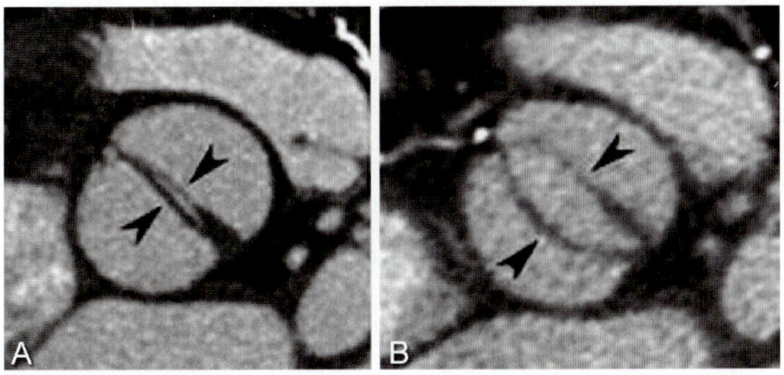

Fig. 14.111: *MRI. Bicuspid aortic valve with regurgitation and minimal restriction of motion. (A) diastolic image in short axis of the aortic valve demonstrates a linear closure of the aortic valve with only two leaflets (arrowheads). A small regurgitant orifice is visible between the mildly thick leaflets. The more anterior leaflet is in the position that would typically be occupied by the right and left coronary leaflets. (B) Systolic image in short axis of the aortic valve demonstrates a "fish-mouth"-shaped opening of the two leaflets (arrowheads) that is typical for a bicuspid valve. The overall aortic valve area is minimally restricted (2 cm² by planimetry)*

or young adults in whom bicuspid aortic valve is suspected on clinical grounds (particularly those with symptoms or findings that suggest infective endocarditis) (Fig. 14.106).

Medical Care

No specific medical care is required for individuals with bicuspid aortic valve unless they have progressive deterioration or infection. Serial follow-up evaluations are important for early recognition of potential complications (valve insufficiency, valve stenosis, progressive aortic root dilation) and the prevention of possible bacterial endocarditis.

Surgical Care

Surgery specifically for bicuspid aortic valve is not necessary unless progressive complications ensue (valve insufficiency, valve stenosis, progressive aortic root dilatation, possible bacterial endocarditis).

The patient with known bicuspid aortic valve no longer requires antibiotic prophylaxis for invasive dental or noncardiac surgical procedures. If endocarditis has occurred on a bicuspid aortic valve, antibiotic prophylaxis is recommended.

For noncardiac procedures, preoperative cardiac evaluation may be appropriate, particularly for patients with aortic stenosis or insufficiency. The patient with simple, uncomplicated bicuspid aortic valve should not require special anesthetic precautions, other than bacterial endocarditis prophylaxis when appropriate.

Diet

Because hypercholesterolemia and other coronary artery disease risk factors may accelerate the sclerosis and deterioration of a congenitally bicuspid aortic valve, a heart-healthy diet is recommended for all patients, not only those with recognized risk factors. This diet should limit fat calories to no more than 30% of total calories. Calories from saturated fats should be limited to no more than 10% of total.

Activity

Patients with normally functioning bicuspid aortic valves (i.e. no stenosis or insufficiency) do not require activity restrictions. They may participate in organized competitive sports activities after echocardiography or MRI to assess for dilated aorta.

Patients who develop valve insufficiency or stenosis from a congenitally bicuspid aortic valve may require restrictions from strenuous competitive sports. Patients with aortic valve insufficiency should avoid strenuous isometric activity, such as weight lifting, rope climbing, and pull-ups.

Medication

Patients with bicuspid aortic valve are at increased risk for infective endocarditis. Prophylactic antibiotics are no longer required for dental or surgical procedures as recommended by the American Heart Association but are recommended to prevent recurrence if an episode of endocarditis has occurred.

Complications

Overall complication rates in patients with bicuspid aortic valves vary. In general, bicuspid aortic valve may be a common reason for acceleration of the normal aging process (e.g. valve sclerosis, calcification). Four specific complications are related to the congenitally bicuspid aortic valve.

1. *Aortic Stenosis*

Sclerosis of the bicuspid aortic valve generally begins in the second decade of life, and calcification becomes more concerning during and after the fourth decade of life. The presence of coronary risk factors (e.g. smoking, hypercholesterolemia) may accelerate these processes. Approximately 50% of adults with severe aortic stenosis have a congenitally bicuspid valve.

Historically, rheumatic fever was the most common cause of aortic stenosis. With significantly decreasing incidence of rheumatic fever in developed nations, bicuspid aortic valve is the most common cause of aortic stenosis in adults and is probably the most common etiology of valve insufficiency as well. Acute rheumatic fever and its recurrences are still a major problem in developing countries, and, in these areas, long-term effects of rheumatic fever are still more significant than bicuspid valve in the etiology of aortic stenosis and insufficiency. Rheumatic aortic valve damage can be confirmed only at surgery or autopsy by the presence of Aschoff bodies.

2. *Aortic Insufficiency*

Most cases of severe aortic insufficiency are related, either directly or indirectly, to a congenitally bicuspid valve. Numerous factors may contribute to development of aortic valve insufficiency. These include cusp prolapse, erosion of irregular commissure lines, aortic root dilatation (particularly at the sinotubular junction or supra-aortic ridge), infective endocarditis, and systemic hypertension (particularly with coarctation).

3. *Infective Endocarditis*

The risk of developing infective endocarditis on a bicuspid aortic valve is 10–30% over a lifetime. Bicuspid aortic valve is the second most common congenital etiology for infective endocarditis in infants and children; overall, approximately 25% of endocarditis infections develop on a bicuspid valve.

4. *Aortic Root Dissection*

Findings on histologic studies of the aortic root in individuals with bicuspid aortic valve are controversial. Enlargement of the root is often attributed to poststenotic dilatation. However, the root may dilate without significant valve stenosis, and abnormal histology with broken elastic fibers and other findings suggestive of Marfan syndrome has been identified in numerous studies.

The risk of aortic root dissection is much higher for individuals with Marfan syndrome (approximately 40%) than for those with bicuspid aortic valve (approximately 5%). However, because bicuspid aortic valve is more prevalent in the general population, this disorder is more commonly associated with aortic root dissection.

A population-based, retrospective cohort study assessed the complications of patients with bicuspid aortic valve living in Olmsted County, Minnesota. Of the 416 patients studied over a mean follow-up of 16 years, reported incidence of aortic dissection was low (2 of 416), but it was significantly higher than in the general population.

Prognosis

Overall prognosis for the individual with bicuspid aortic valve is good. Reviews and reports in the past have emphasized the fairly benign course for patients with bicuspid valves. However, more recent reports on the natural history of these valves suggest numerous more serious problems and an acceleration of normal valvular wear and tear. These problems may not develop until adulthood. Routine and regular follow-up for the child or adolescent with bicuspid aortic valve is recommended.

Patient Education

Patient and family education should emphasize the fairly benign course for the child with bicuspid aortic valve.

Older children and adolescents should begin to be made aware of the accelerated aging processes (i.e. progressive stenosis), with particular attention to coronary risk factors.

The importance of bicuspid aortic valve as a potential substrate for infective endocarditis should be emphasized. Good oral and dental hygiene is important.

Most young individuals with bicuspid aortic valve should not require restrictions in physical activity or sports participation unless they have stenosis or insufficiency. Routine examination is recommended prior to sports participation at least once.

The condition can be associated with a heart murmur located at the right second intercostal space. Often there will be differences in blood pressures between upper and lower extremities. The diagnosis can be assisted with echocardiography or magnetic resonance imaging (MRI).

Most patients with bicuspid aortic valve whose valve becomes dysfunctional will need careful follow-up and potentially valve replacement at some point in life. Regular echocardiography and MRI may be performed. For diagnosed patients, genetic testing is done to allow for future offspring with the disease to be monitored and treated early in life.

Patients with bicuspid aortic valve should be followed by a cardiologist or cardiac surgeon with specific interest in this valve pathology.

If the valve is normally functioning or minimally dysfunctional, average lifespan is similar to that of those without the anomaly.

SUBVALVULAR AORTIC STENOSIS

Anatomy

Subaortic membrane is a fibrous membrane below the aortic valve that may involve the ventricular septum, the anterior leaflet of the mitral valve, and the aortic valve itself. It may be associated with other structural anomalies of the aortic valve, such as bicuspid aortic valve, and other abnormalities of the left ventricular outflow tract, such as in atrioventricular canal or tunnel subaortic stenosis (Fig. 14.112).

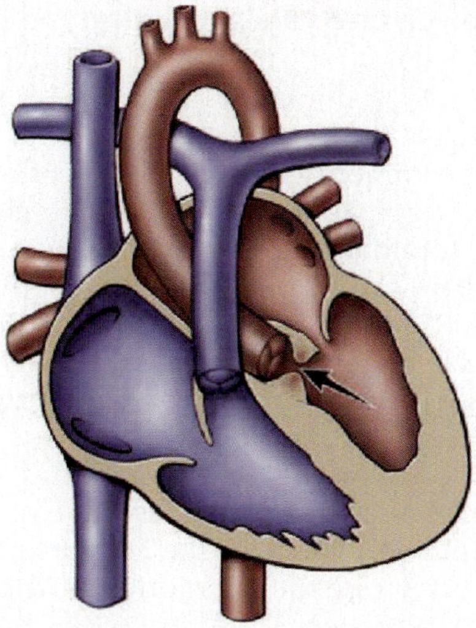

Fig. 14.112: *Anatomy showing location of subvalvular aortic stenosis (arrow)*

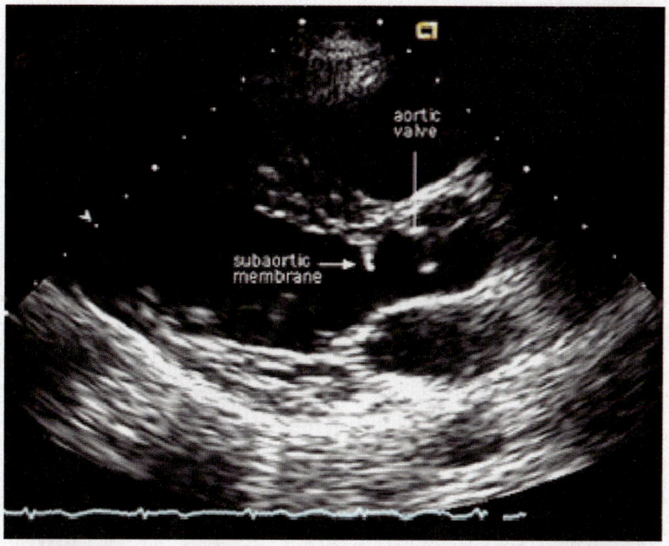

Fig. 14.113: *Subvalvular stenosis in transthoracic LAX view demonstrating a membrane in the out flow tract of the aorta below the aortic valve*

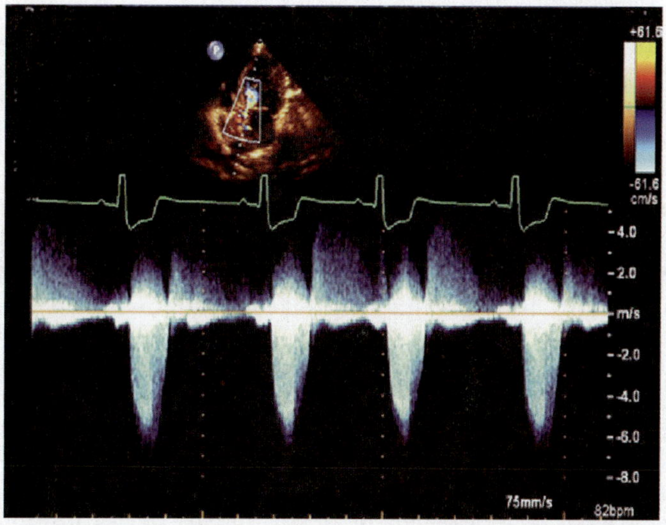

Fig. 14.114: *Left parasternal two dimensional five chamber apical echocardiographic view from a patient with severe subaortic stenosis. There is evidence of severe stenosis with a velocity of 6 m/s (144 mmHg) and aortic insufficieny during diastole*

Physiology and Pathology

The subaortic stenosis causes problems in several different ways. It may obstruct left ventricular outflow and cause subaortic stenosis. The resultant effects are essentially the same as valvular aortic stenosis: left ventricular hypertrophy from the pressure overload, myocardial ischemia (too little blood flow to the heart which may cause a heart attack) heart failure, and sudden death.

In addition, a subaortic membrane may alter left ventricular outflow dynamics and harm the aortic valve without any significant obstructive component. The abnormal flows cause aortic insufficiency (a leaking aortic valve) and permanent structural damage to the aortic valve.

There may be other effects from subaortic membrane as well including permanent damage to the mitral valve and direct damage to the aortic valve if the membrane grows up into the aortic valve itself.

The abnormal flow characteristics that initiate the growth of a subaortic membrane may allow the regrowth of the membrane, even after complete resection.

Echocardiography: It is helpful in the diagnosis of subaortic membrane in relationship with surrounding anatomy of LVOT and native aortic valve (Figs 14.113 and 14.114).

Cineangiography: It can evaluate both aortic annulus and subaortic lesions in the presence of subaortic stenosis (Fig. 14.115).

Surgical Indications and Approach

Surgery is indicated when (a) the subaortic stenosis becomes hemodynamically significant, that is, when the gradient increases to the point that there is a significant pressure load on the left ventricle or (b) when there is any evidence that the aortic valve is involved, that is, by presence of any aortic insufficiency whatsoever.

Surgery for subaortic membrane requires complete removal of the membrane and frequently may involve resection of septal muscle as well.

Fixed subaortic stenosis occurs when fibromuscular tissue develops in the left ventricular outflow tract and obstructs flow. Subaortic stenosis is rarely seen in infancy, but typically develops and becomes more severely obstructive in childhood. It presents usually as an asymptomatic ejection systolic murmur with a suprasternal thrill, but without an ejection click.

Echocardiographic studies have suggested that subaortic stenosis may be caused by localized tissue proliferation in response to flow disturbance in the left ventricular outflow tract. The progressive development of increasingly severe left ventricular outflow tractobstruction and aortic valve regurgitation are the main concerns. Fixed lesions causing

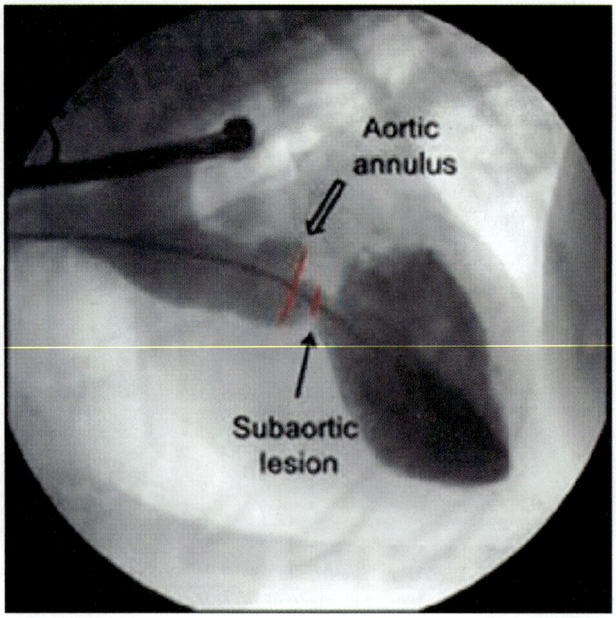

Fig. 14.115: *Cineangiogram showing subaortic stenosis*

important obstruction require surgical resection; the management of mild to moderate obstruction is controversial, but requires as a minimum careful serial echocardiographic assessment to detect progression.

SUPRAVALVULAR AORTIC STENOSIS

Supravalvular aortic stenosis (SVAS) is a fixed form of congenital left ventricular outflow tract (LVOT) obstruction that occurs as a localized or diffuse narrowing of the ascending aorta beyond the superior margin of the sinuses of valsalva. It accounts for less than 7% of all fixed forms of congenital LVOT obstructive lesions. SVAS may occur sporadically, as a manifestation of elastin arteriopathy, or as part of Williams syndrome (also known as Williams-Beuren syndrome), an autosomal dominant genetic disorder. The sporadic form of SVAS is the most common (>50%) presentation. There is no known risk factor to account for these cases. A less common presentation of SVAS is a familial form caused by autosomal dominant inheritance. Like the sporadic form, it is not a part of Williams syndrome.

Patients with SVAS usually become symptomatic during childhood, but cases associated with Williams syndrome are usually identified during infancy. The diagnosis of Williams syndrome can be established with cytogenic analysis which means that this diagnosis can be made in utero using chorionic villus tissue. Therefore, SVAS can be detected prenatally, particularly in patients with Williams syndrome if it is revealed with fetal echocardiography.

The anatomic diagnosis of SVAS can reliably be made from 2-dimensional (2D) echocardiography that uses multiple views, including parasternal, apical long-axis, and suprasternal (see Workup). Cardiac catheterization or MRI may be indicated to evaluate the coronary artery or aortic arch anatomy. Surgery is the primary treatment for SVAS. The choice of procedure varies with the type and severity of the stenosis.

Anatomy (Fig. 14.116)

SVAS has three commonly recognized morphologic forms. An external hourglass deformity of the aorta with a corresponding luminal narrowing at a level just distal to the coronary artery ostia is present in 50–75% of patients. In approximately 25% of patients, a fibrous diaphragm is present just distal to the coronary artery ostia. In fewer than 25% of patients, a diffuse narrowing along a variable length of ascending aorta is present.

Similarly, the following three anatomic subtypes of coronary lesions have been recognized in SVAS:

- Circumferential narrowing of the left coronary ostium
- Ostial obstruction due to fusion of the aortic cusp to the supravalvular ridge
- Diffuse narrowing of the left coronary artery.

Pathophysiology

The origins of the coronary arteries proximal to the obstruction site have the same systolic pressure as the left ventricle (LV). Consequently, they become dilated and tortuous over time, with hypertrophy and intimal thickening. These changes predispose them to premature atherosclerosis. The hemodynamic consequences of coronary artery changes are increased total mean coronary flow but significantly decreased diastolic coronary flow which is the major determinant of the development of myocardial ischemia.

Concentric LV hypertrophy caused by SVAS exacerbates the problem of myocardial ischemia. In most patients, the jet of blood flow from SVAS has a preferential trajectory

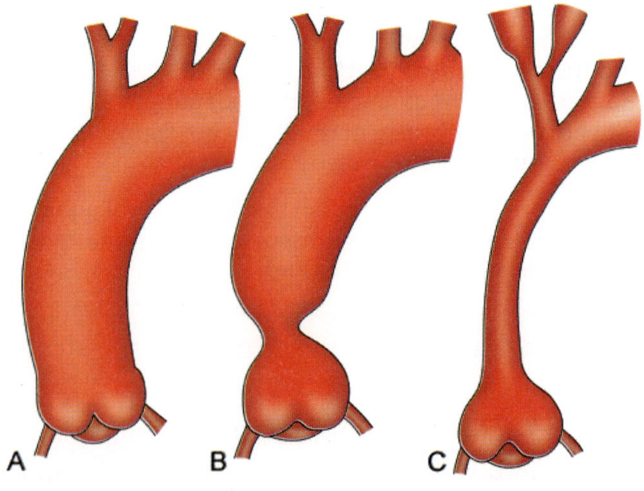

Fig. 14.116: *The anatomic types of supravalvular aortic stenosis: (A) normal; (B) and (C) two forms of supravalvular stenosis. The difference between these two forms is in the length of the obstruction, which sometimes involves virtually all of the ascending aorta. Note the obstructions in the innominate and common carotid arteries as they arise from the aortic arch. Other obstructions such as coarctation of the aorta, renal artery stenosis, and pulmonary artery stenosis, are found in some patients*

into the brachiocephalic vessels, the so-called Coanda effect; this accounts for a marked increase in the right upper extremity systolic pressure relative to the left. Complications of SVAS also include progressive coronary osteal stenosis, infective endocarditis and sudden death.

Historical Background

Symptoms caused by SVAS usually develop in childhood. Rarely, symptoms develop in infancy; in some cases, symptoms develop in the second or third decade of life.

Most pediatric patients present because of a heart murmur or the features of Williams syndrome. Patients with Williams syndrome may also develop systemic hypertension and involvement of joints, peripheral pulmonary artery stenosis, coarctation of aorta, and mitral insufficiency.

Dyspnea on exertion, angina, and syncope develop in the course of the disease if SVAS is untreated. These symptoms indicate at least a moderate degree of LVOT obstruction. Because of the coronary artery involvement, angina may arise early and more often than in other obstructive LVOT lesions. Because of the risk of sudden death in SVAS, the development of angina and syncope should prompt immediate investigation.

Etiological Factors

The precise etiology of SVAS is unknown. The disease's high association with Williams syndrome, a genetic disorder caused by a hemizygous deletion or mutation of the elastin gene at band 7q11 suggests that defective connective tissue formation contributes to its pathology.

Patients with the sporadic form of SVAS may have associated peripheral pulmonary artery stenosis. There is no known risk factor for sporadic SVAS. As previously stated, a less common presentation of SVAS is a familial form caused by autosomal dominant inheritance.

Physical Examination

The physical examination focuses on upper extremity pulses, the precordium, heart sounds, and heart murmurs (Fig. 14.117).

Asymmetrical Upper Extremities Pulses

Discrepancies between carotid pulsations and upper extremity pulses and blood pressure are the characteristic clinical findings in SVAS. The discrepancies occur because the jet of blood flow from SVAS has a preferential trajectory into the brachiocephalic (innominate) artery (i.e. Coanda effect).

Precordium: The precordium is usually hyperdynamic, and the apex of the heart is displaced laterally and inferiorly because of ventricular hypertrophy. A thrill in the suprasternal notch is usually felt because of the trajectory of the blood flow jet from SVAS heart sounds.

The first heart sound is generally normal. A narrowly split, single, or paradoxically split second heart sound and a fourth heart sound are present in severe SVAS.

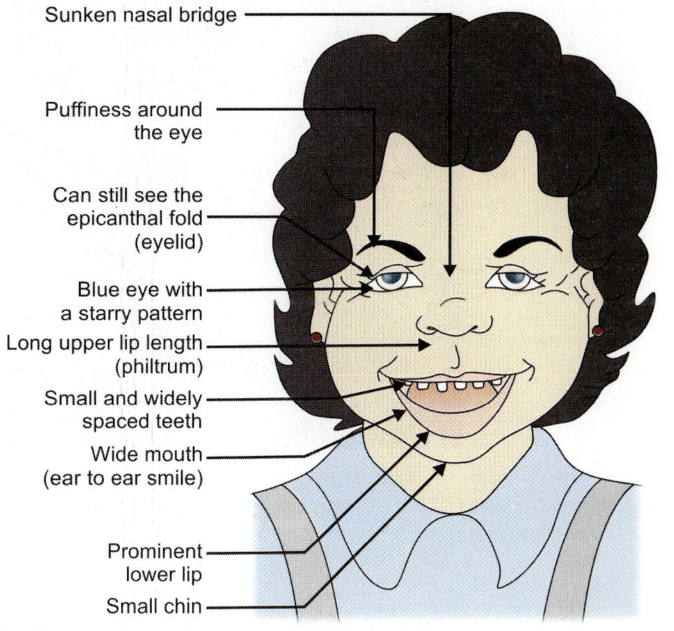

Fig. 14.117: *Various structural abnormalities in William syndrome as depicted on the face*

Heart Murmurs

The characteristic systolic murmur of SVAS is crescendo-decrescendo in shape, low pitched, and best heard at the base of the heart, sited higher than in valvular aortic stenosis. It mainly radiates to the right carotid artery and tends to peak during the last two-thirds of ventricular systole if the obstruction is severe. A high-pitched, short, early diastolic aortic regurgitation murmur is uncommon in SVAS, and an ejection click is absent.

Diagnositic Considerations

Supravalvular aortic stenosis (SVAS) should be considered in the differential diagnosis of children or infants presenting with a suspicious murmur or with signs of syncope, fatigue, angina, exercise intolerance, or left ventricular hypertrophy or dysfunction. Additionally, a cardiac evaluation should be performed with this diagnosis in mind in an infant or child with Williams syndrome. It should be differentiated from valvular and subvalvular aortic stenosis. This differentiation can be made through the use of pulse wave echocardiography to delineate the level of obstruction and through measurements of the aorta above the level of the sinotubular junction. Cardiac catheterization or MRI is frequently indicated after the diagnosis of SVAS is made in order to evaluate for coronary involvement or stenosis of the arch vessels.

Laboratory Investigations

SVAS produces abnormalities that are evident on electrocardiography (ECG) and chest radiography. These include increased left ventricular voltages from left ventricular hypertrophy. ST and T wave changes may be present if there is coronary involvement. Additionally, if right ventricular outflow tract obstruction is present, there

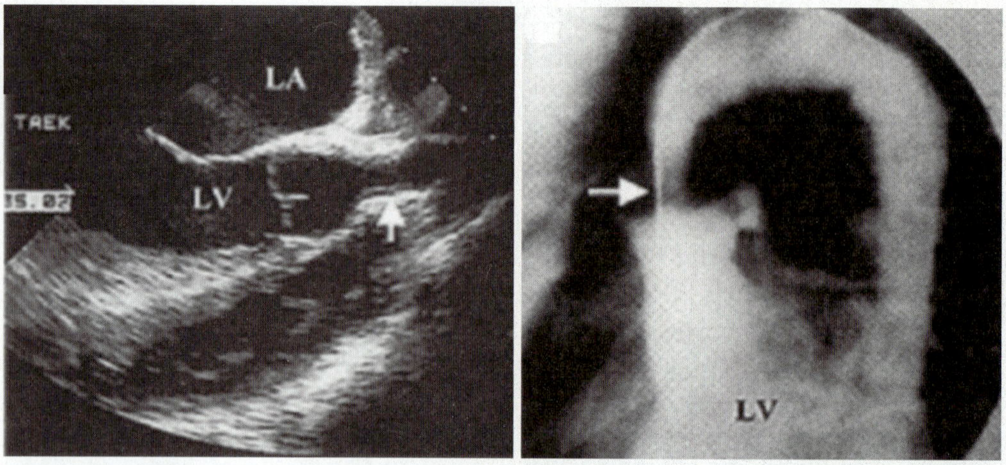

Fig. 14.118A and B: *(A) TEE showing supravalvular aortic stenosis, discrete type. (B) Left ventricular catheter angiogram demonstrates a discrete narrowing of the ascending aorta at the sinotubular junction, just above the sinuses of Valsalva (arrow). The distal ascending aorta and transverse aortic arch are relatively normal in size*

may be voltage criteria for right ventricular hypertrophy. The principal diagnostic test, however, is echocardiography. Cardiac catheterization along with angiography is indicated to evaluate the severity of the lesion and to confirm the coexisting anomalies prior to surgery if they cannot be accurately assessed with other modalities. MRI may be appropriate to evaluate for stenosis of the arch vessels or for better delineation of the anatomy if a catheterization is not being performed.

Echocardiography (Figs 14.18A and B; 14.119)

The anatomic diagnosis of SVAS can reliably be made from 2D echocardiography that uses multiple views, including parasternal, apical long-axis, and suprasternal In SVAS with hourglass deformity and diffuse hypoplasia, the diameter of the ascending aorta is smaller than that of the aortic root. In SVAS with fibrous diaphragm, the external ascending aortic diameter is normal although an echogenic membrane is commonly observed above the sinuses of valsalva.

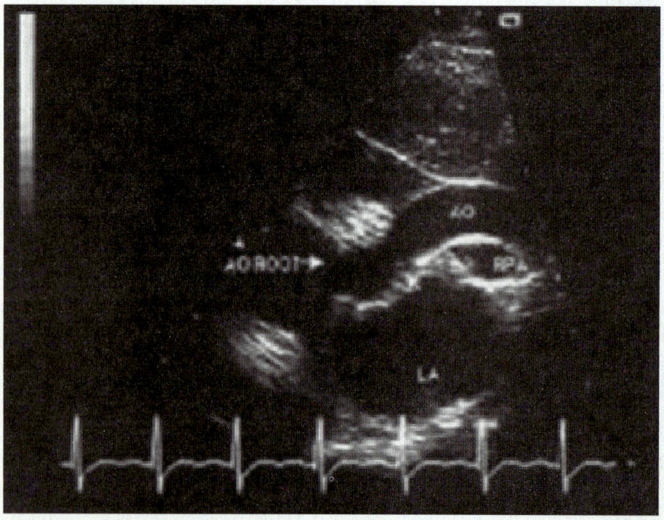

Fig. 14.119: *Two dimensional suprasternal echocardiographic image of supravalvular aortic stenosis*

Turbulent color flow mapping indicates the site of hemodynamically significant obstruction and can reveal coronary ostial stenosis, the incidence of which is high in SVAS.

Doppler peak gradient overestimates and, therefore, does not predict catheter-measured gradient well in patients with SVAS and may not be reliable in assessing its severity and guiding the need for intervention.

Cardiac Catheterization

A retrograde aortic catheterization with an end-hole catheter can be used to localize the site of obstruction by showing the pressure gradient above the aortic valve on pullback tracing. Blade balloon angioplasty has been effective for associated peripheral pulmonary artery stenosis when conventional balloon angioplasty fails.

Complications include blood vessel rupture, tachyarrhythmias, bradyarrhythmias, and vascular occlusion. Postcatheterization precautions are for hemorrhage, vascular disruption after balloon dilation, pain, nausea and vomiting, and arterial or venous obstruction from thrombosis or spasm.

Cardiac asystole and mortality due to coronary events have been reported during catheterization and during the postprocedure period. Cardiac catheterization should therefore be performed only if clearly indicated and should be done undergeneral anesthesia, which should be undertaken with close supervision and administered by an experienced anesthesiologist.

Chest Radiography

On chest radiography, the cardiac silhouette may be variably increased, and the ascending aorta may be asymmetrically dilated. The presence of both findings indicates hemodynamically significant SVAS.

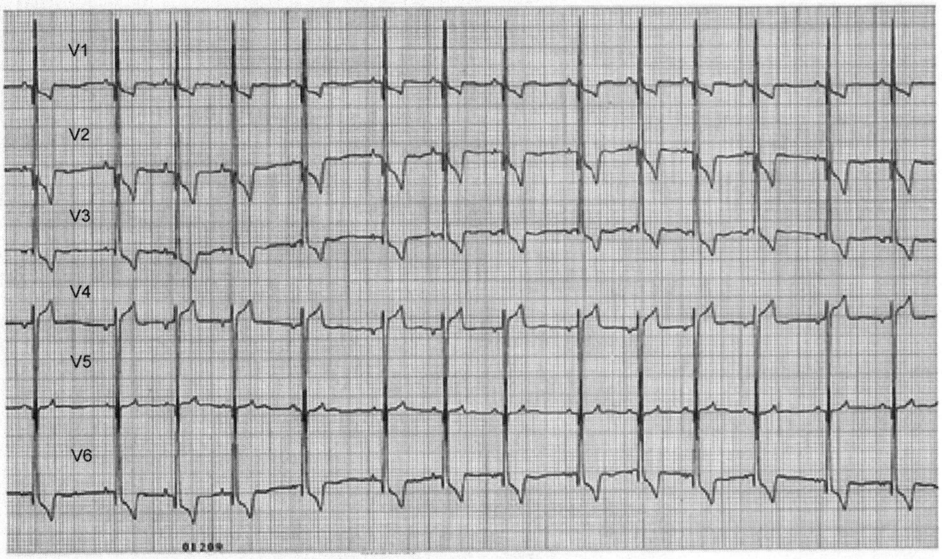

Fig. 14.120: *Supra valvular aortic stenosis. Six lead ECG recording from a boxer with severe aortic stenosis. Notice the increased R wave amplitude and S-T segment depression consistent with left ventricular hypertrophy and myocardial hypoxia, respectively*

Electrocardiography

ECG usually reveals left ventricular hypertrophy, depending on the severity of stenosis. ST/T segment changes may be present with involvement of coronary ostia and the coronary arteries. Right ventricular hypertrophy may be present if there is associated right ventricular outflow tract obstruction (Fig. 14.120).

Cineangiography

A biplane left ventriculogram and an aortogram can reveal the morphology of supravalvular narrowing, stenosis of the arch vessels, aortic root abnormalities, and dilated coronary arteries (see the image below). Right ventricular or pulmonary arterial angiography should be performed simultaneously in order to discern the presence of peripheral pulmonary artery stenosis, particularly in Williams syndrome (Fig. 14.121).

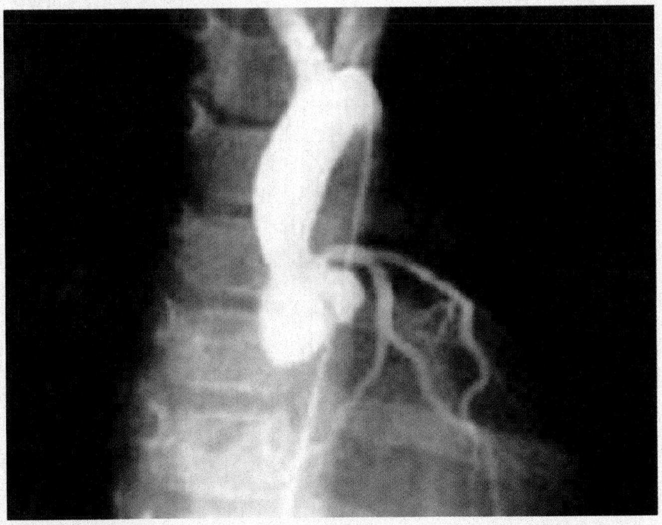

Fig. 14.121: *Aortogram of a patient with supravalvular aortic stenosis and dilated sinus of valsalva*

Magnetic Resonance Imaging

Although magnetic resonance imaging (MRI) can provide high definition of SVAS, obtaining an MRI in infants and young children may require sedation, which carries a risk of sudden death. Therefore, this study should be undertaken with close supervision and administered by an experienced anesthesiologist. MRI may be particularly useful in delineating aortic arch anatomy and evaluating for stenosis of the arch vessels (Figs 14.122A to D).

Computed Tomography

Multislice computed tomography (CT) scanning with angiography can generate high-resolution images of aortic valve lesions within seconds. However, this test exposes the pediatric patient to radiation (Fig. 14.123).

Histologic Findings

Myocardial hypertrophy, coronary intimal hyperplasia, and atherosclerotic changes can be observed in most cases of SVAS. Subendocardial fibrosis may be present in severe cases of SVAS. Abnormal deposition of elastin in arterial walls of patients with SVAS has been seen which leads to the increased proliferation of arterial smooth muscle cells, resulting in the formation of hyperplastic intimal lesions.

Genetic Evaluation

Obtain a genetic evaluation for patients with SVAS to confirm the diagnosis of Williams syndrome, which is often associated with SVAS. Molecular diagnosis of Williams syndrome can be made by fluorescent in situ hybridization (FISH) using Williams probe.

Differential Diagnoses

1. Subvalvular aortic stenosis
2. Valvular aortic stenosis
3. Hypertrophic cardiomyopathy

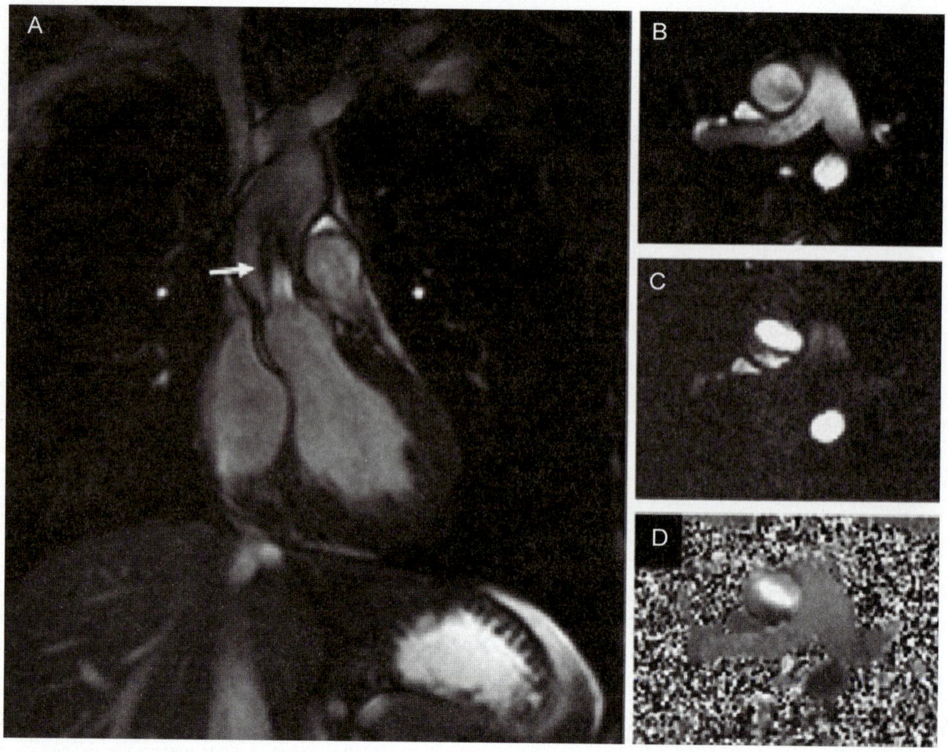

Fig. 14.122A to D: *Magnetic resonance imaging. Williams syndrome and supravalvular aortic stenosis. A flame-shaped area of signal dephasing results from turbulence beyond the affected level in A (arrow). (B-D) Magnitude and phase-sensitive images at the level of the stenosis. An elevated peak velocity of 281 cm/s was confirmed on flow quantification*

Prognosis

In one series, the actuarial survival rate following operative repair of SVAS was approximately 85% at 15 years. Overall survival including operative mortality, was 98% at 10 years and 97% at 20 years and at 30 years.

Postoperatively in this study, 73% of patients were in class I of the New York Heart Association's (NYHA) functional classification, and 27% were in NYHA functional class II. Most patients did not require reoperation.

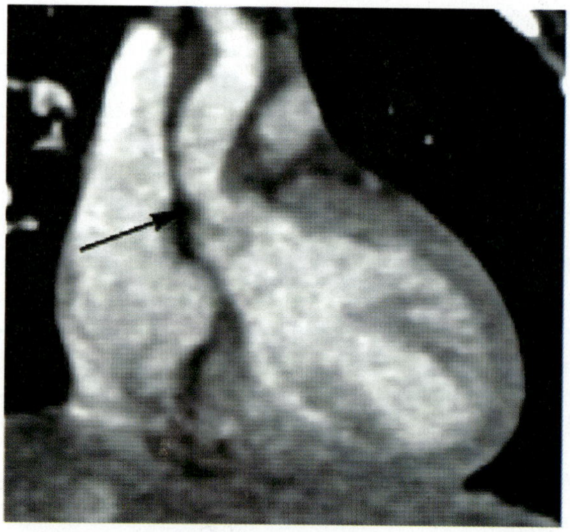

Fig. 14.123: *Multidetecter CT showing supravalvular aortic stenosis (arrow)*

Prognosis is influenced by the presence of genetic disorders, coronary artery lesions, and associated obstructive lesions of pulmonary arteries. SVAS is a progressive lesion, whereas peripheral pulmonary artery stenosis remains unchanged or decreases in severity over time. The mortality rate is higher in patients with diffuse SVAS than in those with the localized form.

The risk of sudden cardiac death including in patients who have undergone surgery, is 1 case per 1,000 patient years and is 25–100 times higher than in the normal population. Patients with SVAS are vulnerable to cardiac arrest or significant hemodynamic instability during induction of anesthesia and cardiac catheterization.

Anatomic abnormalities that predispose individuals with SVAS and Williams syndrome to sudden death include coronary artery stenosis and severe biventricular outflow tract obstruction. The mechanisms for sudden death for both anatomic subgroups are believed to include myocardial ischemia, decreased cardiac output, and arrhythmia.

Patient Education

Preoperative recommendations for restriction of physical activities should be followed (see Activity). Physical activity restrictions are not required postoperatively if no residual lesion is present and the pressure gradient is less than 20 mmHg across the LVOT, which is similar to the preoperative recommendation. In general, persons with SVAS should have risk stratification for coronary artery disease early in adult life because SVAS may predispose the coronary artery to premature atherosclerotic changes.

Surgical Intervention

Children and adolescents with catheter peak-to-peak (or Doppler mean) gradient of 50 mmHg or more should have surgical intervention. The choice of procedures in these patients is similar to that indicated for valvular aortic stenosis.

Children and adolescents with catheter peak-to-peak (or Doppler mean) gradient of 30–50 mmHg may be considered for surgical intervention if they are symptomatic, with angina, syncope, or dyspnea on exertion (class I). Asymptomatic patients who have developed ST/T-wave changes over the left precordium on ECG at rest or with exercise should also be considered for surgical intervention (class I).

Surgical resection of the supravalvular obstruction and patch aortoplasty and multiple-sinus reconstructions (inverted bifurcated patch plasty and three-sinus reconstruction) are the procedures of choice for the fibrous diaphragm and hourglass deformities.

Associated coronary artery involvement is addressed with the following measures which are performed at the same time as aortoplasty:

- Patch aortoplasty encompassing the left main ostium for circumferential narrowing of the left main ostium
- Excision of the fused leaflet from the aortic wall for ostial obstruction caused by a fusion of the aortic cusp to the supravalvular ridge
- Bypass grafting for diffuse narrowing of the left main coronary artery.

In patients who have SVAS with diffuse narrowing, the ascending aorta and the arch of the aorta can be reconstructed using an aortic allograft or a pulmonary autograft.

Surgical treatment of associated abnormalities of aortic valve and aortic arch vessels should be undertaken at the same time to optimize the overall surgical outcome.

Standard postoperative care and precautions for pediatric cardiac patients are also required for patients with SVAS. Postoperative complications include aortic insufficiency (in 25% of patients).

Activity: Exercise recommendations for children with SVAS are as follows:

- Mild stenosis (< 20 mmHg), normal ECG findings, no symptoms—full sports participation
- Moderate stenosis (21–49 mmHg), mild left ventricular hypertrophy (LVH), no symptoms—low static or moderately dynamic sports participation
- Severe stenosis (> 50 mmHg) or moderate degree of stenosis with symptoms—no competitive sports participation (only recreational)
- Coronary artery stenosis or abnormal anatomy—no competitive sports participation (only recreational).

Additional Management

Williams syndrome, which is found in many children with SVAS, may be associated with infantile hypercalcemia with some risk of nephrocalcinosis, osteosclerosis with progressive joint limitation and abnormal gait, and neurodevelopmental delay. These children require multidisciplinary support. Use a coordinated management approach. They are also at risk of higher mortality than the normal population is because of cardiac and noncardiac causes. No published reports have documented the outcome of pregnancy in postoperative patients with SVAS. Address pregnancy on an individual basis, taking into account the type of lesion and surgical procedure performed, the presence of residual lesion, and the associated cardiac and noncardiac conditions and syndromes.

Long-term Monitoring

Follow-up care is recommended for all patients with SVAS, whether or not their condition has been surgically corrected. Infants and children with SVAS require follow-up at 3-month to 6-month intervals; older children require follow-up at 6-month to 12-month intervals. Rapid progression of SVAS may occur preoperatively. Detailed cardiac examination and ECG should be performed at the follow-up visit. An echocardiogram may be indicated based on physical examination or ECG findings. Changes in intensity of the murmur.

CONGENITAL MITRAL STENOSIS (Fig. 14.124)

Congenital mitral valve stenosis is rare, but is almost always the result of chordal and papillary muscle malformations, and associated with other cardiac abnormalities. Surgical intervention of the mitral valve in this situation is difficult. Normally, there is no pressure difference between the left atrium and the left ventricle during diastole, even during exercise. Any pressure gradient suggests obstruction, the degree of obstruction being crudely proportional to the

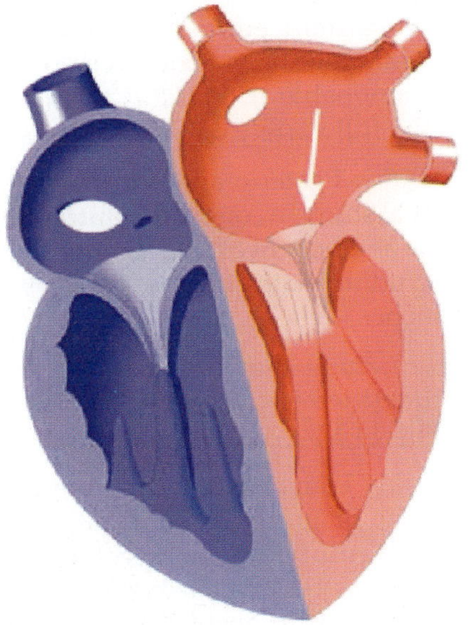

Fig. 14.124: *Diagram showing narrowed mitral valve (arrow) in patient with congenital mitral stenosis, the mitral valve is defective in form, with a blockage or narrowing that makes it difficult for blood to enter the left ventricle*

gradient. Left atrial hypertension is transmitted to the pulmonary veins and the pulmonary capillaries where if oncotic pressure is exceeded, pulmonary edema develops. Thus, the maximal imaginable pressure in the left atrium may be as high as 30–40 mmHg in the worst case, and at that level it is associated with dyspnea (diastolic pressures, as well as the best available estimation of blood flow across the valve, is needed) as the child grows, upgrading to a larger valve is difficult and sometimes impossible. Various solutions, none completely satisfactory, have been suggested. Excising the mitral valve and inserting a prosthesis above the valve ring have been tried, as has the insertion of a conduit from the left atrium to the left ventricle. For these reasons, surgery for congenital mitral stenosis is delayed until the child is larger if possible, it is avoided in infancy. Puncture of the atrial septum to gain access to the left atrium is undertaken, even though the targeted left atrium may not be particularly large. Generally, good quality pressure tracings of the left atrium and left ventricle, which can be overlaid for precise comparison, are obtained. Usually, angiography with left atrial injection not only confirms the echocardiographic findings but provides further confidence in deciding on a plan of surgical management. A contrast agent with as low osmolality as is available should be selected when high left atrial pressures are discovered. Any suggestion that the patient has a supravalvular membrane or cor triatriatum (sometimes confused with valvular mitral stenosis) must be diligently pursued because those lesions are readily corrected. For these reasons, surgery for congenital mitral stenosis is delayed until the child is larger if possible, it is avoided in infancy. Only when it is certain that there is no alternative to valve replacement surgery, even though it is anticipated that valvuloplasty might offer a possible solution. Correction of associated defects that cause increased mitral valve flow, such as a patent ductus arteriosus or ventricular septal defect, may reduce the transvalvular gradient enough to relieve symptoms. Rheumatic mitral stenosis is a different problem and, in pure form, is amenable to balloon valvuloplasty or, if necessary, to the full variety of surgical possibilities.

Chest radiography: Posterio-anterior view of chest along with barium meal study in congenital mitral stenosis would be helpful in the assessment of enlarged LA and pulmonary vasculature including main pulmonary artery and its apical and basal branches (Figs 14.125 and 14.126).

Electrocardiography: It shows features of RVH, right-axis deviation, bifid P wave due to left atrial enlargement (M pattern) (Fig. 14.127).

Echocardiography: Transthoracic 2D, color Doppler views are exellent in the diagnosis of congenital mitral stenosis and TEE though minimally invasive is helpful in the diagnosis of other associated cardiac malformations such as ASD,VSD and LA thrombosis/clot (Figs 14.128A–D to 14.131A and B).

Cardiac catheterization: It can visualise the path of percutaneous balloon catheter and pressure differences in LA and LV before and after valvoplasty (Figs 14.132A and B).

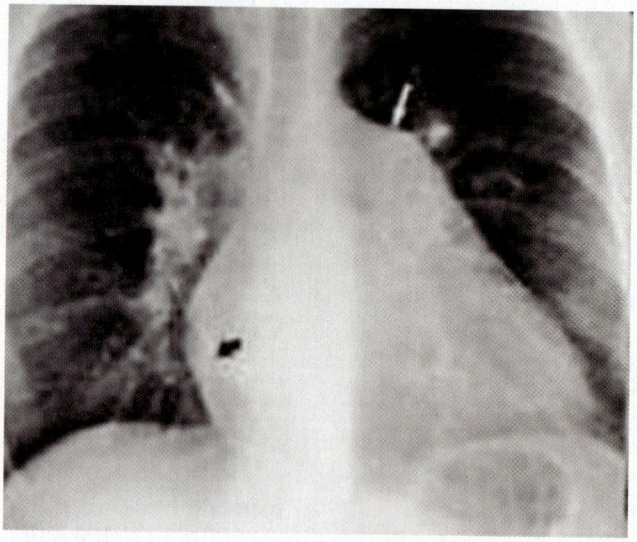

Fig. 14.125: *Pulmonary artery hypertension in mitral stenosis. Large main (white arrow) and hilar pulmonary arteries plus dilated upper lobe vessels resulting from pulmonary arterial and venous hypertension. The left side of the heart-lung interface is mainly the large right ventricle which has rotated the normal-sized left ventricle posteriorly. Note the double density of the left atrium (black arrow)*

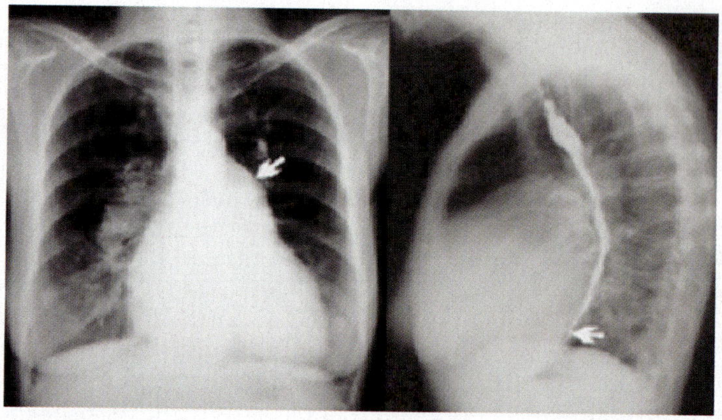

Fig. 14.126: *Prominence of main pulmonary artery due to raised pulmonary artery pressure (left) PA view and enlargement of the left atrium as a consequence of increased pressure in the chamber can be imaged using a chest radiograph.in lateral position with barium contrast study (right)*

Medical management: It can be managed with low sodium diet, diuretics, digioxin in patients with CCF and those with atrial fibrillation, additional aspirin or Warfarin should be added. Infective endocarditis should be treated accordingly.

Surgical intervention: It should be done in cases with other associated cardiac anomalies with valvular repair or replacement and closure of ASD or VSD as the case may be.

Ballon valvoplasty: It can be done in emergency situation and ultimately valve can either repaired or replaced as per recommedations of consulting cardiologist/surgeon.

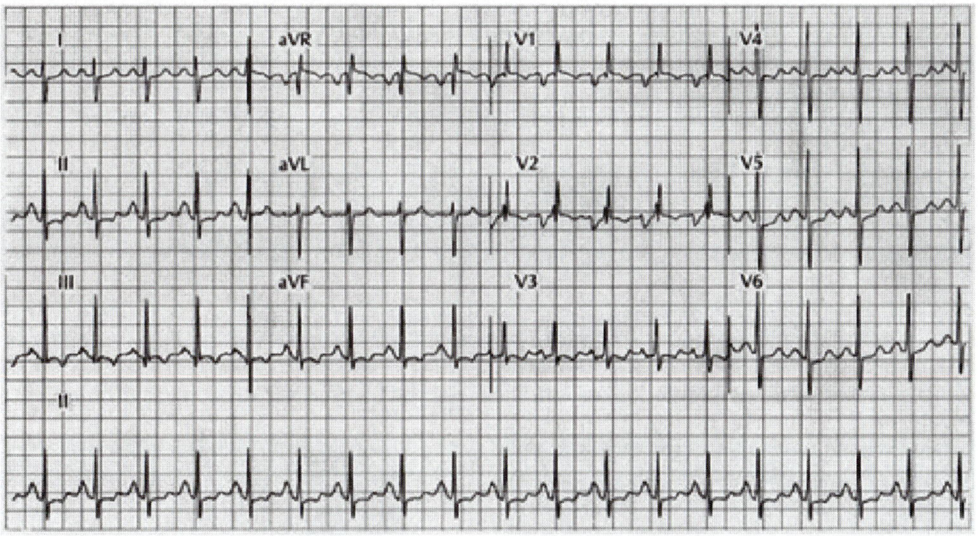

Fig. 14.127: *This ECG from a 6 year with severe mitral stenosis shows multiple abnormalities. The rhythm is sinus tachycardia. Right axis deviation and a tall R wave in lead V1 indicate right ventricular hypertrophy. The prominent biphasic P wave in lead V1 indicates left atrial enlargement. The tall P waves in lead II may indicate concomitant right atrial enlargement. Nonspecific ST-T changes and incomplete right bundle branch block are also present. The combination of right ventricular hypertrophy and left atrial enlargement is highly suggestive of mitral stenosis*

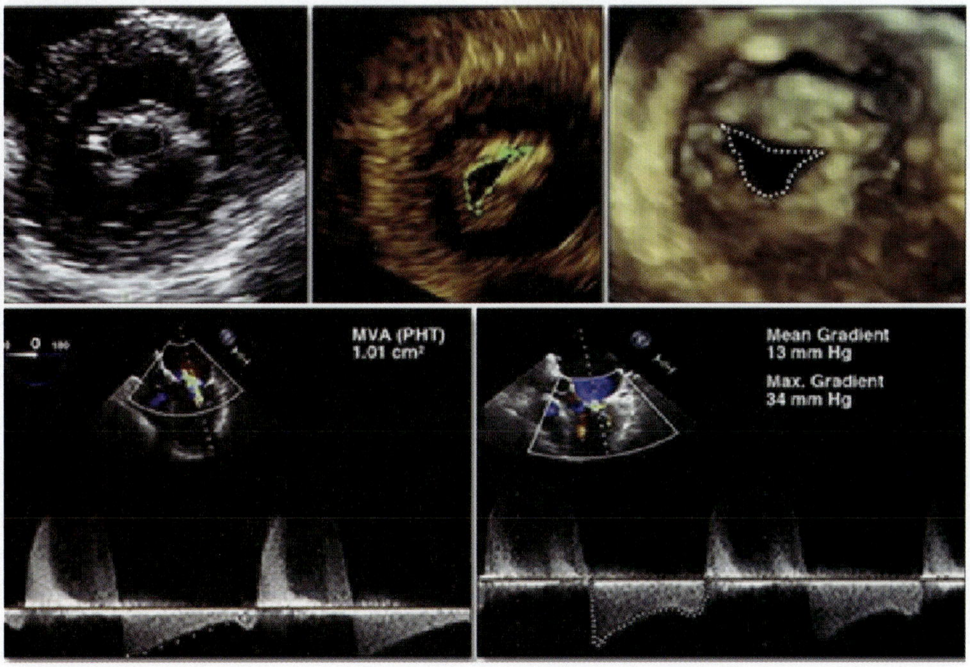

Fig. 14.128A to E: *Different methods to evaluate the MVA and assessment of Doppler gradients. (A) A planimetric measurement in a transthoracic short-axis view is shown. (B) Using three dimensional transesophageal echocardiography (TEE), the planimetry is done in a post-processing step. (C) The direct delineation of the MVA (mitral valve area) in a 3D TEE image (left ventricular aspect) is demonstrated. (D) The MVA is assessed by using pressure half-time (PHT), which is 218 ms (calculated valve area: 1.01 cm^2) . (E) Mean and maximal Doppler gradients are obtained by tracing the Doppler diastolic mitral flow profile*

COR TRIATRIUM (Fig. 14.133)

Definition: When a membranous diaphragm divides the left atrium into two chambers, the proximal chamber accepting the pulmonary veins and the distal chamber comunicating with the mitral valve and left atrial append age, cor triatriatum is said to be present.

Pathology: Normally during cardiogenesis, the common pulmonary vein is absorbed into, and becomes part of, the left atrium. Incomplete absorption, leaving obstructing tissue at the line of connection between the left atrium and the common pulmonary vein, results in cor triatriatum. The degree of obstruction is variable, ranging from being barely detectable to being severe. Often the dividing tissue in the

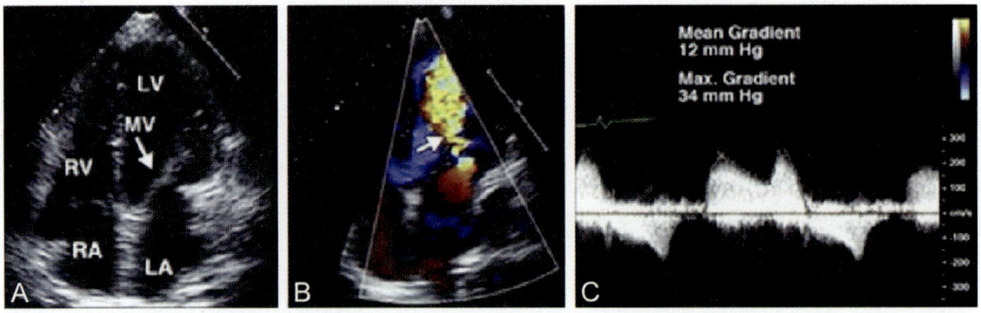

Fig. 14.129A to C: *Congenital mitral stenosis. (A) In the four chamber transthoracic view, the thickened and restrictive mitral leaflets are visible. (B) The accelerated flow through the stenotic mitral valve is shown. (C) Doppler gradients are shown to be increased*

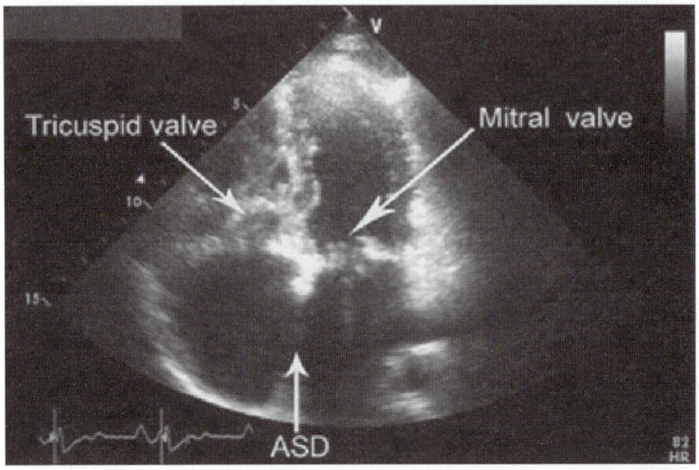

Fig. 14.130: *Apical four chamber view showing congenital mitral stenosis with ASD*

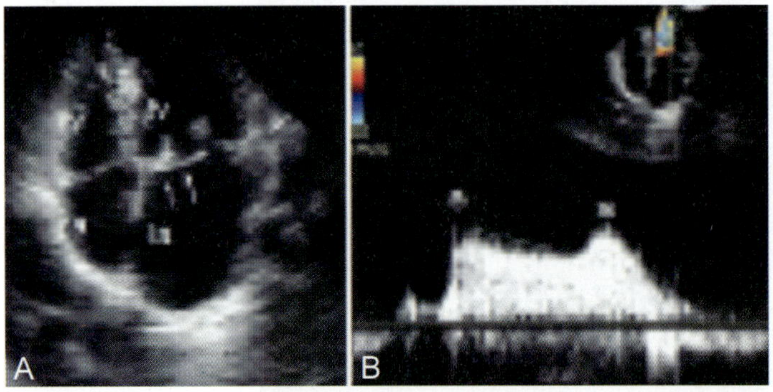

Fig. 14.131: *Congenital mitral stenosis. Transthoracic echocardiograms. (A) Apical four chamber view. This diastolic frame shows a dilated LA and and supravalvular stenosing ring (arrows) that is adherent to the mitral valve. (B) Contineous wave Doppler studies demonstrated increased peak early (e) and late atrial (a) diastolic flow velocities and decreased EF slope*

left atrium is a flexible diaphragm, sometimes bulging, downward like a windsock into the region of the mitral valve. The foramen ovale and the left atrial appendage communicate with the left atrium and provide a means to distinguish between cor triatriatum and obstructing supravalvular rings. Atrial defects may communicate between the right atrium and either the proximal or distal

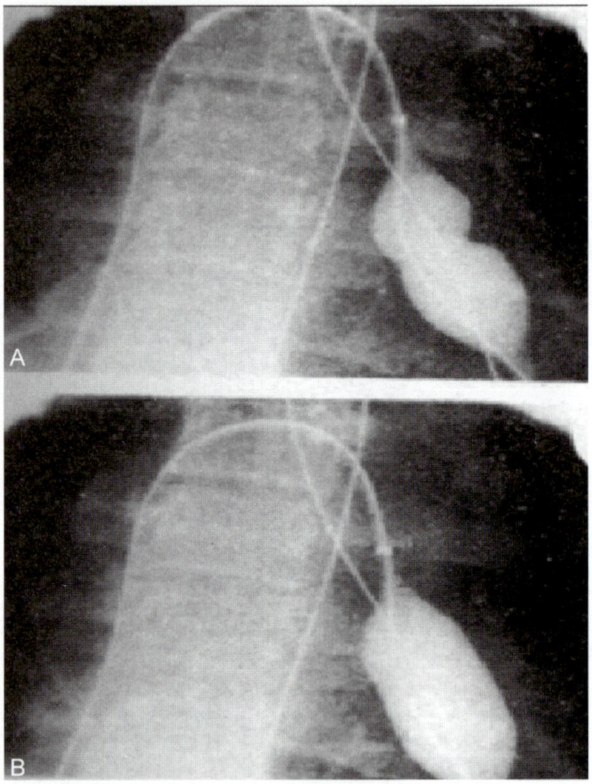

Fig. 14.132A and B: *Transseptal dilatation of stenosed MV by balloon valvoplasty*

left atrial chamber. Cor triatriatum may be associated with a variety of other cardiac lesions although 40% of the time it is a pure and uncomplicated problem.

Sometimes one or two, right or left, pulmonary veins are anomalously located and may enter the systemic venous circulation by various routes.

Physiology: The physiologic abnormalities associated with cor triatriatum are a direct function of the size of the orifice between the pulmonary venous chamber and the left atrium. When there is sufficient obstruction to raise the pulmonary venous pressure, there is pulmonary hypertension that may reach or exceed systemic levels. With elevated right heart pressure, right-to-left shunting through a foramen ovale may result in cyanosis. In this case, as with mitral stenosis, the cardiac output may be limited and may

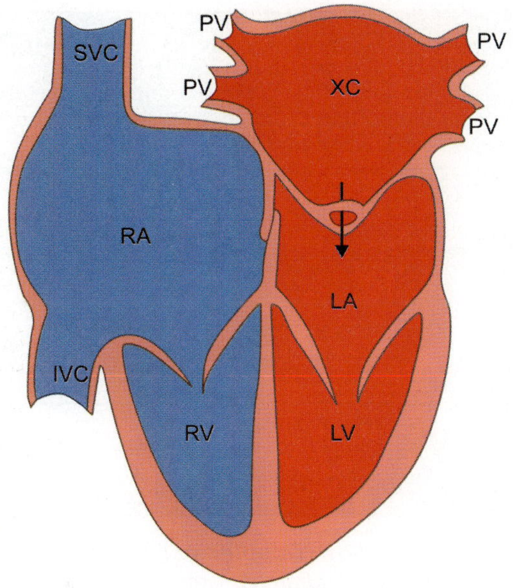

Fig. 14.133: *The upper chamber (XC) of this partition receives blood from the pulmonary veins, and the distal chamber communicates with the mitral valve. The orifice diameter of the windsock ranges from less than 3 mm to about 1 cm. In a minority of cases, a patent foramen ovale or an atrial septal defect allows communication with the right atrium. Right ventricular hypertrophy and dilation are almost always present, and right atrial dilation occurs 25% of the time. Current theories suggest that the defect occurs because the common pulmonary vein fails to incorporate into the left atrium during cardiac embryogenesis*

not increase with exercise. Pulmonary edema is often a clinical problem. In most regards, the clinical picture and course of patients with cor triatriatum are comparable to those for infants with mitral stenosis. When there are anomalous pulmonary veins, there is differential pulmonary vascular pathology. In the part of the lungs communicating with a severely obstructing membrane there is reflex pulmonary vascular change. The pulmonary vein draining into the systemic venous circulation, offering less resistance, may carry a large part of the total pulmonary flow. However, when there is anomalous pulmonary venous drainage of a single lobe, there is persistence of the (fetal vascular muscle and pulmollnary hypertension. If there is more than one anomalous pulmonary vein, it is possible that the available vascular space of one lung can manage nearly the entire cardiac output without pulmonary hypertension. In this case, there would be greatly difierent blood flow in the two lungs, drained by the two different routes.

Clinical manifestations: Many patients with cor triatriatum develop symptoms early in infancy, although some other asymptomatic forms of heart disease are discovered during echocardiographic studies. When there is mild obstruction there are no symptoms and, if this is an isolated lesion, there is no reason to suspect disease. With severe obstruction there may be pulmonary edema, pulmonary hypertension, and respiratory symptoms, such as tachypnea or dyspnea, early in infancy. Cor triatriatum should be suspected whenever there is unexplained pulmonary edema.

On physical examination there is often little to discern. The second heart sound is accentuated, specifically the pulmonary component of the second heart sound. With pulmonary hypertension, there may be a diastolic murmur of pulmonary regurgitation. Usually, there is no diastolic rumbling murmur at the apex. Why there is a diastolic rumble with valvular mitral stenosis and usually not in patient with cor triatriatum is a matter of some interest. Perhaps the lack of muscular contraction of the common pulmonary venous segment acconts for the presystolic murmur. Possibilly, the major reason diastolic murmurs are not heard is that this disease is dominantly a lesion of infancy when the heart rate is fast and auscultation is not easy.

Electrocardiography (Fig. 14.134)

There is right ventricular hypertrophy and P-pulmonale in patients who are symptomatic with cor triatriatum.

Chest X-ray: There is evidence of pulmonary edema and Kerley B lines are present when the degree of obstruction is severe. Usually, the heart is not enlarged (Fig. 14.135).

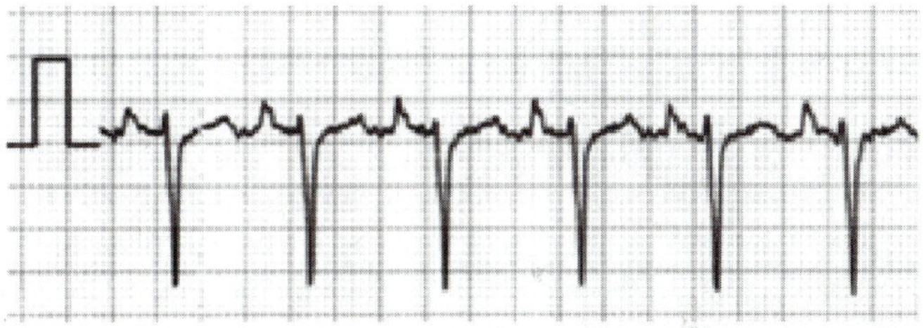

Fig. 14.134: *ECG showing small R waves (0.2 mV) and deep S waves (1.8 mV) and P-pulmonale are observed in the ECG tracing (lead II) recorded from the patient with cor triatriatum. These features are consistent with right ventricular hypertrophy (paper speed = 50 mm/s; 10 mm = 1 mV)*

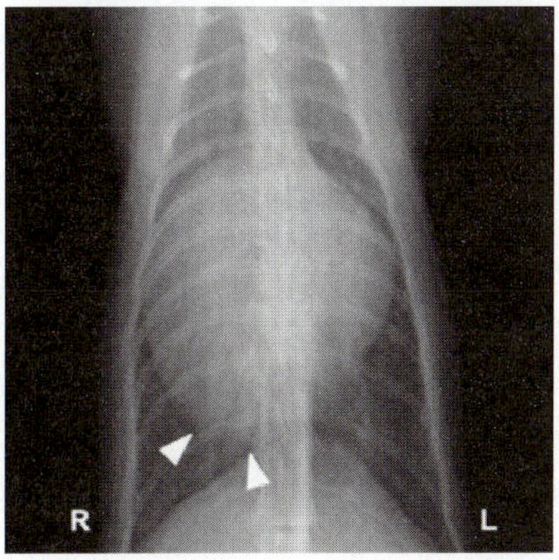

Fig. 14.135: *Dorsoventral shows extreme cardiac enlargement and dilation of the pulmonary vasculature. The cardiac apex is shifted to the right of midline (arrow heads) from the patient with cor triatriatum*

Echocardiography

Obstruction to left ventricular filling also occurs at the atrial level, usually because of a fibrous membrane that impedes the flow of blood through the chamber. These membranes may be located in the middle of the atrium, effectively partitioning the left atrium into two chambers (a condition known as cor triatriatum) or they may occur at or near the level of the mitral annulus (a supravalvular stenosing ring). Such membranes are readily detected and localized with two dimensional echocardiography. Distinguishing between these two entities (and differentiating both from mitral valve stenosis) is best accomplished using the parasternal long-axis and apical four chamber views. The membrane is visualized as a linear, echogenic structure extending from the antero-superior to the posterolateral wall . In most cases, the superior "chamber" receives the pulmonary veins and the inferior "chamber" is associated with the atrial appendage and mitral valve (which is usually normal). The obligatory perforation connecting two chambers is most often posterior and may be multiple. This communication is often difficult to record with echocardiography. Color Doppler imaging may permit localization of the opening in the membrane so that the pressure gradient can be assessed with pulsed Doppler (Figs 14.136 and 14.137).

Transesophageal echocardiography has also been used for the evaluation of this entity. The transesophageal echocardiogram, performed in the operating room, allows visualization of the defect within the membrane. The insertion of all four pulmonary veins and their site of entrance relative to the membrane also are recorded, as are the degree of obstruction to left ventricular filling and the associated mitral regurgitation. Finally, the presence and severity of pulmonary hypertension are assessed.

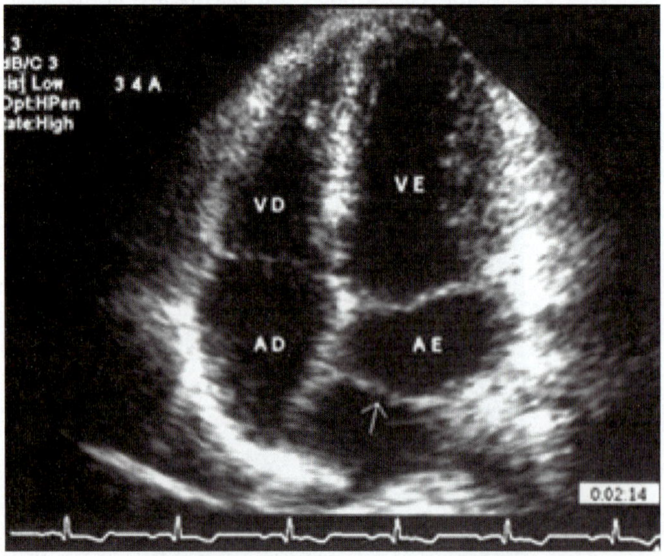

Fig. 14.136: *Apical four chamber view shows diaphragm-like membrane (arrow) dividing the LA into a posterosuperior chamber receiving the pulmonary veins and an anteroinferior chamber connected to the left atrial appendage (LAA) and draining into the left ventricle via the mitral valve*

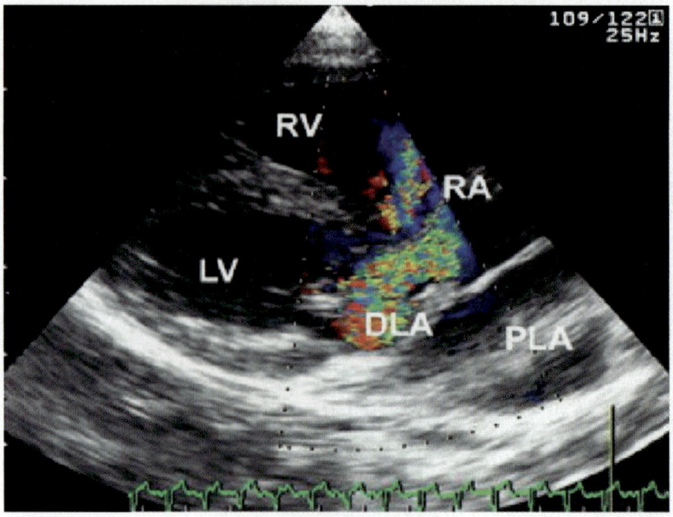

Fig. 14.137: *Color-flow Doppler echocardiography (right parasternal long-axis four chamber view) shows turbulent systolic flow in the DLA and the RA. PLA, proximal left atrium; DLA, distal left atrium in patient with cor triatrium*

In contrast to cor triatriatum, these membranes are closer to the mitral valve and may actually adhere to the valve leaflets. Distinguishing between valvular mitral stenosis and a supravalvular ring is best accomplished with two-dimensional and Doppler echocardiography. Absence of anterior leaflet doming excludes the possibility of rheumatic mitral stenosis and the presence of the supravalvular membrane was detected from the apical window. Using color Doppler, the identification of flow acceleration and turbulence at the level of the annulus rather than the leaflet tips is an additional clue to distinguish a supravalvular ring from mitral valve stenosis. Continuous wave Doppler can then be used to assess the severity of the obstruction. The proximity of the membrane to the valve can lead to leaflet damage, the result of high-velocity turbulent flow. Leaflet thickening and mitral regurgitation may develop as a consequence. Caution must be used when diagnosing a supravalvular stenosing ring with echocardiography. Differentiating between a thickened and calcified mitral annulus and a stenosing ring may be difficult, leading to both false-positive and false-negative results. Associated anomalies are seen frequently with both cor triatriatum and supravalvular stenosis. Atrial septal defect and persistent left superior vena cava are especially common and are readily detected with echocardiography. These entities may also occur in association with aortic coarctation and subaortic stenosis (Shone's complex).

Management: The obstructing membrane of cor triatriatum should be resected if the infant is symptomatic. Asymptomatic patients without significant obstruction are managed expectantly. Often a membrane of cor triatriatum is removed when surgical procedures are being carried out for other cardiac defects. Ordinarily, removal of the obstructing membrane is curative.

PULMONARY VALVE STENOSIS

Definition (Fig. 14.138)

This is a congenital anomaly consisting of a dome-shaped or conical pulmonary valve with a narrow outlet at its apex. Pathology additional characteristics of the anomaly include the following:

- No separate leaflets are usually definable in the valve.
- Poststenotic pulmonary artery dilatation is usually present.
- Secondary pulmonary infundibular hypertrophy may be present.

Clinical Manifestations

History

Pulmonary valve stenosis occurs equally often in both sexes. Most patients are asymptomatic and have normal growth and development. There is frequently a history of a heart murmur that has been heard since birth. With severe stenosis and limitation of cardiac output, patients may have increased fatigue and breathlessness on exertion. Exertional chest discomfort, perhaps from right ventricular myocardial ischemia, may occur in patients with severe stenosis.

Physical Examination

The arterial pulse is usually normal but the jugular venous pulse has a prominent a wave. There is a right ventricular lift or heave along the left sternal edge, together with a loud midsystolic, spindle-shaped systolic murmur that tends to radiate upward and to the left and may be associated with a palpable thrill. There may be pulmonic ejection click along the left upper sternal border that may decrease or disappear during inspiration and increase during expiration. The pulmonic component of the second heart sound is either diminished and delayed or absent.

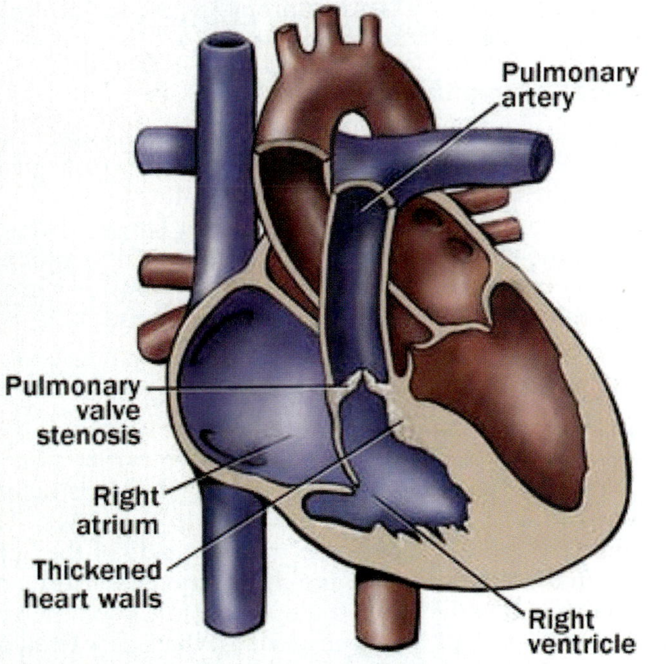

Fig. 14.138: *Diagram showing anatomical features of pulmonary valve stenosis*

Diagnostic Tests

Chest X-ray

The chest X-ray may show right ventricular hypertrophy and prominence of the main pulmonary artery and the left pulmonary artery, but the right pulmonary artery is usually small (Fig. 14.139).

Electrocardiogram

The electrocardiogram usually shows normal sinus rhythm. Evidence of right ventricular and right atrial hypertrophy is usually present in patients with significant stenosis (Fig. 14.140).

Differential Diagnosis

The differential diagnosis includes infundibular pulmonary stenosis, peripheral pulmonary stenosis, aortic stenosis, atrial septal defect, and ventricular septal defect.

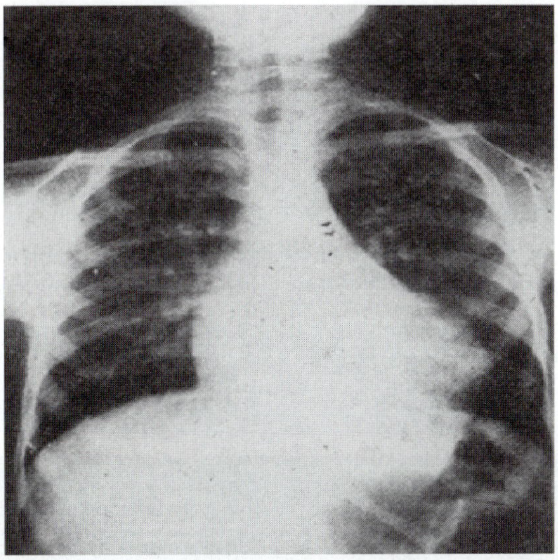

Fig. 14.139: *X-ray chest (PA view) showing right ventricular hypertrophy smaU main pulmonary artery shadow and pulmonary oligaemia in pulmonary valvular stenosis*

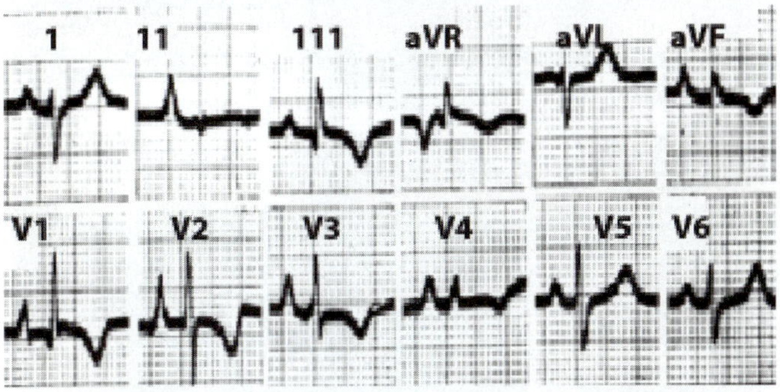

Fig. 14.140: *ECG showing right-axis deviation, right ventricular hypertrophy and right atrial hypertrophy (P-pulmonale) in uncomplicated pulmonic stenosis*

Laboratory Evaluation

Echocardiography

The echocardiogram may be normal with mild stenosis but usually demonstrates a prominent "a dip" with moderate or severe stenosis. Doppler echocardiography permits an estimation of the systolic pressure difference across the pulmonary valve (Fig. 14.141).

Cardiac Catheterization

Cardiac catheterization remains the procedure of choice for a definitive diagnosis, providing measurement of the systolic pressure differences between the pulmonary artery and right ventricle and the cardiac output. The degree of stenosis is sometimes classified on the basis of the peak-to-peak pressure differences (Figs 14.42A to C):

1. Mild (Less than 50 mmHg)
2. Moderate (50–100 mmHg)
3. Severe (100 mmHg or more).

Cardiac catheterization also assists in ruling out the presence of other lesions.

Natural History and Prognosis

Most patients survive into adulthood. Patients with mild gradients usually do not progress in severity after the third decade of life. Some patients may develop infundibular stenosis, right-to-Ieft shunt through a patent foramen ovale, tricuspid regurgitation, or endocarditis.

Medical Treatment

Prophylaxis against infective endocarditis is important. Asymptomatic patients may be followed by obtaining an electrocardiogram and chest film every 2 years, whereas symptomatic patients should be so checked every 6 months, or even more frequently until surgery is performed.

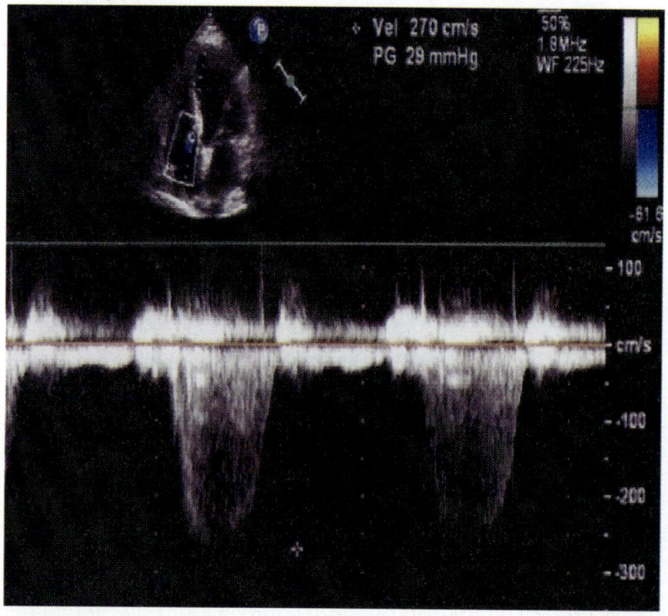

Fig. 14.141: *2D Doppler echoscan at pulmonary valve showing increased pulmonary flow velocity in pulmonic valvular stenosis*

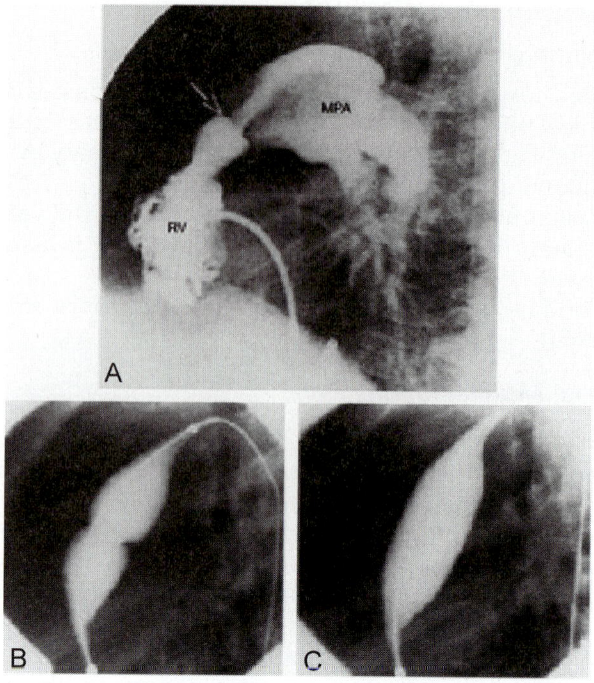

Fig. 14.142: *(A) Lateral view of a right ventricular (RV) angiogram demonstrating the typical features of valvular pulmonary stenosis with doming of the pulmonary valve (arrow) and a narrow jet of contrast entering the dilated main pulmonary artery (MPA). (B) An 18 mm balloon is inflated across the 14 mm annulus. A moderate waist is seen at 1 atm of pressure. (C) The waist is eliminated at 4 atm*

Balloon Valvoplasty and Placement of Stent

It can be done safely in patients with simple cases of pulmonary valvular stenosis without other associated congenital heart defects. An appropriate pulmonary valve stent can be placed after valvoplasty.

Surgical Intervention

Surgery is indicated in patients with cyanosis, heart failure, "failure to thrive", or syncope or in the presence of a peak-to-peak pressure gradient across the pulmonary valve of 100 mmHg or more. The indications for surgery are less clear if the gradient is 60–100 mmHg, but surgery is probably indicated if the gradient is 60 mmHg or more at rest and increases significantly during exercise.

PULMONARY ATRESIA

Pulmonary atresia is a congenital malformation of the pulmonary valve in which the valve orifice fails to develop. The valve is completely closed thereby obstructing the outflow of blood from the heart to the lungs. The pulmonary valve is located on the right side of the heart between the right ventricle and the pulmonary artery. In a normal functioning heart, the opening to the pulmonary valve has three flaps that open and close like one way doors. As these flaps open and close they allow blood to flow forward into the pulmonary artery and on to the lungs where the blood becomes oxygenated, and prevent

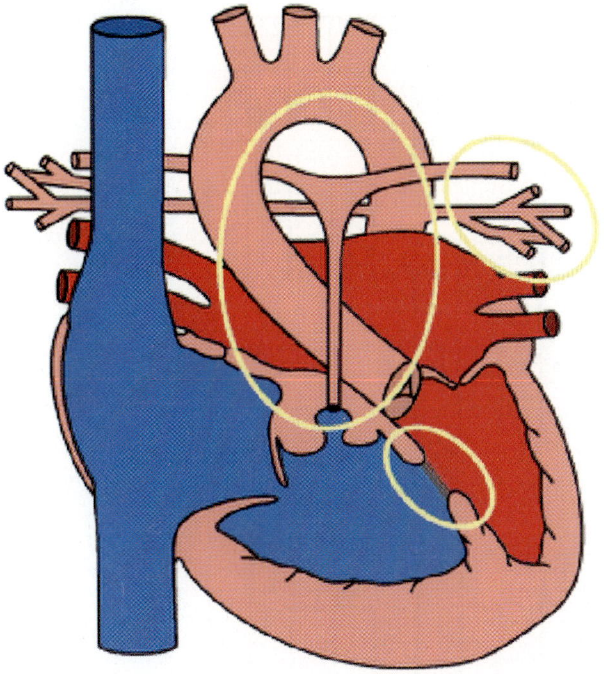

Fig. 14.143: *Anatomical structures in pulmonary atresia with VSD*

backward flow into the right ventricle. With the disease pulmonary atresia, the flap-like openings are completely covered by a layer of tissue, thus preventing the ability of blood flow to the lungs to become oxygenated. The body requires oxygenated blood for survival. Pulmonary atresia is not threatening to a developing fetus however, because the mother's placenta provides the needed oxygen since the baby's lungs are not yet functional. Once the baby is born its lungs must now provide the oxygen needed for survival, but with pulmonary atresia there is no opening on the pulmonary valve for blood to get to the lungs and become oxygenated and the only source of pulmonary blood flow is a patent ductus arteriosus. Due to this, the newborn baby is blue in color and pulmonary atresia can usually be diagnosed within hours or minutes after birth (Fig. 14.143).

Classification

There are two types of pulmonary atresia.

Pulmonary Atresia with Intact Ventricular Septum (PA-IVS)

PA-IVS is a rare congenital lesion. This lesion can be diagnosed during the fetal stage of life by using fetal echocardiography, which is a test that uses sound waves to look at the structure of an unborn baby's heart. PA-IVS involves complete blockage of the pulmonary valve located on the right side of the heart. This blockage thus prevents the flow of blood to the lungs. Because of this lack of blood flowing through the right side of the heart, the structures on that side, such as the pulmonary valve and the tricuspid valve, are abnormally small. The genetic cause of PA-IVS is unknown. It is rare, occurring in around 4–6 cases per every 100,000 live births.

Pulmonary atresia with Ventricular Septal Defect (PA-VSD)

This lesion is identified by underdevelopment of the right ventricle. The Ventricular Septal Defect (VSD) is a second opening in the ventricular wall, which provides a way out for blood in the right ventricle. When this second opening does not exist, very little blood goes to the right ventricle, which is what causes it to be underdeveloped in PA-IVS. This defect can also be determined before birth. Out of all congenital cardiac malformations, it is estimated that PA-VSD occurs in 2.5–3.4% of the cases. The genetic cause of PA-VSD is not known; it is found however, that children whose parents have PA-VSD are at a higher risk for congenital heart lesions.

Etiology

Doctors are unsure of the cause of congenital heart defects, but there are some medical conditions that have been found to increase the risk of having a baby with a heart defect such as congenital heart disease in the mother, father, brother, or sister of the baby, a diabetic mother, use of drugs or alcohol or over the counter prescriptions during pregnancy. These conditions do not mean that the baby will definitely be born with a heart defect, but that it runs a higher chance. Sometimes, babies are born without any of these conditions; the cause is unknown.

Laboratory Investigations

Chest radiography: X-ray chest PA view usually shows marked right ventricular hypertrophy, abscence of impression of main pulmonary artery and olegemic lung fields (Fig. 14.144).

Electrocardiogram: It reveals left axis deviation, right atrial enlargement (peaked P waves in lead 11) with left ventricular hypertrophy (Fig. 14.145).

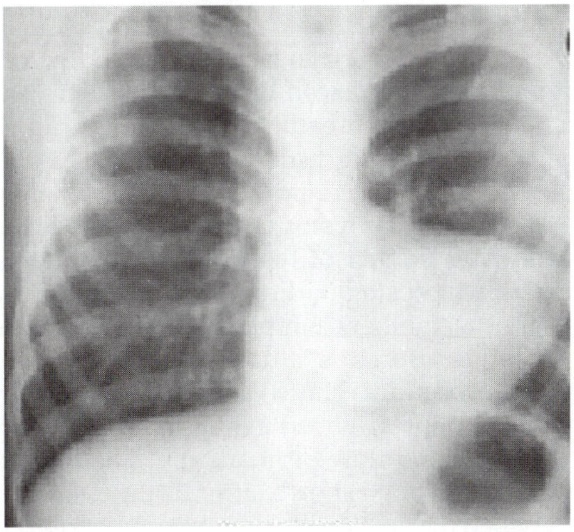

Fig. 14.144: *X-ray chest PA view shows marked RVH with absence of pulmonary bay in a patient with pulmonary atresia with intact IVS*

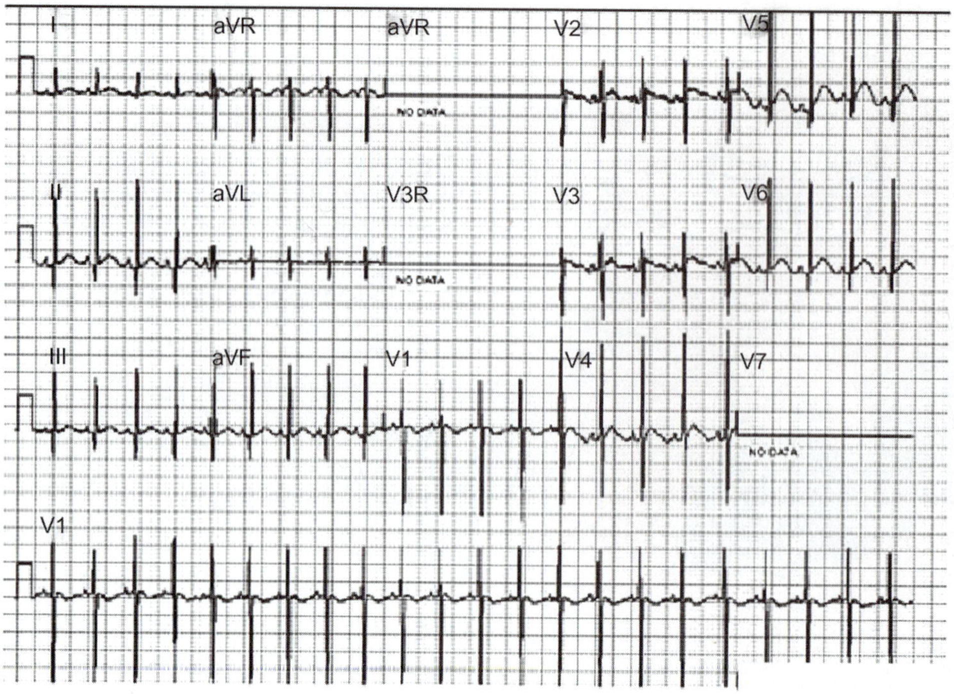

Fig. 14.145: *Pulmonary atresia with intact IVS: electrocardiogram 9-day-old infant with pulmonary atresia, intact ventricular septum with tracing showing left-axis deviation for age (68°), right atrial enlargement (peaked P waves in lead II), and left ventricular hypertrophy*

Echocardiography: In pulmonary atresia with intact ventricular septum, apical four chamber view shows severely hypoplastic right ventricle and atresic pulmonary valve (Figs 14.146; 14.147A and B).

Computerized axial tomography and MRI: This noninvasive imaging technique is helpful in demonstratiing the anatomical defects in different categories of pulmonary atresia such as pulmonary atresia with intact IVS or pulmonary atresia with VSD or other associated anomalies (Figs 14.148 and 14.149).

Medical Treatment

At first, the child will need to be admitted to the intensive care unit and possibly placed on oxygen and a ventilator that will help the child breathe. Also, IV medications that assist the heart and lung function may be given. An IV medication called prostaglandin E1 is used for treatment of pulmonary atresia, as it stops the ductus arteriosus from closing, allowing mixing of the pulmonary and systemic circulations. But, prostaglandin E1 can be dangerous as it can cause apnea. Another example of preliminary treatment is heart catheterization to evaluate the defect or defects of the heart; this procedure is much more invasive. Ultimately, however, the patient will need to have a series of surgeries to improve the blood flow permanently. The first surgery will likely be performed shortly after birth. A shunt can be created between the aorta and the pulmonary artery to help increase blood flow to the lungs. As the child grows, so does the heart and the shunt may need revised in order to meet the body's requirements.

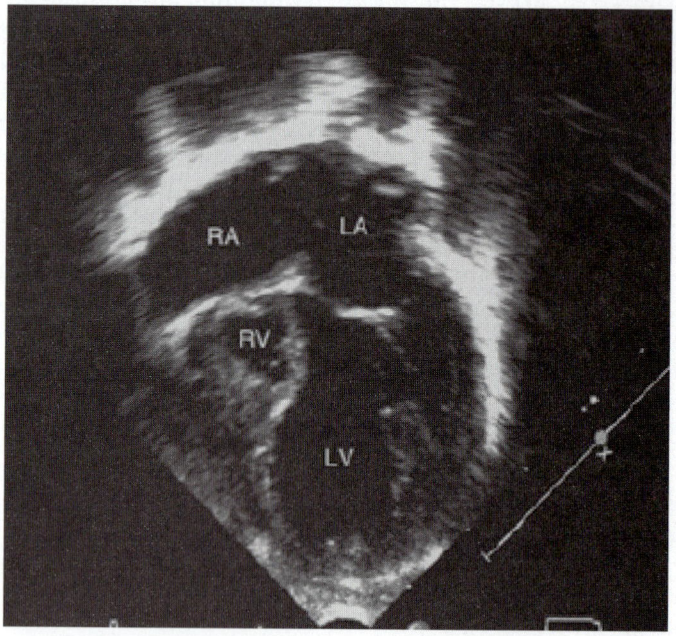

Fig. 14.146: *Pulmonary atresia with intact ventricular septum. Apical four-chamber echocardiogram image in this newborn demonstrates the severely hypoplastic right ventricle (RV), too small to support any effective pulmonary blood flow, and requiring a single-ventricle palliative approach. A severely hypoplastic but patent tricuspid valve was present in this patient. LA, left atrium; LV, left ventricle; RA, right atrium*

The type of surgery recommended depends on the size of the right ventricle and the pulmonary artery.

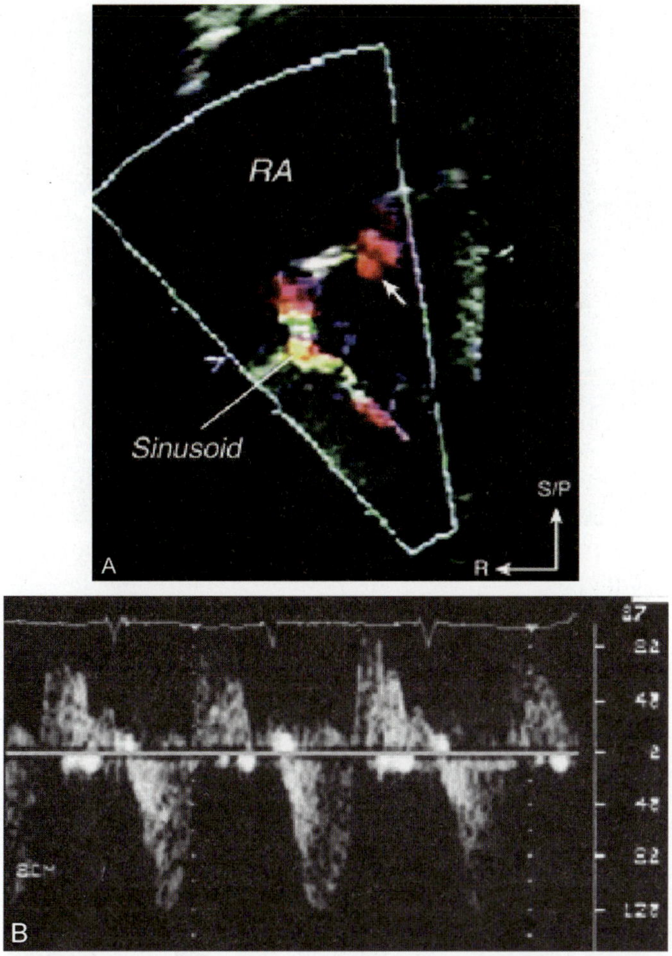

Fig. 14.147: *Echocardiographic assessment of pulmonary atresia with intact ventricular septum and RV-to-coronary artery communication. (A) Color Doppler flow mapping of the fistula. Tricuspid valve patency is confirmed by the presence of tricuspid inflow (arrow). (B) Pulsed wave Doppler evaluation of the sinusoid demonstrates flow toward the apex in diastole and from the RV toward the coronary artery in systole. RA, right atrium*

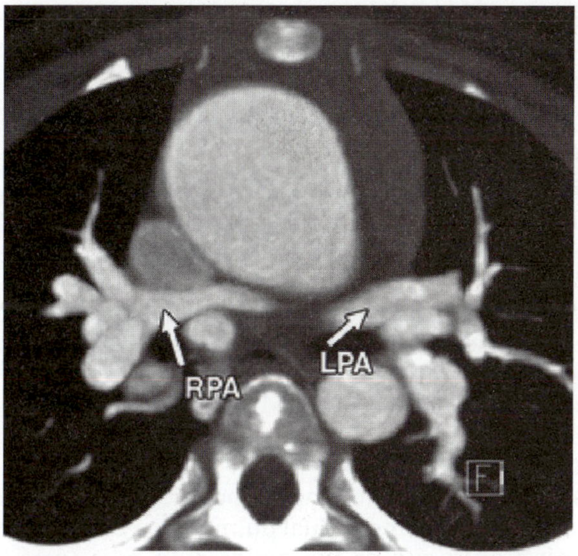

Fig. 14.148: *64-MDCT in evaluation of pulmonary atresia with ventricular septal defect 5-year-old girl with effort intolerance of 6 months' duration, found to have pulmonary atresia with ventricular septal defect. RPA, right pulmonary artery; LPA, left pulmonary artery. Thick maximum-intensity-projection axial image shows nonconfluent right and left pulmonary arteries (arrows)*

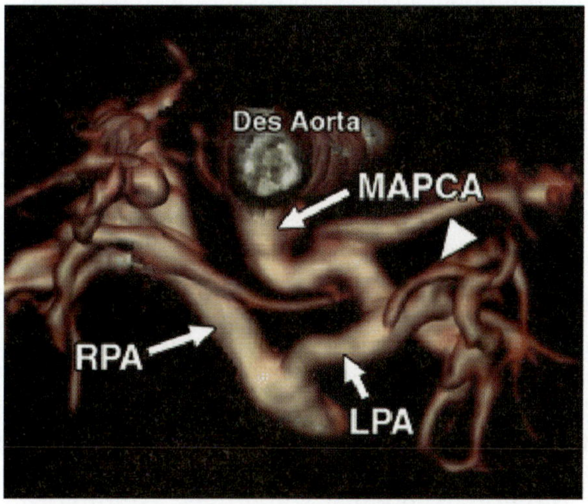

Fig. 14.149: *Type B pulmonary atresia with ventricular septal defect in 30-day-old boy with feeding difficulty and cardiac murmur. Oblique superior view volume-rendered image shows large major aortopulmonary collateral artery (MAPCA) reinforcing left pulmonary artery (LPA) and having separate branch (arrowhead) independently supplying left lung. RPA; right pulmonary artery*

If they are normal in size and the right ventricle is able to pump blood, open heart surgery can be performed to make blood flow through the heart in a normal pattern.

If the right ventricle is small and unable to act as a pump, doctors may perform another type of operation called the Fontan procedure. In this three-stage procedure, the right atrium is disconnected from the pulmonary circulation. The systemic venous return goes directly to the lungs, by-passing the heart.

Prognosis

The outcome varies for every child. If the condition is left uncorrected it may be fatal, but the prognosis has greatly improved over the years for babies with pulmonary atresia. Some factors that affect how well the child does include how well the heart is beating, the condition of the blood vessels that supply the heart, and how leaky the other heart valves are. Most cases of pulmonary atresia can be helped with surgery. If the patient's right ventricle is exceptionally small, many surgeries will be needed in order to help stimulate normal circulation of blood to the heart.

If uncorrected, babies with this type of congenital heart disease may only survive for the first few days of life while the fetal shunts between left and right circulations remain patent. However, there are cases of uncorrected pulmonary atresia in which the baby has survived.

Many children with pulmonary atresia will go on to lead "normal" lives. Patients are usually seen regularly throughout their lifetime by a cardiologist to be sure that their heart is functioning properly. They have an increased risk of endocarditis.

PULMONARY VENOUS STENOSIS

Stenosis of normally positioned pulmonary veins is a rare problem that may occur as an isolated phenomenon or in association with other defects, usually postoperatively. The stenosis is usually at the junction of the pulmonary vein and the left atrium. Later, the vein itself may become involved, becoming hypoplastic and even atretic. Subsequently, other veins may become involved. This disease should not be confused with the obstructions that occur at baffle sites in Senning operations or at the anastomotic site of repaired total anomalous pulmonary veins. At the same time, these operations have preceded the development of individual pulmonary vein obstruction. Although only one or two veins may be affected, the problem is often progressive, the stenoses becoming more severe and sometimes spreading to affect all the pulmonary veins. Based on presently available information, it is possible that most of these patients have an acquired problem. Some most certainly do, and in others there is no way to be confident. Good documentation of the absence of pulmonary vein disease in patients who subsequently develop pulmonary vein stenosis has been recorded. With progression of involvement of a single vein and later involvement of other veins, the hemodynamics may be confusing. A single obstructed vein may or may not have an elevated pulmonary arteriolar wedge pressure. When there is involvement of more than one vein, there may be pulmonary hypertension simply because of obstruction of some veins results in excessive blood flow in others (Figs 14.150 to 14.153).

Clinical Manifestations

Clinically, the symptoms of pulmonary venous hypertension are dyspnea and tachypnea. There is nothing that points to this diagnosis on physical examination other than evidence of pulmonary edema. The electrocardiogram shows right ventricular hypertrophy. The chest X-ray may show pulmonary edema, sometimes asymmetric, and Kerley B lines.

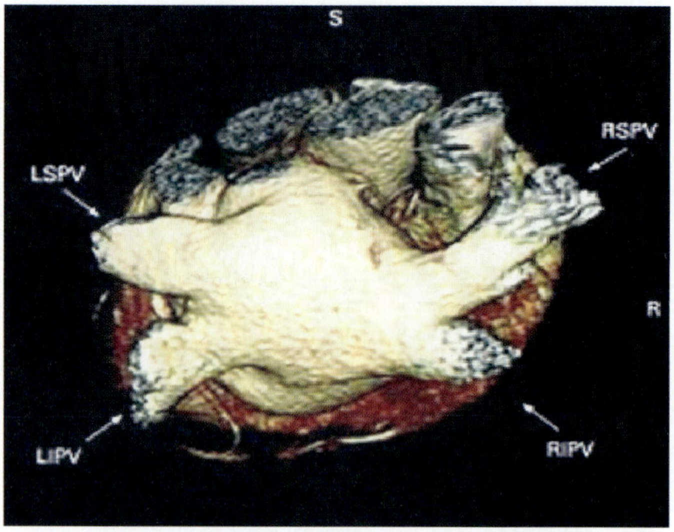

Fig. 14.150: *CT angiography in the anatomy of pulmonary venous system*

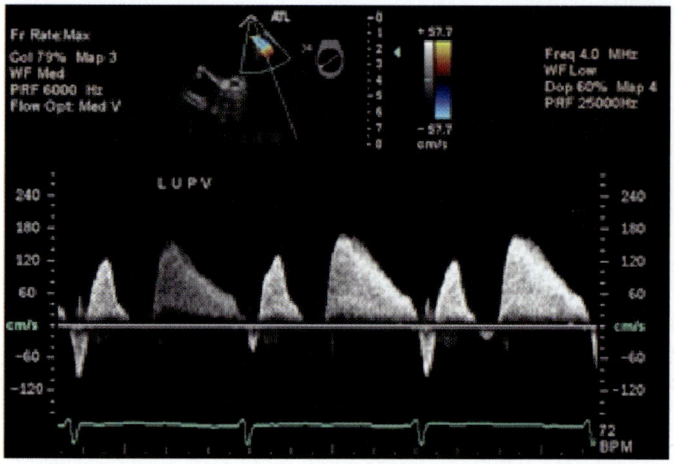

Fig. 14.151: *Pulsed wave echo of left upper pulmonary vein stenosis*

Echocardiographic examination: The extra parenchymal pulmonary veins may show turbulence at the point of entry of the veins into the left atrium. At cardiac catheterization

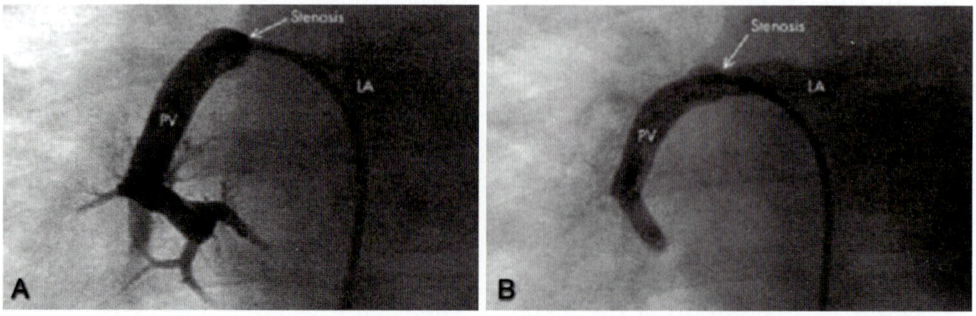

Fig. 14.152A and B: *Angiogram of the right lower pulmonary vein (PV) in anteroposterior projection before (A) and after (B) cutting balloon angioplasty of a discrete stenosis at the junction between the left atrium (LA) and PV. Note the hypoplastic smaller peripheral vessels*

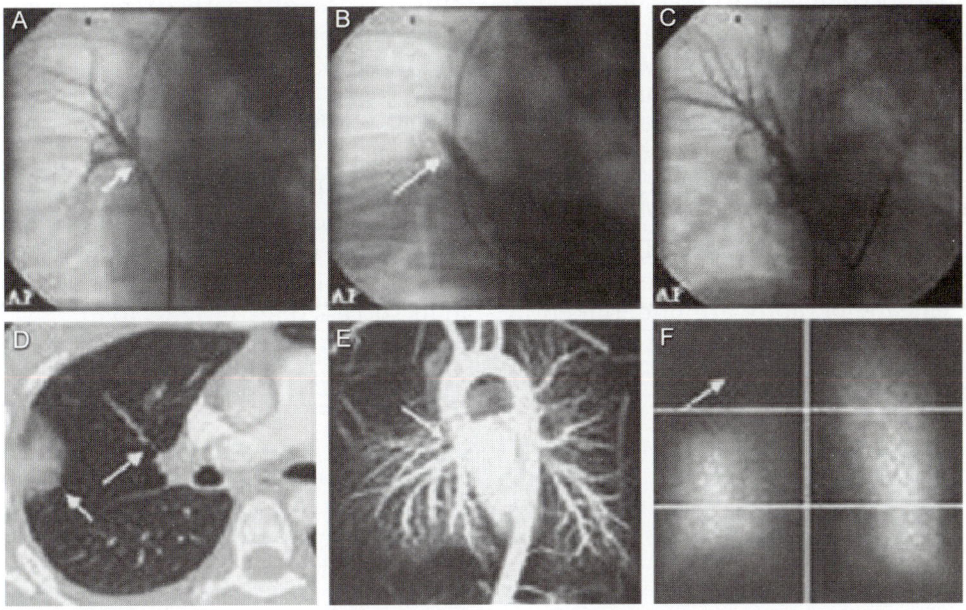

Fig. 14.153A to F: *Images of a right superior pulmonary vein stenosis (A) Angiographic view of the high grade stenosis (arrow). (B) Balloon dilatation (arrow). (C) Result after dilatation and stenting. (D) Preinterventional computed tomographic scanning of the stenosis (arrow) including infiltration in the dependent lung lobe (arrow). (E) Three dimensional magnetic resonance reconstruction of the stenosis (arrow). (F) Lung scan showing perfusion deficit in the right upper field (arrow)*

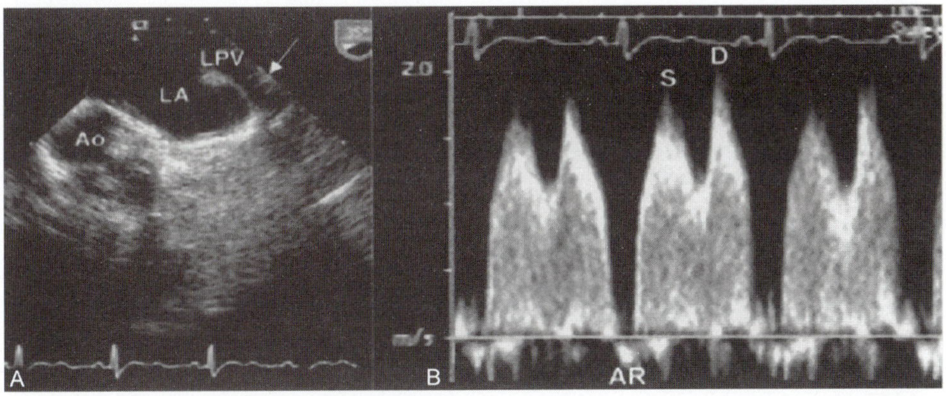

Fig. 14.154: *Pulmonary vein stenosis induced by radiofrequency ablation for atrial fibrillation. Left upper pulmonary vein stenosis (arrow) is seen by two dimensional echocardiography (A), and the peak velocities of pulmonary venous systolic (S) and early diastolic (D) waves are markedly increased (B). Ao, ascending aorta; AR, pulmonary venous atrial reversal wave; LA, left atrium; LPV, left upper pulmonary vein*

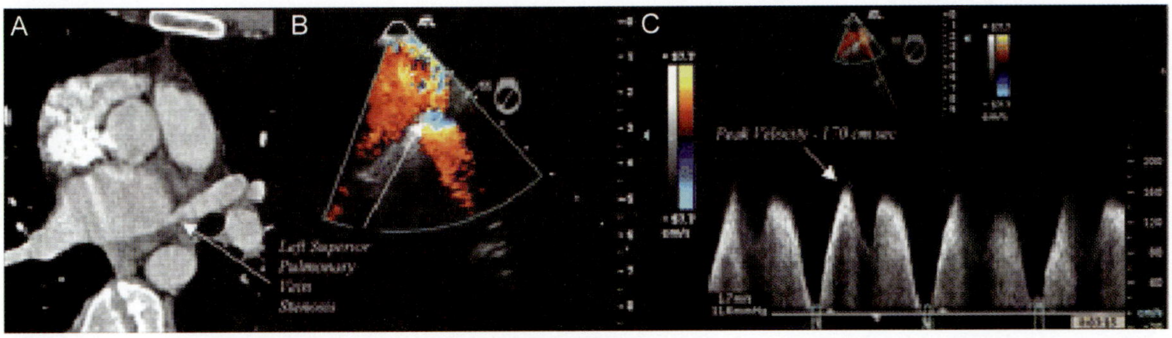

Fig. 14.155: *Transoesophageal echocardiography can identify significant pulmonary vein stenosis: (A) CT scan with ostial narrowing in the left superior pulmonary vein; (B) Significant ostial narrowing with turbulence and aliasing of the color Doppler identifies significant pulmonary vein stenosis on transoesophageal echocardiography; and (C) Pulsed-wave Doppler of pulmonary venous inflow >100 cm/s confirms hemodynamically significant stenosis*

there is right ventricular and pulmonary hypertension and, usually, elevated pulmonary arteriolar wedge pressure, although this is not necessarily found right-to-left shunting through a foramen ovale and arterial oxygen unsaturation because of pulmonary edema may be seen. Naturally occurring venous stenosis is usually a fatal disease.

Cardiac Catheterization and Angiography

Routine cases are investigated with 2D and 3D transesophageal echocardiography, but rarely, cardiac catheterization and cineangiography are undertaken in difficult cases and particularily when balloon dilation and stent implantation are the treatment of choice (Figs 14.152A and B; 14.155).

Surgical Intervensions

Surgical attempts to relieve pulmonary venous obstruction have rarely been successful. Similarly, dilating veins with balloon catheters has been unsuccessful. Although insertion of a stent in a pulmonary vein may be worth trying in this almost universally fatal disease, one has little confidence in its success (Figs 14.153A to F).

COARCTATION OF THE AORTA

Definition, Pathology and Pathophysiology

Coarctation of the aorta is a focal narrowing of the distal aortic arch due to an abnormality of the media. In infants, the lesion forms opposite or proximal to the ductus arteriosus. In adults, the lesion usually forms distal to the ligamentum arteriosum. The obstruction to flow through the ductus results in hypertension proximal to the lesion with left ventricular hypertrophy and relative hypotension and delayed pulses distal to the lesion, and prominent collateral formation. Coarctation may be associated with a bicuspid aortic valve, a hypoplastic aortic arch, endocardial fibroelastosis, ventricular septal defect, patent ductus arteriosus, or stenosis of the aortic valve. It may occur in Turner's syndrome (Figs 14.156; 14.157A and B).

Clinical Manifestations

History

Infants with coarctation may suffer from heart failure and failure to thrive, but young adults with coarctation are usually asymptomatic, reaching clinical attention due to hypertension and its complications, or by recognition of associated cardiac abnormalities. Occasionally, fatigue, dyspnea, or leg claudication develop. Heart failure may develop during middle life.

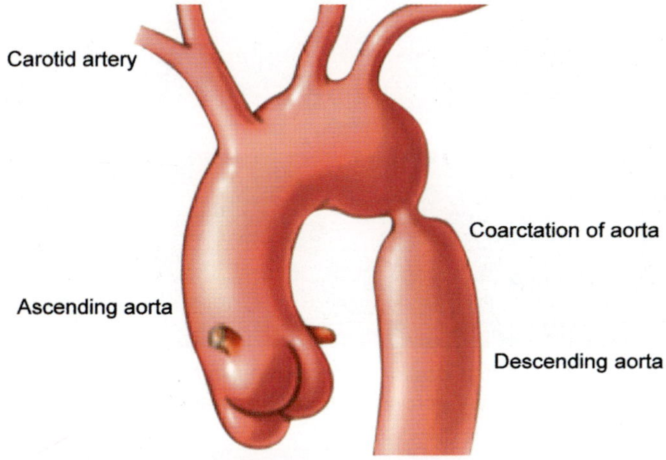

Fig. 14.156: *Diagram showing coarctation of aorta*

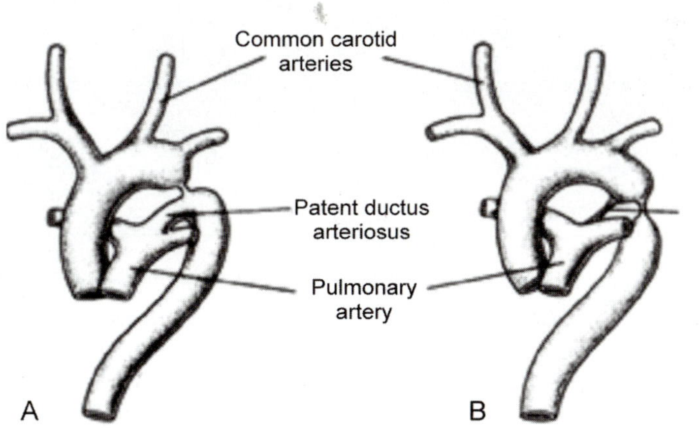

Fig. 14.157: *Coarctation of the aorta: (A) preductal type, (B) postductal type. The caudal part of the body is supplied by large hypertrophied intercostal and internal thoracic arteries*

Physical Examination

Coarctation is associated with mild to moderate hypertension of the upper extremities, prominent upper extremity pulses, and delayed, weak lower extremity pulses. A higher blood pressure in the upper extremities compared to the lower extremeties is diagnostic. Signs of left ventricular hypertrophy are common. The aortic component of the second heart sound is frequently prominent. An early systolic ejection click is suggestive of a bicuspid aortic valve. This click is usually heard best at the apex. A medium-pitched systolic murmur in the interscapular region may be present. A continuous murmur heard over the back may represent collateral arterial flow.

Diagnostic Tests

Chest X-ray

The chest film usually shows mild cardiomegaly with left ventricular prominence. The left atrium may be prominent. The "figure 3" pattern seen in the left upper portion of the aorta represents the slight dilatation of the aorta, the indentation at the coarctation site, and poststenotic dilatation of the descending aorta. The reverse of these indentations, i.e. the "E sign", can be seen on barium swallow. Notching of the ribs begins to develop in late childhood (Fig. 14.158).

Electrocardiogram

If hypertension is mild and bicuspid aortic stenosis is not present, the electrocardiogram may be normal. With time,

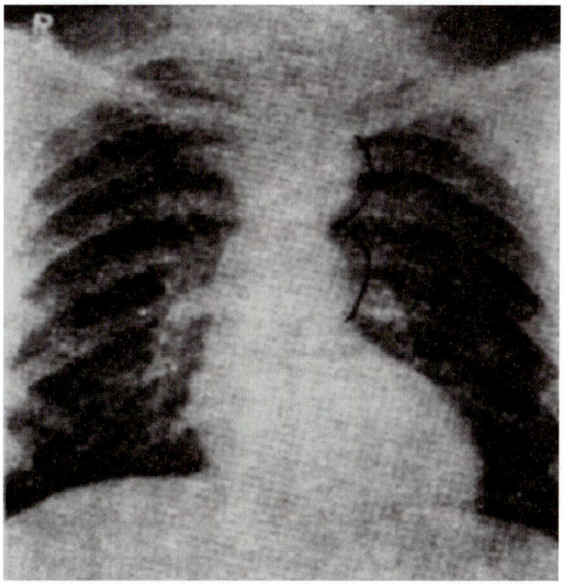

Fig. 14.158: *Photograph of X-ray chest PA view showing classic 3 or inverted E sign in patient with coarctation of aorta*

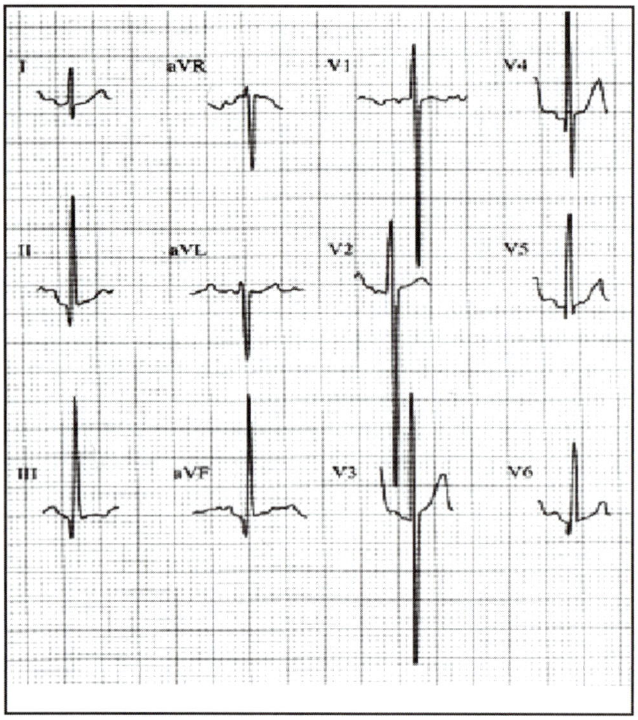

Fig. 14.159: *ECG showing deep S wave in V1-V3 indicating LVH in an infant with congenital coarctation of aorta*

left ventricular hypertrophy and left axis deviation develop, as well as ventricular ectopy (Fig. 14.159).

Differential Diagnosis

In older people, coarctation must be distinguished from other causes of hypertension as well as other causes of left ventricular hypertrophy, such as left ventricular outflow tract obstruction.

Laboratory Evaluation

Echocardiography (Figs 14.160 and 14.161)

Echocardiography may be helpful in the assessment of left ventricular hypertrophy to rule out other causes of left ventricular hypertrophy and heart failure or associated defects such as bicuspid aortic valve.

Computerized axial tomography and MRI: These noninvasive imaging are very contributory in delineation of cardiac anatomy and implanted devices (Figs 14.162A and B to 14.165A and B).

Cardiac Catheterization (Figs 14.166A and B)

Cardiac catheterization and aortography is essential to establish the site and length of coarctation, to measure the pressure gradient across the coarctation, to assess left ventricular function, and to rule out associated congenital defects such as aortic stenosis.

Natural History and Prognosis

The median length of life of people surviving childhood without surgical repair is about 30 years. Coarctation of

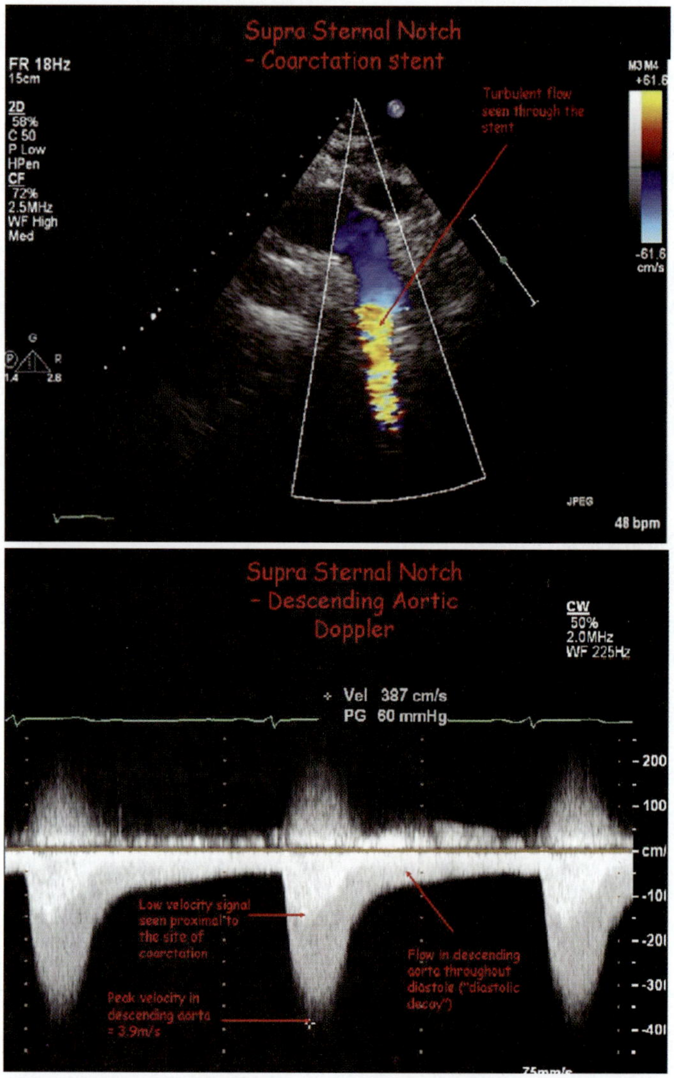

Fig. 14.160: *Color Doppler echocardiography shows signature of enhanced velocity across coarctation of aorta*

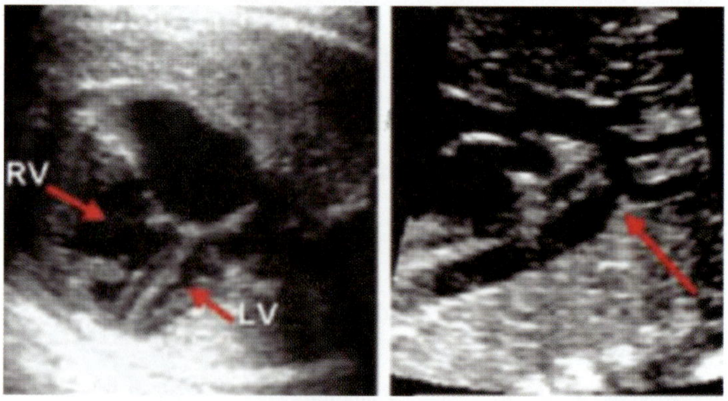

Fig. 14.161: *Coarctation may be a postnatal event, and this limits prenatal diagnosis in many cases. It should be suspected when the right ventricle is enlarged (right ventricle to left ventricle ratio of more than 1.3). Narrowing of the isthmus, or the presence of a shelf is often difficult to demonstrate because in the fetus aortic arch and ductal arch are close and are difficult to distinguish. In most cases, coarctation can only be suspected in utero and a certain diagnosis must be delayed until after birth*

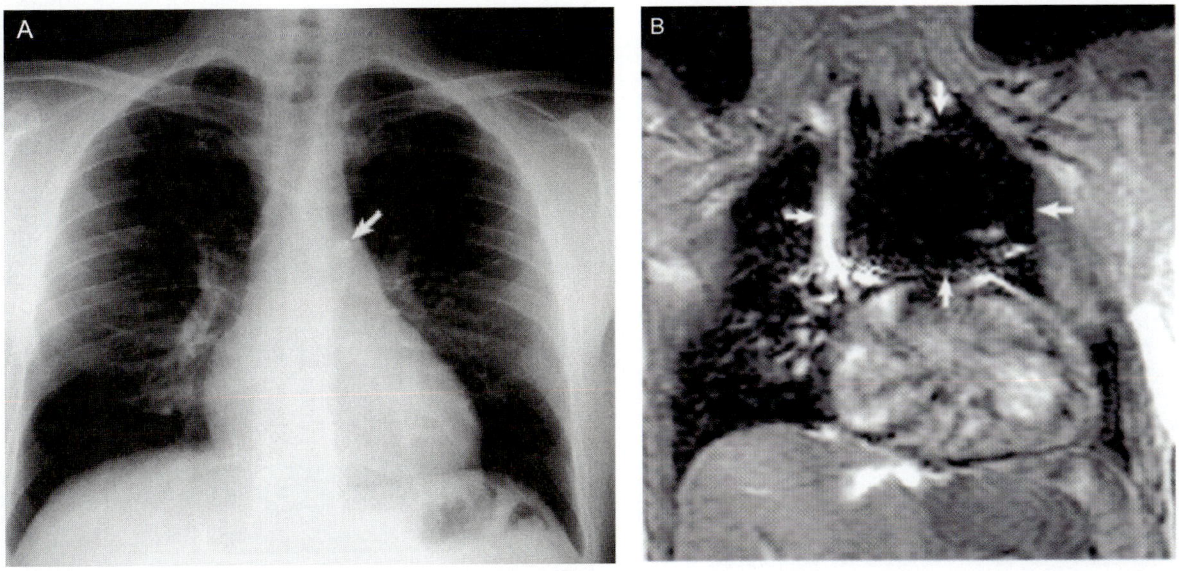

Fig. 14.162: *Image artifacts due to a stainless steel endovascular coil. (A) Chest radiogram showing a single coil used for closure of a patent ductus arteriosus. (B) Gradient echo image in the coronal plane showing a large imaging artifact (8–10 cm in diameter) due to the coil*

the aorta may be associated with aortic dissection, heart failure, and premature atherosclerosis. Intracranial hemorrhage may result from aneurysm formation in the circle of Willis. Endocarditis may occur at the site of coarctation, the aortic valve, or the mitral valve. Patients with associated endocardial fibroelastosis usually die of heart failure by age 30–40 years.

Treatment

Medical

Medical therapy includes restriction from strenuous sports and severe isometric exercises, antihypertensive therapy, and avoidance of pregnancy. Endocarditis prophylaxis is recommended.

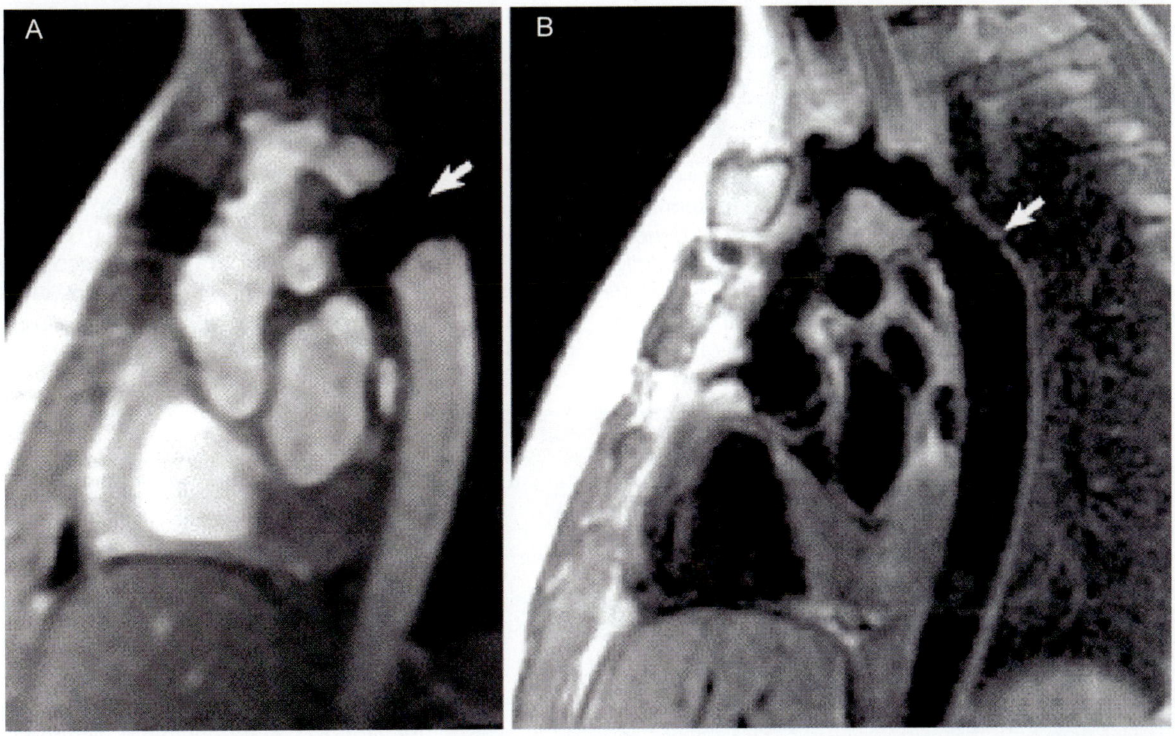

Fig. 14.163A and B: *Image artifact (arrow) due to an endovascular stent placed in the aortic isthmus for treatment of recurrent coarctation of the aorta. (A) Gradient echo image; (B) fast spin echo with double inversion recovery showing a markedly reduced image artifact*

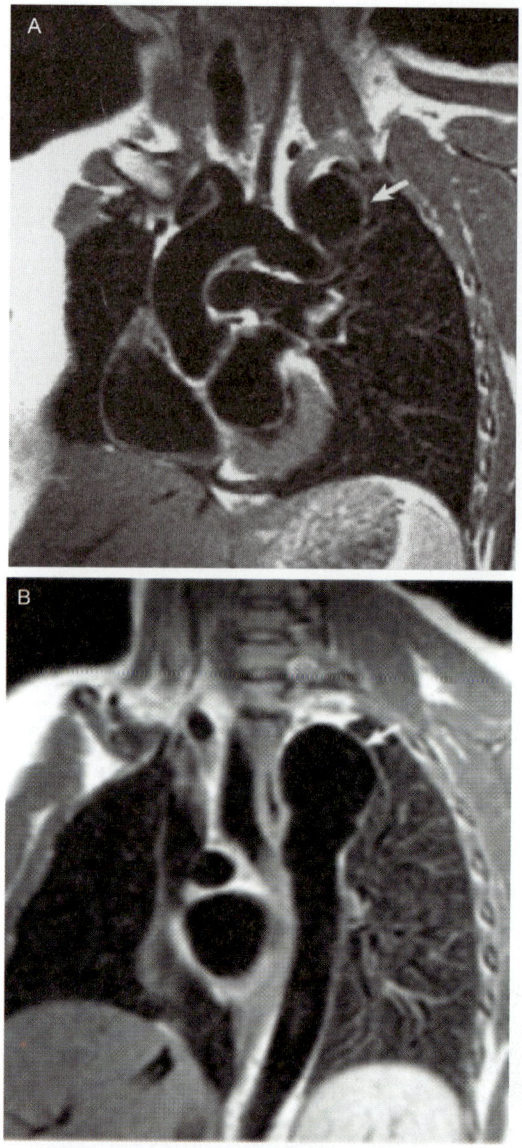

Fig. 14.164A and B: *MRI at 27-weeks gestation in a patient with unrepaired coarctation of the aorta. (A) Fast spin echo with double inversion recovery image in the coronal plane showing a mildly elongated transverse aortic arch and a large aneurysm in the left upper hemithorax (arrow); (B) oblique view of the descending aorta showing a large aneurysm of the aortic isthmus (arrow)*

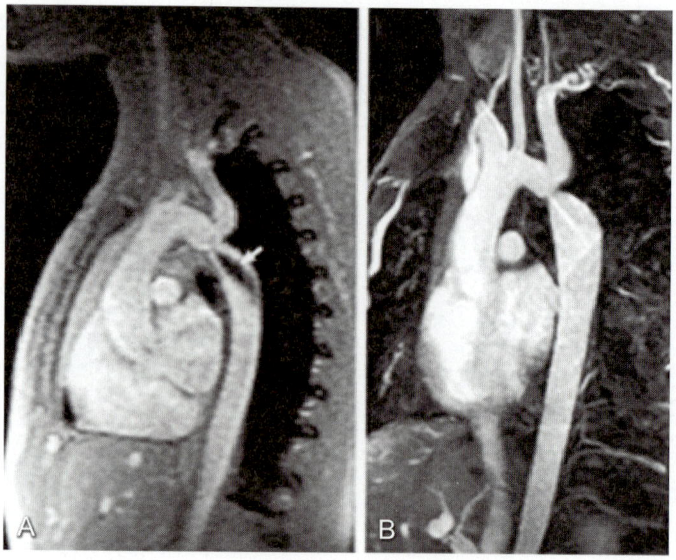

Fig. 14.165: *MRI evaluation of aortic coarctation. (A) Systolic frame from a cine MR sequence showing a turbulent jet at the coarctation site (arrow); (B) gadolinium-enhanced 3D MRA subvolume MIP image of the aorta*

Balloon Angioplasty and Stent Placement

Gruntzig's technique of balloon angioplasty was adopted by Sos Singer and Sperling and their associates to enlarge coarcted aortic segments in a postmortem specimen, post-surgical recoarctation and native coarctation, respectively. This is followed by a report of successful use of this technique in a sizeable population of patients with native aortic coarctation by Lababidi subsequently, the procedure was adopted by other groups of workers.

Surgery

Older children and adults should undergo operative repair of coarctation with resection and reanastomosis or patch angioplasty. Surgical correction of the defect does not, however, ensure that the blood pressure will return to normal. If coarctation recurs with a pressure gradient greater than 30 mmHg, reoperation is recommended.

Coartation of aorta can also be repaired with successful implantation of appropriate stents (Figs 14.166 to 14.168A and B).

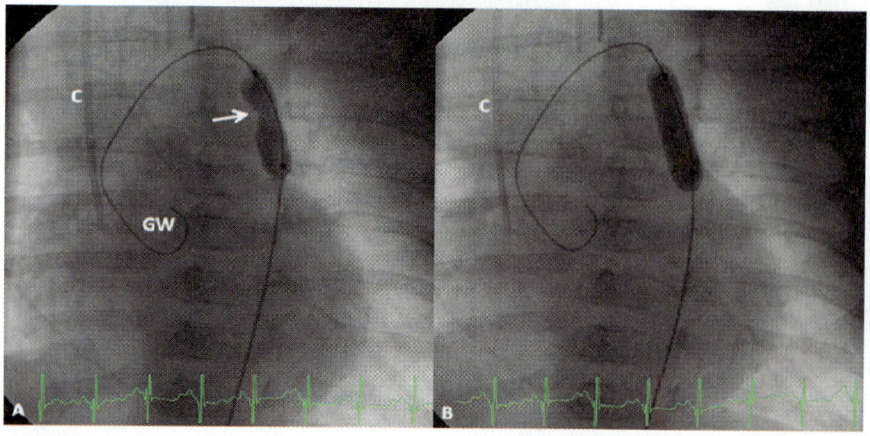

Fig. 14.166A and B: *Balloon dilatation catheter positioned across the aortic coarctation in 20° left anterior oblique view showing waisting of the balloon (arrow) during the initial phases of balloon inflation (A). Note complete disappearance of the waisting of the balloon (B) after complete balloon inflation. C, catheter in the superior vena cava; GW, guidewire.*

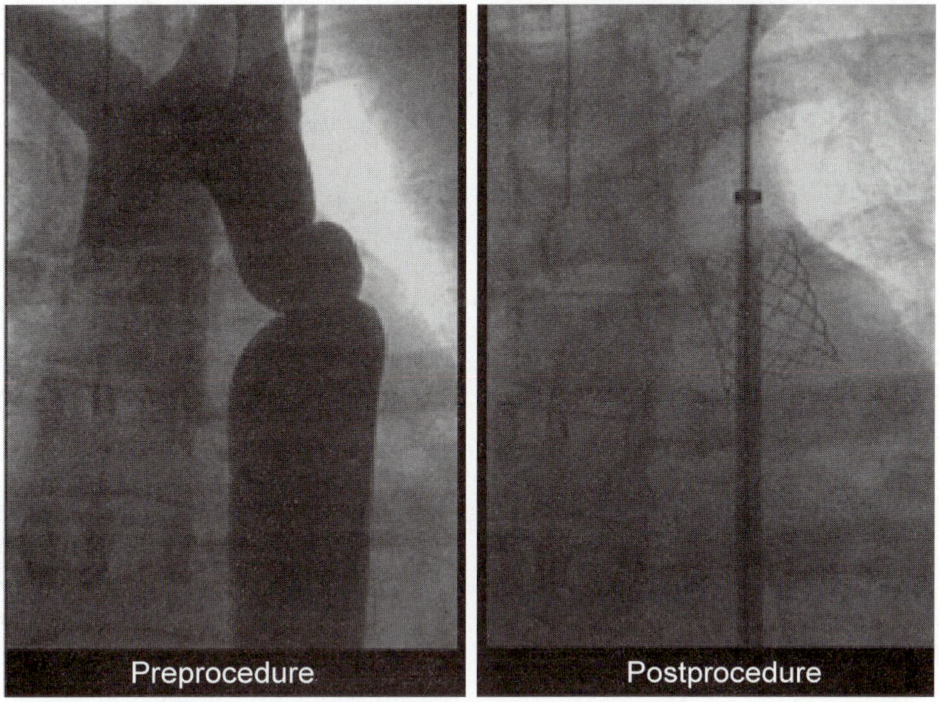

Fig. 14.167: *Stent placement is considered by some the treatment of choice to replace surgery in older children and adults with coarctation. Studies have shown excellent results in the short and intermediate term*

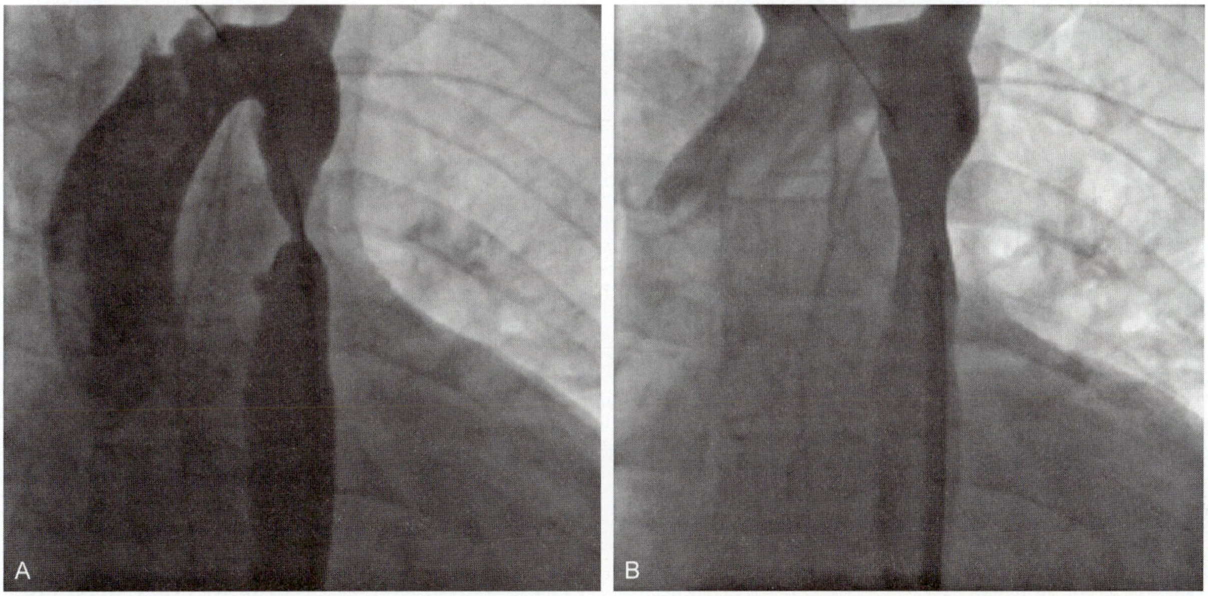

Fig. 14.168: *Repair of coarctation with transcatheter stent placement. (A) Catheter angiogram demonstrates severe discrete coarctation of the aorta in this 18-year-old patient with upper-extremity hypertension. (B) Similar angiogram after transcatheter balloon dilation and stent placement demonstrates significant improvement of the coarctation*

TETRALOGY OF FALLOT

Definition, Pathology and Pathophysiology

Tetralogy of Fallot is a complex consisting of (Fig. 14.169):
1. A large ventricular septal defect
2. An obstruction to pulmonary outflow
3. Biventricular origin of the aorta over the VSD (overriding aorta)
4. Right ventricular hypertrophy.

It is believed that the complex is due to a congenital displacement of the conal septum resulting in the infundibular stenosis and the VSD, as well as right ventricular hypertrophy, and an overriding aorta. A similar clinical picture occurs whether the right ventricular outflow tract obstruction is due to infundibular or to pulmonary valve stenosis.

Tetralogy may be associated with right-sided aortic arch, atrial septal defect, or coronary anomalies. The pathophysiology of tetralogy of Fallot is determmed by the ratio of resistance to flow through the systemic circuit versus resistance to flow through "the VSD and across the right ventncular outflow tract. If right ventricular outflow tract resistance is high, right-to-left shunting across the VSD predominates. If right ventricular outflow tract obstruction is mild, however, right-to -Ieft shunting is mild (acyanotic tetralogy of Fallot). Infundibular stenosis may be dynamic, increasing with conditions of increased myocardial contractility. Exercise decreases systemic vascular resistance, resulting in increased right-to-left shunting and potentially causing syncope. Squatting increases systemic vascular resistance, thereby decreasing right-to-left shunting.

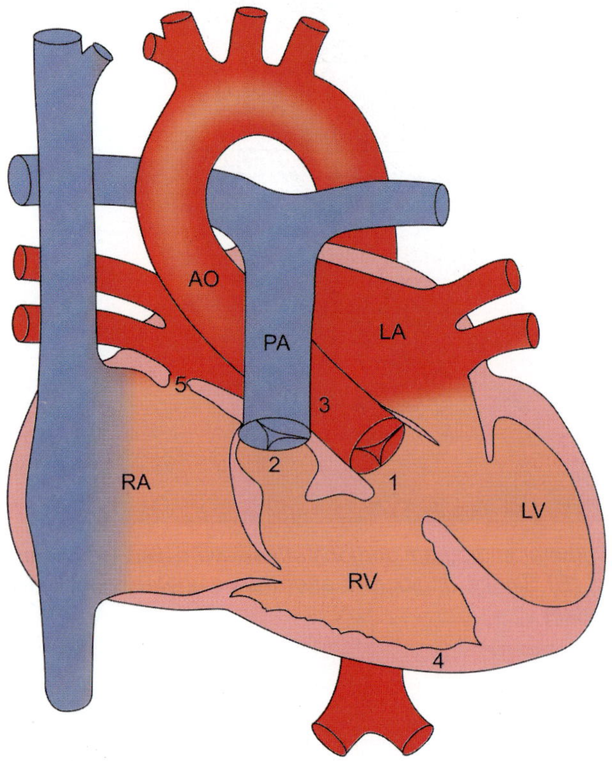

Fig. 14.169: *Structural abnormalities in tetralogy of Fallot 1. ventricular septal defect, 2. valvular and infundibular pulmonary stenosis, 3. overriding aorta, 4. right ventricular hypertrophy, 5. atrial septal defect (optional)*

Clinical Manifestations

History

Tetralogy of Fallot and Eisenmenger's syndrome are the most common forms of cyanotic congenital heart disease found in adults. The condition is usually recognized as cyanosis in childhood, but if right ventricular outflow tract obstruction develops slowly, cyanosis may develop later in life. Dyspnea and fatigability usually force the patient to restrict activity. Cyanotic or hypoxic spells may occur, and may be precipitated by infection, heat or exertion. Syncope may result from a cyanotic spell or from ventricular arrhythmias. Squatting relieves exertional dyspnea and is very suggestive of tetralogy.

Signs and Symptoms

The clinical features of tetralogy of Fallot are directly related to the severity of the anatomic defects. Infants often display the following:
1. Difficulty with feeding
2. Failure to thrive
3. Episodes of bluish pale skin during crying or feeding (i.e. "Tet" spells)
4. Exertional dyspnea, usually worsening with age.

Physical Examination

1. Most infants are smaller than expected for age
2. Cyanosis of the lips and nail bed is usually pronounced at birth
3. After age 3–6 months, the fingers and toes show clubbing
4. A systolic thrill is usually present anteriorly along the left sternal border
5. A harsh systolic ejection murmur (SEM) is heard over the pulmonic area and left sternal border
6. During cyanotic episodes, murmurs may disappear
7. In individuals with aortopulmonary collaterals, continuous murmurs may be auscultated

The following may also be noticed:
1. RV predominance on palpation
2. A bulging left hemithorax
3. Aortic ejection click
4. Squatting position (compensatory mechanism)
5. Scoliosis (common)
6. Retinal engorgement
7. Hemoptysis.

Laboratory Tests

Hemoglobin and hematocrit values are usually elevated in proportion to the degree of cyanosis. Patients with significant cyanosis have the following, in association with a tendency to bleed:
1. Decreased clotting factors
2. Low platelet count

3. Diminished coagulation factors
4. Diminished total fibrinogen
5. Prolonged prothrombin and coagulation times
6. Arterial blood gas (ABG) results are as follows:
   - Oxygen saturation varies.
   - pH and partial pressure of carbon dioxide (pCO_2) are normal unless the patient is critically sick.

The hemoglobin and hematocrit should be evaluated periodically to rule out polycythemia and relative anemia. Uric acid levels may be associated with polycythemia. Because bleeding may be associated with polycythemia, platelet and coagulation studies should be considered if surgery is planned.

Imaging Studies

Chest Radiography (Fig. 14.170)

1. Often normal initially
2. Diminished vascularity in the lungs and diminished prominence of the pulmonary arteries gradually become apparent
3. The classic boot-shaped heart (coeur en sabot) is the hallmark of the disorder.

Electrocardiogram (Fig. 14.171)

The electrocardiogram generally shows right ventricular hypertrophy, usually with a right atrial abnormality.

Echocardiography has the following attributes:
1. Color-flow Doppler echocardiography accurately diagnoses ductus arteriosus, muscular VSD, or atrial septal defect (Figs 14.172 to 14.74A and B)
2. The coronary anatomy can be revealed with some degree of accuracy

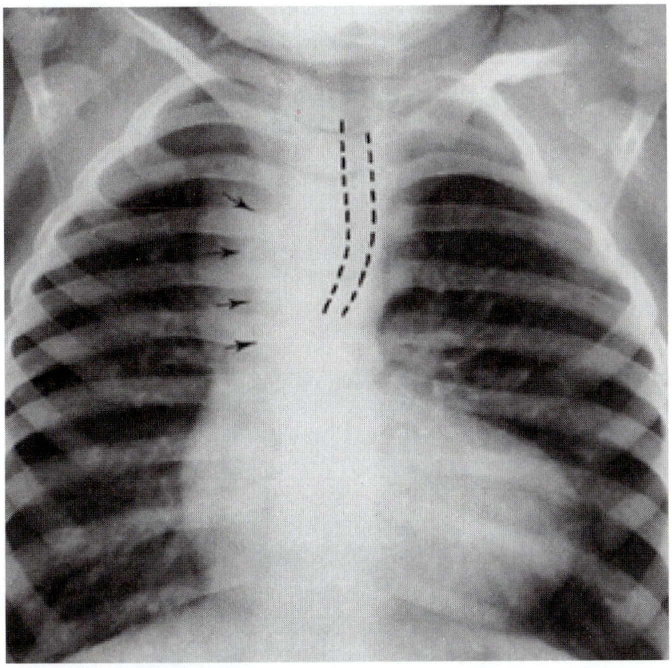

Fig. 14.170: *X-ray chest (PA view) showing right ventricular hypertrophy SmaU main pulmonary artery shadow and pulmonary oligaemia inTOF (typically described as" boot-shaped heart"*

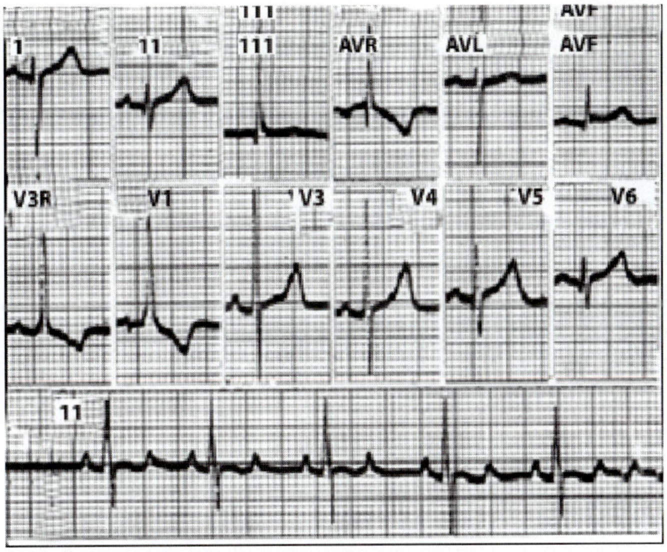

Fig. 14.171: *ECG showing right axis deviation, right ventricular hypertrophy and P-pulmonale (RAH) in TOF*

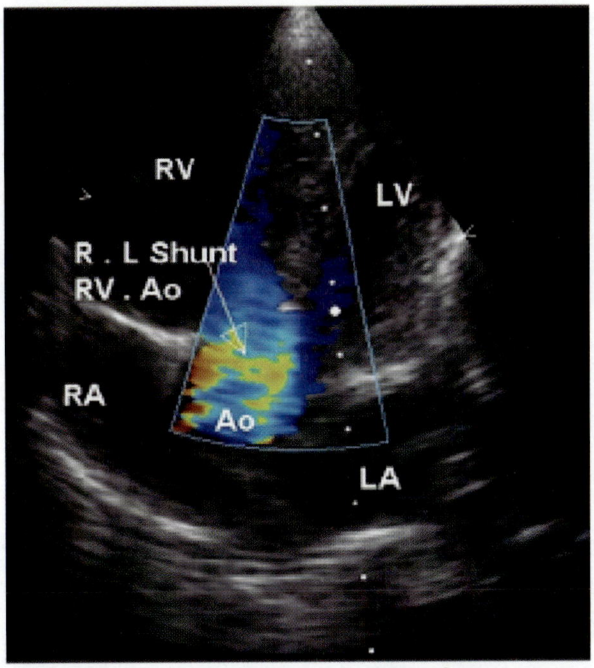

Fig. 14.172: *Apical five chamber view in tetralogy of fallot with color flow mapping (Colour Doppler imaging) in systole with right to left shunt across the VSD. Blue stream moving from right ventricle across the VSD to the aorta is clearly visualized in this frame. There is also a blue stream from the left ventricle to the aorta*

3. Valvular alterations can be detected with ease
4. In many institutions, echocardiography is the only diagnostic study used before surgery.

MRI has the following attributes (Figs 14.175A and B, 14.176):
1. Provides good delineation of the aorta, RVOT, VSDs
2. RV hypertrophy, and the pulmonary artery and its branches (Fig. 14.176)

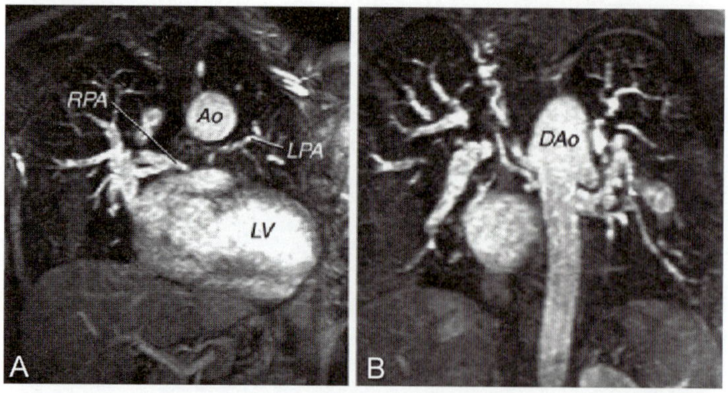

Fig. 14.173: *Preoperative MRI in a 13-year-old boy with TOF, pulmonary atresia, and discontinuous pulmonary arteries. (A) Gadolinium-enhanced 3D MRA subvolume MIP in the coronal plane showing discontinuity between the right (RPA) and left pulmonary arteries (LPA). (B) Subvolume MIP image of the descending aorta (DAo) showing multiple aortopulmonary collaterals*

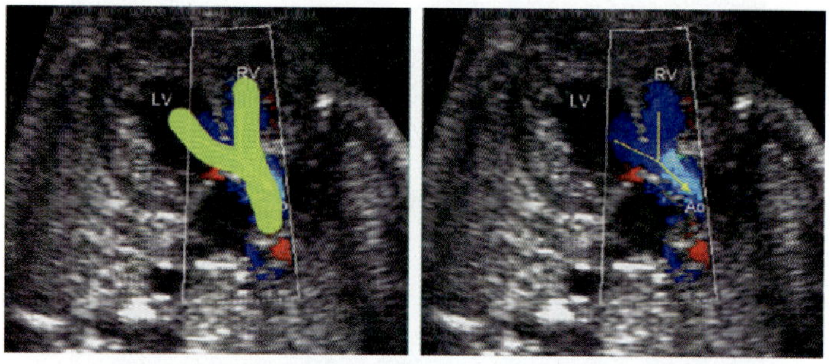

Fig. 14.174: *Fetal ultrasonography: five chamber view in a fetus with tetralogy of Fallot (TOF), demonstrating the systolic perfusion from both the right and left ventricle (RV, LV) into the overriding aorta (Y-shape)*

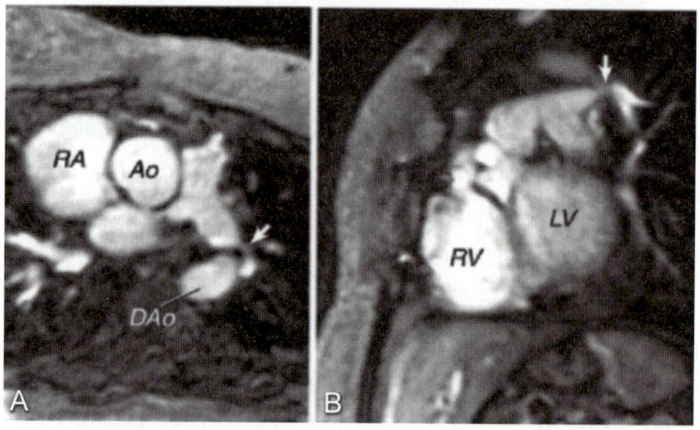

Fig. 14.175A and B: *Postoperative MRI after TOF repair in a patient who has undergone a previous Potts shunt. (A) Gadolinium-enhanced 3D MRA subvolume MIP in the axial plane showing severe left pulmonary artery stenosis (arrow) at the site of the previous Potts shunt. (B) Oblique sagittal subvolume MIP image showing the superior-inferior aspect of the left pulmonary artery stenosis (arrow)*

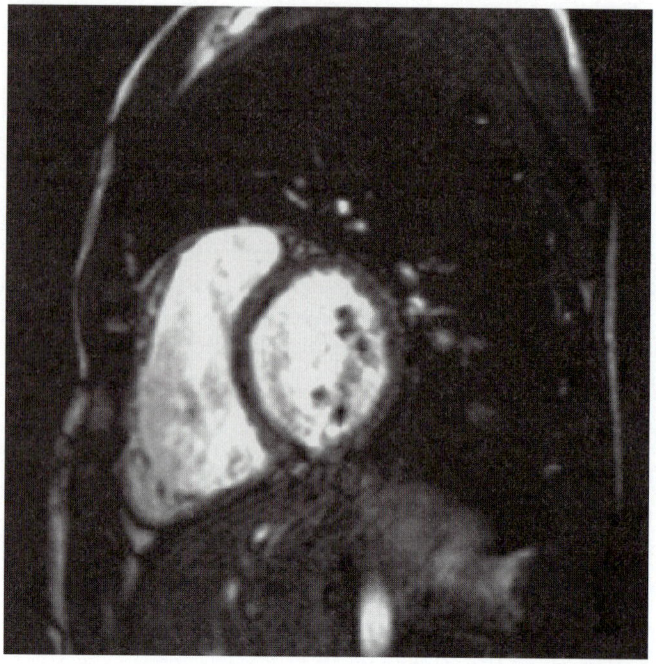

Fig. 14.176: *Cardiac magnetic resonance image in a 24-year-old late after tetralogy of Fallot repair in the first year of life, with transannular right ventricular outflow tract patch. Oblique short-axis image demonstrates the severely dilated right ventricle relative to the left ventricle. By off-line volumetric analysis utilizing a series of three dimensional cut planes, this patient's right ventricular end-diastolic volume was 200 mL/m²*

3. Can also be used to measure intracardiac pressures, gradients, and blood flows.

Cardiac catheterization is extremely useful in any of the following instances (Fig. 14.177):

1. The anatomy cannot be completely defined by echocardiography

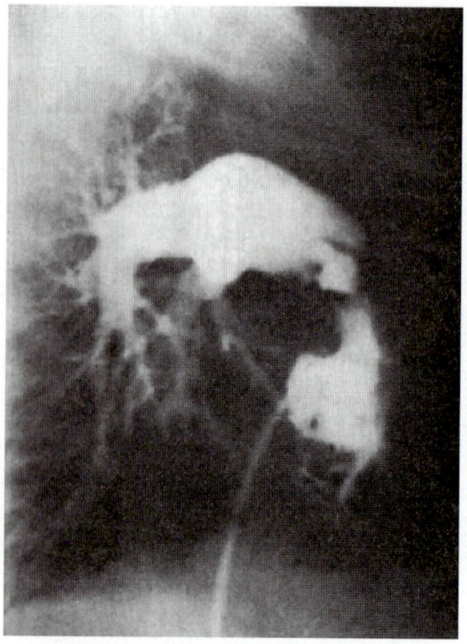

Fig. 14.177: *Cineangiogram shows a catheter in the right ventricle demonstrating severe infundibular stenosis*

2. Disease in the pulmonary arteries is a concern
3. Pulmonary vascular hypertension is possible
4. Assessment of the pulmonary annulus size and pulmonary arteries
5. Assessment of the severity of RVOTO
6. Location of the position and size of the VSD
7. Ruling out possible coronary artery anomalie.

Differential Diagnosis

Tetralogy of Fallot must be distinguished from other forms of cyanotic congenital heart disease, particularly Eisenmenger's syndrome. With Eisenmenger's syndrome, the systolic murmur is usually less prominent, S2 may not be single, and the pulmonic component of the second heart sound (P2) is loud. Tetralogy of Fallot must be distinguished from isolated pulmonary stenosis, which is not associated with cyanosis. In the newborn, it must be distinguished from tricuspid atresia, transposition of the great arteries, severe pulmonary stenosis or atresia with an intact ventricular septum, and truncus arteriosus.

Natural History and Prognosis

The prognosis of uncorrected tetralogy of Fallot is poor, with survival past 30 years being unusual. Complications Include sudden death, stroke and brain abscess, polycythemia resulting in bleeding, thrombosis, gout and endocarditis.

Management

Acute treatment for hypercyanosis is as follows:

1. Place the baby on the mother's shoulder with the infant's knees tucked up underneath; this provides a calming effect, reduces systemic venous return, and increases systemic vascular resistance (SVR)
2. Oxygen is of limited value, as the primary abnormality is reduced pulmonary blood flow
3. Morphine sulfate, 0.1–0.2 mg/kg intramuscularly (IM) or subcutaneously (SC), may reduce the ventilatory drive and decrease systemic venous return
4. Phenylephrine, 0.02 mg/kg IV, is used to increase SVR
5. Dexmedetomidine infusion has been used, but requires caution and careful titration
6. General anesthesia is a last resort
7. Most infants with tetralogy of Fallot require some type of surgical procedure.

Surgical Intervention

It is preferably done at or about 12 months of age. Primary correction is the ideal operation and is usually performed under cardiopulmonary bypass. Palliative procedures (e.g. placement of the modified Blalock-Taussig shunt) may be necessary in patients with contraindications to primary repair, which include the following (Fig. 14.178):

1. The presence of an anomalous coronary artery
2. Very low birth weight
3. Small pulmonary arteries
4. Multiple VSDs
5. Multiple coexisting intracardiac malformations

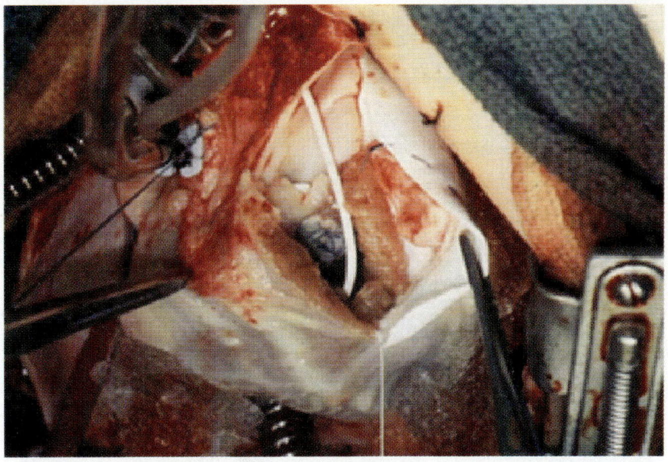

Fig. 14.178: *This image shows a closed ventricular septal defect and closure of right ventriculotomy with Gore-Tex*

DOUBLE OUTLET RIGHT VENTRICLE

Double-outlet right ventricle is said to be present when both great arteries arise completely or nearly completely above the right ventricle (Fig. 14.179).

Prevalence

Among critically ill infants, it is found to be in the order of 0.032 per 1,000 live births. The diagnosis of double-outlet right ventricle depends greatly on how much one or the other great vessel overrides the right ventricle.

Pathophysiology (Fig. 14.180)

Double-outlet right ventricle is not a single cardiac anomaly or even a part of a complex of anomalies. It is a term that is used to describe the position of the great arteries found in association with a variety of cardiac anomalies that can be

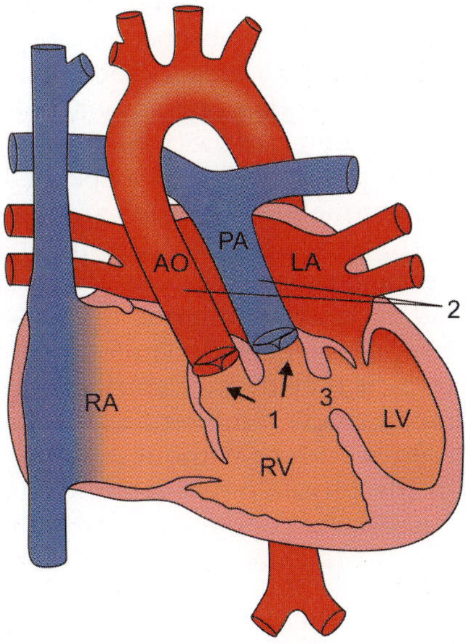

Fig. 14.179: *Diagram showing double outlet right ventricle featuring. 1. Double-outlet right ventricle, 2. Transposed great arteries, 3. Ventricular septal defect*

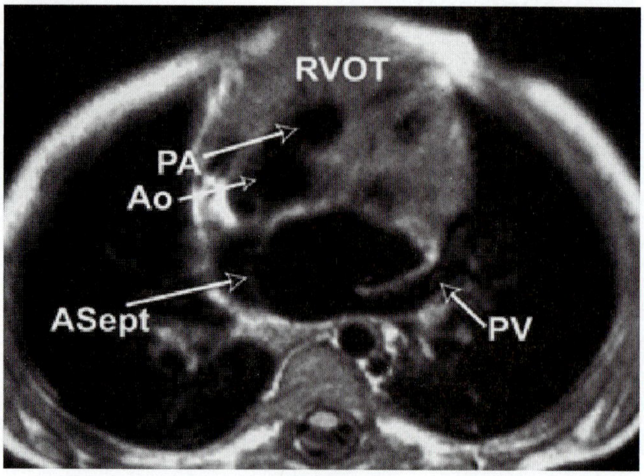

Fig. 14.180: *Heterotaxy syndrome, polysplenia, and a double-outlet right ventricle in a 1½-year-old boy. Axial MR image shows the side-by-side origins of the aorta (Ao) (posterior, right) and the main pulmonary artery (PA) (anterior, left), both of which arise from the right ventricular outflow tract (RVOT). The left superior pulmonary vein (PV) is seen entering the left-sided atrium. ASept, atrial septum*

viewed, physiologically, as ventricular septal defects, tetralogy of Fallot, transposition of the great arteries, single ventricle, or atrioventricular atresia. Pulmonary stenosis is common in patients with double-outlet right ventricle of all types. The relation of the great arteries to each other is often side-by-side and parallel, with the aorta on the right or left, anterior or posterior, often resembling transposition of the great .arteries. A variety of atrioventricular valvular abnormalities and outflow valve and subvalvular obstructions are encountered. Interrupted aortic arch and coarctation of the aorta are often seen. Hypoplasia or stenosis of the aortic valve is often encountered when there is coarctation of the aorta, although subvalvular aortic stenosis may be seen in the absence of coarctation. Any malfunction of the atrioventricular or semilunar valves may be present, with various types of pulmonary stenosis being the most common. A defect of the common atrioventricular canal is frequently present, with its associated mitral and tricuspid valve abnormalities There is a gradation of defects ranging from subaortic.The relationship between the ventricular defect and the great arteries, the relative outflow obstruction, and the relative systemic to pulmonary artery resistance determine the hemodynamic situation. Double-outlet right ventricle may mimic ventricular septal defect, tetralogy of Fallot, single right ventricle, or transposition of the great arteries with or without pulmonary stenosis. Depending on the physiology, the child may have the problems of cyanosis, of congestive heart failure, or both. Some degree of arterial un saturation is almost always present.

Clinical Manifestations

The patient may have the symptoms of congestive heart failure, cyanosis, or no symptoms at all.

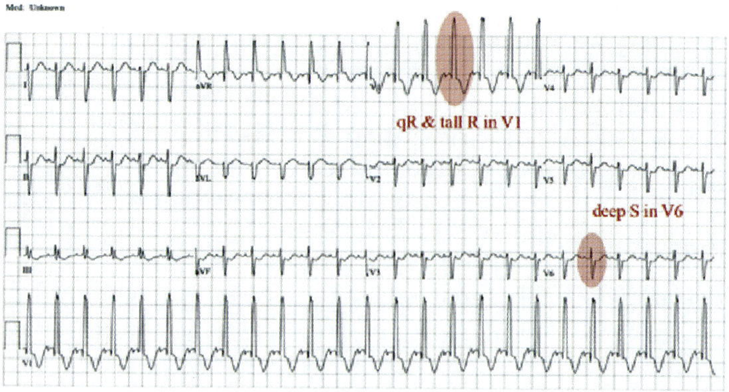

Fig. 14.181: *The RV will be hypertrophied with right-axis deviation and possible RAE in patient with DORV*

Electrocardiography (Fig. 14.181)

There is no characteristic electrocardiographic pattern, although virtually all have a pattern compatible with right ventricular hypertrophy.

Chest X-ray

Similarly, there is no characteristic chest X-ray. The size of the heart and the amount of pulmonary vascularity are dependent on the hemodynamics and may range from a relatively small heart with decreased pulmonary vascularity to a large heart with increased pulmonary vascular markings (Fig. 14.182).

Echocardiography

The diagnosis is usually apparent from the subxiphoid view. The criterion for diagnosis is alignment of both great arteries, totally or predominantly, with the right ventricle.

- Bilateral conus is often, but not invariably, present.
- Parasternal long- and short-axis views are also useful for detecting the alignment of the great arteries and for detecting subarterial conal muscle. Because there are a

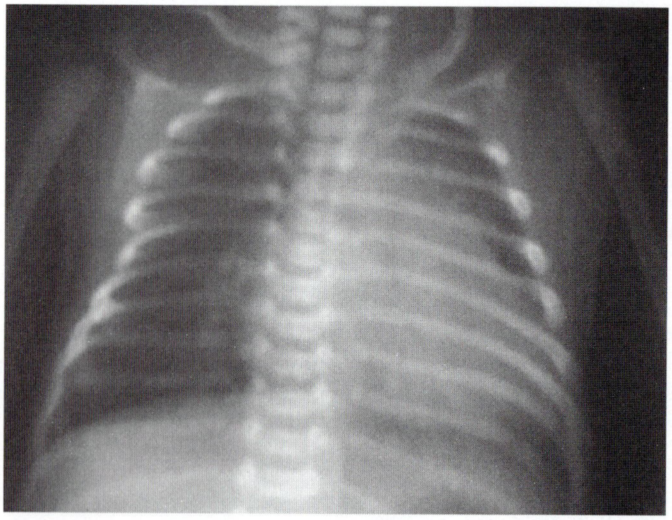

Fig. 14.182: *Chest radiograph showing a mildly enlarged heart with symmetrically slightly increased pulmonary vasculature.in a neonate with double-outlet right ventricle*

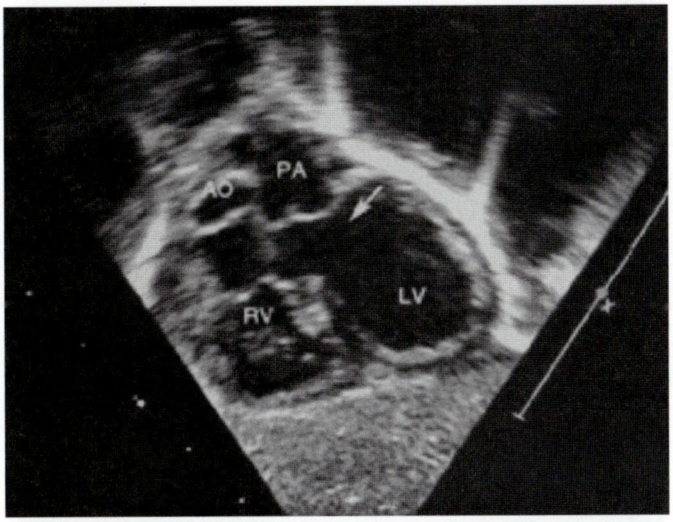

Fig. 14.183: *Double-outlet right ventricle. Subxiphoid short-axis echocardiogram image in this infant with Taussig-Bing type double-outlet right ventricle demonstrates both great vessels arising from the right ventricle (RV). The ventricular septal defect is subpulmonary in location (arrow), with the aorta (AO) rightward of the pulmonary artery (PA). LV, left ventricle*

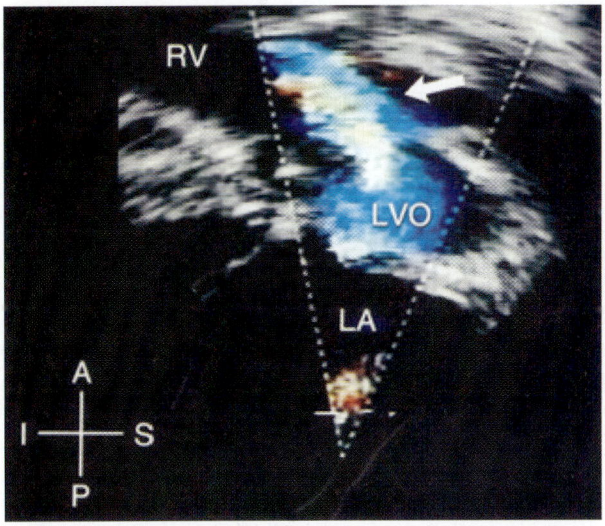

Fig. 14.184: *Echocardiography in DORV. The subxiphoid view allows to characterize the origin of both great vessels emerging from the RV, and also their relationship to one another. In addition to the anatomy mentioned before it allows the evaluation of the subpulmonic conus, the severity of the pulmonary stenosis and the relationship of the VSD to the aortic valve*

large number of anatomic variations and associated intracardiac lesions, a thorough examination of all segments of the heart is mandatory (Figs 14.183 to 14.185).

Cardiac Catheterization

Before cardiac surgery is undertaken, cardiac catheterization is scheduled to confirm the echocardiographic findings and the clinical understanding of the hemodynamics. The patients usually have some degree of arterial oxygen unsaturation and have the hemodynamics of tetralogy of Fallot, single right ventricle, transposition of the great arteries, dominant left-to-right shunt, or pulmonary vascular obstructive disease. The wide variety of physiologic possibilities are unraveled by the usual techniques. The information obtained from the echocardiogram may suggest the best positioning of the patient in order to demonstrate the origins of the great vessels and the location of the ventricular defects. Often these are seen best in a biplane angiogram in anteroposterior and straight lateral views, since the great arteries often are side-by-side with the semilunar valves at the same level.

Treatment Options for Double-Outlet Right Ventricle

Medications may be necessary early on to help the heart to function better prior to and after surgical intervention. However, double-outlet right ventricle requires open heart surgery. Surgeons have a variety of methods to repair this heart defect, depending on the anatomy (structure) of the child's heart.

Sometimes they use a patch made of a synthetic fiber called Dacron to create a tunnel (called a baffle) through the VSD (the hole between the right and left ventricles). The tunnel connects to the aorta. This means all of the

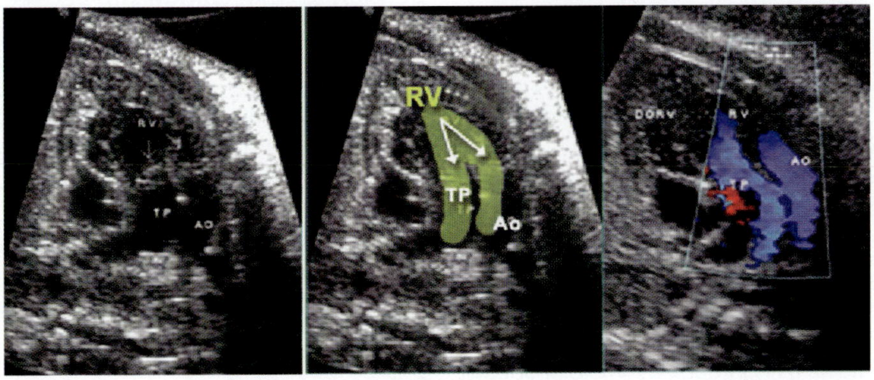

Fig. 14.185: *Fetal ultrasonography. Double-outlet right ventricle (DORV) with both the aorta (AO) and pulmonary trunk (TP) arising from the right ventricle. Color Doppler demonstrates blood flow from the right ventricle into both vessels and the flow is not turbulent because there is no stenosis*

oxygenated blood from the left ventricle is channeled through the right ventricle into the aorta, without mixing with the deoxygenated blood in the right ventricle.

In other cases, surgeons reverse the double-outlet right ventricle by detaching the aorta from the right ventricle and reattach it to the left ventricle, move the coronary arteries to the new aorta and close the VSD. This surgery is called the arterial switch.

In other cases, the left or right ventricle will be too small or malformed to ever function correctly. Surgeons will reconfigure the heart and circulatory system so that the heart functions with one ventricle (pumping chamber), instead of two. This is called Fontan circulation and requires three open heart surgeries, called staged reconstruction: Norwood procedure, hemi-Fontan or Glenn operation and Fontan procedure.

Ventricular septal defect with pulmonary stenosis, to tetralogy of Fallot, to double-outlet right ventricle with pulmonary stenosis. There is a similar range of clinical problems extending from subpulmonary ventricular septal defect with varying degrees of overriding of the pulmonary artery (transposition of the great arteries) to double-outlet right ventricle. Another anatomic spectrum ranges from a single right ventricle giving rise to both great vessels, to a single right ventricle with a hypoplastic left ventricle, to a double-outlet right ventricle with a small left ventricle that is, nevertheless, of sufficient size to permit a two-ventricle repair (Figs 14.186 and 14.187).

Ventricular Septal Defect

A ventricular septal defect is almost always present, although rarely there is none, the pulmonary venous blood

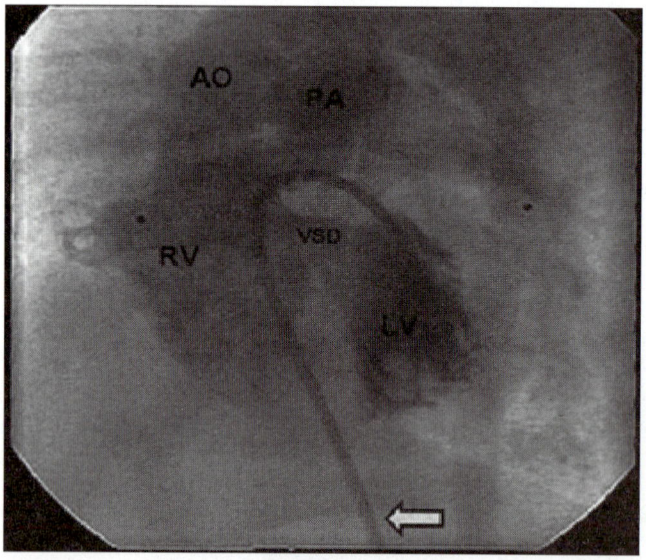

Fig. 14.186: *This is an angiogram obtained during catheterization of a patient with double-outlet right ventricle (DORV) with transposition of the great arteries. Injection of contrast though the catheter (arrow) into the left ventricle (LV) shows that blood is directed toward the right ventricle (RV) through a remote or doubly committed ventricular septal defect (VSD). The aorta (AO) is anterior to the pulmonary artery (PA) and both clearly arise from the RV*

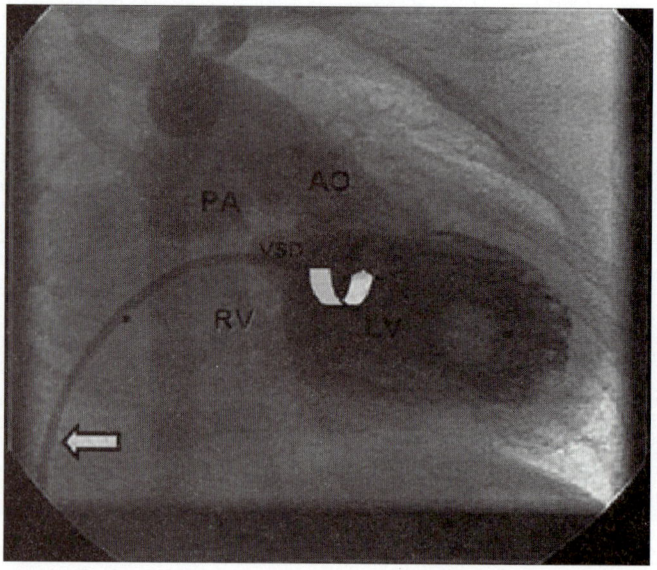

Fig. 14.187: *This is an angiogram obtained during catheterization of a patient with double-outlet right ventricle (DORV) with transposition of the great arteries. Blood fills the aorta (AO) and pulmonary artery (PA) almost simultaneously, which is another indicator of a remote or doubly committed ventricular septal defect (VSD) (curved arrow). LV indicates the left ventricle, RV indicates the right ventricle, and the small arrow to the left indicates the catheter*

reaching the right ventricle by shunting left-to-right through an atrial septal opening. The ventricular defect may be subaortic, subpulmonary, uncommitted (both subaortic and subpulmonary), or remote (muscular or endocardial cushion type) The subaortic and subpulmonary defects rarely lie immediately below the corresponding semilunar valve without intervening conal tissue. The subpulmonary and the subaortic ventricular defects have the same location and that it is the variation in distribution of conal tissue that determines the great artery with which the ventricular defect is associated. Because of variations in location of infundibular tissue (conal tissue), anteriorly or posteriorly, malalignment of the ventricular septal defect is directly related to the presence of subaortic stenosis on the one hand and pulmonary stenosis on the other. Another factor that determines the relationship between the ventricular defect and the great arteries is the relative rightward or leftward position of the great arteries themselves. The location of the ventricular defect relative to the great arteries determines pulmonary arterial growth have been reported. This approach is not yet widely accepted for the most part, transcatheter therapies for adults with TOF are limited to patients who have undergone the surgical possibilities. As in most other complex groups of cardiac anomalies, some ventricular defects have a tendency to get smaller with time. This must be considered in the clinical management of these children.

Pulmonary Stenosis

Almost 3 of 4 of patients with double-outlet right ventricle have some degree of pulmonary stenosis, even, rarely, pulmonary atresia. The stenosis is usually subvalvular and is derived from conal tissue. Because extreme degrees of aortic override seen in patients with tetralogy of Fallot may resemble the anatomy seen in double-outlet right ventricle, at times it may not be possible to distinguish between the two. Usually, however, the presence of mitral-aortic valvular continuity establishes the diagnosis of tetralogy of Fallot, whereas absence of mitral-aortic continuity characterizes double-outlet right ventricle. The majority of patients in whom this question arises have tetralogy of Fallot; and the diagnosis of double-outlet right ventricle with subaortic ventricular septal defect and subvalvular pulmonary stenosis is most often not correct.

Transposition of the Great Arteries

When there is a subpulmonary ventricular defect that delivers left ventricular blood to the pulmonary artery, the hemodynamics and the anatomy resemble those of transposition of the great arteries. The distinction between double-outlet right ventricle and transposition of the great arteries can be made if there is mitral-pulmonary valvular continuity. When continuity can be confidently said to be present, the patient has transposition of the great arteries; when it is not, the diagnosis is double-outlet right ventricle. Although this distinction is readily described, it not always obvious to the angiographer who may not have obtained the perfect view or to the echocardiographer who was in a hurry. The Taussig-Bing anomaly is a specific variation of this problem, which includes the hemodynamics and usual anatomy of transposed great arteries but in which both arteries arise from the right ventricle. There is a subpulmonary ventricular defect, no pulmonary stenosis, and absence of mitral-pulmonary valvular continuity. The level of the semilunar valves is the same and the great vessels are parallel.

Other Associated Anomalies

Virtually every other cardiac anomaly can be found asociated with double-outlet right ventricle. Mitral atresia, mitral stenosis, and straddling atrioventricular valves are common. Some babies with mitral atresia and a hypoplastic left ventricle do surprisingly well, because there may be no aortic valve obstruction and an aorta of normal size receives normal amounts of blood flow from the right ventricle. Supero-inferior ventricles (upstairs-downstairs ventricles) are often associated with the origin of both great arteries from the upper right ventricle. This interesting relationship may become modified with growth, the ventricles assuming a more nearly normal position if the child survives. Inverse ventricles are common, as are viscera heterotaxy, polysplenia and asplenia. The great arteries may be normally related to each other, or in a position reminiscent of tetralogyof Fallot, or as situated in D- or L-transposition of the great arteries. Most often the great artefes are side-by-side, with the plane of the valves being identical. Continuity between the mitral valve and the adjacent semilunar valve is absent and is thought by most to represent the sine qua non of this diagnosis. Conal musculature is usually seen under both great arteries, but it may be absent under one or the other, or both. In cases without bilateral conal tissue, there is usually continuity between the adjacent great artery and the tricuspid valve; most of these children have mitral atresia.

Management

The initial decision in management concerns the ultimate goal. Can a two ventricle repair be imagined? Are the ventricles of reasonable size? Or is the only realistic possibility a Fontan type of palliation? If a two-ventricle repair is possible, is there pulmonary stenosis and will a conduit be required? In very small infants, because of expected rapid growth, the use of conduits is avoided if reasonably possible. At the same time, a shunting procedure, which will require surgical takedown later, is scarcely better than a reparative procedure with a conduit that needs replacement later. When the ventricular septal defect is closed, will the circulation be transposed and, if so, will an arterial switch be possible (i.e. is the coronary anatomy favorable for an arterial switch)? Sometimes placement of the ventricular patch can cure the patient and sometime placement of the patch and surgery for pulmonary stenosis provides a satisfactory result. Immediate survival is dependent on the anatomy of the defect (Fig. 14.188).

Course

The long-range course depends on the anatomy and the surgical procedures used. In general, these patients face shorter survival and more complicating problems than their

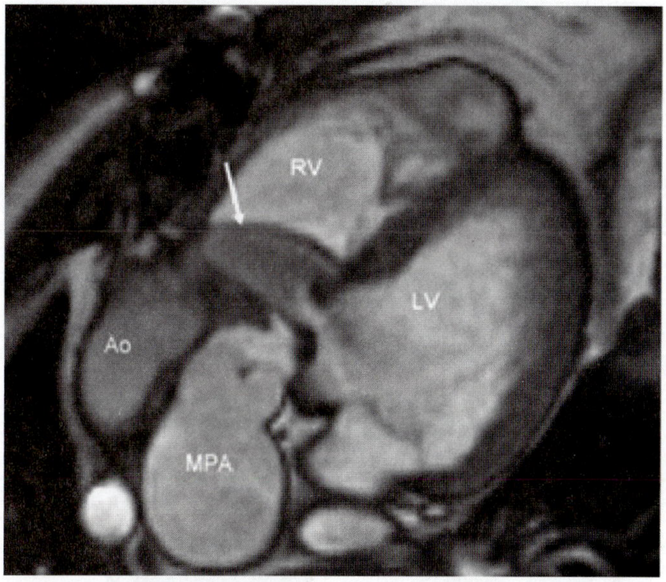

Fig. 14.188: *Rastelli repair of a double-outlet right ventricle. A baffle (arrow) is placed to divert flow from the LV through the VSD to the anterior aortic valve, coursing directly through the RV. Usually, this requires placement of a conduit from the RV to the pulmonary artery. In this case, RV flow circled around either side of the baffle. Ao, aorta; LV, left ventricle; RV, right ventricle; MPA, main pulmonary artery*

counterparts without the added feature of double-outlet right ventricle. Rhythm problems are common.

DOUBLE-INLET LEFT VENTRICLE

Double-inlet left ventricle is a congenital defect (the baby is born with it) in which the left and right atria (plural for atrium) of the heart are connected to the same ventricle. In some cases, one of the ventricles of the heart may be extremely small (Fig. 14.189).

Babies with double inlet left ventricle have an intact left ventricle (the pumping chamber of the heart that pumps blood to the body) and a small right ventricle (the pumping chamber that pumps blood to the lungs). Both atria supply blood to the left ventricle. As a result, oxygen-rich blood and oxygen-poor blood are combined. This mixture of blood flows to the baby's lungs and body. Double-inlet left ventricle is also called common ventricle or single ventricle.

Aetiology of DILV

The cause of double-inlet left ventricle is unknown, but the defect is likely to occur early in a pregnancy while the baby's heart is developing.

Symptoms of Double-inlet Left Ventricle

Symptoms of double inlet left ventricle usually appear in the early weeks of a baby's life and include:

1. Blue skin (cyanosis)
2. Failure to gain weight normally
3. Trouble breathing
4. Swollen legs or abdomen
5. Pale skin
6. Poor feeding
7. Sweating
8. Fast heartbeat
9. Heart murmur (an unusual heart sound)
10. Fluid buildup around the lungs
11. Heart failure.

Many babies with double-inlet left ventricle have other abnormalities in the heart or the main arteries. These abnormalities can block the flow of blood to the lungs.

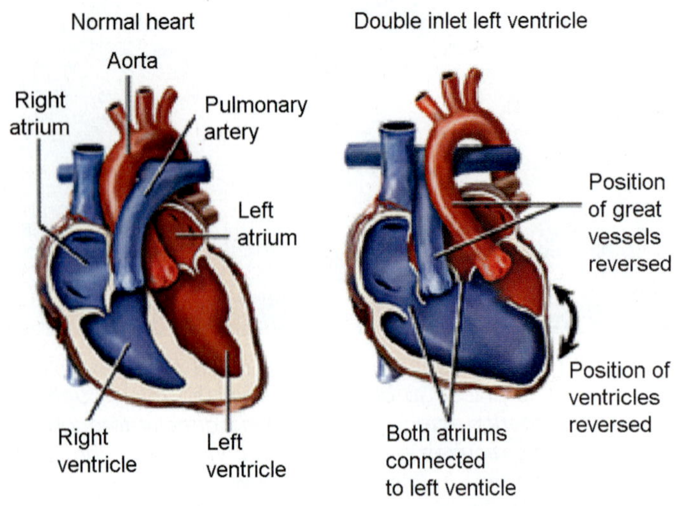

Fig. 14.189: *Anatomical structures in double-inlet left ventricle*

Diagnosis in DILV (Figs 14.190 to 14.192; 14.193)

The doctor will perform a physical examination and listen to the baby's heartbeat with a stethoscope in order to hear if there is a heart murmur. The doctor may also order various tests, including:

An electrocardiogram to measure the heart's electrical activity Cardiac catheterization (a thin tube is inserted into a vein and advanced to the heart to observe how the heart is functioning)—echocardiogram, or ultrasound imaging of the heart—magnetic resonance imaging, a test that produces very clear pictures, or images, of the human body with a large magnet, radio waves, and a computer.

Surgical Management in DILV

With surgery, blood circulation through the body and into the lungs can be improved. Surgeries most commonly performed to treat double inlet left ventricle lead up to a surgery called the Fontan procedure. If blood flow to the pulmonary artery is restricted, a small tube called a shunt can be surgically placed from an artery attached to the aorta to the pulmonary artery. If there is too much blood flow to the lungs, the surgeon may perform a pulmonary artery banding, which protects the pulmonary arteries from high blood pressure.

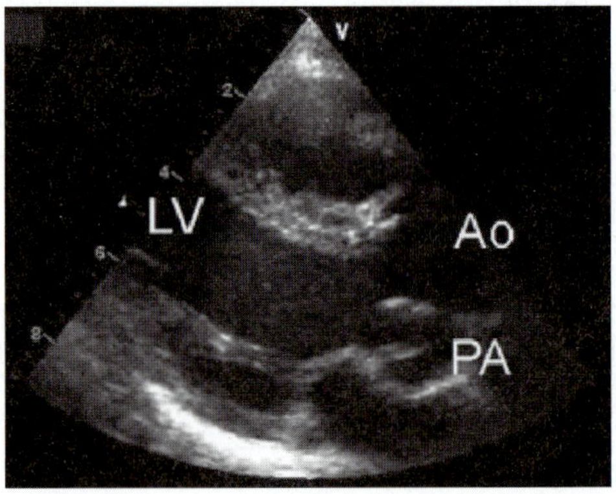

Fig. 14.190: *Echocardiography, parasternal long-axis view. Both great arteries are committed to the left ventricle (LV). The aorta (Ao) is malpositioned anteriorly and to the right of the stenotic pulmonary artery (PA). The ventricular septal defect has been closed*

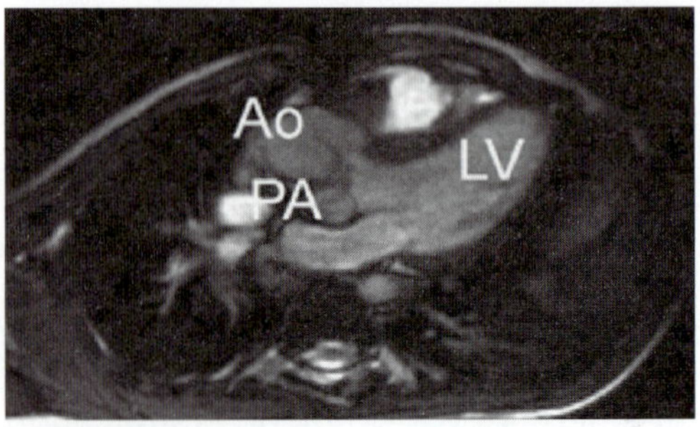

Fig. 14.191: *Magnetic resonance imaging, axial scan, gradient echo. The intracardiac anatomy is visualized in detail. There is mild subaortic stenosis. The pulmonary artery (PA) has been transsected. Residual flow is detected across the pulmonary valve. LV, left ventricle; Ao, aorta.*

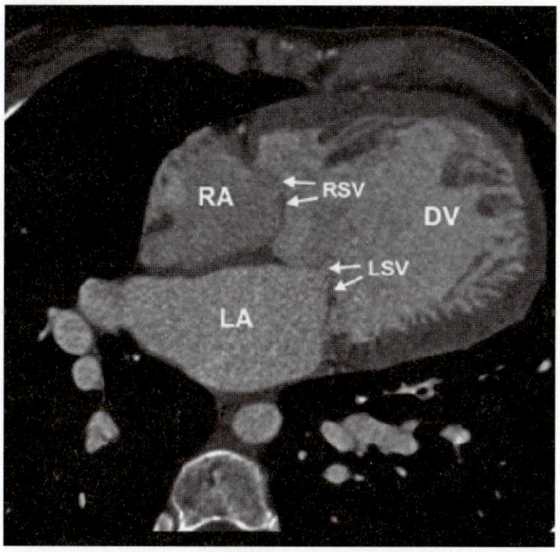

Fig. 14.192: *Double-inlet left ventricle with d-transposition of the great arteries, observed at ECG-gated CT performed to supplement postoperative echocardiography in a patient after surgical banding of the common pulmonary artery. Thin-section reformatted image along the long axis of the heart shows connection of the left atrium (LA) and right atrium (RA) through a left-sided valve (LSV) and a right-sided valve (RSV), respectively, to a dominant ventricle (DV), morphologic left ventricle*

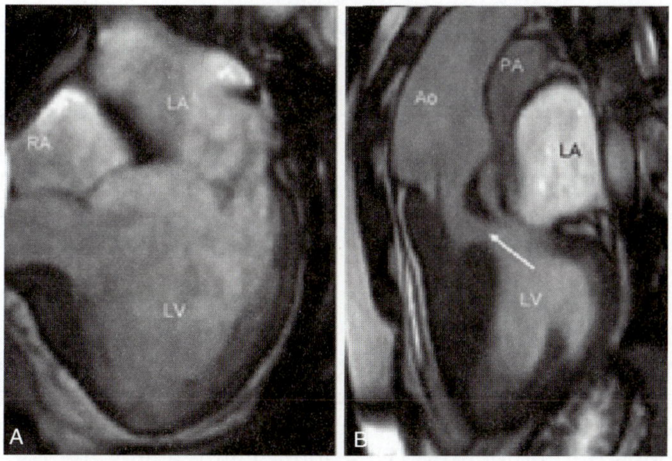

Fig. 14.193A and B: *(A) Double inlet left ventricle, one of the most common forms of a functional single ventricle. The RV is hypoplastic. Usually, these patients also have transposition of the great arteries with an anterior aorta (B), and the LV outflow is through the VSD (arrow). Patient shown has pulmonary stenosis. Most such patients have now been palliated with a Fontan procedure. Ao, aorta; PA, pulmonary artery; LA, left atrium; LV, left ventricle; RA, right atrium*

The first surgery may have to be performed within the first few days of the baby's life. The baby usually goes home after the first surgery. A pediatric cardiologist will decide when the baby should undergo the second surgery. The follow-up surgery (or initial surgery if the baby was not operated on in the first few days of life) is called the Hemi-Fontan or Glenn shunt procedure. This operation usually is performed when the baby is 4-6 months old. The baby's skin still may appear blue after the first operation(s). The Fontan procedure usually is done when a child is 3 to 6 years old. After the final stage of surgery, the child no longer will have blue skin. Although the Fontan procedure does not result in normal blood circulation in the body, it does improve the circulation and allows the child to grow.

A child may need additional types of surgeries for related defects or to extend survival while waiting for the Fontan procedure. The patients may require pacemaker therapy who have complication of complete A-V dissociation.

Medications

1. Digoxin to help with heart contractions
2. ACE inhibitors to lower blood pressure
3. Anticoagulants to prevent blood clots
4. Diuretics to remove extra fluid from the body
5. In addition, children with double inlet left ventricle have to take antibiotics before dental treatment in order to prevent endocarditis (infection of the heart lining).
6. In the most severe cases of double inlet left ventricle, a surgeon may recommend a heart transplant.

Prognosis (outlook) for children who have double-inlet left ventricle?

Factors that affect how well a baby with double-inlet left ventricle does include:

1. How severe the defect is?
2. The overall condition of the baby when the diagnosis is made.
3. Genetic syndromes
4. Many babies with double-inlet left ventricle live to adulthood as a result of advances in surgical procedures.
5. Many people with double-inlet left ventricle need regular followups. In addition, they can face various complications and their physical activity can be limited.

DOUBLE-OUTLET LV

Double-outlet left ventricle (DOLV) is a rare congenital cardiac malformation in which both great arteries originate entirely or predominantly from the morphologic left ventricle. DOLV occurs most commonly in the form of atrial situs solitus with atrioventricular (AV) concordance. Ventricular septal defect (VSD) is most commonly subaortic, and 90% of these patients have associated pulmonary stenosis. In most cases, there is a right anterior position of the aorta relative to the pulmonary artery. Most patients with DOLV will have pulmonary outflow obstruction and present soon after birth with cyanosis. DOLV with two well-developed ventricles is conventionally treated surgically by VSD closure, closure of the native left ventricle-to-pulmonary outflow, and placement of a right ventricle-to-pulmonary artery extracardiac conduit. However, pulmonary root translocation may be used as an alternative to biventricular repair of DOLV. Patients with DOLV and functionally single-ventricle or AV valve atresia will require a Fontan procedure (Figs 14.194A and B).

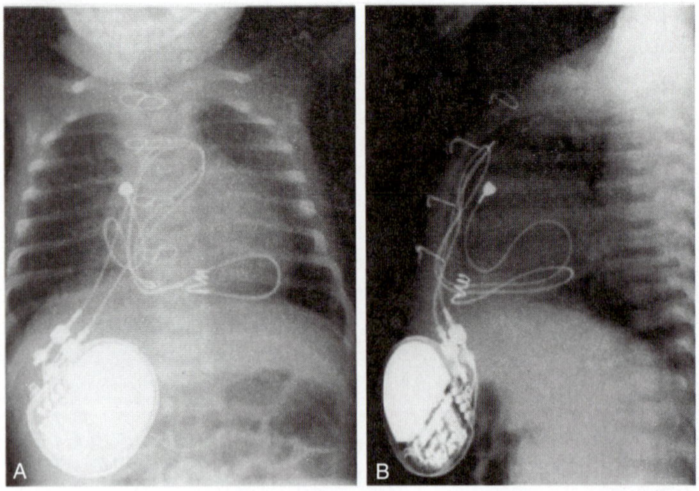

Fig. 14.194A and B: *Infant with double-inlet left ventricle and pulmonary atresia with complete AV block, status postbilateral patent ductus arteriosus ligation, shunt placement, and dual chamber pacemaker implantation. The anteroposterior projection (A) and the lateral projection (B) show a steroid eluting epicardial lead on the atrium a screw-in epicardial lead on the ventricle*

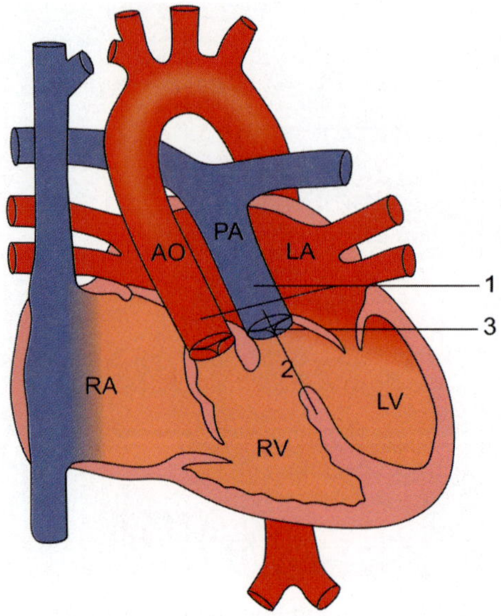

Fig. 14.195: *Transposition of the great arteries (aka d-TGA), Taussig-Bing anomaly (VSD + TGA + PA overriding the IVS) 1.Transposition of the great arteries; 2.Ventricular septal defect (one component of Taussig-Bing anomaly); 3.Overriding pulmonary artery (the second component of Taussig-Bing anomaly)*

Management

Double outlet left ventricle is an extremely rare anomaly. Until recently, the diagnosis was usually established by angiography or at postmortem. There are only a few reports describing the echocardiographic findings in this lesion. The patient reported here underwent surgery at the age of four years, when an aortic homograft was placed between the right ventricle and the pulmonary trunk. This biventricular repair had to be changed into a Fontan-type procedure, 15 years later since the hypoplastic right ventricle did not grow adequately.

Dextrotransposition of the Great Vessels (DTGV)

Historical Background

Infants with transposition of the great arteries (TGA) are usually born at term, with cyanosis apparent within hours of birth (Fig. 14.195).

The clinical course and manifestations depend on the extent of intercirculatory mixing and the presence of associated anatomic lesions.

Transposition of the great arteries with intact ventricular septum: prominent and progressive cyanosis within the first 24 hours of life is the usual finding in infants.

Transposition of the great arteries with large ventricular septal defect: infants may not initially manifest symptoms of heart disease, although mild cyanosis (particularly when crying) is often noted. Signs of congestive heart failure (tachypnea, tachycardia, diaphoresis, and failure to gain weight) may become evident over the first 3–6 weeks as pulmonary blood flow increases.

Transposition of the great arteries with ventricular septal defect and left ventricular outflow tract obstruction: infants often present with extreme cyanosis at birth, proportional to the degree of left ventricular (pulmonary) outflow tract obstruction. The clinical history may be similar to that of an infant with tetralogy of Fallot.

Transposition of the great arteries with ventricular septal defect and pulmonary vascular obstructive disease: Progressively advancing pulmonary vascular obstructive disease can prevent this rare subgroup of patients from developing symptoms of congestive heart failure, despite a large ventricular septal defect. Most often, patients present with progressive cyanosis, despite an early successful palliative procedure.

Etiology

Etiology for transposition of the great arteries is unknown and is presumed to be multifactorial. Embryology likely involves abnormal persistence of the subaortic conus with resorption or underdevelopment of the subpulmonary conus (infundibulum). This abnormality aligns the aorta anterior and superior with the right ventricle during development.

Physical Examination

Newborns with transposition of the great arteries are usually well developed, without dysmorphic features. Physical findings at presentation depend on the presence of associated lesions.

1. ***Transposition of the great arteries with intact ventricular septum:*** Infants typically present with progressive central (perioral and periorbital) cyanosis. Other than cyanosis, the physical examination is often unremarkable.
2. ***Transposition of the great arteries with large ventricular septal defect:*** Cyanosis may be mild initially, although it is usually more apparent with stress or crying. Upon presentation, infants often have an increased right

ventricular impulse, a prominent grade 3–4/6 holosystolic murmur, third heart sound, mid-diastolic rumble, and a gallop rhythm. Hepatomegaly may be present.

3. ***Transposition of the great arteries with ventricular septal defect and left ventricular outflow tract obstruction:*** Cyanosis is prominent at birth, and the findings are similar to those of infants with tetralogy of Fallot. A single, or narrowly split, diminished second heart sound and a grade 2–3/6 systolic ejection murmur may be present. Hepatomegaly is rare. Transposition of the great arteries with ventricular septal defect and pulmonary vascular obstructive disease: progressive pulmonary vascular obstructive disease is not always evident from physical examination findings. Cyanosis is usually present and can progress despite palliative therapy in the newborn period.

No murmur (despite the ventricular septal defect) or early short systolic ejection sounds are heard. The second heart sound is often single, with increased intensity.

In later childhood or adolescence, a high-pitched, blowing, early decrescendo diastolic murmur of pulmonary insufficiency and a blowing apical murmur of mitral insufficiency are evident.

Differential Diagnoses

1. Pulmonary atresia with intact ventricular septum
2. Tetralogy of fallot with absent pulmonary valve
3. Tetralogy of fallot with pulmonary atresia
4. Total anomalous pulmonary venous connection
5. Tricuspid atresia
6. Truncus arteriosus.

Laboratory Studies

A hyperoxia test (for cyanotic congenital heart disease) may be indicated in patients with transposition of the great arteries (TGA). In a patient with arterial hypoxemia, an ABG measurement is obtained on 100% oxygen for 10 minutes. Pulmonary disease (not cyanotic congenital heart disease) is suspected if the partial pressure of oxygen increases to more than 150 mmHg with oxygen.

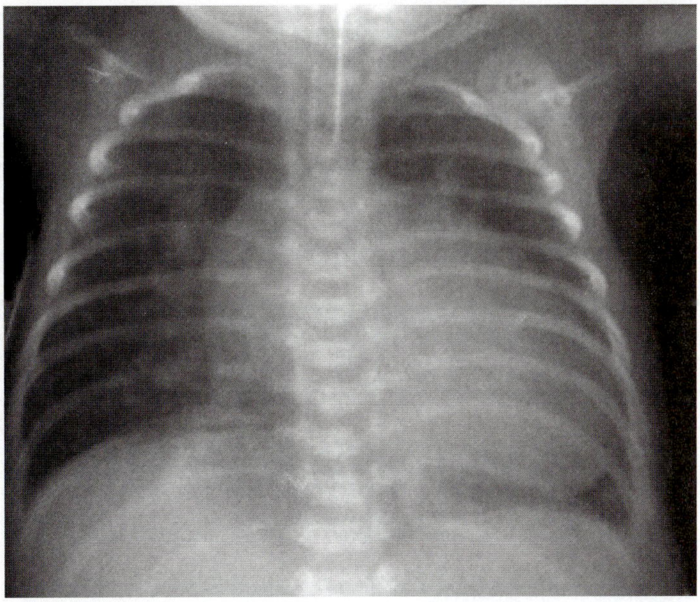

Fig. 14.196: *Photograph X-ray chest PA view showing right ventricular type of cardiomegaly, narrow base, absence of pulminary conus and almost an egg shaped heart as seen in D-transposition of great arteries with pulmonic stenosis*

Chest Radiography (Fig. 14.196)

The chest radiograph may appear normal in newborns with transposition of the great arteries and intact ventricular septum but may demonstrate the classic "egg on a string" appearance in approximately one-third of patients. With a ventricular septal defect, cardiomegaly usually occurs with increased pulmonary arterial vascular markings.

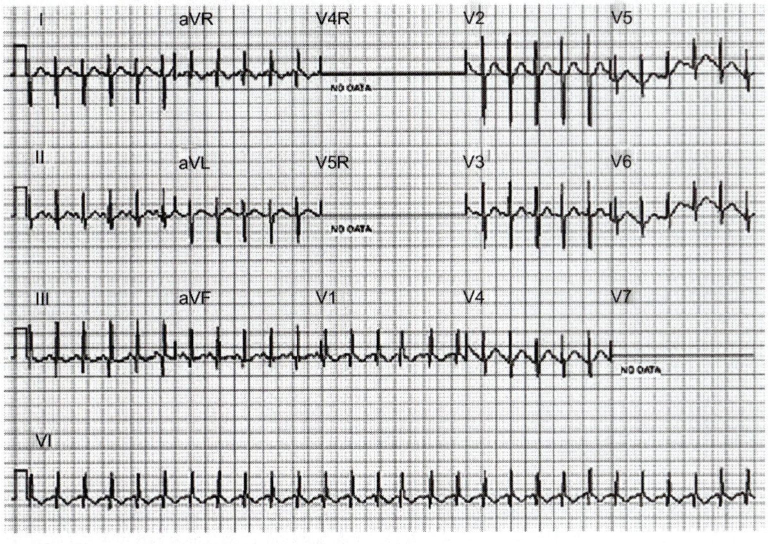

Fig. 14.197: *d-TGA: electrocardiogram- obtained from a 3-day-old neonate. The tracing demonstrates right-axis deviation and right ventricular predominance*

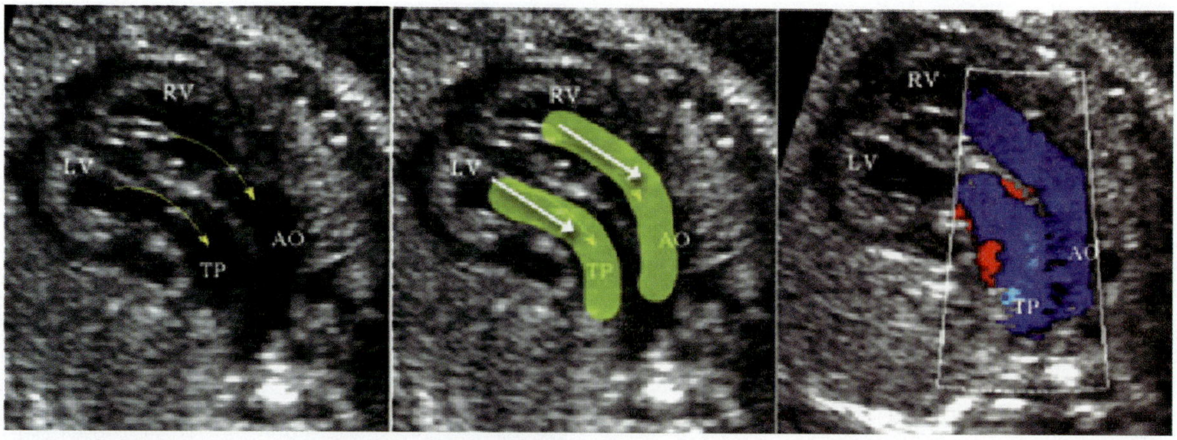

Fig. 14.198: *Fetal ultrasonography demonstrates transposition of the great arteries with abnormal connection of the right ventricle (RV) with the aorta (AO) and the left ventricle (LV) with the pulmonary trunk (TP). Both great arteries show a parallel course*

Electrocardiography

It reveals right axis deviationand right ventricular dominance (Fig. 14.197).

Echocardiography

Echocardiographic images should be diagnostic of transposition of the great arteries by demonstrating the bifurcating pulmonary artery arising posteriorly from the left ventricle in the parasternal long-axis view.

The parasternal short-axis view shows the relationship of the great arteries to one another. The aorta is usually anterior and rightward of the pulmonary artery in cross-section.

Most associated anatomic lesions including atrial septal defects, ventricular septal defects, and patent ductus arteriosus, are also diagnosed readily by echocardiography.

The coronary artery anatomy needs to be ascertained and may be abnormal in nearly one-third of patients. The coronary artery origins and branching pattern are often delineated by echocardiography (Figs 14.198 and 14.199).

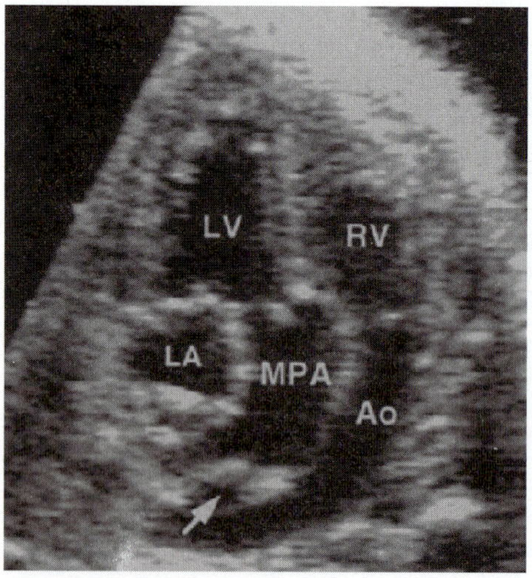

Fig. 14.199: *Prenatal echocardiogram at 28 weeks in patient who had persistent pulmonary hypertension postnatally. Image demonstrates transposed great arteries, as well as a severely narrowed ductus arteriosus at pulmonary artery end (arrow)*

Computerized Axial Tomography

It reveals intracardiac anatomy including atrioventricular concordance and ventriculoarterial discordance (Fig. 14.200).

Cardiac Catheterization

Diagnostic cardiac catheterization is usually reserved for the subgroup of patients for whom echocardiography does not adequately delineate the anatomy. Suspected coronary artery abnormalities and additional ventricular septal defects may be confirmed or better delineated by cardiac catheterization with angiography. In addition, cardiac catheterization may be necessary to improve left-to-right shunting. Postcatheterization precautions include

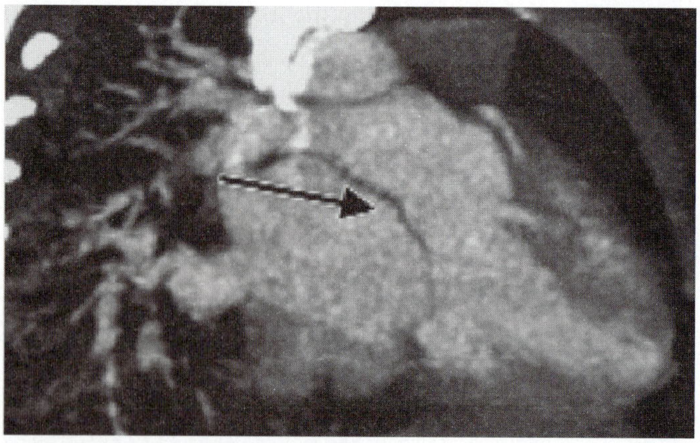

Fig. 14.200: *D-transposition of the great vessels. coronal oblique images from thoracic CT. The pulmonary artery arises from the left ventricle and mitropulmonary valvular continuity is seen. It also showed S,D,D-TGV, with atrioventricular concordance and ventriculoarterial discordance. Figure shows D-transposition of the great vessels. coronal oblique images from thoracic CT. The pulmonary artery arises from the left ventricle and mitropulmonary valvular continuity is seen. It also showed S,D,D-TGV, with atrioventricular concordance and ventriculoarterial discordance*

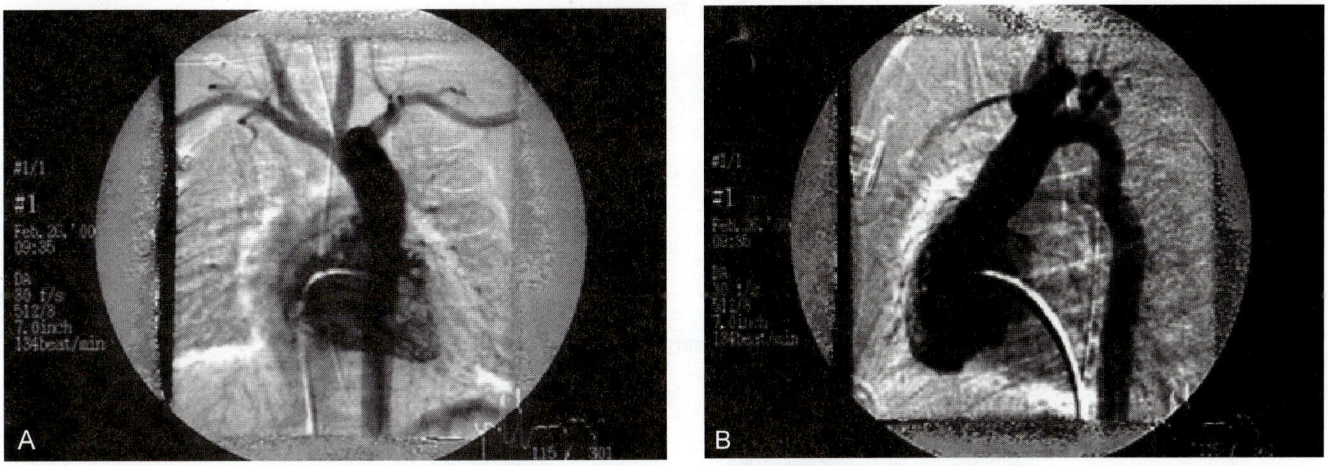

Fig. 14.201A and B: *Both upper and bottom panels show right ventricular angiogram in a patient with transposition of the great arteries. The aorta arises directly from the right-sided anterior right ventricle [(10° left anterior oblique (LAO)]*

hemorrhage, vascular disruption after balloon dilation, pain, nausea and vomiting, and arterial or venous obstruction from thrombosis or spasm (Figs 14.201A and B).

Complications may include rupture of blood vessel, tachyarrhythmias, bradyarrhythmias, and vascular occlusion.

Medical Treatment

Initial treatment consists of maintaining ductal patency with continuous intravenous (IV) prostaglandin E1 infusion to promote pulmonary blood flow, increase left atrial pressure, and promote left-to-right intercirculatory mixing at the atrial level. This is particularly important in patients with severe left ventricular outflow tract stenosis or atresia. Prostaglandin therapy may or may not benefit the patient with simple transposition of the great arteries (TGA) and an intact ventricular septum without left ventricular outflow tract obstruction.

Cardiac catheterization depending on the degree of restriction at the atrial septum and the timing of operative repair, is indicated for a balloon atrial septostomy in severely hypoxemic patients with an inadequate atrial level communication and insufficient mixing. The balloon atrial septostomy is used to increase the atrial level shunt and to improve mixing. For the ill neonate, metabolic acidosis should be corrected with fluid replacement and bicarbonate administration. Mechanical ventilation may be necessary if pulmonary edema develops in concert with severe hypoxemia. Ultimately, the patient requires surgical repair or palliation early in life.

Surgical Intervention (Figs 14.202 and 14.203)

Surgical approach depends on the age of the patient at presentation, the presence of associated congenital cardiac lesions, and the experience of the cardiothoracic surgeon with a given surgical technique. Most full-term neonates with uncomplicated transposition of the great arteries can undergo an arterial switch procedure in one operation, with minimal mortality.

Transposition of the great arteries with intact ventricular septum: The ideal operation is an arterial switch procedure. It represents an anatomic repair and establishes ventriculoarterial concordance. This procedure should be performed when the infant is younger than 4 weeks as the left ventricle may not be able to handle systemic pressure postoperatively if left too long in the low-pressure, low-resistance pulmonary circuit. Rarely, however, depending on the particular coronary artery anatomy (e.g. intramural coronary artery), coronary artery translocation may not be feasible, and an arterial switch is not recommended. In this subgroup, an atrial level switch (Senning or Mustard procedure) has lower surgical and short-term morbidity and mortality.

Transposition of the great arteries with ventricular septal defect: The preferred operation is an arterial switch procedure with ventricular septal defect closure. If the ventricular septal defect is large and nonrestrictive and coronary artery anatomy makes an arterial switch operation inadvisable, a Rastelli-type intracardiac repair may be feasible. With the Rastelli-type procedure, waiting until the infant is older and larger may be preferred because of the need for a right ventricle—pulmonary artery conduit in the Rastelli operation. If the infant has excessive congestive heart failure (with growth failure), it may be advisable to either proceed with reparative surgery or, if not feasible, band/ligate the main pulmonary artery and place an aortopulmonary shunt during the newborn period to restrict pulmonary blood flow.

Transposition of the great arteries with ventricular septal defect and left ventricular outflow tract obstruction: An arterial switch operation may not be feasible due to pulmonary (left ventricular outflow tract) stenosis or atresia. If the ventricular septal defect is nonrestrictive and not too remote from the aorta, a Rastelli intracardiac repair could be possible. Because the Rastelli procedure necessitates a conduit from the right ventricle to the pulmonary artery, delaying repair until the infant is older and larger may be preferable. In this case, placing an

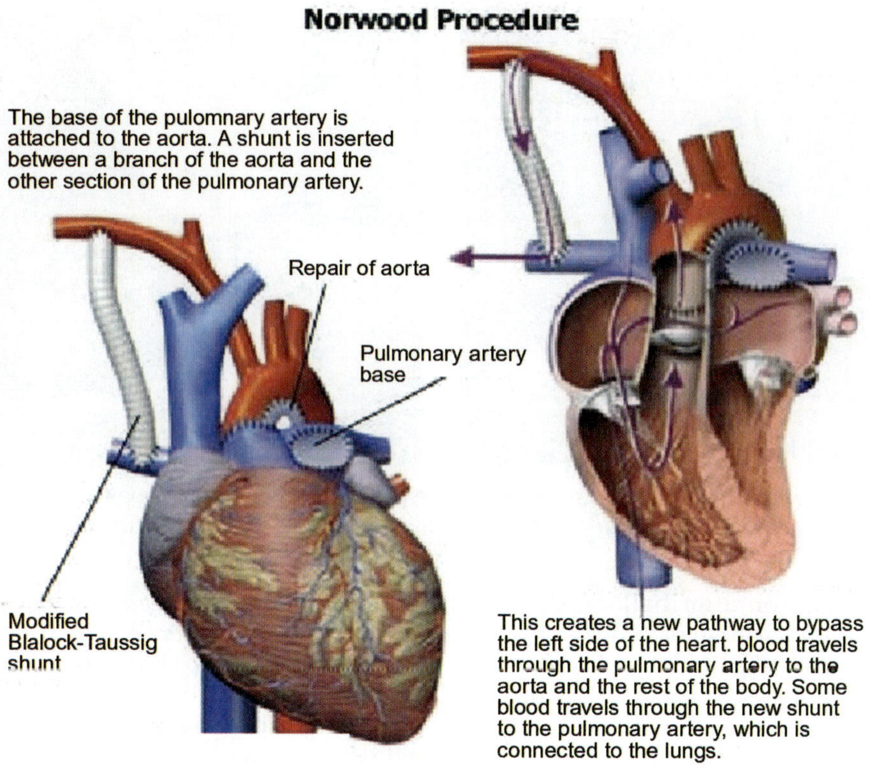

Fig. 14.202: *Diagram showing Norwood procedure in transposition of the great arteries*

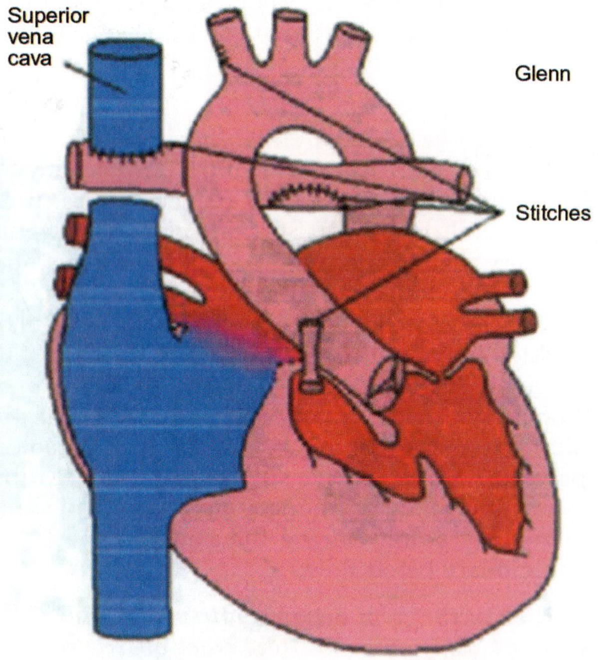

Fig. 14.203: *The bidirectional Glenn procedure involves anastomosis of the SVC to the pulmonary artery*

aortopulmonary shunt during the newborn period may be necessary to establish adequate pulmonary blood flow while waiting.

Transposition of the great arteries with ventricular septal defect and pulmonary vascular obstructive disease: These patients might not be appropriate surgical candidates because of the progressive increase in pulmonary vascular resistance. This is a small subgroup of patients whose conditions are not often diagnosed until after a palliative or reparative procedure is performed.

Norwood Procedure

The Norwood operation establishes a single outlet from the single ventricle by anastomosing the hypoplastic ascending aorta to the main pulmonary artery, producing a so-called neoaorta and connecting the distal pulmonary artery to a systemic shunt, usually a modified Blalock-Taussig shunt Often, an atrial septectomy is required to allow complete mixing at the atrial level (Fig. 14.202).

Glenn Procedure

The bidirectional Glenn procedure involves anastomosis of the SVC to the pulmonary artery. It includes takedown of a previously placed shunt and repair of any branch pulmonary artery stenosis. The term bidirectional refers to the fact that the right pulmonary artery remains in continuity with the left pulmonary artery; this contrasts with the classic Glenn procedure, which involves anastomosis of the SVC to a right pulmonary artery that has been disconnected from the main and left pulmonary arteries. The bidirectional Glenn procedure is now done at 4–6 months of age (Fig. 14.203).

Fontan procedure: The Fontan procedure is the final palliative procedure, providing direct connection of flow from the SVC and inferior vena cava (IVC) to the pulmonary circuit. Initially, this was a one-stage procedure that involved attaching the RA to the pulmonary artery or RV outflow tract and was performed in patients older than 4 years.

Current practice is to stage the anastomosis of SVC and IVC to the pulmonary circuit, with the final stage, total cavopulmonary artery anastomosis, occurring at 2–3 years of age. The IVC is connected to the pulmonary artery either by a lateral tunnel placed in the RA to direct blood from the IVC to the proximal SVC stump, which is then attached to the pulmonary artery or by an extracardiac conduit connecting the IVC to the pulmonary artery directly. With any of these routes of flow, a small communication (fenestration) may be made between the caval blood flow conduit and the functional left atrium. Pulmonary blood flow is achieved by passive venous return without assistance of a ventricular pumping chamber. Any mild alteration of pulmonary pressure or resistance will impair adequacy of pulmonary blood flow.

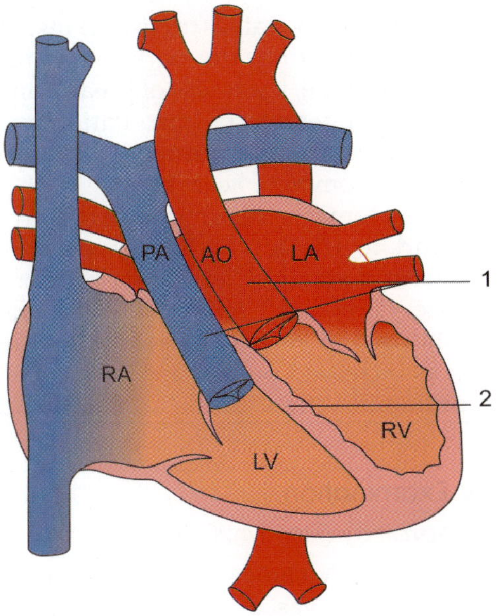

Fig. 14.204: *Congenitally corrected transposition of the great Arteries (l-TGA) 1. Congenitally corrected TGA (AV and VA discordance), 2. Intact ventricular septum, 3. No associated lesions (thus, the term "isolated")*

Congenitally Corrected Transposition of the Great Arteries (ccTGA)

Ventricular inversion or ccTGA is arare congenital anomaly that occurs in less than 1% of children with congenital cardiovascular defects. Among these patients, it is equally rare to have no other associated structural abnormalities. The natural history of ccTGA is gradual congestive failure caused by systemic atrioventricular (AV) valve insufficiency and systemic ventricular dysfunction, even in the absence of other associated malformations. The presence of associated defects and conduction abnormalities contributes to a further decrease in life expectancy without intervention. Life expectancy is good but does not reach normal.

Anatomy

1. The defining feature of this congenital abnormality of cardiac looping is AV and ventriculoarterial discordance. Blood flows from the right atrium across a mitral valve into a right-sided, morphologic left ventricle that is related to the pulmonary artery, which typically is more posterior and rightward than usual. Pulmonary venous return is normal to the left atrium but then flows across an anatomic tricuspid valve into a left-sided, morphologic right ventricle, which is related to an anterior and leftward aorta (Fig. 14.204).
2. ***The anatomic coronary arteries***, like the AV valves, follow their respective ventricles. The left-sided coronary artery resembles the anatomic right coronary artery as it courses in the AV groove and gives rise to infundibular and marginal branches. The right-sided coronary artery resembles the morphologic left coronary artery, which branches into the anterior descending and circumflex arteries.
3. ***The conduction system*** likewise follows the respective ventricle as the right-sided, morphologic left ventricle depolarizes first. Accessory AV nodal tissue is located anteriorly with respect to normal and His bundle must traverse anterior to the pulmonary artery and along the superior margin of a ventricular septal defect (VSD) if present. There is increased risk for acquired complete heart block in this lesion because of the abnormally placed AV node and its extended course. As a result of this abnormal course, approximately 30% of adolescents and adults have complete heart block, the rate of which increases at 2% per year without surgical intervention. Accessory pathways have been described and are typically left sided in the presence of an Ebstein anomaly-like malformation of the left-sided (tricuspid) AV valve. Some patients have evidence of preexcitation, which may predispose them to supraventricular tachycardia.
4. ***Isolated ccTGA is the exception:*** Associated lesions are common and are considered in the diagnotic evaluation. They include VSD, pulmonary outflow obstruction, or abnormalities of the left-sided, systemic tricuspid valve. Up to 90% of patients have some abnormality of the tricuspid valve in some form (i.e. dysplastic or Ebstein-like tricuspid valves).

Clinical Presentation

1. Because physiologic blood flow is preserved, patients may have no symptoms through adulthood in the absence of other structural lesions or associated complications. This scenario is rare, however, because associated lesions commonly dictate the clinical features.
2. Without associated structural abnormalities, failure of the systemic, morphologic right ventricle with various

degrees of systemic AV valve (tricuspid) insufficiency is the norm. In this setting, the patient has nonspecific descriptions of fatigue, shortness of breath, and exercise intolerance or congestive failure. Patients may have syncope or presyncope caused by conduction abnormalities or complete heart block.

In the usual anatomic configuration of ccTGA, the aorta is anterior and to the left, which produces a chest radiograph with a straight left heart border. The left pulmonary artery is not well defined. The chest radiograph may appear normal or reflect the presence of associated lesions, such as increased pulmonary flow from a VSD or decreased pulmonary flow in the setting of pulmonary stenosis.

Laboratory Examination

Chest Radiography (Fig. 14.205)

Chest X-ray (PA) view shows left sided ascending aorta and normal pulmonary vasculature in uncompicated cases.

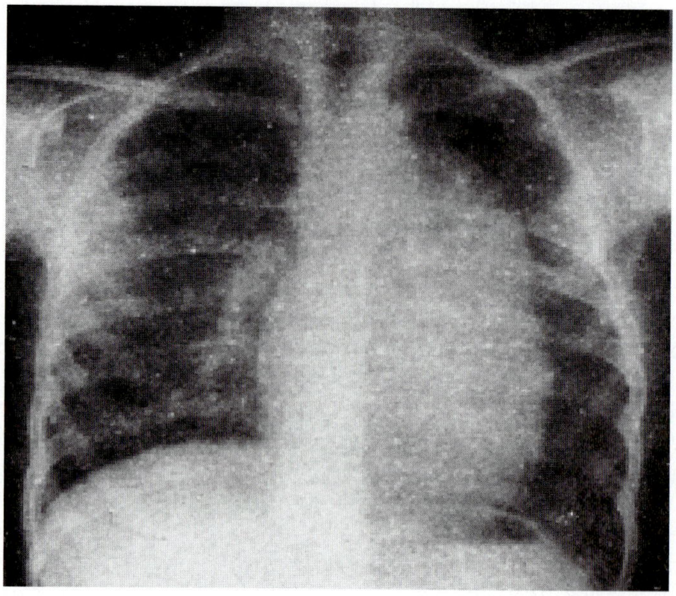

Fig. 14.205: *Photograph of X-ray chest PA view showing left-sided ascending aorta in patient with ccTGA*

Electrocardiogram (ECG): The typical electrocardiogram (ECG) shows a left axis deviation. Among pediatric patients, there is lossof the usual Q waves in the precordial leads, with deep Q waves in leads II and aVF. A variety of AV node conduction abnormalities may manifest with time and progress to complete heart block (Fig. 14.206).

Echocardiography: In most instances, the diagnosis can be made with echocardiography. The essential findings of AV and ventriculoarterial discordance must be demonstrated. Close attention must be paid to the morphologic details of each chamber (Figs 14.207A and B, 14.208).

a. The morphologic right ventricle is identified on the basis of its triangular shape, the presence of trabeculations, an inferiorly placed AV valve, and absence of AV valve attachments to the interventricular septum.
b. The morphologic left ventricle is identified on the basis of its bullet shape, smooth wall, more superiorly positioned AV valve, and presence of AV valve attachments to the interventricular septum. In the case of ccTGA, these relationships are preserved but reversed.
c. Continuity is lacking between the left-sided (tricuspid) AV valve and aorta but is present between the right-sided (anatomic mitral) valve and pulmonary artery. The left-sided AV valve is displaced inferiorly relative to the right-sided (mitral) valve and may appear malformed or have the characteristics of Ebstein anomaly.
d. Apical four-chamber and subcostal images are particularly helpful. Comparable transesophageal images may be needed for adult patients. The aortic arch typically lies to the left of midline in the sagittal plane and can often be visualized from the high left parasternal

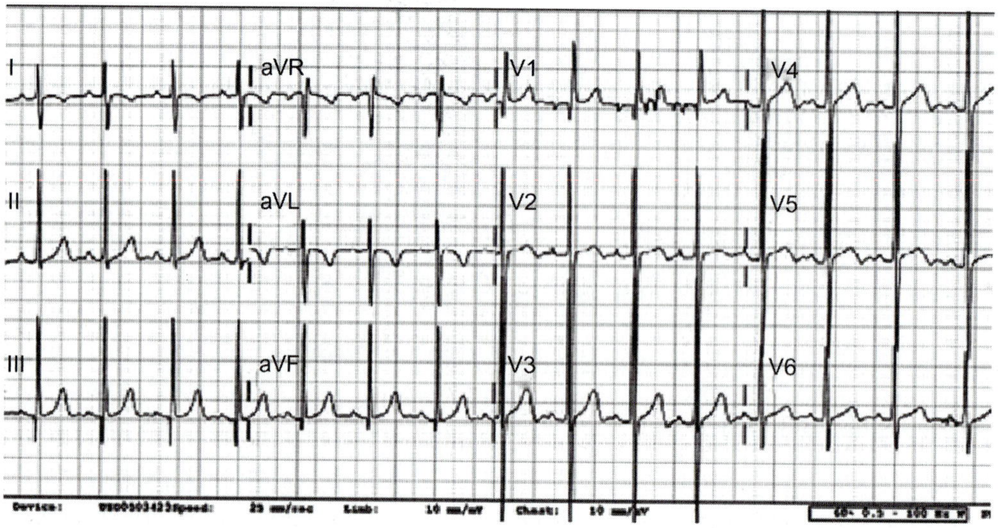

Fig. 14.206: *Corrected TGV. The electrocardiogram shows a qR pattern in lead V1, with absence of Q waves in leads V5 and V6, demonstrating abnormal ventricular depolarization*

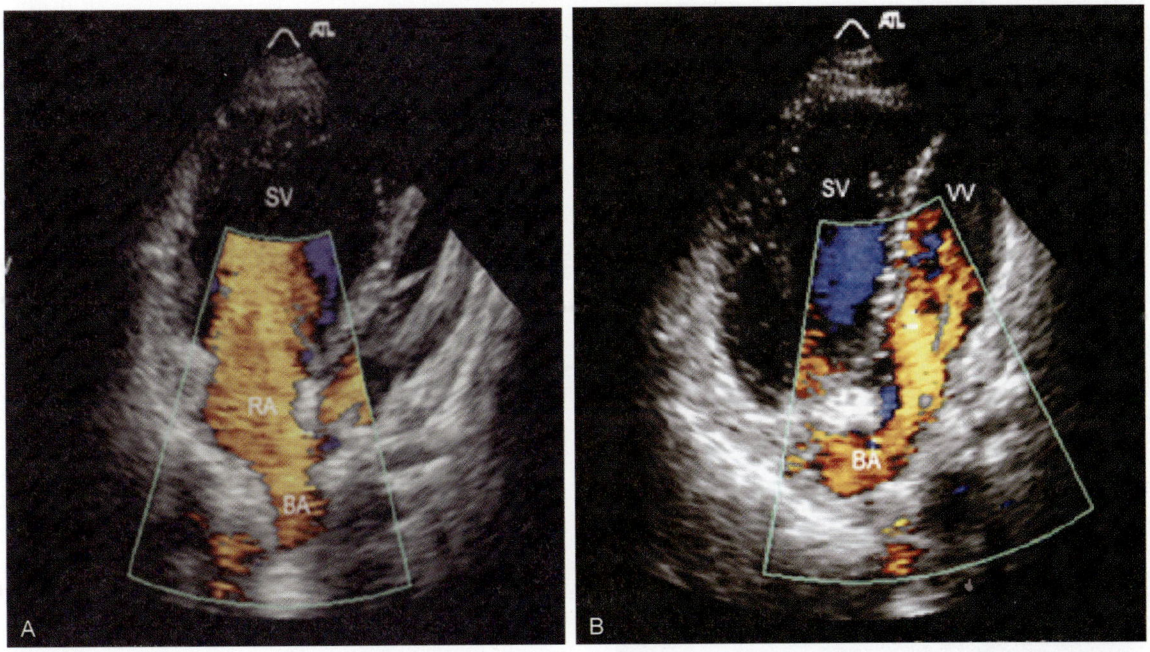

Fig. 14.207: *(A) Modified apical image of D-transposition after baffle (Mustard) procedure. Pulmonary venous blood flows through a baffle (BA) to enter the right atrium (RA) and the systemic ventricle (SV), which is a morphologic right ventricle. The SV ejects into the aorta. There is no evidence of baffle stenosis. (B) Modified apical image from the same patient showing vena caval blood flow through a BA into the left atrium and venous ventricle (VV), which is a morphologic left ventricle. The venous ventricle ejects into the pulmonary artery. Again, there is no evidence of baffle stenosis*

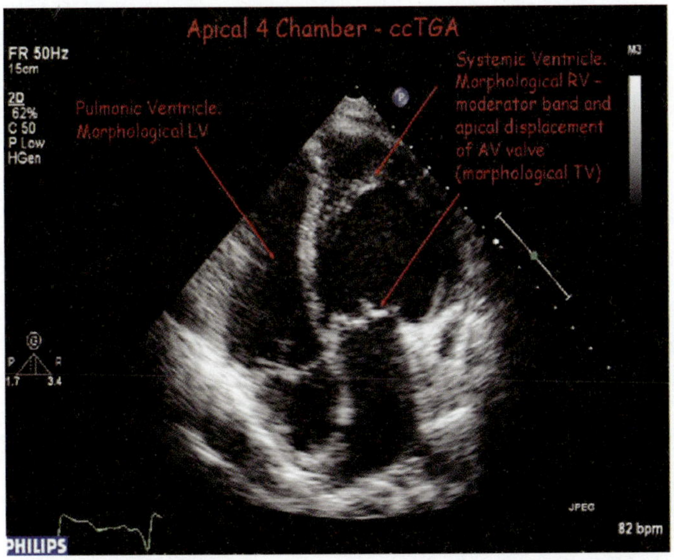

Fig. 14.208: *Congenitally corrected TGA is the condition in which the atria are in the normal position (atrial situs solitus), and receive the appropriate venous return however there is double discordance, in that the atria are connected to the opposite ('wrong') ventricle (LA to RV, RA to LV) and the ventricles are connected to the "wrong" great artery (RV to aorta, LV to PA). This results in a morphological right ventricle supporting the systemic circulation and the morphological left ventricle supporting the pulmonary circulation. The aorta lies in a leftward position relative to the PA. The heart postion in the chest is usually normal (levocardia) or midline (mesocardia), but in 20% it is right-sided (dextrocardia). Associated lesions are most commonly VSD, PS or pulmonary atresia, and tricuspid valve abnormalities*

position. Because variations in great vessel position occur, the spatial orientation must be clarified.

e. Associated defects (e.g. systemic AV valve insufficiency, VSD, outflow tract obstruction) with ccTGA must be excluded or defined.

Computerized Axial Tomography (Fig. 14.209)

It clearly defines the anatomy of ccTGV with anterior position of the aorta arising from the RV and main pulmonary artery from LV.

Cardiac catheterization: It is unnecessary for the diagnosis of ccTGA but may be helpful in preoperative planning with regard to the hemodynamic significance of associated lesions. In rare instances, ccTGA is diagnosed by catheterization but was not recognized during routine echocardiography. An unusual arterial catheter course is caused by the anterior and leftward position of the aorta in most instances (Figs 14.210A and B). The left-sided coronary artery typically arises from the posterior sinus and assumes a right coronary branching distribution, whereas the right-sided coronary artery arises from the anterior and rightward sinus and assumes a typical left coronary branching distribution. Because the ventricular septum often lies in the sagittal plane, ventriculography is usually best performed in the straight postero-anterior and lateral projections.

Therapy

Medical management is dictated primarily by the as sociated malformations. In the rare case of isolated ccTGA,

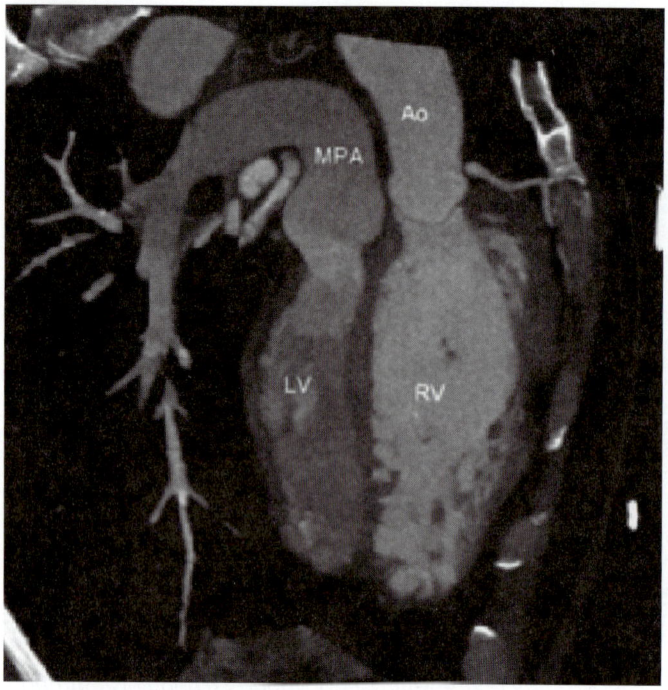

Fig. 14.209: *CT scan showing congenitally corrected transposition of the great arteries. Note the anterior position of the aorta arising from the right ventricle and the main pulmonary artery arising from the left ventricle*

the risk for development of conduction abnormalities is cumulative over time. Permanent pacemaker placement often is needed. The systemic AV valve and ventricle also show signs of failure that necessitate initiation of anticongestive measures in the form of diuretics and afterload reduction. Associated lesions such as pulmonary stenosis or atresia, severe systemic AV valve regurgitation, or VSD may likewise contribute to the medical treatment of these patients but often also necessitate surgical intervention. Periodic Holter monitoring is warranted because of the increased risk for acquired conduction abnormalities (Figs 14.212A and B).

Surgery

a. Infants and children who are brought to medical attention early often need surgical intervention in the form of relief of pulmonary outflow tract obstruction or placement of palliative shunts depending on the associated lesions.
b. For selected children, a double switch procedure may be performed but may necessitate a period of retraining of the left ventricle by means of pulmonary artery banding. The results of this operation are generally less favorable in older patients, in whom the right ventricle has been the systemic ventricle for a longer period. The double switch procedure consists of baffling atrial blood to the appropriate ventricle (i.e., oxygenated blood diverted from the left atrium rightward to the right-sided left ventricle and vice versa). Arterial switch is performed in the same operation to restore physiologic AV and anatomic ventriculoarterial concordance. The intermediate-term results of this procedure are encouraging, but long-term results have yet to be determined (Fig. 14.213).
c. Adult patients with symptoms of progressive systemic AV valvular insufficiency may need valve repair or replacement. Most centers that have reported results with this procedure have found improved functional status after surgical treatment and acceptable risks. The timing of surgical intervention among patients with less severe symptoms is a topic of debate.

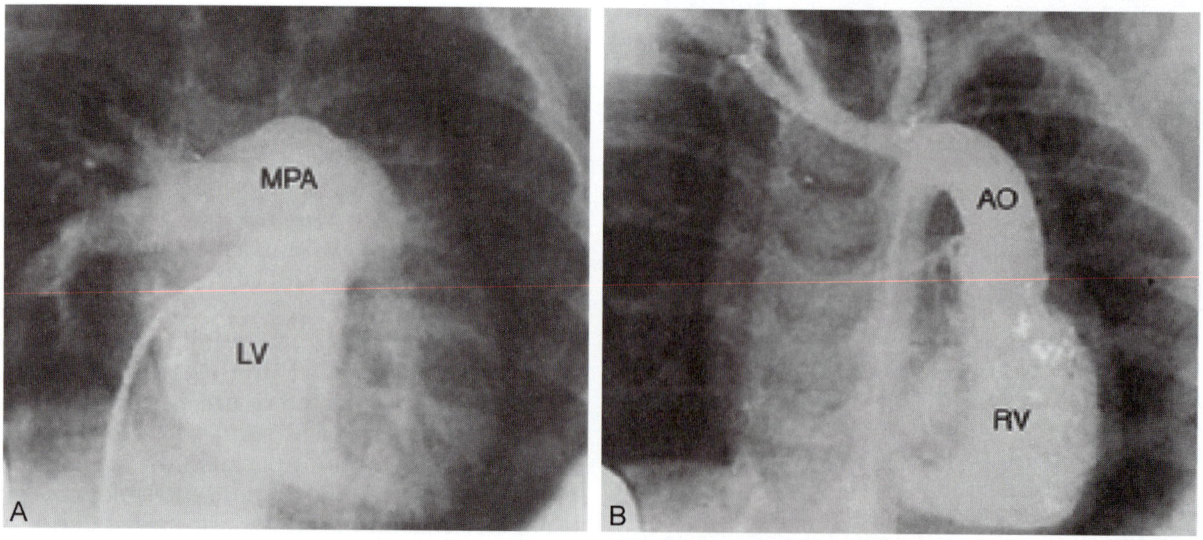

Figs 14.210A and B: *(A) Posteroanterior view of the left ventricular (LV) angiogram in a child with corrected transposition of the great arteries. The main pulmonary artery (MPA) arises from the smooth-walled left ventricle, which receives the systemic venous blood. (B) Posteroanterior view of the right ventricular angiogram (RV). The ascending aorta (AO) arises to the left of the pulmonary artery from the more heavily trabeculated right ventricle, which receives the pulmonary venous blood. The ventricular septum, seen here perpendicular to the frontal plane, is intact*

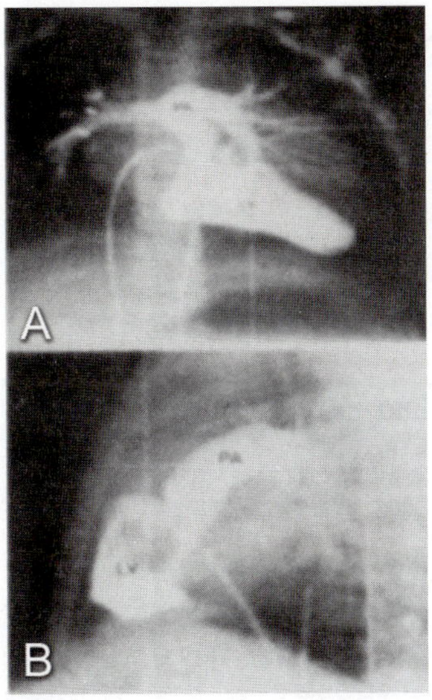

Figs 14.211A and B: *(A) Anteroposterior and (B) lateral views of a left ventricular (pulmonary ventricular) angiogram in a child with ccTGA. The finely trabeculated right-sided anatomic left ventricle empties into a right ward, posterior pulmonary artery PA, pulmonary artery; LV, left ventricle*

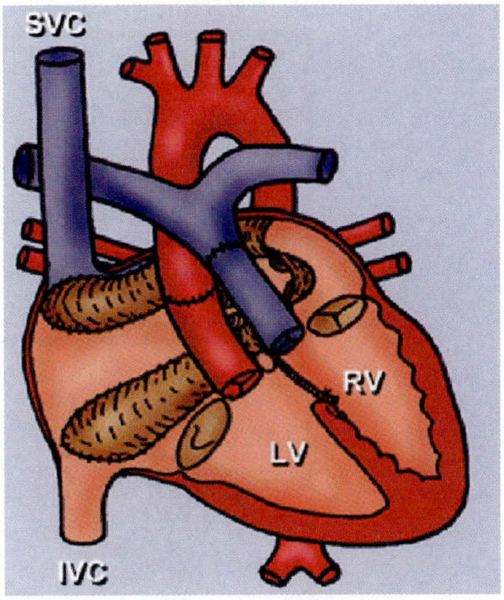

Fig. 14.213: *"Double-switch" operation for C-TGA using the Mustard atrial baffle technique and arterial switch procedure. The VSD has been closed with a patch. Venous blood from the superior and inferior vena cava (SVC, IVC) is directed to the RV and then to the pulmonary trunk, and pulmonary venous blood is directed to the LV and then to the aorta*

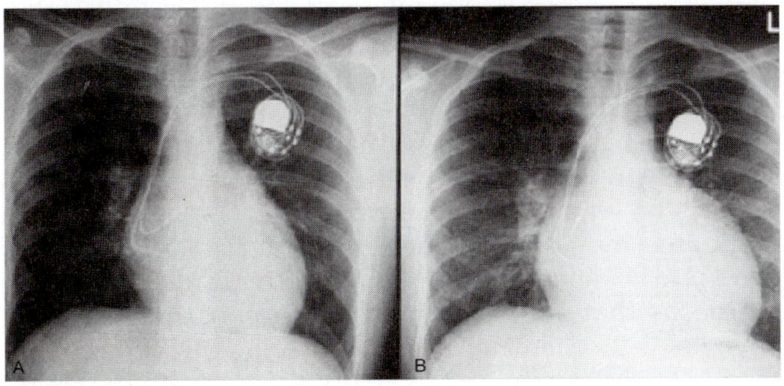

Figs 14.212A and B: *(A) Chest radiograph of a 16-year-old young man with C-TGA just after implantation of an endocardial pacemaker. Reportedly, his ejection fraction was 40%, and he had moderate systemic AV valve regurgitation. (B) Chest radiograph 18 months later at the time of referral. His systemic ventricular ejection fraction was 15%, and he had severe psystemic AV valve regurgitation. Cardiac transplantation was the only viable surgical option because referral was too late for conventional operation. (Reproduced with courtesy from the American College of Cardiology Foundation.)*

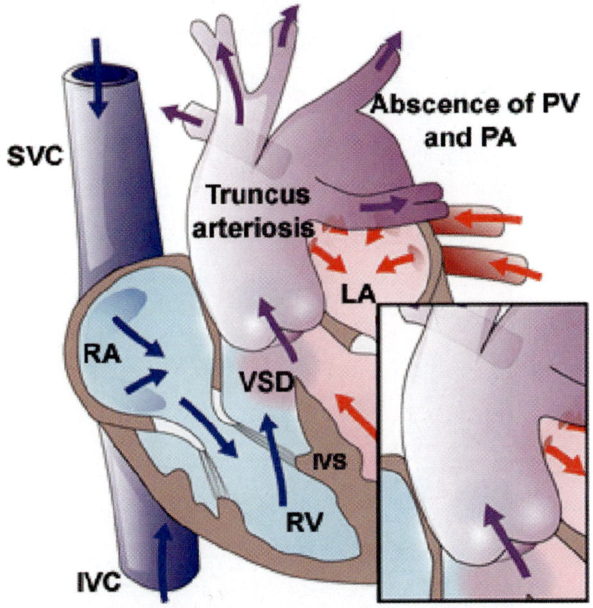

Fig. 14.214: *Illustration showing anatomy and circulation in truncus arteriosus*

TRUNCUS ARTERIOSUS (Figs 14.214 to 14.216)

History

Historical presentation of patients with truncus arteriosus (TA) who are not diagnosed before the onset of symptoms typically consists of the following:

1. Poor feeding
2. Diaphoresis
3. Tachypnea
4. Cyanosis

Etiology

As with most forms of congenital heart disease, the causes of truncus arteriosus are unknown. In experimental animal models, truncus arteriosus has been linked to abnormal development of cells from the neural crest that normally inhabit the outflow region of the developing heart. This is thought to be an important etiologic factor in at least some cases of human truncus arteriosus also.

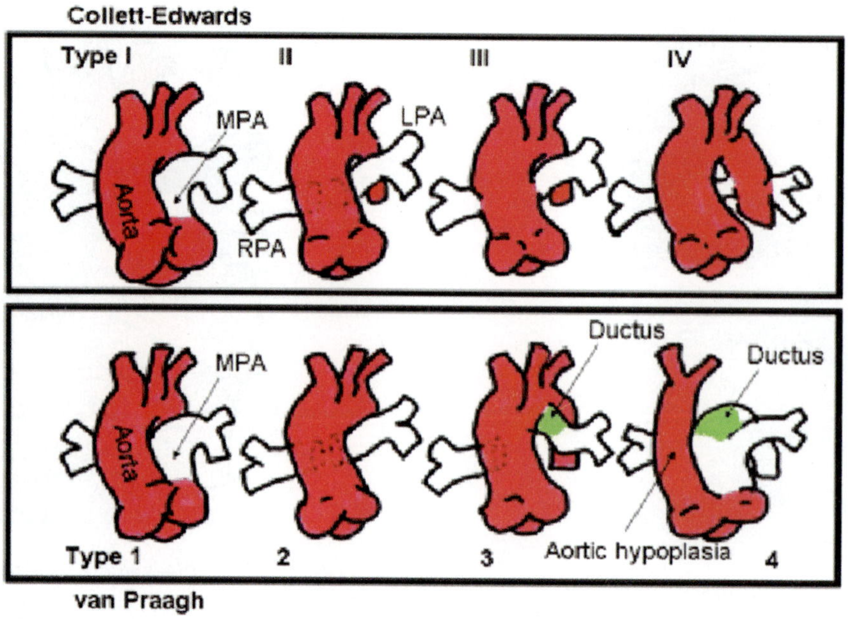

Fig. 14.215: *Collett-Edwards and Van Praagh classification systems for persistent truncus arteriosus. Ao, aorta; MPA, main pulmonary artery; LPA, left pulmonary artery; RPA, right pulmonary artery. (Modified from St. Louis, JD. Persistent truncus arteriosus. Critical Heart Disease in Infants and Children. Philadelphia, Mosby, 2006, p. 690.)*

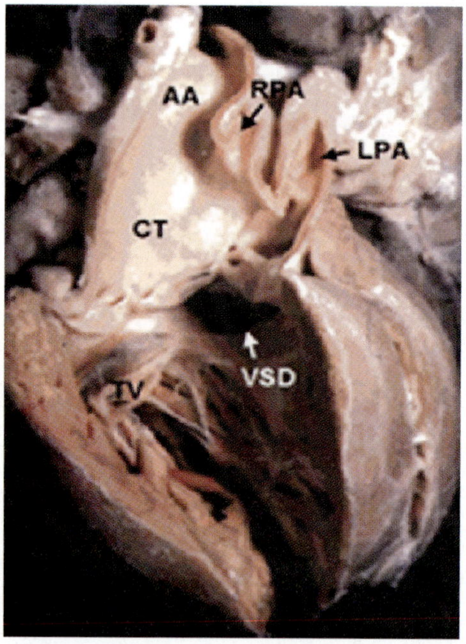

Fig. 14.216: *Pathologic specimen with truncus arteriosus (TA), viewed through the opened right ventricle and truncal valve. The common trunk (CT) can be seen giving off the ascending aorta (AA) as well as the left (LPA) and right (RPA) pulmonary arteries. The truncal valve straddles the ventricular septal defect (VSD). The tricuspid valve (TV) also is labeled. (Photograph courtesy of Robert H. Anderson, MD).*

As with various other congenital cardiac anomalies of the conotruncal region, a substantial number of patients with truncus arteriosus (approximately 30–40%) have microdeletions within chromosome band 22q11.2, which contains a number of characterized genes. This particular type of chromosomal deletion is thought to affect migration or development of cardiac neural crest cells and may contribute to the pathogenesis of truncus arteriosus in certain cases. Patients with truncus arteriosus and anomalies of the branch pulmonary arteries, such as stenosis or separate origin from the undersurface of the aortic arch, may have a higher incidence of association with band 22q11 deletion. Other specific features of truncus arteriosus that may be related to chromosomal deletion have yet to be characterized. The specific gene product or products responsible for cardiovascular anomalies in individuals with a 22q11 deletion has not been identified definitively in humans, although one of the genes in the 22q11.2 band, TBX1, has been shown to be involved pharyngeal arch and conotruncal development. Extensive research regarding truncus arteriosus and band 22q11 association is being conducted.

For the most part, other factors that may cause truncus arteriosus in humans have not been clearly identified. Other sporadic chromosomal and genetic abnormalities have been reported in humans with truncus arteriosus, including duplication of chromosome arm 8q and mutation of the NKX2.6 and GATA6 genes.

Several other genes have been associated with truncus arteriosus in transgenic mouse models including Tbx20, ALK2, Cited2, and Semaphorin 3c, but so far these genes have not been implicated in human truncus arteriosus.

Several studies found that children of mothers with significant diabetes mellitus during pregnancy had an increased incidence of truncus arteriosus (as well as other conotruncal malformations); however, this is not widely recognized as a significant risk factor.

Although certain teratogens (e.g. retinoic acid, bis-diamine) have been found to predispose to truncus arteriosus in animal models, no evidence suggests that these or others contribute importantly to this anomaly in humans.

DiGeorge syndrome or velocardiofacial syndrome, of ten included together as variations of CATCH-22 syndrome, are present in approximately 30–35% of patients with truncus arteriosus; most of these patients have deletions in band 22q11.

The most common noncardiac anomalies in patients with truncus arteriosus are those typically found in association with CATCH-22 syndrome, such as velopharyngeal insufficiency, cleft palate, and thymic and parathyroid dysfunction. Other noncardiac anomalies found sporadically in patients with truncus arteriosus include renal abnormalities, vertebral and rib anomalies, and anomalies of the alimentary tract.

Symptoms

These vary and may be more or less pronounced, depending on specific anatomic features and age at presentation. For example, patients with significant truncal valve regurgitation tend to present earlier with more profound symptoms of congestive heart failure.

Physical Examination

Patients with truncus arteriosus often present with cyanosis and are typically found to have decreased systemic arterial oxygen saturation. Cyanosis may not be evident, especially in very young neonates in whom pulmonary vascular resistance remains elevated. Even in slightly older neonates and young infants, pulmonary overcirculation and streaming of left and right ventricular outflow into the aorta and pulmonary arteries, respectively, may occasionally result in systemic oxyhemoglobin saturation well above 90%. Symptoms and signs of congestive heart failure are probably more common findings than cyanosis in patients presenting early in life.

Symptoms of failure typically manifest as pulmonary vascular resistance falls and pulmonary overcirculation increases.With progressively increasing pulmonary blood flow and, consequently, myocardial work, the initial symptoms of congestive heart failure (e.g. poor feeding, diaphoresis, mild lethargy) become more evident as failure to thrive ensues.

Patients occasionally present in extremis, with the usual high output failure exacerbated by significant regurgitation of the truncal valve. Patients with associated interruption of the aortic arch may exhibit a shocklike picture of cardiovascular collapse during ductal closure, although the arterial duct frequently remains patent in patients with truncus and interrupted arch, even without pharmacologic therapy.

Differential Diagnoses

- Acidosis, metabolic
- Aortopulmonary septal defect
- Double-outlet right ventricle, normally related great arteries
- Double-outlet right ventricle, with transposition
- Hypoplastic left heart syndrome
- Shock and hypotension in the newborn
- Tetralogy of fallot with absent pulmonary valve
- Tetralogy of fallot with pulmonary atresia
- Total anomalous pulmonary venous connection
- Transposition of the great arteries.

Laboratory Studies

Routine laboratory studies in the neonate with truncus arteriosus generally aid in determining therapeutic strategy rather than diagnosis.

An important exception in some cases is an arterial blood gas measurement, which helps to evaluate the degree of acidosis on presentation and may aid in differentiating cardiac disease from primary pulmonary pathology when performed before and after administration of 100% inspired oxygen (hyperoxia test).

Note that a hyperoxia test may be misleading in patients with truncus arteriosus and torrential pulmonary blood flow, both because of severe mismatch between pulmonary and systemic blood flow and, in some cases, because of streaming of left and right ventricular outflow into the systemic and pulmonary arterial systems, respectively.

Measurement of serum electrolytes including total and ionized calcium, is important in patients with truncus arteriosus, given the common association with DiGeorge syndrome, which frequently may include hypoparathyroidism and hypocalcemia.

Chest Radiography

Upon presentation, obtain a chest radiograph in most patients with truncus arteriosus.

Cardiomegaly and increased pulmonary vascular markings are typically present, and fullness in the region of the truncal root may possibly be discerned. In patients with a right aortic arch, this radiographic finding in association with increased pulmonary vascular markings suggests truncus arteriosus (Fig. 14.217).

Echocardiography

Echocardiography with cross-sectional and Doppler flow analysis is sufficient to confirm diagnosis of truncus arteriosus and fully characterize the various anatomic features in most patients. A full complement of echocardiographic views is necessary to ensure complete and accurate definition of the anatomy and potential associated anomalies.

Using subcostal coronal and parasternal long-axis images is the best way to demonstrate the single arterial trunk arising from the ventricles, with variable override of the ventricular septum. These views also demonstrate the thickness and mobility of the truncal valve leaflets. In general, the subcostal coronal view allows delineation of the pulmonary arterial origin(s) from the common trunk, although additional views are helpful to more completely characterize the pulmonary arterial anatomy. Morphology of the truncal valve and origins and course of the proximal coronary arteries are best observed from the parasternal short-axis window.

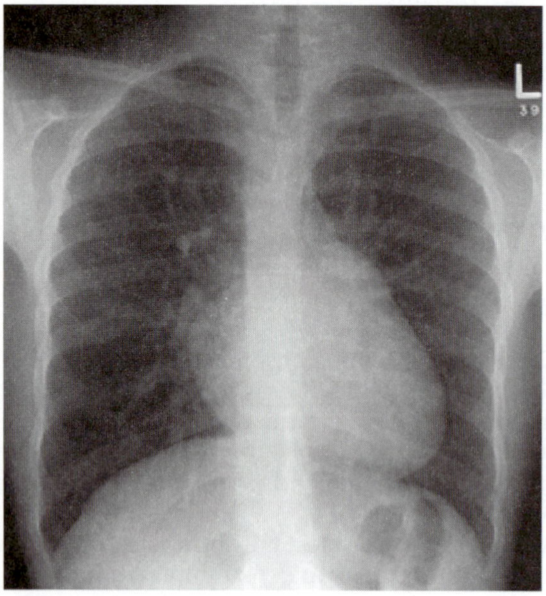

Fig. 14.217: *Cardiomegaly and prominent pulmonary artery chest radiograph of a young patient with truncus arteriosus type 1*

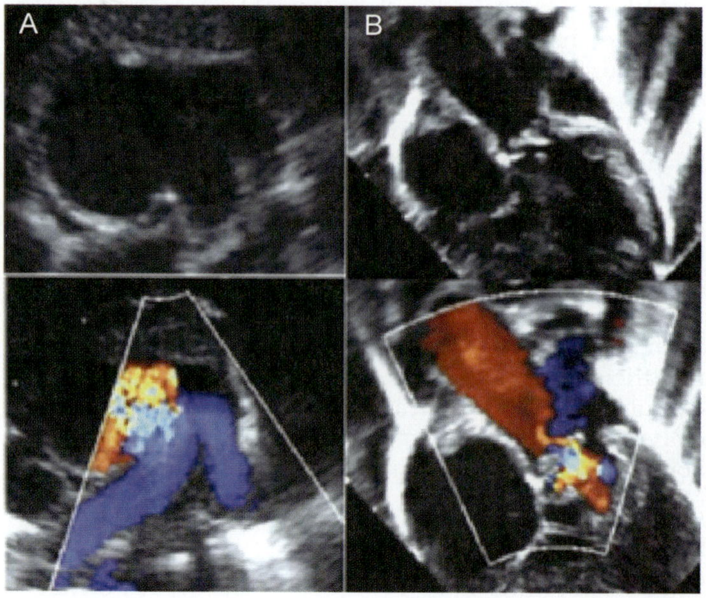

Figs 14.218A and B: *(A) Suprasternal frontal view of truncus arteriosus. Notice that the branch pulmonary arteries come off the truncus without evidence of a clear main pulmonary artery; this is consistent with truncus type 2. (B) Subcostal left anterior oblique view of the truncus. 2D imaging is consistent with a thick truncal valve and the pulmonary arteries are seen coming off the trunk. Color Doppler over the truncal valve shows flow acceleration*

Doppler color imaging from these windows is critical to evaluate pulmonary arterial flow and regurgitation or stenosis of the truncal valve. Imaging from the high parasternal and suprasternal notch views is necessary to define the aortic arch and provide additional perspective on the anatomy of the central pulmonary arteries. Standard approaches to imaging of the ventricular masses, atrioventricular valves, and atriums are important for full characterization of their structure and function (Figs 14.218 to 14.220).

Increasingly, diagnosis of truncus arteriosus and other complex heart defects is made by prenatal echocardiography. Prenatal echocardiography is generally accurate and sensitive for the diagnosis of truncus arteriosus, although the precise diagnosis may be difficult to

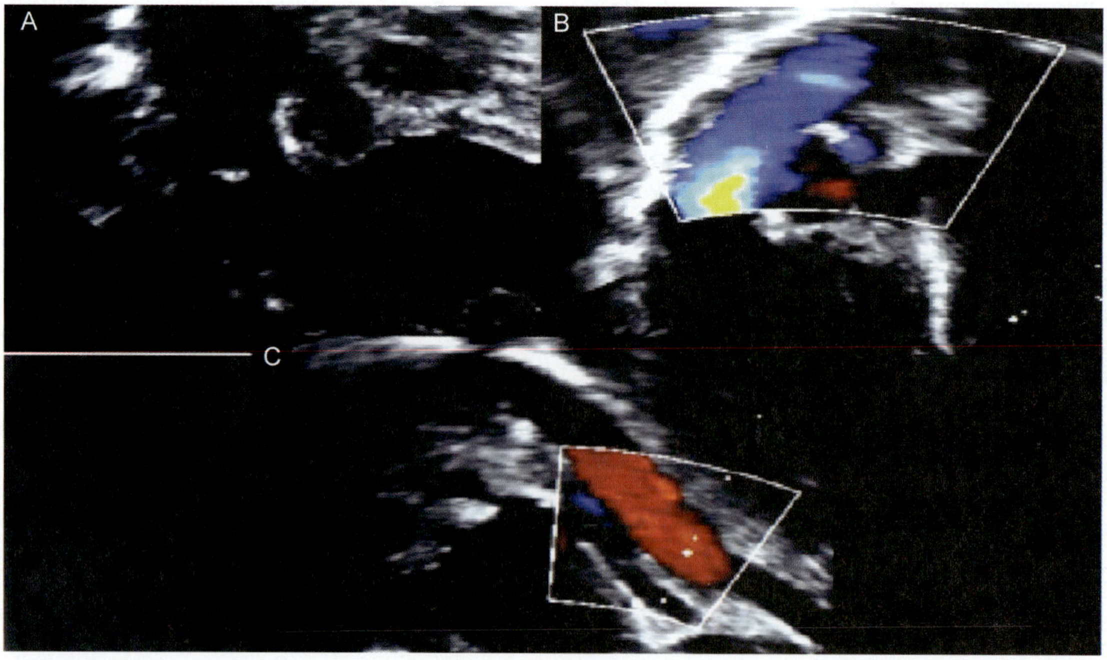

Fig. 14.219: *Subcostal views of a Damus–Kaye–Stansel. (A and B) focus on the proximal anastomosis between the aorta and the pulmonary artery. (B) Shows color in the proximal anastomosis, confirming it is unobstructed. (C) Subcostal sagittal view. It nicely delineates the descending aorta. Color in the descending aorta is laminar, confirming the absence of obstruction*

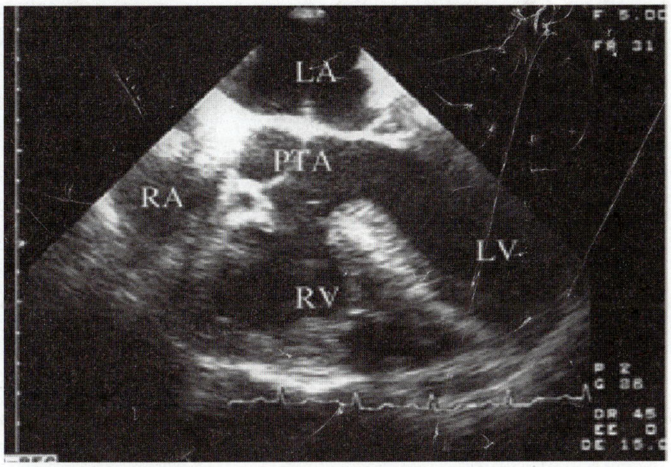

Fig. 14.220: *Transesophageal echocardiogram revealed a hypertrophied right ventricle, normal function in the left ventricle, absence of pulmonary valve and artery, a single great vessel (persistent truncus arteriosus) overriding both ventricles and a large single subtruncal ventricular septal defect. LA, left atrium; LV, left ventricle; RA, right*

distinguish from similar anomalies, such as tetralogy of Fallot or double-outlet right ventricle with pulmonary atresia, or aortic atresia with a ventricular septal defect (Fig. 14.221).

Computerized axial tomography and MRI: These are rarely necessary in patients with truncus arteriosus. MRI modality provides excellent imaging for characterizing anatomy, and may be especially useful in reconstructing complex pulmonary arterial anatomy in older patients with truncus arteriosus (Fig. 14.223).

Electrocardiography (Fig. 14.221)

Electrocardiographic (ECG) findings in young infants with truncus arteriosus do not distinguish this lesion from others on the differential diagnosis. A normal sinus rhythm, normal intervals, and either a normal QRS axis or minimal right-axis deviation are generally observed. Biventricular hypertrophy is a characteristic finding. In patients with substantial pulmonary overcirculation, left ventricular forces are especially prominent with evidence of left atrial enlargement.

Procedures

Cardiac Catheterization

Standard angiographic images from the truncal root can aid in the assessment of coronary arterial anatomy if echocardiography is inadequate, and in the assessment of regurgitation through the truncal valve.

Cardiac catheterization is generally not required prior to repair in neonates and young infants with truncus arteriosus. Catheterization is an important tool for evaluating some of the most common anatomic problems in patients with repaired truncus arteriosus, such as obstruction of the surgical reconstructed right ventricular outflow tract, branch pulmonary arterial stenosis, truncal valve regurgitation, and, in patients repaired later in life, pulmonary vascular obstructive disease.

Transcatheter balloon dilation: Treatment of pulmonary outflow tract or pulmonary arterial obstruction with transcatheter balloon dilation or stenting is an effective therapy for these problems in many patients.

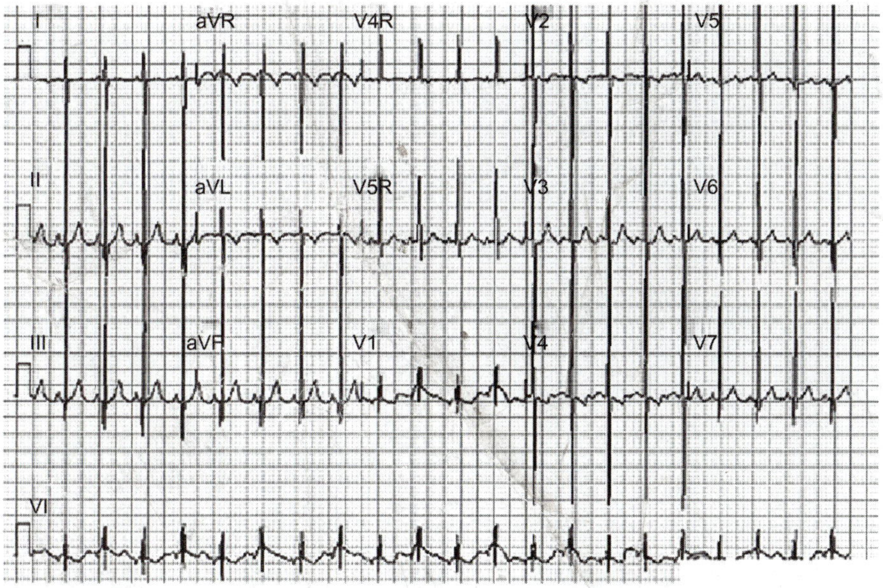

Fig. 14.221: *Truncus arteriosus: electrocardiogram obtained in a 4-month-old infant with type II truncus arteriosus. The tracing shows normal sinus rhythm, right atrial enlargement (peaked P wave in lead II), right ventricular hypertrophy (tall R wave V4R), right ventricular strain (flat or upright T waves in anterior chest leads), and left ventricular hypertrophy (tall R waves in lateral chest leads)*

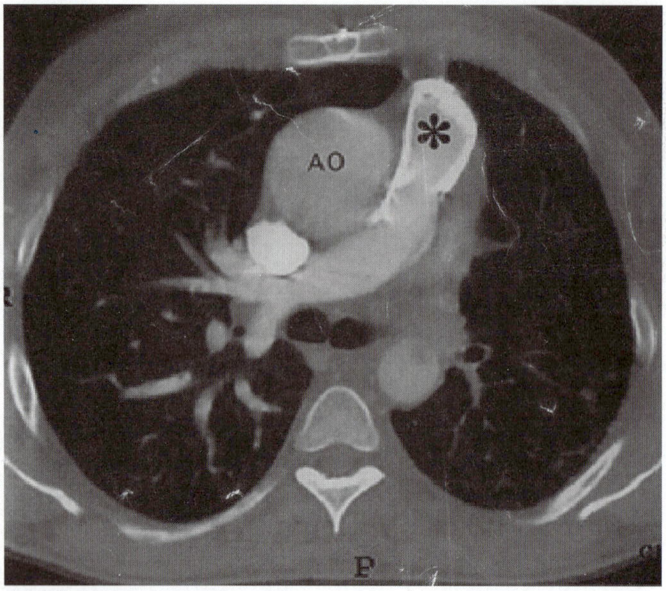

Fig. 14.222: *Interruption of the left pulmonary artery in a 36-year-old man who was born with a persistent truncus arteriosus (surgically repaired in childhood). Axial CT angiogram obtained at the level of the carina shows interruption of the left main pulmonary artery. The left lung is mildly hypoplastic with decreased vascularity. Note the calcified conduit (*) that connects the right ventricle to the main pulmonary artery and an aneurysmal ascending aorta (AO)*

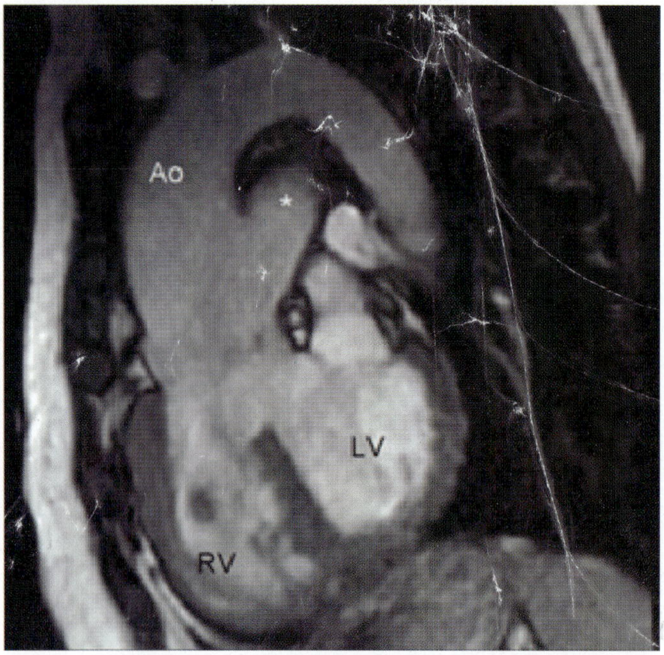

Fig. 14.223: *MRI showing unrepaired truncus arteriosus and a large outlet VSD. Lack of unobstructed pulmonary blood flow at systemic pressure means the patient has developed Eisenmenger physiology. The pulmonary arteries can arise in varying locations off the ascending aorta. Here, both arise from a single ostium (asterisk) and then divide to right and left out of plane (type 1). Note the RV hypertrophy. Ao, aorta; LV, left ventricle; RV, right ventricle*

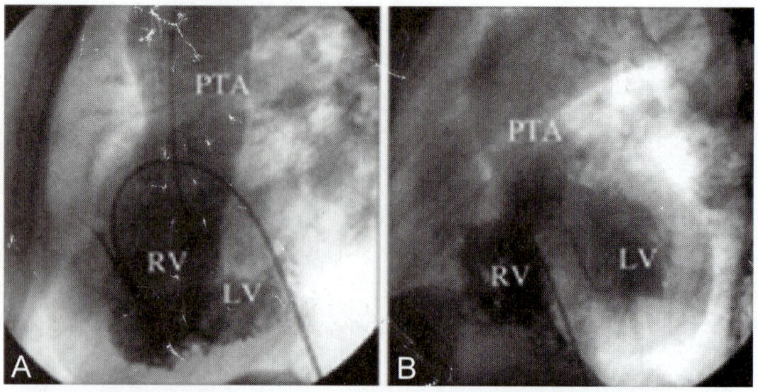

Figs 14.224A and B: *(A) Right ventriculogram in left anterior oblique projection. (B) Left ventriculogram in right anterior oblique projection. Angiography revealed biventricular hypertrophy with normal systolic function in both ventricles, a single and dilated truncal artery overriding both ventricles, a quadricuspid truncal valve with moderate insufficiency, a large subtruncal ventricular septal defect and absence of pulmonary valve and arteries (either from the right ventricle or from the truncus). LV, left ventricle; RV, right ventricle; PTA, persistent truncus arteriosus*

Differential Diagnosis

The differential diagnosis includes pericardial effusion, pulmonary atresia, atrial septal defect, congenital tricuspid regurgitation, and Uhl's malformation.

Medical Care

Medical care before surgical repair depends on clinical presentation. Most neonates with truncus arteriosus display some evidence of congestive heart failure; they are usually The electrocardiogram is seldom normal. The usual rhythm is normal sinus, but 25–30% of patients at some time have atrial tachycardia. atrial flutter, or atrial fibrillation. About 5–25% have preexcitation, usually a type B Wolff-Parkinson- White syndrome, which may be present intermittently. Tall, peaked, "Himalayan" P waves are characteristic, and the PR interval is usually prolonged in the absence of preexcitation. Most patients have right bundle-branch block due to the late activation of the "atrialized" right-ventricle. Q waves may be present In the precordial leads VI to V4.

Natural History and Prognosis

Most patients die by the age of 25 years. Patients may have progressive symptoms of heart failure, paradoxical embolism, brain abscess, or cardiac arrhythmia, many of which can cause sudden death.

Management

Management includes antibiotic prophylaxis against infective endocarditis, treatment of heart failure with digitalis and diuretlc and control of atrial and ventricular arrhythmias. Surgical intervention is possible, but it may not eliminate cardiac arrhythmia and death may still occur. Intravenous prostaglandin is often administered in patients with truncus arteriosus upon presentation because the differential diagnosis includes numerous anomalies with duct-dependent systemic or pulmonary blood flow. However, it is beneficial only in patients with associated interruption of the aortic arch or aortic coarctation. Other preoperative medications are not generally indicated, although specific circumstances may dictate afterload reducing agents, inotropic medications, or antiarrhythmics. Full-term and premature newborns with truncus arteriosus may be at increased risk for necrotizing enterocolitis, either preoperatively or postoperatively, and appropriate evaluation should be undertaken in any newborn exhibiting signs or symptoms of necrotizing enterocolitis.

Surgical Care

Indications

Truncus arteriosus invariably requires operative repair. Symptoms typically develop in the early neonatal period, indicating that complete repair is required at this point.

Techniques

Surgical management of truncus arteriosus has undergone significant evolution over the past 30 years. Complete repair was first performed in 1967, but until neonatal and early infant repair became routine in the 1980s, palliative pulmonary artery banding was common, with complete repair performed at an older age. At most centers, primary complete repair in the neonate and young infant has become the accepted standard.

Currently, surgical management consists of complete primary repair, with closure of the ventricular septal defect, committing the common arterial trunk to the left ventricle, and reconstruction of the right ventricular outflow tract.

In patients with both branch pulmonary arteries arising from the common trunk, the standard method of right ventricular outflow tract reconstruction entails removing the central pulmonary arteries from the common trunk en bloc and placing a valved conduit from the right ventricle proximally to the central pulmonary arteries distally. Also, the most common type of conduit used is a cryopreserved valved aortic or pulmonary allograft. Before allograft conduits became widely available, other forms of pulmonary outflow reconstruction were used. These alternative forms remain in use in areas where the cost and availability of conduits prohibit routine use of modern techniques. Such alternatives include xenograft valves housed in synthetic tube grafts, direct anastomosis of the pulmonary arteries to the right ventriculotomy, or autologous flaps of pulmonary or aortic tissue augmented with synthetic patch material. In patients with one pulmonary artery arising from the common trunk and one from the underside of the aortic arch, the pulmonary arteries are disconnected separately; they are then anastomosed together before being anastomosed to the conduit or are anastomosed to the conduit independently. Coexisting anomalies are repaired as appropriate with cardiopulmonary bypass, cardioplegia, and sometimes deep hypothermic arrest, depending on anatomic features and the preference of the surgeon. When the truncal valve is abnormal and repaired at the time of the initial truncus repair, outcomes appear to be significantly worse that when early truncal valve repair is not necessary.

Consultations

Unless specific associated anomalies or problems are identified, consultations are not generally necessary.

Band 22q11 deletion is present in approximately one-third of patients with truncus arteriosus, and consultation with a geneticist may be appropriate in some of these patients. Although patients with this chromosomal anomaly may have subtle associated abnormalities that are more likely to be identified if an experienced clinical geneticist is consulted, no evidence suggests that outcomes or management considerations differ in patients with or without chromosomal deletion. When a chromosome 22q11 deletion is identified, comprehensive evaluation for associated conditions is indicated including an otolaryngologist to evaluate for submucosal cleft palate, an immunologist to evaluate for immunodeficiency, and early intervention services for evaluation of learning and speech. Consult a cardiologist before beginning, changing, or discontinuing cardiac medications in these patients.

Diet

No special dietary considerations are indicated in patients with truncus arteriosus, other than a diet that might be dictated by associated conditions.

Resume enteral feeding once the patient is hemodynamically stable. Resume oral feedings when the patient has been removed from mechanical ventilatory support and is adequately alert to take oral feedings safely. In patients with deletion in band 22q11, velopharyngeal insufficiency or cleft palate is frequently present, and oral feedings should be resumed with the aid of feeding specialists.

Activity

Specific restrictions on activity are not indicated in patients with truncus arteriosus. Patients with repaired truncus arteriosus and either residual defects or regurgitation of the right ventricle to pulmonary artery conduit may have limited exercise capacity best addressed on an individual basis.

EBSTEIN'S ANOMALY OF TV

Definition

In Ebstein's anomaly abnormal attachments of the posterior and septal leaflets of the tricuspid valve to the wall of the right ventricle below the atrioventricular junction produce a zone of "atrialized right ventricle" between the right atrium and the right ventricle. A patent foramen ovale or atrial septal defect is present in many cases. Other defects may be present. These include coarctation of the aorta, ventricular septal defect, stenosis of the pulmonary valve, and pulmonary atresia (Fig. 14.225).

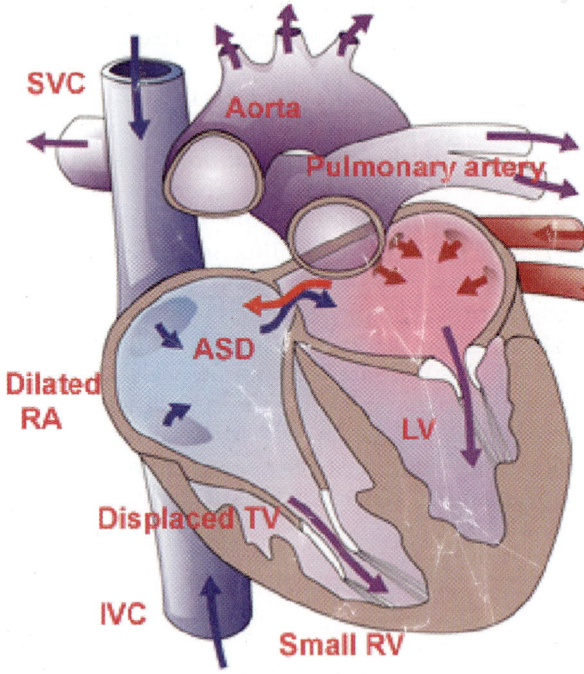

Fig. 14.225: *Ebstein's malformation of the tricuspid valve is characterized by displacement of the septal and posterior leaflets of the tricuspid valve downward into the right ventricle (RV) to varying degrees*

Pathology

Abnormal attachments of the septal and posterior tricuspid valve leaflets are characteristic. The displaced leaflets are often dysplastic and occasionally adherent to the right ventricular wall. With severe displacement of the leaflets, the functional right ventricle is significantly decreased in size. The "atrialized" portion of right ventricle is often very thin-walled. The deformed tricuspid valve is usually incompetent and occasionally stenotic.

Clinical Manifestations

History

A history of transient neonatal cyanosis is occasionally obtained. Dyspnea, cyanosis, fatigue, palpitations, and syncope are the most common symptoms. Some patients are asymptomatic until adolescence or adulthood. Cyanosis, which may be intermittent or persistent, occurs in more than one-half of patients. Chest pain of varying characteristics and of uncertain etiology may occur. Brain abscess and paradoxic embolus occur, but infective endocarditis is uncommon.

Physical Examination (Fig. 14.226)

Growth and development are usually normal, although cyanosis is relately common. Initially, it may only be induced by cold, effort, or arrhythmia. There is usually no abnormal right ventricular lift or heave. The first and second heart sounds are usually both widely split. The pulmonic component of the second heart sound (P2) is occasionally in audible. Often there are loud third (S3) and fourth (S4) heart sounds. Characteristically, there is a scratchy, harsh, grade 3 to 4 early systolic murmur that is heard loudest between the left sternal border and the apex.

Imaging of Ebstein Anomaly

Chest radiographs can reveal the following:

1. Normal findings
2. Cardiomegaly (Fig. 14.227)
3. Small aortic root and main pulmonary artery shadow
4. Decreased pulmonary vasculature
5. Large right atrium.

Echocardiography (Figs 14.228 to 14.230)

M-mode

1. Paradoxical septal motion
2. Dilated right ventricle
3. Delayed closure of tricuspid valve leaflets more than 65 milliseconds after mitral valve closure.

Two Dimensional

1. Apical displacement of the septal leaflet of tricuspid leaflet of greater than 8 mm/m^2—most specific sign
2. Abnormalities in morphology and septal attachment of the septal and anterior tricuspid leaflets
3. Ecentric leaflet coaptation
4. Dilated right atrium
5. Dilated right ventricle with decreased contractile performance

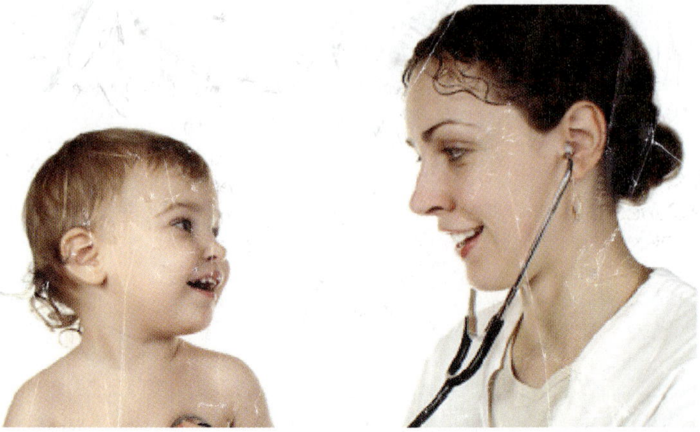

Fig. 14.226: *Doctor in conducting physical examination in a patient with Ebstein anomaly*

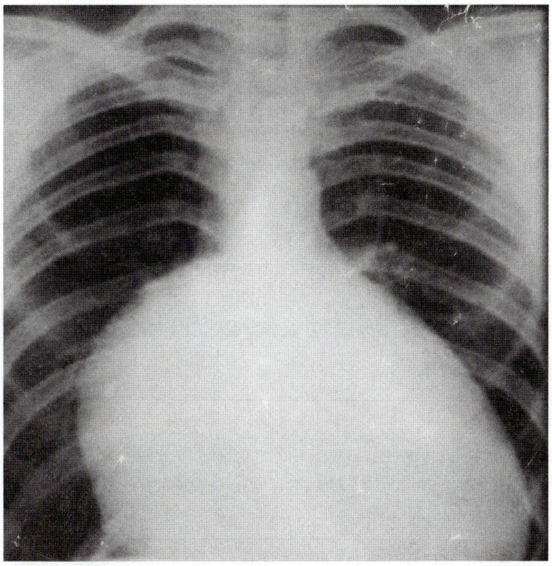

Fig. 14.227: *Ebstein's anomaly showing the classic appearance of cardiomegaly, small aortic knuckle, small pulmonary arteries giving the appearance of underfilled lungs, dilated inferior vena cava and huge right atrium. The right ventricular outflow is prominent and pushed to the left by the dilated right atrium, which is dilated due to tricuspid regurgitation*

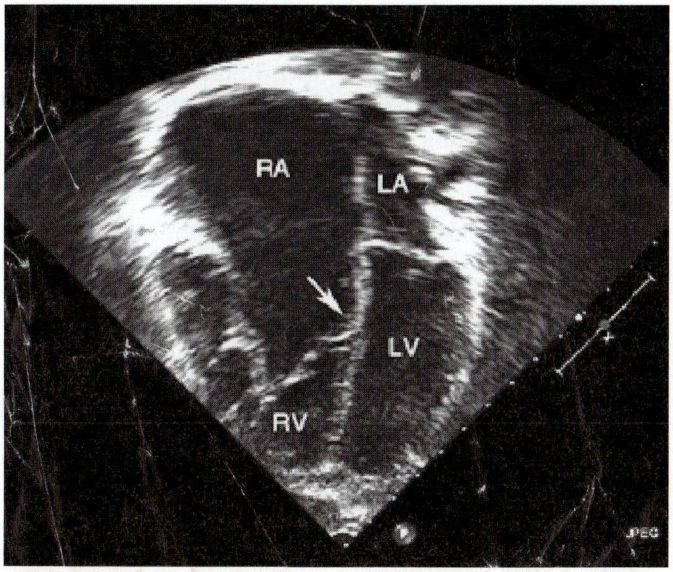

Fig. 14.228: *Ebstein anomaly of the tricuspid valve. Apical four chamber echocardiogram in a patient with Ebstein anomaly demonstrates severe apical displacement of the septal leaflet of the tricuspid valve (arrow), with resulting "atrialization" of a large portion of the right ventricular sinus. The anterior leaflet of the tricuspid valve is large (often described as "sail-like") and has multiple attachments to the apex and anterior right ventricular wall (RV). LA, left atrium; LV, left ventricle, RA, right atrium*

6. Various left heart structural abnormalities (described recently in up to 39% of patients with Ebstein abnormality)

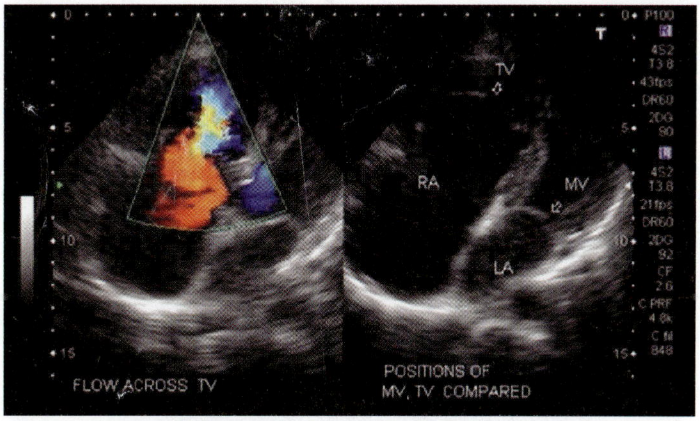

Fig. 14.229: *This patient presented with dyspnea and palpitation. Echocardiography and Color Doppler imaging of the heart revealed apically displaced tricuspid valve with resultant atrialization of a major part of the right ventricle. There was also evidence of tricuspid regurgitation (image on left-color Doppler). The right ventricle and the right atrium appear enlarged. These ultrasound images suggest Ebstein anomaly with tricuspid regurgitation*

Doppler Studies

1. Varying degrees of tricuspid regurgitation
2. Excludes associated shunts
3. Assessment of severity and surgical options by echocardiography
4. Functional right ventricular area less than 35% of total right ventricular area or an atrialized to functional right ventricular ratio greater than 0.5 associated with unfavorable prognosis
5. Functional right ventricular size
6. Degree of septal leaflet displacement
7. Amount of leaflet tethering
8. Magnitude of leaflet deformity and dysplasia

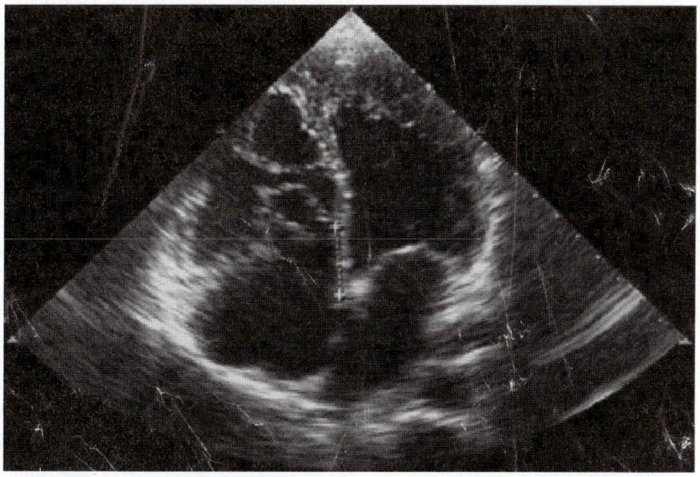

Fig. 14.230: *Apical four chamber view shows displacement of TV into RV with apical aneurysm due to noncompact cardiomyopathy in a patient with Ebstein's anomaly*

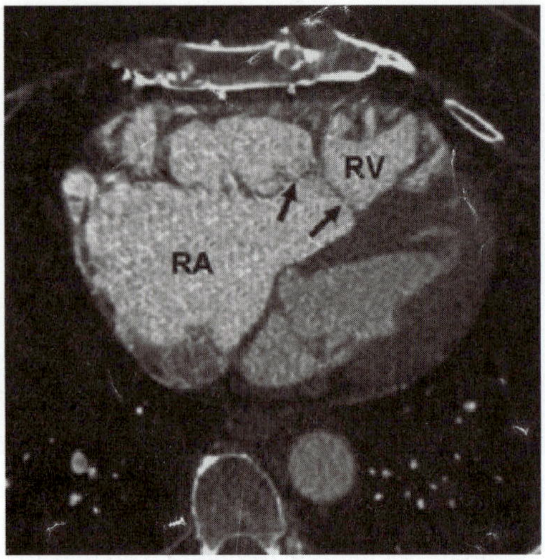

Fig. 14.231: *Ebstein's anomaly in a 18-year-old man in whom CMR evaluation was precluded by claustrophobia. Axial MDCT imaging showing displacement of the tricuspid valve leaflets (arrows) deep into the "atrialized" right ventricle. RA, right atrium; RV, right ventricle*

9. Aneurysmal dilatation of right ventricular outflow tract (right ventricular outflow tract-to-aortic root ratio of > 2:1 on parasternal short-axis view)
10. Moderate-to-severe tricuspid regurgitation

MRI: It is currently not used routinely; it may become a useful noninvasive modality in the future (Fig. 14.231).

Electrocardiography

Twelve-lead

1. Rhythm
2. Usually normal sinus findings
3. Intermittently SVT, paroxysmal SVT, atrial flutter, atrial fibrillation, ventricular tachycardia
4. Abnormal P waves consistent with right atrial enlargement
5. *PR interval:* Most commonly prolonged
   May be normal or short in patients with WPW syndrome
6. *QRS complex:* RBBB
7. Low voltage in many patients.

Cardiac Catheterization (Fig. 14.234)

Rarely performed today: Confirms echocardiographic findings. Can reveal right ventricular electrical activity on the intracardiac ECG with simultaneous right atrial pressure and waveform when the catheter is withdrawn from the right ventricle, back across the tricuspid valve into the right atrium.

Electrophysiologic Studies

Patients with Ebstein anomaly, 25–30% have accessory pathways, and 5–25% have evidence of preexcitation on the surface ECG.

Electrophysiologic (EP) studies in patients with tachyarrhythmias can delineate accessory conduction pathways and guide ablative therapy. Right-sided pathways are more common. Fifty percent of the patients have multiple pathways.

Medical Care

Ebstein anomaly presents with a spectrum of congenital abnormalities of the tricuspid valve and the right ventricle. The age of presentation with symptoms is variable, and a wide range of treatment options is available. Treatment of Ebstein anomaly is complex and dictated mainly by the severity of the disease itself and the effect of accompanying congenital structural and electrical abnormalities.

Treatment options include medical therapy, radiofrequency ablation and surgical therapy.

1. Antibiotic prophylaxis for infective endocarditis
2. Medical therapy for heart failure—angiotensin-converting enzyme (ACE) inhibitors, diuretics, and digoxin

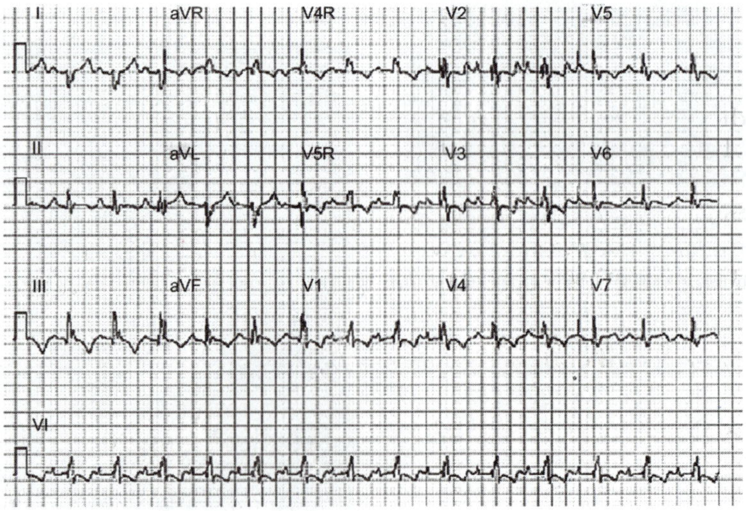

Fig. 14.232: *Ebstein's Anomaly: electrocardiogram obtained in a 13-year-old adolescent with Ebstein's anomaly of the tricuspid valve. The tracing demonstrates right-axis deviation, right atrial enlargement, first-degree heart block (PR interval 232 msec), and complete right-bundle branch block*

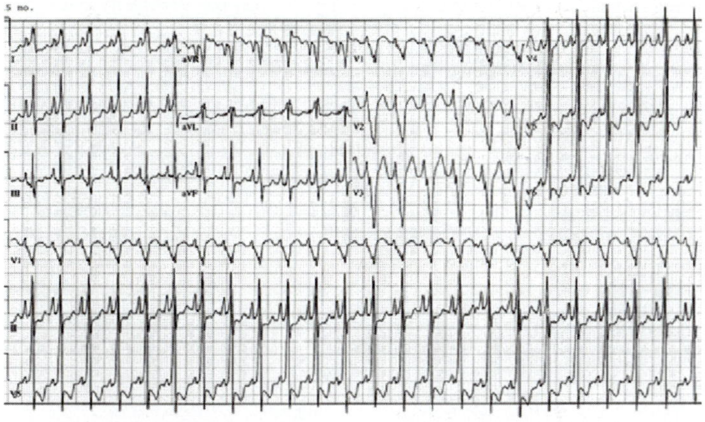

Fig. 14.233: *ECG showing right lateral accessory pathway (AP) in a patient with Ebstein anomaly*

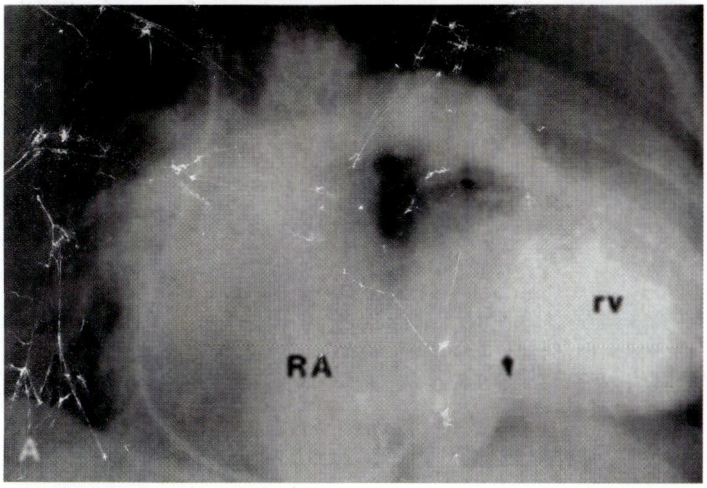

Fig. 14.234: *A, anterior projection right ventricular angiogram in a patient with Ebstein's anomaly. The cavernous right atrium (RA) is seen with a notch inferiorly (arrow) at the attachment of the congenitally displaced and incompetent tricuspid valve. Note the relatively small right ventricle (rv)*

3. Arrhythmia treatment—medical treatments such as antiarrhythmic drugs or radiofrequency ablation of the accessory pathways
4. Curative therapy of SVT with radiofrequency ablation is currently the treatment of choice. The success rate is lower than that in patients without significant structural heart disease.

Factors associated with lower likelihood of success include the following:
1. Accessory pathways located along the atrialized right ventricle
2. Multiple accessory pathways
3. Complex geometry of the pathways
4. Abnormal morphology of the endocardial action potentials in this region.

Surgical Care

Surgical care includes correction of the underlying tricuspid valve and right ventricular abnormalities, correction of any associated intracardiac defects, palliative procedures in early days of life as a bridge to more definitive surgical treatment later, and surgical treatment of associated arrhythmias. Complete repair of Ebstein anomaly in symptomatic neonates has been shown to be feasible, with good early and late survival and excellent functional status. In patients <50 years of age with Ebstein anomaly, surgery is associated with good long-term survival and improved functional status, although long-term survival might be improved by performing surgery earlier.

The trend is to perform surgery earlier rather later in the course of heart failure. Indications for surgery are generally as follows:
1. New York Heart Association (NYHA) class I-II heart failure with worsening symptoms or with a cardiothoracic ratio of 0.65 or greater
2. NYHA class III-IV heart failure
3. History of paradoxical embolism
4. Significant cyanosis with arterial O_2 saturation of 80% or less and/or polycythemia with hemoglobin of 16 g/dL or more
5. Arrhythmias refractory to medical and radiofrequency ablation.

Various approaches are available to treat structural abnormalities. Tricuspid valve repair is preferred over valve replacement, and bioprosthetic valves are preferred over mechanical prosthetic valves. The atrialized portion of the right ventricle can be resected surgically, and the markedly dilated, thin-walled right atrium can be resected. Associated septal defects may be closed.

Palliative procedures include creation of atrial septal defect, closure of tricuspid valve with plication of the right atrium, and maintenance of pulmonary blood flow through aortopulmonary shunt. Palliative procedures usually are reserved for severely ill infants with otherwise dire prognosis. Left ventricular dysfunction should not be considered a contraindication to tricuspid valve surgery. In these patients, although early mortality is greater with tricuspid valve surgery, the late results are favorable and left ventricular function seems to improve postoperatively.

Functional status improves after surgery. Surgical treatments of arrhythmias include the following:
1. Ablation of the accessory pathways
2. Maze procedure for atrial arrhythmias
3. Cardiac transplantation is appropriate in selected patients.

Medication

Ebstein anomaly requires drug treatment for cardiovascular consequences resulting from tricuspid atrialization of the right ventricle, valvular regurgitation, and septal defects. Patients may require antibiotic prophylaxis for bacterial endocarditis. Treatment of SVT is typically by radiofrequency ablation rather than drug therapy. CHF is treated with ACE inhibitors, diuretics and digoxin.

TRICUSPID ATRESIA

In this type of cardiac anomaly, there is an agenesis of the tricuspid valve. The right atrioventricular endocardial cushion fuses into the right wall with the result that tricuspid valve does not develop. An atrial septal defect is a must for survival since it allows systemic venous return to reach the left atrium. The blood reaches the lungs either through a ventricular septal defect or a patent ductus arteriosus.Tricuspid atresia may be associated with transposition of great vessels.The pulmonary stenosis may or may not be present.

Anatomy (Figs 14.235 and 14.236)

The pathologic anatomy of tricuspid atresia is best understood by reviewing variations in valvular morphology, as follows:

The most common type of tricuspid atresia is muscular It is characterized by a dimple or a localized fibrous thickening in the floor of the right atrium at the expected site of the tricuspid valve. The muscular variety accounts for 89% of cases.

In the membranous type (6.6%), the atrioventricular portion of the membranous septum forms the floor of the right atrium at the expected location of the tricuspid valve. This particular type appears to be associated with absent pulmonary valve leaflets. Minute valvular cusps are fused together in the valvular type (1%).

In the Ebstein type (2.6%), fusion of the tricuspid valve leaflets occurs; attachment is displaced downward, and plastering of the leaflets to the right ventricular wall occurs. This variant is rare but well documented.

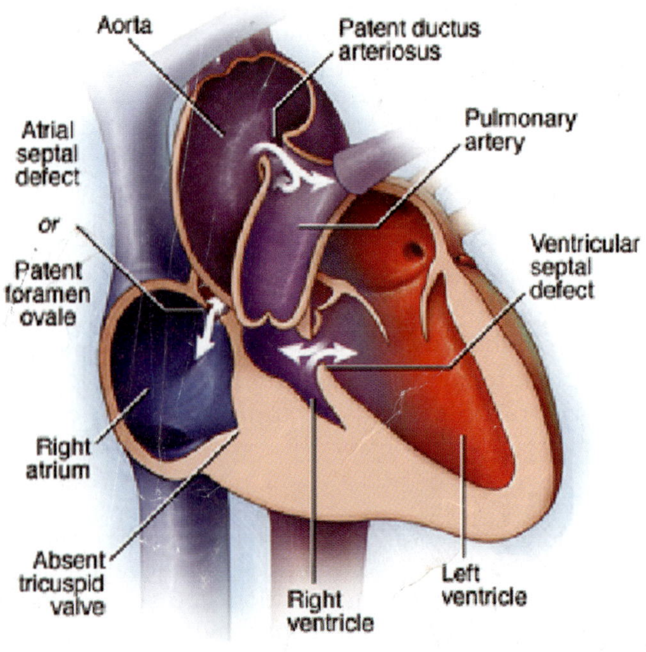

Fig. 14.235: *Diagram showing structural abnormalities in tricuspid atresia*

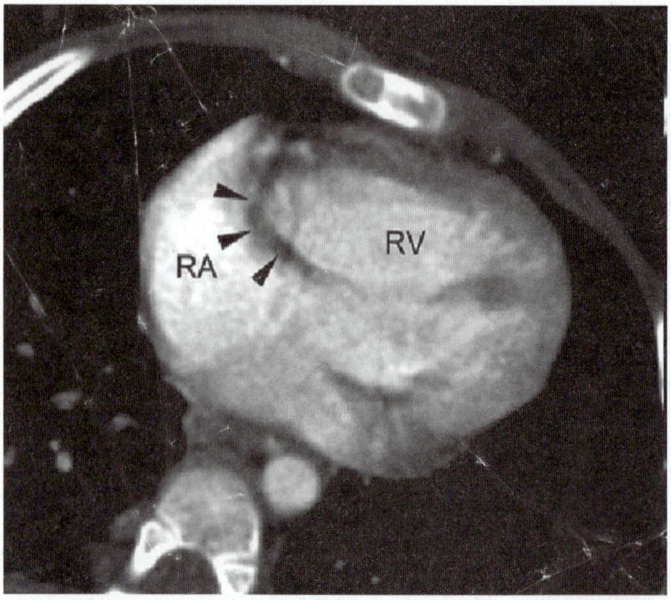

Fig. 14.236: *Tricuspid atresia. CT scan shows fatty tissue (arrowheads) between the right atrium (RA) and the right ventricle (RV), which prevents any direct connection between the two compartments. This case represents the more common type of tricuspid atresia*

The atrioventricular canal type is extremely rare (0.2%). In this type, a leaflet of the common atrioventricular valve seals off the only entrance into the right ventricle.

In the final type, unguarded with a muscular shelf (0.6%), the atrioventricular junction is unguarded, but the inlet component of the morphologic right ventricle is separated from its outlet by a muscular shelf.

The right atrium is enlarged and hypertrophied. An interatrial communication is necessary for survival. This communication most commonly is a stretched patent foramen ovale. Sometimes, an ostium secundum or an ostium primum atrial septal defect (ASD) is present. In rare cases, the patent foramen ovale is obstructive and may form an aneurysm of the fossa ovalis, which is sometimes large enough to produce mitral inflow obstruction. The left atrium may be enlarged, especially when the pulmonary blood flow is increased. The mitral valve is morphologically normal; it is rarely incompetent and has a large orifice. The left ventricle is enlarged and hypertrophied but often morphologically normal.

The ventricular septal defect (VSD) is usually small; however, it can be large, or several VSDs may be present. The ventricular septum is rarely intact. When present, the VSD may be conoventricular or perimembranous in type (inferior to the septal band), it may be of conal septal malalignment type (between the limbs of the septal band), or it may be of the muscular or atrioventricular canal type. Muscular VSDs are the most common defects and are usually restrictive; they produce subpulmonary stenosis in patients with normally related great arteries and simulate subaortic obstruction in patients with transposition of the great arteries.

The right ventricle is small and hypoplastic, and its size largely depends on the anatomic type. In patients with a large VSD or transposition of the great arteries, the size of the right ventricle may be larger, but, even in these patients, the right ventricle is smaller than normal. In patients with pulmonary atresia and normally related great arteries, the right ventricle is small and may escape detection. However, it is a true right ventricle in most patients; it is composed of a sharply demarcated infundibulum with septal and parietal bands and a sinus with trabeculae, which may communicate with the left ventricle by means of a VSD. By definition, the inflow region is absent although papillary muscles may occasionally be present.

The great artery relationship is variable and forms the basis of a major classification. Obstruction to the pulmonary outflow tract is present in most cases of tricuspid atresia and is used in the scheme of classification. The aorta is either normal or slightly larger than normal. In 30% of patients, various associated cardiac defects are present; aortic coarctation and persistent left superior vena cava are particularly notable.

Associated cardiac defects in tricuspid atresia are as follows:
- D-transposition of the great arteries
- L-transposition of the great arteries
- Double-outlet right ventricle
- Double-outlet left ventricle
- Other malpositions of the great arteries

Truncus Arteriosus

Defects that may need attention before or during palliative or total surgical correction are as follows:
- Absent pulmonary valve
- Aneurysm of the atrial septum
- Anomalous origin of the coronary arteries from the pulmonary artery
- Anomalous origin of the left subclavian artery
- Anomalous origin of the right subclavian artery
- Aortopulmonary fistula
- Coarctation of the aorta
- Common atrium
- Cor triatriatum dexter
- Coronary sinus septal defect
- Double aortic arch
- Double-outlet left atrium
- Hemitruncus
- Hypoplastic ascending aorta and/or aortic atresia
- Ostium primum ASD
- Parchment right ventricle
- Patent ductus arteriosus
- Persistent left superior vena cava
- Right aortic arch
- Subaortic stenosis
- Total anomalous pulmonary venous connection
- Tubular hypoplasia of the aortic arch
- Valvular aortic stenosis.

Other associated defects are as follows:
- Juxtaposition of the atrial appendages
- Anomalous entry of coronary sinus into the left atrium

Subtypes

Tricuspid atresia is classified according to the morphology of the valve, the radiographic appearance of pulmonary vascular markings, and the associated cardiac defects.

Van Praagh and associates (1971) initially proposed a classification based on the morphology of the atretic tricuspid valve. He and others later modified and expanded the classification, as described in tricuspid atresia.

Astley and associates (1953) proposed a classification based on pulmonary vascular markings on a chest radiograph: Group A are cases with decreased pulmonary vascular markings, and group B are those with increased pulmonary vascular markings. Dick et al (1975) added a third group, group C, to describe cases with a transition from increased to decreased pulmonary vascular markings. This type of classification has some clinical value although a more precise definition than these can often be made by using noninvasive 2-dimensional (2D) and Doppler echocardiography.

In 1906, Kuhne first proposed a classification based on great-artery relationships, which Edwards and Burchell expanded in 1949. Keith, Rowe, and Vlad popularized this classification in 1967. Other investigators have offered various other classifications. These are reviewed in detail in the American Heart Journal and Tricuspid Atresia. Although these classifications are generally good, their exclusion of some variations in great-artery relationships and the lack of consistency in subgroups are problematic. Therefore, the authors propose the following new, comprehensive-yet-unified classification:

The principle grouping continues to be based on the following interrelationships of the great arteries:
- Type I—Normally related great arteries
- Type II—D-Transposition of the great arteries
- Type III—Great artery positional abnormalities other than D-transposition of the great arteries
  - Subtype 1— L-transposition of the great arteries
  - Subtype 2—Double outlet right ventricle
  - Subtype 3—Double outlet left ventricle
  - Subtype 4—D-malposition of the great arteries (anatomically corrected malposition)
  - Subtype 5—L-malposition of the great arteries (anatomically corrected malposition)
- Type IV—Persistent truncus arteriosus.

All types and subtypes are subdivided into the following subgroups:
- Subgroup a—Pulmonary atresia
- Subgroup b—Pulmonary stenosis or hypoplasia
- Subgroup c—No pulmonary stenosis (normal pulmonary arteries).

After the above categorization, the status of the ventricular septum (intact or VSD) and the presence of other associated malformations are described.

This unified classification includes all the previously described abnormalities in the positions of the great arteries and can be further expanded if new variations are revealed. This classification maintains uniformity of the subgroups and preserves the basic principles of classification that Kuhne, Edwards and Burchell, and Keith, Rowe, and Vlad devised.

History

Symptoms of tricuspid atresia manifest early in life. Nearly one half of patients have symptoms on first day of life, and 80% are symptomatic by the first month of life. The clinical features largely depend on the magnitude of pulmonary blood flow. The two known presentations are decreased pulmonary blood flow and increased pulmonary blood flow:

- Cyanosis occurs in the first few days of life in infants with pulmonary oligemia.
- The lower the pulmonary flow, the earlier the infant becomes cyanotic.
- Hyperpnea and acidosis are also present if the pulmonary blood flow is markedly decreased.
- Most infants have the type Ib defect. If pulmonary atresia is present (subgroup a), early cyanosis appears as the ductus begins to close.
- Hypercyanotic episodes are not common in the neonate but can be present later in infancy.
- Patients with pulmonary plethora present with symptoms of dyspnea, fatigue, difficulty feeding, and perspiration, which are suggestive of congestive heart failure.
- Cyanosis is minimal if present.
- Other presenting symptoms include failure to thrive and recurrent respiratory tract infection.
- Most symptoms develop within several weeks of life, although patients occasionally present in the first week of life.
- Most patients have type IIc (i.e. transposition without pulmonary stenosis, but with ventricular septal defect [VSD]; some have type Ic (i.e. normally related great arteries and no pulmonary stenosis and a VSD).
- Coarctation of the aorta may be present in patients with a type II defect; in these patients, the onset of cardiac failure is early.
- Patients with rare, late-appearing cyanosis may present with exercise intolerance and a cardiac murmur.

Physical Examination

The physical findings for pulmonary oligemia and pulmonary plethora are discussed separately.

- Patients with pulmonary oligemia may have central cyanosis, tachypnea or hyperpnea, normal pulses, and prominent a waves in the jugular venous pulse (in the presence of clinically significant interatrial obstruction). No hepatomegaly is observed.
- A quiet precordium and no thrills are found on palpation.
- Upon auscultation, the second heart sound is single, and a holosystolic type of murmur at the lower sternal border, suggestive of VSD, is heard. Diastolic murmurs are usually not heard. In patients with pulmonary atresia, the holosystolic murmur is not present, and a continuous murmur of patent ductus arteriosus is occasionally heard.
- Clinical signs of heart failure are not observed.
- Patients with pulmonary plethora usually have tachypnea, tachycardia, minimal cyanosis (if any), decreased femoral pulse (if aortic coarctation is present), prominent neck venous pulsations, and hepatomegaly.
- Prominent a waves in the jugular veins and/or presystolic hepatic pulsations may be observed if interatrial obstruction is severe.
- Increased and hyperdynamic precordial impulses may be palpated. The second heart sound may be single or split, and a third heart sound at the apex may be heard.
- Additional auscultatory findings include holosystolic murmur of VSD at the left lower sternal border and mid-diastolic rumble at the apex.
- Clinical signs of congestive heart failure are usually evident.
- Problems related to chronic cyanosis, such as clubbing, polycythemia, relative anemia, stroke, brain abscess, coagulation abnormalities and hyperuricemia,[52] are similar to those observed in other cyanotic congenital heart defects.
- The risk for bacterial endocarditis is similar to that for other cyanotic cardiac defects.
- Atrial arrhythmias (flutter and/or fibrillation) may be observed in older children and adolescents with long-standing cyanosis, a systemic-to-pulmonary artery shunt, or left ventricular volume overloading or in those who previously underwent a classic Fontan operation.
- Tricuspid atresia may be associated with cat's-eye syndrome, Christmas disease, and asplenia syndrome.
- Extracardiac anomalies often involving GI or musculoskeletal systems may be present in as many as 20% of patients.

Laboratory Studies

The following studies are indicated in tricuspid atresia:

- Pulse oximetry and arterial blood gas determination
- Estimation of systemic arterial oxygen saturation by means of pulse oximetry, which is readily available in most outpatient and inpatient settings, is a useful adjunct in the clinical assessment. Arterial oxygen saturations less than 70–80% are of concern and lead one to expedite intervention to relieve pulmonary oligemia.
- ABG determinations provide accurate information regarding PO_2, the partial pressure of carbon dioxide (PCO_2), and base deficit. This test provides data about blood oxygen values (i.e., PO_2), ventilatory status (i.e., PCO_2), and metabolic status (i.e., base deficit). However, this is an invasive test and is not reliable if the child is agitated or crying during blood sampling. If an arterial line is already in place, blood gas analysis is valuable.

Hemoglobin and hematocrit measurements: Whereas the oxygen saturation measurement gives the value at one point in time, the level of hemoglobin indicates the degree and duration of hypoxemia. A rapid increase in hemoglobin suggests severe or long-standing hypoxemia.

Routinely obtain RBC indices to ensure that no relative iron-deficiency anemia is present. Microcytosis and hypochromia suggest iron deficiency and warrant treatment with iron supplements.

IMAGING STUDIES

Chest Radiography (Figs 14.237)

Chest radiography is a useful adjunct in the evaluation of any congenital heart defect, including tricuspid atresia. The radiographic features are also useful in evaluating the pulmonary blood flow and categorizing them into pulmonary oligemia and pulmonary plethora groups.

If the pulmonary blood flow is decreased, the heart is normal in size or only mildly enlarged. If pulmonary blood flow is excessive, moderate-to-severe cardiac enlargement is observed. The cardiac silhouette has been characterized in the literature as egg, bell, square, or boot shaped (coeur en sabot). However, in the experience of the author and of others, no consistent pattern is diagnostic of tricuspid atresia. Concavity in the region of the pulmonary artery segment is observed in patients with pulmonary oligemia and a small pulmonary artery or pulmonary atresia. The right atrial border may be prominent, especially if interatrial obstruction is present. With a restrictive atrial septal defect (ASD), the right atrial shadow may be prominent.

A right aortic arch, which is frequently observed in patients with tetralogy of Fallot (25%) or truncus arteriosus (40%), is present in only 8% of patients with tricuspid atresia. In rare types of tricuspid atresia (type III, subtypes 1 and 5), an unusual contour of the left border of the heart secondary to leftward and anterior displacement of the ascending aorta is present.

Chest radiography is also useful in depicting the position of the heart; visceroatrial situs; and abnormalities of lungs, diaphragm, or vertebrae.

The most useful aspect of chest radiography is that it allows for the differentiation of decreased and increased pulmonary vascular markings. This distinction is often all that is necessary to establish a diagnosis after history taking, physical examination, and electrocardiography are performed.

Echocardiography

2D echocardiography reveals a small right ventricle and an enlarged right atrium, left atrium, and left ventricle. In the most common muscular type of tricuspid atresia, a dense band of echoes is observed where the tricuspid valve is usually located (*see* the image below). The anterior leaflet of the detectable atrioventricular valve is attached to the left side of the interatrial septum. These echocardiographic features are best demonstrated in the apical and subcostal 4-chamber views. The size of the left atrium and the size and function of the left ventricle can be assessed with M-mode echocardiography. Repeated measurements during follow-up are useful in evaluating left ventricular function (Figs 14.238 and 14.239).

Subcostal four chamber two dimensional echocardiographic view of a neonate with tricuspid atresia shows an enlarged left ventricle (LV), a small right ventricle (RV), and a dense band of echoes where the tricuspid valve echo should be. Atrial and ventricular septal defects and the mitral valve are also seen. Note the attachment of the anterior leaflet of the detectable atrioventricular valve to the left side of the interatrial septum. Reprinted from Rao, Fetal and Neonatal Cardiology, 1990, with permission from Elsevier Science. Demonstration of ASDs and ventricular septal defects (VSDs) by means of 2D echocardiography is essential, and shunting across the defects can be documented by using Doppler echocardiography. Semilunar valves can be similarly identified as pulmonic or aortic by following the great vessels until the bifurcation of the pulmonary artery or the arch of the aorta is seen. Coarctation of the aorta, which is more frequent in patients

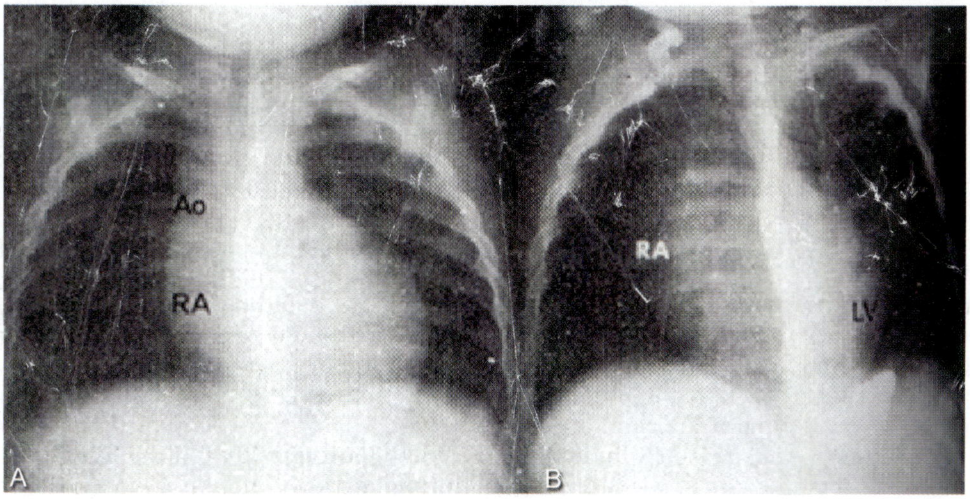

Fig. 14.237: *Chest X-ray in a patient with tricuspid atresia demonstrating the following features: (A) Reduced pulmonary blood flow, prominent aortic root (AO) and right atrium (RA) (B) The left anterior oblique projection on the right side shows distinctive humped appearance of the anterior cardiac silhouette due to right atrial (RA) enlargement in the absence of a right ventricle. The left ventricle (LV) is enlarged. A right aortic arch may be observed in some cases*

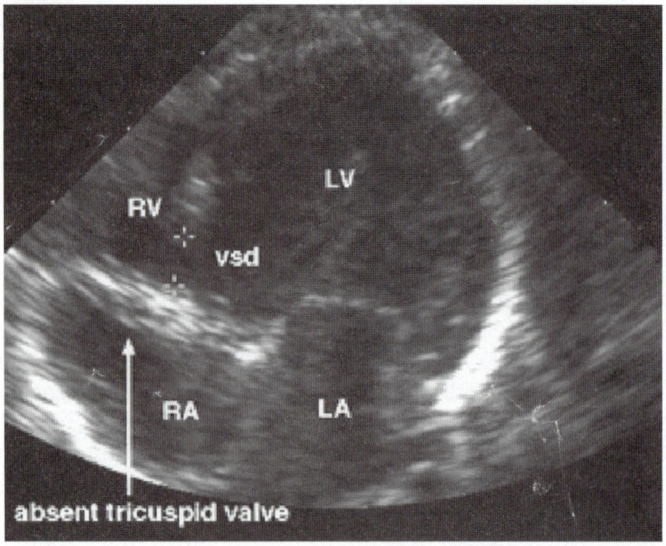

Fig. 14.238: *TTE four chamber view shows abscence of tricuspid valve (arrow), a VSD (astrex) and a small RV in a newborn with tricuspid atresia*

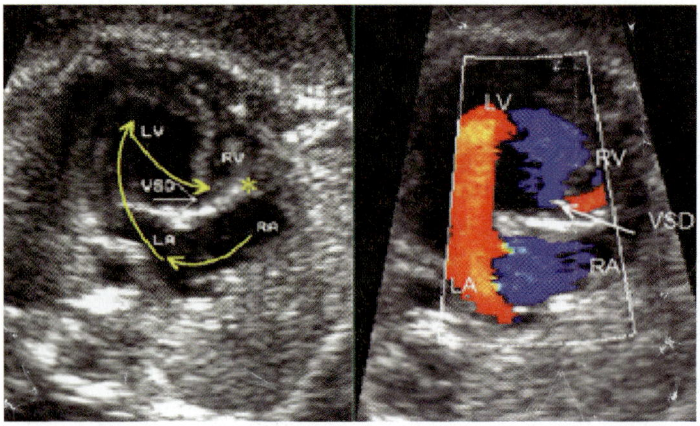

Fig. 14.239: *Tricuspid atresia (*) and ventricular septal defect (VSD). Arrows show the direction of flow; due to the atresia of the tricuspid valve, blood entering the right atrium cannot enter directly into the right ventricle and it flows to the left atrium, left ventricle and across the VSD to the hypoplastic right ventricle (right)*

with tricuspid atresia type II, may be demonstrated in the suprasternal notch view.

Doppler echocardiography is useful for demonstrating the degree of obstruction across the ASD or VSD, for detecting stenosis of the right ventricular outflow tract and pulmonary valve, and for showing aortic coarctation.

Contrast echocardiography with an injection of agitated sodium chloride solution or other contrast material demonstrates sequential opacification of the right atrium, left atrium, left ventricle, and, subsequently, the right ventricle although the study is not required for diagnosis.

Radionuclide Scanning

Radioisotopic scanning studies may be used to identify and quantitate a right-to-left shunt, to demonstrate cardiac

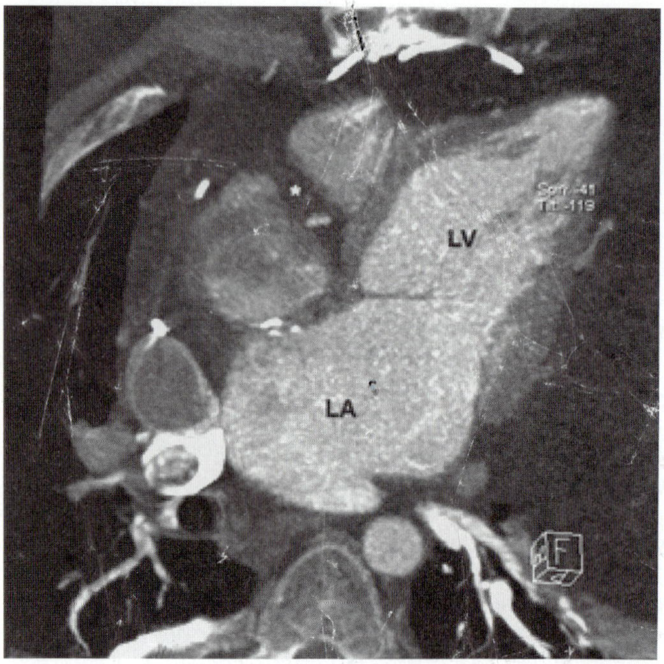

Fig. 14.240: *An oblique axial view shows the anatomy of an adolescent with tricuspid atresia who has undergone palliative repair with an extracardiac Fontan. Note the floor of the right atrium is completely separate from the ventricular mass (asterisk). LA indicates left atrium; LV, left ventricle*

anatomy by means of nuclear angiography, and to quantitate relative perfusions to both lungs.

However, pulse oximetry, blood gas analysis, and echocardiography are preferred because they are more simple and less cumbersome than nuclear scanning for demonstrating a right-to-left shunt and cardiac anatomy.

Quantitative pulmonary perfusion scans are useful if stenosis of a branch pulmonary artery is suspected, especially after a Fontan operation (Fig. 14.240).

Electrocardiography: In an infant with cyanosis, electrocardiographic findings are virtually diagnostic of tricuspid atresia. Electrocardiography reveals right atrial hypertrophy, an abnormal and superiorly oriented major QRS vector, the so-called left axis deviation in the frontal plane, left ventricular hypertrophy, and decreased right ventricular forces (Fig. 14.241).

Right atrial hypertrophy, manifested by tall and peaked P waves (> 2.5 mm) in lead II and right chest leads may be present in 75% of patients with tricuspid atresia. In the so-called P-tricuspidale with a double peak, spike and dome configuration may be present. The initial tall peak is related to right atrial depolarization, and the second small peak is presumed to be secondary to left atrial depolarization. Regardless of the P wave configuration, its duration is prolonged, which may be caused by right atrial enlargement.

An abnormal superior vector (left axis deviation 0° to –90° in the frontal plane) is present in most patients with tricuspid atresia (*see* the image below). This abnormal vector is present in 80% of patients with tricuspid atresia

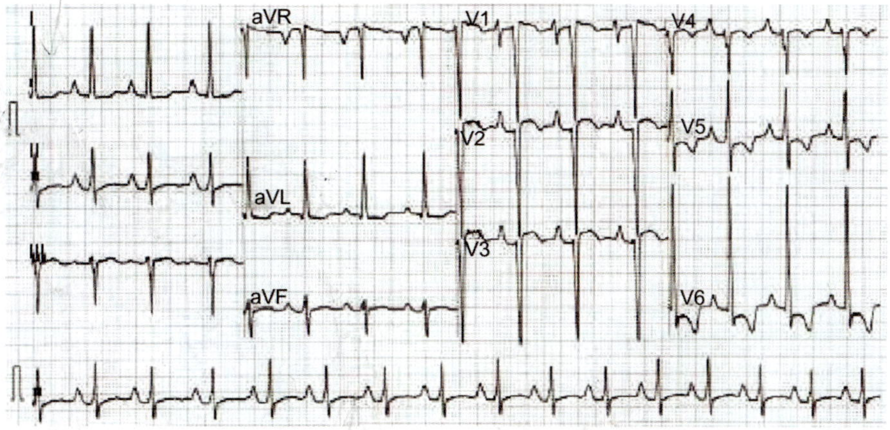

Fig. 14.241: *Electrocardiography in tricuspid atresia reveals right atrial hypertrophy, an abnormal and superiorly oriented major QRS vector, the so-called left axis deviation in the frontal plane, left ventricular hypertrophy, and decreased right ventricular forces. Right atrial hypertrophy, manifested by tall and peaked P waves (P-tricuspidale) in lead II and right chest leads may be present in 75% of patients with tricuspid atresia. In the so-called P-tricuspidale with a double peak, spike and dome configuration may be present*

type I (normally related great arteries) but only 50% of patients with tricuspid atresia type II or III. Normal (0° to +90°) or right axis deviation (+90° to ± 180°) is present in a minority of patients, mainly those with tricuspid atresia type II or III.

Numerous mechanisms have been postulated to explain the abnormal superior vector, including destructive lesions on the left anterior bundle, fibrosis of the left-bundle branch, a long right-bundle branch along with an early origin of left-bundle branch, a small right ventricle, and a large left ventricle. Data from ventricular activation studies suggest that the superior vector is likely due to the interaction of several factors. The most crucial findings are right-to-left phase asynchrony of ventricular activation, right-to-left ventricular disproportion, and asymmetric distribution of the left ventricular mass favoring the superior wall.

Regardless of the abnormality in the frontal-plane vector, left ventricular hypertrophy is observed in most patients. This usually manifests as increased amplitude of S waves in leads V1 and V2 and R waves in V5 and V6. ST–T-wave changes indicative of left ventricular strain are present in 50% of patients. The pattern of left ventricular hypertrophy is related to the anatomic nature of the lesion and left ventricular overload, and it is secondary to a lack of opposition to the left ventricular electrical forces by the small right ventricle. Biventricular hypertrophy is occasionally observed; when such a pattern is present, it is usually tricuspid atresia type II or III with a good-sized right ventricle. Decreased R waves in leads V1 and V2 and S waves in leads V5 and V6 are secondary to a hypoplastic right ventricle.

Procedures

Cardiac Catheterization

Indications: Perform cardiac catheterization if noninvasive evaluation provides insufficient data to address the management issues. Catheterization may be indicated before planned surgical correction is performed to provide the surgeon with important anatomic detail. Accurate data about the pulmonary-artery anatomy, size, and pressures and about left ventricular end-diastolic pressure (LVEDP), size, and function are needed before a Fontan procedure can be performed (Figs 14.242 and 14.243).

Perform a methodic evaluation of Choussat criteria [i.e., normal vena caval drainage, normal right atrial volume, mean pulmonary artery pressure < 15 mm Hg, pulmonary vascular resistance (PVR) < 4 U/m^2, pulmonary artery–to–aortic root diameter ratio >0.75, normal left ventricular

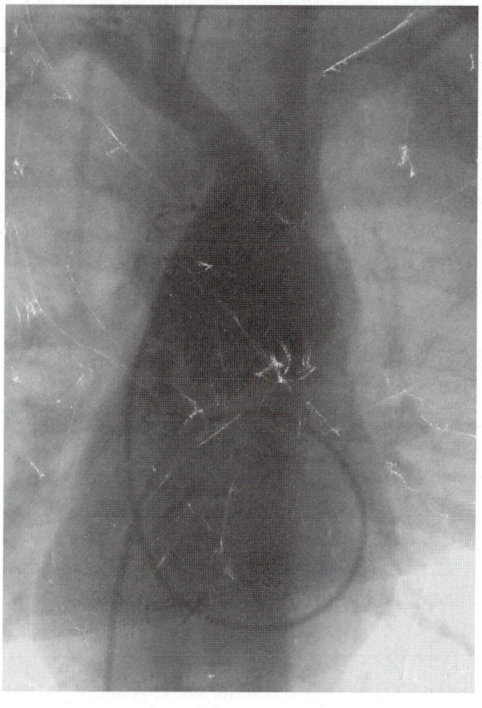

Fig. 14.242: *Aortogram in tricuspid atresia and discordant ventriculoarterial connections after Norwood stage II procedure. Note distorted arch (PA tube orientation)*

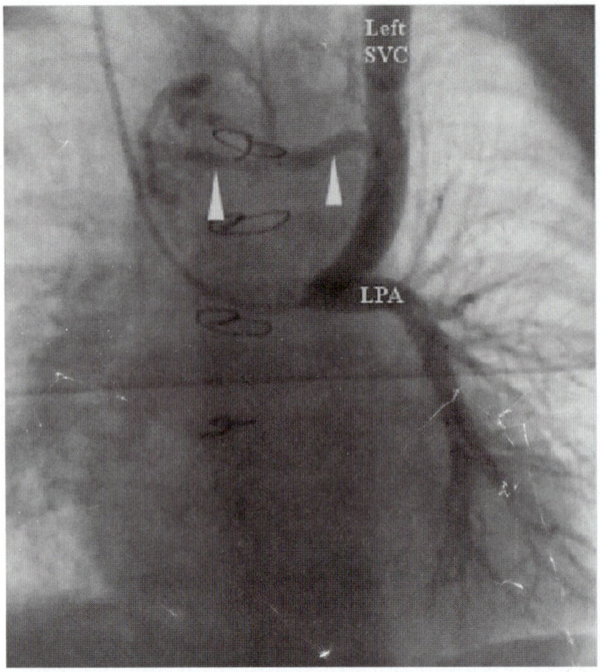

Fig. 14.243: *Bilateral bidirectional Glenns (bilateral bidirectional cavopulmonary shunts). Arrow indicates veno-venous malformation*

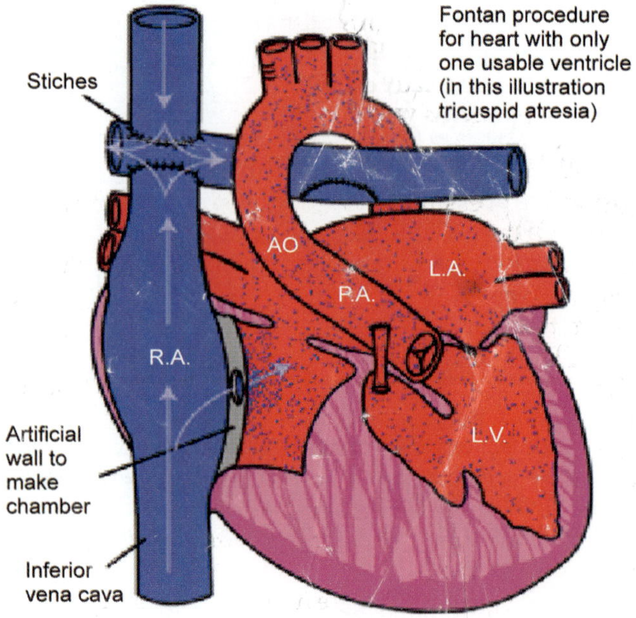

Fig. 14.244: *Diagram describing Fontan circulation in tricuspid atresia*

function (ejection fraction >0.60), no mitral insufficiency, and undistorted pulmonary arteries]. However, exceptions to most of these criteria have been made. Introduction of the bidirectional Glenn procedure before the Fontan procedure has changed the rigid adherence to some of these criteria (Fig. 14.244).

Also, cardiac catheterization is indicated as an integral part of transcatheter therapeutic intervention, which may be necessary in some patients.

Catheter insertion: The percutaneous femoral venous route is preferred because it facilitates access into the left side of the heart. The percutaneous jugular venous route may be used when a bidirectional Glenn procedure was already performed or if infrahepatic interruption of the inferior vena cava with azygos or hemiazygos continuation is present. Percutaneous femoral arterial access is also used to define aortic coarctation and subaortic stenosis, to visualize collateral vessels to the lungs, or to aid in performing balloon coarctation angioplasty or coil occlusion of aortopulmonary collateral vessels.

The course of the catheter in the right side of the heart is abnormal. The right ventricle cannot be directly entered from the right atrium because of the atretic tricuspid valve. Instead, the catheter can be easily advanced into the left atrium through the interatrial defect, especially when femoral venous access is used. From the left atrium, the left ventricle can be entered across the mitral valve. In neonates, further catheter manipulation to enter a great vessel or the right ventricle is usually unnecessary; hemodynamic and angiographic information is usually adequate. Cardiac catheterization in neonates is rarely needed for diagnostic purposes. With the availability of balloon-tipped catheters and various catheters and guide wires, the right ventricle may be catheterized through the VSD. In patients with normally related great vessels (type I), the aorta and pulmonary artery may also be catheterized from the left and right ventricles, respectively. In patients with transposed great vessels (type II), the aorta and pulmonary artery may also be catheterized from the right and left ventricles, respectively.

The course of a retrograde arterial catheter is normal in patients with tricuspid atresia type I, whereas it traverses anteriorly as it enters the right ventricle from the aorta in patients with tricuspid atresia type II. In patients with corrected transposition (type III, subtypes 1 and 5), the catheter courses anteriorly and to the left.

Oxygen Saturations

Oxygen saturation in the vena cavae is decreased. The extent of this reduction is proportional to the systemic arterial desaturation and the degree of congestive heart failure. A step up in right atrial oxygen saturation is not ordinarily observed because of the obligatory right-to-left shunt. In some patients, a step up in oxygen saturation may be observed and explained on the basis of instantaneous pressure differences between the atria. The oxygen saturation in the pulmonary veins is usually normal, with a step down in saturations in the left atrium secondary to obligatory right-to-left shunt at the atrial level. Oxygen saturation in the left ventricle is also decreased and may reflect a better admixture of the pulmonary venous and systemic venous returns. The left atrial, left ventricular, right ventricular, pulmonary arterial, and aortic saturations are similar, reflecting complete admixture of systemic and pulmonary venous returns in the left atrium. The aortic oxygen saturation is always lower than normal and proportional to the Qp:Qs. The oxygen saturations are generally lower in patients with a type I defect than those in patients with a type II defect. This difference appears to be related to the relatively high prevalence of pulmonary oligemia in patients with a type I defect.

Intracardiac Pressures

Right atrial pressure is normal or slightly elevated and depends on the LVEDP. The a waves are usually prominent. Interatrial obstruction results in giant a waves in the right atrial pressure recording. A mean atrial pressure difference of more than 5 mmHg indicates interatrial obstruction. If the LVEDP is markedly elevated, the interatrial pressure difference may be eliminated, even in the presence of considerable interatrial obstruction.

The left ventricular end-diastolic and left atrial pressures are usually normal. They increase with increasing Qp:Qs and diminishing left ventricular function. Prominent left atrial v waves may be observed with a high Qp:Qs and mitral insufficiency.

The peak systolic pressure in the left ventricle is usually normal but may be elevated in subaortic obstruction and aortic coarctation. Aortic systolic pressure is normal unless aortic coarctation is present. Aortic diastolic pressure may be decreased because of diastolic runoff secondary to a patent ductus arteriosus or a surgical aortopulmonary shunt. In patients with type II (transposition) defects, perform careful pressure pullback recordings across the aortic valve and across the VSD. A pressure gradient between the ventricles (across the VSD) indicates subaortic obstruction due to spontaneous shrinkage of the VSD.

In patients with normally related great arteries (type I), the systolic pressure in the right ventricle is proportional to the size of the VSD; the larger the VSD, the higher the pressure. Of course, pulmonary stenosis influences the right ventricular pressure. In patients with transposition of the great arteries (type II), the right ventricular pressure is at a systemic level.

Pulmonary artery pressure is usually normal in patients with tricuspid atresia type I; however, in those with tricuspid atresia type I with a large VSD, it may be elevated depending on the size of the VSD. In tricuspid atresia type II, the pulmonary pressures are high unless a clinically significant subvalvular or valvular pulmonary stenosis is present.

Because of the importance of pulmonary artery pressure in the overall treatment of patients with tricuspid atresia, every attempt should be made to measure pulmonary artery pressure. Pulmonary venous wedge pressure should be measured to estimate pulmonary artery pressure if all methods of catheterizing the pulmonary artery fail.

Calculation of systemic and pulmonary blood flows and shunts.

Calculation of systemic and pulmonary blood flows and shunts are made using the Fick principle, either by measuring oxygen consumption (preferred) or by assuming it from the tables of normal values. Detailed methods and formulas for calculation may be found in tricuspid atresia. The Qp:Qs and PVR are particularly critical calculations.

The reliability of Qp:Qs is not adversely influenced by not measuring the oxygen consumption.

A PVR of more than 4 U/m^2 is a contraindication for Fontan operation.

Mair, et al suggested that the preoperative catheterization index (PI) is useful for predicting poor results after Fontan surgery. The index is calculated as PVR + [LVEDP/(PI + SI)], where LVEDP is in millimeters of mercury, PI = the pulmonary flow index in liters per minute per meters squared, PVR is in units per meters squared, and SI is the systemic flow index in liters per minute per meters squared. An index of less than 4 U/m^2 is associated with an overall lower mortality rate. Although it has some limitations, this index reflects the importance of PVR and left ventricular function in the preoperative selection of patients for Fontan surgery.

Cineangiography: Lack of direct anatomic continuity between the right atrium and right ventricle is the hallmark angiographic finding of tricuspid atresia. After tricuspid atresia is demonstrated, the ventricular anatomy, type and size of VSDs, ventriculoarterial connections, pulmonary artery anatomy, sources of pulmonary blood flow, and associated defects should be defined (Figs 14.245 and 14.246).

Right Atrial Angiography

Selective cineangiography from the superior vena cava or right atrium demonstrates successive opacification of the left atrium and left ventricle without opacification of the right ventricle. The negative shadow between the right atrium and the left ventricle, called the right ventricular window, corresponds to the unfilled right ventricle. These features are best illustrated on a posteroanterior view. Although initially thought to be pathognomonic for tricuspid atresia, these signs may be present in a number of other conditions, including pulmonary atresia or severe

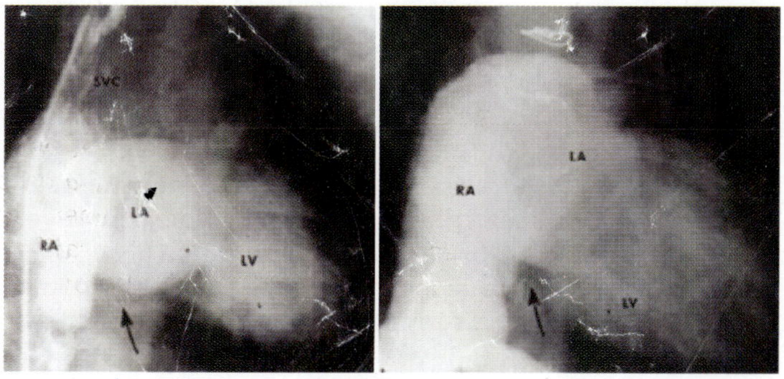

Fig. 14.245: *Selected cineangiographic frames from superior vena caval (SVC) and right atrial (RA) frontal angiography in two patients. Note sequential opacification of the left atrium (LA) and left ventricle (LV) without opacification of the right ventricle. The RA on the right, the LA superiorly, and the LV on the left form a nonopacified right ventricular window (arrow). This is a classic appearance of the muscular variety of tricuspid atresia. (From Rao PS. Tricuspid atresia: anatomy, imaging, and natural history. In: Brawnwald E, Freedom RM, eds. Atlas of Heart Disease: Congenital Heart Disease. Vol 12. Philadelphia, PA: Current Medicine; 1997:14.1 with permission.)*

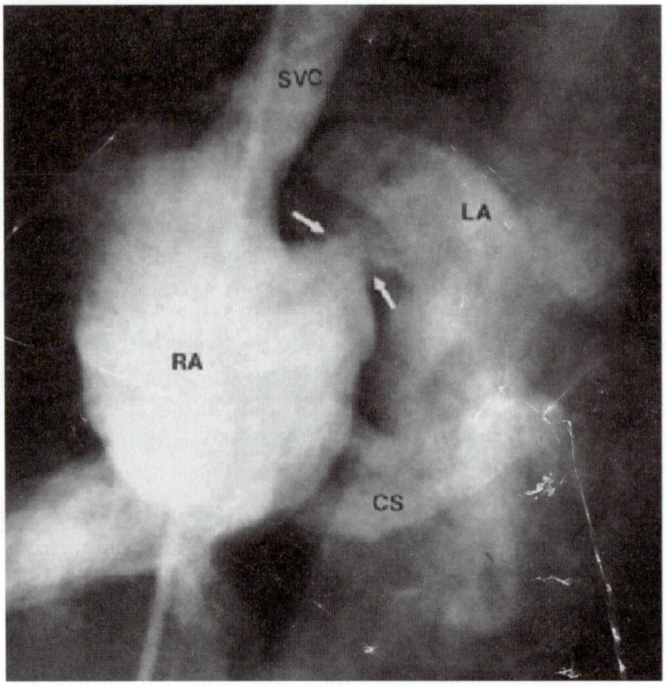

Fig. 14.246: *Selective superior vena caval (SVC) injection for a fourr-chamber projection (hepatoclavicular) shows tricuspid atresia and filling of the left atrium (LA) through a somewhat restrictive atrial septal defect (arrows). Note the retrograde filling of the coronary sinus (CS). RA = right atrium. (From Schwartz DC, Rao PS. Angiography in tricuspid atresia. In: Rao PS, ed. Tricuspid Atresia. 2nd ed. Mt Kisco, NY: Futura Publishing Co; 1992:223, with permission.)*

pulmonary stenosis with intact ventricular septum, tetralogy of Fallot with ASD (pentalogy), total anomalous venous return to coronary sinus, and cor triatriatum dexter.

The size and location of the interatrial communication is optimally visualized on hepatoclavicular or lateral views. Opacification of the left atrium through an obstructed patent foramen ovale may produce the onionskin or waterfall appearance.

During right atrial angiography, contrast material refluxes normally into the vena cavae and hepatic veins and does not indicate interatrial obstruction. However, dense opacification of the coronary sinus (Fig. 14.46) suggests interatrial obstruction. Aneurysmal formation of the atrial septum may also suggest a restrictive atrial defect.

Right atrial angiography is useful in demonstrating the size and position of the right atrial appendage and morphologic variants of the atretic tricuspid valve.

Left Ventricular Angiography

Selective left ventricular angiography demonstrates a finely trabeculated, morphologically left ventricle, which is typical in most cases of tricuspid atresia. The left ventricle is slightly enlarged, and its size is proportional to pulmonary blood flow. The size and position of the VSDs, the presence of mitral insufficiency, and the origin and relative positions of the great vessels should also be evaluated.

Left ventriculography is initially performed in posteroanterior and lateral views. Left anterior oblique, hepatoclavicular, or long axial oblique views may also be used, depending on the structure that needs greater definition. Particular attention is needed to define the size of the VSD in type II (transposition) because of the potential for development of subaortic obstruction.

Right ventriculography: In cases of type II (transposition), right ventricular cineangiography can be accomplished by passing a catheter antegrade from the left ventricle or retrograde from the aorta. Right ventriculography may improve assessment of the size of the right ventricle compared with left ventriculography. This information was of considerable importance in the past, when incorporation of the right ventricle into the Fontan circuit and its potential for growth were serious considerations. However, this issue is not longer as important since the advent of total cavopulmonary connection.

Aortography: Aortography should be performed in patients with tricuspid atresia type II because of a high incidence of aortic arch anomalies, particularly aortic coarctation. An anterograde or retrograde approach via the femoral artery may be used. In addition, aortography is used to define sources of pulmonary blood flow and the origin and distribution of the coronary arteries.

Medical Management

Medical management during the process of identification, transfer to a pediatric cardiology center, initial workup, and cardiac catheterization (if needed) and during and after palliative surgery or procedures includes maintenance of a neutral thermal environment, normal acid-base balance, normoglycemia, and normocalcemia with appropriate monitoring and correction, if necessary. Unless associated pulmonary parenchymal pathology is present, the fraction of inspired oxygen (FIO_2) administered should be no more than 0.4. Neonates who have low arterial PO_2 and O_2 saturation and ductal-dependent pulmonary blood flow should receive an intravenous infusion of PGE1 0.03–0.1 mcg/kg/min to open the ductus arteriosus or to maintain its patency. This is followed by an aortopulmonary shunt

In the infant who presents with signs of congestive heart failure (type Ic or IIc), anticongestive therapy with digoxin, diuretics, and afterload reduction should be promptly given.

In patients with severe aortic coarctation, which is particularly observed in those with type II disease, ductal dilation with an infusion of PGE1 may improve systemic perfusion. Surgical repair of the coarctation should follow. Some cardiologists use balloon angioplasty to relieve the aortic obstruction.

If interatrial obstruction is present, it should be relieved by means of balloon atrial septostomy. On occasion, blade or surgical septostomy is necessary. For patients presenting after infancy, the treatment approach is similar to that described above, except that PGE1 is not effective in opening the ductus.

Medical Management after Palliation

The management issues in tricuspid atresia are similar to those in other cyanotic congenital heart defects and are discussed in tricuspid atresia.

Hemoglobin should be periodically measured, and anemia and polycythemia, when present, should be treated.

Patients should receive antibiotic prophylaxis before undergoing any bacteremia-producing surgery or procedures.

The risks of stroke and brain abscess are similar to those in other cyanotic heart defects. When such a problem develops, appropriate neurologic or neurosurgical consultation and treatment is indicated.

Routine well-child care, including immunizations, by the primary care physician is suggested. Administration of polyvalent pneumococcal vaccine and influenza vaccine and immunization against respiratory syncytial virus should be considered. Issues such as physical and emotional development, genetic counseling, vocational training and rehabilitation, pregnancy, and contraception are addressed similarly to those in other cyanotic heart defects.

The development of hyperuricemia, gout, and uric acid nephropathy in adolescents and adults with long-standing cyanosis and polycythemia is similar to that in other cyanotic heart defects. Timely palliative and corrective surgery may prevent such complications.

Catheter Intervention

In the neonate, obstruction at the level of the atrial septum may be treated with conventional Rashkind balloon atrial septostomy. In infants and children, the interatrial septum may be too thick to be torn with balloon septostomy; therefore, Park blade septostomy should precede the Rashkind procedure. In most patients, obstruction to pulmonary blood flow is at the ventricular septal defect (VSD) level or in the subpulmonary region. In some patients, the obstruction is at the pulmonary valve. In such patients, balloon pulmonary valvuloplasty may be useful in improving pulmonary blood flow and oxygen saturation.

If progressive cyanosis develops after a previous Blalock-Taussig shunt and if the hypoxemia is due to a stenotic shunt, balloon dilatation may be used to improve oxygen saturation. However, if the patient is of sufficient size and age to undergo a bidirectional Glenn procedure, this procedure should be performed instead of balloon angioplasty of a narrowed Blalock-Taussig shunt.

If severe aortic coarctation is present, particularly in patients with tricuspid atresia type II, balloon angioplasty may be useful in relieving aortic obstruction and may help achieve better control of congestive heart failure.

If clinically significant branch pulmonary artery stenosis is present before bidirectional Glenn or Fontan conversion or after a Fontan procedure is performed, balloon angioplasty or placement of intravascular stents is recommended.

Development of aortopulmonary collateral vessels has been increasingly observed in recent studies. Before the final Fontan conversion, occlusion of these vessels in the catheterization laboratory, usually by means of coil embolization, is recommended to reduce left ventricular volume overloading and, probably, the duration of chest-tube drainage. After a Fontan procedure, some patients may have recurrent pleural effusion, liver dysfunction, plastic bronchitis or protein-losing enteropathy. In these patients, rule out obstructive lesions in the Fontan circuit, then puncture of the atrial septum by using a Brockenbrough technique followed by static balloon atrial septal dilatation or stent implantation may be beneficial. Patients who undergo a fenestrated Fontan operation or who have a residual atrial defect despite correction may have clinically significant right-to-left shunting that causes severe hypoxemia. These residual atrial defects may be closed by using transcatheter techniques Some patients may develop systemic venous-to-pulmonary venous collateral vessels following Fontan operation, causing arterial desaturation. These vessels should be defined and closed by coils, plugs, or devices, depending on the size, location, and accessibility.

Surgical Intervention

Surgical management may be broadly grouped into palliative and corrective therapies.

Palliative surgery: Palliative therapy depends on the hemodynamic disturbance the associated cardiac anomalies produce and may be discussed in terms of decreased pulmonary flow, increased pulmonary flow, or intracardiac obstruction.

Decreased Pulmonary Blood Flow

Pulmonary blood flow may be increased by surgical creation of an aortopulmonary shunt. After Blalock and Taussig (1945) initially described subclavian artery-to-ipsilateral pulmonary artery anastomosis in 1945, other procedures have been described, including Potts shunt (descending aorta-to-left pulmonary artery anastomosis), Waterston-Cooley shunt (ascending aorta–to–right pulmonary artery anastomosis), central aortopulmonary fenestration or expanded polytetrafluoroethylene shunt, modified Blalock-Taussig shunt (Gore-Tex interposition graft between the subclavian artery and the ipsilateral pulmonary artery), Glenn shunt (superior vena cava-to-right pulmonary artery anastomosis, end-to-end), formalin infiltration of the wall of ductus arteriosus, enlargement of the VSDs, and stent implantation into the ductus (Fig. 14.247).

Modified Blalock-Taussig shunt with an interposition Gore-Tex tube graft between the subclavian artery and the ipsilateral pulmonary artery, which de Leval et al described, has stood the test of time and is currently the procedure of choice for palliation in pulmonary oligemia.

Because the site of obstruction to pulmonary flow in most patients with tricuspid atresia is at the VSD, resection of the septal muscle to enlarge the VSD, which Annechino et al advocate, appears to be a logical choice because it addresses rather than bypasses the site of obstruction. However, this resection is an open-heart surgical procedure

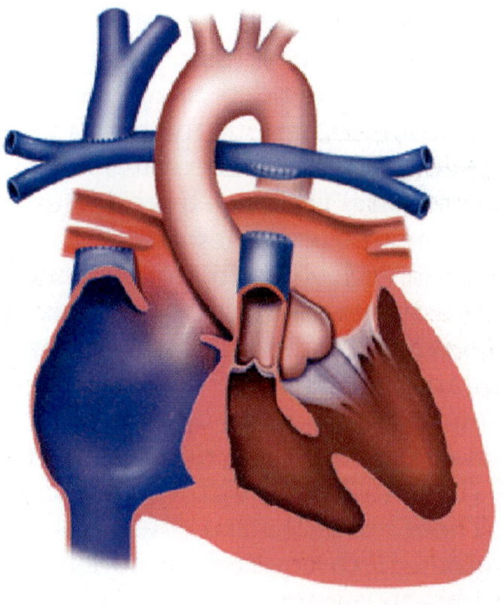

Fig. 14.247: *Diagram shows bidirectional Glenn shunt and atrial septectomy in setting of tricuspid atresia and VSD*

and more cumbersome than the modified Blalock-Taussig shunt in augmenting the pulmonary blood flow; it has not been routinely used. In the rare patient with predominant obstruction at the pulmonary valve, balloon pulmonary valvuloplasty may be used to increase the pulmonary blood flow. Stenting the arterial duct is an attractive nonsurgical option; however, because of limited experience, it is not currently a first-line therapeutic option.

In summary, a number of palliative procedures are available to augment pulmonary blood flow, but the modified Blalock-Taussig shunt is the recommended procedure of choice in most, if not in all, patients with tricuspid atresia with pulmonary oligemia.

Increased Pulmonary Blood Flow

Patients with increased pulmonary blood flow are likely to have type Ic or type IIc defects without associated pulmonary stenosis. Congestive heart failure is likely to occur in these patients. In patients with tricuspid atresia type II (transposition of the great arteries), pulmonary artery banding should be performed after stabilization with anticongestive measures. Banding not only improves congestive heart failure but also helps achieve normal pulmonary artery pressure so that bidirectional Glenn and Fontan procedures can safely be performed later. If associated aortic coarctation is present, it must be relieved. Pulmonary artery banding stimulates more ventricular hypertrophy, which may further reduce the size of the VSD, thus increasing subaortic obstruction.

In patients with tricuspid atresia type I (normally related great arteries), aggressive anticongestive measures should promptly be undertaken. Because natural history studies suggest that the VSD spontaneously closes or becomes smaller with time and the patients with pulmonary plethora develop pulmonary oligemia, banding of the pulmonary artery is generally not recommended in this group of patients. However, if symptoms are not relieved after optimal anticongestive therapy and some delay, pulmonary-artery banding should be performed. Patients with no pulmonary-artery banding should receive careful follow-up and monitoring of pulmonary artery pressure.

Absorbable pulmonary artery bands have been used for palliation in such infants. By restricting the pulmonary blood flow, the absorbable polydioxanone band decreases pulmonary artery pressure and initially helps abate symptoms of heart failure. As the VSD spontaneously closes, the pulmonary artery band is resorbed and does not produce the severe pulmonary oligemia that might have been associated with a conventional nonabsorbable band. This is an ingenious approach although it is likely to be helpful in a limited number of patients.

Intracardiac obstruction which may occur at the level of patent foramen ovale and VSD.

Interatrial Obstruction

Because the entire systemic venous return must pass through the patent foramen ovale, it should be large enough to allow unimpeded egress of systemic venous blood. Because of the compliant right atrium and proximal systemic veins, evaluating interatrial obstruction is difficult. Clinical signs of systemic venous congestion and presystolic hepatic and jugular venous pulsations suggest obstructed atrial septum. A mean atrial pressure difference of more than 5 mmHg and prominent a waves in the right atrial pressure wave are generally considered diagnostic of clinically significant obstruction.

Balloon atrial septostomy usually promptly improves presystolic hepatic and jugular pulsations and decreases interatrial pressure difference. Blade atrial septostomy is occasionally necessary, especially in older infants and children. Surgical atrial septostomy is needed even less frequently. However, surgical septostomy to allow unrestricted flow across the atrial system may be performed concurrently with bidirectional Glenn procedure.

Interventricular Obstruction

Spontaneous closure of the VSD can occur, causing interventricular obstruction. Functional VSD closure in tricuspid atresia type I results in cyanotic spells, similar to those in tetralogy of Fallot Initial management is similar to that of tetralogy of Fallot and includes knee-chest positioning, humidified oxygenation, and the administration of morphine sulfate 0.1 mg/kg. If the patient's condition is unresponsive, beta-blockers (propranolol, esmolol) or intravenous pressors (methoxamine, phenylephrine) are administered to increase systolic blood pressure by 10–20%. Concurrent correction of anemia or metabolic acidosis should also be undertaken. If no improvement occurs, emergency surgical palliation with a Blalock-Taussig type of shunt may be necessary. If the infant's condition improves clinically, elective surgery, Blalock-Taussig shunting, or a bidirectional Glenn or Fontan procedure may be performed, depending on the patient's age and weight and the status of pulmonary arteries and left ventricle.

Partial or complete anatomic closure of the VSD can also occur in patients with type I, causing pulmonary oligemia. The management is as described in the decreased pulmonary blood flow section above.

In patients with tricuspid atresia type II, spontaneous closure of the VSD produces subaortic obstruction. This obstruction should be relieved or bypassed as soon as it is detected because it produces left ventricular hypertrophy, which, in turn, increases the risk at the time of Fontan operation. The VSD, right ventricle, and aortic valve may be bypassed with an anastomosis of the proximal stump of the divided pulmonary artery to the ascending aorta (Damus-Kaye-Stansel procedure) directly or by means of a prosthetic conduit at the time of bidirectional Glenn or Fontan conversion. Alternatively, the conal septal muscle may be resected to enlarge the VSD; this is a direct approach in relieving the subaortic obstruction. However, development of heart block, inadequate relief of obstruction, and spontaneous closure of the surgically enlarged or created VSD remain major concerns.

Corrective Surgery

After Fontan and Kreutzer's initial description of the physiologically corrective operation for tricuspid atresia, corrective surgery was widely adapted by most workers in the field. The concept was even extended to treat other cardiac defects with a functionally single ventricle. The originally described Fontan operation consisted of the following:

- Superior vena cava-to-right pulmonary artery end-to-end anastomosis (Glenn procedure).
- Anastomosis of the proximal end of the divided right pulmonary artery to the right atrium directly or by means of an aortic homograft.

Closure of the Atrial Septal Defect

Insertion of a pulmonary valve homograft into the inferior vena caval orifice. Ligation of the main pulmonary artery to completely bypass the right ventricle. Kreutzer performed anastomosis of the right atrial appendage and pulmonary artery directly or by using a pulmonary homograft and closed the ASD. A Glenn procedure was not performed, and a prosthetic valve was not inserted into the inferior vena cava.

Fontan's concept was to use the right atrium as a pumping chamber; therefore, he inserted a prosthetic valve into the inferior vena cava and right atrial–pulmonary artery junction. Kreutzer's view was that the right atrium may not function as a pump and that the left ventricle functions as a suction pump in the system. Numerous modifications to the aforementioned procedures were made by these and other workers in the field, as Chopra and Rao reviewed in the American Heart Journal (1992). When their review was published, the four major types of Fontan-Kreutzer procedures used were right atrium-to-pulmonary artery anastomosis with or without a valved conduit and right atrium-to-right ventricular connection with and without a valved conduit.

On the basis of immediate-term and intermediate-term results, direct atriopulmonary anastomoses (i.e., without a conduit) appears to be the best procedure for patients with type I defects who have a small (<30% of normal) right ventricle and for all patients with type II (transposition) defects. Right atrial-to-right ventricular valved conduit (preferably homograft) anastomosis appears to be most suitable for patients with type I defects who have good-sized (>30% of normal) right ventricles and a trabecular component. During the time of Chopra and Rao's review, several other emerging concepts were noted, including bidirectional cavopulmonary anastomosis, fenestrated Fontan, and total cavopulmonary connection.

Bidirectional cavopulmonary anastomosis is a modified Glenn procedure in which the upper end of the divided superior vena cava is anastomosed end-to-side to the right pulmonary artery without disconnecting the latter from the main pulmonary artery. Thus, the superior vena cava blood is diverted into both the right and left pulmonary arteries.

Haller et al (1996) studied experimental bidirectional cavopulmonary connection in animal models, and Azzolina et al (1972) first described its clinical use. Others later applied this technique to palliate complex heart defects with decreased pulmonary blood flow. Hemodynamic advantages of the bidirectional Glenn procedure are improved effective pulmonary blood flow, decreased total pulmonary blood flow, and reduced left ventricular volume overloading. Preserved continuity of the pulmonary artery is another advantage and may help enable a low-risk Fontan procedure. When right and left superior vena cavae are present, bilateral bidirectional Glenn shunting should be performed, especially if the bridging innominate vein is absent or small.

Fenestrated Fontan operation is another procedure used in tricuspid atresia.

Many cardiologists and surgeons have modified the criteria Choussat et al outlined. Patients not meeting these criteria are at higher risk for a poor prognosis after a Fontan operation than patients who do. For the high-risk group, several workers have advanced the concept of leaving a small ASD open to facilitate decompression of the right atrium. Laks et al advocated closure of the atrial defect by constricting the preplaced suture in the postoperative period, whereas Bridges et al used a transcatheter closure technique later.

Clinically significant decreases in the postoperative pleural effusions and systemic venous congestion and higher cardiac output have been noted after a fenestrated Fontan procedure. The duration of hospitalization appears to be decreased. However, these beneficial effects are at the expense of mild arterial hypoxemia.

Although the fenestrated Fontan procedure was initially conceived for patients at high risk, it has since been used in patients with modest or even low risk. Although rare, reports of cerebrovascular or other systemic arterial embolic events occurring after a fenestrated Fontan operation tend to contraindicate the use of fenestrations in patients with low or usual risk. Some data indicate that routine fenestration is not necessary.

Total Cavopulmonary Connection

On the basis of their hemodynamic studies, de Leval et al (1988) concluded that the right atrium is not an efficient pump. Flow in nonvalved circulation generates turbulence with consequent net decrease in flow, and energy losses are significant in the nonpulsatile chambers, corners, and obstructions. Using these principles, they designed and performed total cavopulmonary diversion in which the upper end of the divided superior vena cava is anastomosed end-to-side to the top of the undivided right pulmonary artery (bidirectional Glenn), and the inferior vena caval blood is routed via an intra-atrial tunnel into the cardiac end of the superior vena cava, which, in turn, is connected end-to-side to the undersurface of the right pulmonary artery.

Technical simplicity, maintenance of low right atrial and coronary sinus pressures, and reduction in right atrial thrombi are advantages of the procedure. Subsequent experimental work by Sharma et al indicated that complete or minimal offset between the orifices of the superior and inferior vena cavae into the right pulmonary artery decreases energy losses.

Although the total cavopulmonary connection was initially devised for patients with complex atrial anatomy and/or systemic venous anomalies, it has since been used extensively for all types of cardiac anatomy with one functioning ventricle and irrespective of venous anomalies.

Current Surgical Interventions

The patient's age, weight, and anatomic and physiologic status determine the types of surgery recommended. The overall objective is to achieve a total cavopulmonary connection.

In the neonates and young infants with pulmonary oligemia, classic or modified Blalock-Taussig shunting is undertaken to improve the pulmonary oligemia.

In patients aged 6 months to 1 year, Blalock-Taussig shunting and bidirectional Glenn procedure are the choices. The author prefers the bidirectional Glenn operation at this age. Some clinicians perform bidirectional Glenn procedures in patients as young as 3 months; however, the probability of failure is increased at this young age presumably because of pulmonary vascular reactivity.

For children aged 1–2 years, the bidirectional Glenn procedure is preferable.

For patients older than 2 years, total cavopulmonary connection may be performed, but most authorities suggest staging by using an initial bidirectional Glenn operation followed by Fontan conversion in 6–12 months.

At the time of bidirectional Glenn surgery, any narrowing of the pulmonary artery should be repaired. Issues related to subaortic obstruction and mitral valve regurgitation should also be addressed.

Before Fontan conversion, cardiac catheterization should be undertaken to ensure normal anatomy and pressure of the pulmonary artery as well as normal left ventricular end-diastolic pressure (LVEDP). At the same time, aortopulmonary collaterals should be evaluated by means of selective subclavian artery and descending thoracic aortic angiography. If collateral vessels are present, they should be occluded with coils. Some authors question routine use of pre-Fontan catheterization and suggest prospective evaluation of this issue.

At the time of Fontan conversion, most surgeons currently prefer extracardiac conduit diversion of inferior vena caval blood into the right pulmonary artery. Some workers prefer a lateral tunnel Fontan procedure. To address the growth issue related to extracardiac Fontan surgery, some surgeons use autologous or bovine pericardial roll grafts. In patients with associated transposition of the great arteries, early banding of the pulmonary artery, relief of aortic coarctation (if present), and bypassing (by means of a Damus-Kaye-Stansel procedure) or resecting the subaortic obstruction should be incorporated into the management plan.

Emerging Therapies

Two-stage cavopulmonary connection is currently recommended for achieving Fontan circulation. Konertz, et al proposed a staged surgical-catheter approach. They initially perform a modified hemi-Fontan that is later completed by transcatheter method. This approach reduces the total number of operations required.

The modified hemi-Fontan operation involves the usual bidirectional Glenn technique. The lower end of the divided superior vena cava is anastomosed to the undersurface of the right pulmonary artery. The superior vena cava is then banded around a 16-gauge catheter with 6-0 prolene suture slightly above the cavoatrial junction. A lateral tunnel with a Gore-Tex baffle is created to divert the inferior vena caval blood toward the superior vena cava. The baffle is then fenestrated with 3–5 holes 5 mm wide. Thus, the first stage achieves a physiologic bidirectional Glenn condition (Fig. 14.243).

At the time of the second stage, the transcatheter stage, the superior vena caval constriction is dilated with a balloon, and fenestrations are closed with devices or by placement of covered stent.

The original physicians and other workers have performed these procedures in a limited number of patients, and preliminary data suggest that the usual post-Fontan complications, such as pleural effusion and ascites, have not occurred with this approach.

HYPOPLASTIC LEFT HEART SYNDROME

Hypoplastic left heart syndrome is a complex and rare heart defect present at birth (congenital). In hypoplastic left heart syndrome, the left side of the heart is critically underdeveloped.

If your baby is born with hypoplastic left heart syndrome, the left side of the heart can't effectively pump blood to the body, so the right side of the heart must pump blood both to the lungs and to the rest of the body (Fig. 14.248).

Medication to prevent closure of the connection (ductus arteriosus) between the right and the left sides, followed by either surgery or a heart transplant, is necessary to treat hypoplastic left heart syndrome. With advances in care, the outlook for babies born with hypoplastic left heart syndrome is better now than in the past.

Symptoms

Babies born with hypoplastic left heart syndrome usually are seriously ill immediately after birth. Hypoplastic left heart syndrome symptoms include:

1. Grayish-blue skin color (cyanosis)
2. Rapid, difficult breathing
3. Poor feeding
4. Cold hands and feet
5. Being unusually drowsy or inactive.

In a baby with hypoplastic left heart syndrome, if the natural connections between the heart's left and right sides (foramen ovale and ductus arteriosus) are allowed to close, he or she may go into shock and may die. Signs of shock include:

1. Cool, clammy skin that may be pale or gray

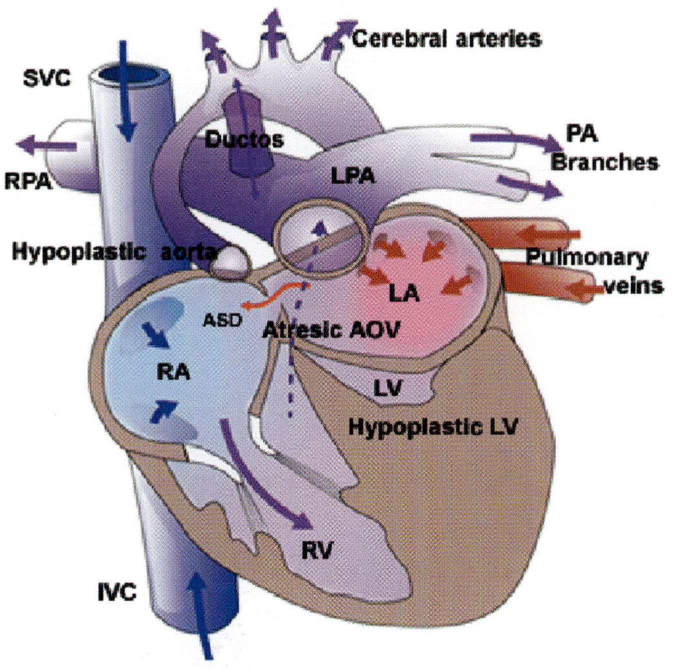

Fig. 14.248: *Illustration explaining disturbed anatomy and circulation in hypoplastic left heart syndrome*

2. A weak and rapid pulse
3. Abnormal breathing that may be either slow and shallow or very rapid
4. Dilated pupils
5. Lackluster eyes that seem to stare
6. A baby who is in shock may be conscious or unconscious.

When to See a Doctor

It's more likely that your baby would be diagnosed with hypoplastic left heart syndrome either before birth or soon after. However, you should seek medical help if you notice that your baby has the following symptoms:

1. Grayish-blue skin color
2. Rapid, difficult breathing
3. Poor feeding
4. Cold hands and feet
5. Being unusually drowsy or inactive.

If your baby has any of the following signs of shock, call at your local emergency number right away:

1. Cool, clammy skin that may be pale or gray
2. *A weak and rapid pulse:* Abnormal breathing that may be either slow and shallow or very rapid
3. Dilated pupils in the eyes
4. Lackluster eyes that seem to stare.

Etiology

Hypoplastic left heart syndrome occurs during fetal growth when the baby's heart is developing. The cause is unknown. However, if your family has one child with hypoplastic left heart syndrome, the risk of having another with the same condition is increased.

Pathophysiology

In hypoplastic left heart syndrome, the left side of the heart can't properly supply blood to the body because the lower left chamber (left ventricle) is too small or in some cases it may not even exist. In addition, the valves on the left side of the heart (aortic valve and mitral valve) don't work properly, and the main artery leaving the heart (aorta) is smaller than normal.

For the first several days of life, the right side of the heart can pump blood both to the lungs and to the rest of the body through a natural opening (foramen ovale) between the upper chambers of the heart (atria) or through a blood vessel that connects the pulmonary artery directly to the aorta (ductus arteriosus). When the foramen ovale and the ductus arteriosus are open, they are referred to as being "patent".

If the ductus arteriosus and the foramen ovale close—which they normally do after the first day or two of life—the right side of the heart has no way to pump blood out to the body. However, many infants with hypoplastic left heart syndrome also have another heart defect, a hole in the wall between the upper chambers of the heart (atrial septal defect), that allows the right side of the heart to continue pumping blood to the body even if the ductus arteriosus or foramen ovale closes.

Risk Factors

If you already have a child with hypoplastic left heart syndrome, you are at a higher risk of having another baby with this condition.

Beyond family history, there are no clear risk factors for hypoplastic left heart syndrome.

Complications

Without surgery, hypoplastic left heart syndrome is fatal, usually within the first week or two of life.

With treatment, many babies survive, although most will have complications later in life. Some of the complications include:

1. Tiring easily when participating in sports or other exercise
2. Heart rhythm abnormalities (arrhythmias)
3. Fluid buildup in the lungs, abdomen, legs and feet (edema)
4. Formation of blood clots that may lead to a pulmonary embolism or stroke
5. Developmental problems related to the brain and nervous system
6. Need for additional heart surgery or transplantation.

Tests and Diagnosis

Before Birth

It's possible for a baby to be diagnosed with hypoplastic left heart syndrome while it's still in the womb. Your doctor may be able to identify the condition on a routine ultrasound examination during the second trimester of pregnancy.

After Birth

After your baby is born, his or her doctor may suspect a heart defect, such as hypoplastic left heart syndrome if your baby has grayish-blue skin or has trouble breathing. Your baby's doctor may also suspect a heart defect if he or she hears a heart murmur—an abnormal whooshing sound caused by turbulent blood flow.

Doctors typically use an echocardiogram to diagnose hypoplastic left heart syndrome. This test uses high-pitched sound waves that bounce off your baby's heart to produce moving images that can be viewed on a video screen. In a baby with hypoplastic left heart syndrome, the echocardiogram reveals a smaller than normal left ventricle and aorta. Because this test can track blood flow, it also shows blood moving from the right ventricle into the aorta. In addition, an echocardiogram can identify associated heart defects, such as an atrial septal defect.

Laboratory Studies

The following studies are indicated in hypoplastic left heart syndrome (HLHS)

CBC Count

Measure hemoglobin levels, because severe neonatal anemia can cause high-output congestive heart failure (CHF) and cardiogenic shock. The hemoglobin level is usually normal in hypoplastic left heart syndrome.

Obtain a total WBC count with differential. Sepsis can cause symptoms of shock. The WBC count is typically normal.

Electrolytes

Electrolyte abnormalities may be present in infants with poor oral intake secondary to CHF. Use carbon dioxide and bicarbonate to assess acid-base status.

Electrolyte levels are usually normal. The carbon dioxide level may be low if a metabolic acidosis is present. The carbon dioxide level may be high if respiratory failure sets in.

BUN/Creatinine

Infants with critical illness and significantly reduced systemic perfusion may show evidence of renal failure.

The creatinine level may be transiently elevated.

Liver Function Tests

Infants with critical illness and significantly reduced systemic perfusion and CHF may show evidence of hepatocellular damage.

Aspartate aminotransferase (AST) and alanine aminotransferase (ALT) levels may be transiently elevated.

ABG and Lactic Acid

Assessing acid-base status is paramount, especially to rule out metabolic acidosis. Most infants have some evidence of metabolic acidosis, which should be immediately corrected. This is usually secondary to decreased systemic perfusion. Appropriate intervention to augment systemic flow should be promptly undertaken. Elevated levels of serum lactic acid generally precede a fall in pH, as acidosis develops. Assessment of PaO_2 and $PaCO_2$ is important for respiratory management and manipulation of pulmonary vascular resistance by mechanical ventilation and the addition of supplemental inhaled nitrogen. The PaO_2 is optimally 30–45 mmHg, and the $PaCO_2$ is ideally 45–50 mmHg.

Karyotype

Chromosomal analysis is indicated for infants with dysmorphic features. Nearly 25% of infants have chromosomal abnormalities.

Imaging Studies

Chest Radiography

Cardiomegaly and increased pulmonary vascular markings are typically present. Marked pulmonary edema may be noted in infants with obstructed pulmonary venous return, usually due to markedly restrictive patent foramen ovale (Figs 14.249).

Although the radiography findings are not specific for the condition, the presence of a large heart with increased pulmonary vascular markings in a mildly cyanotic neonate

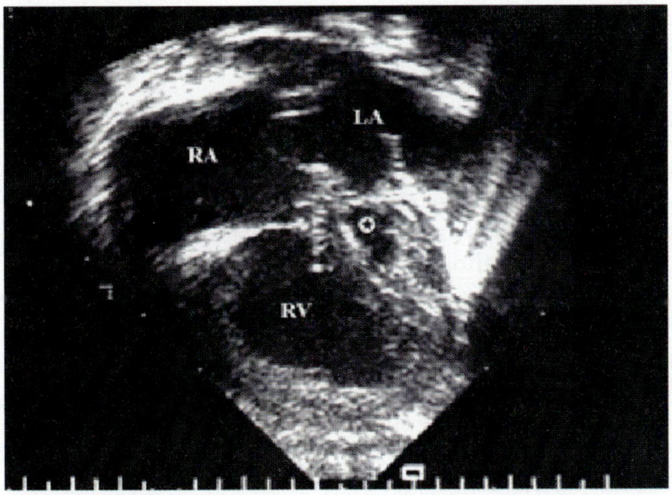

Fig. 14.249: *This echocardiographic still frame shows a four-chamber view of the heart in a patient with hypoplastic left heart syndrome (HLHS). A large right ventricle (RV) and hypoplastic left ventricle (star) are seen. RA, right atrium; LA, left atrium*

should always prompt inclusion of hypoplastic left heart syndrome in the differential diagnosis.

Electrocardiography (Fig. 14.250)

Electrocardiography typically reveals sinus tachycardia, right-axis deviation, right atrial enlargement, and right ventricular hypertrophy with a qR configuration in the right precordial leads. A paucity of left ventricular forces is noted in the left precordial leads. ST-T wave changes suggestive of myocardial ischemia may be present in some patients

Echocardiography

Echocardiography is the test of choice for diagnosing hypoplastic left heart syndrome. Two-dimensional imaging clearly shows the hypoplastic left ventricle and ascending aorta. The right atrium, tricuspid valve, right ventricle, and main pulmonary artery are larger than usual (Figs 14.249 to 14.254A-E).

Other structural abnormalities should be excluded.

Doppler and color Doppler imaging are also important.

Evaluate tricuspid regurgitation, which is a preoperative risk factor for the Norwood procedure (Fig. 14.255), and blood flow across the atrial septum. High-velocity Doppler jet across the atrial septum indicates restrictive interatrial communication. Observe retrograde blood flow from the ductus arteriosus into the transverse aortic arch and ascending aorta.

Evaluate the aortic arch and thoracic aorta for evidence of coarctation.

Two-dimensional and doppler echocardiographic features are sufficiently characteristic of hypoplastic left heart syndrome such that cardiac catheterization and angiography are no longer necessary for diagnosis of this anomaly. Variability of the chamber and vessel size is seen in hypoplastic left heart syndrome.

Ultrasonography of the Head and Abdomen

Ultrasonography of the head was thought to be necessary only if the infant has had a significantly long period in shock with potentially poor cerebral perfusion. However, at most institutions, routine head ultrasonography to exclude central nervous system abnormality and abdominal ultrasonography to evaluate kidneys are performed prior to the Norwood procedure or cardiac transplantation.

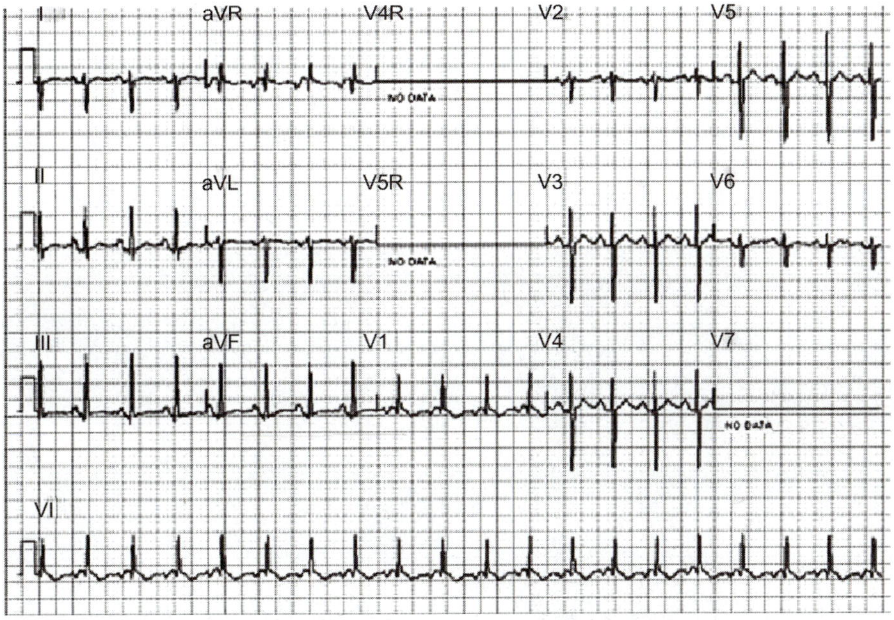

Fig. 14.250: *Hypoplastic left heart syndrome. Electrocardiogram obtained in an 18-day-old neonate, with Norwood stage 1 operation at 2 days of age. The tracing shows right atrial enlargement, right ventricular hypertrophy, and diminished lateral left ventricular forces*

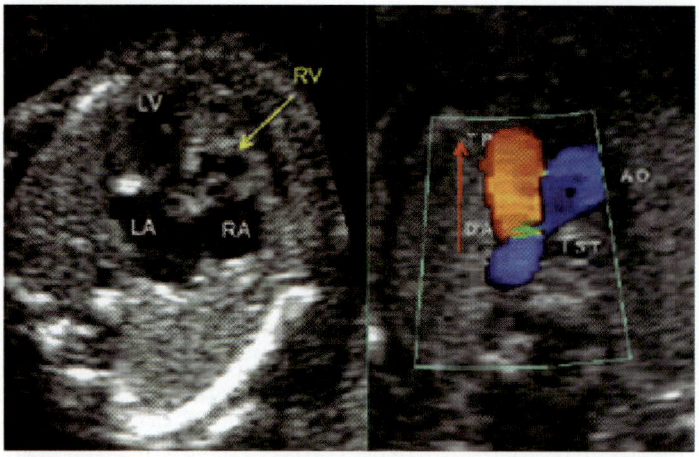

Fig. 14.251: *Hypoplastic right ventricle (arrow) in a fetus with pulmonary atresia and intact ventricular septum (a). Color doppler of the four chamber view with asymmetric flow between the left heart and right heart. Pulmonary valve atresia can be diagnosed using color Doppler by visualizing the great vessels - aorta (Ao) and pulmonary trunk (TP) - in the upper thorax and demonstrating the retrograde flow from the descending aorta across the ductus arteriosus toward the pulmonary valve*

A significant prevalence of abnormalities is observed using ultrasonography of the head and abdomen.

Procedures

Cardiac catheterization (pre–Norwood procedure): Routine diagnostic catheterization is not necessary because two-dimensional and Doppler echocardiography can provide the necessary anatomic and hemodynamic data. However, a focused catheterization may become necessary to resolve any echocardiographic discrepancies that may be deemed important in surgical management.

If catheterization is performed, the features reflect the pathophysiology described above.

Oxygen saturation data indicate moderate-to-severe systemic venous desaturation, with a step-up at the level of right atrium secondary to left to right shunt across the atrial septum. The oxygen saturations in the right ventricle, pulmonary artery and aorta are similar reflecting common mixing in the right atrium. Mild systemic arterial desaturation is usually present unless severe pulmonary edema is noted.

The right atrial pressure is mildly elevated, and the left atrial pressure is moderate to severely elevated, unless a large atrial septal defect is present. The right ventricular and pulmonary arterial systolic pressures are at systemic level. If the ductus arteriosus is constricted, these pressures are higher than those in the aorta.

Angiography

Although not necessary in all cases, reveals hypoplasia of the mitral valve, left ventricle and aorta. The ascending aorta is perfused in a retrograde fashion and serves as a common coronary artery, supplying both the right and left coronary arteries.

Perform interventional catheterization with blade/balloon atrial septostomy or static dilatation of the atrial septum to relieve pulmonary venous hypertension if blood flow from left atrium to right atrium is severely restricted at the atrial septum. Because of marked hypoplasia of the left atrium, conventional Rashkind balloon or Park blade atrial septostomy may not be possible. In such situations, static dilatation of the atrial septum may be performed. If the atrial septum is extremely thick with a markedly restrictive atrial septum, stent implantation to keep the atrial septum open may become necessary.

When hybrid procedures are contemplated, stenting of the ductus, atrial septum, or both may become necessary.

Cardiac catheterization [pre-bidirectional Glenn (stage II) procedure]

- Perform routine catheterization before the operation to obtain hemodynamic data and several important angiograms.
- Calculate pulmonary vascular resistance to ensure the patient's suitability for the stage II procedure.
- Perform angiography in the right ventricle to show ventricular function and tricuspid regurgitation.
- Perform angiography in the transverse aortic arch near the shunt to show pulmonary artery size and distribution and to rule out recurrent aortic coarctation or significant

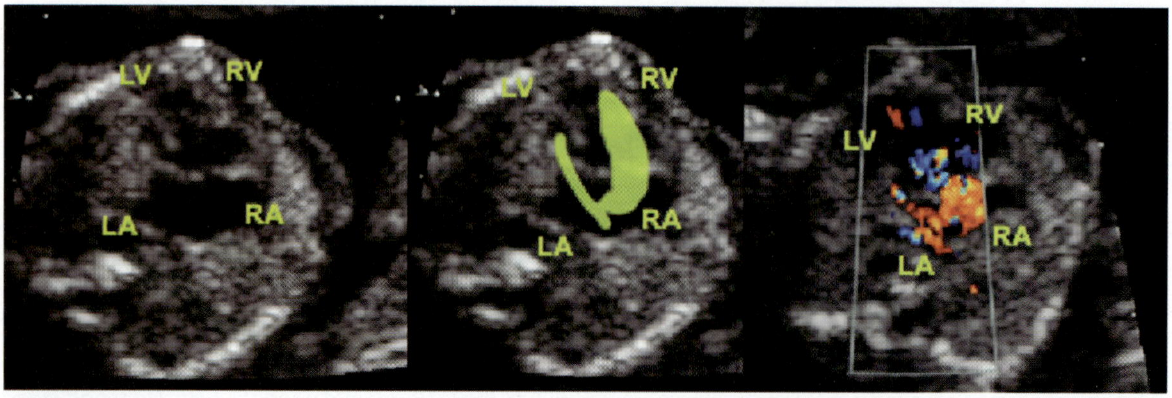

Fig. 14.252: *Hypoplastic left heart syndrome—the left ventricle diminutive, with color doppler there is an assimetric color perfusion of the chambers*

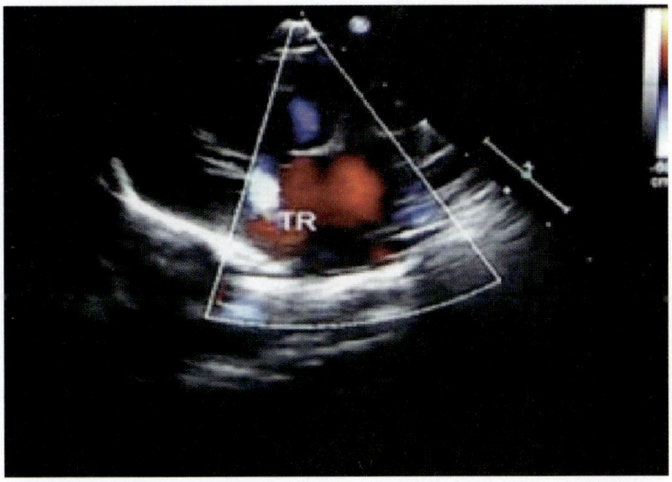

Fig. 14.253: *Color Doppler echo showing TR jet in hypoplastic left heart syndrome*

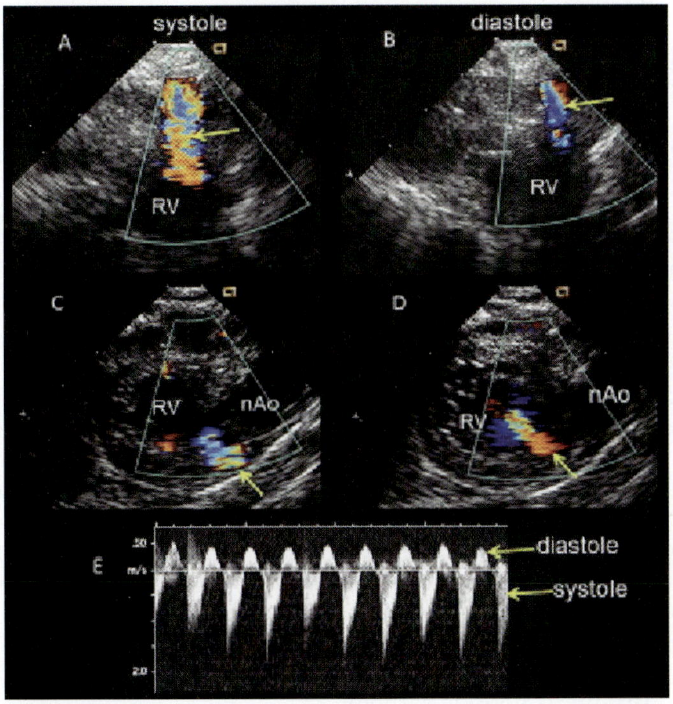

Figs 14.254A to E: *Color Doppler flow mapping and pulsed-wave Doppler blood flow analysis of the Sano right ventricle (RV)-to-pulmonary artery conduit obtained by TEE using the micro-TEE transducer (Micro-TEE) in a patient with hypoplastic left heart (HLH) after Norwood-Sano procedure. (A) Short-axis plane view color Doppler flow map of systolic antegrade flow within the Sano conduit. (B) Short-axis plane view color Doppler flow map of diastolic retrograde flow within the Sano conduit. (C) Sagittal plane view color Doppler flow map of systolic antegrade flow into the Sano conduit at its connection to the RV. (D) Sagittal plane view color Doppler flow map of diastolic retrograde flow into the RV from the Sano conduit at its connection to the RV. (E) Sagittal plane view pulsed-wave Doppler flow analysis at the connection of the Sano conduit to the RV, demonstrates systolic antegrade flow and diastolic retrograde flow. nAo, neo-aorta*

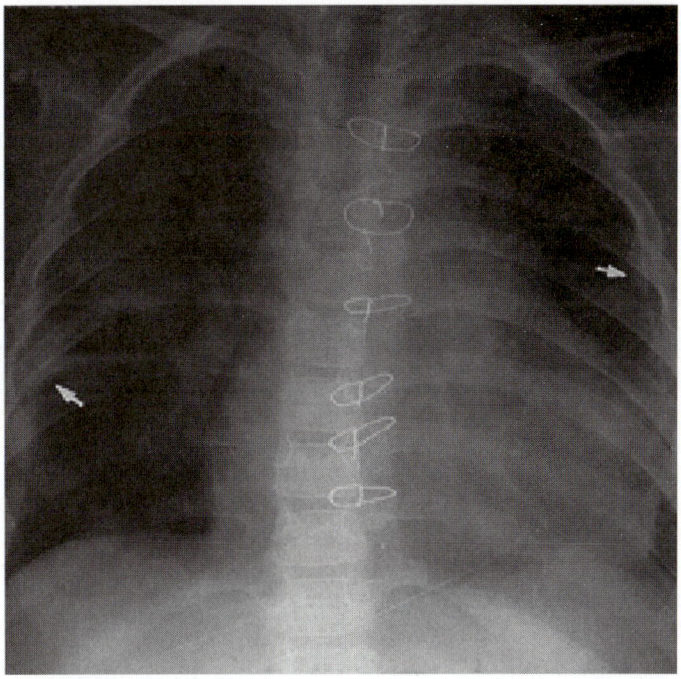

Fig. 14.255: *Chest radiograph obtained in a 3-year-old boy with HLHS who had undergone a modified Norwood procedure and creation of a bidirectional cavopulmonary shunt demonstrates a moderately enlarged, globular cardiac silhouette and slightly prominent pulmonary vasculature but no pulmonary edema*

aortopulmonary collateral vessels. If collateral vessels are found, they may be occluded with coils at the same catheterization.

Pre-Fontan (Stage III) Procedure

- Routine catheterization before completing the operation is generally recommended.
- Measure pulmonary artery pressure and calculate pulmonary vascular resistance and perform right ventricular angiography.
- Delineate pulmonary artery anatomy by performing angiography at the superior vena cava–pulmonary artery anastomosis via an internal jugular approach.
- Recurrent coarctation of the aorta and significant collateral vessels are excluded again.
- Descending aortography and selective right and left subclavian artery angiography to identify any collateral vessels to lungs is recommended.
- Postcatheterization complications include hemorrhage, vascular disruption after balloon dilation, pain, nausea and vomiting, and arterial or venous obstruction from thrombosis or spasm but are rare.

Catheter Intervention

In the neonate, obstruction at the level of the patent foramen ovale (atrial septum) may be treated with conventional Rashkind balloon atrial septostomy. However, because the left atrium is small, Rashkind septostomy may not be feasible. In addition, the septum may be too thick to be torn by balloon septostomy; therefore, Park blade septostomy may be necessary and should precede the Rashkind procedure. However, hypoplastic left atrium may preclude blade septostomy. Static dilatation of the atrial septum with a balloon angioplasty catheter may be used and may not only relieve the obstruction but also keep some restriction, such that no rapid fall in the pulmonary vascular resistance occurs. In some patients, the atrial septum may be intact or have a tight patent foramen ovale that may not even allow passage of a catheter. In such situations, puncture of the atrial septum by a Brockenbrough technique or radiofrequency perforation of the atrial septum followed by static balloon atrial septal dilatation or, preferably, stent implantation may become necessary. If progressive cyanosis develops after a previous Blalock-Taussig shunt, and if the hypoxemia is due to a stenotic shunt, balloon dilatation may be used to improve oxygen saturation. However, if the patient is of sufficient size and age to undergo a bidirectional Glenn procedure, this procedure should be performed instead of balloon angioplasty of a narrowed Blalock-Taussig shunt.

If severe aortic coarctation is present, particularly after Norwood procedure, balloon angioplasty may be useful in relieving aortic obstruction and may help to achieve reduce right ventricular afterload.

If significant branch pulmonary artery stenosis is present before a bidirectional Glenn or Fontan conversion or after a Fontan procedure, balloon angioplasty or placement of intravascular stents is recommended.

Development of aortopulmonary collateral vessels has been increasingly observed in recent studies. Before the final Fontan conversion, occlusion of these vessels in the catheterization laboratory, usually by means of coil embolization is recommended to reduce left ventricular volume overloading and, probably, the duration of chest tube drainage following surgery.

Following completion of Fontan procedure, some patients may develop recurrent pleural effusion, liver dysfunction, plastic bronchitis or protein-losing enteropathy. In these patients, following exclusion of obstructive lesion in the Fontan circuit, puncture of the atrial septum by a Brockenbrough technique followed by static balloon atrial septal dilatation or stent implantation may be beneficial.

Patients who have undergone a fenestrated Fontan operation or have a residual atrial defect, despite correction, may have significant right-to-left shunting causing severe hypoxemia. These residual atrial defects may be closed using transcatheter techniques.

Medical Care

Prenatal diagnosis of hypoplastic left heart syndrome (HLHS) by fetal echocardiography is possible. When the HLHS is identified, it is advisable to have the baby deliver at an institution where tertiary care (Fig. 14.256) including neonatal cardiac surgery, is performed routinely. There was some suggestion in the past that elective cesarean delivery may provide better outcomes. A recent study examining

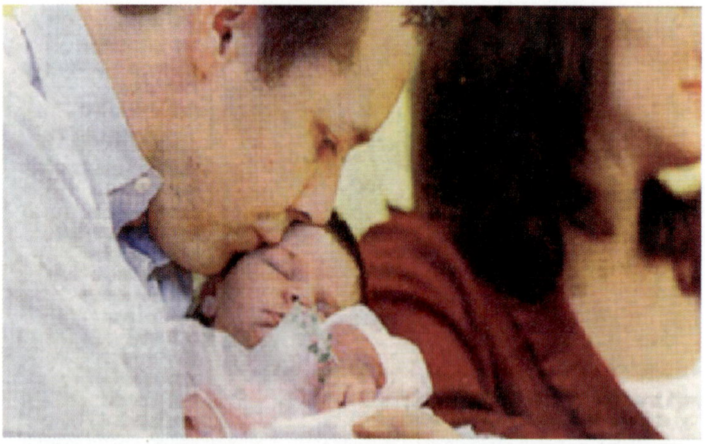

Fig. 14.256: *Photograph of a newborn baby, Grace out of US national couple mother Angela VanDer-worken of Virginia who became Worlds first baby to receive intrauterine stent for the treatment of HLHS when this baby was 7 months old in the womb of the mother. This surgery was performed by the team of experts under chief surgeon Dr James Lock at children and women hospital Boston*

this issue found that there was no hemodynamic advantage for elective cesarean delivery section over vaginal delivery.

Successful preoperative management depends on providing adequate systemic blood flow while limiting pulmonary overcirculation.

Open the Ductus Arteriosus

Blood flow to the systemic circulation (coronary arteries, brain, liver, kidneys) depends on flow through the ductus arteriosus. If a diagnosis of hypoplastic left heart syndrome is suspected, start prostaglandin E1 infusion immediately to establish ductal patency and ensure adequate systemic perfusion.

If the diagnosis is made prenatally or when the infant is relatively asymptomatic, a smaller dose of prostaglandin E1 may be sufficient to keep the ductus arteriosus patent while limiting its side effects.

A larger dose of prostaglandin E1 is often required to reopen the ductus arteriosus if an infant has cardiovascular collapse and shock due to ductal closure.

Ideally, prostaglandin E1 is administered centrally via an umbilical venous catheter.

Correct Metabolic Acidosis

- Metabolic acidosis indicates inadequate cardiac output to meet the metabolic demands of the body. Acidosis adversely affects the myocardium.
- Correction of metabolic acidosis with sodium bicarbonate infusion is essential in early management. This therapy is futile if the ductus arteriosus remains constricted.
- Manipulate pulmonary vascular resistance. The pulmonary vascular resistance of a newborn is slightly less than the systemic vascular resistance and begins to fall soon after birth. In the patient with hypoplastic left heart syndrome, decreased pulmonary vascular resistance causes increased pulmonary blood flow and

an undesirable obligatory decrease in systemic blood flow. Increased alveolar oxygen decreases pulmonary vascular resistance, leading to increased pulmonary blood flow. Therefore, oxygen should not be administered unless pulmonary parenchymal disease or pulmonary edema, causing severe hypoxemia, is present. The oxygen should be discontinued once these abnormalities resolve. Consequently, most infants should remain in room air with acceptable oxygen saturation (pulse oximeter) in the low 70s. An exceptional circumstance is the infant with severe hypoxemia caused by pulmonary venous hypertension. Achieving a slightly higher $PaCO_2$, in the range of 45–50 mmHg, can increase pulmonary vascular resistance. This can be accomplished by intubation, sedation, mechanical hypoventilation, or the addition of nitrogen or carbon dioxide (FIO_2 of 15–19%) to the infant's inspired gas via the endotracheal tube or hood. Intubation is not preferred. However, intubation and ventilation along with measures to balance pulmonary and systemic flows may improve tricuspid regurgitation.

Serial blood gas analysis is necessary. Initially, an umbilical arterial catheter is useful to obtain frequent blood samples. Although administration of subambient inspired oxygen to balance systemic and pulmonary blood flows is an attractive concept and should be applied during stabilization of the neonate, it should not be pursued for long periods because severe pulmonary hypertension may complicate the postoperative course. However, this does not seem to adversely affect the pulmonary vasculature on long-term follow-up.

Inotropes

Inotropic support is indicated only in severely ill neonates with concurrent sepsis or profound cardiogenic shock and acidosis.

The administration of inotropes can adversely affect the balance between pulmonary and systemic vascular resistance. If needed, wean from inotropic support as soon as the infant is clinically stable.

Diuretics

Consider diuretics to manage pulmonary overcirculation before surgery. Agents commonly used to include furosemide and spironolactone.

Antibiotics

Antibiotics are indicated if the infant is at risk for antepartum infection. Discontinue antibiotics after obtaining negative blood cultures.

Surgical Care

Sinha and associates, Caylor and colleagues and Dotty and associates proposed various palliative operations; however, survival was not feasible until Norwood and associates demonstrated that a multistage operative approach could be used to treat hypoplastic left heart syndrome. After Fontan and Kreutzer's initial description of the physiologically corrective operation for tricuspid atresia, corrective surgery was widely adapted to treat this entity. The concept was extended to treat other cardiac defects with a functionally single ventricle including hypoplastic left heart syndrome.

The originally described Fontan operation consisted of the following:

Superior Vena Cava-to-right Pulmonary Artery End-to-end Anastomosis (Glenn Procedure)

Anastomosis of the proximal end of the divided right pulmonary artery to the right atrium directly or by means of an aortic homograft.

Closure of the Atrial Septal Defect

Insertion of a pulmonary valve homograft into the inferior vena caval orifice, ligation of the main pulmonary artery, thus completely bypassing the right ventricle (Fig. 14.257).

Kreutzer performed anastomosis of the right atrial appendage and pulmonary artery directly or via a pulmonary homograft and closed the atrial septal defect. A Glenn procedure was not performed, and a prosthetic valve was not inserted into the inferior vena cava. Fontan's concept was to use the right atrium as a pumping chamber; therefore, he inserted prosthetic valves into the inferior vena cava and right atrial pulmonary artery junction. Kreutzer's view was that the right atrium may not function as a pump and that the left ventricle functions as a suction pump in the system. Numerous modifications to the

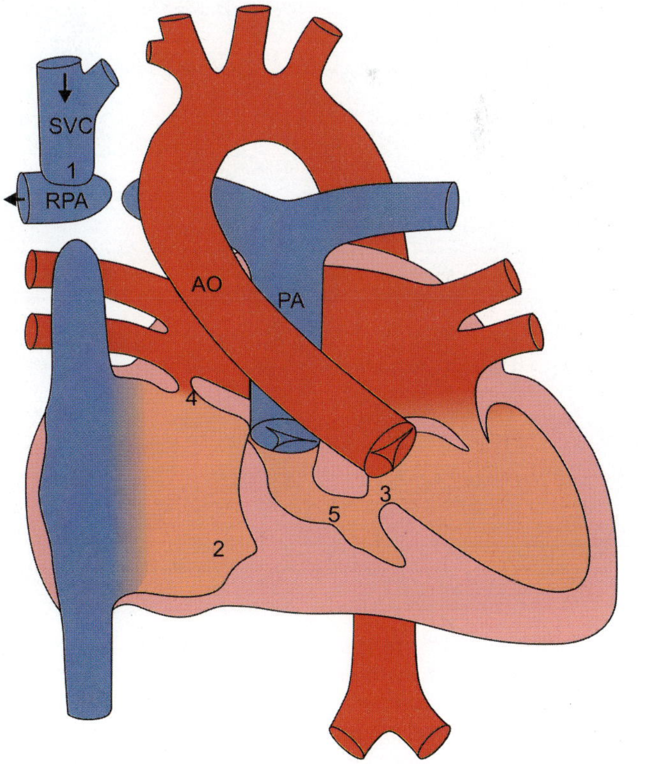

Fig. 14.257: *Diagram showing classic Glenn anastomosis (not a bidirectional Glenn) postoperative superior vena cava to right pulmonary artery (Glenn anastomosis)*

aforementioned procedures were undertaken by these and other workers in the field (*see* Tricuspid Atresia). Currently, staged total cavopulmonary connection is the procedure of choice.

The goal of surgical reconstruction of hypoplastic left heart syndrome is to eventually separate the pulmonary and systemic circulations by achieving a Fontan circulation. The right ventricle remains the systemic ventricle while blood passively flows to the lungs. This ultimate reconstruction is accomplished in the following three stages:

Norwood Procedure (Stage I) (Fig. 14.258)

This procedure is usually performed during the first weeks of life after the infant has been stabilized in the neonatal intensive care unit (ICU). The goals of the procedure are:

1. To establish reliable systemic circulation without the ductus arteriosus
2. To provide enough pulmonary blood flow for adequate oxygenation while simultaneously protecting the pulmonary vascular bed in preparation for stages II and III.

The Norwood procedure includes:

1. Performing an atrial septectomy to provide unrestricted blood flow across the atrial septum
2. Ligating the ductus arteriosus
3. Creating an anastomosis between the main pulmonary artery and the aorta to provide systemic blood flow

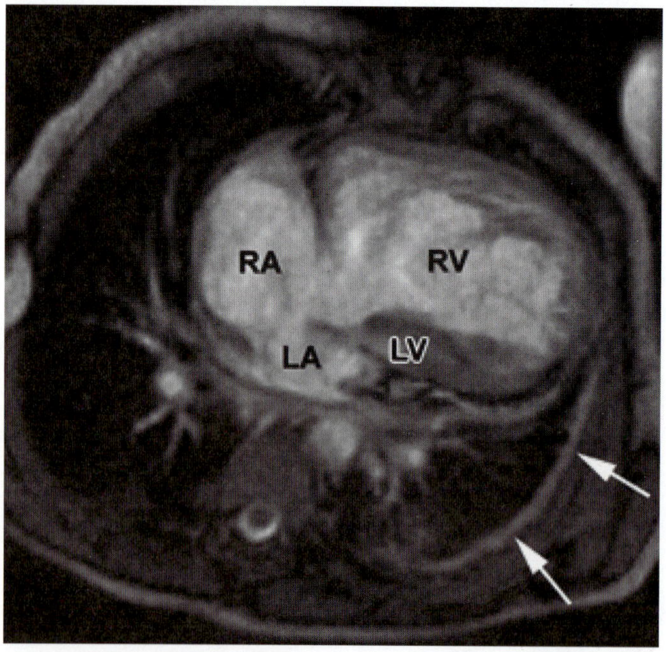

Fig. 14.258: *Aortic stenosis in an 11-month-old boy with hypoplastic left heart syndrome. The patient had undergone a Norwood stage I procedure and bidirectional cavopulmonary anastomosis (Norwood stage II procedure). Horizontal long-axis cine image shows a hypoplastic left ventricle (LV) and thickening of the left pleura (arrows), findings that are indicative of a transpleural collateral blood supply to the left lung. LA, left atrium; RA, right atrium; RV, right ventricle.*

4. Eliminating coarctation of the aorta and
5. Placing an aorta-to-pulmonary artery shunt (usually a modified Blalock-Taussig shunt) to provide pulmonary circulation.

More recently, connecting a Gore-Tex graft from the right ventricular outflow tract to the pulmonary artery (Sano operation) has been advocated instead of conventional modified Blalock-Taussig (BT) shunt; some surgeons have shown better results with the Sano procedure than with the conventional Norwood approach. However, prospective randomized studies from a single institution, as well as multiple institutions, compared the techniques and have not found significant advantage of Sano over Blalock-Taussig shunt or vice versa.

Upon hospital discharge, most infants remain on digoxin to augment cardiac function, on diuretics to help manage right ventricular volume overload, and on aspirin to prevent thrombosis of the shunt. If tricuspid regurgitation is present, use afterload reduction with captopril. Oxygen saturation is typically 70–80% in room air.

Bidirectional Glenn Procedure (Stage II)

This procedure is performed approximately 6 months after the Norwood procedure. Before surgery, perform a cardiac catheterization to assess right ventricular function, pulmonary artery anatomy, and pulmonary vascular resistance. If results are favorable, schedule elective surgery. The bidirectional Glenn procedure includes creating an anastomosis between the superior vena cava and the right pulmonary artery, end-to-side so that venous return from the upper body can flow directly into both lungs. In the hemi-Fontan, the superior vena cava-right atrial junction is closed with a patch that is removed during the next stage. Blood from the inferior vena cava continues to drain into the right atrium. The aorta-to-pulmonary artery shunt that was placed at stage I is ligated.

When both right and left superior vena cavae are present, bilateral bidirectional Glenn shunts should be performed, especially if the bridging innominate vein is absent or small. At the time of bidirectional Glenn, repair of pulmonary artery narrowing, if present, should be undertaken. Issues related to tricuspid valve regurgitation, restrictive atrial septum and any other abnormalities should also be addressed.

At discharge, infants usually remain on digoxin, diuretics, aspirin, and captopril for the reasons mentioned above.

Fontan Procedure (Stage III)

The Fontan procedure is performed approximately 12 months after the bidirectional Glenn procedure. Again, catheterization is necessary to ensure that the child is a candidate for surgery (Fig. 14.259).

Completion of the Fontan procedure includes directing blood flow from the inferior vena cava to the pulmonary arteries either via a lateral tunnel procedure or via an extracardiac conduit. Extracardiac conduit diversion of inferior vena caval blood into the right pulmonary artery

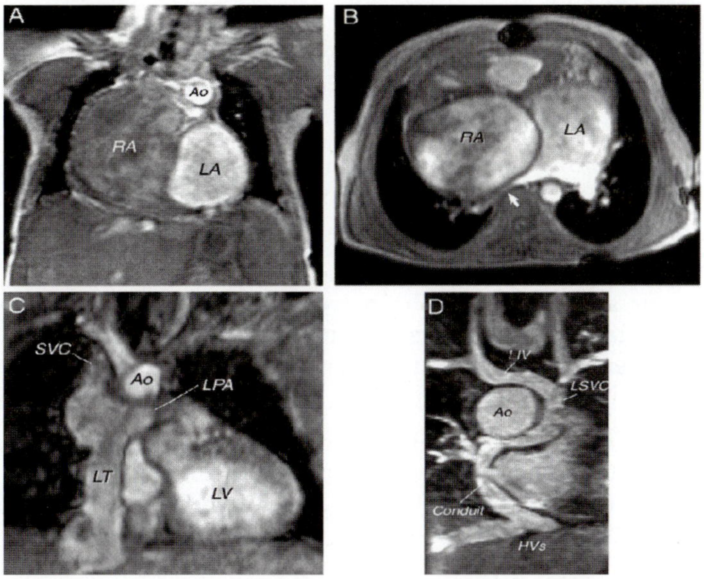

Figs 14.259A to D: *MRI evaluation of Fontan pathways. (A) Cine MRI in the coronal plane in a patient with atriopulmonary Fontan anastomosis. Note the giant right atrium (RA) with low signal intensity due to low flow velocity. (B) Cine MRI in the axial in the same patient showing compression of the right pulmonary vein between the giant right atrium and the spine (arrow). (C) Cine MRI in a patient with a lateral tunnel (LT) and total cavopulmonary anastomosis. (D) Gadolinium-enhanced 3D MRA subvolume MIP image in a patient with an extracardiac conduit between the hepatic veins (HVs) and the right pulmonary artery*

is currently preferred by most surgeons. To address the growth issue related to extracardiac Fontan, some surgeons use autologous pericardial roll grafts. At the conclusion of the procedure, systemic venous blood returns to the lungs passively without passing through a ventricle. Choussat et al's criteria have been modified by many cardiologists and surgeons. Patients violating these criteria are at a higher risk for poor prognosis following Fontan operation than patients within the limits set by Choussat. In this high-risk group, the concept of leaving a small atrial septal defect open to facilitate decompression of the right atrium has been advanced. Laks et al advocated closure of the atrial defect by constricting the preplaced suture in the postoperative period, whereas Bridges et al used a transcatheter closure technique. Although the fenestrated Fontan was initially conceived for high-risk patients, it has since been used in patients with modest or even low risk. Rare reports of cerebrovascular or other systemic arterial embolic events following the fenestrated Fontan procedure tend to contraindicate its use in non–high-risk patients. Some studies suggest routine fenestration is unnecessary.

At discharge, most children remain on digoxin, diuretics, aspirin, and captopril if necessary. In an uncomplicated case, most of these medications can be weaned over 6 months following the Fontan operation. Some cardiologists advocate using aspirin indefinitely. Routine use of more aggressive anticoagulation with Coumadin is debated. When warfarin and aspirin regimens were compared, no difference in thrombotic complications between the groups was detected. Similar early uncontrolled studies indicated similar finding; thus, most pediatric cardiologists use aspirin for prevention of thrombotic events in children. Use of more potent drugs such clopidogrel (plavix) may be reasonable in adolescents and adults.

Heart transplantation is another surgical option. The infant must remain on prostaglandin E1 infusion to keep the ductus arteriosus patent while waiting for a donor heart to become available. Approximately 20% of infants listed for heart transplantation die while waiting for a suitable donor organ. After successful cardiac transplantation, infants require multiple medications for modulation of the immune system and prevention of graft rejection. Perform frequent outpatient surveillance to identify rejection early and prevent lasting damage to the transplanted heart. Periodic endomyocardial biopsy usually is performed for more precise monitoring.

Emerging therapies include the following:

Catheter-assisted Fontan

Following Norwood procedure, 2-stage cavopulmonary connection is currently recommended for achieving Fontan circulation. Konert et al proposed a staged surgical-catheter approach; they initially perform a modified hemi-Fontan procedure that is later completed by transcatheter methodology. This reduces the total number of operations required.

The modified hemi-Fontan procedure involves the usual bidirectional Glenn procedure. The lower end of the divided superior vena cava is anastomosed to the undersurface of the right pulmonary artery. The superior vena cava is then banded around a 16-gauge catheter with 6-0 Prolene slightly above the cavoatrial junction. A lateral tunnel with a Gore-Tex baffle is created, diverting the inferior vena caval blood toward the superior vena cava. The Gore-Tex baffle is then fenestrated with 3–5 mm holes. Thus, the first stage achieves a physiologic bidirectional Glenn procedure.

At the time of the second stage (the transcatheter stage), the superior vena caval constriction is balloon dilated, and fenestrations are closed with devices or by placement of covered stent. These procedures have been performed in a limited number of patients, and preliminary data suggest that the usual post-Fontan operation complications, such as pleural effusion and ascites, have not occurred with this approach. Additional experience is reported; however, scrutiny of results of larger experience and longer-term follow-up and ready availability of covered stents are necessary for routine application of this innovative approach. To the authors knowledge, this approach is not well documented in patients with hypoplastic left heart syndrome.

Sano's Modification of the Norwood Procedure

Because of high mortality that Sano and his associates observed with the conventional Norwood procedure, they performed right ventricular outflow-to-pulmonary artery Gore-Tex graft anastomosis to provide for the pulmonary blood flow instead of conventional modified aorto-pulmonary shunt. Significant improvement was demonstrated in both immediate and late mortality with this modification. A multi-institutional study comparing the results of these two types of stage I palliation of hypoplastic left heart syndrome suggested no significant difference between the groups.

Other hybrid approaches: Again, because of high mortality following stage I Norwood reconstruction, several groups have performed bilateral banding of the branch pulmonary arteries via median sternotomy and implant stent in the ductus arteriosus. Maintaining ductal patency with long-term prostaglandin infusion instead of ductal stenting is advocated by some. At the time of the second stage, aortic arch reconstruction, atrial septectomy, and bidirectional Glenn shunt are performed. This is followed by Fontan conversion. Although reduction of early mortality is theoretically feasible, larger experience with this approach than is currently available is necessary prior to general adaptation of this method of management of hypoplastic left heart syndrome (Figs 14. 254A to D).

Prevention by Fetal Intervention

Fetal echocardiography studies have shown development of hypoplastic left heart syndrome in fetuses initially found to have severe/critical aortic stenosis or absent of markedly restrictive patnet foramen ovale. Some data suggest that fetal intervention to relieve aortic valve stenosis (by balloon aortic valvuloplasty) or creation of atrial septal defects (by percutaneous septostomy), both under the guidance of ultrasonography), may promote normal development of the left ventricle or confer benefit following birth. Further research into this type of approach is needed.

Treatments and Drugs

Treatment for hypoplastic left heart syndrome involves either a three-step surgical procedure or a heart transplant. If the diagnosis has been made before the baby is born, doctors usually recommend delivery at a hospital with a cardiac surgery center.

Before Surgery

Your baby's doctor may recommend several options to help manage the condition before surgery or transplant. They include:

Medication: The medication alprostadil (Prostin VR Pediatric) helps dilate the blood vessels and keeps the ductus arteriosus open.

Breathing assistance: If your baby has trouble breathing, he or she may need help from a breathing machine (ventilator), which ensures adequate oxygen delivery. Intravenous fluids. Your baby will receive fluids through a tube inserted into a vein.

Atrial septostomy: This procedure is used to create an opening between the heart's upper chambers (atria) if the foramen ovale closes. If your baby already has an atrial septal defect, an atrial septostomy may not be necessary.

Follow-up Care

After surgery or a transplant, your baby will need lifelong follow-up care with a heart doctor (cardiologist) who specializes in congenital heart disease, to monitor his or her heart health. Some medication may be necessary to regulate heart function. If your baby receives a heart transplant, antirejection medication will be necessary for the rest of his or her life to combat rejection of the new heart. Your child's cardiologist may recommend taking antibiotics before certain dental or other procedures to prevent infections, especially if the heart hasn't been fully repaired yet or if there are small defects that remain after repair. In some cases, he or she may also recommend that your child limit physical activity.

Prevention

There's no known way to prevent hypoplastic left heart syndrome. If you have a family history of heart defects, or if you already have a child with a congenital heart defect, before getting pregnant consider talking with a genetic counselor and a cardiologist experienced in congenital heart defects.

TOTAL ANOMALOUS PULMONARY VENOUS CONNECTIONS (TAPVC)

Embryology

The pulmonary veins may make abnormal connections at either supracardiac, cardiac or infracardiac levels.

At supracardiac levels, pulmonary veins drain either into innominate veins or superior vena cava. At cardiac level, it may drain either in right atrium or coronary sinus. At infracardiac level, it may drain either in IVC, hepatic or portal veins. This defect may be partial or complete. In order to sustain life, in such cases left to right shunt is most essential and hence atrial septal defect is an integral part of the anomaly (Fig. 14.260).

Haemodynamics

The oxygenated pulmonary venous blood is diverted to he right atrium. All chambers of the heart have identical oxygen saturations. In the earlier stages there is no cyanosis but when the pulmonary vascular resistance rises cyanosis may develop (Figs 14.261A to D).

Clinical History and Physical Examination

1. *Patients with Pulmonary Vein Obstruction*

Pulmonary venous obstruction occurs in virtually all patients with subdiaphragmatic drainage and in approximately 50% of patients with supracardiac drainage. Patients with obstruction develop symptoms early, usually at age 24–36 hours including tachypnea, tachycardia, and cyanosis. Signs of pulmonary hypertension progress with decreasing pulmonary blood flow and worsening cyanosis. Natural history is that of progressive clinical deterioration and early death in the first week or month of life depending on the degree of pulmonary venous obstruction.

Physical examination findings include severe cyanosis with significant respiratory distress. Cardiac impulse is prominent anteriorly, but, usually, the heart is not clinically enlarged. The pulmonary component of the second heart sound is increased, and a gallop may be present. A murmur usually is not present, yet a systolic murmur over the pulmonary area or a tricuspid insufficiency murmur at the mid and lower left sternal border may be observed. Peripheral pulses are usually normal after birth but may decrease as heart failure progresses. Liver enlargement commonly occurs, especially in total anomalous pulmonary venous connection (TAPVC) type III, subdiaphragmatic drainage.

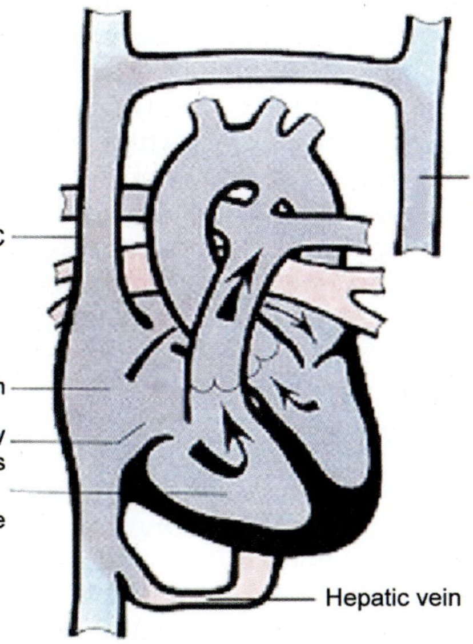

Fig. 14.260: *Diagram explains the anatomy and altred structures in TAPVC*

2. *Patients without Pulmonary Venous Obstruction*

Patients with unobstructed pulmonary venous flow present with symptoms more similar to a very large atrial septal defect. Mild failure to thrive with greater respiratory effort than normal with activity or recurrent respiratory infections may be present. Often, chest radiography in patients with respiratory infections reveals significant cardiac enlargement.

Physical examination findings suggest right ventricular volume loading with increase in right ventricular impulse, a wide split-second sound (usually with normal-intensity pulmonary closure), and pulmonary outflow murmur with or without a tricuspid diastolic murmur. Cyanosis infrequently occurs in the first year of life.

Reverse difference cyanosis has been reported in the newborn period in total anomalous pulmonary venous connection to the superior vena cava (SVC). In this setting highly saturated blood in the SVC streams preferentially from right ventricle across ductus arteriosus to descending aorta; lower saturated blood in inferior vena cava streams across the foramen ovale to the left heart and aorta, resulting in higher saturation in the foot than in the right hand.

If a restriction develops in the foramen ovale, some degree of pulmonary hypertension is more likely, with earlier onset of tachypnea, louder pulmonary closure sound, more prominent right ventricular impulse, and a greater likelihood of systemic and pulmonary venous congestion.

Laboratory Studies

Assess and improve (as possible) the oxygenation, acid-base status, and hemogram status in newborns or young infants with total anomalous pulmonary venous connection (TAPVC) in preparation for surgery.

Imaging Studies

Chest radiography

In patients with total anomalous pulmonary venous connection with pulmonary venous obstruction, chest radiographs reveal a normal heart size with a diffuse reticular pattern fanning out from the hilum. When the pulmonary veins are unobstructed, the heart is enlarged (right atrial and right ventricular enlargement), and pulmonary markings reveal active increase in size of the pulmonary hilar and midzone vessels (Fig. 14.262).

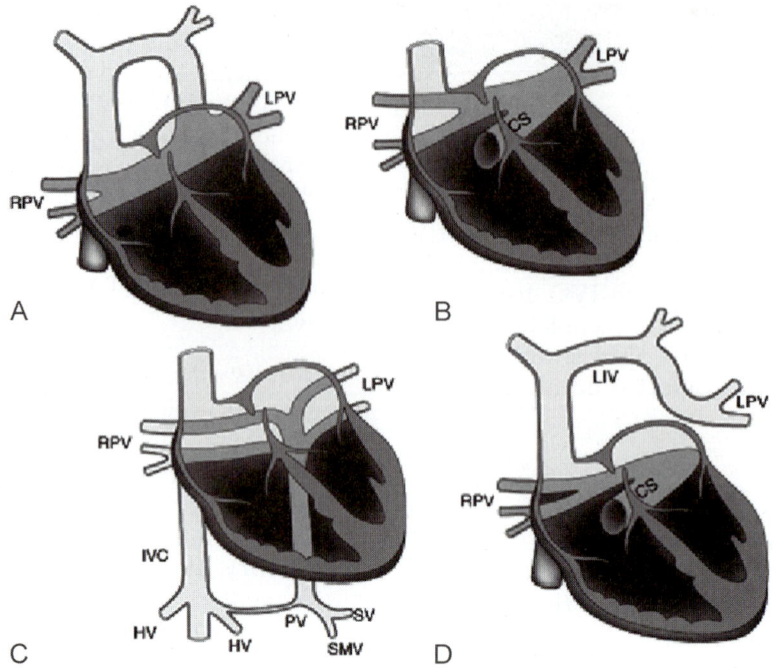

Fig. 14.261A to D: *Total anomalous pulmonary venous connection: variants. (A) Supracardiac. Both right (RPV) and left (LPV) pulmonary veins join a common pulmonary venous confluence behind the heart that drains via a vertical vein to the undersurface of the left innominate vein and then to the right atrium. (B) Cardiac. The pulmonary venous confluence connects to the coronary sinus (CS) and then to the right atrium via the coronary sinus ostium. (C) Infradiaphragmatic. The pulmonary venous confluence drains inferiorly via a vertical vein to the portal vein (PV) or hepatic veins (HV) and then to the right atrium. (D) Mixed connections. Left pulmonary veins drain to the left innominate vein (LIV) and right pulmonary veins to the coronary sinus in this example. SV, splenic vein; SMV, superior mesenteric vein*

Echocardiography

Echocardiographic findings, which are usually definitive, have been vital in pin pointing the exact cardiac defect.

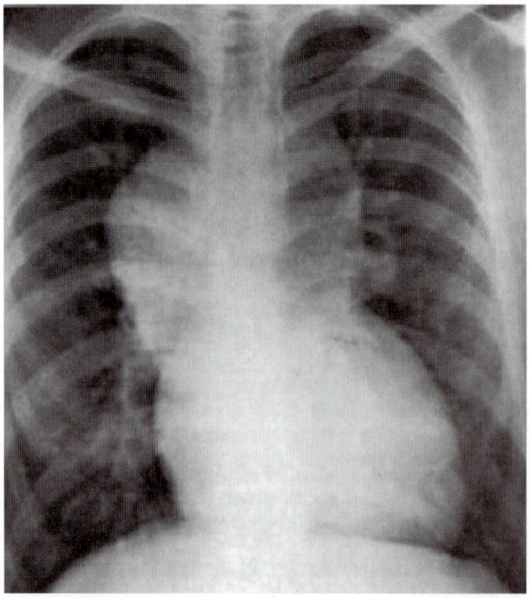

Fig. 14.262: *X-ray chest PA view shows classic "Snowman" or "figure of 8" pattern of enlarged supracardiac veins,TAPVR due to an anomalous connection tol eft SVC, left innominate veins, and right SVC.*

Hyaline membrane disease may demonstrate similar findings initially. In this setting, ECG helps identify right ventricular hypertrophy in patients with total anomalous pulmonary venous connection, especially in premature babies, particularly because premature babies usually have a greater level of left ventricular force (Figs 14.263; 14.264A and B).

Echocardiography of the precordium in patients with total anomalous pulmonary venous connection reveals right ventricular and pulmonary artery volume loading with flattened or paradoxic septal motion on M-mode imaging. Apical and subcostal four chamber views usually best identify individual pulmonary veins and their confluence in patients with total anomalous pulmonary venous connection. Then, using multiple views, the common pulmonary vein can usually be tracked to its point of entry to the systemic venous system or to the coronary sinus.

Subcostal long- and short-axis views can also help to evaluate size and flow patterns across the foramen ovale.

Total anomalous pulmonary venous connection may be difficult to diagnose, especially in an ill newborn on a ventilator if views of the atrial septum are difficult to obtain or if the common pulmonary vein is small or at an obtuse angle to the left atrial back wall. The addition of color Doppler ultrasonography greatly aids in the diagnosis of individual pulmonary veins and in analysis of the abnormal flow pattern across the atrial septal defect.

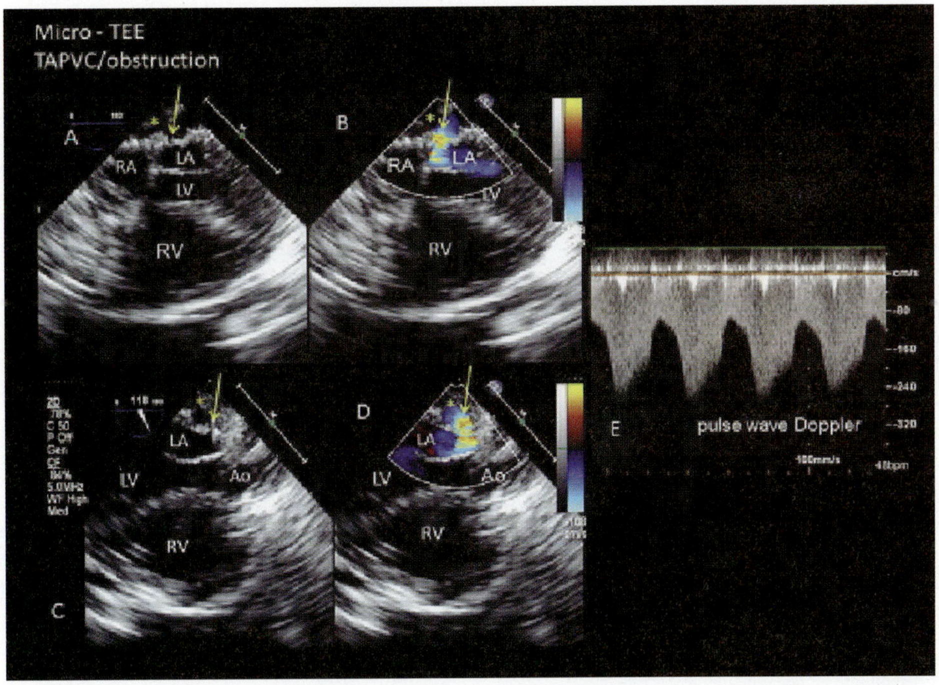

Fig. 14.263: *Transesophageal echocardiograms using the micro-TEE transducer (micro-TEE) in a patient with total anomalous pulmonary venous connection (TAPVC) with residual stenosis at the anastomosis of the pulmonary venous confluence (asterisk) to the left atrium (LA) (arrow). (A) Four chamber two dimensional echocardiographic view. (B) Four chamber color Doppler flow map. (C) Long-axis two dimensional echocardiographic view. (D) Long-axis color Doppler flow map. (E) Obstructive pattern pulsed-wave Doppler echocardiogram. Ao, Aorta; LV, left ventricle; RA, right atrium.*

Color-flow mapping may be helpful in finding individual pulmonary veins and confirming whether they enter the left atrium. Color-flow ultrasonography may also be used to assess directional flow at the foramen ovale. In patients with total anomalous pulmonary venous connection, flow across the atrial septum predominantly occurs from the right to left. Altogether, echocardiography with additional color Doppler can help to make the diagnosis in the vast majority of patients with total anomalous pulmonary venous connection. In patients with pulmonary inflow obstruction, further diagnostic studies may be needed.

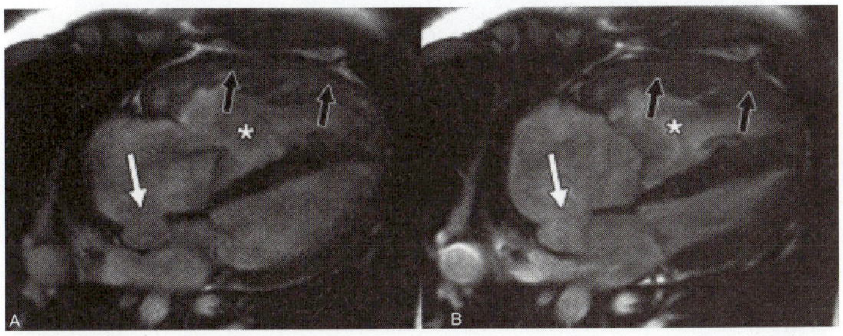

Fig. 14.264A and B: *Images in 16-year-adolescent with cyanosis secondary to total anomalous pulmonary venous return (type II, drainage into coronary sinus) and large ASD. Diastolic (A) and systolic (B) image frames from double-oblique four-chamber cine SSFP MR imaging sequence (2.4/1.2; flip angle, 65°) show the large ASD (white arrows). An enlarged right ventricle (*) with right ventricular myocardial hypertrophy (black arrows) can also be appreciated*

With fetal echocardiography, an attempt should be made to see the individual pulmonary veins, but most consistent diagnostic findings in total anomalous pulmonary venous connection have involved a confluence (chamber) behind the left atrium or a vertical vein.

MRI (Figs 14.265 to 14.267)

It serves to confirm the diagnosis in patients with total anomalous pulmonary venous connection (especially in those with associated lung disease).

Selective pulmonary vein or pulmonary artery angiography: this may precisely reveal a vessel's anatomy.

Electrocardiography (Fig. 14.268)

ECG reveals significant right ventricular hypertrophy in most of these patients, usually with a qR pattern in the right chest leads by age 5–7 days. Right atrial enlargement rarely occurs in these younger patients.

Procedures

In some patients with multiple sites of pulmonary venous connection, cardiac catheterization serves to better define sites of pulmonary venous obstruction when other associated cardiac defects are present (i.e. pulmonary atresia), and to directly measure foramen ovale size when surgery is delayed (Figs 14.269A and B; 14.270).

Complications

Early in the postoperative period in patients with obstructed total anomalous pulmonary venous connection

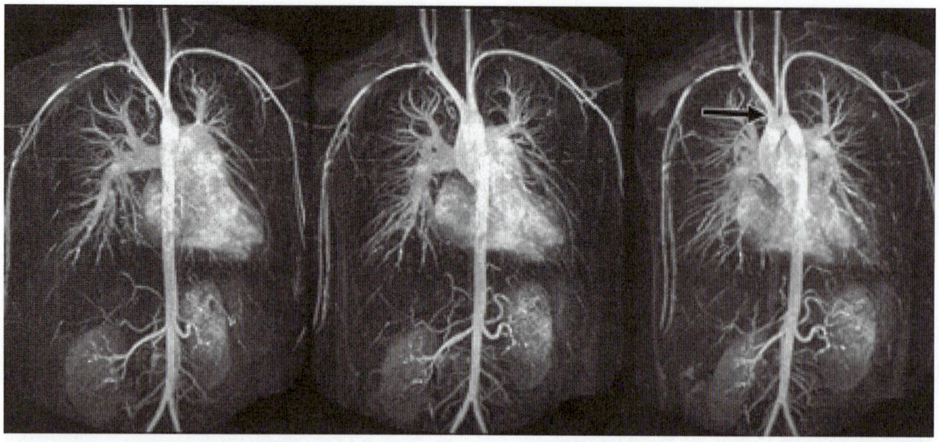

Fig. 14.265: *Images in patient with cyanosis secondary to total anomalous pulmonary venous return (type II, drainage into coronary sinus) and large ASD.Coronal MIPs from high-spatial-resolution MR angiography, flip angle, 30°) in anterioposterior projection and with ±15° rotation. Branching of right and left carotid arteries from brachiocephalic artery (arrow), which can merely be suspected with the time-resolved image series, is clearly visualized. Diastolic (left) and systolic (right) image frames from double-oblique four-chamber cine SSFP MR imaging sequence (2.4/1.2; flip angle, 65°) show the large ASD (white arrows). An enlarged right ventricle (*) with right ventricular myocardial hypertrophy (black arrows) can also be appreciated*

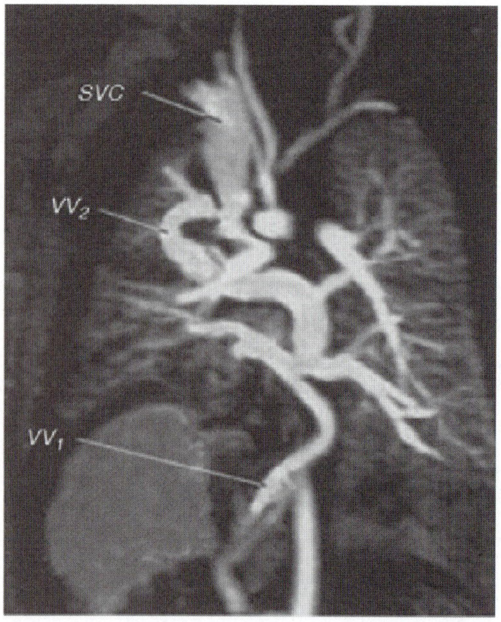

Fig. 14.266: *Maximal-intensity projection coronal plane image of gadolinium-enhanced three dimensional magnetic resonance angiogram in a newborn with obstructed mixed-type total anomalous venous connection. There is infradiaphragmatic connection by means of a vertical vein (VV-1) to the portal vein, as well as supracardiac stenotic connection to the right superior vena cava (SVC) via an additional vertical vein (VV-2). (Courtesy of Tal Geva, MD)*

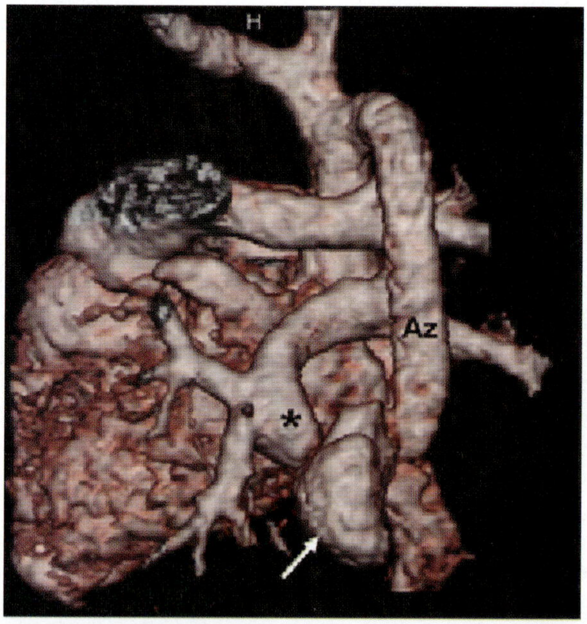

Fig. 14.267: *Volume-rendered technique of computed tomography angiogram in the left posterior oblique view. This provides an overview of the descending common chamber (*), dilatation (white arrow) and drainage into azygos vein (Az)*

(TAPVC), the pulmonary arteries may be hypoplastic and respond poorly to the vasodilators.

The complication of pulmonary venous obstruction occurs later in 5–10% of patients and is usually evident in the first 6 months following surgery. This obstruction is more easily treated surgically if it involves only the pulmonary venous confluence and anastomosis area. Sutureless marsupialization with pericardium has seemed to help to improve surgical results. If the pulmonary venous obstruction involves intimal fibrotic hyperplasia of individual pulmonary veins extending deeper back into the veins then surgery may not be successful. Surgical mortality remains higher in repair of mixed form of total anomalous pulmonary venous connection, especially in patients with

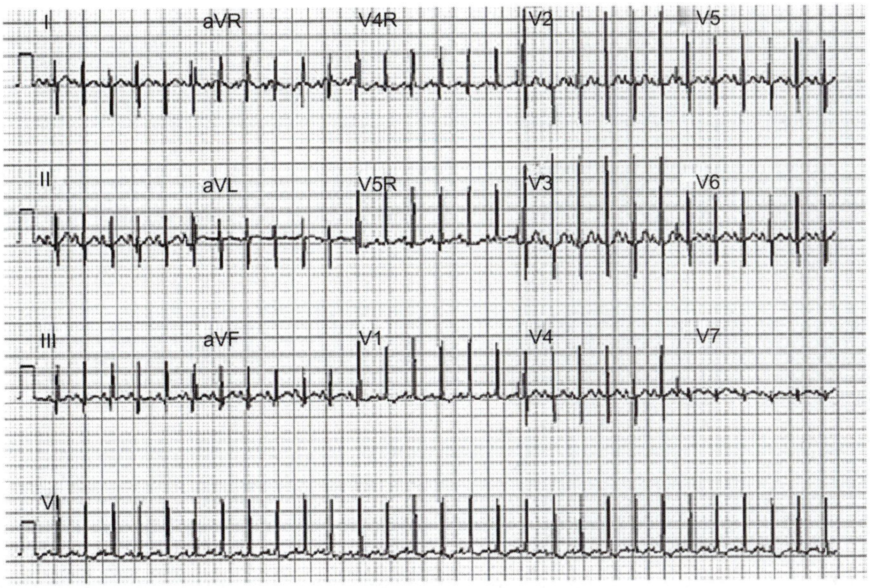

Fig. 14.268: *TAPVR: electrocardiogram obtained in a 10-days old infant with total anomalous pulmonary venous return to the coronary sinus. The tracing shows right atrial enlargement (peaked P waves in lead II) and right ventricular hypertrophy*

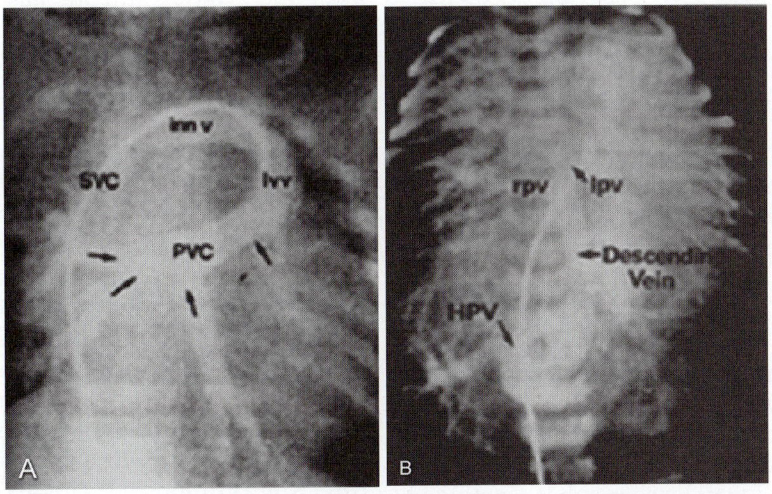

Figs 14.269A and B: *Contrast angiography showing contrast material entering into pulmonary artery (PA) showing return of pulmonary venous blood (B) Left-sided vertical vein with subsequent opacification of the right SVC (RSVC) in patient with total anomalous pulmonary venous connection*

more complex patterns of pulmonary venous connection, which have persistently small or thickened individual pulmonary veins.

Medical Treatment

No catheter-corrective treatment is possible for total anomalous pulmonary venous connection (TAPVC), although atrial septostomy is used in some patients when the foramen ovale is restricted and corrective surgery is delayed for some reason. Catheter placement of a ***stent*** has been reported for pretreatment of obstructed vertical vein prior to surgery. If a vertical vein is left patent postoperatively and significant shunt persists it may be possible to close this vessel with an ***Amplatzer PDA device***.

Surgical repair is used as treatment for total anomalous pulmonary venous connection whenever it best serves the individual patient. Stabilizing the patient prior to surgery as much as possible from a cardiovascular and metabolic standpoint is important. In a newborn with obstructive total anomalous pulmonary venous connection, stabilization often involves mechanical ventilation, correction of acidosis, inotropic support, and administration of prostaglandin E1 for patency of patent ductus arteriosus and, in patients with total anomalous pulmonary venous connection type III, for patency of the ductus venous.

Nitric oxide may be useful as a pulmonary dilator postoperatively in patients experiencing episodic pulmonary hypertension that is affecting cardiac output.

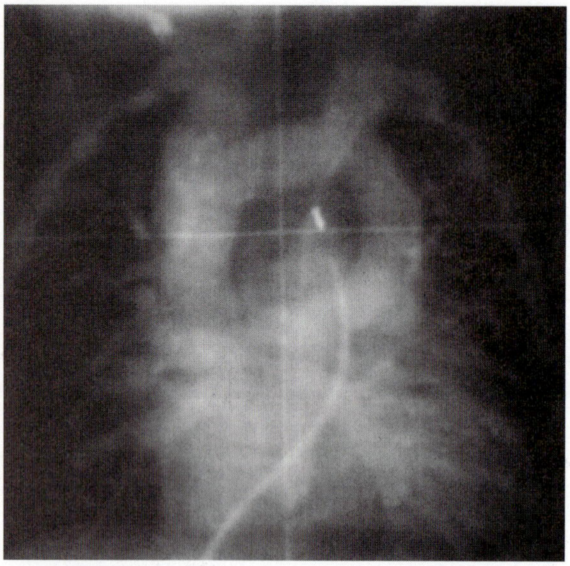

Fig. 14.270: *Type I TAPVR frontal view obtained with angiocardiography in a neonate shows the aberrant cardiovascular anatomy: the upper left heart is bordered by the vertical vein; the superior part of the heart, by the left innominate vein; and the upper part of the right heart, by the dilated superior vena cava*

Reports indicate that magnesium sulfate is a useful pulmonary vasodilator in these patients. Extracorporeal membrane oxygenation (ECMO) may be life-saving in some patients. If transesophageal echocardiography is used intraoperatively in infants with pulmonary vein obstruction, waiting for probe insertion until after chest is opened may be safer.

Pulmonary Vasodilators

When sustained severe cyanosis or severe hypercyanotic episodes occur in patients with obstructed total anomalous pulmonary venous connection postoperatively, treatment with one or more pulmonary vasodilators may be helpful. The pulmonary vascular bed may be somewhat reactive in the postoperative period, resulting in episodic pulmonary hypertension and low cardiac output. Although this should improve over time, interim therapy with pulmonary vasodilator agents may be useful in this setting. Vasodilators that are specific for the pulmonary vasculature are rare; however, inhaled nitric oxide may be a good agent in this setting. Therefore, the following three vasodilators can be used to treat-elevated pulmonary vascular resistance in the postoperative period. Note that this therapy is controversial in the preoperative patient with known pulmonary venous obstruction.

Nitric Oxide, Inhaled (INOmax)

Stimulates guanylate cyclase to form cyclic GMP, which causes relaxation of vascular smooth muscle. Because it can be delivered by inhalation directly to alveolar units and is rapidly inactivated by hemoglobin, it is the most selective of currently available pulmonary vascular dilators (except for oxygen).

Magnesium Sulfate

Reportedly useful in patients with obstructed TAPVC who have hypercyanotic episodes to decrease pulmonary vascular resistance and decrease pulmonary vascular reactivity. Mechanism of action is believed to be direct action on vascular muscle cells but may also increase formation or release of NO. $MgSO_4$ has systemic and pulmonary vascular dilating effects, and use of a slow infusion of lower-dose $MgSO_4$ is wise to avoid systemic hypotension.

Alprostadil IV (Prostin VR)

Prostaglandin E1 (PGE1) that causes dilation of vascular smooth muscle in the ductus arteriosus, systemic arteries, and pulmonary vascular muscles. In obstructed TAPVC, PGE1 is usually used as a pulmonary vascular dilator, but its effects on the ductus arteriosus and ductus venosus can be very important (e.g. in subdiaphragmatic connection, PGE1 can help to dilate the ductus venosus and improve pulmonary venous flow. In other types of connection with obstruction, PGE1 can dilate pulmonary arteries and increase pulmonary flow or dilate the ductus arteriosus and systemic arteries and increase right-to-left shunting and worsen cyanosis). PGE1 is readily available and easily administered, preferably via a large vessel. Care must be taken to observe its effects in the complex circulation of TAPVC.

Each 1 mL ampule contains 500 mcg/mL.

Surgical Intervention

The goal of surgery is to redirect pulmonary vein flow entirely to the left atrium. In patients with a supracardiac or infracardiac connection, the common pulmonary vein is opened wide and connected side to side to the left atrium. The foramen ovale is closed, and the ascending or descending vein is usually ligated. In a cardiac connection (to right atrium or coronary sinus), the atrial septum is resected partially and a new septum is surgically created, directing pulmonary veins to the left atrium. A coronary sinus may be separately tunneled to the right atrium or left to drain with the pulmonary veins to the left atrium.

Newborns or patients in early infancy with obstructed total anomalous pulmonary venous connection (TAPVC) frequently have pulmonary edema with varying degrees of increase in pulmonary arterial and venous resistance. Pulmonary edema is probably treated best with surgical relief of the pulmonary venous obstruction, but diuretics and assisted ventilation with high fraction of inspired oxygen (FIO_2) and end-expiratory pressure are often helpful preoperatively and postoperatively.

Prognosis

Most reports indicate an early mortality rate of less than 10%. Most patients survive surgery without late cardiovascular problem manifestations. An increased incidence of neurodevelopmental difficulties has been reported, with fine motor function, visual-motor integration, and attention difficulties noted.

UNIVENTRICULAR HEART (SINGLE VENTRICLE)

Pathophysiology

A functional single ventricle may result from hypoplastic left heart syndrome (aortic atresia, mitral atresia, or both), tricuspid atresia, pulmonary atresia with intact ventricular septum, or an unbalanced ASD resulting in hypoplasia of either the RV or LV (Fig. 14.271).

History

Neonates with single ventricle and subpulmonary stenosis become cyanotic but are usually without other symptoms.

Neonates with single ventricle and aortic obstruction may have rapid breathing, lethargy and poor feeding.

Physical Examination

Cyanosis is present in patients with subpulmonary stenosis.

Poor peripheral perfusion is evident in patients with single ventricle with aortic obstruction.

If aortic obstruction involves coarctation or interruption, then a difference in blood pressure is observed between the right arm and a lower extremity, unless the right subclavian artery is aberrant.

The first heart sound is normal.

The second heart sound is frequently single.

A systolic ejection murmur is present in those with subpulmonary stenosis as well as those with aortic obstruction.

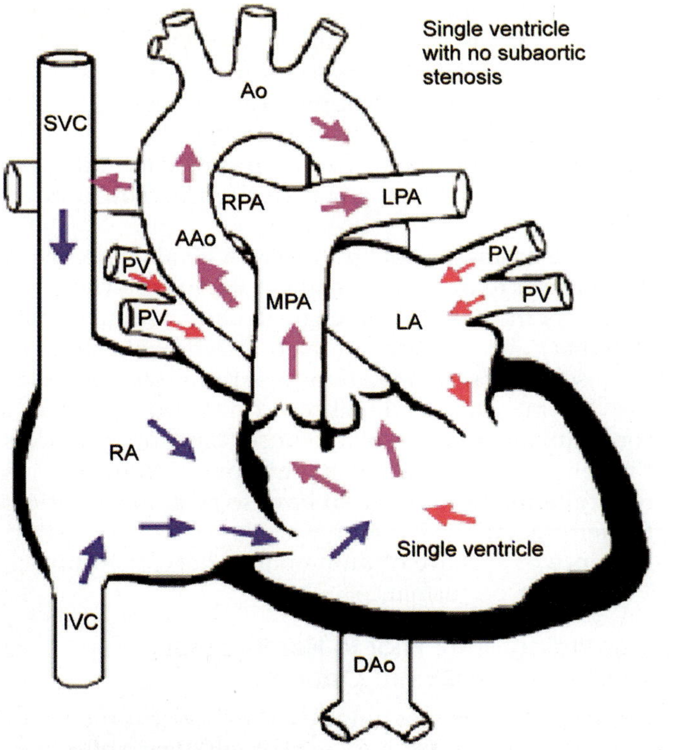

Fig. 14.271: *Illustration shows anatomical and circulatory disturbances in single ventricle.*

Causes

The cause of single ventricle in humans is unknown.

So far, at least 10 targeted single-gene disruptions in mice have produced a right ventricular (RV) hypoplasia phenotype reminiscent of single left ventricle (LV). These disruptions include global nulls in Nkx2.5; Isl1; Mef2c; dHand (also known as Hand2); Fog-2; Fgf8 hypomorph; Foxh1; TGFβ2; Bop; and Has2. The Fog -2 null also displays a common atrioventricular orifice situated almost entirely over the future LV (i.e., common-inlet ventricle). Whether hypomorphic alleles of the homologous mutations in the human produce a single ventricle phenotype but do not result in embryonic lethality remains to be shown. Ventricular-specific misexpression of Tbx5 and myocardial-specific inactivation of GATA4 cause single ventricle.

Differential Diagnoses

- Aortic stenosis, valvular
- *Corrected transposition of the great arteries:* Surgical perspective
- *Double-outlet right ventricle:* Surgical perspective
- Heterotaxy, asplenia
- Heterotaxy, polysplenia
- Hypoplastic left heart syndrome
- Hypoplastic left heart syndrome and the staged. Norwood procedure
- Neonatal sepsis
- Protein-losing enteropathy
- Pulmonary stenosis, valvular.

Laboratory Studies

No specific laboratory blood tests are required in the preoperative workup for single ventricle, although, in the near future, affordable whole-genome sequencing will likely be helpful. An ABG measurement is frequently helpful in distinguishing between cases of single ventricle with subpulmonary stenosis and those cases of single ventricle with arch obstruction, aortic stenosis, or both. For example, when prostaglandin E1 has not been administered, a PaO_2 of greater than 50 mmHg lessens the likelihood that a newborn with single ventricle has significant subpulmonary stenosis. However, this PaO_2 is perfectly consistent with the presence of arch obstruction.

Following Fontan operation, fecal alpha1-antitrypsin measurement is crucial in surveillance for the complication of protein-losing enteropathy (PLE). Abnormalities in serum total protein and albumin are relatively late clues to PLE; because the liver is the sole site of endogenous albumin production, a low serum albumin level signifies the liver's inability to compensate for poor protein intake or excessive protein loss. Prolongation in the prothrombin time (a measure of hepatic synthetic function) abnormally elevated gamma-glutamyl-transpeptidase, and a reduction in alkaline phosphatase levels (largely a reflection of osteoblastic activity in preadolescent children) are likely early clues to hepatic dysfunction, biliary dysfunction, and reduced bone formation, respectively.

Imaging Studies

Echocardiography (Figs 14.272 to 14.274)

Two-dimensional echocardiography is diagnostic for single ventricle. The presence or absence of subpulmonary stenosis, arch obstruction, and aortic stenosis can also be determined. The particular atrioventricular connection and ventriculoarterial alignment is also revealed in a straightforward manner.

The two most common forms of single ventricle are L-looped single left ventricle (LV) with transposition of the great arteries and subpulmonary stenosis and D-looped single LV with transposition of the great arteries and subpulmonary stenosis. The third most common form is L-looped single LV with transposition of the great arteries and aortic arch hypoplasia. The fourth most common form is D-looped single LV with normally aligned great arteries (i.e. aorta from LV and pulmonary artery from outlet chamber), which is sometimes referred to as a Holmes heart.

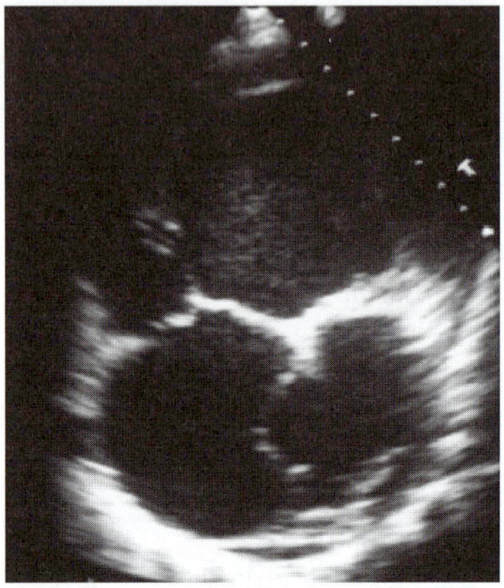

Fig. 14.272: *Apical four chamber view, single ventricle interatrial aneurysm*

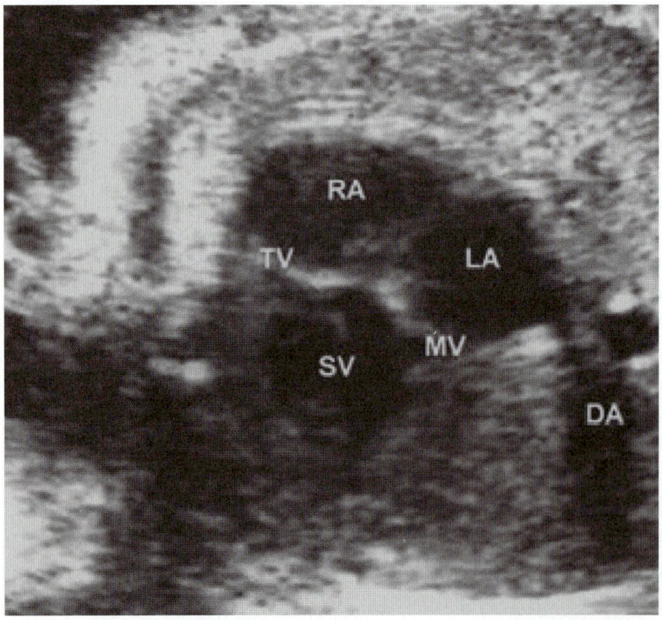

Fig. 14.273: *Fetal heart .The four chamber view only reveals three chambers including the left atrium (LA), right atrium (RA) and the single ventricle (SV). Both atrioventricular valves (TV, tricuspid valve, MV, mitral valve) are seen opening in the single ventricle*

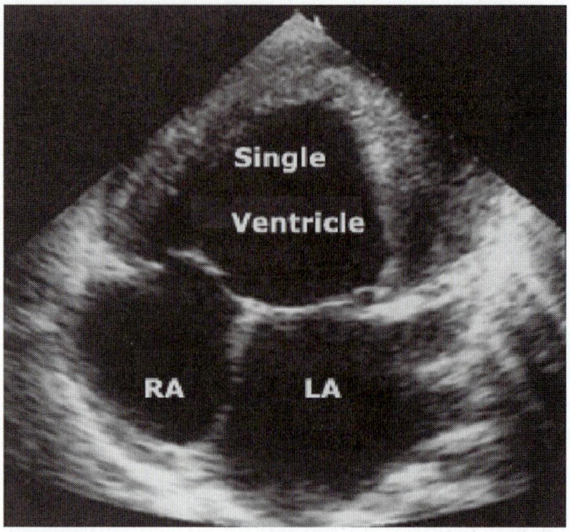

Fig. 14.274: *Four chamber apical image showing single ventricle. LA, left atrium; LV, left ventricle; RA, right atrium; RV, right ventricle.*

In single LV with transposition of the great arteries and aortic arch obstruction, the (sub) aortic stenosis that frequently coexists is due to a narrowing at the communication between the LV and the rudimentary right ventricle (outlet chamber). This orifice is frequently referred to as a bulboventricular foramen or outlet foramen. Echocardiography prior to initial surgery:

1. Initial identification of single ventricle
2. Presence or absence of subpulmonary stenosis
3. Presence or absence of arch obstruction
4. Presence or absence of narrowing of communication between normal-sized ventricle and rudimentary ventricle
5. Presence or absence of straddling AV valve (i.e. the AV valve closer to the outlet chamber having attachments to the rim of the outlet foramen or actually within the outlet chamber): the presence of such attachments should be an absolute contraindication to surgical enlargement of the outlet foramen which might otherwise be contemplated in cases of late-onset "subaortic stenosis".
6. Presence or absence of atrioventricular valve regurgitation, which would have to be palliated prior to Fontan operation
7. Presence or absence of pulmonary artery distortion
8. Ventricular performance.

Echocardiography Prior to Hemi-Fontan (or Bidirectional Glenn) Operation

1. Presence or absence of pulmonary artery distortion, either congenital or created inadvertently by prior pulmonary artery surgery
2. Presence or absence of second superior vena cava

Chest Radiography (Figs 14.275 and 14.276)

Chest radiography findings vary. In cases with pulmonary stenosis, the cardiac silhouette is normal to mildly enlarged. Pulmonary vascularity is not increased.

In cases with arch obstruction, the cardiac silhouette is usually at least mildly enlarged. Pulmonary vascularity usually is increased.

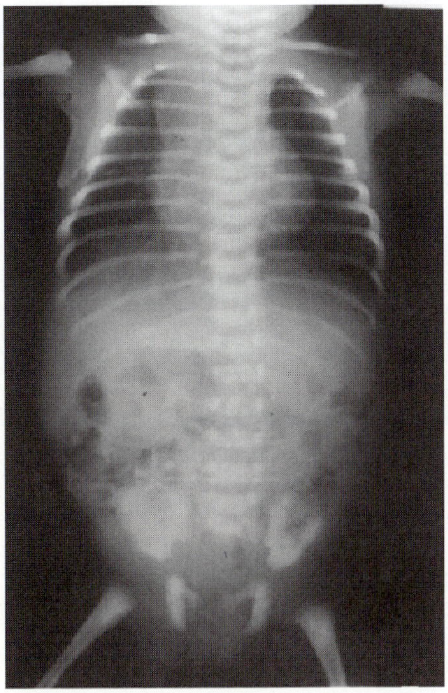

Fig. 14.275: *The radiograph shows a functioning heart with a single atrium and a single ventricle, as well as a degree of sacral dysgenesis*

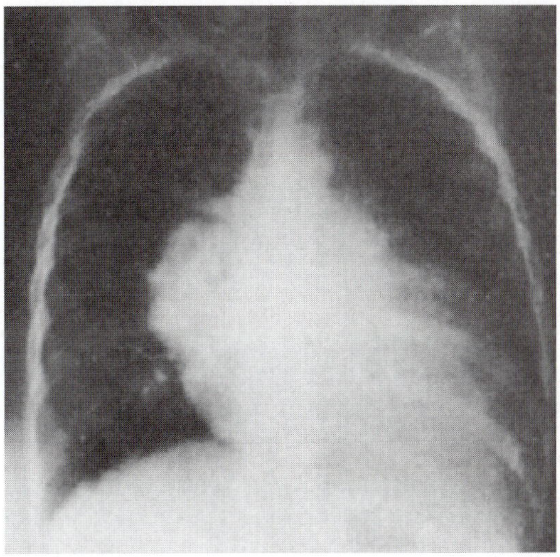

Fig. 14.276: *Photograph X-ray chest PA view showing cardiomegaly with enlargement of right atrium due to progressive tricuspid regurgitation in patient with single ventricle*

Other Tests

Electrocardiography: Common findings include septal q wave in the right precordial leads (in cases of L-looped single LV) and a monotonous R/S pattern over the anterior precordium (Fig. 14.277).

Holter monitoring: This is useful after a hemi-Fontan operation (or bidirectional Glenn operation) and is particularly helpful after a Fontan operation for surveillance of supraventricular arrhythmias and conduction block.

Procedures

Cardiac catheterization is largely reserved for evaluating candidacy for Fontan operation, characterizing post-Fontan hemodynamics, and managing supraventricular arrhythmic complications (Figs 14.278 and 14.279).

Postcatheterization precautions include hemorrhage, vascular disruption after balloon dilation, pain, nausea and vomiting, and arterial or venous obstruction from thrombosis or spasm.

Complications may include rupture of blood vessel, tachyarrhythmias, bradyarrhythmias and vascular occlusion.

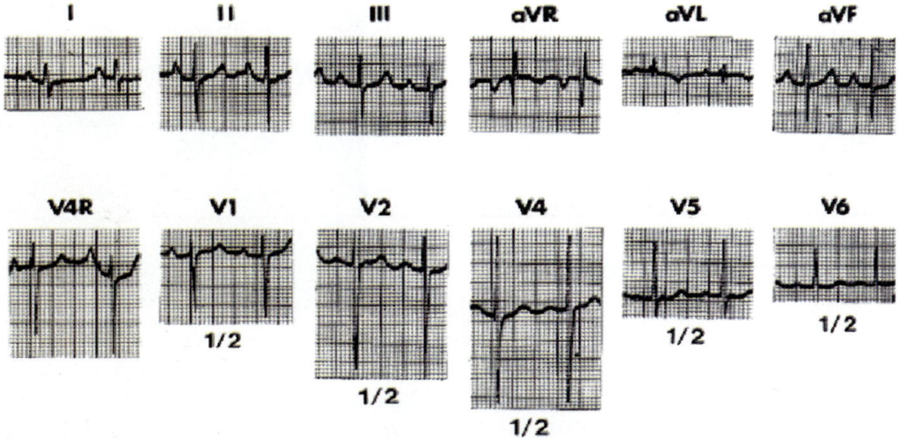

Fig. 14.277: *ECG showing Q waves in V1 and no Q waves in V6 and precordial leads, stereotype RS complex in most or all precordial leads, Ist degree AV block pulmonary stenosis in a single ventricle of 6-year-old girl*

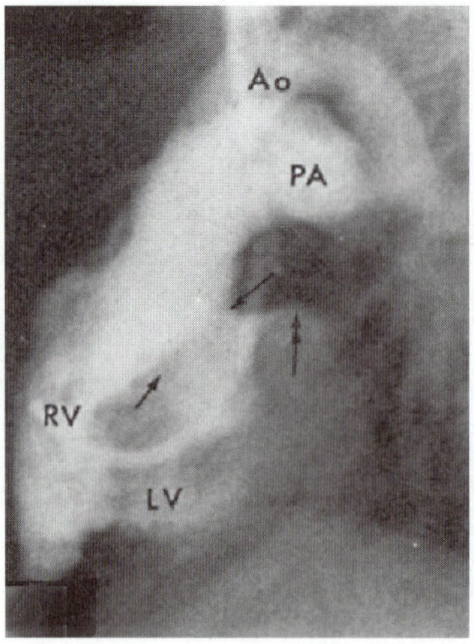

Fig. 14.278: *Single ventricle. A lateral view shows the anteriorly situated right ventricle (RV) communicating with the left ventricle (LV) via a ventricular septal defect (single arrows). (PA, pulmonary artery; Ao, aorta.)*

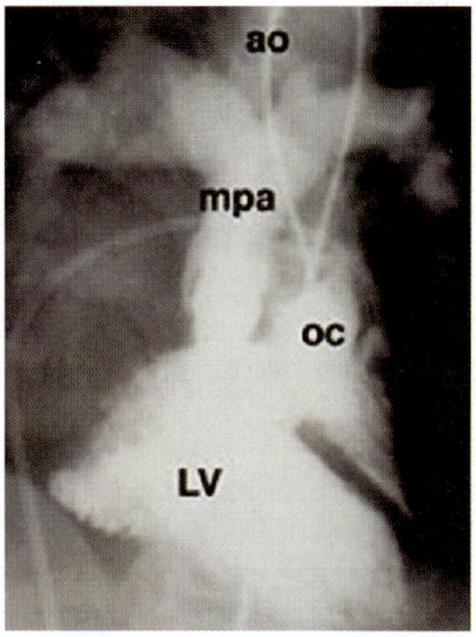

Fig. 14.279: *Cranially angulated frontal angiogram of an L-looped single left ventricle. Abbreviations are as follows: ao, aorta; mpa, main pulmonary artery; oc, outlet chamber (rudimentary right ventricle).*

Medical Management

Evaluation as an inpatient in an intensive care setting is advised for patients with single ventricle. Intravenous prostaglandin E1 is indicated in patients with severe arch obstruction and is frequently indicated in patients with subpulmonary stenosis. The need for introduction of an arterial line and assisted ventilation can be judged best from the initial ABG measurement.

Surgical Intervention

Because the pulmonary vascular resistance gradually falls over the first few months of life, conversion to a cavopulmonary or atriopulmonary circulation cannot be safely accomplished in the first few days of life.

If subpulmonary stenosis is present, its severity dictates whether a systemic-to-pulmonary artery shunt is needed after ductal closure. If aortic arch obstruction is present instead, the most widely adopted approach is to reestablish unobstructed aortic arch flow and to limit pulmonary blood flow (Figs 14.280 to 14.282).

As a way of limiting pulmonary blood flow, banding of the pulmonary artery has given way to other methods because most patients with arch obstruction have a narrow bulboventricular foramen.

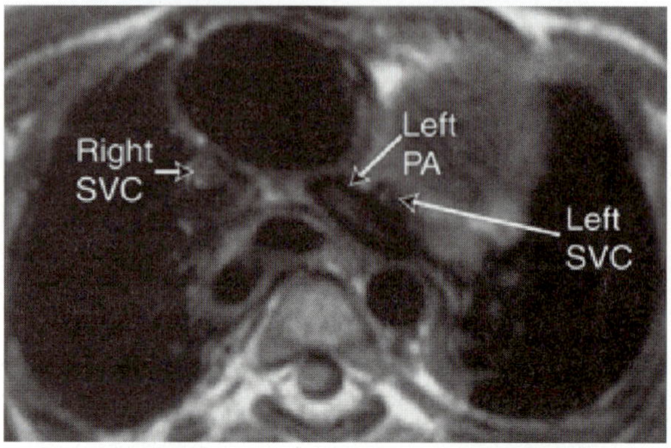

Fig. 14.280: *Heterotaxy and a single ventricle in a 4½-year-old boy who underwent a bidirectional Glenn procedure. MR imaging was performed to evaluate the pulmonary and hepatic veins before additional corrective surgery. Axial MR image shows the left superior vena cava (SVC) entering the left pulmonary artery (PA). The right superior vena cava is still proximal to the right pulmonary artery*

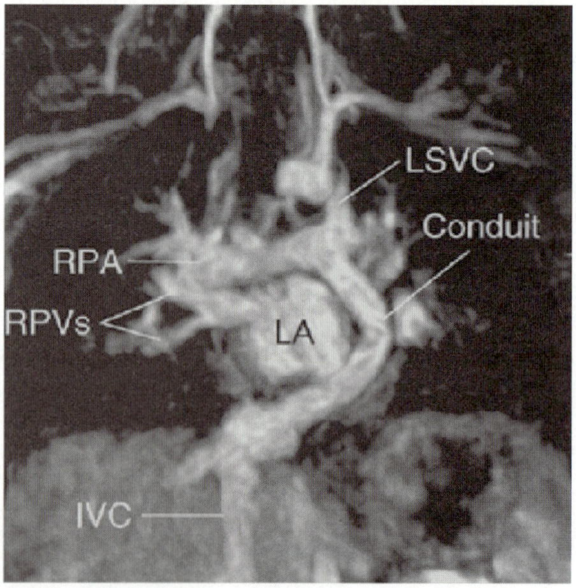

Fig. 14.281: *Single ventricle; maximum-intensity projection image of gadolinium-enhanced three-dimensional magnetic resonance angiogram in a patient with extracardiac Fontan by cardiac magnetic resonance imaging. IVC, inferior vena cava; LA, left atrium; LSVC, left superior vena cava; RPA, right pulmonary artery; RPVs, right pulmonary veins*

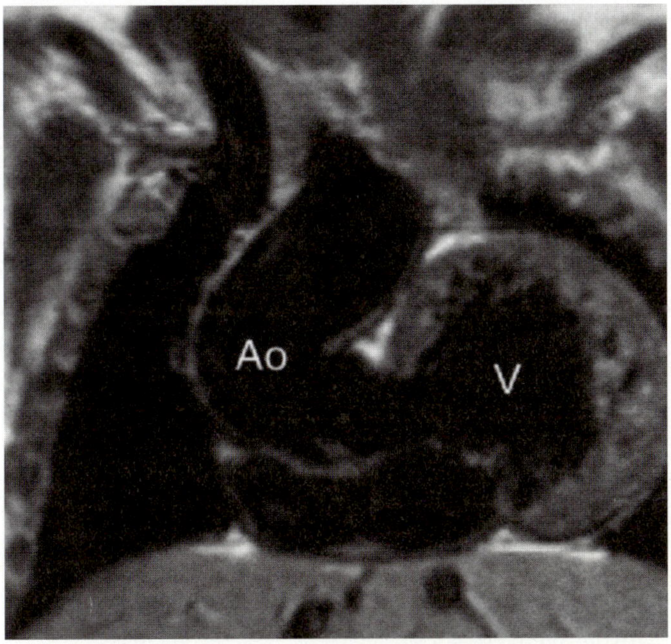

Fig. 14.282: *Heterotaxy and a single ventricle in a 4½-year-old boy who underwent a bidirectional Glenn procedure. MR imaging was performed to evaluate the pulmonary and hepatic veins before additional corrective surgery. (A) Coronal MR image shows a single ventricle (V) that gives rise to a "tucked" aorta (Ao). The pulmonary artery has been disconnected from the heart and is in continuity with the bidirectional Glenn anastomosis. The coronary sinus is absent. (B) Axial MR image shows bilateral superior venae cavae (SVC) with turbulent flow. Ao = aorta. (C) Axial MR image shows the left superior vena cava (SVC) entering the left pulmonary artery (PA). The right superior vena cava is still proximal to the right pulmonary artery. (D) Sagittal MR image shows a hepatic venous confluence (HV) entering the left atrium (LA). (E) Sagittal MR image shows a second hepatic venous confluence (HV) entering the right atrium (RA), which is anterior to the left atrium (LA). Ao, aorta. (F) Axial MR image shows the right and left superior pulmonary veins (PV) entering the left atrium (LA). There is a large atrial septal defect (double-headed arrow). ASept, atrial septum, RA; right atrium. Surgery involved completion of a Fontan procedure.*

Although it may not be initially restrictive, the bulboventricular foramen tends to reduce in diameter over time and may precipitously reduce in caliber following volume-unloading procedures, including pulmonary artery banding (as well as the hemi-Fontan and Fontan operations).

To avoid the possibility of hemodynamically important aortic stenosis, a Norwood-type reconstruction (proximal pulmonary artery-to-aorta anastomosis) is currently favored. Enlarging the bulboventricular foramen by resection of muscle is hazardous because of the proximity of the conduction system and the frequent presence of atrioventricular valve attachments to the rim.

Creation of a cavopulmonary circulation is more safely accomplished in stages over 1–2 years because acute volume unloading is associated with an acute increase in ventricular wall thickness. This wall thickness increase markedly alters the diastolic performance of the single ventricle and can limit cardiac output. Because the cardiac output falls by a lesser amount, the hemi-Fontan procedure results inthan the nonfenestrated "complete Fontan" procedure. The less-than-complete Fontan is currently viewed as the most favorable balance of nearly normal arterial oxygen saturation and the lowest frequency of effusive complications. Thus, even the so-called "final" stage commonly takes the form of a fenestrated Fontan, in which virtually all of the vena caval blood is routed to the pulmonary arteries. A solitary hole 4–5 mm in diameter or multiple holes 2–3 mm in diameter are placed in whatever structure separates the systemic venous pathway from the pulmonary venous pathway. In the latter style, eventual spontaneous closure is the rule; however, some of these patients subsequently develop protein-losing enteropathy and return for surgical creation of a stable fenestration 5 mm in diameter.

An alternative less-than-complete Fontan involves partial hepatic vein exclusion. One hepatic vein, typically the left anterior hepatic vein, can be excluded from the systemic venous pathway when the baffle is placed. This excluded hepatic vein drains into the pulmonary venous pathway. Unfortunately, most patients with partial hepatic vein exclusion eventually return with right hepatic vein-to-left hepatic vein collaterals.

Cardiac transplantation is considered for patients who have undergone the Fontan operation and have developed serious complications and for patients whose hemodynamics make them poor candidates for Fontan operation.

EISENMENGER'S SYNDROME

Definition, Etiology and Pathology

Eisenmenger's syndrome consists of pulmonary hypertension at systemic level due to high pulmonary vascular resistance with reversal or bidirectional shunts at the aortopulmonary, ventricular, or atrial level. Pulmonary vascular obstructive disease refers to the development of intimal fibrosis of smaller pulmonary arteries and arterioles that increases the pulmonary vascular resistance, necessitating higher proximal pulmonary artery pressures to maintain pulmonary flow. Eisenmenger's complex refers to development of the Eisenmenger's syndrome in association with a VSD (Fig. 14.283).

History

Symptoms related specifically to pulmonary hypertension result from the inability to increase pulmonary blood flow in response to physiologic stress. Other symptoms are caused by various multisystem complications associated with cyanotic congenital heart disease. The Dana Point studies offer clinical aspects and diagnostic options, medical treatments, and surgical options.

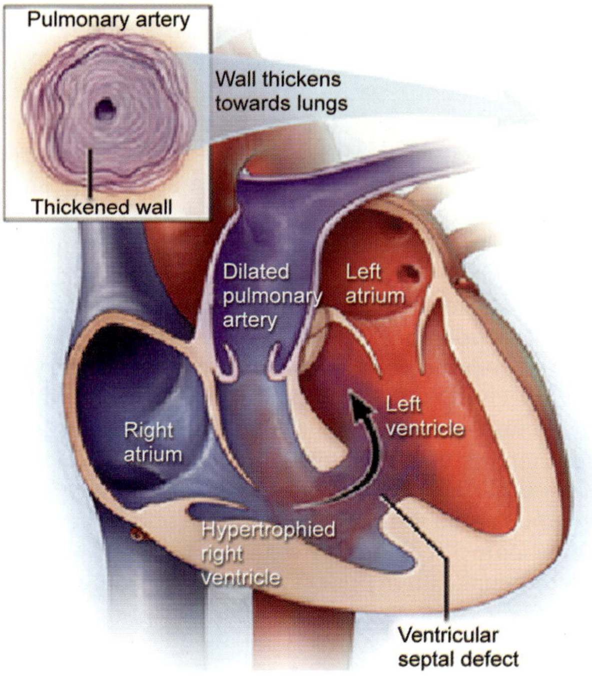

Fig. 14.283: *Diagram explaining the pathogenesis in Eisenmenger syndrome is most often a complication of having a hole (shunt) between two chambers of your heart. Here, a hole between the heart's main pumping chambers (ventricular septal defect) causes increased blood flow to the pulmonary arteries. Eventually, the shunt irreparably damages the walls of your lung's arteries (pulmonary arteries). Eisenmenger syndrome occurs when the pressure in the pulmonary arteries becomes so high that it causes oxygen poor (blue) blood to flow from the right to left ventricle and then to the body, causing cyanosis. The high pressure also causes the walls of your heart's ventricle to thicken (hypertrophy)*

Symptoms

Symptoms of pulmonary hypertension include the following:
- Breathlessness
- Fatigue
- Lethargy
- Severely reduced exercise tolerance with a prolonged recovery phase
- Presyncope
- Syncope

Symptoms of heart failure include the following:
- Exertional dyspnea
- Orthopnea
- Paroxysmal nocturnal dyspnea
- Edema
- Ascites
- Anorexia
- Nausea

Symptoms of erythrocytosis include the following:
- Myalgias
- Muscle weakness
- Anorexia
- Fatigue
- Lassitude
- Paresthesias of the digits and lips
- Tinnitus
- Blurred or double vision
- Scotomata
- Headache
- Dizziness
- Slowed mentation
- Decreased alertness
- Irritability

Symptoms of a tendency toward bleeding include the following:
- Mild mucocutaneous bleeding
- Epistaxis
- Menorrhagia
- Pulmonary hemorrhage

Symptoms of vasodilation include the following:
- Presyncope
- Syncope

Symptoms of cholelithiasis include the following:
- Right upper quadrant pain
- Biliary colic
- Fever
- Pale stools
- Jaundice

Symptoms of nephrolithiasis include the following:
- Renal colic
- Secondary gout
- Joint pain and swelling

Additional symptoms include the following:

Paradoxical embolus can cause symptoms of localized vascular insufficiency end-organ ischemia.

Hypertrophic osteoarthropathy can cause long bone pain and tenderness.

Retinal complications include episodes of transient visual loss and spontaneous hyphemas. Patients who develop Eisenmenger syndrome may be asymptomatic for long periods of time. The elevated pulmonary vascular resistance (PVR) prevents pulmonary overcirculation and the symptoms of heart failure. This can result in a delay in diagnosis.

In the first weeks of life when the PVR begins to fall toward adult levels, an infant with a large atrial septal defect (ASD), ventricular septal defect (VSD), or patent ductus arteriosus (PDA) may present with congestive heart failure symptoms due to the large left-to-right shunt. This may simply be reflected by poor weight gain.

Infants with the same defects who maintain a high PVR have less left-to-right intracardiac shunting and less pulmonary blood flow. Therefore, developing Eisenmenger physiology may remain undetected in infants with a high PVR and relatively large defects because they lack a loud systolic murmur and/or diastolic rumble and the symptoms of heart failure.

Patients may have a period of poor weight gain, reflecting congestive heart failure, that improves as pulmonary pressures increase and overcirculation decreases. Clues to the diagnosis may include only dyspnea upon exertion and exercise intolerance. These symptoms become increasingly evident with advancing age, particularly at adolescence, and may progress to lethargy and syncopal episodes.

Erythrocytosis secondary to chronic cyanosis is an adaptation to low levels of circulating oxyhemoglobin and is present in most patients. Excessive polycythemia may result in hematocrit levels of greater than 65% and hyperviscosity syndrome. Hyperviscosity may lead to thromboembolic events, cerebrovascular complications, gout, chest pain from pulmonary infarction, and hemoptysis. Most of the symptoms are nonspecific and are confirmed if they are relieved by phlebotomy.

Any of the multitude of multisystem complications that occur in patients with congenital heart disease may be present.

Cyanosis and clubbing eventually result from arterial desaturation. Prior to the development of the Eisenmenger's syndrome, the cardiac examination is dominated by the physical findings of the specific left-to-right shunt. As Eisenmenger's syndrome develops, however, findings of pulmonary hypertension dominate the cardiac examination resulting in a prominent jugular venous a wave, right ventricular lift, loud pulmonic component of the second sound (P2), and murmurs of pulmonary regurgitation or tricuspid regurgitation. The second heart sound (S2) may be single or may have fixed splitting with a loud pulmonic component.

Physical Examination

Cardiovascular findings include the following:

1. Central cyanosis (differential cyanosis in the case of a PDA)
2. Clubbing (Figs 14.284 and 14.285)

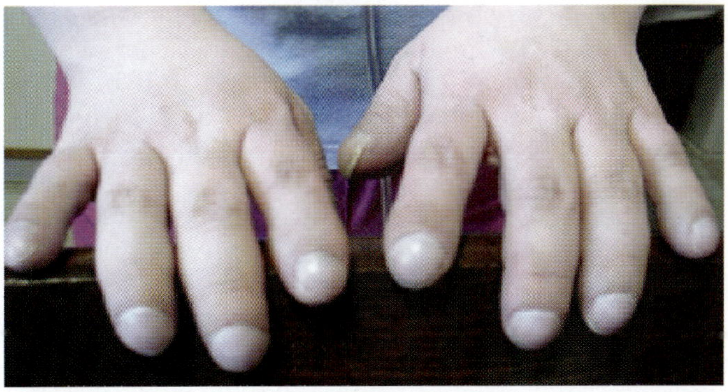

Fig. 14.284: *Showing nail clubbing of fingers in a patient with Eisenmenger's syndrome. First described by Hippocrates, clubbing is also known as "Hippocratic fingers"*

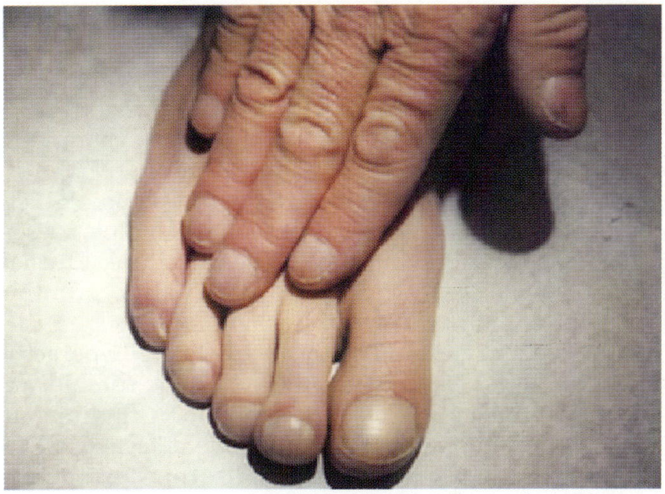

Fig. 14.285: *A patient with unrepaired large PDA, Eisenmenger's syndrome, and right-to-left shunting at the ductal level producing differential cyanosis. The transcutaneous oxygen saturation in the fingers was 92% and in the toes 84%. The central hematocrit was 65%. Clubbing is more apparent in the toes than in the fingers*

3. Jugular venous pulse wave may be A-wave dominant, and, in the presence of a significant tricuspid regurgitation, the V wave may be prominent; central venous pressure may be elevated.
4. Precordial palpation reveals a right ventricular heave and, frequently, a palpable S2.
5. Loud P2
6. High-pitched early diastolic murmur of pulmonic insufficiency
7. Right-sided fourth heart sound
8. Pulmonary ejection click
9. *Single S2:* As the pulmonary vascular resistance progressively rises, the holosystolic murmur of a nonrestrictive VSD shortens and softens, first becoming early systolic in timing before disappearing entirely as the shunt is reversed.
10. The continuous murmur of a PDA disappears when Eisenmenger physiology develops; a short systolic murmur may remain audible.

Other signs of Eisenmenger syndrome include the following:
- *Respiratory signs*—include cyanosis and tachypnea
- *Hematologic signs*—include bruising and bleeding; funduscopic abnormalities related to erythrocytosis include engorged vessels, papilledema, microaneurysms, and blot hemorrhages
- *Abdominal signs*—include jaundice, right upper quadrant tenderness, and positive Murphy sign (acute cholecystitis)
- *Vascular signs*—include postural hypotension and focal ischemia (paradoxical embolus)
- *Musculoskeletal signs*—include clubbing, tenderness over the metacarpal or metatarsal joints (hypertrophic osteoarthropathy), and joint effusions
- *Cutaneous signs*—the skin demonstrates fewer urate deposits than are commonly observed in primary gout
- *Ocular signs*—include conjunctival injection, rubeosis iridis, and retinal hyperviscosity changes.

Clinical Findings in Progressing Disease

Examination findings vary with the progression of the disease. Early in life, infants with a large systemic-to-pulmonary communication may demonstrate mild pulmonary overcirculation with symptoms of cor pulmonale. Initially, cyanosis is absent, and infants present with the signs and symptoms of heart failure. Physical examination may reveal tachypnea, nasal flaring, grunting, retractions and tachycardia.

An ausculatory examination may reveal a hyperactive precordium, systolic flow murmur, diastolic rumble, and hepatosplenomegaly. Cardiac examination findings are determined by the underlying anatomic defects. Delayed capillary refill may be present indicating low cardiac output. As the PVR increases, the pulmonary circulation receives less blood flow, with gradually advancing pulmonary artery pressure. Symptoms of congestive heart failure wane. The right ventricle may become hypertrophied, and the chest, when examined, may be asymmetrical, with a right ventricular heave and a palpable P2 (i.e. a pulmonary closure sound that is so forceful that it can be felt).

As pulmonary resistance increases over time, a relative decrease in the left-to-right intracardiac shunting occurs, initially with periods of subclinical right-to-left and bidirectional shunting, followed by frank cyanosis, clubbing and polycythemia (giving a ruddy appearance to the skin).

A hallmark of Eisenmenger syndrome is this seemingly improved clinical condition, despite the lack of change in therapy for congestive heart failure (Fig. 14.286). It represents a physiologically normalized condition caused by the progressively worsening pulmonary vascular obstructive disease (PVOD), with resolution of pulmonary overcirculation and heart failure.

Diagnostic Considerations

Conditions to consider in the differential diagnosis of Eisenmenger syndrome include the following:
1. Idiopathic pulmonary hypertension
2. Persistent newborn pulmonary hypertension
3. Pulmonary infarction
4. Respiratory failure
5. Tetralogy of Fallot with absent pulmonary valve
6. Tetralogy of Fallot with pulmonary atresia
7. Total anomalous pulmonary venous connection
8. Transposition of the great arteries
9. Tricuspid atresia
10. Truncus arteriosus
11. Ventricular septal defect (VSD)
12. Pulmonary atresia with VSD
13. Single ventricle with pulmonary stenosis.
14. Tetralogy of Fallot.

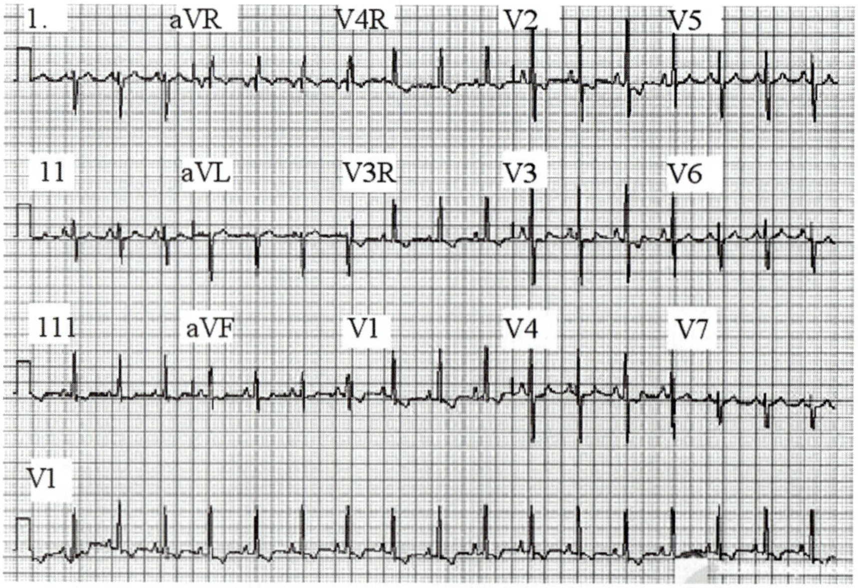

Fig. 14.286: *The tracing shows right axis deviation, right atrial enlargement, right ventricular hypertrophy, and right ventricular strain (inverted T waves in the anterior leads) in a patient with Eisenmenger syndrome*

Differential Diagnoses

1. Pulmonary hypertension, primary
2. Tetralogy of fallot.

Laboratory Studies

1. ***Complete blood count (CBC) findings include the following:***
- Erythrocytosis increases hematocrit and hemoglobin concentration
- Phlebotomy-related iron deficiency decreases the mean corpuscular volume and mean corpuscular hemoglobin concentration
- The red cell mass is increased with erythrocytosis
- Bleeding time is prolonged by platelet dysfunction.

2. ***Biochemical profile findings include the following:***
- Increased conjugated bilirubin
- Increased uric acid
- Urea and creatinine are sometimes elevated
- Urinary biochemical analysis reveals proteinuria
- Erythrocytic hypoglycemia is an artifactually low blood glucose level caused by increased in vitro glycolysis in the setting of increased red cell mass.

3. ***Iron study findings include the following:***
- Reduced serum ferritin due to phlebotomy-related iron store reduction
- Increased total iron binding capacity.

4. ***Additional findings include the following:***
- Pulse oximetry-cyanosis and decreased saturations may be present
- Arterial blood gas (ABG): Reduced resting partial pressure of carbon dioxide ($PaCO_2$) due to resting tachypnea and reduced partial pressure of oxygen (PaO_2) due to right-to-left shunting; mixed respiratory and metabolic acidosis
- Brain natriuretic peptide (BNP): BNP may be a marker for prognosis in pulmonary arterial hypertension (PAH).

Chest Radiography (Fig. 14.287)

In the early stages, chest radiography reveals a typical appearance of increased pulmonary flow with right ventricular or biventricular enlargement, right atrial or biatrial enlargement, pulmonary vascular plethora, and an enlarged main pulmonary artery.

Advancing pulmonary vascular disease appears as a normal cardiac silhouette with dilated main and branch pulmonary arteries without evidence of pulmonary overcirculation. In patients with severe pulmonary vascular disease, radiography reveals a normal-sized heart, pruning of the pulmonary vasculature (i.e. diminished distal/peripheral pulmonary vascularity), pulmonary infarction, and/or calcification of a patent ductus arteriosus (PDA).

Computerized Axial Tomography and MR

Magnetic resonance imaging (MRI) can be used for the following:
- Estimation of the magnitude of the right-to-left shunt
- Anatomical definition (in some cases) (Figs 14.288 to 14.291).

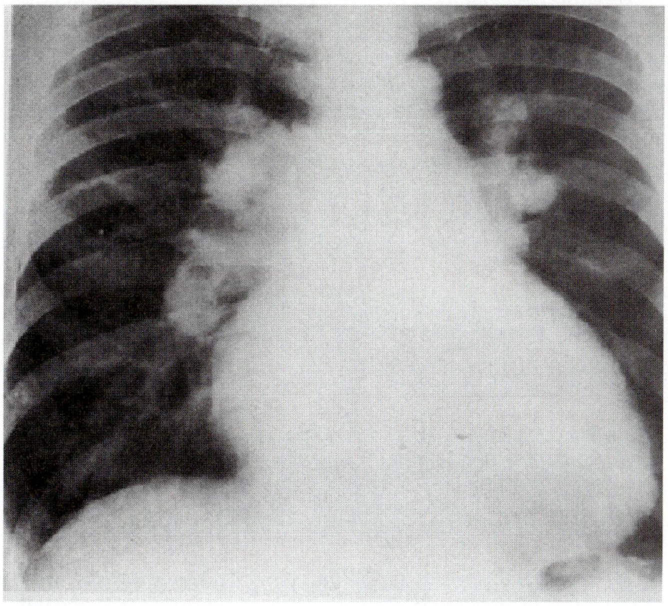

Fig. 14.287: *Atrial septal defect, with elevated pulmonary vascular resistance. Secundum atrial septal defect. There is a larked disparity between the size of the hilar arteries and the peripheral pulmonary vessels, indicating an increase in pulmonary vascular resistance. The right ventricular pressure was almost at systemic levels as seen in Eisenmenger's syndrome*

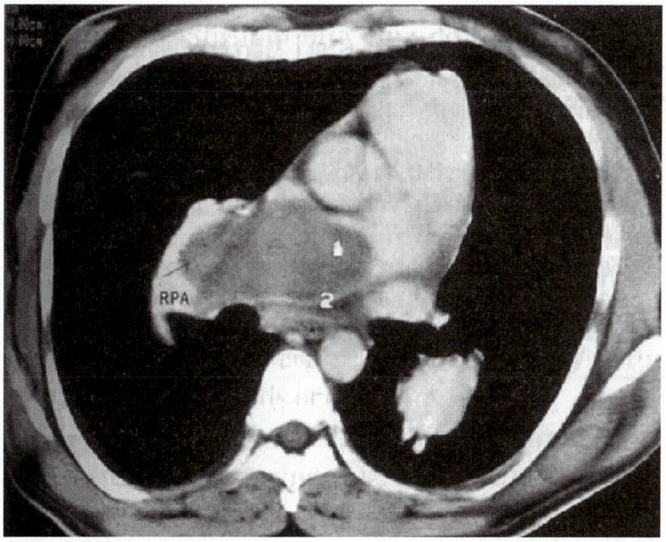

Fig. 14.288: *CT scan of the thorax with contrast injection showing the large MPA lied RPA and a thrombus in the RPA (arrow) in Eisenmenger syndrome*

Echocardiography

Two dimensional (2D) transthoracic imaging can reveal the particular features of the structural cardiac defect responsible for the shunt. Coexistent structural abnormalities can also be identified (Figs 14.292A and B; 14.92A to D; 14.294A to C).

Color-flow Doppler interrogation is useful for demonstrating the direction of intracardiac blood flow.

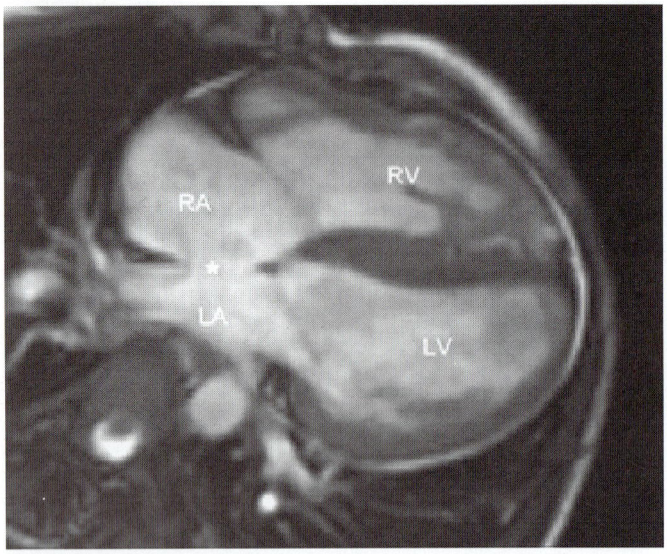

Fig. 14.289: *Secundum ASD (asterisk) in a 17-year-old patient with pulmonary arterial hypertension and cyanosis (Eisenmenger syndrome). Note the RV and RA are not as dilated as the previous patient, but the RV is hypertrophied. Bidirectional shunting across the defect was present. Although the rims were suitable for transcutaneous closure, the procedure was contraindicated given the high pulmonary vascular resistance. The patient was referred for pulmonary vasodilator therapy. LA, left atrium; LV, left ventricle; RA, right atrium; RV, right ventricle*

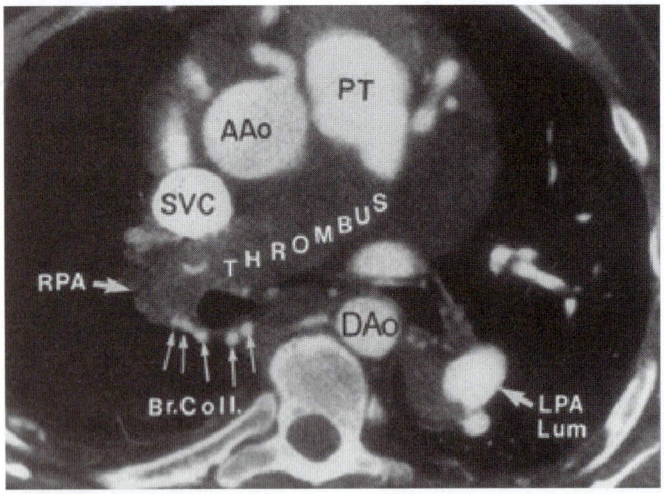

Fig. 290: *Transaxial section from the pulmonary CTA of a 34-year-old man with Eisenmenger syndrome and a nonrestrictive VSD. Massive thrombus extended from a virtually occluded pulmonary trunk (PT) into both the right pulmonary artery (RPA) and left pulmonary artery (LPA). Five vertical arrows, bronchial collateral arteries (Br Coll). SVC, superior vena cava*

Pulsed and continuous wave doppler measurements permit quantification of the intracardiac shunt, right ventricular pressures, and estimation of pulmonary artery systolic/diastolic and mean pressures by means of the modified Bernoulli equation. Echocardiography can also be used to identify surgical systemic-to-pulmonary shunts.

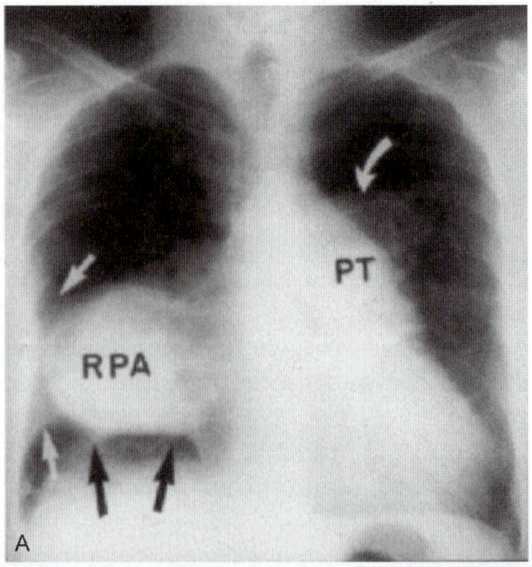

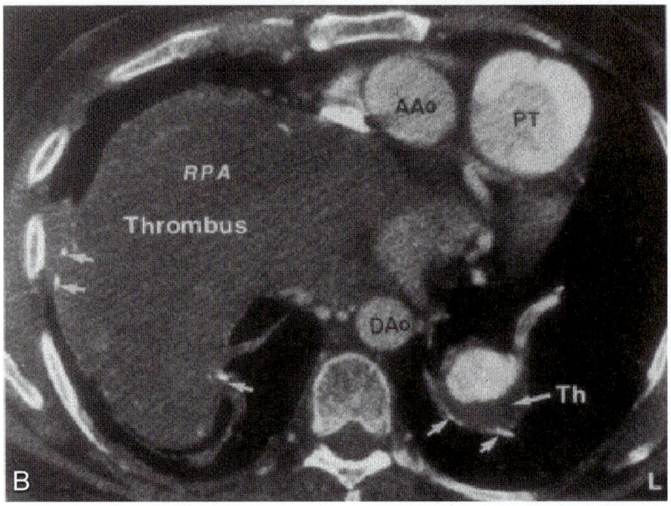

Figs 14.291A and B: *Posteroanterior chest X-ray from a patient with Eisenmenger syndrome and a nonrestrictive perimembranous VSD. (A) An aneurysmal right pulmonary artery (RPA) compressed the middle lobe bronchus causing atelectasis (paired white arrows) and elevation of the right hemidiaphragm (paired black arrows). The pulmonary trunk (PT) and left pulmonary artery (curved white arrow) are also aneurysmal. (B) A transaxial section from the pulmonary CTA of the same patient showing massive thrombus completely occluding the aneurysmal RPA. Extension of thrombus into the right and left branches caused asphyxic death. There is a paucity of calcification (arrows) in the wall of the aneurysmal RPA. An enlarged left intrapulmonary artery also contained thrombus (Th) and a thin rim of calcification (paired arrows). AAo = ascending aorta; DAo = descending aorta.*

The addition of supine bicycle ergometry can demonstrate increased right-to-left shunting with exercise.

Transesophageal Echocardiography

Transesophageal echocardiography is useful for imaging posterior structures including the atria and pulmonary veins.

Electrocardiography (Fig. 14.286)

Electrocardiographic findings are almost always abnormal in Eisenmenger syndrome. They include the following:

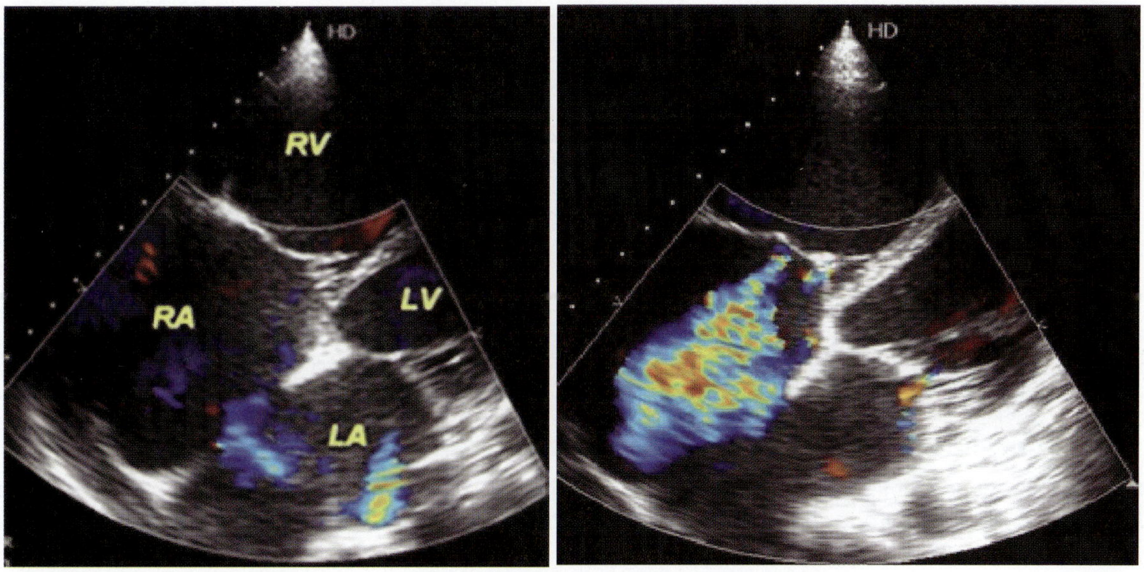

Figs 14.292A and B: *Upper panel Color Doppler echocardiography shows reversal of flow across ASD secundum lower panel shows gross TR with raised pulmonary artery pressure in an adolescent with Eisenmenger syndrome*

signs of right heart hypertrophy, in addition to abnormalities associated with the underlying defect

1. Frontal plane QRS right axis deviation
2. Tall monophasic R wave in V1, deep S wave in V6, ± ST and T wave abnormalities
3. P pulmonale.

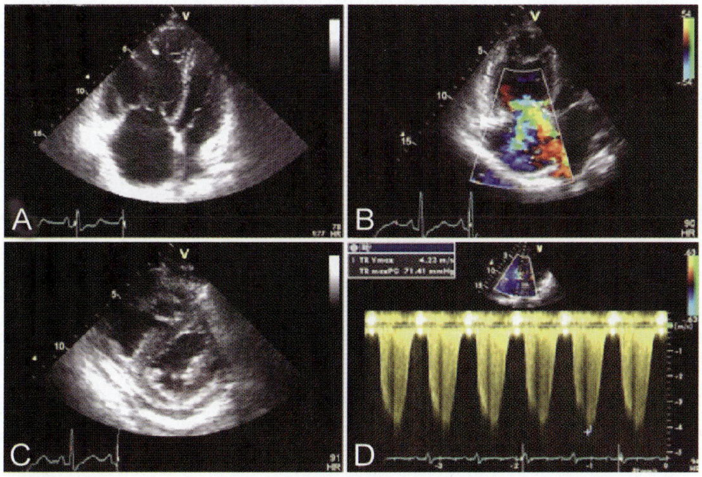

Figs 14.293A to D: *Color Doppler echocardiography in pulmonary hypertension as seen in Eisenmenger syndrome (A-D) echocardiography in a patient with portopulmonary PAH. (A and B) apical four chamber view and parasternal short-axis view showing an enlarged and hypertrophic right ventricle and a flattened interventricular septum, compromising the left ventricle. Pericardial effusion is present, a predictor of worse outcome. (C and D) Significant tricuspid regurgitation with a flow velocity of 4.23 m/sec in accordance with a pulmonary artery pressure of 71.4 mmHg + right atrial pressure)*

Six-minute Walk Test Versus Cardiopulmonary Exercise Test

The 6-minute walk test (6MWT), which requires minimal equipment and subspecialty experience, is simpler than the more formal and involved traditional cardiopulmonary exercise test (CPET).

Moreover, the 6MWT is better tolerated in younger children, who often will not comply with the multiple leads, facemask, or other equipment needed for a CPET.

The 6MWT may be effective in patients with a walk distance of less than 300 m. In patients above the 300 m threshold, however, a CPET should be considered.

Cardiac Catheterization

Cardiac catheterization can be of value, after collecting clinical and noninvasive data, to confirm and/or demonstrate the following:

1. Severity of PAH
2. Conduit patency and pressure gradient
3. Coexisting coronary artery anomalies (rare)
4. Degree of shunting

Cardiac catheterization permits the examination of the intracardiac structure and exclusion of potentially reversible causes of pulmonary hypertension, as well as assessment of ventricular function (systolic and diastolic), examination of the intracardiac shunt, determination of pulmonary artery pressure and flow, and calculation of pulmonary vascular resistance (PVR).

Approach Considerations

The treatment of Eisenmenger syndrome varies widely and depends on the patient's age, degree of cyanosis, and subsequent polycythemia. Asymptomatic patients require periodic evaluation with anticipation of potential needs. All patients with intracardiac right-to-left shunts have potential for the following:

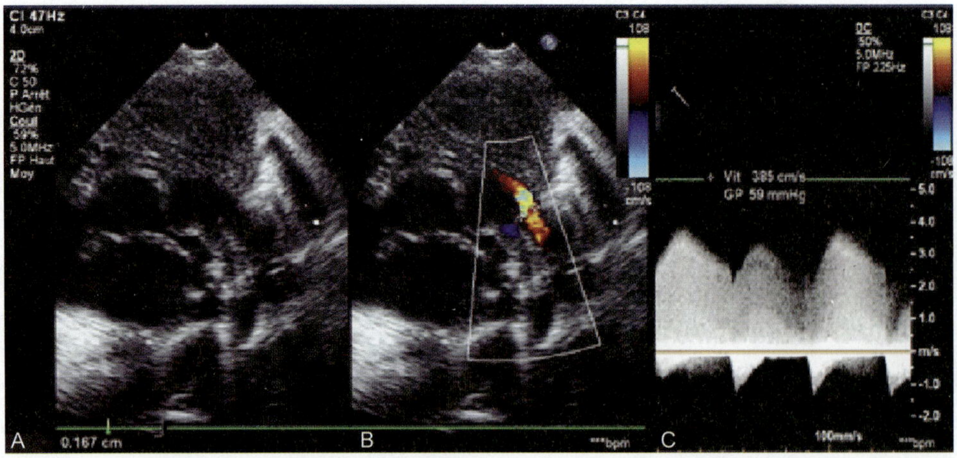

Figs 14.294A to C: *Echocardiogram showing patent ductus arteriosus. (A) two dimensional image of patent ductus arteriosus. (B) colour Doppler flow showing retrograde flow in the pulmonary trunk. (C) spectral Doppler of continuous ductal flow, enabling measurement of a systolic pressure gradient of 59 mmHg*

1. Syncope, paradoxical embolus, stroke, brain abscess and sudden death
2. Polycythemia, hemoptysis and pulmonary infarction
3. Congestive heart failure
4. *Endocarditis:* Much of the therapy currently used for Eisenmenger syndrome has been studied in the treatment of idiopathic pulmonary arterial hypertension (IPAH). Numerous review articles are available on the subject. Because of the similarities between these entities, therapies found useful in patients with IPAH are very attractive for use in.
5. Eisenmenger physiology
6. *Fluid balance and climate control:* Patients should avoid sudden fluid shifts or dehydration, which may increase right-to-left shunting. They should also avoid very hot or humid conditions, which may exacerbate vasodilation, causing syncope and increased right-to-left shunting.
7. *Right heart failure:* Right heart failure is often present in patients with Eisenmenger syndrome, but limited treatment options are available for this complication. Typically, digoxin and diuretics have been used. Diuretics, specifically loop diuretics, are used for symptomatic relief of congestion. However, diuretics should be used cautiously in these patients, given their preload-dependent state.
8. *CNS events:* Central nervous system (CNS) events can occur secondary to paradoxical embolus, CNS venous thrombosis, intracranial hemorrhage, or brain abscesses in the setting of endocarditis. Endocarditis prophylaxis, the use of air filters with all intravenous catheters during hospital admissions, and adequate management of hyperviscosity can help to decrease these potentially fatal complications.

Surgical Intervention

Surgical palliation or repair should be performed early in patients with congenital heart disease to prevent progression to Eisenmenger syndrome. No surgical care is available to correct the congenital cardiac defect that caused the pathologic pulmonary vascular changes once Eisenmenger syndrome has developed to the irreversible stage.

For patients with systemic or suprasystemic pulmonary artery pressures and impending right ventricular failure, creation of an atrial septal defect (ASD) can be palliative. For example, a patient with an increased pulmonary vascular resistance (PVR) secondary to pulmonary vein obstruction may benefit from a surgical ASD to serve as "pop-off" for the right ventricle.

Heart-lung transplantation and single or bilateral, sequential lung transplantation with or without repair of relatively simple congenital cardiovascular anomalies, are viable transplant procedures and are the only surgical options for a patient with Eisenmenger syndrome.

Inpatient Care

Patients do not require hospitalization for therapeutic erythropheresis but may need attention for infectious disease complications and/or other hematologic concerns. Initiation of vasodilator therapy may require inpatient hospitalization and observation.

Follow-up

Patients should follow-up at a specialized cardiology clinic within 2 weeks of discharge from inpatient care and every 3 months when stable.

Transfer

Nonurgent transfers are made to a tertiary facility because this disease, by nature, is a chronic and terminal condition.

Air Travel

For patients with Eisenmenger syndrome, air travel carries the risk of deep venous thrombosis, especially since this group of patients is predisposed to thrombotic events, and compromised oxygen delivery at high altitudes. Nonetheless, a study comparing the 10-year air travel history of 48 acyanotic patients with that of 53 patients with Eisenmenger syndrome found no major adverse events in either group. (One patient in the Eisenmenger group had a probable transient ischemic attack and another required supplemental oxygen after exposure to ambient cigarette smoke in flight.) This study indicated that patients with Eisenmenger syndrome can fly frequently and safely. It is recommended, however, that these patients avoid dehydration and inactivity during travel.

Tobacco and Alcohol Use

Smoking is absolutely contraindicated in patients with Eisenmenger syndrome because of the deleterious effects on the heart, blood vessels and lungs.

Alcohol may exacerbate myocardial dysfunction, hypovolemia, and worsening hyperviscosity and can result in systemic hypotension with an exacerbation of the right-to-left shunt.

Oxygen Therapy

The use of oxygen supplementation in patients with Eisenmenger syndrome is controversial. It has been shown to have no impact on exercise capacity and survival in adult patients with this condition.

Some patients, however, may benefit from nocturnal supplementation although oxygen therapy is most useful as a bridge to heart-lung transplant.

Air travel appears to be safe as long as the airplanes are adequately pressurized. Supplemental oxygen during commercial air travel is often recommended, but limited data exist regarding this issue.

Pulmonary Vasodilator Therapy

Studies of patients with IPAH have shown an imbalance between vasoconstrictors (endothelin, thromboxane) and vasodilators (prostacyclin, nitric oxide) in the pulmonary vasculature, and current therapy is directed at correcting this imbalance. Vasodilator studies for IPAH (most of which have been performed in adults) have revealed a significant improvement in exercise tolerance, 6-minute walk distance, or New York Heart Association (NYHA) class. Subgroups, as well as smaller studies, have shown improvement in pulmonary hypertension caused by congenital heart disease.

The pathophysiology of pulmonary hypertension in patients with Eisenmenger syndrome is somewhat similar to that of IPAH; both are associated with a neurohormonal imbalance of endogenous pulmonary vasodilators and vasoconstrictors. This imbalance leads to vascular remodeling, intimal fibrosis, and increased pulmonary vascular resistance (PVR). Therefore, in the management of patients with Eisenmenger syndrome, the use of pulmonary vasodilating agents that have been shown to be useful in the management of patients with IPAH is conceptually appealing; data support this use.

Prostacyclins

Long-term prostacyclin therapy was shown to improve hemodynamics (decrease in mean pulmonary artery pressure, improvement in cardiac index, decrease in PVR) and the quality of life in patients with congenital heart disease and pulmonary arterial hypertension (PAH).

Another study evaluated epoprostenol infusion in adolescents with congenital heart disease and Eisenmenger physiology. The report showed improved oxygenation (from 69% to 85%) and improvement in a 6-minute walk test (6 MWT) distance (from 48 yd to 375 yd).

Epoprostenol requires a continuous intravenous infusion via a central catheter because of its short half-life (5 min). Patients must carry a portable pump in a waist pack and must maintain the drug at a cool temperature during the infusion. It has been shown to improve pulmonary pressure, 6MWT distance, oxygenation, and quality of life in patients. New therapies my allow discontinuation of this cumbersome medication.

Treprostinil is a prostacyclin analogue that is administered by continuous subcutaneous infusion. Data on its use in children with pulmonary hypertension are limited.

Iloprost is an inhaled prostacyclin administered intermittently 6–9 times daily via nebulizer and is approved for adults with IPAH. Preliminary evidence suggests that it may have efficacy in children with pulmonary hypertension due to cardiac lesions; however, it may cause bronchospasms, and its use may be limited.

Endothelin Receptor Antagonists

Bosentan, an endothelin receptor antagonist that has been approved for patients with IPAH, was the second vasodilator to be evaluated in patients with Eisenmenger syndrome. In a small, retrospective study of 9 patients with congenital heart disease and Eisenmenger syndrome, bosentan therapy resulted in improved oxygen saturation (from 79% to 88%) and improved NYHA class.

A larger, multicenter, prospective study by Schulze-Neick et al also demonstrated the effectiveness of bosentan. In this study, bosentan titrated to 125 mg and taken orally twice daily was associated with improvement in 6MWT distance (362–434 m), improvement in NYHA class (3.1–2.4), and a decrease in systolic pulmonary artery pressure (111–106 mmHg)

A multicenter, prospective, double-blind, placebo-controlled study [the Bosentan Randomized Trial of Endothelin Antagonist Therapy-5 (BREATH-5) study] found that bosentan reduced the mean pulmonary arterial pressure and improved exercise capacity and World Health Organization (WHO) class. The study tested the effect of bosentan titrated to 125 mg bid in 54 patients with Eisenmenger syndrome. A longer follow-up study in the BREATH-5 population (up to 40 week) showed that bosentan remained safe and had a positive impact on patients with Eisenmenger syndrome. Data have been emerging on the use of bosentan in children.

Ambrisentan, which has been approved for IPAH, is a specific endothelium receptor-1 type A antagonist. Data on its use in Eisenmenger syndrome are limited. A retrospective study that examined the outcomes of patients with Eisenmenger syndrome who were treated with pulmonary vasodilators versus those who were not showed that treatment with prostacyclin analogues and/or endothelin receptor antagonists delayed the need for transplantation.

Phosphodiesterase Inhibitors

Sildenafil, another vasodilatory agent, was originally used for erectile dysfunction but has since been approved by the US Food and Drug Administration (USFDA) for IPAH. It acts as an inhibitor of phosphodiesterase 5, resulting in an increase in cyclic guanosine monophosphate (cGMP) and vascular relaxation. It works synergistically with inhaled nitric oxide.

Studies suggest that sildenafil is safe and effective in patients with Eisenmenger syndrome. In a randomized, placebo-controlled study of 20 patients with PAH (10 patients with Eisenmenger syndrome and 10 with IPAH), sildenafil improved the patients' NYHA class, 6 MWT distance, and exercise duration. Furthermore, sildenafil therapy resulted in a decrease in systolic pulmonary arterial pressure from 98 mmHg to 78 mmHg. The effects of the drug were similar for the two patient populations in this study.

In a study by Chau et al., sildenafil improved hemodynamics and symptoms in patients with pulmonary hypertension secondary to Eisenmenger syndrome and a similar group of patients with idiopathic arterial hypertension.

In a study from India, another phosphodiesterase inhibitor, tadalafil, was shown to be safe and effective in 16 symptomatic patients with Eisenmenger syndrome. Tadalafil improved oxygen saturation (84–89% at 12 weeks), and the mean WHO class (2.31–1.25). It has been approved by the FDA for the once-daily treatment of patients with group 1 PAH.

Nitric Oxide Replacement

Innovative home nitric oxide delivery devices have been described and have been used on a compassionate basis in patients with severe pulmonary hypertension.

In summary, vasodilator therapy improves symptoms in patients with Eisenmenger syndrome and should be used routinely in the management of this patient population. However, a single medical therapy has not been consistently shown to reduce mortality in patients with Eisenmenger syndrome.

Endocarditis

Patients with Eisenmenger syndrome are at very high risk for endocarditis. Endocarditis prophylaxis should be emphasized, and patients should be given repeat instructions about this issue. For standard, general prophylaxis for dental, oral, respiratory tract, esophageal, genitourinary, and gastrointestinal procedures, refer to the American Heart Association recommendations for the prevention of bacterial endocarditis.

Infective endocarditis prophylaxis (nonchemotherapeutic) includes the following:

1. Encourage good oral hygiene: Soft-bristle toothbrushing twice a day; mouthwash or hydrogen peroxide rinses; soft, conical, rubber gum stimulator; and semiannual dental visits
2. Skin care advice should include using a nonabrasive cleanser and avoidance of squeezing skin
3. Nail biting should be avoided.

Erythrocytosis

Erythrocytosis is almost always present in patients with Eisenmenger syndrome. This can result in symptoms of hyperviscosity including visual disturbances, fatigue, headache, dizziness and paresthesias. Routine phlebotomy is not usually recommended for this condition, except in the presence of hyperviscosity symptoms. Before initiating phlebotomy, dehydration must be ruled out, since it can falsely increase the hematocrit level. Phlebotomy should always be performed with concomitant fluid replacement.

Repeated phlebotomy can result in iron deficiency anemia. Patients with iron deficiency have an apparently normal hematocrit level and a low mean corpuscular volume (MCV). The iron-deficient erythrocytes are less deformable than normal erythrocytes, and this lack of deformability can worsen hyperviscosity.

A small study found that iron deficiency was associated with a higher risk of adverse outcome in patients with Eisenmenger syndrome.

To manage erythrocytosis, first rule out dehydration. Then, if the patient has symptoms of hyperviscosity and the hematocrit level is greater than 65%, venesect 250–500 mL of blood and replace it with an equivalent volume of isotonic sodium chloride (or 5% dextrose if in heart failure).

Thrombotic and Bleeding Complications

Patients with Eisenmenger syndrome are prone to thrombotic events as part of their hyperviscosity. At the same time, they are susceptible to bleeding because their platelets are dysfunctional. Therefore, patients who have a hematocrit level greater than 65% and are undergoing noncardiac surgery should receive phlebotomy and concomitant fluid replacement in order to decrease the risk of thrombotic and bleeding events.

Anticoagulation

Silversides et al reported that the incidence of proximal pulmonary artery thrombus in patients with Eisenmenger syndrome is 21%. However, although an increased risk of thrombosis is observed in patients with Eisenmenger syndrome, an increased risk of bleeding and pulmonary hemorrhage is also recognized. Thus, anticoagulation is still not routinely recommended for these patients.

A small study found that oral anticoagulation is a factor in iron deficiency in patients with Eisenmenger syndrome.

The results suggested that patients with Eisenmenger syndrome who are receiving anticoagulation therapy should be rigorously monitored for iron deficiency. In patients with low oxygen saturation, careful iron substitution is indicated to avoid hemoglobin levels that are too high.

Contraception, Pregnancy, and Genetic Counseling

Among pregnant women with Eisenmenger syndrome, the fetal mortality rate is approximately 25% and the maternal mortality rate is about 50%. Pregnancy should therefore be avoided by women with Eisenmenger syndrome. Tubal ligation is strongly recommended for this patient group.

If patients refuse tubal ligation, hormone therapy (controlled release levonorgestrel or norethindrone and ethinyl estradiol preparations) is preferred over intrauterine devices, which can cause significant menorrhagia and potentially increase the risk of endocarditis. Therapeutic abortion is recommended for women in the early stages of pregnancy.

The risk of congenital heart defects in offspring of women with Eisenmenger syndrome is approximately 10%, although, depending on the primary natural cardiac defect, it is sometimes higher. Fetal echocardiography is recommended for pregnant patients or siblings.

For resuscitation in the event of massive, acute bleeding, replace losses with fresh frozen plasma, cryoprecipitate, and platelets.

Maternal Considerations in Pregnancy

Despite the fact that more women with congenital heart disease than ever before are reaching reproductive age, maternal mortality rates in patients with congenital heart disease have not improved in the last 50 years and pregnancy is absolutely contraindicated in the Eisenmenger syndrome.

Although the maternal mortality rate in Eisenmenger syndrome ranges from 23–52% in different series, most experienced physicians estimate that the mortality rate is in excess of 50%. The most critical time is postpartum, and the majority of deaths occur in the first week.

Factors that increase the risk of a peripartum death include the following:

1. Congestive heart failure
2. Sudden increases in pulmonary vascular resistance (PVR) or decreases in systemic vascular resistance (SVR)
3. Bleeding/anemia
4. Hematocrit greater than 60%
5. Oxygen saturation less than 80%
6. Syncope
7. Excessive straining should be avoided during the second stage of labor. Therefore, assisted delivery usually is recommended. Cesarean delivery, however, carries a higher mortality rate and should be reserved for obstetric indications, such as cephalopelvic disproportion.
8. The use of anticoagulants is controversial. The rationale for anticoagulation is that the risk of clotting during pregnancy is increased when associated with preexisting cyanosis. However, reports indicate that anticoagulation has contributed to mortality in several patients.

If anticoagulants are used, a suggested protocol is heparin until 12 hours predelivery, then warfarin from 48 hours postdelivery to the end of the puerperium. At the minimum, ensure proper leg care, use of elastic bandages, sufficient hydration, and early mobilization to prevent deep venous thrombosis.

Fetal Considerations

The main risks to the fetus include arterial oxygen desaturation, hypoxemia and polycythemia. The fetal mortality rate ranges from 7.8–28%, and only 15% of babies are born at term.

Transplantation

1. *Heart-lung Transplantation*

Heart-lung transplantation is the procedure of choice if repair of the underlying cardiac defect is not possible in Eisenmenger syndrome. This procedure was performed successfully for the first time in 1981. Since then, the outcome has improved due to better immunosuppressive therapy, new antiviral agents, and improved patient selection.

Reported actuarial survival rates are 68% at 1 year, 43% at 5 years, and 23% at 10 years. The main complications are infection, rejection, and obliterative bronchiolitis.

2. *Bilateral Lung Transplantation*

Repair of the underlying cardiac defect is required, but bilateral lung transplantation is considered the preferable procedure if the cardiac defect is simple.

Bilateral lung transplantation is better than single-lung transplantation in terms of mortality, New York Heart Association functional class, cardiac output, and postoperative pulmonary edema.

Advantages of this procedure over heart-lung grafting include no transplant coronary artery disease or cardiac rejection. Bilateral lung transplantation may be considered as an option in current times of donor organ shortage, although exact indications have yet to be defined.

Outcomes

Excellent results can be obtained with transplantation, with return to normal pulmonary function. However, several donor-specific issues complicate the use of transplantation. Fewer donors are acceptable for lung or heart-lung donation than heart donation alone.

In addition, the strategy for transplanting organs from oversized donors is limited in heart-lung transplantation. A weight mismatch of over 20% is generally a contra-indication for heart-lung transplants.

Five-year and 10-year survival rates are markedly lower in patients who receive heart-lung transplantation than they are in those who undergo heart transplantation alone.

Corrective Surgery

Repair of the primary defect is contraindicated in the context of established severe pulmonary arterial hypertension (PAH). However, corrective surgery may be possible in certain cases if a significant degree of left-to-right shunting remains and if responsiveness of the pulmonary circulation to vasodilator therapy can be demonstrated. Limitations include a transient, dynamic right ventricular outflow tract obstruction, and exact indications for this approach have not yet been defined.

Diet and Activity

Diet

Patients with right-sided congestive heart failure should follow a no-salt-added or salt-restricted diet. However, sodium restriction must be balanced against the need to maintain intravascular volume.

Attention to weight control is important because excess weight places additional strain on the cardiovascular system. In addition, significant obesity is a contraindication to transplantation.

Activity

Intense athletic activities carry the risk of sudden death in patients with Eisenmenger syndrome. Patients should not participate in competitive sports. In certain patients, an exercise prescription can be individualized based on exercise testing that documents a level of activity that meets the following three criteria:

1. Oxygen saturations remain greater than 80%
2. No symptomatic arrhythmias occur
3. No evidence of symptomatic ventricular dysfunction is present.

Scuba diving is contraindicated in any patients with an intracardiac shunt. Even patients with a predominant left-to-right shunt run the risk of transient right-to-left shunts and air embolism.

Deterrence and Prevention

Prevention of Eisenmenger syndrome is critical. When recognized in a timely fashion, congenital cardiac defects can be effectively treated with minimal morbidity and mortality. Eisenmenger syndrome is, by definition, an untreated lesion that has progressed to the point of inoperability.

Many congenital heart defects can be identified in utero when families receive appropriate prenatal care. Continued perinatal care and routine follow-up with a qualified pediatrician lead to the identification of most lesions that are not identified prenatally.

Complications of Eisenmenger syndrome can be discouraged with the following measures:

1. Patients should receive instruction regarding infective endocarditis risk reduction
2. Patients should avoid situations that exacerbate vasodilation
3. Patients should avoid abrupt, strenuous, or isometric exercise
4. Activities that may result in further oxygen desaturation, symptomatic arrhythmias, or right ventricular dysfunction should be restricted
5. Steady-state exercise should be stopped at the onset of symptoms
6. Good dental hygiene should be followed to prevent infectious concerns, such as infective endocarditis and brain abscess.

Consultations

In the course of therapy, the following consultations may be appropriate:

Hematologist: To assist with therapeutic phlebotomy, coagulopathy, and bleeding diatheses secondary to hyperviscosity, polycythemia, and platelet dysfunction or thrombocytopenia.

Nephrologist: To assist with patients who are hyper-uricosuric and, ultimately, to assist with management problems in patients with congestive heart failure, poor cardiac output, decreased renal blood flow, and coincident renal insufficiency in its terminal stages.

Infectious disease specialist: Management of potential bacteriologic complications (e.g. endocarditis, brain abscess).

Surgeon: Placement of central venous access devices for use in long-term treatment of endocarditis or therapeutic phlebotomies.

Cardiologist: For optimal inpatient and outpatient treatment of patients who require a cardiologist with a special interest in congenital cardiology; enrollment in clinical trials may be required for access to newer treatment modalities.

Cardiothoracic surgeon: Evaluation for heart-lung transplantation or lesion repair with lung transplantation.

MARFAN SYNDROME AND CARDIOVASCULAR ABNORMALITIES

Cardiovascular (heart and blood vessel) problems are common in people with Marfan syndrome. In fact, 9 out of 10 people with Marfan syndrome experience cardiovascular problems. The most serious problem is enlargement of the aorta (the main blood vessel that carries blood away from the heart). Heart valves can also be affected. Less often, people have problems in blood vessels other than the aorta.

Types of Cardiovascular Problems

1. Aortic dilation and aortic aneurysms
2. Aortic dissection
3. Mitral valve prolapse
4. Aortic regurgitation
5. Aortic dilation and aortic aneurysms

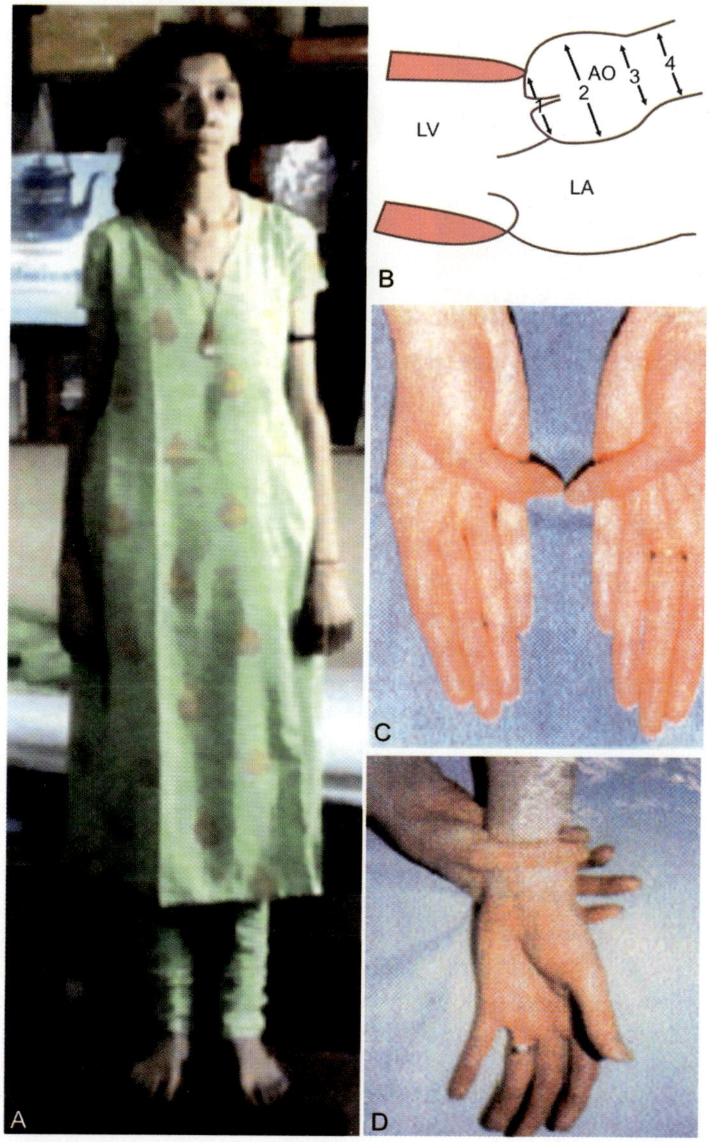

Fig. 14.295: *20-year-old female adolescent with Marfanoid syndrome, (A) clinically, tall, thin body with long upper extremities, and pectus excavatum; (B) Aortic dimension; (C) and (D) show arachnodactyly*

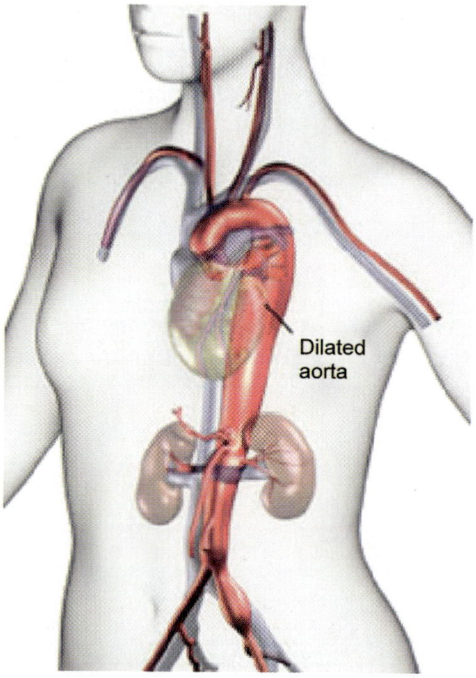

Fig. 14.296: *Diagram showing thoracic aortic aneurysm in Marfanoid syndrome*

These are very serious cardiovascular problems because a significantly enlarged aorta is at risk for dissection (tear) or rupture. Aortic dilation (enlarged aorta) and aortic aneurysms (bulging sides of the aorta) can occur along any segment of the aorta. For most people with Marfan syndrome, the problem starts in the aortic root (aortic segment closest to the heart).

Doctors use a person's age, height, and weight to determine whether the aorta is enlarged. For this reason, people with Marfan syndrome should talk with their doctors about what size aorta is within normal limits for them.

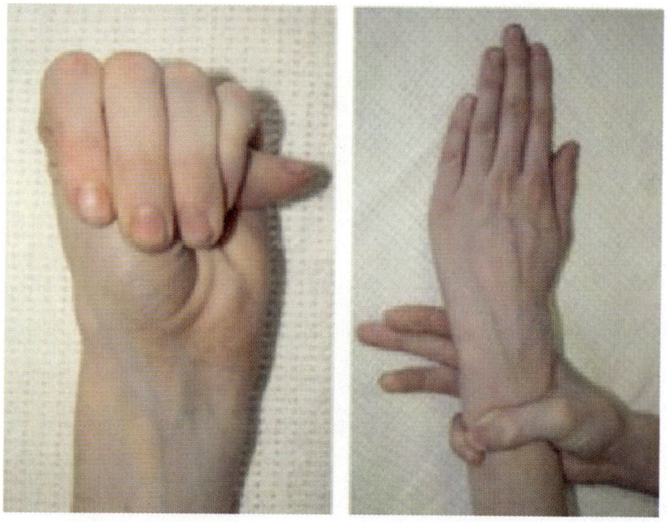

Fig. 14.297: *Photograph showing the "thumb and wrist sign" in Marfan syndrome*

Skin Elasicity in Marfan syndrome

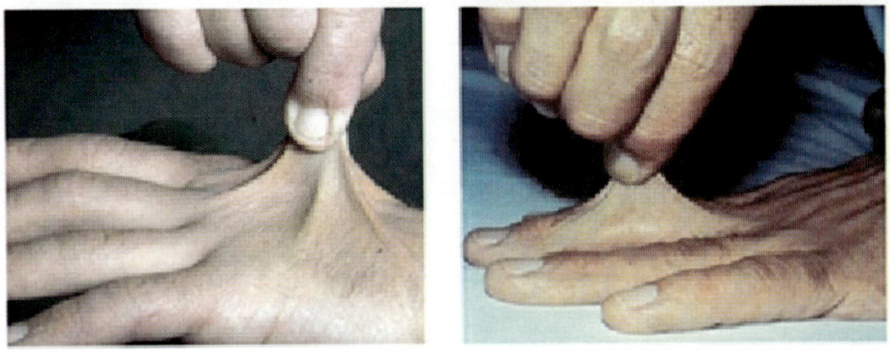

Hand mobility in Marfan syndrome

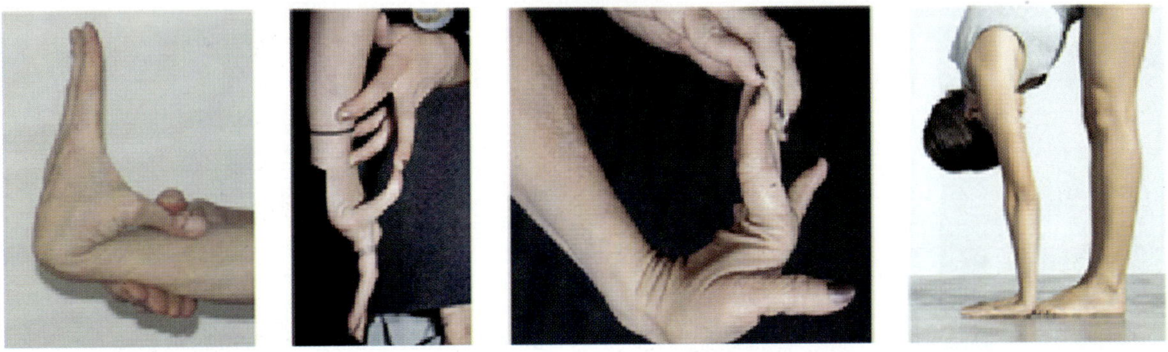

Fig. 14.298: *Diagrams showing extreme flexibility of both fingers and wrist in Marfan syndrome*

Aortic Dissection

This happens when there is a tear between layers of the aorta. Most people know when this happens because of severe pain in the center of their chest, abdomen (stomach), or back. The pain may be "severe", "sharp", "tearing", or "ripping" and may travel from the chest to the back and/or abdomen. Sometimes, the pain is less severe, but a person still has a feeling that "something is very wrong". If a dissection is suspected, a person needs to go to a hospital emergency room right away. There are two types of aortic dissection:

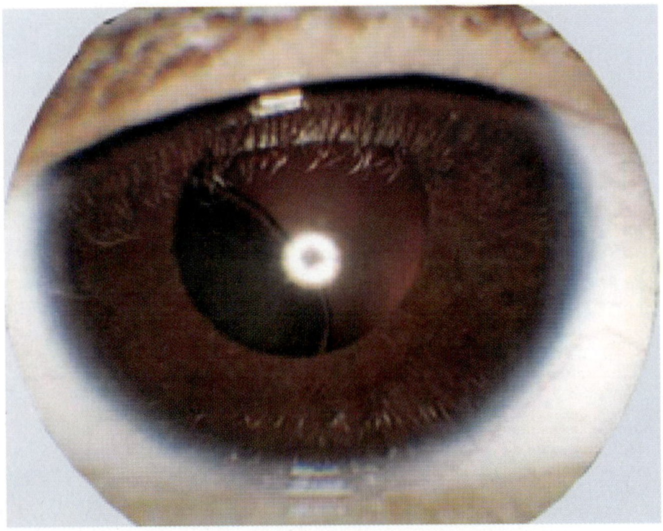

Fig. 14.299: *Photograph showing ectopia lentis in Marfan syndrome*

1. *Dissection of the ascending aorta:* This is the most common dissection in Marfan syndrome. It is life-threatening (people can die if not treated right away). If this kind of dissection happens, people need immediate surgery.
2. *Descending aortic dissection:* This can often be managed just with medication and monitoring (watching). People only need surgery if they have serious complications. These include loss of blood flow to vital organs or an aorta that is severely dilated.

Mitral Valve Prolapse

This is a "billowing" (motion) of the mitral valve when the heart contracts. Symptoms can include irregular or rapid heartbeats and shortness of breath. Some people also have mitral valve regurgitation (leaking of the mitral valve). A small amount of leaking is often not a problem, but a person may need surgery if the mitral valve leaks a lot.

Aortic Regurgitation

This is when the aortic valve does not fully close and blood leaks back into the heart. The only symptoms a person may

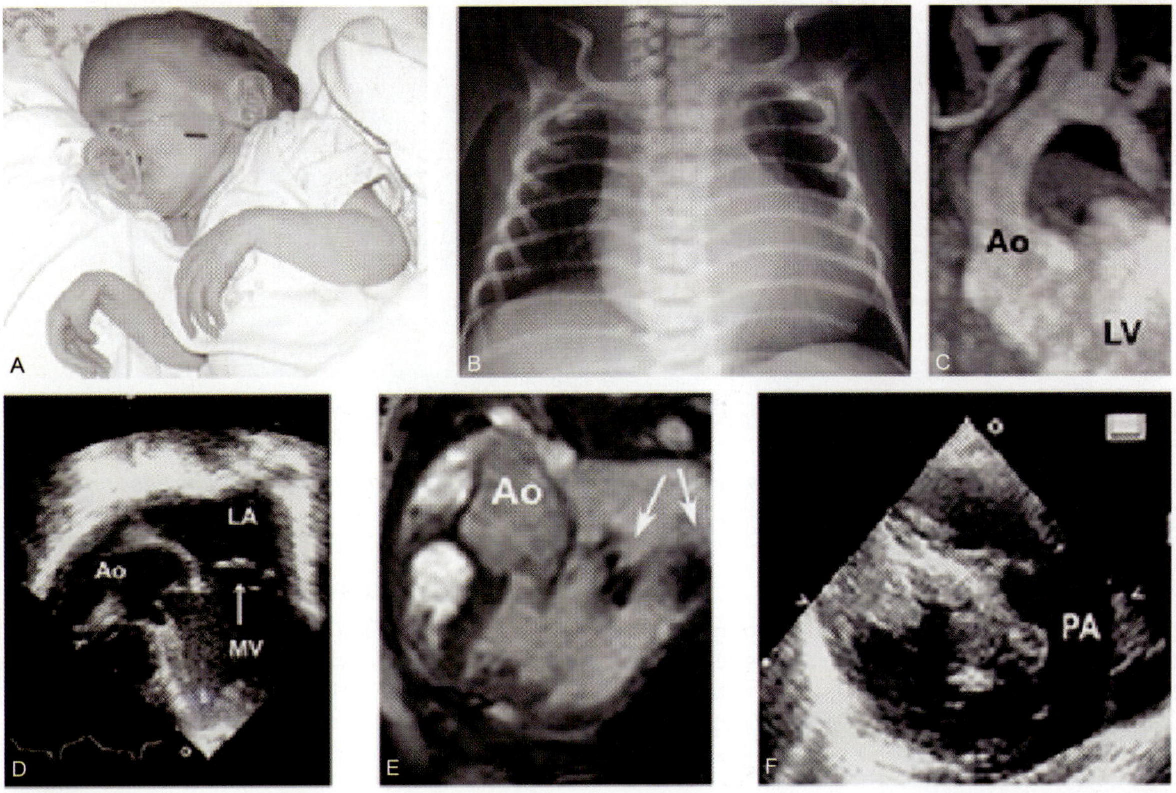

Fig. 14.300: *Neonatal Marfan syndrome: the patient had dolichocephaly, frontal bossing, deep sunken eyes and simplified ears as well as redundant skin at the neck and pronounced arachnodactyly (A). Chest X-Ray at birth demonstrates cardiomegaly, thin ribs, scoliosis and eventration of the right hemidiaphragm (B). Magnetic resonance angiogram (MRA) demonstrates a markedly dilated aortic root at the sinuses of Valsalva, while the ascending aorta, aortic arch and major arch branches are of normal caliber (C). two-dimensional echocardiography from the four-chamber view and short-axis parasternal view demonstrate a dilated aortic root, prolapsing mitral valve and dilated pulmonary trunk, respectively (D and F). Magnetic resonance imaging from bright-blood cine loops demonstrate a complex, regurgitant jet characterized by dark signals on the left atrial side of the mitral valve (white arrows in e) during mid-systole. The aortic root, left ventricle, left atrium and pulmonary trunk are all markedly dilated (C-F). Close-up view of the mitral valve upon opening the left ventricle. The leaflets are irregular, bumpy and show myxoid degeneration. Ao, aorta; PA, pulmonary artery; LV, left ventricle; LA, left atrium; MV, mitral valve*

have are forceful heartbeats and shortness of breath during light activity. Aortic regurgitation often happens because of aortic dilation (when the aorta is so enlarged that the valves cannot fully come together).

Laboratory Studies

Because no common mutations have been identified, genetic testing includes screening the entire FBN1 gene. DNA testing cannot exclude a diagnosis of Marfan syndrome.

Molecular studies of the fibrillin gene should be performed in patients in whom Marfan syndrome is suspected.

By 1998, 137 FBN1 mutations had been characterized in patients with Marfan syndrome. Mutations are distributed throughout the FBN1 gene.

Most mutations are missense mutations, small in-frame deletions, or insertions that alter a single peptide of about 3000 amino acids.

All mutations described to this point are predicted to produce a mutant fibrillin-1 protein.

Mutation analysis can identify the exact mutation in the fibrillin gene, and linkage analysis can be used to track an abnormal fibrillin gene within a family.

Sequencing of the entire gene for the purpose of detecting mutations is tedious and expensive. Mutations detected using sequencing may represent normal variations, resulting in both false-positive and false-negative results.

Molecular diagnosis is commercially available by sequencing of entire coding region or select exons, by mutations scanning, by performing targeted mutation analysis, by conducting linkage analysis, and by sequencing RNA.

A comprehensive clinical and molecular description of a large series of pediatric cases with a FBN1 mutation. Besides lethal neonatal Marfan syndrome, which represents a genuine entity, most clinical manifestations of Marfan syndrome increase with age, highlighting the limited usefulness of international criteria for diagnosis in early infancy and emphasizing the value of FBN1 mutation screening, which not only confirms the diagnosis but also facilitates determination of prognosis and timely management.

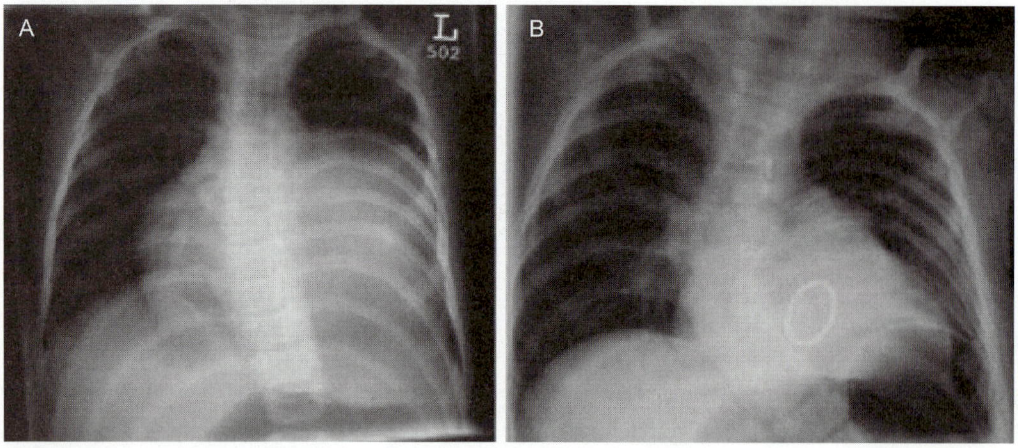

Fig. 14.301: *Chest X-ray (A) showing huge dialation of thoracaic aorta and almost normal aortic shadow after repair of aneurysm (B)*

Imaging Studies

Advances in noninvasive diagnostic imaging modalities have had a profound influence on case management. These studies provide accurate detection and quantification of the severity of cardiovascular disease, aiding in the appropriate timing of surgical intervention.

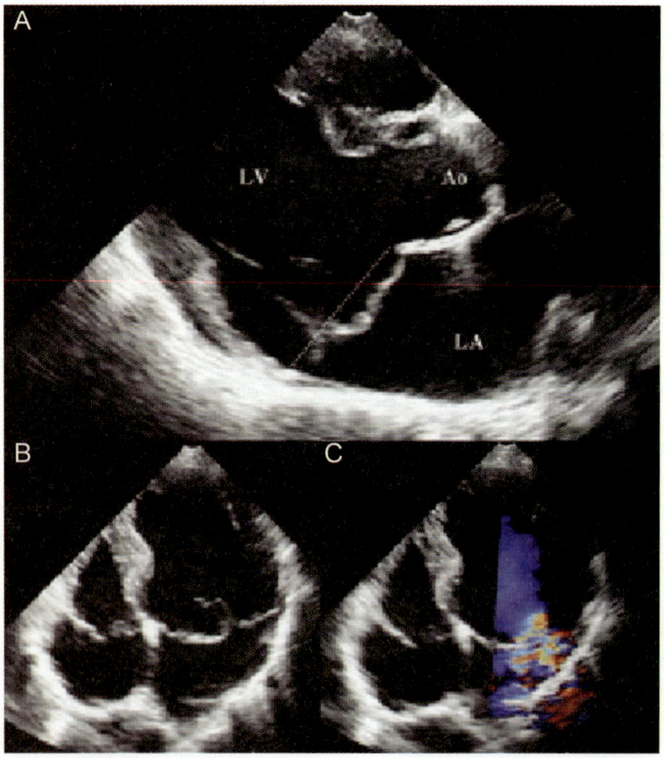

Fig. 14.302: *Mitral valve prolapse. (A) Echocardiographic parasternal long-axis view showing the mitral leaflets prolapsing more than 2 mm above the plane of the mitral annulus (dotted line) during systole in a child with Marfan syndrome. (B) Echocardiographic apical four-chamber view showing bileaflet prolapse in the same patient. (C) Colour Doppler view showing moderate mitral regurgitation. Ao: aorta; LA: left atrium; LV: left ventricle*

Chest Radiography

It should be focused on apical blebs. Chest radiographs may also be of value in detecting a thoracic aortic dissection by demonstrating enlargement of the aortic and cardiac silhouette.

Pelvic radiography is required only if a positive finding of protrusio acetabula is needed for the diagnosis.

Echocardiography

Cross-sectional echocardiography is a common tool in the diagnosis and management of aortic root dilatation. The upper limit of the normal aortic root size is 1.9 cm/m^2 of body surface area and is independent of the patient's sex. Standard echocardiography is valuable in assessing mitral valve prolapse, left ventricular size and function, left atrial size, and function of the tricuspid valve.

Transesophageal echocardiography depicts the distal ascending and descending aorta. It also improves assessment of the prosthetic valves.

Doppler echocardiography is useful in detecting and grading the severity of aortic and mitral regurgitation.

CT and MRI

MRI is the best choice for assessing chronic dissection of any region of the aorta. It should be performed in any patient at any age who has an aortic root dimension of more than 150% of the mean for their body surface area or a ratio of actual to predicted aortic root dimension of more than 1.5.

CT or MRI of the lumbosacral spine may be needed to detect dural ectasia. The following MRI and CT criteria for dural ectasia in adults have been proposed:

Presence of dural ectasia requires one major criterion or both minor criteria.

Major criterion: Sagittal width of the dural sac at S1 or below that is greater than the sagittal width of the dural sac above L4.

Minor criterion: Nerve root sleeve at L5 of more than 6.5 mm in diameter or scalloping at S1 of more than 3.5 mm.

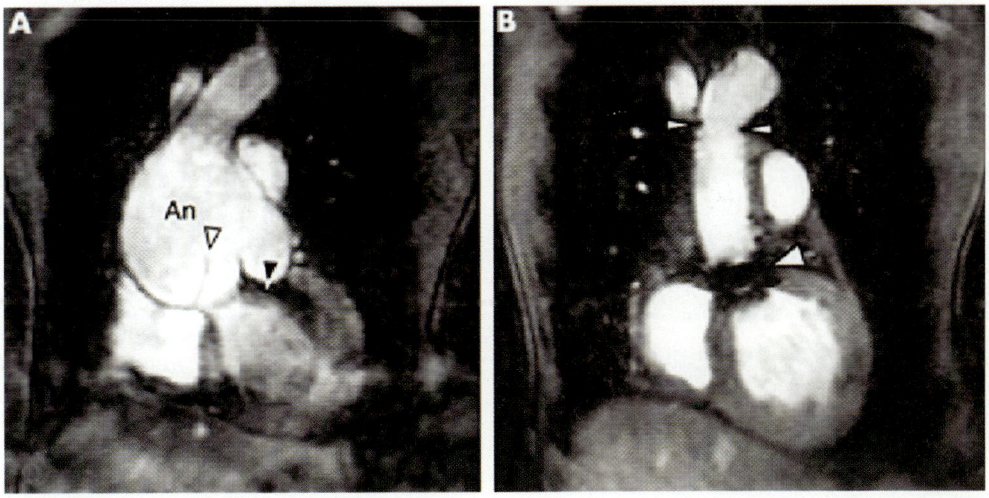

Fig. 14.303: *MRI imaging in aortic aneurysm (A) and almost normal-sized aorta after operation (B)*

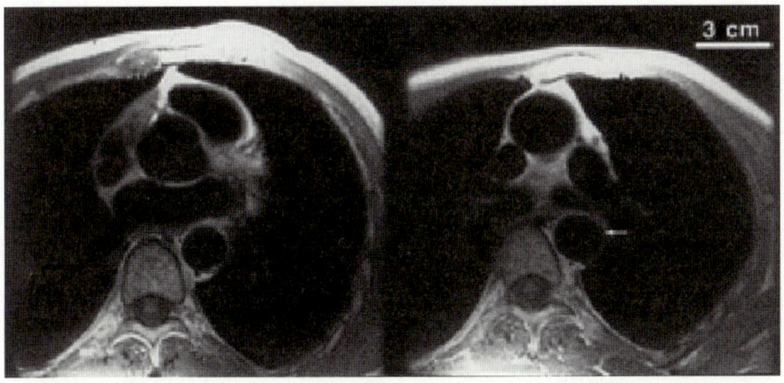

Fig. 14. 304: *Magnetic resonance imaging and asymptomatic aortic dissection*

Aortography

Many still consider this procedure the criterion standard for diagnosing acute aortic dissection.

However, the sensitivity is not 100%, and aortography has associated risks.

Other Tests

1. An ambulatory electrocardiogram should be obtained in patients with symptomatic palpitations, syncope, or near syncope or a baseline ECG that shows major rhythm or conduction disturbance.
2. Measure blood pressure.
3. Upon slit-lamp examination, the patient's pupils should be dilated and checked for lens dislocation and any sign of retinal tears.
4. Histologic findings.

Immunohistologic evaluation of the skin for abnormal fibrillin has been reported but is not widely available in the United States. This is partly due to the high incidence of false-positive results in patients with other connective-tissue disorders who have symptoms and signs of Marfan syndrome. Electron microscopy of fibrillin from cultured fibroblasts has shown a substantial increase in fraying of microfibrils in patients with Marfan syndrome. In neonatal Marfan syndrome, electron microscopy of fibrillin strands reveals only beads that are not strung together in the usual necklace like pattern, resulting in poor elastic tissue strength.

Management of Cardiovascular Problems

Cardiovascular (heart and blood vessel) problems are common in people with Marfan syndrome. In fact, cardiovascular problems affect about 9 out of every 10 people diagnosed with Marfan syndrome. It is important that people with Marfan syndrome know about cardiovascular problems and ways to prevent or manage them.

Medical Management

General measures for patients with Marfan syndrome are as follows:

1. Moderate restriction of physical activity
2. Endocarditis prophylaxis
3. Echocardiography at annual intervals
4. Beta-blocking treatment
5. Beta-blocker therapy should be considered at any age if the aorta is dilated, but prophylactic treatment may be more effective in those with an aortic diameter of less than 4 cm.
6. Risk factors for aortic dissection include:

Aortic diameter greater than 5 cm, aortic dilatation extending beyond the sinus of Valsalva, rapid rate of dilatation (45% per year, or 1.5 mm per year in adults), and family history of aortic dissection.

At least annual evaluation should be offered and should include clinical history, examination and echocardiography.

In children, serial echocardiography at 6-month to 12-month intervals is recommended, and the frequency depends on the aortic diameter (in relation to body surface area) and the rate of increase.

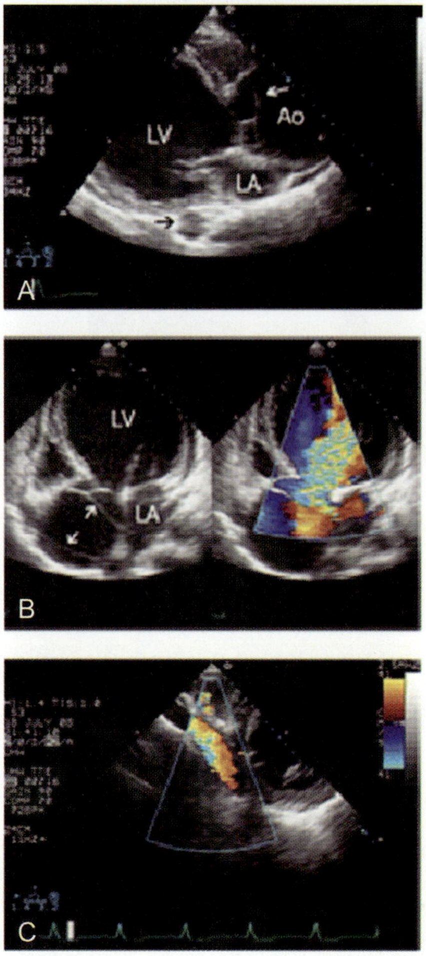

Fig 14.305: *Transthoracic echocardiography in a patient with Marfan's syndrome and type A dissection. (A) Parasternal long-axis view. There is severe dilatation of the aorta and a linear echo is seen just above the aortic valve (white arrow). Note the normal caliber and appearance of the descending thoracic aorta, posterior to the left atrium (black arrow). LV, left ventricle; LA, left atrium; Ao, aorta. (B) Apical five-chamber view. The dilated aortic root, with two reflections of the intimal flap, (white arrows) is seen. Severe aortic regurgitation (right panel) is seen with colour flow mapping. (C) Subcostal view. Normal caliber, no dissection flap and normal flow are seen*

Prophylactic aortic root surgery should be considered when the aortic diameter at the sinus of Valsalva is more than 5 cm.

Counseling for pregnancy is as follows:

- Fifty percent risk for transmitting a pathogenic mutation to offspring
- High-risk pregnancy with aortic root diameter of more than 40 mm or previous cardiovascular surgery or severe heart disease
- Prepartum aortic root replacement with diameters of more than 40 mm
- Serial echocardiography until 3 months postpartum
- Medication in Marfan syndrome

Beta-blockers

Beta-adrenergic receptor antagonists have gained acceptance as potential agents for delaying aortic expansion and for delaying the progression to rupture or dissection.

The rate of surgical interventions has substantially declined during the past decade of beta-blockade use.

Beta-blocker therapy retards aortic growth in children and adolescents with Marfan syndrome.

A recent study concluded that data are not sufficient to recommend or discourage the use of beta-blockers in children with congestive heart failure.

Calcium antagonist also retards aortic growth, but a recommended dose has not been established. The optimal age to begin beta-blockade therapy has not been determined. Some investigators begin therapy during infancy, but others wait until the aortic diameter exceeds the 95th percentile or a rapid rate of dilation is observed.

In asymptomatic patients, the elastic properties of the aortic root appear to have a heterogeneous response after long-term treatment with atenolol.

The stiffness index and distensibility are most likely to be useful when the baseline end-diastolic aortic root diameter is more than 40 mm. More experience is needed to determine the optimal dose of beta-blockers to minimize growth of the aortic root.

ACE Inhibitors

ACE inhibitors reduce central arterial pressure and conduit arterial stiffness and may be useful in Marfan syndrome. This approach received support by a short-term, non-randomized study comparing enalapril with beta-blockade in which stiffness and rate of dilatation improved with the ACE inhibitors. Another study of patients with Marfan syndrome maintained on beta-blockade examined the impact of adding an ACE inhibitor, perindopril, compared with placebo. Over a 24-week period, those receiving the ACE inhibitor had a reduction in aortic stiffness and less absolute change in aortic root dimensions.

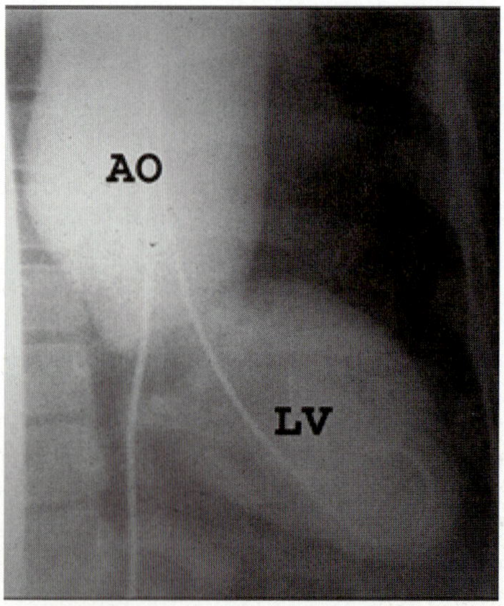

Fig. 14.306: *Venticulography huge dilatation of ascending aorta in Marfan syndrome*

Matrix Metalloproteinases (MMPs)

Syndromes that resemble Marfan syndrome, especially in the potential for aneurysm and dissection, were found to be due to mutations in genes encoding TGFβ receptors.

The potential importance of MMPs was stimulated by studies of non-Marfan syndrome abdominal aortic aneurysm in humans and thoracic aortic aneurysm in mice engineered to have Marfan syndrome, in both of which levels of MMP-2 and MMP-9 were raised.

Doxycycline administration to a mouse model of Marfan syndrome suppressed MMPs and improved aortic wall architecture and stiffness compared with atenolol.

Other Therapies

1. Anticoagulant medications such as warfarin are needed after artificial heart-valve placement.
2. Intravenous antibiotic therapy is required during cardiac and noncardiac procedures to prevent bacterial endocarditis.
3. Progesterone and estrogen therapy have been used to induce puberty and reduce the patient's ultimate height if hormonal treatment is begun before puberty, but no conclusive data are yet available to show whether this therapy reduces scoliosis.
4. Conservative treatment of protrusio acetabuli mostly involves physiotherapy by forcible stretching (stress fractures of the femoral neck due to stretching are documented, weight extension on an abduction frame, local heating, and re-education concerning daily activities.
5. Myopia is treatable with refraction.
6. Patients with flat feet may wear shoes with adequate arch support, although custom orthotics may be required. Guidelines for the diagnosis and treatment of pediatric flat foot have been established.
7. Psychological counseling is helpful for families coping with feelings of denial, anger, blame, depression, or guilt.

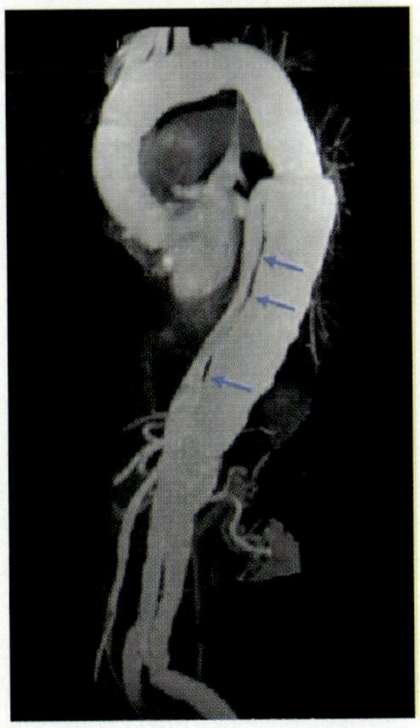

Fig. 14.307: *MRI of type B aortic dissection (blue arrows) in a patient with Marfan. Previous aortic root graft replacement is noted*

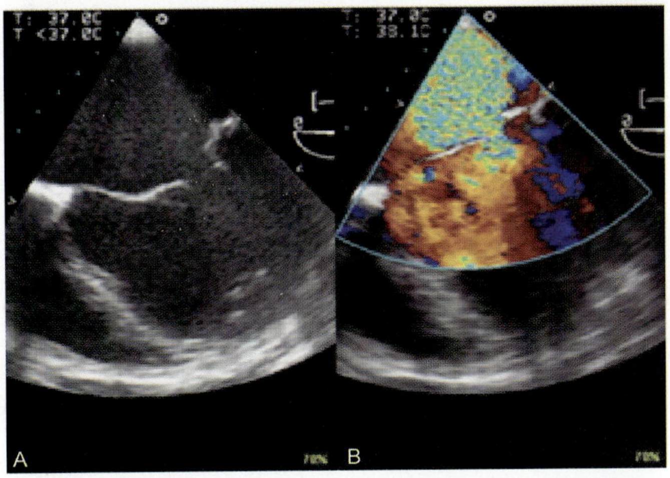

Fig. 14.308: *Transesophageal echocardiogram: 2D (A) and color Doppler flow (B) from a 27 year-old man, with Marfan syndrome. Note severe mitral valve regurgitation from: annulus dilatation, lengthening of the chordae tendineae and a redundancy of the leaflets, especially of the posterior one*

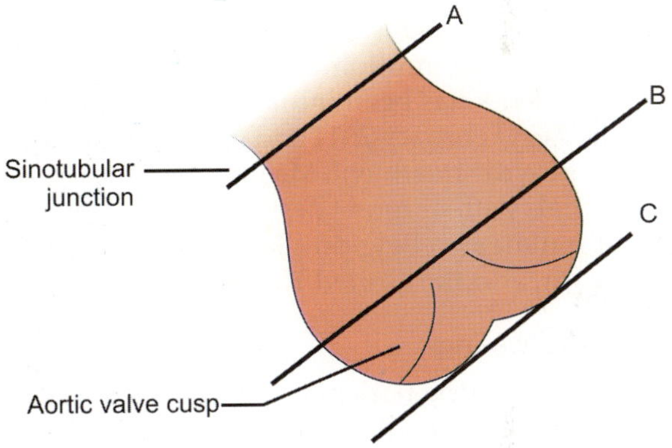

Fig. 14.309: *Preoperative assessment of aortic valve anatomy and area of operation*

Future Therapeutic Strategies

The current criterion standard for treatment of aortic aneurysm in Marfan syndrome is the preventive administration of beta-blockers. However, beta-blockers do not prevent surgery at a later age. The discovery that TGFβ antagonism can rescue aortic aneurysm in C1039G/+ mice prompted the idea to test the efficacy of losartan, a widely used angiotensin II type I receptor (AT1) antagonist, because of its antihypertensive properties and ability to counteract TGFβ in animal models of chronic renal disease and cardiomyopathy.

Thus, TGFβ antagonism is a general strategy against aneurysm progression in patients with Marfan syndrome and other disorders of the TGFβ-signaling network.

Proof of the above principle was obtained by treating Marfan mice with TGFβ-neutralizing antibody by intraperitoneal injection.

In a preliminary observational study, 17 pediatric Marfan syndrome patients with progressive aortic

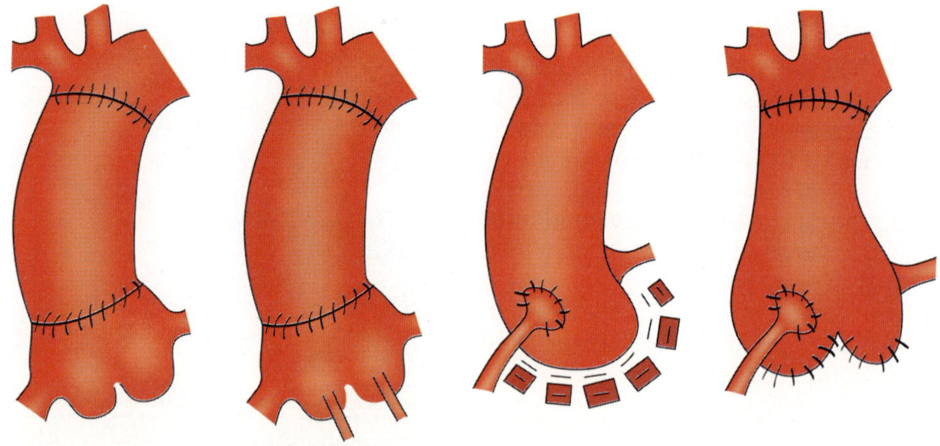

Fig. 14.310: *Stepwise approach in surgical intervention in the treatment of Marfan syndrome*

enlargement despite optimal medical therapy were given an angiotensin receptor blocker agent and were followed for 12–42 months. Patients had a significant decrease in rate of change of aortic root dimension. This study provides the first evidence for a significant benefit of angiotensin receptor blocker use over current therapies in reducing aortic root dilation in severe pediatric Marfan syndrome.

Currently a large, randomized clinical trial in Marfan syndrome patients has been initiated and included a total of 608 patients in February 2011 and compares atenolol with losartan for a 3-year treatment. Meanwhile, a nearly a dozen additional trials with different designs and inclusion criteria have been initiated in Belgium, France, Italy, the Netherlands, Taiwan, and the United Kingdom.

Genetic Counseling

Recurrence risk for the patient's siblings is small if neither parent is affected. Gonadal mosaicism is reported as the cause of multiple affected offspring being born to unaffected parents. Risk is 50% if one parent is affected.

Recurrence risk for the patient's offspring is 50% if the spouse is normal. Fifty percent homozygous Marfan syndrome was reported in case of an affected spouse. Compound heterozygosity at the FBN1 locus was confirmed at the molecular level; the affected child had a severe phenotype, leading to early death. During counseling, the variability of the disease should be emphasized because an affected child may be more or less affected than the parent.

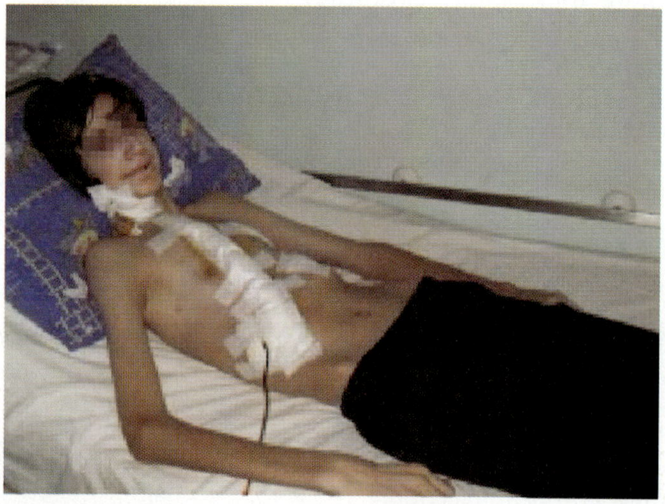

Fig. 14.311: *An adolescent is being observed in ICU after operative intervention in Marfan syndrome*

Surgical Intervention

Indications in Children

1. If possible, surgery should be delayed until adolescence

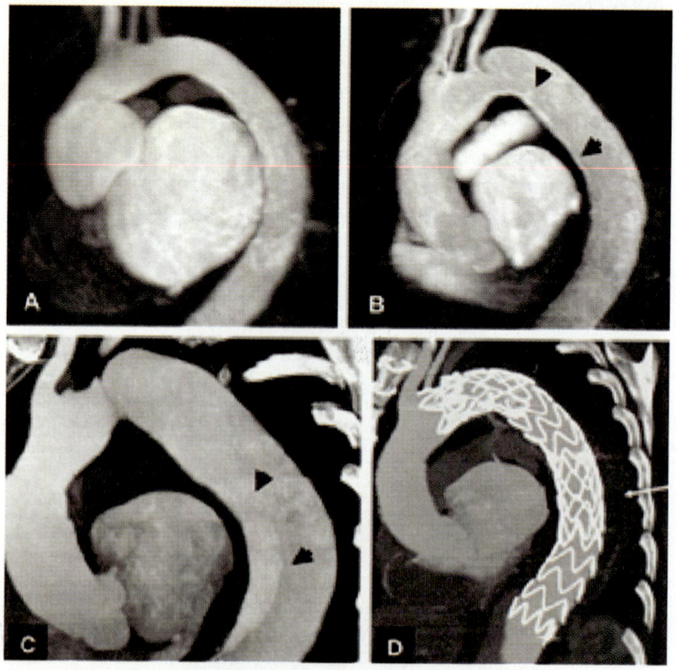

Fig. 14.312: *MR MIP (A-B) and MDCT MIP (C-D) images before (A-C) and after (D) EVT. Image of the aorta before (A) and after (B-C) heart transplant and dissection: a substantial aortic luminal enlargement is seen during 3 years of follow-up (A-C), intimal flap is shown (arrowhead). Endovascular stent graft placed in the descending thoracic aorta (D) with complete thrombosis of the false lumen (arrow)*

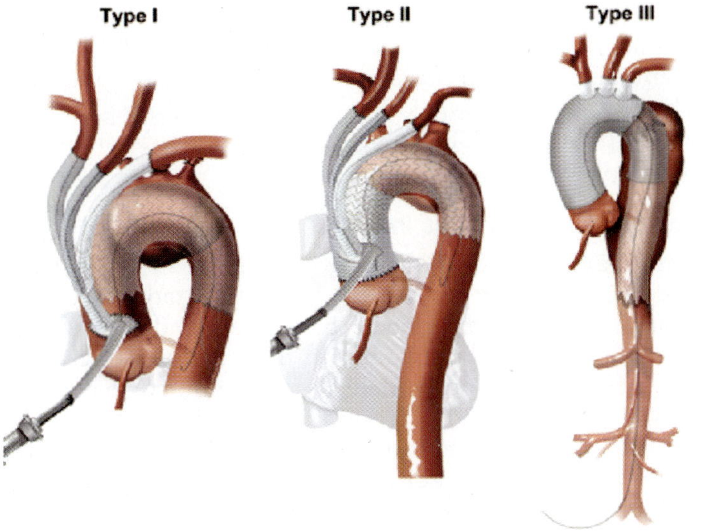

Fig. 14.313: *Hybrid aortic arch repair types I, II and III*

2. Aortic root diameters with similar thresholds as in adults
3. Aortic root diameters outside the upper confidence interval deviate upward from the perused centile on follow-up echocardiograms.

Cardiovascular Surgery

Cardiovascular surgery can substantially prolong survival. Prophylactic and emergency cardiovascular surgery is needed for treatment of aortic and mitral regurgitation, aortic aneurysm and aortic dissection. Emergency surgical replacement of the aortic root is indicated for survivors of acute proximal aortic dissection.

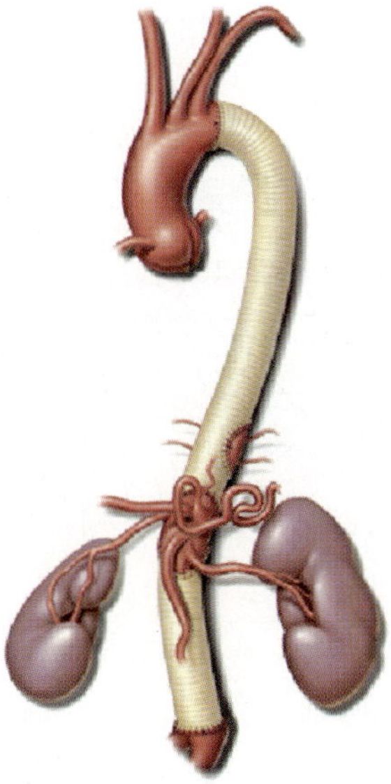

Fig. 14.314: *Completed aortic reconstruction. The completed extent II repair. Note the proximal anastomosis located just distal to the left subclavian artery; the intercostal patch incorporating two pairs of intercostal arteries; the single visceral patch incorporating the celiac axis, superior mesenteric artery, and both renal arteries; and the distal anastomosis at the aortic bifurcation*

The ascending aorta is usually replaced when the aorta exceeds 55–60 mm in diameter. Composite valve-graft replacement is performed, in which the dilated aortic segment is replaced by a prosthetic valve sewn into a tube graft with reimplantation of the coronary ostia (modified Bentall procedure). Composite valve-graft replacement of the aortic root has low rates of morbidity and mortality, produces excellent long-term results, and is currently the treatment of choice for proximal dissection or clinically significant annuloaortic ectasia in patients with Marfan syndrome.

An aortic valve-sparing procedure is evolving for patients with an aortic aneurysm and favorable characteristics of the aortic valve and annulus. The advantages of this procedure include the avoidance of anticoagulation and a lowered risk of thromboembolism and endocarditis. The aortic valve-sparing procedure is still controversial because of concerns that it poses a risk of progressive valvular degeneration and annular dilation. Additional long-term data are required before routine use of this procedure can be recommended.

Consultations

Consultations may include the following:
- Clinical geneticist
- Cardiologist
- Ophthalmologist
- Cardiovascular surgeon
- Orthopedic surgeon
- Orthodontics surgeon
- Psychologist
- Diet
- No special diet is needed.

Activity

In general, patients can remain fully active unless their symptoms limit them. Patients should be discouraged from participating in demanding sports because several highly trained athletes with unrecognized Marfan syndrome have suddenly died from ruptured aortic aneurysms.

Competitive and contact sports are potentially dangerous because of underlying aortic weakness and dilatation, valvular insufficiency, ocular abnormalities, and skeletal problems. Patients should avoid blows to the head (e.g. in boxing, high diving) and to protect themselves against blows to the globe (racquet sports) with cushioned spectacles.

To protect against pneumothorax, patients should avoid the rapid decompression associated with quick ascents in elevators, scuba diving, and flying in unpressurized aircraft.

Patients should avoid activities involving isometric work such as weightlifting, climbing steep inclines, participating in gymnastics, and performing pull-ups. These exercises cause excessive elevations of systolic blood pressure and may lead to sudden death.

Nonstrenuous activities and sports (e.g. golf, walking, fishing) are recommended. Appropriate exercise is physically and emotionally beneficial.

DEXTROCARDIA AND LEVOCARDIA

In this condition, the heart is found to be placed in the right hemithorax, the apex pointing to the right. True dextrocardia is apart of total situs inversus and is known as "Mirror Image Dextrocardia with Situs Inversus". Since there is no alteration in the circulation and hence is a benign condition per se. Structural cardiac defects do occur with dextrocardia but are far less common in true dextrocardia as compared to dextrocardia without situs inversus. A syndrome of true dextrocardia, bronchiectasis, abnormal paranasal sinuses, along with bronchial cilliary mucosal defects and male infertality is termed as Kartagener's syndrome.

Clinical Examination

The apical impulse is on the right side of the chest and the heart sounds are louder on the right side. Liver dullness is on the left side and stomach tympany can be elicited on the right side. When a patient drinks a glass of water or an aerated drink, gurgling sounds can be heard in the right hypochondrium suggestive of a right-sided stomach. Fluoroscopy with barium bolus can also prove this.

Electrocardiogram

It is characteristic of dextrocardia in which lead I is a mirror image of the normal tracing. The P wave is invertedin lead I and upright in lead aVR. The leads II and III are interchanged and so are leads aVR and aVL. The limb leads thus prove atrial inversion whereas ventricular inversion is proved by chest leads. The normal leads V5, V6 show rS complexes whereas right-sided chest leads, i.e. V5R, V6R show qR complexes. The prognosis depends on the presence or absence of associated cardiac defects.

In dextroversion, the abdominal viscera are in normal position but the heart is rotated along its axis so that the apex points to the right. The atria are not transposed but the ventricles may be inverted. It is always accompanied with serious congenital cardiac malformations like single ventricle, transposition of great vessels and tricuspid atresia. A tetralogy of Fallot is rare. The clinical picture is dominated by the associated cardiac anomalies. It carried a bad prognosis and majority of patients die during infancy. When pulmonary stenosis is present, it can be managed with a shunt procedure.

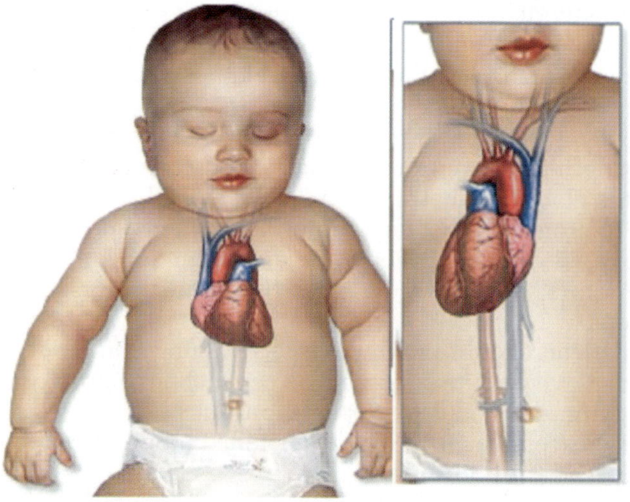

Fig 14.315: *Normally placed heart in the thorax (left) dextrocardia (right)*

Levocardia with Situs Inversus

The heart is in its normal anatomic position but the abdominal viscera are totally or partially transposed. The heart is grossly malformed. The congenital defects which are found to be associated with this condition are atrio-ventricularis communis defect with pulmonary stenosis, single ventricle with transposition of great vessels, persistent truncus arteriosus and anomalies of systemic and pulmonary venous return. There may be asplenia or polysplenia. Such patients are predisposed to over-whelming infections due to lack of defense mechanism which is usually offered by a normal spleen in a healthy person. The clinical findings are of the associated cardiac defects. The electrocardiographic changes are according to the associated cardiac defects. The chest radiograph confirms the normal position of the heart. The liver is often bilobed and symmetrical. The location, size and shape of the liver and spleen can be demonstrated by radioisotope scanning techniques. The prognosis is usually bad and majority of the patients succumb in their early infancy. When associated with pulmonic stenosis, creation of a shunt operation is usually of much benefit.

Criscross Heart

It is one of the rarest form of cardiac malformations which is characterized by an atrioventricular spatial relation that

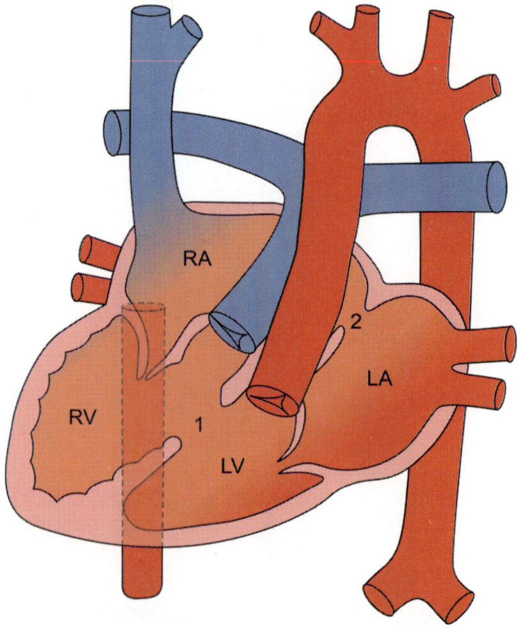

Fig. 14.316: *Dextrocardia with ASD & VSD. 1. Ventricular septal defect; 2. Atrial septal defect; 3 Dextrocardia; 4.Situs solitus of the atria; 5. Normal atrioventricular connection; 6. Normally connected great arteries (normal VA connection); 7. Left aortic arch; 8.Ventricular septal defect and 9. Atrial septal defect*

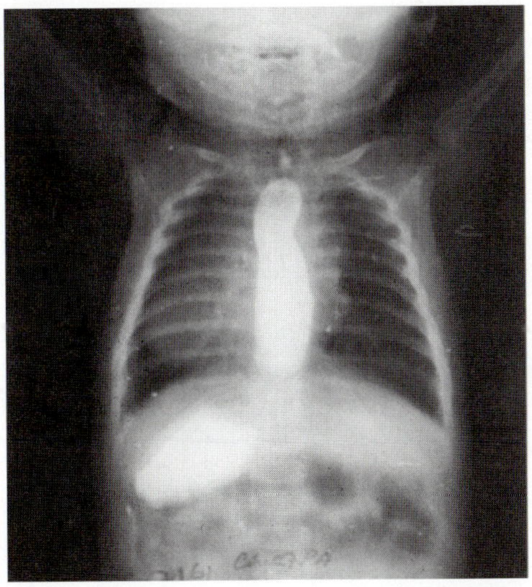

Fig. 14.317: *X-ray chest (PA view) showing apex of the heart in the right hemithorax and stomach lies on the right side as seen with barium meal study and liver is on the left side in a child with dextrocardia with situs inversus*

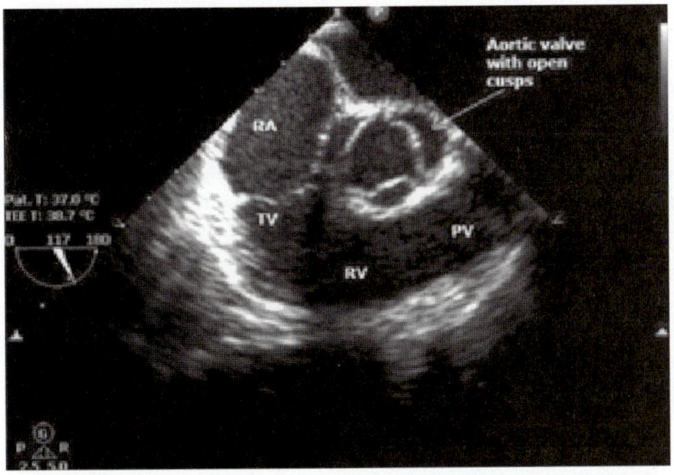

Fig. 14.318: *Transesophageal echocardiogram mid esophageal AV short-axis view in mirror image dextrocardia*

positions or apparently appears to place each ventricle in a contralateral position with respect to its associated atrium. These patients have situs solitus and atrioventricular concordance (d-loop) in which major portion of the right ventricle cavity lies in a left and superior position and the left ventricle is positioned in a right and inferior directions. This relationship has also been named as "upstairs and down stairs" heart or the superoinferior heart. Atrioventricular discordance is invariably found in about 1/3rd of the cases. Majority of them have ventriculoarterial discordance in which case, these may be D-transposition, L-transposition or double outlet right ventricle. A large VSD is found in many of these cases. The other defects which are encountered are, pulmonic stenosis (valvular or subvalvular), straddling of either of the AV valves triscuspid valve hypoplasia resulting into either TR or TS or both, This leads to very high mortality and death is almost certain either soon of the birth or a few days later.

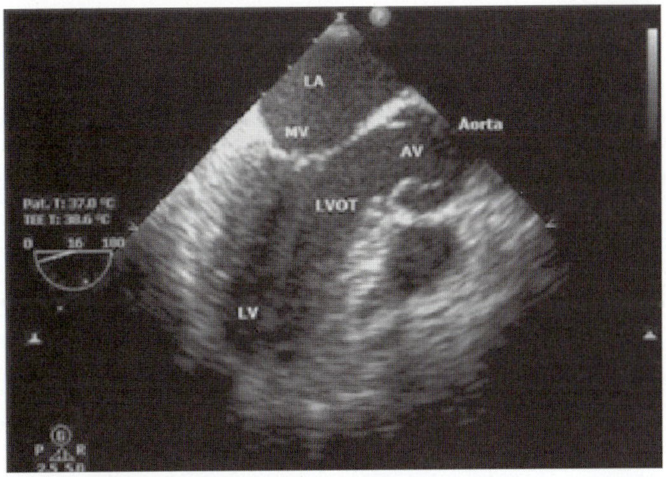

Fig. 14.319: *Transesophageal echocardiogram mid-esophageal long-axis view in mirror image dextrocardia*

This anomaly is managed according to the types and number of associated cardiac defects.

Ectopia Cordis

It may be defined as that situation in which the heart l lies outside the thoracic cavity. It is one of the rarest form of cardiac abnormality. The heart is devoid of its coverings and lies on the anterior chest wall with its apex directed cephalad and at times it may kiss the chin of the baby. The great vessels of the heart are seen through a cleft in the sternum. It is recognised into two forms:

1. Thoracic (frequent)
2. Abdominal (most uncommon).

The various other associated cardiac malformations which are observed in ectopia cordis of thoracic variety

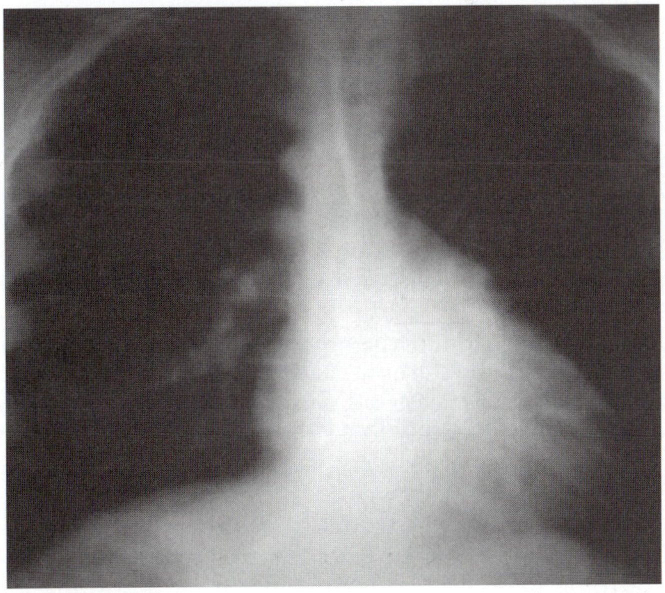

Fig. 14.320: *Levocardia with situs inversus. Note the prominence of the shadow at the high right-sided cardiac border. Discordance of the apex of the heart and visceral situs is often associated with structural defects*

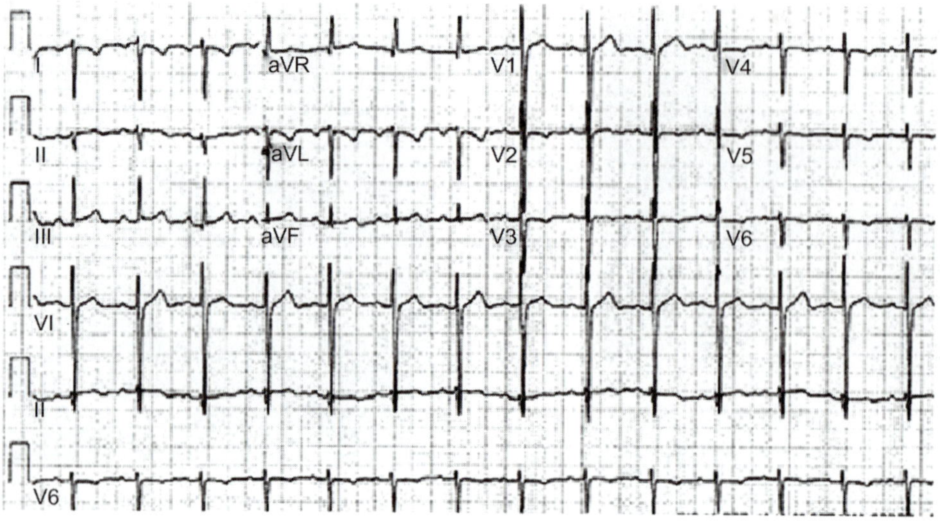

Fig. 14.321: *The dextrocardia ECG findings include: (1) Predominantly negative P wave, QRS complex, and T wave in lead I (2) Low voltage in leads V3-V6 (since these leads are placed on the left side of the chest)*

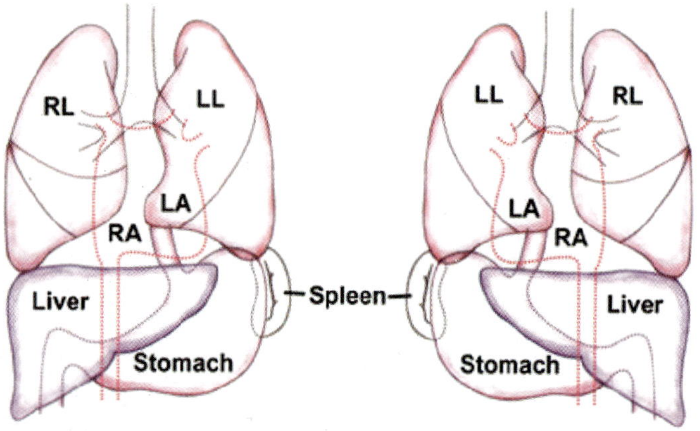

Fig. 14.322: *Normal organ placement (left) and liver and spleen in a reverse order in levocardia (right)*

are: VSD, single ventricle, transposition of GV, coarctation of aorta, pulmonary atresia and severe pulmonary stenosis. The patient usually die soon after birth due to kinking of the great arteries or veins, cardiac temponade as a result of repositioning of the heart and to the related intracardiac malformations. Such cases need differentiation from isolated cleft of the sternum. In this condition, heart can be seen to pulsate beneath a covering of skin or cutaneous tissue which apparently looks like a scar tissue. The heart may protrude anteriorly and superiorly with crying but true ectopia or displacement of heart does not take place. Both types of ectopia cordis (thoracic and abdominal) should be distinguished from Cantrell's Pentalogy. This syndrome in its fullest form consists of the following malformations:

1. A midline supraumbilical abdominal wall defect.
2. A defect of the lower sternum.
3. A deficiency of the anterior diaphragm.
4. A defect of the diaphragmatic pericardium.
5. A congenital intracardiac malformation usually a VSD.

Only a few cases with ectopia cardis associated with mild intracardiac malformations, survive after successful management of the malposition.

Anomalous Origin of Left Coronary Artery from Pulmonary Artery (ALCAPA)

Origin of the left coronary artery from the pulmonary artery is a rare, but important anomaly because early death is often the natural outcome. At present, with early diagnosis and surgery, it appears that the child may be completely cured.

Physiology

Before birth, the pulmonary artery pressure equals systemic pressure, allowing for satisfactory myocardial perfusion from the pulmonary artery via the anomalous coronary. With birth and falling pulmonary artery pressure, the antegrade perfusion of the left coronary gradually falls, the circulation being taken over by collateral vessels from the right coronary. In many patients the flow in the left coronary artery reverses and, effectively, a coronary artery steal develops from the myocardium to the pulmonary artery. The size of this left-to-right shunt is rarely enough to be a significant hemodynamic burden except that it deprives the myocardium of perfusion.

Sometime in the first weeks of reversed coronary flow, myocardial ischemia becomes sufficient to be recognizable on an electrocardiogram. The heart enlarges and congestive heart failure becomes manifest. With ischemic damage to the left papillary muscles, mitral regurgitation is often added to an already deteriorating situation. If for any reason, the patient maintains sysemic pressure in the pulmonary arteries, this sequence of events will not occur and the left coronary will be perfused by blood originating from the pulmonary artery.

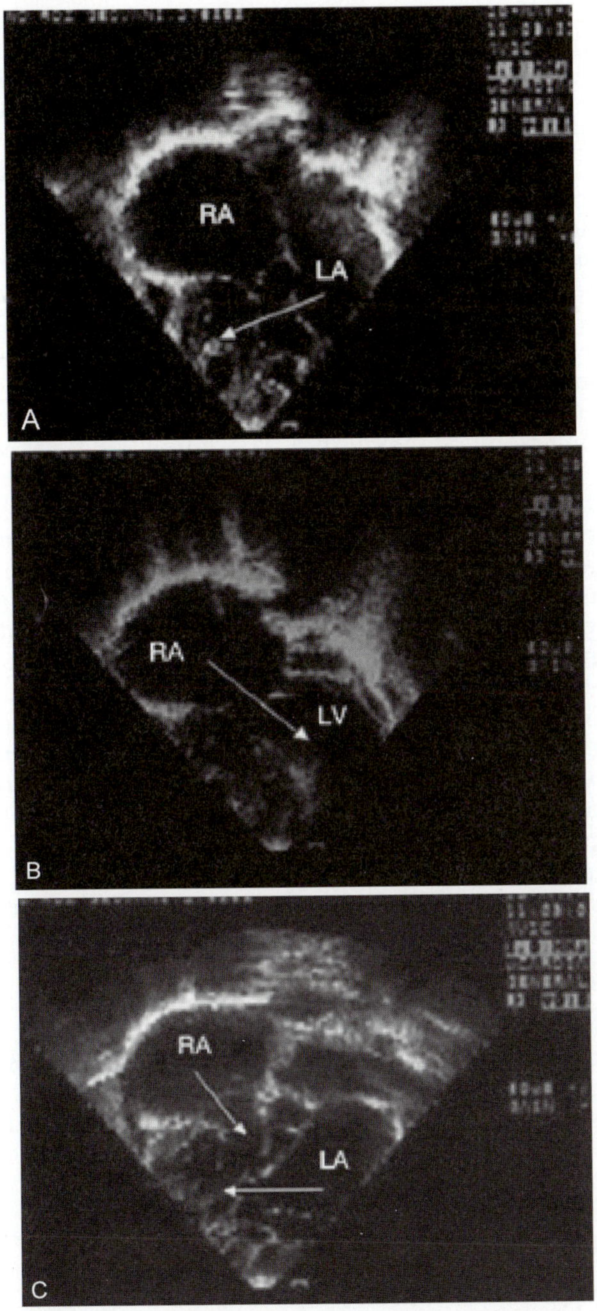

Fig. 14.323: *Two-dimensional echocardiography of patient four-chamber apical view. (A) left atrium (LA) connected to a right-sided morphologic right ventricle (RV) with atrioventricular discordance and straddling mitral valve. (B) right atrium (RA) connected to a left-sided morphologic left ventricle (LV). (C) atrioventricular crossover with vertically oriented ventricles*

Despite the fact that this blood may have substantially lower oxygen saturation than that from the right coronary, evidences of myocardial ischemia are not seen.

Some patients with uncorrected anomalous origin of the left coronary from the main pulmonary artery survive to adulthood. Rarely, the right coronary artery arises from the pulmonary artery even more rarely, both coronary arteries arise from the pulmonary artery.

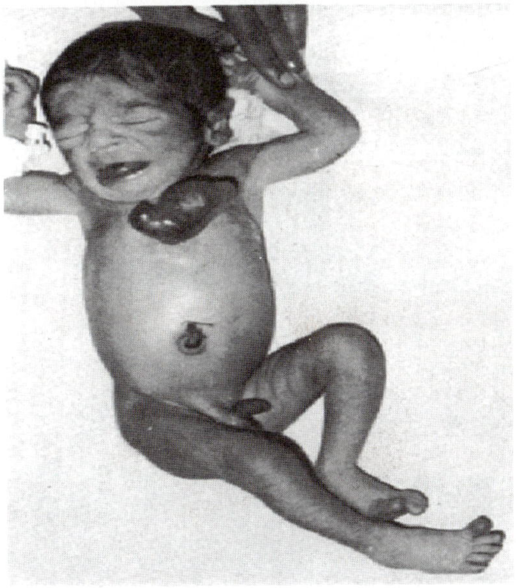

Fig. 14.324: *Photograph showing thoracic type of ectopia cordis (arrow) in a newborn baby*

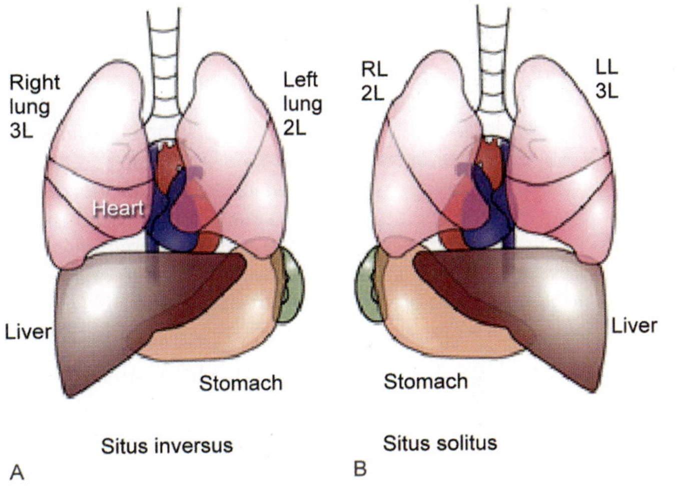

Fig. 14.325: *Anatomical arrangement of structures in normal heart (B) and classical dextrocardia (A)*

Clinical Manifestations

These patients seem to be normal at birth; approximately 60% of the patients developed congestive heart failure weeks, later. Occasionally, a history of irritability, perhaps related to angina, is elicited. But, this is more of a retrospective explanation than a useful fact. Older patients are discovered because of the systolic murmur of mitral regurgitation or because of chest X-ray showing cardiomegaly.

Electrocardiography

The electrocardiogram almost always shows evidence of anterolateral myocardial infarction in the symptomatic patient.

Chest radiography: The heart is enlarged, sometimes grossly enlarged without an increase in pulmonary

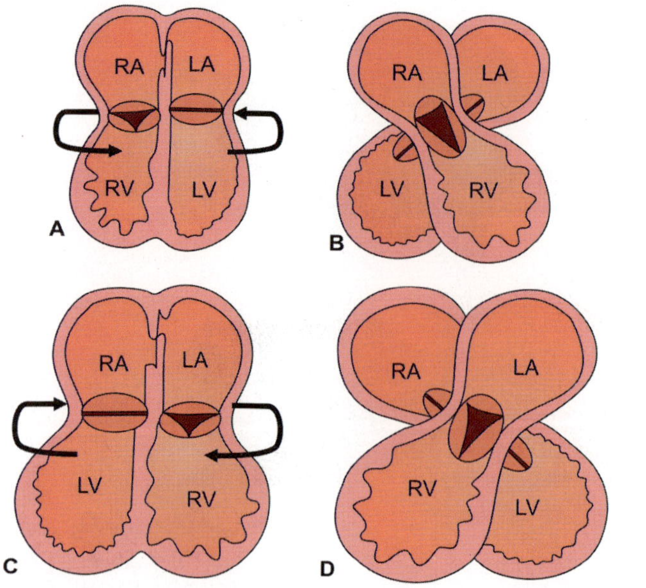

Fig. 14.326: *Anterior view (from the observer). Diagram of the cardiac chambers illustrating the etiologic mechanism (ventricular twist) that causes criss-cross heart. (A) atrioventricular (AV) concordance; ventricular twist is counterclockwise. (B) AV concordance with discordant spatial relationship: right-sided morphologic right atrium (RA) connected to a left-sided morphologic right ventricle (RV) and left-sided morphologic left atrium (LA) connected to a right-sided morphologic left ventricle (LV). (C) AV discordance; ventricular twist is clockwise. (D) AV discordance with concordant spatial relationship: right-sided morphologic RA connected to a left-sided morphologic LV and left-sided morphologic LA connected to a right-sided morphologic RV. This disorder can be interpreted as the crossing of systemic and pulmonary venous blood without mixing in the AV valves*

vascularity. The X-ray is characteristic of primary myocardial disease and, in the past, caused frequent confusion with other forms of primary myocardial disease.

Echocardiography: An enlarged, poorly functioning left ventricle is characteristic. Evidences of mitral regurgitation may be documented and differential enlargement of the right coronary versus the left may be demonstrable. In recent years, identification of the origin of the left coronary artery from the pulmonary artery has usually been possible. As a rule, all patients with unexplained myocardial disease should have the origin of the coronary arteries identified.

Parasternal short-axis view best demonstrates the origins of the coronary arteries from the aorta. An anomalously connecting left coronary artery passes near to the usual left sinus of Valsalva of the aortic root before connecting with the pulmonary root. The closer the vessel passes to the aorta, the more difficult it may be to establish the diagnosis by imaging alone. Scanning in a parasternal, long-axis view may demonstrate more clearly the orifice of the coronary artery in the pulmonary root.

Doppler color flow mapping has proved to be extremely valuable for demonstrating both the flow from the left coronary into the pulmonary root and the direction of flow in the left coronary artery. It requires clear imaging of the coronary ostium in the pulmonary root, demonstration of flow from the coronary artery into the pulmonary root, and documentation of retrograde flow in the left coronary artery and branches for the diagnosis of anomalous left coronary artery. Similarly, documentation of anterograde flow in the left coronary artery and branches by Doppler color flow mapping excludes anomalous left coronary artery. With careful imaging, coupled with Doppler color flow mapping, a highly accurate diagnosis or exclusion of the diagnosis is possible.

Cardiac Catheterization

At cardiac catheterization, the findings are those of a dilated cardiomyopathy. Left ventricular dysfunction, as evidenced by an elevated left ventricular end-diastolic pressure and elevated left atrial pressure, is usually

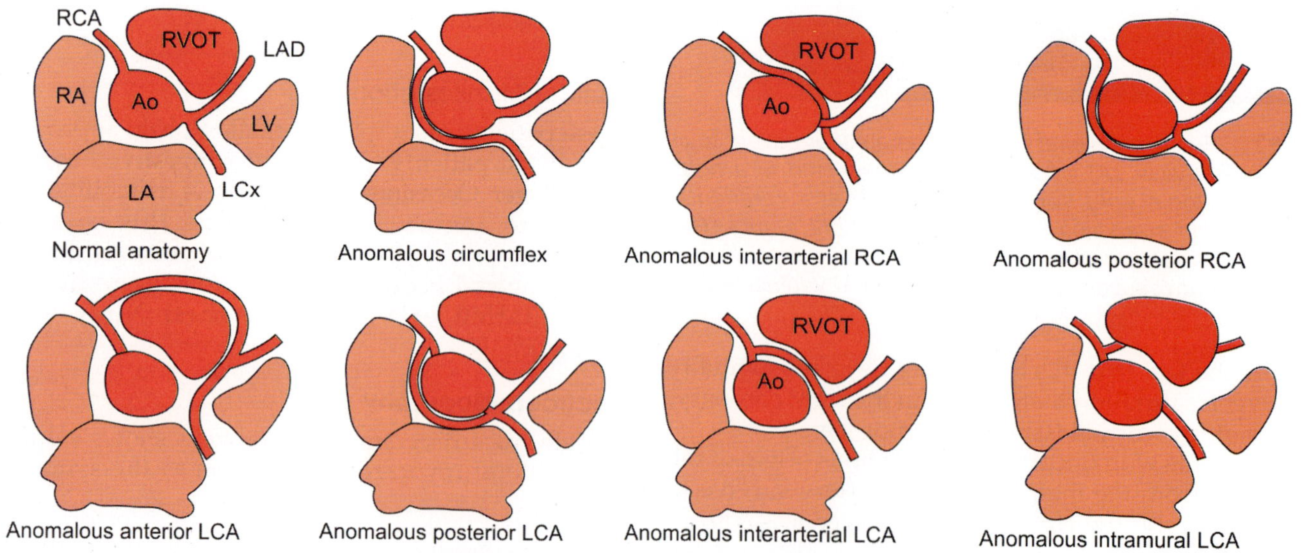

Fig. 14.327: *Different anomalies of coronary arteries*

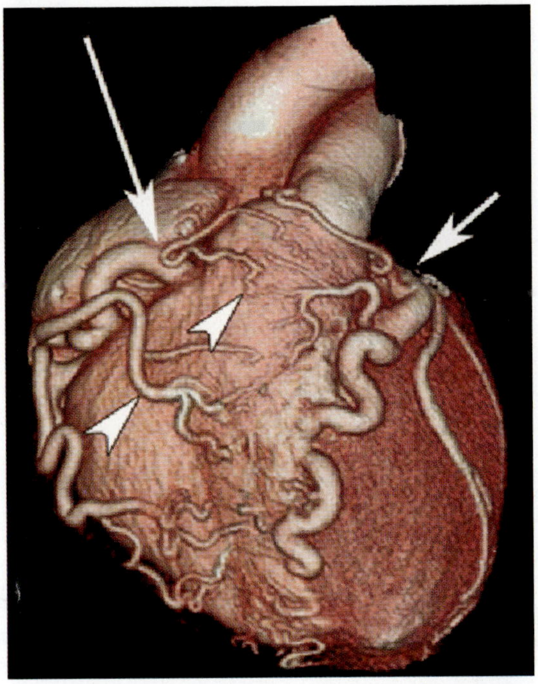

Fig. 14.328: *Three dimensional volume-rendered multidetector CT angiogram shows dilated intercoronary collateral arteries (arrow heads), which connect the tortuous RCA (long arrow) to the LCA (short arrow)*

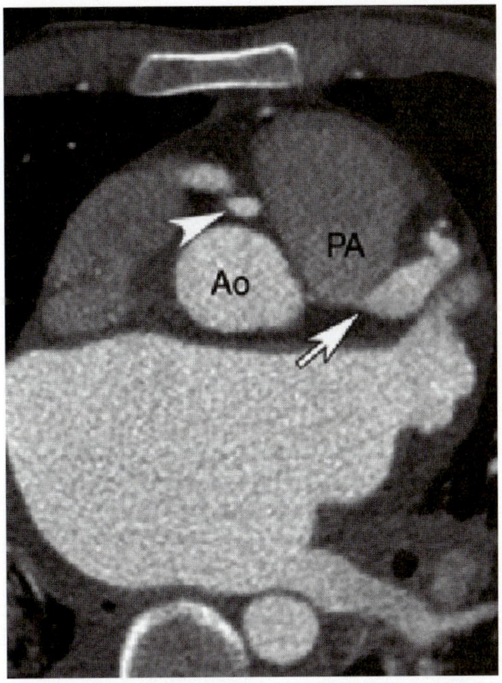

Fig. 14.330: *ALCAPA syndrome in a patient. Axial multidetector CT angiogram shows the origin of the LCA (arrow) from the main pulmonary artery (PA) and the dilated RCA (arrow head). Ao, aorta*

demonstrable. The diagnosis is established when an angiogram of the aortic root shows a large right coronary artery with opacification of the left coronary system, and even of the main pulmonary artery Angiograms with the contrast injected into the pulmonary artery have not been successful unless a balloon is inflated in the pulmonary artery and contrast material is injected proximal to the balloon.

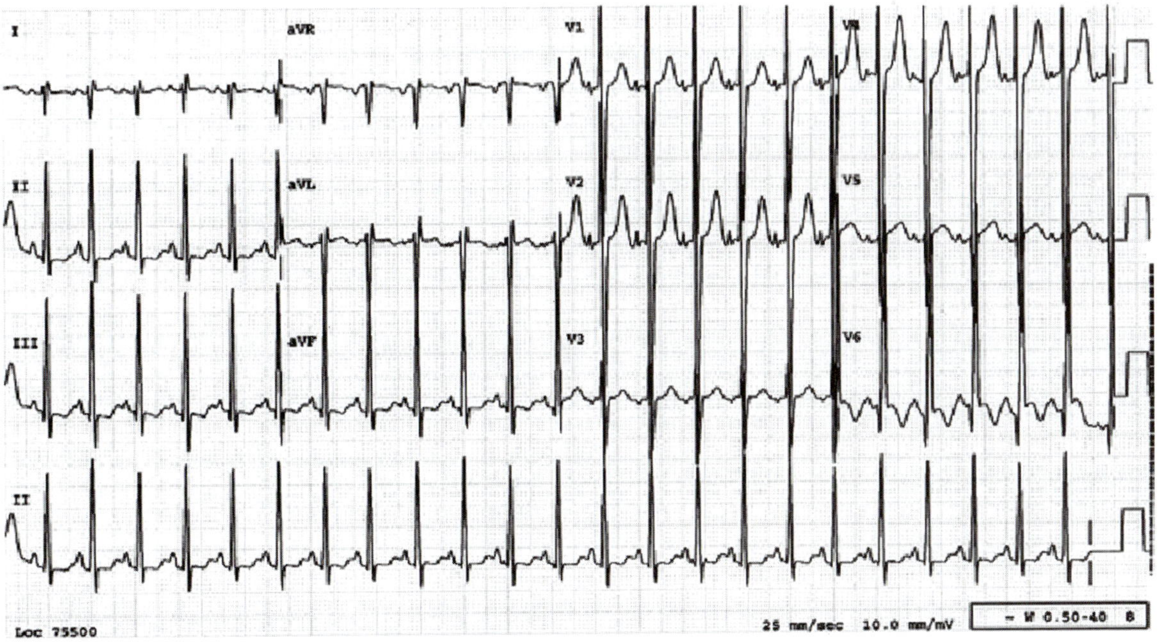

Fig. 14.329: *ST elevation in leads 1, aVL ,V1-V3 and T inversion in leads 1, aVL, V5-V6 in anomalous origin of the left coronary artery from the pulmonary artery (ALCAPA)*

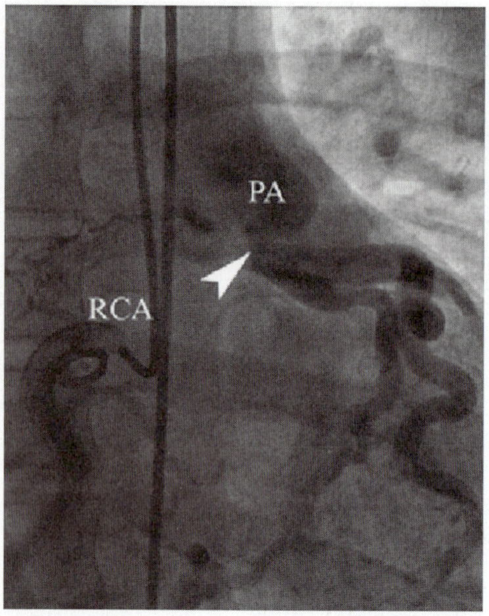

Fig. 14.331: *ALCAPA syndrome in a 15-year-old girl. Coronary angiogram obtained with a single RCA injection shows a tortuous and dilated RCA as well as an equally tortuous and dilated LCA. The LCA opacifies the main pulmonary artery (PA). The connection of the LCA with the main pulmonary artery (arrowhead) and the resultant steal phenomenon are the main diagnostic features of ALCAPA syndrome*

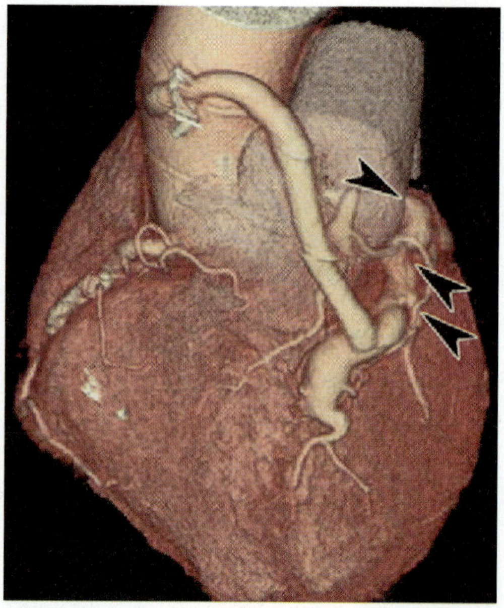

Fig. 14.332: *ALCAPA syndrome in a patient who underwent ligation of an LAD artery arising from the pulmonary artery and placement of a venous bypass graft from the aorta to the proximal LAD artery distal to the ligation. Volume-rendered CT image shows the venous graft and a patent proximal LAD artery (arrowheads). Note the dilated left main coronary artery (arrowhead). Ao, aorta.*

Computerized Cardiac Scan (MD/CT)

Currently, this type of imaging technique is found be very helpful in profiling coronary arteries and other intracardiac defects of the heart with good index of certainity.

Management

Delaying surgery while waiting for the child to grow is no longer justifiable. Once the diagnosis has been recognized and the infant stabilized with anticongestive medications, surgery is undertaken to correct the coronary circulation. Formerly, ligation of the left coronary artery at its source from the pulmonary artery was used to eliminate the left-to-right shunt and prevent a steal from the myocardium. Although this surgery is often successful, the initial and late mortality are significant. A variety of methods to connect the left coronary artery to the aorta have been tried with varying success. One of the most satisfactory has been the operation proposed by Takeuchi. However, it is accomplished, the desired effect is perfusion of the left coronary from the aorta. With survival, the evidences of myocardial infarction may disappear, the heart size may return to normal, the child becomes asymptomatic, and measures of myocardial function improve. Revision of the operative connections may be needed. Close follow-up of these patients is necessary until the long-term outcome is established.

Course

The remarkable improvements in the electrocardiogram, the echocardiographic measures of function, and the patient are surprisingly impressive, suggesting that the infant myocardium has a capacity for repair after ischemia and infarction that exceeds that seen in the adult. It is too early to be confident that these patients are truly cured.

Among older patients any evidence of cardiac embarrassment may be a reason to connect the coronary artery to the aorta. The reports of sudden death in these patients are sufficient to encourage surgery to provide a two-coronary system wherever possible.

CONGENITAL AV BLOCKS

The most common causes of congenital heart block include anatomic cardiac defects (particularly ventricular inversion or atrioventricular canal defects) and fetal exposure to maternal antibodies related to connective tissue disease (primarily systemic lupus erythematosus). Often, it is first diagnosed in utero when a slow fetal pulse is detected on routine obstetrical evaluation. Fetal echocardiography can be performed to rule out structural cardiac defects and to record an M-mode tracing that views simultaneous atrial and ventricular wall motion. Third-degree block is readily diagnosed as the faster atrial motion is completely dissociated from the slow ventricular contraction. If block is seen in the absence of structural defects, maternal testing for antinuclear antibody titers should be performed. It is estimated that as many as 60% of mothers will have clinical and/or serologic evidence of connective tissue disease in this setting. Congenital heart block is usually well tolerated

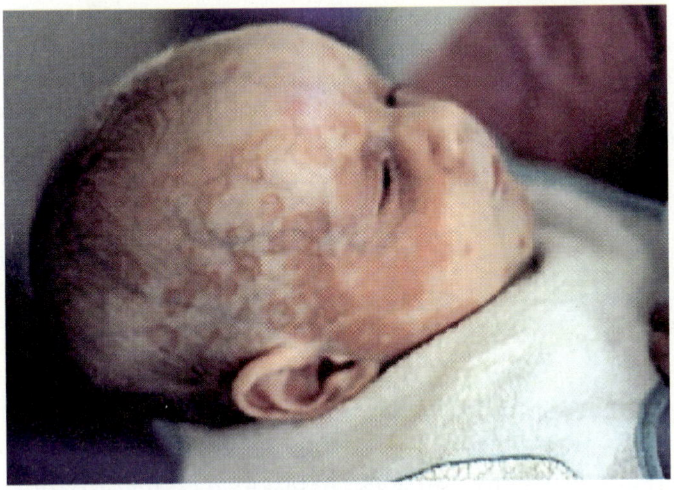

Fig. 14.333: *Typical cutaneous manifestations of lupus contracted through mother and had complete heart block after birth*

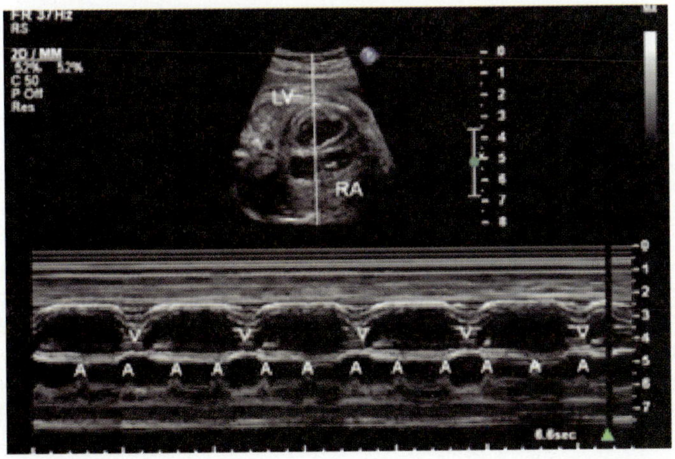

Fig. 14.334: *Fetal complete heart block. M-mode tracing from a four chamber view with the transducer beam through the RA and the LV. There are regular atrial contractions (A) with a normal heart rate of 125 bpm and independent ventricular contractions (V) with a heart rate of 50 bpm*

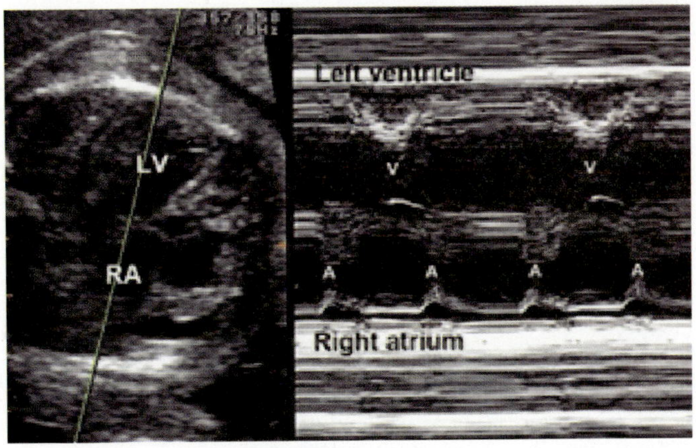

Fig. 14.335: *Fetal 2.1 AV block. M-mode tracing from a four chamber view with the transducer beam through the RA and the LV. There are regular atrial contractions (A) with a normal heart rate of 125 bpm and independent ventricular contractions (V) with a heart rate of 50 bpm*

in utero, but there are well described instances of fetal hydrops and even fetal death. Unfortunately treatment for a distressed fetus is difficult because in utero pacing techniques are not yet perfected. At present, the only safe course for a hydrops infant is early delivery and immediate pacing but this option is frequently limited by fetal lung maturity.

Fortunately, in most cases the fetus adapts well to slow heart rates and will usually come to term without difficulty. Delivery should be performed at a center with pediatric cardiology back-up, because abrupt extrauterine decompensation may occur occasionally even if the fetus did well in uterus.

Emergency pacemaker placement will stabilize such infants promptly. For the vast majority of newborns with congenital heart block, the transition to extrauterine life is smooth unless complicated by prematurity, lung disease, or anatomic cardiac defects.

Although the short-term prognosis for most of patients with congenital block is generally good. Certainly, all symptomatic patients should be treated promptly with pacing and pacemaker implant should also be considered in advance of symptoms for any patient thought to risk for sudden events. Potential risk factors for poor outcome have been sought in multiple studies and have included:

1. Resting ventricular rate lie below 55/min for neonates,
2. Resting ventricular rate below 50/min for older patients,
3. Prolonged Q-T interval
4. Wide QRS escape rhythm
5. Ventricular ectopy
6. Advanced cardiomegaly and/or ventricular dysfunction.

It remains uncertain which of these factors is the single best predictor of the need for prophylactic pacer insertion, but given the low risk and high reliability of modern pacer technology, the threshold for recommending the procedure should be low. If none of the above factors is present, it appears reasonable to follow the patient conservatively, particularly the very young child in whom small body size may complicate pacemaker implantation.

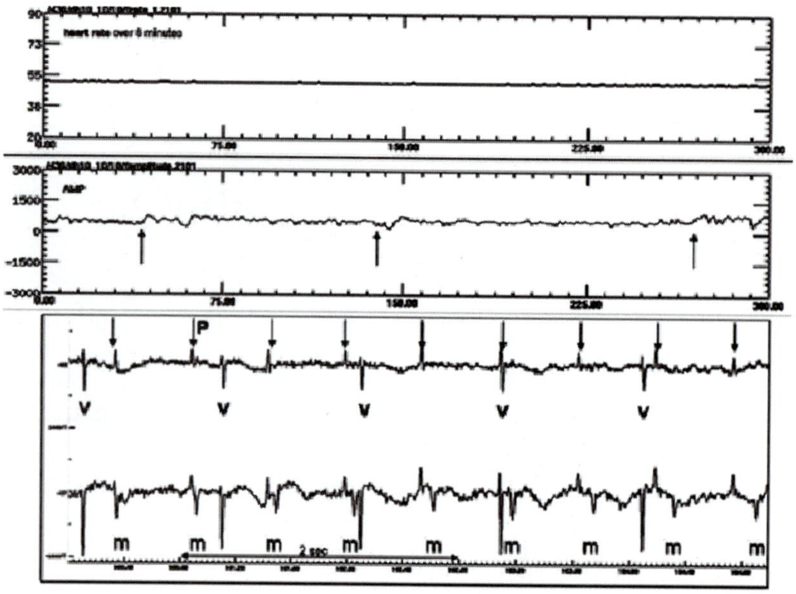

Fig. 14.336: *FMCG recording from a 24-week GA fetus with complete heart block. Note in the top two tracings that the rate is stable at about 52 beats/minute during 5 minutes. There is no reactivity of the ventricular rate with the fetal movement, denoted by the upward-facing arrows in the actogram tracing. In the lower tracing, the maternal QRS is marked "m", fetal QRS "V", and the fetal P waves with the downward-facing arrows. Note complete atrioventricular dissociation. The QRS duration is not prolonged in this case, but due to the non-reactivity and low rate, this fetus will require pacing after birth*

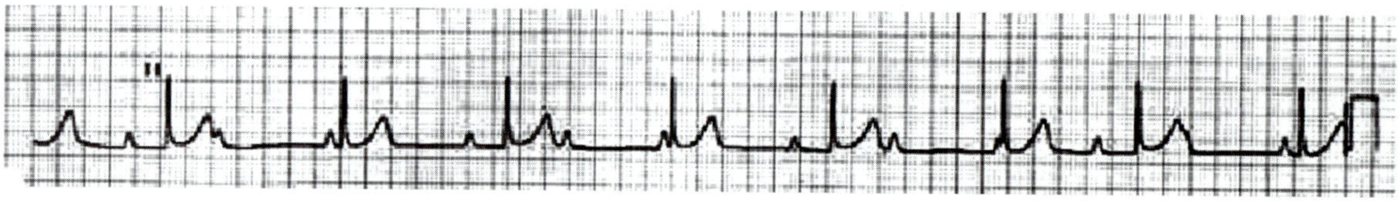

Fig. 14.337: *ECG of a neonate showing bradycardia with variable PR interval in complete heart block*

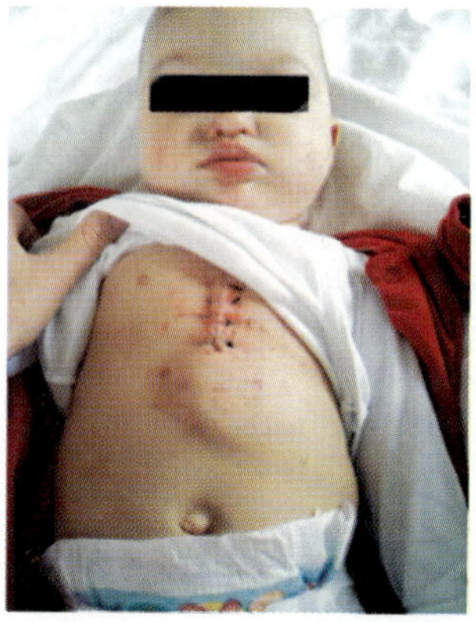

Fig. 14.338: *Dual chamber pacemaker with epicardial electrodes implanted through a median sternotomy in a newborn with complete heart block*

Physical Examination

The fetus may be monitored with ultrasonography for varying degrees of heart block and hydrops fetalis. In the newborn, the findings may range from asymptomatic to signs of congestive heart failure and low cardiac output.

The most typical physical finding is a low heart rate for age. Because the block is usually complete and the escape rhythm is usually junctional in origin, a regular rhythm at 60–80 beats per minute (bpm) is often found. Auscultation demonstrates a variable first heart sound caused by the AV asynchrony.

Congenital AV block may be associated with findings of low cardiac output or congestive heart failure. Low cardiac output may manifest with physical findings of irritability or lethargy, cool skin, mottling, or cyanosis.

Congestive heart failure may manifest with tachypnea and hepatomegaly. If congestive heart failure has been present prenatally, marked edema may be part of the complex of hydrops fetalis.

Children with neonatal lupus can present with rash, as well as with neurologic and hepatic manifestations. The rash can occur some days after birth and is worsened with sun exposure. Annular or elliptical erythematous plaques can be present on the skin of face, scalp, and extremities. It usually resolves without scarring but can be associated with residual hypopigmentation or, rarely, telangiectasias. Children with structural heart disease may manifest symptoms and signs related to the specific congenital heart defect. Patients with heterotaxia syndrome may be cyanotic. Patients with L-transposition of the great arteries may be completely asymptomatic or may demonstrate a murmur.

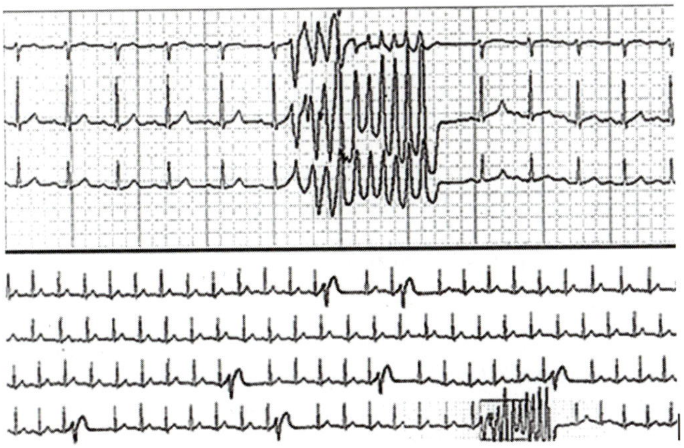

Fig. 14.339: *Holter monitoring shows in upper three tracings the onset of rapid polymorphic ventricular tachycardia that occurs near the peak of the T-wave. The QT interval is normal, and this has been referred to as short-coupled torsade de pointes. These patients frequently have premature ventricular contractions that are also short-coupled as noted on the bottom strip (recorded for a more prolonged period). This arrhythmia does not occur frequently enough to evaluate various forms of therapy in a randomized controlled trial, but there are many reports in the literature confirming its lethal nature.*

Approach Considerations

After birth, electrocardiography (ECG) is recommended to assess for CAVB and to assess the QT interval that can be prolonged. ECG and Holter ambulatory ECG monitoring are routinely performed initially and periodically in patients with complete CAVB.

Holter Monitoring (Ambulatory ECG)

It is recommended to determine if the AV block is intermittent or persistent and to evaluate for associated arrhythmias.

Exercise Testing

It is performed on a regular basis in patients who are capable, usually in patients older than age 7 years. Electrophysiologic testing is not routinely performed in patients with CAVB, although it provides information regarding pathophysiology and prognosis in certain cases.

Chest radiography: It can reveal cardiomegaly and pleural effusions. Heterotaxia can be suspected in presence of visceroatrial discordance. One should look for a midline liver, rightward stomach bubble, and dextrocardia. Looking at lead placement in temporary and permanent pacemakers is helpful.

Consultations

The mother should consult with a rheumatologist to begin monitoring for possible autoimmune disease. Consultation with a rheumatologist is also advised for the infant, particularly if other manifestations of neonatal lupus erythematosus are present.

Genetic consultation is recommended for children with first-degree relatives with structural heart disease or those with storage disorder or cardiomyopathy.

Pediatric cardiology consultation is necessary for every case.

Laboratory Studies

In patients with CAVB, routine electrolyte assays should be performed to assess for metabolic derangements (especially hyperkalemia), and a complete blood count (CBC) should be obtained to assess for anemia, neutropenia, and thrombocytopenia.

Neonatal assessment should include a measurement of anti-Ro and anti-La antibody levels, preferably using an enzyme-linked immunosorbent assay (ELISA) in the mother. Assessment for other organ and/or tissue damage

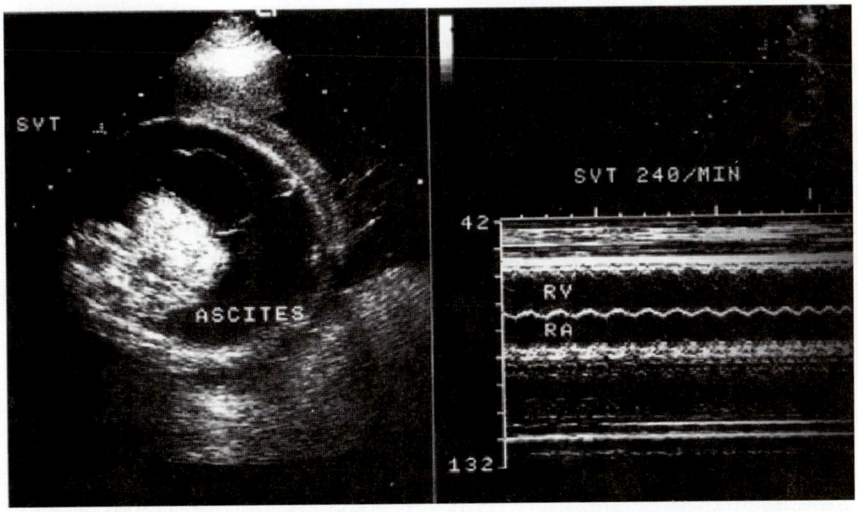

Fig. 14.340: *Transverse section per abdomen echocardiogram of the foetus showing severe form of foetal hydrops (left) secondary to heart failure due to sustained atrioventricular re-entry tachycardia which is demonstrated by the M-mode recording of the foetal heart rate (right) with 1.1 A-V conduction*

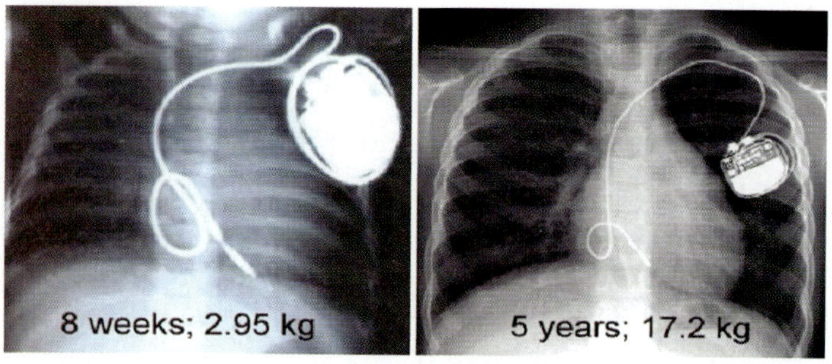

Fig. 14.341: *Left panel shows lead position in a baby with congenital complete heart block who was born prematurely with hydrops. A transvenous endocardial pacemaker was implanted at the age of 8 weeks when she weighed 2.95 kg. At 5 years of age (weight 17.2 kg), she still has the initial lead and generator (right panel). The redundant loop of lead formed in the right atrium has not yet been taken up and will allow generator replacement without the need for lead advancement*

should include a platelet assessment to rule out thrombocytopenia and an assessment of liver enzymes to rule out alloimmune hepatitis.

If inflammatory disease is suspected, workup for various infectious etiologies [e.g., human immunodeficiency virus (HIV)] should be performed. Cardiac troponins and pro-brain natriuretic peptide (BNP) levels can be helpful in assessing the severity of the disease.

If hypertrophic cardiomyopathy is suspected, evaluation for lysosomal storage diseases should be included.

Preductal and post-ductal saturations by pulse oximetry should be performed. Check for hypoxemia and acidosis using ABG findings. Also, check lactic acid for perfusion. A hyperoxia test is very helpful in differentiating lung disease-related hypoxemia versus hypoxemia due to a cyanotic heart disease. One can evaluate for Heinz bodies on peripheral smear for evaluation of asplenia that is seen with heterotaxia syndromes.

Ultrasonography

It should be performed initially and in periodic follow-up care in affected fetuses, infants, and children to assess ventricular function and size and to rule out congenital or acquired cardiac malformations or valve dysfunction.

Children of mothers with the anti-Ro and anti-La antibodies should undergo regular fetal ultrasonographic assessments including detailed fetal echocardiography to identify conduction delay, bradycardia and ventricular function. All children, regardless of fetal findings, should undergo an electrocardiogram after birth to check the conduction intervals. Children with first-degree or second-degree AV block have been known to progress to third-degree CAVB.

Mothers with the autoimmune antibodies or those with one affected child should undergo regular fetal ultrasonographic assessments including detailed fetal echocardiography, to identify subsequent affected pregnancies starting early, at 16 weeks' gestation. Fetal echocardiography can reveal varying degrees of AV block. Fetal monitoring should be performed to look for bradycardia, fetal distress and hydrops fetalis.

Fetal echocardiography is geared toward looking for early heart block, bradycardia, arrhythmias, pericardial effusion, cardiomegaly, valvular insufficiency (especially tricuspid regurgitation), decreasing contractile function, and abnormal venous and arterial pulsations.

Approach Considerations

Pharmacologic Therapy

Little evidence suggests that the administration of steroids or immunoglobulins or the performance of plasmapheresis in the mother can reverse third-degree AV block in the fetus. However, these therapies may be helpful in early first- and second-degree heart block and in reducing associated myocardial dysfunction.

Regular and close monitoring for heart block and transplacental therapy with fluorinated steroids (dexamethasone) and beta-sympathomimetics have been used by some centers with satisfactory results at the first evidence of heart block and bradycardia with hydrops, respectively. Prophylactic therapy is not currently indicated because these medications can have maternal and fetal side effects.

Children with CAVB due to heart disease may need to be on prostaglandin therapy to keep the ductus patent.

In patients with CAVB, prophylactic antibiotic therapy during and following surgery appears to reduce the incidence of pacemaker system infections, although current studies do not reach statistical significance because of the relative rarity of this complication (approximately 1%).

Hydrops Fetalis

Therapy for hydrops fetalis can be challenging in utero and after birth. A staged approach with stabilization of the patient, drainage of the effusions, the use of intravenous inotropes (dopamine) and chronotropes (isoproterenol), and placement of a pacemaker has shown some success. Some centers recommend cesarean and preterm delivery for fetuses with CAVB and hydrops fetalis.

Bradycardia

In the perinatal period, fetal bradycardia may be an incidental finding. However, when persistent bradycardia is identified in the third trimester, emergency delivery is sometimes inappropriately carried out without differentiating acute causes of bradycardia related to fetal distress from the more chronic condition of isolated CAVB.

Pacemaker Therapy

The medical care of congenital atrioventricular block (CAVB) is currently focused on identifying the optimal timing of pacemaker therapy to ensure a positive outcome. Additional care is aimed at identifying and treating the associated conditions that arise. Patients who present with symptoms as fetuses or newborns may require earlier pacing than do those who present with symptoms later in childhood. Fetuses with hydrops fetalis secondary to maternal autoimmune disease have successfully received pacing in utero; however, this has not prevented fetal demise.

Symptoms referable to bradycardia are an indication for pacing in complete CAVB. Because severe symptoms (e.g. syncope) occasionally arise suddenly or sudden cardiac death can occur, additional risk factors identified from monitoring have been recommended as indications for pacing.

Temporary pacing can be achieved transcutaneously, transesophageally, or transvenously. However, permanent pacemaker placement is eventually needed in most children with CAVB. Major criteria for pacing based on ECG or Holter monitoring include an average heart rate of less than 50 bpm, a nighttime or sleeping average heart rate of less than 45 bpm, or pauses secondary to AV block that are longer than 3 seconds.

In the setting of borderline major criteria, other criteria that may influence the decision for timing of pacemaker implantation include cardiomegaly, a high atrial rate, junctional instability (e.g. junctional exit block), a broad complex escape rhythm, diminished ventricular response to exercise, QT prolongation, and complex ventricular ectopy.

When criteria are met, surgical implantation of an epicardial pacemaker should be performed, with knowledge of the implications of pacing in children and recognition of the lifelong need for pacing and pacemaker lead access. Multiple backup pacing systems at the time of surgery (e.g. temporary transvenous pacing, transthoracic pacing units) are helpful to avoid the extremes of bradycardia that may be associated with anesthesia and pacemaker surgery.

Venous obstruction, small patient size, and actual or potential right-left shunting are relative contraindications for transvenous pacing. Fortunately, epicardial pacing leads have greatly improved and allow for successful pacing system insertion under these conditions. Some centers are using neonatal endocardial pacing systems.

In children older than the neonatal period, an endocardial pacing with transvenous approach is possible. The risk of venous occlusion appears to correlate with the ratio of available transvenous lead body sizes and the patient's body surface area. Exceeding this ratio may lead to a high incidence of venous obstruction.

In addition, imaging of the subclavian-innominate venous channels before pacemaker lead placement is helpful for transvenous lead placement. The course of the lead should be evaluated in 2 planes to avoid inadvertent lead placement into the foramen ovale, an unroofed left superior vena cava to coronary sinus, or left-sided circulation via the subclavian artery. Either a subcutaneous or subpectoral pocket may be formed inferior to the clavicle.

Major lawsuits related to pacing in congenital atrioventricular block (CAVB) have arisen primarily because of inadvertent placements of pacing leads into the left-sided circulation. This complication can be recognized at or immediately following system placement using complementary radiographic views, usually lateral and posteroanterior (PA) or anteroposterior (AP).

Follow-up

Routine pacemaker follow-up visits should be maintained according to national or international guidelines. Transtelephonic pacemaker monitoring may allow for improved follow-up care and longer intervals between outpatient visits.

Activity

Patients with permanent pacing systems should be restricted from activities that result in repeated intentional direct trauma to the pacemaker area (e.g. martial arts). Patients with permanent pacing systems should be restricted from exposure to high magnetic fields, such as direct magnetic resonance imaging (MRI) exposure.

Medication

Intrauterine treatments used for CAVB include chronotropic agents, inotropic agents, steroids, and plasmapheresis. In general, medications are not necessary in children with complete CAVB. Emergency use of chronotropic medications with or without inotropic agents, may be helpful in fetuses and newborns with hydrops fetalis, congestive heart failure, or low cardiac output.

Some investigators have suggested the use of immunosuppressive agents in fetuses and newborns to potentially slow or halt progressive CAVB in utero. This is currently being evaluated as a prospective study.

The use of steroids or immunoglobulins may be helpful in early first- and second-degree heart block and in reducing associated myocardial dysfunction.

Corticosteroids

Corticosteroids have antiinflammatory properties and cause profound and varied metabolic effects. They modify the body's immune response to diverse stimuli. It may be helpful in early first- and second-degree heart block and in reducing associated myocardial dysfunction.

Blood Products

These agents are used to improve the clinical aspect of the disease. It may reduce associated myocardial dysfunction.

Immune globulin intravenous (Gamunex, Octagam, Gammaplex, Gammagard).

This provides an antibody-mediated blockade of Fas-Fas ligand interactions involved in the epidermal necrosis of toxic epidermal necrolysis-like cutaneous lupus erythematosus.

LONG QT SYNDROME

Patients with a prolonged QT interval are more prone to the risk of recurrent syncope and sudden death due to ventricular tachycardia or ventricular fibrillation. The idiopathic long QT syndrome ventricular fibrillation. The idiopathic long QT syndrome may be either autosomal recessive or autosomal dominant.

Genetic Basis of LQTS

After each heartbeat, the heart recovers electrically and prepares itself for the next beat through what is known as repolarization. This process relies on the normal function of multiple ion channels in the cells of the heart muscle. These channels are pores or tiny openings that allow for the passage of certain ions like sodium or potassium.

There are specific genes in the body that lead to the development of the ion-channels. Congenital LQTS is linked to mutations of these genes and leads to their abnormal function. The electrical activity of the heart becomes disturbed and requires a longer time to recover. Thus, patients with congenital LQTS have a prolonged repolarization stage, or QT interval.

Scientific discoveries dating back to the 1990s have identified specific genes that encode the ion channels in the cells of the heart muscle. Although progress is being made, there are still many patients and families with LQTS for whom no mutation has been found. There are almost certainly other LQTS genes that have not yet been discovered. Prolongation of the QT interval may be:

a. Acquired by patients having electrolyte-imbalance
b. Taking antiarrhythmic drugs
c. Taking psychotropic drugs
d. Having myocarditis
e. Myocardial ischemia
f. Snus node disease or
g. Central nervous system disease
h. Consuming liquid protein diets

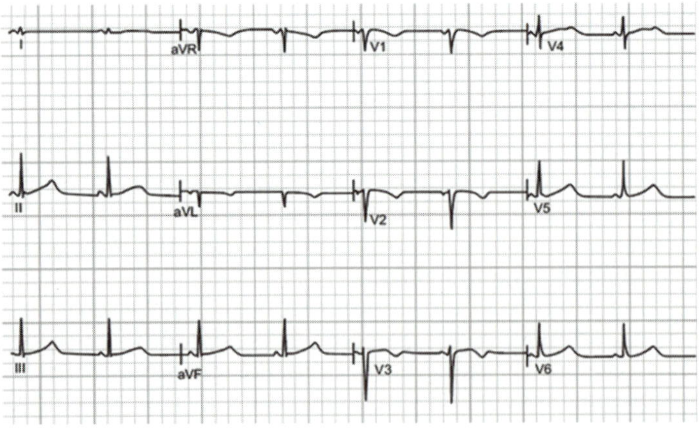

Fig. 14.342: *The 12-lead EKG of a 13-year-old girl with long QT syndrome with the clinical presentation of recurrent syncopes. The QTc is 645 ms, with typical biphasic T waves in V2 and V3*

Diagnosis in LQTS

- If you have unexplained fainting episodes or seizures, a family history of unexplained sudden death at a young age, or LQTS runs in your family, you might have LQTS.
- An ECG will often show the prolonged QT interval.
- Some patients with LQTS have a normal or borderline QT interval on an ECG performed at rest and may require additional tests for diagnosis, such as the ECG with stress test (administered on a treadmill) and/or a 24-hour Holter monitor.

Treatment in LQTS

Treatment is available and may include:

- Beta-blocker medications which substantially reduces the risk of fainting and sudden death. These medications must be taken daily.
- Patients who have experienced high-risk signs of LQTS such as cardiac arrest, or fainting in spite of beta-blocker use, may be advised additional treatment such as an implantable defibrillator or pacemaker.

Medications to Avoid in LQTS

Certain medications may prolong the QT interval and should be avoided by patients with LQTS or a family history of LQTS symptoms. It is associated with a specific type of ventricular arrhythmia, torsade de pointes, which is characterized by the cycles of alternating electrical polarity of the QRS complex peaks that oscillate or twist around the isoelectric line. The alternating cycles may be interrupted by periods of rapid tachycardia and polarity. The rhythm rate varies from 160 to 280 beats per minute and most often is between 200 and 250 beats per minute. Assessment and treatment of ventricular tachyarrhythmias present extraordinary challenges to the clinician. Moreover, the prognosis for patients is quite variable with these characteristically sudden-onset, unpredictable, and transitory arrhythmias. In some patients, ventricular ectopic activity may be benign and without sequelae, but in other patients, comparable ectopy is a harbinger of ventricular fibrillation and sudden cardiac death.

Short QT Syndrome

Short QT syndrome is a genetic disease of the electrical system of the heart. It consists of a constellation of signs and symptoms, consisting of a short QT interval interval on EKG (300 ms) that doesn't significantly change with heart rate, tall and peaked T waves, and a structurally normal heart. Short QT syndrome appears to be inherited in an autosomal dominant pattern, and a few affected families have been identified. Short QT syndrome is inherited in an autosmal dominant patterns. Individuals with short QT syndrome frequently complain of palpitations and may have syncope (loss of consciousness) that is unexplained. Mutations in the KCNH2, KCNJ2, and KCNQ1 genes cause short QT syndrome. These genes provide instructions for making proteins that act as channels across the cell membrane. These channels transport positively charged atoms (ions) of potassium into

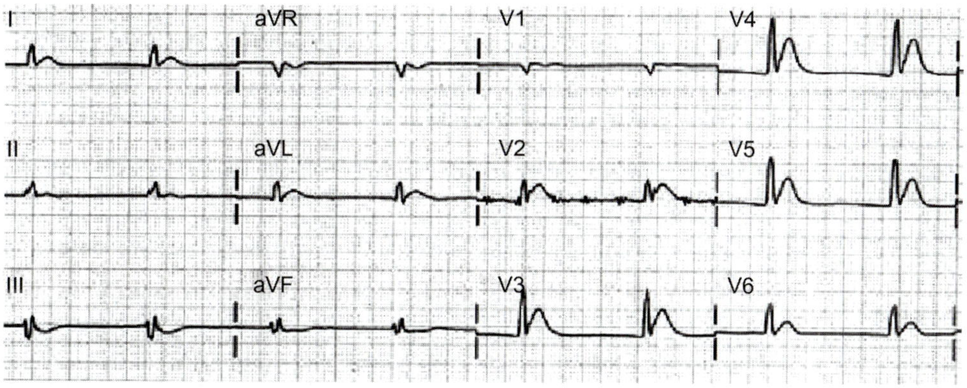

Fig. 14.343: *Electrocardiogram of a patient with short QT syndrome. Observe the tall-peaked T waves. QT interval (260 ms) in a patient with hypercalcaemia*

and out of cells. In cardiac muscle, these ion channels play critical roles in maintaining the heart's normal rhythm. Mutations in the KCNH2, KCNJ2, or KCNQ1 gene increase the activity of the channels, which changes the flow of potassium ions between cells. This disruption in ion transport alters the way the heart beats, leading to the abnormal heart rhythm characteristic of short QT syndrome. Short QT syndrome appears to have an autosomal dominant pattern of inheritance. Due to the autosomal dominant inheritance pattern, most individuals will have family members with a history of unexplained or sudden death at a young age (even in infancy), palpitations, or atrial fibrillation. Short QT syndrome is associated with an increased risk of sudden cardiac death, most likely due to ventricular fibrillation.

Diagnosis: The diagnosis of short QT syndrome consists of characteristic history and findings on EKG and electrophysiologic testing. There are currently no set guidelines for the diagnosis of short QT syndrome.

Electrocardiogram: The characteristic findings of short QT syndrome on EKG are a short QT interval, typically 300 ms, that doesn't significantly change with the heart rate. Tall, peaked T waves may also be noted. Individuals mayalso have an underlying atrial rhythm of atrial fibrillation.

Brugada Syndrome

In 1992, Brugada and colleagues described a clinical syndrome consisting of apparently healthy adults presenting with syncope or sudden death. Their ECGs showed coved ST segment elevation and negative T waves in leads VI and V2 (V3) in the absence of RBBB pattern This ECG pattern has become to be known as the "Brugada-ECG". These patients were thought to have no evidence of structural heart disease, and were at high risk for recurrent syncope or sudden death. In 15–20% of patients a genetic defect in the cardiac sodium channel was found. It has been proposed that there is a premature termination of the epicardial action potential with loss of the phase-2 dome pattern. The ECG changes are believed to be due to regional epicardial, endocardial voltage gradient during the plateau phase of the action potential. This voltage gradient may give rise to VT due to phase-2 reentry caused by inhomogeneity of the voltage in adjacent areas of the myocardium. In patients with the Brugada syndrome, syncope and sudden death are due to polymorphic VT. Since the original descripion, it has been observed that the "Brugada-ECG"-type ST segment elevation in V1 in the right precordial leads can be:

i. Cove shaped, ST segment
ii. Saddle-shaped ST segment.

There has been a recent attempt to standardize this diagnostic ECG feature as follows:

- *Type I :* Coved-shaped right precordial ST elevation, in more than one right precordial lead (VI-V3), of > 2 mm followed by a negative T wave
- *Type II:* Saddle-shaped ST elevation
- *Type III:* ST elevation of < 2 mm.

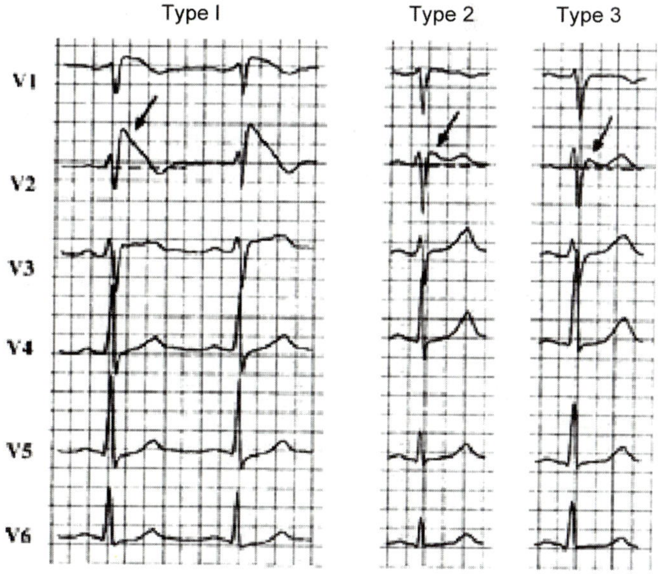

Fig. 14.344: *Precordial ECG leads (25 mm/s; 10 mm/mV) of different ECG patterns in Brugada syndrome. Type I: coved ST segment elevation in leads VI and V2 (and V3) followed by a negative T wave. Type II: saddle back-type ST segment elevation <2 mm. Type III: saddle back-type ST segment elevation <2 mm*

Only type I is said to be diagnostic of Brugada syndrome. These ST elevations are sensitive to heart rate and the effects of autonomic stimulation. Furthermore, sodium channel-blocking antiarrhythmic drugs such as procainamide or lecainide have been shown to "provoke" these ECG changes in patients with otherwise normal baseline ECG, and have been proposed as a screening tool in patients suspected to have the Brugada syndrome. However, the sensitive, specificity and reproducibility of this drug provocation are not well established. Of interest, certain gene mutations are sensitive to temperature with regard to their phenotypic expression. Indeed, Brugada-type ECG changes have been seen in patients only during febrile illness . Some speculate that seizures during febrile illness may be related to self-terminating ventricular arrhythmias due to a temperature sensitive mutation in the sodium channel, giving rise to the "Brugada syndrome".

Patients with resuscitated sudden death or syncope or with a family history of premature sudden death and typical type I Brudaga. ECG changes are at increased risk of recurrent events, and should be considered for ICD therapy. Asymptomatic patients who have an unprovoked typical Brudaga ECG (type I) are also at increased risk for arrhythmic events, but the magnitude of the risk is unclear. In one study, the event rate over a mean of 24 months follow up was 8% in these patients. Those presenting with typical Brugada ECG (type I) only after drug exposure or those presenting with nondiagnostic right precordial ECG abnormalities (type II, type III) are believed to be at low risk. The role of electrophysiologic study and prognostic value of inducible VF remain controversial.

Management in Brugada Syndrome

At present, implantation of an automatic implantable cardiac defibrillator (ICD) is the only treatment proven effective in treating ventricular tachycardia and fibrillation and preventing sudden death in patients with Brugada syndrome. No pharmacologic therapy has been proven to reduce the occurrence of ventricular arrhythmias or sudden death.

Patients with Brugada syndrome and a history of cardiac arrest must be treated with an ICD. In contrast, asymptomatic patients with no family history of sudden cardiac death can be managed conservatively with close follow-up, and ICD implantation is not recommended. Patients with intermediate clinical characteristics present the greatest challenge.

ENDOCARDIAL FIBROELASTOSIS

The term endocardial fibroelastosis (EFE) was introduced by Weinberg and Himmelfarb in 1943 Endocardial fibroelastosis refers to a pronounced, diffuse thickening of the ventricular endocardium and presents as unexplained heart failure in infants and children. The disease can be primary or secondary to various congenital heart diseases, most notably hypoplastic left heart syndrome, aortic stenosis, or atresia. The two pathologic forms of primary endocardial fibroelastosis include dilated, which is most common, and contracted. Primary endocardial fibroelastosis is not associated with any significant structural anomaly of the heart. Secondary endocardial fibroelastosis is associated with other congenital heart diseases. Once regarded as a common cause of unexplained heart failure, endocardial fibroelastosis is now considered rare.

Pathophysiology

Endocardial fibroelastosis is characterized by diffuse endocardial thickening and myocardial dysfunction. The endocardial thickening is believed to be caused by persistent and increased wall tension in the ventricles, possibly secondary to damaged myocardium, mitral regurgitation, or both. However, endocardial fibroelastosis changes are progressive with age. The disease is usually sporadic, but familial cases have been reported (10%). Observations that favor a viral etiology include a clinical presentation similar to that of chronic myocarditis, findings of myocarditis or myocardial fibrosis in affected patients, a higher incidence following epidemics of coxsackievirus B infection, demonstration of persistent viral infection with molecular studies, and experimental production of the disease in animal models by viral infections of the myocardium. A phenotypic resemblance to dilated cardiomyopathy has been noted.

Dilated endocardial fibroelastosis is characterized by a markedly enlarged globular heart, mainly involving the left ventricle (LV) and left atrium (LA). The LV endocardium is opaque, glistening, milky white, and diffusely thickened to about 1–2 mm. The thickening is most marked in the outflow tract.

Papillary muscles arise more superiorly on the ventricular wall with thickened and shortened chordae tendineae, the characteristic rolled-free edge of mitral leaflets. Papillary muscles and trabeculae carneae are flattened and partially incorporated in the fibrotic process, giving a smooth appearance to the lining of the cavity; thus, the papillary muscles exert an undesirable lateral traction on the chordae tendineae and mitral cusps, leading to faulty leaflet opposition.

Although the endocardium is thickened, the ventricular wall (myocardium) thickness is within the reference range. Endocardial thickening extends to the LA, right ventricle, and right atrium. Microthrombi may adhere to the endocardium. The right ventricle is anteriorly displaced to the right, and its cavity is usually flattened. The pulmonary artery may be enlarged, but the aorta and coronary arteries appear normal in caliber. In approximately 50% of patients, the mitral and aortic valves are involved, often producing marked deformity and either valvular regurgitation or stenosis.

The less common contracted type of primary endocardial fibroelastosis is associated with a relatively hypoplastic or normal LV size. The right and left atria and the right ventricle are markedly enlarged and hypertrophied, with minimal or no endocardial sclerosis. An early event in fetal life is believed to result in dilated endocardial fibroelastosis, which later morphoses into a contracted type. This suggests that the dilated type could appear as two different diseases while remaining a single disease. Secondary endocardial fibroelastosis, associated with cardiac malformations, is attributed to the cardiac hypertrophy and consequent imbalance in the myocardial oxygen supply-demand relationship. Resultant fibroelastotic thickening is often focal and less severe.

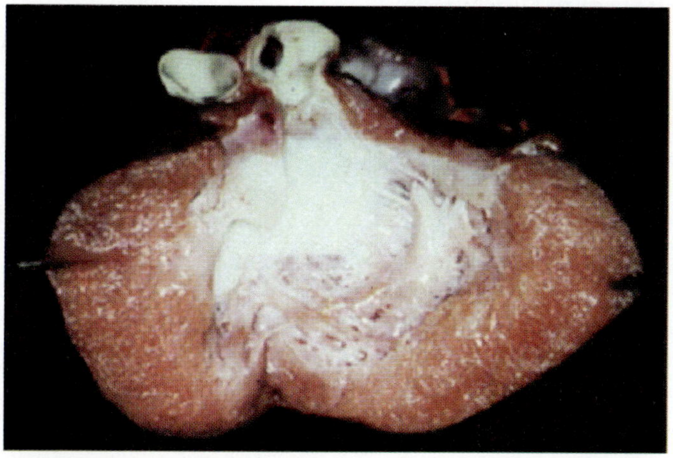

Fig. 14.345: *Specimen of the heart of patient with severe endocardial fibroelastosis and aortic stenosis. Note the anastomosis between the outflow conduit and the ascending aorta*

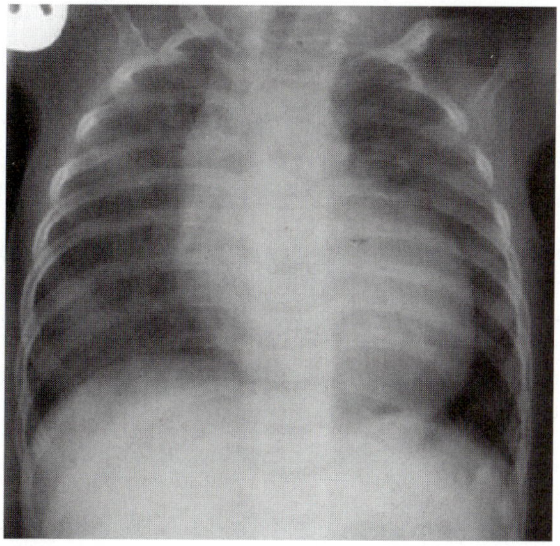

Fig. 14.346: *Chest radiograph, anteroposterior view, showing cardiomegaly and pulmonary venous congestion in a 6-month-old infant with endocardial fibroelastosis (EFE)*

Acute congestive heart failure (CHF) becomes progressive CHF that results in death within weeks, usually within the first 6 months of life. In a subgroup of individuals who survive from a few months to several years, a more chronic course is common. Such patients respond to medications used to treat CHF. A variable cyclical clinical course ensues, with CHF recurrences related to respiratory or other intercurrent infections or to progression of disease. Remissions can occur with intensification of medical therapy.

History

Symptoms of endocardial fibroelastosis (EFE) include feeding difficulty, excessive sweating, breathlessness, failure to thrive, and wheezing.

Onset may acute enough to produce cardiogenic shock or sudden death; it is a recognized cause of sudden death in infancy.

Approximately, 20% of patients have a history of frequent or recent respiratory tract infections.

Episodes of severe sudden abdominal pain may indicate coronary insufficiency.

The contracted form of endocardial fibroelastosis presents with features of left-sided obstructive disease and acute left ventricular failure.

Endocardial fibroelastosis is one of the recognized causes of nonimmune hydrops fetalis.

Physical Examination

Endocardial fibroelastosis manifests as the classic features of heart failure.

Tachypnea during feeding and grunting respirations with subcostal or intercostal retractions have been reported. Fine expiratory wheezes or rales in the lung bases are common. The following may be present upon admission:

- Pallor
- Peripheral cyanosis
- Fever
- Leukocytosis
- Anemia
- Rash.

Thromboembolic episodes may lead to sudden death, myocardial infarction, cerebrovascular events, or even pulmonary embolism. The usual physical findings are as follows:

Cardiomegaly with normal-to-faint first and second heart sounds, a gallop rhythm with an audible third heart sound, apical pansystolic murmur of mitral regurgitation, and hepatosplenomegaly.

Clinically, detectable pleural or pericardial effusions (rare).

Causes

Possible causative factors include intrauterine viral infection (mumps, coxsackievirus B), subendocardial ischemia, impaired lymphatic drainage of the heart, and systemic carnitine deficiency. Using polymerase chain reaction (PCR) analysis, Ni et al reported that the mumps

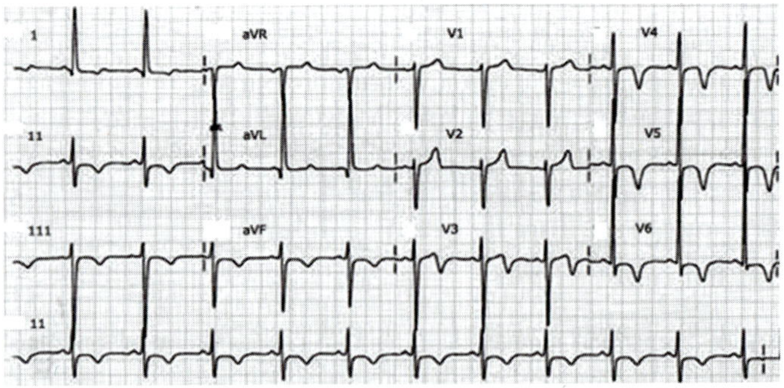

Fig. 14.347: *ECG shows marked clockwise rotation, high voltage of QRS. T invertion over the left precordium (left ventricular hypertrophy) in a 17-months-old girl with endocardial fibroelastosis*

viral genome persisted in the myocardium of children with endocardial fibroelastosis; however, this requires further study. The authors suggested cause and effect and speculated that the disease disappeared after the initiation of the measles-mumps-rubella (MMR) vaccination.

Nine patients with familial endocardial fibroelastosis were reported in 4 families, and inheritance patterns included X-linked recessive, autosomal dominant, and autosomal recessive. Recently, mutation of the gene G4.5 (tafazzin) has been associated with familial X-linked endocardial fibroelastosis and Barth syndrome and has been reported to result in morphologic changes in the fetal heart as early as 18 weeks' gestation.

Dilated (primary) endocardial fibroelastosis occurs when the heart is otherwise normal and no other cause of unexplained heart failure including systemic carnitine deficiency is demonstrable. Dilated endocardial fibroelastosis (secondary) is associated with aortic stenosis or atresia and includes coarctation of the aorta, ventricular septal defect, anomalous origin of left coronary artery from the pulmonary artery, myocardial injury from any cause, and metabolic or carnitine deficiency. Contracted endocardial fibroelastosis (secondary) is associated with hypoplastic left heart syndrome.

Differential Diagnoses

- Anomalous left coronary artery from the pulmonary artery
- Cardiomyopathy, dilated
- Cardiomyopathy, restrictive
- Carnitine deficiency
- Glycogen-storage disease type I
- Glycogen-storage disease type II
- Hypoplastic left heart syndrome
- Mucopolysaccharidosis type IH
- Mucopolysaccharidosis type II
- Mucopolysaccharidosis type III
- Mucopolysaccharidosis type IS
- Mucopolysaccharidosis type IV
- Mucopolysaccharidosis type VI
- Mucopolysaccharidosis type VII
- Myocarditis, viral
- Neonatal lupus and cutaneous lupus erythematosus in children

Laboratory Studies

Blood tests in endocardial fibroelastosis (EFE) include the following:

- Serum electrolyte levels
- BUN and creatinine levels
- CBC count
- Blood culture tests indicated for management of acute episodes
- Autoantibody profile including anti-Ro and anti-La.

Chest Radiography

- Chest radiograph in shows cardiomegaly and pulmonary venous congestion in a 6-month-old infant with endocardial fibroelastosis (EFE).
- Chest radiograph, left lateral view, shows enlarged heart in 6-month-old infant.
- Cardiomegaly and cardiothoracic ratios exceed 0.65 in 50% of patients.
- Cardiac enlargement (CE) is present in some patients at birth. In others, the heart size is normal during the first few weeks to the first few months of life, but CE subsequently develops.
- The shape of the cardiac silhouette varies although it is often globular.
- Pulmonary venous congestion is common.
- Left lower lobe atelectasis secondary to dilated left atrium (LA) is found in 25% of patients.

Echocardiography

- LA and left ventricular (LV) dimensions are increased.
- LV, septal, and posterior wall (PW) excursions are reduced.
- The ejection fraction (EF) is reduced.
- Mitral valve (MV) motion is abnormal.
- Echogenicity along the endocardium of the LV (diagnostic clue) is dense.
- Suggestive indicators include increased endocardial echo brightness and globular shape of the LV.
- The echocardiograph may depict a normalization of the shortening fraction and the LV dimensions when the clinical condition improves following medical therapy.
- A varying degree of mitral regurgitation is common.
- Fetal echocardiography
- This is a valuable tool for early identification, particularly of the secondary type.
- One of the congenital malformations (e.g. aortic stenosis) is often demonstrated at the initial study. The endocardial fibroelastosis becomes obvious in repeat studies.

Electron Beam CT Scanning

Recently, electron beam CT has been reported to be useful in the early diagnosis of endocardial fibroelastosis because of its demonstration of calcification and fibrosis of the ventricles, especially at the apex.

MRI: It helps in identifying the presence of endocardial fibroelastosis. MRI that uses perfusion and myocardial delayed enhancement can be useful in establishing the diagnosis. Endocardial fibroelastosis gives the endocardial surface a rim of hypointense signal in the perfusion sequences and a rim of hyperintense signal in the myocardial delayed-enhancement sequences.

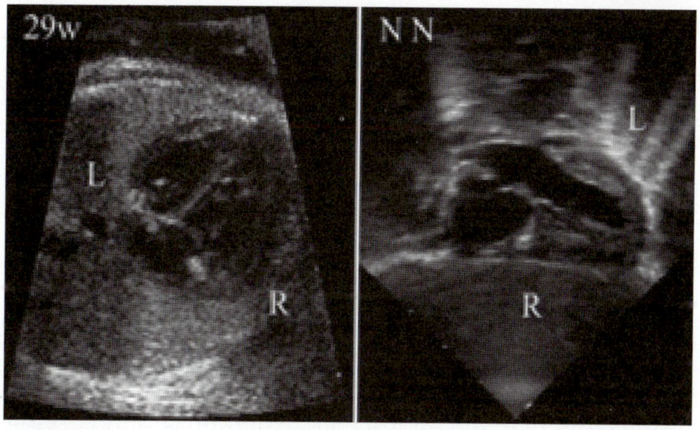

Fig. 14.348: *Fetal ultrsonography. Left: Echographic appearance of heart of case 29 weeks of gestation. Both mitral and tricuspid annuli appear markedly thickened. Multiple hyperechogenic foci are also visible in left (L) and right (R) ventricles. Right: Appearance of heart on echocardiogram recorded few hours after birth. Except for hyperechogenicity around tricuspid annulus, heart appears normal*

Other Tests

Holter ECG (24 hour): This is useful in documenting ambient arrhythmias.

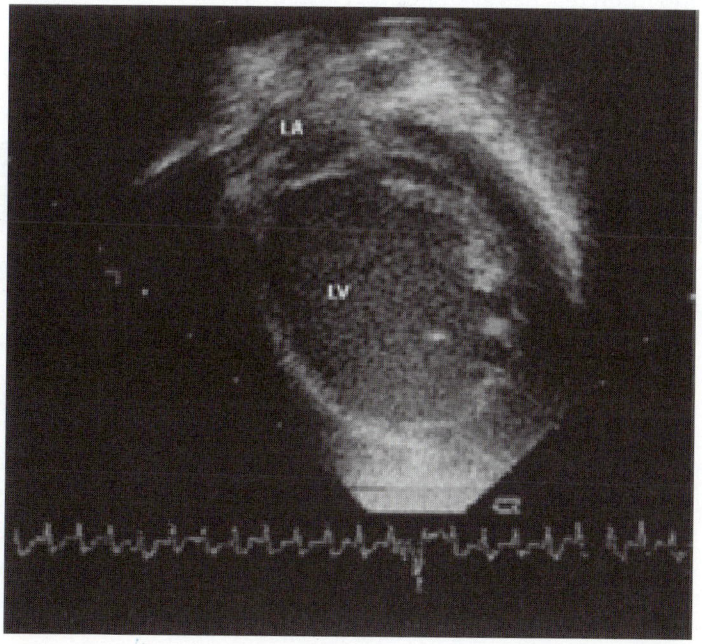

Fig. 14.349: *Transthoracic echocardiogram at the time of hospital admission for congestive heart failure demonstrating a dilated left ventricle (LV) with areas of endocardial fibroelastosis along the endocardial surface of the LV, mitral valve, and papillary muscles. LA, left atrium*

Electrocardiography

Tall R waves, deep Q waves, and T-wave inversion or flattening in the left precordial or inferior lead have been reported. Findings depict LV hypertrophy in more than 75% of patients. In the first few weeks of life, right axis deviation and isolated right ventricular hypertrophy are more common. Pulmonary hypertension may develop in patients who survive for a long period and appears as biventricular hypertrophy on electrocardiography.

Patterns of left, right, or biatrial enlargement are evident in 50% of patients.

Conduction or rhythm abnormalities include Wolff-Parkinson-White syndrome, left bundle-branch block, supraventricular and ventricular arrhythmias, and varying degrees of atrioventricular block. Low-voltage tracings in the initial stage of heart failure and in the terminal phase are noted in 5% of patients. Occasionally, an infarct pattern appears, pointing to extensive myocardial fibrosis and necrosis.

Procedures

Cardiac Catheterization

Cardiac chambers and pulmonary arteries contain elevated pressures consistent with heart failure. Generally, systolic pulmonary artery pressure is not more than 50% of systemic pressure. Marked pulmonary hypertension may be seen in older children.

The constrictive type of endocardial fibroelastosis is rare and is associated with a left-sided atrioventricular obstructive pattern, with very high LA pressures from an early age. A diastolic gradient can be detected across the mitral valve (MV). Pulmonary artery pressure is elevated and often reaches systemic levels in this type of endocardial fibroelastosis.

Postcatheterization precautions include hemorrhage, vascular disruption after balloon dilation, pain, nausea and vomiting, and arterial or venous obstruction due to thrombosis or spasm.

Complications may include blood vessel rupture, tachyarrhythmias, bradyarrhythmias, and vascular occlusion.

Angiocardiographic Findings

- Marked dilation of the LV cavity
- Reduced EF with little or no LV wall thickening
- Dyskinetic LV contraction
- Mitral regurgitation (common)
- In the contracted type, dilated right ventricle, right atrium, and pulmonary artery with slow clearance of the contrast from the left side of the heart.

Digital subtraction angiography: This may reveal an avascular rim between the opacified LV cavity and the ventricular walls perfused by the coronary arteries. The contrast void rim can be identified even in ordinary cineangiographic films.

Biopsy: In cases in which the diagnosis is unclear, myocardial biopsy can be helpful.

Medical Care

The treatment of endocardial fibroelastosis (EFE) is essentially the same as that of chronic cardiac failure; its acute exacerbations are often precipitated by respiratory infections.

Early and prolonged treatment with digoxin is suggested. Continue therapy for several years after the symptoms disappear; cessation of drug administration may result in acute cardiac failure, even when heart size has returned to normal.

Other measures for acute failure and exacerbations of failure may be required, and precipitating factors, such as infection and anemia, require attention.

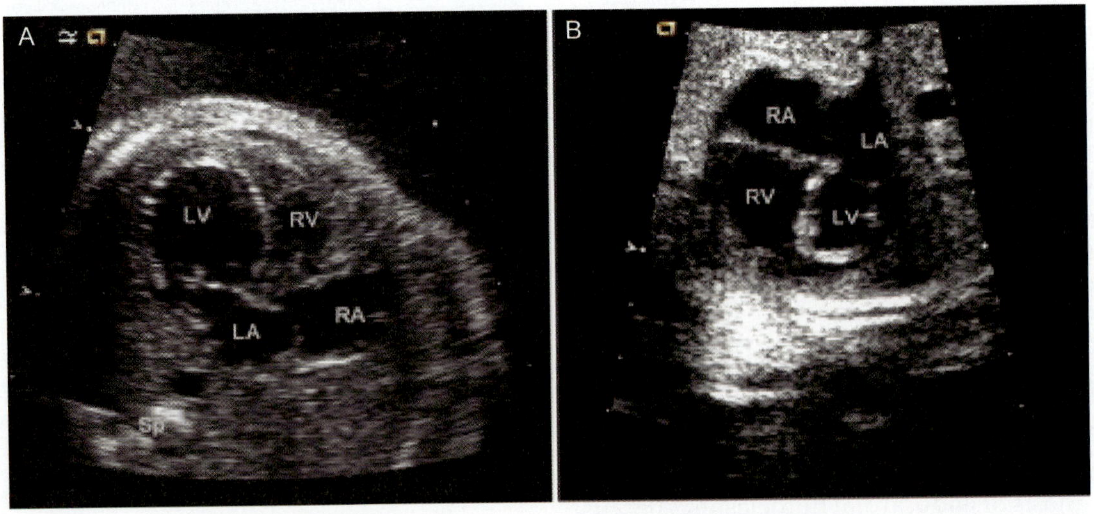

Fig. 14.350: *Fetal echocardiograms (A) Four chamber view of a fetal echocardiogram at 20 weeks' gestation demonstrates a dilated left ventricle with echo bright endocardium suggestive of endocardial fibroelastosis. The position of the atrial septum suggests abnormal left atrial to right atrial shunting in utero. (B) Four chamber view of a fetal echocardiogram in the same fetus imaged at 33 weeks' gestation demonstrates that the left ventricle has become hypoplastic. The echo bright endocardium is even more evident. LA, left atrium; LV, left ventricle; RA, right atrium; RV, right ventricle; Sp, spine*

Anticoagulation may be required in the presence of thromboembolic complications.

Case reports in the literature cite resolution of antenatally diagnosed endocardial fibroelastosis associated with positive anti-Ro and anti-La antibodies with corticosteroid therapy.

Surgical Care

Both pericardial poudrage and mitral valve (MV) replacement have had disappointing results.

Cardiac transplantation may be recommended for patients with end-stage disease.

Medication

If the patient is asymptomatic and his or her heart size is normal, provide early, adequate, and prolonged therapy with digitalis and diuretics for at least 2–3 years, with gradual discontinuation.

Early and prolonged treatment with digoxin is suggested. Anticoagulants may be required in the presence of thromboembolic complications.

Antibiotics for endocarditis prophylaxis are administered to patients with certain cardiac conditions, such as endocardial fibroelastosis, before procedures that may cause bacteremia are performed. For more information, see Antibiotic Prophylactic Regimens for Endocarditis.

Diuretics

These agents are used to eliminate retained fluid and to lower preload.

Furosemide (Lasix)

Inhibits reabsorption of fluid from ascending limb of Henle loop in renal tubule. IV administration has a venodilator action. Lowers preload even before diuresis sets in. DOC in acute heart failure and in exacerbations of chronic heart failure. Used for long-term management of chronic heart failure.

Spironolactone (Aldactone)

Potassium-sparing diuretic that acts on distal convoluted tubule of kidney as an aldosterone antagonist. It has synergistic action with furosemide.

ACE inhibitors

These agents reduce afterload and decrease myocardial remodeling, which worsens chronic heart failure.

Captopril (Capoten) accepted as an essential part of any antifailure therapy; promotes symptomatic improvement and enhances survival.

Cardiac Glycosides

Digoxin (lanoxin) improves myocardial contractility, reduces heart rate, and lowers sympathetic stimulation in chronic heart failure.

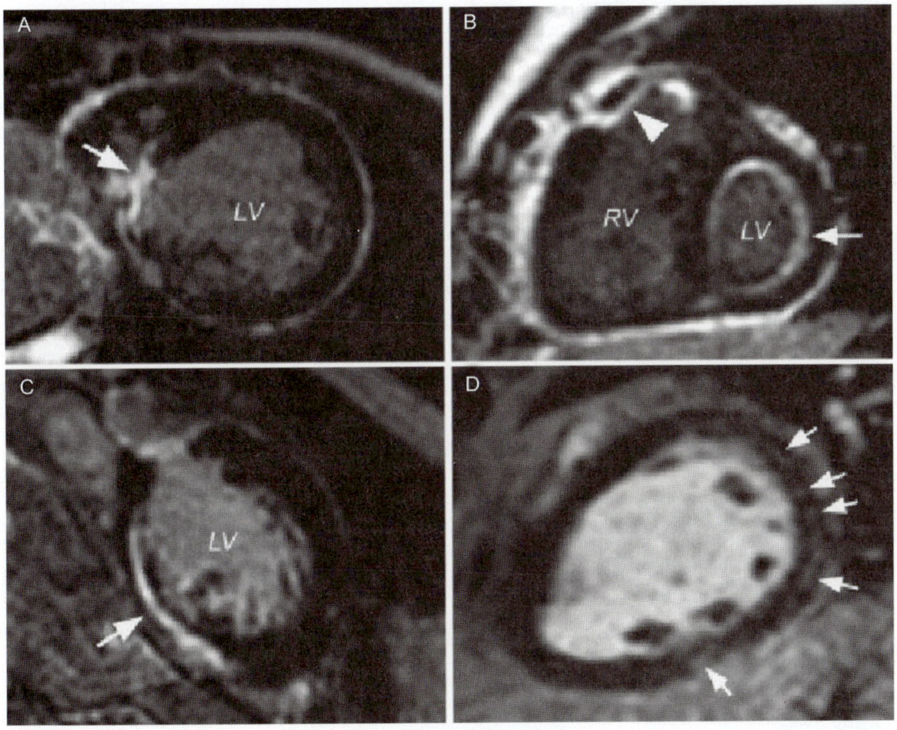

Fig. 14.351: *Locations and patterns of LGE late after fontan operation (A) The arrow points to a transmural late gadolinium enhancement (LGE) lesion involving the ventricular septum. (B) The arrowhead points to a primary subendocardial lesion with transmural extension in the free wall of the primary ventricle, whereas the full arrow identifies endocardial fibroelastosis. (C) The arrow points to a subepicardial LGE lesion in the free wall of the primary ventricle. (D) Speckled pattern (arrows) in the free wall of the primary ventricle. LV, left ventricle; RV, right ventricle*

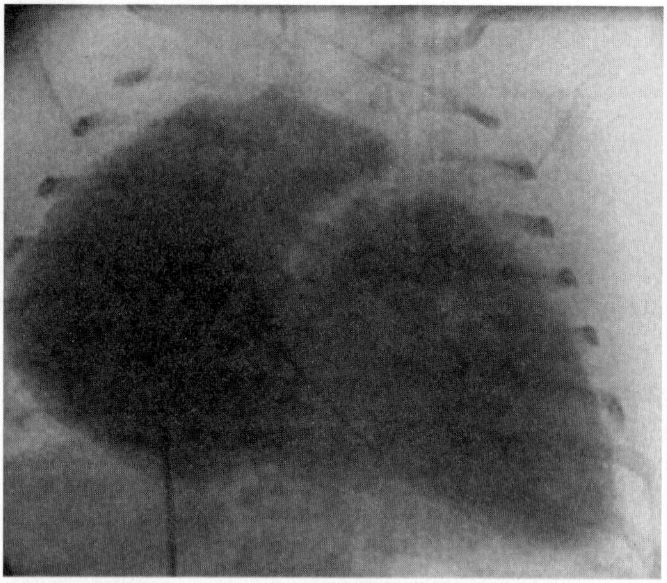

Fig. 14.352: *Digitized reproduction of preoperative angiography from a patient with endocardial fibroelastosis demonstrating severe bilateral enlargement of the heart caused by tricuspid insufficiency and right ventricular failure*

Oral Anticoagulants

These agents prevent recurrence of thromboembolic episodes of cardiac origin.

Warfarin (Coumadin)

Prevents thrombus formation within cardiac chambers and venous circulation by antagonizing effects of vitamin K.

Complications

- Resistant cardiac failure
- Recurrent chest infections
- Severe failure to thrive
- Cardiac cirrhosis
- Cerebral, coronary, and pulmonary thromboembolism
- Persistent collapse of left lower lobe or entire left lung.

Prognosis

Primary endocardial fibroelastosis prognosis is relatively poor although the condition is not universally fatal. The prognosis is worse if onset of heart failure occurs earlier.

Congestive heart failure (CHF) may be present.

Acute CHF becomes progressive CHF and terminates in death within weeks, usually within the first 6 months of life. In patients who survive from a few months to several years, a more chronic course is common. Such patients respond to medications for CHF. A variable cyclical clinical course ensues, with CHF recurrence related to respiratory or other intercurrent infections or to progression of disease. Remissions can occur through intensification of medical therapy.

Progressive CHF causes deteriorating conditions that lead to death in one-third of patients. One-third of the patients survive and may experience persistent symptoms or show residual ECG abnormalities or evidence of cardiomegaly. Some believe that approximately one third of patients completely recover, although others are skeptical. Early diagnosis and prompt persistent administration of digitalis may result in clinical improvement and reversion of the ECG and cardiac enlargement (CE) to normal. Poor prognostic signs of CHF include:

1. Presentation in the newborn period
2. Recurrent episodes of CHF despite adequate therapy, especially if episodes recur more than 6 months after initial onset of symptoms.

VASCULAR RINGS

Vascular rings are unusual congenital anomalies that occur early in the development of the aortic arch and great vessels. The primary symptomatology associated with vascular rings relates to the structures that are encircled by the ring, chiefly the trachea and esophagus. Prompt diagnosis and treatment of these congenital abnormalities can be life-saving.

Historical Background

The first vascular ring described was a double aortic arch noted by Hommel in 1737. Bayford reported retroesophageal right subclavian artery in 1794 after performing an autopsy on a woman who had experienced dysphagia for years and died of starvation. Maude Abbott described 5 cases of double aortic arch in 1932 and made the suggestion that surgical intervention should be undertaken in such cases. Finally, in 1945, Gross used the term vascular ring in the New England Journal of Medicine publication that he wrote after performing the first successful division of a double aortic arch. Since that time, numerous reports of successful treatment have occurred, and the forms of aortic arch anomalies causing this problem have been well delineated.

Etiology

The various forms of this anomaly occur very early in embryologic development. They result from the abnormal or incomplete regression of 1 of the 6 embryonic branchial arches. Several recent papers report the close association of band 22q11 deletion with anomalies of the aortic arch as well as other congenital cardiac abnormalities.

Early in normal development, both a dorsal and a ventral aortic arch are present. The 2 arches are connected by 6 embryonic branchial arches, as depicted in the image below. The third, fourth, and sixth embryonic arches are the most crucial in the development of the aortic arch and several of its major branches, as well as the ductus arteriosus and the main pulmonary arteries.

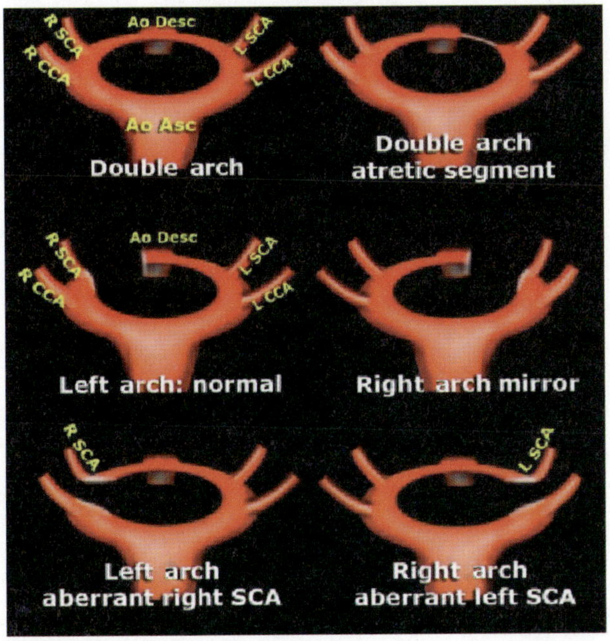

Fig. 14.353: *Diagrams showing self-explained embryological development of aortic arches leading to various vascular anomalies of aorta, pulmonary and systemic vessels*

Embryology

Embryonic aortic arch with dorsal and ventral arches and 6 branchial arches on right and left.

In normal development, each primitive arch either progresses into a functional vascular structure or involutes as follows:

- The right and left first and second arches become a portion of the arterial supply to the face.
- The third arches develop into the carotid arteries.
- The dorsal aorta between the third and the fourth arches involutes.
- The fourth arches are the primary contributors to the aortic arch itself, with the proximal right fourth arch developing into the proximal right subclavian artery. The distal portion of the right fourth arch involutes at the

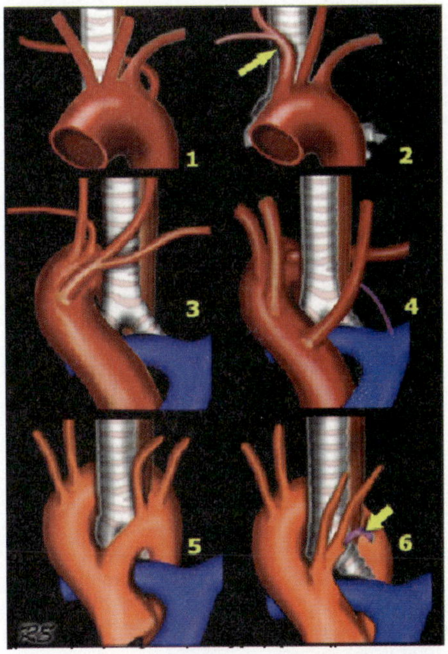

Fig. 14.354: *Showing overview of arch anomalies. 1. Aberrant Right subclavian artery, • Most common arch, • anomaly, • Not a true ring, • Usually asymptomatic, • Sometimes dysphagia lusoria when dilated suvclavian artery compresses esophagus posteriorly; 2. Innominate artery compression syndrome. In children the brachiocephalic (innominate) artery is located more to the left and may compresses the trachea anteriorly; 3. Right Arch Mirror Image, • Mirror-image variety of the left arch, • Asymptomatic, • Associated congenital heart disease in 98%, mostly tetralogy of Fallot; 4. Right arch with aberrant left subclavian, • Left subclavian artery is the last branch, • Obstructing anomaly; 5. Double aortic arch, • Complete ring encircles esophagus and trachea, • Four vessel sign; 6. Double arch with atretic segment, • Left arch is very small and has atretic posterior segment, • Still a four vessel sign*

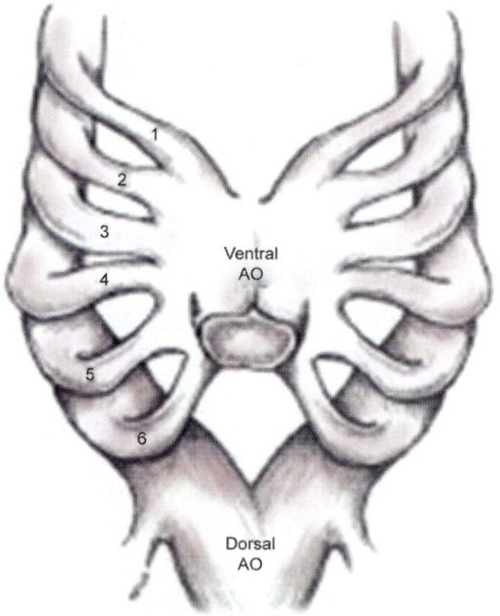

Embryonic aortic arch with dorsal and ventral arches and 6 branchial arches on right and left.

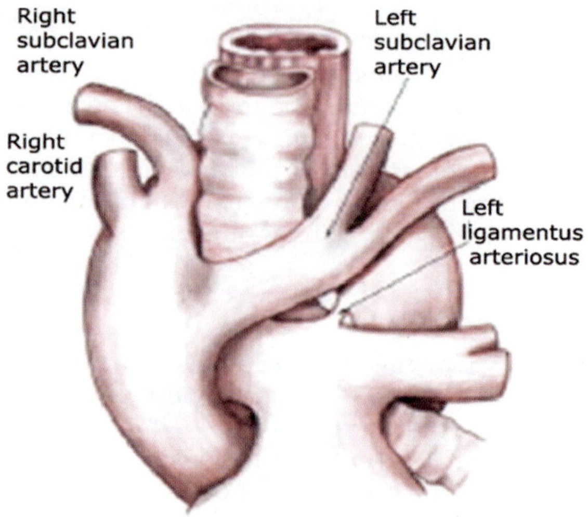

Right aortic arch with mirror-image branching and retroesophageal ligamentum arteriosum.

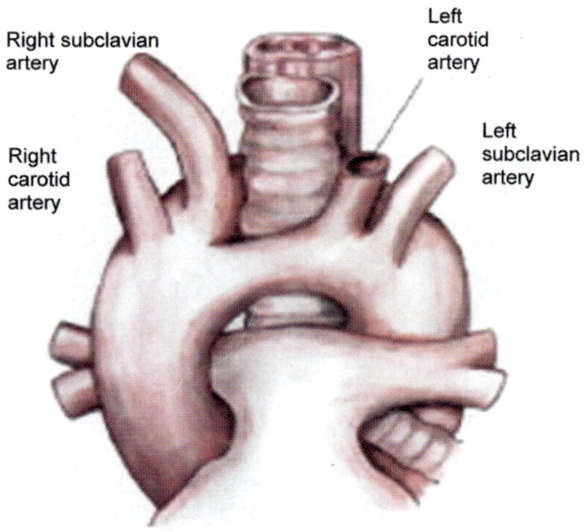

Double aortic arch.

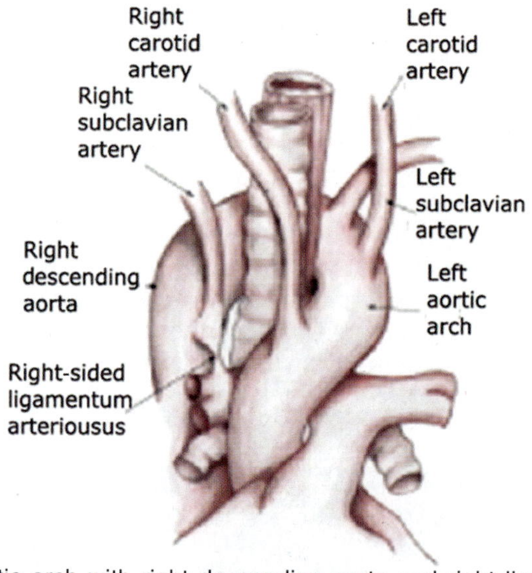

Left aortic arch with right descending aorta and right ligamentum arteriosum.

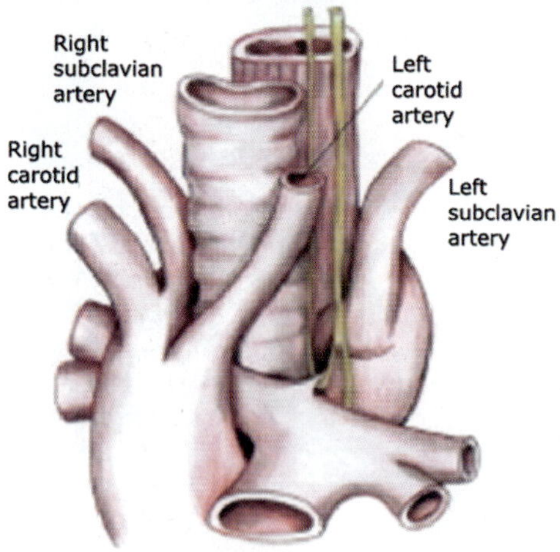

Right aortic arch with aberrant left subclavian artery and left ligamentum arteriosum.

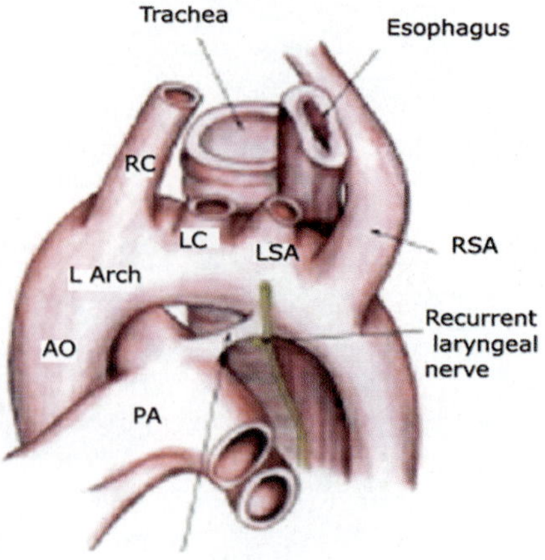

Retroesophageal right subclavian artery with left aortic arch and left ligamentum arteriosum.

Fig. 14.355: *Illustrations showing different anomalies of aortic arches* point where it joins the dorsal arch. The left fourth arch remains as the aortic arch in normal development.

- The fifth arches involute bilaterally.
- The ventral right sixth arch becomes the proximal right pulmonary artery. The ventral portion of the left sixth arch develops into the left pulmonary artery, while the dorsal portion becomes the ductus arteriosus.
- The entire left and the distal right subclavian arteries arise from the seventh segmental arterial branches of the dorsal aorta.
- Abnormal arch development results when one or more of the necessary involutions or other changes in embryonic arch structures does not occur.

Double Aortic Arch

The classic double aortic arch anatomy develops when involution of the distal right fourth arch does not take place. The fourth right and left arches both persist and join the left-sided descending thoracic aorta. The right and left aortic arches encircle the trachea and esophagus. In about 30% of cases of double aortic arch, the small, or less dominant, of the arches is atretic but remains in continuity with the descending aorta, maintaining the complete ring. The double aortic arch forms a ring around the trachea and esophagus, compressing both of these structures. Tracheoesophageal compression typically results in early symptoms. This type of defect is rarely associated with intracardiac defects.

Right Aortic Arch—Associated Abnormalities

In cases of individuals in whom the left fourth branchial arch involutes and the right remains, a right aortic arch is present. Right aortic arch occurs less frequently than 1 in 100,000 times in the general population and may exist in the absence of any other anomalies. Its presence is suggestive of the existence of an associated anomaly. About

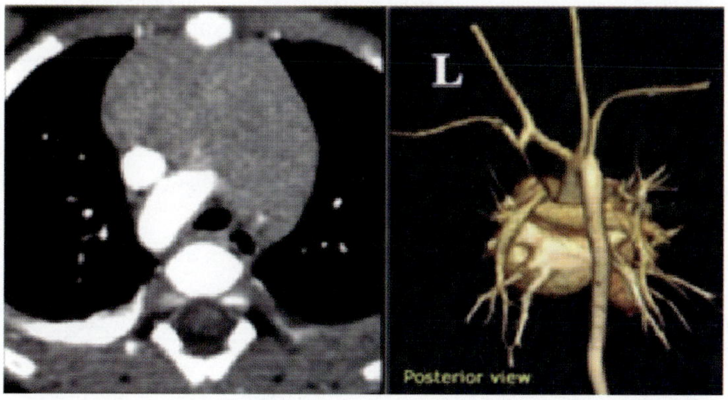

Fig. 14.356: *Right arch mirror image. This is the mirror-image variety of the left arch. On the left a 2-year-old girl with wheezing and coughing. Study the images and then continue. Axial CT-images are viewed from the feet while the illustrations above are viewed from above. On the axial image, there is a right arch On the volume rendered image, there is mirror image branching of the brachiocephalic arteries, no aberrant subclavian artery, so this is a right arch mirror image*

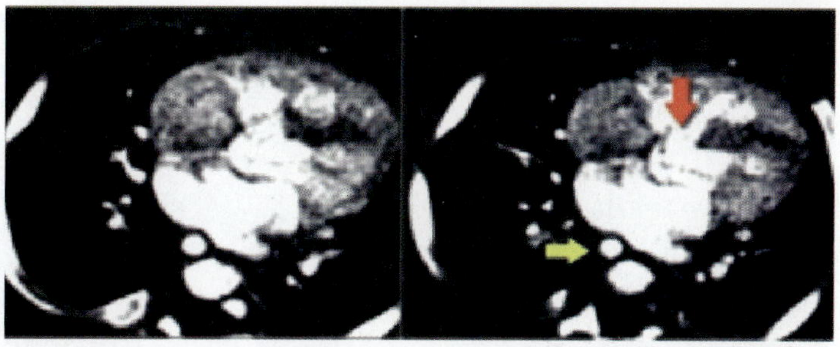

Fig. 14.357: *Mirror image aortic arch (yellow arrow) and a VSD (red arrow). This anomaly is asymptomatic because there is no obstructing ring. Almost all of these patients however come to our attention because they have associated congenital heart disease in 98% of cases. This patient had a mirror image aortic arch and a VSD*

30% of patients with tetralogy of Fallot have an associated right aortic arch.

Persistence of the right arch with involution of the left creates a situation in which the origins of the left subclavian artery and ductus arteriosus can vary. Several of these configurations can produce a vascular ring.

Right Aortic Arch with Aberrant Left Subclavian Artery and Left Ligamentum Arteriosum

In this anomaly, the right arch first gives off the left carotid artery, which travels anterior to the trachea (see image below). It then gives off the right carotid, followed by the right subclavian artery, and, lastly, the left subclavian artery, which courses in a retroesophageal position and gives rise to the ligamentum arteriosum from its base. The ligamentum arteriosum connects the left subclavian or descending aorta to the left pulmonary artery. The trachea and esophagus are surrounded by the ascending aorta anteriorly, the aortic arch on the right, the descending aorta posteriorly, and the ligamentum arteriosum and left pulmonary artery on the left. Almost 10% of these defects are associated with an intracardiac defect.

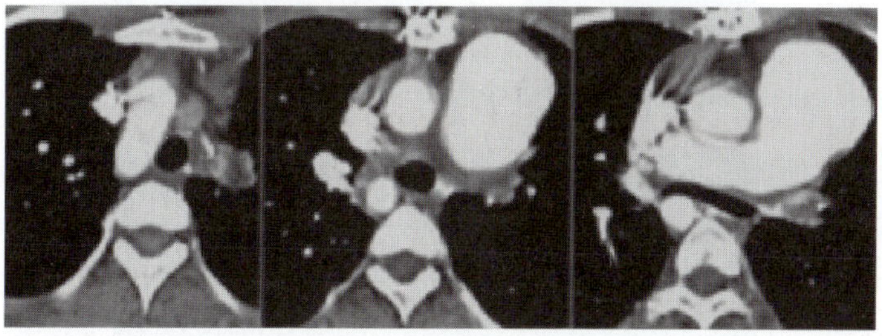

Fig. 14.358: *Mirror image aortic arch in patient operated for tetralogy of Fallot. On the left, an adult who was operated in his childhood for a tetralogy of Fallot (pulmonary stenosis, right ventricular hypertrophy, VSD, overriding aorta). At surgery, the VSD was patched and the pulmonary outflow tract was enlarged. Notice that there is also a right arch. In the ER, you will see these patients because they age and get chest pain like many adults do and so you will see these anomalies more frequently*

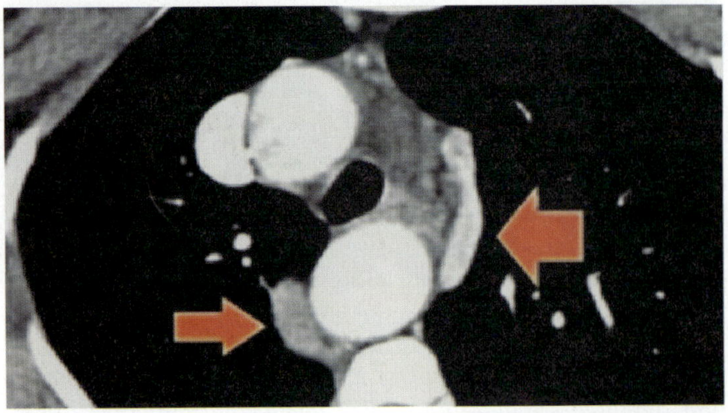

Fig. 14.359: *Right arch with aberrant left subclavian.On the left, a patient with a right arch with an aberrant left subclavian (indicated by the yellow arrow).There is a right arch and the left subclavian artery is the last branch of the aortic arch, indicating that this is an aberrant left subclavian. Medially to the left subclavian artery, we see the left common carotid that originates from the right side and has an oblique course to the left*

Right Aortic Arch with Mirror-image Branching and Retroesophageal Ligamentum Arteriosum

In these cases, only partial resorption of the distal left fourth arch occurs. The first brachiocephalic vessel originating from the right arch is the left innominate artery, which, in turn, branches into a left carotid and left subclavian artery. These vessels course anterior to the trachea.

Following these, a right carotid artery and then a right subclavian artery arise. The ligamentum arteriosum is the final structure arising from the arch in this sequence. It originates from an area called Kommerell diverticulum, which represents the nonresorbed remnant of the left fourth arch and is situated at the point of merger between the right arch and the proximal descending thoracic aorta. The ligamentum passes leftward and behind the esophagus and then travels anteriorly to join with the left pulmonary artery and complete the ring, as depicted in the image below. More commonly, in cases of right aortic arch with mirror-image branching, the ligamentum arteriosum travels from the mirror-image innominate or left subclavian artery to the left pulmonary artery. A complete ring is not present in these cases. This type of vascular ring has a more than 90% association with intracardiac defects.

Vascular Rings Associated with Left Aortic Arch

Two extremely rare complete rings occur in the presence of a left aortic arch, and both are associated with a right-sided descending thoracic aorta.

Left Aortic Arch with Right Descending Aorta and Right Ligamentum Arteriosum

The first arch vessel to exit the left aortic arch is the right common carotid, which passes anterior to the trachea. The left carotid is next, followed by the left subclavian artery. The right subclavian artery arises more distally as a branch of the proximal right-sided descending aorta. The ligamentum arteriosum arises from the base of the right

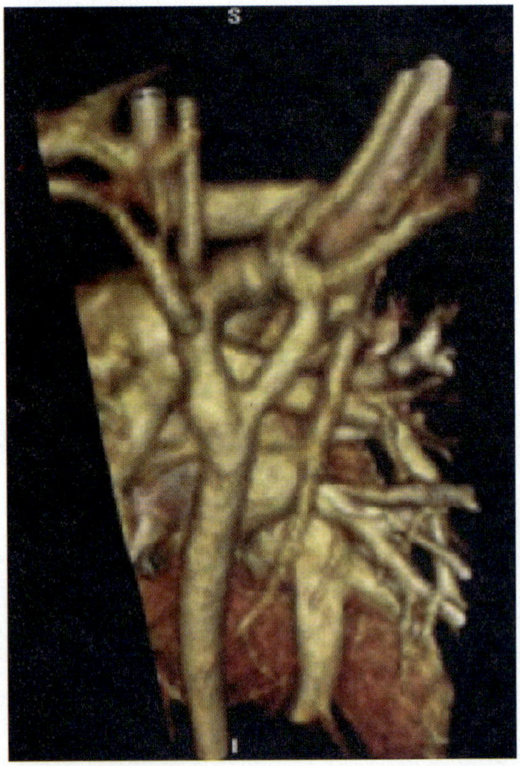

Fig. 14.360: *Double aortic arch. Posterior image from a 3D volume rendered MR angiogram demonstrating a double aortic arch with the left and right arches joining posteriorly. The left and right arches give rise to the left and right common carotid and subclavian arteries, respectively*

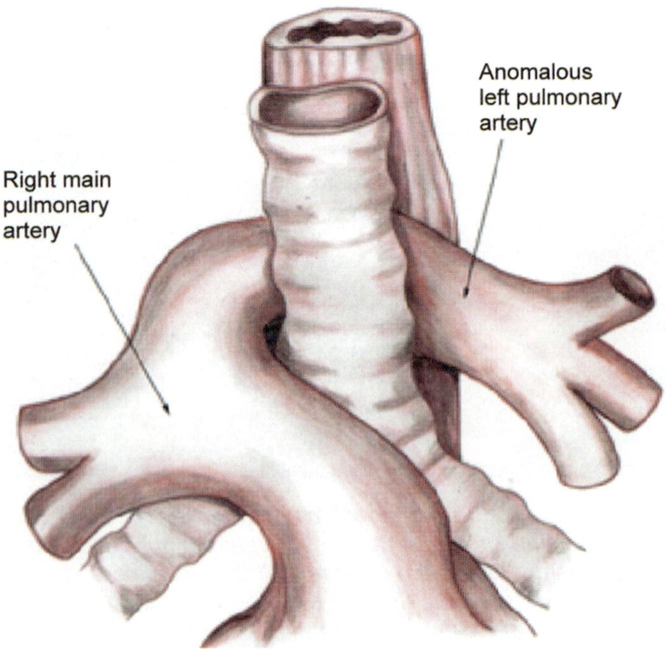

Fig. 14.361: *Aberrant left pulmonary artery or pulmonary artery sling*

subclavian artery or a nearby diverticulum and travels to the right pulmonary artery (see image below).

Left Aortic Arch, Right Descending Aorta, and Atretic Right Aortic Arch

The brachiocephalic vessels arise from the left-sided arch in a normal arrangement. The left arch passes behind the esophagus to join a right-sided descending aorta. An atretic right arch is present and completes the ring.

Arch Abnormalities Producing Compression Symptoms without an Anatomic Ring

Anomalous Innominate Artery

The actual prevalence of this abnormality is widely debated. This is because, in as many as 90% of cases in which symptomatic tracheal compression is produced by the innominate artery, the vessel is noted angiographically to have a normal origin from the aorta. When an anatomic abnormality is noted in these cases, the innominate artery appears to originate from a more distal and leftward position on the arch than normal. As it takes its course from left to right, it crosses the trachea anteriorly and in doing so may produce compression of the trachea.

Retroesophageal Right Subclavian Artery with Left Aortic Arch and Left Ligamentum Arteriosum

This is the most common of the arch vessel anomalies, occurring in about 0.5% of the population. In these cases, the right subclavian artery does not arise from an innominate trunk with the right carotid artery but originates as the last brachiocephalic branch from the descending aorta and takes a retroesophageal route to its destination, as depicted in the image below. A normally positioned ligamentum arteriosum is present on the left. If a right ligamentum arteriosum were present instead of one on the left, its course would proceed from the base of this anomalous right subclavian artery to the right pulmonary artery and a complete ring would exist. Instead, no true vascular ring is present in these cases. Most patients are symptomatic, but the occasional patient may present with dysphagia.

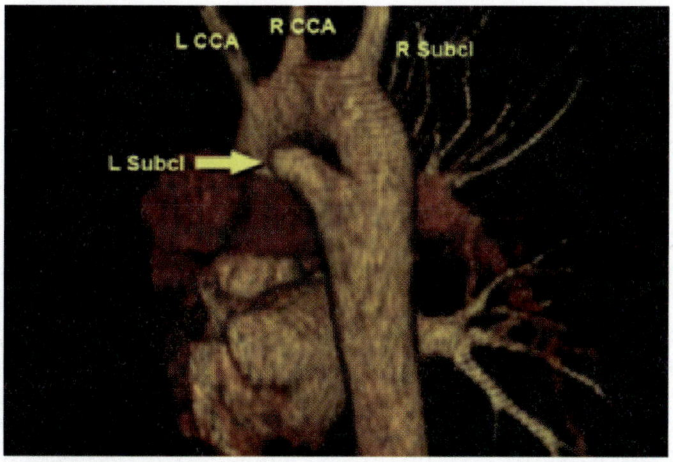

Fig. 14.362: *Posterior oblique view: right arch with aberrant left subclavian (yellow arrow)*

Anomalous Left Pulmonary Artery or Pulmonary Sling

This abnormality occurs when the left main pulmonary artery arises as a branch of the right pulmonary artery instead of originating from the main pulmonary artery. This is believed to be an abnormality related to sixth aortic arch development. In this anomaly, the left pulmonary artery leaves the right and courses in a position cephalad to the right mainstem bronchus, proceeding around the right side of the trachea (see image below). It then travels between the trachea and esophagus as it goes to the left lung.

Aberrant Left Pulmonary Artery or Pulmonary Artery Sling

This lesion is often associated with hypoplasia and other abnormalities of the tracheal and bronchial cartilages. Most patients are symptomatic by 1 month after birth. Respiratory symptoms predominate, as the most severe compression is on the trachea. More than 50% of infants also have severe tracheobronchial anomalies such as tracheomalacia, stenosis, webs, or complete tracheal rings. Intracardiac defects are also seen in 20% of these infants.

Pathophysiology

In spite of the significant variability in this group of structural abnormalities of the aortic arch, they all possess a common feature. They all produce some degree of compression on the major airway structures and/or the esophagus. The location and severity of compression varies with the configuration of the lesion. Individuals with anomalies producing more severe compression are likely to present earlier in life.

Tracheal or tracheobronchial malacia and stenosis may develop in association with some of these lesions in the areas where the greatest degree of compression exists. This is particularly true in cases of anomalous left pulmonary artery.

Other congenital cardiac anomalies may be present in association with aortic arch anomalies.

The presence of a right aortic arch should always raise the suspicion of additional congenital cardiac disease. Right aortic arch has been reported in as many as 34% of cases of tetralogy of Fallot. Other intracardiac lesions found in association with a right aortic arch include double-outlet right ventricle, truncus arteriosus, ventricular septal defect with pulmonary atresia, transposition of the great vessels, tricuspid atresia, and absent left pulmonary artery.

Anomalous left pulmonary artery has also been associated with other cardiac defects in as many as 50% of cases. These include the aforementioned lesions as well as persistent left superior vena cava, atrial septal defect, and ventricular defect. Complete tracheal rings (congenital absence of the membranous trachea) resulting in tracheal stenosis are another anomaly reported in as many as 50% of infants with anomalous left pulmonary artery. The combination of these 2 lesions is often termed the ring-sling complex.

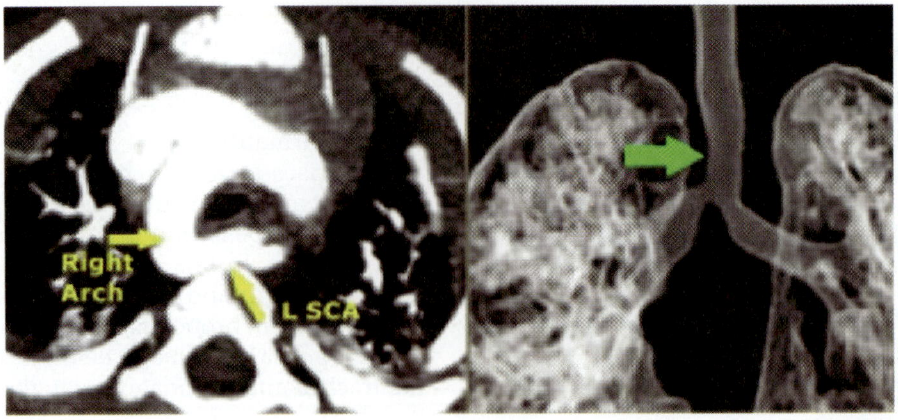

Fig. 14.363: *Right arch with aberrant left subclavian.On the left images of a symptomatic child. On the axial image there is a right arch with the left subclavian artery that comes off on the posterior side and runs behind the trachea and the esophagus. The compression of the trachea is demonstrated on the volume rendered view (arrow)*

Clinical Manifestations

Symptoms and physical findings produced by vascular rings are primarily those of airway or esophageal compression. Individuals with a narrow or tight ring have a significant degree of constriction of one or both of these structures and present very early in life.

The vast majority of patients with a vascular ring present with symptoms in infancy or very early in childhood. However, a small number of patients do not manifest symptoms until later in life, and others remain entirely asymptomatic. Common symptoms include stridor, cyanosis, wheezing, respiratory distress, apnea, and/or a characteristic high-pitched, brassy cough. Additional findings include a history of asthma, recurrent pneumonia, or evidence of dysphagia or difficulty with feedings. In some cases, airway symptoms are worsened or aggravated by feedings. Intercostal retractions during respiration are observed in some infants with severe obstruction. Others may try to maintain a position in which the head is hyperextended to improve breathing and minimize the obstruction. Air-trapping and evidence of pulmonary hyperinflation may also be present in one or both lungs in severe cases.

Symptoms of airway obstruction predominate in patients who present in infancy or the first few years of life. Dysphagia and symptoms related to the esophagus are the more likely presenting findings in older children and adults with vascular rings. Esophageal compression is usually posterior. Symptoms that are present soon after birth may include slow breast or bottle feeding, fatigue with feeding, frequent regurgitation, and aspiration pneumonias. In most cases, workup is initiated when solid foods are introduced, which causes more pronounced dysphagia.

The double aortic arch is the anomaly that usually produces the most severe airway compression in the youngest patients. The second most common configuration, right aortic arch and left ligamentum arteriosum with retroesophageal left subclavian artery, displays a spectrum of severity. Some individuals present in infancy or very early in childhood while others do not present until adulthood.

Although patients with associated cardiac lesions may have additional symptoms secondary to that abnormality, symptoms of airway compression related to the constricting vascular ring are usually most prominent.

Finally, note that some patients with a complete vascular ring have minimal symptoms or remain asymptomatic. In such cases, the abnormal arch anatomy is often discovered incidentally when the patient is undergoing diagnostic studies for another problem.

Conversely, if left aortic arch with associated retroesophageal right subclavian artery is incidentally found during diagnostic studies for symptoms of dysphagia, the clinician should not believe that this vascular abnormality, which is not a true vascular ring, is the source of the symptoms. Additional investigation for the true cause should be pursued. This arch abnormality, previously believed to be responsible for dysphagia symptoms and for which the term dysphagia lusoria was coined long ago, is rarely responsible for esophageal symptoms.

Surgical Indications

Surgical division of a vascular ring is indicated in all symptomatic patients. To avoid serious complications such as sudden death or significant tracheal or bronchial damage, surgery should not be delayed, especially in patients with symptoms of airway compression.

Double Aortic Arch

Visualization through a left thoracotomy incision shows a normally positioned left, or anterior, arch exiting the pericardium and joining the left-sided descending thoracic aorta after giving off the left subclavian artery. The ligament arteriosum is positioned normally. The posterior, or right, arch joins the descending thoracic aorta at the same level as the anterior arch but reaches that point from an extreme posterior course behind the esophagus. Often, the posterior arch is visible only after circumferential dissection of the aorta at the level of its junction with the anterior arch.

Right Aortic Arch with Retroesophageal Left Subclavian Artery and Left Ligamentum Arteriosum

The arch travels to the right and behind the esophagus, joining the left-sided descending aorta. As it takes this course, it gives off the left carotid artery first. Then, it sequentially gives off the right carotid, the right subclavian, and the left subclavian arteries. This last branch often has a retroesophageal position. The ligamentum arteriosum courses from the base of the left subclavian artery to the left pulmonary artery.

Through a left thoracotomy, the structures visible in normal position are the descending thoracic aorta and the distal portion of the left subclavian artery. These structures can be traced proximally to identify the site where the left subclavian artery exits the right arch as it joins with the descending aorta. The ligamentum arteriosum can be found at the base of the subclavian artery and traced towards the pulmonary artery.

Right Cortic Arch with Mirror-image Branching and Retroesophageal Ligamentum Arteriosum

In the rightward and retroesophageal course, the aortic arch gives off a left innominate artery, which in turn branches into the left carotid and subclavian arteries. The right carotid artery then branches from the arch, followed by the right subclavian. The ligamentum arteriosum exits distal to this point from the area of Kommerell diverticulum and courses to the left pulmonary artery. As viewed through a left thoracotomy, the descending thoracic aorta is visible and can be traced proximally to the area of its merger with the right aortic arch, which joins it from behind the esophagus. In this area, the ductus diverticulum and ligamentum arteriosum can be found.

Left Aortic Arch with Right Descending Thoracic Aorta and Right Ligamentum Arteriosum

The arrangement of this anomaly is the mirror image of right aortic arch with retroesophageal left subclavian artery and left ligamentum arteriosum. Approaching through a right thoracotomy, structures are identified and traced in the same manner.

Left Aortic Arch with Right Descending Aorta and Atretic Right Arch

In a retroesophageal position, the left arch passes to the left of the trachea to join the right descending thoracic aorta. The surgical view is via right thoracotomy. At the level of this junction and immediately superior to a right ligamentum arteriosum, an atretic right arch is found. The brachiocephalic vessels in this case exit the left arch in a normal sequence.

Anomalous Innominate Artery

The brachiocephalic vessels exit the left arch in the normal sequence. The innominate artery may be more distally positioned and leftward on the arch than normal.

Retroesophageal Right Subclavian Artery with Left Aortic Arch and Left Ligamentum Arteriosum

Rather than an innominate artery exiting the arch as the normal first brachiocephalic branch, the right carotid is the first brachiocephalic vessel. It is followed by the left carotid and then the left subclavian artery. The right subclavian artery is the last brachiocephalic branch to exit the arch, and it takes a course rightward and posterior to the esophagus. The ligamentum arteriosum is normally positioned on the left.

Anomalous Left Pulmonary Artery

Instead of the normal pulmonary artery configuration in which the main pulmonary artery gives rise to both the right and left pulmonary arteries, the main pulmonary artery continues behind the ascending aorta and rightward as the right pulmonary artery, which then gives off the left pulmonary artery. The left pulmonary artery passes from right to left between the trachea and the esophagus in its course to the left lung. The ligamentum arteriosum takes a course from the junction of the main and right pulmonary arteries posteriorly to the aorta.

Contraindications

Individuals who are asymptomatic from a vascular ring may not require surgical intervention.

In patients with vague symptoms of difficulty swallowing, the clinician should not regard the presence of a left aortic arch with retroesophageal right subclavian artery as the definitive cause of the patient's symptoms. Reports of surgical division of anomalous retroesophageal right subclavian artery for treatment of such symptoms appear in older surgical literature. This was found to be ineffective treatment because the majority of these patients continued to have symptoms. Currently, the presence of this anomaly is believed not to cause such symptoms, and the clinician should continue further diagnostic studies.

Cases of anomalous innominate artery with evidence of tracheal compression do not require surgical treatment if the patient has few or no symptoms. Only about 10% of these patients require surgery.

Imaging Studies

Chest Radiography

Because children usually present with symptoms of respiratory difficulty, chest radiography is always the first and most commonly performed test.

Look for the position of the aortic arch, which is usually identifiable on the plain chest radiograph. The identification of a right aortic arch on chest radiograph in a child with airway difficulties, respiratory distress or dysphagia should alert the clinician to the likelihood of a vascular ring.

An ill-defined arch location is often observed in patients with double aortic arch. Such a finding should raise the suspicion of an arch anomaly in a symptomatic child.

Other radiographic findings that may be noted with vascular rings include compression of the trachea and hyperinflation and/or atelectasis of some of the lobes of either lung.

A specific finding associated with anomalous left pulmonary artery is hyperinflation of the right lung.

In general, chest radiography is not very sensitive in the diagnosis of vascular rings.

Barium Esophagram

Most authorities consider barium esophagram to be the most important study in patients with a suspected vascular ring, and it is diagnostic in the vast majority of cases.

Double aortic arch produces bilateral and posterior compressions of the esophagus, which remain constant regardless of peristalsis. The right indentation is usually slightly higher than the left, and the posterior compression is usually rather wide and courses in a downward direction as it goes from right to left.

Patients having one of the anomalies in which the right subclavian artery takes a retroesophageal course have a posterior defect slanting upward from left to right. The posterior defect in these cases is usually not as broad as that found in double aortic arch.

An anomalous left pulmonary artery produces a characteristic defect in the anterior wall of the esophagus at the level of the tracheal bifurcation. No posterior compression is present with this anomaly.

Cases of abnormally located innominate artery causing tracheal compression have normal findings on esophagram.

Echocardiography and Color-flow Doppler

Echocardiographic studies have been increasingly used for the diagnosis of a vascular ring.

This study has replaced pulmonary angiography at many centers to determine the presence of an anomalous left pulmonary artery. It is also extremely useful in the diagnostic workup of associated congenital cardiac defects.

Some limitations in diagnosis using this study exist. Structures without a lumen, such as a ligamentum arteriosum or an atretic arch, have no blood flow and are difficult to identify with color-flow echocardiography. Also, identification of compressed midline structures and their relationship to encircling vascular anomalies may be difficult to detect, especially for the less experienced echocardiographer.

Computerized Tomography Scan, Magnetic Resonance Imaging, and Digital Subtraction Angiography

These expensive radiological studies are rarely necessary to evaluate vascular rings.

Computerized tomography (CT) scan, magnetic resonance imaging (MRI), and digital subtraction angiography (DSA) can be useful diagnostic tools because they reveal the positions of vascular, tracheobronchial, and esophageal structures and their relationships to one another.

Although these modalities provide excellent delineation of all of the associated structures, they should be reserved for cases in which the results of barium esophagram do not provide a clear diagnosis. MRI has been proposed as an excellent substitute for angiography.

All of these studies have drawbacks. CT scan and DSA expose the patient to radiation and require intravenous contrast. MRI requires patients to remain very still, so very young patients who are unable to understand verbal instructions require sedation. This may be particularly risky in young children with existing airway compromise. The expense encountered with these investigations must also be considered.

Aortic Angiography and Cardiac Catheterization

In the past, diagnostic aortography was performed in selected cases to delineate the anomalous arch vasculature.

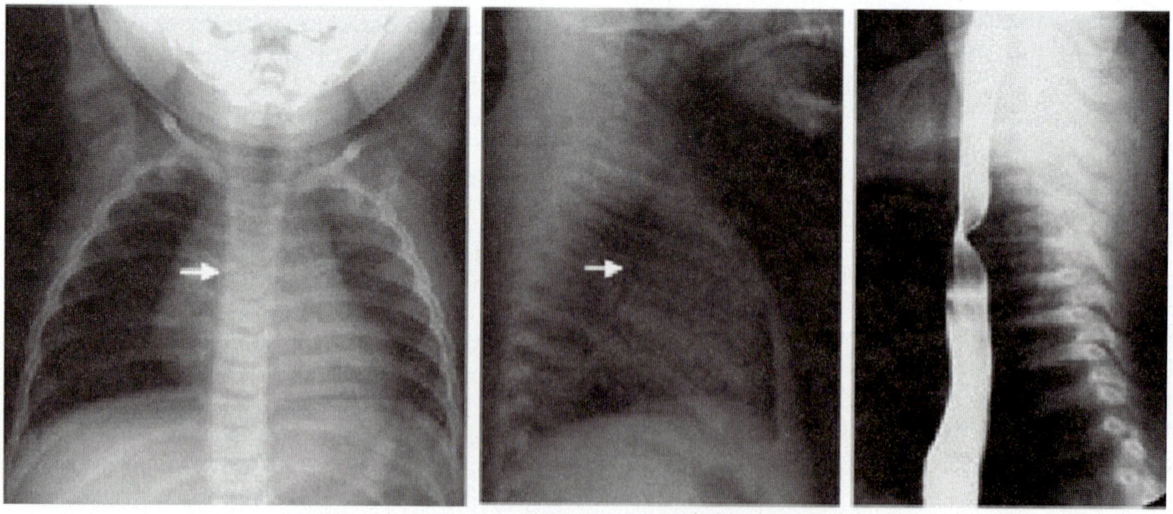

Fig. 14.364: *(Left) Anterior-posterior radiograph of the chest in child with a right aortic arch. Note: Displacement of the trachea towards the left indicating a right aortic arch. (Center) Lateral radiograph of the chest demonstrating narrowing and anterior displacement of the trachea by the aberrant left subclavian artery which passes behind it. (Right) Lateral esophagram showing posterior impression of the esophagus by the aberrant left subclavian artery*

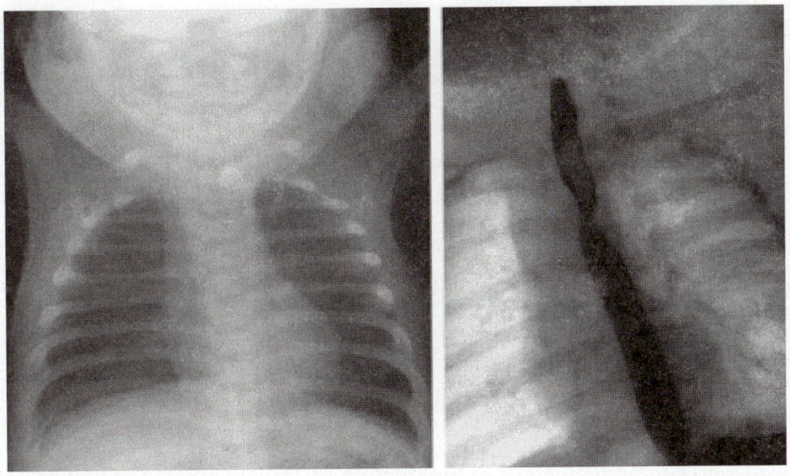

Fig. 14.365: *Anterior–posterior (AP) radiograph of the chest in a child with a double aortic arch. Note: Indistinct view of the trachea on the AP view. AP esophagram showing compression of the upper thoracic esophagus by the double aortic arch: the more inferior (caudad) indentation is due to the left aortic arch and the more superior (cephalad) indentation is due to the right aortic arch*

It is generally agreed at present that, in the vast majority of cases, this study adds very little to the information obtained from a barium esophagram. If additional studies are required, echocardiography, CT scan, or MRI can usually provide the required information. However, reported cases exist of rare arch anomalies in which aortography was the only study from which the correct anatomic configuration was identified.This study may be required in cases in which the diagnosis and arch configuration remains in question after other less invasive studies fail to provide a definitive answer.

Cardiac catheterization is useful in cases in which associated cardiac abnormalities are known or suspected.

Diagnostic Procedures

Bronchoscopy

This diagnostic study has been used in the evaluation of children with symptoms of airway obstruction or compression. It is most commonly used in the diagnosis of an abnormally placed innominate artery or pulmonary sling but is rarely required in the diagnosis of the various types of complete vascular ring.

In the presence of a vascular ring, pulsatile external tracheal compression is easily observed. Note that compression of the airway by a vascular structure in the pediatric patient does not represent an unyielding obstruction and should not pose a problem for passage of the bronchoscope.

In cases of an abnormally placed innominate artery, obvious pulsation is observed in the anterior wall of the trachea corresponding to the area of compression.

Medical Therapy

No medical therapy exists for the definitive treatment of vascular rings. Preoperatively, the patient should be given adequate nutritional support as well as general respiratory care and appropriate treatment of any respiratory tract infection. Surgery should not be delayed in the presence of

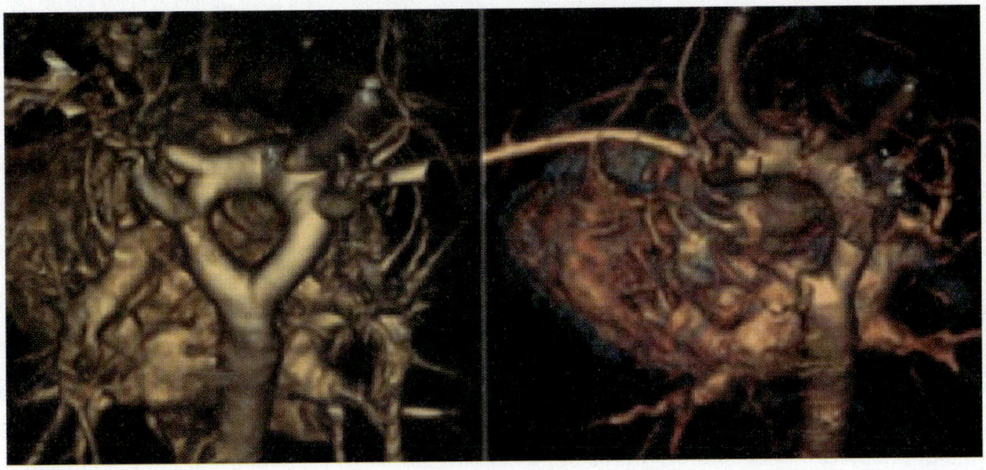

Fig. 14.366: *Pre and postoperative reconstructions of a double aortic arch. On the left preoperative and postoperative MDCT studies of a 2-month-old female infant with double aortic arch presenting with stridor and repeated apnea. The smaller left arch is partially resected (Image courtesy of Dr. W. Chu)*

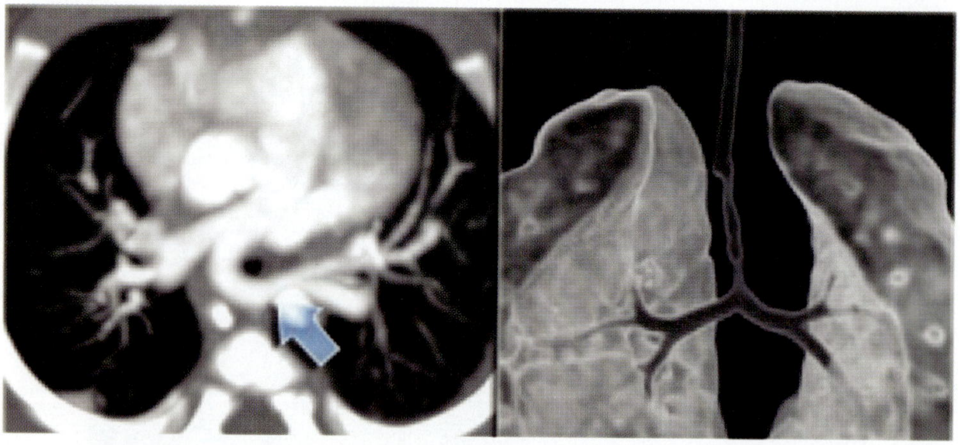

Fig. 14.367: *Pulmonary sling with long segment stenosis of the trachea on the left images of a child with wheezing and dyspnea. The left PA comes off the right PA and runs between the esophagus (with nasogastric tube) and the trachea. Some of these patients also have long segment stenosis in the trachea because of cartilagenous rings (Courtesy J. Schoef)*

a respiratory tract infection, because the division of the ring allows more adequate and complete clearing of respiratory secretions.

Surgical Intervention

Surgical division of symptomatic vascular rings is the only appropriate form of therapy. Surgery should be performed promptly after the diagnosis is made, especially in patients with stridor, apnea, or other symptoms of respiratory distress. Delay in operative intervention can result in complications of a serious nature. Left thoracotomy is the surgical approach of choice for the division of a vascular ring in the majority of cases. Anomalous left pulmonary artery has been corrected using the left thoracotomy approach in the past. More recently, the use of median sternotomy and cardiopulmonary bypass has been shown to produce better long-term results. The extremely rare configurations associated with left aortic arch and right descending thoracic aorta are the lesions that should be approached via a right thoracotomy for division of the ring.

Division of a Double Aortic Arch

The left chest is entered through the fourth intercostal space. The mediastinal pleura is opened, and the components of the vascular ring are visualized.

The right, or posterior, arch does not require mobilization unless it is the lesser of the 2 arches and is to be divided. In such cases, the proximal descending aorta should be reflected anteriorly to visualize the area where the right arch enters.

In cases of double aortic arch, the nondominant, or smaller, arch is divided. If one arch is atretic, it is the obvious choice for division. A likely site for division of the minor, or atretic, arch is at its point of juncture with the descending aorta.

Division of the chosen arch should be performed between applied vascular clamps. Prior to actual division,

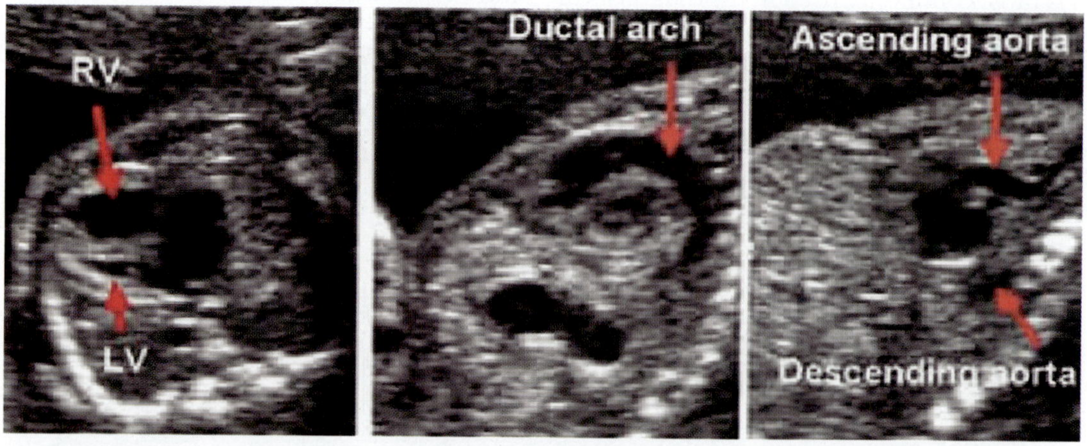

Fig. 14.368: *Fetal ultrasonography. Interrupted aortic arch should always be considered when intracardiac lesions diverting blood flow from the left to the right heart are encountered (aortic stenosis and atresia in particular). Isolated interruption of the aortic arch is often encountered with enlargement of the right ventricle (right ventricle to left ventricle ratio of more than 1.3). As the sonographic access to the arch is difficult, the diagnosis is not always possible. The characteristic finding of an ascending aorta more vertical than usually, and the impossibility to demonstrate a connection with the descending aorta suggests the diagnosis*

the strength of the right and left carotid and the radial pulses should be evaluated with the vascular clamps applied. Diminution or absence of the pulse in one or several of these areas indicates that division of the arch at the chosen location would result in interruption of blood flow to that area. In such cases, another site for division should be chosen.

Perfusion to the lower extremities should be assessed prior to division of 1 of 2 equal-sized patent arches.

The ends of the divided arch should be oversewn with fine, nonabsorbable vascular suture.

The ligamentum arteriosum and any other fibrous bands around the trachea or esophagus in that area should be divided as well.

Identify and avoid the recurrent laryngeal and vagus nerves. Closure of the mediastinal pleura is not performed to avoid the development of adhesive scarring in the already affected area of the trachea and esophagus.

Division of a vascular ring in cases with right aortic arch anatomy.

In cases of complete vascular rings with right aortic arch anatomy, the primary structure to be divided is the ligamentum arteriosum.

After left thoracotomy, the anatomy should be dissected out and clearly visualized.

The vagus and recurrent nerves should be visualized and preserved.

The ligamentum is divided between vascular clamps and the ends oversewn. After ligamentum division, any associated fibrous or adhesive bands in the area are also divided.

In cases of right aortic arch with mirror-image branching and retroesophageal ligamentum arteriosum, a prominent or aneurysmal Kommerell diverticulum may be present. If so, it should be resected over a partially occluding vascular clamp and primarily oversewn or mobilized with adjacent descending aorta so that it may be pexed or transfixed to nearby vertebral fascia. If left alone, these diverticula can contribute to the compression on the trachea and esophagus. A few authors have advocated division of the aberrant left subclavian artery in these cases as well, but this is very rarely indicated for relief of the symptoms caused by the ring and may cause symptoms of subclavian steal later.

Repair of Anomalous Left Pulmonary Artery

In the past, this abnormality was approached through either a right or a left thoracotomy. Presently, many centers utilize a median sternotomy approach with the aid of cardiopulmonary bypass. Others continue to report excellent results performing the corrective surgery using a left thoracotomy.

In cases using median sternotomy and bypass, aortic and single right atrial cannulation is employed. The infant is cooled to 32°C so that the normal cardiac rhythm is maintained.

The left pulmonary artery is identified at its junction with the right and is dissected out as far to the left as possible, taking care to avoid injury to the membranous portion of the trachea. Its origin is often on the posterior surface of the right pulmonary artery and to the right of the trachea.

The pericardium is opened on the posterior left side near the site where the ligamentum arteriosum meets the pulmonary artery. The left pulmonary artery is identified in this area and freed from surrounding adhesions.

A partially occluding clamp is placed on the right pulmonary artery at the site of its junction with the left, which is then transected. The orifice left in the right pulmonary artery is closed primarily with fine interrupted polypropylene sutures.

The partial occluding clamp is released and replaced on the main pulmonary artery posteriorly where an arteriotomy is made. The location of the clamp on the main pulmonary artery is critical so that the left pulmonary artery is without deformity after the anastomosis.

The divided left pulmonary artery is brought through the path created for it behind the trachea and into the pericardium through the left-sided pericardial opening. It is sewn to the arteriotomy with interrupted fine polypropylene sutures.

Tracheal anomalies associated with anomalous left pulmonary artery.

As many as 50% of patients with aberrant left pulmonary artery may have the associated anomaly of complete tracheal rings. In these infants, the membranous portion of the trachea is congenitally absent. This abnormality results in tracheal stenosis/malacia and significantly adds to the morbidity of surgery.

Diagnosis of Tracheal/Bronchial Malacia is Made Using Rigid Bronchoscopy

The choice of repair depends upon the length of the trachea involved and may involve resection and end-to-end anastomosis in cases with short segment involvement to a variety of tracheoplasty procedures for long segment abnormalities.

When tracheal stenosis secondary to complete tracheal rings is found in association with an aberrant pulmonary artery, the two abnormalities may be repaired during the same operative procedure. The approach for this is median sternotomy, and cardiopulmonary bypass is used.

Congenital Cardiac Defects Associated with Anomalous Left Pulmonary Artery

Intracardiac defects are commonly associated with an anomalous left pulmonary artery. Depending on the type of intracardiac pathology, the surgeon must use discretion in deciding to correct or palliate the cardiac defect at the same setting or at a later time.

Anomalous Innominate Artery

Tracheal compression from an aberrant innominate artery is most often approached via an anterolateral right thoracotomy. The right lobe of the thymus is removed, avoiding injury to the phrenic nerve. The pericardium immediately beneath this area is opened, and the innominate artery is identified near its junction with the aorta.

The treatment of this condition simply involves tacking the innominate artery to the posterior sternal surface. The innominate artery is affixed to the posterior periosteal layer of the sternum using interrupted polypropylene sutures with pledgets. The sutures are each passed through the adventitia of the innominate artery and then through the periosteal layer of the sternum. Usually about 3 sutures are used and placed at intervals along the length of the artery, with the most proximal one placed at the junction of the innominate artery and the aorta. When these sutures are tied, the innominate artery is pulled away from the anterior surface of the trachea, relieving the compression.

Left Aortic Arch with Right Descending Aorta Lesions

These are extremely rare lesions, but they are the lesions that must be approached via a right thoracotomy.

Division of the ring in these cases is accomplished by dividing the right-sided ligamentum arteriosum.

Patients having this anomaly often have associated congenital cardiac defects and commonly receive extensive preoperative workup.

Follow-up

Most patients are essentially asymptomatic within a few weeks after surgery and can resume activity and feedings as tolerated.

A small group continues to have some symptoms postoperatively; however, these findings are less prominent than those noted preoperatively in the majority of cases. These patients should show gradual improvement over 6-12 months, and most eventually become asymptomatic. This group may require closer follow-up in the immediate postoperative outpatient period so that early diagnosis and treatment of common forms of pediatric airway infections that result in epiglottitis or tracheobronchitis may be performed.

Patients who undergo more extensive surgery, especially tracheal reconstruction, require long-term follow-up. They may require bronchoscopy at regular intervals for elimination of encroaching granulation tissue and for tracheal or bronchial stenosis.

Patients who have associated congenital cardiac disease require regular follow-up with a pediatric cardiologist.

Complications

Serious surgical complications are rare in most reported surgical series of vascular ring division. Most complications associated with these problems occur in the preoperative setting and may even occur before the diagnosis is known. The majority of these are related to airway obstruction. Postoperatively, atelectases and pneumonias can and do occur. Pain from the thoracotomy incision can be long-lasting in some patients and can hamper breathing efforts.

Complications related to surgery itself are uncommon in most cases. Injury to the phrenic, vagus, or recurrent laryngeal nerve may occur. Disruption of the thoracic duct is also possible. Late vascular complications, such as subclavian steal, may be noted in cases in which division of a brachiocephalic vessel, such as a retroesophageal subclavian artery, was deemed necessary.

Rare cases in which symptoms of airway obstruction persist may require resection of a severely malacotic segment of trachea or bronchus or a more complex tracheoplasty procedure.

One series reported two very rare cases in which a vascular ring that was originally identified as right arch with retroesophageal left subclavian artery and left ligamentum arteriosum was divided via left thoracotomy with no postoperative improvement in symptoms. These patients were described as having a circumflex aorta in which it appeared that the posterior arch itself made up a portion of the obstructing ring. Additional surgery was required in these patients. A second procedure was performed via median sternotomy with cardiopulmonary bypass support in which the posteriorly positioned aortic arch was divided at the point where it traveled around the right side of the trachea and esophagus. The divided leftward portion was brought anterior to the trachea and esophagus on the left and reanastomosed to the portion from which it was originally divided. Fortunately, such cases are extremely rare.

Outcome and Prognosis

About 95% of patients who undergo surgical correction of a vascular ring survive long term, and most of these are soon relieved of their symptoms. In those infants with no intracardiac or extracardiac defects, surgery for vascular rings carries essentially no mortality.

Among those with less optimal long-term results are patients with an anomalous left pulmonary artery with and without complete tracheal rings and those with severe associated congenital cardiac defects. In those patients with a severely deformed trachea or tracheomalacia, additional reconstruction procedures may be required in the future.

A number of patients continue to show evidence of some pulmonary function abnormalities years after surgery. Several studies report that measured pulmonary function studies show some degree of airway obstruction in as many as 50% of patients 7–8 years postoperatively. Also, a large number of patients appear to have a pronounced bronchial responsiveness to histamine.

Congenital Absence of the Pericardium

Congenital absence of the pericardium is a rare condition. With contemporary imaging techniques, an increase of incidental pericardial defects has arisen. Significant concern comes from potential life-threatening complications.

Pericardial defects are rare. They are associated with other congenital abnormalities in 30–50% of patients, mostly cardiac and pulmonary in nature (atrial septal defect, patent ductus arteriosus, tetralogy of Fallot, bronchogenic cysts and pulmonary sequestrations). Chest wall abnormalities have also been described. Pericardial absence is classified as a left or right defect. It is divided secondarily as being

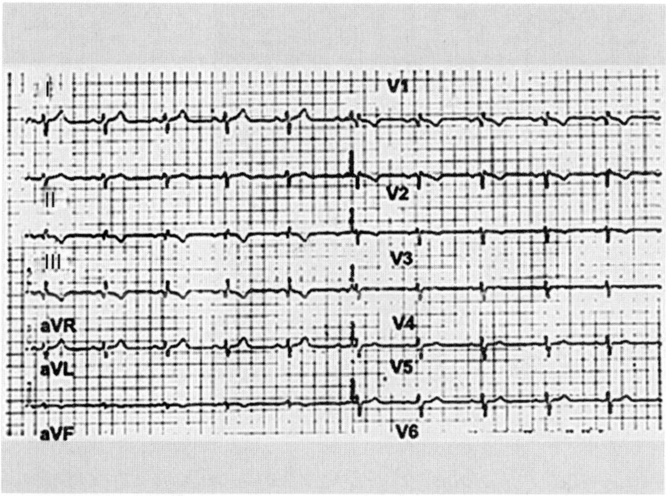

Fig. 14.369: *ECG showing right-axis deviation with incomplete right bundle-branch block and poor R wave progression in the precordial leads in patient with abscence of pericardium*

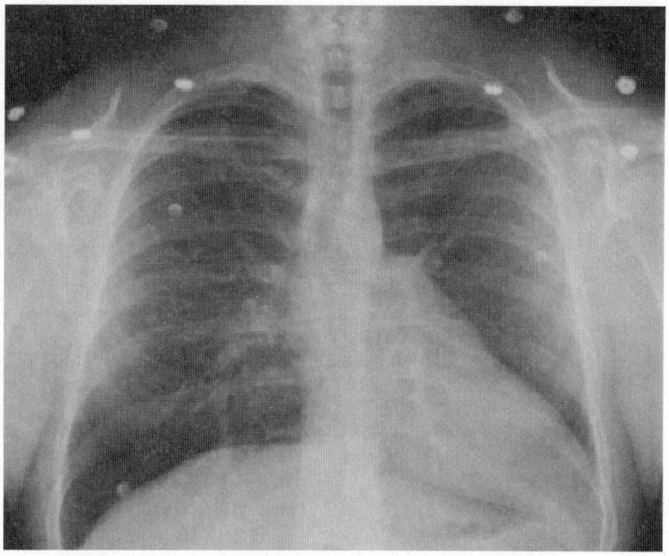

Fig. 14.371: *X-ray chest PA view showing "snoopy sign". Left cardiac border straightening and elongation (snoopy sign), lung tissue between aorta and pulmonary artery*

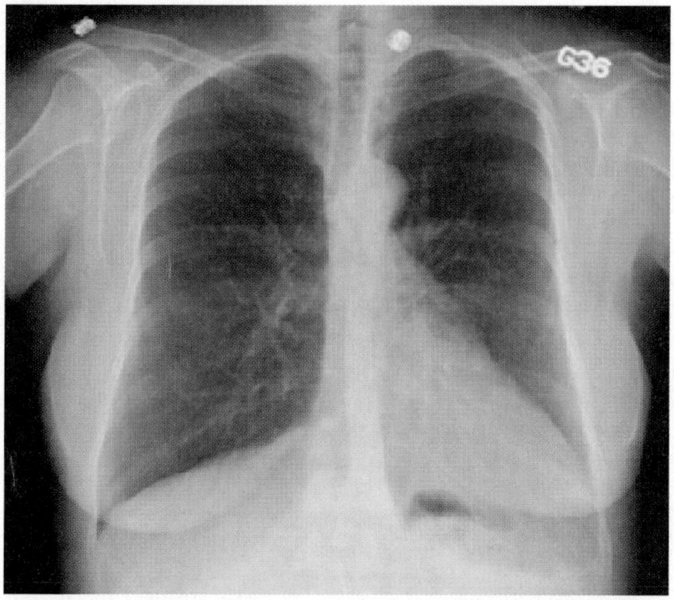

Fig. 14.370: *Posteroanterior chest roentgenogram showing the leftward displacement of the heart and rectification of the left heart border, suggestive of left pericardial absence*

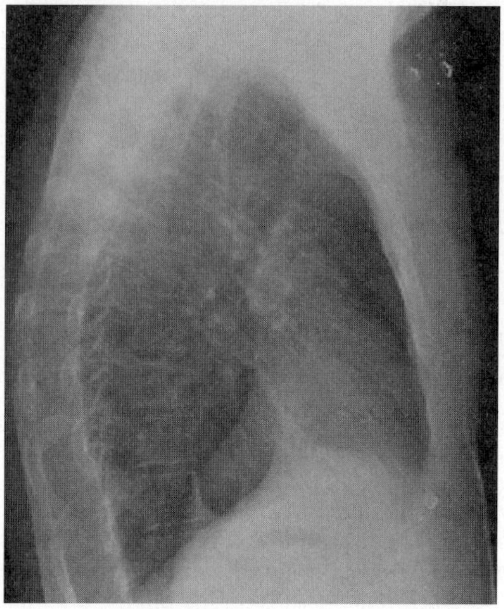

Fig. 14.372: *X-ray chest PA view showing prominent anterior clear space*

total or partial. The most commonly reported pericardial defect is by far left-sided, with left total defects more frequent than the left partial defects. Right-sided and bilateral absence have seldom been reported. The suspected etiology of a pericardial defect is the premature atrophy of the left common cardinal vein (duct of Cuvier). The consequent reduced blood supply to the left pleuropericardial membrane results in pericardial agenesis.

The clinical presentation is nonspecific. In most reported cases, the defect was discovered incidentally in an asymptomatic patient . For subjects who present with symptoms, atypical chest pain, dyspnea, trepopnea and palpitations are most commonly encountered. A physical examination may reveal a laterally displaced apex and systolic murmurs and clicks of undetermined origin. Patients may also present with complications clearly related to the defect. Most commonly cited are herniation and incarceration of the myocardium, predominantly the left atrial appendage. Ventricular herniation has also been described. Other complications include torsion of the great vessels secondary to increased cardiac mobility within the chest cavity, coronary artery compression by the edge of the pericardial defect, and cardiac traction due to adherence of the epicardium to other chest structures in the absence of the pericardial and pleural membranes. All these complications have been associated with presentations

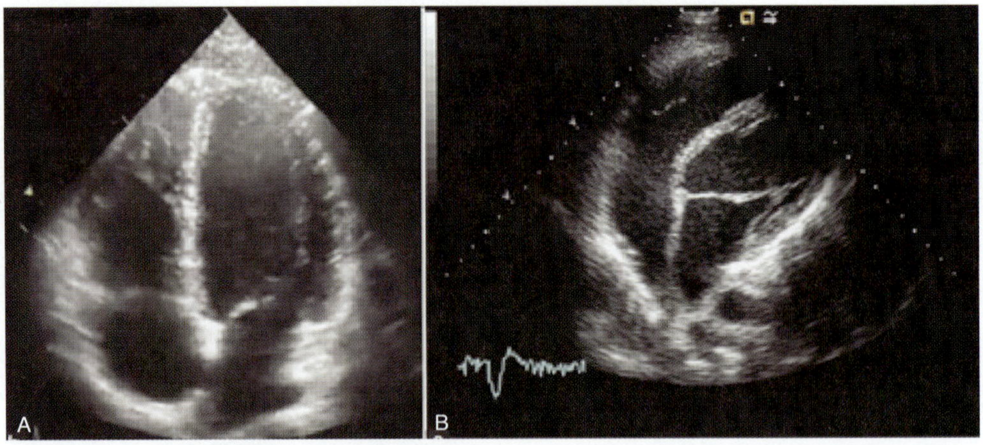

Fig. 14.373: *(A) A normal 2-D echo with interventricular septum pointing toward the probe, (B) 2D echo in a patient with congenital absence of pericardium, with left ventricle flopped to the left side and interventricular septum pointing to the left side*

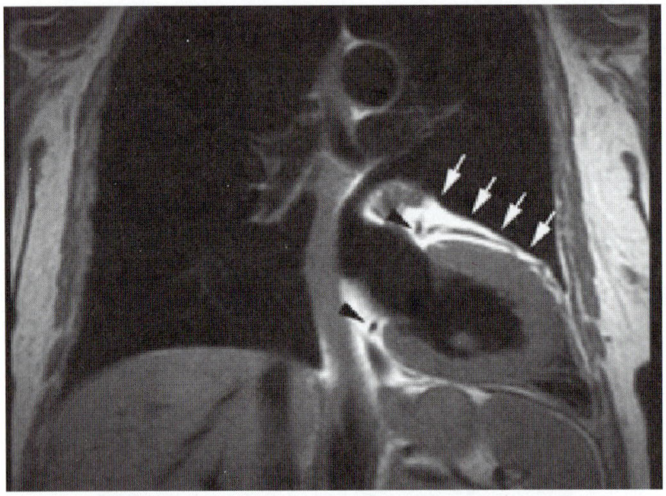

Fig. 14.374: *T1-weighted cardiac magnetic resonance image in the coronal view indicating the left anterior descending coronary artery coursing within epicardial fat (white arrows). In this imaging sequence, the pericardium would normally be inferred from a dark stripe sandwiched between bright epicardial and pericardial fat. The absence of pericardium here results in a single layer of fat, known to be epicardial because of the coursing coronary artery. Also note the normal positions of the left main and right coronary arteries in this patient (black arrowheads)*

varying from chest pain to infarction, syncope, tricuspid regurgitation and sudden death.

With such a wide range of nonspecific symptoms, diagnostic testing is the basis for raising suspicion and confirming the pericardial defect. ECG, chest X-ray, echocardiography , and even coronary angiography, may all serve as a basis for clinical suspicion, showing features mostly resulting from levoposition of the heart.

Laboratory Investigations and Imaging Studies

Electrocardiogram usually presents typical findings. The most common observation is right axis deviation with incomplete right bundle-branch block and poor R wave progression in the precordial leads in patient with abscence of pericardium.

Radiography include levoposition of the heart, confirmed by the absence of the right heart border projecting on the right of the vertebral column, as well as left cardiac border straightening and elongation ("Snoopy sign"), and the deep or very well-defined aortopulmonary window caused by the absence of pleura allowing lung to invaginate into this space.

Echocardiographic findings are also related to cardiac levoposition and increased mobility within the chest cavity. These include unusual echocardiographic windows, marked change in cardiac position with changing patient position on the examination table (cardioptosis) and with the cardiac cycle (swinging heart), abnormal septal motion, and false-positive appearance of right cavity dilation.

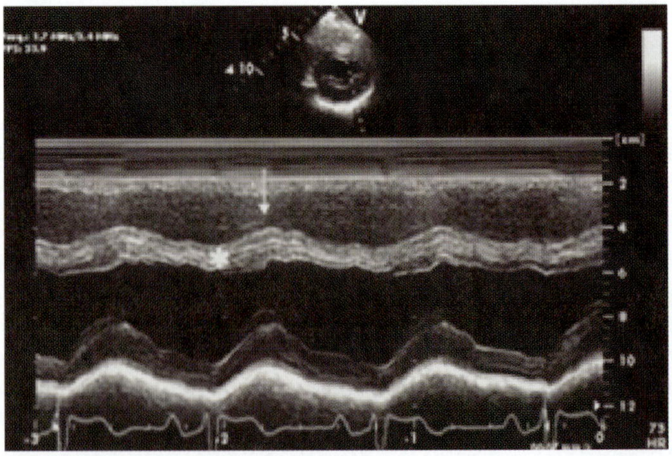

Fig. 14.375: *Transthoracic echocardiogram: parasternal short-axis M-mode was consistent with paradoxical motion of the septum. Septum (asterisk) moved anteriorly during systole and posteriorly (arrow) during diastole with the posterior wall demonstrating an exaggerated movement during systole as seen in congenital abscence of pericardium*

CMR or CT: These modalities not only confirm the diagnosis, they also delineate the extent of the defect, which provides important information in the subsequent management of patients. Furthermore, advanced imaging allows exclusion of complications associated with the pericardial defect. CMR is the gold standard because it exquisitely visualizes the pericardium while providing additional information critical to decision making, most notably whether significant focal infarction has occurred. Delayed-enhancement CMR can detect infarction as light as 1.6 g, representing roughly 1.5% of the LV myocardial mass, even when no underlying function defect is identified. The features of congenital absence of the pericardium observed on CMR include left-sided shift of the heart, lung interposition between the aorta and pulmonary artery, as well as the precise location and extent of the pericardial absence.

Therapeutic options are chiefly based on small, retrospective series. It is recommended that patients presenting with complications be treated surgically . For patients in whom no complications have arisen, various strategies are proposed. A common approach is to estimate the risk of life-threatening complications (mostly herniation) based on the size of the pericardial defect. Total left defects, because they carry very little risk, usually warrant no surgical treatment. Left partial pericardial defects are more complex and controversial. While some authors consider all partial pericardial defects to be high-risk, irrespective of defect size, others divide the risk according to the size of the defect.

Treatment

Complete cases of pericardial absence require no intervention unless complications occur. Patients with debilitating symptoms may benefit from pericardioplasty. However, in partial defects, when herniation occurs or is threatened, extension of the defect by the pericardiectomy, or pericardioplasty may be preformed 2, 8 but in straight back syndrome therapy is directed toward specific coexisting conditions (e.g. MVP).

Conclusion

Although congenital absence of the pericardium and straight back syndrome seem to be unrelated, it is important to know their similarities: usually asymptomatic, basal systolic murmurs, right bundle-branch block in ECG, levoposition of heart in postero-anterior chest X-ray. Furthermore we want to propose that echocardiography of the patient with straight back syndrome could have abnormal view and paradoxical septal motion probably due to clockwise rotation of heart. Not knowing these issues lead us to misdiagnose patient as congenital absence of pericardium primarily.

Using this size-related approach, asymptomatic, large partial pericardial defects are not surgically treated because they are considered to carry a low risk of complications compared with complete defects.

Small- and moderate-sized left pericardial defects are considered for prophylactic surgery by some, while others suggest treating only symptomatic patients. Watchful waiting appears to entail a good prognosis in such asymptomatic patients.

BIBLIOGRAPHY

1. Acar P, Dulac Y, Roux D, et al. Comparison of transthoracic and transesophageal three-dimensional echocardiography for assessment of atrial septal defect diameter in children. Am J Cardiol. 2003;91:500.
2. Alano MA, Ngougmna E, Ostrea EM Jr, et al. Analysis of nonsteroidal antiinflammatory drugs in meconium and its relation to persistent pulmonary hypertension of the newborn. Pediatrics. 2001;107:519.
3. Alexi-Meskishvili V, Ishino K, Dahnert I, et al. Correction of complete atrioventricular septal defects with the double-patch technique and cleft closure. Ann Thorac Surg. 1996;62:519.
4. Anderson PA, Sleeper LA, Mahony L, et al. Contemporary outcomes after the Fontan procedure: a Pediatric Heart Network multicenter study. J Am Coll Cardiol. 2008;52:85-98.
5. Aoki M, Forbess JM, Jonas RA, et al. Result of biventricular repair for double-outlet right ventricle. J Thorac Cardiovasc Surg. 1994;107:338-349.
6. Aram DM, Ekelman BL, Ben-Shachar G, et al. Intelligence and hypoxemia in children with congenital heart disease: fact or artifact? J Am Coll Cardiol. 1985;6:889.
7. Bacha EA, Almodovar M, Wessel DL, et al. Surgery for coarctation of the aorta in infants weighing less than 2 kg. Ann Thorac Surg. 2001;71:1260.
8. Bacha EA, Cao QL, Galantowicz ME, et al. Multicenter experience with perventricular device closure of muscular ventricular septal defects. Pediatr Cardiol. 2005;26:169.
9. Bailey LL, Nehlsen-Cannarella SL, Doroshow RW, et al. Cardiac allotransplantation in newborns as therapy for hypoplastic left heart syndrome. N Engl J Med. 1986;315: 949-951.
10. Bando K, Turrentine MW, Ensing GJ, et al. Surgical management of total anomalous pulmonary venous connection. Thirty-year trends. Circulation. 1996;94:II12-II26.
11. Beekman RH, Tuuri DT. Acute hemodynamic effects of increasing hemoglobin concentration in children with a right to left ventricular shunt and relative anemia. J Am Coll Cardiol. 1985;5:357.
12. Beekman RH. Coarctation of the aorta. In: Emmanouilides GC, Riemenschneider TA, Allen HD, Gutgesell HP, eds. Moss and Adams Heart Disease in Infants, Children and Adolescents. 5th ed. Baltimore, MD: Williams & Wilkins; 1995:1111.
13. Behrendt DM, Aberdeen E, Waterson DJ, et al. Total anomalous pulmonary venous drainage in infants. I. Clinical and hemodynamic findings, methods, and results of operation in 37 cases. Circulation. 1972;46:347-356.
14. Belli E, Serraf A, Lacour-Gayet F, et al. Surgical treatment of subaortic stenosis after biventricular repair of double-outlet right ventricle. J Thorac Cardiovasc Surg. 1996;112:1570-1578.
15. Bell-Thomson J, Jewell E, Ellis FH Jr, et al. Surgical technique in the management of patent ductus arteriosus in the elderly patient. Ann Thorac Surg; 1980;30:80.

16. Belmont JW. Recent progress in the molecular genetics of congenital heart defects. Clin Genet. 1998;54:11.
17. Bengur AR, Snider AR, Serwer GA, et al. Usefulness of the Doppler mean gradient in evaluation of children with aortic valve stenosis and comparison to gradient at catheterization. Am J Cardiol. 1989;64:756.
18. Benson DW, Sharkey A, Fatkin D, et al. Reduced penetrance, variable expressivity, and genetic heterogeneity of familial atrial septal defects. Circulation. 1998;97:2043.
19. Bergersen LJ, Perry SB, Lock JE. Effect of cutting balloon angioplasty on resistant pulmonary artery stenosis. Am J Cardiol. 2003;91:185-189.
20. Beuren AJ, Apitz J, Harmjanz D. Supravalvular aortic stenosis in association with mental retardation and a certain facial appearance. Circulation. 1962;26:1235.
21. Bharati S, Lev M. The surgical anatomy of the heart in tubular hypoplasia of the transverse aorta (preductal coarctation). J Thorac Cardiovasc Surg. 1986;91:79.
22. Blalock A, Taussig H. The surgical treatment of malformation of the heart in which there is pulmonary stenosis or pulmonary atresia. JAMA. 1945;128:129.
23. Brochu MC, Baril JF, Dore A, et al. Improvement in exercise capacity in asymptomatic and mildly symptomatic adults after atrial septal defect percutaneous closure. Circulation. 2002;106:1821.
24. Brown JW, Ruzmetov M, Okada Y, et al. Surgical results in patients with double outlet right ventricle: a 20-year experience. Ann Thorac Surg. 2001;72:1630-1635.
25. Burke RP, Wernovsky G, van der Valde M, et al. Video-assisted thoracoscopic surgery for congenital heart disease. J Thorac Cardiovasc Surg. 1995;109:499.
26. Calder AL, Peebles CR, Occleshaw CJ. The prevalence of coronary arterial abnormalities in pulmonary atresia with intact ventricular septum and their influence on surgical results. Cardiol Young. 2007;17:387-396.
27. Cameron JW, Rosenthal A, Olson AD. Malnutrition in hospitalized children with congenital heart disease. Arch Pediatr Adolesc Med. 1995;149:1098.
28. Campbell M. Natural history of coarctation of the aorta. Br Heart J. 1970;32:633.
29. Carminati M, Butera G, Chessa M, et al. Transcatheter closure of congenital ventricular septal defects: results of the European Registry. Eur Heart J. 2007;28:2361.
30. Carpentier A, Chauvaud S, Mace L, et al. A new reconstructive operation for Ebstein's anomaly of the tricuspid valve. J Thorac Cardiovasc Surg. 1988;96:92-101.
31. Castaneda AR, Jonas RA, Mayer JE, et al. Anomalies of the pulmonary veins. In: Castaneda AR, Jonas RA, Mayer JE, Hanley FL, eds. Cardiac Surgery of the Neonate and Infant. Philadelphia, PA: Saunders; 1994:160.
32. Castaneda AR, Jonas RA, Mayer JE, et al. D-transposition of the great arteries. In: Castaneda AR, Jonas RA, Mayer JE, Hanley FL, eds. Cardiac Surgery of the Neonate and Infant. Philadelphia, PA: Saunders; 1994:437.
33. Castaneda AR, Jonas RA, Mayer JE, et al. Tetralogy of Fallot. In: Castaneda AR, Jonas RA, Mayer JE, Hanley FL, eds. Cardiac Surgery of the Neonate and Infant. Philadelphia, PA: Saunders; 1994:215.
34. Celermajer DS, Cullen S, Sullivan ID, et al. Outcome in neonates with Ebstein's anomaly. J Am Coll Cardiol. 1992;19:1041-1046.
35. Cetta F, Feldt RH, O'Leary PW, et al. Improved early morbidity and mortality after Fontan operation: the Mayo Clinic experience, 1987 to 1992. J Am Coll Cardiol. 1996;28:480-486.
36. Chandar JS, Wolff GS, Garson A Jr, et al. Ventricular arrhythmias in postoperative tetralogy of Fallot. Am J Cardiol. 1990;65:655.
37. Chang CW, Chiu SN, Wu ET, et al. Transcatheter closure of a ruptured sinus of Valsalva aneurysm. Circ J. 2006;70:1043.
38. Chin AJ, Sanders SP, Sherman F, et al. Accuracy of subcostal two-dimensional echocardiography in prospective diagnosis of total anomalous pulmonary venous connection. Am Heart J. 1987;113:1153-1159.
39. Clagett O, Kirklin JW, Edwards JE. Anatomic variations and pathologic changes in coarctation of the aorta: a study of 124 cases. Surg Gynecol Obstet. 1954;98:103.
40. Clyman RI. Ibuprofen and patent ductus arteriosus. N Engl J Med. 2000;343:728.
41. Coceani F, Olley PM. Roll of prostaglandins prostacyclin and thromboxanes in the control of prenatal patency and postnatal closure of the ductus arteriosus. In: Prostaglandins in the Perinatal Period. New York, NY: Grune & Stratton; 1980:109.
42. Cohen LS, Friedman JM, Jefferson JW, et al. A reevaluation of risk of in utero exposure to lithium. JAMA. 1994;271:146-150.
43. Connelly MS, Liu PP, Williams WG, et al. Congenitally corrected transposition of the great arteries in the adult: functional status and complications. J Am Coll Cardiol. 1996;27:1238-1243.
44. Cowley CG, Rosenthal A. Congenitally corrected transposition of the great arteries: the systemic right ventricle. Prog Pediatr Cardiol. 1999;10:31-35.
45. Daebritz S, Del Nido PJ. Surgical management of common atrioventricular canal. Prog Pediatr Cardiol. 1999;10:161.
46. Dall'Agata A, McGhie J, Taams MA, et al. Secundum atrial septal defect is a dynamic three-dimensional entity. Am Heart J. 1999;137:1075.
47. Danielson GK, Driscoll DJ, Mair DD, et al. Operative treatment of Ebstein's anomaly. J Thorac Cardiovasc Surg. 1992;104:1195-1202.
48. Dawes G. Foetal and Neonatal Physiology: A Comparative Study of the Changes at Birth. Chicago, IL: Year Book; 1968.
49. Dobell AR, Van PR. The Holmes heart: historic associations and pathologic anatomy. Am Heart J. 1996;132:437-445.
50. Donnelly JE, Brown JM, Radford DJ. Pregnancy outcome and Ebstein's anomaly. Br Heart J. 1991;66:368-371.
51. Donofrio MT, Jacobs ML, Norwood WI, et al. Early changes in ventricular septal defect size and ventricular geometry in the single left ventricle after volume-unloading surgery. J Am Coll Cardiol. 1995;26:1008-1015.
52. Driscoll DJ, Mottram CD, Danielson GK. Spectrum of exercise intolerance in 45 patients with Ebstein's anomaly and observations on exercise tolerance in 11 patients after surgical repair. J Am Coll Cardiol. 1988;11:831-836.
53. Driscoll DJ, Wolfe RR, Gersony WM, et al. Cardiorespiratory responses to exercise of patients with aortic stenosis, pulmonary stenosis, and ventricular septal defect. Circulation. 1993;87:I102.
54. Duncan BW, Mee RB, Mesia CI, et al. Results of the double switch operation for congenitally corrected transposition of the great arteries. Eur J Cardiothorac Surg. 2003;24:11-19.

55. Edwards JE. Classification of congenital heart disease in the adult. In: Roberts WC, ed. Congenital Heart Disease in Adults. Philadelphia, PA: Davis; 1979:1.
56. Egito ES, Moore P, O'sullivan J, et al. Transvascular balloon dilation for neonatal critical aortic stenosis: early and midterm results. J Am Coll Cardiol. 1997;29:442.
57. Elkins RC, Knott-Craig CJ, Ward KE, et al. The Ross operation in children: 10-year experience. Ann Thorac Surg. 1998;65:496.
58. Ensing GJ, Schmidt MA, Hagler DJ, et al. Spectrum of findings in a family with nonsyndromic autosomal dominant supravalvular aortic stenosis: a Doppler echocardiographic study. J Am Coll Cardiol. 1989;13:413.
59. Ewart AK, Morris CA, Atkinson D, et al. Hemizygosity at the elastin locus in a developmental disorder, Williams syndrome. Nat Genet. 1993;5:11.
60. Fernandes SM, Sanders SP, Khairy P, et al. Morphology of bicuspid aortic valve in children and adolescents. J Am Coll Cardiol. 2004;44:1648.
61. Fineman JR, Soifer SJ, Heymann MA. Regulation of pulmonary vascular tone in the perinatal period. Annu Rev Physiol. 1995;57:115.
62. Fischbach P, Law I, Serwer GA. Congenitally corrected l-transposition of the great arteries: abnormalities of atrioventricular conduction. Prog Pediatr Cardiol. 1999; 10:37-43.
63. Fischbein CA, Rosenthal A, Fischer EG, et al. Risk factors of brain abscess in patients with congenital heart disease. Am J Cardiol. 1974;34:97.
64. Fletcher SE, Nihill MR, Grifka RG, et al. Balloon angioplasty of native coarctation of the aorta: midterm follow-up and prognostic factors. J Am Coll Cardiol. 1995;25:730.
65. Fontan F, Baudet E. Surgical repair of tricuspid atresia. Thorax. 1971;26:240-248.
66. Fredriksen PM, Chen A, Veldtman G, et al. Exercise capacity in adult patients with congenitally corrected transposition of the great arteries. Heart. 2001;85:191-195.
67. Freed MD, Heymann MA, Lewis AB, et al. Prostaglandin E1 infants with ductus arteriosus-dependent congenital heart disease. Circulation. 1981;64:899.
68. Freedom RM, Culham J, Moes CA. Angiocardiography of Congenital Heart Disease. New York, NY: Mcmillan; 1989.
69. Freedom RM. Congenitally corrected transposition of the great arteries: definitions and pathologic anatomy. Pediatr Cardiol. 1999;10:3-16.
70. Fu YC, Bass J, Amin Z, et al. Transcatheter closure of perimembranous ventricular septal defects using the new Amplatzer membranous VSD occluder: results of the U.S. phase I trial. J Am Coll Cardiol. 2006;47:319.
71. Fulton D, Fyler DC. D-transposition of the great arteries. In: Keane JF, Lock JE, Fyler DC, eds. Nadas' Pediatric Cardiology. 2nd ed. Philadelphia, PA: Hanley & Belfus; 2006:645.
72. Fyler DC. Aortic outflow abnormalities. In: Fyler DC, ed. Nadas' Pediatric Cardiology. Philadelphia, PA: Hanley & Belfus; 1992:506.
73. Fyler DC. Report of the New England Regional Infant Cardiac Program. Pediatrics. 1980;65:375.
74. Gardiner H, Celermajer D, Sorensen K. Arterial reactivity is significantly impaired in normotensive young adults after successful repair of aortic coarctation in childhood. Circulation. 1954;89:1745.
75. Gathman GE, Nadas AS. Total anomalous pulmonary venous connection: clinical and physiologic observations of 75 pediatric patients. Circulation. 1970;42:143-154.
76. Gatzoulis MA, Till JA, Somerville J, Redington AN. Mechanoelectrical interaction in tetralogy of Fallot. QRS prolongation relates to right ventricular size and predicts malignant ventricular arrhythmias and sudden death. Circulation. 1995;92:231-237.
77. Gaynor JW, Mahle WT, Cohen MI, et al. Risk factors for mortality after the Norwood procedure. Eur J Cardiothorac Surg. 2002;22:82-89.
78. Gentles TL, Calder AL, Clarkson PM, et al. Predictors of long-term survival with Ebstein's anomaly of the tricuspid valve. Am J Cardiol. 1992;69:377-381.
79. George B, Kaplan S. Single ventricle and subaortic obstruction. Prog Pediatr Cardiol. 1994;3:167-176.
80. Gersony WM, Hayes CJ, Driscoll DJ, et al. Bacterial endocarditis in patients with aortic stenosis, pulmonary stenosis, or ventricular septal defect. Circulation. 1993;87:I121.
81. Gersony WM, Peckham GJ, Ellison RC, et al. Effects of indomethacin in premature infants with patent ductus arteriosus: results of a national collaborative study. J Pediatr. 1983;102:895.
82. Gersony WM. Long-term follow-up of operated congenital heart disease. Cardiol Clin. 1989;7:915.
83. Geva T. Indications and timing of pulmonary valve replacement after tetralogy of Fallot repair. Semin Thorac Cardiovasc Surg Pediatr Card Surg Annu. 2006;9:11-22.
84. Gidding SS, Stockman JA III. Effect of iron deficiency on tissue oxygen delivery in cyanotic congenital heart disease. Am J Cardiol. 1988;61:605.
85. Graham TP Jr, Bernard YD, Mellen BG, et al. Long-term outcome in congenitally corrected transposition of the great arteries: a multi-institutional study. J Am Coll Cardiol. 2000;36:255-261.
86. Graham TP Jr, Bricker JT, James FW, et al. 26th Bethesda conference: recommendations for determining eligibility for competition in athletes with cardiovascular abnormalities. Task Force 1: congenital heart disease. J Am Coll Cardiol. 1994;24:867.
87. Hagler DJ, Edwards WD. Univentricular atrial ventricular connection. In: Emmanouilides GC, Riemenschneider TA, Allen HD, Gutgesell HP, eds. Moss and Adams Heart Disease in Infants, Children and Adolescents. 5th ed. Baltimore, MD: Williams & Wilkins; 1995:1278.
88. Hagler DJ. Double outlet right ventricle and double outlet left ventricle. In: Emmanouilides GC, Allen HD, Gutgesell HP, Clark EB, Driscoll DJ, eds. Moss and Adams Heart Disease in Infants Children and Adolescents. 6th ed. Philadelphia, PA: Lippincott Williams & Wilkins; 2001:1102.
89. Hall JG. CATCH 22. J Med Genet. 1993;30:801.
90. Hamilton W, Hattajee C, Dalen J. Atrial septal defect secundum: clinical profile with psychologic correlates. In: Roberts WC, eds. Adult Congenital Heart Disease. Philadelphia, PA: Davis; 1987:395.
91. Hanley FL, Fenton KN, Jonas RA, et al. Surgical repair of complete atrioventricular canal defects in infancy. Twenty-year trends. J Thorac Cardiovasc Surg. 1993;106:387.
92. Harrild DM, Berul CI, Cecchin F, et al. Pulmonary valve replacement in tetralogy of Fallot: impact on survival and ventricular tachycardia. Circulation. 2009;119: 445-451.

93. Hart EM, Garson A Jr. Psychosocial concerns of adults with congenital heart disease. Employability and insurability. Cardiol Clin. 1993;11:711.
94. Hawkins JA, Minich LL, Tani LY, et al. Late results and reintervention after aortic valvotomy for critical aortic stenosis in neonates and infants. Ann Thorac Surg. 1998;65:1758.
95. Healy J. An anatomic survey of anomalous pulmonary veins: their clinical significance. J Thorac Cardiovasc Surg. 1952;23:433.
96. Heath D, Edwards JE. The pathology of hypertensive pulmonary vascular disease: a description of six grades of structural changes in the pulmonary arteries with special reference to congenital cardiac septal defects. Circulation. 1958;18:533.
97. Henriksson P, Varendh G, Lundstrom NR. Haemostatic defects in cyanotic congenital heart disease. Br Heart J. 1979;41:23.
98. Hernandez F, Rochkind R, Cooper H. The intracavitary electrocardiogram in the diagnosis of Ebstein's anomaly. Am J Cardiol. 1958;1:181-190.
99. Heymann MA, Rudolph AM. Effects of congenital heart disease on fetal and neonatal circulations. Prog Cardiovasc Dis. 1972;15:115.
100. Hill SL, Hijazi ZM, Hellenbrand WE, et al. Evaluation of the AMPLATZER vascular plug for embolization of peripheral vascular malformations associated with congenital heart disease. Catheter Cardiovasc Interv. 2006;67:113.
101. Hoffman JI, Christianson R. Congenital heart disease in a cohort of 19,502 births with long-term follow-up. Am J Cardiol. 1978;42:641.
102. Hovels-Gurich HH, Seghaye MC, Ma Q, et al. Long-term results of cardiac and general health status in children after neonatal arterial switch operation. Ann Thorac Surg. 2003;75:935-943.
103. Hraska V, Duncan BW, Mayer JE Jr, et al. Long-term outcome of surgically treated patients with corrected transposition of the great arteries. J Thorac Cardiovasc Surg. 2005;129:182-191.
104. Hraska V, Krajci M, Haun C, et al. Ross and Ross-Konno procedure in children and adolescents: mid-term results. Eur J Cardiothorac Surg. 2004;25:742.
105. Ilbawi MN, DeLeon SY, Backer CL, et al. An alternative approach to the surgical management of physiologically corrected transposition with ventricular septal defect and pulmonary stenosis or atresia. J Thorac Cardiovasc Surg. 1990;100:410-415.
106. Ing FF, Starc TJ, Griffiths SP, et al. Early diagnosis of coarctation of the aorta in children: a continuing dilemma. Pediatrics. 1996;98:378.
107. Jacobs ML, Blackstone EH, Bailey LL. Intermediate survival in neonates with aortic atresia: a multi-institutional study. The Congenital Heart Surgeons Society. J Thorac Cardiovasc Surg. 1998;116:417-431.
108. Jacobs ML, Rychik J, Rome JJ, et al. Early reduction of the volume work of the single ventricle: the hemi-Fontan operation. Ann Thorac Surg. 1996;62:456-461.
109. John Sutton MG, Tajik AJ, McGoon DC. Atrial septal defect in patients ages 60 years or older: operative results and long-term postoperative follow-up. Circulation. 1981; 64:402.
110. Keane JF, Driscoll DJ, Gersony WM, et al. Second natural history study of congenital heart defects. Results of treatment of patients with aortic valvular stenosis. Circulation. 1993;87:I16.
111. Keane JF, Fyler DC. Total anomalous pulmonary venous return. In: Keane JF, Lock JE, Fyler DC, eds. Nadas' Pediatric Cardiology. 2nd ed. Philadelphia, PA: Saunders Elsevier; 2006:773.
112. Keane JF, Fyler DC. Tricuspid valve problems. In: Keane JF, Lock JE, Fyler DC, eds. Nadas' Pediatric Cardiology. 2nd ed. Philadelphia, PA: Saunders Elsevier; 2006:761.
113. Keane JF, Lock JE, Fyler DC. Nadas—Pediatric Cardiology. Philadelphia, PA: Saunders Elsevier; 2006.
114. Keith J. Foetal and neonatal physiology: a comparative study of the changes at birth. In: Keith JD, Rowe RD, Vlad P, eds. Heart Disease in Infancy and Childhood. 3rd ed. New York, NY: MacMillan; 1978:3.
115. Kinsella JP, Abman SH. Recent developments in inhaled nitric oxide therapy of the newborn. Curr Opin Pediatr. 1999;11:121.
116. Kirjavainen M, Happonen JM, Louhimo I. Late results of Senning operation. J Thorac Cardiovasc Surg. 1999;117:488-495.
117. Kirklin JK, Barratt-Boyes BG. Congenitally corrected transposition of the great arteries. In: Kirklin JK, Barratt-Boyes BG, eds. Cardiac Surgery. New York, NY: Churchill Livingstone; 1993:1511.
118. Kirklin JK, Barratt-Boyes BG. Double outlet right ventricle. In: Kirklin JK, Barratt-Boyes BG, eds. Cardiac Surgery. 2nd ed. New York, NY: Churchill Livingstone; 1993:1469.
119. Kirklin JW, Barratt-Boyes BG. Congenital aortic stenosis. In: Kirklin JW, Barratt-Boyes BG, eds. Cardiac Surgery. 2nd ed. New York, NY: Churchill Livingstone; 1993:1195.
120. Kirklin JW, Blackstone EH, Kirklin JK, et al. Surgical results and protocols in the spectrum of tetralogy of Fallot. Ann Surg. 1983;198:251-265.
121. Kirklin JW. Atrio ventricular canal defect. In: Kirklin JW, Barratt-Boyes BG, eds. Cardiac Surgery. 2nd ed. New York, NY: Churchill Livingstone; 1993:693.
122. Kiziltan HT, Theodoro DA, Warnes CA, et al. Late results of bioprosthetic tricuspid valve replacement in Ebstein's anomaly. Ann Thorac Surg. 1998;66:39-45.
123. Knauth AL, Gauvreau K, Powell AJ, et al. Ventricular size and function assessed by cardiac MRI predict major adverse clinical outcomes late after tetralogy of Fallot repair. Heart. 2008;94:211-216.
124. Knauth AL, Lock JE, Perry SB, et al. Transcatheter device closure of congenital and postoperative residual ventricular septal defects. Circulation. 2004;110:501.
125. Knott-Craig CJ, Overholt ED, Ward KE, et al. Repair of Ebstein's anomaly in the symptomatic neonate: an evolution of technique with 7-year follow-up. Ann Thorac Surg. 2002;73:1786-1792.
126. Konduri GG, Kim UO. Advances in the diagnosis and management of persistent pulmonary hypertension of the newborn. Pediatr Clin North Am. 2009;56:579.
127. Kreutzer J, Perry SB, Jonas RA, et al. Tetralogy of Fallot with diminutive pulmonary arteries: preoperative pulmonary valve dilation and transcatheter rehabilitation of pulmonary arteries. J Am Coll Cardiol. 1996;27:1741-1747.
128. Kulik TJ. Inhaled nitric oxide in the management of congenital heart disease. Curr Opin Cardiol. 1996;11:75-80.

129. Laborde F, Folliguet T, Batisse A, et al. Video-assisted thoracoscopic surgical interruption: the technique of choice for patent ductus arteriosus. Routine experience in 230 pediatric cases. J Thorac Cardiovasc Surg. 1995;110:1681.
130. Lacour-Gayet F, Zoghbi J, Serraf AE, et al. Surgical management of progressive pulmonary venous obstruction after repair of total anomalous pulmonary venous connection. J Thorac Cardiovasc Surg. 1999;117:679-687.
131. Lacro R. Dysmorphology. In: Fyler DC, ed. Nadas' Pediatric Cardiology. Philadelphia, PA: Hanley & Belfus; 1992:37.
132. Lang P, Fyler DC. Hypoplastic left heart syndrome, mitral atresia and aortic atresia. In: Keane JF, Lock JE, Fyler DC, eds. Nadas' Pediatric Cardiology. 2nd ed. Philadelphia, PA: Saunders Elsevier; 2006:715.
133. Langley SM, Winlaw DS, Stumper O, et al. Midterm results after restoration of the morphologically left ventricle to the systemic circulation in patients with congenitally corrected transposition of the great arteries. J Thorac Cardiovasc Surg. 2003;125: 1229-1241.
134. Lev M, Liberthson RR, Joseph RH, et al. The pathologic anatomy of Ebstein's disease. Arch Pathol. 1970;90:334-343.
135. Levine J, Geva T. Echocardiographic evaluation of AV canal malformation. Prog Pediatr Cardiol. 1999;10:137.
136. Lewin MB, McBride KL, Pignatelli R, et al. Echocardiographic evaluation of asymptomatic parental and sibling cardiovascular anomalies associated with congenital left ventricular outflow tract lesions. Pediatrics. 2004;114:691.
137. Lewis F, Winchell P, Bashour F. Open repair of atrial septal defects: results in sixty-three patients. J Am Med Assoc. 1957;165:922.
138. Liebman J, Cullum L, Belloc NB. Natural history of transposition of the great arteries. Anatomy and birth and death characteristics. Circulation. 1969;40:237-262.
139. Lillehei CW, Cohen M, Warden HE, et al. Direct vision intracardiac surgical correction of the tetralogy of Fallot, pentalogy of Fallot, and pulmonary atresia defects: report of first ten cases. Ann Surg. 1955;142:418-442.
140. Lind J, Wegelius C. Human fetal circulation: changes in the cardiovascular system at birth and disturbances in the post-natal closure of the foramen ovale and ductus arteriosus. Cold Spring Harb Symp Quant Biol. 1954;19:109.
141. Losay J, Touchot A, Serraf A, et al. Late outcome after arterial switch operation for transposition of the great arteries. Circulation. 2001;104:I121.
142. Lucas RV Jr, Lock JE, Tandon R, Edwards JE. Gross and histologic anatomy of total anomalous pulmonary venous connections. Am J Cardiol. 1988;62:292-300.
143. Lundstrom U, Bull C, Wyse RK, et al. The natural and "unnatural" history of congenitally corrected transposition. Am J Cardiol. 1990;65:1222-1229.
144. Mahle WT, McBride MG, Paridon SM. Exercise performance after the arterial switch operation for D-transposition of the great arteries. Am J Cardiol. 2001;87:753-758.
145. Mahoney LT, Truesdell SC, Krzmarzick TR, et al. Atrial septal defects that present in infancy. Am J Dis Child. 1986;140:1115.
146. Mainwaring R, Lamberti J, Moore J. The bidirectional Glenn Fontan procedures: integrated management of the patient with a functionally single ventricle. Cardiol Young. 1996;6:198-207.
147. Makikallio K, McElhinney DB, Levine JC, et al. Fetal aortic valve stenosis and the evolution of hypoplastic left heart syndrome: patient selection for fetal intervention. Circulation. 2006;113:1401.
148. Marianeschi SM, McElhinney DB, Reddy VM, et al. Alternative approach to the repair of Ebstein's malformation: intracardiac repair with ventricular unloading. Ann Thorac Surg. 1998;66:1546-1550.
149. Marino BS, Wernovsky G, McElhinney DB, et al. Neo-aortic valvular function after the arterial switch. Cardiol Young. 2006;16:481-489.
150. Marshall AC, Tworetzky W, Bergersen L, et al. Aortic valvuloplasty in the fetus: technical characteristics of successful balloon dilation. J Pediatr. 2005;147:535.
151. Masura J, Lange PE, Wilkinson JL, et al. US/International Multicenter Trial of Atrial Septal Catheter Closure using the Amplatzer Septal Occluder: initial results [abstract]. J Am Coll Cardiol. 1998;131:57A.
152. Matitiau A, Geva T, Colan SD, et al. Bulboventricular foramen size in infants with double-inlet left ventricle or tricuspid atresia with transposed great arteries: influence on initial palliative operation and rate of growth. J Am Coll Cardiol. 1992;19:142-148.
153. Mavroudis C, Backer CL, Muster AJ, et al. Taussig-Bing anomaly: arterial switch versus Kawashima intraventricular repair. Ann Thorac Surg. 1996;61:1330-1338.
154. Mayer JE Jr, Bridges ND, Lock JE, et al. Factors associated with marked reduction in mortality for Fontan operations in patients with single ventricle. J Thorac Cardiovasc Surg. 1992;103:444-451.
155. McCrindle BW. Independent predictors of immediate results of percutaneous balloon aortic valvotomy in children. Valvuloplasty and Angioplasty of Congenital Anomalies (VACA) Registry Investigators. Am J Cardiol. 1996;77:286.
156. McElhinney DB, Lock JE, Keane JF, et al. Left heart growth, function, and reintervention after balloon aortic valvuloplasty for neonatal aortic stenosis. Circulation. 2005;111:451.
157. McElhinney DB, Marshall AC, Wilkins-Haug LE, et al. Predictors of technical success and postnatal biventricular outcome after in utero aortic valvuloplasty for aortic stenosis with evolving hypoplastic left heart syndrome. Circulation. 2009;120:1482.
158. Mitchell SC, Korones SB, Berendes HW. Congenital heart disease in 56,109 births. Incidence and natural history. Circulation. 1971;43:323.
159. Moak JP, Gersony WM. Progressive atrioventricular valvular regurgitation in single ventricle. Am J Cardiol. 1987;59:656-658.
160. Moore P, Egito E, Mowrey H, et al. Midterm results of balloon dilation of congenital aortic stenosis: predictors of success. J Am Coll Cardiol. 1996;27:1257.
161. Murphy JG, Gersh BJ, Mair DD, et al. Long-term outcome in patients undergoing surgical repair of tetralogy of Fallot. N Engl J Med. 1993;329:593-599.
162. Murphy JG, Gersh BJ, McGoon MD, et al. Long-term outcome after surgical repair of isolated atrial septal defect. Follow-up at 27 to 32 years. N Engl J Med. 1990;323:1645.
163. Najm HK, Coles JG, Black MD, et al. Extended aortic root replacement with aortic allografts or pulmonary autografts in children. J Thorac Cardiovasc Surg. 1999;118:503.
164. Nakanishi T, Matsumoto Y, Seguchi M, et al. Balloon angioplasty for postoperative pulmonary artery stenosis in

transposition of the great arteries. J Am Coll Cardiol. 1993;22:859-866.
165. Narayanan M, Cooper B, Weiss H, et al. Prophylactic indomethacin: factors determining permanent ductus arteriosus closure. J Pediatr 136:330:2000.
166. Newfeld EA, Wilson A, Paul MH, et al. Pulmonary vascular disease in total anomalous pulmonary venous drainage. Circulation. 1980;61:103-109.
167. Nihill MR. Clinical management of patients with pulmonary hypertension. In: Emmanouilides GC, Riemenschneider TA, Allen HD, Gutgesell HP, eds. Moss and Adams Heart Disease in Infants, Children and Adolescents. 5th ed. Baltimore, MD: Williams & Wilkins; 1995:1695.
168. Nollert G, Fischlein T, Bouterwek S, et al. Long-term survival in patients with repair of tetralogy of Fallot: 36-year follow-up of 490 survivors of the first year after surgical repair. J Am Coll Cardiol. 1997;30:1374-1383.
169. Nora JJ, Nora AH. Maternal transmission of congenital heart diseases: new recurrence risk figures and the questions of cytoplasmic inheritance and vulnerability to teratogens. Am J Cardiol. 1987;59:459.
170. Nora JJ. Causes of congenital heart diseases: old and new modes, mechanisms, and models. Am Heart J. 1993;125:1409.
171. Norwood WI, Hougen TJ, Castaneda AR. Total anomalous pulmonary venous connection: surgical considerations. Cardiovasc Clin. 1981;11:353-364.
172. Norwood WI, Lang P, Hansen DD. Physiologic repair of aortic atresia-hypoplastic left heart syndrome. N Engl J Med. 1983;308:23-26.
173. Ohlsson A, Walia R, Shah S. Ibuprofen for the treatment of patent ductus arteriosus in preterm and/or low birth weight infants. Cochrane Database Syst Rev. 2005;CD003481.
174. Ohye RG, Gomez CA, Ohye BJ, et al. The Ross/Konno procedure in neonates and infants: intermediate-term survival and autograft function. Ann Thorac Surg. 2001;72:823.
175. Omeish A, Hijazi ZM. Transcatheter closure of atrial septal defects in children & adults using the amplatzer septal occluder. J Interv Cardiol. 2001;14:37.
176. Oosterhof T, van SA, Vliegen HW, et al. Preoperative thresholds for pulmonary valve replacement in patients with corrected tetralogy of Fallot using cardiovascular magnetic resonance. Circulation. 2007;116:545-551.
177. Paridon SM, Mitchell PD, Colan SD, et a. A cross-sectional study of exercise performance during the first 2 decades of life after the Fontan operation. J Am Coll Cardiol. 2008;52:99-107.
178. Perron J, Moran AM, Gauvreau K, et al. Valved homograft conduit repair of the right heart in early infancy. Ann Thorac Surg. 1999;68:542-548.
179. Perry LW, Neill CA, Ferencz C. Infants with congenital heart disease: the cases. In: Ferencz C, Rubin JD, Loffredo CA, Magee CA, eds. Epidemiology of Congenital Heart Disease: The Baltimore-Washington Infancy Study 1981-1989. Mount Kisco, NY: Futura; 1993:33.
180. Petrossian E, Reddy VM, McElhinney DB, et al. Early results of the extracardiac conduit Fontan operation. J Thorac Cardiovasc Surg. 1999;117:688-696.
181. Phornphutkul C, Rosenthal A, Nadas AS, et al. Cerebrovascular accidents in infants and children with cyanotic congenital heart disease. Am J Cardiol. 1973;32:329.
182. Pierpont ME, Basson CT, Benson DW Jr, et al. Genetic basis for congenital heart defects: current knowledge: a scientific statement from the American Heart Association Congenital Cardiac Defects Committee, Council on Cardiovascular Disease in the Young: endorsed by the American Academy of Pediatrics. Circulation. 2007;115:3015.
183. Pollock JC, Jamieson MP, McWilliam R. Somatosensory evoked potentials in the detection of spinal cord ischemia in aortic coarctation repair. Ann Thorac Surg. 1986;41:251.
184. Ponce FE, Williams LC, Webb HM, et al. Propranolol palliation of tetralogy of Fallot: experience with long-term drug treatment in pediatric patients. Pediatrics. 1973;52:100-108.
185. Porstmann W, Wierny L. Percutaneous transfemoral closure of the patent ductus arteriosus: an alternative to surgery. Semin Roentgenol. 1981;16:95.
186. Pretre R, Tamisier D, Bonhoeffer P, et al. Results of the arterial switch operation in neonates with transposed great arteries. Lancet. 2001;357:1826-1830.
187. Prieto LR, Foreman CK, Cheatham JP, et al. Intermediate-term outcome of transcatheter secundum atrial septal defect closure using the Bard Clamshell Septal Umbrella. Am J Cardiol. 1996;78:1310.
188. Quaegebeur JM, Jonas RA, Weinberg AD, et al. Outcomes in seriously ill neonates with coarctation of the aorta. A multiinstitutional study. J Thorac Cardiovasc Surg. 1994;108:841.
189. Quaegebeur JM, Sreeram N, Fraser AG, et al. Surgery for Ebstein's anomaly: the clinical and echocardiographic evaluation of a new technique. J Am Coll Cardiol. 1991;17:722-728.
190. Rabinovitch M. Pathophysiology of pulmonary hypertension. In: Emmanouilides GC, Riemenschneider TA, Allen HD, Gutgesell HP, eds. Moss and Adams Heart Disease in Infants, Children and Adolescents. 5th ed. Baltimore, MD: Williams & Wilkins; 1995:1659.
191. Radford DJ, Graff RF, Neilson GH. Diagnosis and natural history of Ebstein's anomaly. Br Heart J. 1985;54:517-522.
192. Rashkind W, Cuaso C. Transcatheter closure of patent ductus arteriosus. Pediatr Cardiol. 1979;1:3.
193. Rastelli GC, Ongley PA, Kirklin JW, et al. Surgical repair of the complete form of persistent common atrioventricular canal. J Thorac Cardiovasc Surg. 1968;55:299.
194. Reich JD, Auld D, Hulse E, et al. The Pediatric Radio-frequency Ablation Registry's experience with Ebstein's anomaly. Pediatric Electrophysiology Society. J Cardiovasc Electrophysiol. 1998;9:1370-1377.
195. Rhodes LA, Colan SD, Perry SB, et al. Predictors of survival in neonates with critical aortic stenosis. Circulation. 1991;84:2325.
196. Roberson DA, Silverman NH. Ebstein's anomaly: echocardiographic and clinical features in the fetus and neonate. J Am Coll Cardiol. 1989;14:1300-1307.
197. Rogers HM, Edwards JE. Incomplete division of the atrioventricular canal with patent inter-atrial foramen primum, persistent common atrioventricular ostium: report of five cases and review of the literature. Am Heart J. 1948;36:28.
198. Rooklin AR, McGeady SJ, Mikaelian DO, et al. The immotile cilia syndrome: a cause of recurrent pulmonary diseases in children. Pediatrics. 1980;66:526-531.

199. Rose V, Izukawa T, Moes CA. Syndromes of asplenia and polysplenia. A review of cardiac and non-cardiac malformations in 60 cases with special reference to diagnosis and prognosis. Br Heart J. 1975;37:840.
200. Rosenthal A, Dick M. Tricuspid atresia. In: Emmanouilides GC, Riemenschneider TA, Allen HD, Gutgesell HP, eds. Moss and Adams Heart Disease in Infants, Children and Adolescents. 5th ed. Baltimore, MD: Williams & Wilkins; 1995:902.
201. Ross EA, Perloff JK, Danovitch GM, et al. Renal function and urate metabolism in late survivors with cyanotic congenital heart disease. Circulation. 1986;73:396.
202. Rudolph AM, Heymann MA. Cardiac output in the fetal lamb: the effects of spontaneous and induced changes of heart rate on right and left ventricular output. Am J Obstet Gynecol. 1976;124:183.
203. Rudolph AM, Heymann MA. Circulatory changes during growth in the fetal lamb. Circ Res. 1970;26:289.
204. Rudolph AM, Heymann MA. The circulation of the fetus in utero. Methods for studying distribution of blood flow, cardiac output and organ blood flow. Circ Res. 1967;21:163.
205. Rudolph AM. Fetal and neonatal pulmonary circulation. Annu Rev Physiol. 1979;41:383.
206. Saalouke MG, Shapiro SR, Perry LW, et al. Isolated partial anomalous pulmonary venous drainage associated with pulmonary vascular obstructive disease. Am J Cardiol. 1977;39:439.
207. Sagin-Saylam G, Somerville J. Palliative mustard operation for transposition of the great arteries: late results after 15-20 years. Heart. 1996;75:72-77.
208. Sakakibara S, Konno S. Congenital aneurysm of the sinus of Valsalva. Anatomy and classification. Am Heart J. 1962;63:405.
209. Sano T, Riesenfeld T, Karl TR, et al. Intermediate-term outcome after intracardiac repair of associated cardiac defects in patients with atrioventricular and ventriculoarterial discordance. Circulation. 1995;92:II272-II278.
210. Satur CR, Walker DR, Dickinson DF. Day case ligation of patent ductus arteriosus in preterm infants: a 10 year review. Arch Dis Child. 1991;66:477.
211. Schmaltz AA, Neudorf U, Winkler UH. Outcome of pregnancy in women with congenital heart disease. Cardiol Young. 1999;9:88.
212. Schott JJ, Benson DW, Basson CT, et al. Congenital heart disease caused by mutations in the transcription factor NKX2-5. Science. 1998;281:108.
213. Schreiber C, Cook A, Ho SY, et al. Morphologic spectrum of Ebstein's malformation: revisitation relative to surgical repair. J Thorac Cardiovasc Surg. 1999;117:148-155.
214. Schuurmans FM, Pulles-Heintzberger CF, Gerver WJ, et al. Long-term growth of children with congenital heart disease: a retrospective study. Acta Paediatr. 1998;87:1250.
215. Seward JB, Tajik AJ. Transesophageal echocardiography in congenital heart disease. Am J Card Imaging. 1990;4:215.
216. Shaffer EM, Snider AR, Beekman RH, et al. Sinus of Valsalva aneurysm complicating bacterial endocarditis in an infant: diagnosis with two-dimensional and Doppler echocardiography. J Am Coll Cardiol. 1987;9:588.
217. Sherwood MC, Rockenmacher S, Colan SD, et al. Prognostic significance of clinically silent coronary artery fistulas. Am J Cardiol. 1999;83:407-411.
218. Shim D, Fedderly RT, Beekman RH III, et al. Follow-up of coil occlusion of patent ductus arteriosus. J Am Coll Cardiol. 1996;28:207.
219. Siassi B, Blanco C, Cabal LA, et al. Incidence and clinical features of patent ductus arteriosus in low-birthweight infants: a prospective analysis of 150 consecutively born infants. Pediatrics. 1976;57:347.
220. Silverman NH. Anomalous pulmonary venous connections. In: Silverman NH, ed. Pediatric Echocardiography. Baltimore, MD: Williams & Wilkins; 1993:179.
221. Snider AR, Serwer GA, Ritter S. Abnormalities in ventricular connection. In: Snider AR, Serwer GA, Ritter S, eds. Echocardiography in Pediatric Heart Disease. St. Louis, MO: Mosby; 1990:317.
222. Snider AR, Serwer GA. Echocardiography and Pediatric Heart Disease. Chicago, IL: Year Book; 1990.
223. Starnes VA, Pitlick PT, Bernstein D, et al. Ebstein's anomaly appearing in the neonate. A new surgical approach. J Thorac Cardiovasc Surg. 1991;101:1082-1087.
224. Steele PM, Fuster V, Cohen M, et al. Isolated atrial septal defect with pulmonary vascular obstructive disease—long-term follow-up and prediction of outcome after surgical correction. Circulation. 1987;76:1037.
225. Stellin G, Vida VL, Milanesi O, et al. Surgical treatment of complete A-V canal defects in children before 3 months of age. Eur J Cardiothorac Surg. 2003;23:187.
226. Strong WB. Introduction: pediatric cardiology exercise testing. Pediatr Cardiol. 1999;20:1.
227. Takach TJ, Reul GJ, Duncan JM, et al. Sinus of Valsalva aneurysm or fistula: management and outcome. Ann Thorac Surg. 1999;68:1573.
228. Talner NS. Heart failure. In: Emmanouilides GC, Riemenschneider TA, Gutgesell HP, eds. Moss and Adams Heart Disease in Infants. 5th ed. Baltimore, MD: Williams & Wilkins; 1995:1746.
229. Teitel DF, Iwamoto HS, Rudolph AM. Effects of birth-related events on central blood flow patterns. Pediatr Res. 1987;22:557.
230. Termignon JL, Leca F, Vouhe PR, et al. "Classic" repair of congenitally corrected transposition and ventricular septal defect. Ann Thorac Surg. 1996;62:199-206.
231. Territo M, Rosov N, Perloff J. Cyanotic congenital heart disease: hematologic management, renal function and urate metabolism. In: Perloff JK, Child JS, eds. Congenital Heart Disease in Adults. Philadelphia, PA: Saunders; 1991:93.
232. Therrien J, Barnes I, Somerville J. Outcome of pregnancy in patients with congenitally corrected transposition of the great arteries. Am J Cardiol. 1999;84:820-824.
233. Tkebuchava T, von Segesser LK, Vogt PR, et al. Congenital coronary fistulas in children and adults: diagnosis, surgical technique and results. J Cardiovasc Surg (Torino). 1996;37:29-34.
234. Turanlahti MI, Laitinen PO, Sarna SJ, et al. Nitric oxide, oxygen, and prostacyclin in children with pulmonary hypertension. Heart. 1998;79:169.
235. UK Collaborative ECMO Trail Group. UK collaborative randomised trial of neonatal extracorporeal membrane oxygenation. Lancet. 1996;348:75.
236. Urrutia-S CO, Falaschi G, Ott DA, et al. Surgical management of 56 patients with congenital coronary artery fistulas. Ann Thorac Surg. 1983;35:300-307.

237. van Praagh R, Weinberg P, Smith S. Malpositions of the heart. In: Adams F, Emmanouilides GC, Riemenschneider TA, eds. Moss' Heart Disease in Infants, Children and Adolescents. Baltimore, MD: Williams & Wilkins; 1989:530.
238. van Praagh R. Segmental approach to diagnosis. In: Fyler DC, ed. Nadas' Pediatric Cardiology. Philadelphia, PA: Hanley & Belfus; 1992:27.
239. van Praagh S, Santini F, Sanders SP. Cardiac malpositions with special emphasis on visceral heterotaxy (asplenia and polysplenia syndromes). In: Fyler DC, ed. Nadas' Pediatric Cardiology. Philadelphia, PA: Hanley & Belfus; 1992:589.
240. van Son JA, Danielson GK, Huhta JC, et al. Late results of systemic atrioventricular valve replacement in corrected transposition. J Thorac Cardiovasc Surg. 1995;109: 642-652.
241. van Son JA, Edwards WD, Danielson GK. Pathology of coronary arteries, myocardium, and great arteries in supravalvular aortic stenosis. Report of five cases with implications for surgical treatment. J Thorac Cardiovasc Surg. 1994;108:21.
242. van Son JA, Falk V, Black MD, et al. Conversion of complex neonatal Ebstein's anomaly into functional tricuspid or pulmonary atresia. Eur J Cardiothorac Surg. 1998;13:280-284.
243. van Son JA, Reddy VM, Haas GS, et al. Modified surgical techniques for relief of aortic obstruction in [S,L,L] hearts with rudimentary right ventricle and restrictive bulboventricular foramen. J Thorac Cardiovasc Surg. 1995;110:909-915.
244. Varvarigou A, Bardin CL, Beharry K, et al. Early ibuprofen administration to prevent patent ductus arteriosus in premature newborn infants. JAMA. 1996;275:539.
245. Vavuranakis M, Bush CA, Boudoulas H. Coronary artery fistulas in adults: incidence, angiographic characteristics, natural history. Cathet Cardiovasc Diagn. 1995;35: 116-120.
246. Velvis H, Schmidt KG, Silverman NH, Turley K. Diagnosis of coronary artery fistula by two-dimensional echocardiography, pulsed Doppler ultrasound and color flow imaging. J Am Coll Cardiol. 1989;14:968-976.
247. Waldman JD, Czapek EE, Paul MH, et al. Shortened platelet survival in cyanotic heart disease. J Pediatr. 1975;87:77.
248. Warnes CA. Congenitally corrected transposition: the uncorrected misnomer. J Am Coll Cardiol. 1996;27:1244-1245.
249. Watson H. Natural history of Ebstein's anomaly of tricuspid valve in childhood and adolescence. An international co-operative study of 505 cases. Br Heart J. 1974;36: 417-427.
250. Wernovsky G, Mayer JE Jr, Jonas RA, et al. Factors influencing early and late outcome of the arterial switch operation for transposition of the great arteries. J Thorac Cardiovasc Surg. 1995;109:289-301.
251. Wernovsky G. Transposition of the great arteries. In: Allen HD, Gutgesell HP, Clark EB, Driscoll DJ, eds. Moss and Adams Heart Disease in Infants Children and Adolescents. 6th ed. Philadelphia, PA: Lippincott Williams & Wilkins; 2001:1027.
252. Williams JC, Barratt-Boyes BG, Lowe JB. Supravalvular aortic stenosis. Circulation. 1961;24:1311.
253. Williams WG, Quaegebeur JM, Kirklin JW, et al. Outflow obstruction after the arterial switch operation: a multiinstitutional study. Congenital Heart Surgeons Society. J Thorac Cardiovasc Surg. 1997;114:975-987.
254. Wilson NJ, Clarkson PM, Barratt-Boyes BG, et al. Long-term outcome after the mustard repair for simple transposition of the great arteries. 28-year follow-up. J Am Coll Cardiol. 1998;32:758-765.
255. Wilson W, Taubert KA, Gewitz M, et al. Prevention of infective endocarditis: guidelines from the American Heart Association: a guideline from the American Heart Association Rheumatic Fever, Endocarditis, and Kawasaki Disease Committee, Council on Cardiovascular Disease in the Young, and the Council on Clinical Cardiology, Council on Cardiovascular Surgery and Anesthesia, and the Quality of Care and Outcomes Research Interdisciplinary Working Group. Circulation. 2007;116:1736.
256. Yetman AT, Rosenberg HC, Joubert GI. Progression of asymptomatic aortic stenosis identified in the neonatal period. Am J Cardiol. 1995;75:636.
257. Yoo S, Burrows P, Moes CA. Evaluation of coronary arterial patterns in complete transposition by laidback aortagraphy. Cardiol Young. 1996;6:149-155.
258. Zalzstein E, Moes CA, Musewe NN, et al. Spectrum of cardiovascular anomalies in Williams-Beuren syndrome. Pediatr Cardiol. 1991;12:219.
259. Zamora R, Rao PS, Lloyd TR, et al. Intermediate-term results of phase I Food and Drug Administration Trials of buttoned device occlusion of secundum atrial septal defects. J Am Coll Cardiol. 1998;31:674.

15 Recognition and Management of Acute Rheumatic Fever

Rheumatic fever is a diffuse inflammatory disease having a delayed non-suppurative after effect of pharyngeal infection with beta-hemolytic group A streptococci. It characteristically tends to recur. Though its name is more familiar with joint involvement but its heart complications are important, to the physician with regards to its morbidity and mortality. This disease is being noticed infrequently in developed countries but its higher incidence almost remained the same in developing countries for the last 2–3 decades (6–15%) as compared to 1% in USA.

Rheumatic fever (RF) is a systemic illness that may occur following group A beta-hemolytic streptococcal (GABHS) pharyngitis in children. RF and its most serious complication, rheumatic heart disease (RHD), are believed to result from an autoimmune response; however, the exact pathogenesis remains unclear. Studies in the 1950s during an epidemic on a military base demonstrated 3% incidence of RF in adults with streptococcal pharyngitis not treated with antibiotics. Studies in children during the same period demonstrated an incidence of only 0.3%. Cardiac involvement is reported to occur in 30–70% of patients with their first attack of RF and in 73–90% of patients when all attacks are counted.

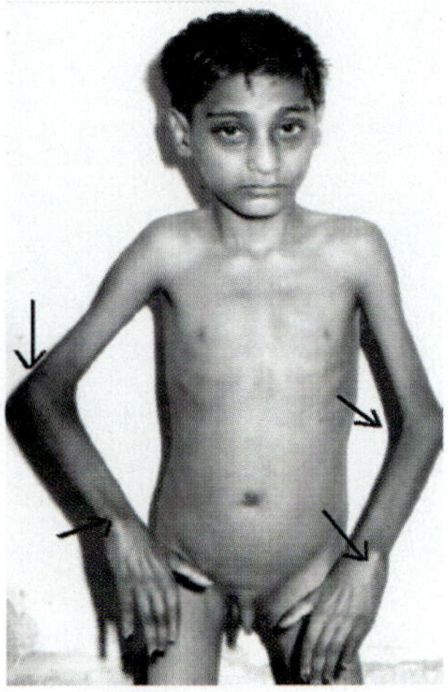

Fig. 15.1: *Swelling (arrows) over the wrist, elbows hands and fingers in a young child with acute rheumatic fever*

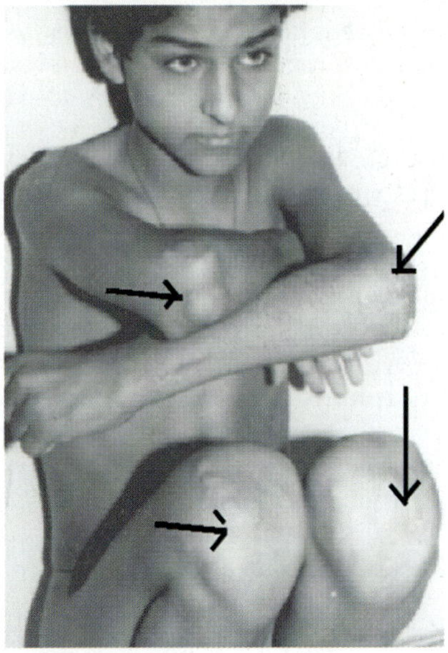

Fig. 15.2: *Subcutaneous nodules (arrows) in a young child with acute rheumatic fever*

Pathophysiology: RF develops in children and adolescents following pharyngitis with GABHS. The organisms attach to the epithelial cells of the upper respiratory tract and produce a battery of enzymes, which allows them to damage and invade human tissues. After an incubation period of 2–4 days, the invading organisms elicit an acute inflammatory response, with 3–5 days of sore throat, fever, malaise, headache, and elevated leukocyte count. In a small percent of patients, infection leads to RF several weeks after the sore throat has resolved. Only infections of the pharynx initiate or reactivate RF.

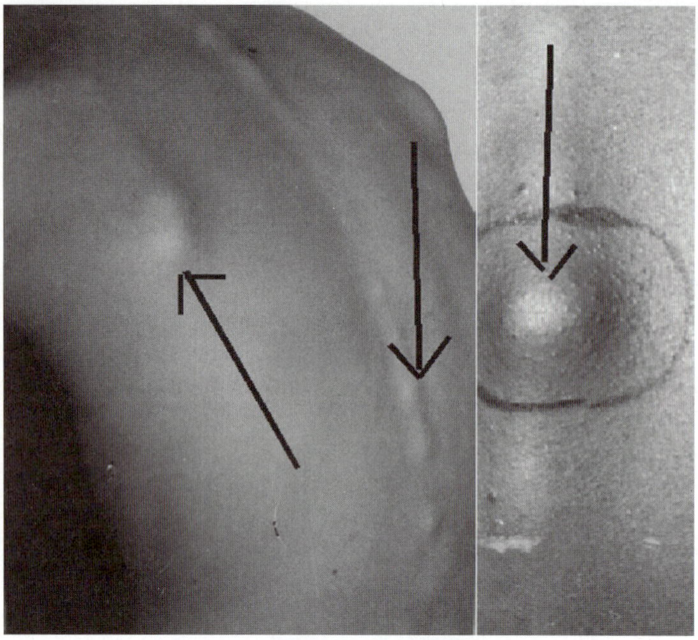

Fig. 15.3: *Subcutaneous nodules (arrows) over the scapulae and spine in a young child with acute rheumatic fever*

Direct contact with oral or respiratory secretions transmits the organism, and crowding enhances transmission. Patients remain infected for weeks after symptomatic resolution of pharyngitis and may serve as a reservoir for infecting others. Penicillin treatment shortens the clinical course of streptococcal pharyngitis and more importantly prevents the major sequelae.

GABHS organisms are gram-positive cocci, which frequently colonize the skin and oropharynx. These organisms may cause suppurative diseases (e.g. pharyngitis, impetigo, cellulitis, myositis, pneumonia, puerperal sepsis). GABHS organisms also may be associated with nonsuppurative diseases (e.g. RF, acute poststreptococcal glomerulonephritis). Group A streptococci (GAS) elaborate the cytolytic toxins, streptolysins S and O. Of these 2 toxins, streptolysin O induces persistently high antibody titers that provide a useful marker of GAS infection and its nonsuppurative complications. GAS, as identified using the Lancefield classification, has a group A carbohydrate antigen in the cell wall that is composed of a branched polymer of L-rhamnose and N-acetyl-D-glucosamine in a 2:1 ratio. Surface proteins on the cell wall of the organism may subserotype GAS. The presence of the M protein is the most important virulence factor for GAS infection in humans. More than 90 M serotypes have been identified, some of which have a long terminal antigenic domain (i.e. epitopes) similar to antigens in various components of the human heart. Rheumatogenic strains often are encapsulated mucoid strains, rich in M proteins, and resistant to phagocytosis. These strains are strongly immunogenic, and anti-M antibodies against the streptococcal infection may cross-react with components of heart tissue (i.e. sarcolemmal membranes, valve glycoproteins).

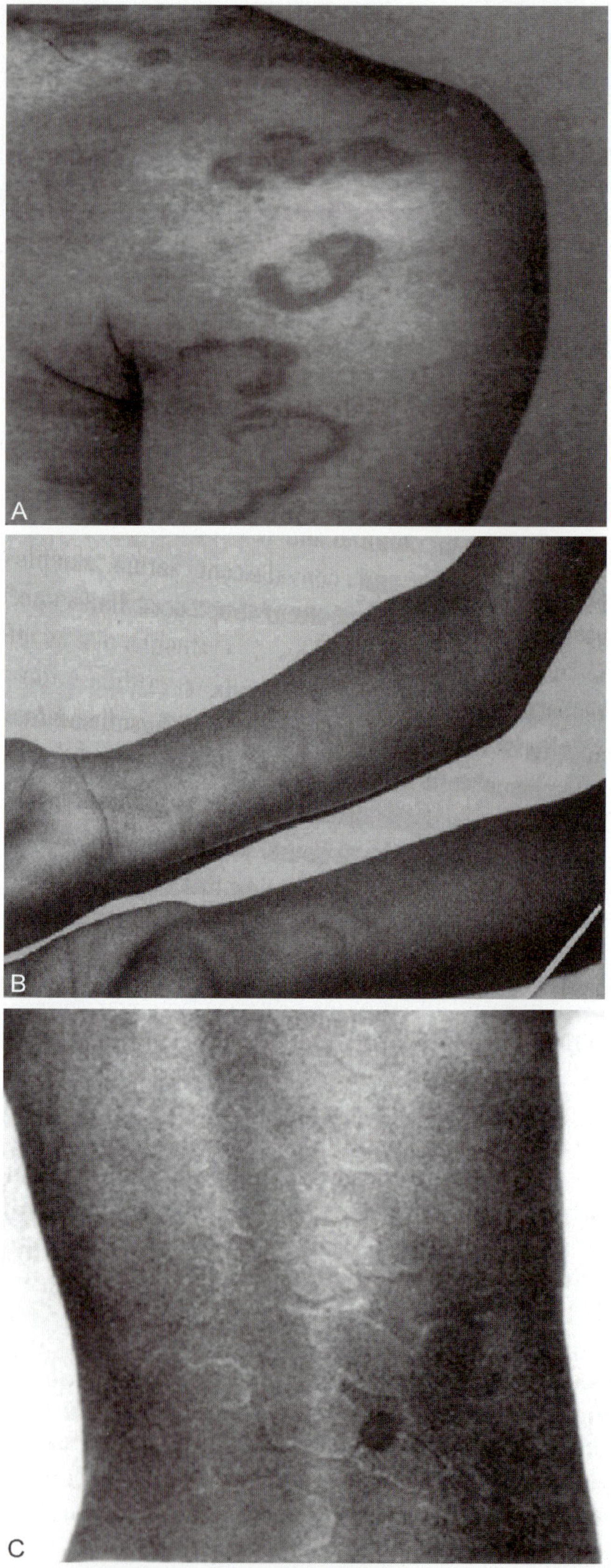

Fig. 15.4A to C: *(A) shoulder and upper arm areas (B) Forearm and (C) back area erythema marginatum. The rash is classically flat to slightly elevated, erythematous and annular (ring-like) in appearance*

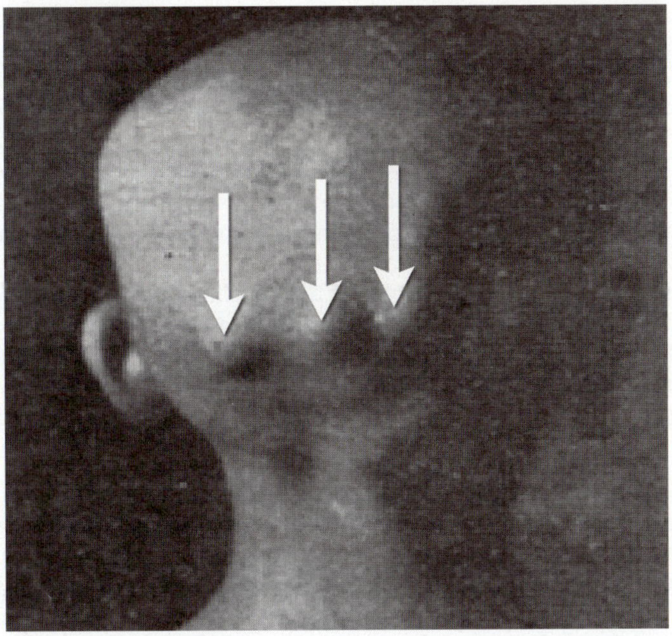

Fig. 15.5: *Rheumatic nodules over the occipit of a young child with acute rheumatic fever*

Acute RHD often produces a pancarditis, characterized by endocarditis, myocarditis, and pericarditis. Endocarditis is manifested as mitral and aortic valve insufficiency. Severe scarring of the valves develops during a period of months to years after an episode of acute RF, and recurrent episodes may cause progressive damage to the valves. The mitral valve is affected most commonly and severely (65–70% of patients); the aortic valve is affected second most commonly (25%). The tricuspid valve is deformed in only 10% of patients, almost always in association with mitral and aortic lesions, and the pulmonary valve rarely is affected. Severe valve insufficiency during the acute phase may result in congestive heart failure (CHF) and even death (1% of patients). Whether myocardial dysfunction during acute RF is related primarily to myocarditis or is secondary to CHF from severe valve insufficiency is not known. When pericarditis is present, it rarely affects cardiac function or results in constrictive pericarditis.

Chronic manifestations occur in adults with previous RHD from residual and progressive valve deformity. RHD is responsible for 99% of mitral valve stenosis in adults, and it may be associated with atrial fibrillation from chronic mitral valve disease and atrial enlargement.

Incidence

RF is now uncommon among children in the US. Incidence of RF and RHD has decreased in the US and other industrialized countries during the past 80 years. Prevalence of RHD in the US is now less than 0.05 per 1000 population, with rare regional outbreaks reported in Tennessee in the 1960s and in Utah, Ohio and Pennsylvania in the 1980s. In the early 1900s, incidence was reportedly 5–10 cases per 1000 population. Decreased incidence of RF has been attributed to the introduction of penicillin or a change in the virulence of the streptococci.

In developing countries, in contrast to trends in the US, RF and RHD have not decreased in developing countries. Retrospective studies in developing countries demonstrate the highest incidence for cardiac involvement and the highest recurrence rates of RF. Worldwide, an estimated 5–30 million children and young adults have chronic RHD, and 90,000 patients die from this disease each year.

Mortality morbidity: RHD is the major cause of morbidity from RF, and it is the major cause of mitral insufficiency and stenosis in the United States and in rest of the world. Variables that correlate with severity of valve disease are the number of previous attacks of RF, the length of time between the onset of disease and start of therapy, and sex (the prognosis for females is worse than for males). Insufficiency from acute rheumatic valve disease resolves in 70–80% of patients if they adhere to antibiotic prophylaxis.

Race: Native Hawaiians and Maori (both of Polynesian descent) have a higher incidence of RF. Incidence of RF in these patients is 13.4 per 100,000 hospitalized children per year, even with antibiotic prophylaxis of streptococcal pharyngitis. Otherwise, race (when controlled for socioeconomic variables) has not been documented to influence the disease incidence.

Sex: RF occurs in equal numbers in males and females. Females with RF fare worse than males and have a slightly higher incidence of chorea.

Age: RF is principally a disease of childhood, with a median age of 10 years; however, RF also occurs in adults (20% of cases).

History: Acute RF is a systemic disease. Thus, patients may present with a large variety of symptoms and complaints.

History of an antecedent sore throat 1–5 weeks prior to onset is present in 70% of older children and young adults. Only 20% of younger children can recall an antecedent sore throat.

Other symptoms on presentation may include fever, rash, headache, weight loss, epistaxis, fatigue, malaise, diaphoresis and pallor. Patients also may have chest pain with orthopnea or abdominal pain and vomiting. Finally, history may reveal symptoms more specific to RF.

- Migratory Joint Pain
- Nodules Under the Skin

Increased irritability and shortened attention span with personality changes, such as pediatric autoimmune neuropsychiatric disorder associated with streptococcal infections (PANDAS)

- Motor dysfunction
- History of previous RF.

Patients with previous RF are at a high risk of recurrence. Highest risk of recurrence within 5 years of the initial episode. Greater risk of recurrence with younger age at the time of the initial episode. Generally, recurrent attacks similar to the initial attack (however, risk of carditis and severity of valve damage increase with each attack).

Physical criteria: Revised in 1992, the modified Jones criteria provide guidelines for making the diagnosis of RF. The Jones criteria require the presence of two major or one major and two minor criteria for the diagnosis of RF. Having evidence of previous GAS pharyngitis is also necessary. These criteria are not absolute, and the diagnosis of RF can be made in patients with only confirmed streptococcal pharyngitis.

Major Diagnostic Criteria

- Carditis
- Polyarthritis
- Chorea
- Subcutaneous nodules
- Erythema marginatum.

Minor Diagnostic Criteria

- Fever
- Arthralgia
- Prolonged PR interval on electrocardiogram
- Elevated acute-phase reactants (APRs), which are erythrocyte sedimentation rate and C-reactive protein.

Patients presenting late to medical attention months after the onset of RF may have insufficient support to fulfill the criteria. Newly ill patients with a history of RF, especially RHD, who have supporting evidence of a recent GAS infection and who manifest either a single major or minor criteria: distinguishing recurrent carditis from preexisting significant RHD may be impossible. Evidence of previous GAS pharyngitis (One of the following must be present).

Positive throat culture or rapid streptococcal antigen test elevated or rising streptococcal antibody titer.

Major Clinical Manifestations

Arthritis: Polyarthritis is the most common symptom and frequently is the earliest manifestation of acute RF (70–75%). Characteristically, the arthritis begins in the large joints of the lower extremities (i.e. knees, ankles) and migrates to other large joints in the lower or upper extremities (i.e. elbows, wrists). Affected joints are painful, swollen, warm, erythematous, and limited in their range of motion. The pain is out of proportion to clinical findings. The arthritis reaches maximum severity in 12–24 hours and persists for 2–6 days (rarely more than 4 weeks, but has been reported to persist 44 days) at each site and is migratory but not additive. The arthritis responds rapidly to aspirin, which decreases symptoms in affected joints and prevents further migration of the arthritis. Polyarthritis is more common and more severe in teenagers and young adults than in younger children. Patients suffering multiple attacks may exhibit destructive arthritis (Jaccoud arthritis).

Carditis: Pancarditis is the most serious complication and the second most common complication of RF (50%). In advanced cases, patients may experience of dyspnea, mild-to-moderate chest discomfort, pleuritic chest pain, edema, cough, or orthopnea. On physical examination, carditis is most commonly revealed by a new murmur and tachycardia that is out of proportion to the fever. New or changing murmurs traditionally have been considered necessary for a diagnosis of rheumatic valvulitis. The murmurs of acute RF are from valve regurgitation, and the murmurs of chronic RF are from valve stenosis (Fig. 15.11).

Frequently examine patients in whom the diagnosis of acute RF is made due to the progressive nature of the disease. Some cardiologists have proposed that evidence of new mitral regurgitation from Doppler echocardiography, even in the absence of accompanying auscultatory findings, may be sufficient for making the diagnosis of carditis, particularly if the echo findings resolve along with other manifestations of RF. This criterion for carditis is not accepted uniformly and remains specifically excluded in the 1992 revised Jones criteria because of insufficient data.

Congestive heart failure: It may develop secondary to severe valve insufficiency or myocarditis. Physical findings associated with heart failure include tachypnea, orthopnea, jugular venous distention, rales, hepatomegaly, a gallop rhythm, and peripheral swelling and edema. A pericardial friction rub indicates that pericarditis is present. Increased cardiac dullness to percussion, muffled heart sounds, and a paradoxical pulse are consistent with pericardial effusion and impending pericardial tamponade. Confirm this clinical emergency with ECG, echocardiogram and evacuate the effusion by pericardiocentesis if it is producing hemodynamic compromise (Fig. 15.7).

In the absence of a family history of Huntington's chorea or findings consistent with systemic lupus erythematosus, the diagnosis of acute RF is almost certain. A long latency period exists between streptococcal pharyngitis (1–6 months) and the onset of chorea, and a history of an antecedent sore throat frequently is not obtained. Patients with chorea often do not demonstrate other Jones criteria.

Sydenham's chorea: It also known as Saint Vitus' dance or chorea minor, this extrapyramidal disorder is characterized by purposeless and involuntary movements of face and limbs, muscular hypotonia and emotional lability.

a. Initial manifestations include difficulty in writing, talking, or walking. Handwriting may deteriorate; speech may change to an explosive and halting tone; and the patient may become uncoordinated and easily frus trated.

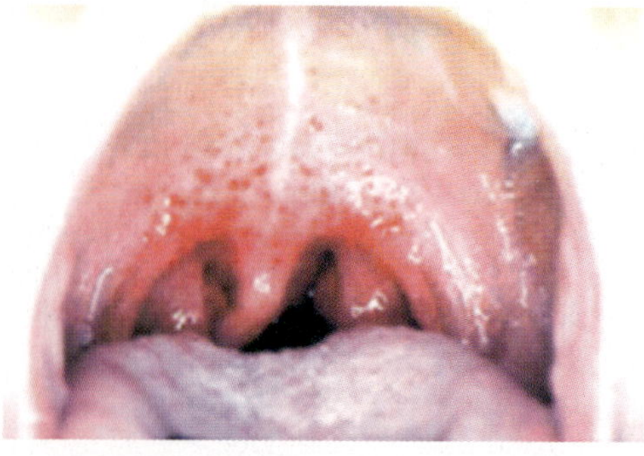

Fig. 15.6: *Acute throat infection with group A beta-hemolytic streptococcoi*

b. Symptoms tend to be more evident when the patient is under stress or awake and usually disappear during sleep.

c. Sydenham's chorea is a delayed manifestation of RF, usually appearing 3 months or more after an upper airway infection; it is often the sole manifestation of acute RF. Chorea has been reported in up to 30% of the patients. Most cases tend to follow a benign course with complete resolution of symptoms in 2–3 months although cases in which symptoms persisted for more than 2 years have been reported.

d. It is important to differentiate the symptoms of Sydenham's chorea from tics, athetosis, conversion reactions, hyperkinesia, and behavioral abnormalities. Chorea is slightly more common in females than males. Chorea also is known as rheumatic chorea.

Described poststreptococcal movement disorders have included pediatric autoimmune neuropsychiatric disorder associated with *Streptococcus* (PANDAS), and Tourette syndrome. Daily handwriting samples can be used as an indicator of progression or resolution of disease. Complete resolution of the symptoms typically occurs, with improvement in 1–2 weeks and full recovery in 2–3 months; however, incidents have been reported in which symptoms wax and wane for several years.

The PANDAS disorder appears to have a relapsing-remitting symptom complex characterized by obsessive-compulsive personality disorder. Patients with Sydenham chorea and obsessive-compulsive symptoms tend to show aggressive, contamination, and somatic obsessions and checking, cleaning, and repeating compulsions. Neurologic abnormalities include cognitive defects and motoric hyperactivity. The symptoms may also include emotional lability, separation anxiety, and oppositional behaviors, and they are prepubertal in onset. Some have proposed that the streptococcal infection triggers the formation of antibodies that cross-react with the basal ganglia of genetically susceptible hosts in a manner similar to the proposed mechanism for Sydenham chorea and causes the symptom complex.

Erythema marginatum: This characteristic rash, also known as erythema annulare, occurs in 5–13% of patients with acute RF. Erythema marginatum begins as 1–3 cm diameter, pink-to-red nonpruritic macules or papules located on the trunk and proximal limbs but never on the face. The lesions spread outward to form a serpiginous ring with erythematous raised margins and central clearing. The rash may fade and reappear within hours and is exacerbated by heat. Thus, if the lesions are not observed easily, they can be accentuated by the application of warm towels, a hot bath, or the use of tangential lighting. The rash occurs early in the course of the disease and remains long past the resolution of other symptoms. Erythema marginatum has also been reported in association with sepsis, drug reactions, and glomerulonephritis (Fig. 15.4).

Subcutaneous Nodules

Subcutaneous nodules are now an infrequent manifestation of RF. The frequency has declined during the past several years to 0–8% of patients with RF. When present, the nodules appear over the extensor surfaces of the elbows, knees, ankles, knuckles, scalp, and spinous processes of the lumbar and thoracic vertebrae (attached to the tendon sheath). The nodules are firm, nontender, and free from attachments to the overlying skin, and they range from a few millimeters to 1–2 cm. The nodules number from 1–12, with a mean of 3–4. Histologically, the nodules contain areas resembling the Aschoff bodies observed in the heart. Subcutaneous nodules generally occur several weeks into the disease and resolve within a month. They are strongly associated with severe rheumatic carditis, and in the absence of carditis, question the diagnosis of subcutaneous nodules (Figs 15.2, 15.3 and 15.5).

Other Clinical Manifestations

Abdominal pain: Abdominal pain usually occurs at the onset of acute RF, resembles other conditions with acute microvascular mesenteric inflammation, and may mimic acute appendicitis.

Arthralgias: Patients may report arthralgias upon presentation. In the history, determining if the patient has taken aspirin or nonsteroidal anti-inflammatory drugs (NSAIDs) is important because these may suppress the full manifestations of the disease. Arthralgia cannot be considered a minor manifestation if arthritis is present.

Epistaxis: Epistaxis may be associated with severe protracted rheumatic carditis.

Fever: Fevers greater than 39°C with no characteristic pattern are present initially in almost every patient with acute RF. The fever may be low grade (38.0–38.5°C) in children with mild carditis or absent in patients with pure chorea. The fever decreases without antipyretic therapy in approximately 1 week, but low-grade fevers persist for 2–3 weeks.

Rheumatic pneumonia: Patients present with the same signs as an infectious pneumonia. Differentiate rheumatic pneumonia from respiratory distress related to CHF.

Causes: RF is believed to result from an autoimmune response; however, the exact pathogenesis remains unclear.RF only develops in children and adolescents following GABHS pharyngitis, and only infections of the pharynx initiate or reactivate RF (Fig. 15.6).

At least some rheumatogenic strains of GAS have antigenic domains similar to antigens in components of the human heart, and some authors have proposed that anti-M antibodies against the streptococci may cross-react with heart tissue, causing the pancarditis that is observed in RF. So-called molecular mimicry between streptococcal and human proteins is felt to involve both the B and T cells of peripheral blood, with infiltration of the heart by T cells. Some believe that an increased production of inflammatory cytokines is the final mechanism of the autoimmune reaction that causes damage to cardiac tissue in RHD. An insufficiency of interleukin-4 (IL-4)—producing cells in the valve tissue may also contribute to the valve lesions.

- Streptococcal antigens, which are structurally similar to those in the heart, include hyaluronate in the bacterial capsule, cell wall polysaccharides (similar to glycoproteins in heart valves), and membrane antigens that share epitopes with the sarcolemma and smooth muscle.

Differentials

Differential diagnosis to be considered:

- Arthritis and/or arthralgias
- Rheumatoid arthritis
- Reactive arthritis
- Dermatomyositis
- Erythema nodosum
- Henoch-Schönlein purpura
- Lupus erythematosus in infants and children
- Poststreptococcal syndrome
- Huntington chorea
- Chorea gravidum
- Periarteritis nodosa
- Erythema marginatum
- Subcutaneous nodules.

Controversy exists as to whether the entity of poststreptococcal reactive arthritis (PSRA) is along the clinical continuum of RF or is a separate clinical entity. PSRA is characterized by objective arthritis in the setting of a vigorous immune response to streptococcal antigens; however, the arthritis is nonmigratory and poorly responsive to aspirin. Children with PSRA do not fulfill modified Jones criteria. Most pediatric rheumatologists treat PSRA with the same antibiotic prophylaxis provided to individuals with RF.

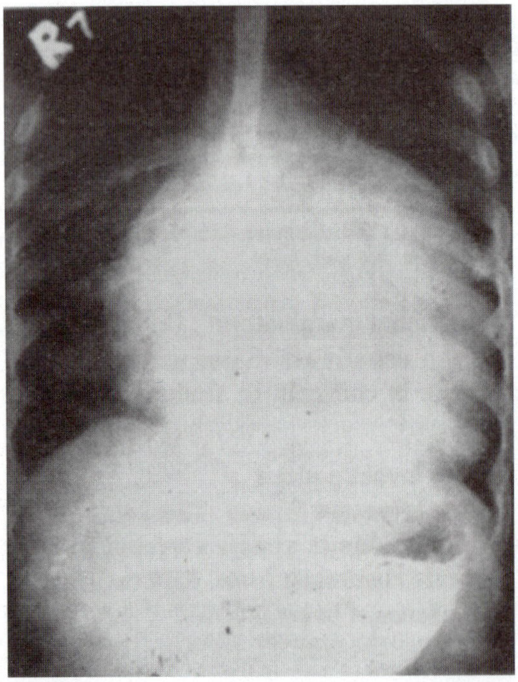

Fig. 15.7: *Photograph of X-ray chest PA view showing diffuse cardiomegaly in patient with acute carditis and CHF as a result of acute RF*

Drug reaction (e.g. oral contraceptive pills, phenytoin, haloperidol, amitriptyline, metoclopramide, fluphenazine) on 5.

Lab Studies

Throat Culture

Throat cultures for GABHS infections usually are negative by the time symptoms of RF or RHD appear.

Make attempts to isolate the organism prior to the initiation of antibiotic therapy to help confirm a diagnosis of streptococcal pharyngitis and to allow typing of the organism if it is isolated successfully.

Rapid Antigen Detection Test

This test allows rapid detection of GAS antigen, allowing the diagnosis of streptococcal pharyngitis to be made and antibiotic therapy to be initiated while the patient is still in the physician's office.

- This test reportedly has a specificity of greater than 95% but a sensitivity of only 60–90%. Thus, obtain a throat culture in conjunction with the rapid antigen detection test.
- Antistreptococcal antibodies.

Clinical features of RF begin when antistreptococcal antibody levels are at their peak. Thus, these tests are useful for confirming previous GAS infection. Antistreptococcal antibodies are particularly useful in patients who present with chorea as the only diagnostic criterion. Sensitivity for recent infections can be improved by testing for several antibodies. Check antibody titers 2 weeks apart to detect a rising titer. The most common extracellular antistreptococcal antibodies tested include antistreptolysin O (ASO) and anti-DNase B, antihyaluronidase, antistreptokinase, antistreptococcal esterase, and antinicotinamide adenine dinucleotide (anti-NAD). Antibody tests for cellular components of GAS antigens include antistreptococcal polysaccharide, antiteichoic acid antibody, and anti-M protein antibody.

In general, the antibodies to extracellular streptococcal antigens rise during the first month after infection and then plateau for 3–6 months before returning to normal levels after 6–12 months. When the ASO titer peaks (2–3 weeks after onset of RF), the sensitivity of this test is 80–85%.

The anti-DNase B has a slightly higher sensitivity (90%) for revealing RF or acute glomerulonephritis. Antihyaluronidase frequently is abnormal in patients with RF with a normal ASO titer, may rise earlier, and persists longer than elevated ASO titers during incidents of RF.

Acute-phase reactants: C-reactive protein and erythrocyte sedimentation rate are elevated in individuals with RF due to the inflammatory nature of the disease. Both tests have high sensitivity but low specificity for RF.Heart reactive antibodies: tropomyosin is elevated in persons with acute RF. Rapid detection test for D8/17: This immunofluorescence technique for identifying the B-cell marker

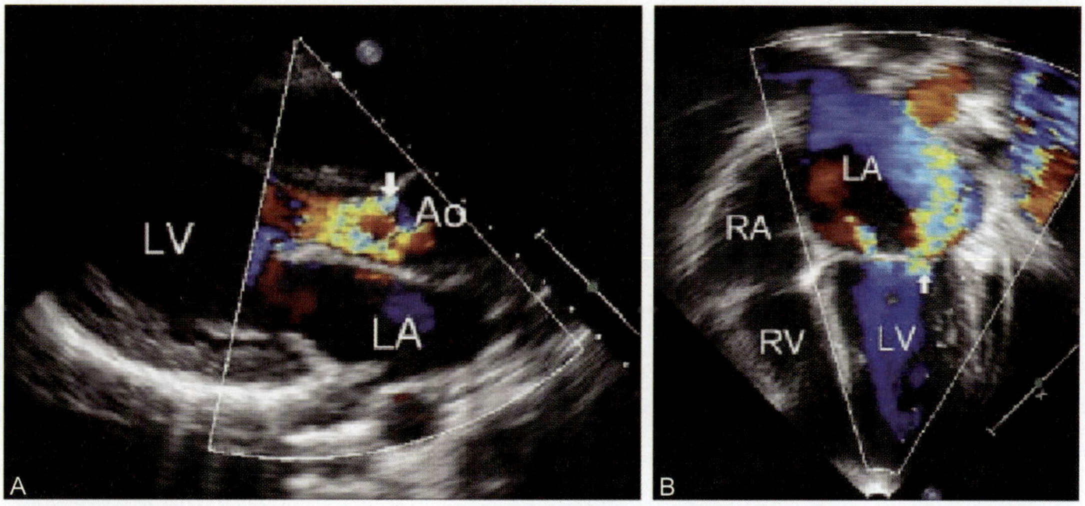

Fig. 15.8: *Two dimensional color and spectral Doppler echocardiographic studies of patients with rheumatic heart disease show moderate to severe aortic valve insufficiency with no stenosis (A, arrow) and bowing of the anterior mitral leaflet with severe insufficiency and no stenosis (B, arrow)*

D8/17 is positive in 90% of patients with RF, and it may be useful for identifying patients who are at risk of developing RF.

Imaging Studies

Chest Radiography (Fig. 15.7)

Cardiomegaly, pulmonary congestion, and other findings consistent with heart failure may be observed on chest radiograph in individuals with RF. When the patient has fever and respiratory distress, the chest radiograph helps differentiate between CHF and rheumatic pneumonia.

Echocardiography (Fig. 15.8)

In individuals with acute RHD, echocardiography identifies and quantitates valve insufficiency and ventricular dysfunction. In persons with mild carditis, Doppler evidence of mitral regurgitation may be present during the acute phase of disease but resolves in weeks to months.

In contrast, patients with moderate-to-severe carditis have persistent mitral and/or aortic regurgitation. The most important echocardiographic features of mitral regurgitation from acute rheumatic valvulitis are annular dilatation, elongation of the chordae to the anterior leaflet, and a posterolaterally directed mitral regurgitation jet.

During acute RF, the left ventricle frequently is dilated in association with a normal or increased fractional shortening. Thus, some cardiologists believe that valve insufficiency (e.g. from endocarditis), rather than myocardial dysfunction (e.g. from myocarditis), is the dominant cause of heart failure in individuals with acute RF. In individuals with chronic RHD, echocardiography tracks the progression of valve stenosis and may help to determine the time for surgical intervention. The leaflets of affected valves become thickened diffusely, with fusion of the commissures and chordae tendineae. Increased echodensity of the mitral valve may signify calcification.

Other Tests

Electrocardiography (Figs 15.9 and 15.10)

Sinus tachycardia most frequently accompanies acute RHD. Alternatively, some children develop sinus bradycardia from increased vagal tone. No correlation exists between bradycardia and severity of carditis.

First-degree atrioventricular (AV) block (prolongation of PR interval) is observed in some patients with RHD. This abnormality may be related to localized myocardial inflammation involving the AV node or to vasculitis involving the AV nodal artery. First-degree AV block is a nonspecific finding and should not be used as a criterion for the diagnosis of RHD. Its presence does not correlate with the development of chronic RHD.

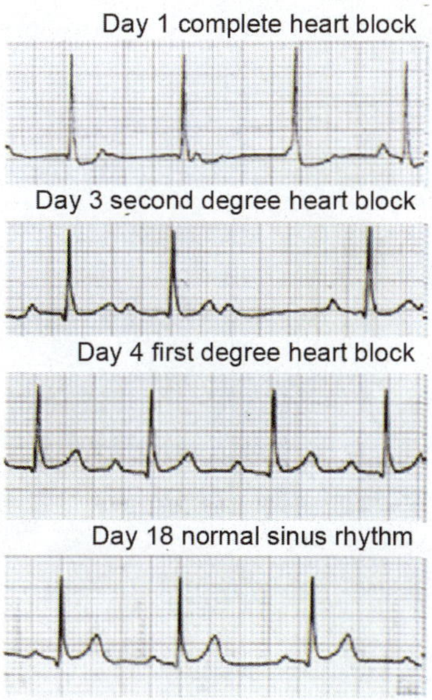

Fig. 15.9: *Serial ECG changes in acute rheumatic fever with carditis*

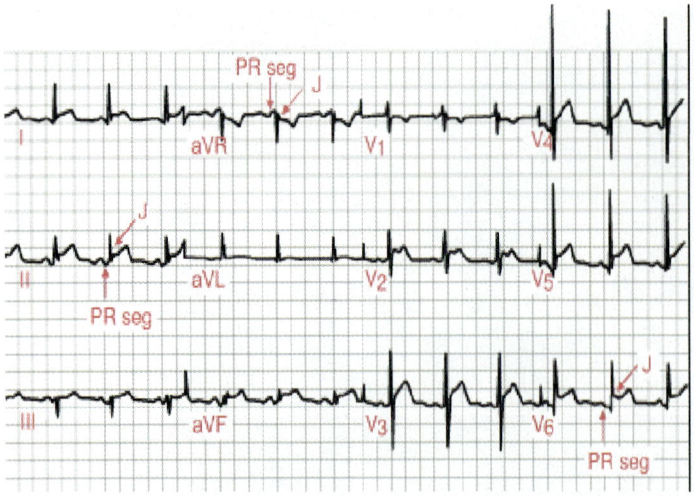

Fig. 15.10: *Acute pericarditis in acute rheumatic fever Stage 1 J points, except aVR and V1, are elevated. T waves are essentially normal. PR segments, except aVR and V1, are depressed. PR deviations are commonly absent in one limb lead (here, aVL).*

Second-degree (i.e. intermittent) and third-degree (i.e. complete) AV block with progression to ventricular standstill have been described. However, heart block in the setting of RF typically resolves with the rest of the disease process. In individuals with acute pericarditis, ST segment elevation may be present, most marked inleads II, III, aVF, and V4 through V6. Finally, patients with RHD may develop atrial flutter, multifocal atrial tachycardia, or atrial fibrillation from chronic mitral valve disease and atrial dilation.

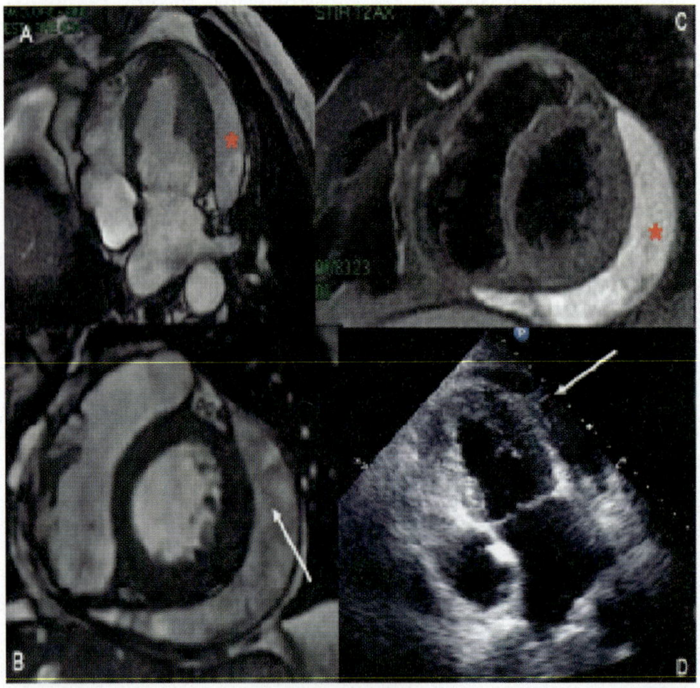

Fig. 15.11: *MRI imaging in various views showing loculated pericardial effusion in acute rheumatic carditis*

Procedures

Cardiac catheterization: This study is not indicated in acute RF due to availability of noninvasive methods.

Histologic findings: Pathologic examination of the insufficient valves may demonstrate verrucous lesions at the line of closure. Aschoff bodies (perivascular foci of eosinophilic collagen surrounded by lymphocytes, plasma cells, and macrophages) are found in the pericardium, perivascular regions of the myocardium and endocardium. The Aschoff bodies assume a granulomatous appearance with a central fibrinoid focus. Sand eventually are replaced by nodules of scar tissue. Anitschkow cells are plump macrophages within Aschoff bodies. In the pericardium, fibrinous and serofibrinous exudates may produce an appearance of "bread and butter" pericarditis.

Medical Management

Direct medical therapy toward eliminating the GAS pharyngitis (if still present), suppressing inflammation from the autoimmune response, and providing supportive treatment of CHF. A recent metaanalysis has supported a protective effect against rheumatic fever when penicillin is used following the diagnosis of GAS pharyngitis. Oral penicillin V remains the drug of choice for treatment of GAS pharyngitis. When oral penicillin is not feasible or dependable, a single dose of intramuscular benzathine penicillin G is therapeutic. For patients who are allergic to penicillin, administer erythromycin or a first-generation cephalosporin. Other options include clarithromycin for 10 days, azithromycin for 5 days, or a narrow-spectrum (first-generation) cephalosporin for 10 days. As many as 15% of penicillin-allergic patients are also allergic to cephalosporins. Do not use tetracyclines and sulfonamides to treat GAS pharyngitis.

Table 15.1: *Treatment of acute rheumatic fever*

Treatment and prophylaxis of group A, hemolytic, streptococcal infection:
Benzathine penicillin, 1.2 millions units intramuscularly every month
Suppression therapy
With no heart involvement:
Aspirin 100 mg/kg/day in four divides doses
Reduce dose if salicylate level exceeds 25 mg/100 mL
Reduce dose if symptoms of salicylism (tinnitus)
Reduce dose by 25% after 1 week if good clinical response and continue for 6–8 weeks, tapering the dose in the last 2 weeks.
With valvar involvement:
Prednisone, 2.0 mg/kg/day for 2 weeks, then taper for 2 weeks.
With good response being aspirin 75 mg/kg/day in the 3rd week and continue until the 8th week, tapering in the final 2 weeks.
Increase supppressive dose if symptoms return or sedimentation rate rises.

For recurrent GAS pharyngitis, a second 10-day course of the same antibiotic may be repeated. Alternate drugs include narrow-spectrum cephalosporins, amoxicillin-clavulanate, dicloxacillin, erythromycin, or other macrolides.

GAS carriage is difficult to eradicate with conventional penicillin therapy. Thus, oral clindamycin (20 mg/kg/d PO in three divided doses for 10 days) is recommended.

In general, antimicrobial therapy is not indicated for pharyngeal carriers of GAS. Exceptions include the following:

1. Outbreaks of RF or poststreptococcal glomerulonephritis
2. Family history of RF
3. During outbreaks of GAS pharyngitis in a closed community
4. When tonsillectomy is considered for chronic GAS carriage
5. When multiple episodes of documented GAS pharyngitis occur within a family despite appropriate therapy
6. Following GAS toxic shock syndrome or necrotizing fasciitis in a household contact.

Treatment of the acute inflammatory manifestations of acute RF consists of salicylates and steroids. Aspirin in anti-inflammatory doses effectively reduces all manifestations of the disease except chorea, and the response typically is dramatic. If rapid improvement is not observed after 24–36 hours of therapy, question the diagnosis of RF.

Attempt to obtain aspirin blood levels from 20–25 mg/dL, but stable levels may be difficult to achieve during the inflammatory phase because of variable GI absorption of the drug. Maintain aspirin at anti-inflammatory doses until the signs and symptoms of acute RF are resolved or resolving (6–8 weeks) and the acute phase reactants (APRs) have returned to normal.

Anti-inflammatory doses of aspirin may be associated with abnormal liver function tests and GI toxicity, and adjusting the aspirin dosage may be necessary.

When discontinuing therapy, withdraw aspirin gradually over weeks while monitoring the APRs for evidence of rebound. Chorea most frequently is self-limited but may be alleviated or partially controlled with phenobarbital or diazepam.

If moderate-to-severe carditis is present as indicated by cardiomegaly, CHF, or third-degree heart block, add oral prednisone to salicylate therapy.

Continue prednisone for 2–6 weeks depending on the severity of the carditis, and taper prednisone during the last week of therapy.

Discontinuing prednisone therapy after 2–4 weeks, while maintaining salicylates for an additional 2–4 weeks, can minimize adverse effects; include digoxin and diuretics, afterload reduction, supplemental oxygen, bed rest, and sodium and fluid restriction as additional treatment for patients with acute RF and CHF. The diuretics most commonly used in conjunction with digoxin for children with CHF include furosemide and spironolactone.

Initiate digoxin only after checking electrolytes and correcting abnormalities in serum potassium.

The total loading dose is 20–30 mcg/kg PO qd, with 50% of the dose administered initially, followed by 25% of the dose 8 and 16 hours after the initial dose. Maintenance doses typically are 8–10 mcg/kg/day PO in two divided doses. For older children and adults, the total loading dose is 1.25–1.5 mg PO, and the maintenance dose is 0.25–0.5 mg PO qd. Therapeutic digoxin levels are present at trough levels of 1.5–2 ng/mL.

Afterload reduction (using ACE inhibitor captopril) may be effective in improving cardiac output, particularly in the presence of mitral and aortic insufficiency. Start these agents judiciously. Use a small, initial test dose (some patients have an abnormally large response to these agents), and administer only after correcting hypovolemia.

When heart failure persists or worsens during the acute phase after aggressive medical therapy, surgery is indicated to decrease valve insufficiency.

Preventive and prophylactic therapy is indicated after RF and RHD to prevent further damage to valves. Primary prophylaxis (initial course of antibiotics administered to eradicate the streptococcal infection) also serves as the first course of secondary prophylaxis (prevention of recurrent RF and RHD).

An injection of 0.6–1.2 million units of benzathine penicillin G intramuscularly every 4 weeks is the recommended regimen for secondary prophylaxis. Administer the same dosage every 3 weeks in areas where RF is endemic, in patients with residual carditis, and in high-risk patients.

Although oral penicillin prophylaxis is also effective, data from the World Health Organization indicate that the recurrence risk of GAS pharyngitis is lower when penicillin is administered parentally.

Table 15.2: *Recommended prophylaxis against recurrent group A streptococcal Infection*

Regime	Drug	Dose
Standard	Penicillin G benzathine	1.2 milion units IM q 3–4 wk* ≤ 27 kg: 600,000 units IM q 3–4 wk*
Alternatives (e.g. for patients unwilling to receive injections)	Sulfadiazine some	≤ 27 kg 500 mg PO once/day
For patients all ergic to penicillin and sulfadiazine some trade names No US trade name	Erythromycin some	250 mg PO bid

* In developing countries, IM prophylaxis q 3 wk.

The duration of antibiotic prophylaxis is controversial. Continue antibiotic prophylaxis indefinitely for patients at high risk (e.g. health care workers, teachers, daycare workers) for recurrent GAS infection. Ideally, continue prophylaxis indefinitely, because recurrent GAS infection and RF can occur at any age; however, the American Heart Association currently recommends that patients with RF without carditis receive prophylactic antibiotics for 5 years or until aged 21 years, whichever is longer. Patients with RF with carditis but no valve disease should receive prophylactic antibiotics for 10 years or well into adulthood, whichever is longer. Finally, patients with RF with carditis and valve disease should receive antibiotics at least 10 years or until aged 40 years.

Patients with RHD and valve damage require a single dose of antibiotics 1 hour before surgical and dental procedures to help prevent bacterial endocarditis. Patients who had RF without valve damage do not need endocarditis prophylaxis. Do not use penicillin, ampicillin, or amoxicillin for endocarditis prophylaxis in patients already receiving penicillin for secondary RF prophylaxis (relative resistance of oral streptococci to penicillin and aminopenicillins). Alternate drugs recommended by the American Heart Association for these patients include oral clindamycin (children: 20 mg/kg; adults: 600 mg) and oral azithromycin or clarithromycin (children: 15 mg/kg; adults: 500 mg). Additional guidelines for endocarditis prophylaxis in patients who are allergic to penicillin or who are unable to receive oral antibiotics.

Control measures for patients with GAS pharyngitis are as follows: hospitalized patients: place hospitalized patients with GAS pharyngitis or pneumonia on droplet precautions, as well as standard precautions, until 24 hours after initiation of appropriate antibiotics.

Exposed persons: People in contact with patients having documented cases of streptococcal infection first should undergo appropriate laboratory testing if they have clinical evidence of GAS infection and should undergo antibiotic therapy if infected.

School and childcare centers: Children with GAS infection should not attend school or childcare centers for the first 24 hours after initiating antimicrobial therapy.

Surgical Management

When heart failure persists or worsens after aggressive medical therapy for acute RHD, surgery to decrease valve insufficiency may be lifesaving. Approximately 40% of patients with acute RF subsequently develop mitral stenosis as adults. Mitral valvulotomy, percutaneous balloon valvuloplasty, or mitral valve replacement may be indicated in patients with critical stenosis. Valve replacement appears to be the preferred surgical option for patients with high rates of recurrent symptoms after annuloplasty or other repair procedures.

Indications for Mitral Valvotomy in Children

1. Dyspnoea Gr. II or more
2. Hemoptysis, more than one severe attack
3. Pulmonary edema, and acute hemoptysis
4. Systemic emboli
5. Physical signs of severe MS. 2-OS interval of less than 0.07–0.08 seconds and a long full length diastolic murmur on phonocardiography.
6. Signs of pulmonary hypertension.
7. EKG: RAD greater than 110 prominent R VI and S in V6′
8. Radiologic evidence of severe pulmonary venous or arterial hypertension or RV enlargement.
9. EF slope less than 15 mm/sec on echocardiography.
10. MV diameter less than 1.0 CM2 on 2-D Echo and Doppler pressure I/2 time, calculations.
11. Cardiac cath; PCWP greater than 20 mmHg. and gradient across MV greater than 10 mmHg or MV area less than 1.0 cm^2.
12. Onset of atrial fibrillation.

Diet

Advise nutritious diet without restrictions except in patients with CHF, who should follow a fluid-restricted and sodium-restricted diet. Potassium supplementation may be necessary because of the mineralocorticoid effect of corticosteroid and the diuretics, if used.

Activity

Initially, place patients on bed rest, followed by a period of indoor activity before they are permitted to return to school. Do not allow full activity until the APRs have returned to normal. Patients with chorea may require a wheelchair and should be on homebound instruction until the abnormal movement.

Treatment and Prevention of GAS Pharyngitis

Treatment and prevention of GAS pharyngitis outlined here are based on the current recommendations of the Committee on Infectious Disease (American Academy of Pediatrics). Medical therapy is directed toward elimination of GAS pharyngitis (if still present), suppression of inflammation from the autoimmune response, and supportive treatment of CHF. Attempts are being made to produce vaccines against GAS infection. Antibiotics for endocarditis prophylaxis are administered to patients with certain cardiac conditions, such as carditis caused by rheumatic fever, before procedures that may cause bacteremia.

Further Outpatient Care

Patients usually demonstrate significant improvement after initiation of anti-inflammatory therapy; however, do not allow patients to resume full activities until all clinical symptoms and laboratory values have returned to normal. Emphasize the importance of prophylaxis against recurrent streptococcal pharyngitis and RF. Each recurrent episode of rheumatic carditis produces further valve damage and the likelihood of valve replacement. Patients should remain on antibiotic prophylaxis at least until the early third decade of life. Many physicians believe lifelong prophylaxis is appropriate.

Monitor patients routinely for the signs and symptoms of mitral stenosis, pulmonary hypertension, arrhythmia, and CHF.

Complications

Potential complications include:

- CHF from valve insufficiency (acute RF) or stenosis (chronic RF).
- Associated cardiac complications include atrial arrhythmias, pulmonary edema, recurrent pulmonary emboli, infective endocarditis, thrombus formationand systemic emboli.

Prognosis

The manifestations of acute RF resolve during a period of 12 weeks in 80% of patients and may extend as long as 15 weeks in the remaining 20% of patients.

RF was the leading cause of death in patients aged 5–20 years in the US 100 years ago. At that time, the mortality rate was 8–30% from carditis and valvulitis but decreased to a 1-year mortality rate of 4% by the 1930s. Following the development of antibiotics, the mortality rate decreased to nearly 0% by the 1960s in the US. However, the mortality rate has remained 1–10% in developing countries. The development of penicillin also has affected the likelihood of developing chronic valvular disease after an episode of acute RF. Prior to penicillin, 60–70% of patients developed valve disease; since the introduction of penicillin, 9–39% of patients develop valve disease.

In patients who developed murmurs from valve insufficiency from acute RF, numerous factors (e.g. severity of initial carditis, presence or absence of recurrences, amount of time since episode of RF) affected the likelihood that valve abnormalities and the murmur would disappear. The type of treatment and the promptness of its initiation did not affect the likelihood that the murmur would disappear. In general, incidence of residual RHD at 10 years was 34% in patients without recurrences but was 60% in patients with recurrent RF. In patients in whom the murmur disappeared, it did so within 5 years in 50%. Thus, a significant number of patients experience resolution of valve abnormalities even 5–10 years after their episode of RF.

The importance of preventing recurrences of RF is evident.

Patient Education

- Emphasize measures that minimize further damage to the valves of the heart.
- Timely evaluation and treatment of pharyngitis in children help prevent RF.
- Secondary prophylaxis of patients with previous RF and valve involvement with penicillin injections every 3–4 weeks decrease the recurrence of RHD.
- Additional prophylactic antibiotics prior to dental and surgical procedures decrease the likelihood of bacterial endocarditis.

BIBLIOGRAPHY

1. Abernethy M, Bass N, Sharpe N, et al: Doppler echocardiography and the early diagnosis of carditis in acute rheumatic fever. Aust N Z J Med 1994 Oct; 24(5): 530–5.
2. Asbahr FR, Garvey MA, Snider LA, et al: Obsessive-compulsive symptoms among patients with Sydenham chorea. Biol Psychiatry 2005 May 1; 57(9): 1073-6.
3. Carapetis JR, McDonald M, Wilson NJ: Acute rheumatic fever. Lancet 2005 Jul 9–15; 366 (9480): 155–68.
4. The natural history of rheumatic fever and rheumatic heart disease. Ten-year report of a cooperative clinical trial of ACTH, cortisone, and aspirin. Circulation 1965 Sep; 32(3): 457–76.
5. Cotran RS, Kumar V, Collins T: Rheumatic fever. In: Robbins Pathologic Basis of Disease. 6th ed. WB Saunders Co; 1999: 570–73.
6. Dajani A, Taubert K, Ferrieri P, et al: Treatment of acute streptococcal pharyngitis and prevention of rheumatic fever: a statement for health professionals. Committee on Rheumatic Fever, Endocarditis, and Kawasaki Disease of the Council on Cardiovascular Disease in the Young, the American. Pediatrics 1995 Oct; 96(4 Pt 1): 758–64.
7. Dajani AS, Taubert KA, Wilson W, et al: Prevention of bacterial endocarditis. Recommendations by the American Heart Association. Circulation 1997 Jul 1; 96(1): 358–66.
8. Ellis NM, Li Y, Hildebrand W, et al: T cell mimicry and epitope specificity of cross-reactive T cell clones from rheumatic heart disease. J Immunol 2005 Oct 15; 175(8): 5448–56.
9. Fae KC, Oshiro SE, Toubert A, et al: How an autoimmune reaction triggered by molecular mimicry between streptococcal M protein and cardiac tissue proteins leads to heart lesions in rheumatic heart disease. J Autoimmun 2005 Mar; 24(2): 101–9.
10. Guidelines for the diagnosis of rheumatic fever: Jones Criteria, 1992 update. Special Writing Group of the Committee on Rheumatic Fever, Endocarditis, and Kawasaki Disease of the Council on Cardiovascular Disease in the Young of the American Heart Asso. JAMA 1992 Oct 21; 268 (15): 2069–73.
11. Guilherme L, Fae K, Oshiro SE, Kalil J: Molecular pathogenesis of rheumatic fever and rheumatic heart disease. Expert Rev Mol Med 2005 Dec 8; 7(28): 1–15.
12. Karademir S, OGuz D, Senocak F, et al: Tolmetin and salicylate therapy in acute rheumatic fever: Comparison of clinical efficacy and side-effects. Pediatr Int 2003 Dec; 45(6): 676–9.
13. Massell BF, Fyler DC, Roy SB: The clinical picture ofrheumatic fever. Diagnosis, immediate prognosis, course and therapeutic implications. Am J Cardiol 1958; 1: 436–39.
14. Narula J, Virmani R, Reddy KS: Rheumatic Fever. American Registry of Pathology. Washington, DC: 1999.
15. Pickering LK: Rheumatic Fever. 2000 Red Book: Report of the Committee on Infectious Diseases. 25th ed. Elk Grove Village, Ill: American Academy of Pediatrics; 2000.
16. Robertson KA, Volmink JA, Mayosi BM: Antibiotics for the primary prevention of acute rheumatic fever: a meta-analysis. BMC Cardiovasc Disord 2005 May 31; 5(1): 11.
17. Swedo SE, Leonard HL, Garvey M, et al: A case of pediatric autoimmune neuropsychiatric disorders associated with

streptococcal infections. Am J Psychiatry 1998 Nov; 155(11): 1592–8.
18. Veasy LG, Wiedmeier SE, Orsmond GS, et al: Resurgence of acute rheumatic fever in the intermountain area of the United States. N Engl J Med 1987 Feb 19; 316(8): 421–7.
19. Walker KG, Lawrenson J, Wilmshurst JM: Neuropsychiatric movement disorders following streptococcalinfection. Dev Med Child Neurol 2005 Nov; 47(11): 771–5.
20. Bisno AL. Group A streptococcal infections and acute rheumatic fever. N Engl J Med 1991;325:783–793.
21. Dajani AS, Ayoub E, Bierman FZ, et a!. Guidelines for the diagnosis of rheumatic fever: Jones criteria. Updated 1993. Circulation 1993;87:302–307.
22. Ferrieri P. Proceedings of the Jones Criteria Workshop. Circulation 2002;106:2521–2523.
23. American Heart Association. Treatment of acute streptococcal pharyngitis and prevention of rheumatic fever. Pediatrics 1995;96:758–764.
24. da Silva NA, de Faria Pereira BA. Acute rheumatic fever. Pediatr Rheumatol 1997;23: 45–568.
25. Stollerman GH. Rheumatic fever. Lancet 1997;349:935–942.
26. Stollerman GH. Rheumatic fever in the 21st century. Clin Infect Dis 2001;33: 806–814.
27. Dajani AS. Rheumatic fever. In: Braunwald. E, ed. Heart disease: a textbook of car-diovascular medicine, 5th ed. Philadelphia: WB Saunders, 1997:1769–1775.

16 Recognition and Management of Valvular Heart Disease

Chronic rheumatic valvular dysfunctions can lead to very high morbidity and mortality among patients unless they are helped with either reconstructive surgery or replacement of an artificial valve. Two types of artificial valves which are available today have their own limitations and till date there is no ideal valve which could closely resemble with natural valve in terms of cost and postoperative long-term out come. Recently, attempts have been made in constructing artificial heart valves with the help of stem cell modification and genetic engineering techniques though long-term follow-up is still awaited (Fig. 16.1).

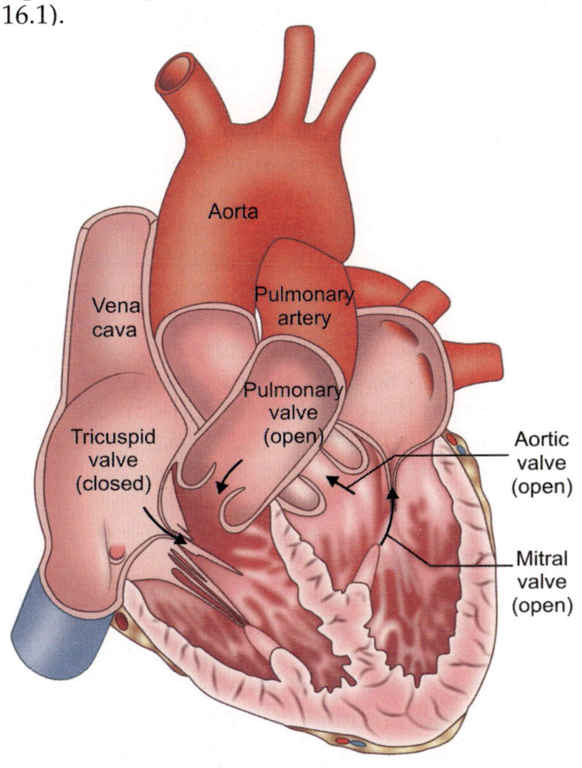

Fig. 16.1: *Anatomical placement of four native valves in human body*

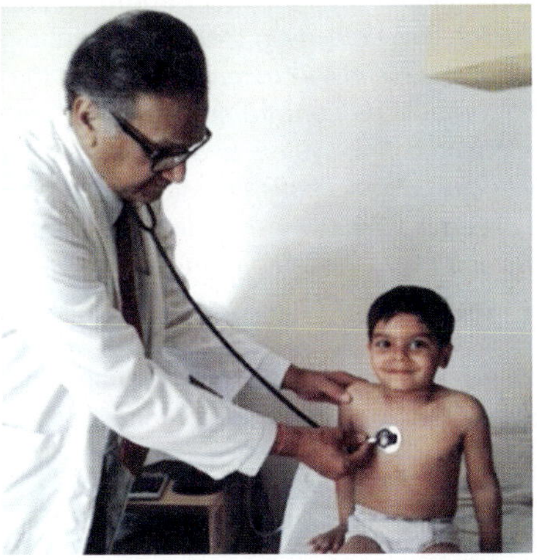

Fig. 16.2: *Cardiologist is examining a young child with valvular heart defect*

Synthetic valve do give rise to bleeding disorders due to anticoagulants and predispose to thromboembolic phenomenon and infection leading to vital organ dysfunctions.

Although tissue valves do not need anticoagulants but still it could be the seat of infections and are often rejected in mismatched cases. Undoubtedly, tissue valve is preferable in pregnant women and younger children where anticoagulants may pose life-threatening complications. The life-span of this valve, is shorter than the synthetic valve due to its rapid degeneration.

In developing countries, rheumatic process is so extensive that often more, than one valves (multivalvular) are affected which further complicates the final management of the patients besides the cost implications among poor patients.

Sincere efforts are still continued to manufacture such a valve which could satisfy all the properties of an ideal

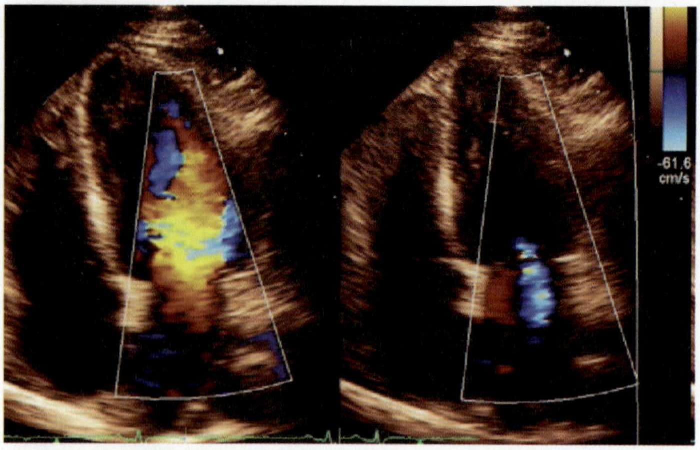

Fig. 16.3: *Colour Doppler of mitral flow on echocardiography with colour flow mapping (CFM) from the apical four chamber view. The left frame is in diastole when the mitral valve is open and there is a forward flow from the left atrium into the left ventricle. The flow is predominantly reddish, though there is an area of variance in the middle with yellowish and greenish colour. This indicates that the flow velocity in that region is above the Nyquist limit, which in this case is 61 cm/s as seen from the colour bar at the top right corner. The right frame shows the mitral valve in a closed position indicating systole and there is a small regurgitant jet of high velocity which is bluish mosaic coloured. Bluish colour indicates a reverse flow away from the transducer. The flow is from the left ventricle to the left atrium. The jet area is quite small compared to that of the left atrium, indicating that the volume of regurgitation is low. There is no significant dilatation of the left atrium or the left ventricle as the regurgitation is not sufficient to produce volume overloading of the left-sided chambers*

valve and come within the reach of low socio-economic strata of people where a large segment of population is affected every year particularly in developing countries of South-East Asia.Valvular heart disease is an important cause of cardiac morbidity in developed countries despite a decline in the prevalence of rheumatic disease in those countries. Valvular heart disease can give rise to stenosis, regurgitation or a combination of lesions at one or more valves. The more common significant anomalies currently encountered are mitral regurgitation, caused by mitral valve prolapse; aortic stenosis, caused by a congenital bicuspid valve or by senile valvular calcification; and aortic regurgitation, caused by a bicuspid aortic valve or dilatation of the aorta. Valvular lesions can occur as a result of pathologic changes in the valve leaflets or supporting structures (i.e. the chordae or papillary muscles). Ventricular or aortic enlargement can also produce valvular regurgitation as a result of annular dilatation and inadequate leaflet coaptation in the absence of any specific valve pathology. Valvular heart disease tends to progress over time as degenerative changes are superimposed on the primary pathology. Iatrogenic causes of valvular disease are increasingly recognized (Fig. 16.3).

Etiology

Congenital disorders: Anomalies in the development of valve cusps are common at the aortic or pulmonary positions. The normal configuration of these valves is tricuspid. Stenosis is the rule when only one cusp develops, whereas bicuspid valves may be stenotic or regurgitant Congenital anomalies of the atrioventricular valves are uncommon; the most common abnormality is congenital cleft mitral valve. Valvular abnormalities can be seen in specific developmental syndromes, such as pulmonary stenosis in rubella syndrome and supravalvular aortic stenosis in Williams syndrome.

Myxomatous Degeneration

Myxomatous degeneration most often involves the mitral or tricuspid valve. In this condition, leaflet tissue, particularly chordal tissue, is abnormally extensible and weak. The affected valves are therefore more likely to prolapse, leading to significant regurgitation. Chordal rupture is common and may precipitate a rapid clinical deterioration from sudden severe regurgitation. The precise abnormality in valvular tissue is unknown but is thought to involve the structural proteins, such as collagen A familial tendency is often noted in this disease. Inherited connective tissue diseases such as Marfan syndrome produce valvular abnormalities similar to those found in myxomatous degeneration.

Rheumatic Heart Disease

Rheumatic heart disease remains the most common cause of mitral stenosis and a frequent cause of aortic regurgitation. It is the most common cause of multivalvular heart disease. Isolated outbreaks of rheumatic fever continue to be reported in the United States, even in affluent communities rheumatic heart disease remains a significant problem in immigrants, especially those from Latin America and Southeast Asia. Rheumatic fever appears to cause valvular heart disease by an autoimmune phenomenon whereby antibodies against streptococcal antigens cross-react with valvular tissue. Valvular involvement can present acutely as a result of edema of valvular tissue. Progressive fibrosis, superimposed calcification, and scarring with retraction of leaflet tissue lead to valvular stenosis, incompetence, or both. The interval between the occurrence of rheumatic fever and clinical manifestations varies, as does the degree of involvement. Both mitral and aortic valves are usually involved.

Degenerative Disease

Degenerative calcificationcan occure in aortic stenosis among the elderly and in patients with renal dysfunction; it results from calcium deposition on the body of the valvular leaflets rather than on the commissures. Factors found to promote degenerative valvular changes are increasing age, a low body mass index, hypertension, and hyperlipidemia. Histologic changes that simulate atheroma and involve lipid deposition and inflammatory cell infiltration of the leaflets have been described in patients with early degenerative changes in the aortic leaflets. Even mild degenerative changes in the aortic valve have been reported to be adverse prognostic factors.

Calcification of the mitral annulus is common in the elderly; it is more common in women than in men and can produce mitral regurgitation. Occasionally, mitral annular calcification extends onto the valvular leaflets, causing stenosis.

Endocarditis

Endocarditis usually occurs on previously abnormal valves, although overwhelming sepsis can infect normal valves. The predominant hemodynamic manifestation of endocarditis is valvular regurgitation. Contributory causes of endocarditis include leaflet prolapse (resulting from a large vegetation), leaflet perforation, and chronic scarring of infected tissue. In rare cases, large vegetations lead to valvular stenosis.

Coronary Artery Disease

Mitral regurgitation is common in coronary artery disease; it has a number of causal mechanisms. Acute ischemia or infarction of a papillary muscle or of the wall to which the papillary muscle is attached leads to impaired leaflet coaptation and mitral regurgitation. Regurgitation can be severe and can vary with the severity of the ischemia. Papillary head rupture or, more rarely, muscle rupture, leads to catastrophic regurgitation that is often fatal.

Connective Tissue Disease

Libman-Sacks endocarditis consists of noninfected warty vegetations involving predominantly the mitral valve; it is characteristic of systemic lupus erythematosus (SLE) Significant regurgitation and stenosis rarely occur acutely but are seen with scarring from chronic disease. Valvular involvement in rheumatoid arthritis is common and leads to valvular thickening but is usually not of hemodynamic significance. Aortitis in ankylosing spondylitis may produce significant aortic regurgitation.

Iatrogenic Causes of Valvular Heart Disease

Iatrogenic causes include radiation therapy, the use of serotonin agonists such as methysergide, and the use of anorexiants such as fenfluramine and phentermine in combination. Radiation leads to scarring and calcification of valvular leaflets many years after the initiating radiation. The effects of both methysergide and anorexiant agents on valvular tissue often simulate rheumatic disease, but regurgitation rather than stenosis predominates as the hemodynamically severe lesion. Serotonin is also thought to play a role in the valvulopathy produced by anorexiants; the precise mechanism by which this occurs remains to be established.

Other Causes of Valvular Heart Disease

Amyloid disease causes valvular thickening but rarely causes significant stenosis. The carcinoid syndrome most often involves the valves on the right side of the heart and leads to stenosis or incompetence of the tricuspid or pulmonary valve.

Secondary Involvement

Left ventricular dilatation can cause dilatation of the mitral annulus and, thereby, mitral regurgitation. Common secondary causes of mitral regurgitation include coronary artery disease, aortic valvular disease, and dilated cardiomyopathy. Similarly, tricuspid regurgitation results from right ventricular enlargement secondary to pulmonary hypertension or an atrial septal defect. Dilatation of the ascending aorta, especially involving the annulus of the aortic valve, can lead to aortic regurgitation. This conditionis seen in hypertension and in aneurysms of the ascending aorta.

Assessment and Management

Valvular heart disease often remains asymptomatic for many years, but once symptoms develop, survival is reduced if the lesion is not corrected. The evaluation of symptoms can require a stress test or stress echocardiogram in addition to a careful history. Characterization of the lesions and assessment of hemodynamic severity are often possible on physical examination but are aided by additional testing, such as Doppler echocardiography and cardiac catheterization. Doppler echocardiography measures the flow velocity across a narrowed valve. By use of the modified Bernoulli equation, the pressure gradient (P), measured in mmHg, may be estimated from the flow velocity (v), which is measured in m/sec: P = 4v2. Therefore, if the peak velocity recorded across the aortic valve by Doppler echocardiography is 4 m/sec, then the peak pressure gradient will be estimated as $4(4^2)$ or 64 mmHg. The effects of valvular heart disease on chamber size and function are best assessed serially by echocardiography or, at the time of cardiac catheterization, by ventriculography. In cases of stenotic lesions, intervention is rarely required until symptoms occur. Indications for intervention in regurgitant lesions are more complex; such indications include significant symptoms or, in the absence of symptoms, increasing ventricular size, overt ventricular contractile dysfunction, or both.

All patients with even mild valvular heart disease require prophylaxis against endocarditis at the time of dental procedures or other procedures that can produce significant bacteremia. The prophylactic regimens recommended by the American Heart Association have been revised.

Despite the increase in intravascular volume, pregnancy is usually well tolerated in previously asymptomatic patients with valvular heart disease.

Patients with hemodynamically significant valvular heart disease should generally avoid participation in competitive sports. Reference should be made to the recommendations of the American College of Cardiology for more information about specific lesions. Valvular heart disease is a chronic disease requiring periodic examination and follow-up, even in asymptomatic patients and in those who have had corrective surgical or other procedures. Patients with prosthetic valves should be seen at least yearly.

SPECIFIC VALVULAR LESIONS

MITRAL STENOSIS

Clinical Manifestations

A. *Symptoms*

1. ***Dyspnea*** on exertion is usually the first symptom. It may progress from grade 1 to 4 in severe cases in which case it may be accompanied by orthopnea or paroxysmal nocturnal dyspnea. Acute pulmonary edema is a grave and dreaded complication of mitral stenosis.
2. ***Palpitation*** on exertion is also a frequent symptom, representing an increased awareness by the patient of her precordial impulse, which in turn may be due to the hypertrophied right ventricle. At times, when the onset of a palpitation is sudden, it may be a manifestation of a transient paroxysmal atrial tachycardia or atrial fibrillation.
3. ***Cough*** is usually brought on by exertion. Some patients develop a chronic bronchitis precipitated by chilly weather, which is very similar to the usual idiopathic chronic bronchitis.
4. ***Chest pain:*** Noncardiac localised in left inframammary region is common in neurotic individuals. True angina pectoris can also occur, especially in patients with severe pulmonary hypertension or associated with coronary artery disease in elderly group of patients.
5. ***Hemoptysis*** is frequent, and often the presenting complaint. It is usually the result of rupture of congested veins in the bronchial mucosa, but occasionally it may be the presenting symptom of pulmonary infarction.
6. ***Embolic phenomenon*** results in blocking of a cerebral artery presenting as a sudden stroke, of the splenic or renal artery manifesting with acute abdominal pain, or of a peripheral limb artery with acute pain and other manifestations of ischemia. Obstruction of the aortic bifurcation by a large embolus is a particularly serious complication.
7. Due to compression of the left recurrent laryngeal nerve by a dilated and tense main pulmonary artery, it may lead to paralysis of left vocal cord presenting as hoarseness of the voice (Ortner's syndrome).

B. *Physical Examination*

i. The patients may have a typical mitral facies with pinkish purple patches on the cheeks.
ii. The pulse is usually normal, but may be weak if stroke volume is reduced.
iii. A prominent "a" wave may be present in the jugular venous pulse of patients in sinus rhythm with pulmonary hypertension (Figs 16.3 and 16.4).
iv. A palpable first heart sound (S1) suggests a pliable anterior mitral valve leaflet. A right ventricular heave and a palpable pulmonic component of the second heart sound (P2) suggests pulmonary hypertension.
v. Aloud first heart sound (S1) occurs because the valve is fibrotic but pliable and higher than normal left ventricular systolic pressure is required to close it.
vi. The opening snap (OS) is best heard at the apex and is as a result of the sudden tensing and deceleration of the mitral valve leaflets when they are fully open. It usually suggests that the valve is still pliable and not rigidly calcified. The duration of the interval between the aortic component of the second heart sound and the opening snap correlates inversely with left atrial pressure.
vii. A low-pitched diastolic rumble which is produced by blood flow across the narrowed mitral valve can be best heard at the apical region, often best heard with the patient in the left lateral decubitus position. The duration of the rumble roughly corrlates with increasing severity of mitral stenosis. It may be masked by noisy respirations or by low cardiac output and may be accentuated by increasing cardiac output with exercise. One may encounter a palpable diastolic thrill at the apex.
viii. There may be an apical holosystolic murmur of associated rheumatic mitral regurgitation.
ix. There may be a holosystolic murmur of tricuspid regurgitation from right ventricular dilatation along the lower left sternal border.
x. There could be a mixture of murmurs produced as a result of involvement of their respective valves, such as aortic, tricuspid and pulmonary inorigion. Normally, the cross-sectional area of the mitral valve is at least 4 cm^2. Mitral stenosis leads to a reduction in valve area and is considered severe when the valve area is less than 1 cm^2. To maintain flow through the valve, leftatrial pressure rises, leading to an increase in the pressure gradient across the valve and to increased pulmonary venous and capillary pressures, with resultant dyspnea. Flow through the stenotic valve is dependent on the duration of diastole. Tachycardia shortens diastole disproportionately and causes a further elevation in left atrial pressure and can precipitate symptoms even in patients with relatively mild stenosis. Elevated left atrial pressure contributes to left atrial enlargement, which in turn predisposes the patient to atrial fibrillation, atrial thrombus formation, and thromboembolism, all of which are common complications of mitral stenosis. Severe mitral stenosis is often associated with an increase in pulmonary arterial pressure, leading to right-sided heart failure and secondary tricuspid and pulmonary incompetence. In patients with severe pulmonary hypertension, cardiac output at rest is reduced; this output reduction can cause a relatively low pressure gradient across the mitral valve even in patients with severe stenosis.

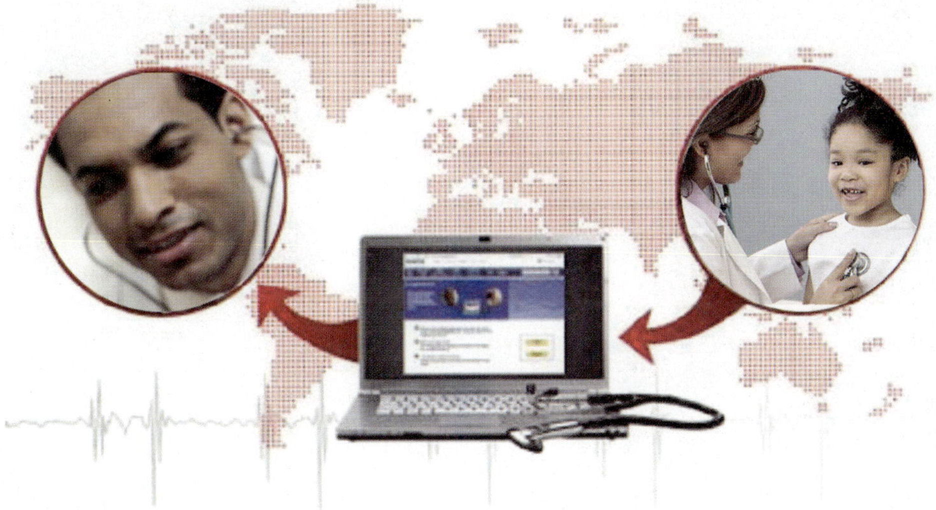

Fig. 16.4: *A teleauscultation system: just when we thought auscultation couldn't get any more sophisticated than with the Littmann 3,200 bluetooth stethoscope and the heart sounds analyzed by the cardioscan software, Zargis-Medical proves us wrong. They have just launched the ZargisTelemed platform, which streams the heart and lung sounds to anywhere in the world. The sounds are transmitted in real-time either over the internet or a private network allowing for remote diagnosis and expert opinions. It can be installed on a private server or accessed from Zargis' servers. The software is integrated with the cardioscan heart sounds analysis software and the Zargis StethAssist heart and lung sounds visualization software*

Diagnosis

Mitral stenosis is often asymptomatic at presentation and for many years thereafter. Symptomatic patients often present with dyspnea, but they can also present with angina, right-sided heart failure, atrial arrhythmia, or embolism. The physical findings in mitral stenosis depend on the severity of the stenosis, the mobility of the valve, and the rhythm. The principal sign is a rumbling diastolic murmur that is best heard at the apex with the stethoscope bell. Such a murmur is accentuated by having the patient lie on the left side and by using provocative maneuvers, such as exercise to increase the heart rate. In sinus rhythm, the murmur increases in intensity with atrial contraction (presystolic accentuation). Increased severity of stenosis is associated with a longer murmur and a thrill. With a pliable valve, an opening sound (OS) is heard, and the sudden closure of the stenotic valve at end diastole gives rise to a loud first heart sound that lends a tapping quality to the apex beat. When the valve calcifies and becomes less mobile, the opening snap and loud first heart sound disappear. A loud pulmonary component of the second heart sound is heard with pulmonary hypertension. The signs and symptoms of mitral stenosis are simulated by left atrial myxoma. In this condition, functional mitral stenosis results from prolapse of a mobile tumor arising from the interatrial septum into the mitral valve opening.

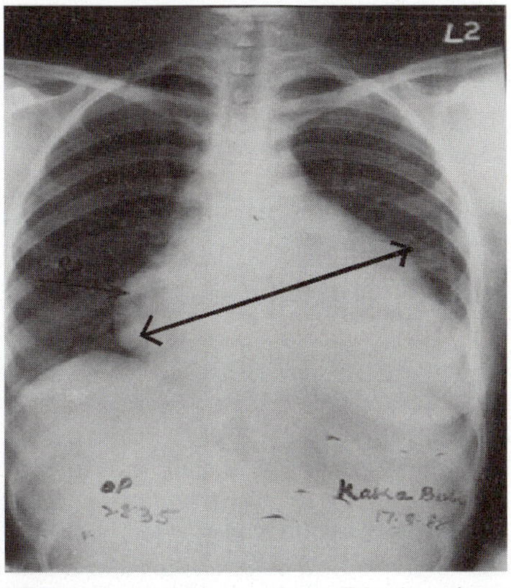

Fig. 16.5: *Photograph of X-ray chest PA view (arrow) showing mild to moderate enlargement of LA in rheumatic MS*

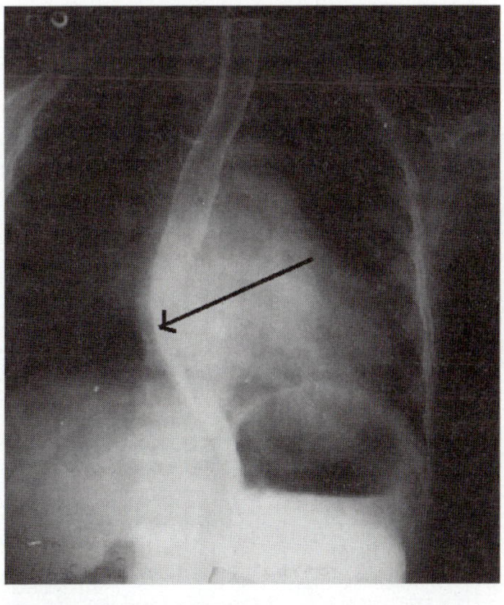

Fig. 16.6: *Photograph of barium meal study (arrow) showing indentation of barium filled esophagus in moderate enlargement of LA in rheumatic MS*

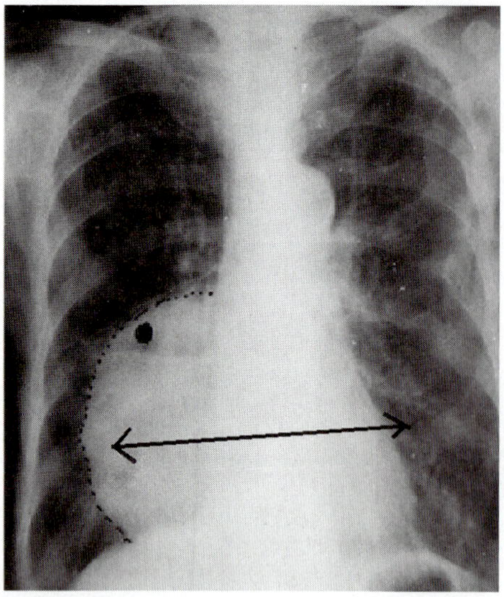

Fig. 16.7: *Photograph of X-ray chest PA view (arrow) showing massive enlargement of RA in rheumatic organic TS in patient with RHD, MS, MR, AS, AR*

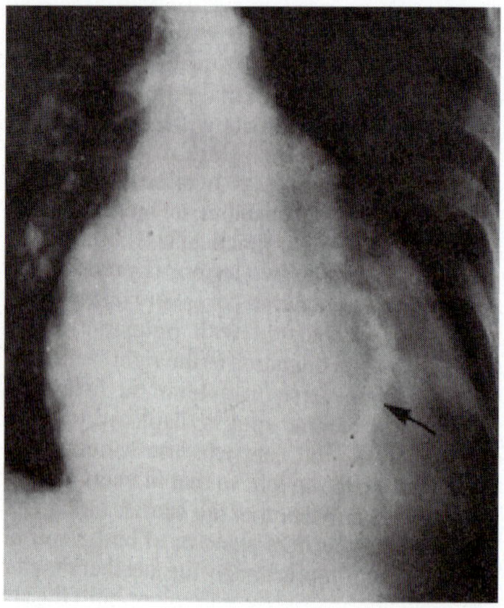

Fig. 16.9: *Calcification of mitral annulus as indicated by broad and curved density (arrow) in chronic mitral valve disease*

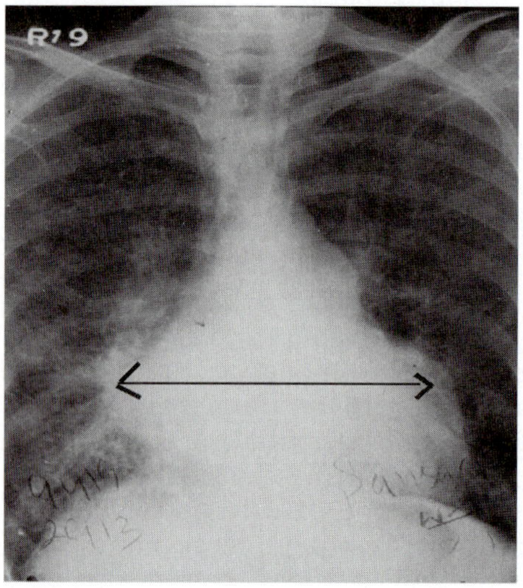

Fig. 16.8: *Photograph of X-ray chest PA view (arrow) showing moderate enlargement of RA in patient with rheumatic MS, TR and PAH*

Imaging Studies

Electrocardiography: It can reveal can reveal left atrial enlargement if the patient is in sinus rhythm. P mitral, indicating left atrial enlargement, right ventricular hypertrophy. It can also show cardiac arrhythmias such as sinus tachycardia, atrial fibrillation and digioxin-related dysarryhthmias (Fig. 16.15).

Chest radiography: Left atrial enlargement, mitral valve calcification, and signs of pulmonary congestion can all be present on chest X-ray (Figs 16.5 to 16.14).

Doppler echocardiography is the test of choice in confirming the diagnosis, establishing the severity of stenosis, detecting complications, and determining the most appropriate treatment. Echocardiography also allows accurate differentiation of mitral stenosis from a left atrial myxoma.

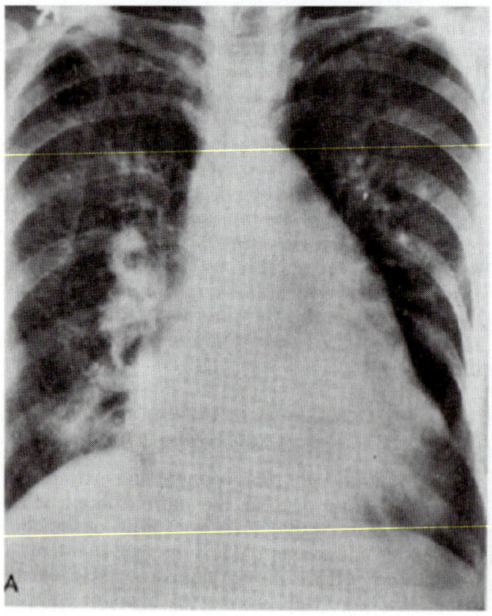

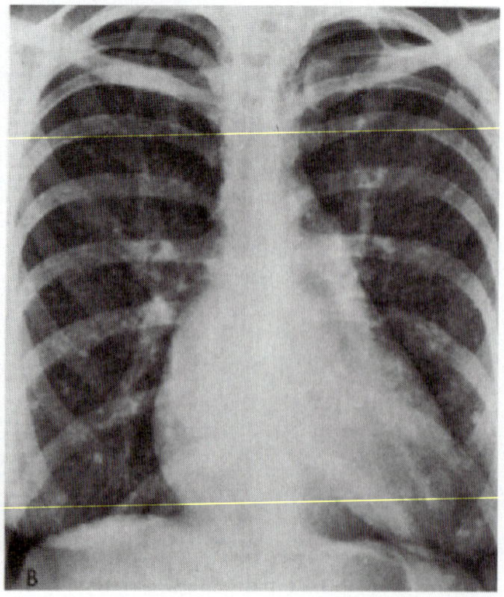

Fig. 16.10: *(A) Pulmonary hemosidrosis; lower lungs are studded with small nodules of moderate radiodensity. The LA and LV are enlarged Kerley B-lines are present in the lateral basal portions of lungs, (B) Showing pulmonary ossifications. Sccattered calcific nodules of differing size and shape are present in the lower lungs in a patient with chronic mitral stenosis*

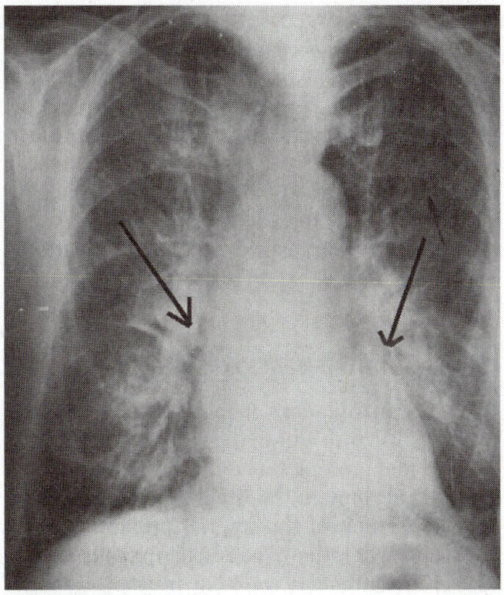

Fig. 16.11: *Interstitial pulmonary edema as indicated by indistinct haze in the perihilar region (arrow) in patient with critical mitral stenosis*

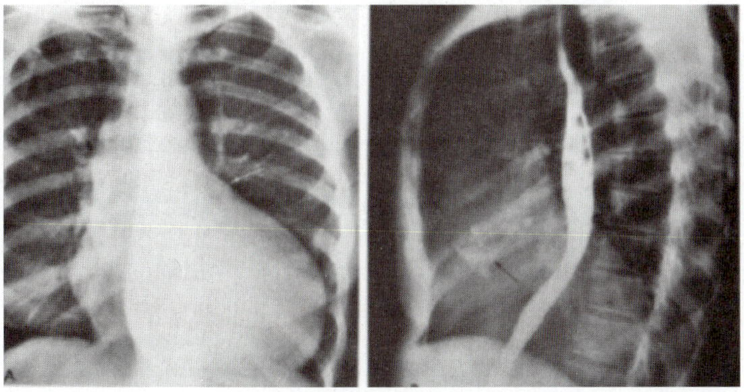

Fig. 16.12: *Dilatation of the left ventricle in aortic valve disease. (A) Frontal view: The cardiac silhouette is elongated downward and to the left, indicating left ventricular enlargement. There is slight prominence of the left atrial appendage (arrow). The esophagus is displaced medially. (B) Lateral view: the left ventricle is markedly enlarged and extends posterior to the esophagus. The aortic valve is densely calcified (arrow). The indentation on the anterior wall of the midesophagus is caused by the moderately dilated left atriumin patient with chronic aortic valvular stenosis*

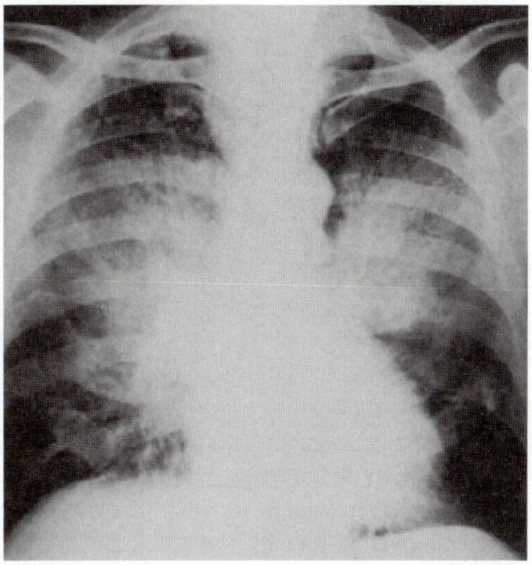

Fig. 16.13: *Photograph of X-ray chest PA view showing pulmonary edema as indicated by the presence of hazy areas of increased density in the central portion of each lung. Air filled bronchi are visualised within the density indicating that it represents consolidation of lung*

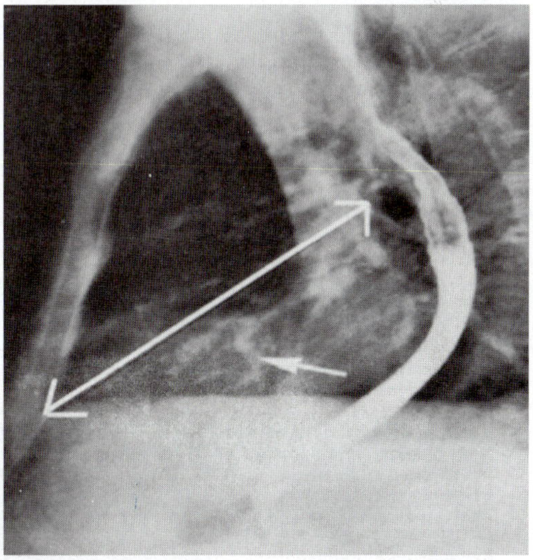

Fig. 16.14: *Photograph of X-ray chest PA view showing (lateral view) showing mitral valve calcification (white arrows). The valvular calcification (arrow) lies below the line drawn from the left bronchus to the anterior costophrenic sinus localizing it to the mitral valve. The aortic valve in this view lies more anteriorly above the line*

Typically, the stenotic mitral valve leaflets are thicker and less mobile than normal. The severity of stenosis is determined by measuring the pressure gradient across the valve with Doppler echocardiography and by calculating the valve area. Mitral stenosis should be suspected if the mean gradient exceeds 5 mmHg; the pressure can exceed 20 mmHg in severe stenosis. Valve area is measured by tracing the smallest opening of the valve in cross-section This method is the most accurate way of defining the severity of stenosis although it is technically demanding and sometimes impossible to perform. The valve area can also be calculated by Doppler echocardiography. Such evaluation is made on the basis of an empirical formula that calculates the time it takes for the pressure gradient to fall to half its initial value (the pressure half-time). Valve area is estimated as 220 divided by the pressure half-time. Pulmonary arterial (systolic) pressure (PAP) can be determined from the tricuspid regurgitant velocity (TRv) and the estimated right atrial pressure (RAP) (usually estimated as 5 mmHg) by the following equation: PAP = 4(TRv)2+ RAP. If the tricuspid regurgitant velocity is 3 m/sec, and RAP is estimated to be 5 mmHg, then the estimated PAP is 4(32) + 5 = 41 mmHg (Figs 16.16 to 16.20).

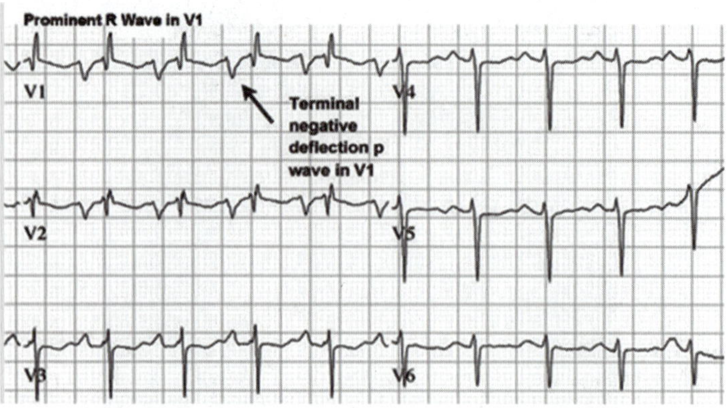

Fig. 16.15: *ECG trace shows terminal negative deflection of P wave in V1 due to LA enlargement and right ventricular hypertrophy in a young patient with chronic mitral valvular stenosis*

Transesophageal echocardiography is more useful than transthoracic echocardiography in excluding atrial thrombus and determining the severity of mitral regurgitation and is usually performed if balloon valvuloplasty is contemplated. Cardiac catheterization is rarely needed to establish the diagnosis but is used to confirm the severity of stenosis. The valve gradient is the difference between the left atrial pressure or the pulmonary arterial wedge pressure and the left ventricular diastolic pressure. Valve area can be calculated from the pressure gradient and the cardiac output.

Treatment

Once symptoms develop in mitral stenosis, the chance of survival decreases without surgical or balloon dilatation or valve replacement. In the absence of symptoms, management is directed at preventing recurrence of rheumatic fever.

Medical therapy: Patients in atrial fibrillation require heart-rate control with a beta-blocker (e.g., atenolol, 50 mg q.d.), digoxin (0.125 to 0.25 mg q.d.), or both. Systemic anticoagulation with warfarin is definitely indicated to prevent thromboembolism under the following situations when

1. Atrial fibrillation is present
2. There is a history of embolism, or
3. A thrombus is detected in the atrium.

Anticoagulation should be considered for patients with paroxysmal atrial fibrillation, a dilated left atrium (> 50 mm in diameter on echocardiography), or severe atrial stasis (as evidenced by swirling echoes or smoke in the left atrium on echocardiography). Regarding symptomatic patients for whom surgical intervention poses a relatively high risk, the judicious use of diuretics and drugs to control heart rate (i.e. digoxin, calcium channel blockers, or beta blockers) may allow symptomatic relief without the need for surgical intervention.

Surgical Intervention (Fig. 16.18)

Intervention to increase valve area is indicated before the onset of symptoms of dyspnea in the following patients: women with severe stenosis who wish to become pregnant but are unlikely to tolerate the volume load of pregnancy, patients who experience recurrent thromboembolic events, and patients who have severe pulmonary hypertension. A number of interventions are currently available to increase the valve area in mitral stenosis. These interventions include:

1. Percutaneous balloon valvuloplasty (Figs 16.21 and 16.36) performed in the cardiac catheterization laboratory

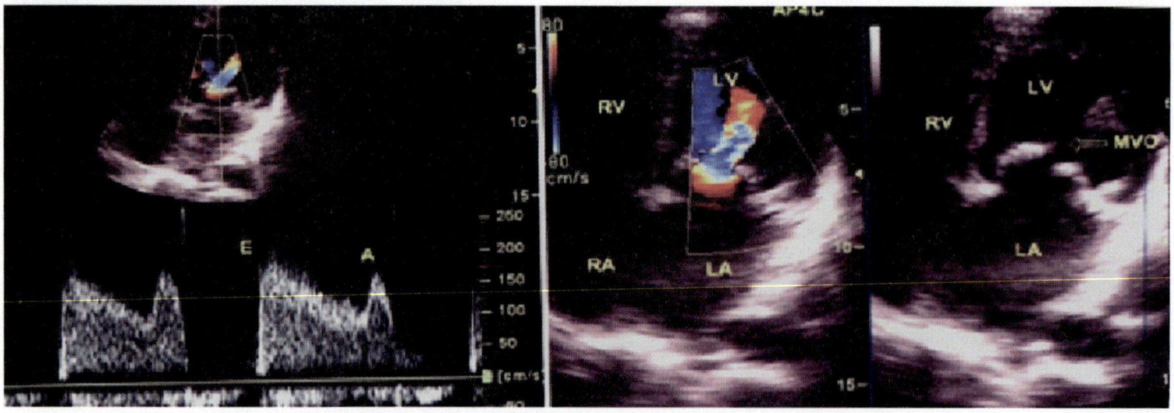

Fig. 16.16: *Left panel shows pulse Doppler tracing with an early diastolic E wave and a late diastolic A wave (during atrial systole). In normal persons, there will be a gap between the two waves when the atrial and ventricular diastolic pressures are equal (diastasis). Diastasis is absent in mitral stenosis as the pressures do not equalise—left atrial pressure is always higher and there is a gradient through out diastole. Mitral valve area can be estimated from the downward slope of the E wave. The slope becomes more flat as the severity of the mitral stenosis increases. The A wave is absent in atrial fibrillation. Right panel shows two pictures, one with colour flow mapping and another without. The colour flow mapping shows the turbulent flow from left atrium to left ventricle through the stenosed mitral valve. The domed mitral leaflets in the open position with a narrow orifice is visible in the frame without colour flow mapping. Both images are in the apical four chamber view. RA, right atrium; LA, left atrium; LV, left ventricle; RV, right ventricle; MVO, mitral valve orifice*

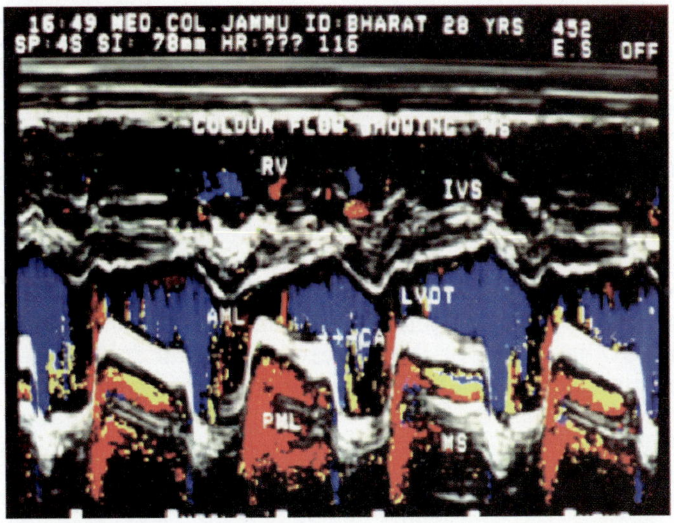

Fig. 16.17: *Color flow M-mode showing markedly thickened anterior and posterior mitral leaflets with paradoxical movement of posterior leaflet in patient with rheumatic mitral native valvular stenosis along with dilated and hypertrophied RV*

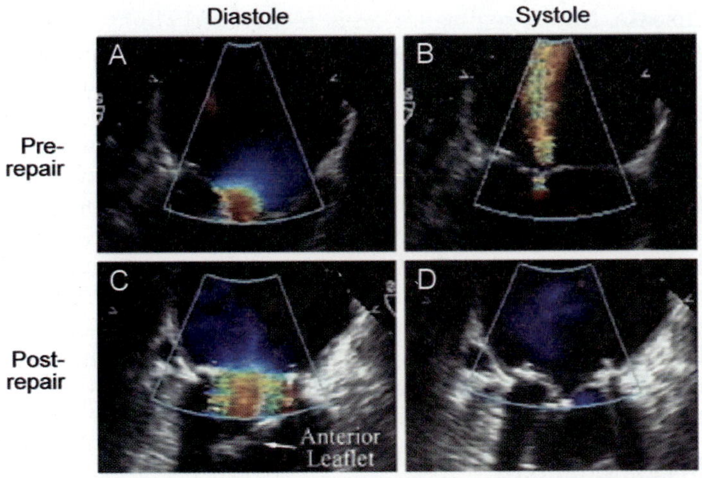

Fig. 16.18: *A patient with long-standing rheumatic mitral stenosis and regurgitation undergoing a rheumatic repair. (A and B) On pre-bypass echo, the stenotic and insufficient mitral valve is demonstrated. (C and D) After insertion of an autologous pericardial patch into the posterior leaflet, decalcifying commissurotomy, resection of the submitral apparatus to the anterior leaflet, and reattachment of the mobile anterior leaflet to both papillary muscles with adjustable ACR, the valve is fully competent with insignificant gradient. A full rigid ring also is placed (AnnuloFlow, Sorin Group). These types of more comprehensive ACR repairs for rheumatic valves have been quite stable in the intermediate-term*

2. Surgical commissurotomy
3. Replacement of the mitral valve with a prosthesis.

Balloon valvuloplasty is performed by inflating a specially designed balloon catheter in the mitral orifice to split the fused commissures. Excellent symptomatic relief is obtained in suitable patients.This intervention is currently the initial choice in mitral stenosis. Typically, the

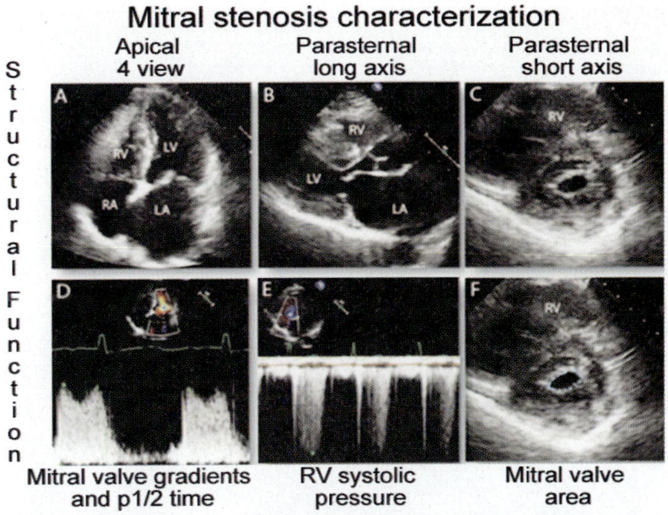

Fig. 16.19: *Two dimensional and Doppler echocardiography in mitral stenosis. Traditionally 2D echocardiography has provided structural information regarding the morphology of the mitral valve in mitral stenosis. In addition chamber size, and ventricular function is assessed by echocardiography. Doppler methods provide hemodynamic functional information regarding the mitral valve in mitral stenosis. Peak and mean mitral valve gradients, pressure half time derived mitral valve area and systolic pulmonary pressure are usually recorded in these patients. RV: right ventricle; LV, left ventricle; RA, right atrium; LA, left atrium*

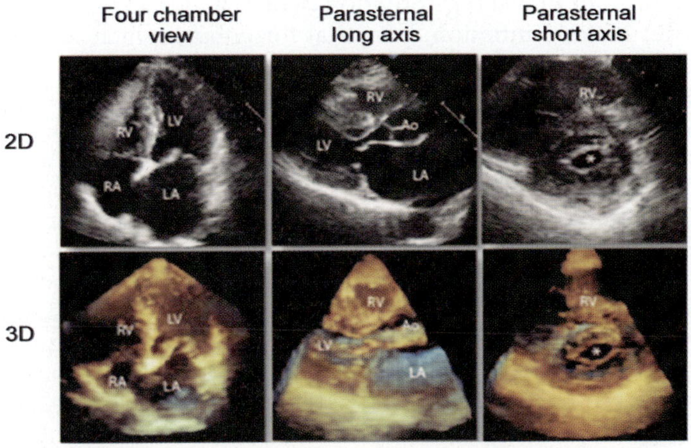

Fig. 16.20: *Comparison of 2D and 3D transthoracic echocardiography in mitral stenosis. The most useful views to evaluate patients with mitral stenosis include the apical four chamber view as well as the parasternal long and short-axis views. This figure illustrates the added value of 3D imaging in better characterizing the mitral valve apparatus. The third dimension increases the anatomic detail of the leaflets, commissures and subvalvular tissue.RV: right ventricle; LV, left ventricle; RA, right atrium; LA, left atrium; Ao, Aorta*

mitral valve area doubles in size from 1.0 to 2.0 cm^2 with a concomitant reduction in the pressure gradient.

Complications of balloon mitral valvuloplasty include:

- Severe mitral regurgitation (3%)

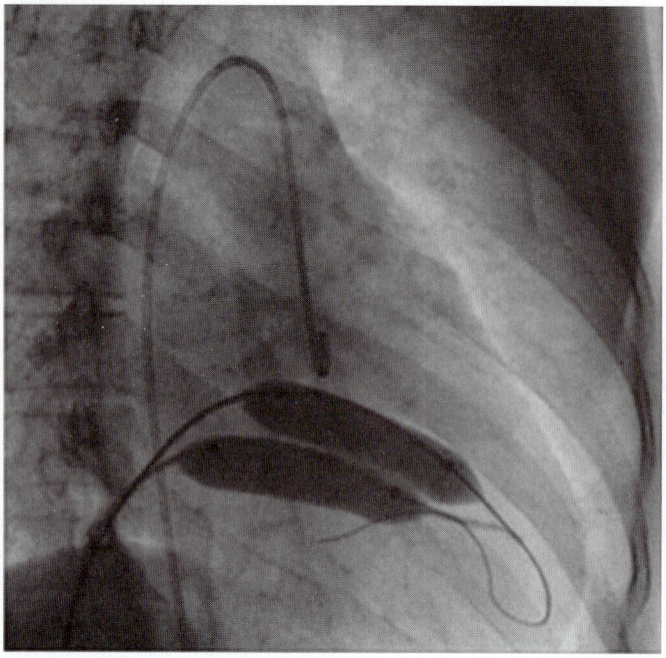

Fig. 16.21: *Percutaneous double balloon valvuloplasty of mitral valve*

- Thromboembolism (3%)
- Residual atrial septal defect with significant shunting (10–20%). Mortality associated with the procedure is less than 1%.

Contraindications to balloon mitral valvuloplasty include significant mitral regurgitation, which will likely increase after balloon inflation; left atrial thrombus, which can be dislodged at the time of the procedure; and significant subvalvular involvement or leaflet calcification, each of which increases the risk of complications and limits the degree of dilatation produced.

Surgical commissurotomy is now usually performed under direct vision after cardiopulmonary bypass. Surgical commissurotomy may be feasible when balloon valvuloplasty is impossible, such as in patients with significant mitral regurgitation, subvalvular stenosis, or atrial thrombus. A number of studies comparing surgical commissurotomy with balloon commissurotomy have shown equivalent immediate and medium-term (3–4 years) results regarding increase in valve area, improvement in symptoms, and freedom from repeat intervention in appropriately selected patients. However, commissurotomy, whether effected by a balloon or surgically, is a palliative procedure, and in most cases further intervention is eventually required. Repeat commissurotomy is sometimes feasible; but most often, mitral valve replacement is also necessary is heavily scarred or calcified or if severe mitral regurgitation is present. Morbidity and mortality are higher with prosthetic replacement than with either surgical or balloon commissurotomy.

MITRAL REGURGITATION

Mitral regurgitation leads to volume overload of the left ventricle, which must increase in size to achieve a normal stroke output to accommodate the leakage of blood back into the left atrium. Progressive left ventricular dilatation eventually leads to an increase in afterload, contractile impairment, reduction of cardiac output, and heart failure. In acute mitral regurgitation (such as can occur with chordal rupture, ischemia, or endocarditis), left atrial and pulmonary venous and arterial pressures increase quickly, giving rise to dyspnea and, often, acute pulmonary edema. In more chronic forms of mitral regurgitation, an increase in left atrial pressure is often offset by a concomitant increase in atrial compliance; and hence, symptoms appear late in the course of the disease. Left atrial enlargement predisposes the patient to atrial fibrillation and atrial thromboembolism. In long-standing mitral regurgitation, pulmonary hypertension can develop, which in turn leads to tricuspid regurgitation and right-sided heart failure.

DIAGNOSIS

Clinical Manifestations

In most patients, mitral regurgitation remains asymptomatic for many years. Dyspnea, fatigue from low cardiac output, and edema occur late in the course of the disease. Mitral regurgitation is recognized clinically by a systolic murmur at the apex, radiating to the axilla and increasing on expiration. In patients with a posteriorly directed jet of mitral regurgitation, the murmur is heard well at the back. In more severe cases, the murmur lasts throughout systole, the first and second heart sounds are soft or difficult to hear, and a third heart sound is present. A midsystolic click can be present in myxomatous disease; in less severe cases, this click can precede the murmur. The murmur can also be confined to late systole, with papillary muscle dysfunction. Mitral regurgitant murmurs caused by ischemia can be variable in duration and intensity, depending on the degree of ischemia and the loading conditions.

Imaging Studies

1. ***2D and 2D doppler echocardiography:*** Doppler echocardiography is the noninvasive method of choice in confirming the presence of mitral regurgitation.

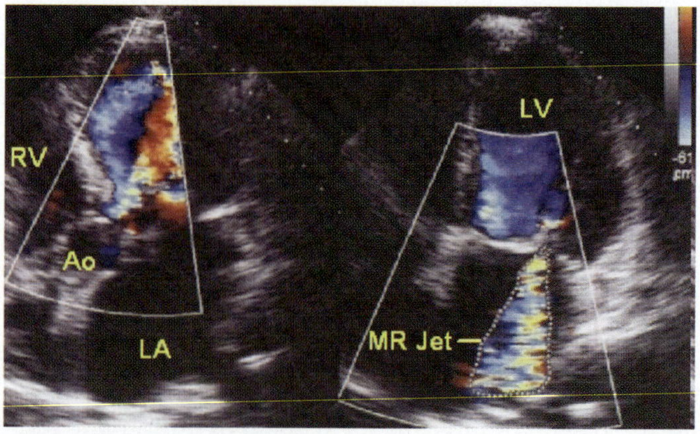

Fig. 16.22: *Colour doppler echocardiogram in RHD, showing moderate mitral regurgitation*

Echocardiography is used to diagnose the mechanism of the regurgitation (e.g. prolapse or annular dilatation); color-flow mapping is used to provide a semiquantitative assessment of severity based on the size and penetration of the left atrium by the regurgitant jet. Additionally, echocardiography can be used to assess the effects of the regurgitation on left ventricular size and function. Quantitative measurements of regurgitation, such as the regurgitant volume, regurgitant fraction [(regurgitant volume plus stroke volume) (Fig. 16.22) divided by regurgitant volume], and regurgitant orifice area (the area through which the valve leaks), are now possible with newer Doppler techniques. These techniques are useful in determining the true severity of the lesion and following it over time. Left ventricular size and volume, as well as contractile function assessed by the ejection fraction, are used to determine the need for surgical intervention.

However, asymptomatic mitral regurgitation is more difficult to assess and manage than other valvular lesions because in this condition, the true contractile function of the left ventricle is difficult to determine with conventional measures such as the ejection fraction. These measurements of contractility are confounded by the increase in ventricular preload caused by the extra volume of blood in the left atrium and the variable effect on afterload. Afterload is increased by left ventricular dilatation, but this effect is offset as the ventricle ejectsmuch of its blood into a relatively low pressure system (the left atrium). The left ventricular ejection fraction can appear falsely elevated in mitral regurgitation and usually falls after surgical correction. An ejection fraction of less than 60% should be considered abnormally low in patients with mitral regurgitation.

2. ***Transesophageal echocardiography*** is very sensitive in the detection of mitral regurgitation and is used mainly in those patients who are difficult to evaluate by the transthoracic approach. Contrast ventriculography is used to determine the severity of mitral regurgitation in patients undergoing cardiac catheterization. This procedure involves injecting radiopaque contrast medium into the left ventricle and assessing the extent and duration of opacification of the left atrium. In patients undergoing hemodynamic monitoring, large systolic V waves on the pulmonary arterial wedge tracing raise the suspicion of acute severe mitral regurgitation, as can occur in acute ischemia, but such V waves can occur in the absence of severe regurgitation.
3. ***Stress echocardiography*** is useful in detecting latent left ventricular dysfunction not evident on a resting study. Failure of the left ventricular ejection fraction to increase on exercise or of the left ventricular end-systolic volume to decrease on exercise is predictive of incipient left ventricular dysfunction and should be considered an indication for early surgery.

Other echocardiographic indices that have been associated with a less favorable surgical outcome include an absolute end-systolic dimension that is greater than 4.5 cm or that is greater than 2.6 cm/m^2 when indexed for body surface area; an end-systolic volume of greater than 50 mL/m^2; and a resting ejection fraction of less than 60%. Surgical referral should be considered if ventricular size and function approach these indices. Serial echocardiographic evaluation should be performed at least yearly and should be performed more frequently as ventricular dilatation progresses in patients with severe asymptomatic mitral regurgitation. Studies indicate a better long-term survival rate in patients with severe mitral regurgitation when surgery is performed early. Symptomatic severe mitral regurgitation is considered an indication for surgical intervention if the valve is primarily involved.

Treatment

In the management of asymptomatic mitral regurgitation, it should be borne in mind that left ventricular dysfunction is often latent and that, once present, the dysfunction cannot be corrected by operative intervention.Therefore, it is important to refer patients for surgery before the onset of true left ventricular dysfunction even in the absence of symptoms. Unfortunately, no load-independent measure of contractile function is readily available.

Surgical Intervention (Fig. 16.18)

Symptomatic patients with ischemic mitral regurgitation often require mitral valve surgery in addition to revascularization. Mitral regurgitation secondary to left ventricular dilatation often improves with afterload reduction, and surgical intervention is not usually indicated. Patients with moderately severe left ventricular dysfunction (ejection fraction < 35%) and significant mitral regurgitation were thought in the past to be poor surgical candidates because of high operative risk. However, recent research has shown that there is acceptable risk associated with operations in these patients. Symptoms usually improve, but a survival benefit associated with surgery in this group has not yet been shown. Patients who are not considered suitable for surgery because of left ventricular dysfunction often benefit from afterload reduction and diuretics. However, in patients who have primary asymptomatic mitral regurgitation with preserved left ventricular function, afterload reduction has not been shown to delay surgery or improve left ventricular function in the few small studies that have addressed this issue; afterload reduction is not currently recommended to treat such patients. Afterload reduction is beneficial for stabilizing patients with hemodynamically significant acute mitral regurgitation in preparation for surgery. Mitral valve repair is currently the technique of choice in the surgical management of mitral regurgitation because the operative mortality is lower, ventricular function is better preserved, and long-term complications such as thromboembolism and infection are lower with repair than with replacement Valve repair is most likely to be feasible in patients with myxomatous disease, especially if such disease involves the posterior leaflet, and is least likely to be successful in patients with rheumatic disease and endocarditis. Valve repair is accomplished by use of a variety of techniques, depending on the mechanism and etiology of the regurgitation. Such techniques include partial leaflet resection, chordal shortening or transfer, and insertion of an annuloplasty ring to reduce the size of the annulus. Long-term failure of repair occurs at a rate of 1–2% a year but is higher in patients with rheumatic disease. If mitral valve repair is not possible, a mitral prosthesis is implanted. Chordal and papillary muscle preservation is increasingly being employed when a mitral prosthesis is inserted, because preserving the muscles has been shown to help conserve left ventricular function after surgery.

MITRAL VALVE PROLAPSE

Mitral valve prolapse is a common condition in which the mitral valve leaflets are displaced in systole into the left atrium. It is usually caused by myxomatous degeneration of the valve and can occur in some form in up to 3% of the general population; it is more common in young females. In the majority of cases, mitral valve prolapse represents a benign abnormality; in a minority, mainly older men, significant mitral regurgitation results from rupture of a chord or from endocarditis and requires surgical intervention. Mitral valve prolapse is associated with low body weight, low blood pressure, and thoracic skeletal abnormalities such as pectus excavatum.

Patients with mitral valve prolapse have a slightly increased risk of stroke, myocardial ischemia, and sudden death. Ventricular extrasystoles are common and can be symptomatically troublesome. Other arrhythmias, such as ventricular or supraventricular tachycardia, are reported but are uncommon.

Diagnosis

Mitral valve prolapse has been associated with multiple nonspecific symptoms, such as atypical chest pain, presyncope, anxiety, and panic attacks. These symptoms are more commonly reported in younger females. A causal relation between these symptoms and mitral valve prolapse has not been established.

A midsystolic click at the mitral area during cardiac auscultation is often the finding that first brings mitral valve prolapse to the attention of the examiner. The click has been

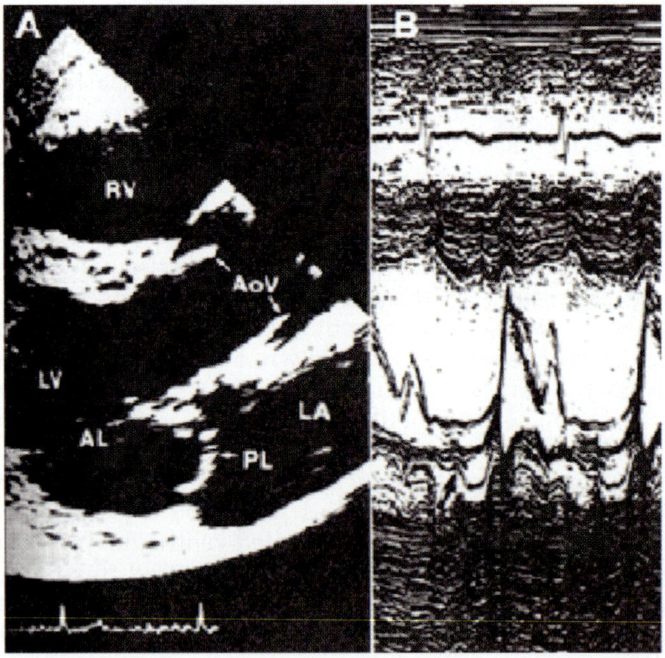

Fig. 16.23: *Echocardiogram from a patient with mitral valve prolapse. (A) Parasternal long-axis view in systole show the posterior leaflet (PL) of the mitral valve with superior displacement (bowing) into the left atrium (LA), i.e. arching posteriorly above the level of the atrioventricular groove and behind the normal coaptation point of the left atrium. (B) M-mode study shows abrupt posterior displacement in midsystole (arrow) of the posterior mitral leaflet. There are multiple echoes arising in the area of the valve during systole as a result of the redundancy of the leaflets. These findings are characteristic of mitral valve proplapse. LV, left ventricle; AL, anterior leaflet of mitral valve; RV, right ventricle; AoV, aortic valve*

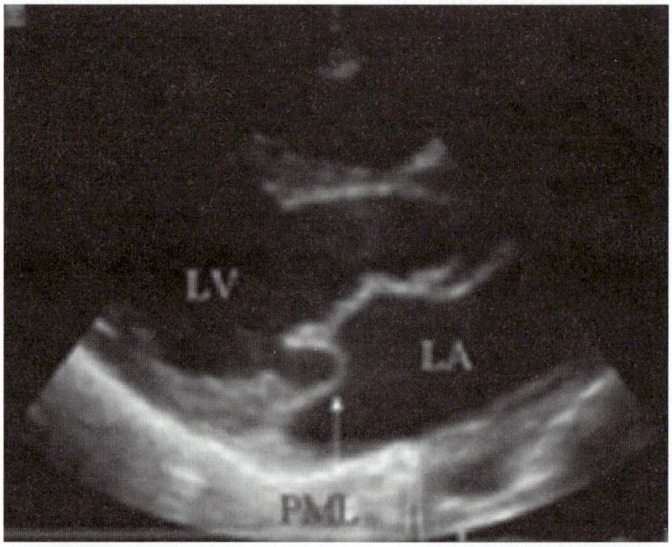

Fig. 16.24: *Two dimensional echocardiographic long-axis parasternal view of mitral valve prolapse. MV, mitral valve; LV, left ventricle; LA, left atrium; RV, right ventricle; Ao aorta*

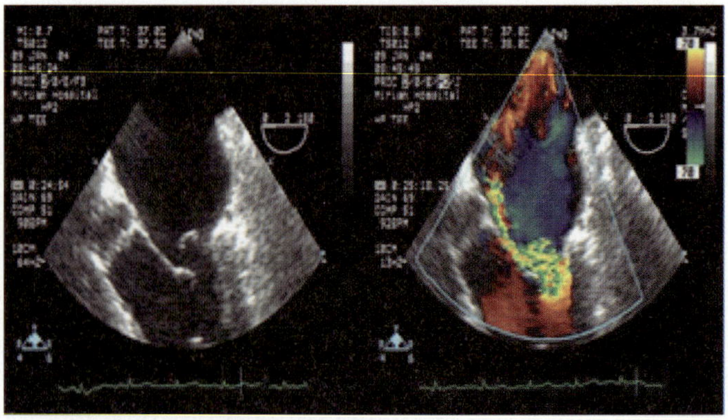

Fig. 16.25: *TEE showing posterior mitral valve prolapse with associated mitral regurgitation*

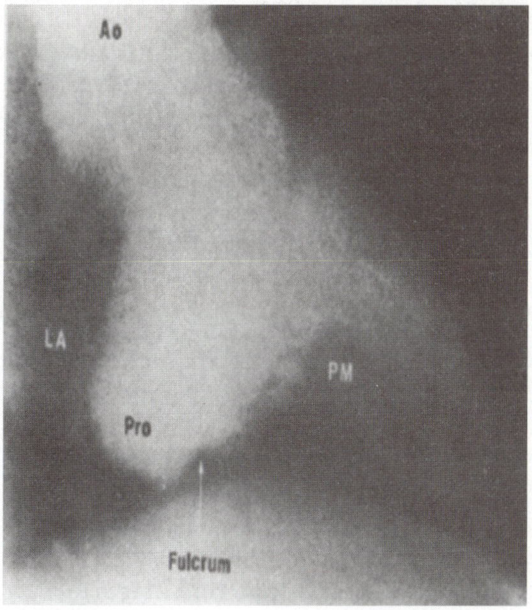

Fig. 16.26: *Systolic frame of left ventricular angiogram depicting prolapse (pro) of the mitral valve . The postero-medial commissural scallop of the posterior mitral leaflet extends posteriorly and inferiorly to the fulcrum*

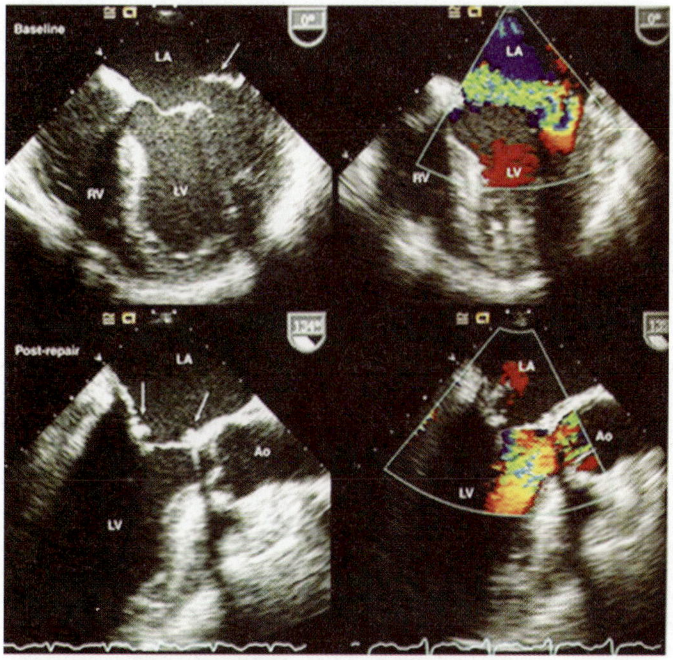

Fig. 16.27: *Mitral valve repair. 2D (left) and color Doppler (right) intraoperative TEE images were taken in a patient with myxomatous mitral valve defect before (top) and after (bottom) mitral valve repair, before repair severe mitral prolapse with partial flail leaflet segment and moderate to severe MR in the four chamber view. After repair, the long-axis view shows the annuloplasty ring (arrows). Regurgitation was not detected after successful repair*

attributed to tensing of the redundant valvular tissue with cardiac contraction. A late systolic murmur can follow the click. Maneuvers that reduce intracardiac volume, such as having the patient stand or perform the valsalva maneuver, cause the click to occur earlier in systole and cause an increase in the duration of the murmur. The typical auscultatory findings and their response to these maneuvers are sufficient to make a diagnosis of mitral valve prolapse. Two-dimensional echocardiography is the method of choice to confirm the diagnosis. Apparent systolic displacement beyond the annular plane is possible with both M-mode and two dimensional approaches because the annulus is nonplanar and saddle-shaped. The possibility of a false positive diagnosis can be minimized by seeking systolic displacement of the leaflets in a parasternal long-axis view. Myxomatous mitral valve leaflets frequently are thicker, are more redundant, and have longer chordae than normal as seen on echocardiography. Doppler echocardiography is used to detect and quantify associated regurgitation (Figs 16.23–16.26).

Treatment

Asymptomatic mitral valve prolapse requires no specific treatment. Periodic examination is indicated to detect any progression in the severity of mitral regurgitation.

Prophylaxis for endocarditis is indicated if both a click and a murmur are present but is not indicated in the absence of mitral regurgitation. Symptomatic ventricular ectopy often responds to beta-blockade. Many patients with atypical chest pain and other nonspecific symptoms improve when they are reassured of the relatively benign nature of the condition. Empirical treatment with small doses of beta-blockers can also provide symptomatic relief. Mitral regurgitation should be treated as described earlier (Fig. 16.27).

AORTIC STENOSIS

The normal aortic valve is 3–4 cm^2 in area when fully open. Aortic stenosis is considered severe when the valve area is 1 cm^2 or less and is considered critical when the area is less than 0.75 cm^2. Aortic stenosis causes concentric left ventricular hypertrophy as a compensatory mechanism that maintains cardiacoutput at rest despite the increased pressure gradient across the valve. Eventually, this compensatory mechanism is overcome, causing the left ventricle to fail and dilate and the resting cardiac output to decline.

Diagnosis

There is a variable relation between the severity of stenosis and symptoms. Many patients with critical aortic stenosis are asymptomatic whereas patients in states of volume overload, may have symptoms with stenosis of lesser severity. Dyspnea is often the presenting feature; it reflects increased left atrial pressure and pulmonary venous hypertension from the increased left ventricular pressure in systole and the diastolic ventricular dysfunction imposed by left ventricular hypertrophy. Angina is common even in the absence of significant obstruction in the epicardial coronary blood vessels because of impaired supply of blood to the subenocardium in the hypertrophied left ventricle.

Exertional syncope also occurs with stenosis and can result from the inability to increase cardiac output sufficiently to supply both skeletal muscle and the cerebral vasculature, resulting in impaired cerebral blood supply, or from abnormal baroreceptor reflexes. Serious arrhythmia can also cause syncope and, in severe aortic stenosis, even sudden death. Fatigue is common because of low cardiac output.

In severe aortic stenosis, the carotid pulse typically is reduced in intensity and has a slow delayed upstroke.

Aortic stenosis gives rise to a systolic murmur that is heard over the aortic area and that can radiate to the carotid arteries and to the apex. In severe stenosis, the murmur peaks later in systole and can be associated with a thrill. A fourth heart sound is usually present. In mobile congenitally abnormal valves, an ejection click can precede the murmur. Severe calcific aortic stenosis is often associated with a diminished intensity of the aortic component of the second heart sound. Although the physical findings are important in alerting the clinician to the presence of aortic valve disease, the degree of hemodynamic severity is more reliably determined with Doppler echocardiography.

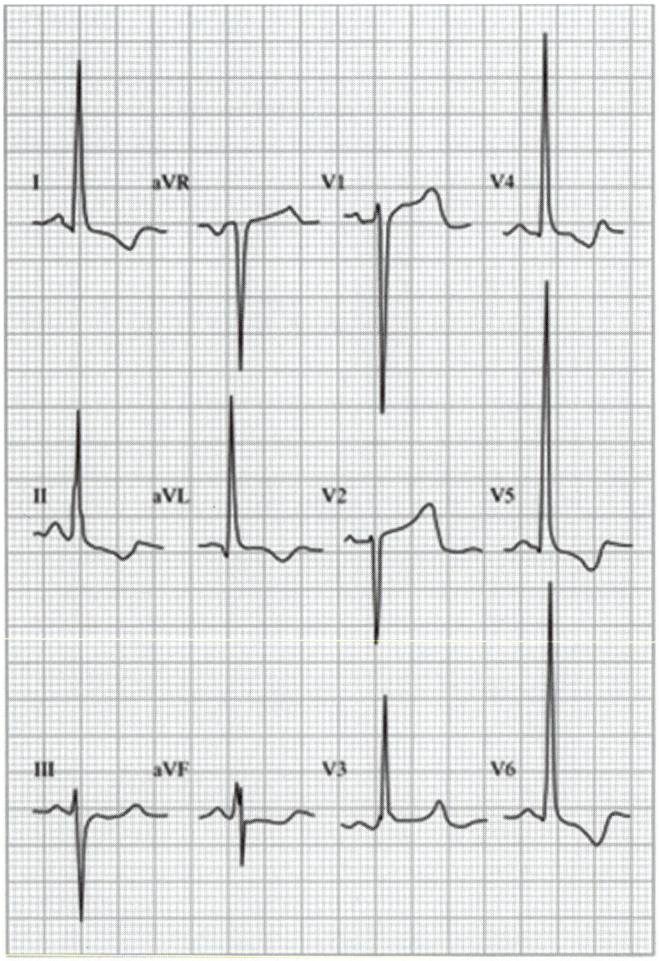

Fig. 16.28: *ECG showing deep S waves in V1-V2 and tall R waves in V4-V6 as voltage criteria of LVH in patient with aortic stenosis*

Imaging Studies

Electrocardiography: There is left ventricular hypertrophy and left atrial enlargement may be the only diagnostic features on surface electrocardiography in significant valvular aortic stenosis. However, ECG trace may be normal in milder lesions (Fig. 16.28).

Chest radiography: X-ray chest (PA view) shows left ventricular hypertrophy pattern, prominent LA shadow and enlarged ascending aorta on right hemithorax (Fig. 16.12).

Simultaneous recording of basal phonocardiogram along with M-mode echocardiography: It shows prominent aortic valvular ejection click in systole. It is followed by a crescendo-decrescendosystolic ejection murmur that ends well before a loud A2 (Fig. 16.31).

Doppler echocardiography is used to determine the mechanism and the hemodynamic severity of the stenosis as well as the effects on left ventricular size and function. In aortic stenosis, the opening of the aortic valve is reduced, as seen on the echocardiogram. Continuous wave Doppler echocardiography is used to measure the peak velocity across the valve and thus the aortic pressure gradient; the mean pressure gradient across the valve is often 50 mmHg or more in patients with severe aortic stenosis. However, the pressure gradient is determined not only by the degree of stenosis but also by flow through the valve and can be relatively low despite severe aortic stenosis if cardiac output is reduced. In most instances, therefore, the valve

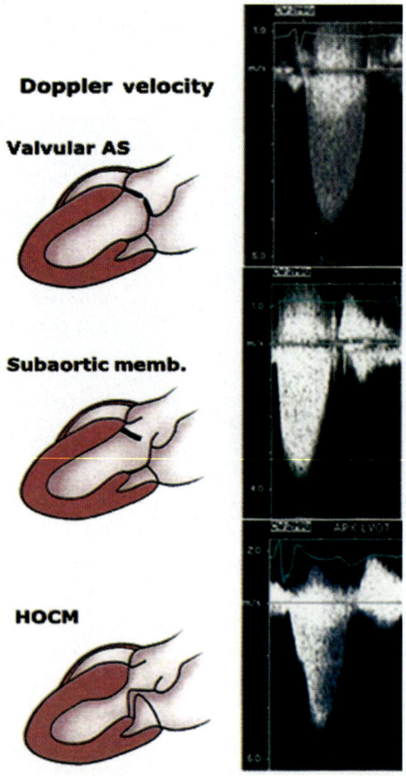

Fig. 16.29: *Ilustrations showing CW Doppler study in different types of LV outflow obstructions*

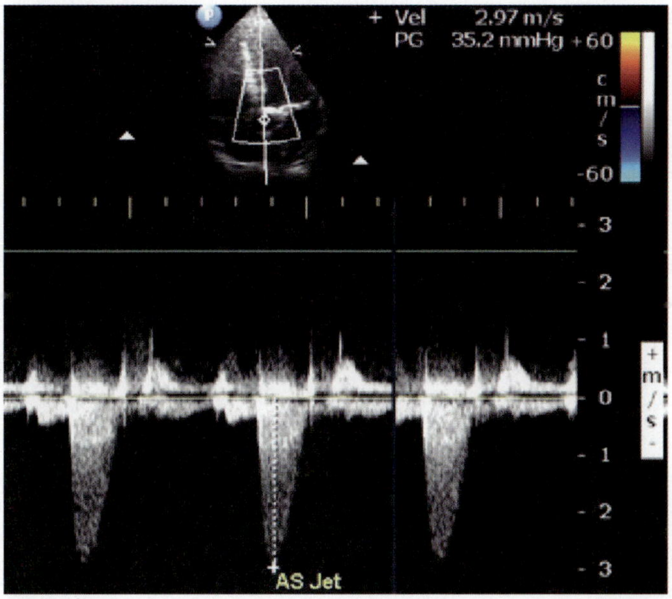

Fig. 16.30: *Color flow-guided evaluation of aortic stenosis jet from apical five chamber view with continuous wave Doppler interrogation*

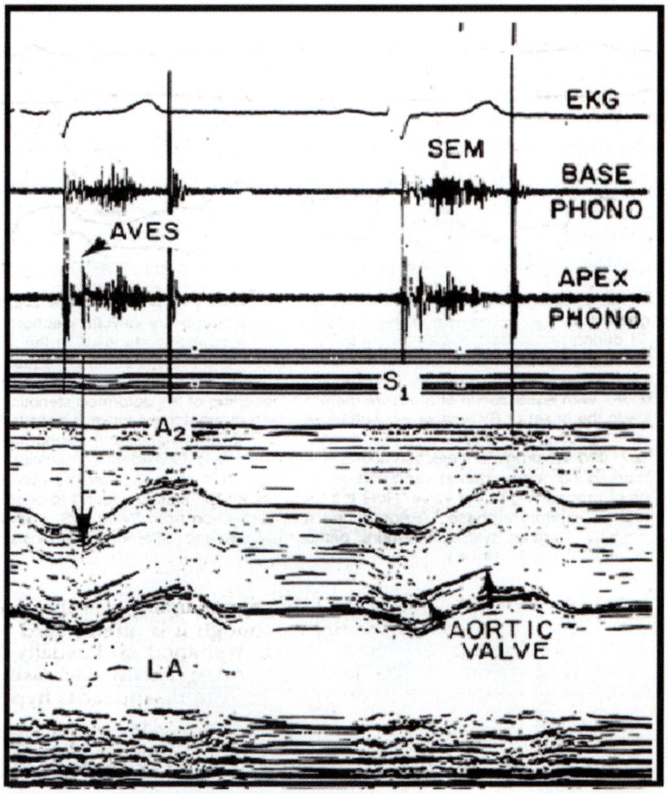

Fig. 16.31: *Simultaneous recordings of base, apex cardiograms and aortic valve echocardiogram showing a prominent aortic valvular ejection click (AVES) is recorded at the apex and is coincident with the maximal excursion of the aortic valve in early systole. It is followed by a crescendo-decrescendo SEM that ends well before a loud A2 in young patient with valvular aortic stenosis*

area as well as the pressure gradient should be calculated. The valve area is estimated readily from the flow through the valve and the pressure gradient across the valve (Figs 16.29, 16.30, 16.34).

Cardiac Catheterization

Cardiac catheterization, the pressure difference across the aortic valve between the left ventricle and the aorta is measured directly. Valve area can be calculated from the cardiac output and the pressure gradient. Because Doppler echocardiography and invasive measurements of aortic valve severity have been shown to agree when both are performed by an experienced personel.

Cardiac catheterization is now used less often as the primary diagnostic tool in assessing aortic stenosis. It is used to confirm the echocardiographic findings in patients being considered for surgery or when there is significant discrepancy between the clinical findings and the echocardiographic findings (Figs 16.32 and 16.33).

Treatment

Aortic stenosis is a progressive disease, and patients with the disease can remain asymptomatic for many years. The rate of progression varies greatly but increases with age, associated coronary artery disease, and the severity of the stenosis. Progression to symptoms or intervention is likely within 2 years in older patients with severe asymptomatic aortic stenosis. Once symptoms become manifest, the survival rate without surgical treatment is reduced; mean survival is 5 years in patients with angina, 3 years in patients with syncope, and 2 years or less in patients with heart failure. Operative mortality increases with severe symptoms, advanced age, and the presence of left ventricular dysfunction.

The onset of symptoms, therefore, is the major indication for surgical intervention. Left ventricular dysfunction

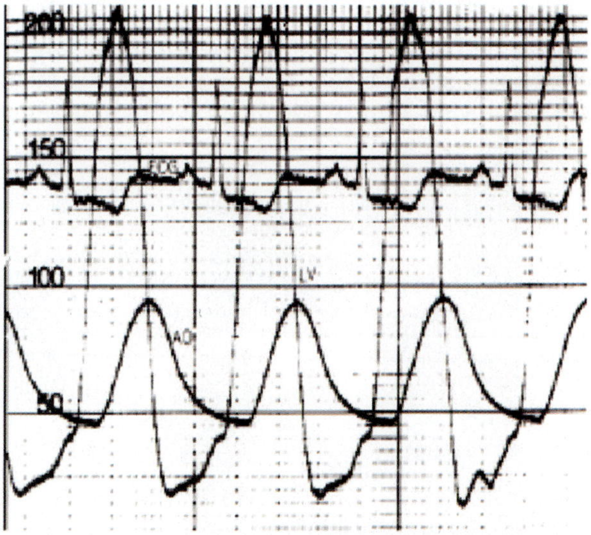

Fig. 16.32: *Simultaneous tracing of ECG and hemodynamic Pressure recording across aorta and LV showing marked gradient between LV and aorta in patient with moderately severe AS*

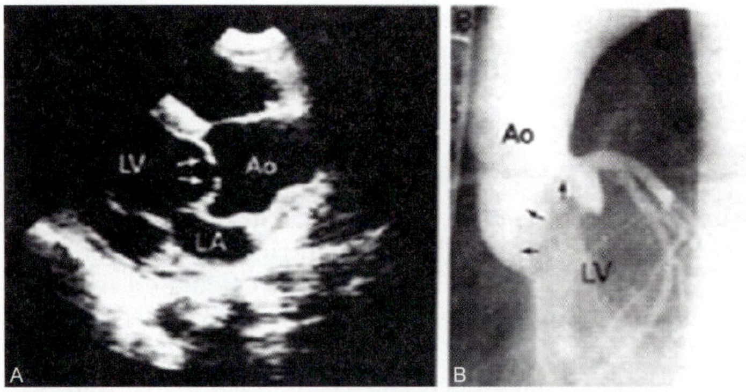

Fig. 16.33: *(A) 2D echocardiographic study with the transducer in the long-axis parasternal position demonstrating leaflet doming and thickening. (B) Aortogram from the same patient showing doming of the aortic valve leaflets. The negative shadow in the proximal aortic root (Ao) is caused by a jet of nonopacified blood from the left ventricle (LV) as it exits through the stenotic aortic valve*

attributable to aortic stenosis is another indication for intervention because it demonstrates failure of compensatory mechanisms and incipient symptoms. Sudden death can occur with aortic stenosis, but this is rare in the absence of symptoms. Patients should be instructed to report the onset of any symptoms and should undergo regular follow-up evaluations with physical examination and Doppler echocardiography. Doppler examination should be performed at least yearly and should be performed more frequently in patients with severe stenosis and in older patients. Surgical relief of aortic stenosis usually leads to relief of symptoms and improvement in left ventricular function when such function was abnormal preoperatively.

Aortic valve surgery in the advancing is associated with an increased mortality but provides excellent palliation of symptoms; surgery should be considered for such patients provided they are otherwise viable candidates. Patients with severe left ventricular dysfunction resulting from aortic stenosis should also be considered for surgery because significant improvement in ventricular function

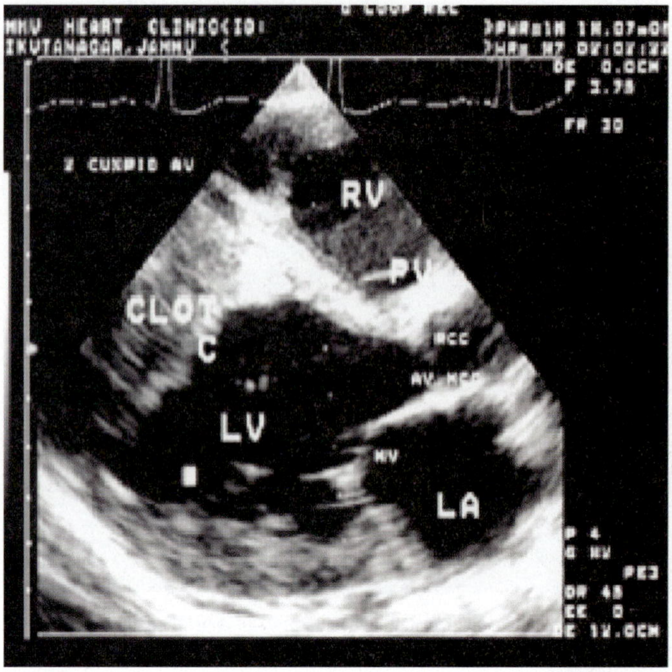

Fig. 16.34: *2D LAX view of LV showing dilated LV cavity with apical clot in patient with severe type of aortic stenosis*

and symptoms often results, and without surgery the survival rate in these patients is poor.

Surgical intervention: Surgical intervention for patients with aortic stenosis usually involves insertion of a prosthesis or a human valve. In congenital aortic stenosis, valve repair or commissurotomy can be feasible, although significant aortic regurgitation can result. Balloon valvuloplasty has proved disappointing in the long-term treatment of adult calcific aortic stenosis. Valve area typically increases from 0.5 cm^2 to 0.8 cm^2 and is associated with improvement of symptoms in the majority of cases. However, stenosis recurs in as many as 50% of patients within 6 months, and fewer than 25% survive more than 3 years.

Balloon valvuloplasty is now indicated in the palliative treatment of patients with aortic stenosis who are not

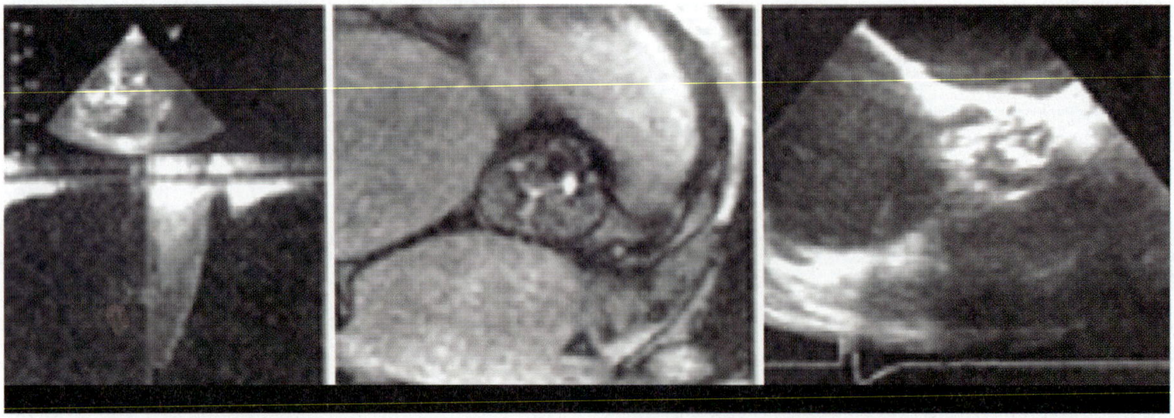

Fig. 16.35: *(A) Showing enhanced Doppler flow velocity in calcified aortic stenosis, (B) MRI scan showing calcified tricuspid morphology of aortic valve, (C) TEE showing calcified native aortic valve*

surgical candidates because of significant comorbidity; it is also used to stabilize critically ill patients for whom surgery is planned at a later stage. Balloon dilatation is effective in young patients with congenital aortic stenosis (Fig. 16.37).

AORTIC REGURGITATION

Aortic regurgitation causes a volume overload of the left ventricle. In chronic aortic regurgitation, the volume overload is well tolerated for years. The left ventricle dilates to accommodate the increased volume load and thereby maintains a normal resting cardiac output. Unlike mitral regurgitation, the left ventricle in aortic regurgitation must expel all of the increased volume of blood into the systemic circulation; severe enlargement of the left ventricle is common. Because of a compensatory increase in ventricular compliance, left ventricular diastolic pressure often remains in the normal range despite the increase in ventricular size. The ventricle hypertrophies to maintain normal wall stress.

Eventually, compensatory mechanisms fail, and contractile impairment and increased diastolic pressure result in elevated left atrial and pulmonary venous pressures and symptoms. Acute aortic regurgitation can develop as a result of sudden disruption of the valve apparatus with endocarditis or aortic dissection. This condition is poorly tolerated because the left ventricle is unable to dilate fast enough to compensate for the volume load. Left ventricular diastolic pressure rises rapidly and leads to pulmonary congestion and edema. Cardiac output falls, and shock and even death can follow (Table 16.1).

Diagnosis

In chronic aortic regurgitation, symptomatic presentation occurs late in the course of disease; dyspnea and fatigue are the usual findings. Angina can occur in the absence of coronary artery disease because of the increased demand for oxygen caused by severe left ventricular enlargement and hypertrophy together with the reduced supply of oxygen resulting from the underperfusion of the coronary arteries. Such underperfusion is caused by the low diastolic pressure characteristic of this condition.

The cardinal physical sign of aortic regurgitation is a diastolic murmur that is high pitched and best heard with the diaphragm of the stethoscope with respiration suspended in expiration. The murmur is loudest immediately after aortic valve closure; it progressively diminishes in intensity throughout diastole, paralleling the decline in the pressure gradient between the aorta and the left ventricle. The murmur is best heard on the left of the sternal border in disease of the aortic cusps and on the right of the sternal border in disease of the aortic root. Even in the absence of significant stenosis, an aortic systolic murmur is audible, reflecting the increased flow through the valve. Severe chronic aortic regurgitation is characterized by a wide pulse pressure and an elevated systolic pressure caused by the increased stroke output; also characteristic is a reduction in the diastolic pressure, which occurs as blood leaks back into the left ventricle

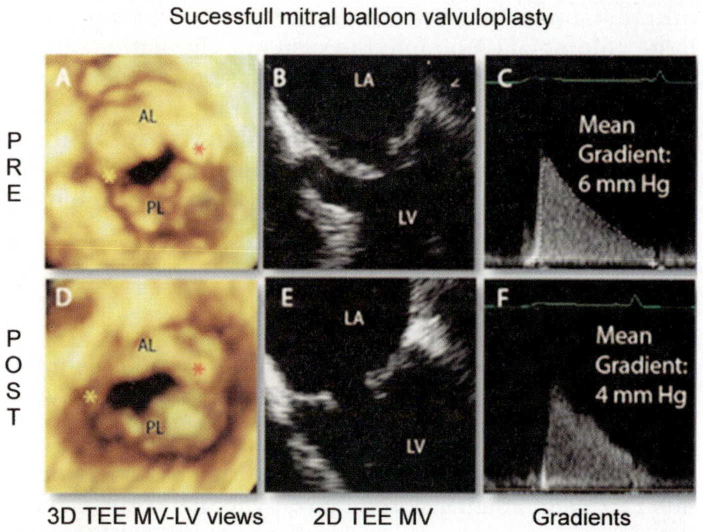

Fig. 16.36: *Panels A and D depict the mitral valve orifice as seen from the LV. Note the commissural fusion and the small mitral orifice in the preprocedure image (Panel A). In panel D, were the commissures are now split and the arealof the mitral orifice has increased. Panels B and E illustrate the 2D TEE views of the mitral valve pre- and postprocedure. Note the increased leaflet distance postprocedure. Panels C and F illustrate the transmitral Doppler gradients pre and postprocedure. The preprocedure gradients had already diminished under general anesthesia and the postprocedure gradients showed only a mild drop despite good bicommissural splitting. This is not uncommon to see in the immediate postprocedure studies and is probably related to decreased left atrial compliance, therefore to gage procedural success; we rely mostly on the 3D visualization of the mitral orifice size and commissural splitting. Yellow asterisk: lateral commissure; red asterisk: medial commissure*

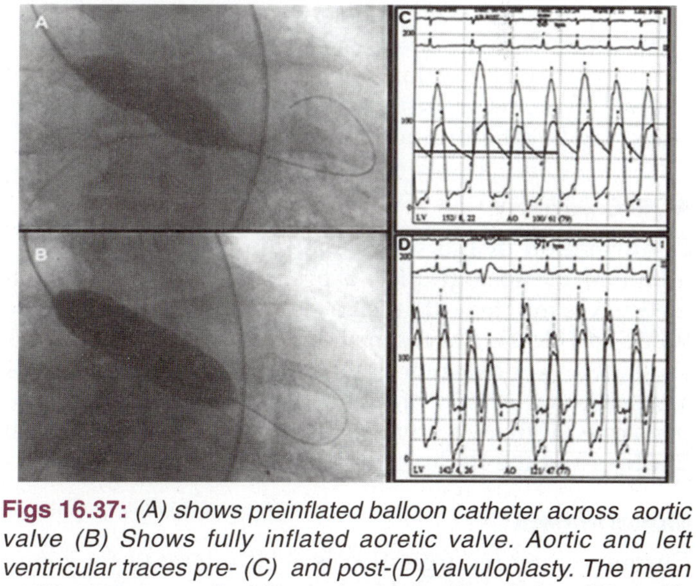

Figs 16.37: *(A) shows preinflated balloon catheter across aortic valve (B) Shows fully inflated aoretic valve. Aortic and left ventricular traces pre- (C) and post-(D) valvuloplasty. The mean aortic pressure gradient has reduced significantly from 50 mmHg to 25 mmHg*

throughout diastole. If the aortic regurgitant jet hits the mitral valvular leaflet, it can cause partial closure of the valve, creating an apical diastolic murmur that simulates mitral stenosis (Austin Flint murmur). The ejection of a large volume of blood into the systemic circulation and its rapid leak backward into the heart cause many peripheral circulatory manifestations that confirm rather than establish the diagnosis. Acute aortic regurgitation can be more difficult to recognize because the murmur is often short, and the reduced cardiac output leads to reduced intensity of the murmur.

Imaging Studies

Chest Radiography

Marked cardiomegaly and prominence of the ascending aorta are often present on chest X-ray in patients with chronic severe aortic regurgitation.

Electrocardiography: It shows left ventricular hypertrophy and LA enlargement in chronic aortic valvular regurgitation.

1. ***Echocardiography*** (Figs 16.38 to 16.40) 2D Doppler echocardiography confirms the mechanism and severity of aortic regurgitation and its effect on left ventricular size and function. Regurgitant volume and fraction can be quantified by echocardiographic Doppler techniques. More often, the severity of regurgitation is graded on the basis of several qualitative and semiquantitative measures including the dimensions of the regurgitant jet in the left ventricular outflow tract and of the ventricular cavity, as determined by color flow Doppler mapping, and the presence of diastolic flow reversal in the descending thoracic aorta, as determined with pulsed wave Doppler echocardiography. In severe aortic regurgitation, early closure of the mitral valve and diastolic mitral regurgitation can occur as a result of the increased pressure in the left ventricle in diastole.
2. ***Stress ventriculography and echocardiography:*** These have both been used to determine the response of the left ventricle to the effects of exercise: a significant fall in left ventricular ejection fraction or an increase in end-systolic volume suggests incipient contractile dysfunction and can be an indication for early surgical intervention.

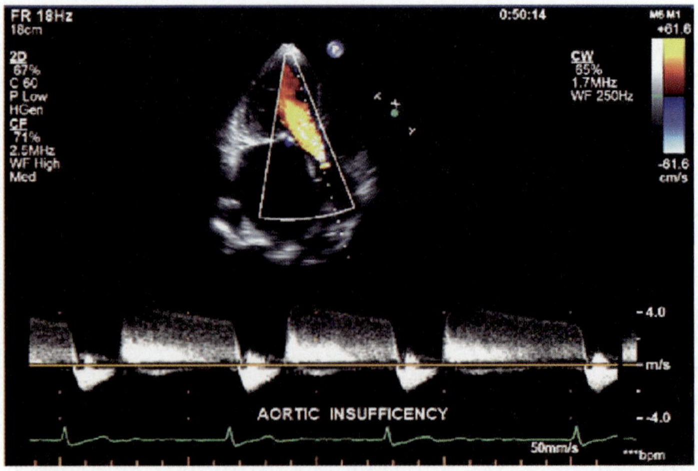

Fig. 16.38: *Color Doppler tracing in aortic regurgitation*

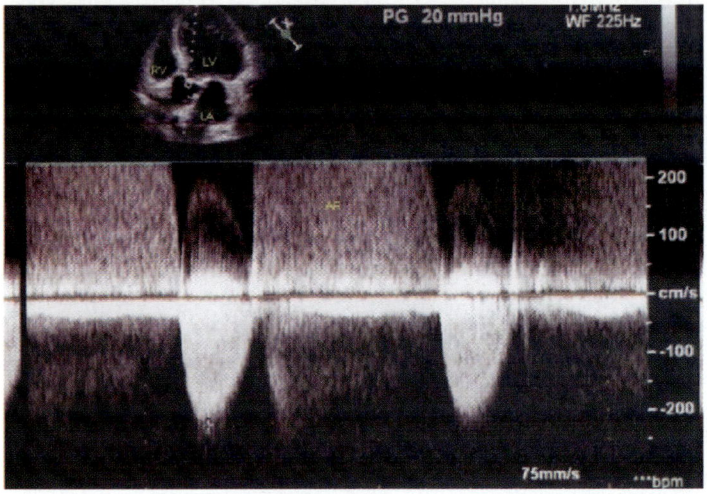

Fig. 16.39: *Doppler tracing in aortic regurgitation (bottom) in apical five chamber view (top)*

AORTOGRAPHY

Confirmation of the severity of aortic regurgitation is obtained by aortography, a process in which contrast medium is injected into the aortic root and the retrograde filling and clearing of contrast dye from the left ventricle is examined. Aortography is the current gold standard for assessing the severity of aortic regurgitation; it should be performed if there is any discrepancy between the clinical findings and the findings on Doppler echocardiography.

Management

Chronic aortic regurgitation is well tolerated for many years. Operative mortality is increased and long-term survival reduced if the left ventricle is greatly enlarged or if left ventricular dysfunction has been present for more than 1 year. Left ventricular dysfunction that is present for a shorter period is likely to improve and even resolve after surgery. Several studies have shown that asymptomatic patients with normal left ventricular function can be safely followed for a long period (up to 11 years in one study) when serial physical examination and Doppler echocardiographic examination are performed at least yearly and then performed more frequently as left ventricular dilatation progresses.

Surgery is indicated when symptoms develop. In asymptomatic patients, surgery is indicated when resting left ventricular function declines or if severe left ventricular dilatation (end-systolic dimension > 5 cm; end-diastolic dimension = 7 cm) occurs.

Medical Treatment

Evidence suggests that these dimensions should be normalized for body size and that surgery should be considered at an earlier stage. Afterload reduction with vasodilators such as hydralazine, captopril, and nifedipine has been shown to reduce regurgitant volume and ventricular size in aortic regurgitation. Treatment with nifedipine, 20 mg twice a day, has been shown to delay the

Table 16.1: *Physical signs associated with hyperdynamic pulse in chronic aortic regurgitation*

Physical sign	*Description*
Water-hammer or corrigan's pulse	Rapid upstroke followed by quick collapse
DeMusset's sign	Head bob with each heartbeat
Traube's sign	Pistol shot sound heard over the femoral arteries in both systole and diastole
Muller's sign	Systolic pulsation of the uvula
Duroziez's sign	Systolic murmur over the femoral artery when compressed proximally and diastolic murmur when compressed distally or systolic-diastolic murmur with increasing compression over femoral artery
Quincke's sign	Capillary pulsations visible in the lunula of the nailbed
Hill's sign	Popliteal cuff systolic pressure exceeding brachial cuff systolic pressure by >60 mmHg
Becker's sign	Arterial pulsations visible in the retinal arteries and pupils

Table 16.2: *Indications for aortic valve replacement in severe chronic aortic regurgitation*

Indication	*Class*
Patients with NYHA functional class III or IV symptoms and preserved left ventricular (LV) systolic function, defined as normal ejection fractinal rest (ejection fraction ≥ 0.50)	I
Patients with NYHA functional class II symptoms and preserved LV systolic function (ejection fraction ≥0.50) but with progressive LV dilatation or declining ejection fraction at rest on serial studies or declining effort tolerance on exercise testing	I
Patients with Canadian Heart Association functional class II or greater angina with or without coronary artery disease	I
Asymptomatic or symptomatic patients with mild to moderate LV dysfunction at rest (ejection fraction 0.25– 0.49)	I
Patients undergoing coronary artery bypass surgery or surgery on the aorta or other heart values	
Patients with NYHA functional class II symptoms and preserved LV systolic function (ejection fraction ≥ 0.50 at rest) with stable LV size and systolic function on serial studies and stable exercise tolerance	IIa
Asymptomatic patients with normal LV systolic function (ejection fraction >0.50) but with severe LV dilatation (end-diastolic dimension >75 mm or end-systolic dimension >55 mm)	IIa
Patients with severe LV dysfunction (ejection fraction <0.25)	IIb
Asymptomatic patients with normal systolic function at rest (ejection fraction >0.50) and progressive LV dilatation when the degree of dilatation is moderalelly severe (end-diastolic dimension 70–75 mm, end-systolic dimension 50–55 mm)	IIb
Asymptomatic patients with normal systolic function at rest (ejection fraction >0.50) but with a decline in ejection fraction during	III
Exercise radionuclide angiography	IIb
Stress echocardiography	III
Asymptomatic patients with normal systolic function at rest (ejection fraction >0.50) LV dilatation when degree of dilatation is not severe (end-diastolic dimension < 70 mm, end-systolic dimension <50 mm)	III

NYHA, New York Heart Association.

Adapted from Bonow HO, Carabello B, de leon AC Jr, et al. Guidelines for the management of patients with valvular heart disease; a report of the American College of Cardiology/American Heart Association Task Force on Practice Guidelines (Committee on Management of Patients with Valvular Heart Disease). J AM Coll Cardiol 1998;32:1496.

need for surgical intervention in chronic asymptomatic aortic regurgitation but has not been widely used for this indication. Acute severe aortic regurgitation necessitates urgent surgery. Intravenous vasodilatation with sodium nitroprusside or another vasodilator can reduce the regurgitant volume and help to stabilize the patient awaiting surgery.

Surgical Intervention (Table 16.2)

Surgical intervention in aortic regurgitation is usually undertaken to improvement in symptoms and left ventricular size. Although the operative risk is increased when severe left ventricular dilatation or dysfunction is present, significant improvement in symptoms and ventricular function often occurs after surgery; the prognosis without surgery is very poor. Aortic regurgitation usually requires insertion of a prosthesis or a human valve. Occasionally, repair is feasible, especially in prolapsing bicuspid valves when the aortic ring is dilated.

TRICUSPID VALVE AND PULMONARY ARTERY DISEASE

Tricuspid regurgitation is most often secondary to right ventricular dilatation and is the most common valvular

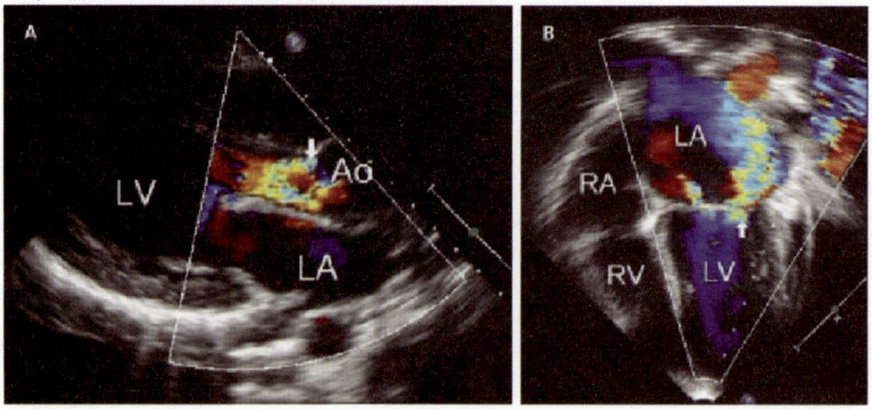

Fig. 16.40: *Two dimensional color and spectral Doppler echocardiographic studies of patients with rheumatic heart disease show moderate to severe aortic valve insufficiency with no stenosis (A, arrow) and bowing of the anterior mitral leaflet with severe insufficiency and no stenosis (B, arrow)*

problem of the right heart. Tricuspid regurgitation is recognized on physical examination by the characteristic large V waves in the jugular venous pulse and by a systolic murmur heard at the base of the xiphisternum that increases on inspiration.

In severe cases, pulsatile hepatomegaly is present. Doppler echocardiography allows rapid detecion in the assessment of the severity of the regurgitation (Figs 16.41 and 16.42).

Presentation often includes fatigue from reduced forward output and peripheral edema. Severe tricuspid regurgitation is usually treated with surgical repair. If a repair is not possible, a bioprosthesis is usually implanted because of the increased risk of thrombosis of a mechanical prosthesis at this position. Secondary tricuspid regurgitation can improve if the primary condition leading to pulmonary hypertension is treated and leads to a decrease in right heart size.

Tricuspid stenosis occurs in approximately 5–10% of patients with severe mitral stenosis. The characteristic physical findings are a large A wave in the jugular venous pressures and a diastolic murmur over the tricuspid area. Doppler echocardiography and right heart catheterization are both used to assess severity. The mean gradient across the tricuspid valve is typically greater than 5 mmHg. In patients with significant stenosis, either balloon dilatation or surgical repair or replacement is indicated (Figs 16.43 to 16.45).

Congenital Pulmonary Stenosis

It occurs in isolation or as part of various syndromes and is usually detected before adulthood. Significant pulmonary stenosis is treated with balloon dilatation or surgery. Significant pulmonary insufficiency is rare but can occur with a carcinoid tumor or endocarditis or secondary to pulmonary hypertension. Pulmonary allograft implantation is indicated for severe cases (Figs 16.46 to 16.49 and 16.51).

PROSTHETIC VALVES

Prostheses can be classified into two groups:

1. Mechanical
2. Biologic each having different properties, problems and indications.

Mechanical Prostheses

Mechanical prostheses are of two main types: ball-in-cage and tilting-disk. The Starr-Edwards valve is the prototypical ball-in-cage valve that has been implanted with various modifications since the 1960s. Tilting-disk vales can consist of one or two leaflets. Single-leaflet models include the Björk-Shiley and Medtronic-Hall valves. The most commonly implanted bileaflet models are the St. Jude valve and the CarboMedics valve. The major advantage of mechanical prostheses is durability. Mechanical prostheses can remain functional for decades and are used especially in young or middle-aged patients to reduce the need for reoperation. Their chief disadvantage is the associated risk of thromboembolism, which necessitates long-term anticoagulation and carries a risk of hemorrhage. An increased incidence of subsequent infection, hemolysis,

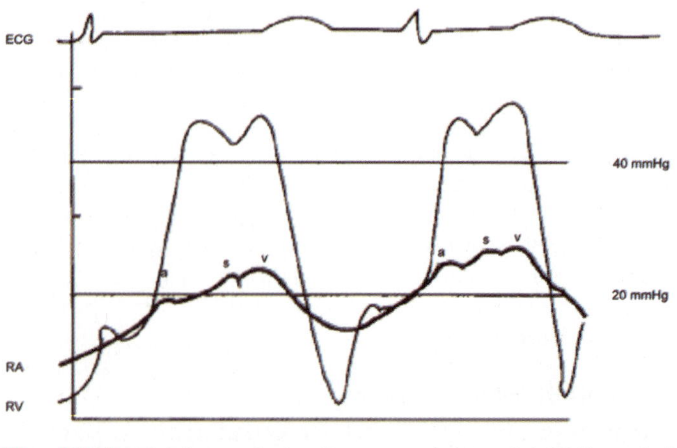

Fig. 16.41: *Tracings of simultaneous right atrial (RA) and right ventricular (RV) pressure in a patient with tricuspid regurgitation*

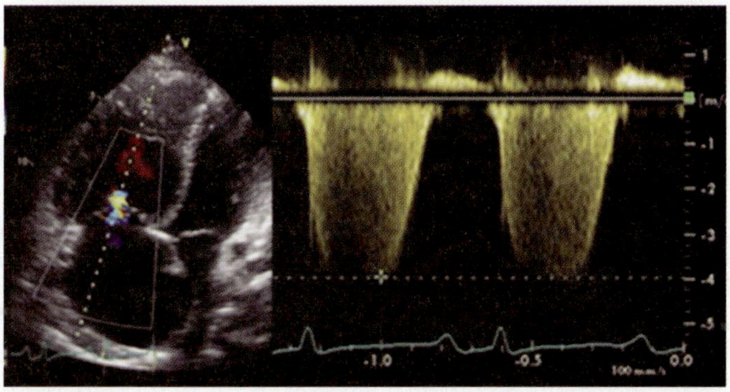

Fig. 16.42: *(Left) 2D apical 4C view showing tricuspid regurgitation jet into right atrium. (Right) continuous wave (CW)-color Doppler showing tricuspid regurgitant jet*

thrombosis of the valve, and mechanical failure is another problem associated with mechanical prostheses.

Bioprostheses

Three classes of biologic valves are currently available. A xenograft is a prosthesis fashioned from animal tissue. Most xenografts consist of modified porcine valves that are preserved in glutaraldehyde and mounted on a stent prostheses have also been constructed of pericardium and other biologic materials. Stentless bioprostheses are under investigation and are postulated to improve the effective size of the prosthetic valve opening. Allografts (homografts) are human valves that have been harvested postmortem and either cryopreserved or treated with antibiotics. An autograft is a valve from the patient's own body that is moved to a different anatomic site. The most common autograft is the pulmonary valve inserted at the aortic position. A pulmonary allograft is inserted in its place. Patients with biologic valves have a lower risk of thromboembolism than those with mechanical prostheses and do not usually require long-term anticoagulation. Biologic valves are indicated for patients in whom anticoagulation is inappropriate. Xenografts are less durable than mechanical prostheses. Xenografts are not usually inserted in patients younger than 60 years because of the poor survival record in this group. Allografts and autografts are alternatives to mechanical prosthetic implantation at the aortic or pulmonary positions in younger patients. Insertion of these valves is technically more demanding and is not widely done. No long-term survival benefit of allografts over xenografts has been demonstrated. Autografts have proved to be durable and have the potential to grow in situ. They are used in the management of pediatric and adolescent patients with aortic valve disease. Both allografts and autografts result in a low reinfection rate when used in the treatment of prosthetic aortic endocarditis and are considered the valve replacement of choice for this condition (Fig. 16.50).

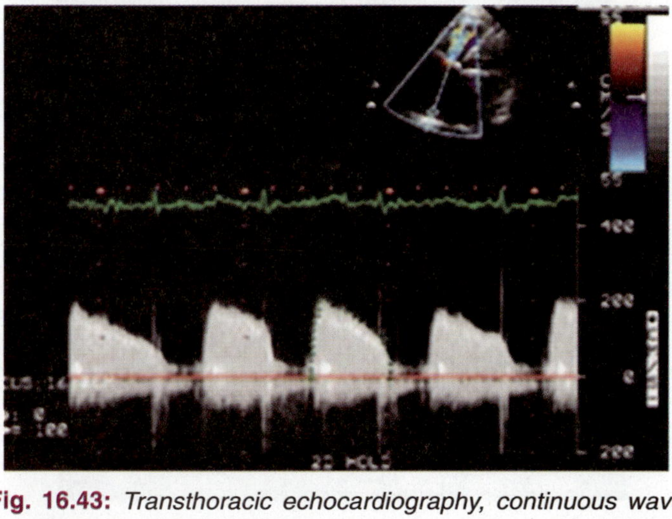

Fig. 16.43: *Transthoracic echocardiography, continuous wave Doppler at the level of tricuspid valve in a patient with tricuspid stenosis*

Problems and Complications of Valve Prostheses

Thromboembolism

Systemic anticoagulation with warfarin or dicumarol decreases the incidence of, but does not eliminate the occurrence of, thromboembolism with mechanical valves. The incidence of thromboembolic events is lowest in patients younger than 50 years, lower with aortic prostheses than with mitral or multiple prostheses, and lower with bileaflet disk valves than with single-leaflet valves. Hemorrhagic events are more common in older patients. Anticoagulation is generally monitored using the international normalized ratio (INR). Studies have indicated that the level of anticoagulation required to prevent thromboembolism is less than was previously thought. A large study of anticoagulation in patients with mechanical prostheses has suggested that an INR of between 2.5 and 4.0 is desirable in most instances and minimizes hemorrhagic and thromboembolic complications. The appropriate INR for an individual patient will vary depending on the history of embolic or bleeding events; age; and type, position, and number of prostheses. Antiplatelet agents such as aspirin (81 mg q.d.) or clopidogrel may be added to the anticoagulation regimen in patients who have sustained recurrent thromboembolic

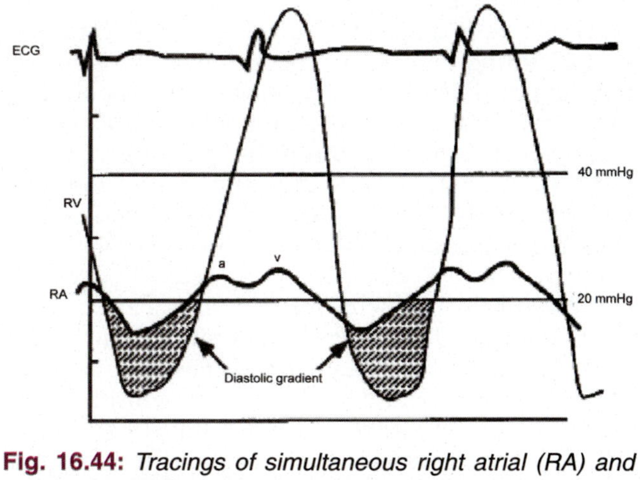

Fig. 16.44: *Tracings of simultaneous right atrial (RA) and right ventricular (RV) pressure waveforms in a patient with tricuspid stenosis*

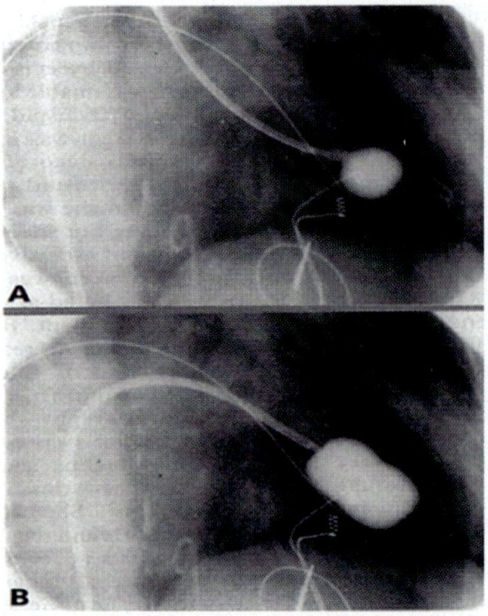

Fig. 16.45: *The Inoue balloon was used for dilatation of tricuspid stenosis in an adolescent. The valve was reached by an over-the-wire approach with a 0.025 exchange length guidewire. The Inoue stylet would not reach the tricuspid orifice because the right atrium was so large. The Inoue balloon's special dilatation characteristics allowed good positioning at the tricuspid orifice. After dilatation to 27.5 mm, the pressure drop across the valve was reduced from 12–5 mmHg. Further dilatation at 30 mm, however, created moderately severe tricuspid reflux without a further reduction of gradient. The Inoue balloon is suitable for dilatation of tricuspid stenosis but small increments in dilatation size may be required for optimal reduction in gradient without creating significant reflux*

events despite adequate anticoagulation. Thromboembolic risk with xenografts is greatest in the first 3 months after surgery. During this period, oral anticoagulation medications are recommended for high-risk patients (e.g. those with mitral prostheses or paroxysmal atrial fibrillation); for patients who are not at high risk, aspirin, 325 mg/day, is recommended.

Valvular Thrombosis

Acute thrombosis of a mechanical valve is more common with a single tilting-disk valve. The incidence is highest at the tricuspid position, followed by the mitral position, and is least common at the aortic position. Thrombosis of left-sided valves can lead to acute pulmonary edema and systemic thromboembolism. Reduced motion of the disk or ball is characteristic of valvular thrombosis and can be demonstrated with transesophageal echocardiography or fluoroscopy. There is usually an increased pressure gradient across the valve. Acute thrombosis of a mechanical valve is an indication for emergency surgery to remove the thrombus and to implant another prosthesis. In patients who are not surgical candidates or who are considered at high operative risk, thrombolysis has been used successfully to increase valve opening and motion and reduce the valve gradient. Success rates greater than 70% have been reported in a number of series. Thromboembolism is the most common complication of thrombolysis in this setting and occurs in 12–22% of patients. Further episodes of valvular thrombosis after initial successful thrombolysis have been reported.

Valve Failure (Fig. 16.46)

In mechanical prostheses, failure of one of the mechanical parts is rare but can have catastrophic consequences. Failure is most common with tilting-disk valves, particularly with the Björk-Shiley single-leaflet tilting-disk valve, which is no longer available commercially in the United States. Failure of the outlet strut in several of these models led to embolization of the disk and acute valve failure, with high morbidity and mortality. Prophylactic repeat surgery has been recommended for certain groups of patients in whom the failure rate is highest. Advanced imaging techniques designed to detect sites of potential strut fractures are currently in development.

Valve failure is expected with bioprostheses and allografts. Fortunately, degeneration is a slow process in biologic prostheses and is usually present for years before significant hemodynamic consequences are seen. Leaflet calcification can give rise to stenosis, whereas cusp degeneration can lead to perforation, with resultant regurgitation. Bioprosthetic degeneration is managed in the same way as stenosis or regurgitation of a native valve. Repeat surgery is indicated for significant symptoms or progressive ventricular enlargement or dysfunction.

Failure of either a mechanical or a biologic prosthesis can occur because of failure of the sutures holding the valve in place. Sutures can fail because of associated infection, but they can also fail spontaneously. A St. Jude valve in which the sewing ring was impregnated with silver nitrate

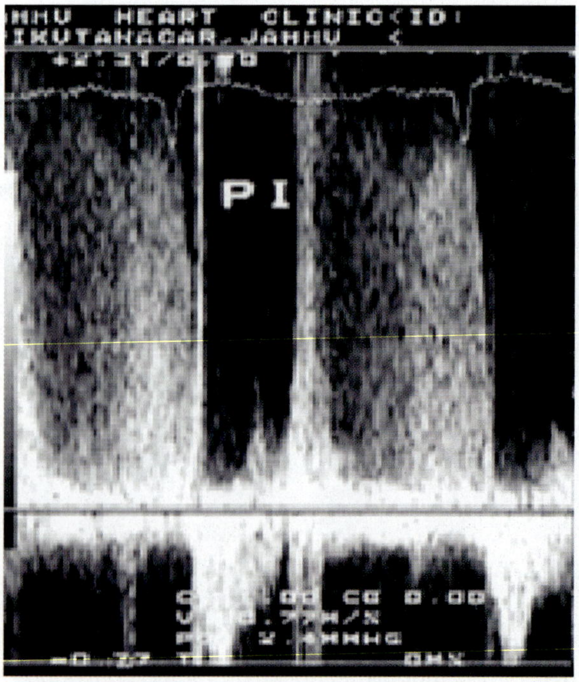

Fig. 16.46: *Doppler echoscan showing severe type of pulmonary regurgitation in patient with pulmonary valvular insufficiency*

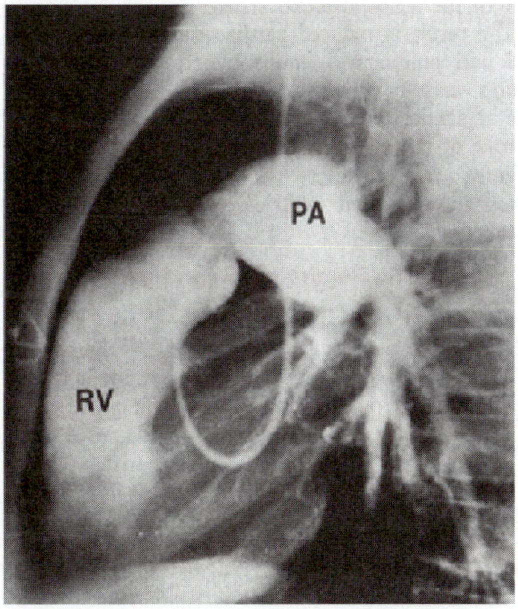

Fig. 16.47: *Contrast medium has been injected into the main pulmonary artery (PA) and regurgitation back into an enlarged right ventricle (RV) in patient with pulmonic valvular regurgitation*

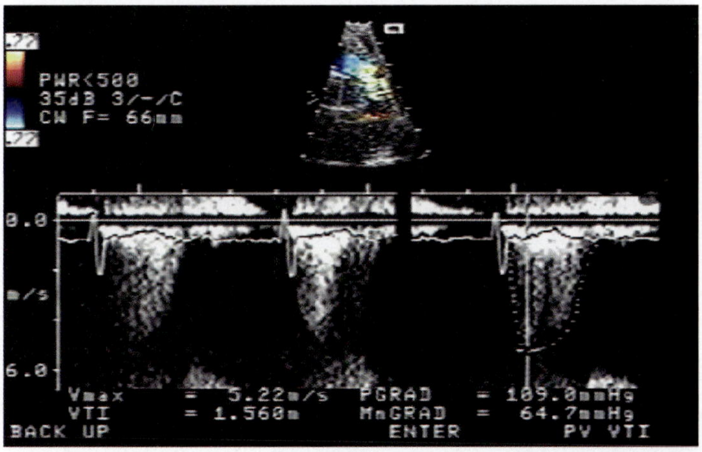

Fig. 16.48: *Pulmonic stenosis. Echocardiogram of a patient with severe pulmonic stenosis. This image shows a Doppler scan of the peak velocity (5.2 m/s) and gradients (peak 109 mmHg, mean 65 mmHg) across the valve*

to reduce the likelihood of infection was recalled because of a high incidence of paravalvular leak. The paravalvular leak resulting from suture failure can begin as a relatively mild lesion, but progression is common. In severe instances, partial or complete dehiscence can result in a characteristic rocking motion of the valve, as revealed by echocardiography. Paravalvular leaks are often accompanied by significant hemolysis as red blood cells are destroyed at the site of increased shear stress. Hemodynamically significant paravalvular leaks are considered an indication for reoperation.

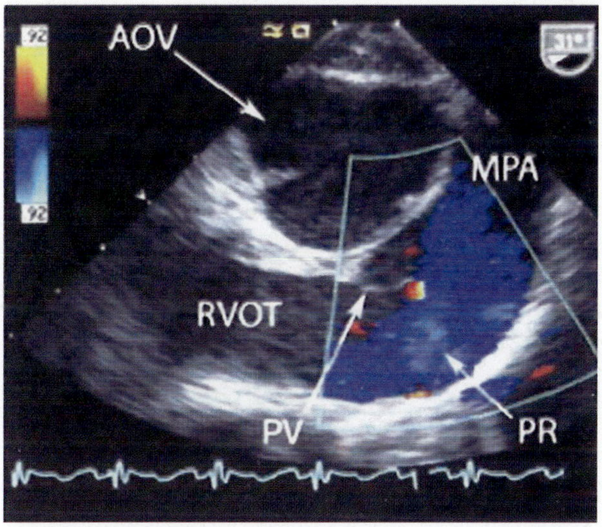

Fig. 16.49: *Preoperative echocardiogram demonstrating severe pulmonary valve regurgitation located anteriorly through the gap created by the transannular patch. (AOV, aortic valve; MPA, main pulmonary artery; PR, pulmonary regurgitation; PV, pulmonary valve; RVOT, right ventricular outflow tract.)*

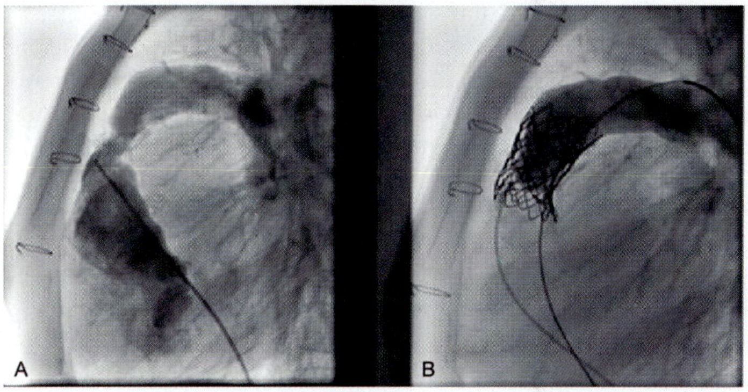

Fig. 16.50: *The implantation of the percutaneous pulmonary valve was performed with excellent results (A) severe stenosis of the homograft. (B) resolution of the stenosis, no regurgitation*

Infection

There is an increased risk of endocarditis with mechanical prostheses and xenografts, compared with native valves or allografts. Prosthetic valve endocarditis is often associated with abscess formation. Prosthetic vegetation and abscess formation are best evaluated by using transesophageal echocardiography, which should be performed if a diagnosis of prosthetic valve endocarditis is being considered. Prosthetic valve endocarditis is extremely difficult to eradicate with medical treatment alone; operative intervention is usually required.

Inherent or Acquired Prosthetic Stenosis

All prosthetic valves are inherently stenotic, but in an appropriately selected prosthesis, the degree of stenosis is mild and not of clinical significance. Occasionally, a smaller than desirable prosthesis is implanted because the native

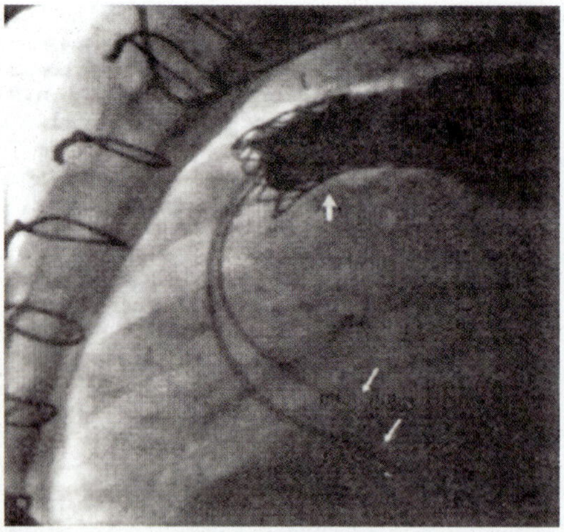

Fig. 16.51: *Double balloon (arrows) across PV for dilatation of valve in patient with pulmonic stenosis*

valve annulus is small. In such cases, patients can manifest symptoms and signs of valvular stenosis and have severely increased pressure gradients across the valve, especially during exercise. In severe cases, explantation of the prosthesis and annular reconstruction may be necessary to accommodate a prosthesis of sufficient size. In some patients with mechanical prostheses, ingrowth of a fibrous pannus can impede blood flow and lead to hemodynamic stenosis, requiring reoperation.

Anorexiant-Induced Valvular Disorder

Drugs that suppress appetite (anorexiants) have been reported to cause a valvular disorder similar to that caused by ergot derivatives and carcinoid syndrome. This finding was first reported in 1997, and a number of large studies since then have confirmed an increased prevalence of valvular disorders in populations treated with fenfluramine, dexfenfluramine, phentermine, or a combination of these drugs Over 18 million prescriptions were filled for these drugs in 1996 alone. The precise pathophysiology of the valvular disorder is still unclear. All of these anorexiants affect central serotininergic receptors. A causal relation of serotonin in this disorder is also suggested by the disorder's similarity to carcinoid disease, in which serotonin is also implicated as a causative factor. Initial reports suggested a high prevalence of valvular disease in patients treated with these anorexiants, and they were withdrawn from the market in September 1997. The prevalence of clinically symptomatic valve-related disease in patients receiving these drugs has been reported to be 1 in 1,000.

Anorexiant-drug valvulopathy affects mainly the aortic and mitral valve. Leaflet thickening, restricted leaflet motion, chordal thickening, and valve regurgitation without stenosis are the most common abnormalities seen. Although valvular disease severe enough to warrant surgery has been reported, in many instances the valvular lesion appears to be mild or moderate in severity. Factors thought to increase the likelihood of more severe disease are longer duration of treatment with anorexiant therapy, use of drug combinations, and higher dosages of drugs. Patients who received less than 3 months of treatment appear to have a relatively low likelihood of significant valvular disease. Studies also suggest that the valvular lesions may not progress and may even regress after discontinuance of the drug. Patients exposed to anorexiants should undergo a thorough cardiovascular examination for signs of mitral or aortic regurgitation. Echocardiography is indicated if the physical findings suggest valvular disease or if the duration of treatment has been more than 3 months. Patients with evidence of valvular disease on echocardiography should be followed serially and receive prophylactic antibiotics for dental and other procedures associated with significant bacteremia.

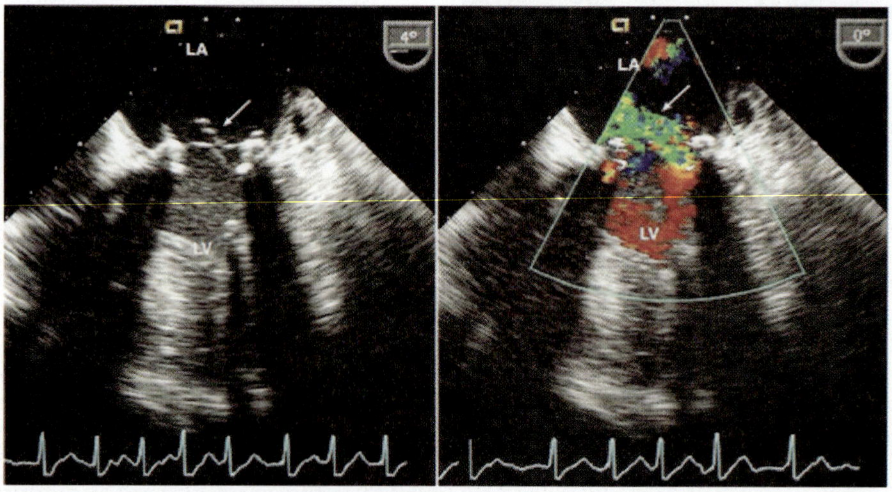

Fig. 16.52: *Bioprosthetic valve structural failure. TEE echocardiography showing a stented tissue mitral valve prosthesis with a flail leafed row, due to endocarditis on 2D imaging (left). Color flow shows an eccentric jet of regurgitation through the valve with a wide vena contracta with severe prosthetic regugitation (right)*

BIBLIOGRAPHY

1. Rose AG: Etiology of valvular heart disease. Curr Opin Cardiol 11:98, 1996.
2. Tamura K, Fukuda Y, Ishizaki M, et al: Abnormalities in elastic fibers and other connective-tissue components of floppy mitral valve. Am Heart J 129:1149, 1995.
3. Devereux RB: Recent developments in the diagnosis and management of mitral valve prolapse. Curr Opin Cardiol 10:107, 1995.
4. Feldman T: Rheumatic heart disease. Curr Opin Cardiol 11:126, 1996.
5. Otto CM, Lind BK, Kitzman DN, et al: Association of aortic valve sclerosis with cardiovascular mortality and morbidity in the elderly. N Engl J Med 341:142, 1999.
6. Roldan CA, Shively BK, Crawford MH: An echocardiographic study of valvular heart disease associated with systemic lupus erythematosus. N Engl J Med 335:1424, 1996
7. Connolly HM, Crary JL, McGoon MD, et al: Valvular heart disease associated with fenfluramine-phentermine. N Engl J Med 337:581, 1997.
8. Gardin JM, Schumacher D, Constantine G, et al: Valvular abnormalities and cardiovascular status following exposure to dexfenfluramine or phentermine/fenfluramine. JAMA 283:1703, 2000.
9. Dajani AS, Taubert KA, Wilson W, et al: Prevention of bacterial endocarditis: recommendations by the American Heart Association. JAMA 277:1794, 1997.
10. Oakley CM: Valvular disease in pregnancy. Curr Opin Cardiol 11:155, 1996.
11. Bonow RO, Carabello BA, de Leon AC, et al: ACC/AHA guidelines for the management of patients with valvular heart disease. Circulation 98:1949, 1998.
12. Faletra F, Pezzano A, Fusco R, et al: Measurement of mitral valve area in mitral stenosis: four echocardiographic methods compared with direct measurement of anatomic orifices. J Am Coll Cardiol 28:1190, 1996.
13. Dajani AS, Taubert K, Ferrieri P, et al: Treatment of streptococcal pharyngitis and prevention of rheumatic fever. Pediatrics 96:758, 1995.
14. Gohlke-Burwolf C, Acar J, Oakley C, et al: Guidelines for prevention of thromboembolic events in valvular heart disease: study group of the working group on valvular heart disease of the European Society of Cardiology. Eur Heart J 16:1320, 1995.
15. Elliott JM, Tuzcu EM: Recent developments in balloon valvuloplasty techniques. Curr Opin Cardiol 10:128, 1995.
16. Palacios IF, Tuzai ME, Weyman AE, et al: Clinical follow-up of patients undergoing percutaneous mitral balloon valvotomy. Circulation 91:671, 1995.
17. Dean LS, Mickel M, Bonan R, et al: Four-year follow-up of patients undergoing percutaneous balloon mitral commissurotomy: a report from the National Heart, Lung and Blood Institute Balloon Valvuloplasty Registry. J Am Coll Cardiol 28:1452, 1996.
18. Orrange SE, Kawanishi DT, Lopez BM, et al: Actuarial outcome after catheter balloon commissurotomy in patients with mitral stenosis. Circulation 95:382, 1997.
19. Reyes VP, Raju BS, Wynne K, et al: Percutaneous balloon valvuloplasty compared with open surgical commissurotomy for mitral stenosis. N Engl J Med 331:961, 1994.
20. Gupta A, Lokhandwada YY, Satoskar PR, et al: Balloon mitral valvotomy in pregnancy: maternal and fetal outcome. J Am Coll Surg 187:409, 1998.
21. Pathan AZ, Mahdi NA, Leon MN, et al: Is redo percutaneous mitral balloon valvuloplasty (PMV) indicated in patients with post-PMV mitral stenosis? J Am Coll Cardiol 34:49, 1999.
22. Pu M, Vandervoort PM, Greenberg NL, et al: Impact of wall constraint on velocity distribution in proximal flow convergence zone. J Am Coll Cardiol 27:706, 1996.
23. Leung DY, Griffin BP, Stewart WJ, et al: Left ventricular function after valve repair for chronic mitral regurgitation: predictive value of preoperative assessment of contractile reserve by exercise echocardiography. J Am Coll Cardiol 28:1198, 1996.
24. Enriquez-Sarano M, Schaff HV, Orszulak TA, et al: Congestive heart failure after surgical correction of mitral regurgitation: a long-term study. Circulation 92:2496, 1995.
25. Gaasch WH, John RM, Aurigemma GP: Managing asymptomatic patients with chronic mitral regurgitation. Chest 108:842, 1995.
26. Ling LH, Enriquez-Sarano M, Seward JB, et al: Early surgery in patients with mitral regurgitation due to flail leaflets: a long-term outcome study. Circulation 96:1819, 1997.
27. Ling LH, Enriquez-Sarano M, Seward JB, et al: Clinical outcome of mitral regurgitation due to flail leaflet. N Engl J Med 335:1417, 1996.
28. Bach DS, Bolling SF: Improvement following correction of secondary mitral regurgitation in end stage cardiomyopathy with mitral annuloplasty. Am J Cardiol 78:966, 1996.
29. Bolling SF, Pagani FD, Deeb GM, et al: Intermediate term outcome of mitral reconstruction in cardiomyopathy. J Thorac Cardiovasc Surg 115:381, 1998.
30. Rosario LB, Stevenson LW, Solomon SD, et al: The mechanism of decrease in dynamic mitral regurgitation during heart failure treatment: importance of reduction of regurgitant orifice size. J Am Coll Cardiol 32:1819, 1998.
31. Levine HJ, Gaasch WH: Vasoactive drugs in chronic regurgitant lesions of the mitral and aortic valves. J Am Coll Cardiol 28:1083, 1996.
32. Enriquez-Sarano M, Schaff HV, Orszulak TA, et al: Valve repair improves the outcome of surgery for mitral regurgitation: a multivariate analysis. Circulation 91:1022, 1995.
33. Grossi EA, Galloway AC, Miller JS, et al: Valve repair versus replacement for mitral insufficiency: when is a mechanical valve still indicated? J Thorac Cardiovasc Surg 115:389, 1998.
34. Stewart WJ: Choosing the "golden moment" for operation in the era of valve repair for mitral regurgitation. American College of Cardiology Heart House Learning Center Highlights 10:2, 1995.
35. Gillinov AM, Cosgrove DM, Lytle BW, et al: Reoperation for failure of mitral valve repair. J Thorac Cardiovasc Surg 113:467, 1997.
36. Corin WJ, Sutsch G, Murakami T, et al: Left ventricular function in chronic mitral regurgitation: preoperative and postoperative comparison. J Am Coll Cardiol 25:113, 1995.
37. Oakley CM: Management of valvular stenosis. Curr Opin Cardiol 10:117, 1995.
38. Otto CM, Burwash IG, Legget ME, et al: Prospective study of asymptomatic valvular aortic stenosis: clinical, echocardiographic, and exercise predictors of outcome. Circulation 95:2262, 1997.

39. Tseng EE, Lee CA, Cameron DE: Aortic valve replacement in the elderly: risk factors and long-term results. Ann Surg 225:793, 1997.
40. Wang A, Harrison JK, Bashore TM: Balloon aortic valvuloplasty. Prog Cardiovasc Dis 40:27, 1997.
41. Dolan MS, Castello R, St. Vrain JA, et al: Quantitation of aortic regurgitation by Doppler echocardiography: a practical approach. Am Heart J 129:1014, 1995.
42. Bonow RO: Chronic aortic regurgitation: role of medical management and optimal timing of surgery. Cardiol Clin 16:449, 1998.
43. Klodas E, Enriquez-Sarano M, Tajik AT, et al: Aortic regurgitation complicated by extreme left ventricular dilation: long-term outcome after surgical correction. J Am Coll Cardiol 27:670, 1996.
44. Scognamiglio R, Rahimtoola SH, Fasoli G, et al: Nifedipine in asymptomatic patients with severe aortic regurgitation and normal left ventricular function. N Engl J Med 33:689, 1994.
45. Vongpatanasin W, Hillis LD, Lange RA: Prosthetic heart valves. N Engl J Med 335:407, 1996.
46. Zellner JL, Kratz JM, Crumbly AS, et al: Long-term experience with the St Jude Medical valve prosthesis. Ann Thorac Surg 68:1210, 1999.
47. Cohn LH, Collins JJ, Rizzo RJ, et al: Twenty-year follow up of the Hancock modified orifice porcine aortic valve. Ann Thorac Surg 66(6 suppl):S30, 1998.
48. Banbury MK, Cosgrove DM, Lytle BW, et al: Long-term results of the Carpentier-Edwards pericardial aortic valve: a 12-year follow up. Ann Thorac Surg 66(6 suppl):S73, 1998.
49. Walther T, Falk V, Langebartels G, et al: Prospectively randomized evaluation of stentless versus conventional biological aortic valves: impact on early regression of left ventricular hypertrophy. Circulation 100(19 suppl):II6, 1999.
50. Ross DN: Evolution of the homograft valve. Ann Thorac Surg 59:565, 1995.
51. Chambers JC, Somerville J, Stone S, et al: Pulmonary autograft procedure for aortic valve disease: long-term results of the pioneer series. Circulation 96:2206, 1997.
52. Milano A, Guglielmi C, DeCarlo M, et al: Valve-related complications in elderly patients with biological and mechanical aortic valves. Ann Thorac Surg 66(6 suppl):S82, 1998.
53. Lupinetti FM, Warner J, Jones TK, et al: Comparison of human tissues and mechanical prostheses for aortic valve replacement in children. Circulation 96:321, 1997.
54. Cannegieter SC, Rosendaal FR, Wintzen AR, et al: Optimal oral anticoagulant therapy in patients with mechanical heart valves. N Engl J Med 333:11, 1995.
55. Heras M, Chesebro JH, Fuster V, et al: High risk of thromboemboli early after bioprosthetic cardiac valve replacement. J Am Coll Cardiol 25:1111, 1995.
56. Binder T, Baumgartner H, Maurer G: Diagnosis and management of prosthetic valve dysfunction. Curr Opin Cardiol 11:131, 1996.
57. Barbetseas J, Nagueh SF, Pitsavos C, et al: Differentiating thrombus from pannus formation in obstructed mechanical prosthetic valves: an evaluation of clinical, transthoracic and transesophageal echocardiographic parameters. J Am Coll Cardiol 32:1410, 1998.
58. Kallewaard M, Algra A, Defauw J, et al: Prophylactic replacement of Bjork-Shiley convexo-concave valves at risk of strut fracture: Bjork-Shiley Study Group. J Thorac Cardiovasc Surg 115:577, 1998.
59. O'Neill WW, Chandler JG, Gordon RE, et al: Radiographic detection of strut separations in Björk-Shiley convexo-concave mitral valves. N Engl J Med 333:414, 1995.
60. Garcia MJ, Vandervoort PM, Stewart WJ, et al: Mechanism of hemolysis with mitral prosthetic regurgitation: a study using transesophageal echo and fluid dynamic simulation. J Am Coll Cardiol 27:399, 1996.
61. Chan WS, Anand S, Ginsberg JS: Anticoagulation of pregnant women with mechanical heart valves: a systemic review of the literature. Arch Intern Med 160:191, 2000.
62. Weyman AE: The left ventricular outflow tract. Principles and Practice of Echocardiography, 2nd ed., rev. Weyman AE, Ed. Lea & Febiger, Philadelphia, 1994.
63. Currie PJ, Seward JB, Reeder GS, et al: Continuous wave Doppler echocardiographic assessment of severity of calcific aortic stenosis: a simultaneous Doppler-catheter correlative study in 100 adult patients. Circulation 71:1162, 1985.
64. Jick H, Vasilakis C, Weinnarich LA, et al: A population based study of appetite suppressant drugs and the risk of cardiac valve regurgitation. N Engl J Med 339:719, 1998.
65. Weissman NJ, Tighe JF, Gottdiener JS, et al: An assessment of heart-valve abnormalities in obese patients taking dexfenfluramine, sustained-release dexfenfluramine, or placebo. N Engl J Med 339:725, 1998.
66. Jick H: Heart valve disorders and appetite-suppressant drugs. JAMA 283:1738, 2000.
67. Weissman NJ, Tighe JF, Gottdiener JS, et al: Prevalence of valvular-regurgitation associated with dexfenfluramine three to five months after discontinuation of treatment. J Am Coll Cardiol 34:2088, 1999.
68. Griffin BP, Stewart WJ. Echocardiography in patient selection, operative planning, and intraoperative evaluation of mitral valve repair. In: Otto CM, ed. The practice of clinical echocardiography, 2nd ed. Philadelphia: WB Saunders, 2002:417–434.
69. Grossman W. Profiles in valvular heart disease. In: Bairn DS, Grossman W, eds. Cardiac catheterization, angiography and intervention, 5th ed. Baltimore: Williams & Wilkins, 1996:735–756.
70. Meier DJ, Landolfo CK, Starling MR. Role of echocardiography in the timing of sur-gical intervention for chronic mitral and aortic regurgitation. In: Otto CM, ed. The practice of clinical echocardiography, 2nd ed. Philadelphia: WB Saunders, 2002: 389–416.
71. Reid CL. Echocardiography in the patient undergoing catheter balloon mitral com-missurotomy. In: Otto. CM, ed. The practice of clinical echocardiography, 2nd ed. Philadelphia: WB Saunders, 2002:435–450.
72. Stewart WJ. Intraoperative echocardiography. In: Topol EJ, ed. Textbook of cardiovascular medicine. Philadelphia: Lippincott-Raven Publishers, 1998:1492–1525.
73. Weyman AE. Left ventricular inflow tract. I. The mitral valve. In: Weyman AE, ed. Principles and practice of echocardiography, 2nd ed. Philadelphia: Lea & Febiger,1994:391–470.
74. Enriquez-Sarano M, Schaff HV, Orszulak TA, et al. Valve repair improves the out-come of surgery for mitral regurgitation: a multivariate analysis. Circulation 1995;91:1022–1028.

75. Enriquez-Sarano M, Tajik AJ, Schaff HV, et al. Echocardiographic prediction of survival after surgical correction of organic mitral regurgitation. Circulation 1994;90: 830–837.
76. Enriquez-Sarano M, Tajik AJ, Schaff HV, et al. Echocardiographic prediction of left ventricular function after correction of mitral regurgitation: results and clinical implications. JAm Coll Cardiol 1994;24:1536–1543.
77. Farhat MB, Ayari M, Maatouk F, et al. Percutaneous balloon versus surgical closed and open mitral commissurotomy: seven year follow-up results of a randomized trial. Circulation 1998;97:245–250.
78. Freed LA, et al. Prevalence and clinical outcome of mitral-valve prolapse. N Engl J Med 1999:341:1–7.
79. Gillinov AM, et al. Durability of mitral valve repair for degenerative disease. J Thorac Cardiovasc Burg 1998;116: 734–743.
80. Gorlin R, Gorlin G. Hydraulic formula for calculation of area of stenotic mitral valve, other cardiac values and central circulatory shunts. Am Heart J 1951;41:1.
81. Hatle L, Brubakk A, Tronsdal A, Angelsen B. Noninvasive assessment of pressure drop in mitral stenosis by Doppler ultrasound. Br Heart J 1978;40:131–140.
82. Leung DY, Griffm BP, Stewart WJ, et al. Left ventricular function after valve repair for chronic mitral regurgitation: predictive value of preoperative assessment of contractile reserve by exercise echocardiography. J Am Coll Cardiol 1996;28: 1198–1205.
83. Levine RA, et al. Three-dimensional echocardiographic reconstruction of the mitral valve, with implications for the diagnosis of mitral valve prolapse. Circulation 1989;80:589–598.
84. Ling LH, Enriquez-Sarano M, Seward JB, et al. Clinical outcome of mitral regurgitation due to flail leaflet. N Engl J Med 1996;335:1417–1423.
85. Marks AR, et al. Identification of high-risk and low-risk subgroups of patients with mitral-valve prolapse. N Engl J Med 1989;320:1031–1036.
86. Reyes VP, Raju BS, Wynee J, et al. Percutaneous balloon valvuloplasty compared with open surgical commissurotomy for mitral stenosis. N Engl J Med 1994;331:961–967.
87. Wilkins GT, Weyman AE, Abascal VM, et al. Percutaneous balloon dilatation of the mitral valve: an analysis of echocardiographic variables related to outcome and the mechanism of dilatation. Br Heart J 1988;60:299–308.
88. Carabello BA. Mitral valve disease. Curr Probl Cardiol 1993;18:426–478.
89. Carabello BA, Crawford FA. Valvular heart disease. N Engl J Med 1997;337:32–41.
90. Irvine T. Assessment of mitral regurgitation. Heart 2002;88:iv11-iv19.
91. Stewart WJ. Choosing the golden moment for mitral valve repair. J Am Coll Cardiol 1994;24:1544–1546.
92. Thomas JD. How leaky is that mitral valve? Simplified Doppler methods to measure regurgitant orifice area. Circulation 1997;95:548–550.
93. Thomas JD. Doppler echocardiographic assessment of valvular regurgitation. Heart 2002;88:651–657.
94. Alpert JS, Sabik J, Cosgrove DM III. Mitral valve disease. In: Topol EJ, ed. Textbook of cardiovascular medicine, 2nd ed. Philadelphia: Lippincott-Raven Publishers, 2001:483–509.
95. Braunwald E. Valvular heart disease. In: Braunwald E, ed. Heart disease: a textbook of cardiovascular medicine, 5th ed. Philadelphia: WB Saunders, 1997:1007–1076.
96. Carabello B, Grossman W. Calculation of stenotic valve orifice area. In: Baim DS, Grossman W, eds. Cardiac catheterization, angiography and intervention, 5th ed. Baltimore: Williams & Wilkins, 1996:151–166.
97. Scully HE, Armstrong CS. Tricuspid valve replacement: fifteen years of experience with mechanical prosthesis and bioprosthesis. J Thorac Cardiovasc Burg 1995; 109:103521041.
98. Van Nooten GJ, Caes FL, Francois KJ, et al. The valve choice in tricuspid valve eplacement: 25 years of experience. Eur J Cardiothorac Burg 1995;9:441–446.
99. Braunwald E.Heart disease: a textbook of cardiovascular medicine, 5th ed. Philadelphia: WB Saunders, 1997:1007–1076.
100. Cheitlin MD, Macgregor JS. Acquired tricuspid and pulmonary valve disease. In: Topol EJ, ed. Textbook of cardiovascular medicine, 2nd ed. Philadelphia: Lippincott-Raven Publishers, 2002:529–548.
101. Weyman AE. Principles and practice of echocardiography, 2nd ed. Philadelphia: Lea & Febiger, 1994:824-862
102. Connolly HM, Crary JL, McGoon MD, et al. Valvular heart disease associated with fenfluramine-phentermine. N Engl J Med 1997;337:581–588.
103. Jick H, Vasilakis C, Weinrauch LA, et al. A population-based study of appetite-suppressant drugs and the risk of cardiac-valve regurgitation. N Engl J Med 1998;339:719–724.
104. Shively BK, Roldan CA, Gill EA, et al. Prevalence and determinants ofvalvulopathy in patients treated with dexfenfluramine. Circulation. 1999;100:2161–2167.
105. Weissman NJ, Tighe JF Jr, Gottdiener JS, et al. Sustained-Release Dexfenfluramine Study Group. An assessment of heart-valve abnormalities in obese patients taking dexfenfluramine, sustained-release dexfenfluramine, or placebo. N Engl J Med 1998;339:725–732.
106. Braunwald E. Valvular heart disease. In: Braunwald E, ed. Heart disease: a textbook of cardiovascular medicine, 5th ed. Philadelphia: WB Saunders, 1997:1059-1061.
107. Cheitlin MD, MacGregor JS. Acquired tricuspid and pulmonary valve disease. In: Topol EJ, ed. Textbook of cardiovascular medicine. Philadelphia: Lippincott-Raven Publishers, 2002:529–548.
108. Bellamy MF, Pellika PA, Klarich KW, et al. Association of cholesterol levels, hydroxymethylglutaryl coenzyme-A reductase inhibitor treatment, and progression of AS in the community. J Am Coll Cardiol 2002;40:1723–1730.
109. Bonow RO, Carabello B, de Leon AC Jr, et al. Guidelines for the management of patients with valvular heart disease: A report of the American College of Cardiology/American Heart Association Task Force on Practice Guidelines (Committee on Management of Patients with Valvular Heart Disease). J Am Coli Cardiol 1998;32:1496.
110. Borer JS, Hochreiter C, Herrold EM, et al. Prediction of indications for valve replacement among asymptomatic or minimally symptomatic patients with chronic aortic regurgitation and normal left ventricular performance. Circulation 1998;97: 525–534.
111. Brener SJ, Duffy CI, Thomas JD, Stewart WJ. Progression of aortic stenosis in 394 patients: relation to changes in myocardial and mitral valve dysfunction. JAm Coli CardiolI995;25:305–310.

112. Connolly HM, Oh JK, Schaff HV, et al. Severe aortic stenosis with low transvalvular gradient and severe left ventricular dysfunction: result of aorti valve replacement in 52 patients. Circulation 2000;101:1940–1946.
113. Currie PJ, Sewaard JB, Chan KL, et al. Continuous wave Doppler echocardiographic assessment of severity of calcific aortic stenosis: a simultaneous Doppler-catheter correlative study in 100 consecutive patients. Circulation 1985;71:1162–1169.
114. Kelly TA, Rothbart RM, Cooper CM, et al. Comparison of outcome of asymptomatic to symptomatic patients older than 20 years of age with valvular aortic stenosis. Am J Cardiol 1988;61:123–130.
115. Khot UN, Novaro GM, Popovic ZB, et al. Nitroprusside in critically ill patients with left ventricular dysfunction and aortic stenosis. N Engl J Med 2003;348: 1756–1763.
116. Novaro GM, Tiong IY, Pearce GL, et al. Effect of hydroxymethylglutaryl coenzyme a reductase inhibitors on the progression of calcific aortic stenosis. Circulation 2001;104:2205–2209.
117. Otto CM, Burwash IG, Legget ME, et al. Prospective study of asymptomatic valvular aortic stenosis: clinical, echocardiographic, and exercise predictors of outcome. Circulation 1997;95:2262–2270.
118. Otto CM, Lind BK, Kitzman DW, et al. Association of aortic-valve sclerosis with cardiovascular morbidity and mortality in the elderly. N Engl J Med 1999;341: 142–147.
119. Pellikka PA, Nishimura RA, Bailey KR, Tajik AJ. The natural history of adults with asymptomatic, hemodynamically significant aortic stenosis. J Am Coll Cardiol 1990;15:1012–1017.
120. Pereira JJ, Lauer MS, Bashir M, et al. Survival after aortic valve replacement for severe aortic stenosis with low transvalvular gradients and severe left ventricular dysfunction. J Am Coll Cardiol 2002;39:1356–1363.
121. Rosenhek R, Binder T, Porenta G, et al. Predictors of outcome in severe asymptomatic aortic valve stenosis. N Engl J Med 2000; 343:611–617.
122. Ross J Jr, Braunwald E. Aortic stenosis. Circulation 1968;37 [Suppl V]:V-61-V-67.
123. Braunwald E. On the natural history of severe aortic stenosis [Editorial]. J Am Coll Cardiol 1990;15:1018–1020.
124. Carabello BA. Timing of valve replacement in aortic stenosis: moving closer to perfection. Circulation 1997;95:2241–2243. Carabello BA, Crawford FA. Valvular heart disease. N Engl J Med 1997;337:32–41.
125. Gaasch WH, Sundaram M, Meyer TE. Managing asymptomatic patients with chronic aortic regurgitation. Chest 1997;111:1702–1709.
126. Carabello BA, Stewart WJ, Crawford FA. Aortic valve disease. In: Topol EJ, ed. Textbook of cardiovascular medicine, 2nd ed. Philadelphia: Lippincott-Raven, 2002: 509–528.
127. Meier DJ, Landolfo CK, Starling MR. Role of echocardiography in the timing of sur-gical intervention for chronic mitral and aortic regurgitation. In: Otto CM, ed. The practice of clinical echocardiography, 2nd ed. Philadelphia: WB Saunders, 2002:389–416.

17

Recognition and Management of Infective Endocarditis

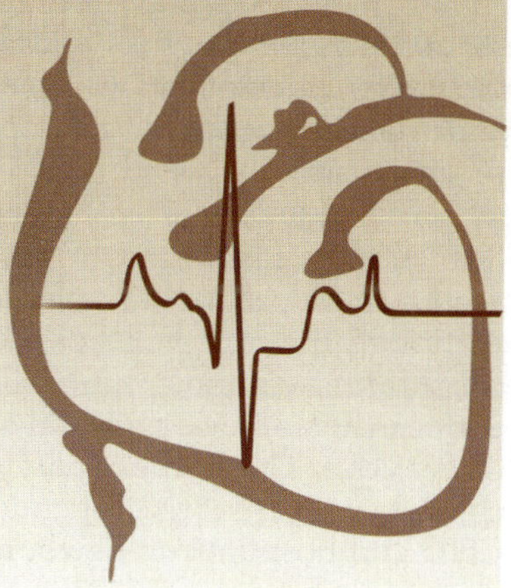

Infective endocarditis (IE) is associated with substantial morbidity and mortality. Although it is relatively rare in children, its incidence may be increasing. The present statement focuses on the features that are particularly relevant to infants and children including important issues for the primary care physician (Fig. 17.1).

The epidemiology of heart disease in children has changed during the past 3 to 4 decades. Because of the increased survival rate of children with congenital heart disease (CHD) and the overall decrease in rheumatic valvular heart disease in developed countries, CHD now constitutes the predominant underlying condition for IE in children over the age of 2 years in these countries. The complexities of management of neonatal and pediatric intensive care unit patients have increased the risks of catheter-related IE. In addition, postoperative IE is a long-term risk after correction of complex CHD.

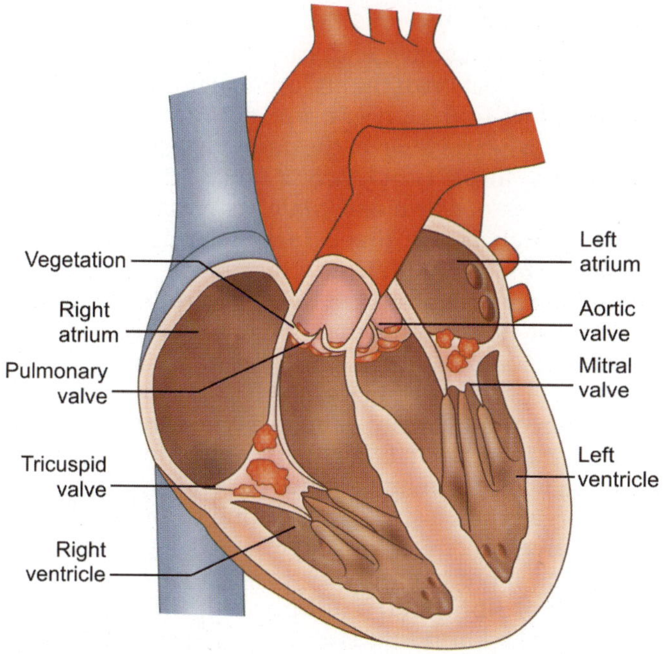

Fig. 17.1: *This cross-sectional view shows vegetations (accumulations of bacteria and blood clots) on the four valves of the heart*

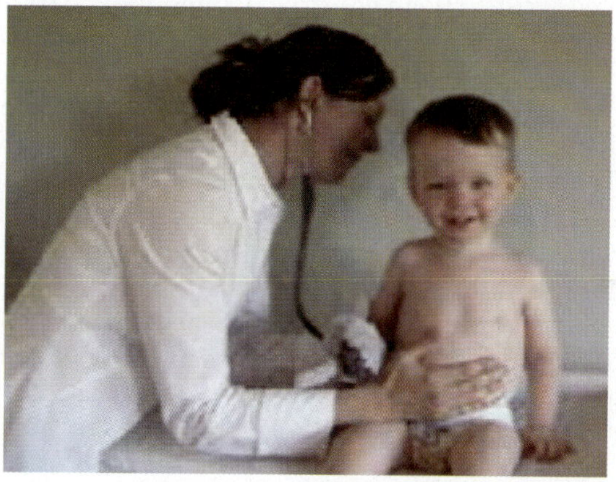

Fig. 17.2: *A young child is being examined by a doctor for physical signs of infective endocarditis*

Proper use of the diagnostic microbiology laboratory is critical in the diagnosis and management of children with IE. Moreover, newer diagnostic guidelines have improved sensitivity for making the diagnosis of clinically definite IE. Advances in noninvasive techniques, such as 2-

Table 17.1: *Localization of organisms according to the condition and site of origin*

Condition	*Location of stream*
Coarctation	Downstream wall
Patent ductus arterosus	Pulmonary artery
A-V fistula	Veins
Aortic insufficiency	Ventricular surface of valves
Mitral insufficiency	Atrial surface of mitral valves
Pulmonary insufficiency	Ventricular surface of pulmonary valve
Tricuspid insufficiency	Atrial surface of tricuspid valve

dimensional echocardiography, have enhanced our ability to diagnose IE. Newer antibiotics that can be used in children with IE have become available, and home intravenous therapy has become an acceptable approach for stable patients who are at low risk for embolization. In addition, approaches to the prevention of endocarditis recently have been modified and are reviewed in the present statement.

IE occurs less often in children than in adults and accounts for >1 in 1280 pediatric admissions per year. Although the reported hospitalization rates for IE vary considerably among published series, the frequency of endocarditis among children seems to have increased in recent years. This is due in part to improved survival among children who are at risk for endocarditis, such as those with CHD and hospitalized newborn infants.

As the prevalence of rheumatic heart disease has declined in developed countries, it has become unusual for patients with IE to have underlying rheumatic heart disease. At the same time, there has been an increase in cases of IE associated with CHD in children. Congenital heart defects, such as ventricular septal defect, patent ductus arteriosus, aortic valve abnormalities, and tetralogy of Fallot, are common underlying conditions. An increasing proportion of children with IE have had previous corrective or palliative surgery for CHD with or without implanted vascular grafts, patches, or prosthetic cardiac valves.

IE in the absence of CHD often is associated with central indwelling venous catheters. In >8–10% of pediatric cases, IE develops without structural heart disease or other identifiable risk factors and usually involves infection of the aortic or mitral valve secondary to *Staphylococcus aureus* bacteremia. Children with congenital or acquired immunodeficiencies but without identifiable risk factors for IE do not seem to be at increased risk for endocarditis compared with the general population. Factors often associated with IE in adults, such as intravenous drug abuse and degenerative heart disease, are not common predisposing factors in children.

In the century and a quarter since William Osler delivered his famed lectures on endocarditis, substantial advancements have occurred in the understanding and treatment of this disease.

Streptococcus viridans is the most common microbial agent responsible for infective endocarditis in children and adults. However, currently, staphylococcal aureus endocarditis is emerging as one of the leading causes of acute infective endocarditis particularily among those patients who are found to be malnourished and have congenital or acquired type of hypogamma-globulinemia with or without associated heart ailment.

Despite the decline in rheumatic heart disease world wide and the use of antibiotic prophylaxis, there is no evidence that the incidence of infective endocarditis is decreasing. In fact, some data suggest it may be increasing. Several factors explain this apparent paradox. First, in industrialized nations, patients are living longer; this results in a higher prevalence of degenerative cardiac disease, which can serve as a nidus for endocardial infection. Second, there is an increase in nosocomial infections which are often caused by species of bacteria or yeasts associated with infective endocarditis. Third, intravenous drug use has increased in industrialized societies. Fourth, increasing application of cardiac surgery has provided new substrates for endocardial infection. Fifth, the increased use of indwelling intravascular lines and implantable devices has resulted in many more catheter-related infections. bacteremias. and device-related infections. Finally, the increased application of echocardiography has probably increased the rate at which infective endocarditis is diagnosed.

These factors have also increased the variety of ways infective endocarditis can present. The classical fever of unknown origin presentation represents a minority of infective endocarditis cases today. Thus. clinicians need to be vigilant about keeping infective endocarditis in mind with some of these more unusual presentations. Gram negative and fungal endocarditis occur most often following cardiac surgery or in debilitated patients. A wide variety of organisms have been implicated in the causation of infective endocarditis. Cardiac malformation is the major factor predisposing to infective endocarditis. With the better survival rate in congenital heart disease, the incidence in this group has shown rather on the increase; whereas with rheumatic heart disease it had shown upward trend in developing countries and concomitant decrease in developed countries of the world. Cardiac defects which are more prone to this infection are tetralogy of Fallot, VSD with aortic regurgitation or obstruction, MVP with MR and those with prosthetic valve. The patients who had undergone recent cardiac surgery are also more prone to infective endocarditis.

Pathogenesis infective endocarditis is a disease caused by microbial infection of the endothelial lining of the heart. The characteristic lesion is a vegetation which usually develops on a heart valve. In the pathogenesis of infectious endocarditis, local turbulence is believed to promote a sterile network of fibrin and platelets on the endocardial surface, which is colonized later by microorganisms entering the bloodstream from a distant site. The infecting microorganisms are protected by the microthrombus from normal host defense mechanisms and from antibiotic penetration, requiring high dose parenteral antimicrobial agents over a long period. Whether the result of colonization of previously damaged heart endothelium or de novo infection of healthy tissues, the lesion is a vegetation whose primary features are a heavy colonization of microorganisms, a stroma consisting primarily of fibrin and a relative paucity of leukocytes. Once established, the vegetations have a tendency to enlarge with further deposition of fibrin and multiplication of the infecting organisms. The fibrin acts as a barrier to leukocytes; yet, it permitis diffusion of essential nutrients from the blood. The high density of infecting organisms and the difficulty for leukocytes to penetrate the nidus of infection partially explains the necessity of prolonged antimicrobials of primarily nature. Its cure usually requires surgical excision of the infected vegetations and valve replacement. Infective endocarditis represents an endothelial infection that usually occurs at sites of endothelial damage, with the superimposed thrombus serving as the nidus. For the nidus to become infected, bacteria must enter the blood stream in sufficient numbers from a break in the epidermal or mucosal surfaces of the body. As the vegetation grows, regurgitation of the affected valve almost always occurs due to destruction, scarring, and retraction of the leaflet Occasionally, chordal involvement results in rupture, causing sudden severe atrioventricular valve regurgitation. Very large vegetations rarely can obstruct the valve orifice. Embolization of vegetations can result in damage to other organs from ischemia or remote infection. Invasion of the valve annulus by the organisms can lead to abscesses and fistulas. Infection of arterial walls due to vegetation embolization would lead to aneurysm formation and rupture, which can be devastating in the central nervous system.

Incidence Osler's portentous words are as relevant now as when originally published. Despite improved preventive strategies, rational antibiotic prescribing, advances in imaging, and increasing use of early life saving cardiac surgery, the incidence of infective endocarditis remains high at 1.7–6.2 per 100,000 person years in the USA and Europe, with a 1 year mortality approaching 40%. The classical patient with infective endocarditis described in textbooks no longer represents the majority of cases in practice. The emergence of staphylococcal infection, often associated with indwelling devices, coexistent medical conditions and resistant to conventional antibiotic regimes, a variety of other atypical organisms, and the persistent syndrome of culture negative endocarditis make diagnosis and treatment as great a challenge as ever.

Diagnostic criteria: The original von Reyn diagnostic criteria for infective endocarditis, based upon clinical and microbiological features, have now been surpassed by the Duke criteria which emphasise the role of echocardiography, the key imaging tool for both diagnosis and assessment of prognosis. Many studies have now demonstrated the superiority of the Duke criteria and a recent scientific statement of the American Heart Association concluded that they should be adopted as the primary diagnostic schema in the clinical evaluation of patients in whom infective endocarditis is suspected. Nevertheless, clear deficiencies remain (Table 17.2).

Major criteria: Two positive blood cultures with atypical microbe. New murmur or echocardiogram finding of oscillating mass, abscess, or prosthetic valve dehiscence.

Minor criteria: Predisposing cardiac condition or IV drug use. Fever is > 35° celsius. Vascular phenomena, such as Osler's nodes, Janeway lesions. Immunologic phenomena, such as splenomegaly. Echocardiograrn consistent with endocarditis, but not meeting major criteria.

Table 17.2: *Duke criteria for the diagnosis of infective endocarditis*

Major criteria
1. Positive blood cultures (>2) with microbe typical for infective endocarditis, or persistently positive blood cultures with compatible microbe
2. Evidence of endocardial involvement: new regurgitant murmur or positive echocardiogram for oscillating mass, abscess, or prosthetic valve dehiscence
Minor criteria
1. Predisposing cardiac condition or intravenous drug use
2. Fever >38.0°C (100.4°F)
3. Vascular phenomena
4. Immunologic phenomena
5. Echocardiogram consistent with endocarditis, but not meeting major criteria
6. Positive blood culture, but not meeting major criteria, or positive serology or molecular test tor compatible microbe
Diagnosis
Definite endocarditis
1. Positive histology, or positive culture from vegetation
2. Two major criteria
3. One major and three minor criteria
4. Five minor criteria
Rejected
1. Firm alternative diagnosis established
2. Resolution after < 4 days of antibiotic treatment. Possible endocarditis (neither definite nor rejected)

Positive blood culture, but not meeting major criteria, or positive serology for a combatable microbe.

Definite diagnosis: Positive histology or positive culture from vegetation. Two major criteria, one major and three minor criteria—all six minor criteria.

Diagnosis rejected: Alternative diagnosis established Resolution of illness after 5–4 days of antibiotics. Possible diagnosis: neither definite nor rejected.

Clinical Presentation

Symptoms and signs malaise: Weight loss, fatigue, night sweats, fever, chills, arthralgias, myalgias. Specific symptoms due to sites of damge, such as dyspnea with heart failure due to severe valvular regurgitation.

Physical Examination (Fig. 17.2 and Table 17.2)

Osler's node, Janeway lesion, petechiae, splinter hemorrhages, Roth spots, blue toe syndrome.

- Fever
- Regurgitant heart murmurs, especially new or Worsemng
- Signs of heart failure
- Signs of stroke
- Splenomegaly
- Four peripheral stigmata of IE
- Janeway lesions
- Roth's spots
- Splinter hemorrhages
- Osler's nodes

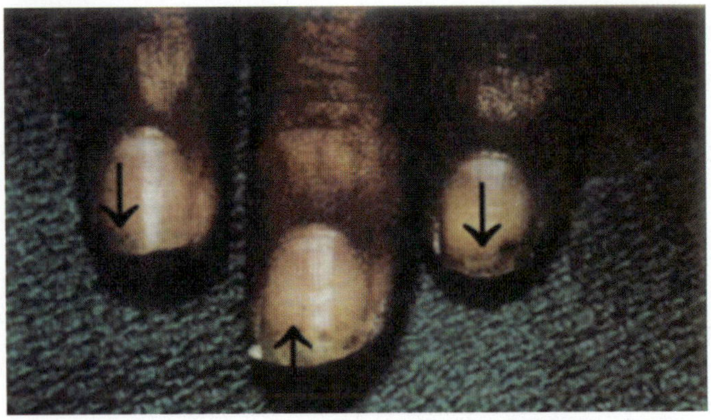

Fig. 17.3: *Suhungual or splinter hemorrahage in patient with infective endocaritis*

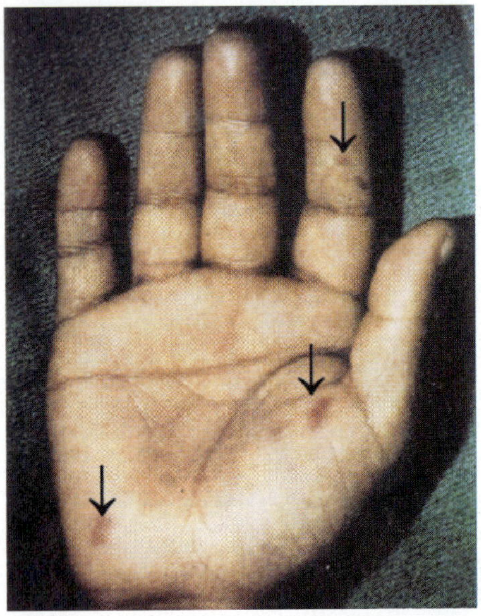

Fig. 17.4: *Janeway lesions on the palm in the same patient*

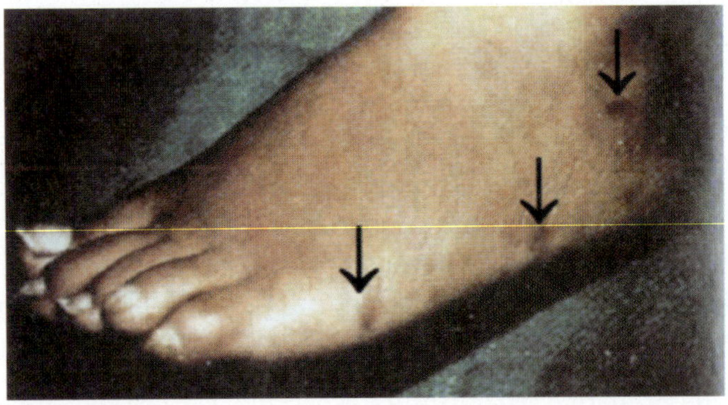

Fig. 17.5: *Janeway lesions on the foot of the same patient*

Differential Diagnosis

1. Fever due to other causes
2. Sepsis not due to infective endocarditis. Valvular lesions on echocardiography that resemble vegetations (e.g. myxomatous valves).

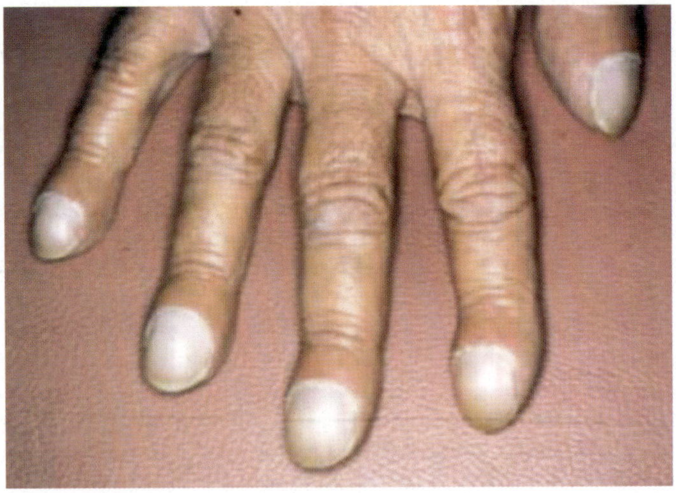

Fig. 17.6: *Clubbing of fingers in infective endocarditis*

Laboratory Tests

Blood cultures: Three from separate venipunctures over 24 hours.

Serologic testing for organisms such as histoplasma, Q fever, brucella.

Rheumatoid factor may be falsely positive leukocytosis, elevated gamma globulins, elevated erythrocyte sedimentation rate, anemia.

Electrocardiography

Aortic valve abscess formation can lead to first second-, or third-degree heart block (Figs 17.19, 17.20 and 17.23).

Increased QRS voltage in acute aortic or mitral regurgitation owing to left ventricular volume increase.

Imaging Studies

Chest X-ray may show cardiomegaly pulmonary edema, or septic pulmonary emboli (right-sided endocarditis) (Fig. 17.18).

Echocardiography

Transesophageal echocardiography is the preferred diagnostic technique because of its high sensitivity and specificity compared with transthoracic echocardiography.

1. Findings that are almost certainly endocarditis include (major criteria) oscillating low-density masses, abscess, fistulas, prosthetic valve dehiscence.
2. Probable endocarditis findings include localized leaflet thickening, nonmobile valve related masses, chordal rupture, aortic leaflet prolapse, paraprosthetic valve regurgitation (minor criteria).
3. Possible endocarditis findings include valve lesions such as diffuse thickening, which could be a substrate for endocarditis, but specific findings are not seen.
4. A negative echocardiographic study does not completely rule out endocarditis, but makes it less likely. If clinical suspicion remains high, a repeat study should be done in 5 days (Figs 17.7 to 17.15).

Diagnostic Procedures

Rarely, cardiac catheterization is done to draw blood cultures in proximity of the valve lesions (Table 17.5).

Medications

Appropriate antibiotic therapy.

Surgery

1. Cardiac surgery, usually to replace the infected valve(s). Absolute indications for valve surgery in endocarditis. Intracardiac abscess or fistula.
2. Left heart failure
3. Endocarditis due to fungi or gram-negative organisms New prosthetic valve paravalve regurgitation, fistula, ascess, or dehiscence.

Monitoring

ECG and blood pressure monitoring as appropriate in the hospital. Repeat blood cultures to assess response to therapy.

Diet and Activity

Restricted activiry: Low-salt diet.

Hospital Discharge Criteria

1. Resolution of problem
2. Sufficient IV therapy to warrant oral antibiotics
3. Successful surgery.

Follow-up

After course of antibiotics, repeat blood cultures and echocardiogram in 2–4 weeks; then careful clinical follow-up at 3-, 6-, then 12-month intervals.

Complications

- Heart failure
- Pulmonary edema
- Pericarditis
- Myocarditis
- Myocardial infarction
- Heart block
- Stroke
- Brain abscess
- Renal failure.

Sudden Death

Osler's or Austrian triad? Osler's or Austrian triad triad consists of endocarditis, pneumonia and meningitis. The most common organism is *Streptococcus pneumoniae*, which is especially prevalent in alcoholic (40%), elderly, and diabetic patients.

The course is fulminant, with rapid valve destruction and abscess formation. The aortic valve is most often, followed by the tricuspid valve.

Infection is usually responsive to penicillin, but resistant strains that require vancomycin are becoming more common.

Prognosis

Despite modern antibiotics and improved surgical techniques, mortaliry rate for patients with infective endocarditis is almost 40%.

Prevention

Antibiotic prophylaxis for invasive procedures/surgery in naturally colonized places such as the mouth, and gastrointestinal tract in patients with the substrate for endocarditis, such as rheumatic valvular disease, audible heart murmurs, or cyanotic congenital heart disease.

Culture Negative Infective Endocarditis and Atypical Organisms

Negative blood cultures occur in 2.5–31% of all cases of infective endocarditis, often delaying diagnosis and the onset of treatment with profound impact on clinical outcome. Moreover, the sensitivity of the Duke criteria, which rely heavily on microbiological indices, is diminished in this setting. Negative cultures arise most commonly as a consequence of prior antibiotic administration, but an increasingly common scenario is infection by fastidious organisms with limited proliferation under conventional culture conditions, or requiring specialized tools for identification. Such pathogens include *Coxiella*, *Legionella*, the HACEK group (*Haemophilus* species, *Actinobacillus actinomycetemcomitans*, *Cardiobacterium hominis*, *Eikenella corrodens*, and *Kingella kingae*), *Chlamydia*, *Bartonella*, *Tropheryma whippelii*, and fungi, including *Candida*, *Histoplasma*, and *Aspergillus species*, and *Torulopsis glabrata*. These organisms may be particularly common in cases of infective endocarditis affecting patients with prosthetic valves, indwelling venous lines, pacemakers, renal failure, and immuno-compromised states.

Modified Criteria and New Diagnostic Techniques

In 1997, Lamas and Eykyn proposed a number of clinical modifications to the Duke criteria to include newly diagnosed splenomegaly or clubbing, elevated inflammatory markers, haematuria, and the presence of central and peripheral venous lines ("the St Thomas modifications"). Simultaneously, recognition of the role of Q fever, a worldwide zoonosis caused by *Coxiella burnetti* and a particularly frequent cause of infective endocarditis in France, increasing prevalence of staphylococcal infection, and widespread use of transoesophageal echocardiography resulted in further modifications; these involved incorporating the acceptance of positive Q fever serology or bacteraemia caused by *Staphylococcus aureus* (regardless of its source) as major criteria and the elimination of minor echocardiographic criteria. A recent study compared these modifications in pathologically proven yet culture negative cases. Only 21% were classified as definite by the original Duke criteria, while 32% were definite by the modified Duke criteria, and the St Thomas modifications classified 62% correctly. Interestingly, the four additional cases identified correctly by the modified Duke criteria were upgraded on account of positive Q fever serology.

Furthermore, careful scrutiny led to identification of the causative organism in almost 50% of culture negative cases, achieved by serology (*C burnetti, Bartonella, Chlamydia psittaci*) in 24%, culture of the excised valve in 14%, microscopy of the excised valve in 5%, and nonvalve culture in 6%.

Histological/immunological techniques: Histological findings are included in the Duke and von Reyn diagnostic criteria and pathological examination of resected valvar tissue or embolic fragments remains the gold standard for the diagnosis of infective endocarditis. Pathological examination may also guide antimicrobial treatment if the causative agent can be identified by means of special stains or immuno histological techniques, and allow distinction from conditions whose echocardiographic features mimic infective endocarditis (for example, myxomas, fibroelastomas, and rheumatoid nodules). It should be noted that specimens are potentially infectious to the examiner, particularly when Q fever is suspected. The pathological hallmark of endocarditis is the demonstration of inflammatory changes in valvar tissue and/or vegetations, characteristically at the site of attachment or base of a vegetation. This finding is not specific, however, and inflammation is also a feature of degenerative and other valve pathology. Electron microscopy has high sensitivity and may help to characterise new microorganisms. However, it is time consuming and expensive and therefore reserved for cases in which other techniques fail to detect an organism. Histological criteria for the diagnosis of endocarditis have been proposed and a variety of specialised stains and immunohistological techniques [immunoperoxidase staining, enzyme-linked immunosorbent assay (ELISA) and immunofluorescent assay (ELIFA), and direct immunofluorescence using fluorescein conjugated monoclonal antibodies] are now available to allow the identification of elusive bacteria and fungi. *C burnetti* and *Bartonella* species are the most common etiological agents in culture negative endocarditis and may be easily detected by serological testing using indirect immunofluorescence or ELISA. Immunological analysis of urine may also allow detection of microorganism degradation products and ELISA detection of *Legionella* species has been described using this technique. However, the incorporation of these techniques into accepted diagnostic criteria awaits prospective validation.

Molecular techniques: Several molecular approaches have been assessed for the detection and identification of pathogens in a wide variety of infectious diseases. The polymerase chain reaction (PCR) utilising nucleic acid target or signal amplification, alone or in combination with sequence analysis, is most widely used and allows rapid and reliable detection of fastidious and nonculturable agents in blood and surgical material of patients with infective endocarditis. It may also be of value when phenotypic characterization is essential following isolation of two or more organisms in separate cultures (most commonly caused by contamination with skin commensals during sampling or polymicrobial infection in intravenous drug abusers). Indeed, the incorporation of such techniques as a major Duke diagnostic criterion has been proposed with widespread support. Specific primers are now available for many bacterial agents including *T whippelii, C burnetti*, and species of *Bartonella, Chlamydia, Brucella, Legionella, Mycobacteria*, and *Mycoplasma*. Future improvements include the possibility of quantitation by real time PCR eliminating the need for gel electrophoresis with faster, more accurate results, and the possibility of investigating common antimicrobial resistance genes enabling a targeted approach to antibiotic treatment.

Laboratory approach for blood sample study: Optimal antiseptic skin preparation is important and at least 10 mL of blood (less in children) should be obtained for each culture. Bacteraemia is usually continuous and there is no rationale for timing blood cultures to coincide with peaks of pyrexia. If there is a history of prior antibiotic treatment, maximum diagnostic yield may be achieved by diluting the culture broth and considering the use of sodium polyanetholsulfonate or a dedicated adsorbent resin, both of which inactivate antimicrobial effects. Multiple separate blood cultures are required and most guidelines recommend at least two, and most usually three sets. Although endocarditis caused by anaerobes is uncommon, blood cultures should be incubated in both aerobic and anaerobic atmospheres to detect organisms such as *Bacteroides* or *Clostridium* species. If all blood cultures remain negative at 5 days but infective endocarditis remains likely on clinical grounds, subculture onto chocolate agar plates may allow identification of an atypical organism, although prolonged culture for up to 2–3 weeks is associated with rising likelihood of contamination. At this stage, therefore, serum should be analysed for antibodies to organisms that cannot be cultured by routine methods, and, if available, antibodies to Gram-positive bacterial cell walls. Excised valves, vegetations or other relevant material should undergo microscopy, culture, histopathology, and relevant molecular techniques (usually PCR) which can also be applied to newly acquired blood samples or the original growth negative blood culture substrate.

Indications for Cardiac Surgery (Tables 17.3 and 17.8)

1. ***Heart failure:*** If heart failure is present, the mortality rate of native valve infective endocarditis is 55–85% in the case of medical treatment only and 10–35% in operated patients. The first indication for cardiac surgery in infective endocarditis is heart failure. It represents more than half of the indications. Heart failure caused by aortic regurgitation is particularly poorly tolerated (heart failure is better tolerated in the case of mitral regurgitation because the left atrium and the pulmonary vascular bed adapt better than the left ventricle to the regurgitant volume), and it progresses faster, thus needing rapid surgery. Not only does heart failure increase the mortality rate if there is no surgery, but it also increases the perioperative mortality rate: from 5–10% in patients without heart failure to 15–35%

in patients with heart failure. Moreover, delaying surgery increases the risk of perivalvar infection.

2. ***No control of infection:*** The first step is to make sure that there is no extra cardiac infectious location. If there is no such extracardiac location, cardiac surgery should be performed if the course of fever and inflammatory syndrome is unfavourable after 1 week of appropriate antibiotic treatment.
3. ***Vegetations and embolic risk:*** The literature on this topic contrasts greatly. The embolism rate varies from 10–50% in different series. Three quarters of embolisms occur before the beginning of antibiotic treatment. The embolic risk decreases greatly and regularly over time, from 15% after 1 week of treatment to 1% after 4 weeks of treatment. In mitral infective endocarditis, embolisms look to be more frequent if vegetations are located on the anterior leaflet than on the posterior leaflet. Embolisms are more frequent when vegetation size is more than 20 mm in some studies, but not in other studies. In a recent study, embolisms were more frequent when the size of the vegetations was more than 10 mm or when vegetations were very mobile. Embolisms should always be looked for not only by clinical means but also by systematic scanners (for example, cerebral, thoraco-abdominal), searching for clinically silent embolisms, especially in spleen and kidneys. Rapid surgery must be performed when there has been an embolic episode and when large and mobile vegetations remain. When there are large and/or mobile vegetations but no embolic event, the medical community is divided. The decision is easier in the case of mitral infective endocarditis when valve repair looks possible, or when there are other arguments for surgery (heart failure, no control of infection, severe valvar and perivalvar lesions, etc).
4. ***Perivalvular infection:*** Infective endocarditis on the aortic valve and prosthetic infective endocarditis are those most commonly associated with perivalvar infection, such as abscesses and intracardiac fistula: 10–40% of aortic valve infective endocarditis and 45–100% of prosthetic infective endocarditis. Occurrence and persistence of conduction disturbances are not very sensitive indicators of perivalvar infection, but they look very specific (85–90%). Rapid surgery is recommended in most cases since the perioperative risk increases with the delay to surgery. However, in large aortic abscesses, a large resection exposes the patient to the risk of postoperative complete atrioventricular block (Table 17.4).
5. ***Valvular obstruction:*** Valvular obstruction is an obvious indication for urgent surgery.
6. ***Unstable prosthesis:*** Dehiscence of an infected prosthesis means that there is perivalvar infection, and haemodynamic deterioration usually occurs quickly. Thus, rapid surgery is recommended.

   Prosthetic infective endocarditis in early prosthetic infective endocarditis > 12 months after valve replacement), most often the microorganism is a *Staphylococcus* and lesions are severe (abscess, prosthesis dehiscence). Redo-surgery is associated with a lower mortality rate than medical treatment alone, and it is most often necessary, although it may be technically difficult. The mortality rate of prosthetic infective endocarditis caused by *Staphylococcus aureus* is about 75% in the case of medical treatment and 25% in the case of combined medical and surgical treatment. Surgery is thus recommended in prosthetic infective endocarditis caused by *S. aureus* when there is an intracardiac complication. Medical treatment only may be sufficient in cases of late infective endocarditis caused by some microorganisms (oral streptococci, organisms from the HACEK group-haemophilus species, actinobacillus *Actinomycetemcomitans*, *Cardiobacterium hominis*, *Eikenella corrodens*, and *Kingella kingae*) if there are no signs of perivalvar infection (Fig. 17.16).
7. ***Fungal infective endocarditis:*** Infective endocarditis caused by *Candida* or *Aspergillus* are often complicated with very large vegetations, infectious metastases, perivalvar infection and embolisms. Amphotericin B poorly penetrates into vegetations. Rapid surgery is thus most often needed.
8. ***Difficult-to-treat microorganisms:*** Surgery is almost always needed in infective endocarditis caused by certain Gram-negative bacilli (for example, *Pseudomonas aeruginosa*, *Achromobacter xylosoxitans*), by *Brucella*, or by highly resistant enterococci.
9. ***Neurological complications:*** The rate of neurological complications varies from 15% to 45% in different series. They mostly are ischaemic cerebral vascular accidents, but also cerebral haemorrhages, ruptured mycotic aneurysms, meningitis and encephalopathy. A cerebral scan must always be performed in infective endocarditis, to look for silent cerebral vascular accidents. In the case of cerebral haemorrhage, an arteriography or an angiomagnetic resonance image must be performed, to look for a mycotic aneurysm. There is a risk of cerebral haemorrhage associated with cardiac surgery because of anticoagulation during and after the procedure.

The risk of cerebral haemorrhage is not increased in the case of a stroke without haemorrhage, but it is greatly increased if the stroke is haemorrhagic. In this case, cardiac surgery should be delayed 2–3 weeks. If there is a ruptured mycotic aneurysm, it must be resected, clipped or embolised before cardiac surgery.

Timing of cardiac surgery: Classically, early surgery was considered to be a greater risk than delayed surgery because of tissue inflammation and the surgery was technically more difficult. In fact, the duration of antibiotic treatment before surgery does not appear to influence the perioperative mortality, nor the rate of recurrent infective endocarditis. Surgery should be rapid in the case of haemodynamic deterioration, where there is no control of infection, or there are large and mobile vegetations. Decision as to the timing of surgery is particularly difficult when there is a neurological complication.

Echocardiography in infective endocarditis since Dillon and colleagues' in 1973 described valvar vegetations by M mode echocardiography, the technique has assumed an increasingly important role in the assessment and management of endocarditis. The development of two dimensional and later transesophageal echocardiography (TEE) has significantly improved the noninvasive detection of vegetations. Moreover, echo-Doppler studies provide clinically important information on the presence and degree of valvar destruction and their haemodynamic consequences, as well as on the existence of perivalvar infection. The diagnostic strategy proposed by Durack and colleagues (the Duke criteria) combined echocardiographic findings with clinical and microbiological data. Three echocardiographic findings were considered to be major criteria for the diagnosis of endocarditis (Fig. 17.8):

1. Presence of vegetations defined as mobile echodense masses implanted in a valve or mural endocardium in the trajectory of a regurgitant jet or implanted in prosthetic material with no alternative anatomical explanation
2. Presence of abscess(s) or (Fig. 17.7)
3. Presence of a new dehiscence of a valvar prosthesis. Abnormal echocardiographic findings not fulfilling those definitions were considered minor criteria. More recently the use of TEE has resulted in better imaging and therefore doubtful findings are not considered minor criteria any longer. Since the definite diagnosis of endocarditis requires the presence of two major criteria, or one major and three minor criteria, it is clear that echocardiography has assumed a crucial role in the diagnosis of the disease, particularly when blood cultures are negative. A negative TEE has an important clinical impact on the diagnosis of endocarditis with a high negative-predictive value ranging from 86–97%. In patients with native heart valves, a negative TEE virtually rules out the diagnosis of infective endocarditis. However, in the study of Sochowski and colleagues. Five out of 65 patients (7.6%) with an initially negative TEE were finally diagnosed with endocarditis: in three of the patients a TEE performed 1–2 weeks after the initial examination showed the presence of vegetations. This study underlines the importance of recognising the phase of the disease in which the study is performed, since vegetations may not be large enough to be visualized when endocarditis is suspected very early on. In common with other diagnostic techniques, specificity of echocardiography is related to the clinical indication and the type of population studied. The technique does not permit differentiation between septic vegetations and other aseptic vegetations present in other situations such as Libman-Sacks endocarditis in systemic lupus erythematosus, and antiphospholipid syndrome or marantic endocarditis. Vegetations persisting after effective treatment must not be interpreted as a clinical recurrence of the disease unless supported by clinical features and bacteriologic evidence. Specificity is influenced mainly by the presence of valvar thickening or calcifications and also by rupture mitral chordae tendinae or Lambl's nodules which can be confused with vegetation images. The usefulness of TEE in patients with suspected endocarditis on a native valve is related to the

Table 17.3: *Indications for surgery in patients with infective endocarditis*

Indication	*Evidence*
Emergency indication for cardiac surgery (same day)	
• Acute AR with early closure of mitral valve	A
• Rupture of a sinus valsalva aneurysm into a right heart chamber	A
• Rupture into the pericardium	A
Urgent indication for cardiac surgery (within 1–2 days)	
• Valvar obstruction	A
• Unstable prosthesis	A
• Acute AR or MR with heart failure, NYHA III–IV	A
• Septal perforation	A
• Evidence of annular or aortic abscess, sinus or aortic true or false aneurysm, fistula formation, or new onset condition disturbances	
• Major embolism-mobile vegetation >10 mm + appropriate antibiotic treatment <7–10 days	B
• Mobile vegetation >15 mm + appropriate antibiotic therapy <7–10 days	C
• No effective antimicrobial treatment available	A
Elective indication for cardiac surgery (earlier is usually better)	
• Staphylococcol prosthetic valve infective endocarditis	B
• Early prosthetic valve infective endocarditis (< months after surgyer)	B
• Evidence of progressive paravalvar prosthetic leak	A
• Evidence of valve dysfunction and persistent infection after 7–10 days of appropriate antibiotic treatment, as indicated by presence of fever or bacteroemia, provided there are no noncardiac causes for infection	A
• Fungal infective endocarditis caused by a mould	A
• Fungal infective endocarditis caused by a yeast	B
• Infection with difficult-to-treat organisms	B
• Vegetation growing larger during antibiotic treatment >7 days	C

results of the TTE. TEE is useful when TTE is negative or inconclusive.

Detection of vegetations: There is no better technique for noninvasive visualisation of vegetations than echocardiography. Overall the detection rate for vegetations by transthoracic echocardiography (TTE) in patients with a clinical suspicion of endocarditis averages around 50%" The diagnostic yield of the technique in the detection of vegetations is influenced by several factors: image quality; echogenicity and vegetation size; vegetation location; presence of previous valvar disease or valvar prosthesis; experience and skill of the examiner; and pretest probability of endocarditis (Figs 17.8 to 17.11).

Native valve endocarditis: The use of harmonic imaging has improved study quality, but not the sensitivity in the visualisation of vegetations. "Vegetation size also affects TTE sensitivity" since only 25% of vegetations < 5 mm and 70% of those between 6 mm and 10 mm are identified. Underlying valve disease may influence the diagnostic accuracy of TTE when a myxomatous mitral valve or sclerotic or calcified valves are present. These limitations have been overcome by TEE owing to its better resolution and multiple study planes. Many studies have compared the sensitivity and specificity of TTE and TEE in the diagnosis of vegetations. In the majority of these studies TTE sensitivity ranges between 40% and 63% and that of transesophgeal echocardiography (TEE) between 90% and 100%. A negative TEE has an important clinical impact on the diagnosis of endocarditis with a high negative predictive value ranging from 86–97%. In patients with native heart valves, a negative TEE virtually rules out the

Table 17.4: *Risk of infective endocarditis associated with pre-existing cardiac disorders*

Prophylaxis for endocarditis recommended

High-risk cardiac condigion
- Prosthetic heart valves
- Previous infective endocarditis
- Cyanotic congenital heart disease (single ventricle states, transposition of the great arteries, tetralogy of Fallot)
- Surgically constructed systemic-pulmonary shunts (e.g. Blalock shunt)

Intermediate-risk cardiac condition
- Mitral valve prolapse with regurgitation
- Acquired valvular dysfunction (e.g. rheumatic heart disease)
- Hypertrophic cardiomyopathy
- Most congenital cardiac malformations (other than those listed above and below

Prophylaxis for endocarditis not recommended

Low-risk cardiac condition (risk no greater than general population)
- Mitral valve prolapse without regurgitation
- Trivial valvular regurgitation on echocardiography without structural abnormality (except mitral valve prolapse)
- Isolated atrial septal defect
- Atherosclerotic plaque
- Coronary disease or previous coronary artery bypass surgery
- Cardiac pacemakers or defibrillators
- Previous Kawasaki's disease or rheumati fever without valvular dysfunction
- Surgically repaired intracardiac lesion, with minimal or no hemodynamic abnormality more than 6 months after operation
- Innocent heart murmur

Adapted from Dajani AS, Tauberi KA, Wilson W, et al. Prevention of bacterial endocarditis: recommendations by the American Heart Association. Circulation 1997;96:358–356.

Table 17.5: *Echocardiographic characteristics of infective endocarditis*

Location	*Findings*
Aortic valve	Shaggy nonuniform thickening in systole or diastole with unrestricted leaflet motion Dense shaggy echoes moving across valve and into LVOT Flail or ruptured cusps Fine diastolic fluttering on anterior mitral leaflet secondary to aortic insufficiency
Mitral Valve	Thick shaggy echoes attached to or moving behind leaflets demonstrat-ingunne stricted motion Systolic flutter of prolapsing segments of mitral valve Fuzzy leaflet echoes in left atrial cavity during systole (differentiate from myxoma)
TV and PV	Shaggy thickening of leaflets, demonstrating unrestrictive motion Mass of echoes moving with leaflets (dependent motion) Rupture of tricuspid chordae tendinae
Prosthetic valve	Thick shaggy collection located behind site of attachment of prosthesis to valve ring Evidence of severe regurgitation

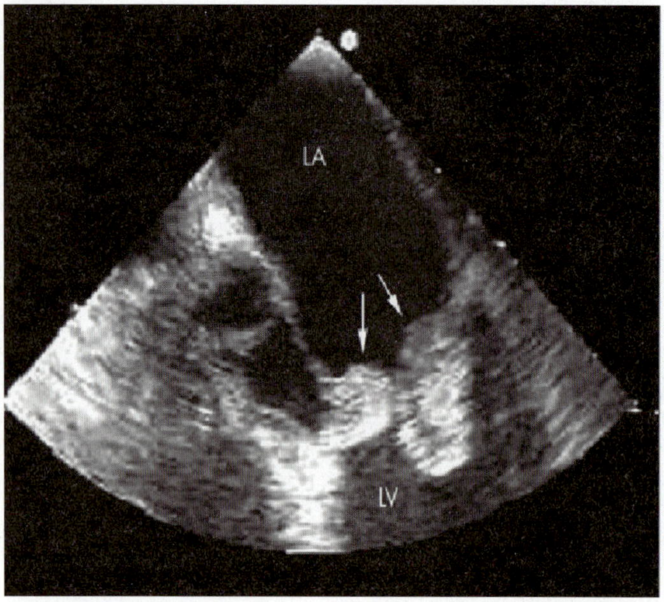

Fig. 17.7: *Large vegetations (arrows) in the mitral valve secondary to fungal endocarditis. LA, left atrium; LV, left ventricle*

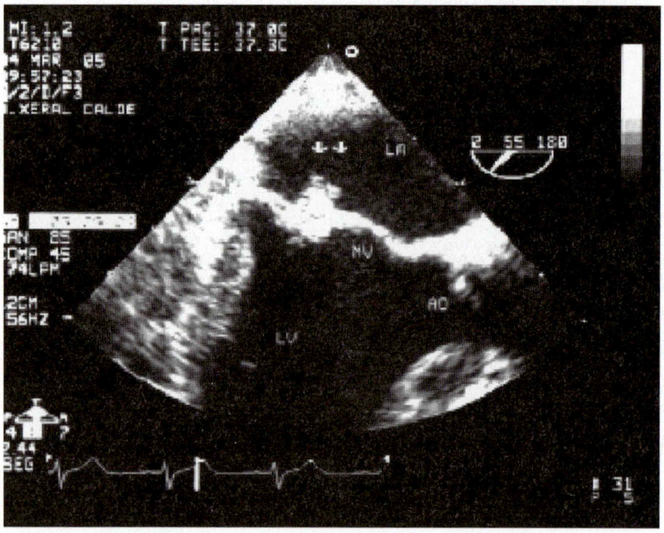

Fig. 17.8: *Longitudinal transesophageal echocardiogram view with zoom showing two native mitral valve vegetations (arrows). MV, mitral valve; LA, left atrium; LV, left ventricle; AO, aortic valve*

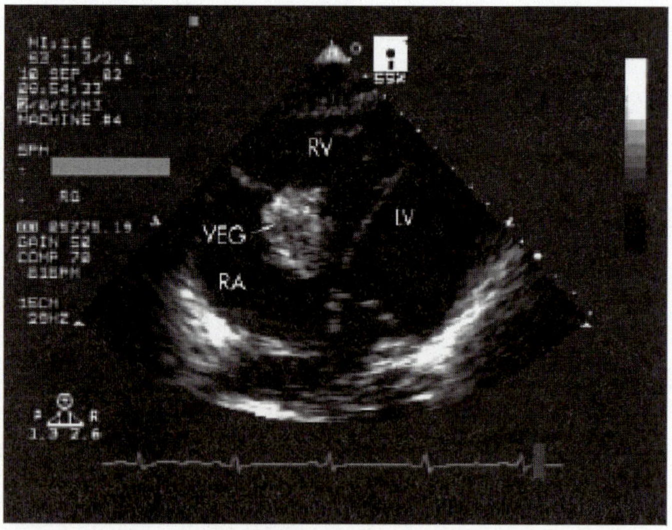

Fig. 17.9: *Large vegetations (arrows) in the tricuspid valve. LA, left atrium; LV, left ventricle*

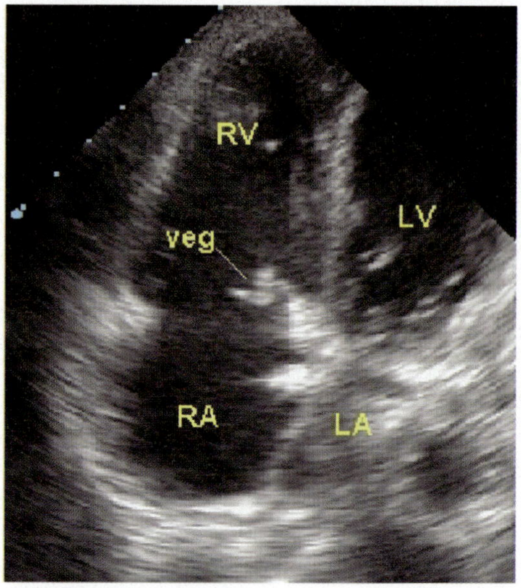

Fig. 17.10: *Apical four chamber view showing vegetation on tricuspid valve*

diagnosis of infective endocarditis. However, in the study of Sochowski and colleagues. Five out of 65 patients (7.6%) with an initially negative TEE were finally diagnosed with endocarditis: in three of the patients a TEE performed 1–2 weeks after the initial examination showed the presence of vegetations. This study underlines the importance of recognizing the phase of the disease in which the study is performed, since vegetations may not be large enough to be visualized when endocarditis is suspected very early on. In common with other diagnostic techniques, specificity of echocardiography is related to the clinical indication and the type of population studied. The technique does not permit differentiation between septic vegetations and other aseptic vegetations present in other situations such as Libman-Sacks endocarditis in systemic lupus erythematosus, and antiphospholipid syndrome or marantic endocarditis. Vegetations persisting after effective treatment must not be interpreted as a clinical recurrence of the disease unless supported by clinical features and bacteriologic evidence. Specificity is influenced mainly by the presence of valvar thickening or calcifications and also by rupture mitral chordae tendinae or Lambl's nodules which can be confused with vegetation images. The usefulness of TEE in patients with suspected endocarditis on a native valve is related to the results of the TTE. TEE is useful when TTE is negative or inconclusive.

Prosthetic valve endocarditis: Vegetations on prosthetic valves are more difficult to detect by TTE than those

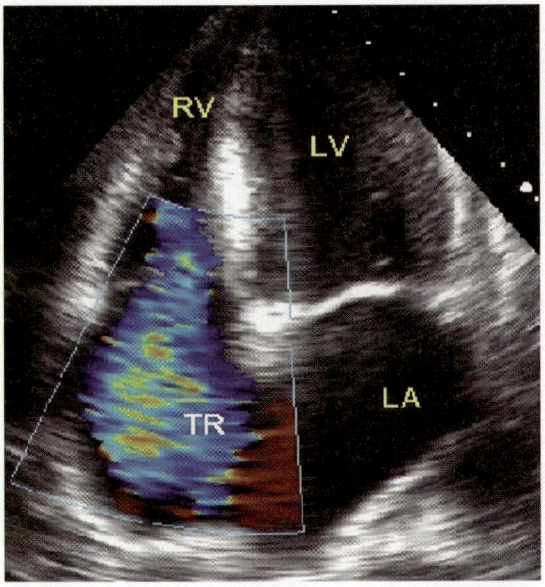

Fig. 17.11: *Tricuspid regurgitation jet due to vegetation on the tricuspid valve*

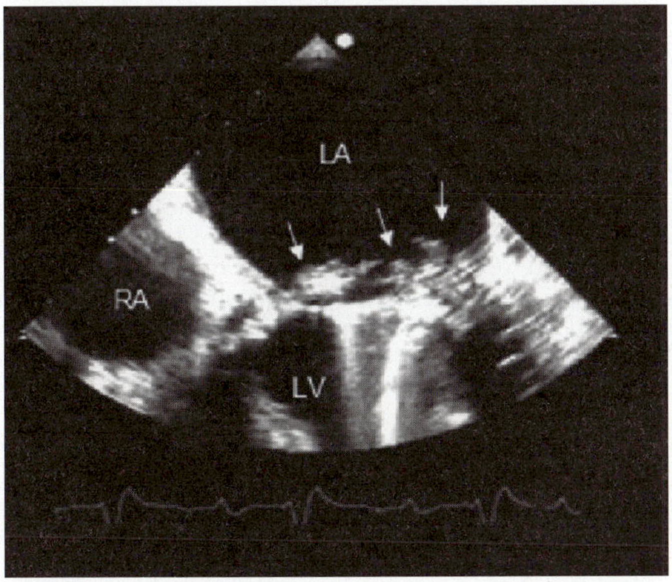

Fig. 17.12: *TEE echocardiography showing vegetations attached to bicuspid aortic valve*

involving native valves, and therefore TEE should always be used if the diagnosis of prosthetic endocarditis is suspected. The sewing ring and support structures of mechanical and bioprosthetic valves are strongly echogenic and may prevent vegetation detection within the valve apparatus or its shadow. The vegetative growth appears as thickening and irregularity of the normally smooth contour of the sewing ring. Both thrombus and pannus have a similar appearance and cannot be distinguished from vegetative material. It is also important to recognize strands to avoid false-positive diagnoses. Strands are commonly observed by TEE on prosthetic valves, particularly in the early postoperative months, especially in mitral prostheses.

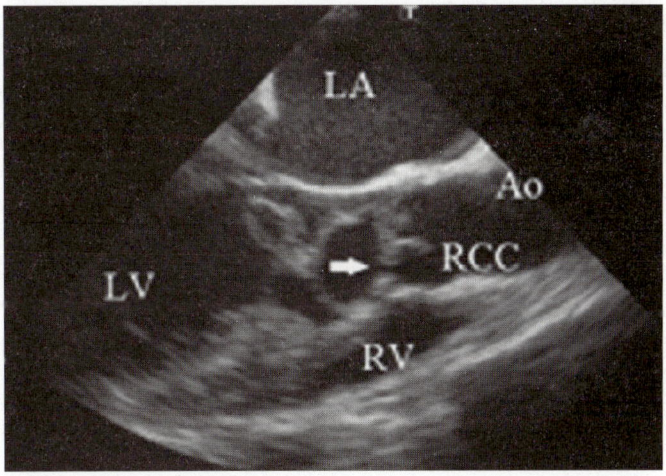

Fig. 17.13: *TEE echocardiography showing vegetations attached to bicuspid aortic valve*

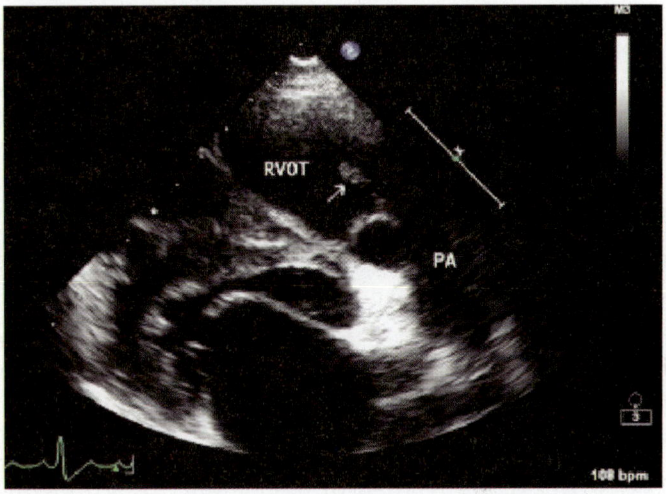

Fig. 17.14: *Two dimensional transthoracic echocardiography showing vegetations attached to the pulmonary valve cusps (arrow). RVOT, right ventricular outflow tract; PA, pulmonary artery*

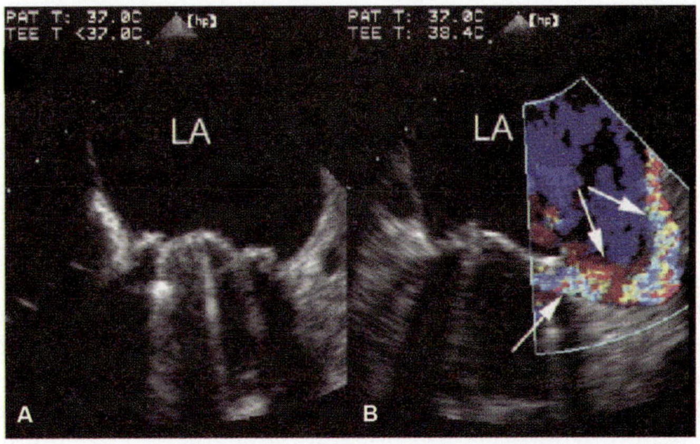

Fig. 17.15: *TEE echocardiography showing vegetations on mitral valve prosthesis*

Table 17.6: *Factors and complications that predispose to a poor outcome*

Congestive heart failure (leading adverse prognostic factor)
Nonstreptococcal disease
Aortic valve involvement
Infection of a prosthetic valve
Older age
Abscess formation
HIV with CD4 count <200
Delayed diagnosis
CNS or coronary embolization
Recurrent infective endocarditis

CNS, central nervous system;
HIV, human immunodeficiency virus

In large series of prosthetic endocarditis, TEE has shown an 86–94% sensitivity and 88–100% specificity for vegetation diagnosis while TTE sensitivity was only 36–69%. Bioprosthetic valve leaflets may become infected with secondary destruction of leaflet tissue. The distinction between wear-and-tear degeneration of tissue valves and endocarditis is often difficult. TEE also led to an improved diagnostic accuracy in the diagnosis of endocarditis on bioprosthetic valves.

RIGHT-SIDED ENDOCARDITIS AND PACEMAKER LEAD INFECTIONS

Staphylococcal endocarditis in injection drug users is now the dominant form of the disease in many urban communities where there is a high incidence of injection drug use and homelessness. Right-sided endocarditis accounts for 10% of all IE in population based surveys' and a higher proportion of IE in injection drug users. Modern echocardiographic techniques have considerably augmented our ability to diagnose IE and to understand its natural history. Despite this, there are many areas in which our understanding of right-sided IE remains incomplete. Right-sided IE has a significant morbidity and mortality that adds a notable economic burden to stretched inner city healthcare facilities. The challenges of caring for this population of patients should not be underestimated and demands a logical and coordinated approach among care providers and physicians from a variety of specialties.

Epidemiology and predisposing factors: Although right sided IE may occur in association with congenital heart disease and instrumentation of the right heart, it is overwhelmingly a disease of injection drug users, at least in Western populations. Among injection drug users presenting with fever, 13% will have echocardiographic evidence of IE. If injection drug users with bacteraemia from an inner city demographic are considered, up to 41% will have evidence of IE. The pathogenic mechanisms that explain the increased prevalence of right-sided IE in injection drug users are not fully elucidated. Damage to the right-sided valves from injected particulate matter in the setting of injected bacterial loads is thought to be important, while subtle abnormalities of immune function may also have a role in pathogenesis. In keeping with the demographic characteristics of injection drug use, this disease occurs most commonly in young males in their 20s and 30s. Before infection the tricuspid valve is usually structurally normal. Reinfection of a tricuspid valve that has been damaged by previous IE accounts for a significant proportion of cases and can add to the difficulty of echocardiographic interpretation. It seems logical that valves previously damaged by infection are more likely than normal valves to become infected. Earlier reports of IE in injection drug users emphasized the dominance of right-sided involvement. The tricuspid valve is most frequently involved followed by the mitral and then the aortic valve. Concurrent involvement of both left and right sided valves is not infrequent. In right-sided IE it is almost always the tricuspid valve that is involved. One study of

Table 17.7: *Complications*

Cardiac complications
- Congestive heart failure (leading cause of death)
- Abscess (pericardial, aortic annular, or myocardial)
- Conduction abnormalities (due to invasive disease)
- Coronary embolism
- Mycotic aneurysm (often clinically silent)
- Valvular regurgitation (cusp/leaflet flail or perforation)
- Valvular stenosis
- Prosthetic dehiscence
- Septal perforation (ventricular septal defect)

Extracardic complications
- Systemic embolism (stroke, renal infarct, splenic infract, or ischemic limb)
- Abscess
- Immune complex deposition (glomerulonephritis)

Table 17.8: *Surgical indications*

Clear indications
- Uncontrolled congestive heart failure due to valve dysfunction
- Unstable prosthesis
- Uncontrolled/uncontrollable infection (e.g. by fungi or resistant enterococcl
- Relapse of prosthetic valve endocarditis after optimal therapy
- Recurrent emboli

Relative indications
- Perivalvular extension of infection (fistula/abscess)
- *S. aureus* endocarditis
- Relapse of native valve endocarditis after optimal antimicrobial theapy
- Culture-negative endocarditis with persistent unexplained fever (<10 d)
- Large vegetations (>10 mm in diameter) with risk of embolization

Adapted from Karchmer AW. Infectious Endocarditis. In: Braunweld E, ed. Heart disease: a textbook of cardiovascular medicine, 6th ed. Philadelphia: WB Saunders, 2002:1723–1748.

Table 17.9: *Circumstances where short course antibiotic treatment for infective endocarditis is not appropriate*

- Confirmed or suspected left-sided endocarditis
- Metastatic sites of infection or empyema
- Cardiac or extracardiac complications
- Methicillin resistant *Staphylococcus aureus* (MRSA)
- Presence of any prosthetic valve
- Vegetation size > 10 mm
- Incomplete response to treatment
- HIV positive and CD4 count <200/mm^3

injection drug users found vegetations involving the tricuspid valve in 127 episodes, the pulmonary valve in four, and both valves in one instance 6. Involvement of other right-sided structures such as the eustachian valve has been reported but is rare.

The dominant infective organism is *Staphylococcus aureus*, in most series accounting for around 70% of infections, with the remainder being caused mainly by streptococcal species or, less frequently, by Gram-negative organisms, fungi or diphtheroids. Pseudomonal infections may have a predilection for multivalve involvement. Infections with unusual organisms and polymicrobial infections do occur, probably as the result of the injection of contaminated diluent, but are relatively unusual. Blood cultures are positive in a high proportion of cases of right-sided IE. When culture negative right-sided IE occurs, it is usually as a result of antibiotic use before the drawing of blood cultures. Bartonella infection has been described as a cause of culture negative IE in a homeless inner city population, and in right-sided IE. Although patterns of drug use in relation to IE have not been extensively studied, cocaine use may be a risk factor, presumably as a consequence of the much higher frequency of injections than in heroin users. The reported prevalence of HIV disease in patients with right-sided IE is variable. In a Spanish series of injection drug users with IE, 76% were HIV positive. In a

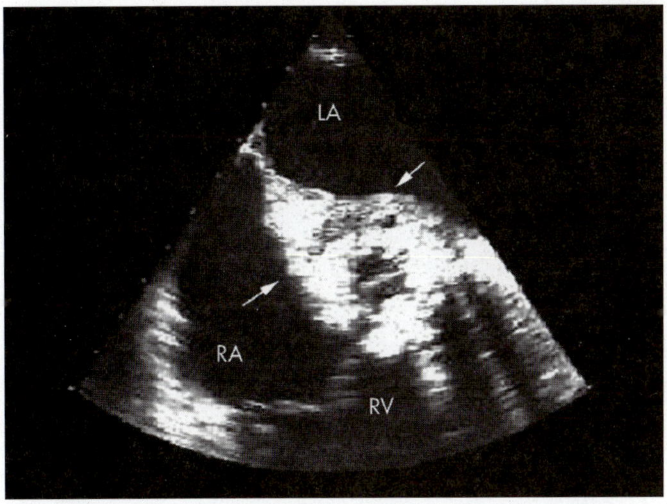

Fig. 17.16: *Vegetations on aortic valve prosthesis*

cohort of injection drug users with IE, those who were HIV positive were more likely to exhibit right-sided involvement. Advanced HIV infection is probably a risk factor for IE.

Clinical manifestations and complications: The presenting clinical features of right and left-sided endocarditis are different. While most patients with right-sided endocarditis will have systolic murmurs, the murmur is clearly pathologic in a minority of cases. Murmurs are, in fact, left-sided and nonspecific in most instances. The usual manifestations are persistent fever, bacteraemia, and multiple pulmonary emboli. Peripheral embolic manifestations are characteristically absent; rather, symptoms and complications arise from the involvement of the pulmonary vasculature by multiple septic pulmonary emboli. chest pain, dyspnoea, cough, and haemoptysis may be presenting feature. When peripheral embolic or

Table 17.10: *Injection drug use and right-sided endocarditis: key points*

- In inner city communities most cases of infective endocarditis (IE) occur in injection drug users; many of these will have right-sided IE caused by staphylococci
- If injection drug users with bacteraemia from an inner city demographic are considered, upto 41% will have evidence of endocarditis
- The conjuction of bacteraemia, fever, and multiple pulmonary infiltrates on chest radiography should always prompt a search for right-sided IE
- A transoesophageal echocardiographic examination is not necessary in may cases of right-sided IE
- Coexistent medical problems such as hepatitis or HIV disease may be present
- Successful treatment of right-sided IE in injection drug users requires a multidisciplinary approach
- Most patients will recover with medical treatment; short course or rarely oral antibiotic treatment may be useful in certain situation

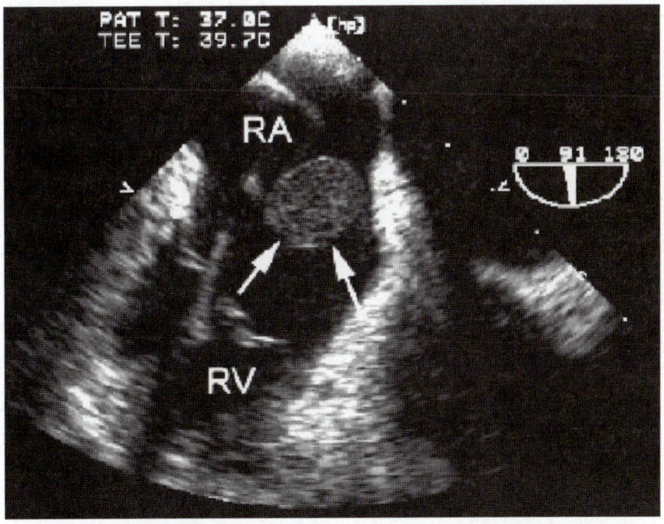

Fig. 17.17: *Endocarditis on a pacemaker or defibrillator lead. Ball-like vegetation on pacemaker lead [vertical echoes seen in right atrium (RA)]. Horizontal echoes between RA and right ventricle (RV) represents the tricuspid valve*

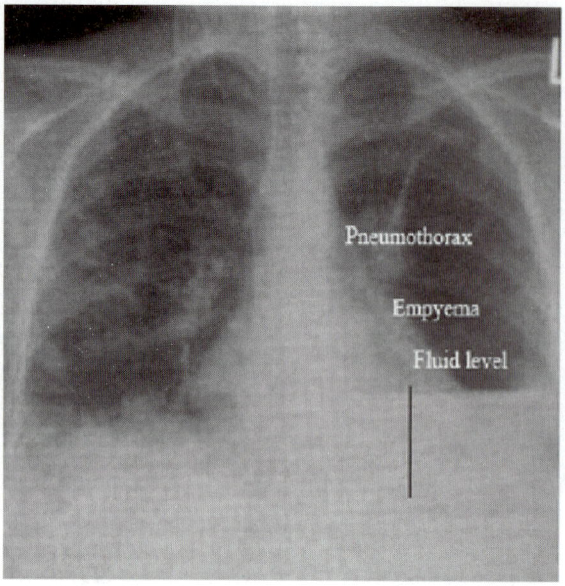

Fig. 17.18: *X-ray chest. PA view in the same patient showing multiple alveolar opacities in the right lung. Abscess formation in the left lung has caused a bronchopleural fistula, pneumothorax and emphysema, hence the air fluid level*

neurologic features occur, either left-sided endocarditis or paradoxical embolism should be considered. The conjunction of bacteraemia, fever, and multiple pulmonary infiltrates on chest radiography should always prompt a search for right-sided endocarditis.

Complications of right-sided endocarditis may be thought of as either cardiac or pulmonary. A variety of complications attributed to septic pulmonary emboli have been described including pulmonary infarction, pulmonary abscesses, bilateral pneumothoraces, pleural effusions, and empyema. Mycotic aneurysms of the pulmonary arteries may be complicated by potentially fatal pulmonary hemorrhage. Multiple pulmonary emboli may result in right-sided chamber dilatation, right heart failure, and a worsening of tricuspid regurgitation. The embolization of vegetations large enough to result in obstruction of a significant portion of the pulmonary arterial circulation has been described but is unusual. Cardiac complications may arise as a consequence of tricuspid valve destruction and severe tricuspid regurgitation with right-sided volume overload, chamber dilatation, and right heart failure. Chronic right atrial dilatation may be a substrate for supraventricular arrhythmias including atrial flutter and fibrillation. Paravalvar abscess formation occurs infrequently. Vasculitis may complicate right-sided IE, but is not a typical feature. Hypoxaemia has been described in right-sided IE when right atrial (Table 17.7).

Diagnosis of Right-Sided Endocarditis

Duke criteria: The Duke system defines a major echocardiographic criterion for IE as the finding of an oscillating intracardiac mass on the valve or supporting structures, in the path of a regurgitant jet, a paravalvar abscess or new dehiscence of a prosthetic valve. Although the sensitivity and specificity of tbe Duke criteria have not been specifically studied in the right-sided endocarditis with finding of anyone of these echocardiographic features involving right heart structures. In the presence of positive blood cultures with atypical organism should be regarded as diagnostic of right-sided endocarditis. There are nonetheless some conceptual difficulties in uncritically applying the Duke criteria to right sided endocarditis. Right-sided murmurs are more difficult to detect. This is especially true of many patients who are injection drug users with their first episode of endocarditis, who will have normal or only slightly elevated right ventricular pressures

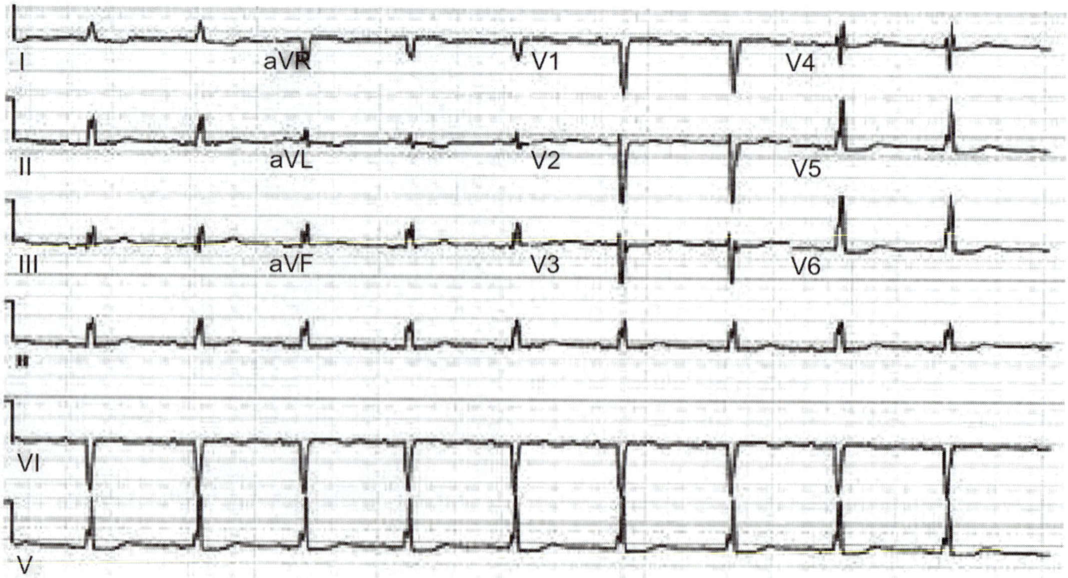

Fig. 17.19: *ECG of a patient with infective endocarditis. Note the first-degree AV block, nonspecific intraventricular conduction delay, and nonspecific ST-T wave abnormalities*

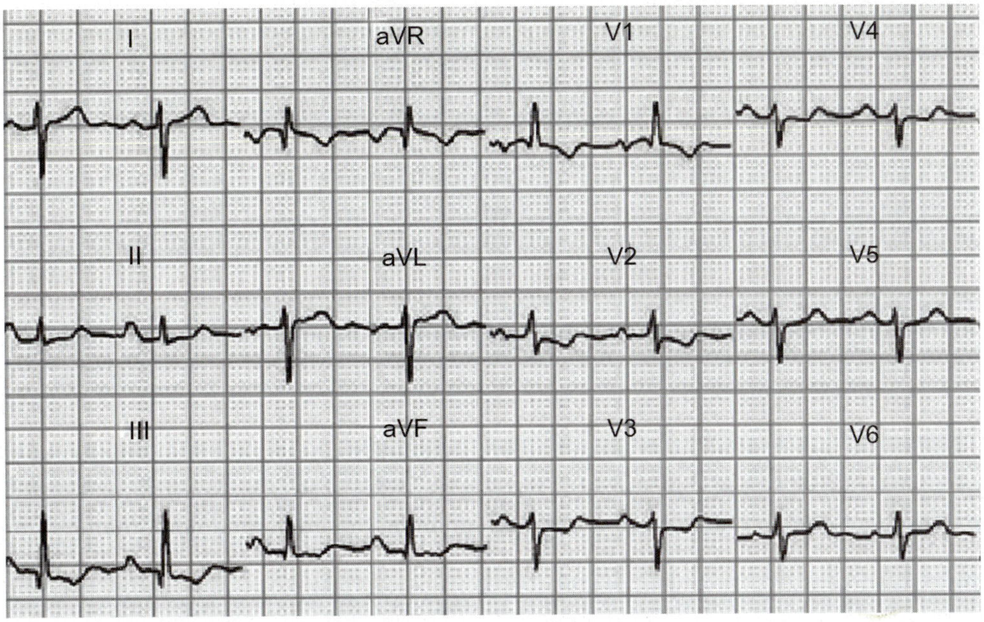

Fig. 17.20: *Pulmonary embolism. S1-Q3 and signs of right-frontal axis are shown in right-sided endocarditis*

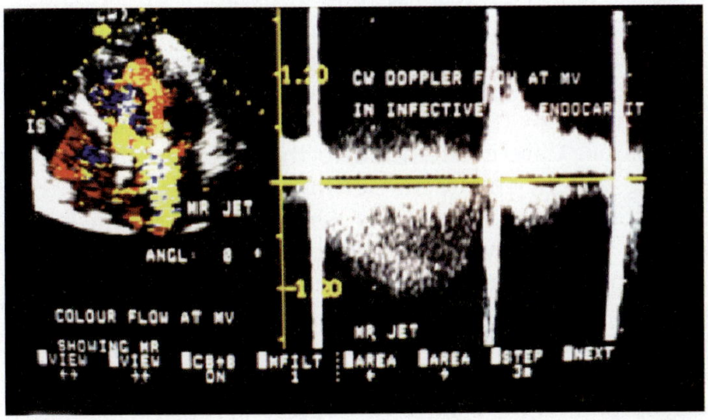

Fig. 17.21: *(Left panel) Color flow apical four chamber left parasternal view and Doppler flow velocity across mitral valve showing mosaic jet of mitral regurgitation into left atrium (aroow) and regurgitant velocity flow on Doppler study (right panel) in patient with infective endocarditis of mitral vale with clinical mitral regurgitant murmur*

and in whom a lower velocity, less turbulent tricuspid regurgitant jet might be anticipated. One should not allow the lack of a murmur, therefore, to preclude further investigation if the clinical suspicion is high. Immunologic and vascular phenomena, which feature as minor criteria in the Duke system, are also less common. Septic pulmonary emboli are listed as a minor criterion in the Duke scheme; it could be argued that this important diagnostic feature is somewhat underweighted in the present Duke criteria. On balance, however, it seems reasonable to continue to use the Duke criteria as a useful diagnostic framework.

Chest X-ray: The chest X-ray is a helpful laboratory aid in diagnosing right-sided endocarditis with 55% of radiographs at presentation showing evidence of pulmonary infiltrates compatible with pulmonary emboli.

Transthoracic echocardiography (TTE): Modern echocardiographic techniques have significantly improved our ability to diagnose right-sided endocarditis and are now the cornerstone of the diagnosis in this disease. In febrile

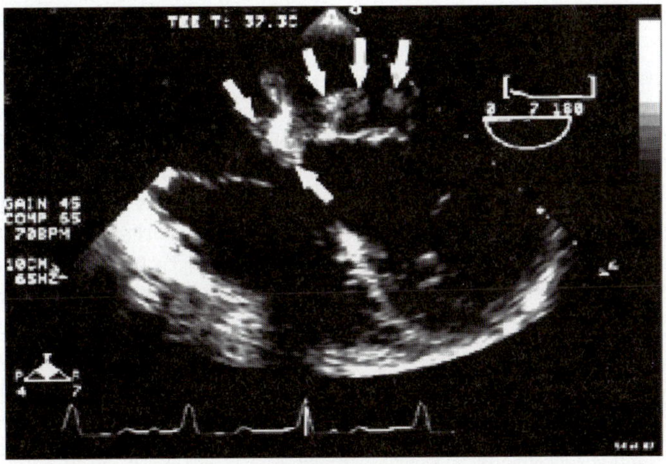

Fig. 17.22: *Transesophageal echocardiogram (TEE) reveals a 1.4-cm vegetation extending from the anterior leaflet, through the trigone, and into the right atrium. A second, 0.9-cm vegetation is visible on the posterior leaflet*

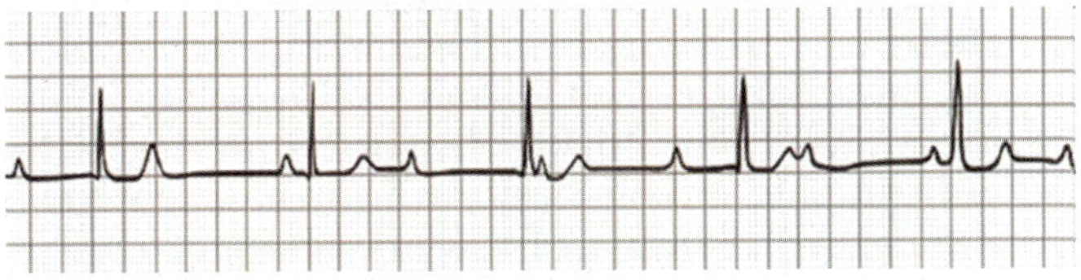

Fig. 17.23: *Complete heart block, there is complete absence of AV conduction–none of the supraventricular impulses are conducted to the ventricles*

Table 17.11: *Standard therapies for susceptible enterococci for resistant and nutritionally variant viridans streptococcus infective endocarditis, and for prosthetic valve endocarditis due to viridans streptococcus or S. Bovis*

Meidcation	*Dosage*	*During of therapy (wk)*
Penicilin G	18–30 million U/24 hr continuously IV or in 6 divided doses	4–6
Plus		
Gentamicin or	1 mg/kg IV or IM every 8 hours	
Ampicilin	12 g/24 hr continuously IV or in 6 divided doses	4–6
Plus		
Gentamicin or,	1 mg/kg IV or IM every 8 hr	
if penicilin allergic:		
Vancomycin	30 mg/kg per 24 hr in 2 divided doses	4–6
Plus		
Gentamicin	1 mg/kg IV or IM every 8 hr	

IM, intramuscular; IV, intravenous

Four-week therapy is recommended for patients with symptoms of less than 3 months duration; 8-weeks therapy is recommended for patients with symptoms of more than 3 months duration.

Adapted from Wilson, WR, Karchmer AW, Dajani AS, et al. Antibiotic treatment of adults with infectious endocarditis due to streptococci, enterococci, and HACEK microorganism. *JAMA* 1995;274:1706–1713.

injection drug users, standard laboratory testing and physical examination without echocardiography were ineffective in detecting the patients with endocarditis. The key echocardiographic finding in right-sided endocarditis is that of vegetation(s) in association with the tricuspid or rarely the pulmonary valve. As with vegetations on the left-sided valves, they tend to be localized to the atrial side of the valve in the path of the regurgitant jet. Tricuspid vegetations are often large and may be in excess of 2 cm, a finding that does not necessarily suggest the presence of fungal endocarditis. On rare occasions, vegetations may be sufficiently large so as to be confused with an intracardiac tumour. Entrapment of an embolised vegetation in the tricuspid chordal apparatus is sometimes seen. Similarly, embolised vegetations have been seen floating free in the right ventricle or pulmonary artery. Occasionally the presence of normal anatomic variants such as Chiari network or prominent eustachian valve may cause diagnostic confusion, more particularly with transthoracic imaging; similarly venous catheters erroneously placed in the right atrium need to be identified and distinguished from vegetations. Right atrial thrombus may be distinguished from vegetation in that it is less likely to lie in the path of the jet and tends to layer on the right atrial wall. Past infection with damage to the tricuspid valve is commonly seen in this group, so the presence of vegetation does not in itself signify the presence of active infection. Extensive valve destruction with failure of leaflet cooptation and severe tricuspid regurgitation is a common sequel to tricuspid endocarditis. Although older or healed vegetations tend to be more echogenic and may even be calcified, this finding cannot reliably distinguish new from old infection. It should be clearly understood that echocardiographic findings need always to be taken in their clinical context. The finding of new or worsening tricuspid regurgitation, which is otherwise unexplained, should always prompt a diligent search for evidence of tricuspid endocarditis in the injection drug using patient.

Transesophageal echocardiography (TEE): Many injection drug users have good thoracic ultrasound windows meaning that high-resolution images can be obtained with transthoracic echocardiographic examination in many patients. This combined with the relative proximity of the tricuspid valve to the ultrasound transducer, means that this valve is often well imaged by the transthoracic technique. Careful attention to the adjustment of sector width, depth, and focus settings will help in accurate identification of vegetations. Under some circumstances higher frequency transducers for example, 4 MHz or broad-band transducers switched to a "resolution setting" may be used to improve spatial resolution. Alternatively use of the "zoom function" (on some machines) may assist with lesion identification. The need for routine transoesophageal echocardiography (TEE) in right-sided endocarditis is therefore questionable. TEE may be useful in detecting paravalvar abscess formation and for diagnosing unusual forms of right-sided endocarditis such as pulmonary valve involvement or infection on the eustachian valve. The rationale for this approach is the simplicity and reduced cost of TTE and the importance of having the TTE information to direct and target a subsequent TEE examination appropriately. If there is a moderate or high suspicion of IE, and the initial TTE is negative, the TTE is repeated after an interval of about 1 week. TEE is then used in those patients in whom diagnostic quality images are not obtained with transthoracic imaging, and those who have negative TTE examinations where the suspicion of endocarditis is moderate or high (especially in the setting of staphylococcal bacteraemia). Occasionally, pacing wires or right-sided prosthetic valves are encountered where there is a suspicion of endocarditis TEE is usually indicated. Rotation of the crystal array and angulation of the probe tip in order to visualize the valves in a number of orientations is mandatory during TEE (Figs 17.9 to 17.11, 17.14, 17.17).

HIV and right-sided endocarditis: Significant immunosuppression (CD4 count < 200/mm) is associated with a higher mortality rate in right-sided IE in HIV infected injection drug users though it is not clear that this increased mortality is as a consequence of the IE. As in non-HIV infected patients with right-sided endocarditis, the involvement of the left-sided valves is predictive of an increased risk of death.

Treatment of right-sided endocarditis (Table 17.11): Short course antibiotic treatment for right-sided endocarditis and management of addiction. The successful management of a complicated case often requires the close cooperation of a cardiologist, an infectious disease physician, and occasionally a cardiac surgeon. The role of physicians in managing intercurrent drug withdrawal and maintaining the patient in hospital has been understated in the past methadone and/or other agents may be needed to control withdrawal symptoms. These patients may be difficult and disruptive and often engender negative attitudes in health care professionals. Their lack of adherence to in hospital treatment is a major practical hurdle and has stimulated interest in developing shorter duration antibiotic regimens. There is reasonable evidence that short course antibiotic treatment for uncomplicated right-sided endocarditis is effective. The benefit of gentamicin in native valve endocarditis lies in earlier defervescence of fever and the sterilisation of blood cultures; there is no proven survival advantage. In the presence of a relative or absolute contraindication to gentamicin, therefore, a 2 weeks course of cloxacillin alone may be adequate. In the event that the patient cannot be persuaded to stay in hospital for the full 2 weeks, a 28 day course of oral treatment with ciprofloxacin and rifampin is prescribed, ideally with administration in a supervised setting such as a drug treatment facility. There are some situations in which short course antibiotic treatment is not appropriate. In general, nonstaphylococcal right-sided endocarditis is treated in a similar fashion to left-sided endocarditis.

Prognosis and surgical treatment of right-sided endocarditis: Right-sided endocarditis is generally regarded as having a relatively benign prognosis and inhospital mortality is less than 10%. Most will survive even if they leave hospital before the full course of treatment has been completed. As follow-up in the injection drug using population is notoriously difficult, few data are available on their long-term outlook. It is clear that there will be a significant late mortality from causes other than IE and right heart failure, such as noncardiac infections, drug overdose, and AIDS related complications. Mortality is higher where there is left-sided involvement. Fortunately,

Table 17.12: *Prophylactic regimens*

Clinical situation	*Antibiotic*	*Dose*
For dental, oral, respiratory tract, or esophageal procedures		
Standard prophylaxis	Amoxicillin	2 g PO 1 hr before procedure
Unable to take oral medications	Ampicillin	2 g IV or IM within 30 min before procedure
Penicillin allergy	Clindamycin	600 mg PO 1 hr before procedure
	or	
	Cephalexin or cephadroxil	2 g PO 1 hr before procedure
	or	
	Azithromycin	500 mg 1 hr before procedure
For genitourinary/gastrointestinal (excluding esophageal) procedure		
High-risk patients	Ampicillin	2 g IM or IV
	plus	
	Gentamicin (within 30 min of starting procedure)	1.5 mg/kg IV or IM (not to exceed 120 mg)
	followed by	
	ampicillin	1 g IM or IV
	or	
	Amoxil (6 hr later)	1 g PO
High-risk patients allergic to penicillin	Vancomycin	1 g IV over 1 –2 hr
	plus	
	Gentamicin (within 30 min starting procedure)	1.5 mg/kg IV or IM (not to exceed 120 mg)
Moderate-risk	Amoxicillin	2 g PO 1 hr before procedure
	or	
	Ampicillin	2 g IV or IM within 30 min of starting procedure
Moderate risk allergic to penicillin	Vancomycin	1 g IV over 1–2 hr completed within 30 min of starting the procedure

IM, intramuscular; IV, intravenous; PO, per oral

Adapted from Dajani AS, Taubert KA, Wilson W. et al. Prevention of bacterial endocarditis; recommendations by the American Heart Association. Circulation 1997;96:358–386.

most patients can be treated medically, with surgery being necessary in only a small minority of cases. Indications for surgical treatment are better defined for left than for right-sided endocarditis. Sepsis, which is uncontrolled despite adequate antibiotic treatment, and intractable right heart failure despite appropriate medical treatment, are the most important indications for surgical intervention. The finding of a paravalvar abscess or fungal endocarditis are usually indications for surgery. Recurrent pulmonary embolism following the initiation of antibiotic treatment may occur and does not in itself represent an indication for surgery. Some authors have felt that large vegetation size (diameter > 10 mm) in the context of persisting fever identifies a set of patients who are likely to benefit from surgery. Others have felt that many of these patients will eventually recover with medical treatment. Very large vegetations (> 20 mm), however, are associated with a poor outcome. Patients may also require an operation to treat concomitant left-sided endocarditis. Enthusiasm for surgery is tempered by the knowledge that the majority of patients will resume injection drug use following hospital discharge. Surgical approaches vary, with valve removal or replacement being the historical, commonly recommended approaches. Both approaches are controversial and there is a lack of controlled trials in the literature upon which to base decision making. Valvectomy may result in permanent damage to the right ventricle and ultimately intractable right heart failure and death. Significant early mortality (11 %) was reported in one group where this approach was used. More recent attention has focused on tricuspid valve vegetectomy or repair. The repair has the advantage of avoiding or minimising the implantation of foreign material in the infected area while preserving the function of the valve. Several different techniques have been used including cusp resection (rendering the valve bicuspid), commissural plication, the use of artificial chordae, and pericardial patch repair of the tricuspid leaflet (sometimes in conjunction with mobilization of the secondary chordae and tricuspid annuloplasty). Where extensive valvar destruction has occurred, replacement of the tricuspid valve may be necessary. When valve replacement is unavoidable our current approach is to use cryopreserved mitral homografts in the tricuspid position, which usually requires the addition of a tricuspid ring to provide annular stability. Reinfection of the valve can be anticipated in some cases; when this occurs, antibiotic treatment may result in a cure of the prosthetic valve endocarditis.

Prevention: It is possible that harm reduction strategies aimed at reducing injection frequency (such as methadone availability) or clean injection strategies (clean injection education, injection rooms, needle exchange programmes or legal heroin) may have a beneficial effect. The clinical suspicion is low. If the clinical suspicion is high TEE should be performed. TEE should also be performed if the results of the TTE are equivocal owing to underlying structural abnormalities or poor acoustic windows. If the TEE is negative, observation or reevaluation of the clinical data are warranted. If the suspicion of endocarditis is high TEE should be repeated after 7–10 days to allow potential vegetations to become more apparent. A repeated negative study should virtually rule out the diagnosis unless TEE images are of poor quality (Table 17.12).

Conclusion: To date, definitive studies of infective endocarditis have been difficult to perform because of its heterogenous nature. Launched in 1999, the International Collaboration on Endocarditis was conceived to develop a large global database of patients whose clinical, echocardiographic, and microbiological findings have been characterized using standard methodology. Modification of the original Duke criteria is now proposed to enhance diagnostic sensitivity, especially in culture negative cases. Increased emphasis on symptoms and signs coupled with improved likelihood of identification of a causative pathogen using serology, additional culture, or newer histological and molecular techniques will improve the sensitivity of the diagnosis and increase therapeutic specificity. These measures, combined with close collaboration and communication between the cardiologist, cardiac surgeon, and microbiologist, are essential to ensure optimal diagnosis and management and a favourable impact on patient outcome.

BIBLIOGRAPHY

1. Cabell CH, Jollis JG, Peterson GE, et al. Changing patient characteristics and the effect on mortality in endocarditis. Arch Intern Med 2002;162:90–4.
2. von Reyn CF, Levy BS, Arbeit RD, et al. Infective endocarditis: an analysis based on strict case definitions. Ann Intern Med 1981;94:505–17.
3. Durack DT, Lukes AS, Bright DK, et al. New criteria for diagnosis of infective endocarditis: utilization of specific echocardiographic findings. Am J Med 1994;96:200–9.
4. Bayer AS, Bolger AF, Taubert KA, et al. Diagnosis and management of infective endocarditis and its complications. Circulation 1998;98:2936–48.
5. Habib G, Derumeaux G, Avierinos JF, et al. Value and limitations of the Duke criteria for the diagnosis of infective endocarditis. J Am Coll Cardiol 1999;33:2023–9.
6. Lamas C, Eykyn SJ. Suggested modifications to the Duke criteria for the clinical diagnosis of native valve and prosthetic valve endocarditis: analysis of 118 pathologically proven cases. Clin Infect Dis 1997;25:713–9.
7. Fournier PE, Casalta JP, Habib G, et al. Modification of the diagnostic criteria proposed by the Duke endocarditis service to permit improved diagnosis of Q fever endocarditis. Am J Med 1996;100:629–33.
8. Li JS, Sexton DJ, Mick N, et al. Proposed modifications to the Duke criteria for the diagnosis of infective endocarditis. Clin Infect Dis 2000;30:633–8.
9. Lamas CC, Eykyn SJ. Blood culture negative endocarditis endocarditis: analysis of 63 cases presenting over 25 years. Heart 2003;89:258–62.
10. Lepidi H, Durack DT, Raoult D. Diagnostic methods. Current best practices and guidelines for histologic evaluation in infective endocarditis. Infect Dis Clin N Am 2002;16:339–61.

11. Houpikian P, Raoult D. Diagnostic methods. Current best practices and guidelines for identification of difficult-to-culture pathogens in infective endocarditis. Infect Dis Clin N Am 2002;16:377–92.
12. Lisby G, Gutschik E, Durack DT. Molecular methods for diagnosis of infective endocarditis. Infect Dis Clin North Am 2002;16:393–412.
13. Millar BC, Moore JE, Mallon P, et al. Molecular diagnosis of infective endocarditis–a new Duke's criterion. Scand J Infect Dis 2001;33:673–80.
14. Moore JE, Millar BC, Yongmin X, et al. A rapid molecular assay for the detection of antibiotic resistance determinants in cause of infective endocarditis. J Appl Microbiol 2001;90:719–26.
15. Grijalva M, Horvath R, Dendis M, et al. Molecular diagnosis of culture negative infective endocarditis: clinical validation in a group of surgically treated patients. Heart 2003;89:263–8.
16. Cabell CH, Abrutyn E. Progress toward a global understanding of infective endocarditis. Early lessons from the International Collaboration on Endocarditis investigation. Infect Dis Clin North Am 2002;16:255–72.
17. F Delahaye, M Celard, O Roth, G de Gevigney, Hopital cardiovasculaire et pneumologique, Lyon, France
18. Correspondence to: Professor Franc;:ois Delahaye, Hopital cardiovasculaire et pneumologique, BP Lyon Montchat, 69394-Lyon Cedex 03, France; francois.delahaye@chu-lyonJr
19. Hoen B, Alia F, Selton-Suty C, et al. Changing profile of infective endocarditis. Results of a 1-year survey in France. JAMA 2002;288:75–81.
20. Olaison L, Pettersson G. Current best practices and guidelines indications for surgical intervention in infective endocarditis. Infect Dis Clin North Am 2002;16:453-75.
21. Di Salvo G, Habib G, Pergola V, et al. Echocardiography predicts embolic events in infective endocarditis. J Am Col Cordial 2001;37:1069–76.
22. Heiro M, Nikoskelainen J, Engblom E, et al. Neurologic manifestations of infective endocarditis: a 17-year experience in a teaching hospital in Finland. Arch Intern Mad 2000;160:2781–7.
23. Alestig K, Hogevik H, Olaison 1. Infective endocarditis: a diagnostic and therapeutic challenge for the new millennium. Scand Infect Dis 2000;32:343–56.
24. ohmann S, Erbel R, Gorge G, et al. Clinical relevance of vegetation localization by transoesophageal echocardiography in infective endocarditis. Fur Heart) 1992; 13:446-52.
25. Choussat R, Thomas D, Isnard R, et al. Perivalvular abscesses associated with endocarditis: clinical features and prognostic factors of overall survival in a series of 233 cases. Perivalvular abscesses French multicentre study. Fur Heart 1999;20:232–41.
26. Blumberg EA, Karalis DA, Chandrasekaran K, et al. Endocarditis-associated paravalvular abscesses. Do clinical parameters predict the presence of abscess? Chest 1995;107:898–903.
27. Knosalla C, Weng Y, Yankah AC, et al. Surgical treatment of active infective aortic valve endocarditis with associated periannular abscess. 11 year results. Fur Heart 2000;21:490–7.
28. Chastre J, T rouillet Jl. Early infective endocarditis on prosthetic valves. Fur Heart 1995;16 (suppl B):32–8.217
29. Gordon SM, Serkey JM, Longworth DL, et al. Early onset prosthetic valveendocarditis: the Cleveland Clinic experience 1992-1997. Ann Thorac Surg 2000;69: 1388–92.
30. John MD, Hibberd PL, Karchmer AW, et al. Staphylococcus aureus prosthetic valve endocarditis: optimal management and risk factors l or death. C/in Infect Dis 1998;26:1302–9.
31. Truninger K, Attenhofer Jost CH, et al. Long term follow up of prosthetic valve endocarditis: what characteristics identify patients who weretreated successfully with antibiotics alone? Heart 1999;82:714–20.
32. Moyer D, Edwards JE. Fungal endocarditis. In: Kaye D, ed. Infective endocarditis. New York: Raven Press, 1992:299–312.
33. Gillinov AM, Shah RV, Curtis WE, et al. Valve replacement in patients with endocarditis and acute neurologic deficit. Ann Thorac Surg 1996;61:1125–30.
34. D'Udekem Y, David TE, Feindel CM, et al. Long-term results of surgery for active infective endocarditis. Fur Cardiothorac Surg 1997;11:46–52.

18 Cardiovascular Manifestations and Complications of HIV Infection and their Management among Children and Adolescents

Cardiac manifestations and complications of human immunodeficiency virus (HIV) infection in children are common. They include cardiac dysfunction, dysrhythmias, cardiac arrest, myocarditis, pericardial disease, cardiac tumors, aortic root dilatation, and cerebral aneurysmal arteriopathy. Serious cardiac events and cardiac death are common among children with acquired immune deficiency syndrome (AIDS); 28% experience serious cardiac events after AIDS is diagnosed. Pericardial effusions in children are commonly associated with pleural fluid and ascites). At fetal echocardiography, fetuses of HIV-positive mothers may have abnormal cardiovascular structure and function (mainly, increased right and left ventricular wall thickness). Congenital cardiovascular malformations that have been observed at imaging in children with HIV infection include atrial and ventricular septal defects, patent ductus arteriosus, valvular pulmonary stenosis, and subaortic stenosis, and a 12.3% rate of cardiovascular malformation has been found. Although this rate is 5 to 10 times higher than that in the general population, it is not higher than that in normal populations that have undergone similar screening. Therefore, the relationship between congenital HIV infection and congenital cardiac or vascular malformation is unclear. Studies published over the past 2–3 years have tracked the incidence and course of HIV infection in relation to cardiac illness in both children and adults. These recent studies show that subclinical echocardiographic abnormalities independently predict adverse outcomes and identify high-risk groups to target for early intervention and treatment.

The World Health Organization (WHO) estimated that the number of people worldwide who were living with the human immunodeficiency virus (HIV) rose in 2004 to the unprecedented level of 39.4 million; the number of those infected with HIV increased in every region, and 4.9 million were newly infected that year. Acquired immune deficiency syndrome (AIDS) was responsible for the deaths of 3.1 million people in 2003. The number of those who have died since the epidemic began exceeds 32 million. In North America alone, 1 million are currently infected with HIV.

Although cardiac involvement in HIV infection was recognized early in the AIDS epidemic, the incidence of this complication and its imaging manifestations have not been fully described in the radiologic literature. Cardiac

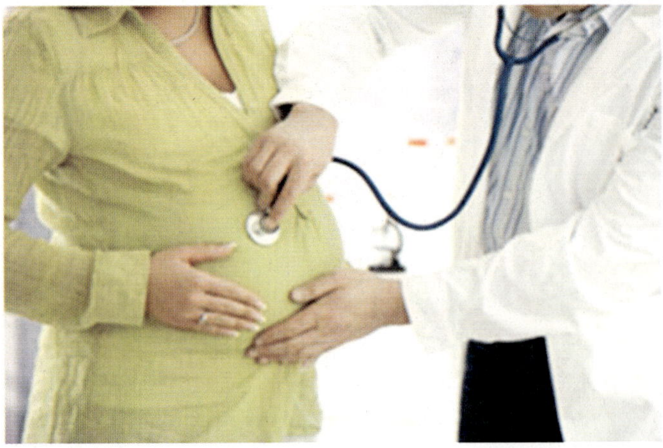

Fig. 18.1: *Doctor is examining young pregnant lady infected with HIV infection*

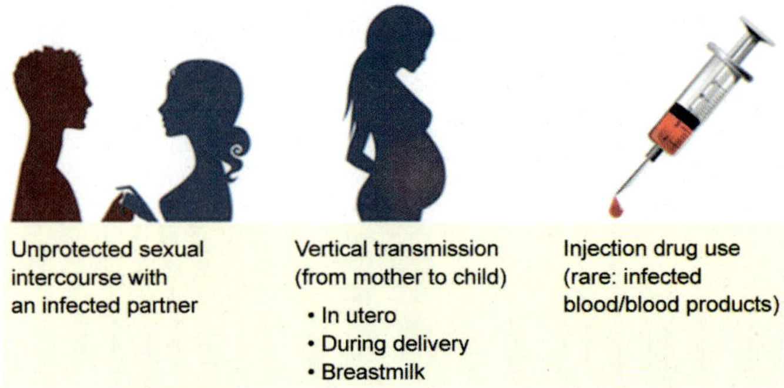

Fig.18.2: *Illustration showing common modes of infection in HIV infection*

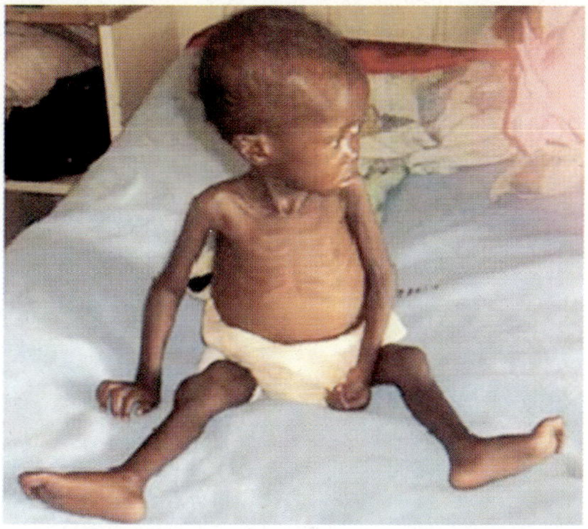

Fig. 18.3: *A young child presenting with protein calorie malnutrition (PCM) in HIV infection.*

involvement in HIV represents a diagnostic and therapeutic challenge for cardiologists, specialists in infective diseases, and radiologists, who should be aware of the resultant imaging manifestations.

According to reports of clinical and autopsy studies, the prevalence of myocardial abnormalities in HIV positive patients ranges from 25% to 75%. The effect of antiretroviral therapy on the incidence and prevalence of HIV-related cardiovascular disease is not clear. Despite fear that the use of new-generation anti-HIV drugs associated with metabolic abnormalities (e.g. dysglycemia and hyperlipidemia) might accelerate the progression of cardiovascular and cerebrovascular disease.

Pericarditis and pericardial effusion: Pericardial effusion is the most common cardiovascular complication of HIV infection. Prior to the introduction of highly active antiretroviral therapy (HAART), the frequency of this complication was estimated to be between 5% and 46%, with an incidence of 11–17% per year. The prevalence of pericardial effusion in children with AIDS is particularly high (68%) and is often associated with cardiac disease. Echocardiograms showed pericardial effusion in 10% of the HIV-infected patients in one study, and fibrinous pericarditis has been identified at autopsy in 9–62% of deceased AIDS patients. The origins of pericardial effusion in patients with HIV and/or AIDS are diverse , but in most cases no etiologic agent has been identified, despite an extensive work-up. In an autopsy series, serous pericardial effusion was more common (59%) than fibrinous pericarditis (3%). In children, serous pericardial effusion has been found more frequently (81.0%) than have serosanguineous and sanguineous (14.3%) or purulent (4.7%) collections. Pericardial effusion in patients with HIV-related disease may be associated with an opportunistic infection or malignancy, but most often no definitive cause is found. An association between pericardial effusion, pleural effusion, and ascites has been reported. The observed pattern may indicate the presence of a generalized serous-effusive process, or polyserositis, that involves pleural and peritoneal as well as pericardial surfaces. Patients with AIDS who are affected by pericardial effusion

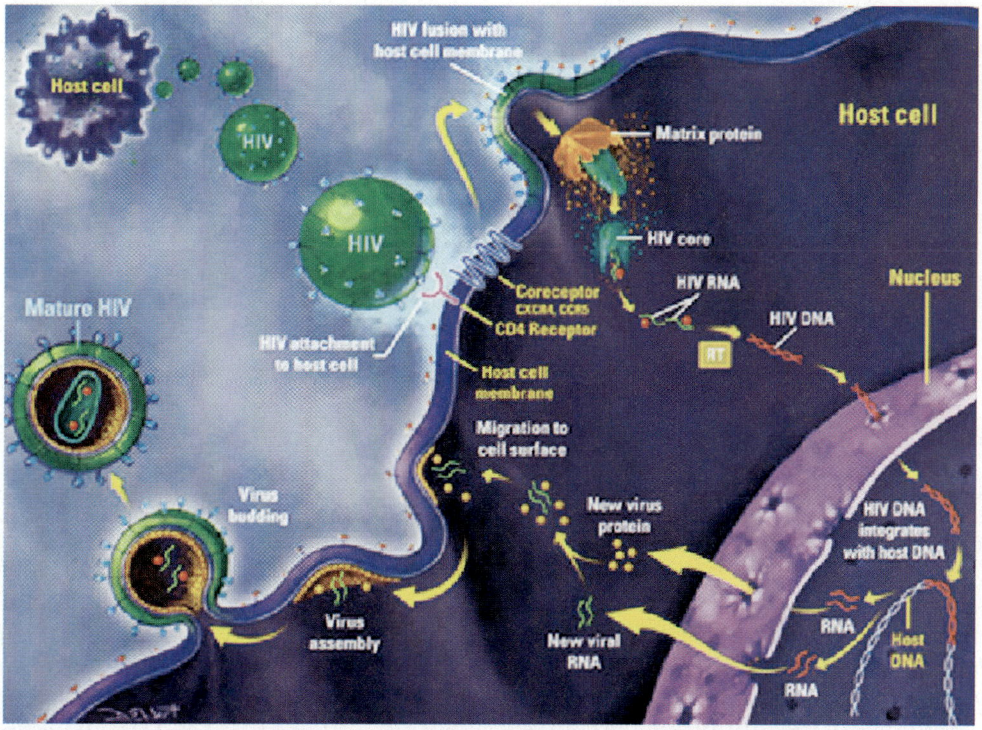

Fig. 18.4: *Potential points of intervention in HIV life cycle. Abbreviations: NRTIs, nucleoside reverse transcriptase inhibitors; NNRTIs, non-nucleoside reverse transcriptase inhibitors. This illustration shows the major sites for potential intervention the major steps in the HIV life cycle*

Table 18.1: *Cardiac conditions associated with HIV infection*

Myocardial disease opportunistic infections		
	Bacterial	*Mycobacterium tuberculosis, mycobactorium,* avium-intracellulare
	Fungal	*Cryptococcus neoformans, Aspergillus fumigatus, Candida albicans, Histoplasma capsulatum, Coccidodes immitus*
	Protozean	*Toxoplasma gondii, Pneumocystis carnii*
	Viral	*Cytomegalovirus, Herpes simplex, Coxsackie B virus*
Direct HIV infection		
Lymphocytic myocarditis		
Noninflammatory		Myocardial necrosis
		Mycovascular spasm
		Cathecholamine excess
Nutritional deficiency (selenium, thiamine) (Fig. 18.2)		
Hypoxic injury		
Drug toxicity		
		Anti-HIV drugs
		Drugs used for opportunistic infections
Arteriopathy		
Cardiomegaly and cardiomyopathy		
		Congestive cardiomyopathy
		Right ventricular hypertrophy/dilatation with pulmonary hypertension:
		Pulmonary infection
		Pulmonary emboli
		HIV plexogenic pulmonary arteriopathy
Neoplasia		
		Kaposi's sarcoma
		Lymphoma
Endocardial disease		
Marantic endocarditis (nonbacterial thrombotic endocarditis)		
Healed infective endocarditis		
Infective endocarditis		
	Bacterial	
	Fungal	
Pericardial disease		
Infectious		
	Bacterial	Tuberculosis (*M. tuberculosis, M. avium-intracellulare), Nocardia asteroides, Klebsiella pneumoniae, Staphylococcus aureus*
	Viral	Herpes simplex, HIV, coxsackie, cytomegalovirus
	Fungal	Histoplasma, cryptococcus
Uraemia		
Neoplastic		Kaposi's sarcoma
		Lymphoma
Fibrinous pericarditis		
Idopathic		
Vascular lesions		
Fibrocalcific degenative arteropathy		

have a total T-cell count that is comparable to that in patients who are not affected by pericardial effusion but they have a significantly lower serum albumin level and lower CD4 count. Although spontaneous resolution of pericardial effusion has occurred in as many as 42% of those affected, the 6-month mortality rate among HIV-positive patients with pericardial effusion (62%) is higher than that among HIV-positive patients without that complication (7%). In HIV-positive patients in whom cardiac tamponade develops, mycobacterial infection is the most common cause worldwide (44%), followed by malignancy (16%) and other bacterial infection (11%). With regard to bacterial infection, *Staphylococcus aureus* is the most common causal agent. There are some differences, depending on the population

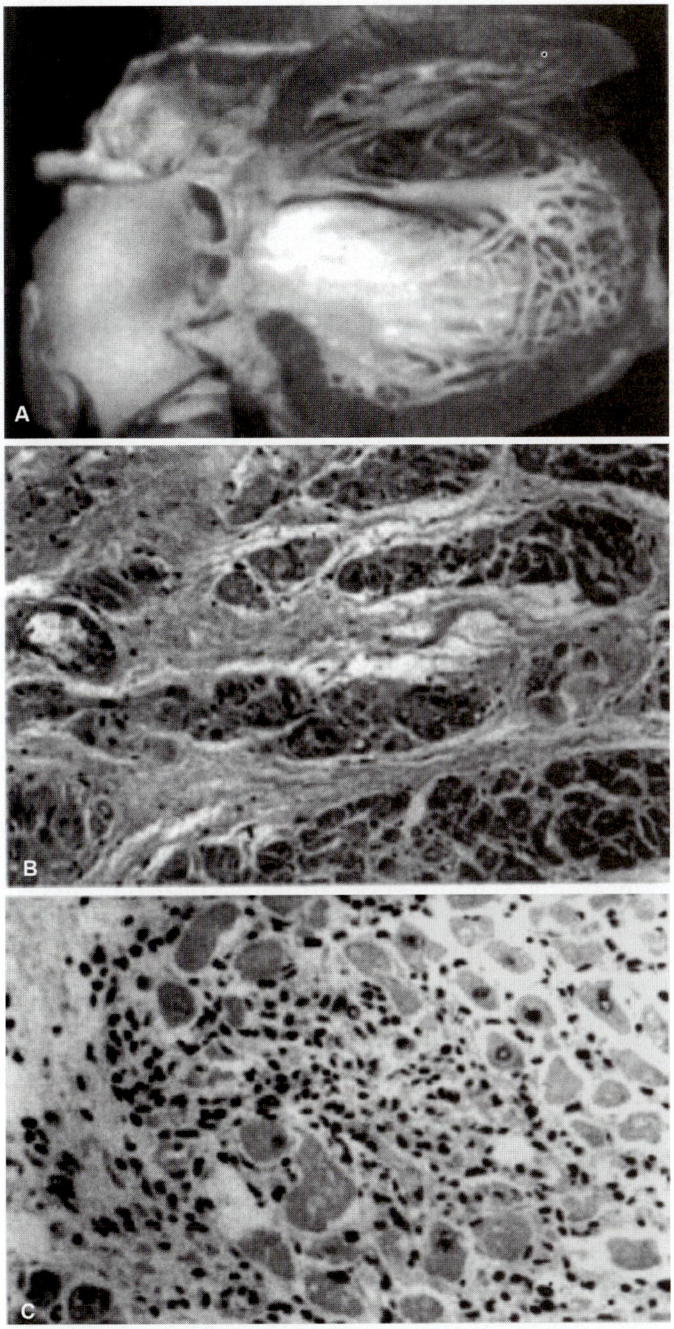

Fig. 18.5: *HIV related cardiomyopathy. (A) The heart is enlarged, principally from ventricular dilatation, and there is mild hypertrophy with diffuse endocardial fibrous thickening. Histological examination (B) may reveal myocyte hypertrophy with increased interstitial collagen or (C) evidence of myocarditis with lymphocytic infiltrate and myocyte necrosis*

of reference. In Africa, for example, in an estimated 70% of patients hospitalized for treatment of pericardial disease, that disease is related to HIV infection, with more than 90% of cases of HIV-related pericardial effusion caused by tuberculosis. Pericardial effusion and tamponade also may be manifestations of cardiac involvement in Kaposi sarcoma. The prognosis for patients with AIDS-related cardiac tamponade is poor, regardless of the method of treatment. Pneumopericardium is a rare complication of AIDS. It occurs when an infection or malignancy of the pericardium produces a fistulous connection to the adjacent esophagus, trachea, or bronchus. The condition may develop in patients with a pericardial infection by a gas-forming organism. Spontaneous pneumopericardium also has been reported.

Myocardial disease: According to various publications, the prevalence of myocardial abnormalities among AIDS patients is 25–75%. Myocardial abnormalities that may occur in HIV-positive patients include myocarditis, dilated cardiomyopathy, ischemic heart disease, and myocardial involvement in Kaposi sarcoma or lymphoma. Hypertrophy of the right ventricle may develop in response to AIDS-related pulmonary disease.

Myocardial dysfunctions: Histopathologic evidence of myocarditis has been found in approximately one-third of AIDS patients at autopsy, but no specific cause was identified in more than 80% of the cases. Common pathogens found in patients with AIDS-related myocarditis include *Toxoplasma gondii*, *Mycobacterium tuberculosis*, and *Cryptococcus neoformans*. Other infective agents that have been reported are *Mycobacterium avium-intracellulare* complex, *Aspergillus fumigatus*, *Candida albicans*, *Coccidioides immitis*, cytomegalovirus, and herpesvirus types 1 and 2 HIV itself has been implicated as a cause of myocarditis. Since cardiac myocytes do not possess CD4 receptors that would allow a virus to attach itself and enter the cell by the usual mechanism, it is not clear how a virus enters the myocytes. Reservoir cells (dendritic cells), as well as infection and injury of myocytes by other cardiotropic viruses, may facilitate the entry of HIV into CD4 receptor-negative cells. Lymphocytic myocarditis was present in 52% of patients who died of AIDS, and it frequently has been found in patients with left ventricular dysfunction. Autoimmune abnormalities and nutritional deficiencies

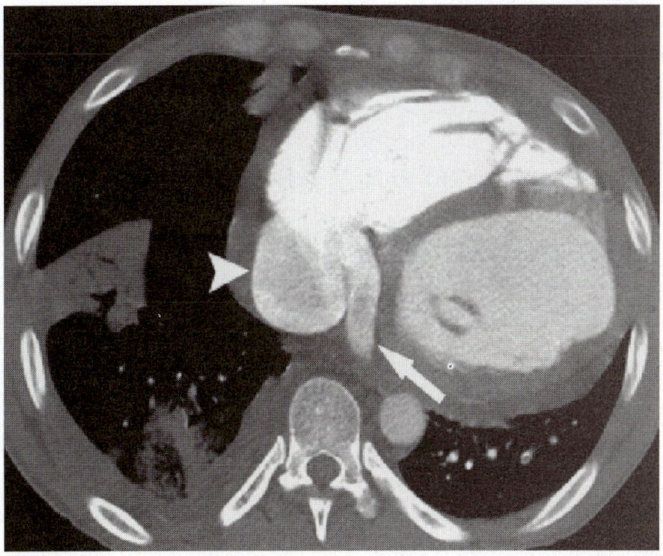

Fig. 18.6: *CT scan showing enlargement of both right and left ventricles in dilated cardiomyopathy*

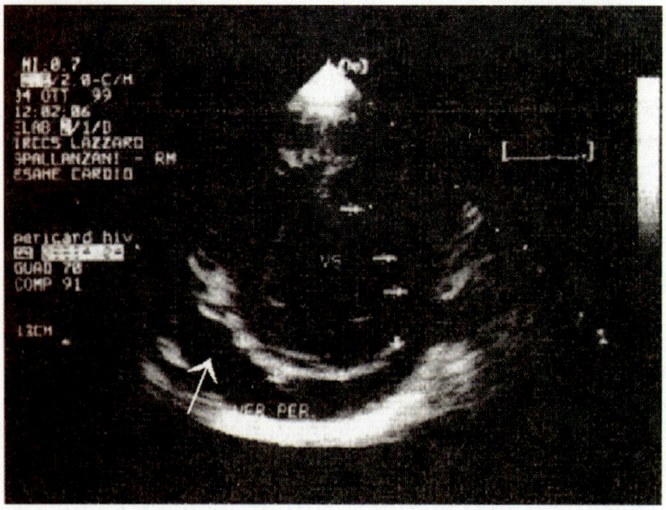

Fig. 18.7: *Echocardiography scan taken in left parasternal short-axis view shows circumscribed pericardial effusion (arrow) induced by mycobacterium avium intracellulare infection in HIV patient*

have been implicated in AIDS-related myocardial disease, and cardiac-specific autoantibodies (anti-myosin) have been found in 30% of patients with HIV-associated cardiomyopathy. An association between the use of zidovudine and cardiomyopathy also has been reported.

Dilated cardiomyopathy: HIV-related disease is now recognized as an important cause of dilated cardiomyopathy, with a prevalence of 8–30%. Prior to the introduction of HAART, the annual incidence of dilated cardiomyopathy was estimated at 15.9 per 1,000 patients with HIV infection. Usually seen in the late stage of AIDS, dilated cardiomyopathy is associated with a low CD4 count (fewer than 400 cells per milliliter) myocarditis due to HIV or another viral agent, such as a group B coxsackievirus (17%), cytomegalovirus (6%), or Epstein-Barr virus (3%), was found in 83% of patients with dilated cardiomyopathy diagnosed on the basis of histopathologic findings. Various studies have shown a correlation between dilated cardiomyopathy and a poor prognosis. In patients with dilated cardiomyopathy, the median survival period is reduced to 101 days, compared with 472 days for patients who are at a similar stage of AIDS, but whose hearts are normal. At gross pathologic examination, hearts with AIDS-related dilated cardiomyopathy reveal a constellation of findings. The left ventricular myocardium may show eccentric hypertrophy with increased wall thickness and chamber dilatation. Conversely, there may be thinning of the ventricular wall, especially of the free wall. In the setting of ventricular wall thinning, endocardial fibroelastosis and apical mural thrombi are common. Pericardial effusion or infective endocarditis may be present, especially in intravenous drug users. The features observed on echocardiograms and CT images acquired with helical scanning reflect the findings at gross pathologic examination and may include abnormal size and shape of the heart, ventricular dilatation, abnormalities of wall morphology and/or motion, and apical rounding. Secondary findings that may result from congestive pathophysiologic change include cephalization of the pulmonary vascular distribution and variable degrees of pulmonary edema and pleural effusion.

HIV endocarditis: Patients with AIDS may develop either infective endocarditis or nonbacterial thrombotic (marantic) endocarditis. Marantic endocarditis has been reported with increasing frequency in HIV-positive patients who are in the advanced or terminal stage of the disease, in whom it is frequently associated with malignancy, inanition, or HIV wasting syndrome. The prevalence of endocarditis in autopsy studies of patients with AIDS has been reported as 10–17%. Any of the cardiac valves may be involved in

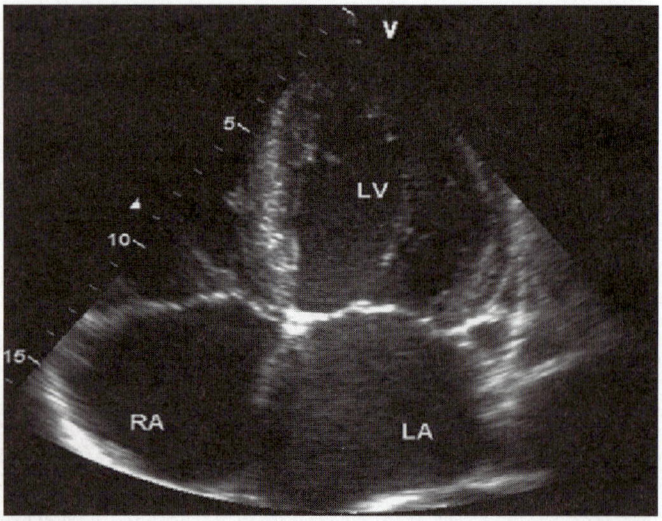

Fig. 18.8: *Two dimensional TTE in apical four chamber view showing enlargement of all four chambers of the heart in DCM caused by HIV disease*

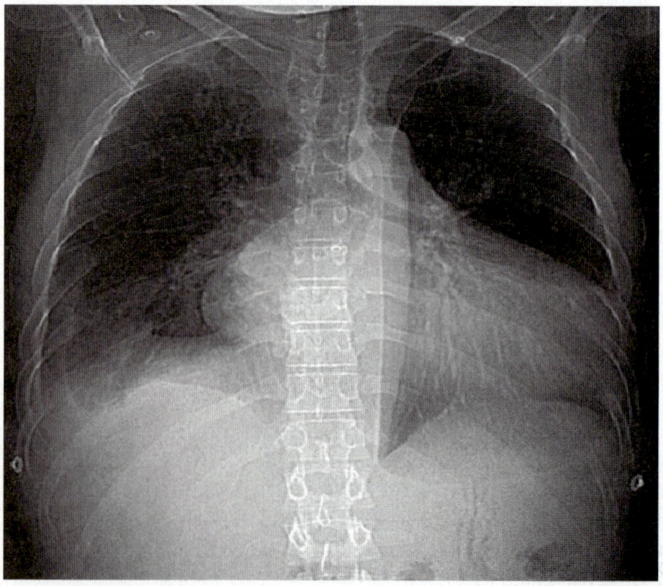

Fig. 18.9: *X-ray chest PA view showing massive enlargement of both right and left ventricles in dilated cardiomyopathy in HIV disease*

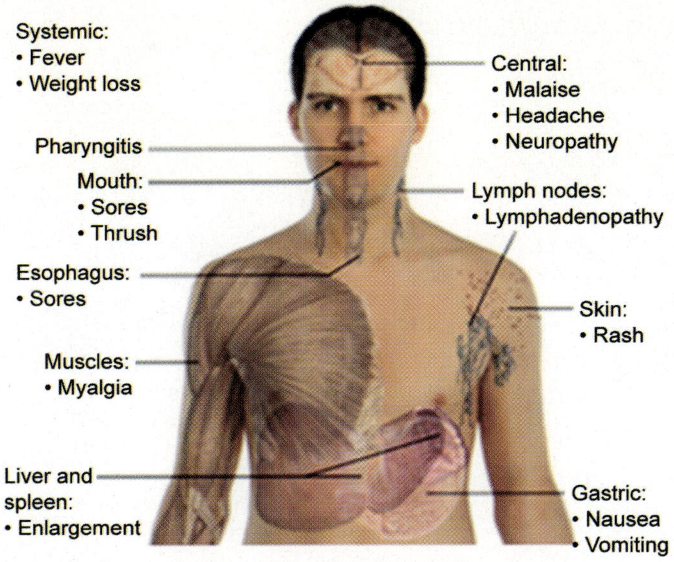

Fig.18.10A: *Illustration showing main symptoms of acute HIV infection*

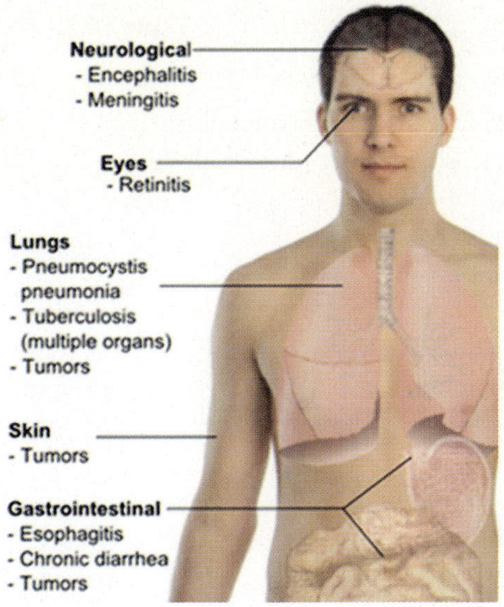

Fig 18.10B: *Illustration showing main symptoms of AIDS infection*

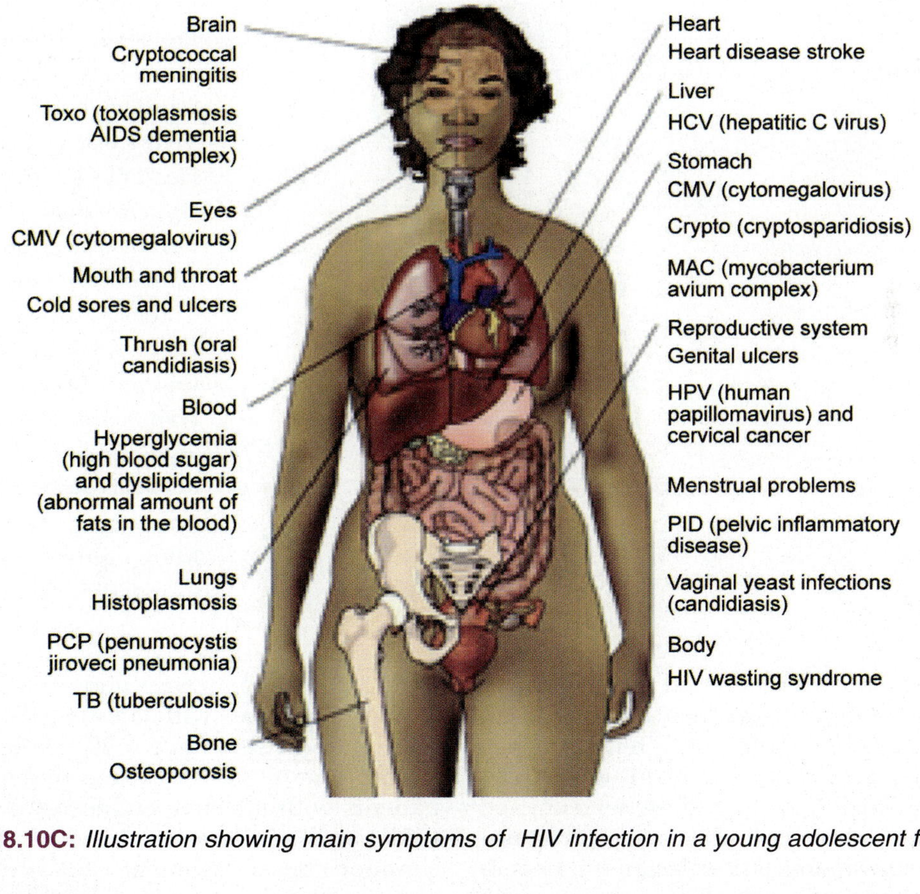

Fig.18.10C: *Illustration showing main symptoms of HIV infection in a young adolescent female*

endocarditis with multivalvular disease being common and tricuspid involvement being strikingly frequent. The condition is not limited to the valves; it also may arise in or involve the endocardial lining or vascular endothelium. The lesions in endocarditis occur singly or in multiples as masses of platelets and red blood cells combined in a fibrin mesh; inflammatory cells also may be present but are not a prominent feature (autopsy has revealed pulmonary and/ or systemic thromboembolism in at least 40% of HIV-positive patients with thrombotic endocarditis. In many

Table 18.2: *Drugs with potential cardiotoxicity used in HIV*

Drug	*Use in HIV*	*Cardiotoxicity*
Nucleoside transcriptase inhibitors	HIV disease	Cardiomyopathy
Nonnucleoside transcriptase inhibitors	HIV disease	Increased coronary vascular risk
Protease inhibitors	HIV disease	Increased coronary vascular risk
Antiinfective drugs	Opportunistic infections	
Eythromycin		Prolonged QT interval
Trimethoprim/sulfamethoxazole		Prolonged QT interval
Clarithromycin		Prolonged QT interval
Peniamidine		Prolonged QT interval Ventricular arrhythmias Orthostatic hypotension
Pyrimethamine		Prolonged QT interval
Fluoroquinolones		Prolonged QT interval
Ganciclovir		Ventricular arrhythmias
Foscarnet		Cardiomyopathy
Psychotropic drugs	Psychotic disorders, depression	
Tricyclic antidepressants		Prolonged QT interval
Phenothiazines		Prolonged QT interval
Antihistamines	Allergic reactions	
Astemizole		Prolonged QT interval
Terfenadine		Prolonged QT interval
Chemotherapy regimens	HIV-related neoplasms	
Anthracylines		Cardiomyopathy (acute/chronic) Ventricular arrhythmias Heart block
Vincristine		Hypertension Coronary heart disease
Interferon-α	Kaposi's sarcoma, Hepatitis C infection	Cardiomyopathy Coronary heart disease
Interleukin-2	HIV disease	Cardiomyopathy Coronary heart disease
Erythropositin-α	Chronic anaemia	Hypertension
Cocaine	Recreational	Hypertension Coronary heart disease (dissection) Cardiomyopathy Myocarditis
Anabolic steroids	Weight gain (recreationa)	Coronary heart disease

cases, embolism is not clinically diagnosed but is found at autopsy. Symptomatic embolic disease may manifest as an ischemic event (in the cerebral, pulmonary, renal, splenic, or mesenteric vessels) or an abscess . In patients with AIDS, infective endocarditis usually occurs in those who engage in nontherapeutic use of intravenous drugs; such drug use is a common risk factor among HIV-infected patients in western societies. Estimates of the prevalence of endocarditis among HIV-positive intravenous drug users vary, with reported values ranging from 6.3% to 34% Patients with infective endocarditis and HIV generally have the same endocarditis-related clinical manifestations as patients without HIV and have a similar survival rate (85% vs 93% for patients with and without HIV, respectively). However, patients with late-stage HIV-related disease and with endocarditis have a 30% higher mortality than do asymptomatic HIV-positive patients. In a series of 34 patients with infective endocarditis, *staphylococcus aureus* (75%) and *streptococcus viridans* (20%) were the most common causal organisms. Less commonly found were *Jaemophilus influenzae, Candida albicans, Salmonella* species, *Aspergillus fumigatus, Histoplasma capsulatum,* and *Cryptococcus neoformans*. The clinical symptoms may include fever, chills, sweating, weight loss, and septic emboli. The course and outcome of infective endocarditis are determined by the degree of damage to the heart, the

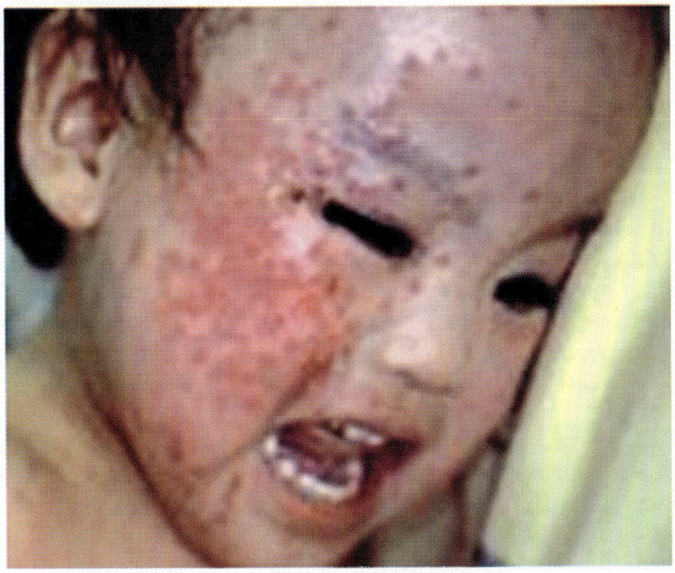

Fig. 18.11A: *Photograph of a young child with facial dermatosis in HIV infection*

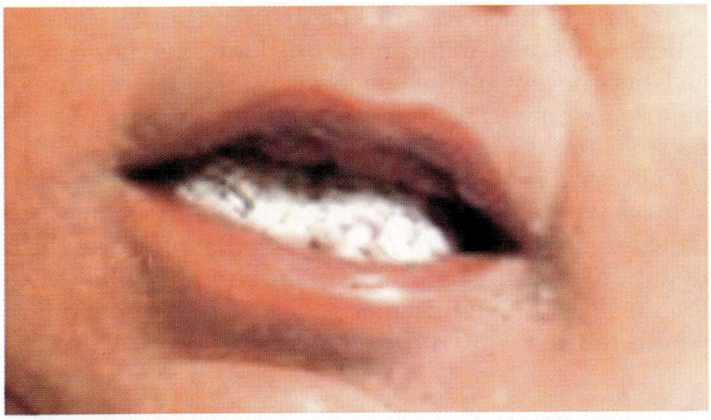

Fig 18.11B: *Photograph of a young child with mouth thrush in HIV infection*

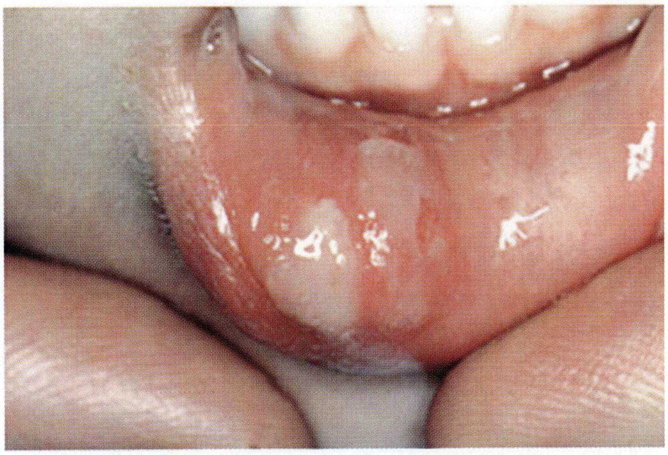

Fig. 18.11C: *Photograph of a young child with mouth ulcers in HIV infection*

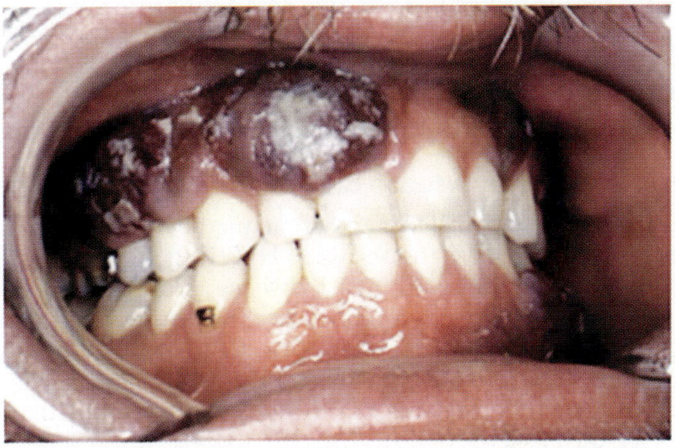

Fig. 18.11D: *Photograph showing intraoral Kaposi's sarcoma in an adolescent boy with HIV infection*

site of infection (right- vs left-sided valves; aortic vs mitral valve), the presence of distant seeding of infection, and the presence of ischemic changes. Peripheral embolization may occur in the presence of any causal organism and in any organ. In left-sided endocarditis, the most serious possible complications are cerebral and myocardial embolization, and the progression of disease may be rapid. Acute valvular insufficiency may develop as the result of the perforation of valve leaflets or rupture of chordae tendineae or papillary muscle and may cause heart failure with a rapid onset and a poor outcome Right-sided endocarditis typically involves the tricuspid valve; the possible pulmonary sequelae include septic emboli, abscess and infarction.

HIV and Cardiovascular Medicine: Key Points

- Approximately, 36 million people worldwide are infected with HIV including over 1 million children
- Significant cardiac disease affects 10–20% of patients infected with HIV and is the cause of death in approximately 5%
- HIV-related cardiomyopathy has a poor prognosis especially in patients with a low CD count or coexistent encephalopathy; pathogenesis is multificatorial and treatment options are limited
- Other frequent cardiac manifestations of HIV infection include opportunistic infection, infective endocarditis (especially affecting intravenous drug users). Pericardial

Table 18.3: *Pediatric HIV infection—immunological categories based on CD4 cell numbers*

Immunological	*<1 year*		*1–5 years*		*6–12 years*	
Category-1 (no immunosuppresion)	≥ 1500 cu mm	≥ 25%	≥ 1000/cu mm	≥ 25%	≥ 500/cu mm	≥ 25%
Category-2 (moderate immunosuppresion)	750–1499/cu mm	15–24%	500–999/cu mm	15–24%	200–499 cu mm	15–24%
Category-3 (severe immunsuppresion)	< 750/cu mm	<15%	<500/cu mm	<15%	<200 cu mm	<15%

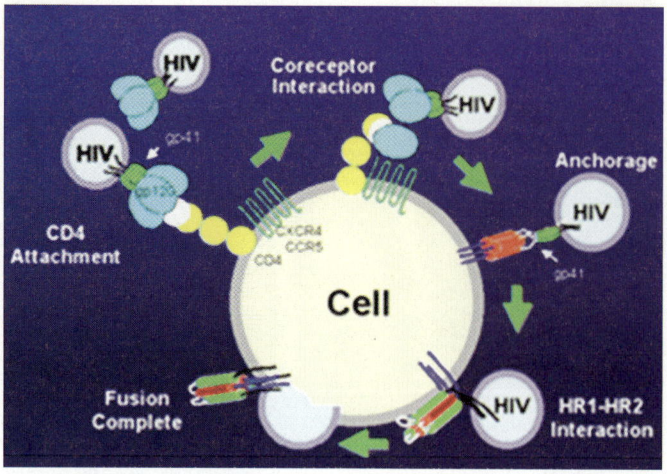

Fig. 18.12: *Showing HIV interaction with CD4 cells*

effusion, neoplasm (Kaposi's sarcoma/lymphoma) and pulmonary hypertension

- Premature vascular disease is an emerging problem especially in patients receiving combination antiretroviral therapy
- Cardiac surgery is well tolerated by patients with HIV/AIDS. The risks of transmission to the surgeon are low.

Ischemic Heart Disease and Coronary Artery Disease

Coronary artery disease and ischemic heart disease have been reported in patients with HIV infection. Both the prevalence of ischemic heart disease and the mortality associated with it apparently are increased among HIV-positive patients. The increased prevalence could be, at least in part, related to an improvement in the overall survival of HIV-positive patients, especially since the introduction of HAART. The origins of the disease appear to be multifactorial and related to the higher incidence of infection with herpesvirus, cytomegalovirus, or HIV-1, as well as to the inclusion in HAART of protease inhibitors, which have been reported to produce lipodystrophy, hyperlipidemia and hyperglycemia. In a retrospective analysis of data from the Frankfurt HIV cohort, which included almost 5,000 patients, a fourfold increase in the annual incidence of myocardial infarction among HIV-infected patients was found after the establishment of HAART with protease inhibitors, compared with the incidence among patients who underwent treatment before the institution of HAART. Histopathologic examination of coronary arteries generally reveals eccentric atheromatous and fibrous plaques, with variable degrees of chronic inflammation and accelerated arteriosclerosis. Unusual proliferation of smooth muscle cells with abundant elastic fibers, as well as diffuse and circumferential involvement of the coronary arteries without any intervening healthy segments, also have been reported.

Vasculitis syndrome with HIV: A range of inflammatory vascular diseases, both infective and noninfective, may occur in the setting of HIV. These include polyarteritis nodosa, Henoch-Schönlein purpura, and drug-induced hypersensitivity vasculitis. In a series of 34 patients with biopsy-documented transmural inflammation of blood vessels, the histopathologic findings included necrotizing arteritis, nonnecrotizing arteritis, neutrophilic inflammatory vascular disease, mononuclear inflammatory vascular disease, and other small-vessel inflammatory changes . Features similar to those in Kawasaki syndrome, coronary arteritis, and Takayasu arteritis also have been described Large-vessel disease may be aneurysmal or occlusive. Aneurysms may be single or multiple and may affect vessels such as the aorta or the common carotid, common iliac, femoral, or popliteal arteries. As many as seven aneurysms have been reported in a single patient. Occlusive disease has been reported in Africa in young HIV-positive patients and is less common than aneurysmal dilatation. In both processes, the main histopathologic features are found in the adventitia, with leukocytoclastic vasculitis of the vasa vasorum and periadventitial vessels, chronic inflammation, and fibrosis. Accelerated atherosclerosis also was found responsible for aortic aneurysm in a young man who had undergone several years of HAART for AIDS. A vast array of pathogens are capable of producing infective vasculitis.

Reports of infective arteritis or aortitis in HIV-positive patients are scarce in the literature. However, large vessels such as the aorta may become infected, and mycotic aneurysms may develop, especially in intravenous drug users. Causative agents include *Salmonella* species, *Mycobacterium tuberculosis*, and *Staphylococcus aureus*. In children with AIDS, arteriopathy with aneurysm may occur in the cerebral circulation, a condition that produces diffuse dilatation of the major arteries of the circle of Willis. Medial fibrosis, loss of the muscularis, destruction of the internal elastic lamina, and intimal hyperplasia are the most

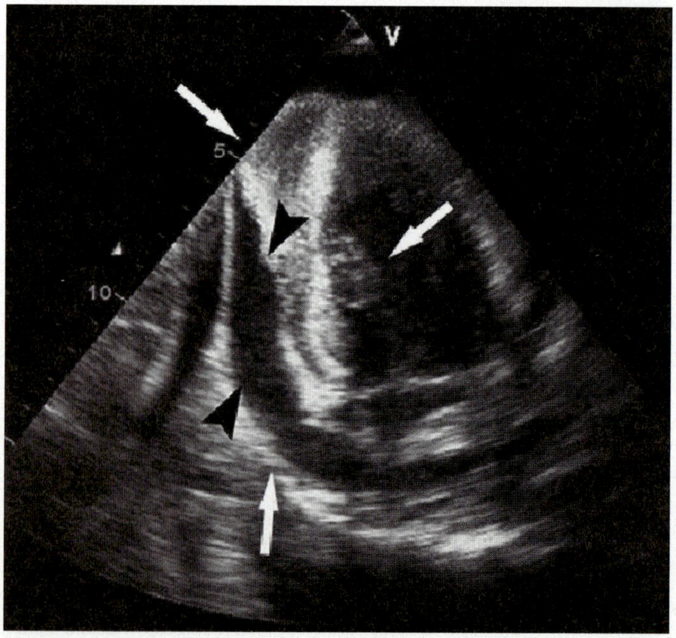

Fig. 18.13: *Short-axis view LV level showing cardiac mass (arrows) associated with pericardial effusion (arrow) in patient with HIV*

common findings. The prognosis is poor, and death occurs shortly after diagnosis.

Systemic arterial hypertension: The prevalence of systemic hypertension among HIV-infected patients is much higher than that in the general population. It has been estimated as 20–25% before the introduction of HAART and as approximately 74% among patients who undergo HAART with protease inhibitors and who subsequently develop lipodystrophy and metabolic syndrome. The lipodystrophic syndrome is characterized by peripheral fat wasting in the arms, legs, and buttocks, as well as by increased fat deposition in the breasts, abdomen, and dorsocervical fat pads. Systemic hypertension in HIV-positive patients seems to have a significant effect on their risk of premature cardiovascular disease: compared with normotensive HIV-positive patients, hypertensive patients have a higher frequency of coronary heart disease (16.1% vs 1.3%) and a higher incidence of myocardial infarction (8.1% vs 0.7%).

Thrombosis and embolism: HIV-infected patients tend to develop coagulation abnormalities due to increased levels of fibrinogen, d-dimer, plasminogen activator inhibitor-1, and tissue-type plasminogen activator antigen. A deficiency of protein S also has been identified. These hematologic abnormalities are associated with both arterial and venous thrombosis, especially in patients who are undergoing therapy with protease inhibitors. In a series of HIV-positive patients with venous or arterial thrombosis, deep vein involvement, most commonly in a lower extremity, and secondary pulmonary emboli accounted for 66% of all thrombotic events. In this cohort, persistent antiphospholipid antibodies were the most common abnormal serologic finding. An association between cigarette smoking and spontaneous thrombosis in HIV patients has been mentioned and was reported to affect 77% of the patients in one series.

Pulmonary arterial hypertension: It has been estimated that the incidence of this complication among HIV-positive patients is several thousand times greater (i.e. 2,500-fold) than that among the general population. Currently, the estimated overall incidence of pulmonary arterial hypertension among HIV-infected individuals is 1 in 200 (0.5%). The prognosis for patients with this complication is grim; mortality is high because of right-heart dysfunction, a condition that causes cardiogenic shock and sudden death in two-thirds of affected patients. Mesa et al reported a 1-year survival rate of 51% among HIV-positive patients with pulmonary arterial hypertension. Pulmonary arterial hypertension is considered an independent predictor of mortality among HIV-positive patients (relative risk). The cause of death may be right-heart failure, cardiogenic shock (64–76%), or respiratory collapse (34%). The exact mechanism by which pulmonary arterial hypertension develops is not clear, although various causal factors have been proposed including genetic predisposition, perivascular inflammation, increased expression of vascular endothelial growth factor A (a potent inducer of the growth of endothelial cells, which increases vascular permeability)

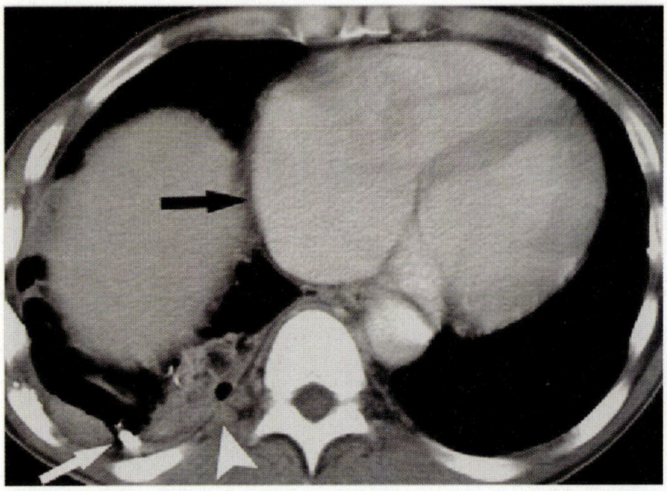

Fig. 18.14: *CT Scan showing infective endocarditis of TV in HIV patient.*

in T cells, increased expression of intrapulmonary platelet-derived growth factor, and HIV-induced release of active endothelial cellular mediators glycoprotein 120, an HIV-1 envelope glycoprotein, has been found to stimulate the production of endothelin 1 and tissue necrosis factor and to chronically increase the expression of endothelin1,a pulmonary vasoconstrictor. In 82% of cases, pulmonary arterial hypertension is due solely to HIV infection. Pulmonary arterial hypertension also has been attributed to recurrent pulmonary infection with secondary pulmonary inflammation and fibrosis, to intravenous drug abuse, and to cirrhosis. The most commonly observed symptoms are progressive shortness of breath (85% of cases), pedal edema (30% of cases) and cough (19% of cases). Findings at histopathologic analysis of lung tissue from patients with the condition are similar to those of primary pulmonary hypertension. The most common finding is plexogenic pulmonary arteriopathy, an abnormality seen in 78–85% of HIV-positive patients with pulmonary arterial hypertension. Less common pathologic findings include medial hypertrophy and intimal fibrosis without plexiform lesions (5% of patients), pulmonary veno-occlusive disease (7% of patients), and thrombotic pulmonary arteriopathy (4% of patients). The imaging findings in these patients also are similar to those observed in primary pulmonary arterial hypertension. They include enlargement of the pulmonary artery trunk (71% of patients), prominence of the central pulmonary arteries, tapering of peripheral vessels, and an enlarged cardiac silhouette secondary to right ventricular and right atrial dilatation (72% of patients). Abnormalities in cardiac morphologic features may be visualized with contrast-enhanced CT. These include right atrial and ventricular dilatation, often with reversal of the curvature of the interatrial and interventricular septa. Dilatation of the right heart chambers is the most common echocardiographic finding (98% of cases), followed by tricuspid regurgitation (64% of cases) and paradoxical septal motion (40% of cases). Other echocardiographic findings are right ventricular wall hypertrophy, septal

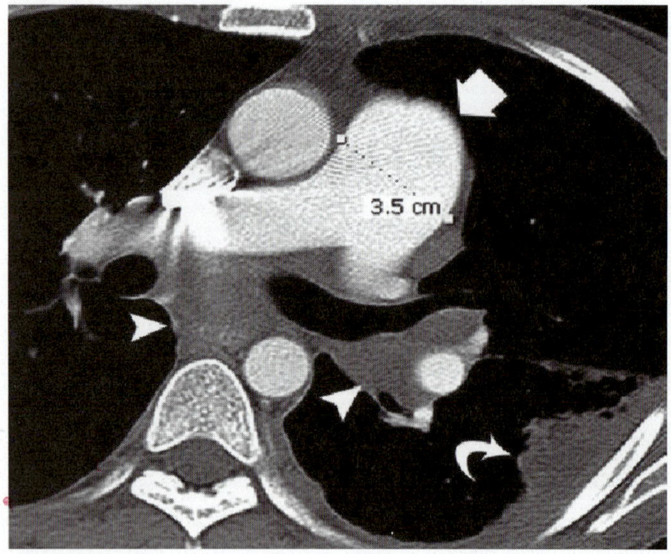

Fig. 18.15: *CT scan showing pulmonary arterial hypertension in patient with HIV disease and pulmonary tuberculosis*

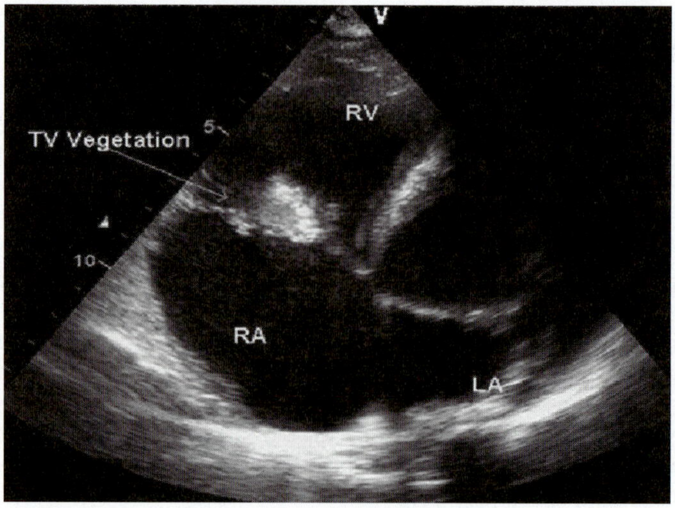

Fig. 18.17: *2-D TTE in Apical 4C oblique view showing TV valve endocarditis caused by HIV disease*

impingement on the left ventricle, and pulmonary valve insufficiency.

Cardiac neoplasms with HIV: Various malignancies are associated with AIDS both in adults and children. Kaposi sarcoma, non-Hodgkin lymphoma, squamous cell carcinoma, Hodgkin disease, and leiomyosarcoma (in children) are the more prevalent malignancies and are found with increasing frequency in patients infected with HIV. Of these malignancies, Kaposi sarcoma and non-Hodgkin lymphoma most often affect the heart. Kaposi sarcoma, which is caused by human herpesvirus 8, is the most common cardiac tumor seen in patients with AIDS. It was probably the first cardiac complication of AIDS to be recognized: Autran et al reported a case of Kaposi sarcoma of the heart in a young Haitian woman with AIDS in 1983. In retrospective autopsy studies in the pre-HAART era, the prevalence of cardiac Kaposi sarcoma in AIDS was estimated as 12–28%. Kaposi sarcoma is a low-grade malignancy that derives from mesenchymal or endothelial cells. The most common AIDS-related neoplasm, it occurs in approximately 30% of patients, mostly in homosexual or bisexual males (relative risk, 178). Cardiac involvement in Kaposi sarcoma in patients with AIDS usually occurs as part of disseminated disease. The epicardium and pericardium are the most frequently involved cardiac structures. Coronary wall infiltration and myocardial involvement also may occur. Pericardial hemorrhage with fatal cardiac tamponade has been described as a complication. In 7% of cases of cardiac tamponade in HIV-infected patients, Kaposi sarcoma was the cause. Isolated Kaposi sarcoma of the heart is rare. Lymphoma is the second most common tumor involving the heart in AIDS patients. Non-Hodgkin lymphoma was added to the group of AIDS-defining illnesses in 1987, after a 60- to 100-fold increase in the rate of lymphoma was observed among patients with HIV. The estimated relative risk of lymphoma for patients with AIDS is 72.8. Lymphoma is the first manifestation of AIDS in up to 4% of new cases. Primary cardiac malignancy associated with HIV infection is generally due to cardiac lymphoma. In 80–90% of cases, the majority of such lesions are high-grade B-cell tumors that consist of large cell immunoblastic or small non-cleaved-cell **(Burkitt or Burkitt-like) lymphomas.** At gross specimen examination, they may appear as a single mass or as multiple firm nodules of white tissue within the myocardium. Any cardiac chamber may be affected, but the right atrium is most commonly involved, followed by the right ventricle, left ventricle, left atrium, and atrial and ventricular septa. Pericardial extension is common. Secondary cardiac involvement in extranodal lymphoma may manifest as a mediastinal mass with extension through the pericardium or as lymphangitic or hematogenous lesions. Chest radiographs of patients with cardiac lymphoma usually show cardiomegaly, pericardial effusion, and signs of congestive heart failure. Echo-

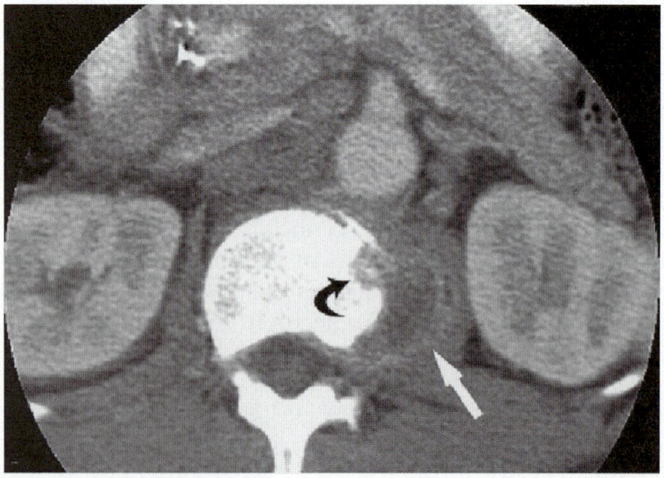

Fig. 18.16: *CT scan showing noncavitory and cavitory septic emboil in the lung in patient with HIV disease*

Table 18.4: *Guidelines for PCP prophylaxis for children born to HIV seropositive mothers*

Age	*Status of child*	*Cortrimoxazole prophylaxis*	*CD4 cell count monitoring*
1. Birth to 6 weeks	Born to HIV Seropositive mother	Not required	At birth and at 4–8 weeks
2. 6 weeks–4 months	Born to HIV Seropositive mother	Given to all babies	Repeat at 3 months
3. 4–12 months	HIV infected or exact status not known	Given to all such babies	Repeat every 3 months
4. 4–12 months	HIV infection ruled out	Stop prophylaxis	Not required
5. 1–5 years	HIV infected	Prophylaxis continued if child is in immne category 3	Repeat every 3 months
6. 6–12 years	HIV infected	Prophylaxis continued if child is in immune category 3	Repeat every 3 months

cardiograms typically depict a hypoechoic cardiac mass with or without pericardial effusion. On unenhanced CT images, the tumors have soft-tissue attenuation equal to or less than that of myocardium. With intravascular administration of an iodinated contrast medium, they show heterogeneous enhancement. MR images depict poorly defined and heterogeneous lesions that, compared with the signal intensity of cardiac muscle, are isointense or slightly hypointense on T1-weighted images, isointense on proton density-weighted images, and isointense to hyperintense on T2-weighted images. The use of an intravenous gadolinium-based contrast medium produces heterogeneous enhancement. These masses are less likely than other cardiac tumors (e.g. sarcomas) to exhibit central necrosis. A significant pericardial effusion has been reported in 50% of patients with pericardial lymphoma. However, the presence of pericardial fluid is not conclusive evidence of pericardial involvement in lymphoma.

Treatment of Pediatric HIV Infection

Basic Principles of Therapy in HIV Children

1. All children with HIV infection should be offered specific ART irrespective of their clinical status, CD4 counts or HIV RNA copy number but economic feasibility is a major consideration in developing countries and only a minority of our patients are able to afford therapy.
2. All drugs which have been approved for adults can be used in children even when specific pediatric pharmacokinetic studies have not been carried out and the effects on growth and development are not clearly defined.
3. Monotherapy is contraindicated because it may result in incomplete suppression of HIV replication thereby allowing the emergence of drug resistance.
4. Early initiation of appropriate therapy (hit hard, hit early!) is advantageous because it slows deterioration of immune function, delays progression of disease, reduces incidence of opportunistic infections and prolongs patient survival
5. ART is most effective in patients who have never received therapy (are treatment naive) and the most potent regimen, appropriate for a given clincial situation, should be initiated rather than keeping it 'in reserve' for future use.
6. Treatment has to continue even after the CD4 T lymphocyte counts have reached normal levels and HIV RNA is undetectable in the blood. In such situations the virus can still be cultured from the lymph nodes and would result in a resurgence of the infection if ART is discontinued. Therapy, therefore, is a life-long commitment.

Recommended Drugs

A large number of antiretroviral drugs are available to the clinician HIV infection is now considered to be a "chronic manageable condition" rather than a "rapidly fatal illness". Prolonged survival is a distinct reality with the advent of triple drug therapy. Nucleoside analogue reverse transcriptase inhibitors (NRTIs) were the first drugs to be used for treatment of HIV infection and are also the least expensive. A combination of 2 NRTIs along with a protease inhibitor (PI) or a non-nucleoside analogue reverse transcriptase inhibitor (NNRTI) is the preferred initial therapy. ddc is believed to be less powerful than ZDV, ddI or 3TC. ZDV and d4T should not be used together.

NNRTIs are being increasingly used in HIV treatment protocols even in children. Unlike most other antiretroviral drugs, NNRTIs are not associated with significant side-effects and do not have restrictions associated with intake of food. Further they need to be taken only once or twice daily and this improves patient compliance. They also freely cross the blood brain barrier. PIs have been in use for more than 5 years now. Nelfinavir and ritonavir were the first PIs to receive FDA approval for use in children. The major problems associated with PIs relate to the expense of therapy and poor patient compliance because of associated side-effects. Most PIs have restrictions related to intake of food and have significant drug-interactions, the most notable of these being with other antiretroviral drugs and antitubercular medications. A number of disturbing and bizarre side-effects have recently been reported in patients on long-term therapy on this group of drugs. These include obesity (protease paunch!), lipodystrophy, gynecomastia, hyperglycemia, hyperlipidemia and perianal abscesses (tails!). It is these side-effects which preclude the continued use of PIs in upto 20–30% of patients.

Initiation of drug therapy: Any one of the following combinations may be started:

1. SZDV + 3TC + PI/NNRTI
2. ZDV + ddI + PI/NNRTI
3. d4T + 3TC + PI/NNRTI
4. d4T + ddI + PI/NNRTIWe prefer using a combination of ZDV and 3TC. Other acceptable NRTI combinations include ZDV + ddI/ddC or d4T + 3TC/ddI.

The role of dual PI based combinations (in addition to 2 NRTIs) as initial therapy is yet to be clearly defined, but may be considered in patients with advanced HIV disease. The only PI which is easily available in India is saquinavir but this is the least powerful of all the PIs.

When to change ART may need to be changed under the following circumstances:

1. **Clinical evidence of disease progression.**
2. **Inadequate virological response** even after 12 weeks of therapy from baseline HIV RNA levels; or repeated detection of HIV RNA in a child who had undetectable levels in response to initial therapy.
3. **Immunological deterioration,** for example, a rapid/substantial decrease in CD4 counts.
4. **Failure of compliance** with the current regimen.

Is there a role for dual/mono NRTI therapy?

Theoretically, any child who requires ART should be given triple drug therapy. However, the cost of this therapy turns out to be prohibitive and very few of our patients are able to afford it. In such situations, we do offer dual NRTI therapy (e.g. with ZDV and 3TC) as it results in significant clinical improvement and virological and immunological recovery and improves the overall quality of life, albeit for a short-term. Development of resistance is a risk associated with such therapy but in children this is to some extent acceptable because under normal circumstances children, unlike adults, would not pass on such resistant strains to other individuals. We never use monotherapy now a days.

Prevention of perinatal transmission: Prevention of perinatal transmission of HIV has been one of the big success stories of HIV treatment. In 1994, the joint French-American placebo-controlled double blind trial (ACTG 076) of ZDV therapy showed that administration of the drug (100 mg five times a day) during the second and third trimesters of pregnancy followed by an intravenous bolus of 2 mg/kg at start of labour and 1 mg/kg/hour thereafter, and oral administration (2 mg/kg/every 6 hours) to the neonate for 6 weeks resulted in a 66% decrease in the rate of perinatal transmission if breastfeeding was not allowed. Subsequent trials conducted in Thailand (breastfeeding not allowed) and in Ivory Coast and Burkina Faso (breast-feeding allowed) have shown that even much shorter courses of ZDV (given for 2–4 weeks before delivery) have resulted in a significant decrease in rates of perinatal transmission (by 38–50%). The cost of such short course ZDV regimens is obviously much less than the original ACTG 076 regimen. An even more promising regimen is the one pertaining to single dose nevirapine (2 tablets of 200 mg each) along with a dose given to the newborn baby (2 mg/kg within 72 hours of birth), which resulted in a 50% reduction in perinatal transmission. It is now clear that if in addition to administration of antiretroviral drug the mother undergoes an elective cesarean section along with douching of the birth canal with virucidal agents, the perinatal transmission rates can be brought down to almost negligible levels (say 1–5%). This is indeed a big change from the perinatal transmission rates of 12–43% reported in early nineties.

Table 18.5: *Showing single tablet antiretriviral medications*

Single-tablet antiretroviral medications

Components	*Brand*	*Dose: each dose contains*	*Meal restrictions*
Tenofovir-emtricitabine-efavirenz	Atripla	1 QD: Tenofovir 300 mg + emtricitabine 200 mg + Efavirenz 600 mg	Take on empty stomach to ↓ side effects
Tenofovir-emtricitabine-rilpivirine	Complera	1 QD: Tenofovir 300 mg + emtricitabine 200 mg + rilpivirine 25 mg	With a meal
Tenofovir-emtricitabine-cobicistat-elvitegravir	Stribild	1 QD: Tenofovir 300 mg + emtricitabine 200 mg + cobicistat 150 mg + elvitegravir 150 mg	With food

Table 18.6: *Showing original and current formulations in antiretroviral medications*

Antiretroviral drug	*Original formulation*		*Current simplest formulation*	
Zidovudine	2 × 100 mg every 4 hours	12/day	300 mg twice daily	2/day
Didanosine	2 × 100 mg twice daily	4/day	400 mg EC once daily	1/day
Stavudine	30/40 mg twice daily	2/day	100 mg XR once daily	1/day
Lamivudine	150 mg twice daily	2/day	300 mg once daily	1/day
Efavirenz	200 mg caps once daily	3/day	600 mg once daily	1/day
Nelfinavir	3 × 250 mg 3 times daily	9/day	2 × 625 mg twice daily	4/day
Saquinavir	3 × 200 mg 3 times daily	9/day	2 × 500 mg + ritonavir 100 mg twice daily	6/day
Amprenavir	8 × 150 mg twice daily	16/day	2 × fosamprenavir 700 mg twice daily	4/day
Lopinavir/ritonavir	3 × 133/33 mg twice daily	6/day	4 × 200/50 mg once daily	4/day

Prophylactic measures in HIV patients: Prophylaxis against opportunistic infections is indicated whenever there is significant immunodeficiency. The most important opportunistic infection is with the fungus *Pneumocystis carinii* for which cotrimoxazole is the preferred drug and definite guidelines are available for its use in children (Table 18.4). The dose is approximately 1–2 mg/kg/day of trimethoprim given at bed-time. Cotrimoxazole perhaps also provides some protection against other bacterial infections which are common in developing countries. Rigid application of the guidelines for cotrimoxazole prophylaxis based on the child's CD4 counts is difficult in our country because of the costs involved in performing the test. Prophylaxis against *Mycobacterium tuberculosis* and fungal infections is given only when there is a specific indication (e.g. contact with an open case of tuberculosis; or culture proven systemic fungal infection). Routine use of isoniazid for all patients with HIV infection is not an acceptable clinical practice. Unusual modes of presentation–the clinician, therefore, has to have a high index of suspicion. We follow the usual immunization schedule in HIV infected children, but inactivated polio vaccine may be preferred to oral polio vaccine. The former, however, is not easily available in India. One should not unnecessarily withhold other live vaccines (e.g. BCG, measles) from such children because the accrued benefits far outweigh the associated risks, specially in developing countries. The immunodeficiency associated with HIV is quantitatively and qualitatively different from that of a child having severe combined immunodeficiency, a syndrome in which live vaccines are strictly contra-indicated. Nutritional rehabilitation is an important aspect of management of such children and requisite efforts must be put in to ensure an adequate intake of food items that are inexpensive and culturally acceptable. The results of such interventions are often very gratifying.

Post-exposure prophylaxis: As the number of HIV infected patients increases it is inevitable that hospital accidents, due to needle-stick injuries and cuts with scalpels/other sharps involving hospital personnel who deal with them, would also show an increase. At our hospital, we encounter 2–4 such accidents every year. The risk of seroconversion following a needle stick injury is believed to be 3/1,000. The site of exposure should be washed with water and detergent and a virucidal agent should be applied. All individuals who have had such accidental pricks/cuts or who have had mucocutaneous exposure to biological fluids

Table 18.7: *Nucleoside and nucleotide reverse transcriptase inhibitors in antiretroviral medications*

Nucleoside and nucleotide reverse transcriptase inhibitors

Generic name	*Trade name*	*Dose*	*Meal restrictions*
Abacavir (ABC)	(Ziagen)	600 mg QD or 300 mg BID	With or without food
Didanosine (ddl)	Videx EC	Weight 60 kg: 400 mg QD (with tenofovir: 250 mg QD)	Take 1/2 hr before or 2 hrs after meal
Emtricitabine (FTC)	Emtriva	200 mg QD	With or without food
Lamivudine (3TC)	Epivir	200 mg QD	With or without food
Stavudine (d4T)	Zerit	40 mg BID (30 mg BID for body weight < 60 kg)	With or without food
Tenofovir DF (TDF)	Viread	300 mg QD	With or without food
Zidovudine (AZT)	Retrovir	300 mg BID or 200 mg TID	With or without food
Abacavir + lamivudine	Epzicom	1 QD; each pill contains abacavir 600 mg + lamivudine 300 mg	With or without food
Tenofovir DF + emtricitabine	Truvada	1 QD; each pill contains tenofovir 300 mg + emtricitabine 200 mg	With or without food
Zidovudine + lamivudine	Combivir	1 BID; each pill contains zidovudine 300 mg + lamivudine 150 mg	With or without food
Zidovudine + lamivudine + abacavir	Trizivir	1 BID; each pill contains zidovudine 300 mg + lamivudine 150 mg + abacavir 300 mg	With or without food

Table 18.8: *Recommended dosing for new antiretroviral agents*

Drug	*Dosing form(s)*	*Recommended dosages for combination therapy*
Darunavir	600, 400 mg tablets	800/100 mg ritonavir once daily[a] 600/100 mg ritonavir twice daily
Etravirine	100 mg tablet	200 mg twice daily
Maraviroc	150 and 300 mg tablets	150 mg twice daily (CYP3A4 inhibitors ± inducers)[b] 300 mg twice daily 600 mg twice daily (CYP3A4 inducers)[c]
Raitegravir	400 mg tablets	400 mg twice daily

CYP, cytochrome P-450

[a] Treatment-naive patients

[b] Includes protease inhibitor (except tipranavir/ritonavir), detavirdine, ketoconazole, itraconazole, clarithromycin or other strong 3A4 inhibitors with or without concomitant 3A4 inducers.

[c] Includes efavirenz, rifampin, cart-bamazepine, phenobarbital, phenyton, excludes nevirapine.

(say over the conjunctiva) should be offered counselling and advised to take a course of ZDV and 3TC for at least 4 weeks, preferably longer. Further, an ELISA test should be performed soon after exposure and repeated thereafter at 6 weeks and 6 months. In situations where the chances of transmission are very high (e.g. patient with high viral load and inoculation involving a hollow bevelled needle) indinavir should be administered along with ZDV and 3TC. Needless to say such accidents are best prevented. One must incorporate stringent precautions (universal precautions) in day to day clinical care. All biological samples must be considered potentially infected. Gloves should be worn during venepunctures and while setting up drips. We use bleaching powder for disinfection of soiled bandages, bed linen, etc.

Role of newer drugs in HIV patients: Triple drug therapy is by no means a panacea as far as treatment of HIV infection is concerned. There is a significant number of patients (say 20–40%) who have to discontinue such therapy due to intolerable side-effects (specially with PIs), treatment related toxicity or treatment failure. A number of new approaches are being tried in such situations. These include use of integrase inhibitors (e.g. AR177) and fusion inhibitors (e.g. T-20). The latter group of drugs prevent fusion of HIV with target cells. Adefovir, a nucleotide analogue, has also shown promising results and is believed to be unique because HIV does not easily develop resistance to it. Even amongst the conventional groups of AR drugs, exciting developments are taking place. Newer NRTIs (e.g. emtricitabine), NNRTIs (DMP 961, DMP 963, AG 1549) and PIs (e.g. AG 1776, ABT 378) are in the stage of trials and may turn out to be clinically useful. Further, chemokines have been isolated which interfere with coreceptors involved in HIV infection (e.g. CCR5, CXCR4). Benzamide comopunds interfere with zinc finger proteins which are necessary for viral packaging and replication. Although curative therapy of HIV infection is still a distant mirage, overall there is far more optimism today than was the case in early nineties. Sources of Information Treatment guidelines for HIV are changing rapidly and regimens which are state of the art today may be considered obsolete within a year. A number of websites are available which provide regular updates. A number of highly effective anti-retroviral drugs are now available for treatment of human immunodeficiency virus (HIV) infection, even in children. HIV infection is no longer considered a rapidly fatal illness, but rather a chronic manageable condition.

Although specific antiretroviral therapy is rather expensive at present and beyond the reach of many patients in developing countries, there is a lot else that one can do for management of such children.

Long-term Effects of Antiretroviral Treatment in Children

Until recently, the prognosis of AIDS was so poor that concerns about long-term effects of drug treatment were minor. However, due to the advent of potent antiretroviral drugs, mortality of persons suffering with the disease has been reduced. Besides, these drugs are also known to reduce disease progression, and incidence of HIV-related disorders. A most important field of research is the possible increase of cardiovascular risk in patients treated with protease inhibitors. The three classes of drugs presently used for people with HIV infection include:

1. Nucleoside reverse transcriptase inhibitors
2. Non-nucleoside reverse transcriptase inhibitors
3. Protease inhibitors.

The current standard of treatment is a protease inhibitor or a non-nucleoside reverse transcriptase inhibitor combined with two nucleoside reverse transcriptase inhibitors, although modifications of this regimen are in constant evolution.

Risk factors pertaining to the usage of these drugs are: Induced **dilated cardiomyopathy** secondary to mitochondrial toxicity.

Hyperlipidaemia, hyperglycaemia, hyperinsulinaemia, and lipodystrophy are frequent adverse effects of potent antiretroviral combination therapy, particularly involving protease inhibitors. Besides, the degree of increase seems to be proportional to the duration of treatment and type of drug. Patients treated with protease inhibitors also are considered to be at a **higher risk of heart attack.**

Drugs used for HIV related diseases may have adverse cardiac effects including cardiomyopathy, QTc prolongation with increased risk of irregular heartbeats and acceleration of coronary disease.

In view of their condition, HIV patients also face difficulties when their cardiac problems require surgery. This is because of concerns that surgeons would be exposed

Table 18.9: *Showing nevirapine therapy for infants*

Nevirapine dosing for infants	
Weight or age of infant	*Nevirapine dose*
Birth to 6 weeks	
Birth weight 2,000–2,499 g	10 mg once daily
Birth weight > 2,500 g	15 mg once daily
> 6 weeks to 6 months	20 mg once daily
> 6 months to 9 months	30 mg once daily
> 9 months to end of breastfeeding	40 mg once daily

This chart outlines appropriate dosing of nevirapine for infants on extended prophylaxis while breastfeeding.
The pharmacokinetics and appropriate dosing of nevirapine for preterm infants with birth weight < 2,000 grams has not been determined: because nevirapine elimination may be longer in preterm infants, initial dosing on a mg per kg body weight basis would be preferred (i.e. 2 mg/kg daily).

Table 18.10: *Recommended neonatal dosing for prevention of mother-to-child transmission of HIV*

All HIV-exposed infants (initiated as soon after delivery as possible)		
Zidovudine (ZDV)	*Dosing*	*Duration*
ZDV	≥ 35 weeks gestation at birth: 4 mg/kg/dose PO twice daily, started as soon after birth as possible and preferably within 6–12 hours of delivery (or, if unable to tolerate oral agents, 3 mg/kg/dose IV, beginning within 6–12 hours of delivery, then every 12 hours)	Birth through 6 weeks
ZDV	≥ 30 to < 35 weeks gestation at birth: 2 mg/kg/dose PO (or 1.5 mg/kg/dose IV), started as soon after birth as possible, preferably within 6–12 hours, advanced to 3 mg/kg/dose PO (or 2.3 mg/kg/dose IV) every 12 hours at age 15 days	Birth through 6 weeks
ZDV	< 30 weeks gestation at birth: 2 mg/kg body weight/dose PO (or 1.5 mg/kg/dose IV) started as soon after birth as possible, preferably within 6–12 hours of delivery, then every 12 hours, advanced to 3 mg/kg/dose PO (or 2.3 mg/kg/dose IV) every 12 hours after age 4 weeks	Birth through 6 weeks
Additional antiretroviral prophylaxis agents for HIV-exposed infants of women who received no antepartum antiretroviral prophylaxis (initiated as soon after delivery as possible)		
In addition to ZDV as shown above, administer	Birth weight 1.5–2 kg: 8 mg/dose PO	3 doses in the first week of life
Nevirapine (NVP)	Birth weight > 2 kg: 12 mg/dose PO	• 1st dose within 48 hours of birth (birth-48 hours) • 2nd dose 48 hours after 1st • 3rd dose 96 hours after 2nd

IV, intravenously; NVP, nevirapine; PO, orally; ZDV, zidovudine.

to significant risk of acquiring HIV infection, during the process. However, with drug-induced preoperative reduction of viral load, use of appropriate precautions, also to combat the event of needlestick injury, surgeons need not fear definite transmission during cardiac surgery.

The heart may indicate an HIV infected patient's overall health, and as role of infection and inflammation in many other cardiovascular diseases is now known, these patients may benefit, even though partially, as would be the case with millions of others. Studies have shown that antiretroviral treatment reduces illness and mortality among children living with HIV in much the same way that it does among adults. A trial in the United States, for example, found that the mortality rate among a sample of infected children was reduced from 5.3% to 0.7% per year after antiretroviral treatment was made widely available. Similar results have been found in developing countries. A study released in 2007, which monitored 586 HIV-positive children receiving antiretroviral treatment in 14 different Asian and African countries, found that 82% were still alive after 2 years.

Some of the most compelling evidence that treatment works in children does not come from studies or statistics, but rather the personal testimonies of those who have witnessed HIV-positive children returning to health after starting treatment:

"You see scrawny, rashy, tired, lethargic kids come in, you start them on treatment and within weeks you've got bounding, podgy, gorgeous growing children. People often don't believe, they're often quite sceptical of the medications, and then you see this transformation and parents are like 'The child's got so much energy!'"—Julie, UK nurse working with children living with HIV.

Starting Antiretroviral Treatment in Children

As with adult treatment, there is ongoing debate about when it is best to start antiretroviral treatment in HIV-positive children. There is a complex balance between the immediate benefits of providing treatment to children who are not showing any symptoms of AIDS-related illness, and concerns about long-term resistance and drug side effects if treatment is started too early. The general view is that treatment should be started when there is a significant risk of progression from HIV to AIDS, although the definition of "significant" is not always clear. Many experts feel that the risk of progression in HIV-positive children under the age of 1 year is so high that they always offer antiretroviral treatment.

To judge whether an HIV-positive person needs to start receiving treatment, a CD4 test is usually carried out. This test measures the number of T-helper cells-white blood cells that are attacked by HIV-in an individual's blood. It can either measure the absolute number of CD4 cells, or the percentage of white blood cells that are CD4 cells, in a sample of blood.

A falling CD4 count is a sign that HIV is progressing, and that the immune system is becoming weaker. In healthy, uninfected adults, absolute CD4 count is usually between 400 and 1,600 cells per millimetre cubed of blood. When a HIV-positive adult's CD4 count falls between 350 and 200, it is usually recommended that they start receiving antiretroviral treatment. For children below the age of six, though, these adult guidelines are generally irrelevant. Children below this age generally have a much higher CD4 level than is usually present in adults, unless their immune system has been damaged by AIDS. The CD4 levels found in children therefore need to be judged in context of their age, which can make it difficult to know exactly when treatment should be started. Since percentage CD4 count generally varies less with age, this type of test is generally recommended in children under the age of 5 years. It is generally agreed across guidelines that a child-aged less than 1 year with a percentage CD4 count below 25% should be started on treatment, whether symptomatic or not. In Europe, it is recommended that asymptomatic HIV positive children be started on treatment if the risk that they will progress to AIDS is higher than 10%, and the risk of death is higher than 5%; this can be determined through an assessment of percentage CD4 count and age. In the US, it is recommended that treatment be at least considered for all HIV positive children under the age of 1 year. In some cases, viral load testing (which measures the amount of HIV in an individual's blood) is used alongside CD4 testing to guide decisions about treatment.

In resource-poor communities, the technology needed for CD4 counts and viral load testing is not always available. In the absence of these facilities, healthcare workers looking after a HIV-positive child sometimes have to make a clinical presumption that treatment needs to be started. The World Health Organisation recommends that if a child has reached a stage of severe or advanced HIV infection, then they need to start treatment. A HIV-positive child may be assumed to have reached these stages if they are suffering from any condition that is strongly associated with AIDS, or if symptoms of oral thrush, severe pneumonia or severe sepsis are present.

Which antiretroviral drugs should be used?

Many of the drugs that are conventionally used to treat adults living with HIV are not available in an appropriate form, or licensed/approved for use in children. Those that are available are often unaffordable in the areas where they are most needed. Where the correct drugs are available, there are a number of different combinations that can work effectively in children. As with adults, antiretroviral therapy with at least three drugs is recommended when treating children, because this prevents HIV from becoming resistant to any single drug. It is usually recommended that this therapy should consist of two nucleoside reverse transcriptase inhibitors (NRTIs) combined with either one non-nucleoside reverse transcriptase inhibitor (NNRTI) or a protease inhibitor (PI). NRTIs form the "backbone" of any treatment regimen for children, and a number of combinations of these drugs are approved for use in paediatric treatment. Equally, there are some combinations that are not recommended, and there are specific advantages and disadvantages attached to all dual NRTI combinations. In developed countries, the two NRTIs are either combined with an NNRTI or a protease inhibitor. In children under 3, the NNRTI used is usually nevirapine, since there is a lack of dosing information available for efavirenz (the only other widely used NNRTI).

In resource-poor communities, NRTI/NNRTI-based combinations are recommended over other combinations, due to their relatively low cost and the availability of appropriate generic drugs. World Health Organisation guidelines for resource-poor communities do not recommend the use of protease inhibitors for initial therapy, because it is felt that they should be saved for second-line treatment if it is needed. The WHO recommends that in resource-poor communities, the two NRTIs should include 3TC (lamivudine), combined with AZT (zidovudine), d4t (stavudine), or ABC (abacavir). A triple NRTI regimen, which avoids the use of an NNRTI, can also be considered as an option for initial therapy in special circumstances. This would be AZT or d4T, combined with both 3TC and ABC.

There are many factors that can influence the choice of drugs for children. Considerations about medications that the mother may have received during pregnancy, the toxicity of certain drugs, and whether the child is still being breastfed, all need to be taken into account when choosing a regimen.

Dosing and Drug Formulations in Children

The dose of antiretroviral drugs given to children is generally based on either weight or body surface area. As children's bodies are constantly changing, drug doses need to be altered to make sure that a child is not given too much, or too little, of a drug. Healthcare workers also need to take into account that children under the age of 6 metabolise drugs faster than adults, so even after adjusting for body weight, they may need to be given higher quantities of ARVs to achieve the same effect that the drugs would have in adults. Information about specific drugs is often limited, and drug manufacturers and expert guidelines use a variety of ways to calculate doses of paediatric ARVs, so there is no uniform dosing system to follow. Because of the complex nature of paediatric dosing, under- or over-dosing can be a serious risk. Dosing is further complicated by the variety of forms that ARVs may take when provided to children, all of which require different measurements. Infants who are too young to swallow tablets ideally need to be provided with ARVs in the form of syrups or powders, but these formulations are expensive and often impractical. Some syrups need to be refrigerated after opening, which requires a reliable electricity supply, and powders need to be mixed with water, which may be unfeasible in areas where clean drinking water is not regularly available. In addition, the unpleasant taste of syrups and powders can make it difficult for children to take their ARVs every day.

In areas where there is a lack of affordable paediatric ARV formulations, clinicians often have no choice but to divide adult fixed-dose combination drugs (FDCs, which combine multiple ARVs into a single tablet) into measures appropriate for children. There is evidence that dividing tablets carries a risk of under- or over-dosing, but equally, a significant 2006 study of eight countries concluded that the use of divided adult FDCs can achieve successful and satisfactory results in children. The World Health Organisation supports this practice in situations where no appropriate paediatric medications are available. Fixed-dose combinations designed specifically for children are in development, but are not yet available.

Compliance in Drug Therapy

Adherence is a major issue in paediatric treatment. Unless a child adheres to a strict treatment regimen, it is likely that treatment failure will occur, and they may become resistant to one or more of the ARVs that they are taking.

There is evidence that adherence problems are common in children. In one US study, for instance, 43% of people caring for a child receiving treatment reported at least one missed dose in the past week. In less developed countries, adherence is an even greater challenge. There are a number of factors that commonly cause adherence problems: inadequate dosing; high pill burden; reluctance among young infants to take syrups and powders due to their unpleasant taste; a lack of willingness among caregivers to inform schools and care-centres that their child is infected, which can lead to them missing out on doses during the day; dietary restrictions; and toxic side effects of drugs. If fixed-dose combinations appropriate for use in children became available, it is likely that adherence would generally improve, since it is much easier to take a single dose every day rather than multiple doses.

Side Effects of Drug Therapy in HIV Patients

Children receiving ARVs can suffer from the same side effects that adults experience. Because children's bodies are still developing, and they are likely to be exposed to treatment for prolonged periods of time, they may be particularly vulnerable to some such complications. Side effects can occur at various stages of a child's course of treatment, and may be acute (occurring directly after drug administration), subacute (within 1 or 2 days after administration), or late (after prolonged drug administration). It can be difficult to distinguish between adverse events caused by ARVs given to a child and complications caused by HIV itself, so care should be taken to exclude other possible causes of illnesses before it is concluded that they are a result of ARVs. The impact of side effects may vary from mild to severe and life-threatening. Some moderate or severe side effects may require drug substitution, or even the discontinuation of treatment. In general, mild side effects do not require such changes, and symptomatic treatment for the side effects may be given. If side effects are regarded as life threatening, all ARVs should be stopped until the child has stabilised.

Support of Nutrition during HIV Treatment

A 7 month old malnourished child malnutrition is common in children living with HIV in developing countries, and is a major cause of death. Ideally, children living with HIV who are asymptomatic need to consume 10% more calories than other children of their age and sex. Children who are symptomatic, or recovering from acute infections, need to consume 20–30% more calories than other children. If a child is suffering from malnutrition, it is recommended that they receive treatment to stabilise their condition before HAART is started. In poorer areas, however, this is not always possible. Even where it is possible to treat malnutrition, recovery from this condition is likely to be slow and limited in HIV-positive children. If a child has not been cured of malnutrition after 6–8 weeks of special feeding or appropriate treatment, it may be decided that HAART should be started despite their condition. In the opposite situation, where a child experiences rapid weight gain as a result of ARVs, nutrition also needs to be monitored carefully. As a child's weight changes, so does the recommended dosage of ARVs that they require, so drug doses need to be constantly reviewed.

Management of Children Co-infected with HIV and Tuberculosis

Tuberculosis presents a serious risk to children's health, particularly if they are suffering from a weak immune system due to HIV infection. Co-infection with HIV and tuberculosis in children is increasingly common in many areas. While the basic principles of TB treatment are the same in HIV-positive children and HIV-uninfected children, the situation is complicated by drug interactions between ARVs and drugs that are used to treat TB. The drug rifampicin, which is commonly used to treat TB, can react negatively with NNRTIs such as nevirapine, as well as with protease inhibitors. Such interactions can lead to subtherapeutic drug levels and an increased risk of toxic side effects. For HIV-positive children who are not yet receiving ARVs, it is recommended that tuberculosis (TB) treatment should ideally be initiated some weeks before ARV treatment, allowing the child to stabilise on this therapy. For children who are diagnosed with TB while already receiving treatment, ARV regimens need to be carefully reviewed, and may need to be adjusted in accordance with official guidelines. In order to avoid late diagnosis of HIV, it has been suggested that all TB-infected children should be considered for an HIV test.

Important Interventions other than Antiretroviral Treatment

Due to their weak immune systems, children living with HIV are very vulnerable to opportunistic infections, and need to be provided with drug prophylaxis to prevent such illnesses. For example, prophylaxis against PCP (one of the most common opportunistic infections in children living with HIV) is recommended for all children born to HIV-positive mothers, starting from about 4–6 weeks after birth. For children who have no access to ARVs, treatment for opportunistic infections may delay the need for antiretroviral treatment.

Cotrimoxazole, an antibiotic that is included in PCP prophylaxis and can help to prevent other infections such as TB, was shown to reduce AIDS-related mortality by 43% and hospital admission rates by 28% among children with HIV in one major Zambian trial. Based on this trial and other evidence, experts agree that cotrimoxazole should be widely provided to all children living with HIV, especially where ARVs are not available. It is also recommended that all children born to HIV-positive mothers should be provided with cotrimoxazole until tests confirm that they are HIV-negative. Cotrimoxazole prophylaxis can be given to a child from 4 to 6 weeks of age. Unfortunately, despite its low cost, few children currently have access to cotrimoxazole in developing countries.

Another important intervention is vaccination or immunisation against common infections. There are some risks associated with providing routine vaccines to children living with HIV, but these risks are far outweighed by the benefits of immunisation. In general, routine vaccines are safe to administer in HIV-positive children, and are recommended. However, it should be noted that "live vaccines" are often not considered safe for use of in HIV-positive children.

Wider Prospectives

There are psychological, as well as technical, issues that need to be considered when providing treatment to children. Children with HIV who have access to treatment can be expected to live longer, healthier lives, so there is a need for sustained emotional support as they carry out their course of treatment. Parents and caregivers need to understand how drugs are administered and stored, and the importance of life-long adherence.

When guidelines are followed carefully, and adequate resources are available, children living with HIV can be treated very effectively. In most cases, however, resources are lacking, and even where they are not, other social and practical barriers can stop them from being treated successfully.

Immunizations

There are a few immunization recommendations regarding HIV-infected children that differ from those for HIV-negative children. Encapsulated bacteria cause considerable illness for HIV-infected children, so Haemophilus influenzae (flu) and pneumococcal conjugate vaccines are important. Varicella vaccine is a live virus vaccine but it can be considered safe for HIV-infected children without immunosuppression. Measles, mumps and rubella vaccine can be safely given to HIV-infected children who do not have severe immunosuppression. Always consult with your pediatrician regarding vaccine administration.

Quick Reading on AIDS Affecting Cardiovascular System

1. How commonly is the heart affected in patients with AIDS?

Cardiac involvement has been reported in 25–50% of patients with AIDS, as defined by echocardiagraphic, endomyocardial biopsy, or autopsy findings. This involvement may cause clinically apparent manifestations in only 10–25% of patients, depending on the stage of disease and whether the patients are hospitalized.

2. List the common lesions in cardiac involvement in AIDS.

Metastatic or primary involvement of Kaposi's sarcoma or other malignant lymphomas involving the myocardium, epicardium, or pericardium myocarditis (infectious, viral, lymphocytic, manifestations), endacarditis, or pericarditis pericardial effusions cardiomyopathy (right, left, or biventricular) vasculitis. Toxic effects of drugs used against infectious complications or anti-HIV drugs.

3. What are the most common clinical manifestations of AIDS when there is heart involvement?

Myocarditis (40–52%) pericarditis (in up to 15% of cases with an effusion in 18–40%), congestive heart failure due to left ventricular dilatatian and dysfunctian (10–42%).

These lesions may present as angina, dyspnea fatigue, and dyspnea on exertion. Also ventricular arrhythmias, endocarditis, and right-heart failure may be presenting abnormalities. Anderson and Virman proposed the use of four clinical categories of AIDS heart disease:

1. Endacardial disease
2. Myocardial disease
3. Pericardial disease
4. Neoplasms.

4. When a patient with HIV infection presents with dyspnea, should he be concerned about a cardiac etiology?

Yes. AIDS patients have multiple symptoms for which the system involved may be unclear. Far example, chest pain, dyspnea, fatigue, edema, and palpitatians are general symptoms which may have multisystem etiologies. Because these patients may not have avert clinical evidence for cardiac disease, only through a heightened awareness of the frequent involvment of the heart will correct diagnosis and management be initiated.

5. Describe the diagnostic work-up for the AIDS patient with dyspnea?

The physical examination may help implicate a pulmonary or cardiac etiology. However, usually this is not sufficient, and a chest X-ray may be inconclusive since old and/or new pulmonary infiltrates do not rule out a cardiac problem. An echo-Doppler study, however, may be very helpful in evaluating a patient for pericardial effusion tamponade, cardiomyopathy valve disease (especially tricuspid regurgitation secondary to pulmonary hypertensian), or segmental wall motion abnormalities. Many of these patients also may have risk factors far coronary artery disease (i.e. male smokers) and ischemia or infarction should be considered; therefore, an electrocardiagram should be routinely obtained.

6. Why is it important to perform an echocardiogram on an AIDS patient with chest pain or shortness of breath?

Because there may be specific findings on the echocardiagram that will change the management, improve the quality of life, and provide symptomatic improvement for the patient. For example, if the patient has a cardiomyapathy, diuretics and angiotensin-converting enzyme (ACE)-inhibitors may markedly alleviate the shortness of breath not, otherwise treated if the patient is diagnosed as having a chronic pulmonary infection. Also, specific antibiotics are indicated for infectious myocarditis and pericarditis, as well as antineoplastic therapy far specific neoplasms. When a pericardial effusion is present, arrangements need to be made for pericardiocentesis and possibly biopsy for specific diagnosis. Tuberculous pericarditis often presents with tamponade and requires urgent drainage.

7. How common is pericarditis in AIDS? What are the common etiologies?

Pericarditis occurs in 5–15% of patients with AIDS and usually presents as chest pain. The causes may be viral disease, bacterial infection, tuberculosis, neoplasm, or fungal infection.

8. How common is endocarditis in AIDS patients?

Endocarditis is not a comman finding in AIDS patients. Because most of the larger studies have been done in centers where the major HIV-positive population is not intravenous drug abusers though, this may be an unidentified area of concern.

9. Which patients develop cardiomyopathy and poor left ventricular function?

This is controversial. One study showed a correlation between the CD4+ counts of < 100/mm³ and the presence of left ventricular (LV) dysfunction. Levy et al showed that patients with CD4+ counts < 100/mm³ and AIDS had the most cases (55%) of LV dysfunction, whereas those with a CD4+ caunt > 100/mm³ and active AIDS or pre-AIDS had approximately the same percentage of cases of LV dysfunction (17% and 16%, respectively). However, in a young population, even these numbers are unexpectedly high. These findings suggest that HIV itself, directly or indirectly, influences the cardiac pathology.

10. What are the suggested therapies for dilated cardiomyopathy and heart failure in HIV-positive patients? What is their prognosis?

Unfortunately, congestive heart failure in HIV-positive patients has been reported to have a rapidly progressive downward course. Despite the poor outcome, however, the heart failure initially responds to conventional therapy with ACE inhibitors and diuretics. Zidavudine therapy does not appear to change the poor outcome or prevent the development of dilated cardiomyopathy.

11. What are the major cardiac malignancies in AIDS?

Two types of malignancies affecting the heart have been described in AIDS. Kaposi's sarcoma and malignant lymphoma, with Kaposi's sarcoma being the more common. Kaposi's sarcoma is found mostly in HIV-positive male homosexuals. Kaposi's sarcoma may involve the epicardium (a comman location), myocardium, and/or pericardium. Malignant cardiac lymphoma may be primary or secondary and is usually high-grade, with Burkitt-like cells (small and noncleaved) or large-cell immunoblastic plasmacytoid types. In such cases, they appear to originate from B cells.

12. Do cardiac abnormalities improve in AIDS patients?

There have been few specific follow-up studies of AIDS-related cardiac findings. In one study, Blanchard et al reported approximately 1 year's follow-up data on AIDS and asymptomatic HIV-positive patients. Over the follow-up, 44% of the AIDS patients and only 5% of the asymptomatic HIV-positive patients died. Echocardiographic abnormalities were common in both groups, but persistent LV dysfunction was more prevalent in the AIDS group and had the grim prognosis of 100% mortality in 1 year. Resolution of cardiac abnormalities was seen with LV dysfunction in 43%, right ventricular enlargement in 44%, and without specific intervention, pericardial effusion resolution in 42%.

13. Why are the cardiac lesions occasionally transient?

This issue needs further study, but it is possible that infectious myocarditis may be the major cause of LV dysfunction and pericarditis and that there is transient occurrence of these cardiopathic agents. The right ventricular transient changes are most likely due to changes in pulmonary hypertension associated with opportunistic pulmonary infections. Therefore, it is important to have patients re-evaluated, especially if symptoms change, as medications may need frequent adjustments. Perform echo-Doppler studies on AIDS patients as symptoms dictate, or electively every year if patients have significant cardiac involvement or advanced disease.

14. What are the clinical manifestations of AIDS myocarditis?

The clinical manifestations of AIDS myocarditis depend on the severity of the inflammatory process, i.e. focal or diffuse, and/or the location of the lesion. For example, if the focus is in the His bundle, the patient presents with conduction abnormalities; diffuse disease presents with full-blown congestive heart failure or with chest pain, shortness of breath, or significant arrhythmias. Most patients have no clinical manifestations or only subtle clinical findings.

15. Do the new drugs for HIV therapy cause additional cardiac side effects?

Yes, the new, highly active antiretroviral therapy (HAART), which has been found to achieve a durable, undetectable viral load, has some physicians worried about drug toxicity. There is special concern about increased risk for hyperlipidemia, diabetes, heart disease and angina.

The concerns are heightened with the assumption that the patient will be on HAART for life. Research now shows that an earlier start is better to achieve the desired HIV levels. Moreover, the side effects are cumulative, with lipid changes being progressive as with fat distribution. Premature atherosclerosis appears to be a side effect, and we should see more clinical evidence of angina and infarction clinical findings levels. Moreover, the side effects are cumulative, with lipid changes being progressive as with fat distribution. Premature atherosclerosis appears to be a side effect, and we should see more clinical evidence of angina and infarction.

BIBLIOGRAPHY

1. AIDS epidemic update. In: Joint United Nations Programme on HIV/AIDS (UNAIDS). Geneva, Switzerland: World Health Organization, 2004; 1–94.
2. Ippolito G, Galati V, Serraino D, Girardi E. The changing picture of the HIV/AIDS epidemic. Ann N Y Acad Sci 2001;946:1–12.
3. d'Amati G, di Gioia CR, Gallo P. Pathological findings of HIV-associated cardiovascular disease. Ann N Y Acad Sci 2001;946:23–45.
4. Lewis W. AIDS: cardiac findings from 115 autopsies. Prog Cardiovasc Dis 1989;32:207–215.
5. Friis-Moller N, Sabin CA, Weber R, et al. Combination antiretroviral therapy and the risk of myocardial infarction. N Engl J Med 2003;349:1993–2003.
6. d'Arminio A, Sabin CA, Phillips AN, et al. Cardio- and cerebrovascular events in HIV-infected persons. AIDS 2004;18:1811–1817.
7. Bozzette SA, Ake CF, Tam HK, Chang SW, Louis TA. Cardiovascular and cerebrovascular events in patients treated for human immunodeficiency virus infection. N Engl J Med 2003;348: 702–710.
8. Rerkpattanapipat P, Wongpraparut N, Jacobs LE, Kotler MN. Cardiac manifestations of acquired immunodeficiency syndrome. Arch Intern Med 2000;160:602–608.
9. Heidenreich PA, Eisenberg MJ, Kee LL, et al. Pericardial effusion in AIDS: incidence and survival. Circulation 1995;92:3229–3234.
10. Hsia J, Ross AM. Pericardial effusion and pericardiocentesis in human immunodeficiency virus infection. Am J Cardiol 1994;74:94–96.
11. Mast HL, Haller JO, Schiller MS, Anderson VM. Pericardial effusion and its relationship to cardiac disease in children with acquired immunodeficiency syndrome. Pediatr Radiol 1992;22:548–551.
12. Himelman RB, Chung WS, Chernoff DN, Schiller NB, Hollander H. Cardiac manifestations of human immunodeficiency virus infection: a two-dimensional echocardiographic study. J Am Coll Cardiol 1989;13:1030–1036.
13. Cammarosano C, Lewis W. Cardiac lesions in acquired immune deficiency syndrome (AIDS). J Am Coll Cardiol 1985;5:703–706.
14. Barbaro G, Fisher SD, Lipshultz SE. Pathogenesis of HIV-associated cardiovascular complications. Lancet Infect Dis 2001;1:115–124.
15. Gowda RM, Khan IA, Mehta NJ, Gowda MR, Sacchi TJ, Vasavada BC. Cardiac tamponade in patients with human immunodeficiency virus disease. Angiology 2003;54:469–474.
16. Longo-Mbenza B, Tonduangu K, Seghers KV, Mubagwa D. HIV infection and pericardial disease invasion in Africa [in French]. Arch Mal Coeur Vaiss 1997;90:1377–1384.
17. Dosios TJ, Theakos NP, Angouras DC, Katsarou OI, Asimacopoulos PJ. AIDS-related cardiac tamponade: is surgical drainage justified? Ann Thorac Surg 2004;78:1084–1085.
18. Kabinoff GS, Gitler B. Pneumopericardium in a patient with AIDS. Tex Heart Inst J 2002;29:51–53.
19. Anderson DW, Virmani R, Reilly JM, et al. Prevalent myocarditis at necropsy in the acquired immunodeficiency syndrome. J Am Coll Cardiol 1988;11:792–799.
20. Kaul S, Fishbein MC, Siegel RJ. Cardiac manifestations of acquired immune deficiency syndrome: a 1991 update. Am Heart J 1991;122:535–544.
21. Barbaro G, Di Lorenzo G, Grisorio B, Barbarini G; for the Gruppo Italiano per lo Studio Cardiologico dei Pazienti Affetti da AIDS. Incidence of dilated cardiomyopathy and detection of HIV in myocardial cells of HIV-positive patients. N Engl J Med 1998;339:1093–1099.
22. Grody WW, Cheng L, Lewis W. Infection of the heart by the human immunodeficiency virus. Am J Cardiol 1990;66:203–206.
23. Baroldi G, Corallo S, Moroni M, et al. Focal lymphocytic myocarditis in acquired immunodeficiency syndrome (AIDS): a correlative morphologic and clinical study in 26 consecutive fatal cases. J Am Coll Cardiol 1988;12:463–469.
24. Reilly JM, Cunnion RE, Anderson DW, et al. Frequency of myocarditis, left ventricular dysfunction and ventricular tachycardia in the acquired immune deficiency syndrome. Am J Cardiol 1988; 62:789–793.
25. Currie PF, Goldman JH, Caforio AL, et al. Cardiac autoimmunity in HIV related heart muscle disease. Heart 1998;79:599–604.
26. Herskowitz A, Willoughby SB, Baughman KL, Schulman SP, Bartlett JD. Cardiomyopathy associated with antiretroviral therapy in patients with HIV infection: a report of six cases. Ann Intern Med 1992;116:311–313.
27. Levy WS, Simon GL, Rios JC, Ross AM. Prevalence of cardiac abnormalities in human immunodeficiency virus infection. Am J Cardiol 1989;63: 86–89.
28. Currie PF, Jacob AJ, Foreman AR, Elton RA, Brettle RP, Boon NA. Heart muscle disease related to HIV infection: prognostic implications. BMJ 1994;309:1605–1607.
29. Anderson DW, Virmani R. Emerging patterns of heart disease in human immunodeficiency virus infection. Hum Pathol 1990;21:253–259.
30. Roldan EO, Moskowitz L, Hensley GT. Pathology of the heart in acquired immunodeficiency syndrome. Arch Pathol Lab Med 1987;111:943–946.

31. Anderson DW, Virmani R. Cardiac pathology of HIV disease. New York, NY: Igaku-Shoin Medical Publishers, 1992.
32. Barbaro G, Di Lorenzo G, Grisorio B, Barbarini G; and the Gruppo Italiano per lo Studio Cardiologico dei Pazienti Affetti da AIDS Investigators. Cardiac involvement in the acquired immunodeficiency syndrome: a multicenter clinical-pathological study. AIDS Res Hum Retroviruses 1998;14: 1071–1077.
33. Guillamon Toran L, Romeu Fontanillas J, Forcada Sainz JM, Curos Abadal A, Larrousse Perez E, Valle Tudela V. Heart pathology of extracardiac origin. I. Cardiac involvement in AIDS [in Spanish]. Rev Esp Cardiol 1997;50:721–728.
34. Nahass RG, Weinstein MP, Bartels J, Gocke DJ. Infective endocarditis in intravenous drug users: a comparison of human immunodeficiency virus type 1-negative and -positive patients. J Infect Dis 1990;162:967–970
35. Cicalini S, Forcina G, De Rosa FG. Infective endocarditis in patients with human immunodeficiency virus infection. J Infect 2001;42:267–271.
36. Huang RM, Naidich DP, Lubat E, Schinella R, Garay SM, McCauley DI. Septic pulmonary emboli: CT-radiographic correlation. AJR Am J Roentgenol 1989;153:41–45.
37. Kuhlman JE, Fishman EK, Teigen C. Pulmonary septic emboli: diagnosis with CT. Radiology 1990; 174:211–213.
38. Paton P, Tabib A, Loire R, Tete R. Coronary artery lesions and human immunodeficiency virus infection. Res Virol 1993;144:225–231.
39. Tabib A, Greenland T, Mercier I, Loire R, Mornex JF. Coronary lesions in young HIV-positive subjects at necropsy [letter]. Lancet 1992;340: 730.
40. Louie JK, Hsu LC, Osmond DH, Katz MH, Schwarcz SK. Trends in causes of death among persons with acquired immunodeficiency syndrome in the era of highly active antiretroviral therapy, San Francisco, 1994–1998. J Infect Dis 2002;186:1023–1027.
41. Rickerts V, Brodt H, Staszewski S, Stille W. Incidence of myocardial infarctions in HIV-infected patients between 1983 and 1998: the Frankfurt HIV-cohort study. Eur J Med Res 2000;5:329–333.
42. Barbaro G, Barbarini G, Pellicelli AM. HIV-associated coronary arteritis in a patient with fatal myocardial infarction. N Engl J Med 2001;344: 1799–1800.
43. Periard D, Telenti A, Sudre P, et al. Atherogenicdyslipidemia in HIV-infected individuals treated with protease inhibitors: the Swiss HIV cohort study. Circulation 1999;100:700–705.
44. Mehta NJ, Khan IA. HIV-associated coronary artery disease. Angiology 2003;54:269–275.
45. Tabib A, Leroux C, Mornex JF, Loire R. Accelerated coronary atherosclerosis and arteriosclerosis in young human-immunodeficiency-virus-positive patients. Coron Artery Dis 2000;11:41–46.
46. Gherardi R, Belec L, Mhiri C, et al. The spectrum of vasculitis in human immunodeficiency virus-infected patients: a clinicopathologic evaluation. Arthritis Rheum 1993;36:1164–1174.
47. Johnson RM, Little JR, Storch GA. Kawasaki-like syndromes associated with human immunodeficiency virus infection. Clin Infect Dis 2001;32: 1628–1634.
48. Shingadia D, Das L, Klein-Gitelman M, Chadwick E. Takayasu's arteritis in a human immunodeficiency virus-infected adolescent. Clin Infect Dis 1999;29:458–459.
49. Chetty R, Batitang S, Nair R. Large artery vasculopathy in HIV-positive patients: another vasculitic enigma. Hum Pathol 2000;31:374–379.
50. Marks C, Kuskov S. Pattern of arterial aneurysms in acquired immunodeficiency disease. World J Surg 1995;19:127–132.
51. Mirza H, Patel P, Suresh K, Krukenkamp I, Lawson WE. HIV disease and an atherosclerotic ascending aortic aneurysm. Rev Cardiovasc Med 2004;5:176–181.
52. Naides SJ. Known causes of vasculitis in man. Cleve Clin J Med 2002; 69(suppl 2):15–19.
53. Brasselet C, Maes D, Tassan S, et al. Extensive mycotic coronary aneurysm detected by echocardiography: apropos of a case [in French]. Arch Mal Coeur Vaiss 1999;92:1229–1233.
54. Gouny P, Valverde A, Vincent D, et al. Human immunodeficiency virus and infected aneurysm of the abdominal aorta: report of three cases. Ann Vasc Surg 1992;6:239–243.
55. Sellami D, Lucidarme O, Lebleu L, Grenier P. Infected aneurysm of abdominal aorta: early CT finding [in French]. J Radiol 2000;81:899–901
56. Dubrovsky T, Curless R, Scott G, et al. Cerebral aneurysmal arteriopathy in childhood AIDS. Neurology 1998;51:560–565.
57. Aoun S, Ramos E. Hypertension in the HIV-infected patient. Curr Hypertens Rep 2000;2:478–481.
58. Sattler FR, Qian D, Louie S, et al. Elevated blood pressure in subjects with lipodystrophy. AIDS 2001;15:2001–2010.
59. Jung O, Bickel M, Ditting T, et al. Hypertension in HIV-1-infected patients and its impact on renal and cardiovascular integrity. Nephrol Dial Transplant 2004;19:2250–2258.
60. Hadigan C, Meigs JB, Rabe J, et al. Increased PAI-1 and tPA antigen levels are reduced with metformin therapy in HIV-infected patients with fat redistribution and insulin resistance. J Clin Endocrinol Metab 2001;86:939–943
61. Witz M, Lehmann J, Korzets Z. Acute brachial artery thrombosis as the initial manifestation of human immunodeficiency virus infection. Am J Hematol 2000;64:137–139.
62. Jacobson MC, Dezube BJ, Aboulafia DM. Thrombotic complications in patients infected with HIV in the era of highly active antiretroviral therapy: a case series. Clin Infect Dis 2004;39: 1214–1222.
63. Kim KK, Factor SM. Membranoproliferative glomerulonephritis and plexogenic pulmonary arteriopathy in a homosexual man with acquired immunodeficiency syndrome. Hum Pathol 1987;18: 1293–1296.
64. Goldsmith GH Jr, Baily RG, Brettler DB, et al. Primary pulmonary hypertension in patients with classic

19 Acute Myocarditis in Children

Myocarditis is an uncommon but significant disease in children. Diagnosis requires a high index of suspicion and understanding of the clinical presentation of this disease. The understanding of the mechanisms of disease-host immune response and host response has improved, but is not completely known. Therapy remains mainly supportive while the use of immunotherapy in children is still controversial. The majority of children will improve; however, a substantial portion of children will die or develop persistent dilated cardiomyopathy leading to necessary heart transplantation.

Myocarditis is defined as inflammation of the myocardium followed by necrosis and/or degeneration of myocytes. The inflammation can be diffuse or focal and is usually due to an infection. Although myocarditis severe enough to be recognized is rare, it is the most common cause of heart failure in otherwise healthy children. In both children and adults, most cases are subclinical; thus, the true incidence of myocarditis in children is unknown. Unfortunately, the clinical features of myocarditis can vary widely, and often no cardiac signs or symptoms occur, complicating recognition. For children in whom the diagnosis is suspected or cardiovascular compromise is severe enough to require admission to the pediatric intensive care unit (PICU), critical care nurses are an essential component in determining management, care, and outcomes.

Incidence of Myocarditis

Myocarditis appears to be more common in children than in adults. Its true incidence, however, is unknown; it is thought that subclinical cases ("silent" myocarditis) occur much more often than do severe cases. Many cases are unrecognized because of the wide range of signs and symptoms and, in some patients, the complete lack of clinical findings. In a postmortem study of children who died without a history suggestive of myocarditis, researchers found evidence of active or healed myocarditis in 17 of 138 cases (12.3%). Of the 17 cases, 15 occurred in children who died suddenly. In postmortem studies in adults, myocardial inflammation occurred in 1–9%.

Etiological Factors

The most common form of myocarditis, endemic in both rural Central and South America, is Chagas' disease, caused by the parasitic protozoan *Trypanosoma cruzi*. In North America, viral infections cause most cases of myocarditis. Enteroviruses, most importantly coxsackievirus B, are the most frequently reported cause of epidemics of viral myocarditis in children. However, more recent reports indicated that adenoviral infection is as common a cause as enteroviral infection is if not more so. Rarely, bacteria, fungi, protozoa, parasites and rickettsiae are causative agents. Myocarditis has also been associated with immune-mediated diseases, collagen vascular diseases and toxins.

Epidemiological Features of Myocarditis

Occurrence of myocarditis can be affected by viral epidemics. An outbreak of coxsackievirus B in Europe in

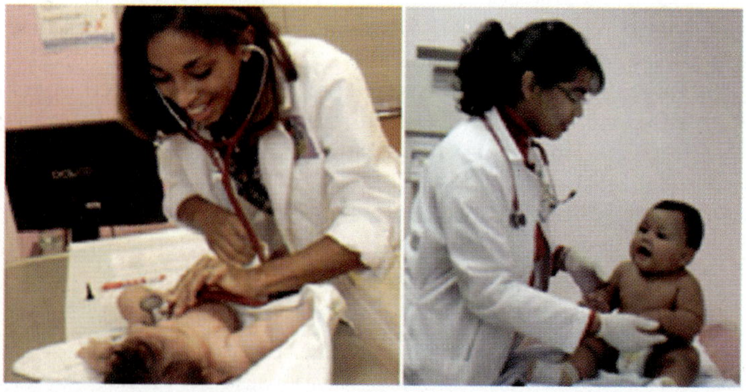

Fig. 19.1: *(Left) doctor is examining an infant who had pyrexia a few days back and has suspicion of acute myocarditis. (Right) medical student is learning to diagnose myocardial infection in the presence of her senior doctor*

Table 19.1: *Aetiology of myocarditis*

Viruses	*Immune-mediated disease*	*Drugs*
Coxsackievirus A	Rheumatoid arthritis	Sulfonamides
Coxsackievirus B	Rheumatic fever	Cyclophosphamide
Echovirus	Ulcerative colitis	Acetazolamide
Adenovirus	Systemic ulcerative colitis	Amphotericin B
Rubella virus		Indomethacin
Measles virus	**Toxins**	Tetracycline
Varicella virus	Ethanol	Phenytoin
Poliovirus	Heavy metals; iron, copper, lead	Penicillin
Mumps virus	Arsenic	
Herpes virus	Bee and wasp stings	**Fungi and yeast**
Epstein-Barr virus	Carbon monoxide	*Aspergillus*
Cytomegalovirus	Scorpion bites	*Candida*
Arbovirus	Spider bites	**Protozoa**
Influenza virus	Snake bites	*Trypanosoma cruzi*
Human immunodeficiency virus	**Physical conditions or agents**	*Toxoplasma gondii*
	Hyperpyrexia	
Bacteria	Electric shock	**Parasites**
Meningococci	Radiation	*Ascaris*
Borrelia burgdorferi (Lyme disease)		*Schistosoma*
Salmonellae		
Mycobacteria		
Streptococci		

1965 correlated with cardiac dysfunction in 5% of infected patients. Incidences were as high as 12% that same year in Scotland, Finland and Austria. Seasonal viral distributions have been recognized for decades (influenza prevalent during winter months; poliovirus and coxsackievirus A and B typically isolated during summer and fall). Myocarditis has been a prominent finding during epidemics of influenza; thus, occurrence may be seasonal.

Age plays a marked role in prevalence. During the neonatal period, myocarditis is usually abrupt, severe, and often fatal, with mortality as high as 75%. Infants infected with coxsackievirus B during the first year of life have a high incidence of myocarditis. Myocarditis has been linked to sudden infant death syndrome because inflammatory infiltrates have been found on autopsies of some victims. Incidence increases again during late childhood and adolescence; the myocarditis usually has a delayed onset and patients recover.

Male predominance has been noted with coxsackievirus B heart disease, particularly in adolescents and adults. In these age groups, two-thirds to three-quarters of patients with myocarditis are male. Male predominance has also been reported with coxsackievirus A myocarditis and poliomyelitis. Whether or not differences between the sexes occur in other viral infections is unknown.

Pathophysiology

Although viral infection is the most common initiator of acute myocarditis, the subsequent autoimmune response plays a lead role in myocyte injury. The principal mechanism of myocardial damage is not just viral replication; it includes cell-mediated immunological reactions.

The pathophysiology of myocarditis has been studied in mice infected with a cardiotropic virus, such as coxsackievirus B. After systemic infection, the virus enters the myocyte, where it replicates in the cytoplasm of the cell. Some replicated viruses then enter the interstitium and are phagocytized by activated macrophages. Macrophage activation is due to both viral particles in the interstitium and the release of interferon-γ by natural killer (NK) cells. The release of interferon-γ is followed by release of proinflammatory cytokines (interleukins 1β and 2 and tumor necrosis factor α). When activated by interleukin 2, NK cells eliminate virally infected myocytes and inhibit virus replication. The significance of the action of NK cells in the pathogenesis of the disease is well established; in animals depleted of NK cells before infection, a more severe myocarditis develops. As noted earlier, myocarditis after infection with coxsackievirus B occurs more often in men. This propensity may be related to differences between the sexes in the activation of NK cells. After infection, myocarditis that develops in female mice is less severe than that in male mice. In one study, after the same infection, male mice were markedly less efficient than female mice in activating NK cells. This decrease in NK-cell activation presumably results in decreased viral clearance with a resultant increase in illness severity. This difference in NK-cell activation may explain the male predominance for the development of clinically significant myocarditis. Unlike NK cells, T cells may contribute to damage in both infected and noninfected myocytes. Activation of T cells results in accumulation of macrophages within the myocyte and production of cell-mediated cytotoxic effects. Although T cells can lyse virus-infected myocytes, the accumulation of macrophages and the concomitant cytotoxic effects create

Table 19.2: *Diagnosis of myocarditis in children*

Assessment	*Finding*
Chest radiography	Cardiomegaly
Electrocardiography	Tachycardia: Sinus or supraventricular Atrioventricular block Low-voltage QRS complexes ST-T wave abnormalities (elevation or depression) Prolonged QT interval Ventricular ectopy
Echocardiography	Impaired ventricular function (left > right) Ventricular dilatation Atrioventricular valve regurgitation[a] Left ventricular thrombi[a]
Laboratory studies	
Serological test	Increased levels of creatine kinase and its MB isoenzyme Increased level of cardiac troponin C Elevated sedimentation rate[a] Increased level of C-reactive protein[s] Increased level of white blood cells, with lymphocytes predominating Viral titers[a] Increased level of immunoglobulin G[a]
Cultures: Blood, stool, cerebrospinal fluid, nasopharyngeal secretions	Presence of virus[a]
Myocardial biopsy	Myocyte destruction, fibrosis, inflammatory cells, lymphocytic infiltrates

[a]May or may not be present.

a fine balance between viral clearance and myocyte damage. Adding to myocyte injury, lysis by T cells is indiscriminate; it occurs in both infected and noninfected cells. The result is necrosis of healthy as well as infected myocytes. Therefore, a percentage of myocardial damage comes from "friendly fire", specifically the patient's own immune response.

Permanent myocardial damage can be the end result of myocarditis. Such damage is thought to be due to an overaggressive immunological activation in which persistent T-cell infiltration leads to long-term tissue destruction and subsequent dilated cardiomyopathy. Infection with enteroviruses plays a major role in chronic forms of dilated cardiomyopathy.

Myocarditis is classified as fulminant, acute, or chronic. Fulminant myocarditis is preceded by a viral prodrome that is followed by sudden onset of severe hemodynamic compromise. Acute myocarditis has a less distinct onset and, initially, less severe compromise but is followed by a worse outcome than fulminant myocarditis. McCarthy et al found that adults with fulminant myocarditis had excellent long-term survival, whereas patients with acute myocarditis had progressive failure that led to death or the need for a heart transplant. Chronic myocarditis can be defined as persistent (lasting >3 months), recurrent and latent.

Diagnosis: It can be challenging. Not only can children have a wide range of nonspecific signs and symptoms, but depending on cognitive development, they may not be able to communicate their symptoms. Despite a variety of invasive and noninvasive studies, myocarditis is a presumptive diagnosis based on history and clinical features.

Clinical History

Clinical features of viral myocarditis are affected by age, sex, and the child's baseline health status. These variables affect the balance between pathogen clearance and degree of inflammation. Older children may have a history of upper respiratory infection; infants may have anorexia, vomiting and lethargy. Often, signs and symptoms are nonspecific or may resemble the signs and symptoms of relatively common diagnoses in children including bronchiolitis, pneumonia, failure to thrive, and gastroenteritis.

Older children may have chest pain (the sole symptom in some patients). Some have abdominal pain. Atypical manifestations such as syncope (KM), seizures, and sudden

Table 19.3: *Signs and symptoms of myocarditis in children*

Subjective	Chest pain Abdominal pain Dyspnea/orthopnea Exercise intolerance Fatigue

Objective	Tachycardia
	Tachypnea
	Wheezing, cough, increased work of breathing
	Alteration in peripheral perfusion
	  Prolonged capillary refill
	  Decreased in pulse quality
	  Extremity coolness
	  Paleness, mottling
	  Decreased urine output
	Murmur[a]
	Gallop
	Rhythm irregularities
	  Ventricular ectopy
	  Atriobentricular block
	  Sinus tachycardia or supraventricular tachycardia
	Hepatomegaly[a]
	Rales[b]
	Hypotension[b]

[a]May or may not be present
[b]Late finding

death also have been reported. A more focused cardiac examination when no signs of congestive heart failure occur may be prompted by patients' reports of chest pain, dyspnea, exercise intolerance, or fatigue. Tachycardia of unknown origin in an otherwise healthy child may be an ominous sign. Newborns and infants unlike older children, are more likely to have circulatory shock.

When myocarditis is suspected, a thorough history is imperative for identifying possible causes. Parents should be asked about exposures to potential infectious agents, pharmacological agents that can cause myocardial inflammation and toxins including illicit drugs (e.g. cocaine). Immunization status should be obtained because several infectious diseases of childhood (diphtheria, poliomyelitis) are potential causes.

Physical Signs and Symptoms (Table 19.3)

During episodes of cardiac compromise, neurohormonal responses activate the sympathetic nervous system and the renin-angiotensin-aldosterone system, resulting in improved contractility, increase in heart rate, vasoconstriction, and fluid and sodium retention. Tachycardia out of proportion for age is common in children with myocardial compromise as the heart attempts to compensate for inadequate oxygen delivery to the tissues. Vasoconstriction occurs to improve preload and maintain blood pressure. This decrease in peripheral perfusion is manifested as cool extremities, described by level of coolness (e.g. cool to midcalf, cool to knee), quality of pulses, capillary refill time (compromise considered at > 3 seconds with the extremity at the level of the heart), decreased urine output (< 1 mL/kg per hour), and changes in mental status. Pulse quality is characterized by using the 0–4 pulse intensity scale (0 = no pulses detected, 4 = bounding). Extremities may appear mottled or pale. Despite these alterations in perfusion, it must be emphasized that vasoconstriction in children will maintain a blood pressure within a normal range for age even when tissue perfusion is inadequate. Hypotension is considered not only a late finding of cardiac failure but also an ominous one (Fig. 19.1).

Often, an S3 (ventricular gallop) occurs because of rapid filling of a noncompliant, poorly contracting left ventricle. Murmurs are less common, although a soft systolic murmur may be heard if mitral or tricuspid insufficiency is present. Heart sounds may be muffled if concomitant pericarditis is present. Rhythm irregularities may be detected, especially supraventricular tachycardia or ventricular ectopic beats as with KM.

Tachypnea is a common sign of myocardial failure in children. Tachypnea is the result of pulmonary edema due to left ventricular failure. Clinical findings can include wheezing, a cough, grunting, nasal flaring, and intercostal retraction. Older children may report orthopnea or inability to catch their breath. Cyanosis is rare. Rales are typically a late sign of pulmonary congestion and may not occur at all in infants.

Hepatomegaly, an indication of venous congestion, may or may not occur. Liver tenderness or absence of a firm edge on palpation below the right costal margin may indicate liver engorgement.

Diagnostic Procedures (Table 19.2)

The diagnostic approach for a child with suspected myocarditis includes strategies to both aid in establishing the diagnosis and rule out disease processes that may mimic myocarditis (e.g. a structural cardiac defect or pericardial effusion). In addition, many of these interventions provide an estimate of myocardial function and can help in establishing clinical interventions (Figs 19.7A to C).

X-ray Chest (Fig. 19.2)

Evidence of cardiomegaly on a chest radiograph is an important clinical finding in myocarditis; however, the degree of heart enlargement depends on the stage of the disease. Subacute or chronic myocarditis is characterized by cardiomegaly; cardiomegaly may or may not occur in children with fulminant myocarditis. In fact, the possibility of myocarditis is often not considered until late when cardiomegaly is evident on chest radiographs. Myocarditis should not be ruled out in infants or children with marked cardiovascular compromise or collapse of unknown cause who do not have evidence of heart enlargement on radiographs.

Electrocardiography (Figs 19.3 and 19.8)

Although not diagnostic, findings on an electrocardiogram are rarely normal in patients with myocarditis. Some children have such mild illness that a conduction disturbance on an electrocardiogram is the only abnormal finding. Sinus tachycardia is a common finding with myocarditis. Low-voltage QRS complexes, ST-T wave abnormalities, or prolonged QT interval may be apparent.

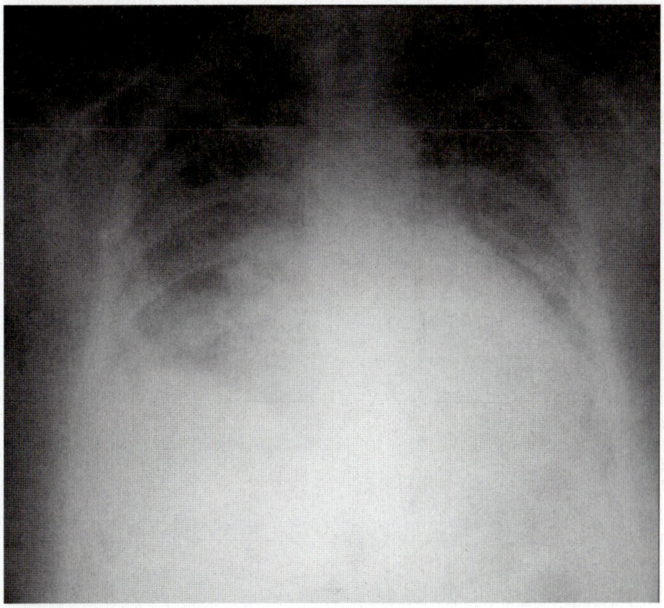

Fig. 19.2: *X-ray chest frontal view showing pulmonary edema in a patient with cardiogenic shock as a result of acute myocarditis in a 12-years-old child*

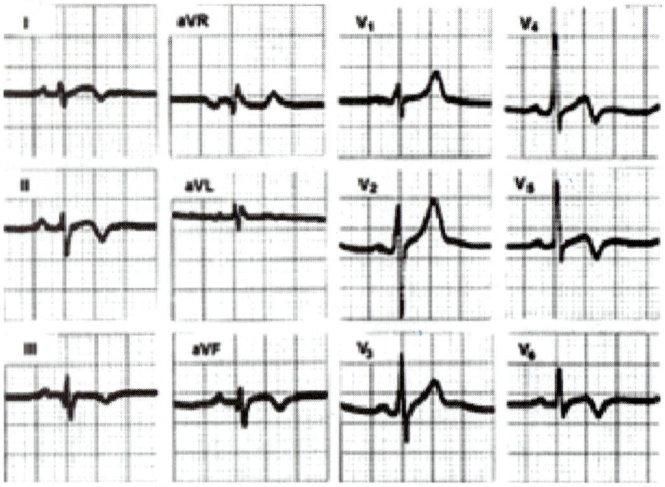

Fig. 19.3: *The T waves are deeply and symmetrically inverted in I, II, III, and V4-6, suggesting a diffuse myocardial process in a young patient with acute viral myocarditis*

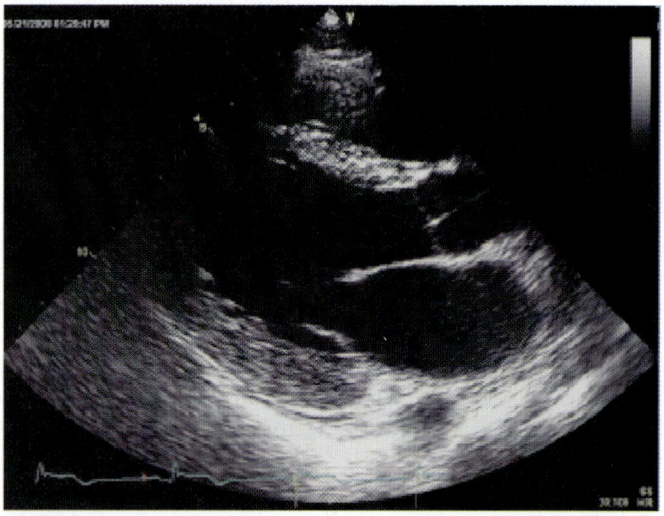

Fig. 19.4: *Two dimensional parasternal long-axis view depicting disproportionate thickening, increased echogenicity, and dyskinesis of the inferolateral wall relative to the septum; findings are consistent with tissue oedema*

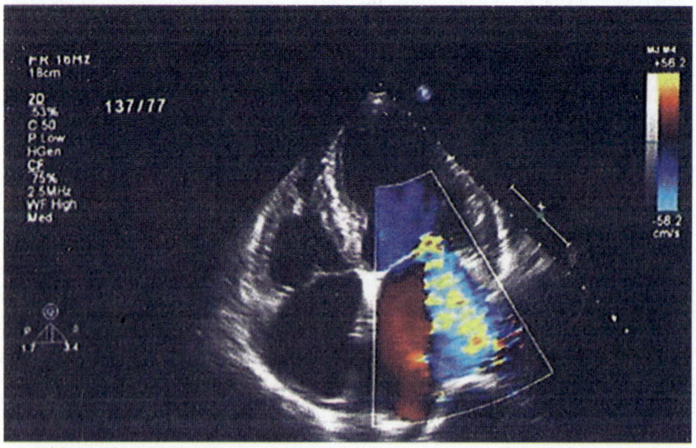

Fig. 19.5: *Color Doppler echocardiography shows MR appears as a systolic regurgitation from the left ventricle to the left atriumin a young patient with acute myocarditis*

Left ventricular hypertrophy with repolarization changes (strain) is typical. Complete atrioventricular block has also been described. Occasionally, evidence of myocardial infarction is seen.

Echocardiography (Figs 19.4 and 19.5)

Findings on echocardiograms are rarely normal in patients with myocarditis. Impaired left ventricular function with dilatation of 1 or more chambers is typical. Echocardiogram showed poor left ventricular systolic function with dilatation and slightly diminished right ventricular function. In the absence of any structural abnormalities, these findings help to establish the diagnosis. Generally, right ventricular function is less compromised than is left ventricular function; atrioventricular valve regurgitation may occur. Occasionally, left ventricular thrombi are found.

Laboratory Tests

Endomyocardial biopsy (Fig. 19.6): Historically, despite its limited sensitivity and specificity and its inherent risks, endomyocardial biopsy has been the reference standard for diagnosing viral myocarditis. Nevertheless, for several reasons, endomyocardial biopsy is used less often in children than in adults. First, biopsy can be associated with significant sampling error. Several tissue specimens (5 or more) are needed because of the focal nature of the disease; many clinicians think that biopsy leads to underestimation of the presence of the disease. Second, borderline myocarditis can result in little to no evidence of myocyte destruction. Third, expert interpretation can vary including variance with other markers of viral infection. Because of the possibility of false-negative results, lack of an endomyocardial biopsy positive for myocarditis does not rule out this disease. For KM, findings on endomyocardial biopsy on hospital day 8 confirmed the diagnosis. Tissue

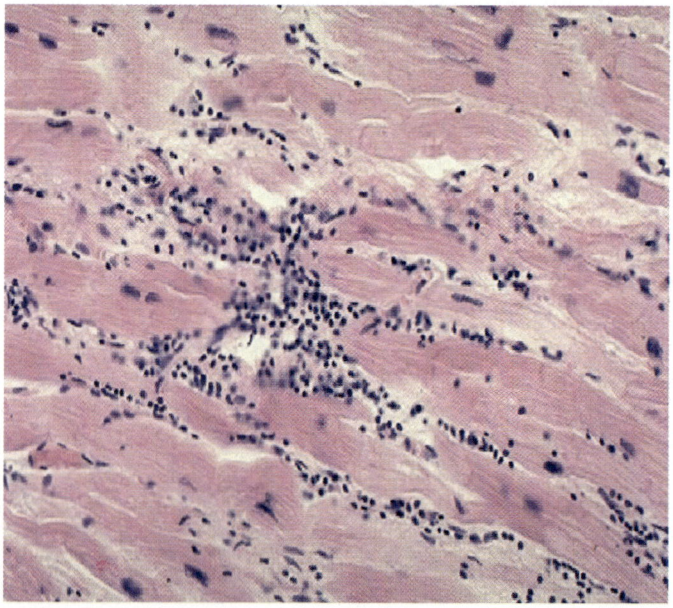

Fig. 19.6: *Histophotograph H/E stain showing interstitial inflammatory infiltrates mostly lymphocytes in acute viral myocarditis*

specimens from the right ventricle had intact myocytes with small foci of lymphocytic infiltrates and extensive areas of myocyte destruction with organizing fibrosis and infiltrates of inflammatory cells most consistent with myocarditis.

Polymerase Chain Reaction (PCR)

Recently, use of less invasive means of diagnosing myocarditis in children has been emphasized.Use of polymerase chain reaction (PCR) and in situ hybridization has increased the sensitivity for diagnosing viral myocarditis.Tracheal aspirates for PCR analysis in intubated children are useful for detecting viral genomes in children with or without myocarditis. Akhtar et al reported that PCR of tracheal aspirates had a sensitivity of 100% for predicting the results of PCR of endomyocardial biopsy specimens, albeit for a small (n = 10) sample size. Although a tracheal aspirate positive for virus is not diagnostic for myocarditis itself, PCR of tracheal aspirates may provide a safer means of identifying a viral cause for illness in children with cardiac decompensation of unknown origin.

Serological studies may reveal an elevation in myocardial enzyme levels [creatine kinase, normal value 25–190 IU/L (to convert to microkatals, multiply by 0.0167); MB isoenzyme of creatine kinase, normal value < 12% of creatine kinase]. In children, the level of cardiac troponin T is a more sensitive indicator of myocardial damage than are myocardial enzyme levels. In healthy children, cardiac troponin levels are typically less than the detection level (< 0.02 ng/mL). Lauer et al reported that 35% of patients with suspected myocarditis also had elevated levels of cardiac troponin; among those, 98% had viral myocarditis confirmed histologically.

Nonspecific laboratory studies; may aid in the diagnosis of viral myocarditis. Elevations in sedimentation rate (> 20 mm/h) and level of C-reactive protein (> 0.05 mg/dL; to convert to nanomoles per liter, multiply by 9.524) may occur. A normal sedimentation rate, however, does not rule out myocarditis. Viral studies may reveal enteroviral or adenoviral antibodies, Esptein-Barr virus, cytomegalovirus, or a fourfold increase in the level of immunoglobulin G but do not definitively establish causation. Levels of immunoglobulin G antibodies to Epstein-Barr virus nuclear antigen were elevated in PCR may also be used to detect viral genomes.

Elevation in white blood cell count with predominance of lymphocytes may suggest viral causes of myocarditis. Cultures of blood, stool, cerebrospinal fluid, or nasopharyngeal secretions are less specific than cultures of tracheal aspirates; Martin et al found that cultures showed growth in only 27% of children with viral myocarditis.

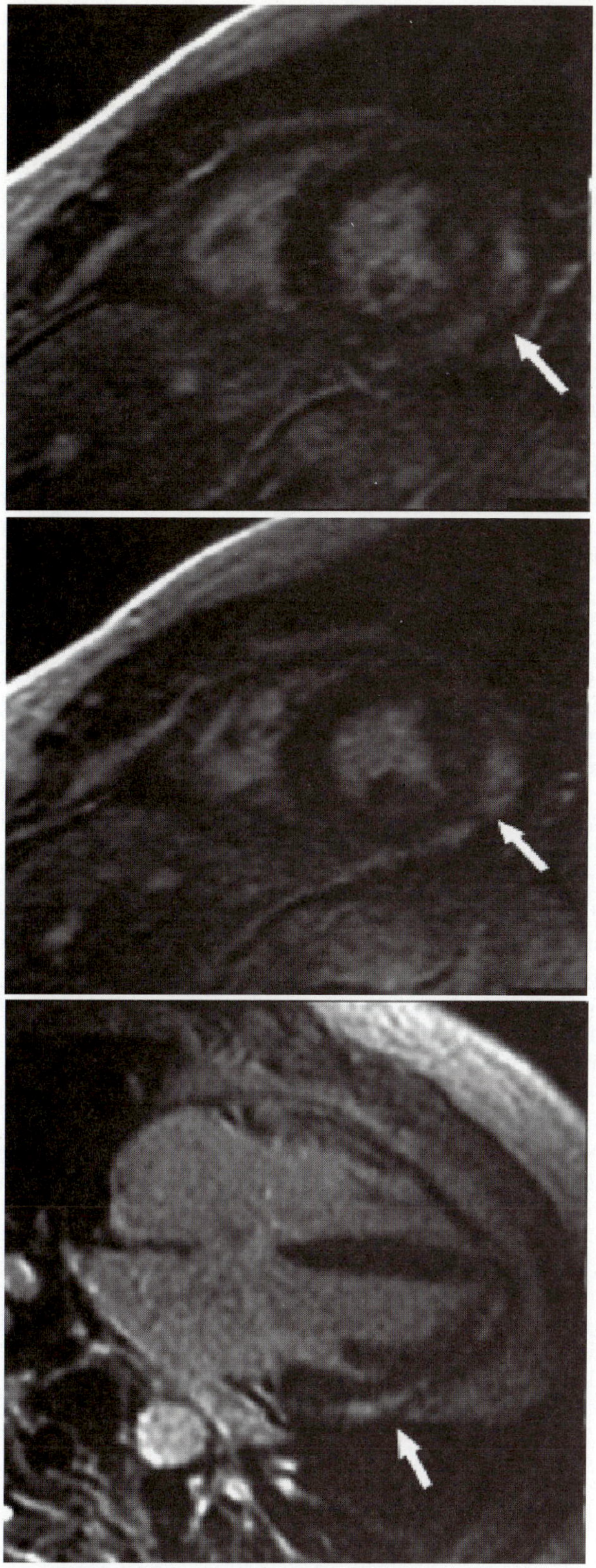

Fig. 19.7: *Cardiac MRI using delayed enhancement. Epicardial delayed enhancement (arrows) can be seen in short-axis (upper and middle) and four chamber (bottom) planes. Myocardial delayed enhancement is seen in epicardial inferolateral and apical segments, involving 50% of left ventricle wall thickness, typical for myocarditis*

Management in Myocarditis

Critical Care

Care of children with clinical features consistent with myocarditis depends on the severity of myocardial dysfunction. Management is designed around supportive measures rather than being aimed at a causative agent. Maintenance of cardiac output with aggressive support of cardiac function is essential. Such support includes initiation and monitoring of inotropic therapy, afterload reduction, arrhythmia management, and adequate tissue oxygenation. Respiratory support may require intubation and mechanical ventilation. Fluid management may include both administration of fluid boluses and diuretic therapy. Monitoring of and interventions to prevent complications should be ongoing.

Inotropic Support (Table 19.5)

When cardiac output is inadequate, a rapid acting inotropic agent is administered. Inotropic agents are administered cautiously because the myocardium is irritable and use of inotropic agents can instigate and/or worsen arrhythmias. One inotropic agent or a combination of such agents, including dopamine, dobutamine, and milrinone, can be administered.

Dobutamine is often used when the primary cause of inadequate tissue perfusion is cardiac in origin. Dobutamine improves contractility and decreases systemic vascular resistance, providing afterload reduction in addition to improving cardiac output. A mild increase in heart rate can occur, although significant tachycardia is unusual. Although dobutamine increases myocardial oxygen demand in adults with congestive heart failure, in children with patent coronary arteries, coronary blood flow and oxygen supply to the heart actually increase.

Dopamine has both inotropic and vasopressor properties and is useful in patients who are in shock with cardiac dysfunction and associated mild to moderate hypotension. Dopamine is not routinely used to tidal volume (pressure ventilation), a decrease in oxygen saturation, and asymmetric chest rise. If the tube migrates into the right main bronchus, the child should immediately be placed back in the previous position and reassessed. Breath sounds should be assessed after any change in body position.

Neck extension increases airway length, potentially causing unintentional extubation because the uncuffed tube

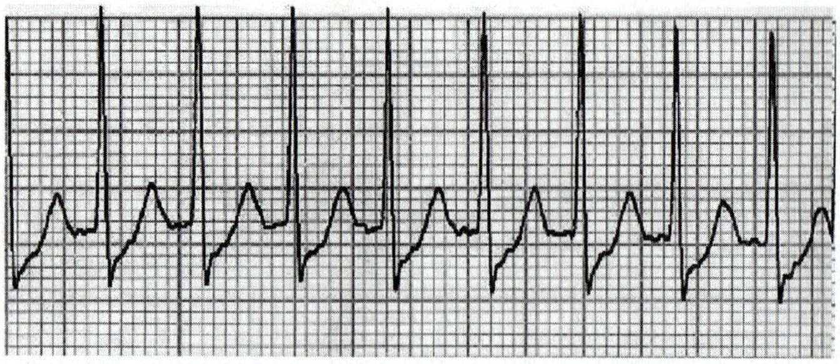

Fig. 19.8: *ECG showing features of supraventricular tachycardia in a patient with myocarditis*

can easily pass upward through the vocal cords. Immediate respiratory distress, decrease in oxygen saturation, marked decrease in or undetectable end-tidal carbon dioxide levels, grunting, or vocalization can indicate possible inadvertent extubation. If dislodgement of the endotracheal tube into the esophagus is suspected, the tube should be removed and bag-valve-mask ventilation performed until reintubation or effective spontaneous breathing occurs.

Although a common practice in intensive care units, endotracheal suctioning should not be performed routinely. Suctioning can be associated with complications including hypoxemia, bradycardia, atelectasis and dysrhythmias. Suctioning should be done on an as-needed basis rather than routinely. Indications for suctioning include to increase in airway pressure, decrease in tidal volume, decrease in oxygen saturation, visualization of secretions in the tube, development of rhonchi, and coughing. Hyperoxygenation may or may not be required before suctioning, depending on the child's arterial oxygenation and tolerance to the procedure. The catheter should not be deeper than the end of the endotracheal tube. Catheters inserted to the point of resistance (carina) cause tissue inflammation and damage. Instillation of normal saline for lavage should be avoided because that practice is not supported by research and may actually be harmful.

Routine bedside nursing interventions such as dressing changes, bathing, weighing, and repositioning all

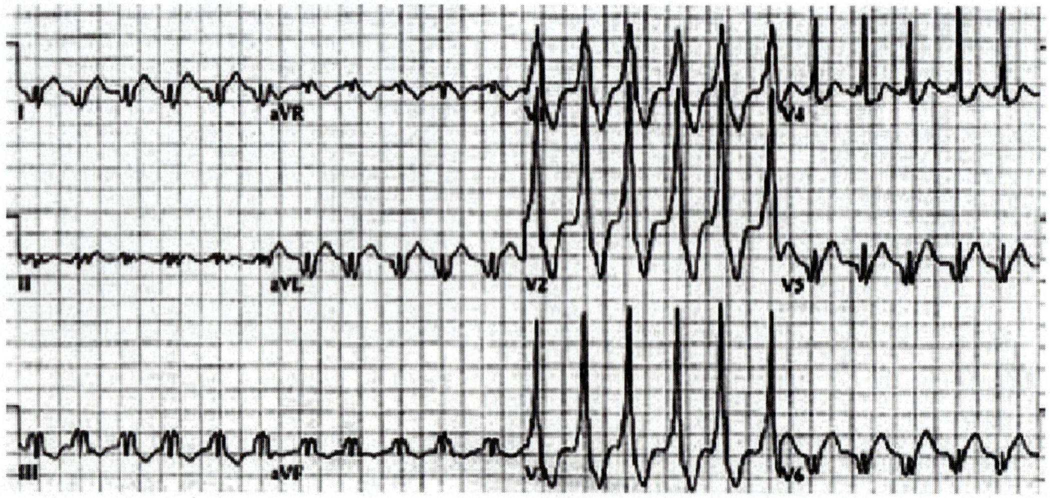

Fig. 19.9: *ECG demonstrating ventricular tachycardia with right bundle-branch block morphologyin a patient with myocarditis*

significantly increase tissue oxygen consumption. Delay in carrying out these procedures may be necessary. Conversely, some or all of these activities may be clustered if tolerated in order to allow longer periods of rest.

Fever increases oxygen consumption 10% for each 1°C elevation in body temperature. Although not all fever is "bad", treatment of fever is recommended in children with cardiopulmonary disease. Attempts should be made to maintain normothermia. Unless contraindicated, antipyretics (acetaminophen, ibuprofen) should be administered. Fever reduction can also be attempted with external cooling, usually by sponging with tepid water.

Pain and anxiety significantly increase oxygen demand and consumption and cause considerable distress for children in the PICU. Assessment and management of pain and anxiety should be ongoing.

Arrhythmias (Table 19.4)

Heart rate and rhythm require monitoring. Arrhythmias are a significant life-threatening complication of myocarditis. Development of bradycardia or tachyarrhythmias is unlikely to be tolerated and requires immediate recognition and treatment.

Infants and small children depend on heart rate for adequate cardiac output because stroke volume is relatively fixed; in young children, bradycardia can rapidly diminish cardiac output. Because chronotropic drugs can induce ventricular tachycardia in patients with viral myocarditis, cardiac pacing is the preferred treatment for life-threatening brady arrhythmias including atrioventricular block.

Transcutaneous or transthoracic pacing is a noninvasive procedure that can be done rapidly. Two electrodes are placed on the patient with the anterior electrode in the V2 to V5 position and the posterior electrode under the scapula to the left of the spine. Electrode adherence should be checked frequently, especially if the child is diaphoretic. If needed for prolonged periods, electrodes should be changed a minimum of every 24 hours to maintain effectiveness of the contact gel.

For ongoing bradyarrhythmias, invasive pacing should be considered. Transvenous leads are placed percutaneously via a large vessel into the right atrium or ventricle. Leads are stiff; nurses must be alert for indications of ventricular perforation including cardiac tamponade. An extra battery should be kept at the bedside of any patient who is pacemaker dependent. Hospital policy should be followed when caring for the insertion site and catheter.

Conversely, an excessively rapid heart rate will decrease ventricular filling time, resulting in inadequate preload and subsequent cardiac output. Tachycardias also result in inadequate coronary artery filling time. Coronary arteries fill and perfuse the myocardium during diastole; the faster the heart rate, the shorter is diastole, leading to a decrease in myocardial oxygen supply during a time of increasing consumption.

Differentiation between sinus tachycardia and supraventricular tachycardia is critical. Typically, sinus tachycardia is heart rate greater than 140/min in children, greater than 160/min in infants, and varies from beat to beat. Heart rate generally remains less than 200/min. Sinus tachycardia can be the result of a variety of factors, including fear, anxiety, fever, pain, intravascular dehydration, and marked vasodilatation. Sinus tachycardia will resolve, or partially resolve with resolution of the inciting factor.

Supraventricular tachycardia is an extremely rapid heart rate (200–280/min); is unresponsive to resolution of fever, pain, hypovolemia, and so on; and has no beat-to-beat variability. Rates of sinus tachycardia and supraventricular tachycardia can overlap, making determination of the type of tachycardia difficult. A 12-lead electrocardiogram may be necessary to differentiate between the two. Once supraventricular tachycardia has been established, rapid treatment with adenosine in the patients with stable hemodynamic status or cardioversion in patients with unstable hemodynamic status is performed. A defibrillator should remain near any child who has myocarditis or recurring supraventricular tachycardia.

Hemodynamic Monitoring

With invasive hemodynamic monitoring, physiological variables specific to cardiovascular function can be monitored and, when coupled with clinical examination, the results provide data for sound clinical decision making.

Arterial Pressure

Continuous blood pressure monitoring via an arterial catheter is preferred in children with severe cardiac dysfunction, particularly those who require infusions of vasoactive agents. Noninvasive measurements may be inaccurate or impossible to obtain because of impaired peripheral perfusion and vasoconstriction. Arterial catheters can be placed peripherally (radial artery) or centrally (femoral artery) and provide a dynamic picture of systolic, diastolic, and mean blood pressures. Because evaluations of interventions and their effectiveness will be based partly on invasive measurement of blood pressure, care must be taken to ensure accuracy of readings. Routinely inspecting for proper transducer placement (phlebostatic axis), zeroing the transducer a minimum of once a shift, inspecting for and eliminating air bubbles in the system, and using noncompliant pressure tubing will help ensure accurate measurements.

Normal blood pressure in children is dependent on age and size. As previously noted, however, children with myocarditis can maintain a blood pressure within normal limits for age until very late in the disease. No single clinical parameter should determine critical care interventions, and

Box 19.1: *Calculation of systolic BP*

As a general rule, for children more than 1 year old, estimated systolic blood pressure norms can be calculated as follows:

50th percentile = 90 mmHg + (2*x age in years*)

5th percentile = 70 mmHg + (2*x age in years*)

Table 19.4: *Shows intravenos antiarrythmic agent*

Drug	*Classification*	*Dose*	*Action*	*Adverse effects*
Adenosine	Antiarrhythmic	0.05–0.1 mg/kg rapid intravenous bolus	Slows conduction time through the atrio-ventricular node, interrupting reentry pathways	Arrhythmias
		Repeat to a maximum of 0.3 mg/kg total		Bradycardia
		Can give 12 mg maximum dose for children who weight >50 kg		Hypotension
Digoxin	Cardiac glycoside	See Table 19.6	Positive inotropic effects Decreases condition through the sinoatrial atrioventricular nodes	Sinus bradycardia Atrioventricular block, Ventricular arrhythmias Hyperkalemia with toxic effect
Amiodarone	Antiarrhythmic given over 5–10 minutes, can be	Loading: 1 mg/kg stimulation	Inhibits adrenergic	Bradycardia, heart block, Sinus arrest, paroxysmal ventricular tachycardia repeated 5 times
		Continuous intravenous infusion at 10–15 mg/kg per day	Decreases atrioventricular node conduction and sinus function	Congestive heart failure, cardiogenic shock, hypotension Pulmonary toxic effects (pneumoritis, fibrosis, acute respiratory distress syndrome)
Lidocaine	Antiarrhythmic	Loading: 1 mg/kg followed by a continuous infusion of 20–50 µg/kg per minute	Suppresses automaticity of the conduction system	Bradycardia, heart block, arrhythmias, hypertension, seizures

this rule is particularly true for blood pressure, unless hypotension is present. Adequacy of tissue perfusion is determined by analysis of clinical findings on bedside examination along with blood pressure. The extremity distal to the arterial catheter should be assessed at least once a shift to monitor for any compromise in perfusion related to catheter placement. Extremity coolness, color changes, delayed capillary refill, and diminishing pulse quality can indicate inadequate perfusion. Numbness, tingling, and motor deficit can also be indicators of impaired circulation. Development or change in any one or more of these variables requires immediate attention and potentially removal of the catheter.

Central Venous Pressure

Central venous pressure (CVP) or right atrial monitoring provides a continual reflection of intravascular volume status and is a good determinant of right ventricular end-diastolic volume, or preload. CVP should be interpreted along with other measures of cardiac function (heart rate, peripheral perfusion, urine output). In critically ill children, the absolute value is not as important as serial measurements and changes in response to interventions.

CVP monitoring should be done via the distal lumen of the catheter. Monitoring can be continual or intermittent, depending on availability of intravenous access. If the distal lumen is being used for continuous intravenous administration of fluids and/or drugs, CVP should be assessed a minimum of once an hour and after any administration of fluid boluses or diuresis. When intermittent CVP monitoring is used, care must be taken to ensure that no cardiotonic medications are infused through the distal port. If such infusions are used, turning the stopcock for pressure readings causes a disruption in the delivery of medication and potential hemodynamic compromise. Ideally, infusions of inotropic or vasoactive agents should be given through the medial or proximal lumen only.

Normal CVP values can vary widely in infants and children, depending on age, disease, concomitant conditions, and critical care therapies. In healthy infants, normal values can range from –2 to +4 mmHg, from 4 to 8 mmHg in those with congenital heart disease, and from 2 to 6 mmHg in those with respiratory disease requiring mechanical ventilation. In this age group, measurements above 8 mmHg are generally indicative of myocardial dysfunction or high intrathoracic pressure. In older children

Table 19.5: *Showing continuous infusion inotropic support*

Drug	*Classification*	*Dose, µg/kg per minute*	*Action*[a]	*Adverse effects*
Dopamine	Sympathomimetic	0.5–2	Dopaminergic: renal vasodilation	Tachyarrhythmias
			Promotion of sodium excretion	Reduced renal blood flow at >5 µ/kg per minute
		5–10	β_1-adrenergic effects	Increased myocardial oxygen demand
		10–15	Mixed α_1–β_1-adrenergic effects	
		>20	Predominately α_1-adrenergic effects	Ectopy
Dobutamine	Sympathomimetic	2–20	Pure β_1-adrenergic effects	Tachycardia Tachyarrhythmias Hypotension
Epinephrine	Sympathomimetic	0.1–1.0	Adrenergic agonist effects, predominately α_1-adrenergic effects	Tachyarrhythmias Ventricular ectopy Hypertension Myocardial ischemia
Milrinone	Phosphodiesterase enzyme inhibitor	May use loading dose of 50–75 µg/kg before infusion	Improves contractillity Afterload reduction	Hypotension Thrombocytopenia ventricular ectopy

[a]α-adrenergic: constriction of veins and arteries; β_1-adrenegic; increased heart rate, contractility; β_2-adrenergic; vasodilatation, bronchodilatation

without underlying disease, a CVP range of 2–6 mmHg is considered normal. Values can vary markedly and should be interpreted along with the child's underlying disease state, concomitant conditions, and critical care therapies.

CVP measurements do not stand alone and must be considered in context of the entire clinical picture. Any changes in intrathoracic pressure will affect CVP values; spontaneous respirations decrease CVP, whereas increased intrathoracic pressure increases CVP. Values lower than expected may or may not indicate hypovolemia; high CVP values may or may not indicate hypervolemia. Elevated CVP values may also occur in patients receiving positive pressure ventilation and with the addition of positive end-expiratory pressure. Conditions that increase pulmonary vascular resistance (hypothermia, hypoxemia, acidosis, severe respiratory disease, underlying pulmonary hypertension) also increase CVP. High CVP values do not necessarily reflect cardiac disease but may be an indication of elevated right ventricular end-diastolic pressure, suggesting right ventricular dysfunction.Variables that affect interpretation of CVP values must be considered when therapies are determined.

Complications of central venous catheters include bloodstream infection (increased risk with multilumen catheters), venous thrombosis, thrombophlebitis, and catheter occlusion. Routine maintenance of the catheter and insertion site should be done per hospital policy.

Pulmonary Artery Pressure

Pulmonary artery catheters can provide valuable information in children with cardiopulmonary failure. The ability to measure pulmonary artery pressures, cardiac output/index, and systemic and pulmonary vascular resistance can provide important data for directing therapies. However, because of potential complications, pulmonary artery catheters tend to be used less often in children than in adults. Pulmonary artery catheters are therefore indicated only when the additional data obtained will enhance clinical decision making.

Hospital-acquired Infections

Hospital-acquired infections are a constant threat for any critically ill child in the PICU. Acquired nosocomial infection coupled with extreme severity of illness in a child with myocarditis significantly increases morbidity and mortality. Nurses' diligence in preventing and monitoring for infection is essential. Within hours of admission, hospital-associated bacteria can be detected on skin and in the respiratory and genitourinary tracts. Invasive devices, antibiotic use, and/or critical care procedures increase the risk of bacterial invasion. Some of the highest rates of hospital-acquired infection occur in PICUs; bloodstream infection and ventilator-associated pneumonia are the most common.

Fever is often the first sign of infection in children; however, infants often have decreases in body temperature because of the immaturity of the brain's temperature-regulating center. Monitoring of temperature changes in this age group can be complicated by the use of radiant warmers, designed to maintain normothermia. Radiant warmer temperature is adjusted according to an infant's skin temperature; consequently, decreases in body temperature related to infection may be masked. Although skin temperature is continuously monitored in infants under a radiant warmer, core body temperature should be monitored a minimum of once an hour, if not continuously, in all age groups. White blood cell count with a differential count should be assessed closely. Leukocytosis (elevation) or leukopenia (decrease) develop in children with infection, depending on age. A normal total white blood cell count is 5,000–10,000 cells/μL but varies depending on the age of the child; the younger the child, the higher the upper range limit. Monitoring trends is as important as getting absolute counts.

The differential count provides the percentage of each subset of white blood cells (eosinophils, neutrophils, basophils, monocytes and lymphocytes) and can aid in differentiating the type of infection. In older infants and children, a "shift to the left", or an excess of immature neutrophils (bands), usually indicates bacterial infection. An increase in the number or percentage of bands along with fever may warrant further workup (e.g. blood cultures for detection of secondary bacterial infection). Coagulase-negative staphylococci are the most common cause of nosocomial bloodstream infections in the PICU. Unlike older children, young infants commonly have neutropenia when infected because of their small storage pools and inability to produce white blood cells at a fast rate.

Pulmonary secretions should be monitored for changes in viscosity, color and amount. Changes in the character of the secretions along with evidence of new pulmonary infiltrates may indicate the development of ventilator-associated pneumonia (the second most common hospital-acquired infection in PICUs) in intubated patients. Although nosocomial urinary tract infections occur less often than do acquired bloodstream or pulmonary infections in children, urine should be routinely examined for color, odor, and changes in opacity, particularly if a child has a urinary catheter in place.

Any invasive catheter is a potential source of infection. Insertion sites should be routinely inspected for edema, redness and drainage. Although central venous catheters are not routinely changed in children, signs of infection at the site may warrant removal of the catheter. Factors increasing the risk for bloodstream infection include multilumen catheters, repeated catheterizations, and certain types of dressing. In order to minimize risk of infection, catheters should be manipulated as little as possible and should be removed as soon as they are no longer needed.

Immobility and alteration in tissue perfusion increase the potential for skin breakdown. Skin should be kept free from exposure to moisture and secretions; moisture-barrier products can be applied to the perineal area. Application of topical moisturizers, with avoidance of products containing perfume or alcohol, aids in maintaining skin hydration. Mouth care, a minimum of every 8 hours, helps to keep oral mucosa clean and moist. In children without a blink response (chemically paralyzed) or with incomplete lid closure, the eyes should be kept moist with artificial tears and/or lubricant as needed. Frequent turning (as tolerated), alleviation of pressure points on bony prominences (use of pillows, stuffed animals), and alternating pressure points related to mechanical devices (oxygen saturation probes, blood pressure cuffs, electrodes) should be performed on a routine basis. Air mattresses or rotating beds can also be used to prevent skin breakdown. Any evidence of altered skin integrity should be immediately addressed.

Prognosis in Myocarditis

The survival rate in children and adults with myocarditis is approximately 80%. Lee et al found that patients who died almost always did so within the first few hospital days. Survival after 72 hours in patients not requiring ECMO is as high as 97%. Some centers have had a 1-year survival rate of 80% in children who required mechanical circulatory support.

Unfortunately, survival to discharge does not imply full recovery. Although Lee et al found that recovery of ventricular function without the need for ongoing cardiac medications or restrictions in physical activity was the norm, some evidence suggests that myocarditis can progress to dilated cardiomyopathy. Viral persistence in the myocardium has been associated with progressive impairment of left ventricular function and is predictive of adverse outcomes. Progression from myocarditis to dilated cardiomyopathy is further supported by the finding of a coxsackievirus B-adenovirus receptor gene present in larger amounts in the myocardium of patients with dilated cardiomyopathy than in healthy hearts. The discovery of this receptor also suggests a role in not only the viral origin of myocarditis but also the occasional "familial" case of myocarditis. Survival in children with dilated cardiomyopathy ranges from 60% to 70% at 1 year to 34–56% at 5 years. Gagliardi et al reported that in children with dilated cardiomyopathy, the first 2 years after diagnosis are the most crucial. Favorable events (nearly complete recovery) and worse outcomes (death or need for a transplant) occur during this period. For children with residual myocardial dysfunction at discharge, diuretics and afterload reducers are considered first-line agents. Diuretics are used for congestive heart failure of any cause because they reduce respiratory signs and symptoms associated with heart failure. Thiazides (diuril, hydrochlorothiazide) are often used; the addition of spironolactone may obviate potassium supplementation. Angiotensin-converting enzyme inhibitors (captopril and enalapril) may also improve chronic signs and symptoms. The use of digoxin in patients with chronic congestive heart failure as a result of myocarditis remains controversial. The poor diastolic function associated with myocarditis is not improved with digoxin. Digoxin also increases the risk of ventricular arrhythmias if myocardial inflammation is still present. If digoxin is used, digitalization should be accomplished during a 24- to 36-hour period with 75% of the usual total loading dose to minimize the possibility of arrhythmia development.

Beta-blockade may improve outcome in children with dilated cardiomyopathy. Carvedilol, a nonselective beta-blocker used in adults, has been examined as an adjunct therapy for management of heart failure in children. Carvedilol may improve congestive heart failure through several mechanisms, including decreased heart rate leading to improved myocardial oxygen consumption and enhanced coronary artery blood flow, improvement in left ventricular ejection fraction, and reduction in neurohormonal vasoconstrictor systems. Carvedilol may also prevent ventricular arrhythmias and sudden death.

Use of carvedilol in children remains controversial. Bruns et al studied the use of carvedilol in 46 children with heart failure in 6 different centers and found improvement in left ventricular function and overall signs and symptoms in 67%. Schwartz and Wessel also examined use of carvedilol in children with heart failure and found no statistically significant effect; left ventricular ejection fraction improved in both the carvedilol and the placebo groups. Although carvedilol is effective in reducing mortality in adults, more research into the use of carvedilol is needed in children with heart failure.

Transplantation is sometimes the only option for children with significant cardiac failure or dilated cardiomyopathy due to myocarditis. Preferably, children are not put on a list for transplantation until they have progressed to the chronic phase of the disease because recovery is possible in even the most severe cases. Transplantation may, however, be considered an option for a child who requires ECMO for more than 10 days and has no clinical signs of improvement.

Summary

Viral myocarditis remains an uncommon but challenging illness. In children, the initial signs and symptoms are often those of common pediatric illnesses and without any obvious cardiac signs. Adding to the challenge is the potential inability of the child to convey precise symptoms or describe location or intensity of pain or discomfort. A history of asthma or congenital heart disease can skew the clinical picture. Although few children actually have viral myocarditis diagnosed and require admission to the PICU, practitioners must maintain a heightened sense of awareness for the "zebra in the herd of horses". Concomitantly, for any previously healthy child with sudden cardiogenic shock, myocarditis must be included in the differential diagnosis. Most children with myocarditis recover without requiring admission to the PICU; only a small percentage progress to development of significant cardiopulmonary compromise that requires intensive cardiopulmonary support and monitoring. Critical care management is aimed at supportive rather than curative measures and depends on the severity of myocardial dysfunction. The most common techniques used in the PICU for children with cardiovascular compromise or collapse include invasive hemodynamic monitoring, infusions of inotropic agents, antiarrhythmics, afterload reducers, mechanical ventilation, prevention of complications, and, when a child is unresponsive to ordinary PICU therapies, extracorporeal life support.

BIBLIOGRAPHY

1. Aretz HT, Billingham ME, Edwards WD, et al. Myocarditis: a histopathologic definition and classification. Am J Cardiovasc Pathol. 1987;1(1):3–14.
2. Batra AS, Lewis AB. Acute myocarditis. Curr Opin Pediatr. 2001;13(3):234–239.
3. Leonard EG. Viral myocarditis. Pediatr Infect Dis J. 2004;23(7):665–666.
4. Mecham N. Acute viral myocarditis in the ED pediatric patient: three case presentations. J Emerg Nurs. 2004; 30(2):179–182.
5. Levi D, Alejos J. Diagnosis and treatment of pediatric viral myocarditis. Curr Opin Cardiol. 2001;16:77–83.
6. Chavda KK, Dhuper S, Makhok A, Chowdjury D. Seizures secondary to a high-grade atrioventricular block as a presentation of acute myocarditis. Pediatr Emerg Care. 2004; 20(6):387–390.
7. Woodruff JF. Viral myocarditis. Am J Pathol. 1980;101(2):427–484.
8. Feldman AM, McNamara D. Medical progress: myocarditis. N Engl J Med. 2000; 343(19):1388–1398.
9. Calabrese F, Rigo E, Milanesi O, et al. Molecular diagnosis of myocarditis and dilated cardiomyopathy in children: clinicopathologic features and prognostic implications. Diagn Mol Pathol. 2002;11(4):212–221.
10. Lee KJ, McCrindle BW, Bohn DJ, et al. Clinical outcomes of acute myocarditis in childhood. Heart. 1999;82(2):226–233.
11. Friedman RA. Myocarditis. In: Garson A, Bricher JT, McNamara DG, eds. The Science and Practice of Pediatric Cardiology. Philadelphia, PA: Lea & Febiger; 1990: 1577–1589.
12. Park MK, Troxler RG. Pediatric Cardiology for Practitioners. 4th ed. St Louis, MO: Mosby; 2002:289–290.
13. Martin AB, Webber S, Fricker FJ, et al. Congenital cardiovascular disease/diabetes: acute myocarditis: rapid diagnosis by PCR in children. Circulation. 1994;90(1):330–339.
14. Baboonian C, McKenna W. Eradication of viral myocarditis: is there hope? J Am Coll Cardiol. 2003;42(3):473–476.
15. Bowles NE, Towbin JA. Molecular aspects of myocarditis. Curr Infect Dis Rep. 2000;2(4):308–314.
16. Pres S, Lipkind RS. Acute myocarditis in infants: initial presentation. Clin Pediatr. 1990;29(2):73–76.
17. Drucker NA, Colan SD, Lewis AB, et al. Gamma-globulin treatment of acute myocarditis in the pediatric population. Circulation. 1994;89(1):252–257.
18. Kawai C. From myocarditis to cardiomyopathy: mechanisms of inflammation and cell death. Circulation. 1999;99(8):1091–1100.
19. Kühl U, Pauschinger M, Noutsias, M, Kapp JF, Schultheiss HP. Diagnosis and treatment of patients with virus induced inflammatory cardiomyopathy. Eur Heart J Suppl. 2002;4 (suppl I):173–180.
20. Drucker NA, Newburger JW. Viral myocarditis: diagnosis and management. Adv Pediatr. 1997;44:141–169.
21. Archard LC, Khan MA, Soteriou BA, Why HJ, Robinson NM, Richardson PJ. Characterization of coxsackie B virus RNA

in myocardium from patients with dilated cardiomyopathy by nucleotide sequencing of reverse transcription-nested polymerase chain reaction products. Hum Pathol. 1998; 29(6):578–584.

22. Fujioka S, Kitaura Y, Ukimara A, et al. Evaluation of viral infection in the myocardium of patients with idiopathic dilated cardiomyopathy. J Am Coll Cardiol. 2000;36(6): 1920–1926.
23. McCarthy RE, Boehmer JP, Hruban RH, et al. Long-term outcome of fulminant myocarditis as compared with acute (non-fulminant) myocarditis. N Engl J Med. 2000; 342(10):690–695.
24. Tobias JD, Deshpande JK, Johns JA, Nichols DG. Inflammatory heart disease. In: Nichols DG, Ungerleider RM, Spevak PJ, et al, eds. 2nd ed. Critical Heart Disease in Infants and Children. Philadelphia, PA: Mosby; 2006:899–925.
25. Slota MC. Clinical assessment of cardiovascular function. In: Slota MC, ed. Core Curriculum for Pediatric Critical Care Nursing. 2nd ed. Philadelphia, PA: WB Saunders Co; 2006:176–185.
26. Craig J, Fineman LD, Moynihan P, Baker AL. Cardiovascular critical care problems. In: Curley MAQ, Moloney-Harmon PA, eds. Critical Care Nursing of Infants and Children. 2nd ed. Philadelphia, PA: WB Saunders Co; 2001:629–631.
27. Hazinski MF. Children are different. In: Hazinski MF. Nursing Care of the Critically Ill Child. 2nd ed. St Louis, MO: Mosby; 1992:1–17.
28. Baughman KL. Diagnosis of myocarditis: death of Dallas criteria. Circulation. 2006; 113(4):593–595.
29. Pophal SG, Sigfusson G, Booth KL, et al. Complications of endomyocardial biopsy in children. J Am Coll Cardiol. 1999; 34(7): 2105–2110.
30. Akhtar N, Ni J, Stromberg D, Rosenthal GL, Bowles NE, Towbin JA. Tracheal aspirate as a substrate for polymerase chain reaction detection of viral genome in childhood pneumonia and myocarditis. Circulation. 1999;99(15):2011–2018.
31. Lauer B, Neiderau C, Kuhl U, et al. Cardiac troponin T in patients with clinically suspected myocarditis. J Am Coll Cardiol. 1997;30(5):1354–1359.
32. Hoffman TM, Wernovsky G, Atz AM, et al. Efficacy and safety of milrinone in preventing low cardiac output syndrome in infants and children after corrective surgery for congenital heart disease. Circulation. 2003;107(7):996–1002.
33. Schwartz SM, Wessel DM. Medical cardiovascular support in acute viral myocarditis in children. Pediatr Crit Care Med. 2006; 7(6)(suppl):S12–S16.
34. American Heart Association. 2006.
35. Matsumori A, Igata H, Ono K, et al. High doses of digitalis increase the myocardial production of proinflammatory cytokines and worsen myocardial injury in viral myocarditis: a possible mechanism of digitalis toxicity. Jpn Circ J. 1999;63(12):934–940.
36. Gagliardi MG, Bevilacqua M, Bassano C, et al. Long-term follow-up of children with myocarditis treated by immunosuppression and of children with dilated cardiomyopathy. Heart. 2004;90(10):1167–1171.
37. Adhoot J, Galindo A, Alejos JC, et al. Use of OKT3 for acute myocarditis in infants and children. J Heart Lung Transplant. 2000; 19(11):1118–1121.
38. Macrae D, Chang AC. Pediatric cardiac intensive care consensus: myocarditis. Paper presented at: Pediatric Cardiac Intensive Care Symposium; December 11, 2005; Miami, FL.
39. Bohn D, Macrae D, Chang AC. Acute viral myocarditis: mechanical circulatory support. Pediatr Crit Care Med. 2006;7(6)(suppl): S21–S24.
40. Weiss WJ. Pulsatile pediatric ventricular assist devices. ASAIO J. 2005;51(5):540–545.
41. Throckmorton AL, Lim DS, McCulloch MA, et al. Computational design and experimental performance testing of an axial-flow pediatric ventricular assist device. ASAIO J. 2005;51(5):629–635.
42. Yong ES, Timmons OD, Uhl MW, et al. Reduction of blood gases in a pediatric ICU (PICU): a process improvement. Paper presented at: 11th Annual Pediatric Critical Care Colloquium; September 1998; Chicago, IL.
43. Thompson A. Pediatric emergency airway management. In: Dieckmann RA, Fiser DH, Selbst SM, eds. Illustrated Textbook of Pediatric Emergency and Critical Care Procedures. Louis, MO: Mosby-Yearbook Inc; 1997:104–115.
44. Curley MAQ, Thompson JE. Oxygenation and ventilation. In: Curley MAQ, Moloney-Harmon, PA. Critical Care Nursing of Infants and Children. 2nd ed. Philadelphia, PA: WB Saunders Co; 2001:233–308.

20 Diagnosis and Management of Dyslipidemia in Children and Adolescents

Dyslipidemia is an important etiologic factor in the development of cardiovascular disease (CVD), which is a leading cause of death worldwide as CVD begins in childhood, and as dyslipidemia is an important risk factor for CVD, screening and treatment of dyslipidemia in adolescents and children becomes an important health matter. This review deals with issues related to screening, diagnosis and treatment of dyslipidemia in children and adolescents (Fig. 20.1).

Dyslipidemia is elevation of plasma cholesterol, triglycerides (TGs), or both, or a low high density lipoprotein level that contributes to the development of atherosclerosis. Causes may be primary (genetic) or secondary. Diagnosis is by measuring plasma levels of total cholesterol, TGs, and individual lipoproteins. Treatment is dietary changes, exercise, and lipid-lowering drugs.

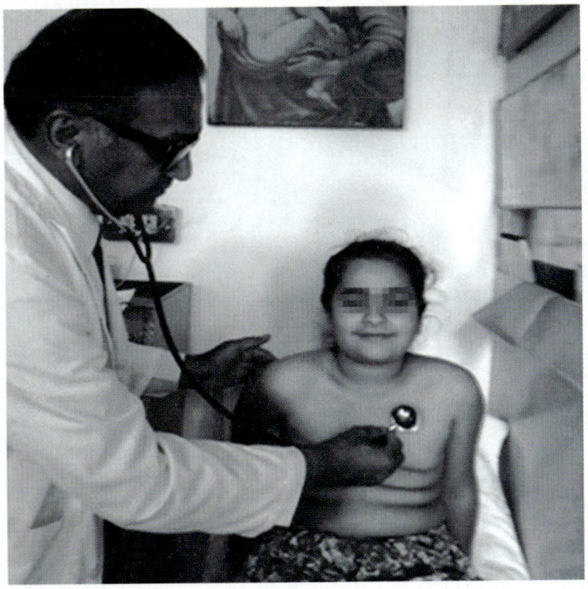

Fig. 20.1: *Doctor is a conducting physical examination in a child with dyslipidemia*

Disturbances in lipid metabolism leads to varying grades of atherosclerotic process in the body, which ultimately ends with fatal cardiovascular, cerebral and renal events. It is therefore important to prevent such complications from childhood period with proper dietic, drugs and exercise programmes.

Cardiovascular disease (CVD) is the leading cause of morbidity and mortality in the industrialized world. It is estimated that 30% of all deaths worldwide can be ascribed to cardiovascular causes, and this number is expected to rise further as the incidence of CVD in the developing world increases because of lifestyle changes.

There is no natural cut-off between normal and abnormal lipid levels because lipid measurements are continuous. A linear relation probably exists between lipid levels and cardiovascular risk, so many people with "normal" cholesterol levels benefit from achieving still lower levels. Consequently, there are no numeric definitions of dyslipidemia; the term is applied to lipid levels for which treatment has proven beneficial. Proof of benefit is strongest for lowering elevated low density lipoprotein (LDL) levels. In the overall population, evidence is less strong for a benefit from lowering elevated TG and increasing low high density lipoprotein (HDL) levels, in part because elevated TG and low HDL levels are more predictive of cardiovascular risk in women than in men. HDL levels do not always predict cardiovascular risk. For example, high HDL levels caused by some genetic disorders may not protect against cardiovascular disorders, and low HDL levels caused by some genetic disorders may not increase the risk of cardiovascular disorders. Although HDL levels predict cardiovascular risk in the overall population, the increased risk may be caused by other factors, such as accompanying lipid and metabolic abnormalities, rather than the HDL level itself.

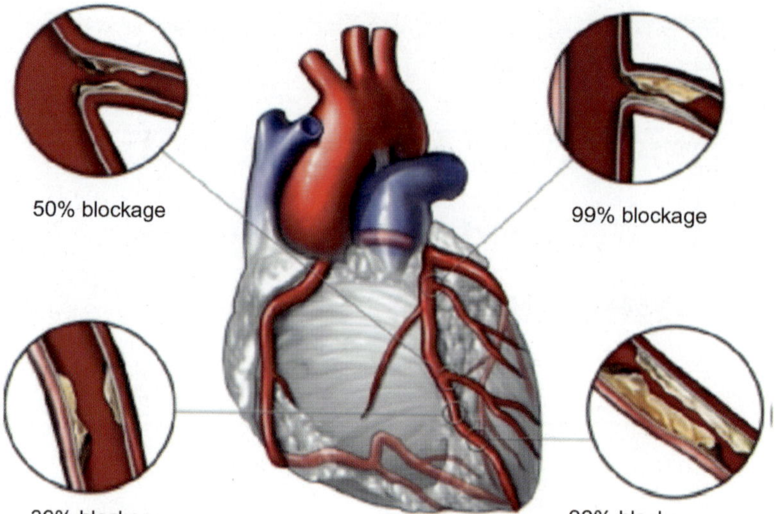

Fig. 20.2: *Diagram of heart and with coronary arteries having different grades of obstruction in patients with dyslipidemia*

Table 20.1: *Showing normal and abnormal plasma values in children and adolescent*

Blood Lipid	*Good*	*Borderline*	*High*
Total cholesterol	200 or less	200–239	240 and above
LDL cholesterol ("Bad cholesterol")	130 or less	130–159	160 and above
Triglycerides	150 or less	150–199	200 and above

Classification

Dyslipidemias were traditionally classified by patterns of elevation in lipids and lipoproteins (A more practical system categorizes dyslipidemias as primary or secondary and characterizes them by increases in cholesterol only (pure or isolated hypercholesterolemia), increases in TGs only (pure or isolated hypertriglyceridemia), or increases in both cholesterol and TGs (mixed or combined hyperlipidemias). This system does not take into account specific lipoprotein abnormalities (e.g. low HDL or high LDL) that may contribute to disease despite normal cholesterol and TG levels (Figs 20.7 and 20.8).

Etiology primary (genetic) causes and secondary (lifestyle and other) causes contribute to dyslipidemias in varying degrees. For example, in familial combined hyperlipidemia, expression may occur only in the presence of significant secondary causes (Table 20.1).

Primary causes: Primary causes are single or multiple gene mutations that result in either overproduction or defective clearance of TG and LDL cholesterol, or in underproduction or excessive clearance of HDL. Primary disorders, the most common cause of dyslipidemia in children, do not cause a large percentage of cases in adults. The names of many reflect an old nomenclature in which lipoproteins were detected and distinguished by how they separated into α (HDL) and β (LDL) bands on electrophoretic gels (Fig. 20.8).

Secondary causes: Secondary causes contribute to most cases of dyslipidemia in adults. The most important secondary cause in developed countries is a sedentary lifestyle with excessive dietary intake of saturated fat, cholesterol, and trans fats. Trans-fats are polyunsaturated or monounsaturated fatty acids to which hydrogen atoms have been added; they are commonly used in many processed foods and are as atherogenic as saturated fat. Other common secondary causes include diabetes mellitus, alcohol overuse, chronic kidney disease, hypothyroidism, primary biliary cirrhosis and other cholestatic liver diseases, and drugs, such as thiazides, β-blockers, retinoids, highly active antiretroviral agents, estrogen and progestins, and

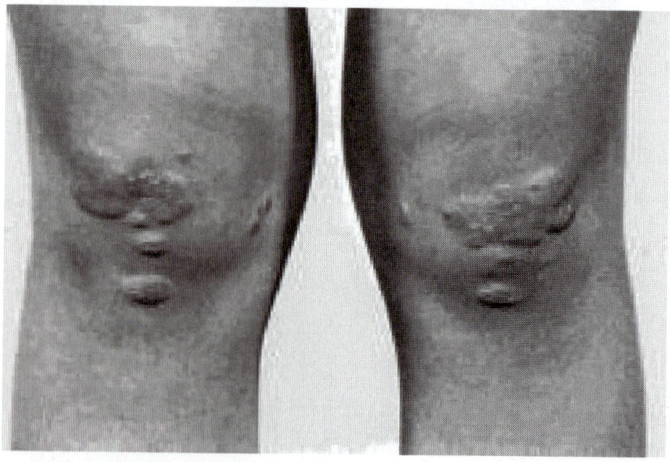

Fig. 20.3: *Tubero-eruptive xanthomata on the knees in a child with dysbeta-lipoproteinemia*

glucocorticoids. Diabetes is an especially significant secondary cause because patients tend to have an atherogenic combination of high TGs; high small, dense LDL fractions; and low HDL (diabetic dyslipidemia, hypertriglyceridemic hyperapo B). Patients with type 2 diabetes are especially at risk. The combination may be a consequence of obesity, poor control of diabetes, or both, which may increase circulating FFAs, leading to increased hepatic VLDL production. TG-rich VLDL then transfers TG and cholesterol to LDL and HDL, promoting formation of TG-rich, small, dense LDL and clearance of TG-rich HDL. Diabetic dyslipidemia is often exacerbated by the increased caloric intake and physical inactivity that characterize the lifestyles of some patients with type 2 diabetes. Women with diabetes may be at special risk for cardiac disease from this form.

Symptoms and Signs

Dyslipidemia itself usually causes no symptoms but can lead to symptomatic vascular disease including coronary artery disease (CAD) and peripheral arterial disease. High levels of TGs [> 1000 mg/dL (> 11.3 mmol/L)] can cause acute pancreatitis. High levels of LDL can cause eyelid xanthelasmas; arcus corneae; and tendinous xanthomas at the achilles, elbow, and knee tendons and over metacarpophalangeal joints. Patients with the homozygous form of familial hypercholesterolemia may have the above findings plus planar or cutaneous xanthomas. Patients with severe elevations of TGs can have eruptive xanthomas over the trunk, back, elbows, buttocks, knees, hands and feet. Patients with the rare dysbetalipoproteinemia can have palmar and tuberous xanthomas. Severe hypertriglyceridemia [> 2,000 mg/dL (> 22.6 mmol/L)] can give retinal arteries and veins a creamy white appearance (lipemia retinalis). Extremely high lipid levels also give a lactescent (milky) appearance to blood plasma.

Symptoms can include paresthesias, dypsnea and confusion.

Diagnosis (Figs 20.3 and 20.5): Serum lipid profile (measured total cholesterol, TG, and HDL-cholesterol and calculated LDL-cholesterol and VLDL), dyslipidemia is suspected in patients with characteristic physical findings

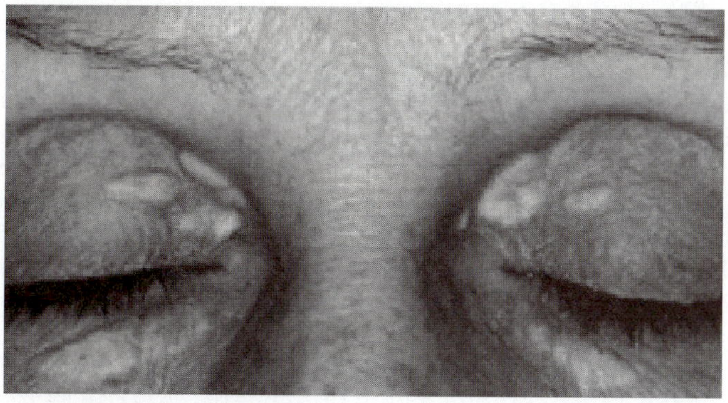

Fig. 20.4: *Xanthelasma in a 18-year-old patient with hypercholesterolemia*

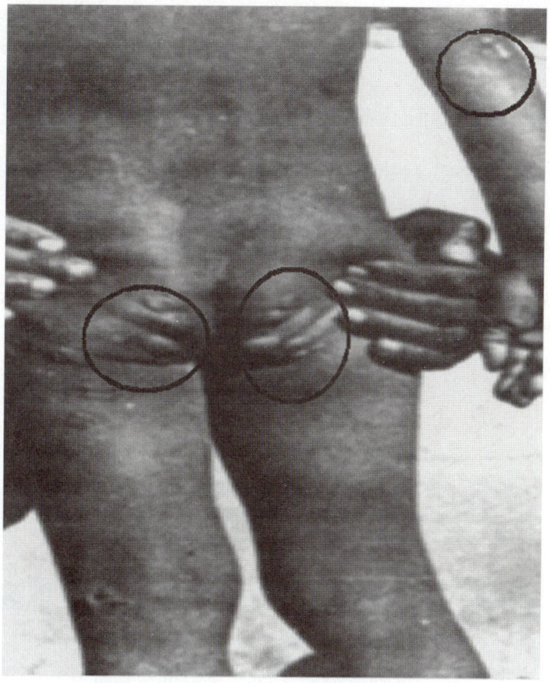

Fig. 20.5: *Tubero-eruptive xanthomata on the gluteal and elbow regions (arrows) in a child with dysbeta-lipoproteinemia*

or complications of dyslipidemia (e.g. atherosclerotic disease). Primary lipid disorders are suspected when patients have physical signs of dyslipidemia, onset of premature atherosclerotic disease (at < 60 year), a family history of atherosclerotic disease, or serum cholesterol > 240 mg/dL (> 6.2 mmol/L). Dyslipidemia is diagnosed by measuring serum lipids. Routine measurements (lipid profile) include total cholesterol (TC), TGs, HDL-cholesterol and LDL-cholesterol.

Lipid profile measurement: TC, TGs, and HDL-cholesterol are measured directly; TC and TG values reflect cholesterol and TGs in all circulating lipoproteins including chylomicrons, VLDL, IDL, LDL, and HDL. TC values vary by 10% and TGs by up to 25% day-to-day even in the absence of a disorder. TC and HDL-cholesterol can be measured in the nonfasting state, but most patients should have all lipids measured while fasting for maximum accuracy and consistency. Testing should be postponed until after resolution of acute illness because TGs increase and cholesterol levels decrease in inflammatory states. Lipid profiles can vary for about 30 days after an acute MI; however, results obtained within 24 hours after MI are usually reliable enough to guide initial lipid-lowering therapy. LDL-cholesterol values are most often calculated as the amount of cholesterol not contained in HDL and VLDL. VLDL is estimated by TG ÷ 5 because the cholesterol concentration in VLDL particles is usually 1/5 of the total lipid in the particle. Thus, LDL-cholesterol = TC [HDL-cholesterol + (TGs ÷ 5)] (Friedewald formula). This calculation is valid only when TGs are < 400 mg/dL and patients are fasting because eating increases TGs. The calculated LDL-cholesterol value incorporates measures of

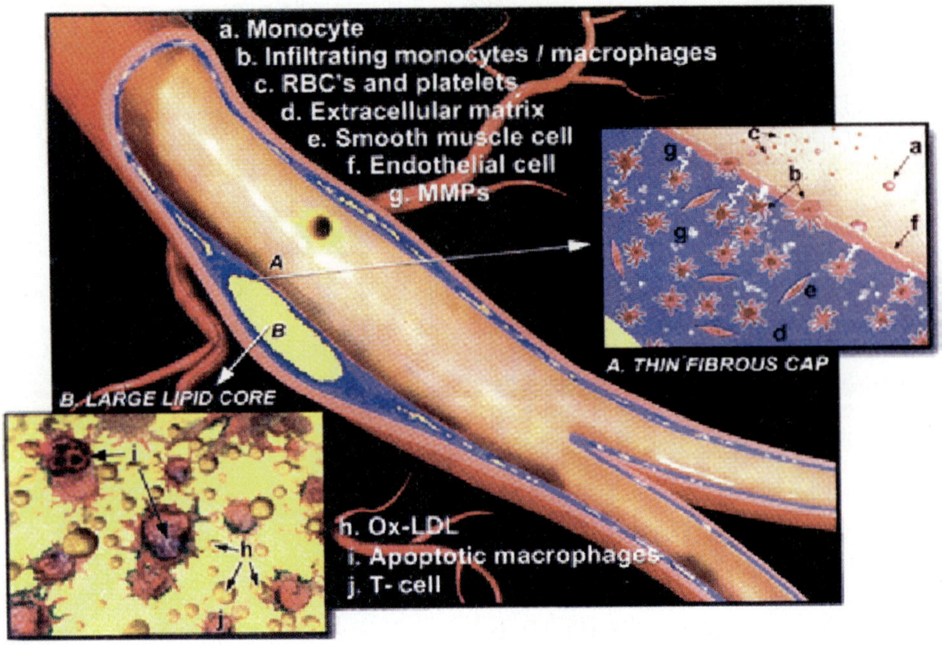

Fig. 20.6: *As how monocytes, RBCs extracellular marix, smooth cells and endothelial cells are held responsible for the genesis of (A) thin fiberous cap and large lipid core (B)*

all non-HDL, nonchylomicron cholesterol including that in IDL and Lp(a). LDL can also be measured directly using plasma ultracentrifugation, which separates chylomicrons and VLDL fractions from HDL and LDL, and by an immunoassay method. Direct measurement may be useful in some patients with elevated TGs, but these direct measurements are not routinely necessary. The role of apo B testing is under study because values reflect all non-HDL cholesterol (in VLDL, VLDL remnants, IDL and LDL) and may be more predictive of CAD risk than LDL alone (Table 20.1).

Other tests: Patients with premature atherosclerotic cardiovascular disease, cardiovascular disease with normal or near-normal lipid levels, or high LDL levels refractory to drug therapy should probably have Lp(a) levels measured. Lp(a) levels may also be directly measured in patients with borderline high LDL-cholesterol levels to determine whether drug therapy is warranted. C-reactive protein and homocysteine measurement may be considered in the same populations (Figs 20.7 and 20.8).

Secondary causes: Tests for secondary causes of dyslipidemia including measurements of fasting glucose, liver enzymes, creatinine, thyroid stimulating hormone (TSH), and urinary protein should be done in most patients with newly diagnosed dyslipidemia and when a component of the lipid profile has inexplicably changed for the worse.

Screening: A fasting lipid profile (TC, TGs, HDL-cholesterol, and calculated LDL-cholesterol) should be obtained in all adults ≤ 20 years and should be repeated every 5 years.

Lipid measurement should be accompanied by assessment of other cardiovascular risk factors, defined as

- Diabetes mellitus
- Cigarette use
- Hypertension.

Family history of CAD in a male 1st-degree relative before age 55 years or a female 1st-degree relative before age 65 years. A definite age after which patients no longer require screening has not been established, but evidence supports screening of patients into their 80s, especially in the presence of atherosclerotic cardiovascular disease. Indications for screening patients < 20 years are atherosclerotic risk factors, such as diabetes, hypertension, cigarette smoking, and obesity; premature CAD in a parent, grandparent, or sibling; or a cholesterol level > 240 mg/dL (> 6.2 mmol/L) or known dyslipidemia in a parent. If information on relatives is unavailable, as in the case of adopted children, screening is at the discretion of the health care practitioner. Patients with an extensive family history of heart disease should also be screened by measuring Lp(a) levels.

Treatment (Table 20.2)

General principles: Treatment is indicated for all patients with cardiovascular disease (secondary prevetion) and for some without (primary prevention). The National Institutes of Health's National Cholesterol Education Program (NCEP) Adult Treatment Panel III (ATPIII) guidelines are the most common reference for deciding which adults should be treated. The guidelines focus primarily on reducing elevated LDL-cholesterol levels and secondarily on treating high TGs, low HDL, and metabolic syndrome. An alternate treatment guide (the Sheffield table) uses TC:HDL ratios combined with presence of CAD risk factors to predict cardiovascular risk, but this approach probably leads to undertreatment. Data from the Third Report of the

Table 20.2: *Different measures in the management of dyslipidemia*

LDL-C ≥130 mg/dL (initial)	• Nutritionist training with <30% calories from fat, <7% calories from saturated fat; cholesterol intake <200 mg/d trans-fat avoidance • Repeat test after 6 mos • If LDL-C ≤130–160 mg/dL, initiate statin with goal <130 mg/dL, ideal target <100 mg/dL
Triglycerides 150–600 mg/dL (initial)	• Decrease intake of simple carbs and fat • Weight loss management if overweigtht
Triglycerides >700–1,000 mg/dL (initial or follow-up)	• Consider fibrates or niacin if patient is aged >10 years

Expert Panel on Detection, Evaluation, and Treatment of High Blood Cholesterol in Adults. National Institutes of Health, National Heart, Lung, and Blood Institute, 2001 and from Grundy SM, Cleeman JI, Merz CNB, et al. Implications of recent clinical trials for the National Cholesterol Education Program Adult Treatment Panel III guidelines. Circulation 110:227–239, 2004.Treatment of children is controversial; dietary changes may be difficult to implement, and no data suggest that lowering lipid levels in childhood effectively prevents heart disease in adulthood. Moreover, the safety and effectiveness of long-term lipid-lowering treatment are questionable. Nevertheless, the American Academy of Pediatrics (AAP) recommends treatment for some children who have elevated LDL-cholesterol levels. Treatment options depend on the specific lipid abnormality, although different lipid abnormalities often coexist. In some patients, a single abnormality may require several therapies; in others, a single treatment may be adequate for several abnormalities. Treatment should always include treatment of hypertension and diabetes, smoking cessation, and in patients with a 10 year risk of MI or death from CAD of ≤ 10% low-dose daily aspirin. In general, treatment options for men and women are the same.

Elevated LDL-cholesterol: In adults, ATPIII guidelines recommend treatment for those with any of the following:

- Elevated LDL-cholesterol levels and a history of CAD
- Conditions that confer a risk for future cardiac events similar to that of CAD itself (CAD equivalents, defined as diabetes mellitus, abdominal aortic aneurysm, peripheral arterial disease, and symptomatic carotid artery disease.

"CAD risk factors ATPIII guidelines recommend that these patients have LDL-cholesterol levels lowered to < 100 mg/dL, but accumulating evidence suggests that this target may be too high and a target LDL-cholesterol <70 mg/dL is an option for patients at very high risk (e.g. patients with known CAD and diabetes, other poorly controlled risk factors, metabolic syndrome, or acute coronary syndrome). When drugs are used, a dose providing at least a 30–40% decrease in LDL-cholesterol is desirable.

For children, the AAP recommends dietary treatment for children with LDL-cholesterol > 110 mg/dL. Drug therapy is recommended for children > 8 years and with either of the following:

Poor response to dietary therapy, LDL-cholesterol ≤ 190 mg/dL, and no family history of premature cardiovascular disease.

LDL-cholesterol 160 mg/dL and a family history of premature cardiovascular disease or risk factors for premature cardiovascular disease. Childhood risk factors besides family history and diabetes include cigarette

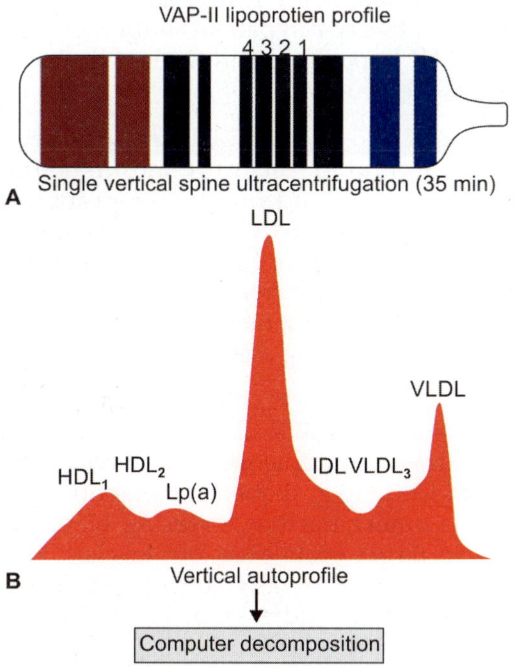

Fig. 20.7: *Diagrammatic depiction of VAP-11 lipoprotein profile*

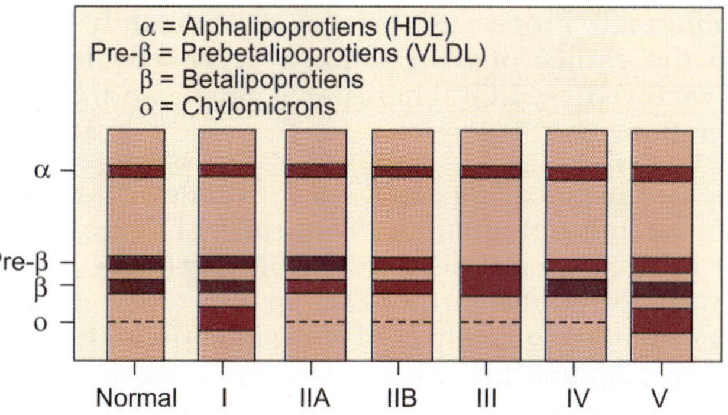

Fig. 20.8: *Finer divisions of lipoproteins*

smoking, hypertension, low HDL-cholesterol (< 35 mg/dL), obesity and physical inactivity. Treatment options to lower LDL-cholesterol in all age groups include lifestyle changes (diet and exercise), drugs, dietary supplements, procedural interventions, and experimental therapies. Many of these options are also effective for treating other lipid abnormalities. Exercise lowers LDL-cholesterol in some people; it is also essential to maintain ideal body weight. Dietary changes and exercise should be the initial approach whenever feasible.

Lifestyle changes can involve diet and exercise. Dietary changes include decreasing intake of saturated fats and cholesterol; increasing the proportion of dietary fiber, and complex carbohydrates; and maintaining ideal body weight. Referral to a dietician is often useful, especially for older people. The length of time for which lifestyle changes should be attempted before beginning lipid-lowering drugs is controversial. In patients at average or low cardiovascular risk, 3–6 mo is reasonable. Generally, 2–3 visits with a patient over 2–3 mo are sufficient to assess motivation and adherence. Drugs are the next step when lifestyle changes are not effective. However, for patients with extremely elevated LDL-cholesterol [> 200 mg/dL (> 5.2 mmol/L)] and those at high cardiovascular risk, drug therapy should accompany diet and exercise from the start.

Statins are the drugs and possibly treatment of choice for LDL-cholesterol reduction; they demonstrably reduce cardiovascular mortality. Statins inhibit hydroxymethylglutaryl CoA reductase, a key enzyme in cholesterol synthesis, leading to upregulation of LDL receptors and increased LDL clearance. They reduce LDL-cholesterol by up to 60% and produce small increases in HDL and modest decreases in TGs. Statins also appear to decrease intra-arterial inflammation, systemic inflammation, or both by stimulating production of endothelial nitric oxide and may have other beneficial effects. Adverse effects are uncommon but include liver enzyme elevations and myositis or rhabdomyolysis. Muscle toxicity without enzyme elevation has also been reported. Adverse effects are more common in older patients, patients with several disorders, and patients taking several drugs. In some people, changing from one statin to another or lowering the dose relieves the problem. Muscle toxicity seems to be most common when some of the statins are used with drugs that inhibit cytochrome P3A4 (e.g. macrolide antibiotics, azole antifungals, cyclosporine and with fibrates, especially gemfibrozil). Properties of statins differ slightly by drug, and the choice of drug should be based on patient characteristics, LDL-cholesterol level, and provider discretion.

Bile acid sequestrants block intestinal bile acid reabsorption, forcing upregulation of hepatic LDL receptors to recruit circulating cholesterol for bile synthesis. They are proven to reduce cardiovascular mortality. Bile acid sequestrants are usually used with statins or with nicotinic acid to augment LDL-cholesterol reduction and are the drugs of choice for children and women who are or are planning to become pregnant. Bile acid sequestrants are safe, but their use is limited by adverse effects of bloating, nausea, cramping and constipation. They may also increase TGs, so their use is contraindicated in patients with hypertriglyceridemia. Cholestyramine and colestipol but not colesevelam interfere with absorption of other drugs—notably thiazides, β-blockers, warfarin digoxin and thyroxine—an effect that can be decreased by administration 4 hours before or 1 h after other drugs.

Cholesterol absorption inhibitors, such as ezetimibe inhibit intestinal absorption of cholesterol and phytosterol. Ezetimibe usually lowers LDL-cholesterol by 15–20% and causes small increases in HDL and a mild decrease in TGs. Ezetimibe can be used as monotherapy in patients intolerant to statins or added to statins for patients on maximum doses with persistent LDL-cholesterol elevation. Adverse effects are infrequent.

Dietary supplements that lower LDL-cholesterol levels include fiber supplements and commercially available margarines and other products containing plant sterols (sitosterol and campesterol) or stanols. The latter reduce LDL-cholesterol by up to 10% without affecting HDL or TGs by competitively displacing cholesterol from intestinal micelles.

Procedural approaches are reserved for patients with severe hyperlipidemia (LDL-cholesterol > 300 mg/dL) that is refractory to conventional therapy, such as occurs with familial hypercholesterolemia. Options include LDL apheresis (in which LDL is removed by extracorporeal plasma exchange), ileal bypass (to block reabsorption of bile acids), liver transplantation (which transplants LDL receptors), and portocaval shunting (which decreases LDL production by unknown mechanisms). LDL apheresis is the procedure of choice in most instances when maximally tolerated therapy fails to lower LDL adequately. Apheresis is also the usual therapy in patients with the homozygous form of familial hypercholesterolemia who have limited or no response to drug therapy.

Future therapies to reduce LDL include peroxisome proliferator-activated receptor agonists that have thiazolidinedione-like and fibrate-like properties, LDL-receptor activators, LPL activators, and recombinant apo E. Cholesterol vaccination (to induce anti-LDL antibodies and hasten LDL clearance from serum) and gene transfer are conceptually appealing therapies that are under study but years away from being available for use.

Elevated TGs: Though it is unclear if elevated TGs independently contribute to cardiovascular disease, they are associated with multiple metabolic abnormalities that contribute to CAD (e.g. diabetes, metabolic syndrome). Consensus is emerging that lowering elevated TGs is beneficial. No target goals exist, but levels < 150 mg/dL (< 1.7 mmol/L) are generally considered desirable. No guidelines specifically address treatment of elevated TGs in children.

The overall treatment strategy is to first implement lifestyle changes including exercise, weight loss, and

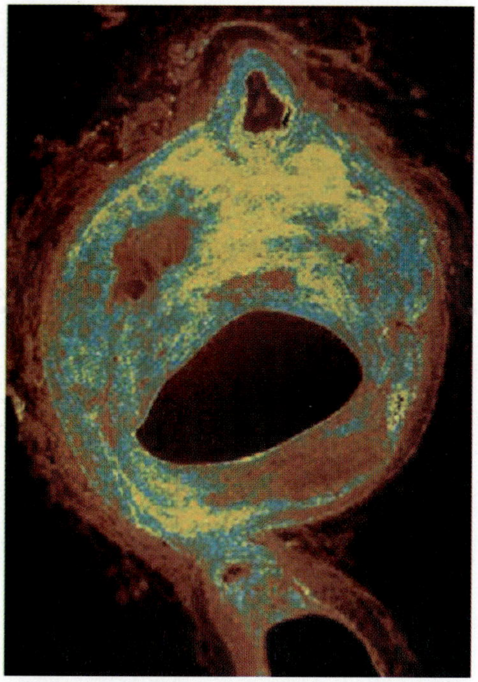

Fig. 20.9: *Patients with arterial plaque (yellow and blue) may cause clot formation*

avoidance of concentrated dietary sugar and alcohol. Intake of 2–4 servings/week of marine fish high in omega-3 fatty acids may be effective, but the amount of omega-3 fatty acids is often lower than needed; supplements may be helpful. In patients with diabetes, glucose levels should be tightly controlled. If these measures are ineffective, lipid-lowering drugs should be considered. Patients with very high TGs should begin drug therapy at diagnosis to more quickly reduce the risk of acute pancreatitis.

Fibrates reduce TGs by about 50%. They appear to stimulate endothelial LPL, leading to increased fatty acid oxidation in the liver and muscle and decreased hepatic VLDL synthesis. They also increase HDL by up to 20%. Fibrates can cause GI adverse effects including dyspepsia, abdominal pain, and elevated liver enzymes. They uncommonly cause cholelithiasis. Fibrates may potentiate muscle toxicity when used with statins and potentiate the effects of warfarin.

Nicotinic acid may also be useful (see Low HDL, below). Statins can be used in patients with TGs < 500 mg/dL if LDL-cholesterol elevations are also present; statins may reduce both LDL-cholesterol and TGs through reduction of VLDL. If only TGs are elevated, fibrates are the drug of choice. Omega-3 fatty acids in high doses [1–6 g/day of eicosapentaenoic acid (EPA) and docosahexaenoic acid (DHA)] can be effective in reducing TGs. The omega-3 fatty acids EPA and DHA are the active ingredients in marine fish oil or omega-3 capsules. Adverse effects include eructation and diarrhea. These may be decreased by giving the fish oil capsules with meals in divided doses (e.g. bid or tid). Omega-3 fatty acids can be a useful adjunct to other therapies.

Low HDL: Treatment to increase HDL-cholesterol levels may decrease risk of death, but data are limited. ATPIII guidelines define low HDL-cholesterol as < 40 mg/dL (< 1.04 mmol/L); the guidelines do not specify an HDL-cholesterol target level and recommend interventions to raise HDL-cholesterol only after LDL-cholesterol targets have been reached. Treatments for LDL-cholesterol and TG reduction often increase HDL-cholesterol, and the 3 objectives can sometimes be achieved simultaneously. No guidelines specifically address treatment of low HDL-cholesterol in children. Treatment includes lifestyle changes such as an increase in exercise weight loss. Alcohol raises HDL-cholesterol but is not routinely recommended as a therapy because of its many other adverse effects. Drugs are useful when lifestyle changes alone are insufficient.

Nicotinic acid (niacin) is the most effective drug for increasing HDL. Its mechanism of action is unknown, but it appears to both increase HDL production and inhibit HDL clearance; it may also mobilize cholesterol from macrophages. Niacin also decreases TGs and, in doses of 1,500–2,000 mg/day, reduces LDL-cholesterol. Niacin produces flushing, pruritus, and nausea; premedication with low-dose aspirin may prevent these adverse effects. Extended-release preparations cause flushing less often. However, most OTC slow-release preparations are not recommended; an exception is polygel controlled-release niacin. Niacin can cause liver enzyme elevations and occasionally liver failure, insulin resistance, and hyperuricemia and gout. It may also increase homocysteine levels. In patients with average LDL-cholesterol and below-average HDL-cholesterol levels, niacin combined with statin treatment may be effective in preventing cardiovascular disorders.

Fibrates increase HDL. Infusion of recombinant HDL (e.g. apoprotein A-1 Milano, an HDL variant in which a cysteine is substituted for an arginine at position 173 allowing for dimer formation) appears promising as a treatment for atherosclerosis but requires further study.

Elevated Lp(a): The upper limit of normal for Lp(a) is about 30 mg/dL (0.8 mmol/L), but values in African-Americans run higher. Few data exist to guide the treatment of elevated Lp(a) or to establish treatment efficacy. Niacin is the only drug that directly decreases Lp(a); it can lower Lp(a) by 20% at higher doses. The usual approach in patients with elevated Lp(a) is to lower LDL-cholesterol aggressively.

Secondary causes: Treatment of diabetic dyslipidemia should always involve lifestyle changes, with statins to reduce LDL-cholesterol, fibrates to decrease TGs, or both drugs. Metformin lowers TGs, which may be a reason to choose it over other oral antihyperglycemic drugs when treating diabetes. Some thiazolidinediones (TZDs) increase both HDL-cholesterol and LDL-cholesterol (probably the less atherogenic large, buoyant type of LDL). Some TZDs also decrease TGs. These antihyperglycemic drugs should not be chosen over lipid-lowering drugs to treat lipid abnormalities in diabetic patients but may be useful

Table 20.3: *Drugs for managing hyperlipidemia*

Type of drug	*Mechanism of action*	*Major effects*	*Example(s)*	*Adverse reactions*
HMG CoA reductase inhibitors (statins)	Inhibits cholesterol synthesis in hepatic cells, resulting in upregulation of hepatic LDL receptors	Lowers LDL cholesterol and triglyceride, raises HDL-C	Atorvastatin, lovastatin, pravastatin, simvastatin, fluvastatin, rosuvastatin	Raised hepatic enzymes, raised CPK, myopathy possibly progressing to rhabdomyolysis
Bile acid-binding resins	Binds intestinal bile acids interrupting enterohepatic recirculation which in turn results in LDL receptor upregulation	Lowers LDL-C, raises triglycerides	Cholestyramine, colestipol, coleveselam	Limited to gastrointestinal tract: gas, bloating, constipation, cramps
Fibric acid derivatives	Probably inhibits hepatic synthesis of VLDL	Mainly lowers triglycerides and raises HDL-C, with less effect on LDL-C	Gemfibrozil, fenofibrate	Dyspepsia, constipation, myositis, anemia
Nicotinic acid (extended release)	Upregulates hepatic LDL receptors	Lowers triglycerides and LDL-C	Niacin	Flushing, hepatic toxicity
Cholesterol absorption inhibitors	Inhibits intestinal absorption of cholesterol and plant sterols	Lowers LDL-C	Ezetimibe	Myopathy, gastrointestinal upset

HDL-C indicates HDL cholesterol; LDL-C, LDL cholesterol; and CPK, creatine phosphokinase.

adjuncts. Patients with very high TG levels and less than optimally controlled diabetes may have better response to insulin than to oral antihyperglycemic drugs. Treatment of dyslipidemia in patients with hypothyroidism, renal disease, liver disease, or a combination of these disorders involves treating the underlying disorders primarily and lipid abnormalities secondarily. Abnormal lipid levels in patients with low-normal thyroid function (high-normal TSH levels) improve with hormone replacement. Reducing the dosage of or stopping drugs that cause lipid abnormalities should be considered.

Monitoring treatment: Lipid levels should be monitored periodically after starting treatment. No data support specific monitoring intervals, but measuring lipid levels 2–3 mo after starting or changing therapies and once or twice yearly after lipid levels are stabilized is common practice. Despite the low incidence of liver and muscle toxicity with statin use (0.5–2% of all users), current recommendations are for baseline measurements of liver and muscle enzyme levels at the beginning of treatment. Many practitioners obtain at least one additional set of liver enzymes 4–12 weeks after beginning treatment and annually thereafter. Statin therapy can be continued unless liver enzymes increase to > 3 times the upper limit of normal. Muscle enzyme levels need not be checked regularly unless patients develop myalgias or other muscle symptoms. If statin-induced muscle damage is suspected, statin use is stopped and CK may be measured. When muscle symptoms subside, a lower dose or a different statin can be tried.

Elevated High-Density Lipoprotein Levels (Fig. 20.10)

Elevated HDL level is HDL-cholesterol > 80 mg/dL (> 2.1 mmol/L). Elevated HDL-cholesterol levels usually correlate with decreased cardiovascular risk; however, high HDL-cholesterol levels caused by some genetic disorders may not protect against cardiovascular disease, probably because of accompanying lipid and metabolic abnormalities. Primary causes are single or multiple genetic mutations that result in overproduction or decreased clearance of HDL. Secondary causes of high HDL-cholesterol include all of the following:

- Chronic alcoholism without cirrhosis
- Primary biliary cirrhosis
- Hyperthyroidism
- Drugs (e.g. corticosteroids, insulin, phenytoin. The unexpected finding of high HDL-cholesterol in patients not taking lipid-lowering drugs should prompt a diagnostic evaluation for a secondary cause with measurements of AST, ALT, and TSH; a negative evaluation suggests a possible primary cause.

Cholesteryl ester transfer protein (CETP) deficiency is a rare autosomal recessive disorder caused by a CETP gene mutation. CETP facilitates transfer of cholesterol esters from HDL to other lipoproteins, and CETP deficiency leads to low-cholesterol LDL and slower HDL clearance. Affected patients display no symptoms or signs but have HDL-cholesterol > 150 mg/dL. Protection from cardiovascular disorders has not been proven. No treatment is necessary.

Familial hyperalphalipoproteinemia is an autosomal dominant condition caused by various unidentified and

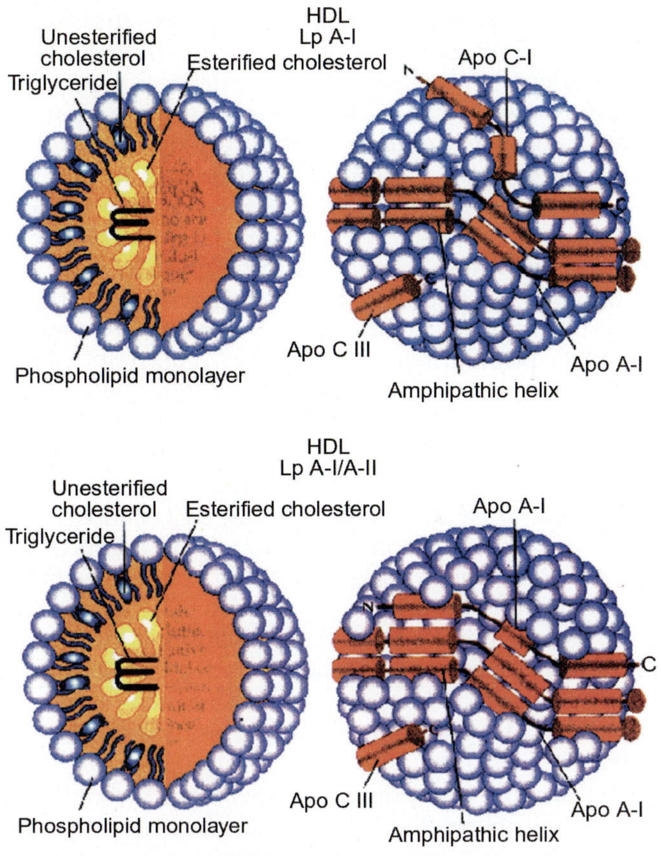

Fig. 20.10: *Diagrammatic representation of ultrastructure of circulating high density lipoprotein in the human body*

known genetic mutations, including those that cause apoprotein A-I overproduction and apoprotein C-III variants. The disorder is usually diagnosed incidentally when plasma HDL-cholesterol levels are > 80 mg/dL. Affected patients have no other symptoms or signs. No treatment is necessary. Many studies have demonstrated that the atherosclerotic process begins in childhood in association with high blood cholesterol levels. Lipid levels show a strong familial aggregation that has both a genetic and environmental component. Monogenic disorders including familial hypercholesterolemia and familial combined hyperlipidemia are expressed in childhood, although adverse diet, polygenic disorders, and environmental causes (including obesity) are the most common causes of high cholesterol levels in children.

Adult patients with diabetes are at significant risk for cardiovascular disease (CVD). Because the combination of diabetes and dyslipidemia accelerates atherogenesis, aggressive lipid management is suggested for such patients. While the American Diabetes Association has stated lipid goals for adults with diabetes, no similar guidelines exist for children. To address this issue, a panel of experts in the areas of pediatric endocrinology, pediatric cardiology, and pediatric nephrology met on the 28th and 29th of July 2002 to hear presentations, review current lipid guidelines for children in general, and formulate a set of recommendations regarding the lipid management of children with diabetes. The panel was asked to develop a consensus position on the following questions.

Systemic Lupus Erythematosus (SLE)

Systemic lupus erythematosus (SLE) is an independent risk factor for atherosclerosis, placing children and adolescents with SLE at great risk for developing cardiovascular sequelae, including myocardial infarction, in adulthood. Dyslipidemia and other traditional cardiac risk factors occur frequently in pediatric SLE and are often under-recognized and under-treated. Two dyslipidemia patterns are evident in pediatric SLE. Active disease is characterized by elevated triglycerides (TG) and low high density lipoprotein (HDL). With SLE treatment HDL and TG often normalize while total cholesterol and low density lipoprotein (LDL) rise. The complex pathophysiology of dyslipidemia in SLE involves cytokines, autoantibodies, disease activity, medications, diet, and physical activity level, as well as other factors. Routine screening for dyslipidemia with fasting lipid profiles is indicated for children and adolescents with SLE. If lipoprotein levels are abnormal, first line therapy involves diet and exercise interventions for a minimum of 6 months. For persistent dyslipidemia, several pharmacologic therapies are available. Hydroxychloroquine, a common treatment for SLE, can improve lipid profiles and should be considered for all patients with SLE. Statins and bile acid sequestrants are typically added first for dyslipidemia, while niacin and fibrates are reserved for refractory disease and optimally prescribed in a multidisciplinary lipid clinic. Future research is needed to further illuminate the mechanisms of dyslipidemia in pediatric SLE with well designed clinical trials to determine the safest and most effective interventions to correct lipid profiles and prevent atherosclerosis (Figs 20.6 and 20.9).

The Atherosclerotic Process in Children

It has become clear that atherosclerotic cardiovascular disease begins in childhood and is progressive. This provides the strongest rationale for aggressive treatment of risk factors in individuals at greater risk for cardiovascular disease at an early age. The earliest pathological abnormality in atherosclerosis is the fatty streak, which is an accumulation of lipid-filled macrophages within the intima of the artery. With increasing age, lipid may continue to accumulate. In response to this lipid accumulation, macrophages and smooth muscle cells proliferate and migrate into the intima and media to form a fibrous plaque lesion. Advanced and complicated fibrous plaques are vulnerable to rupture, which initiates a cascade of events leading to the formation of thrombus. This can lead to occlusion of the artery and subsequent myocardial infarction or stroke. Complications also can occur when there is vascularization of the plaque, which can lead to hemorrhage and swelling within the plaque and occlusion of the arterial lumen. The American Heart Association Committee on Lesions has described the gross and microscopic aspects of the development of atherosclerosis.

Impact on Vascular End Points

Optimally, the screening and management of hyperlipidemia in children should be aimed at making an impact on the atherosclerotic disease process itself, with an aim of preventing cardiovascular morbidity and mortality in adulthood. Although a clinical study spanning childhood through adulthood will likely never be performed, some evidence is now being acquired to suggest an impact on vascular function and structure in children.

A clinical trial of dietary intervention in infancy aimed at altering fat consumption to reduce saturated fat intake (the Special Turku Coronary Risk Factor Intervention Project) evaluated participants at 11 years of age for flow-mediated dilatation as assessed by vascular ultrasound of the brachial artery. The investigators noted greater dilation for boys but not girls in the intervention group relative to the control group, which they attributed to reduced LDL cholesterol levels (Fig. 20.2).

A clinical trial of simvastatin in 50 children with familial hypercholesterolemia was performed by de Jongh and colleagues. After a treatment period of 28 weeks, flow-mediated dilatation as assessed by vascular ultrasound of the brachial artery was noted to have improved to normal levels in the patients treated with 40 mg simvastatin compared with no improvement in the placebo group. Wiegman and colleagues assessed carotid intima-media thickness as part of a clinical trial of pravastatin in children with familial hypercholesterolemia. They noted that those in the placebo group showed progression of intima-media thickness over a 2-year period, whereas those treated with pravastatin demonstrated regression. A further study by Koeijvoets et al in the pravastatin-treated group showed greater intima-media thickness in those children with heterozygous familial hypercholesterolemia who had a null allele for LDL receptor genotype (compared with receptor-defective mutations). The null allele also was associated with higher LDL cholesterol levels. There was a nonsignificant tendency toward less LDL cholesterol lowering in this group also. They concluded that genotyping of patients with familial hypercholesterolemia will identify patients with null alleles who may require more aggressive interventions.

The impact of adjuvant therapies on vascular structure and function also has been explored. Engler and colleagues performed a double-blind randomized crossover trial in 15 children with familial or familial combined hypercholesterolemia, comparing placebo with 500 mg/day vitamin C and 400 U vitamin E given over a 6-week period. Although flow-mediated dilatation as assessed by vascular ultrasound of the brachial artery was similarly reduced at baseline in the diet-only phase and in the placebo phase, it returned toward near normal with intake of the antioxidant vitamins. Nonetheless, it is difficult to make a recommendation for their use because long-term efficacy trials in adults, often with cardiovascular disease or other medical conditions, have not shown benefit.

Engler and colleagues studied 20 hyperlipidemic children in a 6-week crossover clinical trial of docosahexaenoic acid supplementation. Endothelial function as assessed by flow-mediated dilation of the brachial artery was significantly improved while the patients were taking docosahexaenoic acid without affecting biomarkers for oxidative stress, inflammation, or nitric oxide metabolism.

Although not yet studied in children, Engler and colleagues performed a clinical trial in healthy adults of high-flavanoid versus low-flavanoid dark chocolate bars. Those subjects who consumed the high-flavanoid dark chocolate were noted to have improved endothelial function as assessed by brachial artery reactivity. One can imagine the popularity of this therapy in children if proven in a clinical trial.

Although plant sterols have been shown to significantly lower LDL cholesterol levels in hyperlipidemic children, a recent study did not show an impact on endothelial function. De Jongh and colleagues studied 41 children with familial hypercholesterolemia in a crossover clinical trial of a plant sterol spread taken for a 4-week period. Although LDL cholesterol was reduced by a mean of 14%, there was no improvement in flow-mediated dilation of the brachial artery. A similar clinical trial incorporating the plant stanol into low-fat yogurt likewise showed reductions in LDL cholesterol levels without improvement in endothelial function.

These studies give preliminary evidence for an impact on the actual atherosclerotic disease process with treatment of familial hypercholesterolemia in children. Similar studies are required for other types of high-risk lipid abnormalities. Increasingly, these types of indicators will be used as surrogate end-points in clinical trials of atherosclerotic risk reduction therapy in children.

Modifications to the Existing NCEP Guidelines (Table 20.3)

Evidence on drug therapy of high-risk lipid abnormalities, notably familial hypercholesterolemia, in children has been accumulating, showing efficacy and safety similar to those in adults, with some evidence of an impact on the atherosclerotic disease process. The existing guidelines had limitations evident from the time of their publication, which have been magnified by an epidemic of overweight and obesity in children and adolescents, which add an additional risk factor to those youth who may already have a high-risk lipid abnormality. From the above discussion, modifications to the existing guidelines are badly needed and are supported by increased evidence of benefit with availability of effective drugs since the original guidelines were published in 1992.

It should, however, be recognized that the evidence base underlying these recommendations is supported by indirect evidence, evidence extrapolated from studies in adults, studies performed in the setting of familial hypercholesterolemia, and expert consensus. Therefore, these recommendations and their implementation should be the subject of ongoing study and modification. Further refinement of guidelines should incorporate new evidence on multiple risk factor scoring and its association with atherosclerotic pathology. They also should incorporate means to individualize cut points on the basis of gender, race, age, pubertal status, and other potential modulating factors. They should be influenced by further studies on the long-term safety and efficacy of lipid-lowering drug therapy and studies of drug therapy for high-risk conditions and abnormalities other than familial hypercholesterolemia. It must be realized that direct evidence of an impact of interventions during childhood and adolescence on later cardiovascular morbidity and mortality will likely always be lacking. It also must be emphasized that drug therapy should be targeted only toward individuals with high-risk lipid abnormalities or high-risk conditions who have not reached target lipid levels with lifestyle modification and should not be used as a first-line therapy for those whose lipid abnormalities are primarily lifestyle related. Effective lifestyle interventions need to be developed, evaluated, and implemented as the primary modality to reduce overall population risk, to prevent and treat obesity, and to prevent and treat exacerbation of high-risk lipid abnormalities and high-risk conditions.

Dyslipidemia Among Perinatally HIV-Infected Children

Protease inhibitor (PI)-containing regimens have led to improved survival among HIV-infected children. However, adverse effects, including dyslipidemia, may put children at risk for cardiovascular disease.

QUICK QUESTIONS REGARDING DYSLIPIDEMIA IN CHILDREN AND ADOLESCENTS

1. Are there specific lipid abnormalities in children with diabetes?

There are insufficient data available to answer this question. Most reviews speculate that the abnormalities seen in adults with diabetes are also seen in children/adolescents. In children with type 1 diabetes, the pathogenesis of the disease would not suggest the presence of specific lipid abnormalities; however, elevated triglycerides would be expected in patients with poorly controlled blood glucose levels. The Pittsburgh Diabetes Clinic found differences between diabetic patients and their siblings in an HDL subfraction, but other lipid levels were not significantly different.

In children with type 2 diabetes, the patterns seen in adults with type 2 diabetes, i.e. elevated triglycerides, normal to slightly elevated LDL cholesterol levels (with an increase of the small, dense LDL subfraction), and decreased HDL cholesterol levels are also seen. Because severe obesity is associated with the premature onset of type 2 diabetes in adolescence and dyslipidemia is generally found in overweight/obese children, the coexistence of both risk factors should be expected and may contribute to dyslipidemia. Since obesity and dyslipidemia are part of the "metabolic syndrome", as defined by the third report of the National Cholesterol Education Program Adult Treatment Panel (NCEP/ATP III childhood obesity is seen as a risk factor for development of the syndrome in adulthood.

2. Do lipid levels track from childhood to adulthood?

Children and adolescents with high cholesterol levels are more likely than the general population to have high levels when they become adults. In the general population, total cholesterol levels are generally 40 mg/dL higher in adults than in childhood. While most children with high cholesterol levels will also have high levels as adults, some children with high levels will have normal levels as young adults. This is in part related to the dramatic decrease in total cholesterol seen as children progress through puberty. Data from the Bogalusa Heart Study . and the Muscatine study, however, clearly show that cholesterol and other cardiovascular risk factors often persist from childhood to adulthood. For example, the development of obesity in childhood predicts a similarly elevated weight as an adult. The tracking correlation coefficients for dyslipidemia suggest that most but not all children with lipid abnormalities will have them as adults).

3. Does atherosclerosis begin in childhood? Is this related to dyslipidemia?

Autopsy studies demonstrate that aortic and coronary atherosclerosis are commonly seen before age 20 years high serum total cholesterol, LDL cholesterol, very-low-density lipoprotein (VLDL) cholesterol levels, and low HDL cholesterol levels are correlated with the extent of early atherosclerotic lesions in adolescents and young adults. For example, in the Bogalusa studies, antemortum total and LDL cholesterol levels, blood pressure, BMI, and fasting insulin were all positively correlated with aortic and coronary artery fatty streaks and plaques. The Pathobiological Determinants of Atherosclerosis in Youth (PDAY) study reported that LDL cholesterol, severe obesity, and elevated glycohemoglobin levels were significantly correlated with the postmortem diagnosis of coronary atherosclerosis in 15–35-year-olds. In the Muscatine study, increased BMI and blood pressure and decreased HDL correlated with the early development of coronary calcification, considered a marker for atherosclerosis. The prevalence of coronary calcium in adolescents with familial hypercholesterolemia is <25%, and the presence of calcium is more likely in those with the highest BMI.

Identified risk factors contributing to the early onset of CHD in children/adolescents include:

Elevated LDL

Family history of premature (aged <55 years) coronary heart disease, CVD, or peripheral vascular disease

- Smoking
- Hypertension
- HDL < 35 mg/dL

Obesity [≤ 95th percentile weight for height on National Center For Health Statistics (NCHS) growth chart]

- Physical inactivity
- Diabetes.

4. What is the frequency for monitoring lipid levels in children with diabetes?

Monitoring should closely follow recommendations currently made for children in general. That is, lipid levels should be measured initially in children (> 2 years of age) only in the presence of a positive family history (a parental total cholesterol level ≤ 240 mg/dL and/or a cardiovascular event in a parent before age 55 years). The preferred test is the fasting lipid profile. In children with diabetes, we recommend modifications in this protocol based on the type of diabetes and the age of the child.

Type 1 diabetes: In those > 12 years of age (assumed to be pubertal), screening should be done at diagnosis but after glycemic control is achieved and should be repeated every 5 years if the initial screen is normal. In those < 12 years of age (generally prepubertal), in the absence of a parental history of dyslipidemia or early coronary heart disease, there is no clear indication for a screening lipid examination.

Type 2 Diabetes

Children should be screened at diagnosis regardless of age but after glycemic control is achieved. If normal lipid values are obtained, screening should be repeated every 2 years. Optimal lipid levels for children with diabetes are based on a synthesis of current pediatric recommendations and current recommendations for adults with diabetes, which recognize that the presence of diabetes is now considered a coronary heart disease equivalent. Optimal lipid levels for those with diabetes, as defined are in accord with those of the Third Adult Treatment Panel and the American Heart Association (AHA):

- LDL <100 mg/dL
- HDL >35 mg/dL
- Triglycerides < 150 mg/dL.

5. How should elevated lipid levels be treated?

Treatment recommendations, are similar to established pediatric guidelines with modifications in response to the higher CVD risk status of patients with diabetes. For children in general, "borderline" levels of total cholesterol and LDL are defined as 170–199 and 110–129 mg/dL, respectively. "Elevated" levels are >200 mg/dL for total cholesterol and >130 mg/dL for LDL cholesterol. Whereas previous recommendations suggested a progression from AHA step 1 to step 2 diet utilization, more recent recommendations suggest the use of the AHA step 2 diet (dietary cholesterol < 200 mg/day and saturated fat < 7% of total calories) initially upon confirmation of hyperlipidemia. Drug therapy has been recommended in children >10 years of age if, after an adequate trial of dietary therapy, LDL levels remain ≤ 190 mg/dL in those with no CVD risk factors or >160 mg/dL in those with CVD risk factors, such as a positive family history, hypertension, obesity, and diabetes . The goal LDL is <130 mg/dL for children in general and < 100 mg/dL in those with diabetes.

Based on the above considerations, the panel recommends the following for children and adolescents with lipid values greater than the optimal levels, as noted above.

Blood glucose control should be maximized and dietary counseling should be provided. Dietary change has been documented to reduce LDL levels. The use of products such as Benachol margarine and increasing amounts of soluble fiber should be considered as part of the dietary approach. Follow-up fasting lipid profiles should be performed at 3 months and then at 6 months to determine the effects of blood glucose management and dietary change. If treatment goals are achieved, the lipid profile should be repeated yearly. If after 6 months of optimized blood glucose control and dietary intervention, there is no significant improvement in lipid parameters, further intervention is warranted based on LDL levels shown below: LDL 100–129 mg/dL: maximize nonpharmacologic treatment. LDL 130–159 mg/dL: "consider" medication, basing the treatment decision on the child's complete CVD risk profile, including assessment of blood pressure, family history, and smoking status. LDL ≤ 160 mg/dL: begin medication.

Resins (bile acid sequestrants) continue to be generally recommended as first-choice treatments in this age group; however, compliance rates with this class of medications are so low that therapeutic efficacy is lacking. Therefore, statin drugs should also be considered. Despite concerns about using statins in children, there are now trial data indicating efficacy and safety in adolescents. When statins are used, treatment should begin at the lowest available dose and dose increases should be based on LDL levels and side effects. Liver function tests (LFTs) should be monitored and medication should be discontinued if LFTs are greater than three times the upper limit of normal. If there is any persistent complaint of significant muscle pain/muscle soreness, the medication should be discontinued to see if symptoms resolve. Routine monitoring of creatine phosphokinase levels is not felt to be helpful. In addition, the use of statins in sexually active adolescent females must be very carefully considered and the risks explicitly discussed, as these drugs are not approved in pregnancy.

Elevated triglyceride levels are not directly managed with medication. If the tryglyceride level is ≤ 150 mg/dL, one should enhance efforts to maximize blood glucose control and achieve desirable weight. If triglycerides are ≤ 1,000 mg/dL, significantly increased risk of pancreatitis is present, and treatment with a fibric acid medication should be considered.

The cardiovascular risk approach to children with diabetes should be comprehensive. Thus, blood pressure should be regularly measured, anti-tobacco counseling provided, physical activity encouraged, and obesity managed.

6. What additional research needs to be done in this area?

The panel identified a number of critical areas of research:

- Longitudinal tracking of lipid levels in children with type 1 and type 2 diabetes are needed, as well as studies regarding the relationship of glycemic control and exercise to lipid levels.

- Studies are needed on the transition from obesity or insulin resistance to the onset of type 2 diabetes to determine at what point dyslipidemia occurs. Particularly important is an understanding of whether dyslipidemia precedes or is coincident with glucose intolerance.
- Understanding the relationship of noninvasive markers of end organ injury (carotid intimal medial thickening, coronary calcification, flow-mediated vascular resistance, and vascular compliance) to insulin resistance and type 2 diabetes would be helpful.
- The association of hyperlipidemia with other diabetes complications, particularly the development of microalbuminuria, should be addressed.
- The influence of diet on hyperlipidemia and the treatment of obesity (specifically high-versus low-carbohydrate diets) needs clarification.
- The influence of demographic characteristics (e.g. race, gender) on the prognosis of abnormal lipid levels should be studied.

BIBLIOGRAPHY

1. Chen Z, Peto R, Collins R, et al. Serum cholesterol concentration and coronary heart disease in population with low cholesterol concentrations. BMJ 1991;303:276–282.
2. Shepherd J, Cobbe SM, Ford I, et al. Prevention of coronary heart disease with ~ pravastatin in men with hypercholesterolemia. West of Scotland Coronary Prevention Study Group. N Engl J Med 1995;333:1301–1307.
3. Downs JR, Clearfield M, Weis S, et al. Primary prevention of acute coronary events with lovastatin in men and women with average cholesterol levels: results of AFCAPS/TexCAPS. Air Force/Texas Coronary Atherosclerosis Prevention Study. JAMA 1998;279:1615–1622.
4. MRC/BHF Heart Protection Study of cholesterol lowering with simvastatin in 20,536 high-risk individuals: a randomised placebo-controlled trial. Lancet 2002; 360:7–22.
5. Shepherd J, Blauw GJ, Murphy MB, et al. Pravastatin in elderly individuals at risk of vascular disease (PROSPER): a randomised controlled trial. Lancet 2002;360:1623–1630.
6. ALLHAT-LLT investigators. Major outcomes in moderately hypercholes-terolemic, hypertensive patients randomized to pravastatin vs usual care: the Antihypertensive and Lipid-Lowering Treatment to Prevent Heart Attack Trial (ALLHAT-LLT). JAMA 2002;288:2998-3007.
7. Randomised trial of cholesterol lowering in 4444 patients with coronary heart disease: the Scandinavian Simvastatin Survival Study (4S). Lancet 1994;344: 1383–1389.
8. Sacks FM, Pfeffer MA, Moye LA, et al. The effect of pravastatin on coronary events after myocardial infarction in patients with average cholesterol levels. Cholesterol and Recurrent Events Trial investigators. N Engl J Med 1996;335: 1001–1009.
9. Prevention of cardiovascular events and death with pravastatin in patients with coronary heart disease and a broad range of initial cholesterol levels. The Long-Term Intervention with Pravastatin in Ischaemic Disease (LIPID) Study Group. N Engl J Med 1998;339:1349–1357.
10. The effect of aggressive lowering of low-density lipoprotein cholesterol levels and low-dose anticoagulation on obstructive changes in saphenous-vein coronary-artery bypass grafts. The Post-Coronary Artery Bypass Graft Trial Investigators. N Engl J Med 1997;336:153–162.
11. Serruys PW, de Feyter P, Macaya C, et al. Fluvastatin for prevention of cardiac events following successful first percutaneous coronary intervention: a random-ized controlled trial. JAMA 2002;287:3215–3222.
12. Executive Summary of The Third Report of The National Cholesterol Education Program (NCEP) Expert Panel on Detection, Evaluation, And Treatment of High Blood - Cholesterol In Adults (Adult Treatment Panel III). JAMA 2001;285: 2486-2497.
13. Berenson G, Srinivasan S, Bao W, Newman W, Tracy R, Wattigney W, for the Bogalusa Heart Study: Association between multiple cardiovascular risk factors and atherosclerosis in children and young adults. N Engl J Med 338:1650–1656, 1998.
14. Newman W, Freedman D, Voors A, Gard P, Srinivasan S, Cresanta J, Williamson GD, Webber L, Berenson G. Relation of serum lipoprotein levels and systolic blood pressure to early atherosclerosis. N Engl J Med 314:138–144, 1986.
15. Strong J, Malcom G, McMahan CA, Tracy R, Newman W, Herderick E, Cornhill JF, for the Pathobiological Determinants of Atherosclerosis in Youth Research Group (PDAY): Prevalence and extent of atherosclerosis in adolescents and young adults: implications for prevention from the Pathobiological Determinants of Atherosclerosis in Youth Study. JAMA 281:727–735, 1999.
16. Kwiterovich PO Jr: Biochemical, clinical, epidemiologic, genetic, and pathologic data in the pediatric age group relevant to the cholesterol hypothesis. Pediatrics 78:349–362, 1986.
17. Expert Panel on Detection, Evaluation and Treatment of High Blood Cholesterol in Adults: Executive Summary of the Third Report of the National Cholesterol Education Program (NCEP) Expert Panel on Detection, Evaluation, and Treatment of High Blood Cholesterol in Adults (Adult Treatment Panel III). JAMA 285: 2486–2497, 2001.
18. American Diabetes Association: Standards of medical care for patients with diabetes mellitus (Position Statement). Diabetes Care 26:S33–S50, 2003.
19. Orchard T, Forrest KYZ, Kuller L, Becker D: Lipid and blood pressure treatment goals for type 1 diabetes: 10-year incidence data from the Pittsburgh Epidemiology of Diabetes Complication Study. Diabetes Care 24:1053–1059, 2001.
20. Jones KL, Haghi M: Type 2 diabetes mellitus in children and adolescence: a primer. Endocrinologist 10:389–396, 2000.
21. Ludwig DS, Ebbeling CB: Type 2 diabetes mellitus in children: primary care and public health considerations. JAMA 286:1427–1430, 2001.
22. Gidding SS, Leibel RL, Daniels S, Rosenbaum M, Van Horn L, Marx GR: Understanding obesity in youth. Circulation 94:3383–3387, 1996.
23. Reaven GM: Role of insulin resistance in human disease. Diabetes 37:1595–1607, 1988.
24. DeFronzo RA, Ferrannini E: Insulin resistance: a multifaceted syndrome responsible fort NIDDM, obesity, hypertension, and atheroschlotic cardiovascular disease. Diabetes Care 14:173–194, 1992.

25. Arslanian S, Suprasongsin C: Insulin sensitivity, lipids and body composition in childhood: is "syndrome X" present? J Clin Endocrinol Metab 81:1058–1062, 1996.
26. Lauer RM, Clarke WR: Use of cholesterol measurements in childhood for the prediction of adult hypercholesterolemia: the Muscatine Study. JAMA 264:3034–3038, 1990.
27. Orchard T, Donahue R, Kuller L, Hodge P, Drash A: Cholesterol screening in childhood: does it predict adult hypercholesterolemia? The Beaver County experience. J Peds 103:678–691, 1983.
28. Berensen GS, Srinivasan SR, Cresanta JL, Foster TA, Webber LS: Dynamic changes of serum lipoproteins in children during adolescence and sexual maturation. Am J Epidemiol 113:157–170, 1981.
29. McGill H, McMahan A, Zieske A, Malcom G, Tracy R, Strong J, for the Pathobiological Determinants of Atherosclerosis in Youth (PDAY) Research Group: Effects of nonlipid risk factors on atherosclerosis in youth with a favorable lipoprotein profile. Circulation 103:1546–1550, 2001.
30. Gidding S, Chomka E, Bookstein L: Usefulness of electron beam tomography in adolescents and young adults with heterozygous familial hypercholesterolemia. Circulation 98:2580–2583, 1998.
31. Mahoney L, Burns T, Stanford W, Thompson B, Witt J, Rost C, Lauer R: Coronary risk factors measured in childhood and young adult life are associated with coronary artery calcification in young adults: the Muscatine Study. J Am Coll Cardiol 27:277–284, 1996.

21 Atherosclerosis in Children and Adolescents

The atherosclerotic process starts in childhood and studies show its development in fetuses. Clinical manifestation often occurs only in the sixth decade of life. Adolescence is a critical period in the development of atherosclerosis, because fatty streaks may change to transition plaque owing to genetic and environment factors. Healthcare by professionals plays a crucial role in the prevention and treatment of atherosclerosis, identifying poor lifestyle, positive family history of early cardiovascular disease, or other diseases such as dyslipidemia, obesity, arterial hypertension and diabetes. Dyslipidemia in childhood and adolescence should be treating by dietary therapy and change in lifestyle. Children with high-risk lipid abnormalities should be considered for drug treatment.

As has been mentioned earlier the begining of atherosclerotic process takes place from an early childhood and its further progression depends upon many factors such as feeding habits, genetic predisposition, physical activity of the children and prevailing dietary practices. Its diagnosis is very important at an early stage of childhood growth and maturation for the preventon of devastating complications such as premature coronary artery disease and peripheral vasculopathies. Atherosclerosis is a disease of large and medium-sized muscular arteries and is characterized by endothelial dysfunction, vascular inflammation, and the buildup of lipids, cholesterol, calcium, and cellular debris within the intima of the vessel wall. This buildup results in plaque formation, vascular remodeling, acute and chronic luminal obstruction, abnormalities of blood flow, and diminished oxygen supply to target organs.

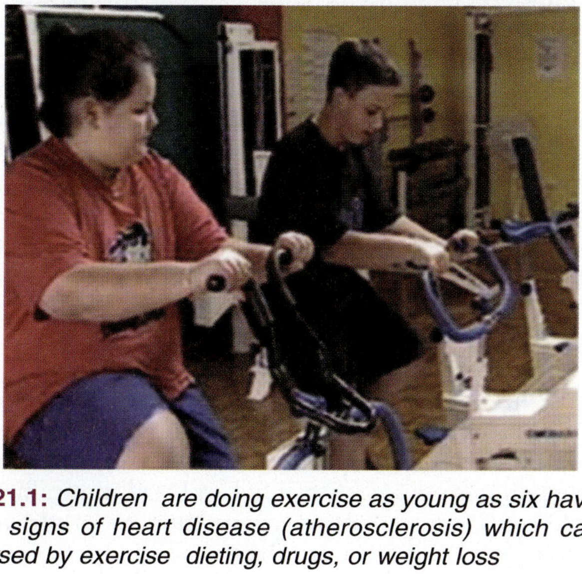

Fig. 21.1: *Children are doing exercise as young as six have the early signs of heart disease (atherosclerosis) which can be reversed by exercise dieting, drugs, or weight loss*

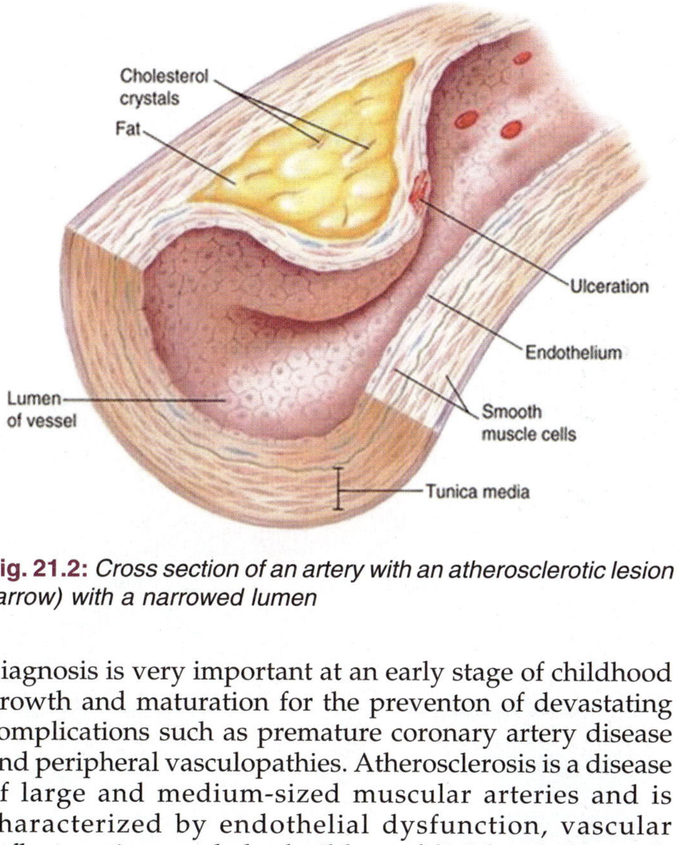

Fig. 21.2: *Cross section of an artery with an atherosclerotic lesion (arrow) with a narrowed lumen*

Pathophysiology: A complex and incompletely understood interaction exists between the critical cellular elements of the atherosclerotic lesion. These cellular elements are endothelial cells, smooth muscle cells, platelets, and

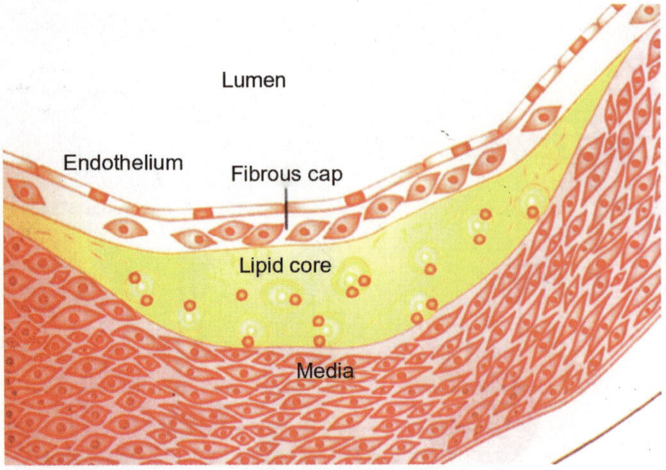

Fig. 21.3: *Lesion in atherosclerosis including development of a fibrous cap that creates a barrier between the lesion and the peripheral blood*

leucocytes. Vasomotor function, the thrombogenicity of the blood vessel wall, the state of activation of the coagulation cascade, the fibrinolytic system, smooth muscle cell migration and proliferation, and cellular inflammation are complex and interrelated biological processes that contribute to atherogenesis and the clinical manifestations of atherosclerosis. The mechanisms of atherogenesis remain uncertain. The "response-to-injury" theory is most widely accepted. Endothelial injury causes vascular inflammation and a fibroproliferative response ensues. Probable causes of endothelial injury include oxidized low-density

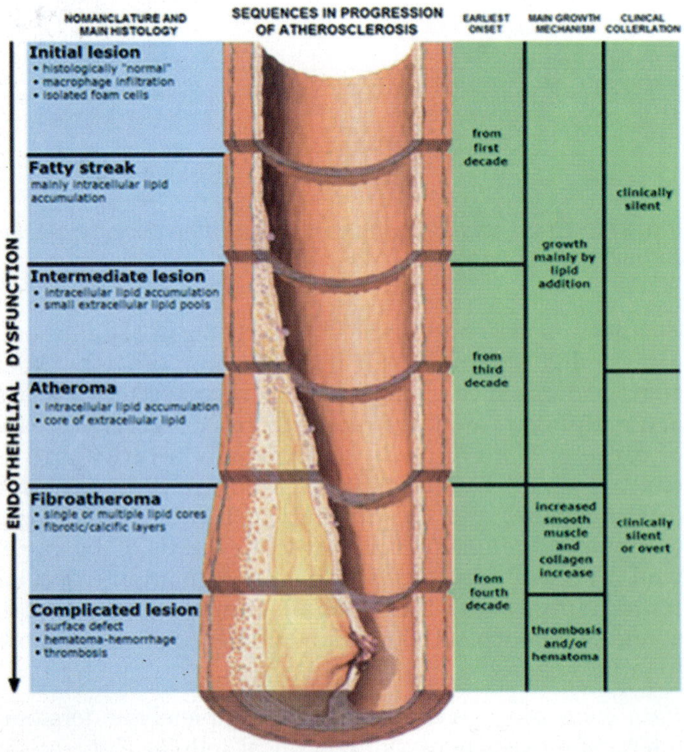

Fig. 21.4: *Demonstrating different stages of endothelial dysfunction in atherosclerosis*

lipoprotein (LDL) cholesterol; infectious agents; toxins, including the byproducts of cigarette smoking; hyperglycemia; and hyperhomocystinemia. Circulating monocytes infiltrate the intima of the vessel wall, and these tissue macrophages act as scavenger cells, taking up LDL cholesterol and forming the characteristic foam cell of early atherosclerosis. These activated macrophages produce numerous factors that are injurious to the endothelium. Elevated serum levels of LDL cholesterol overwhelm the antioxidant properties of the healthy endothelium and result in abnormal endothelial metabolism of this lipid moiety. Oxidized LDL is capable of a wide range of toxic effects and cell/vessel wall dysfunctions that are characteristically and consistently associated with the development of atherosclerosis. These dysfunctions include impaired endothelium-dependent dilation and paradoxical vasoconstriction. These dysfunctions are the result of direct inactivation of nitric oxide by the excess production of free radicals, reduced transcription of nitric oxide synthase messenger RNA (mRNA), and post-transcriptional destabilization of mRNA. The decrease in the availability of nitric oxide also is associated with increased platelet adhesion, increased plasminogen activator inhibitor, decreased plasminogen activator, increased tissue factor, decreased thrombomodulin, and alterations in heparan sulfate proteoglycans. The consequences include a procoagulant milieu and enhanced platelet thrombusformation. Furthermore, oxidized LDL activates inflammatory processes at the level of gene transcription by upregulation of nuclear factor kappa B, expression of adhesion molecules, and recruitment of monocytes/macrophages. The lesions of aterosclerosis do not occur in a random fashion. Hemodynamic factors interact with he activated vascular endothelium. Fluid shear stresses generated by blood flow influence the phenotype of the endothelial cells by modulation of gene expression and regulation of the activity of flow-sensitive proteins. Atherosclerotic plaques characteristically occur in regions of branching and marked curvature at areas of geometric irregularity and where blood undergoes sudden changes in velocity and direction of flow. Decreased shear stress and turbulence may promote atherogenesis at these important sites within the coronary arteries, the major branches of the thoracic and abdominal aorta, and the large conduit vessels of the lower extremities. The earliest pathologic lesion of atherosclerosis is the fatty streak. The fatty streak is observed in the aorta and coronary arteries of most individuals by age 20 years. The fatty streak is the result of focal accumulation of serum lipoproteins within the intima of the vessel wall. Microscopy reveals lipid-laden macrophages, T lymphocytes, and smooth muscle cells in varying proportions. The fatty streak may progress to form a fibrous plaque, the result of progressive lipid accumulation and the migration and proliferation of smooth muscle cells. Platelet-derived growth factor, insulin-like growth factor, transforming growth factorsalpha and beta, thrombin, and angiotensin II are potent mitogens that are produced by activated platelets, macrophages, and dysfunctional

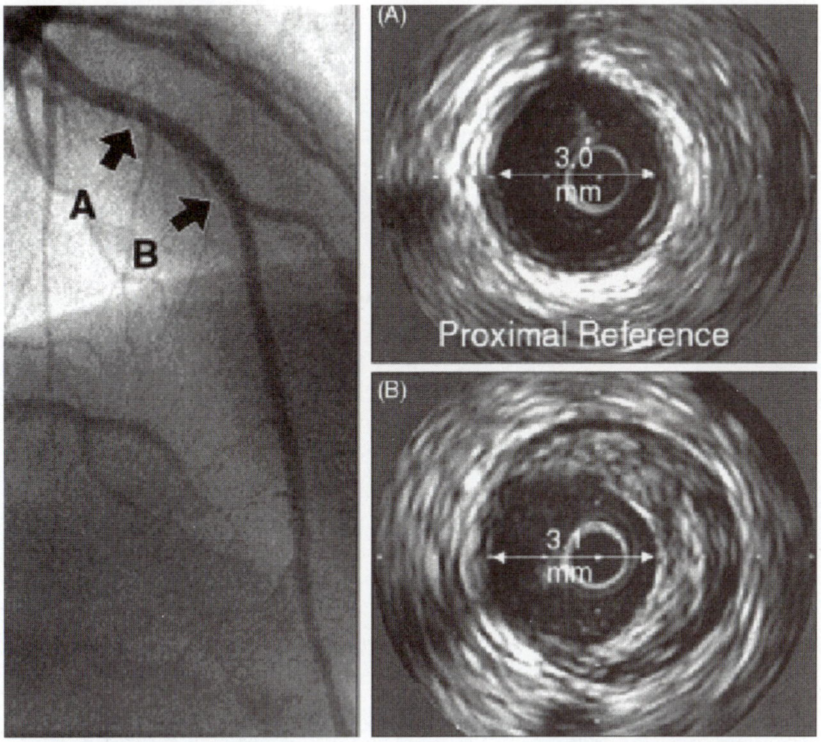

Fig. 21.5: *Angiographic vs. intravascular ultrasound images of coronary atherosclerosis. In the angiogram on the left sections A and B appear indistinguishable, whereas the IVUS images on the right show differing degrees of disease between sections A and B. While both A and B display a similar lumen diameter as a result of remodelling of the arterial wall, it is clear that a substantial crescent-shaped atheroma is present in panel B*

endothelial cells that characterize early atherogenesis, vascular inflammation, and platelet-rich thrombosis at sites of endothelial disruption. The relative deficiency of endothelium-derived nitric oxide further potentiates this proliferative stage of plaque maturation. These smooth muscle cells are responsible for the deposition of extracellular connective tissue matrix and form a fibrous cap that overlies a core of lipid laden foam cells, extracellular lipid, and necrotic cellular debris. Growth of the fibrous plaque results in vascular remodeling, progressive luminal narrowing, blood-flow abnormalities, and compromised oxygen supply to the target organ. Human coronary arteries enlarge in response to plaque formation, and luminal stenosis may only occur once the plaque occupies greater than 40% of the area bounded by the internal elastic lamina. Developing atherosclerotic plaques acquire their own microvascular network called vasa vasorum which are prone to hemorrhage and contribute to progression of atherosclerosis. Denudation of the overlying endothelium or rupture of the protective fibrous cap may result in exposure of the thrombogenic contents of the core of the plaque to the circulating blood. This exposure constitutes an advanced or complicated lesion. The plaque rupture occurs due to weakening of the fibrous cap. Inflammatory cells localize to the shoulder region of the cell proliferation and collagen synthesis. Furthermore, activated macrophages produce matrix metalloproteinases that degrade collagen. These mechanisms explain the predisposition to plaque rupture and highlight the role of inflammation in the genesis of the complications of the fibrous atheromatous plaque. A plaque rupture may result in thrombus formation, partial or complete occlusion of the blood vessel, and progression of the atherosclerotic lesion due to organization of the thrombus and incorporation within the plaque (Figs 21.2 and 21.3).

Incidence

The true frequency of atherosclerosis is difficult, if not impossible, to accurately determine because it is a predominantly asymptomatic condition. The process of atherosclerosis begins in childhood with the development of fatty streaks. These lesions can be found in the aorta shortly after birth and appear in increasing numbers in those aged 8–18 years. More advanced lesions begin to develop when individuals are aged approximately 25 years.

Subsequently, an increasing prevalence of the advanced complicated lesions of atherosclerosis exists, and the organ-specific clinical manifestations of the disease increase with age through the fifth and sixth decades of life. In the United States, approximately 1.5 million myocardial infarctions have chronic coronary artery disease. Of persons older than 50 years, 30% have some evidence of carotid artery disease, and cerebrovascular disease is responsible for over 200,000 deaths per year in developed countries.

The frequency of clinical manifestations of atherosclerosis in Great Britain, west of Scotland in particular, is especially high. The same is true of Finland,

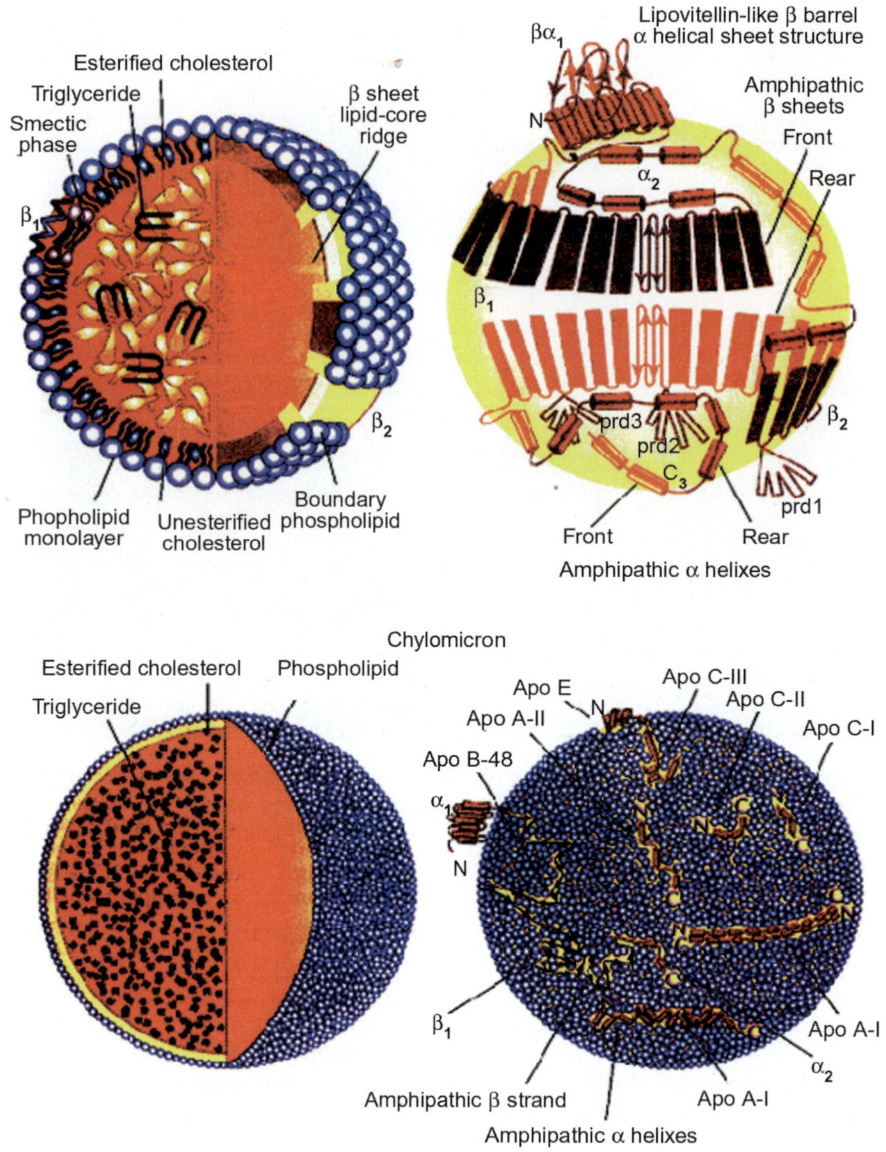

Figs 21.6: *Diagrammatic depiction of ultrastructure of different types of lipid particles responsible for atherosclerotic process in human body*

in particular, and Scandinavia in general. Russia and many of the former states of the Soviet Union have recently experienced an exponential increase in the frequency of coronary heart disease that likely is the result of widespread economic hardship and social upheaval, a high prevalence of cigarette habituation, and a diet high in saturated fats. The frequency of coronary heart disease in the Far East is significantly lower than that documented in the West. Ill-defined genetic reasons for this phenomenon may exist, but significant interest surrounds the role of diet and other environmental factors in the absence of clinical atherosclerotic vascular disease in these populations. The rate of coronary artery disease in ethnic immigrant populations in the United States approaches that of the disease in whites, supporting the role of these putative environmental factors. Atherosclerotic cardiovascular disease is also rare on the African continent, although growing evidence indicates that this too is changing as a result of rapid westernization and urbanization of the traditionally rural and Agrarian African populations.

Mortality/morbidity: Atherosclerosis is the leading cause of death in the developed world, and atherosclerosis is predicted to be the leading cause of death in the developing world within the first quarter of the next century. Atherosclerosis is responsible for more than half of the yearly mortality in the United States, and more than 500,000 people die annually of myocardial infarction alone. This rate of mortality costs the country more than $100 billion a year. More than 50 million people in the United States are candidates for some form of dietary and/or drug treatment to modify their lipid profile. An encouraging decrease in mortality due to coronary heart disease in the developed

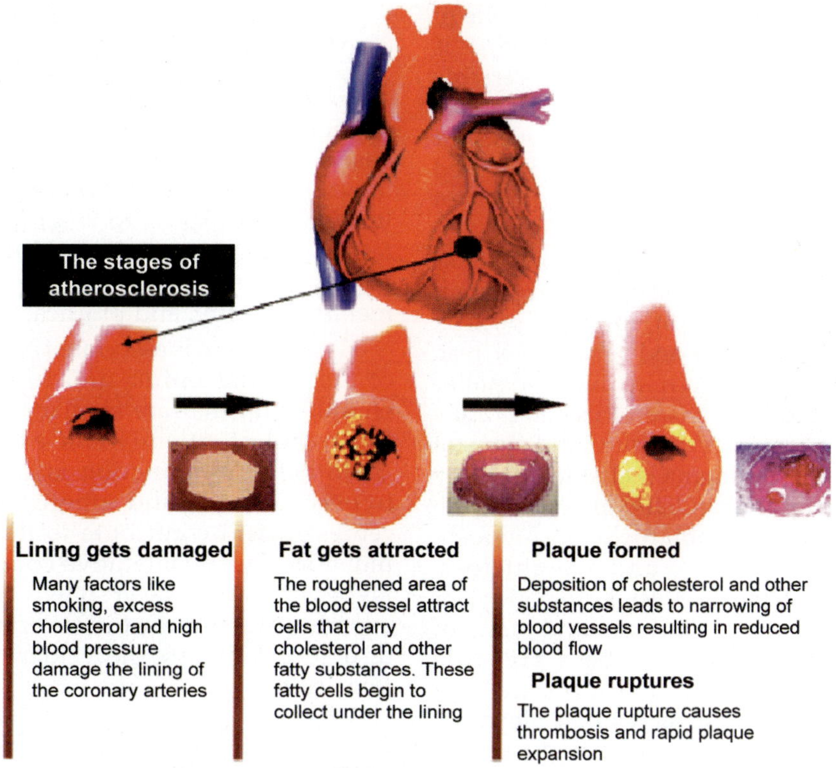

Fig. 21.7: *Different stages of formation of atherosclerosis starting from fatty streaks under the endothelial lining of the affected artery to the rupture of the atherosclerotic plaques and subsequent luminal thrombosis*

world has occurred. Unfortunately, this decrease has not occurred in the developing world, and an exponential increase in tobacco habituation and the adoption of a Western diet high in saturated fats likely predicts the continued increase in death and disability due to coronary heart disease.

Gender Distribution

Atherosclerosis is more common among men than women. The higher prevalence of atherosclerosis in men is thought to be due to the protective effects of the female sex hormones. This sex effect is absent after menopause in women. The incidence of coronary heart disease among women parallels that of men, but women demonstrate an approximately 10-year chronological delay in the onset of clinical manifestations.

Age: Most cases of atherosclerotic vascular disease become clinically apparent in patients aged 40–70 years.

History: The symptoms of atherosclerosis are highly variable. Patients with mild atherosclerosis may present with clinically important symptoms and signs of disease and myocardial infarction, or sudden cardiac death may be the first symptom of coronary heart disease. However, many patients with anatomically advanced disease may have no symptoms and experience no functional impairment. Initially thought to be a chronic, slowly progressive, degenerative disease, it is now apparent that atherosclerosis is a disease with periods of activity and quiescence. Although a systemic disease, atherosclerosis manifests in a focal manner and affects different organ systems in different patients for reasons that remain unclear. Progressive luminal narrowing of an artery due to expansion of a fibrous plaque results in impairment of flow once more than 50–70% of the lumen diameter is obstructed. This impairment in flow results in symptoms of inadequate blood supply to the target organ in the event of increased metabolic activity and oxygen demand. Stable angina pectoris, intermittent claudication, and mesenteric angina are examples of the clinical consequences of this mismatch. Rupture of a plaque or denudation of the endothelium overlying a fibrous plaque may result in exposure of the highly thrombogenic subendothelium and lipid core. This exposure may result in thrombus formation which may partially or completely occlude flow in the involved artery. Unstable angina pectoris, myocardial infarction, transient ischemic attack, and stroke are examples of the clinical sequelae of partial or complete acute occlusion of an artery. Atheroembolism is a distinct clinical entity that may occur spontaneously or as a complication of aortic surgery, angiography, or thrombolytic therapy in patients with advanced and diffuse atherosclerosis. Angina pectoris is characterized by retrosternal chest discomfort that typically radiates to the left arm and may be associated with dyspnea. Angina pectoris is exacerbated by exertion and relieved by rest or nitrate therapy. Unstable angina pectoris describes a pattern of increasing frequency or intensity of episodes of angina pectoris and includes pain at rest. A prolonged episode of angina pectoris that may be associated with diaphoresis is suggestive of myocardial infarction. Stroke, reversible ischemic neurological deficit, and transient ischemic attack are a range of manifestations of impairment of vascular supply to the central nervous system and are characterized by the sudden onset of a focal neurological deficit of variable duration, respectively. Peripheral vascular disease typically manifests as intermittent claudication, impotence, and nonhealing ulceration and infection of the extremities. Intermittent claudication describes calf, thigh, or buttock pain that is exacerbated by exercise and relieved by rest. Intermittent claudication may be accompanied by pallor of the extremity and paresthesias.Visceral ischemia may be occult or symptomatic prior to symptoms and signs of target organ failure. Mesenteric angina is characterized by epigastric or periumbilical postprandial pain and may be associated with hematemesis, hematochezia, melena, diarrhea, nutritional deficiencies, and weight loss. Abdominal aortic aneurysm typically is asymptomatic prior to the dramatic and often fatal symptoms and signs of rupture, although patients may describe a pulsatile abdominal mass. Atheroembolism may present with symptoms of digital necrosis, gastrointestinal bleeding, myocardial infarction, retinal ischemia, cerebral infarction, and renal failure.

Clinical aspects: The physical signs of atherosclerosis provide objective evidence of extracellular lipid deposition, stenosis or dilatation of large muscular arteries, or target organ ischemia or infarction.

Hyperlipidemia: Xanthelasma, tendon xanthomata coronary artery disease—fourth heart sound, tachycardia, hypotension, hypertension.

Cerebrovascular disease: Diminished carotid pulses, carotid artery bruits, focal neurological deficits.

Peripheral vascular disease: Decreased peripheral pulses, peripheral arterial bruits, pallor, peripheral cyanosis, gangrene, ulceration. Abdominal aortic aneurysm—pulsatile abdominal mass, peripheral embolism, circulatory collapse. Atheroembolism—livedo reticularis, gangrene, cyanosis, ulceration (the presence of pedal pulses in the setting of peripheral ischemia suggests microvascular disease and includes cholesterol embolization).

Causes: A number of large epidemiological studies in North America and Europe have identified numerous risk factors for the development and progression of atherosclerosis. The risk factors can be divided into modifiable and nonmodifiable risk factors and include hyperlipidemia, hypertension, cigarette habituation, diabetes mellitus, age, and sex. More recently, a number of novel risk factors have been dentified that add to the predictive value of the established risk factors and may prove to be a target for future medical interventions.

Hyperlipidemia: Hyperlipidemia is an established risk factor for atherosclerosis. Convincing evidence that lowering serum cholesterol reduces the risk of subsequent coronary heart disease events and overall mortality exists.

Hypertension: Hypertension is a risk factor for the development of atherosclerosis, atherosclerotic cardiovascular disease, and stroke. The mechanism by which hypertension causes these effects is not known, and some uncertainty exists as to what the primary and secondary factors are in a typically multifactorial syndrome. These factors may include hyperlipidemia, hypertension, diabetes mellitus, obesity, and physical inactivity.

Hypertension is associated with morphologic alterations of the arterial intima and functional alterations of the endothelium that are similar to the changes observed in hypercholesterolemia and established atherosclerosis. Endothelial dysfunction is a feature of hypertension, hyperlipidemia, and atherosclerosis and is known to represent and contribute to the procoagulant, proinflammatory, and proliferative components of atherogenesis. Hypertension has been shown, in both epidemiologic and experimental studies, to accelerate atherosclerotic vascular disease and increase the incidence of clinical complications (Fig. 21.9).

Diabetes mellitus: An important risk factor for hyperlipidemia and atherosclerosis and commonly associated with hypertension, abnormalities of coagulation, platelet adhesion and aggregation, increased oxidative stress, and functional and anatomic abnormalities of the endothelium and endothelial vasomotion (Fig. 21.9).

Cigarette addiction: A major and modifiable risk factor for atherosclerosis and is associated with an increased relative risk of dying from vascular disease. The mechanisms are complex and likely multifactorial and result in endothelial dysfunction and a relatively hypercoagulable state. This increased relative risk rapidly and significantly is reduced with smoking cessation. The relative risk is reduced to the extent that the incidence of coronary heart disease in people who have recently quit smoking is similar to that of people who have not smoked for at least 2 years.

Biochemical risk factors: The established risk factors noted above successfully predict future cardiac events in about 50–60% of patients. In recent years, a concerted effort to identify and validate new markers of future risk of the clinical consequences of atherosclerosis has been made.

1. *C-reactive protein:* Baseline C-reactive protein (CRP) levels add to the predictive value of lipid parameters in determining the risk of first myocardial infarction in apparently healthy men and women without a history of coronary heart disease. Baseline CRP levels also were found to be predictive of symptomatic peripheral vascular disease in a cohort of healthy men. CRP reflects systemic inflammation, and these results support the hypothesis that chronic inflammation may play a role in the pathogenesis and progression of atherosclerosis.
   Standardization of the CRP assay is required before this test may be clinically useful, and whether this is a truly modifiable risk factor remains unclear. Some early

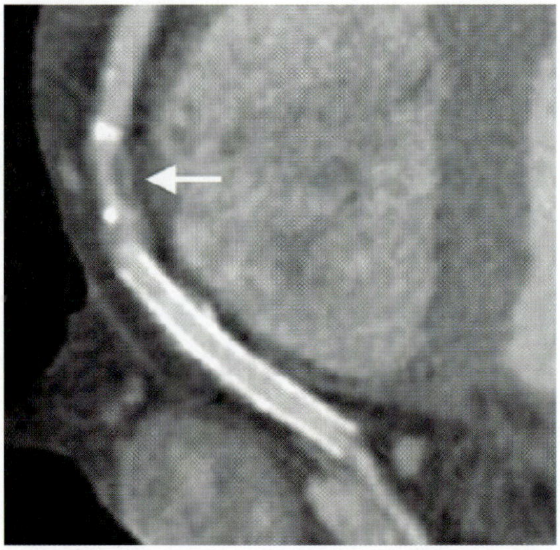

Fig. 21.8: *Contrast-enhanced 16-detector row CT coronary angiography in a patient who has undergone percutaneous transluminal coronary angioplasty with stent placement in right coronary artery (RCA). Colored 3D volume-rendered view from right posterior oblique perspective reveals luminal narrowing (arrow head) of artery proximal to the stent. Maximum intensity projection and multiplanar reformation in oblique coronal planes show patent stent lumen and mixed atherosclerotic lesion (arrow) with calcified and noncalcified components as the cause of high-grade (H 70%) stenosis proximal to the stent*

evidence exists that risk factor modification, particularly the use of aspirin and the hydroxymethylglutaryl coenzyme A (HMG-CoA) reductase inhibitors, may reduce plaque inflammation.

2. *Homocysteine:* Homozygous hyperhomocystinemia is associated with extensive atherosclerosis at an early age. The inherited enzymatic abnormalities of homocysteine metabolism that result in such abnormal levels of the amino acid fortunately are very rare. However, approximately 5–7% of the general population have mild elevations of plasma homocysteine, and recent evidence has confirmed that mild hyperhomocystinemia is an independent risk factor for atherosclerosis. Of the risk for coronary artery disease in the general population, 10% has been estimated as being attributable to homocysteine. Atherogenesis due to hyperhomocystinemia likely is due to oxidative damage to the endothelium followed by platelet activation and thrombus formation. Treatment options for an elevated plasma homocysteine level include folic acid and, possibly, vitamin B_6. A number of clinical trials that will assess the efficacy of this intervention are underway.
3. *Fibrinogen:* Fibrinogen may be elevated in association with risk factors for atherosclerosis including smoking, age, and diet; however, recent evidence suggests that elevated levels of fibrinogen are a strong independent predictor of future cardiovascular events in apparently healthy patients and patients with a prior history of cardiovascular disease. This association may be as strong as the established association between hypercholesterolemia and coronary heart disease.
4. *Lipoprotein (a):* Numerous studies have linked elevated plasma levels of lipoprotein (a), an LDL-like moiety that circulates in the blood attached to apolipoprotein (a), with the development of coronary artery disease. This complex shares structural domains with the fibrinolytic enzyme plasminogen and may render the molecule prothrombotic. The LDL-like moiety is susceptible to oxidation and may be particularly atherogenic. However, the results of prospective studies have been discordant and have not proven the relationship between elevated plasma levels of lipoprotein (a) and coronary artery disease inconclusively. Niacin is known to reduce plasma levels of lipoprotein (a) although whether this truly is a modifiable risk factor remains unclear.

Lab Studies in Dyslipidemias

- ***Lipid profile:*** Elevated LDL cholesterol is a risk factor for atherosclerotic vascular disease. High triglycerides are associated with low high-density lipoprotein (HDL) cholesterol and are a probable risk factor for vascular disease. The National Cholesterol Education Program (NCEP) has issued guidelines for the diagnosis and optimal treatment of hyperlipidemia.
- ***Blood glucose and hemoglobin A1c:*** Routine measurement of blood glucose and hemoglobulin A1c is appropriate in patients with diabetes mellitus. Measuring any number of parameters that may reflect inflammation, coagulation, fibrinolytic status, and platelet aggregability is possible. These measurements may prove to be valuable, but, at this time, how these measurements affect clinical decision-making is unclear, and including them in routine clinical practice is premature.

Imaging Studies (Figs 21.4 to 21.6 and 21.8)

Ultrasonography aids in evaluating brachial artery reactivity and carotid artery intima-media thickness which are measures of vessel wall function and anatomy, respectively. These evaluations remain research techniques at this time but hold promise as reliable noninvasive, and therefore repeatable, measures of disease and surrogate end-points for the evaluation of therapeutic interventions.

Brachial artery reactivity: The loss of endothelium-dependent vasodilation is a feature of even the early stages of atherosclerosis. The availability of high-resolution ultrasonographic systems makes the visualization and measurement of small peripheral conduit vessels, such as the human brachial artery, possible. Flow-mediated dilation of the brachial artery has been pioneered as a means of evaluating the health and integrity of the endothelium. The healthy endothelium dilates in response to an increase in blood flow, whereas vessels affected by atherosclerosis do not dilate and may paradoxically constrict (Fig. 21.12).

Carotid artery intima-media thickness: B-mode ultrasonography of the common and internal carotid arteries is a noninvasive measure of arterial wall anatomy that may be performed repeatedly and reliably in asymptomatic individuals. The combined thickness of the

Table 21.1: *Characteristics of lipid disorders*

Phenotype	*Naked eye appearance*	*Total cholesterol*	*Triglyceride*	*LDL-C*	*HDL-C*	*Electrophoresis*	*Estimated prevalence*	*Mode of inheritance*	*Age of onset*	*Risk of CHO*
Type I	Cream layer, infranted clear or slightly turbid	Normal to moderate elevation	Markedly elevated	Normal	Normal to decreased	Intense band at origin	1×10^5	Recessive	Infancy	None
Type IIa	Clear, possible increased yellow-orange tint	Usually elevated, occasionally within normal range	Normal	Elevated	Normal to decreased	Increased band in β-region	0.1–1%	Dominant	Infancy	60% by age 50 in man 40% by age 50 in women
Familial combined	Clear to slightly turbid	Elevated, occasionally marginally so	Elevated	Elevated	Normal to decreased	Increased β and pre-β band	1.0–1.8%	Apparently dominant	Childhood	Accelerated
Type III	Turbed to opique with thin cream layer occasionally present	Elevated	Elevated	Elevated	Normal to decreased	Broad b-band present	0.1–0.4%	Recessive	Childhood	Heterozygous accelerated; Heterozygous unknown
Type IV	Turtid to opaque	Normal to slightly elevated	Moderate to markedly	Normal	Normal to decreased	Increased pre-β-band	1%	Apparently dominant	Childhood	Controvesial estimates range from no increase to moderate to substan
Type V	Cream layer, infranted turbid to opaque	Slightly to moderately elevated	Marked by elevated	Normal	Normal to decreased	Intense band at origin plus increased	0.1%	Unknown; apparently dominant	Young adulthood	Mild to moderate
Hyperalphalipoproteinemia	Clear	Normal to mode rately to elevated	Normal	Normal	Elevated	Increased α-band	0.8%	Apparently dominant	Infancy	Significantly reduced
Hyperalphalipoproteinemia	Clear	Mild to markedly rately to elevated	Normal	Decreased	Normal	Decreased α-band	0.8%	Apparently dominant	Infancy	Significantly reduced
Hyperalphalipoproteinemia	Clear	Normal decreased, or increased	Normal	Normal	Decreased	Decreased α-band	0.1%	Apparently dominant	Infancy	Increased

intima and media of the carotid artery is associated with the prevalence of cardiovascular risk factors and disease and an increased risk of myocardial infarction and stroke. This association is at least as strong as the associations observed with traditional risk factors (Fig. 21.6).

Medical care: The prevention and treatment of atherosclerosis requires control of the known modifiable risk factors for this disease. This includes the medical treatment of hypertension, hyperlipidemia, diabetes mellitus, and cigarette habituation (Table 20.12).

Hypertension

Hypertension is a risk factor for the development of atherosclerosis, atherosclerotic cardiovascular disease, and stroke. The mechanism by which hypertension causes these effects is not known, and some uncertainty exists as to what the primary and secondary factors are in a typically multifactorial syndrome. These factors may include hyperlipidemia, hypertension, diabetes mellitus, obesity, and physical inactivity.

Dietary and pharmacological treatment of hypertension is associated with a decreased incidence of stroke and, to a lesser degree, atherosclerotic cardiovascular disease.

Hyperlipidemia (Table 21.1)

Convincing evidence that lowering serum cholesterol reduces the risk of subsequent coronary heart disease events and overall mortality exists. The HMG-CoA reductase inhibitors inhibit the rate-limiting step of cholesterol synthesis in the liver. HMG-CoA reductase inhibitors are effective in lowering the serum total cholesterol, LDL cholesterol, and triglyceride levels and in raising the serum HDL cholesterol level, and they have a low incidence of adverse effects, the most common being hepatotoxicity and myopathy. The success of the HMG-CoA reductase inhibitors in reducing circulating lipid levels and improving the clinical and anatomic course of atherosclerosis has focused attention on the management of hyperlipidemia. In addition, an important role remains for other hypolipidemic agents that may be of particular benefit for patients with refractory LDL hypercholesterolemia, hypertriglyceridemia, low HDL cholesterol, and elevated lipoprotein (a).

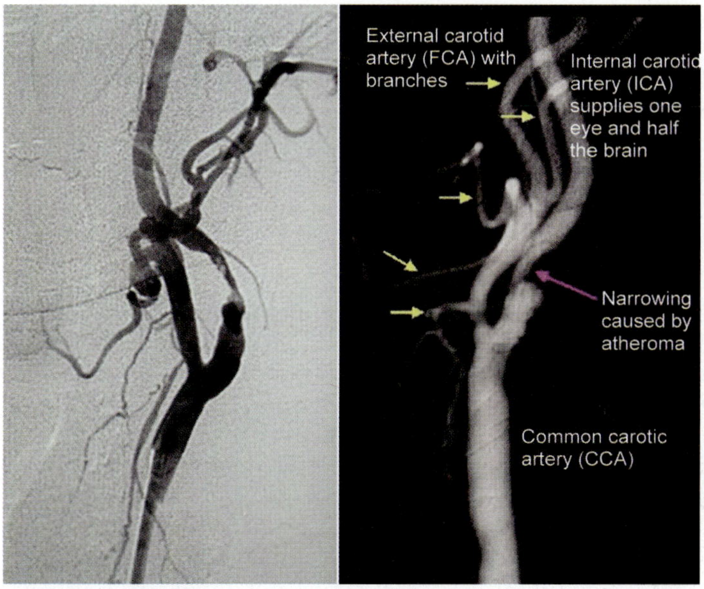

Fig. 21.9: *Formal angiogram and MRI angiograms showing carotid artery narrowing in patient with atherosclerosis (stenosis)*

Secondary Prevention of CAD

The Scandinavian Simvastatin Survival Study (4S) examined the effects of simvastatin on mortality in 4444 patients with established coronary heart disease and elevated total serum cholesterol. A statistically significant 29% reduction in the overall mortality rate (8.2% versus 11.5%) and a 42% reduction in the cardiac mortality rate (5% versus 8.5%) occurred after an average of 5.4 years of follow-up. The cholesterol and recurrent events (CARE) study examined the effects of pravastatin on mortality rates and cardiac events in 1,159 patients with established coronary heart disease and serum cholesterol concentrations that are within the reference range or are mildly elevated. A statistically significant 24% reduction in the incidence of fatal coronary heart disease or nonfatal myocardial infarction (9.9% versus 12.9%) occurred after an average of 5 years of follow-up. A lower total mortality rate (8.6% versus 9.4%) and coronary heart disease mortality rate (4.6% versus 5.7%) occurred in patients receiving pravastatin, although the results were not statistically significant.

The long-term intervention with pravastatin in ischaemic disease (LIPID) trial examined the effects of 40 mg of pravastatin on the incidence of coronary events over a period of 6.1 years in 9,014 patients with known coronary heart disease and a broad range of initial cholesterol levels. The following relative risk reductions occurred: 24% for death from coronary heart disease ($P < 0.001$), 22% for the overall mortality rate ($P < 0.001$), 29% for all cardiovascular outcomes ($P < 0.001$), and 19% for stroke ($P = 0.048$). The effects were similar for all predefined subgroups.

Primary Prevention of Coronary Artery Disease

The West of Scotland Coronary Prevention Study (WOSCOPS) examined the effects of pravastatin on the incidence of nonfatal myocardial infarction and coronary mortality rates in 6,595 men with moderate hypercholesterolemia and no prior history of coronary heart disease. A statistically significant 29% reduction in nonfatal myocardial infarction (4.6% versus 6.5%) and a 30% reduction in death from all cardiovascular causes (1.6% versus 2.3%) occurred after an average of 4.9 years of follow-up. The Air Force/Texas Coronary Atherosclerosis Prevention Study (AFCAPS/TexCAPS) examined the effects of lovastatin on the incidence of a first major coronary event in 5,608 men and 997 women with average total cholesterol and LDL cholesterol and below-average HDL cholesterol levels. A statistically significant 37% reduction in the incidence of the first major coronary event

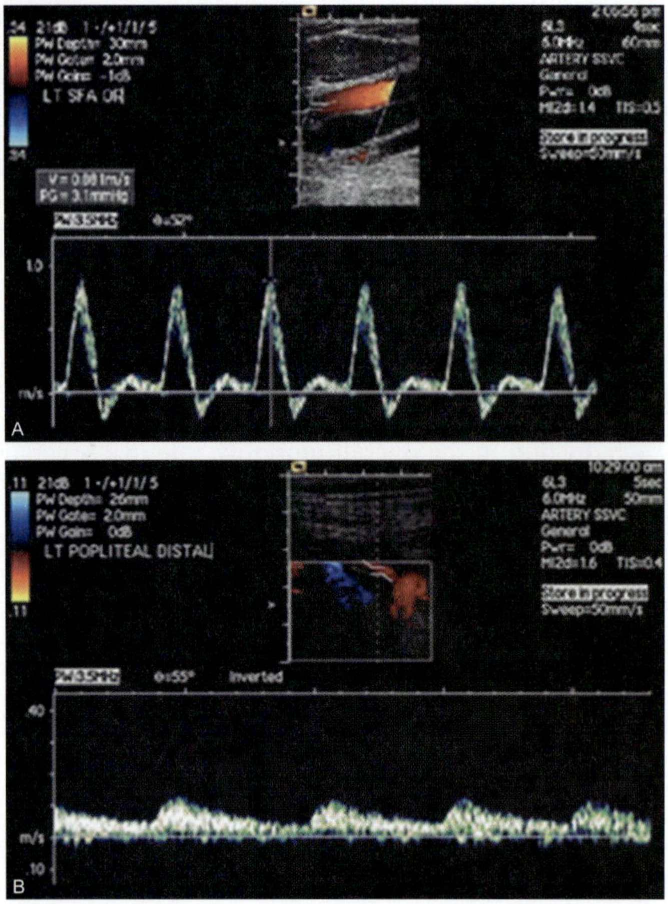

Figs 21.10A and B: *Duplex (vascular) ultrasound images showing a good quality blood flow (A) brachial artery compared to very damped (reduced flow) (B) as evidenced in the "waveforms" at the bottom of each image in a young patient with atherosclerosis*

(4% versus 6.8%) occurred after an average of 5.2 years. Therapy with lipid-lowering agents should be a component of multiple risk factor intervention and only is indicated as an adjunct to diet therapy when the response to a diet restricted in saturated fat and cholesterol has been inadequate. The NCEP guidelines recommend aggressive lipid-lowering therapy for patients at high risk for coronary heart disease. More than 50 million individuals in the United States are candidates for some form of dietary and/ or pharmacological intervention to modify their lipid profile. Pharmacoeconomic studies of implementation of the NCEP guidelines confirm the cost-effectiveness of primary and secondary prevention. Evidence exists that physicians are poorly compliant with these guidelines. For patients with diabetes mellitus, strict control of comorbid risk factors is especially important, and ample evidence exists that this reduces the incidence of the clinical complications of microvascular and macrovascular disease. Cholesterol lowering with the HMG-CoA reductase inhibitors has yielded important reductions in coronary heart disease events in patients with diabetes mellitus. The benefit of strict glycemic control in the prevention of macrovascular disease has been difficult to confirm,

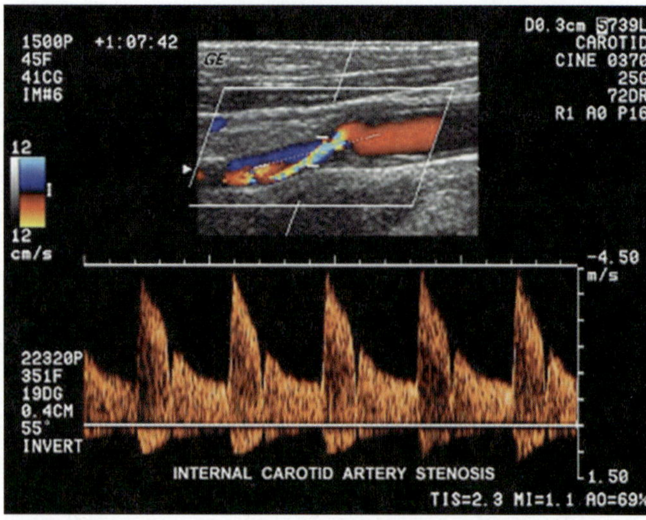

Fig. 21.11: *Vascular ultrasound showing stenosis of internal carotid artery in young person with atherosclerosis*

although this intuitively is beneficial and is known to retard the progression of microvascular disease.

Cigarette Habituation

The risks of cigarette smoking are reduced rapidly and significantly with smoking cessation. The relative risk is so significant that the incidence of coronary heart disease in people who have recently quit smoking is similar to that of people who have not smoked within 2 years.

Diet

The primary treatment of LDL hypercholesterolemia is dietary and includes restriction of caloric intake, saturated fats, and cholesterol. The NCEP and the American Heart Association (AHA) made specific recommendations for dietary therapy for coronary heart disease prevention. The recommended daily intake of nutrients is described by the step I and step II diets and is appropriately tailored to the level of coronary heart disease risk. Moderate alcohol intake is associated with a reduced incidence of coronary heart disease events. The mechanism(s) of this benefit is not well understood. Heavy alcohol intake probably is associated with an increased incidence of coronary heart disease events, as well as cardiomyopathy and arrhythmia and obviously should be discouraged.

Activity: Physical inactivity is a minor modifiable risk factor for coronary heart disease, and regular exercise has been shown to reduce the risk of coronary heart disease in a number of observational epidemiological studies. The mechanisms for this apparent benefit may include an increase in HDL cholesterol and a decrease in body weight, insulin resistance, and blood pressure. The optimal intensity and duration of exercise is not known; however, 20–30 minutes of aerobic exercise of mild-to-moderate intensity (including walking) three times per week probably is appropriate Prevention and treatment of atherosclerosis requires risk factor control, including the medical treatment

Table 21.2: *Guidelines for cardiovascular health promotion in all children and adolescents*

Health promotion goals	*Recommendations*
Diet	
• An overall healthy eating pattern	• Assess diet at every visit
• Appropriate body weight	• Match energy intake with energy needs for normal growth and development
• Desirable lipid profile	• Make appropriate changes to maintain a healthy weight and achieve weight loss when indicated
• Desirable blood pressure	• Advocated consumption of a variety of fruit, vegetables, whole grains, diary products, fish, legumes, poultry, and lean meat. • Fat intake is unrestricted prior to 2 years of age. After age 2, limit foods high in saturated fats (<10% of calories per day) cholesterol (<300 mg per day), and *trans*-fatty acids. • Limit salt intake to <6 g per day • Limit intake of sugar
Smoking	
• No new initiation of cigarette smoking	• Question tobacco use by parents at every visit.
• No exposure to environmental tobacco smoke	• Question tobacco use by children at every visit starting at age 10.
• Complete cessation for those who smoke	• Provide clear, strong, informed, and personalized counseling against initiating of smoking.
Physical activity	
• Be physically active every day	• Assess physical activity at every visit.
• Reduced sedentary time (e.g. television watching, computer, video games, or time on the phone)	• Advise young people to participate in at least 60 minutes of moderate to vigorous physical activity every day • Physical activity should be fun for children and adolescents • For adolescents, resistance training (10–15 repetitions at moderate intensity) can be combined with aerobic activity in an overall activity program • Sedentary time should be limited. For example, limit television time to at most 2 hours per day
Assessment	*Recommendations*
General assessment	
Goals for pediatric care providers	
• Timed, targeted risk factor assessment	• Family history: Update regularity (parents, grandparents, aunts and uncles) with regard to obesity, hypertension dyslipidemia, diabetes, cigratte smoking and cardiovascular disease before age 55 for men and age 65 for women
• Appropriate interpretation of results and communication to families	• Match energy intake with energy needs for normal growth and development
Goals for parents	
• Recognition of risk factor significance for development of cardiovascular disease, especially family history	• Height, weight, BMI: Assess at every examination • Blood pressure: Measure at every examination after age 3 years; chart for age sex/height • Diet and physical activity: Assess at every visit • Cigarette smoking: Evaluate starting at 9–10 years of age.
Specific risk assessment: levels of concern:	
Lipid and Lipoprotein	
• Total cholesterol > 170 mg/dL is borederline; >200 mg/dL is elevated	• Perform targeted screening of fasting lipids in children >2 years of age with a family history of dyslipidemia or premature CVD.
• LDL-C > 110 mg/dL is borderline; > 130 mg/dL is elevated	• For children in whom family history is unknown and other risk factors are present, assess lipid and lipoprotein
• Triglycerides > 150 mg/dL	
• HDL-C <35 mg/dL	• If averaged results of three fasting, lipid profiles are above cut points
Blood pressure	
• Systolic and diastolic blood pressure >90th percentile for age, sex and height	• Known appropriate blood pressure measurement techniques including appropriate cuff size. Interpret blood pressure measurement on the basis of age, sex and height
Body size	
• BMI > 85th percentile is at risk of overweight; 95th percentile is overweight	• Body size should be charted by BMI. • The 95th percentile can be approximated by the age (in years) + 13 for boys and the age (in years) + 14 for girl after age 9 years.

BMI indicates body mass index: CVD, cardiovascular disease; HDL-C, high-density lipoprotein cholesterol, and LDL-C, low-density lipoprotein cholesterol.

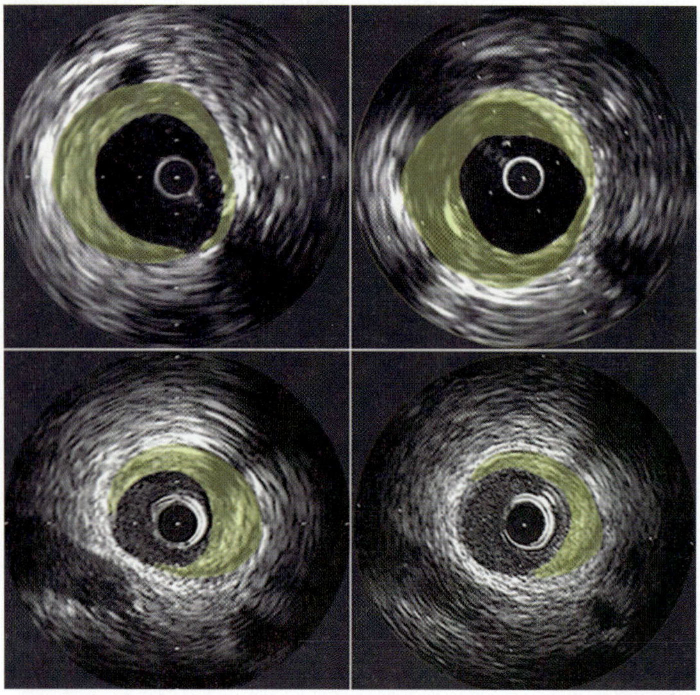

Fig. 21.12: *Representative cross-sectional IVUS images demonstrating plaque progression (top panels) and regression (bottom panels) at matched sites that were studied at baseline (left panels) and follow-up (right panels)*

of hypertension, diabetes mellitus, and cigarette habituation. Advances in the understanding of the vascular biology of atherosclerosis raises the possibility of novel therapies that may address more directly the various aspects of endothelial dysfunction and the role of endothelial dysfunction in atherogenesis. Potential cellular targets include vascular smooth muscle cells, monocyte/macrophage cell lines, platelets and endothelial cells. Evidence exists that antiplatelet agents, antioxidant therapies, amino acid supplementation, angiotensin-converting enzyme inhibitors, and angiotensin receptor blockers may prove to prevent or slow the progression of the disease.

Antiatherosclerotic Pharmacology

HMG-CoA reductase inhibitors: These agents are competitive inhibitors of 3-hydroxy-3-methyl Co-A reductase, an enzyme that catalyzes the rate-limiting step in cholesterol biosynthesis, resulting in upregulation of LDL receptors in response to the decrease in intracellular cholesterol. The HMG-CoA reductase inhibitors are indicated for the secondary prevention of cardiovascular events and for the treatment of hypercholesterolemia and mixed dyslipidemia. A number of HMG-CoA reductase inhibitors are indicated for patients with homozygous familial hypercholesterolemia as an adjunct to other lipid-lowering treatments. However, these agents may be less effective in patients with rare homozygous familial hypercholesterolemia, possibly because these patients are lacking functional LDL receptors, making it more likely to raise serum transaminases.

Pravastatin (pravachol): Effective in reducing circulating lipid levels and improving the clinical and anatomic course of atherosclerosis.

Adult dose: 10–40 mg/d PO hours.

Simvastatin (Zocor): Inhibits cholesterol synthesis and increases cholesterol metabolism.

Adult dose: 5–80 mg/d PO hours.

Lovastatin (Mevacor, altocor): Adjunct to dietary therapy in reducing serum cholesterol. Immediate-release (mevacor) and extended-release (altocor) are available.

Adult dose: Immediate-release: 10–80 mg/d PO qd or divided bid. Sustained-release: 10–20 mg PO hs initially; may increase dose q4wk, not to exceed 60 mg/d.

Fluvastatin (lescol): Used as an adjunct to dietary therapy in decreasing cholesterol levels.

Adult dose: 20–80 mg/d PO qd or divided bid.

Contraindications: Documented hypersensitivity; active liver disease; unexplained elevations in liver function tests; pregnancy; breastfeeding.

Interactions: Toxicity increases when co-administered with triazole antifungals, CNS depressants, macrolide antibiotics, mibefradil, immunosuppressive agents, gemfibrozil and niacin; coadministration with warfarin may increase PT; rifampin, nicotinic acid, bile acid sequestrants, and propranolol may decrease effects.

Precautions: May elevate creatine kinase and transaminase levels; photosensitivity may occur with prolonged exposure to sunlight or tanning equipment.

Atorvastatin (lipitor): Adjunct to dietary therapy in reducing serum cholesterol.

Adult dose: 10 mg PO qd; titrate to maximum 80 mg/d.

Rosuvastatin (Crestor): HMG-CoA reductase inhibitor that in turn decreases cholesterol synthesis and increases cholesterol metabolism. Reduces total-C, LDL-C, and TG levels and increases.

HDL-C level: Used adjunctively with diet and exercise to treat hypercholesterolemia.

Adult dose 5–10 mg PO qd initially; may increase dose if needed, not to exceed 40 mg/d; for marked hypercholesterolemia (i.e. LDL-C >190 mg/dL), initiate with 20 mg/d PO.

Fibric acid derivatives: The precise mechanism of action of this class of drugs is complex and incompletely understood. They increase the activity of lipoprotein lipase and enhance the catabolism of triglyceride-rich lipoproteins which is responsible for an increase in the HDL cholesterol fraction. A decrease in hepatic very low-density lipoprotein (VLDL) synthesis and an increase in cholesterol excretion into bile also appear to occur. The fibrates typically reduce triglyceride levels by 20–50% and increase HDL cholesterol levels by 10–15%. The effect on LDL cholesterol is variable. Levels may be expected to decrease by 10–15%. In patients with marked hypertriglyceridemia, LDL cholesterol levels may increase which likely reflects the ability of the LDL receptor to clear the increased LDL generated by increased VLDL catabolism. Fibrate therapy may also be responsible for a decrease in the clotting ability of platelets and fibrinogen levels which may account for some of the reported clinical benefits. These agents can enhance the synthesis of lipoprotein lipase which can cause triglycerides and very low density lipoprotein levels to decrease.

Fenofibrate (tricor): Adjunct to dietary therapy in treating hyperlipidemias associated with hypertriglyceridemia including type IV and type V. Not proven to be of use in prevention of coronary rtery disease.

Adult dose: 67 mg/d PO.

Gemfibrozil (lopid): Adjunct to dietary therapy in adult patients with type IV and V hyperlipidemias presenting at risk for pancreatitis. Adjunctive therapy in coronary heart disease prevention in patients with type IIb hyperlipidemia (low HDL, elevated LDL and triglycerides) not responding to other agents or diet modifications.

Adult dose: 1,200 mg/d PO divided bid 30 min before breakfast and dinner.

Bile acid sequestrants: The bile acid sequestrants block enterohepatic circulation of bile acids and increase the fecal loss of cholesterol. This results in a decrease in intrahepatic levels of cholesterol. The liver compensates by up-regulating hepatocyte LDL receptor activity. The net effect is a 10–25% reduction in LDL cholesterol, but no consistent effect on triglycerides or HDL cholesterol exists.

Cholestyramine (questran, locholest, prevalite): May use as adjunct in primary hypercholesterolemia. Forms a nonabsorbable complex with bile acids in the intestine, which, in turn, inhibits enterohepatic reuptake of intestinal bile salts.

Adult dose: 4–24 g PO divided bid; not to exceed 24 g/d or 6 doses per d.

Pediatric dose: Not established; suggested dosing is 240 mg/kg/d PO divided bid/tid; not to exceed 8 g/d.

Colestipol (Colestid): Forms a soluble complex after binding to bile acid, increasing fecal loss of bile acid-bound LDL cholesterol.

Adult dose: Granules: 5–30 g/d PO qd or divided bid mixed with liquid.

Antioxidants: Epidemiologic studies have demonstrated an association between increased intakes of antioxidant vitamins, including vitamins C, E, and beta-carotene, and reduced mortality from coronary artery disease. Antioxidants are thought to reduce the oxidation of LDL cholesterol, inhibit lipid accumulation in the arterial wall, and improve endothelial function; however, the results have been inconclusive, and the oxidative modification hypothesis of atherosclerosis has been called into question. Some evidence exists that beta-carotene may, in fact, be deleterious. Dietary supplementation in smokers was evaluated in 2 trials that revealed an increased incidence of lung cancer with a nonsignificant decrease in the incidence of coronary mortality in patients who received beta-carotene. The recently published results of the Heart Outcomes Prevention Evaluation (HOPE) Study and the Gruppo Italiano per lo Studio della Streptochinasi nell'Infarto Miocardico (GISSI) have not provided evidence-based proof of the efficacy or benefit of vitamin E supplementation. Specifically, in patients at high risk of coronary heart disease, treatment with 400 IU or 300 IU of vitamin E respectively for more than 3.5 years had no apparent effect on cardiovascular outcomes. The American College of Cardiology (ACC) and the AHA assign a IIb recommendation to vitamins C and E (IIb recommendation designates conditions for which conflicting evidence or a divergence of opinion about the usefulness/efficacy of a procedure or treatment exists) for the treatment of chronic stable angina pectoris. A statement for healthcare professionals from the AHA concludes that, "The most prudent and scientifically supportable recommendation for the general population is to consume a balanced diet with emphasis on antioxidant-rich fruits and vegetables and whole grains.

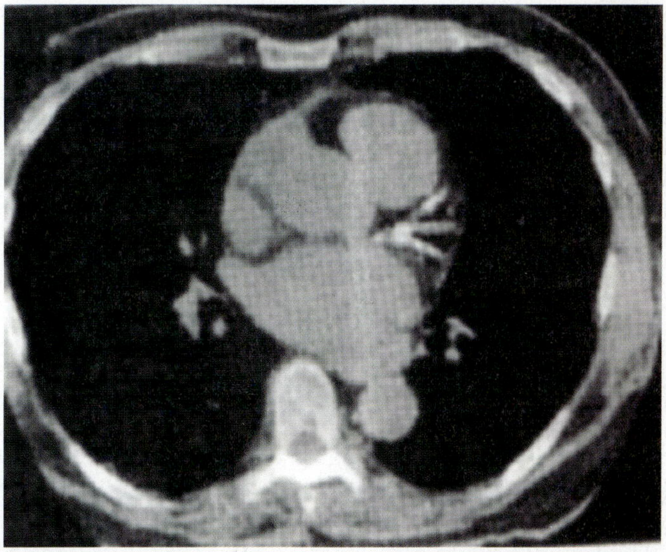

Fig. 21.13: *EBCT shows three-vessels disease involving (LAD,RCA,circumflex) alongwith calcification incorporating CACS=530 in a 20 years asymptomatic old patient with family H/O of premature CAD disease*

Vitamin E (vita-plus E, softgels, aquasol E): Protects polyunsaturated fatty acids in membranes from attack by free radicals.

Adult dose: 60–75 IU/d PO/IM; study doses for the prevention of coronary artery disease have ranged from 400–800 IU/d PO.

Nicotinic acid derivatives: Niacin (vitamin B_3) inhibits the hepatic secretion of VLDL cholesterol. Niacin is effective in most categories of hyperlipidemia. Niacin has been demonstrated to lower LDL cholesterol and triglyceride levels by 32% and 20–50%, respectively, and to raise the HDL cholesterol level by 43%. Niacin lowers lipoprotein (a) levels, which may be of some clinical importance because lipoprotein(a) levels have been associated with coronary heart disease in numerous epidemiological studies. The clinical benefit of lowering lipoprotein(a) levels has not been determined.

Niacin (niaspan, niacor, slo-niacin): Used in tissue respiration, lipid metabolism, and glycogenolysis. Available in immediate- and extended-release formulations. Extended-release formulation may reduce flushing, an unpleasant adverse effect that causes 30–40% of patients to discontinue therapy.

Adult dose: 2–6 g/d PO with food divided tid.

Prognosis

The prognosis of atherosclerosis depends on a number of factors including systemic burden of disease, the vascular bed(s) involved, and the degree of flow limitation. Wide variability exists, and clinicians appreciate that many patients with critical limitation of flow to vital organs may survive many years, despite a heavy burden of disease. Conversely, myocardial infarction or sudden cardiac death may be the first clinical manifestation of atherosclerotic cardiovascular disease in a patient who is otherwise asymptomatic with minimal luminal stenosis and a light burden of disease. Much of this phenotypic variability is likely to be determined by the relative stability of the vascular plaque burden. Plaque rupture and exposure of the thrombogenic lipid core are critical events in the expression of this disease process and determine the prognosis. The ability to determine and quantify risk and prognosis in patients with atherosclerosis is limited by the inability to objectively measure plaque stability and other predictors of clinical events.

Patient Education

The most effective and probably the most cost-efficient means of reducing the burden of disease secondary to atherosclerosis in the general population is primary prevention. The role of diet and exercise in the prevention of atherosclerotic cardiovascular disease has been well established. Education of the general population regarding healthy dietary habits and regular exercise will reduce the prevalence of multiple coronary heart disease risk factors. Medical therapies aimed at improving blood pressure control and various lipid parameters are appropriate for the prevention of first coronary heart disease events if these risk factors are refractory to lifestyle interventions.

Medical/Legal Pitfalls

As previously noted, clinical sequelae of atherosclerosis are hard to predict because of the nonlinear rate of progression of this systemic disease. Address the underlying causes of atherosclerosis in an attempt to slow this process and stabilize the existing plaque burden. Failure to do so results in predictable clinical events in the same or other vascular beds, and this is a common cause of medical/legal error. For example, a patient with limb claudication can be assumed to have significant atherosclerotic plaque burden in multiple vascular beds, including the coronary and cerebral vessels. In evaluating preoperative risk in such a patient, pay particular attention to careful risk stratification and medical or interventional efforts to reduce this risk.

Special Concerns

Familial Hypercholesterolemia

Familial hypercholesterolemia is an autosomal dominant disorder caused by a defect in the gene for the hepatic LDL receptor. In the United States, heterozygous familial hypercholesterolemia occurs in approximately 1 in 500 individuals and typically results in symptomatic coronary heart disease by the fifth decade of life in men and sixth decade of life in women. In the United States, homozygous familial hypercholesterolemia occurs in approximately 1 in 1 million individuals, and total cholesterol may exceed 1,000 mg/dL and result in symptomatic coronary heart disease by the second decade of life. Treatment options include combination drug therapy, although drug therapy alone often is inadequate because of the relative or absolute deficiency of hepatic LDL receptors. Lipid apheresis is an effective means of reducing circulating lipid levels and coronary heart disease events. Liver transplantation has been performed on young patients with severe disease and patients experiencing very early onset of symptomatic coronary artery disease.

BIBLIOGRAPHY

1. Anderson TJ: Assessment and treatment of endothelial dysfunction in humans. J Am Coll Cardiol 1999 Sep; 34(3): 631–8.
2. Arbustini E, Dal Bello B, Morbini P: Plaque erosion is a major substrate for coronary thrombosis in acute myocardial infarction. Heart 1999 Sep; 82(3): 269–72.
3. Burke AP, Farb A, Malcom GT: Coronary risk factors and plaque morphology in men with coronary disease who died suddenly. N Engl J Med 1997 May 1; 336(18): 1276–82.
4. Davies MJ: Stability and instability: two faces of coronary atherosclerosis. The Paul Dudley White Lecture 1995. Circulation 1996 Oct 15; 94(8): 2013–20.
5. Davies MJ: The pathophysiology of acute coronary syndromes. Heart 2000 Mar; 83(3): 361–6.
6. Denke MA, Grundy SM: Dyslipoproteinemias/atherosclerosis: dietary therapy, In: Smith T, ed. Cardiovascular Therapeutics. Philadelphia, Pa: WB Saunders; 1996: 385–402.
7. Diaz MN, Frei B, Vita JA: Antioxidants and atherosclerotic heart disease. N Engl J Med 1997 Aug 7; 337(6): 408–16.
8. Downs JR, Clearfield M, Weis S: Primary prevention of acute coronary events with lovastatin in men and women with average cholesterol levels: results of AFCAPS/TexCAPS. Air Force/Texas Coronary Atherosclerosis Prevention Study. JAMA 1998 May 27; 279(20): 1615–22.
9. Farmer JA, Gotto AM: Dyslipidemia and other risk factors for coronary artery disease. In: Braunwald ed. Heart Disease: A Textbook of Cardiovascular Medicine. 5th ed. Philadelphia, Pa: WB Saunders; 1997: 1126–60.
10. Fuster V: Lewis A. Conner Memorial Lecture. Mechanisms leading to myocardial infarction: insights from studies of vascular biology. Circulation 1994 Oct; 90(4): 2126–46.
11. Gaziano JM: Epidemiology of risk-factor reduction. In: Loscalzo J, Creager MA, Dzau VJ, eds. Vascular Medicine. Boston, Mass: Little, Brown; 1996: 569–586.

12. Gibbons RJ, Chatterjee K, Daley J: ACC/AHA/ACP-ASIM guidelines for the management of patients with chronic stable angina: a report of the American College of Cardiology/American Heart Association Task Force on Practice Guidelines (Committee on Management of Patients With Chronic Stable. J Am Coll Cardiol 1999 Jun; 33(7): 2092–197.
13. Gimbrone MA Jr, Nagel T, Topper JN: Biomechanical activation: an emerging paradigm in endothelial adhesion biology. J Clin Invest 1997 Dec 1; 100 (11 Suppl): S61-5 GISSI: Dietary supplementation with n-3 polyunsaturated fatty acids and vitamin E after myocardial infarction: results of the GISSI-Prevenzione trial. Gruppo Italiano per lo Studio della Sopravvivenza nell'Infarto miocardico. Lancet 1999 Aug 7; 354(9177): 447–55.
14. Glagov S, Weisenberg E, Zarins CK: Compensatory enlargement of human atherosclerotic coronary arteries. N Engl J Med 1987 May 28; 316(22): 1371–5.
15. Haffner SM, Alexander CM, Cook TJ: Reduced coronary events in simvastatin-treated patients with coronary heart disease and diabetes or impaired fasting glucose levels: subgroup analyses in the Scandinavian Simvastatin Survival Study. Arch Intern Med 1999 Dec 13-27; 159(22): 2661–7.
16. Hiro T, Fujii T, Yoshitake S: Longitudinal visualization of spontaneous coronary plaque rupture by 3D intravascular ultrasound. Circulation 2000 Mar 28; 101(12): E114–5.
17. Kannel WB: Contributions of the Framingham Study to the conquest of coronary artery disease. Am J Cardiol 1988 Nov 15; 62(16): 1109–12.
18. Kolodgie FD, Gold HK, Burke AP, et al: Intraplaque hemorrhage and progression of coronary atheroma. N Engl J Med 2003 Dec 11; 349(24): 2316–25.
19. Labarthe DR: Cardiovascular diseases: a global public health challenge. In: Labarthe DR, ed. Epidemiology and Prevention of Cardiovascular Diseases. Gaithersburg, Md: Aspen Publishers, Inc; 1998: 3–16.
20. Lees RS, Cashin-Hemphill L, Lees AM: Non-pharmacological lowering of low-density lipoprotein by apheresis and surgical techniques. Curr Opin Lipidol 1999 Dec; 10(6): 575–9.
21. Levine GN, Keaney JF Jr, Vita JA: Cholesterol reduction in cardiovascular disease. Clinical benefits and possible mechanisms. N Engl J Med 1995 Feb 23; 332(8): 512–21.
22. Libby P: Atherosclerosis. In: Fauci A, et al, eds. Harrison's Principles of Internal Medicine. 14th ed. New York, NY: McGraw-Hill, Inc; 1998: 1345–1352.
23. Libby P: Molecular bases of the acute coronary syndromes. Circulation 1995 Jun 1; 91(11): 2844-50hanging concepts of atherogenesis. J Intern Med 2000 Mar; 247(3): 349–58.
24. Long-Term Intervention with Pravastatin in Ischaemic Disease Study Group: Prevention of cardiovascular events and death with pravastatin in patients with coronary heart disease and a broad range of initial cholesterol levels. The Long-Term Intervention with Pravastatin in Ischaemic Disease (LIPID) Study Group. N Engl J Med 1998 Nov 5; 339(19): 1349–57.
25. Multiple Risk Factor Intervention Trial Research Group: Relationship between baseline risk factors and coronary heart disease and total mortality in the Multiple Risk Factor Intervention Trial. Multiple Risk Factor Intervention Trial Research Group. Prev Med 1986 May; 15(3): 254–73.
26. National Cholesterol Education Program: Summary of the second report of the National Cholesterol Education Program (NCEP) Expert Panel on Detection, Evaluation, and Treatment of High Blood Cholesterol in Adults (Adult Treatment Panel II). JAMA 1993 Jun 16; 269(23): 3015–23.
27. Pate RR, Pratt M, Blair SN: Physical activity and public health. A recommendation from the Centers for Disease Control and Prevention and the American College of Sports Medicine. JAMA 1995 Feb 1; 273(5): 402–7.
28. Ridker P, Libby P: Nontraditional coronary risk factors and vascular biology: the frontiers of preventive cardiology. J Investig Med 1998 Oct; 46(8): 338–50.
29. Ridker PM: Evaluating novel cardiovascular risk factors: can we better predict heart attacks? Ann Intern Med 1999 Jun 1; 130(11): 933–7.
30. Ridker PM, Hennekens CH, Buring JE: C-reactive protein and other markers of inflammation in the prediction of cardiovascular disease in women. N Engl J Med 2000 Mar 23; 342(12): 836–43.
31. Ross R: The pathogenesis of atherosclerosis. In: Braunwald E, ed. Heart Disease: A Textbook of Cardiovascular Medicine. Philadelphia, Pa: WB Saunders; 1997: 1105–1125.
32. Ross R: The pathogenesis of atherosclerosis: a perspective for the 1990s. Nature 1993 Apr 29; 362(6423):801–9.
33. Rosss R: Atherosclerosis: an inflammatory disease. N Engl J Med 1999 Jan 14; 340(2): 115–26.
34. Rubins HB, Robins SJ, Collins D: Gemfibrozil for the secondary prevention of coronary heart disease in men with low levels of high-density lipoprotein cholesterol. Veterans Affairs High-Density Lipoprotein Cholesterol Intervention Trial Study Group. N Engl J Med 1999 Aug 5; 341(6): 410–8.
35. Sacks FM, Pfeffer MA, Moye LA: The effect of pravastatin on coronary events after myocardial infarction in patients with average cholesterol levels. Cholesterol and Recurrent Events Trial investigators. N Engl J Med 1996 Oct 3; 335(14): 1001–9.
36. Salonen JT, Salonen R: Ultrasound B-mode imaging in observational studies of atherosclerotic progression. Circulation 1993 Mar; 87(3 Suppl): II56–65.
37. Scandinavian Simvastatin Survival Study: Randomised trial of cholesterol lowering in 4444 patients with coronary heart disease: the Scandinavian Simvastatin Survival Study (4S). Lancet 1994 Nov 19; 344(8934): 1383–9.
38. Selwyn AP, Kinlay S, Libby P: Atherogenic lipids, vascular dysfunction, and clinical signs of ischemic heart disease. Circulation 1997 Jan 7; 95(1): 5–7.
39. Shepherd J, Cobbe SM, Ford I: Prevention of coronary heart disease with pravastatin in men with hypercholesterolemia. West of Scotland Coronary Prevention Study Group. N Engl J Med 1995 Nov 16; 333(20): 1301–7.
40. Stary HC, Chandler AB, Dinsmore RE: A definition of advanced types of atherosclerotic lesions and a histological classification of atherosclerosis. A report from the Committee on Vascular Lesions of the Council on Arteriosclerosis, American Heart Association. Circulation 1995 Sep 1; 92(5): 1355–74.
41. Topper JN, Gimbrone MA Jr: Blood flow and vascular gene expression: fluid shear stress as a modulator of endothelial phenotype. Mol Med Today 1999 Jan; 5(1): 40–6.
42. Tribble DL: AHA Science Advisory. Antioxidant consumption and risk of coronary heart disease: emphasis

on vitamin C, vitamin E, and beta-carotene: A statement for healthcare professionals from the American Heart Association. Circulation 1999 Feb 2; 99(4): 591–5.
43. Tunstall-Pedoe H, Kuulasmaa K, Amouyel P: Myocardial infarction and coronary deaths in the World Health Organization MONICA Project. Registration procedures, event rates, and case-fatality rates in 38 populations from 21 countries in four continents. Circulation 1994 Jul; 90(1): 583–612.
44. Uehata A, Lieberman EH, Gerhard MD: Noninvasive assessment of endothelium-dependent flow-mediated dilation of the brachial artery. Vasc Med 1997; 2(2): 87–92.
45. Weissberg PL: Atherogenesis: current understanding of the causes of atheroma. Heart 2000 Feb; 83(2): 247–52.
46. Yusuf S, Dagenais G, Pogue J: Vitamin E supplementation and cardiovascular events in high-risk patients. The Heart Outcomes Prevention Evaluation Study Investigators. N Engl J Med 2000 Jan;342(3): 145–53.

22 Hypertension in Children and Adolescents

The development of a national database on normal blood pressure levels throughout childhood has contributed to the recognition of elevated blood pressure in children and adolescents. The epidemic of childhood obesity, the risk of developing left ventricular hypertrophy, and evidence of the early development of atherosclerosis in children would make the detection of and intervention in childhood hypertension important to reduce long-term health risks; however, supporting data are lacking. Secondary hypertension is more common in preadolescent children, with most cases caused by renal disease. Primary or essential hypertension is more common in adolescents and has multiple risk factors including obesity and a family history of hypertension. Evaluation involves a thorough history and physical examination, laboratory tests, and specialized studies. Management is multifaceted. Nonpharmacologic treatments include weight reduction, exercise, and dietary modifications. Recommendations for pharmacologic treatment are based on symptomatic hypertension, evidence of endorgan damage, stage 2 hypertension, stage 1 hypertension unresponsive to lifestyle modifications, and hypertension with diabetes mellitus.

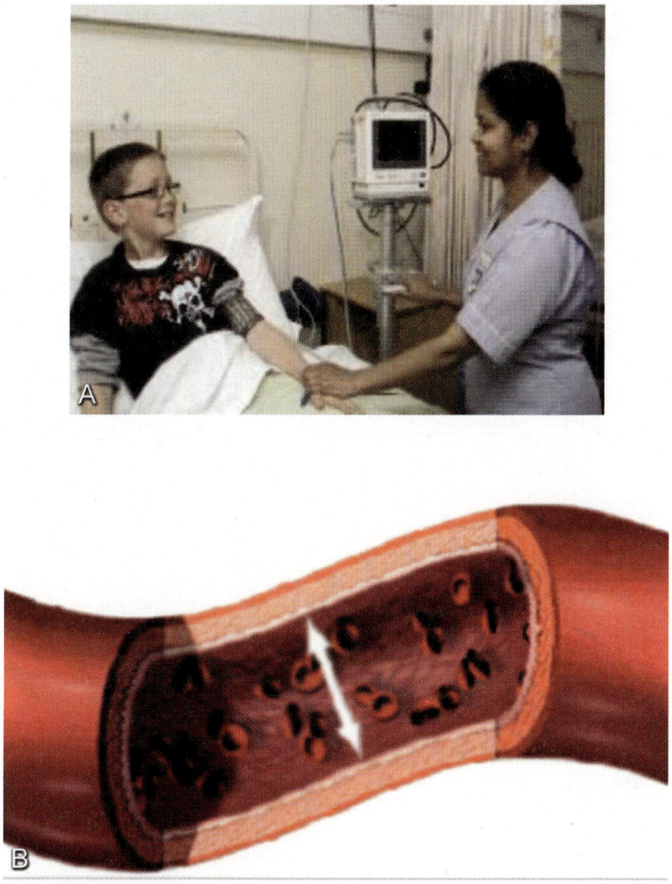

Figs. 22.1A and B: *(A) Measurement of blood pressure of a child admitted in the hospital by the nurse. (B) Diagram explaining exertion of systolic and diastolic forces on the arterial wall which is measured as systolic and diastolic pressures in human beings*

Hypertension is one of the leading causes of cardiovascular mortality and morbidity in the developed countries of the world but its higher incidence with all its complications is also seen in India in both adult and child population. The main reasons of hypertension in children and adolescents are sedentary habits, less knowledge of

Table 22.1: *Causes of childhood hypertension according to age group*

Age	*Causes*
1–6	Renal parenchymal disease; renal vascular disease; endocrine causes; coarctation of the aorta; essential hypertension
6–12 years	Renal parenchymal disease; essential hypertension; renal vascular disease; endocrine causes; coarctation of the aorta; iatrogenic illness
12–18 years	Essential hypertension; iatrogenic illness; renal parenchymal disease; renal vascular disease; endocrine causes; coarctation of the aorta

dietary practices, lack of exercise and genetic predisposition. Arterial blood pressure may be defined as measurement of the pulsating driving force produced by the heart to push the blood through the arteries. Blood pressure which is influenced by the sympathetic nervous system, is dependent on

a. Cardiac output
b. Elasticity of the walls of the arteries
c. Resistance to blood flow through the blood vessels
d. Volume and viscosity of the blood.

Considerable advances have been made in detection, evaluation, and management of high blood pressure (BP), or hypertension, in children and adolescents. Because of the development of a large national database on normative BP levels throughout childhood, the ability to identify children who have abnormally elevated BP has improved. On the basis of developing evidence, it is now apparent that primary hypertension is detectable in the young and occurs commonly. The long-term health risks for hypertensive children and adolescents can be substantial; therefore, it is important that clinical measures be taken to reduce these risks and optimize health outcomes.

The purpose of this report is to update clinicians on the latest scientific evidence regarding BP in children and to provide recommendations for diagnosis, evaluation, and treatment of hypertension based on available evidence and consensus expert opinion of the working group when evidence was lacking. This publication is the fourth report from the National High Blood Pressure Education Program (NHBPEP) Working Group on Children and Adolescents and updates the previous 1996 publication, "update on the 1987 Task Force Report on High Blood Pressure in Children and Adolescents".

This report includes the following information:

- New data from the 1999–2000 National Health and Nutrition Examination Survey (NHANES) have been added to the childhood BP database, and the BP data have been reexamined. The revised BP tables now include the 50th, 90th, 95th, and 99th percentiles by gender, age, and height (Tables 22.1 to 22.3).
- Hypertension in children and adolescents continues to be defined as systolic BP (SBP) and/or diastolic BP (DBP), that is, on repeated measurement, 95th percentile. BP between the 90th and the 95th percentile in childhood had been designated "high normal". To be consistent with the Seventh Report of the Joint National Committee on the Prevention, Detection, Evaluation, and Treatment of High Blood Pressure (JNC 7), this level of BP will now be termed "prehypertensive" and is an indication for lifestyle modifications.
- The evidence of early target-organ damage in children and adolescents with hypertension is evaluated, and the rationale for early identification and treatment is provided.

Table 22.2: *Classification of hypertension in the young by age group*

Age group	*High normal* (90–94th percentile), mmHg	*Significant hypertension* (95–99th percentile), mmHg	*Severe hypertension* (>99th percentile) mmHg
Newborns (SSP)			
7 days	—	96–105	>106
8–30 days		104–109	>110
Infants (<2 years)			
SBP	104–111	112–117	>118
DBP	70–73	74–81	>82
Children			
3–5 years			
SBP	108–115	116–123	>124
DBP	70–75	76–83	>84
6–9 years			
SBP	114–121	122–129	>130
DBP	74–77	78–85	>86
10–12 years			
SBP	122–125	126–133	>134
DBP	78–81	82–89	>90
13–15 years			
SBP	130–135	136–143	>144
DBP	80–85	86–91	>92
Adolescents (16–18 years)			
SBP	136–141	142–149	>150
DBP	84–91	92–97	>98

Table 22.3: *Circumstances under which children <3-years-old should have BP measured*

History of prematurity, very low birth weight, or other neonatal complication requiring intensive care
Congenital heart disease (repaired or nonrepaired)
Recurrent urinary tract infections, hematuria, or proteinuria
Known renal disease or urologic malformations
Family history of congenital renal disease
Solid-organ transplant
Malignancy or bone marrow transplant
Treatment with drugs known to raise BP
Other systemic illnesses associated with hypertension (neurofibromatosis, tuberous sclerosis, etc.)
Evidence of elevated intracranial pressure

- Based on recent studies, revised recommendations for use of antihypertensive drug therapy are provided.
- Treatment recommendations include updated evaluation of nonpharmacologic therapies to reduce additional cardiovascular risk factors. Information is included on the identification of hypertensive children who need additional evaluation for sleep disorders.

Definition of Hypertension

- Hypertension is defined as average SBP and/or diastolic BP (DBP) that is 95th percentile for gender, age, and height on three occasions.
- Prehypertension in children is defined as average SBP or DBP levels that are 90th percentile but <95th percentile.
- The definition of hypertension in children and adolescents is based on the normative distribution of BP in healthy children. Normal BP is defined as SBP and DBP that are <90th percentile for gender, age and height. Hypertension is defined as average SBP or DBP that is 95th percentile for gender, age, and height on at least three separate occasions. Average SBP or DBP levels that are 90th percentile but <95th percentile had been designated as "high normal" and were considered to be an indication of heightened risk for developing hypertension. This designation is consistent with the description of prehypertension in adults. The JNC 7 committee now defines prehypertension as a BP level that is 120/80 mmHg and recommends the application of preventive health-related behaviors, or therapeutic lifestyle changes, for individuals having SBP levels that exceed 120 mmHg[2]. It is now recommended that, as with adults, children and adolescents with BP levels 120/80 mmHg but <95th percentile should be considered prehypertensive.
- The term white-coat hypertension defines a clinical condition in which the patient has BP levels that are >95th percentile when measured in a physician's office or clinic, whereas the patient's average BP is <90th percentile outside of a clinical setting.

Measurement of BP in Children

Children >3 years old who are seen in a medical setting should have their BP measured. The preferred method of BP measurement is auscultation. Correct measurement requires a cuff that is appropriate to the size of the child's upper arm (Figs 22.1, 22.3, 22.4 and 22.12).

- Elevated BP must be confirmed on repeated visits before characterizing a child as having hypertension.
- Measures obtained by oscillometric devices that exceed the 90th percentile should be repeated by auscultation.

Children >3 years old who are seen in medical care settings should have their BP measured at least once during every healthcare episode. Children <3 years old should have their BP measured in special circumstances.

The BP tables are based on auscultatory measurements; therefore, the preferred method of measurement is auscultation. The oscillometric devices are convenient and minimize observer error, but they do not provide measures that are identical to auscultation. To confirm hypertension, the BP in children should be measured with a standard clinical sphygmomanometer, using a stethoscope placed over the brachial artery pulse, proximal and medial to the cubital fossa, and below the bottom edge of the cuff (i.e. 2 cm above the cubital fossa). The use of the bell of the stethoscope may allow softer Korotkoff sounds to be heard better. The use of an appropriately sized cuff may preclude the placement of the stethoscope in this precise location, but there is little evidence that significant inaccuracy is introduced, either if the head of the stethoscope is slightly out of position or if there is contact between the cuff and the stethoscope. Preparation of the child for standard measurement can affect the BP level just as much as technique. Ideally, the child whose BP is to be measured should have avoided stimulant drugs or foods, have been sitting quietly for 5 minutes, and seated with his or her back supported, feet on the floor and right arm supported, cubital fossa at heart level. The right arm is preferred in

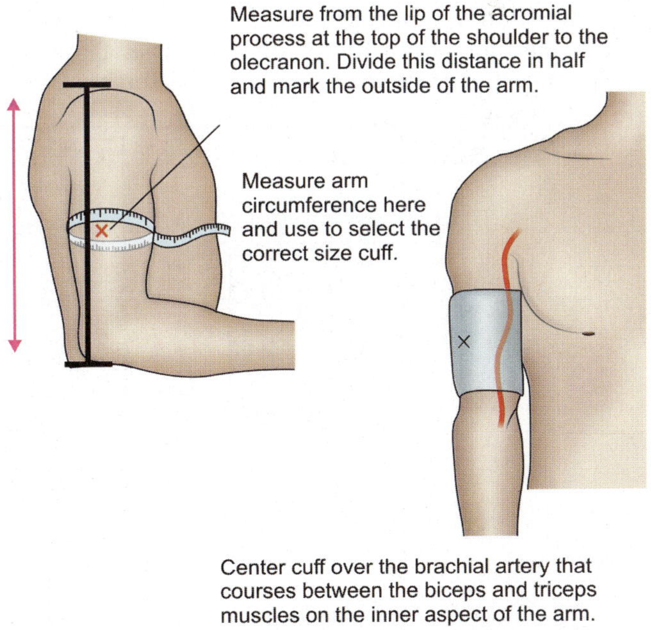

Fig. 22.2: *Measurement of arm circumference and for choosing accurate cuff size in the measurement of blood pressure in the upper arm*

Table 22.4: *Recommended dimensions for BP cuff bladders*

Age range	*Width (cm)*	*Length (cm)*	*Maximum arm circumference (cm)*
Newborn	4	8	10
Infant	6	12	15
Child	9	18	22
Small adult	10	24	26
Adult	13	30	34
Large adult	16	38	44
Thigh	20	42	52

Table 22.5: *Situations in which automated noninvasive ambulatory blood pressure monitoring devices may be useful*

1. "Office" or "white-coat" hypertension; blood pressure repeatedlyelevated in office setting but repeatedly normal out of office
2. Evaluation of drug resistance
3. Evaluation of nocturnal blood pressure changes
4. Episodic hypertension
5. Hypotensive symptoms associated with antihypertensive medications or autonomic dysfunction
6. Carotid sinus syncope and pacemaker syndromes

repeated measures of BP for consistency and comparison with standard tables and because of the possibility of coarctation of the aorta, which might lead to false (low) readings in the left arm. Correct measurement of BP in children requires use of a cuff that is appropriate to the size of the child's upper right arm. The equipment necessary to measure BP in children, ages 3 through adolescence, includes child cuffs of different sizes and must also include a standard adult cuff, a large adult cuff, and a thigh cuff. The latter 2 cuffs may be needed for use in adolescents.

By convention, an appropriate cuff size is a cuff with an inflatable bladder width that is at least 40% of the arm circumference at a point midway between the olecranon and the acromion (see for such a cuff to be optimal for an arm, the cuff bladder length should cover 80–100% of the circumference of the arm. Such a requirement demands that the bladder width-to-length ratio be at least 1:2. Not all commercially available cuffs are manufactured with this ratio. Additionally, cuffs labeled for certain age populations (e.g. infant or child cuffs) are constructed with widely disparate dimensions. Accordingly, the working group recommends that standard cuff dimensions for children be adopted (Tables 22.4 to 22.6, Figs 22.3 and 22.4).

BP measurements are overestimated to a greater degree with a cuff that is too small than they are underestimated by a cuff that is too large. If a cuff is too small, the next largest cuff should be used, even if it appears large. If the appropriate cuffs are used, the cuff-size effect is obviated.

SBP is determined by the onset of the "tapping" Korotkoff sounds (K1). Population data in children and risk-associated epidemiologic data in adults have established the fifth Korotkoff sound (K5), or the disappearance of Korotkoff sounds, as the definition of DBP. In some children, Korotkoff sounds can be heard to 0 mmHg. Under these circumstances, the BP measurement should be repeated with less pressure on the head of the stethoscope. Only if the very low K5 persists should K4 (muffling of the sounds) be recorded as the DBP.

The standard device for BP measurements has been the mercury manometer. Because of its environmental toxicity, mercury has been increasingly removed from healthcare settings. Aneroid manometers are quite accurate when calibrated on a semiannual basis and are recommended when mercury-column devices cannot be obtained.

Auscultation remains the recommended method of BP measurement in children under most circumstances. Oscillometric devices measure mean arterial BP and then calculate systolic and diastolic values. The algorithms used by companies are proprietary and differ from company to company and device to device. These devices can yield results that vary widely when one is compared with

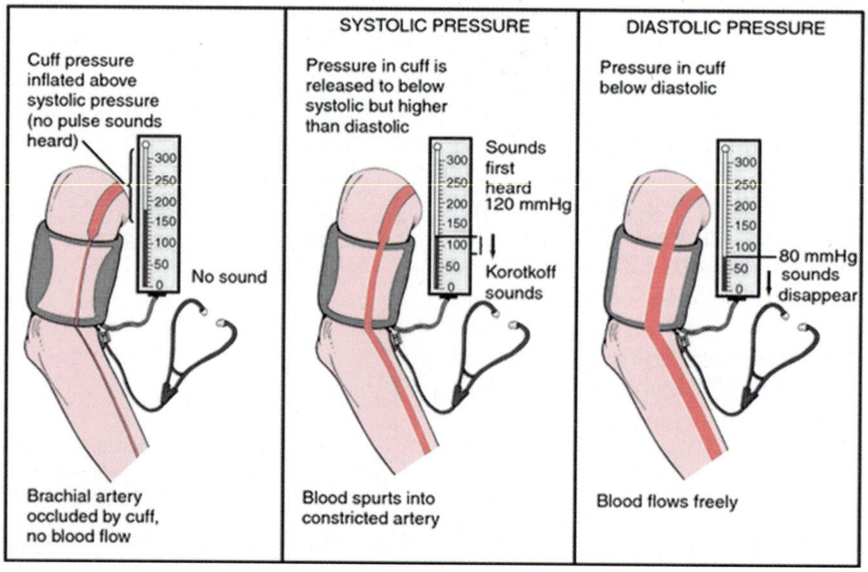

Fig. 22.3: *Technique of measuring systolic and diastolic blood pressure*

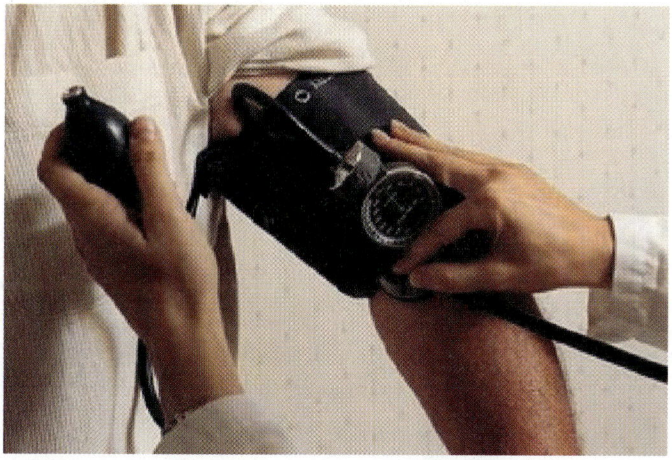

Fig. 22.4: *Measurement of blood pressure by the doctor with aneroid meter type of arm clock*

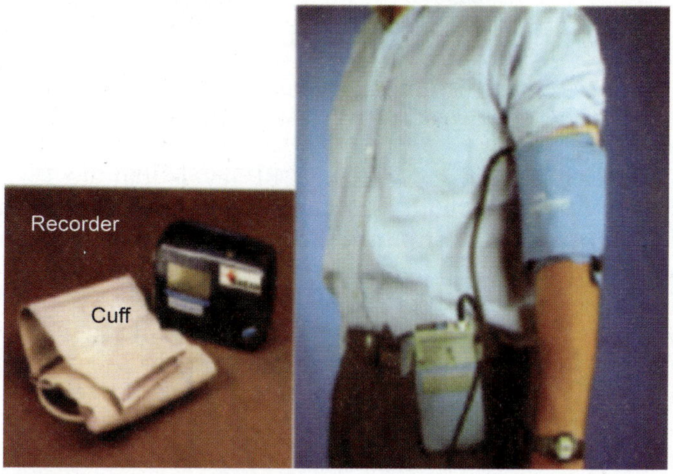

Fig. 22.5: *ABPM instrument fitted in the arm of the patient under investigation*

another, and they do not always closely match BP values obtained by auscultation. Oscillometric devices must be validated on a regular basis. Protocols for validation have been developed,but the validation process is very difficult.

Two advantages of automatic devices are their ease of use and the minimization of observer bias or digit preference. Use of the automated devices is preferred for BP measurement in newborns and young infants, in whom auscultation is difficult, and in the intensive care setting, in which frequent BP measurement is needed. An elevated BP reading obtained with an oscillometric device should be repeated by using auscultation.

Elevated BP must be confirmed on repeated visits before characterizing a child as having hypertension. Confirming an elevated BP measurement is important, because BP at high levels tends to fall on subsequent measurement as the result of (1) an accommodation effect (reduction of anxiety by the patient from one visit to the next) and (2) regression to the mean. BP level is not static but varies even under standard resting conditions. Therefore, except in the presence of severe hypertension, a more precise characterization of a person's BP level is an average of multiple BP measurements taken over weeks to months.

Ambulatory BP Monitoring (ABPM)

ABPM refers to a procedure in which a portable BP device, worn by the patient, records BP over a specified period, usually 24 hours. ABPM is very useful in the evaluation of hypertension in children. By frequent measurement and recording of BP, ABPM enables computation of the mean BP during the day, night, and over 24 hours as well as various measures to determine the degree to which BP exceeds the upper limit of normal over a given time period, i.e., the BP load. ABPM is especially helpful in the evaluation of white-coat hypertension as well as the risk for hypertensive organ injury, apparent drug resistance, and hypotensive symptoms with antihypertensive drugs. ABPM is also useful for evaluating patients for whom more information on BP patterns is needed, such as those with episodic hypertension, chronic kidney disease, diabetes, and autonomic dysfunction. Conducting ABPM requires specific equipment and trained staff. Therefore, ABPM in children and adolescents should be used by experts in the field of pediatric hypertension who are experienced in its use and interpretation (Table 22.5, Figs 22.6–22.10)

Talbe 22.6: *Key recommendations for practice*

Clinical recommendations	*Evidence rating*
Blood pressure should be checked routinely at every visit in children 3 years of age and older	C
Three separate readings of an elevated blood pressure (greater than 90th percentile for age, height, and sex) on separate visits are needed to make the diagnosis of hypertension.	C
Patients diagnosed with primary hypertension should have a comprehensive assessment for cardiovascular risk factors (lipid profile, fasting glucose, body mass index)	C
Non-pharmacologic treatment (e.g. weight loss, dietary modifications, exercise) should be first-line therapy in patients with stage 1 hypertension	C
Pharmacologic treatment should be initiated in patients with stage 2 hypertension, symptomatic hypertension, when end-organ damaged is present (left ventricular hypertrophy, proteinuria); and in stage 1 hypertension when blood pressure is unresponsive to lifestyle changes.	C

C = consensus, disease-oriented evidence, usual practice, expert opinion, or case series. For information about the SORT evidence rating system.

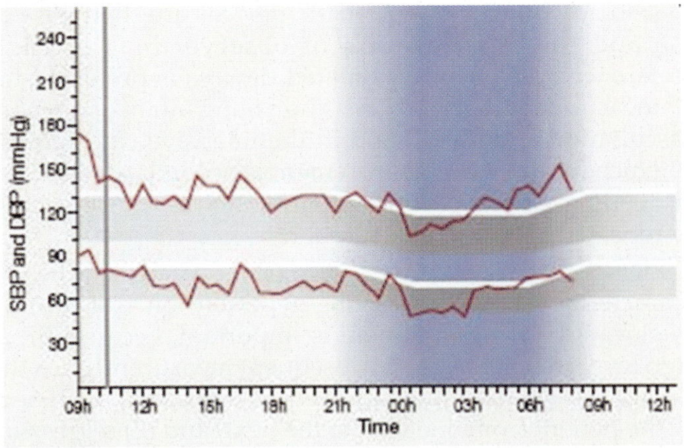

Fig. 22.6: *ABPM suggests white-coat hypertension (175 mmHg/ 95 mmHg) with otherwise normal 24-hour systolic blood pressure (133 mmHg day-time, 119 mmHg night-time) and optimal 24-hour diastolic blood pressure (71 mmHg day-time, 59 mmHg night-time). Normal dipping pattern*

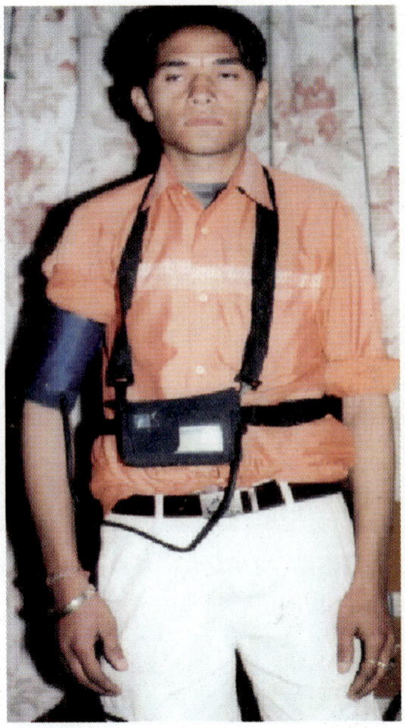

Fig. 22.7: *Fixation of ambulatory blood pressure instrument for recording BP of an adolescent with white coat hypertension*

If the child's BP (systolic or diastolic) is 95th percentile, the child may be hypertensive, and the measurement must be repeated on at least two additional occasions to confirm the diagnosis. Staging of BP, according to the extent to which a child's BP exceeds the 95th percentile, is helpful in developing a management plan for evaluation and treatment that is most appropriate for an individual patient. On repeated measurement, hypertensive children may have BP levels that are only a few mmHg >95th percentile; these children would be managed differently from hypertensive children who have BP levels that are 15–20 mmHg above the 95th percentile. An important clinical decision is to determine which hypertensive children require more immediate attention for elevated BP. The difference between the 95th and the 99th percentiles is only 7–10 mmHg and is not large enough, particularly in view of the variability in BP measurements, to adequately distinguish mild hypertension (where limited evaluation

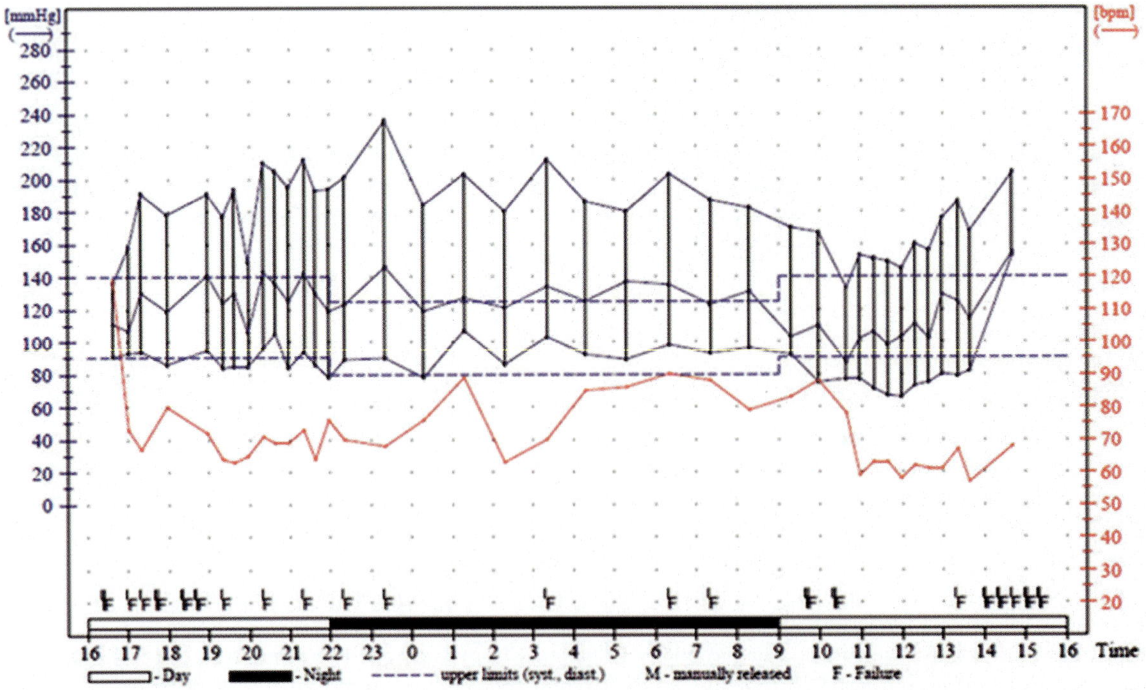

Fig. 22.8: *ABPM. A 24 hour BP monitor test. A blood pressure cuff is fitted to your arm. It is connected to an automated inflating device which records the blood pressure every half an hour during the day and every hour at night. When you return the monitor, the readings are analysed to give a day-time, night-time and 24 hour average for your blood pressure*

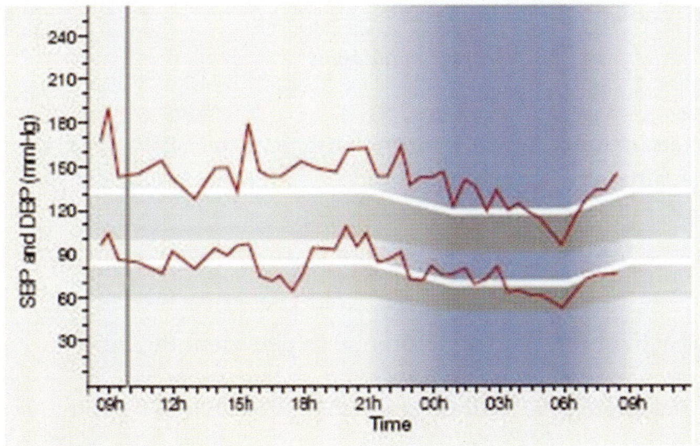

Fig. 22.9: *ABPM suggests mild day-time systolic hypertension (150 mmHg), borderline daytime diastolic hypertension (87 mmHg), borderline night-time systolic hypertension (123 mmHg), and normal night-time diastolic blood pressure (68 mmHg) with a white-coat effect (187 mmHg/104 mmHg). Normal dipping pattern*

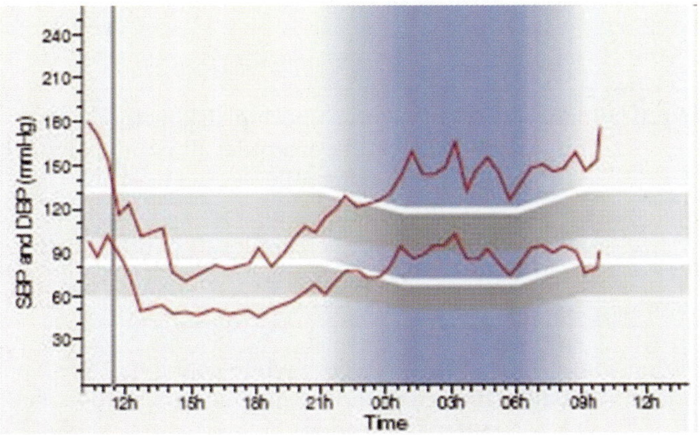

Fig. 22.10: *ABPM suggests low day-time systolic and diastolic blood pressure (100 mmHg/59 mm Hg) and moderate night-time systolic and diastolic hypertension (146 mmHg/89 mmHg) with a white-coat effect (181 mmHg/102 mmHg). Reverse dipping pattern*

is most appropriate) from more severe hypertension (where more immediate and extensive intervention is indicated). Therefore, stage 1 hypertension is the designation for BP levels that range from the 95th percentile to 5 mm Hg above the 99th percentile. Stage 2 hypertension is the designation for BP levels that are >5 mmHg above the 99th percentile. Once confirmed on repeated measures, stage 1 hypertension allows time for evaluation before initiating treatment unless the patient is symptomatic. Patients with stage 2 hypertension may need more prompt evaluation and pharmacologic therapy. Symptomatic patients with stage 2 hypertension require immediate treatment and consultation with experts in pediatric hypertension. These categories are parallel to the staging of hypertension in adults, as noted in the JNC 7.

How to Use BP Tables?

Use the standard height charts to determine the height percentile. Measure and record the child's SBP and DBP. Use the correct gender table for SBP and DBP. Find the child's age on the left side of the table. Follow the age row horizontally across the table to the intersection of the line for the height percentile (vertical column). There, find the 50th, 90th, 95th, and 99th percentiles for SBP in the left columns and for DBP in the right columns.

- BP < 90th percentile is normal.
- BP between the 90th and 95th percentile is prehypertension. In adolescents, BP 120/80 mmHg is prehypertension, even if this figure is <90th percentile.
- BP > 95th percentile may be hypertension.
- If the BP is >90th percentile, the BP should be repeated twice at the same office visit, and an average SBP and DBP should be used.
- If the BP is >95th percentile, BP should be staged. If stage 1 (95–99th percentile plus 5 mmHg), BP measurements should be repeated on two more occasions. If hypertension is confirmed, If BP is stage 2 (>99th percentile plus 5 mmHg), prompt referral should be made for evaluation and therapy. If the patient is symptomatic, immediate referral and treatment are indicated. Those patients with a compelling indication, would be treated as the next higher category of hypertension.

1. Primary Hypertension

Primary hypertension is identifiable in children and adolescents.

Both hypertension and prehypertension have become a significant health issue in the young because of the strong association of high BP with overweight and the marked increase in the prevalence of overweight children.

The evaluation of hypertensive children should include assessment for additional risk factors.

Because of an association of sleep apnea with overweight and high BP, a sleep history should be obtained.

High BP in childhood had been considered a risk factor for hypertension in early adulthood. However, primary (essential) hypertension is now identifiable in children and adolescents. Primary hypertension in childhood is usually characterized by mild or stage 1 hypertension and is often associated with a positive family history of hypertension or cardiovascular disease (CVD). Children and adolescents with primary hypertension are frequently overweight. Data on healthy adolescents obtained in school health-screening programs demonstrate that the prevalence of hypertension increases progressively with increasing body mass index (BMI), and hypertension is detectable in 30% of overweight children (BMI >95th percentile). The strong association of high BP with obesity and the marked increase in the prevalence of childhood obesity indicate that both hypertension and prehypertension are becoming a significant health issue in the young. Overweight children frequently have some degree of insulin resistance (a prediabetic condition). Overweight and high BP are also components of the insulin-resistance syndrome, or

Table 22.7: *Clinical evaluation of confirmed hypertension*

Study or procedure	*Purpose*	*Target population*
Evaluation for identifiable causes		
History including sleep history, family history, risk factors, diet, and habits such as smoking and drinking alcohol; physical examination	History and physical examination help focus subsequent evaluation	All children with persistent BP ≥ 95th percentile
BUN, creatinine, electrolytes, urinalysis, and urine culture	R/O renal disease and chronic pyelonephritis	All children with persistent BP ≥ 95th percentile
CBC	R/O anemia, consistent with chronic renal disease	All children with persistent BP ≥ 95th percentile
Renal U/S or disparate renal size	R/O renal scar, congenital anomaly, percentile	All children with persistent BP ≥ 95th
Evaluation for comorbidity		
Fasting lipid panel, fasting glucose	Identify hyperlipidemia, identify metabolic abnormalities	Overweight patients with BP at 90th–94th percentile; all patients with BP ≥ 95th percentile; family history of hypertension or CVD; child with chronic renal disease
Drug screen	Identify substances that might cause hypertension	History suggestive of possible contribution by substances or drugs.
Polysomnography	Identify sleep disorder in association with hypertension	History of loud, frequent snoring
Evaluation for target-organ damage		
Echocardiogram	Identify LVH and other indications of cardiac involvement	Patients with comorbid risk factors* and BP 90th–94th percentile; all patients with BP ≥ 95th percentile
Retinal examination	Identify retinal vascular changes	Patients with comorbid risk factors and BP 90th–94th percentile; all patients with BP ≥ 95th percentile
Additional evaluation as indicated		
ABPM	Identify white-coat hypertension, abnormal diurnal BP pattern, BP load	Patients in whom white-coat hypertension is suspected, and when other information on BP pattern is needed
Plasma renin determination	Identify low renin, suggesting mineralocorticoid-related disease	Young children with stage 1 hypertension and any child or adolescent with stage 2 hypertension Positive family history of severe hypertension
Renovascular imaging	Identify renovascular disease	Young children with stage 1 hypertension and any child or adolescent with stage 2 hypertension
Isotopic scintigraphy (renal scan)		
MRA		
Duplex Doppler flow studies		
three dimensional CT		
Arteriography: DSA or classic		
Plasma and urine steroid levels	Identify steroid-mediated hypertension	Young children with stage 1 hypertension and any child or adolescent with stage 2 hypertension
Plasma and urine catecholamines	Identify catecholamine-mediated hypertension	Young children with stage 1 hypertension and any child or adolescent with stage 2 hypertension

BUN, blood urea nitrogen; CBC, complete blood count; R/O, rule out; U/S, ultrasound.

* Comorbid risk factors also include diabetes mellitus and kidney disease.

metabolic syndrome, a condition of multiple metabolic risk factors for CVD as well as for type 2 diabetes. The clustering of other CVD risk factors that are included in the insulin-resistance syndrome (high triglycerides, low high-density lipoprotein cholesterol, truncal obesity, hyperinsulinemia) is significantly greater among children with high BP than in children with normal BP. Recent reports from studies that examined childhood data estimate that the insulin-resistance syndrome is present in 30% of overweight children with BMI >95th percentile. Historically, hypertension in childhood was considered a simple independent risk factor for CVD, but its link to the other risk factors in the insulin-resistance syndrome indicates that a broader approach is more appropriate in affected children (Table 22.11).

Primary hypertension often clusters with other risk factors. Therefore, the medical history, physical examination, and laboratory evaluation of hypertensive children and adolescents should include a comprehensive assessment for additional cardiovascular risk. These risk factors, in addition to high BP and overweight, include low plasma high-density lipoprotein cholesterol, elevated plasma triglyceride, and abnormal glucose tolerance. Fasting plasma insulin concentration is generally elevated, but an elevated insulin concentration may be reflective only of obesity and is not diagnostic of the insulin-resistance syndrome. To identify other cardiovascular risk factors, a fasting lipid panel and fasting glucose level should be obtained in children who are overweight and have BP between the 90th and the 94th percentile and in all children with BP >95th percentile. If there is a strong family history of type 2 diabetes, a hemoglobin A1c or glucose tolerance test may also be considered. These metabolic risk factors should be repeated periodically to detect changes in the level of cardiovascular risk over time. Fewer data are available on the utility of other tests in children [e.g. plasma uric acid or homocysteine and Lp(a) levels], and the use of these measures should depend on family history.

Sleep disorders including sleep apnea are associated with hypertension, coronary artery disease, heart failure, and stroke in adults. Although limited data are available, they suggest an association of sleep-disordered breathing and higher BP in children.

Approximately 15% of children snore, and at least 1–3% have sleep-disordered breathing. Because of the associations with hypertension and the frequency of occurrence of sleep disorders, particularly among overweight children, a history of sleeping patterns should be obtained in a child with hypertension. One practical strategy for identifying children with a sleep problem or sleep disorder is to obtain a brief sleep history, using an instrument called BEARS. BEARS addresses five major sleep domains that provide a simple but comprehensive screen for the major sleep disorders affecting children 2–18 years old. The components of BEARS include: bedtime problems, excessive daytime sleepiness, awakenings during the night, regularity and duration of sleep, and sleep-disordered breathing (snoring). Each of these domains has an age-appropriate trigger question and

Table 22.8: *Classification of hypertension in children and adolescents with measurement frequency and therapy recommendations*

	*SBP or DBP percentile**	*Frequency of BP measurement*	*Therapeutic lifestyle changes*	*Pharmacologic therapy*
Normal	<90th	Recheck at next scheduled physical examination	Encourage healthy diet, sleep, and physical activity	—
Prehypertension	90th to <95th or if BP exceeds 120/80 even if <90th percentile up to <95th percentile‡	Recheck in 6 months	Weight-management counseling if overweight; introduce physical activity and diet management†	None unless compelling indications such as chronic kidney disease, diabetes mellitus, heart failure, or LVH exist
Stage 1 hypertension	95–99th percentile plus 5 mmHg	Recheck in 1–2 weeks or sooner if the patient is symptomatic; if persistently elevated on two additional occasions, evaluate or refer to source of care within 1 month	Weight-management counseling if overweight; introduce physical activity and diet management†	Initiate therapy based on indications in Table 22.5 or if compelling indications (as shown above) exist
Stage 2 hypertension	>99th percentile plus 5 mmHg	Evaluate or refer to source of care within 1 wk or immediately if the patient is symptomatic	Weight-management counseling if overweight; introduce physical activity and diet management†	Initiate therapy§

* For gender, age, and height measured on at least 3 separate occasions; if systolic and diastolic categories are different, categorize by the higher value.

‡ This occurs typically at 12 years old for SBP and at 16 years old for DBP.

† Parents and children trying to modify the eating plan to the Dietary Approaches to Stop Hypertension Study eating plan could benefit from consultation with a registered or licensed nutritionist to get them started.

§ More than 1 drug may be required.

includes responses of both parent and child as appropriate. This brief screening for sleep history can be completed in 5 minutes.

In a child with primary hypertension, the presence of any comorbidity that is associated with hypertension carries the potential to increase the risk for CVD and can have an adverse effect on health outcome. Consideration of these associated risk factors and appropriate evaluation in those children in whom the hypertension is verified are important in planning and implementing therapies that reduce the comorbidity risk as well as control BP.

Secondary Hypertension Evaluation (Table 22.9)

- Secondary hypertension is more common in children than in adults.
- Because overweight is strongly linked to hypertension, BMI should be calculated as part of the physical examination.
- Once hypertension is confirmed, BP should be measured in both arms and a leg.
- Very young children, children with stage 2 hypertension, and children or adolescents with clinical signs that suggest systemic conditions associated with hypertension should be evaluated more completely than in those with stage 1 hypertension.

History

The possibility that some underlying disorder may be the cause of the hypertension should be considered in every child or adolescent who has elevated BP. However, the extent of an evaluation for detection of a possible underlying cause should be individualized for each child. Very young children, children with stage 2 hypertension, and children or adolescents with clinical signs that suggest the presence of systemic conditions associated with hypertension should be evaluated more extensively, as compared with those with stage 1 hypertension. Present technologies may facilitate less invasive evaluation than in the past although experience in using newer modalities with children is still limited (Table 22.11).

A thorough history and physical examination are the first steps in the evaluation of any child with persistently elevated BP. Elicited information should aim to identify not only signs and symptoms due to high BP but also clinical findings that might uncover an underlying systemic disorder. Thus, it is important to seek signs and symptoms suggesting renal disease (gross hematuria, edema, fatigue), heart disease (chest pain, exertional dyspnea, palpitations), and diseases of other organ systems (e.g. endocrinologic, rheumatologic).

Past medical history should elicit information to focus the subsequent evaluation and to uncover definable causes of hypertension. Questions should be asked about prior hospitalizations, trauma, urinary tract infections, snoring and other sleep problems. Questions should address family history of hypertension, diabetes, obesity, sleep apnea, renal disease, other CVD (hyperlipidemia, stroke), and familial endocrinopathies. Many drugs can increase BP, so it is important to inquire directly about use of over-the-counter, prescription, and illicit drugs. Equally important are specific questions aimed at identifying the use of nutritional supplements, especially preparations aimed at enhancing athletic performance.

Table 22.9: *Physical findings indicative of a secondary cause for childhood hypertension*

Physical examination finding	*Possible etiologies*
Abdominal bruit	Renal artery stenosis
Abdominal mass	Polycystic kidney disease; hydronephrosis/obstructive renal lesions; neuroblastoma; Wilms' tumor
Acne	Cushing's syndrome
Adenotonsillar hypertrophy	Sleep disorder associated with hypertension
Decreased perfusion of lower extremities	Coarctation of the aorta
Diaphoresis	Pheochromocytoma
Flusing	Pheochromocytoma
Growth retradation	Chronic renal failure
Hirstism	Cushing's syndrome
Joint swelling	Systemic lupus erythematosus
Malar rash	Systemic lupus erythematosus
Moon facies	Cushing's syndrome
Murmur	Coarctation of the aorta
Muscle weakness	Hyperaldosteronism
Obesity (general)	Association with primary hypertension
Obesity (of the face, neck or trunk)	Cushing's syndrome
Tachycardia	Hyperthyroidism; pheochromocytoma; neuroblastoma
Thyromegaly	Hyperthroidism

Adapted with permission for National High Blood Pressure Education Program Working Group on High Blood Pressure in Children and Adolescents. The foruth report on the diagnosis, evaluation, and treatment of high blood pressure in children and adolescents. Pediatrics 2004; 114(2 suppl 4th report):564

Table 22.10: *Physical examination findings suggestive of hypertension*

	*Finding**	*Possible etiology*
Vital signs	Tachycardia	Hyperthyroidism, pheochromocytoma, neuroblastoma, primary hypertension
	Decreased lower extremity pulses; drop in BP from upper to lower extremities	Coarctation of the aorta
Eyes	Retinal changes	Severe hypertension, more likely to be associated with secondary hypertension
Ear, nose, and throat	Adenotonsillar hypertrophy	Suggests association with sleep-disordered breathing (sleep apnea), snoring
Height/weight	Growth retardation	Chronic renal failure
	Obesity (high BMI)	Primary hypertension
	Truncal obesity	Cushing syndrome, insulin resistance syndrome
Head and neck	Moon facies	Cushing syndrome
	Elfin facies	Williams syndrome
	Webbed neck	Turner syndrome
	Thyromegaly	Hyperthyroidism
Skin	Pallor, flushing, diaphoresis	Pheochromocytoma
	Acne, hirsutism, striae	Cushing syndrome, anabolic steroid abuse
	Café-au-lait spots	Neurofibromatosis
	Adenoma sebaceum	Tuberous sclerosis
	Malar rash	Systemic lupus erythematosus
	Acanthrosis nigricans	Type 2 diabetes
Chest	Widely spaced nipples	Turner syndrome
	Heart murmur	Coarctation of the aorta
	Friction rub	Systemic lupus erythematosus (pericarditis), collagen-vascular disease, end stage renal disease with uremia
	Apical heave	LVH/chronic hypertension
Abdomen	Mass	Wilms tumor, neuroblastoma, pheochromocytoma
	Epigastric/flank bruit	Renal artery stenosis
	Palpable kidneys	Polycystic kidney disease, hydronephrosis, multicystic-dysplastic kidney, mass (see above)
Genitalia	Ambiguous/virilization	Adrenal hyperplasia
Extremities	Joint swelling	Systemic lupus erythematosus, collagen vascular disease
	Muscle weakness	Hyperaldosteronism, Liddle syndrome

* Findings listed are examples of physical findings and do not represent all possible physical findings.
Adapted from Flynn JT. *Prog Pediatr Cardiol.* 2001;12:177–188.

Clinical Examination

The child's height, weight, and percentiles for age should be determined at the start of the physical examination.

Because obesity is strongly linked to hypertension, BMI should be calculated from the height and weight, and the BMI percentile should be calculated. Poor growth may indicate an underlying chronic illness. When hypertension is confirmed, BP should be measured in both arms and in a leg. Normally, BP is 10–20 mmHg higher in the legs than the arms. If the leg BP is lower than the arm BP or if femoral pulses are weak or absent, coarctation of the aorta may be present (Tables 22.9, 22.10 and 22.11).

Obesity alone is an insufficient explanation for diminished femoral pulses in the presence of high BP. The remainder of the physical examination should pursue clues found on history and should focus on findings that may indicate the cause and severity of hypertension.

The physical examination in hypertensive children is frequently normal except for the BP elevation. The extent of the laboratory evaluation is based on the child's age, history, physical examination findings, and level of BP elevation. The majority of children with secondary hypertension will have renal or renovascular causes for the BP elevation. Therefore, screening tests are designed to have a high likelihood of detecting children and adolescents who are so affected. These tests are easily obtained in most primary care offices and community hospitals. Additional evaluation must be tailored to the specific child and situation. The risk factors, or comorbid conditions, associated with primary hypertension should be included in the evaluation of hypertension in all children, as well as efforts to determine any evidence of target-organ damage.

Table 22.11: *Causes of resistant hypertension*

Improper blood pressure measurement
Volume overload and pseudotolerance
Excess sodium intake
Volume retention from kidney disease
Inadequate diuretic therapy
Drug-induced or other causes
Nonadherence
Inadequate doses
Inappropriate combinations
Nonsteroidal anti-inflammatory drugs; cyclooxygenase 2 inhibitors
Cocaine, amphetamines, other illicit drugs
Sympathomimetics (decongestants, anorectics)
Oral contraceptives
Adrenal steroids
Cyclosporine and tacrolimus
Erythropoietin Licorice (including some chewing tobacco)
Selected over-the-counter dietary supplements and medicines (e.g. ephedra, ma haung, bitter orange)
Associated conditions
Obesity
Excess alcohol intake
Identifiable causes of hypertension

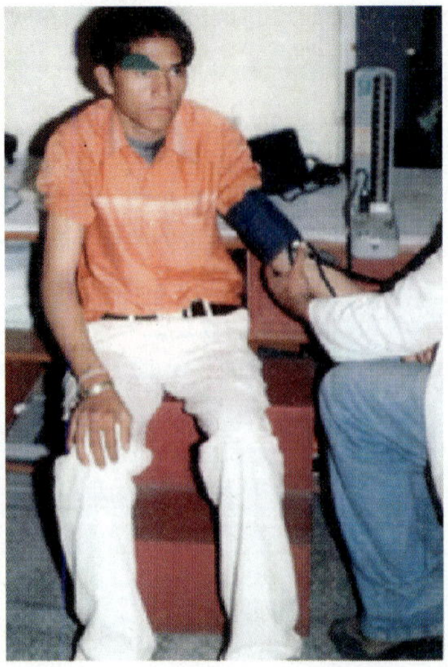

Fig. 22.12: *Measurement of blood pressure in an adolescent by the doctor with mercury manometer with arm keeping at the level of heart*

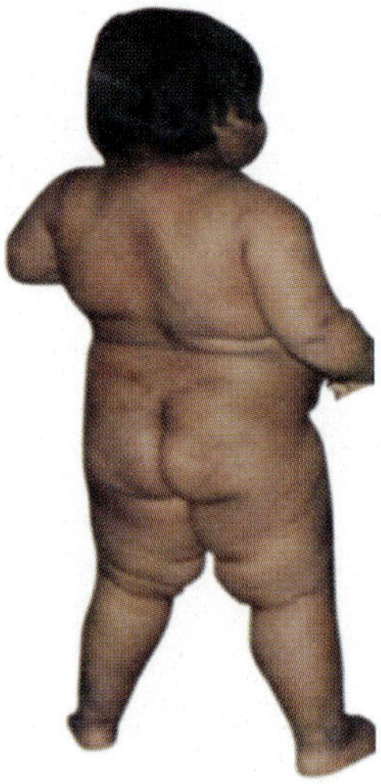

Fig. 22.11: *A young child of 2 years old weighing 30 kg showing significant obesity as a risk factor for future HT*

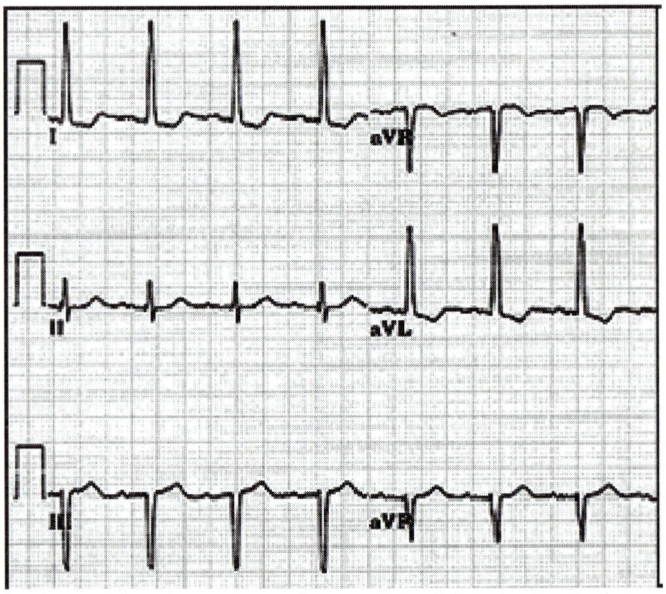

Fig. 22.13: *Voltage criteria for LVH and significant ST segment depression in leads with tall R waves. The voltage criteria include (1) R in aVL >11 mm; (2) R in I + S in III >25 mm and (3) (RI+SIII) - (RIII+SI) >17 mm (Lewis Index) in a young patient with hypertension*

Diagnostic Laboratory and Imaging Studies in Hypertension

Additional diagnostic studies may be appropriate in the evaluation of hypertension in a child or adolescent, particularly if there is a high degree of suspicion that an underlying disorder is present. ABPM is also used to detect white-coat hypertension (Figs 22.13–22.24).

Renin Profiling

Plasma renin level or plasma renin activity (PRA) is a useful screening test for mineralocorticoid-related diseases. With these disorders, the PRA is very low or unmeasurable by the laboratory and may be associated with relative hypokalemia. PRA levels are higher in patients who have renal artery stenosis. However, 15% of children with arteriographically evident renal artery stenosis have normal PRA values. Assays for direct measurement of renin, a different technique than PRA, are commonly used, although extensive normative data in children and adolescents are unavailable.

Table. 22.12: *Antihypertensive drugs for management of severe hypertension in children 1–17 years*

Drug	*Class*	*Dose**	*Route*	*Comments*
Most useful†				
Esmolol	β-blocker	100–500 μg/kg per min	IV infusion	Very short-acting; constant infusion preferred. May cause profound bradycardia. Produced modest reductions in BP in a pediatric clinical trial.
Hydralazine	Vasodilator	0.2–0.6 mg/kg per dose	IV, IM	Should be given every 4 hour when given IV bolus. Recommended dose is lower than FDA label.
Labetalol	α- and β-blocker	Bolus: 0.2–1.0 mg/kg per dose up to 40 mg/dose Infusion: 0.25–3.0 mg/kg per h	IV bolus or infusion	Asthma and overt heart failure are relative contraindications.
Nicardipine	Calcium channel blocker	1–3 μg/kg per min	IV infusion	May cause reflex tachycardia
Sodium nitroprusside	Vasodilator	0.53–10 μg/kg per min	IV infusion	Monitor cyanide levels with prolonged (>72 hour) use or in renal failure; or coadminister with sodium thiosulfate.
Occasionally useful‡				
Clonidine	Central α-agonist	0.05–0.1 mg/dose, may be repeated up to 0.8 mg total dose	po	Side effects include dry mouth and sedation.
Enalaprilat	ACE inhibitor	0.05–0.1 mg/kg per dose up to 1.25 mg/dose	IV bolus	May cause prolonged hypotension and acute renal failure, especially in neonates.
Fenoldopam	Dopamine receptor agonist	0.2–0.8 μg/kg per min	IV infusion	Produced modest reductions in BP in a pediatric clinical trial in patients up to 12 years
Isradipine	Calcium channel blocker	0.05–0.1 mg/kg per dose	po	Stable suspension can be compounded
Minoxidil	Vasodilator	0.1–0.2 mg/kg per dose	po	Most potent oral vasodilator, long-acting.

FDA indicates food and drug administration; IM, intramuscular; IV, intravenous; po, oral.
* All dosing recommendations are based on expert opinion or case series data except as otherwise noted.
† Useful for hypertensive emergencies and some hypertensive urgencies.
‡ Useful for hypertensive urgencies and some hypertensive emergencies.

Renovascular Hypertension

Renovascular hypertension is a consequence of an arterial lesion or lesions impeding blood flow to 1 or both kidneys or to 1 intrarenal segments. Affected children usually, but not invariably, have markedly elevated BP. Evaluation for renovascular disease also should be considered in infants or children with other known predisposing factors such as prior umbilical artery catheter placements or neurofibromatosis. A number of newer diagnostic techniques are presently available for evaluation of renovascular disease, but experience in their use in pediatric patients is limited. Consequently, the recommended approaches generally use older techniques such as standard intraarterial angiography, digital-subtraction angiography (DSA), and scintigraphy [with or without angiotensin-converting enzyme (ACE) inhibition]. As technologies evolve, children should be referred for imaging studies to centers that have expertise in the radiologic evaluation of childhood hypertension (Fig. 22.20).

Electrocardiogram: It is helpful in detecting LVH and associated cardiac arrhythmia computerised renal angioscan (Fig. 22.13).

It may find out intrinsic or pressure induced renal dysfunctions in the genesis of secondary hypertension.

Intraarterial DSA

Intraarterial DSA with contrast is used more frequently than standard angiography, but because of intraarterial injection, this method remains invasive. DSA can be accomplished also by using a rapid injection of contrast into a peripheral vein, but quality of views and the size of pediatric veins make this technique useful only for older children. DSA and formal arteriography are still considered the "gold standard", but these studies should be undertaken only

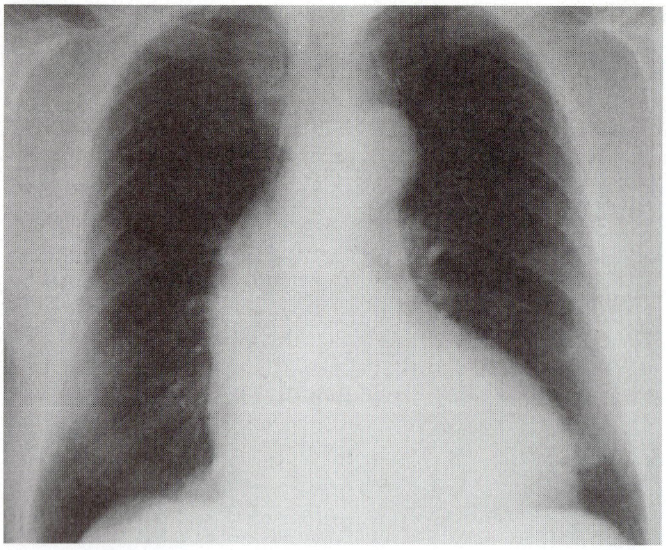

Fig. 22.14: *X-ray PA view showing dilatation of ascending aorta (arrow) and unfolding of aortic knuckle in patient with hypertensive heart disease*

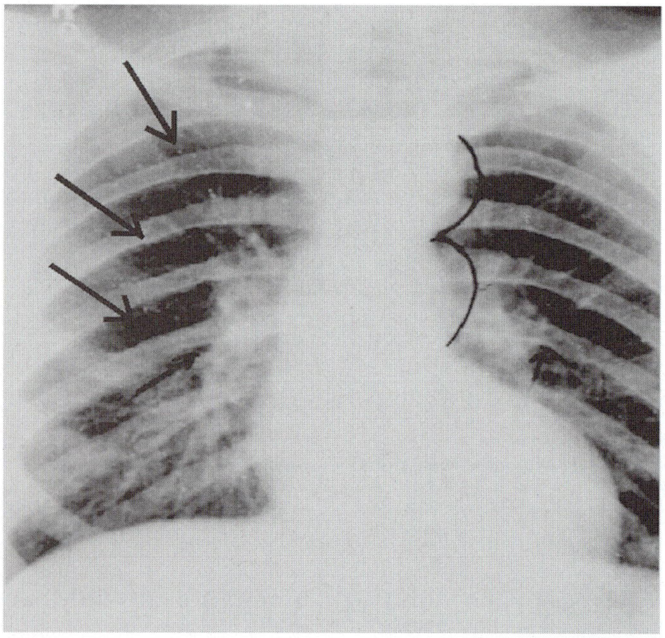

Fig. 22.15: *X-ray chest PA view showing figure of 3 as indicated on film due to enlarged subclavian artery superiorly and dilated descending aorta distally in patient with coarctation of aorta in patient with severe superior hypertension*

when surgical or invasive interventional radiologic techniques are being contemplated for anatomic correction. Newer imaging techniques may be used in children with vascular lesions.

Skiagram of the Chest PA View

(Figs 22.14 to 22.16)

It may be helpful in finding out the basic cause(s) in secondary hypertension such as coarctation of aorta, LVH in systemic hypertension and complications as a result of end organ failure, i.e. pulmonary edema and heart failure.

Magnetic resonance angiography (MRA) is increasingly feasible for the evaluation of pediatric renovascular disease, but it is still best for detecting abnormalities in the main renal artery and its primary branches. Imaging with magnetic resonance requires that the patient be relatively immobile for extended periods, which is a significant difficulty for small children. At present, studies are needed to assess the effectiveness of MRA in the diagnosis of children with renovascular disease. Newer methods, including (Figs 22.17–22.19).

Three dimensional reconstructions of computed tomography (CT) images, or spiral CT with contrast: It seem promising in evaluating children who may have renovascular disease.

Target-organ Abnormalities in Hypertension

Target-organ abnormalities are commonly associated with hypertension in children and adolescents.

Left ventricular hypertrophy (LVH) is the most prominent evidence of target-organ damage. Pediatric patients with established hypertension should have echocardiographic assessment of left ventricular mass at diagnosis and periodically thereafter.

The presence of LVH is an indication to initiate or intensify antihypertensive therapy. Hypertension is associated with increased risk of myocardial infarction, stroke, and cardiovascular mortality in adults, and treatment of elevated BP results in a reduction in the risk for cardiovascular events. Children and adolescents with severe elevation of BP are also at increased risk of adverse outcomes, including hypertensive encephalopathy, seizures, and even cerebrovascular accidents and congestive heart failure. Even hypertension that is less severe contributes to target-organ damage when it occurs

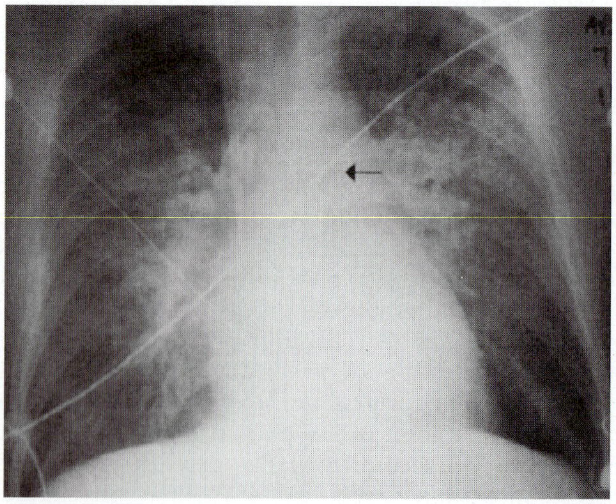

Fig. 22.16: *X-ray chest PA view showing prominent hilar shadows and dilated peripheral veins called as B-lines of kerleys due to acute pulmonary edema in patient with stage 11 hypertension and LVF*

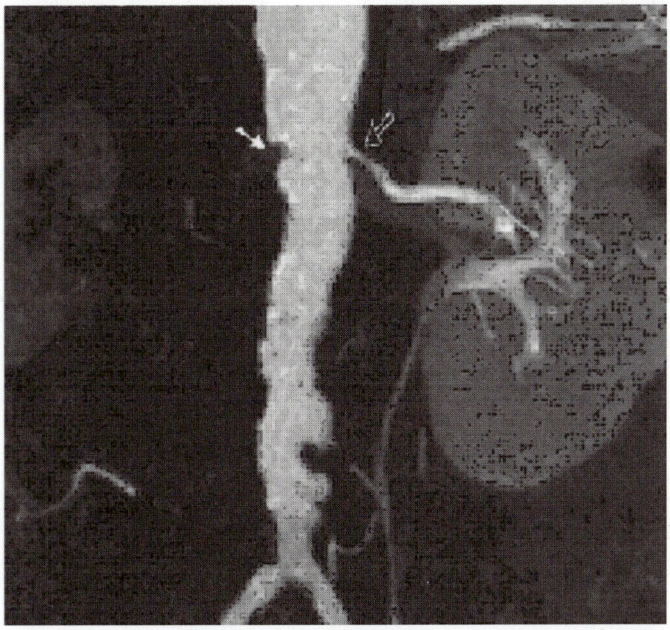

Fig. 22.17: *MIP image from CE-MRA obtained with focus on renal arteries shows occlusion of right renal artery (solid arrow) and mild stenosis of proximal left renal artery (open arrow) in patient with uncontrolled hypertension*

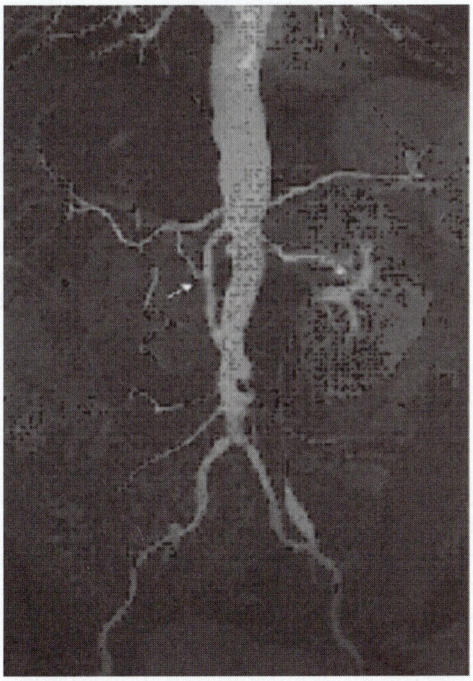

Fig. 22.18: *Coronal maximum intensity projection (MIP) image from contrast-enhanced MR angiography (CE-MRA) shows diffuse atherosclerosis of abdominal aorta with mild stenosis of infrarenal part and proximal right common iliac artery. There is also mild stenosis of origin of right hepatic artery from superior mesenteric artery (arrow) in patient with severe hypertension*

with other chronic conditions such as chronic kidney disease. Two autopsy studies that evaluated tissue from adolescents and young adults who had sudden deaths due

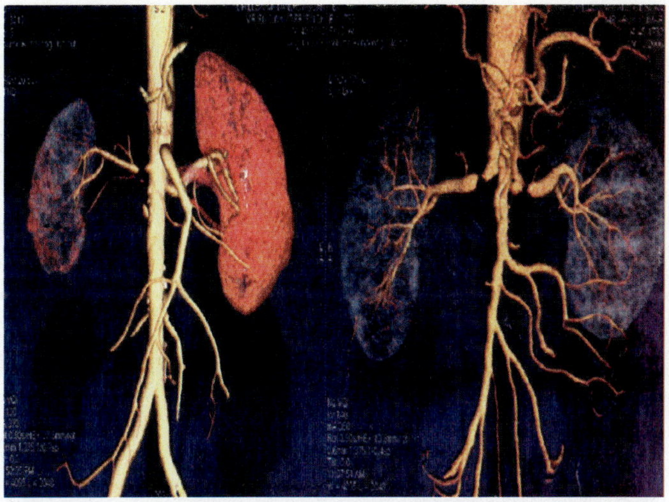

Fig. 22.19: *CT angioscan of kidneys showing bilateral renal artery stenosis in patient with stage 11 type of hypertension with renal failure*

to trauma demonstrated significant relationships between the level of BP, or hypertension, and the presence of atherosclerotic lesions in the aorta and coronary arteries. The exact level and duration of BP elevation that causes target-organ damage in the young has not been established.

One difficulty in the assessment of these relationships is that, until recently, few noninvasive methods could evaluate the effect of hypertension on the cardiovascular system. Noninvasive techniques that use ultrasound can demonstrate structural and functional changes in the vasculature related to BP. Recent clinical studies using these techniques demonstrate that childhood levels of BP are associated with carotid intimal-medial thickness and large artery compliance in young adults. Even healthy adolescents with clustering of cardiovascular risk factors demonstrate elevated carotid thickness, and those with BP levels at the higher end of the normal distribution show decreased brachial artery flow-mediated vasodilatation. Overall, evidence is increasing that even mild BP elevation can have an adverse effect on vascular structure and function in asymptomatic young persons.

LVH is the most prominent clinical evidence of target-organ damage caused by hypertension in children and adolescents. With the use of echocardiography to measure left ventricular mass, LVH has been reported in 34–38% of children and adolescents with mild, untreated BP elevation. Daniels et al evaluated 130 children and adolescents with persistent BP elevation. They reported that 55% of patients had a left ventricular mass index >90th percentile, and 14% had left ventricular mass index >51 g/m^2, a value in adults with hypertension that has been associated with a fourfold greater risk of adverse cardiovascular outcomes. When left ventricular geometry was in hypertensive children, 17% had concentric hypertrophy, a pattern that is associated with higher risk for cardiovascular outcomes in adults, and 30% had eccentric hypertrophy, which is associated with intermediate risk for cardiovascular outcomes.

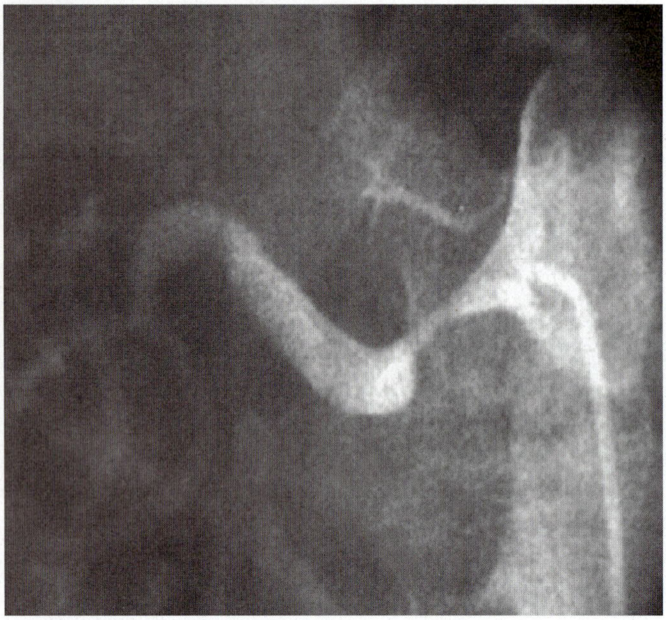

Fig. 22.20: *Renal angiogram showing stenosis of renal artery in patient with hypertensive renal disease*

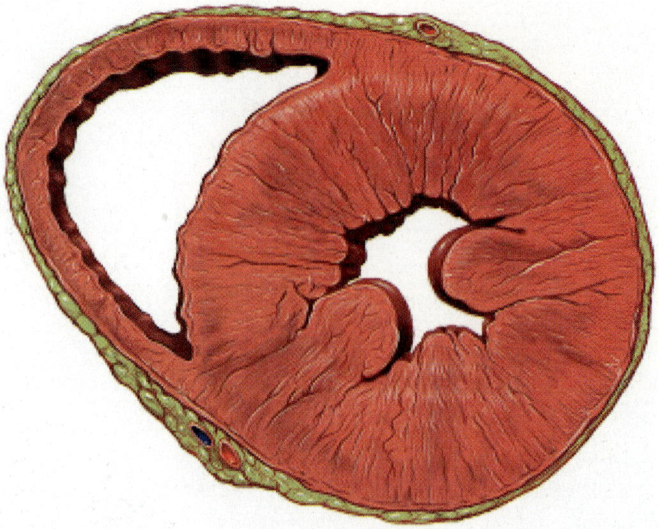

Fig. 22.22: *Morbid anatomy showing left ventricular hypertrophy*

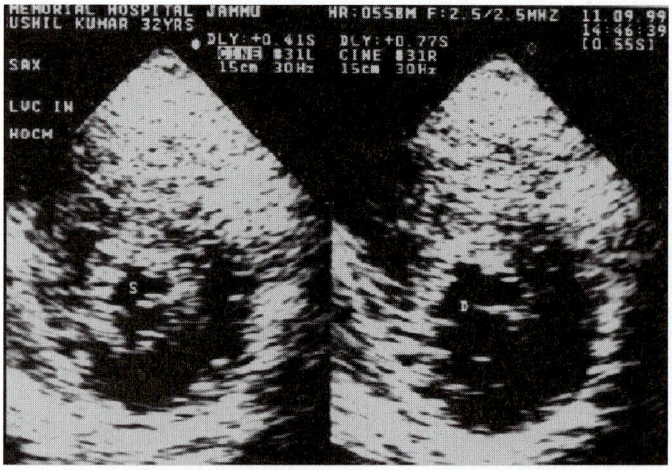

Fig. 22.23: *2D short axis echocardiographic view of LV both during systole (left) and diastole (right) in patient with hypertensive heart disease*

In addition, abnormalities of the retinal vasculature have been reported in adults with hypertension. Few studies of retinal abnormalities have been conducted in children with hypertension. Skalina et al evaluated newborns with hypertension and reported the presence of hypertensive retinal abnormalities in 50% of their patients. On repeat examination after the resolution of hypertension, these abnormalities had disappeared.

Echocardiography is recommended as a primary tool for evaluating patients for target-organ abnormalities by assessing the presence or absence of LVH. Left ventricular mass is determined from standard echocardiographic measurements of the left ventricular end-diastolic dimension, the intraventricular septal thickness, and the thickness of the left ventricular posterior wall and can be calculated as left ventricle mass (Figs 22.21–22.23).

Heart size is closely associated with body size. Left ventricular mass index is calculated to standardize measurements of left ventricular mass. Several methods for indexing left ventricular mass have been reported, but it is recommended that height (m^2) be used to index left ventricular mass as described by de Simone et al. This method accounts for close to the equivalent of the effect of lean body mass and excludes the effect of obesity and BP elevation on left ventricular mass. Some echo laboratories use height as the indexing variable. This calculation is also acceptable and is somewhat easier to use, because fewer calculations are needed.

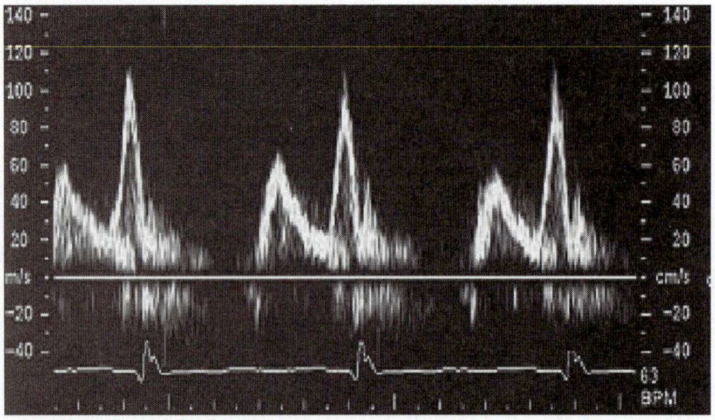

Fig. 22.21: *Dopper echoscan of mitral velocities showing diastolic LV dysfunctions in moderate hypertension in a young person*

Children and adolescents with established hypertension should have an echocardiogram to determine if LVH is present. A conservative cutpoint that determines the presence of LVH is 51 g/m^2. This cutpoint is >99th percentile for children and adolescents and is associated with increased morbidity in adults with hypertension. Other references exist for normal children, but unlike adults, outcome-based standards for left ventricular mass index are not available for children. In interpreting the left ventricular mass index, it should be remembered that some factors such as obesity and hypertension have pathologic effects on the heart, whereas others (such as physical activity, particularly in highly conditioned athletes) may be adaptive.

Ascertainment of left ventricular mass index is very helpful in clinical decision-making. The presence of LVH can be an indication for initiating or intensifying pharmacologic therapy to lower BP. For patients who have LVH, the echocardiographic determination of left ventricular mass index should be repeated periodically.

At the present time, additional testing for other target-organ abnormalities (such as determination of carotid intimal-medial thickness and evaluation of urine for microalbuminuria) is not recommended for routine clinical use. Additional research will be needed to evaluate the clinical utility of these tests.

Lifestyle Changes and Dietic Modifications (Fig. 22.26)

- Weight reduction is the primary therapy for obesity-related hypertension. Prevention of excess or abnormal weight gain will limit future increases in BP.
- Regular physical activity and restriction of sedentary activity will improve efforts at weight management and may prevent an excess increase in BP over time. Dietary modification should be strongly encouraged in children and adolescents who have BP levels in the prehypertensive range as well as those with hypertension.
- Family-based intervention improves success. Evidence that supports the efficacy of nonpharmacologic interventions for BP reduction in the treatment of hypertension in children and adolescents is limited. Data that demonstrate a relationship of lifestyle with BP can be used as the basis for recommendations. On the basis of large, randomized, controlled trials, the following lifestyle modifications are recommended in adults weight reduction in overweight or obese individuals increased intake of fresh vegetables, fruits, and low-fat dairy (the Dietary Approaches to Stop Hypertension Study eating plan) dietary sodium reduction; increased physical activity and moderation of alcohol consumption. Smoking cessation has significant cardiovascular benefits. As information on chronic sleep problems evolves, interventions to improve sleep quality also may have a beneficial effect on BP.

The potential for control of BP in children through weight reduction is supported by BP tracking and weight-reduction studies. BP levels track from childhood through adolescence and into adulthood in association with weight. Because of the strong correlation between weight and BP, excessive weight gain is likely to be associated with elevate BP over time. Therefore, maintenance of normal weight gain in childhood should lead to less hypertension in adulthood (Figs 22.24 and 22.25).

Weight loss in overweight adolescents is associated with a decrease in BP. Weight control not only decreases BP, it also decreases BP sensitivity to salt and decreases other

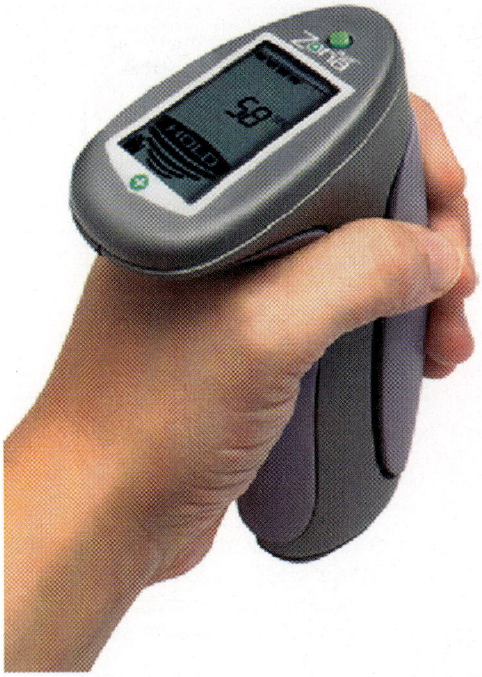

Fig. 22.24: *Innovative high blood pressure device by Brian Klein. The FDA has conditionally approved an investigational device exemption (IDE) for a pivotal clinical trial to evaluate a new patented isometric handgrip therapy technology. A product of Zona Health (Boise, ID), the ZonaRx device was developed for use in the treatment of resistant hypertension (high blood pressure that persists despite treatment by two or more medications). The IDE approval marks the first pivotal trial of isometric handgrip therapy for hypertension treatment. Earlier clinical studies demonstrate that the isometric handgrip therapy could provide "a significant reduction in blood pressure levels for the majority of hypertensive patients"*

cardiovascular risk factors such as dyslipidemia and insulin resistance. In studies that achieve a reduction in BMI of 10%, short-term reductions in BP were in the range of 8–12 mmHg. Although difficult, weight loss, if successful, is extremely effective. Identifying a complication of overweight such as hypertension can be a helpful motivator for patients and families to make changes. Weight control can render pharmacologic treatment unnecessary but should not delay drug use when indicated.

Emphasis on the management of complications rather than on overweight shifts the aim of weight management from an aesthetic to a health goal. In motivated families, education or simple behavior modification can be successful in achieving moderate weight loss or preventing additional weight gain. Steps can be implemented in the primary care setting even with limited staff and time resources. The patient should be encouraged to self-monitor time spent in sedentary activities, including watching television and playing video or computer games, and set goals to progressively decrease these activities to <2 hours per day. The family and patient should identify physical activities that the child enjoys, engage in them regularly, and self-monitor time spent in physical activities (30–60 minutes per day should be achieved). Dietary changes can

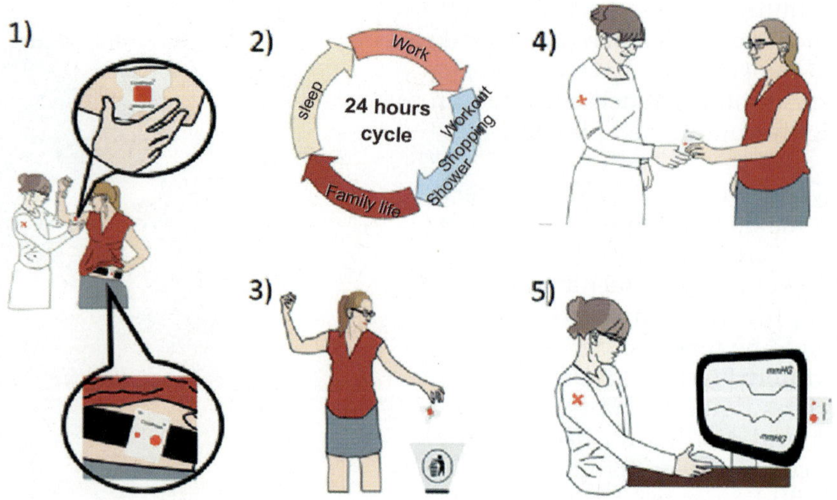

Fig. 22.25: *Steps in using new start-up continuous blood pressure measurement device without a counter-pressure cuff by gene ostrovsky with continuous blood pressure monitor that doesn't rely on a typical pressure cuff, but rather on a patch that has electrodes that sense the changing impedance of tissue around a vessel and convert it into a BP reading. Measuring other characteristics in electrical signal can also identify vascular stiffness and pulse velocity.*

involve portion-size control, decrease in consumption of sugar-containing beverages and energy-dense snacks, increase in consumption of fresh fruits and vegetables, and regular meals including a healthy breakfast. Consultation with a nutritionist can be useful and provide customized recommendations. During regular office visits, the primary care provider can supervise the child's progress in self-monitoring and accomplishing goals and provide support and positive feedback to the family. Some patients will benefit from a more intense and comprehensive approach to weight management from a multidisciplinary and specialized team if available.

Despite the lack of firm evidence about dietary intervention in children, it is generally accepted that hypertensive individuals can benefit from a dietary increase in fresh vegetables, fresh fruits, fiber, and nonfat dairy as well as a reduction of sodium. Despite some suggestion that calcium supplements may decrease BP in children, thus far the evidence is too limited to support a clinical recommendation. Lower BP has been associated in children and adolescents with an increased intake of potassium, magnesium, folic acid, unsaturated fat, and fiber and lower dietary intake of total fat. However, these associations are small and insufficient to support dietary recommendations for specific, individual nutrients.

Sodium reduction in children and adolescents has been associated with small reductions in BP in the range of 1–3 mmHg. Data from 1 randomized trial suggest that sodium intake in infancy may affect BP in adolescence. Similarly, some evidence indicates that breastfeeding may be associated with lower BP in childhood. The current recommendation for adequate daily sodium intake is only 1.2 g/day for 4- to 8-year-olds and 1.5 g/day for older children. Because this amount of sodium is substantially lower than current dietary intakes, lowering dietary sodium from the current usual intake may have future benefit. Reduced sodium intake, with calorie restriction, may account for some of the BP improvement associated with weight loss.

Regular physical activity has cardiovascular benefits. A recent meta-analysis that combined 12 randomized trials, for a total of 1,266 children and adolescents, concluded that physical activity leads to a small but not statistically significant decrease in BP. However, both regular physical activity and decreasing sedentary activities (such as watching television and playing video or electronic games) are important components of pediatric obesity treatment and prevention. Weight-reduction trials consistently report better results when physical activity and/or prevention of sedentary activity are included in the treatment protocol. Therefore, regular aerobic physical activity (30–60 minutes of moderate physical activity on most days) and limitation of sedentary activities to <2 hours per day are recommended for the prevention of obesity, hypertension, and other cardiovascular risk factors. With the exception of power lifting, resistance training is also helpful. Competitive sports participation should be limited only in the presence of uncontrolled stage 2 hypertension.

The scope of hypertension as a public health problem in adults is substantial. Poor health-related behaviors such as physical inactivity, unfavorable dietary patterns, and excessive weight gain raise the risk for future hypertension. The therapeutic lifestyle changes discussed above may have benefit for all children in prevention of future disease, including primary hypertension. Accordingly, appropriate health recommendations for all children and adolescents are regular physical activity; a diet with limited sodium but rich in fresh fruits, fresh vegetables, fiber, and low-fat dairy; and avoiding excess weight gain.

Medical Management of Hypertension

Indications for antihypertensive drug therapy in children include secondary hypertension and insufficient response to lifestyle modifications (Table 22.12).

Recent clinical trials have expanded the number of drugs that have pediatric dosing information. Dosing recommendations for many of the newer drugs are provided.

Pharmacologic therapy, when indicated, should be initiated with a single drug. Acceptable drug classes for use in children include ACE inhibitors, angiotensin-receptor blockers, β-blockers, calcium channel blockers, and diuretics.

The goal for antihypertensive treatment in children should be reduction of BP to <95th percentile unless concurrent conditions are present, in which case BP should be lowered to <90th percentile. Severe, symptomatic hypertension should be treated with intravenous antihypertensive drugs. In adults, hypertension is typically a lifelong condition. Most hypertensive patients will need to remain on medications for the rest of their lives. Usually, adults readily accept this fact, given the known long-term adverse consequences of untreated or undertreated hypertension. In children, however, the long-term consequences of untreated hypertension are unknown. Additionally, no data are available on the long-term effects of antihypertensive drugs on growth and development. Therefore, a definite indication for initiating pharmacologic therapy should be ascertained before a drug is prescribed.

Other indications for use of antihypertensive drugs can be considered depending on the clinical situation. For example, because the presence of multiple cardiovascular risk factors (elevated BP, dyslipidemia, tobacco use, etc) increases cardiovascular risk in an exponential rather than additive fashion, antihypertensive therapy could be considered if the child or adolescent is known to have dyslipidemia.

The number of antihypertensive drugs has increased since the publication of the first task force report on BP control in children. The number of drugs that have been studied systematically in children has increased also, largely because of incentives provided to the pharmaceutical industry under the auspices of the 1997 Food and Drug Administration Modernization Act (FDAMA) and the 2002 Best Pharmaceuticals for Children Act. These developments have had both negative and positive consequences. Chief among the negative consequences is the lack of reliable pediatric data for older, commonly used compounds with expired patent protection. Currently, no incentives exist for industry-sponsored trials of such drugs, and alternative methods of stimulating pediatric studies such as those contained in the Best Pharmaceuticals for Children Act have yet to come to fruition. On the other hand, publication of the results of industry-sponsored clinical trials and single-center case series will provide additional data that can be combined with prior recommendations based on expert opinion and collective clinical experience to guide the use of antihypertensive drugs in children and adolescents who require pharmacologic treatment.

Long-term clinical endpoint data from randomized trials such as the Antihypertensive and Lipid-Lowering Treatment to Prevent Heart Attack Trial support the preferential use of specific antihypertensive drugs in adults However, pediatric clinical trials of antihypertensive drugs have focused only on their ability to lower BP and have not compared the effects of these drugs on clinical endpoints. Therefore, because all classes of antihypertensive drugs have been shown to lower BP in children, the choice of drug for initial antihypertensive therapy resides in the preference of the responsible physician. Some diuretics and β-adrenergic blockers, which were recommended as initial therapy in the first and second task force reports, have a long history of safety and efficacy based on clinical experience in hypertensive children, and these drugs remain appropriate for pediatric use. Similarly, some members of the newer classes of antihypertensive drugs including ACE inhibitors, calcium channel blockers, and angiotensin-receptor blockers, have been studied in children and, based on short-term use, shown to be safe and well-tolerated with satisfactory BP reductions in hypertensive children.

Specific classes of antihypertensive drugs should be used preferentially in certain hypertensive children with specific underlying or concurrent medical conditions. Examples include the use of ACE inhibitors or angiotensin-receptor blockers in children with diabetes and microalbuminuria or proteinuric renal diseases, and the use of β-adrenergic blockers or calcium channel blockers in hypertensive children with migraine headaches. This approach is similar to that outlined in the recent JNC 7 report, which recommends specific classes of antihypertensive drugs for use in adults in certain high-risk categories.

All antihypertensive drugs should be prescribed in a similar fashion. The dose can be increased until the desired BP goal is achieved. Once the highest recommended dose is reached, or if the child experiences side effects from the drug, a second drug from a different class should be added. Consideration should be given to combining drugs with complementary mechanisms of action such as an ACE inhibitor with a diuretic or a vasodilator with a diuretic or β-adrenergic blocker. Because little pediatric experience is available in using fixed-dose combination products, except for bisoprolol/hydrochlorothiazide, routine use of these products in children cannot be recommended at this time.

For children with uncomplicated primary hypertension and no hypertensive target-organ damage, the goal BP should be <95th percentile for gender, age, and height, whereas for children with chronic renal disease, diabetes, or hypertensive target-organ damage, the goal BP should be <90th percentile for gender, age and height. Again, this approach is similar to the recommended treatment of hypertension in adults with additional cardiovascular risk factors or comorbid conditions.

Important adjunctive aspects to the drug therapy of childhood hypertension include ongoing monitoring of target-organ damage as well as BP monitoring, surveillance for drug side effects, periodic monitoring of electrolytes in children treated with ACE inhibitors or diuretics, counseling regarding other cardiovascular risk factors, and continued emphasis of nonpharmacologic measures. It also may be appropriate to consider "step-down" therapy in selected patients. This approach attempts a gradual reduction in the drug after an extended course of good BP control, with the eventual goal of completely discontinuing drug therapy. Children with uncomplicated primary hypertension, especially overweight children who successfully lose weight, are the best candidates for the step-down approach. Such patients require ongoing BP monitoring after the cessation of drug therapy as well as continued nonpharmacologic treatment because hypertension may recur.

Severe, symptomatic hypertension with BP well above the 99th percentile occurs in some children, usually those with underlying renal disease, and requires prompt treatment. Hypertensive emergencies in children are usually accompanied by signs of hypertensive encephalopathy, typically causing seizures. Hypertensive emergencies should be treated by an intravenous antihypertensive that can produce a controlled reduction in BP, aiming to decrease the pressure by 25% over the first 8 hours after presentation and then gradually normalizing the BP over 26–48 hours. Hypertensive urgencies are accompanied by less serious symptoms such as severe headache or vomiting. Hypertensive urgencies can be treated by either intravenous or oral antihypertensives depending on the child's symptomatology.

Hypertensive Pharmacotherapy

The goals of pharmacotherapy are to reduce morbidity and to prevent complications.

- Diuretics—cause diuresis, which decreases plasma volume and edema, thereby decreasing cardiac output and blood pressure.

Hydrochlorothiazide inhibits reabsorption of sodium in distal tubules, causing increased excretion of sodium, water, potassium and hydrogen ions.

Pediatric dose: < 6 months: 2–3 mg/kg/d PO divided bid > 6 months: 2 mg/kg/d PO divided bid

Spironolactone (aldactone)—Used for management of hypertension. May block effects of aldosterone on arteriolar smooth muscles.

Pediatric dose: 1.5–3.5 mg/kg/d PO in divided doses q6-24 hour.

Furosemide (lasix): Increases excretion of water by interfering with chloride-binding cotransport system, which in turn inhibits sodium and chloride reabsorption in ascending loop of Henle and distal renal tubule. Dose must be individualized to patient. Depending on response, administer at increments of 20–40 mg no sooner than 6–8 hours after previous dose until desired diuresis occurs. When treating infants, titrate with 1 mg/kg per dose increments until satisfactory effect achieved.

Pediatric dose: 1–2 mg/kg/dose PO; not to exceed 6 mg/kg/dose; not to administer more often than q6h alternatively, 1 mg/kg IV/IM slowly under close supervision; not to exceed 6 mg/kg.

Alpha 1-adrenergic blockers: Selectively block postsynaptic alpha 1-adrenergic receptors. Dilate arterioles and veins, thus lowering blood pressure.

Prazosin (minipress), terazosin (hytrin): Prazosin treats prostatic hypertrophy. Improves urine flow rates by relaxing smooth muscle, which is caused by blocking alpha 1-adrenoceptors in bladder neck and prostate. When increasing dose, administer first dose of each increment at bedtime to reduce syncopal episodes. Although doses >20 mg/d usually do not increase efficacy, some patients may benefit from as much as 40 mg/d.Terazosin decreases arterial tone by allowing peripheral postsynaptic blockade. It has minimal alpha2 effect.

Pediatric dose: Prazosin: not established; suggested dose is 0.5–7 mg PO tid; Terazosin: not established

Beta-adrenergic blocking agents: Used to treat hypertension as initial agents or in combination with other drugs (e.g. thiazides).

Atenolol (tenormin), metoprolol (lopressor, toprol XL), propranolol (inderal): Atenolol and metoprolol selectively block beta 1-receptors with little or no effect on beta 2 types. Propranolol is a class II antiarrhythmic, nonselective, beta-adrenergic receptor blocker with membrane-stabilizing activity that decreases automaticity of contractions.

Pediatric dose: Atenolol: 1–2 mg/kg/dose PO qd; metoprolol: 1–5 mg/kg/d PO divided bid; propranolol: 0.5 mg/kg/d PO divided bid/qid; increase gradually q3–7d; range is 2–4 mg/kg/d divided bid; not to exceed 2 mg/kg/d.

- Alpha/beta-adrenergic blocking agents; block alpha-, beta1-, and beta2-adrenergic receptor sites, thus decreasing blood pressure.

Labetalol (normodyne, trandate), Ccarvedilol (coreg): Nonselective beta- and alpha-adrenergic blockers. Do not appear to have intrinsic sympathomimetic activity. May reduce cardiac output and decrease peripheral vascular resistance. Use in aortic dissection not advisable when titratable drugs, such as esmolol and nitroprusside, available.

Pediatric dose: Labetalol: not established; suggested dose is 0.4–1 mg/kg/h; not to exceed 3 mg/kg/h carvedilol: not established.

Peripheral vasodilators: Relax blood vessels to improve blood flow, thus decreasing blood pressure.

Hydralazine (apresoline), minoxidil (rogaine loniten): Hydralazine decreases systemic resistance through direct vasodilation of arterioles. Minoxidil relaxes arteriolar smooth muscle, causing vasodilation, which in turn may reduce blood pressure.

Adult dose Hydralazine: 10–20 mg/dose IV/IM q4–6h prn initial; increase to 40 mg/dose if necessary; change to PO as soon as possible; Minoxidil: 5 mg PO qd; increase gradually q3d; 10–40 mg/d PO qd or divided bid maintenance; not to exceed 100 mg/d

Pediatric dose: Not established.

Diltiazem (cardizem, dilacor), verapamil (calan, covera-HS), nifedipine (adalat): During depolarization, inhibits calcium ion from entering slow channels or voltage-sensitive areas of vascular smooth muscle and myocardium.

Adult dose: Diltiazem: cardizem SR: 60–120 mg PO bid; Cardizem CD: 180–240 mg PO qd Dilacor.

Hypertension: 180–240 mg PO qd

Angina: 120 mg/d PO; titrate slowly over 7–14 d up to 480 mg/d prn; not to exceed 540 mg/d; Verapamil: 240–480 mg/d PO divided tid/qid; Nifedipine: 10-30 mg IR cap PO tid; not to exceed 120–180 mg/d; 30–60 mg SR tab PO qd; not to exceed 90-120 mg/d.

Pediatric dose: Diltiazem: not established. Verapamil: nifedipine: 0.25–0.5 mg/kg/dose PO tid/qid prn.

Angiotensin-converting enzyme (ACE) inhibitors: Competitive inhibitors of ACE. Reduces angiotensin II levels, thus decreasing aldosterone secretion.

Captopril (capoten), enalapril (vasotec), lisinopril (zestril), ramipril (altace—prevents conversion of angiotensin I to angiotensin II, a potent vasoconstrictor, resulting in lower aldosterone secretion.

Pediatric dose: Captopril: 6.25–12.5 mg/dose PO q12–24h; not to exceed 6 mg/kg/d; enalapril: not established lisinopril: not established; ramipril: not established.

- ACE inhibitors may increase digoxin, lithium, and allopurinol levels; rifampin decreases levels; probenecid may increase levels; hypotensive effects of ACE inhibitors may be enhanced when administered concurrently with diuretics.
- Angiotensin II receptor antagonists—for patients unable to tolerate ACE inhibitors.

Losartan (cozaar), valsartan (diovan)—nonpeptide angiotensin II receptor antagonists that block vasoconstrictor and aldosterone-secreting effects of angiotensin II. May induce more complete inhibition of renin-angiotensin system than ACE inhibitors, do not affect response to bradykinin, and are less likely to be associated with cough and angioedema.

Adult dose: Losartan: 25–100 mg PO qd/bid; valsartan: 80 mg/d PO; may increase to 160 mg/d if needed

Pediatric dose: Not established

Eprosartan (teveten), olmesartan (benicar): Angiotensin receptor antagonist that binds to AT1 angiotensin II receptor, blocking vasoconstrictor and aldosterone-secreting effects of angiotensin II. May induce a more complete inhibition of renin-angiotensin system than ACE inhibitors and do not affect response to bradykinin and, thus, is less likely to be associated with cough and angioedema. For patients unable to tolerate ACE inhibitors.

Adult dose: Eprosartan (teveten): 400–800 mg PO qd or divided bid. Olmesartan (benicar): 20 mg PO qd initially; may increase to 40 mg/d after 2 wk if further BP reduction required. Note: lower dose in volume- or salt-depleted patients.

Pediatric dose: Not established.

Contraindications: Documented hypersensitivity; bilateral renal artery stenosis and preexisting renal insufficiency; significant aortic/mitral stenosis.

- *Aldosterone antagonists:* Compete with aldosterone receptor sites, reducing blood pressure and sodium reabsorption.

Eplerenone (INSPRA): Selectively blocks aldosterone at the mineralocorticoid receptors in epithelial (e.g. kidney) and nonepithelial (e.g. heart, blood vessels, brain) tissues, thus decreasing blood pressure and sodium reabsorption.

Adult dose: 50 mg PO qd; may increase dose after 4 wk, not to exceed 100 mg/d.

Pediatric dose: Not established.

Alpha-adrenergic agonists: Stimulate presynaptic alpha2-adrenergic receptors in the brain stem, which reduces sympathetic nervous activity.

Methyldopa (aldomet): Stimulates central alpha-adrenergic receptors by a false transmitter, resulting in decreased sympathetic outflow. This results in inhibition of vasoconstriction.

Pediatric dose: 10 mg/kg/d PO divided bid/qid; increase q2d prn to maximum 65 mg/kg/d; not to exceed 3 g/d.

Clonidine (catapres): Stimulates alpha 2-adrenoreceptors in brain stem, activating an inhibitory neuron, which in turn results in reduced sympathetic outflow. These effects result in a decrease in vasomotor tone and heart rate.

Adult dose: 0.1 mg PO bid initial; 0.2–1.2 mg/d divided bid/qid maintenance; not to exceed 1.2 mg/d.

Pediatric dose: Not established.

Catheter-based minimal invasive techniques in the management of severe hypertensionin children and adolescents.

Radiofrequency Catheter Ablation in Hypertension

Catheter-based renal denervation is a minimally invasive procedure involving the application of radiofrequency energy in short bursts along the length of the main renal arteries to ablate the renal nerves that lie within and just beyond the adventitia of the renal artery as they pass to the kidneys. Two-year results from a nonrandomized proof-of-principle cohort study (Symplicity HTN-1) and a larger group of registry patients with resistant hypertension treated by renal denervation have demonstrated substantial reductions in office-based blood pressure without serious adverse events. The symplicity HTN-2 trial randomized patients with resistant hypertension, who met all clinical and anatomic eligibility criteria, to renal denervation or no renal denervation, with both groups maintained for 6 months on unchanged antihypertensive medications. The primary end point, change in office-based systolic blood pressure (SBP) at 6-month follow-up, demonstrated a significant difference in reduction of SBP between the treatment and control groups (33/11 mmHg; P<0.0001). After assessment of the primary end-point, patients in the control group had the option to receive the renal denervation procedure. We now report the 1-year results from the symplicity HTN-2 trial, which includes 6-month outcomes for the crossover control patients who were treated with renal denervation after the primary end-point was assessed (Figs 22.29 and 22.30).

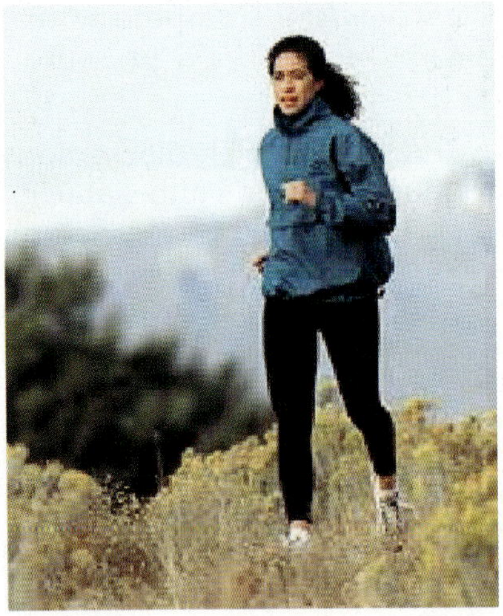

A. Jogging > 10,000 steps in 15 min

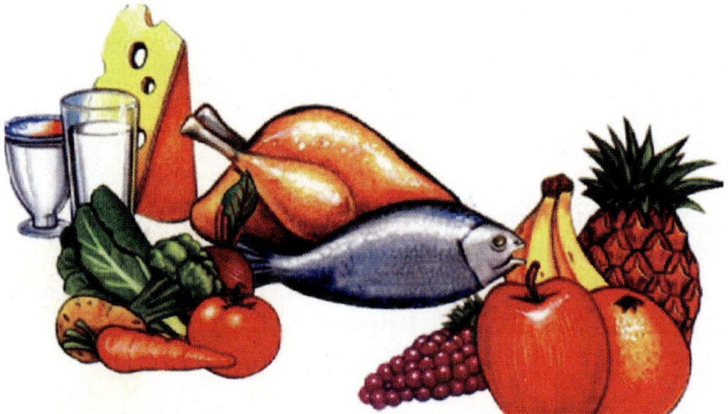

B. Liberal consumption of leafy vegetables, eggs, skimmed milk and fish meat

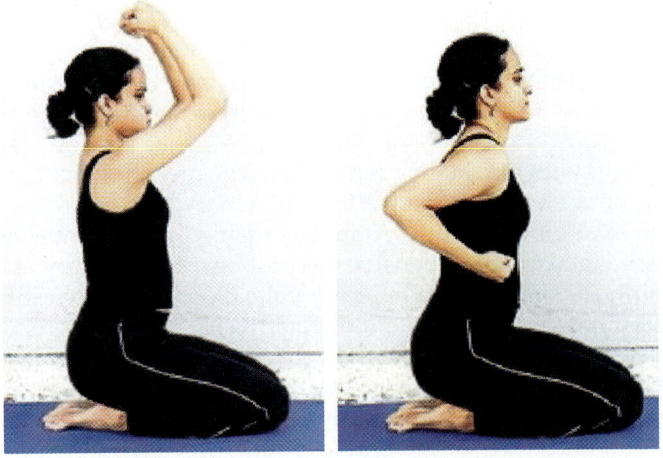

C. Yogic exercises

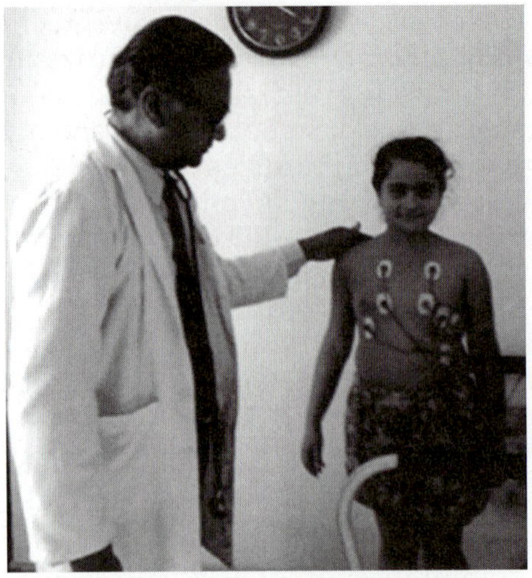

D. Doctor is preparing a young obese child for treadmill exercise

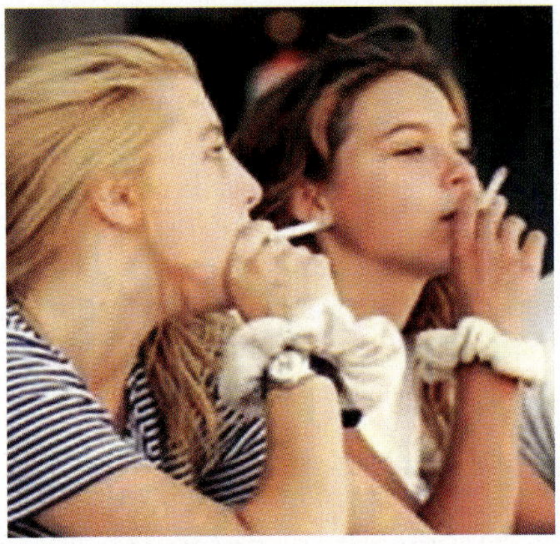

E. Two young girls are in the habit of chronic smoking. They need proper guidance for stopping this habit in order to prevent many health hazards including hypertension in their later life

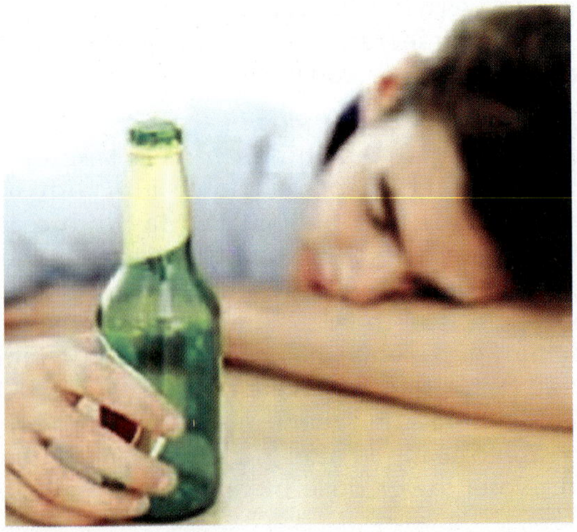

F. Advised abstain from chronic alcoholism. An adolescent is consuming over dose of alcohol with drowsiness

Fig. 22.26(A–F): *Lifestyle changes and physical activities in at prehypertension stage of blood pressure management*

Percutaneous Transluminal Angioplasty (PTA) of the Renal Artery in Severe Hypertension

Percutaneous transluminal angioplasty (PTA) of the renal artery has become an increasingly widespread peripheral vascular intervention for the treatment of renovascular hypertension (HTN). Catheter-based procedures began in 1964 when Charles Dotter initially developed PTA for treating peripheral vascular atherosclerosis. Andreas Gruntzig revolutionized the technique in 1974 when he developed a soft, flexible, double-lumen balloon catheter for use in coronary arteries. PTA has since rapidly evolved into a widely used, versatile, and dependable vascular interventional technique. Excellent results may now be achieved in the renal arteries if patients are well selected and if experienced clinicians perform the procedure (Fig. 22.27).

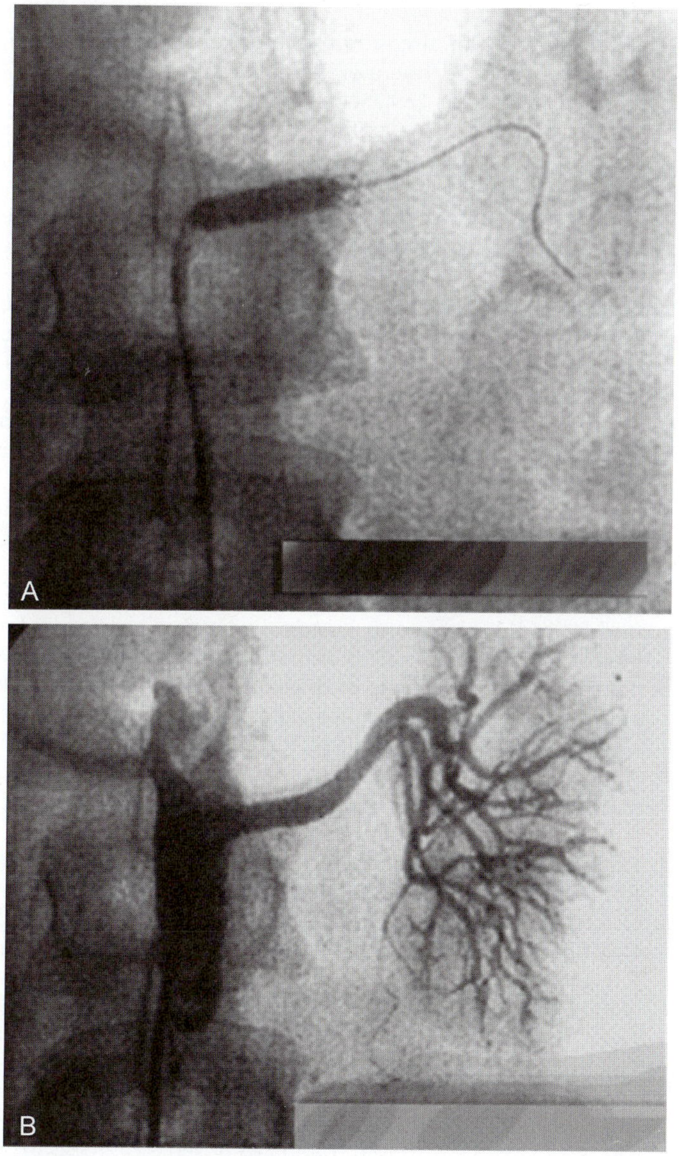

Fig. 22.27: *(A) Balloon catheter across the stenosed renal artery. (B) Fully opened renal artery after successful renal angioplasty in a young patient with resistant severe hypertension*

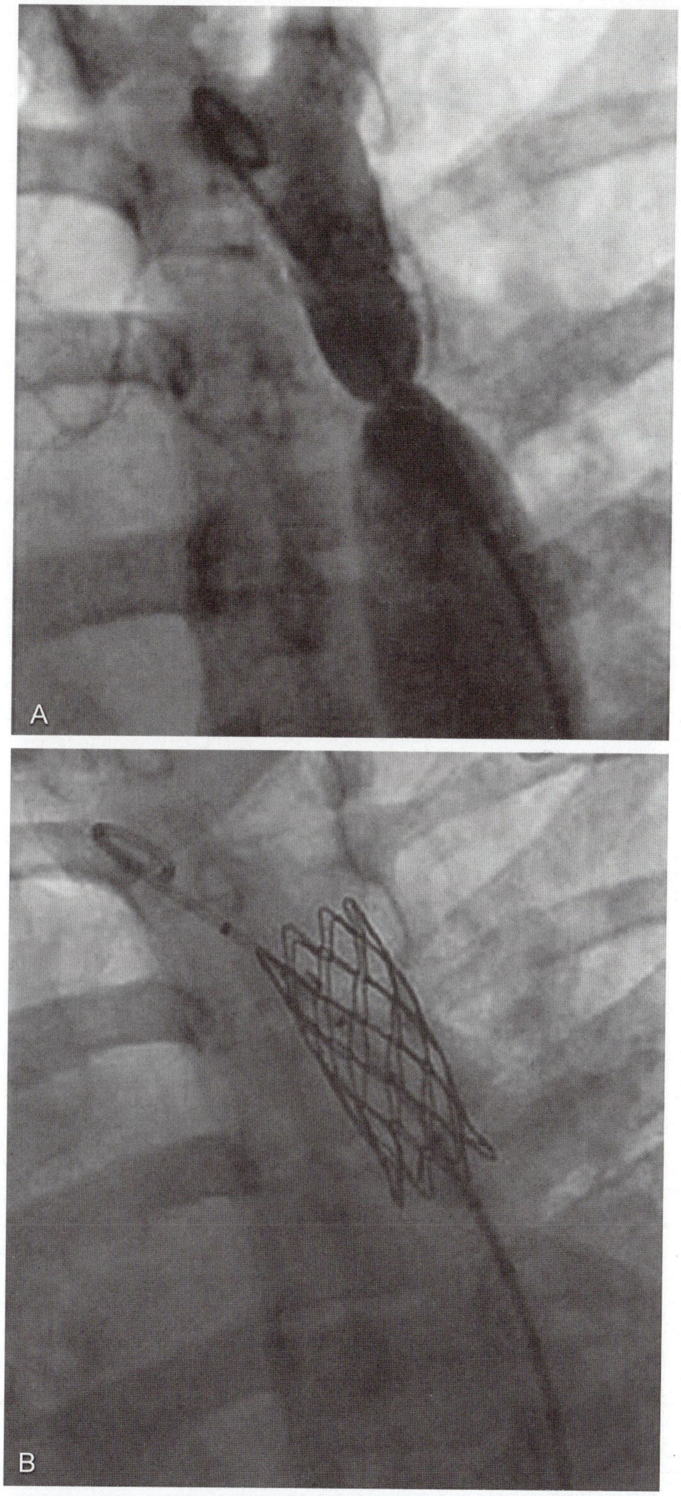

Fig. 22.28: *(A) Preoperative stage angiogram showing coarctation of aorta (B) poststent stage showing fully opened stenosed segment of aorta after successful implantation of valve stent in a young patient with resistant severe superior hypertension*

Coarctation Angioplasty in Surgical Treatment of Severe Hypertension

Significant hypertension or congestive heart failure (CHF) is an indication for intervention. Surgical relief of the aortic

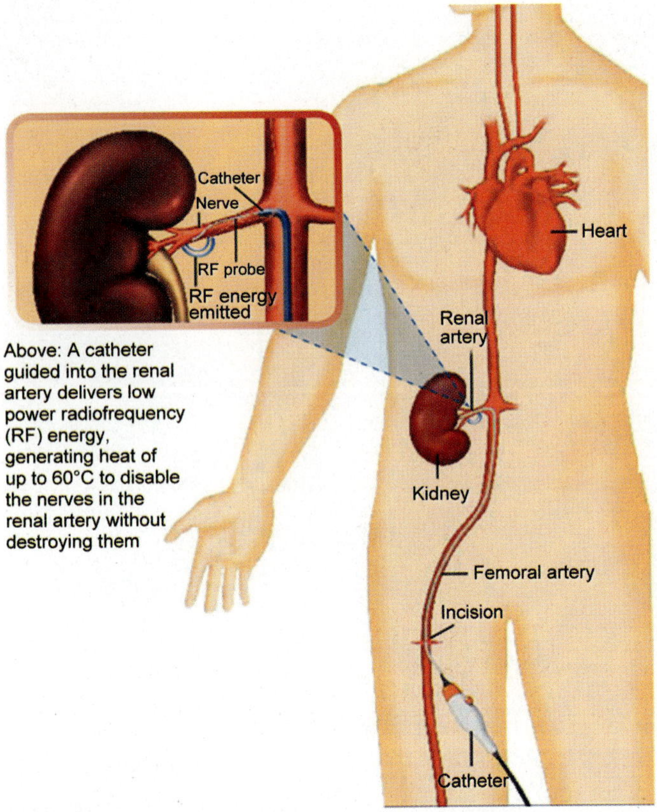

Fig. 22.29: *Technique of renal nerve denervation in treatment of resistant hypertension with symplicity renal denervation system*

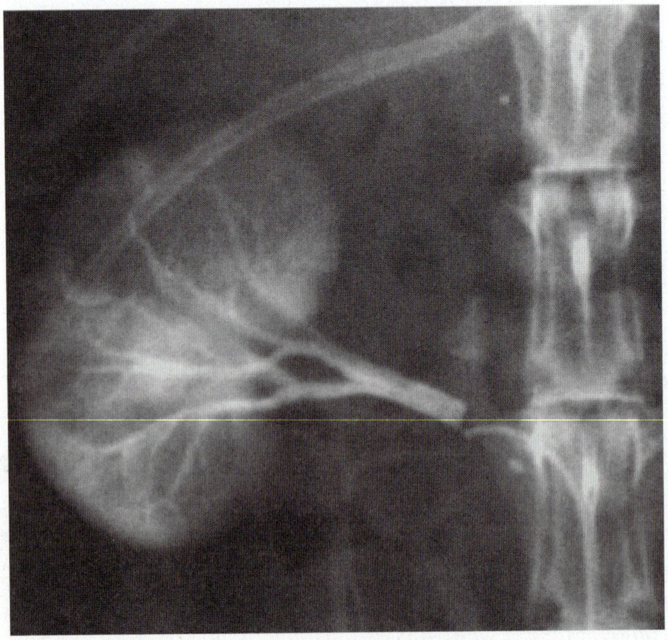

Fig. 22.30: *Renal sympathetic nerve ablation for refractory hypertension*

obstruction and catheter interventional techniques (balloon angioplasty and stents) are available alternatives. Symptomatic neonates and infants should undergo urgent intervention soon after the infant is stabilized. Asymptomatic infants, children, adolescents, and adults should undergo the procedure electively. If neither hypertension nor heart failure is present, elective surgical or balloon therapy in children aged 2–5 years is suggested. Waiting beyond age 5 years for surgery or balloon therapy to relieve aortic obstruction is not advisable because of the evidence of residual hypertension if intervention is performed after age 5 years (Fig. 22.28).

BIBLIOGRAPHY

1. National High Blood Pressure Education Program Working Group on Hypertension Control in Children and Adolescents. Update on the 1987 Task Force Report on High Blood Pressure in Children and Adolescents: a working group report from the National High Blood Pressure Education Program. Pediatrics. 1996;98:649–658.
2. Chobanian AV, Bakris GL, Black HR, et al. The seventh report of the joint national committee on prevention, detection, evaluation, and treatment of high blood pressure: the JNC 7 report. JAMA.2003; 289:2560–2572.
3. Prineas RJ, Jacobs D. Quality of Korotkoff sounds: bell vs diaphragm, cubital fossa vs brachial artery. Prev Med.1983; 12 :715 –719.
4. Londe S, Klitzner TS. Auscultatory blood pressure measurement—effect of pressure on the head of the stethoscope. West J Med.1984; 141 :193 –195
5. Prineas RJ. Blood pressure in children and adolescents. In: Bulpitt CJ, ed. Epidemiology of Hypertension. New York, NY: Elsevier; 2000:86–105. Birkenhager WH and Reid JL, eds. Handbook of Hypertension, Vol. 20.
6. Mourad A, Carney S, Gillies A, Jones B, Nanra R, Trevillian P. Arm position and blood pressure: a risk factor for hypertension? J Hum Hypertens. 2003;17:389–395
7. Netea RT, Lenders JW, Smits P, Thien T. Both body and arm position significantly influence blood pressure measurement. J Hum Hypertens. 2003;17:459–462.
8. Rocchini AP. Coarctation of the aorta and rupted aortic arch. In: Moller JH, Hoffmann U, eds. Pediatric Cardiovascular Medicine. New York, NY: Churchill Livingstone; 2000:570.
9. Gomez-Marin O, Prineas RJ, Rastam L. Cuff bladder width and blood pressure measurement in children and adolescents. J Hypertens. 1992;10:1235–1241.
10. American Heart Association. Home monitoring of high blood pressure. Available at: www.americanheart.org/presenter.jhtml? identifier = 576. Accessed March 18,2004
11. Prineas RJ. Measurement of blood pressure in the obese. Ann Epidemiol. 1991;1:321–336.
12. Ostchega Y, Prineas RJ, Paulose-Ram R, Grim CM, Willard G, Collins D. National Health and Nutrition Examination Survey 1999–2000: effect of observer training and protocol standardization on reducing blood pressure measurement error. J Clin Epidemiol. 2003;56:768–774.
13. Lewington S, Clarke R, Qizilbash N, Peto R, Collins R. Age-specific relevance of usual blood pressure to vascular mortality: a meta-analysis of individual data for one million adults in 61 prospective studies. Lancet. 2002;360:1903–1913.
14. Jones DW, Appel LJ, Sheps SG, Roccella EJ, Lenfant C. Measuring blood pressure accurately: new and persistent challenges. JAMA. 2003;289:1027–1030.

15. Canzanello VJ, Jensen PL, Schwartz GL. Are aneroid sphygmomanometers accurate in hospital and clinic settings? Arch Intern Med. 2001;161:729–731.
16. Butani L, Morgenstern BZ. Are pitfalls of oxcillometric blood pressure measurements preventable in children? Pediatr Nephrol. 2003;18:313–318.
17. Kaufmann MA, Pargger H, Drop LJ. Oscillometric blood pressure measurements by different devices are not interchangeable. Anesth Analg. 1996;82:377–381.
18. Park MK, Menard SW, Yuan C. Comparison of auscultatory and oscillometric blood pressures. Arch Pediatr Adolesc Med. 2001;155:50–53.
19. O'Brien E, Pickering T, Asmar R, et al. Working Group on Blood Pressure Monitoring of the European Society of Hypertension International Protocol for validation of blood pressure measuring devices in adults. Blood Press Monit. 2002;7:3–17.
20. O'Brien E, Coats A, Owens P, et al. Use and interpretation of ambulatory blood pressure monitoring: recommendations of the British hypertension society. BMJ.2000; 320:1128–1134.
21. Sorof JM, Portman RJ. Ambulatory blood pressure measurements. Curr Opin Pediatr. 2001;13:133–137.
22. Simckes AM, Srivastava T, Alon US. Ambulatory blood pressure monitoring in children and adolescents. Clin Pediatr (Phila). 2002;41:549–564.
23. Lurbe E, Sorof JM, Daniels SR. Clinical and research aspects of ambulatory blood pressure monitoring in children. J Pediatr. 2004;144:7–16.
24. Centers for Disease Control and Prevention, National Center for Health Statistics. 2000 CDC growth charts: United States. Available at: www.cdc.gov/growthcharts. Accessed March 18,2004.
25. Task Force on Blood Pressure Control in Children. Report of the Second Task Force on Blood Pressure Control in Children—1987. National Heart, Lung, and Blood Institute, Bethesda, Maryland. Pediatrics. 1987;79:1–25.
26. Sorof J, Daniels S. Obesity hypertension in children: a problem of epidemic proportions. Hypertension. 2002; 40:441–447.
27. Ogden CL, Flegal KM, Carroll MD, Johnson CL. Prevalence and trends in overweight among US children and adolescents, 1999–2000. JAMA. 2002;288:1728–1732.
28. Reaven GM. Insulin resistance/compensatory hyperinsulinemia, essential hypertension, and cardiovascular disease. J Clin Endocrinol Metab. 2003;88:2399–2403.
29. National Cholesterol Education Program. Third report of the Expert Panel on Detection, Evaluation, and Treatment of High Blood Cholesterol in Adults (Adult Treatment Panel III) final report. NIH Publication 02–5215. Bethesda, MD: National Heart, Lung, and Blood Institute, National Cholesterol Education Program; 2002.
30. Sinaiko AR, Steinberger J, Moran A, Prineas RJ, Jacobs DR Jr. Relation of insulin resistance to blood pressure in childhood. J Hypertens. 2002;20:509–517.
31. Cook S, Weitzman M, Auinger P, Nguyen M, Dietz WH. Prevalence of a metabolic syndrome phenotype in adolescents: findings from the Third National Health and Nutrition Examination Survey, 1988–1994. Arch Pediatr Adolesc Med. 2003;157:1–827.
32. Williams CL, Hayman LL, Daniels SR, et al. Cardiovascular health in childhood: a statement for health professionals from the Committee on Atherosclerosis, Hypertension, and Obesity in the Young (AHOY) of the Council on Cardiovascular Disease in the Young, American Heart Association. Circulation. 2002;106:143–160.
33. Quan SF, Gersh BJ. Cardiovascular consequences of sleep-disordered breathing: past, present and future: report of a workshop from the National Center on Sleep Disorders Research and the National Heart, Lung, and Blood Institute. Circulation. 2004;109:951–957.
34. Strohl KP. Invited commentary: to sleep, perchance to discover. Am J Epidemiol. 2002;155:394–395.
35. Marcus CL, Greene MG, Carroll JL. Blood pressure in children with obstructive sleep apnea. Am J Respir Crit Care Med. 1998;157:1098–1103.
36. Enright PL, Goodwin JL, Sherrill DL, Quan JR, Quan SF. Blood pressure elevation associated with sleep-related breathing disorder in a community sample of white and Hispanic children: the Tucson Children's Assessment of Sleep Apnea study. Arch Pediatr Adolesc Med. 2003;157:901–904.
37. Mindell JA, Owens JA. A Clinical Guide to Pediatric Sleep: Diagnosis and Management of Sleep Problems. Philadelphia, PA: Lippincott, Williams & Wilkins; 2003:10
38. Sinaiko AR. Hypertension in children. N Engl J Med. 1996; 335:1968–1973.
39. Flynn JT. Evaluation and management of hypertension in childhood. Prog Pediatr Cardiol. 2001;12:177–188.
40. Hiner LB, Falkner B. Renovascular hypertension in children. Pediatr Clin North Am. 1993;40:123–140.
41. Dillon MJ, Ryness JM. Plasma renin activity and aldosterone concentration in children. Br Med J. 1975;4(5992):316–319.
42. Guzzetta PC, Potter BM, Ruley EJ, Majd M, Bock GH. Renovascular hypertension in children: current concepts in evaluation and treatment. J Pediatr Surg. 1989;24:1236–1240.
43. Watson AR, Balfe JW, Hardy BE. Renovascular hypertension in childhood: a changing perspective in management. J Pediatr. 1985;106:366–372.
44. Dillon MJ. The diagnosis of renovascular disease. Pediatr Nephrol. 1997;11:366–372.
45. Mena E, Bookstein JJ, Holt JF, Fry WJ. Neurofibromatosis and renovascular hypertension in children. Am J Roentgenol Radium Ther Nucl Med. 1973;118:39–45.
46. Shahdadpuri J, Frank R, Gauthier BG, Siegel DN, Trachtman H. Yield of renal arteriography in the evaluation of pediatric hypertension. Pediatr Nephrol. 2000;14:816–819.
47. Binkert CA, Debatin JF, Schneider E, et al. Can MR measurement of renal artery flow and renal volume predict the outcome of percutaneous transluminal renal angioplasty? Cardiovasc Intervent Radiol. 2001;24:233–239.
48. Marcos HB, Choyke PL. Magnetic resonance angiography of the kidney. Semin Nephrol. 2000;20:450–455.
49. Debatin JF, Spritzer CE, Grist TM, et al. Imaging of the renal arteries: value of MR angiography. AJR Am J Roentgenol. 1991;157:981–990.
50. Vade A, Agrawal R, Lim-Dunham J, Hartoin D. Utility of computed tomographic renal angiogram in the management of childhood hypertension. Pediatr Nephrol. 2002;17:741–747.
51. MacMahon S, Peto R, Cutler J, et al. Blood pressure, stroke, and coronary heart disease. Part 1, prolonged differences in blood pressure: prospective observational studies corrected

for the regression dilution bias. Lancet. 1990;335:765–774.
52. Still JL, Cottom D. Severe hypertension in childhood. Arch Dis Child. 1967;42:34–39.
53. Gill DG, Mendes dC, Cameron JS, Joseph MC, Ogg CS, Chantler C. Analysis of 100 children with severe and persistent hypertension. Arch Dis Child. 1976;51:951–956.
54. Johnstone LM, Jones CL, Grigg LE, Wilkinson JL, Walker RG, Powell HR. Left ventricular abnormalities in children, adolescents and young adults with renal disease. Kidney Int. 1996;50:998–1006.
55. Mitsnefes MM, Daniels SR, Schwartz SM, Khoury P, Strife CF. Changes in left ventricular mass in children and adolescents during chronic dialysis. Pediatr Nephrol. 2001; 16:318–323.
56. Mitsnefes MM, Kimball TR, Witt SA, Glascock BJ, Khoury PR, Daniels SR. Left ventricular mass and systolic performance in pediatric patients with chronic renal failure. Circulation. 2003;107:864 –868.
57. Berenson GS, Srinivasan SR, Bao W, Newman WP III, Tracy RE, Wattigney WA. Association between multiple cardiovascular risk factors and atherosclerosis in children and young adults. The Bogalusa Heart Study. N Engl J Med. 1998;338:1650–1656.
58. McGill HC Jr, McMahan CA, Zieske AW, Malcom GT, Tracy RE, Strong JP. Effects of nonlipid risk factors on atherosclerosis in youth with a favorable lipoprotein profile. Circulation. 2001;103:1546–1550.
59. Davis PH, Dawson JD, Riley WA, Lauer RM. Carotid intimal-medial thickness is related to cardiovascular risk factors measured from childhood through middle age: the Muscatine Study. Circulation. 2001;104:2815–2819.
60. Arnett DK, Glasser SP, McVeigh G, et al. Blood pressure and arterial compliance in young adults: the Minnesota Children's Blood Pressure Study. Am J Hypertens. 2001;14: 200–205.
61. Knoflach M, Kiechl S, Kind M, et al. Cardiovascular risk factors and atherosclerosis in young males: ARMY study (Atherosclerosis Risk-Factors in Male Youngsters). Circulation. 2003;108:1064 –1069.
62. Sanchez A, Barth JD, Zhang L. The carotid artery wall thickness in teenagers is related to their diet and the typical risk factors of heart disease among adults. Atherosclerosis. 2000;152:265–266.
63. Barnes VA, Treiber FA, Davis H. Impact of transcendental meditation on cardiovascular function at rest and during acute stress in adolescents with high normal blood pressure. J Psychosom Res. 2001;51:597–605.
64. Belsha CW, Wells TG, McNiece KL, Seib PM, Plummer JK, Berry PL. Influence of diurnal blood pressure variations on target organ abnormalities in adolescents with mild essential hypertension. Am J Hypertens. 1998;11:410–417.
65. Sorof JM, Alexandrov AV, Cardwell G, Portman RJ. Carotid artery intimal-medial thickness and left ventricular hypertrophy in children with elevated blood pressure. Pediatrics. 2003;111:61–66.
66. Hanevold C, Waller J, Daniels S, Portman R, Sorof J. The effects of obesity, gender, and ethnic group on left ventricular hypertrophy and geometry in hypertensive children: a collaborative study of the International Pediatric Hypertension Association. Pediatrics. 2004;113:328–333.
67. Daniels SR, Loggie JM, Khoury P, Kimball TR. Left ventricular geometry and severe left ventricular hypertrophy in children and adolescents with essential hypertension. Circulation. 1998;97:1907–1911.
68. Svardsudd K, Wedel H, Aurell E, Tibblin G. Hypertensive eye ground changes. Prevalence, relation to blood pressure and prognostic importance. The study of men born in 1913. Acta Med Scand. 1978;204:159–167.
69. Skalina ME, Annable WL, Kliegman RM, Fanaroff AA. Hypertensive retinopathy in the newborn infant. J Pediatr. 1983;103:781.
70. Devereux RB, Alonso DR, Lutas EM, et al. Echocardiographic assessment of left ventricular hypertrophy: comparison to necropsy findings. Am J Cardiol. 1986;57:450–458.
71. Sahn DJ, DeMaria A, Kisslo J, Weyman A. Recommendations regarding quantitation in M-mode echocardiography: results of a survey of echocardiographic measurements. Circulation. 1978;58:1072–1083.
72. Daniels SR, Kimball TR, Morrison JA, Khoury P, Witt S, Meyer RA. Effect of lean body mass, fat mass, blood pressure, and sexual maturation on left ventricular mass in children and adolescents. Statistical, biological, and clinical significance. Circulation. 1995;92:3249–3254.
73. de Simone G, Daniels SR, Devereux RB, et al. Left ventricular mass and body size in normotensive children and adults: assessment of allometric relations and impact of overweight. J Am Coll Cardiol. 1992;20:1251–1260.
74. Daniels SR, Kimball TR, Morrison JA, Khoury P, Meyer RA. Indexing left ventricular mass to account for differences in body size in children and adolescents without cardiovascular disease. Am J Cardiol. 1995;76:699–701.
75. He J, Whelton PK, Appel LJ, Charleston J, Klag MJ. Long-term effects of weight loss and dietary sodium reduction on incidence of hypertension. Hypertension. 2000;35:544–549.
76. Sacks FM, Svetkey LP, Vollmer WM, et al. Effects on blood pressure of reduced dietary sodium and the Dietary Approaches to Stop Hypertension (DASH) diet. DASH-Sodium Collaborative Research Group. N Engl J Med. 2001; 344:3–10.
77. Vollmer WM, Sacks FM, Ard J, et al. Effects of diet and sodium intake on blood pressure: subgroup analysis of the DASH-sodium trial. Ann Intern Med. 2001;135:1019–1028.
78. Whelton SP, Chin A, Xin X, He J. Effect of aerobic exercise on blood pressure: a meta-analysis of randomized, controlled trials. Ann Intern Med. 2002;136:493–503.
79. Xin X, He J, Frontini MG, Ogden LG, Motsamai OI, Whelton PK. Effects of alcohol reduction on blood pressure: a meta-analysis of randomized controlled trials. Hypertension. 2001; 38:1112–1117.
80. Ayas NT, White DP, Manson JE, et al. A prospective study of sleep duration and coronary heart disease in women. Arch Intern Med. 2003;163:205–209.
81. Cook NR, Gillman MW, Rosner BA, Taylor JO, Hennekens CH. Combining annual blood pressure measurements in childhood to improve prediction of young adult blood pressure. Stat Med. 2000;19:2625–2640.
82. Lauer RM, Mahoney LT, Clarke WR. Tracking of blood pressure during childhood: the Muscatine Study. Clin Exp Hypertens A. 1986;8:515–537.
83. Lauer RM, Clarke WR. Childhood risk factors for high adult blood pressure: the Muscatine Study. Pediatrics. 1989;84:633–641.

84. Clarke WR, Woolson RF, Lauer RM. Changes in ponderosity and blood pressure in childhood: the Muscatine Study. Am J Epidemiol. 1986;124:195–206.
85. Burke V, Beilin LJ, Dunbar D. Tracking of blood pressure in Australian children. J Hypertens. 2001;19:1185–1192.
86. Figueroa-Colon R, Franklin FA, Lee JY, von Almen TK, Suskind RM. Feasibility of a clinic-based hypocaloric dietary intervention implemented in a school setting for obese children. Obes Res. 1996;4:419–429.
87. Wabitsch M, Hauner H, Heinze E, et al. Body-fat distribution and changes in the atherogenic risk-factor profile in obese adolescent girls during weight reduction. Am J Clin Nutr. 1994;60:54–60.
88. Rocchini AP, Key J, Bondie D, et al. The effect of weight loss on the sensitivity of blood pressure to sodium in obese adolescents. N Engl J Med. 1989;321:580–585.
89. Rocchini AP, Katch V, Anderson J, et al. Blood pressure in obese adolescents: effect of weight loss. Pediatrics.1988;82: 16–23.
90. Sinaiko AR, Gomez-Marin O, Prineas RJ. Relation of fasting insulin to blood pressure and lipids in adolescents and parents. Hypertension. 1997;30:1554–1559.
91. Robinson TN. Behavioural treatment of childhood and adolescent obesity. Int J Obes Relat Metab Disord.1999; 23 (suppl 2):S52–S57.
92. Epstein LH, Myers MD, Raynor HA, Saelens BE. Treatment of pediatric obesity. Pediatrics. 1998;101:554 –570.
93. Barlow SE, Dietz WH. Obesity evaluation and treatment: expert committee recommendations.The Maternal and Child Health Bureau, Health Resources and Services Administration and the Department of Health and Human Services. Pediatrics. 1998;102.
94. Krebs NF, Jacobson MS. Prevention of pediatric overweight and obesity. Pediatrics. 2003;112:424–430.
95. US. Department of Health and Human Services. The Surgeon General's Call to Action to Prevent and Decrease Overweight and Obesity. Rockville, MD: US Department of Health and Human Services, Public 94. Krebs NF, Jacobson MS. Prevention of pediatric overweight and obesity. Pediatrics. 2003;112:424–430.
95. US Department of Health and Human Services. The Surgeon General's Call to Action to Prevent and Decrease Overweight and Obesity. Rockville, MD: U.S. Department of Health and Human Services, Public Health Service, Office of the Surgeon General; 2001.
96. Gutin B, Owens S. Role of exercise intervention in improving body fat distribution and risk profile in children. Am J Human Biol. 1999;11:237–247.
97. Siega-Riz AM, Popkin BM, Carson T. Trends in breakfast consumption for children in the United States from 1965–1991. Am J Clin Nutr. 1998;67:748S–756.
98. Warren JM, Henry CJ, Simonite V. Low glycemic index breakfasts and reduced foodintake in preadolescent children. Pediatrics. 2003; 112.
99. Gillman MW, Hood MY, Moore LL, Nguyen US, Singer MR, Andon MB. Effect of calcium supplementation on blood pressure in children. J Pediatr. 1995;127:186–192.
100. Simons-Morton DG, Hunsberger SA, Van Horn L, et al. Nutrient intake and blood pressure in the Dietary Intervention Study in Children. Hypertension. 1997;29:930–936.
101. Simons-Morton DG, Obarzanek E. Diet and blood pressure in children and adolescents. Pediatr Nephrol. 1997;11:244–249.
102. Miller JZ, Weinberger MH, Christian JC. Blood pressure response to potassium supplementation in normotensive adults and children. Hypertension. 1987;10:437–442.
103. Sinaiko AR, Gomez-Marin O, Prineas RJ. Effect of low sodium diet or potassium supplementation on adolescent blood pressure. Hypertension. 1993;21:989–994.
104. Falkner B, Sherif K, Michel S, Kushner H. Dietary nutrients and blood pressure in urban minority adolescents at risk for hypertension. Arch Pediatr Adolesc Med. 2000;154:918–922.
105. Stern B, Heyden S, Miller D, Latham G, Klimas A, Pilkington K. Intervention study in high school students with elevated blood pressures. Dietary experiment with polyunsaturated fatty acids. Nutr Metab.1980;24:137–147.
106. Goldberg RJ, Ellison RC, Hosmer DW Jr, et al. Effects of alterations in fatty acid intake on the blood pressure of adolescents: the Exeter-Andover Project. Am J Clin Nutr. 1992;56:71–76.
107. Cooper R, Van Horn L, Liu K, et al. A randomized trial on the effect of decreased dietary sodium intake on blood pressure in adolescents. J Hypertens. 1984;2:361–366.
108. Falkner B, Michel S. Blood pressure response to sodium in children and adolescents. Am J Clin Nutr. 1997;65:618S–621.
109. Gillum RF, Elmer PJ, Prineas RJ. Changing sodium intake in children. The Minneapolis Children's Blood Pressure Study. Hypertension. 1981;3:698–703.
110. Howe PR, Cobiac L, Smith RM. Lack of effect of short-term changes in sodium intake on blood pressure in adolescent schoolchildren. J Hypertens. 1991;9:181–186.
111. Geleijnse JM, Hofman A, Witteman JC, Hazebroek AA, Valkenburg HA, Grobbee DE. Long-term effects of neonatal sodium restriction on blood pressure. Hypertension. 1997; 29:913 –917.
112. Martin RM, Ness AR, Gunnell D, Emmett P, Smith GD. Does breast-feeding in infancy lower blood pressure in childhood? The Avon Longitudinal Study of Parents and Children (ALSPAC). Circulation. 2004;109:1259–1266.
113. Wilson AC, Forsyth JS, Greene SA, Irvine L, Hau C, Howie PW. Relation of infant diet to childhood health: seven year follow up of cohort of children in Dundee infant feeding study. BMJ. 1998;316:21–25.
114. Panel of Dietary Intakes for Electrolytes and Water, Standing Committee on the Scientific Evaluation of Dietary Reference Intakes, Food and Nutrition Board, Institute of Medicine. Dietary Reference Intakes for Water, Potassium, Sodium, Chloride, and Sulfate. Washington, DC: National Academies Press; 2004.
115. Kelley GA, Kelley KS, Tran ZV. The effects of exercise on resting blood pressure in children and adolescents: a meta-analysis of randomized controlled trials. Prev Cardiol. 2003; 6:8–16.
116. Scott HW Jr, Bahnson HT. Evidence for a renal factor in the hypertension of experimental coarctation of the aorta. Surgery. Jul 1951;30(1):206–17.
117. Scott HW Jr, Collins HA, Langa AM, Olsen NS. Additional observations concerning the physiology of the hypertension associated with experimental coarctation of the aorta. Surgery. Sep 1954;36(3):445-59.
118. Alpert BS, Bain HH, Balfe JW, Kidd BS, Olley PM. Role of the renin-angiotensin-aldosterone system in hypertensive

children with coarctation of the aorta. Am J Cardiol. Apr 1979;43(4):828–34.

119. Bagby SB. Dissection of pathogenetic factors: I. coarctation hypertension, in Loggie. In: JMH, Horan MJ, Hohn AR, et al Ieds). Proceedings of the NHLBI Workshop on Juvenile Hypertension. Biomedical Informatio Corp. New York, NY: 1984:pp. 253–266.
120. Esler MD, Krum H, Schlaich M et al. Renal sympathetic denervation for treatment of drug-resistant hypertension: one-year results from the Symplicity HTN-2 randomized, controlled trial. Circulation 2012; 126(25):2976–82.
121. Pokushalov E, Romanov A, Corbucci G et al. A randomized comparison of pulmonary vein isolation with versus without concomitant renal artery denervation in patients with refractory symptomatic atrial fibrillation and resistant hypertension. J Am Coll Cardiol 2012; 60(13):1163–70.
122. Brandt MC, Mahfoud F, Reda S et al. Renal sympathetic denervation reduces left ventricular hypertrophy and improves cardiac function in patients with resistant hypertension. J Am Coll Cardiol 2012; 59(10):901–9.
123. Ukena C, Mahfoud F, Kindermann I et al. Cardiorespiratory response to exercise after renal sympathetic denervation in patients with resistant hypertension. J Am Coll Cardiol 2011; 58(11):1176–82.
124. Mahfoud F, Cremers B, Janker J et al. Renal hemodynamics and renal function after catheter-based renal sympathetic denervation in patients with resistant hypertension. Hypertension 2012; 60(2):419–24.
125. Catheter-based renal sympathetic denervation for resistant hypertension: durability of blood pressure reduction out to 24 months. Hypertension 2011; 57(5):911–7.

23 Obesity and Metabolic Syndrome with Cardiovascular Disease in Children and Adolescents

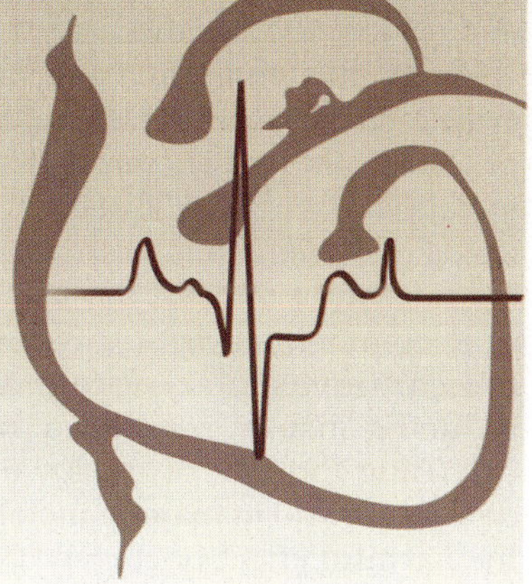

Metabolic syndrome in children represents a potentially serious threat to health in adulthood, yet many parents and caregivers do not have a clear idea of what metabolic syndrome is and why it is dangerous.

It comprises of group of cardiovascular risk factors, including obesity, hypertension, prediabetes, and reduced HDL ("good") cholesterol. Because it is difficult to know when a child is at risk for metabolic syndrome, some doctors fear that children may not be properly diagnosed.

The members of the PMSWG explored the potential for a unified and cohesive definition for metabolic syndrome. The researchers evaluated how current definitions relate to the number of children diagnosed with metabolic syndrome. They found that because of the variety of definitions used by pediatricians. It is difficult to estimate the prevalence of the syndrome among children and adolescents. Additionally, the researchers looked at how well each metabolic risk factor predicts future health issues. Dr John Morrison and colleagues from Cincinnati Children's Medical Center, Cincinnati Jewish Hospital, and Maryland Medical Research Institute collected data from a 25–30 year, study concerning cardiovascular risk factors. They found that metabolic syndrome in children may have a direct link to type 2 diabetes in adulthood. In a related article, Dr Claudio Maffeis and colleagues from the Obesity Study Group of the Italian Society of Pediatric Endocrinology and Diabetology used body mass index (BMI), waist circumference, and weight to height ratios to determine obesity in a group of 974 children. They found that evaluating waist circumference and weight to height ratio measurements may be more accurate in determining metabolic risk than using body mass index alone. These articles demonstrate that symptoms of adult metabolic syndrome begin in childhood and may be directly related to obesity. They also illustrate the need for a clear definition of metabolic syndrome in children. According to Dr Reginald Washington, "once this definition exists, medical providers who care for children will know what to look for in order to identify children who are at risk to develop adult metabolic syndrome". Such a definition could lead to better treatment of childhood metabolic syndrome, which could positively impact the growing obesity epidemic.

Cardiovascular Disease and Metabolic Syndrome

Metabolic syndrome symptoms significantly increase the chances of developing cardiovascular disease, which, if neglected, can lead to a heart attack or stroke.

Having three or more traits of metabolic syndrome raises the risk of coronary death, according to a recent study in Circulation: Journal of the American Heart Association Even one or two symptoms of metabolic syndrome increase the danger of dying from cardiovascular disease.

Diagnosis of Metabolic Syndrome

- A BMI (body mass index) of 30 kg/m^2 or greater which is classed as obesity
- HDL "good" cholesterol less than 40 mg/dL if male or less than 50 mg/dL if female
- Triglycerides greater than or equal to 150 mg/dL if fasting or greater than or equal to 400 mg/dL if not fasting
- Blood pressure greater than or equal to 130/85 mmHg or if the patient was on antihypertension (high blood pressure) medication
- Glucose greater than or equal to 110 mg/dL if fasting or 2-hour postload glucose greater than or equal to 140 mg/dL. Overall, 26% of participants had metabolic syndrome and 19.8% had preexisting cardiovascular disease.
- More attention to the medical management of elevated risk factors is essential to prevent metabolic syndrome, diabetes and their complications.

Insulin resistance-linked obesity is an underlying cause of metabolic syndrome. Insulin is produced in the pancreas and released into the circulatory system where it is crucial to the absorption of glucose by the body's cells. If the cells resist insulin, then both insulin and glucose build up in your blood. Excess insulin leads to weight gain and high blood pressure—both precursors to metabolic syndrome and cardiovascular disease.

As insulin comes in contact with the interior wall of the arteries, it damages the tissue, causing the initial injury that produces plaque. Therefore, having insulin resistance and metabolic syndrome directly cause changes in the blood lipids and overall cardiovascular health that contribute to the formation of heart disease.

Recommendations for reducing the risk of damage to the cardiovascular system are the same as those for reducing insulin resistance, namely decreasing insulin, balancing cholesterol and lowering blood pressure. Action centers around managing metabolic syndrome to minimize the harmful effect of current symptoms and prevent or at least delay the worsening of underlying conditions that can lead to heart disease. This can be done through careful food choices including a balanced, nutritious diet, exercise and weight loss in overweight individuals.

But, there is no one "magic" pill to reverse metabolic syndrome. To address all the symptoms, a complete system is required which includes nutraceuticals (vitamins, herbs and minerals that are disease specific), a realistic exercise program combined with nutritional guidance and a support network that will help you change unhealthy lifestyle choices.

The unique, new Insulite MetaX System, which has been scientifically-designed to help reduce risk factors for cardiovascular disease such as high cholesterol and high blood pressure (hypertension) by balancing glucose and insulin levels. Among the Insulite MetaX System formulations is one called InsulX that includes alpha lipoic acid which increases insulin insensitivity and lowers glucose levels.

Clinical Outcomes of Metabolic Syndrome

ATP III viewed CVD as the primary clinical outcome of metabolic syndrome. Most individuals who develop CVD have multiple risk factors. In 1988, Reaven noted that several risk factors (e.g. dyslipidemia, hypertension, hyperglycemia) commonly cluster together. This clustering he called syndrome X, and he recognized it as a multiplex risk factor for CVD. Reaven and subsequently others postulated that insulin resistance underlies syndrome X (hence the commonly used term insulin resistance syndrome). Other researchers use the term metabolic syndrome for this clustering of metabolic risk factors. ATP III used this alternative term. It avoids the implication that insulin resistance is the primary or only cause of associated risk factors. Although ATP III identified CVD as the primary clinical outcome of the metabolic syndrome, most people with this syndrome have insulin resistance, which confers increased risk for type 2 diabetes. When diabetes becomes clinically apparent, CVD risk rises sharply. Beyond CVD and type 2 diabetes, individuals with metabolic syndrome seemingly are susceptible to other conditions, notably polycystic ovary syndrome, fatty liver, cholesterol gallstones, asthma, sleep disturbances, and some forms of cancer.

Components of Metabolic Syndrome

ATP III1 identified six components of the metabolic syndrome that relate to CVD:

1. Abdominal obesity
2. Atherogenic dyslipidemia
3. Raised blood pressure
4. Insulin resistance ± glucose intolerance
5. Proinflammatory state
6. Prothrombotic state.

These components of the metabolic syndrome constitute a particular combination of what ATP III terms underlying, major, and emerging risk factors. According to ATP III, underlying risk factors for CVD are obesity (especially abdominal obesity), physical inactivity, and atherogenic diet; the major risk factors are cigarette smoking, hypertension, elevated LDL cholesterol, low HDL cholesterol, family history of premature coronary heart disease (CHD), and aging; and the emerging risk factors include elevated triglycerides, small LDL particles, insulin resistance, glucose intolerance, proinflammatory state, and prothrombotic state.

Abdominal obesity is the form of obesity most strongly associated with the metabolic syndrome. It presents clinically as increased waist circumference.

Atherogenic dyslipidemia manifests in routine lipoprotein analysis by raised triglycerides and low concentrations of HDL cholesterol. A more detailed analysis usually reveals other lipoprotein abnormalities, e.g. increased remnant lipoproteins, elevated apolipoprotein B, small LDL particles, and small HDL particles. All of these abnormalities have been implicated as being independently atherogenic.

Elevated blood pressure strongly associates with obesity and commonly occurs in insulin-resistant persons. Hypertension thus commonly is listed among metabolic risk factors. However, some investigators believe that hypertension is less "metabolic" than other metabolic-syndrome components. Certainly, hypertension is multifactorial in origin. For example, increasing arterial stiffness contributes significantly to systolic hypertension in the elderly.

Insulin resistance is present in the majority of people with the metabolic syndrome. It strongly associates with other metabolic risk factors and correlates univariately with CVD risk. These associations, combined with belief in its priority, account for the term insulin resistance syndrome. Even so, mechanisms underlying the link to CVD risk factors are uncertain, hence the ATP III's classification of insulin resistance as an emerging risk factor. Patients with long-standing insulin resistance frequently manifest glucose intolerance, another emerging risk factor. When glucose intolerance evolves into diabetes-level hyperglycemia, elevated glucose constitutes a major, independent risk factor for CVD.

A proinflammatory state, recognized clinically by elevations of C-reactive protein (CRP), is commonly present in persons with metabolic syndrome. Multiple mechanisms seemingly underlie elevations of CRP. One cause is obesity, because excess adipose tissue releases inflammatory cytokines that may elicit higher CRP levels.

A prothrombotic state, characterized by increased plasma plasminogen activator inhibitor (PAI)-1 and fibrinogen, also associates with the metabolic syndrome. Fibrinogen, an acute-phase reactant like CRP, rises in response to a high-cytokine state. Thus, prothrombotic and proinflammatory states may be metabolically interconnected.

Pathogenesis of Metabolic Syndrome

The metabolic syndrome seems to have three potential etiological categories:

1. Obesity and disorders of adipose tissue
2. Insulin resistance
3. Constellation of independent factors (e.g. molecules of hepatic, vascular and immunologic origin) that mediate specific components of the metabolic syndrome. Other factors aging, proinflammatory state, and hormonal changes have been implicated as contributors as well.

1. *Obesity and Abnormal Body Fat Distribution*

ATP III considered the "obesity epidemic" as mainly responsible for the rising prevalence of metabolic syndrome. Obesity contributes to hypertension, high serum cholesterol, low HDL cholesterol, hyperglycemia, and it otherwise associates with higher CVD risk. Abdominal obesity especially correlates with metabolic risk factors. Excess adipose tissue releases several products that apparently exacerbate these risk factors. They include nonesterified fatty acids (NEFA), cytokines, PAI-1, and adiponectin. A high plasma NEFA level overloads muscle and liver with lipid, which enhances insulin resistance. High CRP levels accompanying obesity may signify cytokine excess and a proinflammatory state. An elevated PAI-1 contributes to a prothrombotic state whereas low adiponectin levels that accompany obesity correlate with

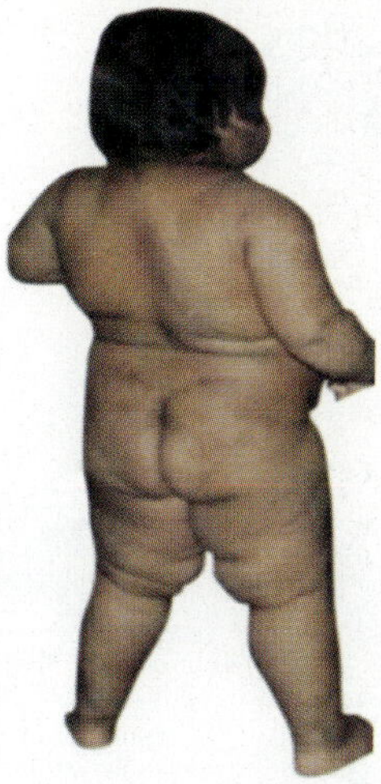

Fig. 23.2: *A defined 2 years obese child weighing 32 kg prone to metabolic syndrome*

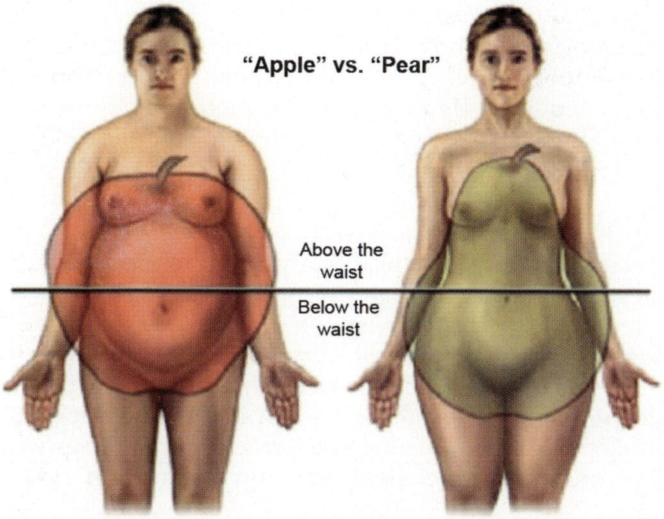

Fig. 23.3: *Types of obesity in childhood and adolescents as one of the factors in metabolic syndrome*

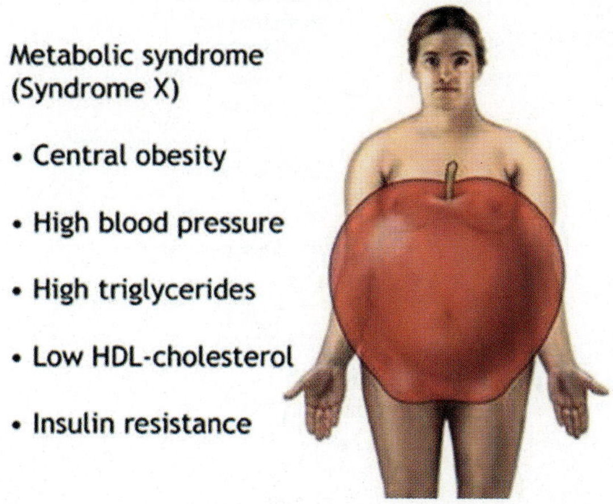

Fig. 23.1: *Physical and biochemical parameters of metabolic syndrome*

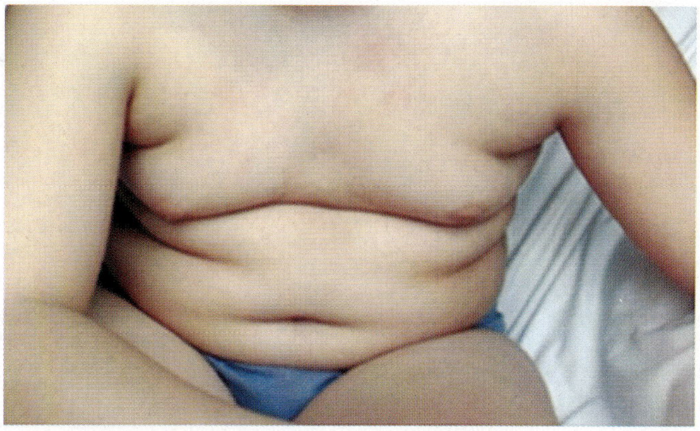

Fig. 23.4: *Fatty folds over breast and abdominal areas in an obese child*

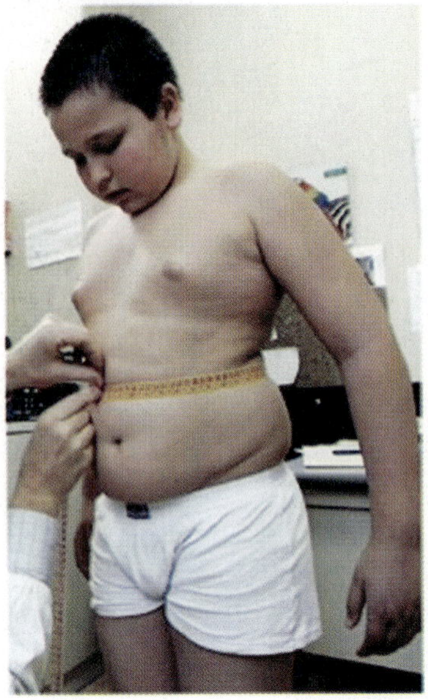

Fig. 23.5: *Measuring abdominal girth in an obese child*

worsening of metabolic risk factors. The strong connection between obesity (especially abdominal obesity) and risk factors led ATP III to define the metabolic syndrome essentially as a clustering of metabolic complications of obesity (Figs 23.1 to 23.5).

2. *Insulin Resistance*

A second category of causation is insulin resistance. Many investigators place a greater priority on insulin resistance than on obesity in pathogenesis. They argue that insulin resistance, or its accomplice, hyperinsulinemia, directly causes other metabolic risk factors. Identifying a unique role for insulin resistance is complicated by the fact that it is linked to obesity. Insulin resistance generally rises with increasing body fat content, yet a broad range of insulin sensitivities exists at any given level of body fat. Most people with categorical obesity [body mass index (BMI) kg/m^2] have postprandial hyperinsulinemia and relatively low insulin sensitivity, but variation in insulin sensitivities exists even within the obese population. Overweight persons (BMI 25–29.9 kg/m^2) likewise exhibit a spectrum of insulin sensitivities, suggesting an inherited component to insulin resistance. In some populations (e.g. South Asians), insulin resistance occurs commonly even with BMI <25 kg/m^2 and apparently contributes to a high prevalence of type 2 diabetes and premature CVD. South Asians and others who manifest insulin resistance with only mild-to-moderate overweight can be said to have primary insulin resistance. Even with primary insulin resistance, however, weight gain seems to enhance insulin resistance and metabolic syndrome. Thus, dissociation of obesity and primary insulin resistance in patients with metabolic syndrome is difficult (Fig. 23.5).

This is not to say that insulin resistance per se does not play a significant role in causation of metabolic syndrome. When insulin-resistant muscle is already overloaded with lipid from high plasma NEFA levels, some excess NEFA presumably is diverted to the liver, promoting fatty liver and atherogenic dyslipidemia. Hyperinsulinemia may enhance output of very-low-density lipoprotein triglycerides, raising triglycerides. Insulin resistance in muscle predisposes to glucose intolerance, which can be worsened by increased hepatic gluconeogenesis in insulin-resistant liver. Finally, insulin resistance may raise blood pressure by a variety of mechanisms.

3. *Independent Factors that Mediate Specific Components of the Metabolic Syndrome*

Beyond obesity and insulin resistance, each risk factor of the metabolic syndrome is subject to its own regulation through both genetic and acquired factors. This leads to variability in expression of risk factors. Lipoprotein

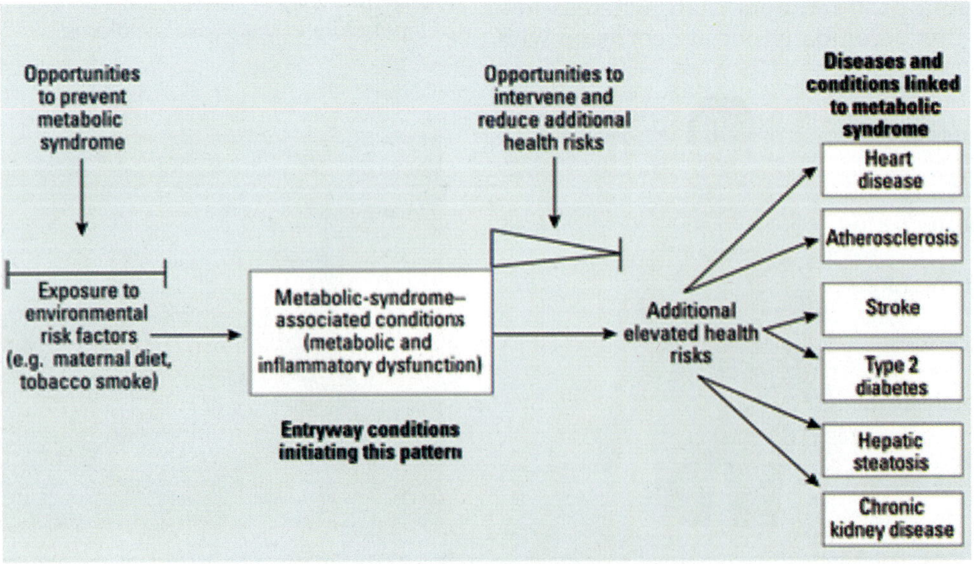

Fig. 23.6: *Prototype of disease in metabolic syndrome*

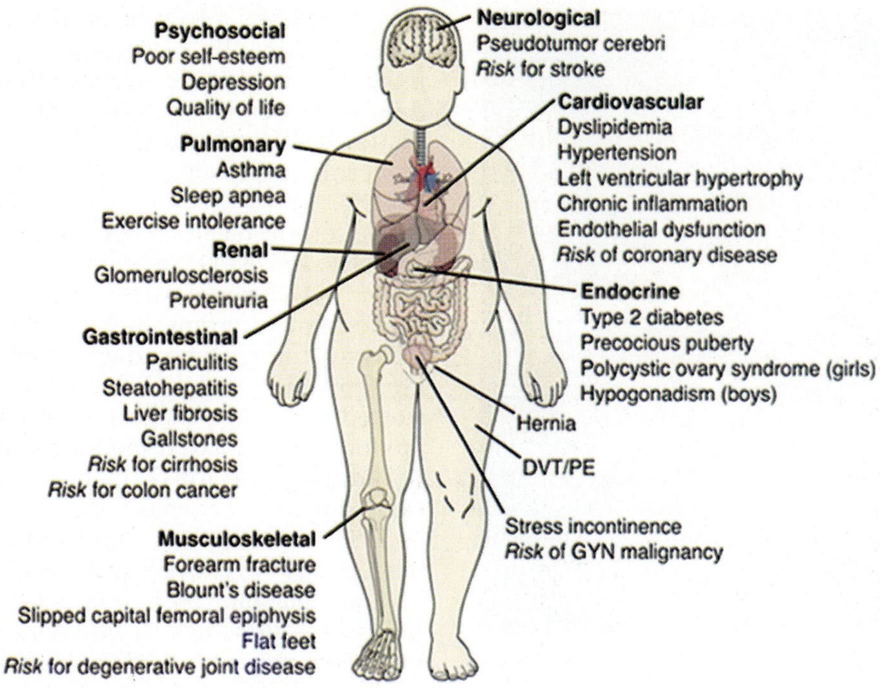

Fig. 23.7: *Depicting various systemic complications in metabolic syndrome*

metabolism, for instance, is richly modulated by genetic variation; hence, expression of dyslipidemias in response to obesity and/or insulin resistance varies considerably. The same holds for blood pressure regulation. Moreover, glucose levels depend on insulin-secretory capacity as well as insulin sensitivity. This variation in distal regulation cannot be ignored as an important factor in causation of metabolic syndrome.

Other Contributing Factors

Advancing age probably affects all levels of pathogenesis, which likely explains why prevalence of the metabolic syndrome rises with advancing age. Recently, a proinflammatory state has been implicated directly in causation of insulin resistance, as well as atherogenesis. Finally, several endocrine factors have been linked to abnormalities in body fat distribution and hence indirectly to metabolic syndrome. Thus, pathogenesis of the metabolic syndrome is complex and ripe with opportunities for further research.

Therapeutic Implications

Obesity and Body Fat Distribution as Targets of Therapy

ATP III recommended that obesity be the primary target of intervention for metabolic syndrome. First-line therapy should be weight reduction reinforced with increased physical activity. Weight loss lowers serum cholesterol and triglycerides, raises HDL cholesterol, lowers blood pressure and glucose, and reduces insulin resistance. Recent data further show that weight reduction can decrease serum levels of CRP and PAI-1. Most of the concerned workers believe that obesity contributes significantly to development of the metabolic syndrome in the general population. They further acknowledged that clinical management should focus first on lifestyle changes particularly weight reduction and increased exercise. Even those who emphasized the role of insulin resistance in the pathogenesis of the metabolic syndrome acknowledged that therapeutic lifestyle changes deserve priority. Some

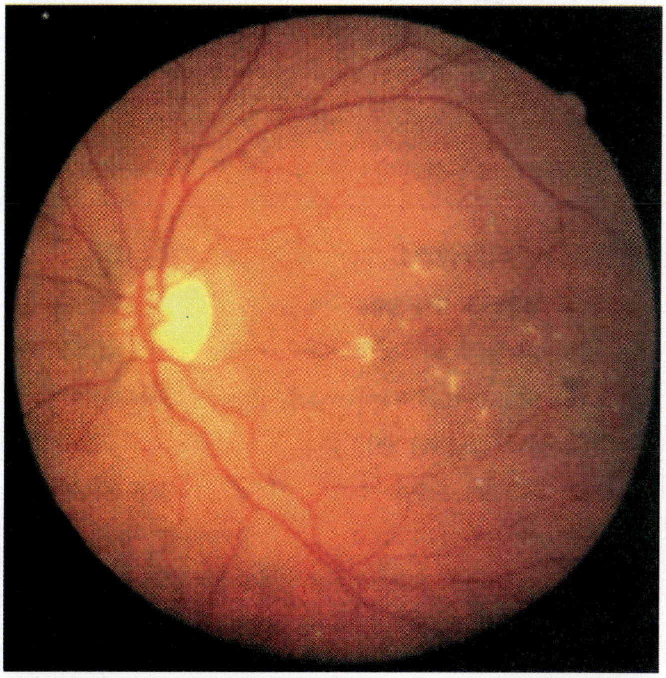

Fig. 23.8A: *Photomicrograph showing ocular fundoscopic appearance of diabetic maculopathy in patient wih metabolic syndrome*

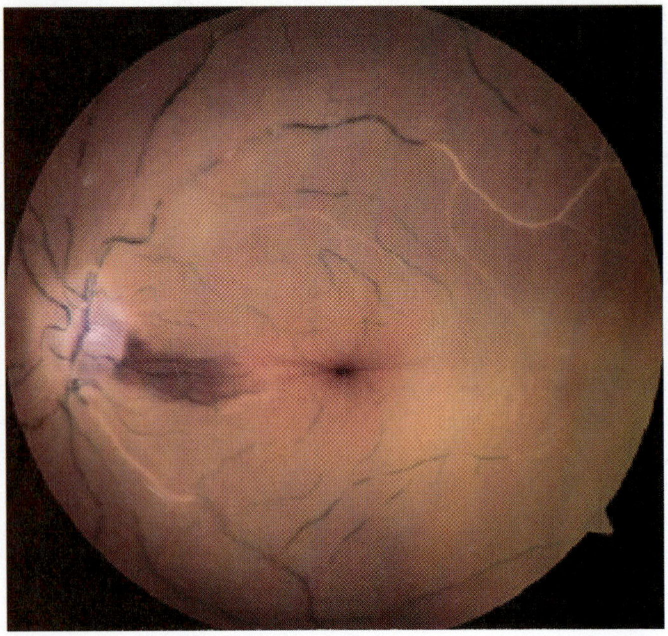

Fig. 23.8B: *Central retinal artery occlusion in a patient with metabolic syndrome*

participants questioned whether such changes could successfully be implemented in clinical practice. Still, the potential for benefit certainly exists; implementation is the challenge.

Insulin Resistance as Target of Therapy

If insulin resistance, whether primary or secondary to obesity, is in the chain of causation of metabolic syndrome, it would be an attractive target. Certainly, weight reduction and increased physical activity will reduce insulin resistance. Insulin resistance as a target has caught the imagination of the pharmaceutical industry, and drug discovery is underway. Two classes of drugs are currently available that reduce insulin resistance. These are metformin and insulin sensitizers such as thiazolidinediones (TZDs).

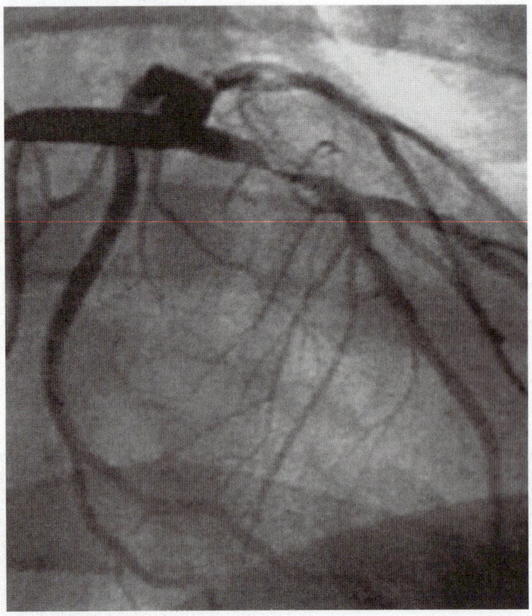

Fig. 23.9: *Coronary angiogram demonstrating 95% stenosis in the proximal left anterior descending coronary artery in a young person with metabolic syndrome*

Metformin has long been used for treatment of type 2 diabetes. In UKPDS, metformin apparently reduced new-onset CHD in obese patients with diabetes. In the Diabetes Prevention Program, metformin therapy prevented (or delayed) onset of type 2 diabetes in persons with IGT. There are, however, no CVD end-point studies on metformin-treated patients with metabolic syndrome. Thus, at present, metformin cannot be recommended for the express purpose of reducing risk for CVD in persons with the metabolic syndrome.

TZDs currently are approved for treatment of type 2 diabetes. They reduce insulin resistance, favorably modify several metabolic risk factors, and reverse abnormal arterial responses. Nonetheless, no clinical trial data yet exist to document benefit in CVD risk reduction. Thus, in spite of promise, TZDs cannot be recommended at present for preventing CVD in patients with either metabolic syndrome or diabetes.

Specific Metabolic Risk Factors as Targets of Therapy

Atherogenic Dyslipidemia

Although statins typically are recognized to be LDL-lowering drugs, they reduce all apolipoprotein B containing lipoproteins. Recent subgroup analyses of statin trials reveal that statins reduce risk for CVD events in patients with metabolic syndrome. Fibrates also favorably modify atherogenic dyslipidemia and may directly reduce atherogenesis. Post hoc analysis of recent fibrate trials strongly suggests that they reduce CVD end-points in patients with atherogenic dyslipidemia and metabolic syndrome. Moreover, clinical studies demonstrate that abnormal lipoprotein patterns are doubly improved by combined statin-fibrate therapy, but just how much this combination reduces CVD events beyond statins alone awaits demonstration with controlled clinical trials (Figs 23.9 to 23.11).

Elevated Blood Pressure

There is full agreement that hypertensive patients with metabolic syndrome deserve lifestyle therapies to reduce blood pressure. In addition, antihypertensive drugs should be used as recommended by hypertension guidelines. No class of antihypertensive drugs has been identified as being uniquely efficacious in patients with metabolic syndrome.

Prothrombotic State

No drugs are available that target PAI-1 and fibrinogen. An alternative approach to the prothrombotic state is antiplatelet therapy. For example, low-dose aspirin reduces CVD events in both secondary and primary prevention. Thus, use of aspirin for primary prevention in patients with

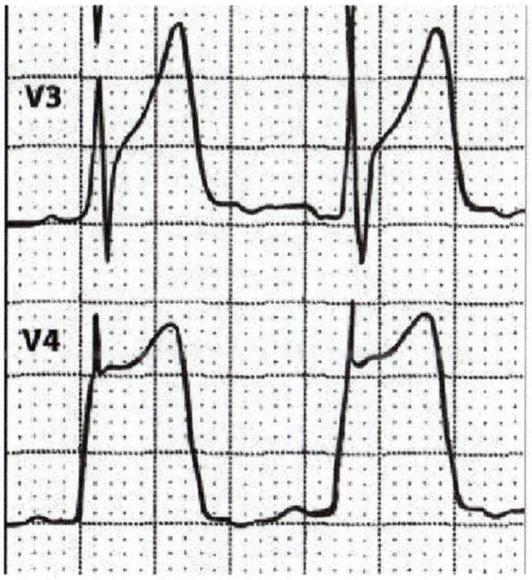

Fig. 23.10: *ECG showing coronary vasospasm (Prinzmetal's angina) localised ST elevation with reciprocal ST depression occurring during episodes of chest pain in a patient with metabolic syndrome*

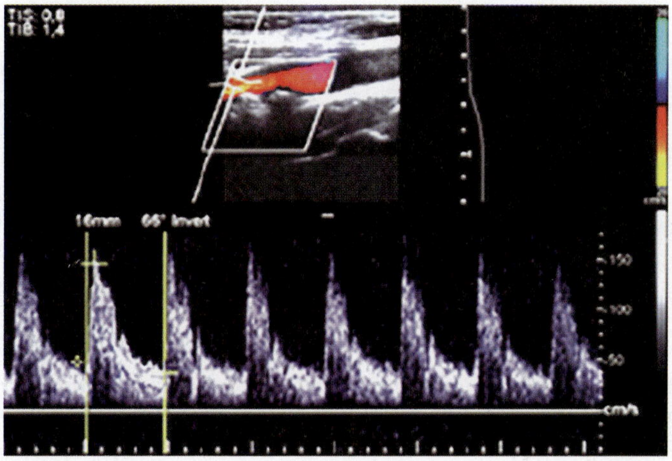

Fig. 23.11: *Doppler ultrasound of right internal carotid artery with calcified and noncalcified plaques showing less than 70% stenosis in an female adolescent with metabolic syndrome*

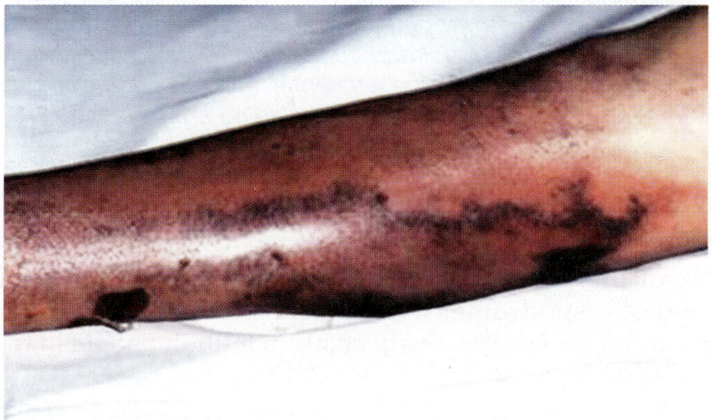

Fig. 23.12: *Leg swelling, change in color of skin and reduced blood flow may be an indication of peripheral arterial disease in metabolic syndrome*

metabolic syndrome is promising. According to current recommendations, low-dose aspirin therapy has a favorable efficacy/side effect ratio when 10-year risk for CHD is 10%.

Proinflammatory State

There is growing interest in development of drugs to dampen the proinflammatory state. Several lipid-lowering drugs will reduce CRP levels which could reflect an anti-inflammatory action.

Hyperglycemia

When patients with metabolic syndrome develop type 2 diabetes, they are at high risk for CVD. All CVD risk factors should be intensively reduced. In addition, glucose levels should be appropriately treated with lifestyle therapies and hypoglycemic agents as needed to keep hemoglobin A1c levels below guideline targets.

Key Points in Metabolic Sydrome

What is metabolic syndrome?

An association between certain metabolic disorders and cardiovascular disease has been known since the 1940s. In the 1980s, this association became more clearly defined and the term metabolic syndrome (also known as syndrome X or the dysmetabolic syndrome) was coined to designate a cluster of metabolic risk factors that come together in a single individual. In more current times, the term metabolic syndrome is found throughout medical literature and in the lay press as well. There are slight differences in the criteria of diagnosis–depending on which authority is quoted. Regardless, the concept of a clustering of risks leading to cardiovascular disease is well accepted (Figs 23.12 and 23.16).

The main features of metabolic syndrome include insulin resistance, hypertension (high blood pressure), cholesterol abnormalities, and an increased risk for clotting. Patients are most often overweight or obese.

Insulin resistance refers to the diminished ability of cells to respond to the action of insulin in promoting the transport of the sugar glucose, from blood into muscles and other tissues. Because of the central role that insulin resistance plays in the metabolic syndrome, a separate article is devoted to insulin resistance. Please see insulin resistance article for more information.

How is metabolic syndrome defined?

The definition of metabolic syndrome depends on which group of experts is doing the defining. Based on the guidelines from the 2001 National Cholesterol Education Program Adult Treatment Panel (ATP III), any three of the following traits in the same individual meet the criteria for the metabolic syndrome:

Abdominal obesity: A waist circumference over 102 cm (40 in) in men and over 88 cm (35 inches) in women (Table 23.1 to 23.4).

Serum triglycerides: 150 mg/dL or above (Figs 23.5 and 23.7).

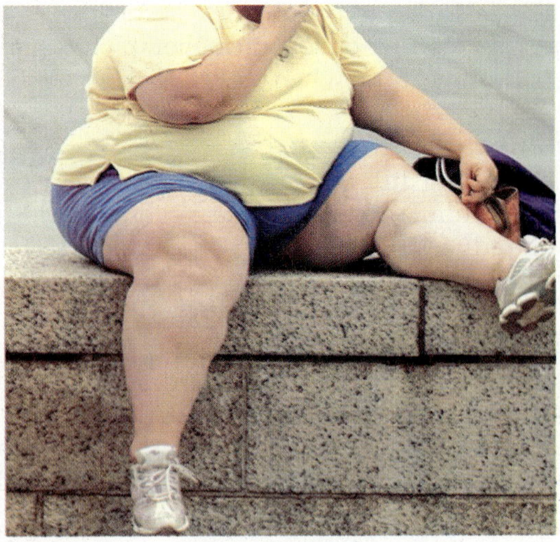

Fig. 23.13: *A young child developed obesity and metabolic syndrome after eating unhealthy diet*

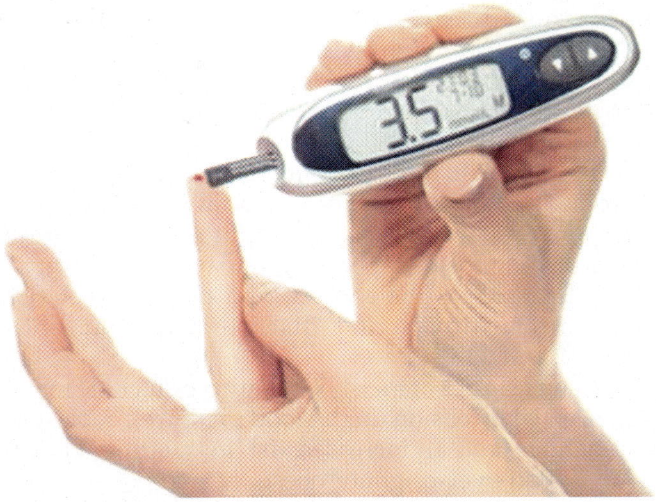

Fig. 23.14: *Measuring the glucose level in blood in patient with metabolic syndrome*

HDL cholesterol 40 mg/dL or lower in men and 50 mg/dL or lower in women.

Blood pressure of 130/85 or more.

Fasting blood glucose of 110 mg/dL or above. (Some groups say 100 mg/dL).

The World Health Organization (WHO) has slightly different criteria for the metabolic syndrome:

High insulin levels, an elevated fasting blood glucose or an elevated post meal glucose alone with at least 2 of the following criteria:

Abdominal obesity as defined by a waist to hip ratio of greater than 0.9, a body mass index of at least 30 kg/m^2 or a waist measurement over 37 inches.

Cholesterol panel showing a triglyceride level of at least 150 mg/dL or an HDL cholesterol lower than 35 mg/dL.

Blood pressure of 140/90 or above (or on treatment for high blood pressure).

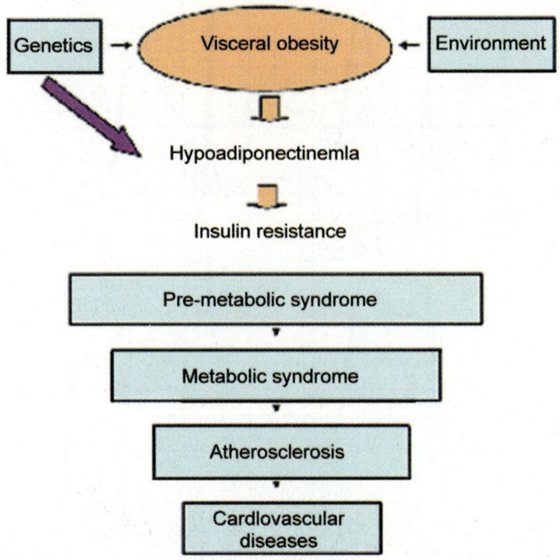

Fig. 23.15: *Role of visceral obesity in the pathogenesis of metabolic syndrome. (From Kadowachi, et al).*

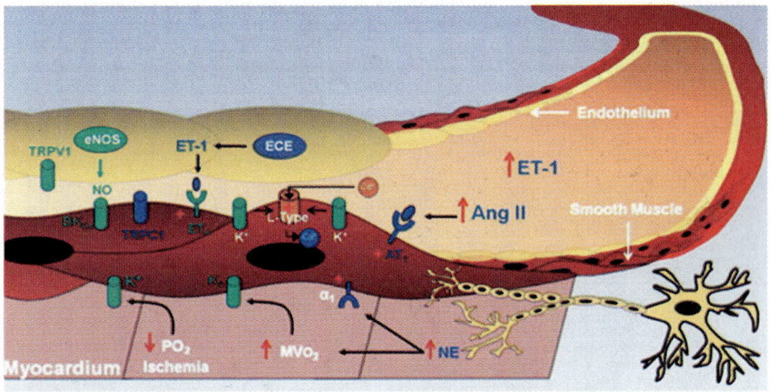

Fig. 23.16: *Schematic diagram illustrating mechanisms by which the metabolic syndrome impairs control of coronary blood flow in response to increases in myocardial oxygen consumption (MVO_2) or a brief coronary artery occlusion (i.e. decrease PO_2/ischemia). Factors, receptors and ion channels that are downregulated in metabolic syndrome are depicted in green. Factors, receptors and pathways that are upregulated in metabolic syndrome are depicted in blue and/or with + symbol. ET-1, endothelin-1; Ang II angiotensin II AT1, angiotensin II type 1 receptor; a1, a1 adrenoceptor; NE, norepinephrine; TRP, transient receptor potential channel; BKCa, large conductance, Ca^{2+} activated K+ channel; ETA, endothelin type A receptor. eNOS, endothelial nitric oxide synthase; ECE, endothelin-converting enzyme*

How common is metabolic syndrome?

Metabolic syndrome is quite common. Approximately, 20–30% of the population in industrialized countries have metabolic syndrome. By the year 2010, the metabolic syndrome is expected to affect 50–75 million people in the US alone.

What causes metabolic syndrome?

As is true with many medical conditions, genetics and the environment both play important roles in the development of the metabolic syndrome.

Table 23.1: *Definition of metabolic syndrome*

IDF	*NCEP*	*WHO*	*AACE*
Diagnosed if glycema is abnormal and 2 further criteria are present	Diagnosed if 3 out of 5 criteria are present	Diagnosed if glycemia is abnormal and 2 further criteria are present	Indicates risk factors
Fasting glycemia 100–125 mg/dL or DM2	Glycemia 110–125 mg/dL	Glucose intolerance, DM2 or insulin resistance due to HOMR-IR	Fasting glycemia 110–125 mg/dL or >140 mg/dL 2 hour after oral GTT
WC ≥ 94 cm MWC ≥ 80 cm W	WC > 102 cm MWC > 88 cm W	BMI > 30 and HWR > 0.9 M and > 0.85 W	BMI ≥ 25 and WC > 102 cm M and WC > 88 cm W
Tg ≥ 150 mg/dL or HDL < 40 M and < 50 W	Tg ≥ 150 mg/dL or HDL < 40 M and < 50 W	Tg ≥ 150 mg/dL or HDL < 35 M and < 39 W	Tg ≥ 150 mg/dL or HDL < 40 M and < 50 W
On treatment for SAH or BP ≥ 130 × 85 mmHg	BP ≥ 130 × 85 mmHg	On treatment for SAH or BP ≥ 160 × 90 mmHg	BP ≥ 130 × 85 mmHg
		Microalbuminuria ≥ 20 mcg/min	

AACE, American College of Endocrinology/American Association of Clinical Endocrinologies; BMI, body mass index; BP, arterial blood pressure; DM2, diabetes mellitus type 2; GTT, oral glucose tolerance test; HOMA, homeostasis model assessment; HWR, hip waist ratio; IDF, international diabetes federation; M, men; NCEP, US National Cholesterol Education Program; SAH, systemic arterial hypertension; Tg, triglycerides; W, women; WC, waist circumference; WHO, world health organization

Table 23.2: *Classification of metabolic syndrome in children and adolescents according to the International Diabetes Federation criteria*

	Age		
Criteria/components	*6 to < 10 years*	*10–16 years*	*> 16 years*
Definition of adioposity	WC ≥ 90th percentile	WC ≥ 90th percentile	WC ≥ 90 cm (men) or ≥ 80 cm (women)
Metabolism glycemic	No set value for diagnosis of metabolic syndrome	Fasting glycemia ≥ 100 mg/dL	Fasting glycemia ≥ 100 mg/dL
Dyslipidemia	No set value for diagnosis of metabolic syndrome	Triglycerides ≥ 150 mg/dL or HDL ≥ 40 mg/dL or taking hypolipemiants	Triglycerides ≥ 150 mg/dL or HDL ≥ 40 (men) or ≥ 50 (women) mg/dL or taking hypolipemiants
Arterial hypertension	No set value for diagnosis of metabolic syndrome	ABP ≥ 130 or 85 mmHg or taking antihypertensives	ABP ≥ 130 or 85 mmHg or taking antihypertensives

ABP, arterial blood pressure.

Genetic factors influence each individual component of the syndrome, and the syndrome itself. A family history that includes type 2 diabetes, hypertension, and early heart disease greatly increases the chance that an individual will develop the metabolic syndrome.

Environmental issues such as low activity level, sedentary lifestyle, and progressive weight gain also

Table 23.3: *Genetic conditions and mutations associated with obesity*

Genetic conditions
- Prader-Willi syndrome
- Bardet-Biedi syndrome
- Carpenter syndrome
- Cohen syndrome
- Alstrom syndrome
- Albright hereditary osteodystrophy (pseudohypoparathyrodism)
- Down syndrome

Single gene mutations
- Leptin (LEP)
- Leptin receptor (LEPR)
- Propiomelanocortin (POMC)
- Melanocortin 4 receptor (MC4R)

Table 23.4: *Criteria for the metabolic syndrome are listed below and can be any three of more*

Criteria list	*Components*
Central obesity	> 90th percentile, age and gender specific
FBG	> 5.6 mmol/L (100 mg/dL) or known type 2 diabetes
Hypertension	> 90th percentile for age, sex and height
TG	> 1.24 mmol/L (110 mg/dL)
HDL-C	< 1.04 mmol/L (40 mg/dL)

*Waist circumference

Source: Cook S, Weitzman M, Auinger P, Nguyen M, Dietz WH. Prevalence of a metabolic syndrome phenotype in adolescents. Arch Pediatr Adolesc Med. 2003;157:821–827. FBG, fasting blood glucose; TG, triglycerides; HDL-C, high density lipoprotein cholesterol.

contribute significantly to the risk of developing the metabolic syndrome.

Metabolic syndrome is present in about 5% of people with normal body weight, 22% of those who are overweight and 60% of those considered obese. Adults who continue to gain 5 or more pounds per year raise their risk of developing metabolic syndrome by up to 45%.

While obesity itself is likely the greatest risk factor, others factors of concern include: women who are post-menopausal, smoking, eating an excessively high carbohydrate diet, lack of activity (even without weight change), and consuming an alcohol-free diet.

Why should I know about metabolic syndrome?

Metabolic syndrome is worth caring about because it is a condition that can pave the way to both diabetes and heart disease, two of the most common and important chronic diseases today. Metabolic syndrome increases the risk of type 2 diabetes (the common type of diabetes) anywhere from 9–30 times over the normal population. That's a huge increase. As to the risk of heart disease, studies vary, but the metabolic syndrome appears to increase the risk 2–4 times that of the normal population. There are other concerns as well that should be mentioned. Metabolic syndrome is associated with fat accumulation in the liver (fatty liver), resulting in inflammation and the potential for cirrhosis. The kidneys can also be affected, as there is an association with microalbuminuria the leaking of protein into the urine, a subtle but clear indication of kidney damage.

Other problems associated with metabolic syndrome include obstructive sleep apnea, polycystic ovary syndrome increased risk of dementia with aging, and cognitive decline in the elderly.

How is metabolic syndrome treated?

The major goals are to treat both the underlying cause of the syndrome, and also to treat the cardiovascular risk factors if they persist. As has been discussed, the majority of people with metabolic syndrome are overweight and lead a sedentary lifestyle.

Lifestyle modification is the preferred treatment of metabolic syndrome. Weight reduction usually requires a specifically tailored multifaceted program that includes diet and exercise. Sometimes, medications may be useful.

Healing Diet for Metabolic Syndrome

A detailed discussion of diet therapies, pros and cons of various diets, etc is beyond the scope of this chapter. However, there is now a trend toward the use of a Mediterranean diet one that is rich in "good" fats (olive oil) and contains a reasonable amount of carbohydrates and proteins (such as from fish and chicken).

The mediterranean diet is palatable and easily sustained. In addition, recent studies have shown that when compared to a low fat diet, people on the mediterranean diet have a greater decrease in body weight, and also had greater improvements in blood pressure, cholesterol levels, and other markers of heart disease all of which are important in evaluating and treating metabolic syndrome (Figs 23.17 to 23.19).

If you're searching for a diet for metabolic syndrome, you'll be happy to learn studies are showing that a mediterranean diet with the addition of low-sugar nuts, is effective at reversing insulin resistance.

Metabolic syndrome is a combination of health conditions-obesity, diabetes or prediabetes symptoms, high blood pressure, large waist circumference, and high cholesterol-that can significantly affect health in a very negative way. Because metabolic syndrome poses such a serious health risk, you may want to aggressively counteract your condition by adopting this healing diet.

What to Eat on a healing diet for metabolic syndrome

1. *Fresh vegetables:* Fill-up on fresh vegetables. Eat them raw, steamed, boiled, sautéed in olive oil, grilled or baked. Don't use butter or cream sauces on them, and avoid all fried vegetables.

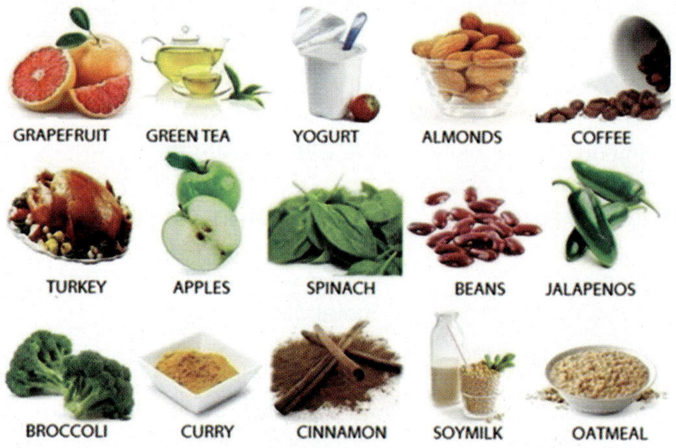

Fig. 23.17: *15 foods that boosts your metabolism*

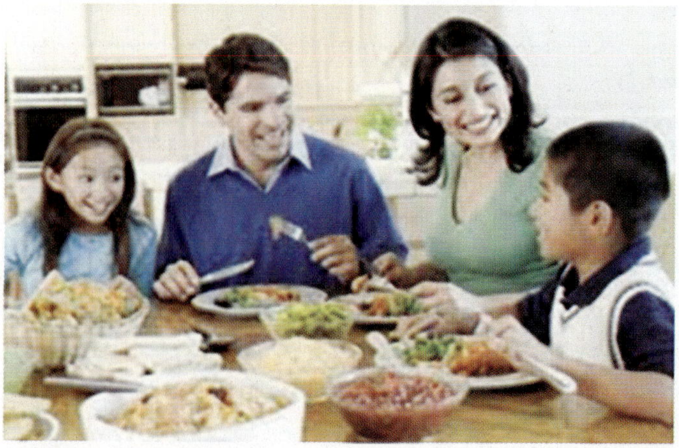

Fig. 23.18: *Family photograph showing enjoying home-cooked healthy food containing various types of fruits and vegetables in the management of childhood obesity*

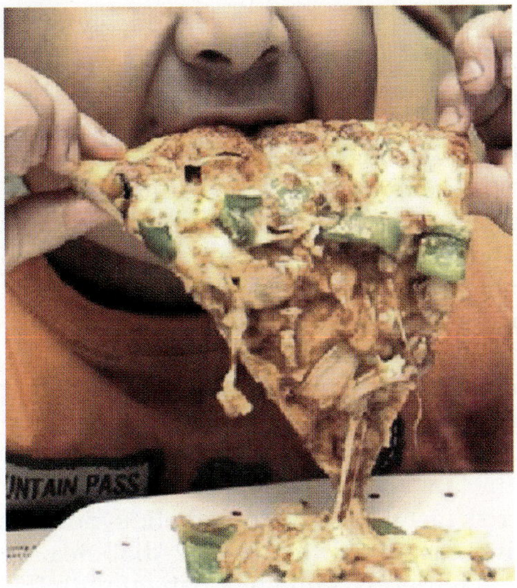

Fig. 23.19: *Big bite the fast food craze makes for a high calorie diet as one of the causes leading childhood obesity*

2. *Fresh fruit:* Eat fresh fruit without any added sugar or dressings. Eat whole fruit and limit fruit juice, since fruit juice is so high in natural sugar. The fiber in the whole fruit helps your body handle the sugar in the fruit.
3. *Whole grains:* Eat your share of whole grains, especially in the forms of brown rice, whole wheat pasta and oats. The fiber from whole grains will help lower cholesterol and fill you up.
4. *Olive oil:* Cook with olive oil as your primary cooking oil. Try olive oil in place of butter on vegetables and bread.
5. *Fish:* Fish should be your primary source of protein on this diet. Try eating salmon, fresh-water fish and seafood several times a week. You can bake, braise, grill, broil, or sauté fish in olive oil, but don't fry it or drench it in creams or butter sauces.
6. *Poultry:* Enjoy chicken, turkey, and other fowl served without the skin and baked, grilled, broiled, or braised, without cream sauces. Skip the gravy.
7. *Low-sugar nuts:* Almonds, Brazil nuts and walnuts are perfect snacks while eating this healing diet. Limit sweeter nuts like peanuts, cashews and pistachios.
8. *Red wine:* A glass of red wine a day is fine on this diet.

What not to eat

1. *Sugar:* Limit sugary foods to a couple times a week, and try to choose foods with a low glycemic-index.
   Processed foods: Avoid processed foods as much as possible. Go for fresh, local, whole foods as often as you can.
2. *Saturated fats:* Stay away from all saturated fats.
3. *Red meat:* Limit red meat to a couple times a month.
4. *Dairy:* Limit dairy to one serving a day. Try to limit dairy to low-sugar dairy products such as sugar-free yogurt. Try to get your calcium from broccoli, leafy greens, and supplements instead of solely from dairy products.

Exercise (Figs 23.20 and 23.21)

A sustainable exercise program, for example, 30 minutes 5 days a week is reasonable to start, providing there is no medical contraindication. (If you have any special concerns in this regard, check with your doctor first). There is a beneficial effect of exercise on blood pressure, cholesterol levels, and insulin sensitivity, regardless of whether weight loss is achieved or not. Thus, exercise in itself is a helpful tool in treating metabolic syndrome.

Cosmetic Surgery for Obesity

Some people may ask: Why not just have liposuction of the abdomen and remove the large amount abdominal fat, which a big part of the problem? Data thus far shows no benefit in liposuction on insulin sensitivity, blood pressure,

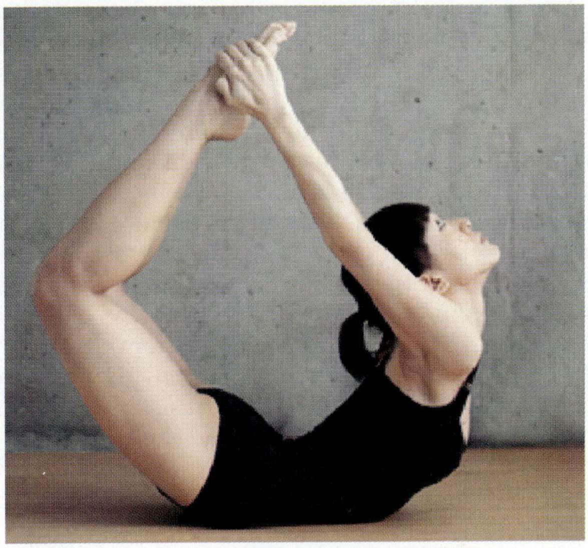

Fig. 23.20: *A young girl performing jogic exercise in childhood obesity*

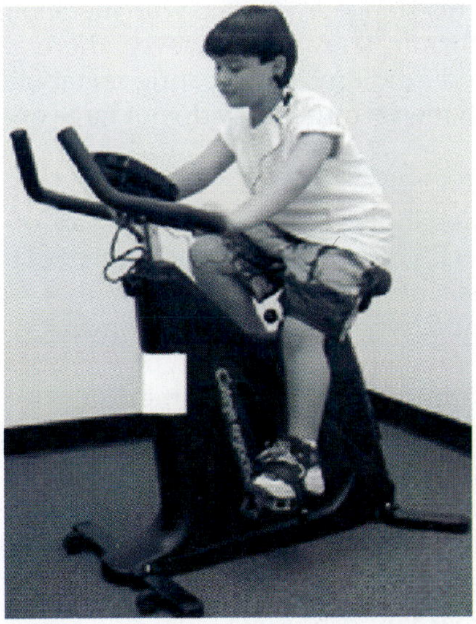

Fig. 23.21: *Cycle exercise programme in childhood obesity*

or cholesterol. As the saying goes, "If is too good to be true, it probably is". Diet and exercise are still the preferred primary treatment of metabolic syndrome.

What if lifestyle changes are not enough to treat metabolic syndrome?

What if changes in lifestyle do not do the trick, what then? Drugs to control cholesterol levels, lipids, and high blood pressure may be considered.

If someone has already had a heart attack, their LDL ("bad") cholesterol should be reduced below 100 mg/dL. (Some experts now say it should be under 70 mg/dL) A person who has diabetes has a heart attack risk equivalent to that of someone who has already one and so should be treated in the same way. What remains controversial is whether metabolic syndrome should be considered a coronary equivalent or not. If you have metabolic syndrome, a detailed discussion about lipid therapy is needed between you and your doctor, as each individual is unique.

Blood pressure goals are generally set lower than 130/80. Some blood pressure medications offer more than simply lowering blood pressure. For example, a class of blood pressure drugs called ACE inhibitors has been found to also reduce the levels of insulin resistance and actually deter the development of type 2 diabetes. This is an important consideration when discussing the choice blood pressure drugs in the metabolic syndrome.

The discovery that a drug prescribed for one condition, and has other beneficial effects is not new. Drugs used to treat high blood sugar and insulin resistance may have beneficial effects on blood pressure and cholesterol profiles. A class of drugs called thiazolidinediones [pioglitazone (Actos) and rosiglitazone (Avandia)] also reduce the thickness of the walls of the carotid arteries.

Metformin (glucophage), usually used to treat type 2 diabetes, also has been found to help prevent the onset of diabetes in people with metabolic syndrome. Indeed, in my practice, I routinely discuss metformin with my patients who have metabolic syndrome. Many of my patients who have insulin resistance associated with metabolic syndrome opt for metformin therapy. However, there are currently no established guidelines on treating metabolic syndrome patients with metformin if they do not have overt diabetes.

Summary

The term "metabolic syndrome" is a way of identifying individuals at high risk for the development of heart disease and diabetes. Intuitively we all know that obesity, high cholesterol, and hypertension are bad omens. We also know that insulin resistance precedes type 2 diabetes, and can itself be an important condition meriting treatment. The final take home message is:

- Find a walk buddy.
- Take a walk during your work break, even if it is just around the building.
- Go to a health food store.
- Look at what you feed your kids.
- Urge them to get outside and play.

It all adds up. Preventing metabolic syndrome really means having a healthy lifestyle.

Conclusions

Most of the workers agreed that CVD is the primary clinical outcome of metabolic syndrome. Additionally, risk for type 2 diabetes is higher, and diabetes is a major risk factor for CVD. ATP III criteria provide a practical tool to identify patients at increased risk for CVD. WHO and AACE criteria require further oral glucose testing if IFG and diabetes are absent. IGT on OGTT denotes greater risk for diabetes than does metabolic syndrome without elevated fasting glucose. Several potential benefits make OGTT in such patients an attractive option for use at the discretion of the physician. First, in the absence of IFG, IGT could count as one metabolic risk factor defining metabolic syndrome, besides carrying increased risk for type 2 diabetes. Moreover, postprandial hyperglycemia in a patient with IFG denotes diabetes, a high-risk condition for CVD.

Regardless of diagnostic criteria used, there is full agreement that therapeutic lifestyle change, with emphasis on weight reduction, constitutes first-line therapy for metabolic syndrome. Drug treatment to directly reduce insulin resistance is promising, but clinical trials to prove reduction of CVD are lacking. In patients in whom lifestyle changes fail to reverse metabolic risk factors, consideration should be given to treating specific abnormalities in these risk factors with drugs. Use of drugs to target risk factors should be in accord with current treatment guidelines.

BIBLIOGRAPHY

1. Metabolic Syndrome Rates in United States Adolescents, from the National Health and Nutrition Examination Survey, 1999-2002" by Stephen Cook, MD, Peggy Auinger, MS, Chaoyang Li, MD, PhD, and Earl S. Ford, MD, MPH.
2. Examining Metabolic Syndrome Definitions in Overweight Hispanic Youth: A Focus on Insulin Resistance" by Gabriel Q. Shaibi, PhD, PT, and Michael I. Goran, PhD.
3. Comparison of Different Definitions of Pediatric Metabolic Syndrome: Relation to Abdominal Adiposity, Insulin Resistance, Adiponectin, and Inflammatory Biomarkers" by SoJung Lee, PhD, Fida Bacha, MD, Neslihan Gungor, MD, and Silva Arslanian, MD.
4. Defining the Metabolic Syndrome in Children and Adolescents: Will the Real Definition Please Stand Up?" by Earl S. Ford, MD, MPH, and Chaoyang Li, MD, PhD.
5. Sensitivity, Specificity, and Predictive Values of Pediatric Metabolic Syndrome Components in Relation to Adult Metabolic Syndrome: The Princeton LRC Follow-up Study" by Terry T-K Huang, PhD, MPH, Tonya R. Nansel, PhD, Allen R. Belsheim, MA, and John A. Morrison, PhD.
6. Childhood Obesity Predicts Adult Metabolic Syndrome: The Fels Longitudinal Study" by Shumei S. Sun, PhD, Ruohong Liang, MS, Terry T-K Huang, PhD, MPH, Stephen R. Daniels, MD, PhD, Silva Arslanian, MD, Kiang Liu, PhD, Gilman D. Grave, MD, and Roger M. Siervogel, PhD.
7. Metabolic Syndrome in Childhood Predicts Adult Metabolic Syndrome and Type 2 Diabetes Mellitus 25 to 30 Years Later"

by John A. Morrison, PhD, Lisa Aronson Friedman, ScM, Ping Wang, PhD, and Charles J. Glueck, MD.

8. Waist-to-Height Ratio, a Useful Index to Identify High Metabolic Risk in Overweight Children" by Claudio Maffeis, MD, Claudia Banzato, MD, and Giorgio Talamini, MD, on behalf of The Obesity Study Group of The Italian Society of Pediatric Endocrinology and Diabetology.
9. Third report of the National Cholesterol Education Program (NCEP) expert panel on detection, evaluation, and treatment of high blood cholesterol in adults (Adult Treatment Panel III). Final report. Circulation. 2002; 106: 3143–3421.
10. Reaven GM. Banting lecture 1988: role of insulin resistance in human disease. Diabetes. 1988; 37: 1595–1607.
11. Ferrannini E, Haffner SM, Mitchell BD, et al. Hyperinsulinaemia: the key feature of a cardiovascular and metabolic syndrome. Diabetologia. 1991;34:416–422.
12. Abbasi F, Brown BW, Lamendola C, et al. Relationship between obesity, insulin resistance, and coronary heart disease risk. J Am Coll Cardiol. 2002; 40: 937–943.
13. Bogardus C, Lillioja S, Mott DM, et al. Relationship between degree of obesity and in vivo insulin action in man. Am J Physiol. 1985; 248(3 pt 1): 286–291.
14. Ford ES, Giles WH, Dietz WH. Prevalence of the metabolic syndrome among US adults: findings from the Third National Health and Nutrition Examination Survey. JAMA. 2002; 287: 356–359.
15. Alberti KG, Zimmet PZ. Definition, diagnosis and classification of diabetes mellitus and its complications. Part 1: diagnosis and classification of diabetes mellitus: provisional report of a WHO consultation. Diabet Med. 1998; 15: 539–553.

24 Recognition and Management of Pericardial Diseases

In children, pericarditis is most likely to occur following surgery to repair congenital (present at birth) heart defects or acquired heart disease. However, other causes may include the following infection (viral, bacterial, fungal, parasitic) chest trauma or injury connective tissue disorders such as systemic lupus erythematosus (SLE).

The presence of a pleural effusion and a pericardial effusion is almost exclusively seen in the children with cardiac abnormalities. Pericardial effusion and cardiac disease should not only be suspected in any child with radiographic signs of cardiomegaly, but be strongly suspected in any child with pleural effusions or ascites, even with a normal cardiac silhouette, especially if they are not responding to conventional medical therapy and their respiratory condition is not improving (Figs 24.1 and 24.2).

Recent advances in the study of pericardial disorders have opened new diagnostic windows to the heart through the pericardial sac with the development of pericardioscopy and thoracoscopy. Specific diagnosis of inflammatory, postinflammatory, autoreactive, or neoplastic pericardial disease can now be made by epicardial and pericardial biopsy and by cytologic analysis of the pericardial fluid. In perimyocarditis, optically guided epicardial biopsy gives more disease-specific results than does endomyocardial biopsy in the same patients. For viral and tuberculous pericarditis, molecular techniques such as polymerase chain reaction and in situ hybridization are available. Immunologic characterization of lymphocytic cells and antibodies demonstrates increased reactivity in viral, autoimmune, and neoplastic disorders of the heart. Doppler echocardiographic features in tamponade are reviewed thoroughly. Advantages and problems of pericardectomy in constrictive disease are noted, and finally, a pragmatic clinical and scientific approach for improved diagnosis of pericardial diseases is outlined.

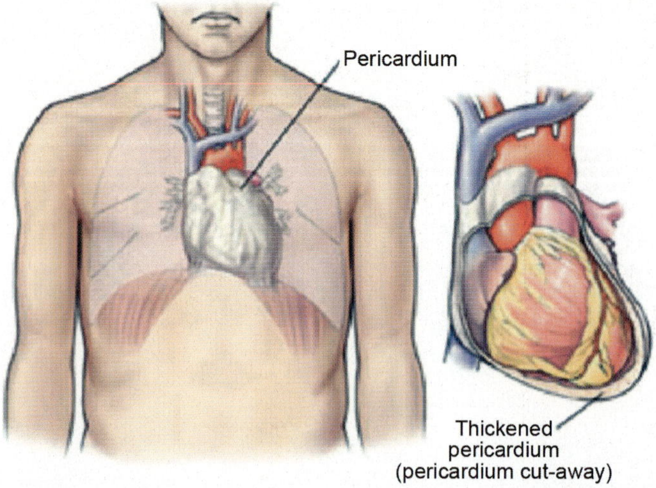

Fig. 24.1: *Anatomy pricardial sac in relation to surrounding vital structures of the heart, particularly myocardium and coronary vessels*

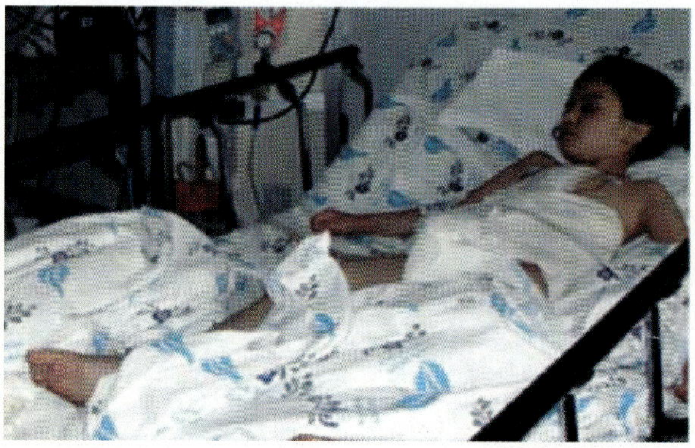

Fig. 24.2: *A child with acute pericarditis in ICU*

Anatomy and Physiology (Fig. 24.1)

The pericardium is composed of the parietal pericardium (an outer fibrous layer) and the visceral pericardium (an inner serous membrane made of a single layer of mesothelial cells). The visceral pericardium is attached to

Table 24.1: *Various etiological factors in different types of pericardial disease*

Idiopathic
Acute idiopathic pericarditis'
Chronic idiopathic effusion
Infectious
Viral
Bacterial
Tuberculosis
Spread from contiguous infection (e.g. pneumonia)
Fungal
Inflammatory
Associated with connective tissue disease
Rheumatiod arthritis
Systemic lupus erythematosis
Other
Post myocardial infarction
Acute after transmural infarct
Partial V complete free wall rupture
Delayed—Dressler syndrome H
Associated with systemic disease
Uremia
Hypothyroidism
Pregnancy
Cirrhosis
Malignancy
Direct tumor involvement
Effusion due to lymphatic obstruction
Miscellaneous
Post-trauma
Post-surgical
Congestive heart failure
Severe pulmonary hypertension, right heart failure.

the epicardial fat and reflects back on itself to form the parietal pericardium. The pericardium normally contains as much as 50 mL of an ultrafiltrate of plasma. Drainage occurs via the thoracic duct and the right lymphatic duct into the right pleural space.

Pericardial physiology includes three main functions. First, through its mechanical function, the pericardium promotes cardiac efficiency by limiting acute dilation, maintaining ventricular compliance with preservation of the Starling curve, and distributing hydrostatic forces. The pericardium also creates a closed chamber with subatmospheric pressure that aids atrial filling and lowers transmural cardiac pressures. Second, through its membranous function, the pericardium shields the heart by reducing external friction and acting as a barrier against extension of infection and malignancy.

Third, through its ligamentous function, the pericardium anatomically fixes the heart.

Absence of pericardium: Partial absence of pericardium is much more common than complete absence. It may be associated with congenital anomalies such as ASD, mitral stenosis, TOF, tricuspid regurgitation, patent ductus arteriosus and Eisenmengerphysiology. Mitral valve prolapse may also be associated in this anomaly. In majority, it does not manifest with any symptom except chest pain due to torsion of the great vessels. Recurrent pulmonary infections may be a significant feature. Physical examination may reveal LV heave in the anterior or mid-axillary line. A systolic murmur may be present and on occasion diastolic murmur has been reported. X-ray chest reveals shift of the heart to the left and its border elongated showing prominent seperation between the aorta and the pulmonary artery. Lucencies caused by interposition of lung may be seen between the pulmonary artery segment

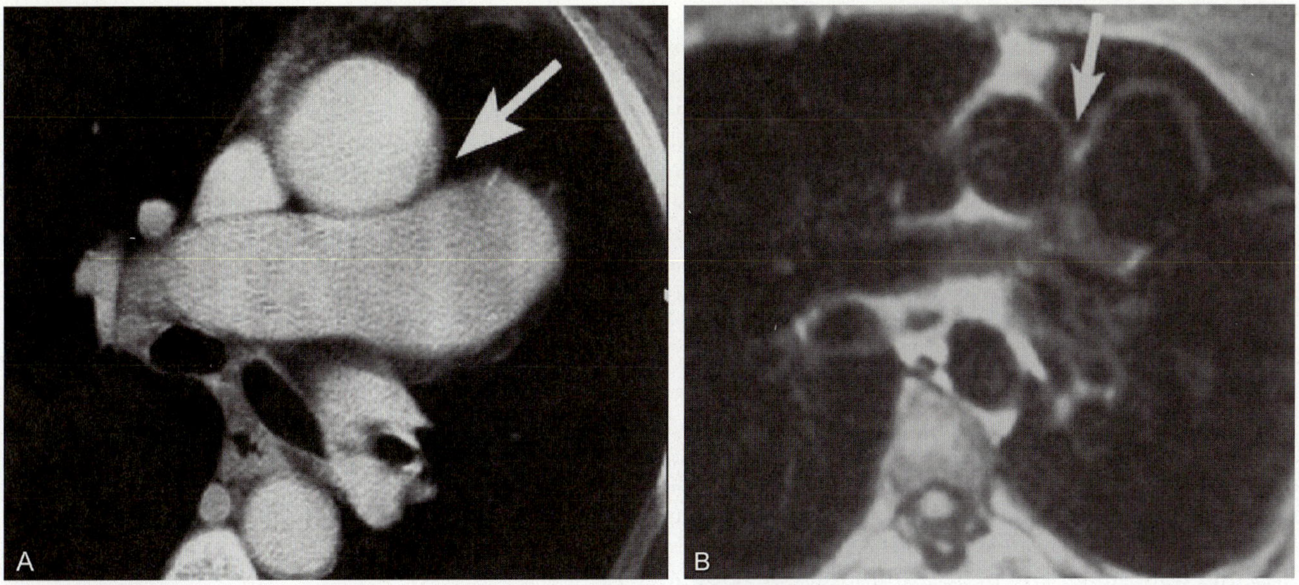

Fig. 24.3: *Congenital absence of the pericardium. Axial contrast-enhanced CT scan (A) and ECG-gated T1-weighted SE image (B) show interposition of lung tissue between the aorta and the main segment of the pulmonary artery (arrow), indicating the absence of the pericardium in this area. Note the rotation of the heart toward the left*

and the aortic knob, and between the left hemidiaphragm and the base of the heart. Electrocardiogram in complete absence of the left side of the pericardium usually shows incomplete RBBB. In the presence of induced or spontaneous pneumothorax, air enters the pericardial space and outlines the percardium. Medium size defects may lead to herniation of the left atrium which may then strangulate and require surgical closure or enlargement of the defect to reduce the herniation and prevent recurrence (Fig. 24.3).

1. ACUTE PERICARDITIS

It may be defined as accumulation of fluid into the pericardial sac of acute or chronic onset due to numberous causes leading to diastolic restriction of filling and a reduction in stroke volume of both the ventricles.

Etiological Factors

Acute pericarditis can be caused by many types off actors such as viral, bacterial, or fungal infections, uremia, acute rheumatic fever, myocardial infarction, collagen vascular diseases such as lupus erythematosus, rheumatoid arthritis, tumor metastases, irradiation and trauma. It can also be caused by drugs, particularly procainamide, hydralazine, minoxidil, anticoagulants, methylsergid, daunorubin, and diphenylhydantoin. Clinically, it can be diagnosed in about 10–20% of the cases after open heart surgery. Acute inflammatory process following acute myocardial infarction may also lead to acute pericarditis which can be diagnosed either clinically or by means of echocardiography. It may occur from 10 days to 2 months later, perhaps due to an autoimmune process. Acute pericarditis process may recurr on account of syndrome of spontaneous recurrences which are thought to represent autoimmune reactions to the initial pericardial injury (Table 24.1).

Clinical Features

Pain may be the dominant clinical feature of acute pericarditis which is usually experienced as a sharp chest pain, that is exacerbated by respiration and lessened by sitting up and learning forward. Usually localised at precordial region but it can be referred at the neck of the left trapezius ridge. Precordial heaviness and breathlessness on exertion may also be encountered. There may be symptoms of a recent upper respiratory tract infection or a flu-like syndrome. The postpericardiotomy syndrome includes pericarditis, pleurisy, pneumonitis, myocarditis and arthralgia.

Pathophysiology (Fig. 24.4)

In most cases of acute pericarditis, the pericardium is acutely inflamed and has an infiltration of polymorphonuclear (PMN) leukocytes and pericardial vascularization. Often, the pericardium manifests a fibrinous reaction with exudates and adhesions. The pericardium may develop a serous or hemorrhagic effusion. A granulomatous pericarditis occurs with tuberculosis, fungal infections, rheumatoid arthritis (RA) and sarcoidosis.

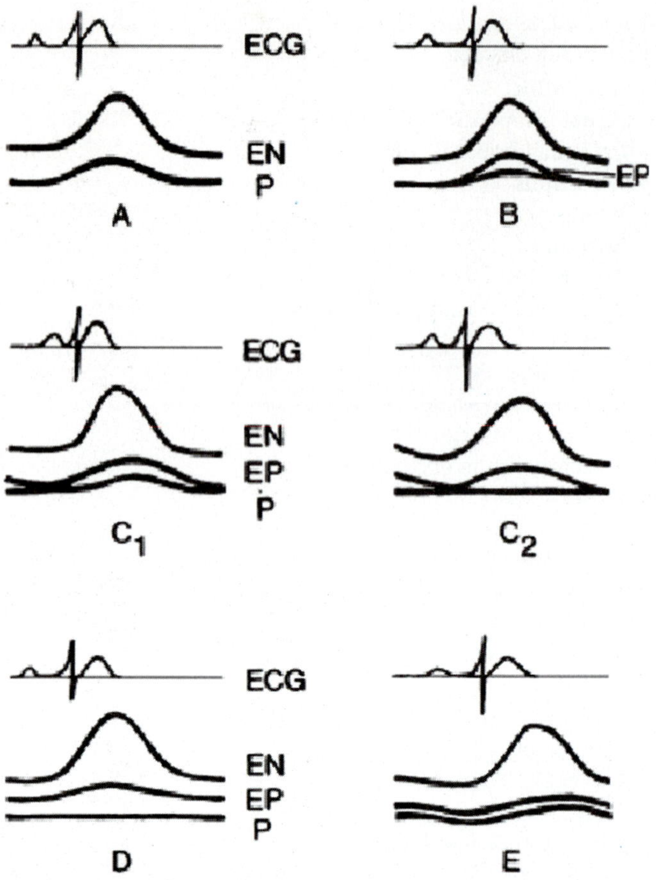

Fig. 24.4: *Horowitz classification of pericardial effusions. Type (A) No effusion; (B) separation of epicardium and pericardium (3–16 mL); (C1) systolic and diastolic separation of epicardium and pericardium (small effusion > 16 mL); (C2) systolic and diastolic separation of epicardium and pericardium with attenuated pericardial motion; (D) pronounced separation of epicardium and pericardium with large echo-free space; (E) pericardial thickening (4 mm)*

Frequency

Epidemiological data on incidence are lacking, likely because acute pericarditis is frequently inapparent clinically, despite its presence in numerous disorders. Lorell notes a diagnosis of acute pericarditis in approximately 1 per 1,000 hospital admissions.

Mortality/Morbidity

Mortality varies greatly depending on etiology. The mortality rate approaches 100% in untreated purulent pericarditis, whereas mortality is virtually nonexistent in acute viral or idiopathic pericarditis.

Morbidity also depends on the etiology and development of complications.

History

- Chest pain is the cardinal symptom. The quality of the pain may be sharped, dull, aching, burning, or pressing. Intensity varies from barely perceptible to severe.

- Pain is usually precordial with referral to the trapezius ridge. It is worse during inspiration when lying flat, or during swallowing and with body motion.
- Dyspnea may be present, especially with tamponade.
- Fever may be present. Abdominal pain occurs infrequently in children (Fig. 24.2).

Physical Examination

A pericardial friction rub is pathognomonic for acute pericarditis. The rub has a scratching, grating sound similar to leather rubbing against leather. Auscultation with the diaphragm of the stethoscope over the left lower sternal edge allows the best detection of the rub. Serial examinations may be necessary for detection. More than 50% of rubs are triphasic. They are composed of:

1. An atrial systolic rub that precedes S1
2. Ventricular systolic rub between S1 and S2 and coincident with the peak carotid pulse
3. An early diastolic rub after S2 (usually the faintest).

The biphasic to-and-fro rub is less common (24%). It can occur with tachycardia and is due to summation of the atrial and early diastolic rub. Monophasic rubs (the ventricular systolic) are the least common but may occur in patients with atrial fibrillation. Especially, when it is monophasic, the pericardial friction rub can be mistaken for a systolic murmur. Pericardial rubs may be differentiated if the rub does not change with usual respiratory or positional maneuvers, if three components are present, and if the findings on the ECG are typical. Tachypnea may be present. Tachycardia may be present. Patients may have fever.

The Beck triad (i.e. hypotension; elevated systemic venous pressure, often with jugular venous distention; muffled heart sounds) may occur in patients with cardiac tamponade, especially from sudden intrapericardial hemorrhage.

Pulsus paradoxus is defined as a 10 mmHg decrease in arterial systolic pressure with inspiration. This decrease is important in patients with more slowly developing tamponade because they may lack findings of the Beck triad.

Etiological Factors

Idiopathic

Between 26% and 86% of cases are idiopathic in nature. No clinical features distinguish idiopathic cases from viral pericarditis. Most likely, most idiopathic cases are undiagnosed viral infections. Seasonal peaks occur in spring and fall (Table 24.1).

Infection

Viral

This is the most common cause of acute pericarditis and accounts for 1–10% of cases. Causative viruses include coxsackievirus B, echovirus, adenoviruses, influenza A and B viruses, enterovirus, mumps virus, Epstein-Barr virus, human immunodeficiency virus (HIV), herpes simplex virus type 1, varicella-zoster virus, measles virus, parainfluenza virus type 2, and respiratory syncytial virus. Viruses, especially coxsackievirus B and influenza, can occur as seasonal epidemics. It is usually a short self-limited disease that lasts 1–3 weeks. Patients may have associated myocarditis. The treatment is based on the symptoms present, with observation for the development of tamponade.

Pericardial involvement is frequent in persons with HIV, but is usually an asymptomatic pericardial effusion of small volume. Persons with advanced HIV infection develop pericardial involvement more frequently, with one study noting right atrial diastolic compression in 5% of cases involving advanced HIV infection. Symptomatic pericarditis occurs in less than 1% of cases involving HIV, and its etiology can include the usual causes, opportunistic infection, Kaposi sarcoma and HIV.

Bacterial

This accounts for 1–8% of cases and causes purulent pericarditis. Bacterial pericarditis develops from direct pulmonary extension, hematogenous spread, myocardial abscess or endocarditis, penetrating injury to chest wall from either trauma or surgery, or a subdiaphragmatic suppurative lesion. Organisms isolated include Gram-positive species such as *Streptococcus pneumoniae* and other *Streptococcus* species and *Staphylococcus*. Isolated gram-negative species include *Proteus*, *Escherichia coli*, *Pseudomonas*, *Klebsiella*, *Salmonella*, *Shigella*, *Neisseria meningitidis*, and *Haemophilus influenzae*. Less common organisms include *Legionella*, *Nocardia*, *Actinobacillus*, *Rickettsia*, and *Borrelia burgdorferi* (*Lyme borreliosis*). Anaerobes also have been isolated in 40% of patients in reviews of the pediatric population. Previously, Pneumococcus was the predominant organism. However, in the antibiotic era, Gram-negative species have become more common.

Purulent pericarditis can develop from previous aseptic pericarditis and is associated with a poorer prognosis, with a mortality rate nearing 100% for untreated persons and a mortality rate of 12–40% for treated patients.

A high percentage of patients develop constrictive pericarditis. Treatment includes appropriate antibiotics for at least 4 weeks and drainage of pericardial fluid.

Some authors have described intrapericardial thrombolytics to assist with drainage. Occasionally, patients require partial to total pericardiectomy.

Tubercular

Tuberculosis accounts for 4% of cases.

- It should be considered in all instances of pericarditis without a rapid course, especially in high-risk groups, such as elderly patients in nursing homes. The diagnostic yield for acid-fast bacilli in pericardial fluid is fairly low (between 30% and 76%).
- Pericardial biopsy has a much better yield (approximately 100%). Elevated adenosine deaminase in pericardial fluid is useful for diagnosing tuberculosis. Studies note greater than 90% sensitivity and specificity with levels higher than 50–70 U/L. High adenosine deaminase values may

indicate a poorer prognosis. Approximately half the patients develop constrictive pericarditis.

- Treatment is with the usual antituberculous chemotherapy. The mortality rate approaches 50%.

Other Infectious Agents

Fungal organisms include *Histoplasma, Blastomyces, Coccidioides, Aspergillus* and *Candida*.

Parasitic organisms include *Entamoeba, Echinococcus* and *Toxoplasma*. Inflammatory disorders.

Rheumatoid Arthritis (RA)

Autopsy studies show a prevalence of 11–50% in patients with RA. Echocardiography studies note pericardial effusions in 50% of patients with RA with nodules and in only 15% of patients with RA without nodules.

Pericardial involvement is usually clinically silent. Diagnosis is made in only 2% of adults and 6% of juveniles.

Rarely, pericarditis precedes the onset of RA. ECG almost never demonstrates typical findings of pericarditis, possibly secondary to masking from RA medications.

Diagnosis is suggested by serous or hemorrhagic pericardial fluid with a glucose level of less than 45 mg/dL, a white blood cell count higher than 15,000/mL with cytoplasmic inclusion bodies, a protein level higher than 5 g/dL, a low total serum hemolytic complement (CH50), a high immunoglobulin G (IgG) level, and a high rheumatoid factor. Cholesterol levels may be high in the fluid of patients with RA who have nodules. Only symptomatic RA pericarditis should be treated. Interestingly, symptomatic disease tends to occur in patients with arthritis, pleuritis, and other complications who are already being treated with antiinflammatory agents such as corticosteroids, gold and antimalarial drugs.

Systemic Lupus Erythematosus

Clinically, evident pericarditis has been reported in 25% of patients with lupus. Autopsy series reveal pericardial involvement in 62%. Pericarditis usually occurs in flare-ups, but it may be the presenting manifestation. In contrast to RA, ECG findings usually demonstrate typical changes of pericarditis. Fluid analysis reveals increased leukocytes of PMN predominance with a high protein level, low-to-normal glucose level, low complement, and, possibly, a pH level of less than 7. In addition, fluid analysis reveals positive autoantibodies, such as the antinuclear antibody or anti-double-stranded DNA. Treat with anti-inflammatory agents and optimization of systemic lupus erythematosus (SLE) treatment. Development of tamponade and constrictive pericarditis is rare.

Scleroderma

Pericarditis is recognized in 5–10% of patients with scleroderma. Autopsy prevalence rate is 70%. Pericardial effusions occur in 40% of patients with scleroderma and can be due to scleroderma, myocardial failure (restrictive cardiomyopathy), and renal failure. Restrictive cardiomyopathy and pericardial constriction can coexist. Usually, pulmonary hypertension, right heart failure, and systolic dysfunction occur. Pericardial fluid has a protein value greater than 5 g/dL, has a low cell count, and does not demonstrate the antibodies found in RA and SLE. These patients have a poor prognosis.

Rheumatic Fever

This occurs more commonly in lower socioeconomic groups and in children. It often accompanies endocarditis and myocarditis with a worse prognosis.

Consider this etiology in any child with pericarditis. In adults, pericarditis may not occur with myocardial or valvular involvement, and it is associated with a better prognosis. It usually appears 7–10 days after onset of fever and arthritis. Often, stage 1 ECG findings are absent. Antistreptolysin O titer is usually greater than 400.

Rarely is a large effusion present. This is not a demonstrated cause of constrictive pericarditis. Pericarditis resolves with antiinflammatory treatment.

Sarcoidosis

Pericarditis is present in autopsies of approximately 25% of these patients. Patients may not have significant myocardial infiltration. It rarely causes cardiac tamponade or constrictive pericarditis.

Other Inflammatory Conditions

- Sjögren syndrome
- Mixed connective-tissue disease
- Reiter syndrome
- Ankylosing spondylitis
- Inflammatory bowel disease
- Wegener granulomatosis
- Vasculitis (e.g. giant cell arteritis, polyarteritis)
- Polymyositis
- Behçet syndrome
- Whipple disease
- Familial mediterranean fever
- Serum sickness
- Metabolic disorders.

Renal Failure

Renal failure accounts for approximately 12% of cases.

In the predialysis era, pericarditis developed in 35–50% of patients with uremia who had chronic renal failure and less commonly in those with acute renal failure. Death often followed in several weeks. With dialysis, the incidence rate is less than 10%. Pericarditis occurs after the onset of dialysis in 8–12% of cases. Some authors suggest that uremic pericarditis is a different entity from dialysis-associated pericarditis. Asymptomatic pericardial effusions can occur in 36–62% of patients with uremia who require dialysis. They are often small to moderate in size, and they can occur secondary to volume overload. They can lead to significant hemodynamic complications during routine dialysis. The presence of a large pericardial effusion that persists for longer than 10 days after intensive dialysis has a high likelihood of causing tamponade.

Treatment

If no improvement is noted after 7–10 days or if the patient has hemodynamic instability, proceed with pericardiocentesis or pericardiectomy. Intensive dialysis is beneficial to most patients with uremia who develop pericarditis prior to dialysis. Dialysis-induced pericarditis fails to respond to more intensive dialysis in 25–33% of patients.

Hypothyroidism: This accounts for as many as 4% of cases. Pericardial involvement usually occurs with severe hypothyroidism. Patients may develop large pericardial effusions, but they rarely develop tamponade. Pericardial fluid is often clear with high protein and cholesterol levels and with few cells. Low ECG voltage is often observed. Myocardial involvement is common. Treatment is hormone replacement.

Cholesterol Pericarditis

Cholesterol pericarditis is also called gold-paint pericarditis. Granulomatous pericarditis has been implicated in some cases. It usually presents with large effusions that are not hemodynamically important. Development of constriction is rare.

Myocardial Infarction

After a transmural infarction, a fibrinous pericardial exudate appears within 24 hours. It begins to organize at 4–8 days, and it completes organization at 4 weeks. If pericardial involvement is confined to the infarct zone, stage 1 ECG findings are often not seen. Positive T waves that last longer than 48 hours after an acute myocardial infarction (AMI) or premature reversal of inverted T waves may indicate pericardial involvement. The pericardial pain occurs less frequently than the friction rub. The rub often is detected on the second or third day after an AMI but may be heard within 24 hours and as late as 10 days.

Prior to thrombolytic therapy, infarct-associated pericarditis ranges from 7–23% of cases. At autopsy, almost all patients were noted to have localized fibrinous pericarditis overlying the area of infarction. With thrombolytic therapy and direct infarct angioplasty, the incidence of infarct-associated pericarditis has decreased to 5–8%.

Overall, pericardial involvement indicates larger infarction, greater incidence of left ventricular dysfunction, and greater mortality. Pericarditis usually heals without consequence. Effusions may occur, but they rarely lead to tamponade. Pericardial involvement does not contraindicate thrombolytic or anticoagulant therapy. Aspirin may be helpful in such cases.

Dressler Syndrome

Pericarditis associated with Dressler syndrome is usually observed 2–3 weeks after a myocardial infarction.

Initially, the syndrome was described in as many as 4% of patients post-AMI. More recent studies suggest a much lower incidence. Dressler syndrome is rarely described with pulmonary embolism. It may be a unique autoimmune-mediated phenomenon to myocardial antigens, or it may merely be an unrecognized postmyocardial infarction pericarditis. ECG findings may demonstrate diagnostic changes of acute pericarditis, especially if the ECG findings normalize after the infarction. Patients may develop pulmonary infiltrates and large pericardial effusions. Because of the risk of hemorrhagic pericarditis, anticoagulant therapy should be stopped. Treatment is with nonsteroidal anti-inflammatory drugs (NSAIDs).

Aortic Dissection

This accounts for 1% of cases. This accounts especially for cases with hemorrhage into the pericardium.

Neoplasm

This accounts for 5–17% of cases. Neplastic disease, particularly advanced, is the most frequent cause of tamponade in the hospital. Symptoms develop over days to weeks. Dyspnea is common and is the most significant symptom. Occasionally, the tumor encases the heart and causes constrictive pericarditis rather than tamponade. Primary neoplasm of the heart and pericardium is rare. Pericardial mesothelioma and angiosarcoma are lethal malignancies with aggressive local spread that respond poorly to treatment. Infants and children can present with a teratoma in the pericardial space. These can often be successfully removed. Most cases are a result of metastatic disease. Autopsy studies have noted that approximately 10% of patients with cancer develop cardiac involvement, and, often, it is clinically silent. The neoplastic cells reach the pericardium through the bloodstream, the lymphatic system, or via local growth.

Lung cancer including adenocarcinoma and squamous and small cell carcinoma, accounts for approximately 33% of cases. Breast cancer accounts for 25%. Leukemia and lymphoma including Hodgkin and non-Hodgkin, account for 15% of cases. Malignant melanoma represents another 5%. Almost all other malignancies, except primary brain, comprise the rest of the cases. Kaposi sarcoma also has become a more prominent cause of neoplastic disease with the AIDS epidemic.

The pericardial carcinoembryonic antigen (CEA) level is often elevated. Cytology findings are positive in 80–90% of breast and lung cancer cases, but the percentage is lower in other malignancies. Obstruction of the lymphatic drainage can cause the pericardial effusion to be more significant than the tumor mass. Initial treatment includes relief of tamponade, confirmation of the diagnosis, and systemic treatment of the neoplasm. Further treatment options include sclerosis of the pericardial space, instillation of chemotherapeutic agents into the pericardial space, local radiation, or pericardiectomy.

Miscellaneous causes including iatrogenic drugs; some medications including penicillin and cromolyn sodium, induce pericarditis through a hypersensitivity reaction. The anthracycline antineoplastic agents, such as doxorubicin and cyclophosphamide, have direct cardiac toxicity and can cause acute pericarditis and myocarditis. Pericarditis can develop from a drug-induced SLE syndrome caused by medications including procainamide, hydralazine, methyldopa, isoniazid, mesalazine and reserpine.

Smallpox vaccination infrequently leads to myocarditis. In a review of a large vaccination program in the US military, approximately 12 per 100,000 vaccinated troops developed myopericarditis within 14 days of vaccination.

Whether this is due to a direct viral cytopathic effect or an immune-mediated phenomenon is unclear. Methysergide causes constrictive pericarditis through mediastinal fibrosis. Dantrolene, phenytoin and minoxidil produce pericarditis through an unknown mechanism. Treatment includes stopping the administration of the offending agent and antiinflammatory therapy as needed.

Irradiation

Pericardial disease is the most common cardiac toxicity. Others are coronary artery disease, conduction disturbance, and myocardial and valvular disease. High incidence occurs with high doses, especially those greater than 4,000 rad. It can present as acute pericarditis with or without effusion; chronic constrictive pericarditis; or effusive-constrictive pericarditis.

Postpericardiotomy Syndrome

This is similar to Dressler syndrome, except that postpericardiotomy syndrome occurs after cardiac surgery. Several series note an incidence rate of 10–40%. Approximately, 1% developes tamponade. Pericardial effusions can occur in the absence of typical features of postpericardiotomy syndrome. In one study, 56% developed pericardial effusions early after cardiac surgery without correlation to pericarditis or tamponade. The effusions were more common after heavy postoperative bleeding. Pericarditis may develop with other cardiac instrumentation including percutaneous transluminal coronary angioplasty (PTCA) and pacemaker implantation. Usually, it is associated with epicardial or pericardial hematoma formation. Treatment is with aspirin or NSAIDs.

Trauma

This accounts for approximately 1% of cases. Pericarditis can develop from penetrating and nonpenetrating cardiac trauma, esophageal rupture or perforation, and pancreatitis.

Laboratory Studies

- CBC count with differential may show leukocytosis.
- Erythrocyte sedimentation rate and C-reactive protein levels are usually elevated.
- BUN and creatinine levels can be measured to evaluate for uremia.
- Evaluate cardiac enzymes for associated myocarditis or myocardial infarction. In a recent study by Imazio and colleagues, an elevated troponin I level was found in 32% of patients with viral or idiopathic pericarditis. In this study, the troponin I level was related to the extent of myocardial inflammation but was not a negative prognostic marker. Further laboratory work may be clinically indicated. Evaluate blood cultures.

  Perform tuberculin testing with sputum for acid-fast bacilli if the illness exceeds 1 week in duration.
- Obtain an antistreptolysin titer.
- Obtain rheumatoid factor, antinuclear antibody, and anti-DNA values, particularly if the illness is prolonged or severe.
- Evaluate thyroid function in patients with severe pericardial effusion.

Imaging Studies

Chest Radiography

A flask-shaped, enlarged cardiac silhouette may be the first indication of a large pericardial effusion. Patients with small effusions (less than a few hundred milliliters) may present with a normal cardiac silhouette. In one study, pleural effusions were seen in 33% of patients. Approximately, 75% of the effusions were left-sided only.

Echocardiography

An echocardiogram is performed if tamponade or pericardial effusion is suspected on clinical or radiographic grounds or if the illness lasts longer than 1 week. It is the procedure of choice for pericardial effusion. M-mode demonstrates persistence of the echo-free space between the parietal pericardium and the epicardium during the cardiac cycle. Fluid is distributed from the posterobasal left ventricle apically and anteriorly, then laterally and posteriorly to the left atrium. Fluid adjacent to the right atrium is an early indicator of an effusion. Other causes of echo-free space that must be considered include pleural effusion, pericardial masses, and epicardial fat. To a limited extent, an echocardiogram can characterize the effusion. Thin fibrous strands within the pericardial space can be seen in acute effusive pericarditis. Shaggy exudate may indicate a potentially difficult pericardiocentesis, but this finding is not diagnostic. Echocardiography can also be used to evaluate for chamber size, tamponade, and ventricular dysfunction.

Computed Tomography

Effusions are easily detected through different X-ray coefficients of fluid and the pericardium. Similarly, the nature of the effusion may be surmised, given the different attenuation coefficients for blood, exudate, chyle, and serous fluid. Hemopericardium may be difficult to assess without intravenous contrast because blood has the same radiodensity as myocardium.

Magnetic resonance imaging: This is a sensitive technique for detecting pericardial effusion and loculated pericardial effusion and thickening.

Other Tests

Electrocardiography (Figs 24.5–24.8)

Classic acute pericarditis evolves through four stages:

Stage 1 accompanies the onset of acute pain and is the hallmark of acute pericarditis. ECG changes to include diffuse concave upward ST elevation, except aVR and V1 (usually depressed). T-waves are upright in the leads with ST elevation, and the PR segment deviates opposite to P-wave polarity.

Stage 2 occurs several days later with the return of the ST segment to baseline, followed by flattening of the T waves.

Stage 3, T-waves become inverted.

Stage 4, the ECG returns to the prepericarditis baseline weeks to months after the onset. The T-wave inversion may persist indefinitely in the chronic inflammation observed with tuberculosis, uremia, or neoplasm. Electrical alternans, the beat-to-beat variability in QRS voltage caused by excessive cardiac mobility, may be seen with an effusion (Fig. 24.5).

Procedures

Cardiac catheterization: This is used for tamponade. It can evaluate constrictive pericarditis versus restrictive cardiomyopathy.

Pericardiocentesis

Blind percutaneous pericardial puncture increases the risk of complication to 5–50% and should be performed only in an emergency. Complications include fatal cardiac laceration. Conversely, pericardiocentesis is relatively safe when guided by echocardiography, especially with large free anterior effusion. One study noted only three minor complications in 117 procedures with ultrasound guidance. In a large study, diagnostic pericardiocentesis led to a diagnosis in only 6% of cases, versus 29% diagnosed with therapeutic pericardiocentesis. As such, pericardiocentesis should not be performed unless tamponade or suspected purulent pericarditis is present. If a pericardiocentesis is performed for drainage, an indwelling catheter should be placed in the pericardial space for continued drainage over several days. If the catheter continues to drain a large amount, a more definitive procedure should be performed. The pericardial fluid should be analyzed for red cells, total protein level, lactic acid dehydrogenase level, adenosine deaminase activity, and culture (ordinary and Loewenstein media). Directly investigate for tuberculous bacilli and perform a cytologic study.

Pericardial window: This procedure, in which only 9 cm^2 or less of pericardium is resected, is used for effusive pericarditis therapy. In critically ill patients, a balloon catheter may be used to create a pericardial window. Some studies note the need for repeat operation in nearly 25% of patients who undergo the procedure at 2 years.

Pericardiectomy: This is used for constrictive pericarditis, effusive pericarditis, or recurrent pericarditis with multiple attacks, steroid dependence, and/or intolerance to other medical management. Studies demonstrate that failure rates are proportional to the amount of pericardium removed (i.e. the more pericardium removed, the less likely the procedure will fail). In effusive pericarditis, the higher failure rate associated with a pericardial window or partial pericardiectomy is likely secondary to the continued fluid production from the remaining pericardium with sealing of the remaining pericardium to the heart. The operative mortality rate was 14% in one series, with a range of 1% for New York Heart Association class 1–2, 10% for class 3, and 46% for class 4. The 5-year survival rate was 80% for class 3–4 and approximately 95% for 1–2. As with pericardiocentesis, studies involving pericardiectomy note a greatly improved diagnostic yield if pericardial biopsy is performed as part of a therapeutic procedure. Diagnostic biopsies yielded 5%, whereas therapeutic biopsies were at 22–54%.

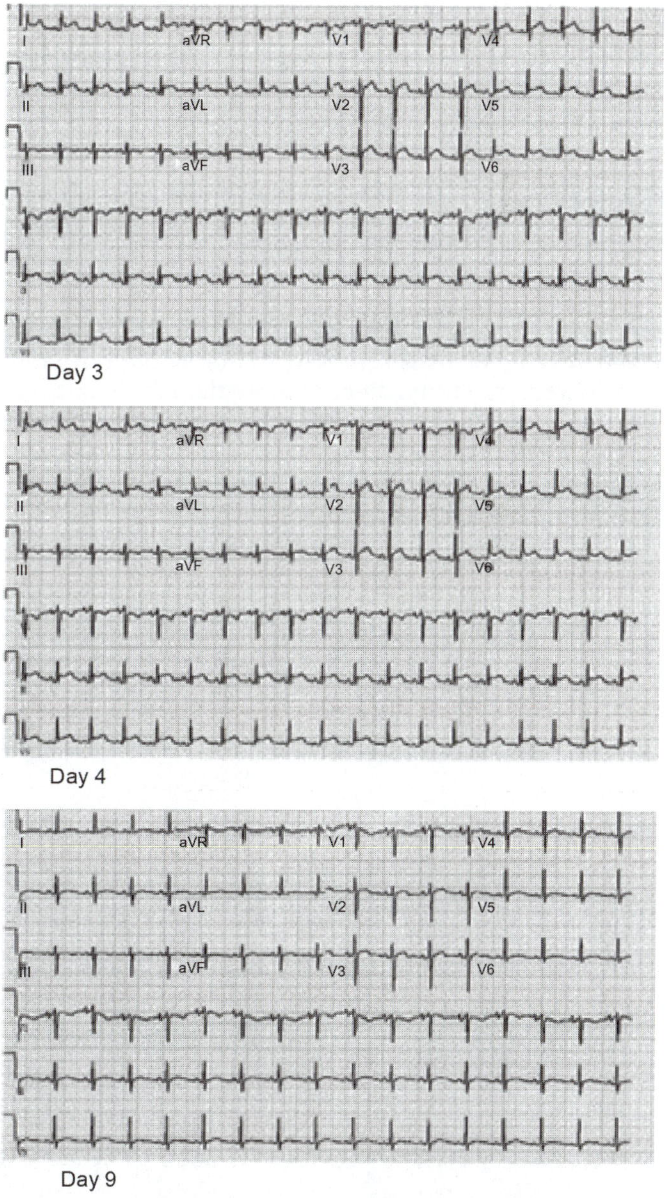

Fig. 24.5: *Serial electrocardiograms obtained during recovery in the ICU that show resolution of the PR and ST segment abnormalities noted previously*

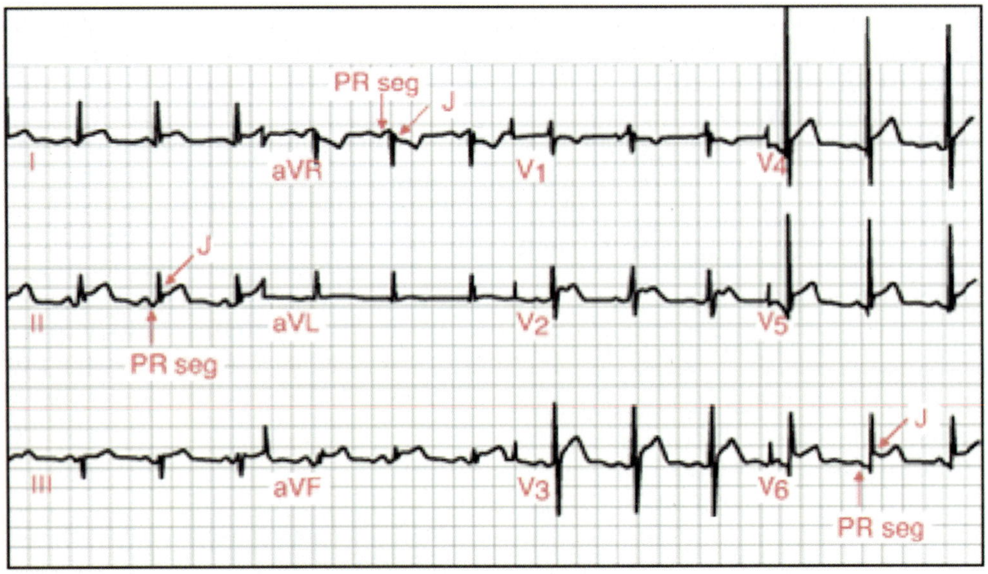

Fig. 24.6: *Acute pericarditis: stage 1 ECG. J points, except aVR and V1, are elevated. T waves are essentially normal. PR segments, except aVR and V1, are depressed. PR deviations are commonly absent in one limb lead (here, aVL)*

Medical Care

Oxygen and a cardiac monitor should be provided. Rule out other life-threatening causes of chest pain, such as myocardial infarction or aortic dissection. Evaluate for evidence of hemodynamic instability. Consider whether further management is safe to continue on an outpatient basis. In a recent study, fever of more than 38°C, subacute onset, immunosuppression, trauma, oral anticoagulation therapy, myopericarditis, severe pericardial effusion, and cardiac tamponade were designated as poor prognostic predictors. Patients without these factors were treated on an outpatient basis without serious complications after a mean follow-up of 38 months. Given an overall lack of specificity of clinical features, several authors describe diagnostic protocols to determine the etiology for pericarditis. Following specific protocols, several authors have determined a specific etiology in 14–22% of patients.

In one study, cardiac tamponade and an unfavorable clinical outcome, with persistence of fever, significant pericardial effusion, or general illness lasting longer than a week, was highly associated with finding a specific etiology. Initial evaluation includes clinical history and

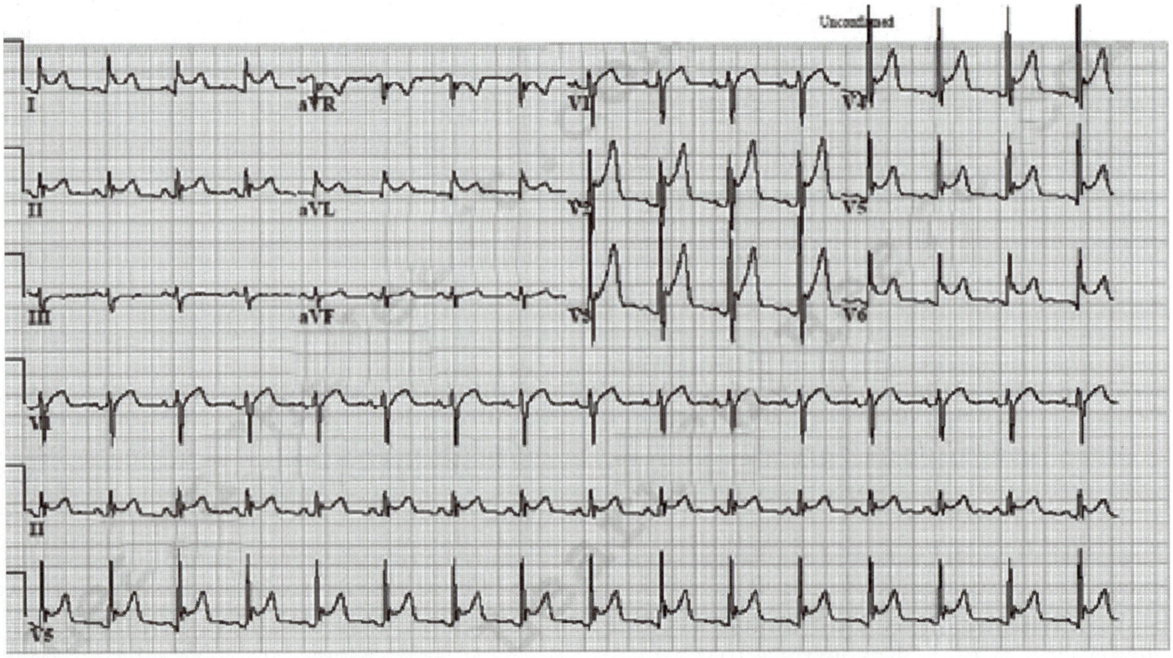

Fig. 24.7: *ECG showing generalised ST elevation in both limb and chest leads in patient with acute pericarditis without reciprocal changes*

physical examination, chest radiograph, ECG, echocardiography as indicated, and initial laboratory work. Consider thoracentesis with adenosine deaminase in addition to conventional studies in patients with a pleural effusion. Pericardiocentesis should be performed on all patients with cardiac tamponade or suspected purulent pericarditis.

Surgical Care

If tamponade recurs after pericardiocentesis, perform a pericardial biopsy with histologic and bacteriologic examinations of the pericardium. If significant clinical activity persists for 3 weeks after admission and without an etiologic diagnosis, some authors recommend pericardial biopsy.

Consultations

Consult a cardiologist or internist for acute and idiopathic cases. In complicated cases, such as tuberculous, purulent uremic etiologies require multidisciplinary involvement including consultations with a cardiologist, cardiac surgeon, and medical subspecialists (e.g. infectious diseases specialist, nephrologist). Treatment for specific causes of pericarditis is directed according to the underlying cause. For patients with idiopathic or viral pericarditis, therapy is directed at symptom relief. NSAIDs are the mainstay of therapy. These agents have a similar efficacy with relief of chest pain in about 85–90% of patients within days of treatment. Colchicine, alone or in combination with an NSAID, can be considered for patients with recurrent or continued symptoms beyond 14 days.

Medication

Nonsteroidal antiinflammatory drugs: These agents are effective for chest discomfort and underlying inflammation.

Indomethacin (indocin): Classic treatment; rapidly absorbed. Metabolism occurs in the liver by demethylation, deacetylation, and glucuronide conjugation.

Adult dose:	50 mg PO q8h
Pediatric dose:	1.5–2.5 mg/kg/d PO divided tid

Ketorolac (toradol): Small studies have documented rapid relief of symptoms with 1–2 doses. Inhibits prostaglandin synthesis by decreasing activity of enzyme, cyclooxygenase, which results in decreased formation of prostaglandin precursors.

Adult dose:	30–90 mg IV/IM, repeat with 30 mg IV/IM in 1 h prn
Pediatric dose:	Not established

Ibuprofen (motrin, advil): Usually, DOC for mild to moderate pain if no contraindications exist. Inhibits

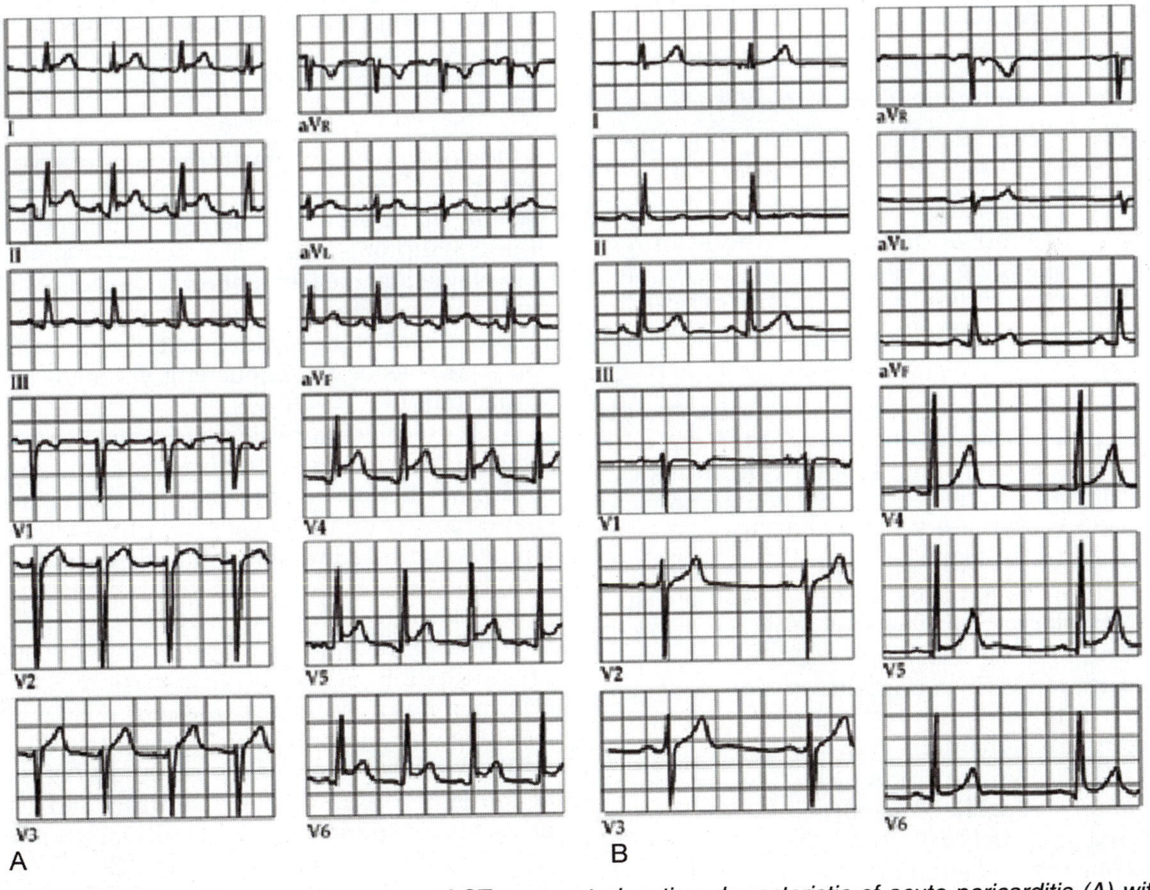

Fig. 24.8: *Electrocardiograms contrast the pattern of ST segment elevation characteristic of acute pericarditis (A) with the normal variant (early repolarization) pattern of ST segment elevation (B). The normal variant pattern is associated with a normal or slow heart rate and has relatively tall R waves and T waves in V4, V5, and V6. The ST segment elevation is less than 25% of the T wave amplitude. In contrast, the acute pericarditis has PR depression and lower T wave amplitude*

inflammatory reactions and pain, probably by decreasing the activity of the enzyme cyclooxygenase, which results in prostaglandin synthesis.

Adult dose: 400–800 mg PO q4-8h

Pediatric dose: <6 months: Not established; 6 months to 12 years: 10–70 mg/kg/d PO divided tid/qid; start at the lower end of dosing range and titrate upward to a maximum of 2.4 g/d > 12 years: administer as in adults

Antiinflammatory agents: These agents reduce the effects of immune reactions.

Colchicine: Used for recurrent pericarditis. Decreases leukocyte motility and phagocytosis observed in inflammatory responses.

Adult dose: 1 mg/d PO

Pediatric dose: < 12 years: not established; > 12 years: administer as in adults

Salicylates: These agents reduce inflammation. Aspirin (anacin, bayer aspirin, ascriptin) used for pericarditis secondary to myocardial infarction. Inhibits prostaglandin synthesis and blocks prostaglandin synthetase action, which prevents formation of the platelet-aggregating thromboxane A2. Full doses are unsafe during pregnancy.

Pediatric dose: Not established

Adult dose: 650 mg PO q6h

Pediatric dose: 60–90 mg/kg/d PO divided q6h.

Complications: Recurrence (can cause significant morbidity, secondary to pain) cardiac tamponade. Constrictive pericarditis. Combination of effusive and constrictive pericarditis.

Prognosis: The prognosis depends on the etiology. Idiopathic and viral etiologies usually have a self-limited course. Purulent, tuberculous and neoplastic pericardial involvement have more complicated courses with worse outcomes.

Medical/legal pitfalls: Avoid NSAIDs and corticosteroids in AMI pericarditis because they may interfere with ventricular healing, remodeling, or both. Pericarditis can be difficult to distinguish from myocardial infarction and repolarization in patients who present with chest pain and ST-segment elevation on ECG.

Aside from clues elicited from the history and physical examination, repolarization does not progress through stages and is uncommonly associated with PR depression. Serial monitoring of ECGs in young patients with chest pain helps differentiate early repolarization from acute pericarditis. An ST-segment–to–T-wave ratio of greater than or equal to 0.25 in V6 can distinguish acute pericarditis from early repolarization. The ST segment in AMI is usually convex, bowing upward with reciprocal changes, as opposed to concave ST segments without reciprocal changes observed in acute pericarditis and repolarization.

Special concerns: Children may present with abdominal pain. The classic feature of chest pain and dyspnea with pericarditis may be subtle and can be confused with other diagnoses, particularly in elderly individuals.

CONSTRICTIVE PERICARDITIS

Although constrictive pericarditis is frequently part of a differential diagnosis, unless the findings are classic, it is not always the leading candidate. The symptoms are nonspecific and may be shared with diseases as diverse as myocardial infarction, aortic dissection, and connective tissue disorders. Constrictive pericarditis is usually a long-term consequence of either acute or chronic forms of pericarditis. The complex pathophysiology, combined with the fact that the condition is most commonly idiopathic, is why having a working knowledge of constrictive pericarditis is important. Constrictive pericarditis occurs when a thickened fibrotic pericardium, of whatever cause, impedes normal diastolic filling. This usually involves the parietal pericardium although it can involve the visceral pericardium. Acute and subacute forms of pericarditis (which may or may not be symptomatic) may deposit fibrin, which may, in turn, evoke a pericardial effusion. This often leads to pericardial organization, chronic fibrotic scarring, calcification, and restricted cardiac filling. The history of constrictive pericarditis is replete with some of the most famous names in medicine. Richard Lower described a patient with dyspnea and an intermittent pulse in 1669. Lancisi first reported on the constrictive syndrome in 1828. Corrigan described the pericardial knock in 1842. Kussmaul described his sign and the associated paradoxical pulse in 1873.

Pathophysiology: The most common forms of constrictive pericarditis can be described as causing an impediment of diastolic filling secondary to a confining pericardium. The clinical symptoms and classic hemodynamic findings can be explained by the fact that early diastolic filling becomes rapid and that elevation and equalization of the diastolic pressures in all of the cardiac chambers restrict late diastolic filling. This leads to venous engorgement and decreased cardiac output.

The constrictive pericarditis is always difficult in distinguishing it from restrictive cardiomyopathy and other syndromes associated with elevated right-sided pressures. They share similar symptoms, physical findings, and hemodynamics. Although obtaining a careful history and performing a physical examination remain the cornerstones of evaluation, technologic advances have facilitated diagnosis, particularly with the appropriate use of Doppler echocardiography, high-resolution computed tomography (CT), magnetic resonance imaging (MRI), and invasive hemodynamic measurement (Table 24.2).

The normal pericardium is composed of two layers: (1) the tough fibrous parietal pericardium and (2) the smooth serous visceral pericardium. Usually, approximately 50 mL of fluid (plasma ultrafiltrate) is present in the intrapericardial space to minimize friction during cardiac motion. In constrictive pericarditis, early ventricular filling during the one-third of diastole is unimpeded, but, afterwards, the stiff pericardium affects flow and hemodynamics. That is, ventricular pressure decreases rapidly early and then increases abruptly to a level that is sustained until systole. All cardiac diastolic pressures become nearly equal. This limits end-diastolic volume, which, in turn, decreases stroke volume and cardiac output.

Incidence

Like many diseases that, in the past, were predominantly infectious in origin, the clinical spectrum of constrictive pericarditis has changed in recent years. In developed countries, the most common etiologies are idiopathic, are presumed viral, or are associated with other medical diseases or postcardiothoracic surgery.

Internationally: In the developing world, infectious etiologies remain more prominent (tuberculosis has the highest total incidence).

Mortality/Morbidity

Scant data exist because the disease is rare.

The underlying disease usually determines the prognosis. Poorer prognoses are associated with malignancy and New York Heart Association (NYHA) class III or IV heart failure symptoms.

Long-term survival after pericardiectomy depends on the underlying cause. Of common causes, idiopathic constrictive pericarditis has the best prognosis (88% survival at 7 year), followed by constriction due to cardiac surgery (66% at 7 year). The worst postpericardiectomy prognosis occurs in postradiation constrictive pericarditis (27% survival at 7 year).

History

Constrictive pericarditis presents with a myriad of symptoms, making a diagnosis based solely on clinical history virtually impossible. Additionally, these symptoms may develop slowly over a number of years such that patients may not be aware of all of their symptoms until questioned.

Dyspnea tends to be the most common presenting symptom and occurs in virtually all patients.

Lower-extremity edema and abdominal swelling and discomfort are other common symptoms. Many may feel that the initial history is more compatible with liver disease (cryptogenic cirrhosis) than with pericardial constriction because of the predominance of findings related to the venous system. Fatigue and orthopnea are common. Chest pain, presumably due to active inflammation, may be present although this is observed in a minority of patients. Nausea, vomiting, and right upper quadrant pain if present, are thought to be due to hepatic congestion, bowel congestion, or both.

Physical Examination

General findings in the early stages, physical findings may be subtle, requiring close examination to avoid missing the diagnosis. In more advanced stages, the patient may appear ill, with marked muscle wasting, cachexia, or jaundice. Constriction should be considered in the presence of otherwise unexplained jugular venous distention, pleural effusion, hepatomegaly, or ascites. Cardiovascular findings. Elevated jugular venous pressures are an almost universal finding (Fig. 24.9).

Avoid examining the patient only in the supine position because venous pressures may be above the angle of the jaw and inadvertently mistaken for normal. Sinus tachycardia is common while the blood pressure is normal or low, depending on the stage of the disease process. The apical impulse is often impalpable, and the patient may have distant or muffled heart sounds.

A pericardial knock, which corresponds with the sudden cessation of ventricular filling early in diastole, occurs in approximately half the cases and may be mistaken for an S3 gallop. However, a knock is of higher frequency than an S3 and occurs slightly earlier in diastole.

A cardiac murmur typically is not present unless concomitant valvular heart disease or a fibrous band that constricts the right ventricular outflow tract is present. Pulsus paradoxicum (paradoxus) is a variable finding (i.e. a decrease in the palpable pulse and systolic pressure more than 10 mmHg during inspiration) a concomitant pericardial effusion with an abnormally elevated pressure exists.

The Kussmaul sign (i.e. elevation of JVP often more than 10 cm with a prominent systolic x descent and abscent y diastolic descent. If the JVP is visible and either remains static or rises with inspiration, it indicates concomitant pericardial constriction It is a common nonspecific finding, but this sign is also observed in patients with right ventricular failure, restrictive cardiomyopathy, right ventricular infarction, and tricuspid stenosis, although, importantly, not in patients with cardiac tamponade.

Gastrointestinal, pulmonary, and other organ system findings, hepatomegaly with prominent hepatic pulsations can be detected in as many as 70% of patients. Other signs that result from chronic hepatic congestion include ascites, spider angiomata, and palmar erythema, which can contribute to the common but erroneous diagnosis of primary liver disease (Table 24.2).

Peripheral edema is a common finding although it may be less prominent in younger patients with competent venous valves.

Etiological Factors

The varied etiologies of constrictive pericarditis parallel those of acute pericarditis which is a common precipitant. All forms of pericarditis may eventually lead to pericardial constriction. Generally, these can be broken down by frequency into common, less common, and rare forms. One of the more difficult distinctions to make is between constrictive pericarditis and restrictive cardiomyopathy.

Because the physical findings may be identical, the physician must rely heavily on the patient's history and other ancillary tests, including CT scan, MRI, echocardiography, and invasive hemodynamic measurements. Although still rare in absolute terms, sarcoidosis, amyloidosis, and hemochromatosis are the most commonly encountered infiltrative processes that lead to restrictive physiology. Cardiac fibrosis is another cause of restrictive cardiomyopathy that is becoming more frequent as cardiac patients with various more common disorders live longer. Congestive heart failure from a number of causes including pressure overload and myocardial, valvular, or atherosclerotic disease, must be excluded.

Cardiac tamponade as a result of hemopericardium, uremia, or malignancy may mimic constrictive pericarditis and is a critical distinction to make. Right-sided valvular abnormalities that increase venous pressure, such as tricuspid stenosis or tricuspid regurgitation, can be confusing upon examination but can usually be diagnosed based on echocardiography. Right atrial tumors such as myxomas can mimic constriction by compressing the tricuspid valve, but these are rare and can be distinguished with echocardiography.

Superior vena cava syndrome and nephrotic syndrome can produce gross edema and ascites but, generally, are easily differentiated, especially with the use of modern imaging modalities.

Cryptogenic cirrhosis is a relatively common presentation, and many patients are mistakenly diagnosed with primary liver disease. Ovarian carcinoma may be another consideration with ascites and edema. The following are common etiologies:

Idiopathic: In many cases, particularly in developed countries, no antecedent diagnosis can be found. These cases are termed idiopathic. Reports by most authors indicate that a high percentage of idiopathic cases of constrictive pericarditis may be related to previously recognized or unrecognized viral pericarditis. Of the viruses, coxsackievirus A and B, other echoviruses, and adenoviruses are most commonly implicated.

Infectious (bacterial): Tuberculosis is the leading cause of constrictive pericarditis in developing nations but represents only a minority of causes in the United States and other developed countries. Bacterial infections that lead to purulent pericarditis are also declining in frequency.

In the past, purulent pericarditis associated with pneumococcal pneumonia was the most common presentation of a bacterial source. However, the widespread use of antibiotics has drastically changed the frequency and spectrum of purulent pericarditis such that the most common presentation now occurs following cardiac surgery.

An increasing number of Gram-positive organisms including multiple resistant strains of staphylococci, may be isolated. Group A and B streptococci and Gram-negative rods (e.g. *Pseudomonas* species, *Escherichia coli*, and *Klebsiella species*) have also been documented.

Radiation-induced: The long-term effects of thoracic and mediastinal radiation therapy (e.g. used in the treament of hematological, breast, and other malignancies) are being increasingly realized. The common features of radiation-induced cardiac complications stem from microcirculation injury with endothelial damage, capillary rupture, and

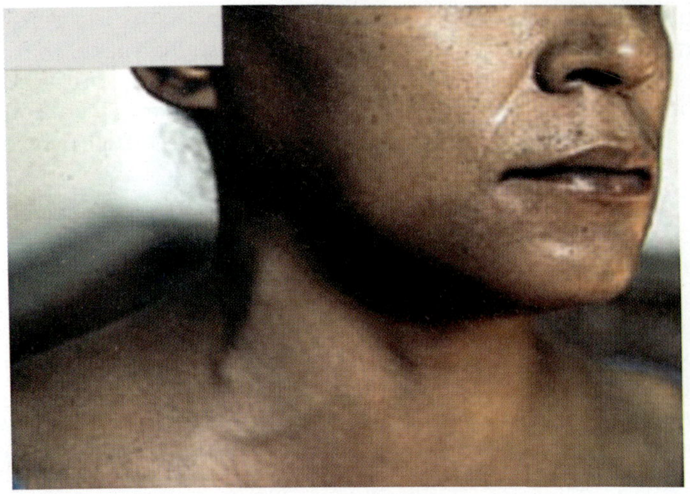

Fig. 24.9: *Raised jugular venous pressure in constrictive pericarditis*

platelet adhesion. This sets up an inflammatory response, which may either resolve or organize to form adhesions between the visceral pericardium and the parietal pericardium which leads to constriction. Generally, radiation-induced constrictive pericarditis presents 5–10 years after radiation therapy and is more likely to present with an associated pericardial effusion.

Postsurgical: Any operative or invasive (catheterization) procedure in which the pericardium is opened, manipulated, or damaged may invoke an inflammatory response, leading to constrictive pericarditis. The most common example is constrictive pericarditis in the setting of previous coronary artery bypass grafting. The following are less common etiologies.

Infectious (fungal): Fungal infections are an uncommon source of constrictive pericarditis in patients who are immunocompetent. Nocardia species can be causative organisms, especially in endemic areas such as the Ohio Valley. *Aspergillus*, *Candida* and *Coccidioides* species are important pathogens in patients infected with HIV and in other immunocompromised hosts.

Neoplasms: Malignant involvement may also manifest as pericardial effusion (with or without tamponade) or as an encased heart with thickening of both visceral and parietal layers, resulting in constrictive physiology. Although many types of neoplasms have been reported, breast and lung carcinomas and lymphomas are the most common metastatic malignancies associated with constrictive pericarditis. Other malignancies that involve the pericardium with relative frequency include melanoma and mesothelioma.

Uremia: Constrictive pericarditis may develop in association with long-term hemodialysis.

Connective tissue disorders: Autoimmune disorders that involve the pericardium are not unusual, typically manifesting as a small pericardial effusion or as an episode of acute pericarditis. Chronic pericardial involvement is less common but can occur in patients with rheumatoid arthritis, usually associated with the presence of subcutaneous nodules. Systemic lupus erythematosus and scleroderma also may lead to constrictive pericarditis, and, in the latter, this carries a poor prognosis.

Drug-induced: Procainamide and hydralazine have been reported to cause constrictive pericarditis through a drug-induced lupus-like syndrome. Methysergide therapy also has been implicated as a cause of constrictive pericarditis.

Trauma: Although uncommon, both blunt and penetrating trauma to the chest wall have been reported to cause constrictive pericarditis, presumably through an inflammatory mechanism.

Myocardial infarction: Post-myocardial infarction constrictive pericarditis has been reported. The patient typically has a history of Dressler syndrome or hemopericardium after thrombolytic therapy. The following are rare etiologies: toxic or metabolic: uremia with chronic hemodialysis can lead to constrictive pericarditis and is usually associated with a pericardial effusion.

Intrapericardial instrumentation: Constrictive pericarditis after implantation of an epicardial pacemaker or automated implantable cardiac defibrillator is a rare but reported phenomenon. Hereditary: Mulibrey nanism is an autosomal recessive disorder characterized by multiple abnormalities including dwarfism, constrictive pericarditis, abnormal fundi, and fibrous dysplasia of the long bones.

Chemical trauma: Constrictive pericarditis following sclerotherapy for esophageal varices is rare.

Chylopericardium: This is a rare cause of constrictive pericarditis. Other problems to be considered:
- Cardiac fibrosis
- Cirrhosis, cryptogenic
- Congestive heart failure (valvular or myocardial).

Laboratory Studies

No laboratory data are diagnostic of constrictive pericarditis. However, as a result of the universal findings of a chronically elevated right atrial pressure and passive congestion of the liver, kidneys, and gastrointetinal tract, resultant abnormalities may be present. These include elevations in both conjugated and unconjugated bilirubin levels and elevated levels as determined by hepatocellular function tests.

Hypoalbuminemia may be a result of both a protein losing enteropathy and proteinuria that may approach nephrotic range. If active or chronic inflammation is present, nonspecific markers, such as an elevated sedimentation rate or a normocytic normochromic anemia, may be present. If an associated collagen vascular disorder is suggested, antinuclear antibody or rheumatoid factor should be measured. Results from a purified protein derivative skin test should be positive in cases of tuberculous pericarditis (unless the patient is anergic).

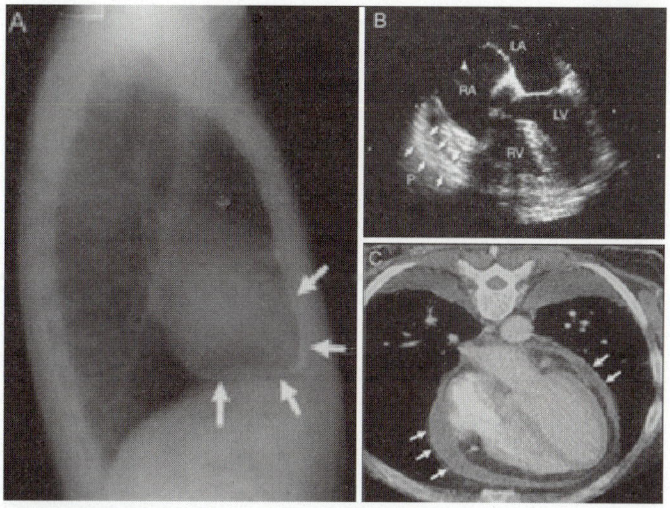

Fig. 24.10: *Chest radiograph, transesophageal echocardiogram (TEE), and cardiac computed tomogram typical of constrictive pericarditis. (A) Pericardial calcification (arrows) on chest radiography is best seen from the lateral view over the right ventricle (RV) and across the diaphragmatic surface of the heart. Pericardial calcification reflects chronicity of constrictive pericarditis and is associated with a higher surgical mortality. (B) Thickness of the pericardium is often difficult to determine by transthoracic echocardiography, but TEE is usually reliable in measuring the pericardial thickness (arrows). (C) Increased pericardial thickness (arrows) can be visualized on computed tomogram of the same patient. LA, left atrium; LV, left ventricle; RA, right atrium*

Expect an elevation in the white blood cell count with an associated left shift in cases of bacterial pericarditis. Cytologically examining the pericardial fluid, if present, helps diagnose a malignant cause (if not otherwise apparent). The levels of brain natriuretic peptide (BNP), a cardiac hormone released in response to increased wall stretch, are often mildly increased in constrictive pericarditis. BNP levels are even higher in restrictive cardiomyopathy and may be useful in differentiating these disorders.

Imaging Studies

Chest Radiography

Although findings are insensitive for the presence of constrictive pericarditis, some classic findings are suggestive of the diagnosis when present within a compatible clinical context. Severe pericardial calcification is common however, it is not specific and does not prove pericardial constriction. If no significant pericardial effusion is present, the cardiac silhouette may appear normal.

The superior vena cava, azygous veins, or both may be dilated. Pleural effusions are common and are usually bilateral. Pulmonary edema is rare and might suggest other cardiac or lung disease (Figs 24.10–24.12, 24.21 and 24.22).

Echocardiography

Echocardiography has been used for many years to help diagnose constrictive pericarditis and, in particular, to

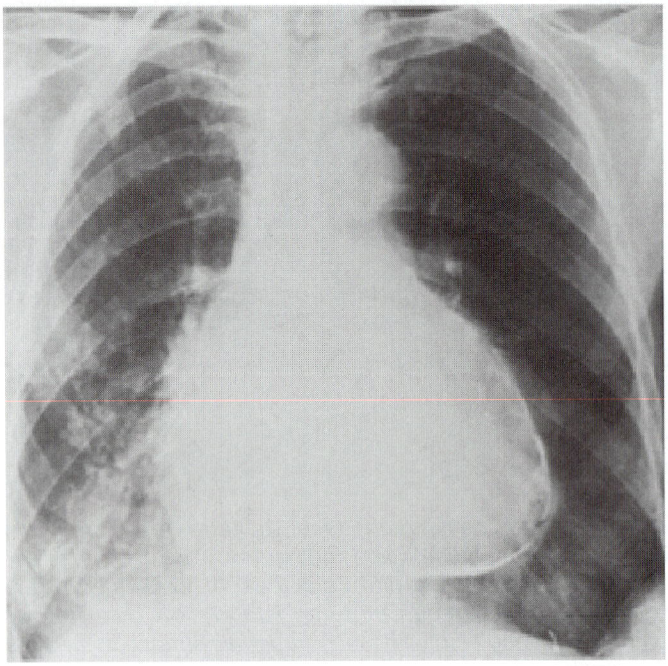

Fig. 24.11: *Extensive pericardial calcifications on chest radiograph (posteroanterior projection). Extensive pulmonary infiltrates caused by tuberculosis can be noted*

differentiate it from restrictive and other cardiomyopathies. Unfortunately, no echocardiographic finding is pathognomonic for constriction. However, when all the echocardiography data are taken together within a clinical context, the likelihood of constriction can usually be accurately assessed.

As a general principle, pericardial imaging by echocardiography is not sensitive and is not considered a reliable technique to visualize the pericardium. Admittedly, the pericardium can be echodense, but this is not always the case.

Transesophageal echocardiography is more reliable than transthoracic echocardiography for helping to detect a thickened pericardium, especially if it is thick or very echogenic, but this is not nearly as accurate as CT or MRI.

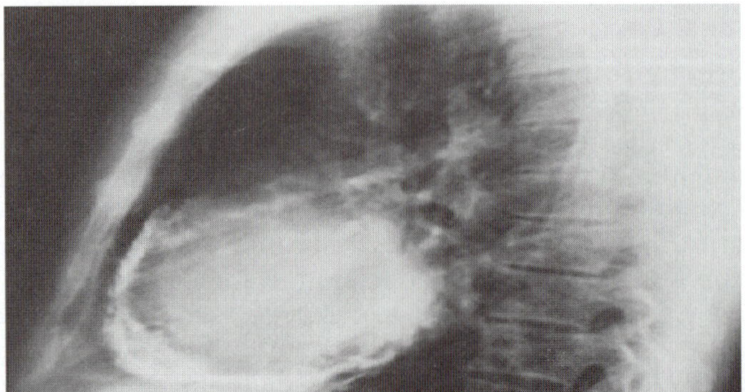

Fig. 24.12: *Extensive pericardial calcifications on chest radiograph (lateral projection). These were caused by tuberculosis*

2D Echocardiography

Two dimensional echocardiography can show evidence of right-sided pressure overload such as atrial septal shifting to the left with inspiration or dilated inferior and superior vena cavae and hepatic veins. These are nonspecific signs that can also occur in right heart failure as a result of other causes (Figs 24.24, 24.25 and 24.28).

Doppler echocardiography provides important hemodynamic information. Early rapid diastolic filling can be imaged by interrogating forward flow at the mitral and tricuspid valve levels. Termed the E (for early filling) and the A (for atrial filling) waves, they may have shortened durations, increased velocity, and rapid decelerations from their peak velocity, reflecting constrictive physiology. These velocities usually decrease with inspiration and increase with expiration. The transtricuspid velocities show an opposite pattern to the transmitral (i.e. increasing with inspiration and decreasing with expiration). The shortened deceleration time from these peak velocities is felt to correspond to the dip-and-plateau hemodynamics seen with limited early diastolic flow. The pulmonary vein Doppler inflow pattern also has respiratory variation, with its diastolic inflow being greater than systolic inflow, which itself may even reverse. These Doppler findings are sensitive when present, but, like many echocardiographic signs, their absence does not exclude constrictive hemodynamics.

Doppler interrogation can be limited if patients cannot adequately vary their respiration or if concomitant myocardial disease, atrial fibrillation, or severe lung disease [e.g. chronic obstructive pulmonary disease (COPD)], which can lead to false-positive findings is present.

Always keep in mind that measurements of diastolic function are load-dependent (i.e. dependent on preload and afterload). If atrial and ventricular filling pressures are low, Doppler interrogation findings may be falsely negative. Likewise, if atrial and ventricular filling pressures are high, respiratory variation may be masked. In such cases, preload may be reduced with either medication or dynamic maneuvers, such as tilting the patient's head up or having the patient sit. These maneuvers may unmask respiratory variation (Figs 24.13–24.15).

Because Doppler transmitral inflow respiratory variation can occur in COPD, other differences must then be examined. For example, the marked increase in inspiratory superior vena cava systolic flow seen in COPD is not seen in constriction. Although technically challenging, Doppler ventricular inflow patterns can help to distinguish constrictive from restrictive cardiac physiology. From a Doppler perspective, constriction limits ventricular filling and enhances ventricular interaction. Conversely, restriction generally limits ventricular distensibility. Put another way, in constriction, presumably normal myocardium is present, but the ventricles are encased together, whereas in restriction, abnormal myocardium is present with no such restraint. Therefore, both physiologies have abnormal early diastolic filling with early atrial ventricular pressure equilibration. The respiratory

Table 24.2: *Differentiation of pericardial constriction from restrictive cardiomyopathy*

Physical examination		
Pulmonary congestion	Usually absent	Usually present
Jugular venous pulse	Prominent Y descent	
Early diastolic sound	Pericardial knock	S3 (low pitched)
Pericardial thickness	> 2 mm (but <2 mm in 15%)	< 2 mm
Echo/Doppler findings LV myocardium	Normal	"Sparkling" mycardium in amyloid
Atrial size	+/− Atrial enlargement	Atrial enlargement
Mitral valve flow pattern	Restricted	Restricted
Respiratory variation in E wave	> 25%	< 20%
Mitral annular diastolic velocity	> 8 cm/s	< 8 cm/s
Biomarker		
B-type natriuretic peptide	< 200 pg/mL	> 600 pg/mL
Hemodynamics		
Y descent	Prominent	Variable
PA systolic pressure	< 50 mmHg	> 60 mmHg
PCW-RA pressure	0	5 mmHg
Reciprocal respiratory variation in right ventricular/left ventricular peak systolic pressure	Present	Absent

PA, pulmonary arterial; PCW, pulmonary capillary wedge; RA, right atrial.

variations are usually greater in constriction than in restriction (probably because of the normal intraventricular septum), usually with greater than 25% changes at the onset of inspiration and expiration. Reflecting this, the deceleration time of the mitral Doppler inflow E wave is usually less than 150 ms with constriction, with a further decrease with inspiration. Unfortunately, when such Doppler findings are not present, the diagnostic reliability decreases. If a concomitant pericardial effusion is present, it may account for some respiratory variation.

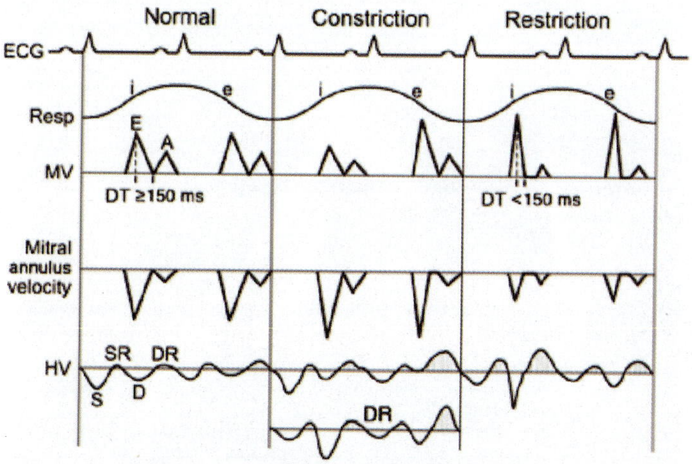

Fig. 24.13: *Schematic diagram of Doppler echocardiographic features in constrictive pericarditis vs. restrictive cardiomyopathy. Schematic illustration of Doppler velocities from mitral inflow (MV), mitral annulus velocity, and hepatic vein (HV). Electrocardiographic (ECG) and respirometer (Resp) recordings indicating inspiration (i) and expiration (e) are also shown. A, atrial filling; D, diastolic flow; DR, diastolic flow reversal; DT, deceleration time; E, early diastolic filling; S, systolic flow; SR, systolic flow reversal. Stippled areas under the curve represent flow reversal*

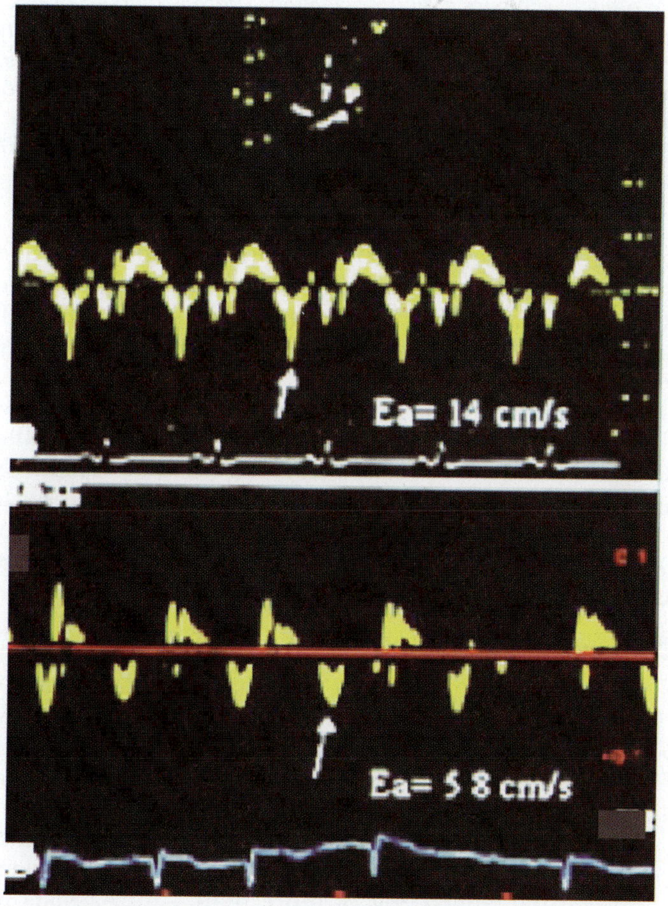

Fig. 24.14: *TDI scans showing typical bounce (arrow) in a patient with constrictive pericarditis, early diastolic longitudinal annular velocity (Ea) recorded by the pulsed Doppler are found normal and helps differentiating this condition from that of restrictive cardiomyopathy*

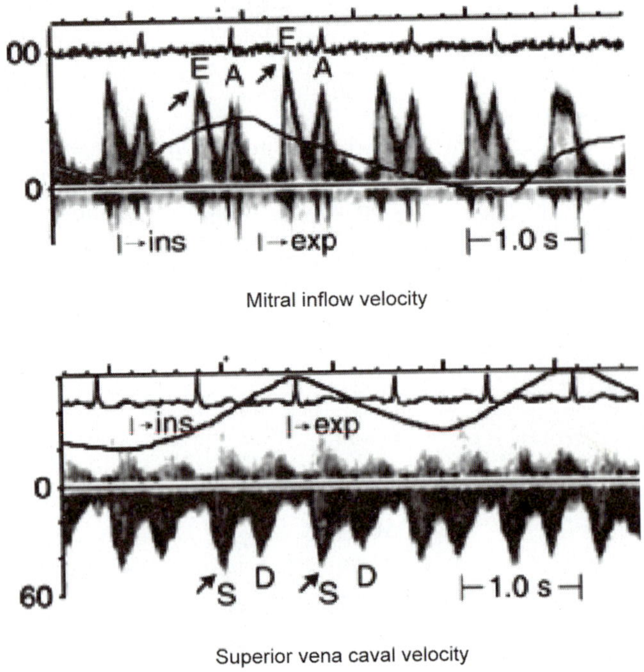

Fig. 24.15: *Doppler mitral flow and superior vena caval velocity in a patient with pericardial constriction. There is marked (>25%) respiratory variation in the peak early diastolic initial flow velocity E [decreased during inspiration (ins) and increased during expiration (exp)]. In contrast, there is less respiratory variation of the flow velocity in the vena cava. S, systole; D, diastole. (Reproduced with permission from Boonyaratavej et al. Copyright 1998, American College of Cardiology Foundation).*

A recent innovation that may improve this differentition is tissue Doppler echocardiography, in which the actual endocardial and epicardial tissue velocities are measured. Because myocardial relaxation itself is preserved in pure constrictive pericarditis, the early relaxation myocardial velocity (Em, also known as Ea) is normal, whereas it is abnormal with restriction (when intrinsic myocardial disease is present). For example, given that a normal Em is more than 10 cm/s, a near-normal (>8 cm/s) Em supports constriction, whereas a much lower Em supports restriction. Only contemporary echocardiography equipment can be used to measure this.

Computed Tomography (Figs 24.17 and 24.23)

Conventional CT scanners may not help adequately visualize the parietal pericardium. However, the parietal pericardium can be visualized well using high-resolution CT. The pericardial thickness, degree of calcification, and distribution of these findings are easily measured.

The normal pericardium is 1–2 mm thick. An abnormal pericardial thickness is considered 3–4 mm thick or thicker.

Pericardial thickening of more than 4 mm assists in differentiating constrictive disease from restrictive cardiomyopathy, and a thickening of more than 6 mm adds even more specificity for constriction. False-negative results may occur if a long-standing thin pericardial scar without appreciable thickening is present. That is, normal pericardial thickness does not exclude pericardial constriction. If the hemodynamics and presentation are otherwise compatible, the diagnosis must still be entertained despite unremarkable pericardial imaging.

Magnetic Resonance Imaging

The development of real-time, high-resolution MRI and the ability to acquire images in 50 ms or less makes MRI the most sensitive method for imaging the pericardium. As can be done with CT scanning, an MRI can be used to measure the pericardium for thickness, calcification, and distribution of abnormalities. A thickened pericardium does not prove that constrictive pericarditis is present; it must be clinically correlated. Likewise, constriction can occur in a scarred fibrous pericardium of normal thickness. Gated MRI has an advantage in determining whether pericardial fluid is hemorrhagic. Obtaining CT scan images may be advantageous compared to performing MRI when calcium levels are significantly elevated (Figs 24.16–24.20).

Other Tests

Electrocardiogram (Figs 24.26 and 24.29)

Chronic pericarditis is not associated with the classic ECG findings seen with acute pericarditis. Findings of acute pericarditis generally include diffuse concave ST-segment elevation that must be distinguished from other causes of ST elevation with PR depression. In most instances of acute pericarditis, the magnitude of the ST elevation is greater than one-fourth of the T-wave height in the lateral V leads. In addition, if a history of these findings exists, the later development of constrictive pericarditis should be

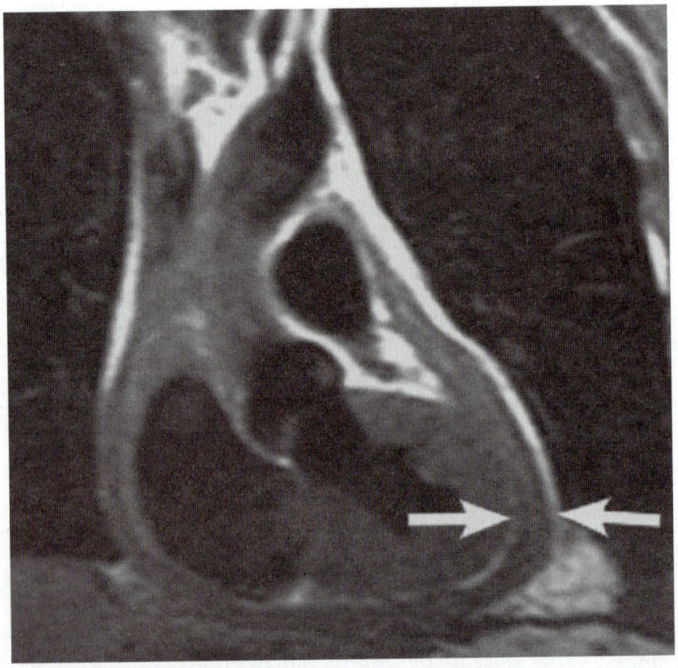

Fig. 24.16: *Constrictive pericarditis in a young lady who presented with symptoms of constriction. Coronal ECG-gated T1-weighted SE image shows abnormally thickened pericardium (arrows) outlined by epicardial and anterior mediastinal fat*

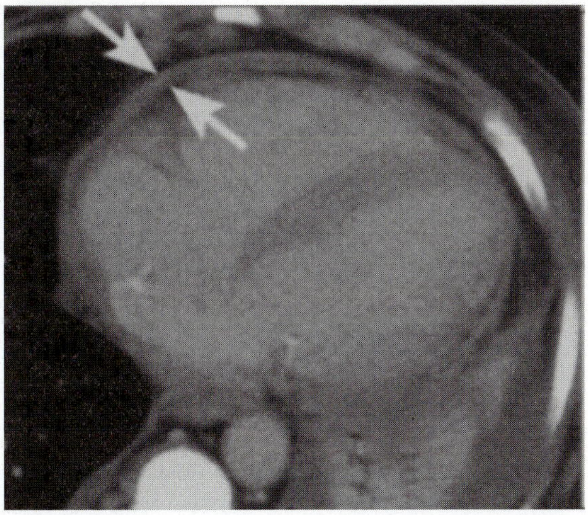

Fig. 24.17: *Constrictive pericarditis in a 20-years-adolescent who presented with symptoms of heart failure after mediastinal irradiation for Hodgkin lymphoma. Axial contrast-enhanced CT scan shows pericardial thickening (arrows)*

considered. Over time, even if chronic pericarditis develops, no specific ECG patterns develop. Inverted T waves may persist, or all ECG findings may resolve to normal. In long-standing cases, atrial fibrillation may occur, but this is certainly nonspecific. If a pericardial effusion develops, a low QRS voltage may be present in the limb and chest leads. This must be distinguished from other causes of low voltage such as long-standing myocardial infarction, pleural effusion, postoperative state, or various cardiomyopathies. When electrical alternans (a beat-to-beat cyclic shift in the QRS axis that may also involve the P and T waves) is present, cardiac tamponade must be considered.

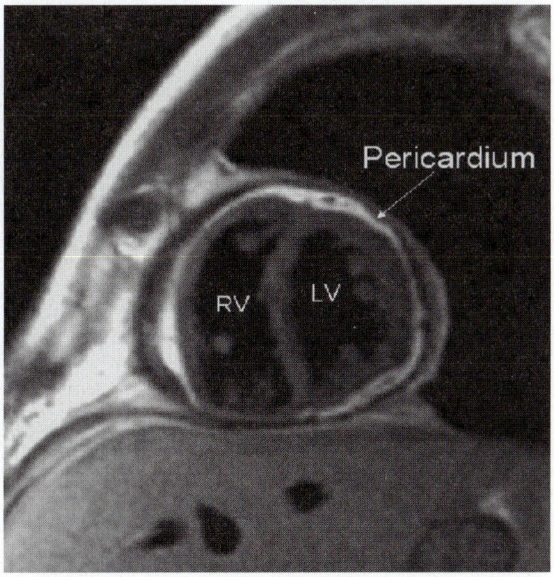

Fig. 24.18: *MRI shows constrictive pericarditis in 13-year-old patient with otherwise structurally normal heart. Infectious workup was negative. (Image courtesy of Tal Geva, MD)*

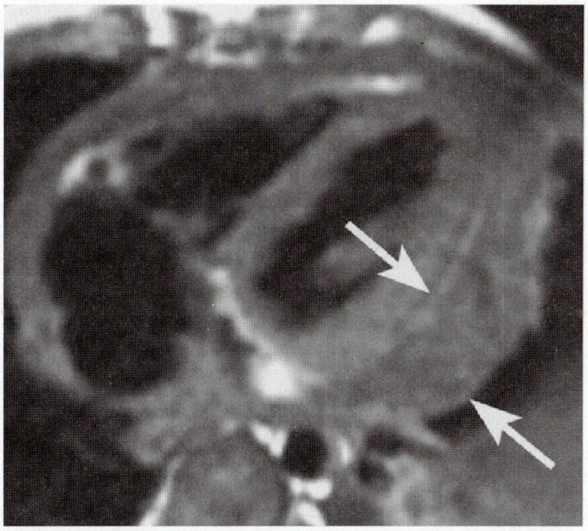

Fig. 24.19: *Effusive constrictive pericarditis secondary to viral infection in a young adolescent with symptoms of heart failure. Axial ECG-gated T1-weighted SE image shows a crescent-shaped area of intermediate signal intensity (arrows) surrounding the ventricles, which indicates either pericardial thickening or pericardial effusion. Axial gadolinium-enhanced fat-saturated T1-weighted SE image shows marked thickening and enhancement in the pericardium (arrows), findings consistent with inflammation. A moderate-sized pericardial effusion is also depicted*

Procedures

Cardiac Catheterization Hemodynamics

Despite best efforts to diagnose constrictive pericarditis using noninvasive testing, the diagnosis may still be uncertain. The differentiation between constrictive pericarditis and restrictive cardiomyopathy is often a major consideration and can be as difficult in the catheterization laboratory as in the echocardiography laboratory (Fig. 24.27).

The hemodynamic changes seen in constrictive pericarditis are based on impaired ventricular diastolic blood flow that leads to an equalization of intraventricular diastolic pressures and an abrupt cessation of ventricular filling after early diastole. The right atrial pressure tracings may show this. Normally, with inspiration, the mean right atrial pressures should decline as returning venous blood flows into the pulmonary vasculature. Failure to do so or an actual pressure increase with inspiration is known as the Kussmaul sign. While this can be seen with constrictive pericarditis, it also can be seen with right heart failure, severe tricuspid regurgitation, or systemic venous congestion. Closer inspection of the atrial waveforms reveals the Y descent becoming exaggerated and, thus, appearing deeper and steeper than its X descent counterpart. This is in contrast to the Y descent in cardiac tamponade, which becomes attenuated or even up-sloping. Measuring right ventricular pressures is vital in determining if a patient has constrictive pericarditis, and a right heart catheterization is included in any hemodynamic evaluation. Traditional teachings have focused on:

1. The equalization of pressures between the two ventricles

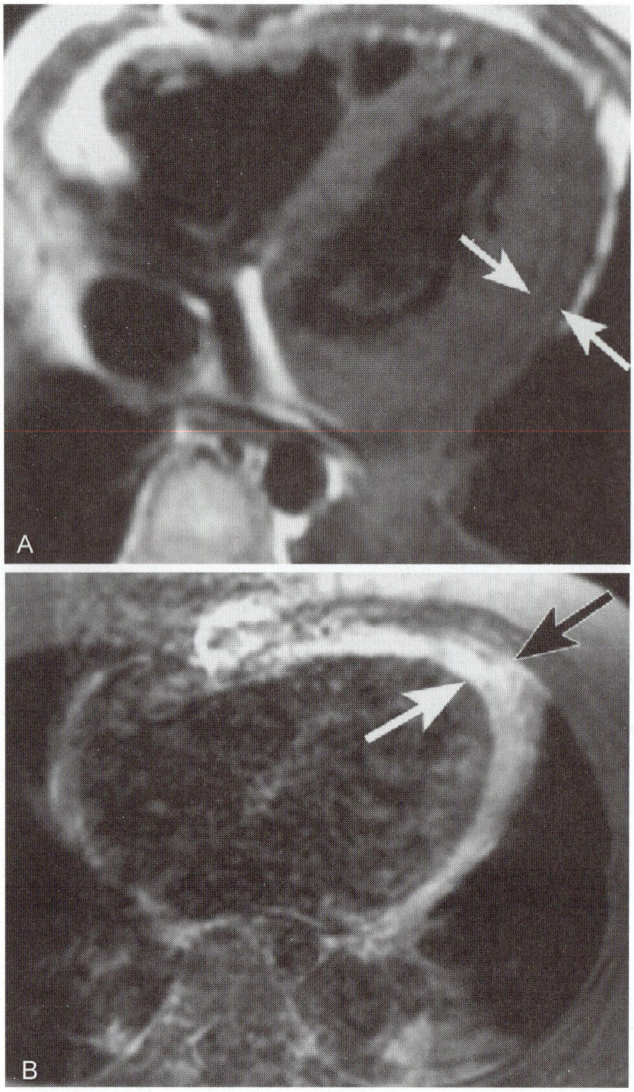

Fig. 24.20: *Inflammatory constrictive pericarditis in an 8-year-old boy with progressive shortness of breath after undergoing surgical repair of an atrial septal defect. Axial ECG-gated T1-weighted SE image (top) and axial gadolinium-enhanced fat-saturated T1-weighted SE image (bottom) show an abnormally thickened pericardium (arrows in A) that enhances after gadolinium administration (arrows in B).*

2. The relationship of the right ventricular systolic to diastolic pressure
3. The pulmonary artery pressures.

Generally, a difference between the left and right ventricular end-diastolic pressures of less than 5 mmHg, a right ventricular diastolic pressure of greater than one-third the right ventricular systolic pressure, or a pulmonary artery pressure of less than 50 mmHg favors a diagnosis of constrictive pericarditis rather than restrictive cardiomyopathy. When making or excluding a diagnosis of constrictive pericarditis, these criteria are neither sensitive nor specific enough to rely on solely. However, the further they are to either extreme, the more reliable they are.

The classic dip-and-plateau (also known as the square-root sign) that has been described in abnormal ventricular diastolic filling patterns can occur in both costrictive and restrictive disorders. In constrictive pericarditis, this pattern represents early rapid ventricular filling followed by a sudden halt in ventricular filling as the pericardium is restrained from the end of the first third of diastole onward. In 1989, a landmark study by Hatle et al (and later by Hurrell et al) was published. It elucidated both the echocardiographic and hemodynamic variations that occur in both right and left ventricular filling patterns during normal respiration with constrictive pericarditis. Using the presence or absence of (1) ventricular pressure interdependence and (2) intrathoracic/intracardiac pressure disossociation, they were able to increase the sensitivity and specificity of hemodynamic testing to greater than 90%. That is, in constrictive pericarditis, with inspiration, the right ventricular inflow is increased, which is believed to cause the interventricular septum to shift toward the left, thus further diminishing left ventricular filling.

As a result of this preload mismatch, stoke volume is augmented in the right ventricle and reduced in the left ventricle. Hemodynamic tracings obtained simultaneously in both ventricles show that the left ventricular pressure falls with inspiration while the right ventricular pressure rises. The opposite is true during expiration. These ventricular pressure responses have been termed discordant. This phenomenon does not occur in congestive heart failure or restrictive disorders. With inspiration, the intrathoracic pressure also drops. This causes a subsequent drop in pulmonary capillary wedge pressure (and mean

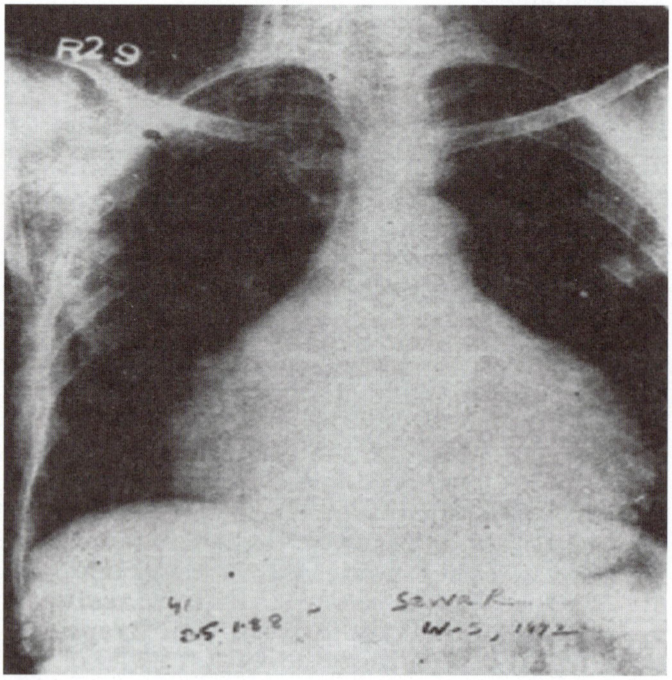

Fig. 24.21: *Photograph of X-ray chest showing money bag appearance of cardiac silhoute in patient with moderate pericardial effusion*

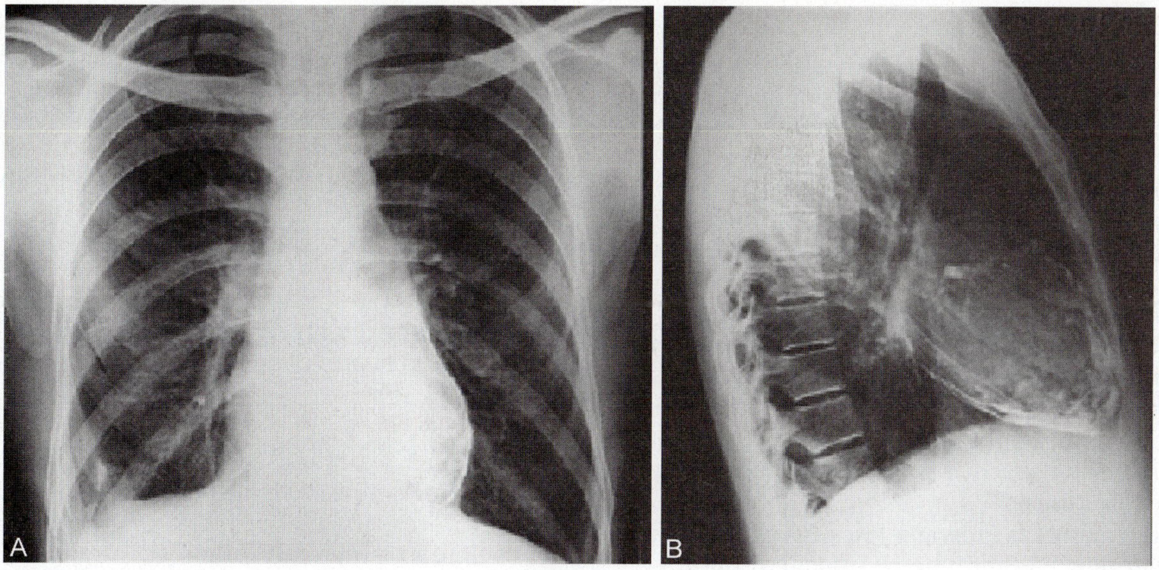

Fig. 24.22: *(A) Chest X-ray, PA view and (B) lateral view, show pericardial calcification along anterior and interior borders*

left atrial pressure). However, because of the constricting pericardium, this drop in pressure cannot be transmitted to the left ventricle during diastole. The result is a decrease in the pressure gradient for filling the left ventricle. This intrathoracic/intracardiac dissociation occurs commonly (although not exclusively) in constrictive pericarditis. This dissociation does occur, although to a much lesser extent, in restrictive cardiomyopathy. Hurrell et al showed a sensitivity of 93% and a specificity of 81% for diagnosing pericardial constriction with this finding.

Although these signs are useful, in practice, uncertainty always exists when attempting to diagnose constrictive pericarditis. Fluid-filled catheters render notoriously poor fidelity tracings, which can lead to a misinterpretation of the data. Irregular rhythms, such as atrial fibrillation, may alter ventricular filling pressures based on the varying RR intervals. Variations in respiration patterns may affect hemodynamics, and patients should be instructed to breathe smoothly and uniformly during hemodynamic recordings. The patient's diastolic filling pressures can affect hemodynamic measurements, and some authors advocate infusing isotonic sodium chloride solution if the patient's left ventricular end-diastolic pressure is less than 15 mm Hg to unmask occult constrictive pericardtis. Conversely, if the filling pressures are too high, the more subtle respiratory variations in pressure may be missed.

Etiologies of diastolic pressure equalization include constrictive pericarditis, restrictive cardiomyopathy, cardiac tamponade, COPD and pneumothorax (pulmonary hyperinflation), dilated cardiomyopathy (if severe, all filling pressures are high), atrial septal defect, and volume depletion (all filling pressures are low).

Pericardial and Endomyocardial Biopsy

Occasionally, direct inspection and pericardial biopsy may be required to diagnose constriction. If constriction is strongly suggested clinically, the pericardium may be thin, and, after careful consideration, direct surgical inspection, biopsy, and pericardectomy may be required to diagnose definitively or to exclude the diagnosis.

Despite the best attempts at diagnosing constrictive pericarditis, confirming the diagnosis may be impossible until surgery. Patients and their families need to be aware of this fact and that, in some cases, surgery may be considered exploratory.

Histologic findings: Pericardial biopsy samples may be examined for malignancy and inflammation by traditional and immunohistologic means. In advanced laboratories, polymerase chain reaction or in situ hybridization may be used to analyze for microbial DNA or RNA. Combined examination of pericardial fluid and biopsy results provides the greatest yield.

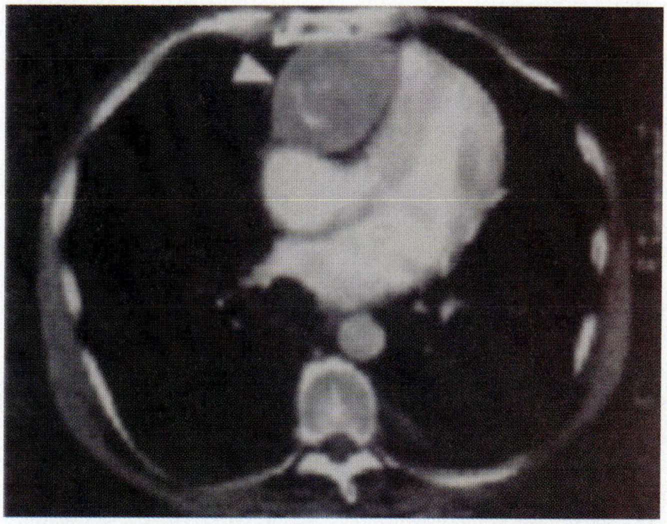

Fig. 24.23: *CAT scan showing localised cardiac tamponade caused by intrapericardial haematoma after 10 years of open heart surgery*

Medical Care

Medical management is generally ineffective in the vast majority of cases unless a prominent inflammatory component is present. This is in contrast with acute pericarditis in which the use of nonsteroidal anti-inflammatory agents, cyclooxygenase-2 inhibitors, colchicine, corticosteroids, or a combination thereof may provide benefit. However, even after optimal therapy of acute pericarditis, over time, the possibility of developing constriction exists. Other medical considerations are as follows:

- Subacute constrictive pericarditis may respond to steroids if treated before pericardial fibrosis occurs.
- Diuretics are commonly used to relieve congestion if ventricular filling pressures are clinically elevated. However, this may decrease cardiac output and requires careful monitoring.
- Any therapy directed toward the causative disease is appropriate, such as antituberculosis medication.
- Complications, such as atrial arrhythmias, require their own therapy as needed. In general, beta-blockers should be avoided because the sinus tachycardia that commonly occurs in constrictive pericarditis is compensatory in nature.

Surgical Treatment

Complete pericardectomy is the definitive therapy and is a potential cure.

Results are generally better if the procedure is performed earlier in the course, when less calcification is present and when the chance of abnormal myocardium or advanced heart failure is reduced.

Some judgment is required because patients who are asymptomatic (NYHA class I) or who have early NYHA stage II symptoms may be clinically stable for years.

Pericardial decortication should be as extensive as possible, especially at the diaphragmatic-ventricular contact regions. The surgical procedure can be long and is often technically complex. Complications may include excessive bleeding and atrial and ventricular arrhythmias.

Poor surgical results are observed in patients with organ failure (especially renal and hepatic), ascites, uncorrected coronary artery disease, myocardial fibrosis, older age, NYHA class IV, or postradiation pericarditis.

The published surgical mortality rates range from 5–15%. Significantly, 80–90% of patients who undergo pericardectomy postoperatively achieve NYHA class I or II. Even though the symptoms following a pericardiectomy are commonly improved, evidence of abnormal diastolic filling (which can be correlated with clinical status) often remains.

A recent study found that some diastolic filling abnormalities remained in a substantial number of patients after pericardectomy for constriction.

In 58 patients who underwent total pericardectomy for constriction, 30% still had some significant symptoms after 4 years. These patients were more likely to have a persistent restrictive or constrictive pattern to their transmitral and transtricuspid Doppler signals as determined by respiratory recording.

Although some improved with time, persistent diastolic filling abnormalities tended to occur in patients who had a longer history of preoperative symptoms, supporting the concept of early operation in patients who are symptomatic. New experimental devices are being investigated to access the pericardial space including in patients without significant effusion.

One is the PerDUCER, which is a percutaneous sheath-needle pericardial access device.

Hopefully, the development of such devices can improve diagnostic and therapeutic options in patients with pericardial disease.

Consultations

A cardiologist can assist with obtaining and interpreting echocardiographic imaging, hemodynamic measurements, and, if necessary, endocardial or pericardial biopsies. Consultation with a cardiothoracic surgeon is appropriate when a pericardial procedure is being considered.

Diet

No specific dietary recommendations are necessary.

Activity

Although no specific restrictions are needed, activity can often be severely limited by symptoms.

Surgical pericardectomy is clearly the treatment of choice for patients with constrictive pericarditis. Diuretics have been used in the early stages of the disease to improve pulmonary and systemic congestion. However, these should be used cautiously because any drop in intravascular volume may cause a corresponding drop in cardiac output.

Pharmacotherapy in Constrictive Pericarditis

Diuretics: These agents may improve pulmonary and systemic congestion. These should be used cautiously because any drop in intravascular volume may cause a corresponding drop in cardiac output.

Furosemide (lasix): Any loop diuretics may be used to treat volume overload. Always start at minimal dose necessary.

Adult dose: 20 mg/d PO/IV
Pediatric dose: Not established.

Complications

Complications arise with failure to diagnose or treat constrictive pericarditis adequately including any existing underlying etiology. Surgical intervention poses separate and significant complication risks.

Prognosis

Long-term prognosis with medical therapy alone is poor. With surgery, the long-term outcome of patients with constrictive pericarditis has been shown to be independently less favorable with advanced age, poor renal function, abnormal left ventricular systolic function, high pulmonary artery systolic pressure, lower serum sodium

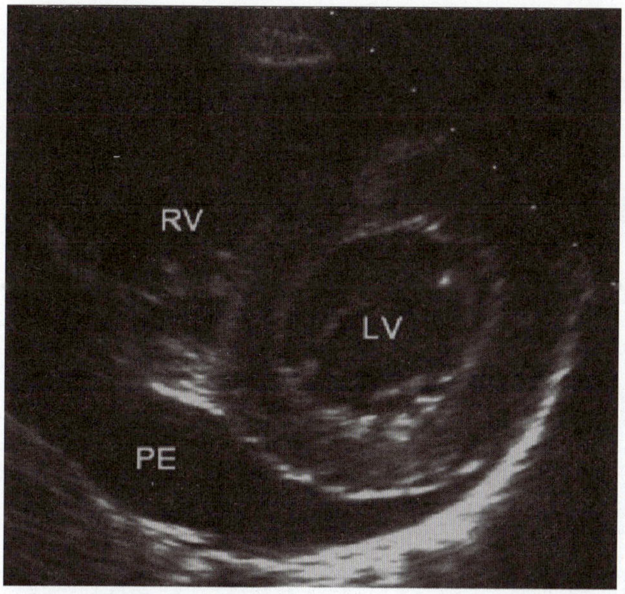

Fig. 24.24: *Pericardial effusion from a parasternal short-axis echocardiographic view. RV indicates right ventricle; LV, left ventricle; PE, pericardial effusion*

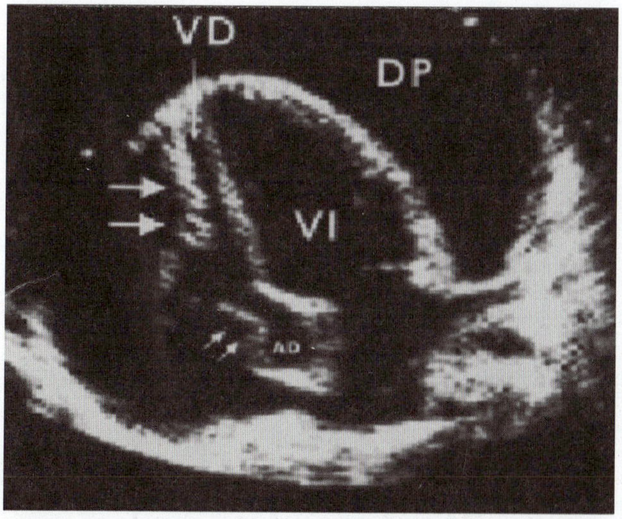

Fig. 24.25: *Two dimensional echocardiogram (four chamber apical plane) showing a significant atrial (small arrows) and right ventricle (large arrows) collapse. The patient showed clinical signs of blockage. The collapse of both cavities is highly specific and has a high positive-predictive value for tamponade. RA indicates right atrium; PE, pericardial effusion; RV, right ventricle; LV, left ventricle*

level, worsening NYHA classification, and, most notably, with a postradiation cause. Pericardial calcification has shown no effect on survival. A recent study showed postpericardiectomy survival rates of 71% and 52% at 5 and 10 years, respectively. Long-term survival after pericardiectomy depends on the underlying cause. Of common causes, idiopathic constrictive pericarditis has the best prognosis, followed by constriction due to cardiac surgery.

PERICARDIAL EFFUSION

Pericardial effusion defines the presence of an abnormal amount and/or character of fluid in the pericardial space. It can be caused by a variety of local and systemic disorders, or it may be idiopathic. Pericardial effusions can be acute or chronic, and the time course of development has a great impact on the patient's symptoms. Treatment varies, and is directed at both removal of the pericardial fluid and alleviation of the underlying cause, which usually is determined by a combination of fluid analysis and correlation with comorbid illnesses.

Pathophysiology: The pericardial space normally contains 15–50 mL of fluid which serves as lubrication for the visceral and parietal layers of the pericardium. This fluid is thought to originate from the visceral pericardium and is essentially an ultrafiltrate of plasma. Total protein levels are generally low; however, the concentration of albumin is increased in pericardial fluids owing to its low molecular weight.

The cause of abnormal fluid production depends on the underlying etiology, but usually it is secondary to injury or insult to the pericardium (i.e. pericarditis). Transudative fluids result from obstruction of fluid drainage, which occurs through lymphatic channels. Exudative fluids occur secondary to inflammatory, infectious, malignant, or autoimmune processes within the pericardium.

Clinical manifestations of pericardial effusion are highly dependent upon the rate of accumulation of fluid in the pericardial sac. Rapid accumulation of pericardial fluid may cause elevated intrapericardial pressures with as little as 80 mL of fluid while slowly progressing effusions can grow to 2 liters without symptoms.

Incidence: Few large studies have characterized the epidemiology of pericardial effusion. Pericardial effusion has been found in 3.4% of subjects in general autopsy studies. Small pericardial effusions often are asymptomatic.

A higher incidence of pericardial effusion is associated with certain diseases. Twenty-one percent of cancer patients have metastases to the pericardium. The most common are lung (37% of malignant effusions), breast (22%), and leukemia/lymphoma (17%). Patients with HIV, with or without AIDS, are found to have increased prevalence, with 41–87% having asymptomatic effusion and 13% having moderate-to-severe effusion.

Mortality/morbidity: Dependent upon etiology and comorbid conditions.

Idiopathic effusions are well tolerated in most patients. As many as 50% of patients with large, chronic effusions were asymptomatic during long-term follow-up.

Pericardial effusion is the primary or contributory cause of death in 86% of cancer patients with symptomatic effusions. Survival rate for patients with HIV and symptomatic pericardial effusion is 36% at 6 months, 19% at 1 year.

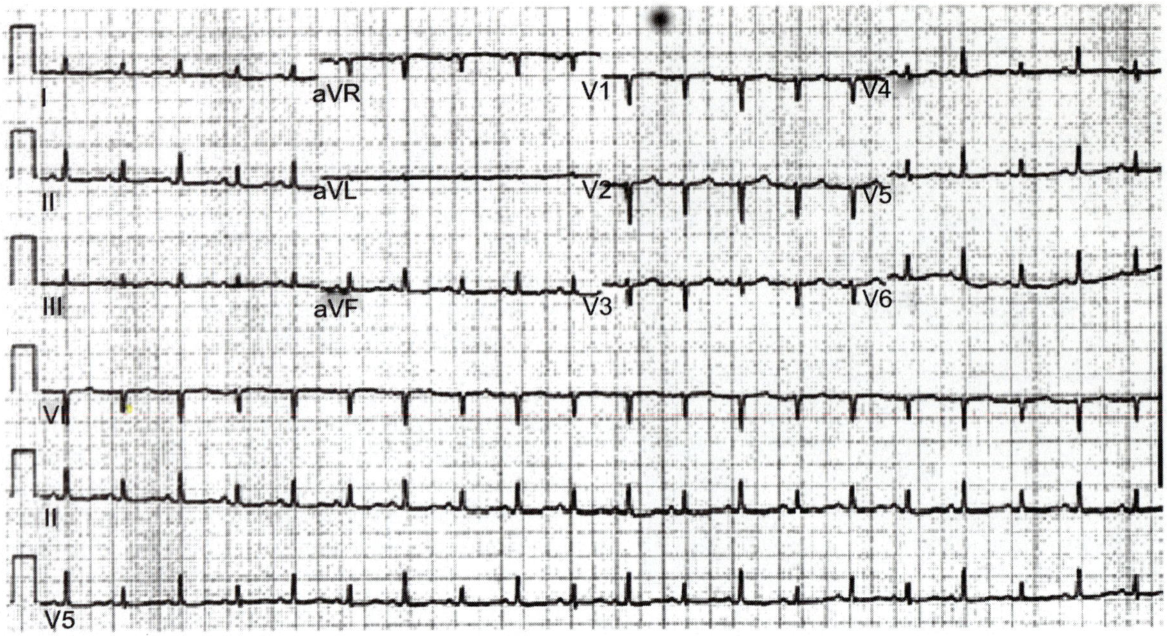

Fig. 24.26: *ECG showing generalised low voltage graph with electrical alterans smaller QRS, flattening of ST segment and T wave inversion in patient with moderate pericardial effusion*

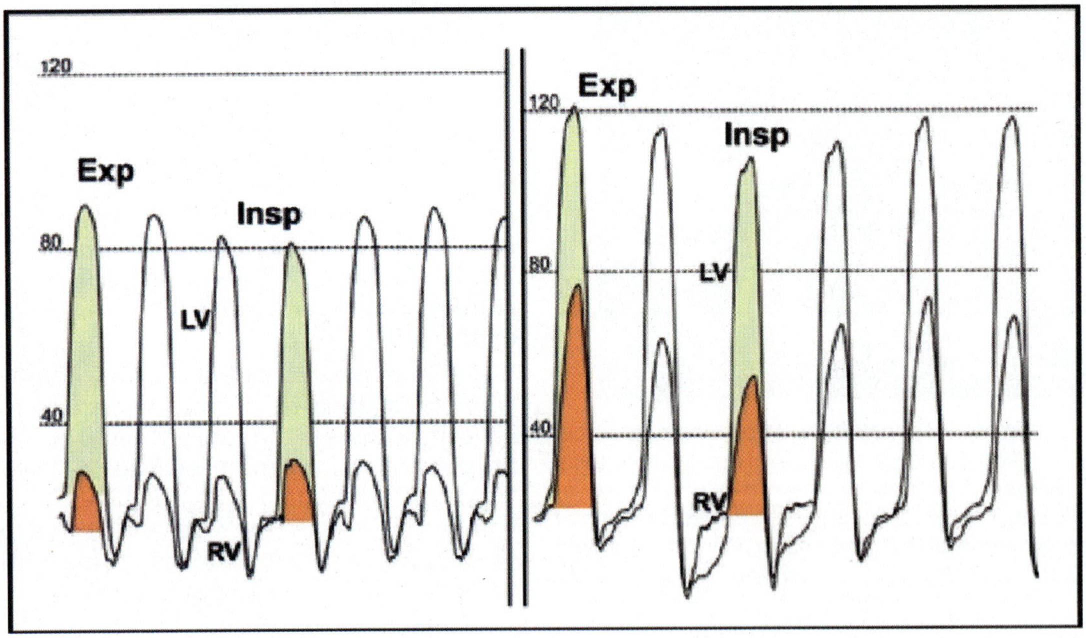

Fig. 24.27: *Ventricular interdependence and respiratory variation in ventricular filling in constrictive pericarditis and restrictive cardiomyopathy. Ventricular interdependence is observed in simultaneous recordings of left ventricular (LV) and right ventricular (RV) pressures. Left, In constrictive pericarditis, inspiration (Insp) induces less filling of the LV, and the area of the LV pressure curve decreases (yellow-shaded area) as compared with expiration (Exp). The opposite changes occur in the RV so that area of the RV pressure curve increases with Insp (orange-shaded area). Ejection time also varies with respiration in opposite directions in LV and RV. This discordant pressure change between the LV and RV occurs in constrictive pericarditis. Right, In restrictive cardiomyopathy, the changes in LV and RV systolic pressures with respiration are concordant. During Insp, the area of the RV pressure curve decreases (orange-shaded area) as compared with Exp. The area of the LV pressure curve (yellow shaded area) is unchanged during Insp as compared with Exp. Note that both patients have early rapid filling and elevation and end-equalization of the LV and RV pressures at end Exp*

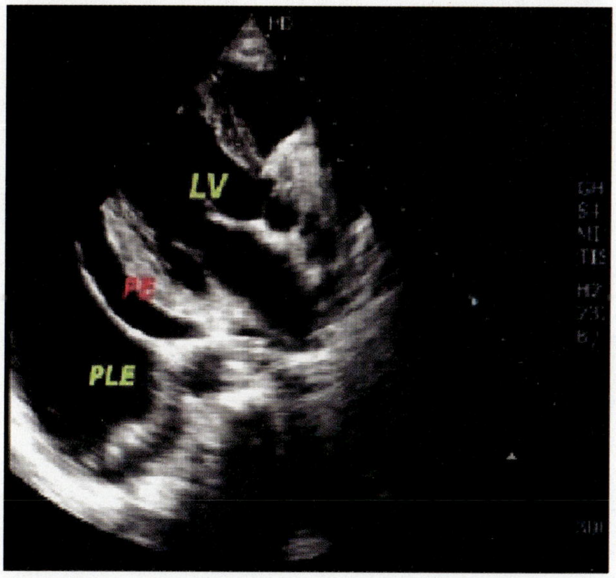

Fig. 24.28: *Echo scan showing both pericardial and pleural effusions in patient with cardiac failure. PLE, pleural efusion and PE, pericardial effusion*

Clinical Presentation

History

1. ***Cardiovascular:*** Chest pain, pressure, discomfort: Characteristically, pericardial pain may be relieved by sitting up and leaning forward and is intensified by lying supine.
2. Light-headedness, syncope
3. Palpitations
4. ***Respiratory:*** Cough, dyspnea, hoarseness
5. ***Gastrointestinal:*** Hiccoughs
6. ***Neurologic:*** Anxiety, confusion.

Physical Examination

Classic Beck triad of pericardial tamponade (hypotension, muffled heart sounds, jugular venous distension).

Pulsus paradoxus: Exaggeration of physiologic respiratory variation in systemic blood pressure, defined as a decrease in systolic blood pressure of more than 10 mmHg with inspiration, signaling falling cardiac output during inspiration.

Pericardial friction rub: The most important physical sign of acute pericarditis may have up to three components per cardiac cycle and is high-pitched, scratching and grating. It can sometimes be elicited only when firm pressure with the diaphragm of the stethoscope is applied to the chest wall at the left lower sternal border. The pericardial friction rub is heard most frequently during expiration with the patient upright and leaning forward.

Widened pulse pressure

Tachycardia

Hepatojugular reflux: This can be observed by applying pressure to the periumbilical region. A rise in the jugular venous pressure (JVP) of greater than 3 cm H_2O for more than 30 seconds suggests elevated central venous pressure. Transient elevation in JVP may be normal.

Respiratory

- ***Tachypnea:*** Decreased breath sounds (secondary to pleural effusions).
- ***Ewart sign:*** Dullness to percussion beneath the angle of left scapula from compression of the left lung by pericardial fluid
- ***Gastrointestinal:*** Hepatosplenomegaly
- ***Extremities***
  - Weakened peripheral pulses
  - Edema
  - Cyanosis.

Etiological Factors

Infectious

- Viral (coxsackievirus A and B, hepatitis, HIV); pyogenic (pneumococci, streptococci, staphylococci, neisseria, legionella species)
- Tuberculous
- Fungal (histoplasmosis, coccidioidomycosis, candida)
- Other infections (syphilitic, protozoal, parasitic)

Noninfectious

- Acute idiopathic
- Uremia
- Neoplasia
- Primary tumors (benign or malignant, mesothelioma)
- Tumors metastatic to pericardium (lung and breast cancer, lymphoma, leukemia)
- Myxedema
- Acute myocardial infarction
- Postirradiation
- Aortic dissection (with leakage into pericardial sac)
- Trauma
- Cholesterol
- Chylopericardium
- Familial mediterranean fever
- Whipple disease
- Sarcoidosis
- Hypersensitivity or autoimmunity related, rheumatic fever
- Collagen vascular disease (systemic lupus erythematosus, rheumatoid arthritis, ankylosing spondylitis, scleroderma, acute rheumatic fever, Wegener granulomatosis)
- Drug-induced (e.g. procainamide, hydralazine, isoniazid, minoxidil, phenytoin, anticoagulants, methys.

Laboratory Studies

Electrolytes: Metabolic abnormalities (e.g. renal failure)

CBC count with differential: Leukocytosis for evidence of infection, as well as cytopenias, as signs of underlying chronic disease (e.g. cancer, HIV).

Cardiac enzymes: Troponin level is frequently minimally elevated in acute pericarditis, usually in the absence of an

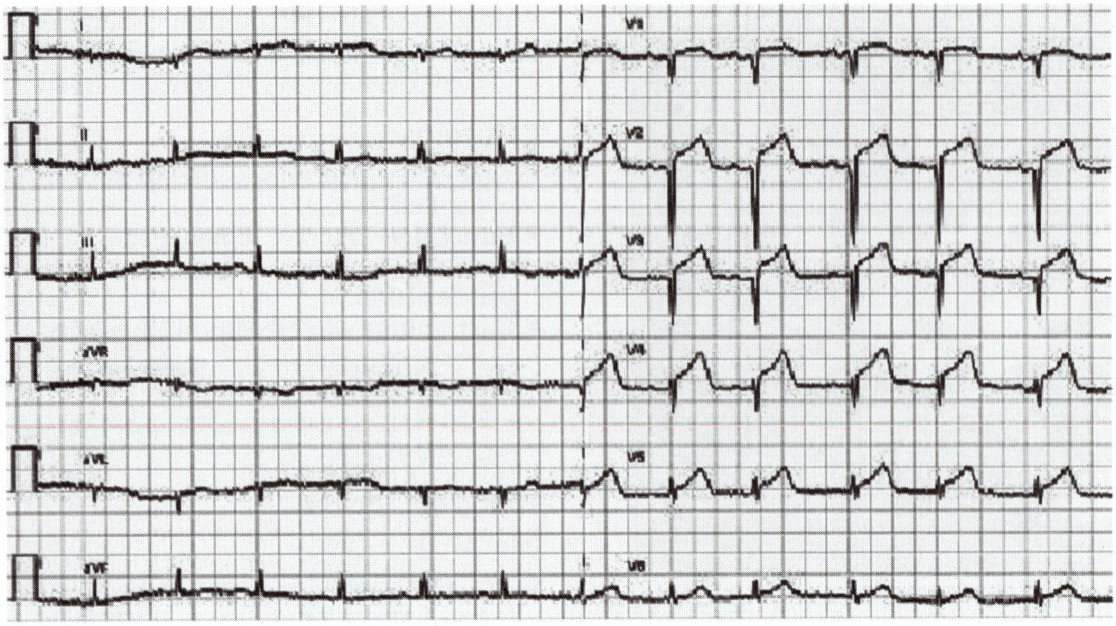

Fig. 24.29: *Mixed constrictive-restrictive cardiomyopathy ECG: sinus rhythm (79/min) with absent progression of R-wave (V1-V4) and omozonal ST elevation*

elevated total creatine kinase level. Presumably, this is due to some involvement of the epicardium by the inflammatory process. Although the elevated troponin may lead to the misdiagnosis of acute pericarditis as a myocardial infarction, most patients with an elevated troponin and acute pericarditis have normal coronary angiograms. An elevated troponin level in acute pericarditis typically returns to normal within 1–2 weeks and is not associated with a worse prognosis.

Thyroid-stimulating hormone: Thyroid-stimulating hormone screen for hypothyroidism.

Rickettsial antibodies: If high index of suspicion of tick-borne disease. Rheumatoid factor, immunoglobulin complexes, antinuclear antibody test (ANA), and complement levels (which would be diminished) in suspected rheumatologic causes.

Pericardial fluid analysis: Routine tests.

Lactic (acid) dehydrogenase (LDH), total protein: The light criteria (for exudative pleural effusion) found to be as reliable in distinguishing between exudative and transudative effusions. Total protein fluid-to-serum ratio >0.5.

LDH fluid-to-serum ratio is > 0.6. LDH fluid level exceeds two-thirds of upper-limit of normal serum level withther indicators suggestive of exudate—specific gravity is > 1.015, total protein is > 3.0 mg/dL, LDH is > 300 U/dL, glucose fluid-to-serum ratio is <1 cell count—elevated leukocytes (i.e. >10,000) with neutrophil predominance suggests bacterial or rheumatic cause although unreliable. Gram stain-specific but insensitive indicator of bacterial infection.

Cultures: These can signal and identifies infectious etiology. Fluid hematocrit for bloody aspirates—hemorrhagic fluid hematocrits usually significantly less than simultaneous peripheral blood hematocrits.

Pericardial fluid: Special tests; viral cultures

Adenosine deaminase; polymerase chain reaction (PCR); culture for tuberculosis; smear for acid-fast bacilli in suspected tuberculosis infection, especially in patients with HIV.

A definite diagnosis of tuberculous pericarditis is based on the demonstration of tubercle bacilli in pericardial fluid or on a histological section of the pericardium. Probable tuberculous pericarditis is based on the proof of tuberculosis elsewhere in a patient with otherwise unexplained pericarditis, a lymphocytic pericardial exudate with elevated adenosine deaminase levels, and/or appropriate response to a trial of antituberculosis chemotherapy.

Imaging Studies

Chest Radiography

Findings include enlarged cardiac silhouette (so called water-bottle heart), pericardial fat stripe. A third of patients have a coexisting pleural effusion. Radiography is unreliable in establishing or refuting diagnosis of pericardial effusion.

Echocardiogram (Transthoracic and TEE) (Fig. 24.32)

This is the criterion standard for noninvasive diagnosis. Pericardial effusion appears as an "echo-free" space between the visceral and the parietal pericardium. Early effusions tend to accumulate posteriorly owing to expandable posterior/lateral pericardium. Large effusions

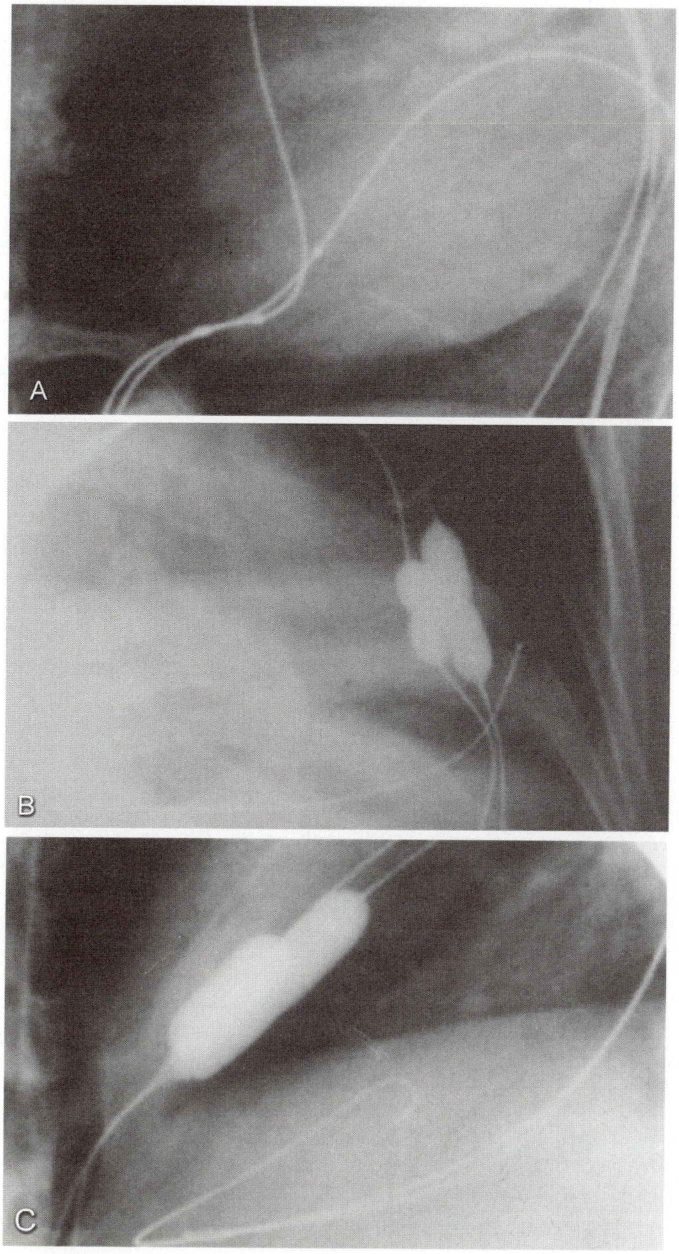

Fig. 24.30: *(A) Two guidewires in the same tract separate from each other after their entrance into the pericardial cavity, so that the pericardial border can be defined clearly under fluoroscopy. (B) Double balloons were straddled over the pericardium. Both balloons were partially inflated and showed a central waist appearance. (C) Fully expanded double balloons creating a pericardial window*

are characterized by excessive motion within the pericardial sac. Severe cases may be accompanied by diastolic collapse of the right atrium and right ventricle (and in hypovolemic patients the left atrium and left ventricle), signaling the onset of pericardial tamponade.

Large pericardial effusions are defined as greater than 1 cm thick on echocardiography, completely surrounding the heart. Small effusions are less than 1 cm and often localized, usually posteriorly.

False-positive echocardiograms can occur in pleural effusions, pericardial thickening, increased pericardial fat (especially the anterior epicardial fat pad), atelectasis, and mediastinal lesions. In patients with pericardial effusion, imaging from low to midposterior thorax can provide additional diagnostic echocardiographic images and should be used in patients in whom conventional images are technically difficult or require additional information.

Transesophageal echocardiography (TEE) is useful in characterizing loculated effusions.

CT Scan

Potentially can determine composition of fluid and may detect as little as 50 mL of fluid. Fewer false-positive results than with echocardiography. Problem: patients must be transported to the CT scanner which may not be possible if the patient's condition is unstable.

MRI

Can detect as little as 30 mL of pericardial fluid. May be able to distinguish hemorrhagic and nonhemorrhagic effusions. More difficult to perform than CT scan acutely, given the length of time the patient must remain in the scanner. Both MRI and CT scan may be superior to echocardiography in detecting loculated pericardial effusions and pericardial thickening.

Other Tests

Electrocardiogram: Early in the course of acute pericarditis, the ECG typically displays diffuse ST elevation in association with PR depression. The ST elevation is usually present in all leads except for aVR, but post-myocardial infarction pericarditis, the changes may be more localized. Classically, the ECG changes of acute pericarditis evolve through four progressive stages: stage I, diffuse ST-segment elevation and PR-segment depression; stage II, normalization of the ST and PR segments; stage III, wide spread T-wave inversions; and stage IV, normalization of the T-waves Patients with uremic pericarditis frequently do not have the typical ECG abnormalities.

Procedures

Transesophageal echocardiography: This procedure is used for diagnostic as well as therapeutic purposes. Support for the use of echocardiographic guidance is increasing, unless emergent treatment is required. Indications include impending hemodynamic compromise (i.e. pericardial tamponade), suspected infectious etiology, and uncertain etiology. Use of a needle that is at least 5 cm long, 16-gauge in diameter, and has a short bevel can minimize the risk of complications and should allow for adequate pericardial drainage. A system allowing placement of a catheter over the needle is preferred. Contrast echocardiography using agitated saline is useful in cases when bloody fluid is aspirated to determine if the needle is in the ventricular cavity. Attaching an ECG electrode to the pericardiocentesis needle is also useful for avoiding myocardial puncture.

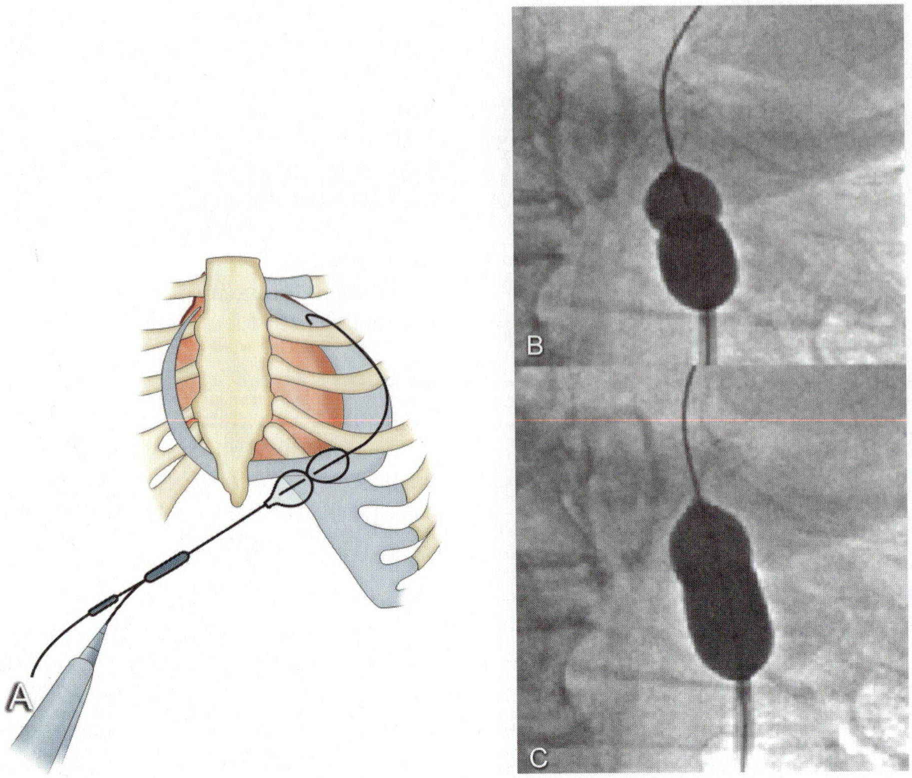

Fig. 24.31: *Steps in single balloon pericardiotomy. (A) Introducer in the pericardium through which contrast has been injected to locate the parietal pericardium. (B) Balloon inserted in the parietal pericardium through a 0.035-inch guide. Before inflating, the introducer is removed slightly. (C) Progressive inflation of the balloon until the notch disappears, observing the typical hour glass image*

Electrical activity will be seen on the monitor when the needle comes into contact with atrial or ventricular myocardium. These changes may be delayed, however, and instill a false sense of security in needle placement; sense of touch and the findings on aspiration should guide the procedure, with the clinician ultimately relying on good clinical sense.

Complications of pericardiocentesis include ventricular rupture, dysrhythmias, pneumothorax, myocardial and/ or coronary artery laceration, and infection. Recurrence rates within 90 days may be as high as 90% in patients with cancer.

Balloon Pericardotomy

A catheter is placed in the pericardial space under fluoroscopy, which, after inflation of the balloon, creates a channel for passage of fluid into the pleural space, where reabsorption occurs more readily. This may be useful for recurrent effusions (Figs 24.30, 24.31).

Pericardial Sclerosis

Several pericardial sclerosing agents have been used with varying success rates (e.g. tetracycline, doxycycline, cisplatin, 5-fluorouracil). The pericardial catheter may be left in place for repeat instillation if necessary until the effusion resolves. Complications include intense pain, atrial dysrhythmias, fever and infection.

Success rates are reported as high as 91% at 30 days.

Pericardioscopy: This procedure is not universally available. It may increase diagnostic sensitivity in cases of unexplained pericardial effusions. It allows for visualization of pericardium and for pericardial biopsies.

Medical Management

Initially, medical care is focused on determination of the underlying etiology.

Aspirin/nonsteroidal antiinflammatory agents (NSAIDs)

Most acute idiopathic or viral pericarditis occurrences are self-limited and respond to treatment with aspirin (650 mg q6h) or another NSAID.

Aspirin may be the preferred nonsteroidal agent to treat pericarditis after myocardial infarction because other NSAIDs may interfere with myocardial healing. Indomethacin should be avoided in patients who may have coronary artery disease.

Colchicine: The routine use of colchicine is supported by recently reported results of the colchicine for acute pericarditis (COPE) trial. In this trial, 120 patients with a first episode of acute pericarditis (idiopathic, acute, postpericardiotomy syndrome, and connective tissue disease) entered a randomized, open-label trial comparing aspirin treatment alone with aspirin plus colchicine (1–2 mg for the first day followed by 0.5–1 mg/d for 3 mo). Colchicine reduced symptoms at 72 hours (11.7% vs 36.7%;

P = 0.03) and reduced recurrence at 18 months (10.7% vs 36.7%; P=0.004; 5 needed treatment). Colchicine was discontinued in 5 patients because of diarrhea. No other adverse events were noted. Importantly, none of the 120 patients developed cardiac tamponade or progressed to pericardial constriction.

Steroids

Steroid administration early in the course of acute pericarditis appears to be associated with an increased incidence of relapse after tapering the steroids. In the COPE trial, steroid use was an independent risk factor for recurrence (odds ratio = 4.3). Also, an observational study strongly suggests that the use of steroids increases the probability of relapse in patients treated with colchicine.

Systemic steroids should be considered only in patients with recurrent pericarditis unresponsive to NSAIDs and colchicine or as needed for treatment of an underlying inflammatory disease. If steroids are to be used, an effective dose (1–1.5 mg/kg of prednisone) should be given, and it should be continued for at least 1 month before slow tapering.

The intrapericardial administration of steroids has been reported to be effective in acute pericarditis without producing the frequent reoccurrence of pericarditis that complicates the use of systemic steroids, but the invasive nature of this procedure limits its use.

Hemodynamic Support

Patients who have effusions with actual or threatened tamponade should be considered to have a true or potential emergency. Most patients require pericardiocentesis to treat or prevent tamponade. However, treatment should be carefully individualized.

Hemodynamic monitoring with a balloon flotation pulmonary artery catheter is useful, especially in those with threatened or mild tamponade in whom a decision is made to defer pericardiocentesis. Hemodynamic monitoring is also helpful after pericardiocentesis to assess both reaccumulation and the presence of underlying constrictive disease. However, insertion of a pulmonary artery catheter should not be allowed to delay definitive therapy in critically ill patients.

Intravenous fluid resuscitation may be helpful in cases of hemodynamic compromise. In patients with tamponade who are critically ill, intravenous positive inotropes (dobutamine, dopamine) can be used but are of limited measures and should not be allowed to substitute for or delay pericardiocentesis.

Antibiotics: Inpatients with purulent pericarditis, urgent pericardial drainage combined with intravenous antibacterial therapy (e.g. vancomycin 1 g bid, ceftriaxone 1–2 g bid, and ciprofloxacin 400 mg/d) is mandatory. Irrigation with urokinase or streptokinase, using large catheters, may liquify the purulent exudate, but open surgical drainage is preferable. The initial treatment of tuberculous pericarditis should include isoniazid 300 mg/day, rifampin 600 mg/day, pyrazinamide 15–30 mg/kg/day, and ethambutol 15–25 mg/kg/day. Prednisone 1–2 mg/kg/day is given for 5–7 days and progressively reduced to discontinuation in 6–8 weeks. Drug sensitivity testing is essential. Uncertainty remains whether adjunctive corticosteroids are effective in reducing mortality or progression to concal intervention is controversial, but many experts recommend a trial of medical therapy for noncalcific pericardial constriction and pericardiectomy in nonresponders after 4–8 weeks of antituberculosis chemotherapy.

Antineoplastic therapy: Systemic chemotherapy, radiation in conjunction with pericardiocentesis has been shown to be effective in reducing recurrences of malignant effusions.

Corticosteroids and NSAIDs are helpful in patients with autoimmune conditions.

Surgical Management

Subxiphoid pericardial window with pericardiostomy. This procedure is associated with low morbidity, mortality, and

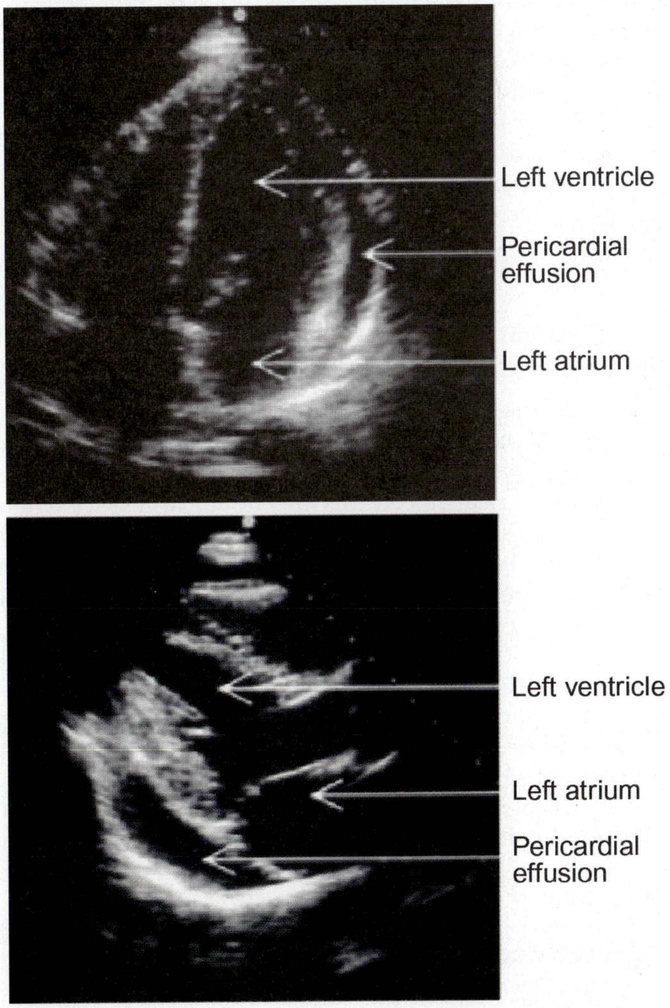

Fig. 24.32: *Pericardial effusion is seen in the two dimensional echocardiogram as an echo-free space outside the cardiac chambers. Two characteristic sites are lateral to the left ventricle in the apical four chamber view (top) and posterior to the left ventricle in the parasternal long-axis view (bottom)*

recurrence rates. It can be performed under local anesthesia. It may be less effective when effusion is loculated. It may replace pericardiocentesis as initial treatment for stable pericardial effusions. A recent study suggests that this may be safer and more effective at reducing recurrence rates than pericardiocentesis. However, only patients who were hemodynamically unstable underwent pericardiocentesis, and no change in overall survival rate was observed.

Thoracotomy

This should be reserved for patients in whom conservative approaches have failed. Thoracotomy allows for creation of a pleuropericardial window, which provides greater visualization of pericardium. Thoracotomy requires general anesthesia and thus has higher morbidity and mortality rates than the subxiphoid approach.

Video-assisted Thoracic Surgery

Video-assisted thoracic surgery (VATS) enables resection of a wider area of pericardium than the subxiphoid approach without the morbidity of thoracotomy.

The surgeon is able to create a pleuropericardial window and address concomitant pleural pathology, which is especially common in patients with malignant effusions.

One disadvantage of VATS is that it requires general anesthesia with single lung ventilation, which may be difficult in otherwise seriously ill patients.

Median sternotomy: This procedure is reserved for patients with constrictive pericarditis. Operative mortality rate is high (5–15%).

MANAGEMENT OF MASSIVE PERICARDIAL EFFUSION AND CARDIAC TAMPONADE

Pericardiocentesis is indicated for clinical tamponade, suspicion of purulent or neoplastic pericarditis, or for symptomatic patients, despite medical treatment for more than 1 week. Pericardiocentesis may not be necessary when the effusion is small and resolving with antiinflammatory treatment. In chronic effusions causing no haemodynamic compromise pericardiocentesis is indicated if additional diagnostic procedures are available (for example, pericardial fluid and tissue analyses, pericardioscopy, and epicardial/pericardial biopsy) to reveal the aetiology of the disease and permit further treatment. Aortic dissection is a major contraindication. Relative contraindications include uncorrected coagulopathy, anticoagulant treatment, thrombocytopenia < 50,000/mm, and small, posterior, and loculated effusions. In acute traumatic haemopericardium and purulent pericarditis, surgical drainage is more appropriate.

1. Pericardiocentesis Procedure

It can be performed either using fluoroscopic (cardiac catheterisation laboratory) or echocardiographic guidance. ECG monitoring from the puncturing needle is not an adequate safeguard. Right heart catheterisation can be performed simultaneously with pericardiocentesis, allowing haemodynamic monitoring and exclusion of effusive-constrictive disease. The subxiphoid approach has been used most commonly, with a long needle with a thin walled (18 gauge) directed towards the left shoulder at a 30° angle to the skin. This route is extrapleural and avoids the coronary, pericardial, and internal mammary arteries. The operator intermittently attempts to aspirate fluid and injects small amounts of contrast medium. After aspiration of the fluid the needle must be promptly replaced with a soft J tip guidewire which, after dilatation, is exchanged for a multiholed pigtail catheter. It is prudent to drain the fluid in stepped amounts of < 1 litre at a time to avoid acute right ventricular dilatation.

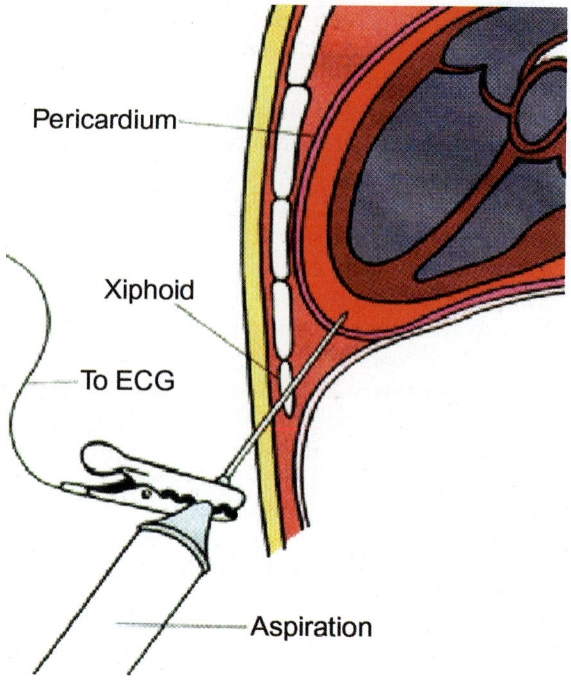

Fig. 24.33: *Steps and proper positioning of pericardiocentesis needle*

Echocardiographic guidance of pericardiocentesis is performed at the bedside. After identification of the shortest route to the effusion by echocardiography the pericardium is entered intercostally (usually in the sixth or seventh rib space in the anterior axillary line). The feasibility of pericardiocentesis is high (93%) in patients with anterior effusion > 10 mm while the rate of success is only 58% with small, posteriorly located effusions. Fluoroscopic and haemodynamic monitoring contribute to a better outcome following the procedure (93.1% v 73.3%) in comparison to emergency pericardial puncture with no imaging control. In addition, fluoroscopic guidance using the epicardial halo phenomenon significantly increased the feasibility of the procedure in patients with small effusions (200–300 mL; 92.6% v 84.9%) and very small effusions < 200 mL; 89.3% v 76.7%) (Fig. 24.33).

Echocardiographic guidance improved efficacy to 96% for pericardiocentesis of loculated pericardial effusion after cardiac surgery and to 99% for rescue pericardiocentesis. The most serious, but rare, complications are lacerations/

perforations of the myocardium and the coronary vessels. In addition, patients can experience air embolism, pneumothorax, arrhythmias (usually vasovagal bradycardia), and puncture of the peritoneal cavity or abdominal viscera. Internal mammary artery fistulas, acute pulmonary oedema, and purulent pericarditis have rarely been reported. The safety of pericardiocentesis was significantly improved with the introduction of echocardiographic or fluoroscopic guidance. Recent large echocardiographic series reported an incidence of major complications of 1.3–1.6%. In a large series of fluoroscopy guided percutaneous pericardiocenteses, cardiac perforations occurred in 0.9%, serious arrhythmias in 0.6%, arterial bleeding in 1.1 %, pneumothorax in 0.6%, infection in 0.3%, and a major vagal reaction in 0.3%. Incidence of major complications was also significantly reduced by utilising fluoroscopic guidance and the epicardial halo phenomenon "Pericardial constriction".

2. Pericardiectomy

Pericardiectomy is the only therapeutic approach that may remove permanent constriction, by aiming to resect the diseased pericardium as far as possible. The indications for surgery should be based upon clinical symptoms, echocardiography findings, CT/MRI, and heart catheterisation. There arc two standard approaches: (1) anterolateral thoracotomy (fifth intercostal space) and (2) median sternotomy (faster access to the aorta and right atrium if extracorporeal circulation becomes necessary). A primary installation of cardiopulmonary bypass cannot, however, be recommended, due to the enhanced diffuse bleeding following systemic heparinisation. If severe calcified adhesions between the peri- and epicardium arc present, or if the epicardium is generally affected ("outer porcelain heart"), surgery carries a high risk of either incomplete success or severe myocardial damage.

An alternative approach in such cases may be "laser shaving" using an Excimer laser. Areas of strong calcification or dense scaring may be left as islands, separated from the other areas, to avoid bleeding. Major complications include acute perioperative cardiac insufficiency (regional bulging or complete dilatation of one or both ventricles) and ventricular wall rupture. Cardiac mortality and morbidity at pericardiectomy is mainly caused by the presurgically unrecognised presence of myocardial atrophy or myocardial fibrosis. Exclusion of patients with extensive myocardial fibrosis and/or atrophy led to the reduction of the mortality rate for pericardiectomy from 50% to 5%. Left ventricular ejection fraction increases due to improved ventricular filling, but complete normalisation of cardiac haemodynamics after the procedure has been reported in only 60% of patients. Postoperative low cardiac output should be treated by fluid substitution and catecholamines, high doses of digitalis, and, in the most severe cases, intraaortic balloon pump. If the indication for surgery is established early, long-term survival after pericardiectomy matches that of an age and sex matched general population.

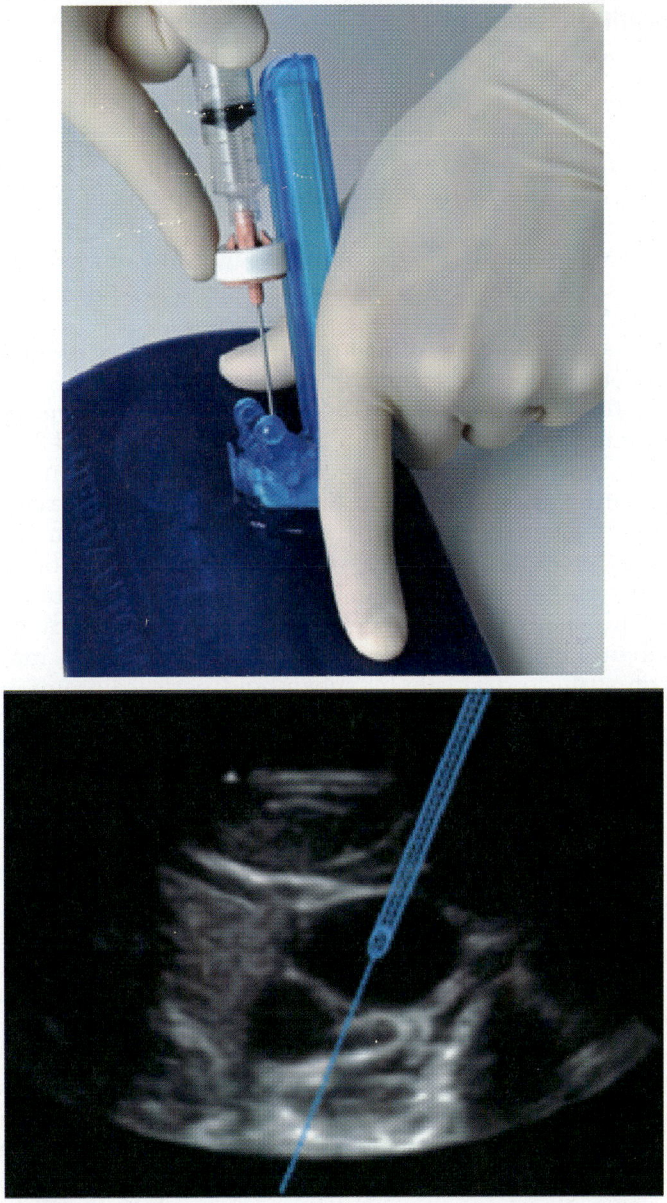

Figs 24.34: *AxoTrack needle guidance ultrasound probe*

3. An AxoTrack-equipped Ultrasound Probe

An AxoTrack-equipped ultrasound probe has an integral needle guide and built-in needle position sensors. Together these project on the ultrasound monitor an enhanced virtual image of the needle as it moves through the tissue toward and into the target vessel. The procedure is performed in three easy steps. First, simply align the on-screen target line with the target vessel displayed on the monitor. Next, insert the needle through the needle guide in the ultrasound probe and advance the needle while observing its progress until the vessel is entered, which can be seen on the monitor and confirmed by the flash of blood in the syringe. Finally, activate the needle lock on the probe to ensure stabilization of the needle before passing the guidewire into the desired vessel. The procedure is completed employing the standard modified Seldinger technique.

Specific Treatment

Viral Pericarditis

In many patients, pericardial viral infection is self-limiting and no specific treatment is necessary. In chronic or reptomatic pericardial effusion and confirmed viral infection, the following specific treatment is under investigation:

1. CMVpericarditis: Hyperimmunoglobulin once daily, 4 mL/kg intravenously on days 0, 4, and 8; 2 mL/kg on day 12 and 16
2. Coxsackie B pericarditis: Interferon alpha 2.5 × 10" IU/m' subcutaneously three times per week
3. *Adenovirus and parvovirus B19 positive myocarditis:* Immunoglobulin 10 g intravenously on days 1 and 3.

Purulent pericarditis is an absolute indication for pericardial drainage and rinsing of the pericardial cavity, combined with high doses of systemic antibiotic treatment. A combination of antistaphylococcal antib instillation of antibiotics (for example, gentamycin) can be useful but is not sufficient. Frequent irrigation of the pericardial cavity with urokinase or streptokinase, using large catheters, may open surgical drainage by subxiphoid pericardiotomy is preferable. Pericardiectomy is required in patients with dense adhesions, loculated and thick purulent effusion, recurrence of tamponade following drainage, as well as persistent symptoms or progression to constriction. Perioperative mortality of up to 8% was reported for pericardiectomy with the total mortality being much higher.

Tuberculous Pericarditis

Tuberculous pericarditis should be promptly treated with a combination of three or four tuberculostatic drugs for 9–12 months, according to standard protocols. "Prednisone should be administered along with antituberculous drugs in relatively high initial doses (1 mg/kg), maintained for 5–7 days, and progressively reduced until discontinued in 6–8 weeks". Corticosteroids reduce the host reaction to mycobacterial infections, minimise exudation, fibrin deposition, and proliferation of tuberculomata, may decrease symptoms and signs, and reduce mortality in tuberculous pericarditis. However, despite combination therapy, some patients develop constriction. If symptoms and signs of constrictive pericarditis remain 6–8 weeks after full tuberculostatic and corticosteroid treatment, pericardiectomy is indicated.

Uraemic Pericarditis

Most patients with uraemic pericarditis respond within 1–2 weeks to haemo- or peritoneal dialysis, with resolution of chest pain and reduction of the pericardia I effusion. To avoid intrapericardial haemorrhage, heparin-free haemodialysis should be used. Patients with pretamponade should undergo pericardiocentesis before haemodialysis since acute fluidremoval with haemodialysis can lead to cardiovascular collapse and tamponade, peritoneal dialysis, which does not require heparinisation, may be therapeutic in pericarditis resistant to intensified haemodialysis, or if heparin-free haemodialysis cannot be performed. However, it can compromise respiratory function because of intraperitoneal fluid accumulation. NSAIDs and systemic corticosteroids have limited success when intensive dialysis is ineffective. Large, non-resolving symptomatic effusions should be treated with instillation of intrapericardial corticosteroids (triamcinolone) after pericardiocentesis or subxiphoid pericardiotomy. Pericardiectomy is indicated only in refractory, severely symptomatic patients.

Postpericardiotomy Syndrome

Treatment of this syndrome is based on administration of an NSAID or colchicine. Preventive application of colchicine before cardiac surgery has also been nvestigated, but it did not reveal significant results because of the relatively small sample size.

Postinfarction Pericarditis

Ibuprofen is the agent of choice. Aspirin, up to 650 mg every 4 hours for 2–5 days, has also been successfully applied. Other nonsteroidal agents risk thinning the infarction zone, corticosteroid treatment is used for refractory symptoms but can delay infarction healing.

Haemopericardium in Aortic Dissection

In patients with aortic dissection with involvement of the ascending aorta (DeBakey type I or II and Stanford type A) pericardiocentesis is contraindicated, because of the risk of intensified bleeding. Surgery should be performed immediately after the diagnosis is established by echocardiography and/or CT/MRI (in tamponade even if no coronary angiography or aortography is available).

Neoplastic Pericarditis

There are no randomised trials comparing the efficacy and safety of different systemic and/or intrapericardial therapeutic modalities in neoplastic pericardial disease. Systemic antineoplastic treatment as baseline therapy and pericardiocentesis to relieve symptoms, establish diagnosis, and enable intrapericardial instillation of cytostatic/sclerosing agents is the common approach. Prevention of recurrences, observed in 40–70% of patients with large malignant pericardial effusion, may be achieved by intrapericardial instillation of sclerosing agents, cytotoxic drugs, immunomodulators, systemic anti-tumour therapy, percutaneous balloon pericardiotomy, radiation therapy or surgical methods. Treatment tailored to the histology and type of tumour in the course of lung (adenocarcinoma) and breast cancer therapy indicate that intrapericardial administration of cisplatin is effective in 83–93% of cases, with no major side effects during the follow-up. Intrapericardial instillation of thiotepa was effective in 83–89% of cases, together with a favourable safety profile of tetracycline as a sclerosing agent controls malignant pericardia effusion in around 85% of cases, but side effects and complications were reported quite frequently: fever (19%), chest pain (20%) and atrial arrhythmias (10%).

Although classic sclerotherapy after intrapericardial instillation of tetracycline, doxycycline, minocycline, and bleomycin is an effective procedure, constrictive pericarditis secondary to fibrosis remains a severe problem in long-term survivors.

Other antineoplastic drugs; (5-fluorouracil and aclarubicine) or immunomodulators (interferon, interleukin-2, OK-432) have been tested only in very small numbers of patients, radiation therapy is very effective (93%) in controlling malignant pericardial effusion in patients with radiosensitive tumours such as lymphomas and leukemias. Although intrapericardial administration of radionuclides has yielded very good results, it is not widely accepted because of the logistical problems associated with their radioactivity. A percutaneous balloon pericardial window creates a pleuropericardial direct communication, which allows fluid to be drained into the pleural space. In patients with large malignant pericardia effusions and recurrent cardiac tamponade, it seems to be effective (90–97%) and relatively safe but has the potential risk of disseminating neoplastic cells. Pericardiectomy is rarely indicated, and mainly used for treating pericardial con, striction or complications of previous procedures.

Management of Chylopericardium

Chylopericardium after thoracic or cardiac surgery is preferably treated by pericardiocentesis and diet. In some cases, after initial drainage the disorder may be resolved through dietary management (medium chain triglycerides) alone. If further production of chylous effusion continues, surgical treatment is mandatory. When conservative treatment and pericardiocentesis fail, pericardioperitoneal shunting by means of a pericardial window is a reasonable option. Alternatively, when the course of the thoracic duct has been precisely identified, ligation and resection of the thoracic duct just above the diaphragm has proved to be the most effective treatment.

Consultations

A cardiologist should be involved in the care of patients with pericardial effusion.

Cardiothoracic surgery may be required for recurrent or complicated cases.

Autoimmune pericardial effusions may respond to treatment with anti-inflammatory medications. In general, selection of an agent depends on the severity of the patient's symptoms and the tolerability and adverse effect profiles of the medications.

Pharmacotherapy in Pericardial Effusion

Nonsteroidal anti-inflammatory drugs are used mostly for patients with active, nonhemorrhagic pericarditis with or without pericardial effusion. NSAIDS have analgesic, anti-inflammatory, and antipyretic activities. The mechanism of action in pericarditis is not known, but NSAIDS may inhibit cyclooxygenase activity and prostaglandin synthesis. Other mechanisms may exist as well, such as inhibition of leukotriene synthesis, lysosomal enzyme release, lipoxygenase activity, neutrophil aggregation, and various cell membrane functions.

Indomethacin (indocin, indometh): Drug of choice in this class, although other NSAIDs (i.e. ibuprofen, naproxen, aspirin) possess some efficacy. Used as initial therapy for mild to moderately severe inflammatory pericardial effusions.

Adult dose: 25–50 mg PO bid/tid; 75 mg SR PO bid; titrate to effectiveness; not to exceed 200 mg/d

Pediatric dose: 1–2 mg/kg/d PO divided bid/qid; not to exceed 4 mg/kg/d or 150–200 mg/d

Corticosteroids: Have anti-inflammatory properties and cause profound and varied metabolic effects. Corticosteroids modify the body's immune response to diverse stimuli.

Prednisone (deltasone, orasone, sterapred): Used for patients with severe inflammatory pericardial effusions or for those in whom initial treatment with NSAIDs has failed.

Other agents may be used if adverse effect profile warrants; dosages should be determined by prednisone equivalents.

Adult dose: 5–60 mg/d PO qd or divided bid/qid; taper over 2 wk as symptoms resolve to 5–10 mg PO qd

Pediatric dose: 4–5 mg/m^2/d PO; alternatively, 0.05–2 mg/kg PO divided bid/qid; taper over 2 weeks as symptoms resolve

Complications

Pericardial Tamponade

It can lead to severe hemodynamic compromise and death. Heralded by equalization of diastolic filling pressures. Treat with expansion of intravascular volume (small amounts of crystalloids or colloids may lead to improvement, especially in hypovolemic patients) and urgent pericardial drainage. Avoid positive-pressure ventilation if possible, as this decreases venous return and cardiac output. Vasopressor agents are of little clinical benefit.

Chronic Pericardial Effusion

Effusions lasting longer than 6 months usually well tolerated.

Prognosis: Most patients with acute pericarditis recover without sequelae. Predictors of a worse outcome include the following: fever greater than 38°C, symptoms developing over several weeks in association with immunosuppressed state, traumatic pericarditis, pericarditis in a patient receiving oral anticoagulants, a large pericardial effusion (>20 mm echo-free space or evidence of tamponade), or failure to respond to NSAIDs. In a recent series of 300 patients with acute pericarditis, 254 (85%) did not have any of the high-risk characteristics and had no serious complications. Of these low-risk patients, 221 (87%) were managed as outpatients and the other 13% were hospitalized when they did not respond to aspirin.

Patients with symptomatic pericardial effusions from HIV/AIDS or cancer have high short-term mortality rates.

Medical/Legal Pitfalls

Failure to consider pericardial effusion as a principal or secondary diagnosis may lead to rapid deterioration and death secondary to cardiac tamponade. Patients with viral cardiomyopathy, especially in the acute setting, may have a similar presentation, with an enlarged heart on chest radiographs. Echocardiography readily distinguishes the difference between enlarged cardiac chambers and a pericardial effusion.

BIBLIOGRAPHY

1. Adler Y, Finkelstein Y, Guindo J, et al: Colchicine treatment for recurrent pericarditis. A decade of experience. Circulation 1998 Jun 2; 97(21): 2183–5.
2. Arunasalam S, Siegel RJ: Rapid resolution of symptomatic acute pericarditis with ketorolac tromethamine: a parenteral nonsteroidal antiinflammatory agent. Am Heart J 1993 May; 125(5 Pt 1): 1455–8.
3. Baljepally R, Spodick DH: PR-segment deviation as the initial electrocardiographic response in acute pericarditis. Am J Cardiol 1998 Jun 15; 81(12): 1505–6.
4. Brook I, Frazier EH: Microbiology of acute purulent pericarditis. A 12-year experience in a military hospital. Arch Intern Med 1996 Sep 9; 156(16): 1857–60.
5. Brosius FC 3d, Waller BF, Roberts WC: Radiation heart disease. Analysis of 16 young (aged 15 to 33 years) necropsy patients who received over 3,500 rads to the heart. Am J Med 1981 Mar; 70(3): 519–30.
6. Callahan JA, Seward JB, Nishimura RA, et al: Two-dimensional echocardiographically guided pericardiocentesis: experience in 117 consecutive patients. Am J Cardiol 1985 Feb 1; 55(4): 476–9.
7. Chen Y, Brennessel D, Walters J, et al: Human immunodeficiency virus-associated pericardial effusion: report of 40 cases and review of the literature. Am Heart J 1999 Mar; 137(3): 516–21.
8. Correale E, Maggioni AP, Romano S, et al: Pericardial involvement in acute myocardial infarction in the post-thrombolytic era: clinical meaning and value. Clin Cardiol 1997 Apr; 20(4): 327–31.
9. Correale E, Maggioni AP, Romano S, et al: Comparison of frequency, diagnostic and prognostic significance of pericardial involvement in acute myocardial infarction treated with and without thrombolytics. Gruppo Italiano per lo Studio della Sopravvivenza nell'Infarto Miocardico (GISSI). Am J Cardiol 1993 Jun 15; 71(16): 1377–81.
10. Dacso CC: Pericarditis in AIDS. Cardiol Clin 1990 Nov; 8(4): 697–9.
11. Eckart RE, Love SS, Atwood JE, et al: Incidence and follow-up of inflammatory cardiac complications after smallpox vaccination. J Am Coll Cardiol 2004 Jul 7; 44(1): 201–5.
12. Fairley CK, Ryan M, Wall PG, Weinberg J: The organisms reported to cause infective myocarditis and pericarditis in England and Wales. J Infect 1996 May; 32(3): 223–5.
13. Fowler NO: Recurrent pericarditis. Cardiol Clin 1990 Nov; 8(4): 621–6.
14. Friman G, Fohlman J: The epidemiology of viral heart disease. Scand J Infect Dis Suppl 1993; 88: 7–10.
15. Ginzton LE, Laks MM: The differential diagnosis of acute pericarditis from the normal variant: new electrocardiographic criteria. Circulation 1982 May; 65(5): 1004–9.
16. Gregoratos G: Pericardial involvement in acute myocardial infarction. Cardiol Clin 1990 Nov; 8(4): 601–8.
17. Hall IP: Purulent pericarditis. Postgrad Med J 1989 Jul; 65(765): 444–8.
18. Hancock EW: Neoplastic pericardial disease. Cardiol Clin 1990 Nov; 8(4): 673–82.
19. Hoit BD: Imaging the pericardium. Cardiol Clin Allen KB, Faber LP, Warren WH: Pericardial effusion: subxiphoid pericardiostomy versus percutaneous catheter drainage. Ann Thorac Surg 1999 Feb; 67(2): 437–40.
20. Artom G, Koren-Morag N, Spodick DH, et al: Pretreatment with corticosteroids attenuates the efficacy of colchicine in preventing recurrent pericarditis: a multi-centre all-case analysis. Eur Heart J 2005 Apr; 26(7): 723–7.
21. Bonnefoy E, Godon P, Kirkorian G, et al: Serum cardiac troponin I and ST-segment elevation in patients with acute pericarditis. Eur Heart J 2000 May; 21(10): 832–6.
22. Braunwald E: Cardiology: how did we get here, where are we today and where are we going?. Can J Cardiol 2005 Oct; 21(12): 1015–7.
23. Braunwald E, ed: Heart Disease: A Textbook of Cardiovascular Medicine. Philadelphia: WB Saunders Company; 1997: 1478–96.
24. Cheitlin MD, Alpert JS, Armstrong WF: ACC/AHA Guidelines for the Clinical Application of Echocardiography. A report of the American College of Cardiology/American Heart Association Task Force on Practice Guidelines (Committee on Clinical Application of Echocardiography). Developed in coll. Circulation 1997 Mar 18; 95(6): 1686–744.
25. Chen Y, Brennessel D, Walters J: Human immunodeficiency virus-associated pericardial effusion: report of 40 cases and review of the literature. Am Heart J 1999 Mar; 137(3): 516–21.
26. Chong HH, Plotnick GD: Pericardial effusion and tamponade: evaluation, imaging modalities, and management. Compr Ther 1995 Jul; 21(7): 378–85.
27. Correale E, Maggioni AP, Romano S, et al: Comparison of frequency, diagnostic and prognostic significance of pericardial involvement in acute myocardial infarction treated with and without thrombolytics. Gruppo Italiano per lo Studio della Sopravvivenza nell'Infarto Miocardico (GISSI). Am J Cardiol 1993 Jun 15; 71(16): 1377–81.
28. Eisenberg MJ, de Romeral LM, Heidenreich PA: The diagnosis of pericardial effusion and cardiac tamponade by 12-lead ECG. A technology assessment. Chest 1996 Aug; 110(2): 318–24.
29. Fagan SM, Chan KL: Pericardiocentesis: blind no more! [editorial; comment]. Chest 1999 Aug; 116(2): 275–6.
30. Feigenbaum, H: Echocardiography. 5th ed. Philadelphia: Lea & Febiger; 1994: 556–74.
31. Flores RM, Jaklitsch MT, DeCamp MM Jr: Video-assisted thoracic surgery pericardial resection for effusive disease. Chest Surg Clin N Am 1998 Nov; 8(4): 835–51.
32. Guberman BA, Fowler NO, Engel PJ: Cardiac tamponade in medical patients. Circulation 1981 Sep; 64(3): 6340.
33. Heidenreich PA, Eisenberg MJ, Kee LL: Pericardial effusion in AIDS. Incidence and survival. Circulation 1995 Dec 1; 92(11): 3229–34.

34. Ilan Y, Oren R, Ben-Chetrit E: Etiology, treatment, and prognosis of large pericardial effusions. A study of 34 patients. Chest 1991 Oct; 100(4): 985–7. 990 Nov; 8(4): 587–600.
35. Imazio M, Demichelis B, Parrini I, et al: Day-hospital treatment of acute pericarditis: a management program for outpatient therapy. J Am Coll Cardiol 2004 Mar 17; 43(6): 1042–6.
36. Imazio M, Demichelis B, Cecchi E: Cardiac troponin I in acute pericarditis. J Am Coll Cardiol 2003 Dec 17; 42(12): 2144–8.
37. Juneja R, Kothari SS, Saxena A, et al: Intrapericardial streptokinase in purulent pericarditis. Arch Dis Child 1999 Mar; 80(3): 275–7.
38. Khan AH: The postcardiac injury syndromes. Clin Cardiol 1992 Feb; 15(2): 67–72.
39. Klacsmann PG, Bulkley BH, Hutchins GM: The changed spectrum of purulent pericarditis: an 86 year autopsy experience in 200 patients. Am J Med 1977 Nov; 63(5): 666–73.
40. Komsuoglu B, Göldelï O, Kulan K, Komsuoglu SS: The diagnostic and prognostic value of adenosine deaminase in tuberculous pericarditis. Eur Heart J 1995 Aug; 16(8): 1126–30.
41. Krainin FM, Flessas AP, Spodick DH: Infarction-associated pericarditis. Rarity of diagnostic electrocardiogram. N Engl J Med 1984 Nov 8; 311(19): 1211–4.
42. Krikorian JG, Hancock EW: Pericardiocentesis. Am J Med 1978 Nov; 65(5): 808–14.
43. Lange RA, Hillis LD: Clinical practice. Acute pericarditis. N Engl J Med 2004 Nov 18; 351(21): 2195–202.
44. Lorell BH: Pericardial Diseases. In: Braunwald E, ed. Heart Disease: A Textbook of Cardiovascular Medicine. 5th ed. Philadelphia, Pa: WB Saunders; 1997: 1478–534.
45. Maisch B: Pericardial diseases, with a focus on etiology, pathogenesis, pathophysiology, new diagnostic imaging methods, and treatment. Curr Opin Cardiol 1994 May; 9(3): 379–88.
46. Maisch B, Pankuweit S, Brilla C, et al: Intrapericardial treatment of inflammatory and neoplastic pericarditis guided by pericardioscopy and epicardial biopsy—results from a pilot study. Clin Cardiol 1999 Jan; 22(1 Suppl 1): 117–22.
47. Mehta M, Jain AC, Mehta A: Early repolarization. Clin Cardiol 1999 Feb; 22(2): 59–65.
48. Mercé J, Sagristà-Sauleda J, Permanyer-Miralda G, Soler-Soler J: Should pericardial drainage be performed routinely in patients who have a large pericardial effusion without tamponade? Am J Med 1998 Aug; 105(2): 106–9.
49. Moder KG, Miller TD, Tazelaar HD: Cardiac involvement in systemic lupus erythematosus. Mayo Clin Proc 1999 Mar; 74(3): 275–84.
50. Moores DW, Dziuban SW Jr: Pericardial drainage procedures. Chest Surg Clin N Am 1995 May; 5(2): 359–73.
51. Mueller XM, Tevaearai HT, Hurni M, et al: Etiologic diagnosis of pericardial disease: the value of routine tests during surgical procedures. J Am Coll Surg 1997 Jun; 184(6): 645–9.
52. Permanyer-Miralda G, Sagristà-Sauleda J, Soler-Soler J: Primary acute pericardial disease: a prospective series of 231 consecutive patients. Am J Cardiol 1985 Oct 1; 56(10): 623–30.
53. Posner MR, Cohen GI, Skarin AT: Pericardial disease in patients with cancer. The differentiation of malignant from idiopathic and radiation-induced pericarditis. Am J Med 1981 Sep; 71(3): 407–13.
54. Rostand SG, Rutsky EA: Pericarditis in end-stage renal disease. Cardiol Clin 1990 Nov; 8(4): 701–7.
55. Sagristà-Sauleda J, Permanyer-Miralda G, Candell-Riera J, et al: Transient cardiac constriction: an unrecognized pattern of evolution in effusive acute idiopathic pericarditis. Am J Cardiol 1987 Apr 15; 59(9): 961–6.
56. Sagristà-Sauleda J, Barrabes JA, Permanyer-Miralda G: Purulent pericarditis: review of a 20-year experience in a general hospital. J Am Coll Cardiol 1993 Nov 15; 22(6): 1661–5.
57. Sagristà-Sauleda J, Permanyer-Miralda G, Soler-Soler J: Tuberculous pericarditis: ten year experience with a prospective protocol for diagnosis and treatment. J Am Coll Cardiol 1988 Apr; 11(4): 724–8.
58. Shabetai R: Acute pericarditis. Cardiol Clin 1990 Nov; 8(4): 639–44.
59. Silva-Cardoso J, Moura B, Martins L, et al: Pericardial involvement in human immunodeficiency virus infection. Chest 1999 Feb; 115(2): 418–22.
60. Soler-Soler J, Permanyer-Miralda G, Sagristà-Sauleda J: A systematic diagnostic approach to primary acute pericardial disease. The Barcelona experience. Cardiol Clin 1990 Nov; 8(4): 609–20.
61. Spodick DH: Pericardial rub. Prospective, Multiple observer investigation of pericardial friction in 100 patients. Am J Cardiol 1975 Mar; 35(3): 357–62.
62. Spodick DH: Differential diagnosis of acute pericarditis. Prog Cardiovasc Dis 1971 Sep; 14(2): 192–209.
63. Spodick DH: Electrocardiogram in acute pericarditis. Distributions of morphologic and axial changes by stages. Am J Cardiol 1974 Apr; 33(4): 470–4.
64. Spodick DH: Diagnostic electrocardiographic sequences in acute pericarditis. Significance of PR segment and PR vector changes. Circulation 1973 Sep; 48(3): 575–80.
65. Spodick DH: Frequency of arrhythmias in acute pericarditis determined by Holter monitoring. Am J Cardiol 1984 Mar 1; 53(6): 842–5.
66. Spodick DH: Arrhythmias during acute pericarditis. A prospective study of 100 consecutive cases. JAMA 1976 Jan 5; 235(1): 39–41.
67. Spodick DH: The normal and diseased pericardium: current concepts of pericardial physiology, diagnosis and treatment. J Am Coll Cardiol 1983 Jan; 1(1): 240–51.
68. Spodick DH: Pericarditis in systemic diseases. Cardiol Clin 1990 Nov; 8(4): 709–16.
69. Stevenson LW, Child JS, Laks H, Kern L: Incidence and significance of early pericardial effusions after cardiac surgery. Am J Cardiol 1984 Oct 1; 54(7): 848–51.
70. Sugiura T, Takehana K, Abe Y, et al: Frequency of pericardial friction rub ("pericarditis") after direct percutaneous transluminal coronary angioplasty in Q-wave acute myocardial infarction. Am J Cardiol 1997 Feb 1; 79(3): 362–4.
71. Tuna IC, Danielson GK: Surgical management of pericardial diseases. Cardiol Clin 1990 Nov; 8(4): 683–96.
72. Wall TC, Califf RM, Harrelson-Woodlief L, et al: Usefulness of a pericardial friction rub after thrombolytic therapy during

acute myocardial infarction in predicting amount of myocardial damage. The TAMI Study Group. Am J Cardiol 1990 Dec 15; 66(20): 1418–21.
73. Weiss JM, Spodick DH: Association of left pleural effusion with pericardial disease. N Engl J Med 1983 Mar 24; 308(12): 696–7.
74. Wenger NK: Pericardial disease in the elderly. Cardiovasc Clin 1992; 22(2): 97–103.
75. Winkler WB, Karnik R, Slany J: Treatment of exudative fibrinous pericarditis with intrapericardial urokinase. Lancet 1994 Dec 3; 344(8936): 1541–2.
76. Wong B, Murphy J, Chang CJ, et al: The risk of pericardiocentesis. Am J Cardiol 1979 Nov; 44(6): 1110–4.
77. Zayas R, Anguita M, Torres F, et al: Incidence of specific etiology and role of methods for specific etiologic diagnosis of primary acute pericarditis. Am J Cardiol 1995 Feb 15; 75(5): 378–82.
78. Appleton CP, Hatle LK, Popp RL: Cardiac tamponade and pericardial effusion: respiratory variation in transvalvular flow velocities studied by Doppler echocardiography. J Am Coll Cardiol 1988 May; 11(5): 1020–30.
79. Bertog SC, Thambidorai SK, Parakh K, et al: Constrictive pericarditis: etiology and cause-specific survival after pericardiectomy. J Am Coll Cardiol 2004 Apr 21; 43(8): 1445–52.
80. Brockington GM, Zebede J, Pandian NG: Constrictive pericarditis. Cardiol Clin 1990 Nov; 8(4): 645–61.
81. Chevers N: Observations on diseases of the orifice and valves of the aorta. Guys Hosp Rep 1842; 7: 387–92.
82. Connolly DC, Mann RJ: Dominic J. Corrigan (1802-1880) and his description of the pericardial knock. Mayo Clin Proc 1980 Dec; 55(12): 771–3.
83. Fowler NO: Constrictive pericarditis: its history and current status. Clin Cardiol 1995 Jun; 18(6): 341–50.
84. Haley JH, Tajik AJ, Danielson GK, et al: Transient constrictive pericarditis: causes and natural history. J Am Coll Cardiol 2004 Jan 21; 43(2): 271–5.
85. Hancock EW: On the elastic and rigid forms of constrictive pericarditis. Am Heart J 1980 Dec; 100(6 Pt 1): 917–23.
86. Hatle LK, Appleton CP, Popp RL: Differentiation of constrictive pericarditis and restrictive cardiomyopathy by Doppler echocardiography. Circulation 1989 Feb; 79(2): 357–70.
87. Hurrell DG, Nishimura RA, Higano ST, et al: Value of dynamic respiratory changes in left and right ventricular pressures for the diagnosis of constrictive pericarditis. Circulation 1996 Jun 1; 93(11): 2007–13.
88. Sengupta PP, Mohan JC, Mehta V, et al: Doppler tissue imaging improves assessment of abnormal interventricular septal and posterior wall motion in constrictive pericarditis. J Am Soc Echocardiogr 2005 Mar; 18(3): 226–30.
89. Senni M, Redfield MM, Ling LH, et al: Left ventricular systolic and diastolic function after pericardiectomy in patients with constrictive pericarditis: Doppler echocardiographic findings and correlation with clinical status. J Am Coll Cardiol 1999 Apr; 33(5): 1182–8.
90. Shabetai R: Constrictive pericarditis. In: Shabetai R, ed. The Pericardium. New York, NY: Grune & Stratton; 1981.
91. Shabetai R: Pericardial Disease: etiology, pathophysiology, clinical recognition, and treatment. New York NY: Churchill Livingstone; 1995:1024–35.
92. Sohn DW, Kim YJ, Kim HS, et al: Unique features of early diastolic mitral annulus velocity in constrictive pericarditis. J Am Soc Echocardiogr 2004 Mar; 17(3): 222–6.
93. Talreja DR, Edwards WD, Danielson GK, et al: Constrictive pericarditis in 26 patients with histologically normal pericardial thickness. Circulation 2003 Oct 14; 108(15): 1852–7.
94. Tuna IC, Danielson GK: Surgical management of pericardial diseases. Cardiol Clin 1990 Nov; 8(4): 683–96.
95. Yazdani K, Maraj S, Amanullah AM: Differentiating constrictive pericarditis from restrictive cardiomyopathy. Rev Cardiovasc Med 2005; 6(2): 61–71.
96. Imazio M, Demichelis B, Cecchi E, et al: Cardiac troponin I in acute pericarditis. J Am Coll Cardiol 2003 Dec 17; 42(12): 2144–8.
97. Imazio M, Bobbio M, Cecchi E, et al: Colchicine in addition to conventional therapy for acute pericarditis: results of the COlchicine for acute PEricarditis (COPE) trial. Circulation 2005 Sep 27; 112(13): 2012–6.
98. Imazio M, Demichelis B, Parrini I, et al: Day-hospital treatment of acute pericarditis: a management program for outpatient therapy. J Am Coll Cardiol 2004 Mar 17; 43(6): 10426.
99. Kasper D, Branunwald E, Fauci A, et al: Harrison's Principles of Internal Medicine. 16th ed. McGraw-Hill Professional; 2005: 1414–1420.
100. Kimberly RP: Treatment. Corticosteroids and anti-inflammatory drugs. Rheum Dis Clin North Am 1988 Apr; 14(1): 203–21.
101. Kocheril AG, Luttmann C, Sadaniantz A: Pneumococcal pericarditis successfully treated with catheter drainage and intravenous antibiotics. Cathet Cardiovasc Diagn 1991 Dec; 24(4): 286–7.
102. Lange RA, Hillis LD: Clinical practice. Acute pericarditis. N Engl J Med 2004 Nov 18; 351(21): 2195–202. Illn 1995 Nov; 10(11): 807–12.
103. Spodick DH: Acute pericarditis: current concepts and practice. JAMA 2003 Mar 5; 289(9): 1150–3.

25 Pulmonary Hypertension in Children and Adolescents

Although pulmonary hypertension (PH) is rare in children, it is being diagnosed more frequently. Pulmonary hypertension may manifest at any age. Symptoms include fatigue (usually the first symptom to develop); difficulty in breathing; dizziness; fainting; swelling in the legs or ankles; chest pain; and a bluish discoloration of the lips. Pulmonary hypertension is an increase in mean pulmonary arterial pressure, which can be caused by or associated with a wide variety of conditions.

Idiopathic pulmonary arterial hypertension is a rare disorder that can be defined as a sustained elevation in pulmonary artery pressure and pulmonary vascular resistance, with normal pulmonary artery wedge pressure, in the absence of a known cause. It is a diagnosis of exclusion after other possible causes of pulmonary hypertension have been excluded. It is a severe and often rapidly progressive illness in many cases.

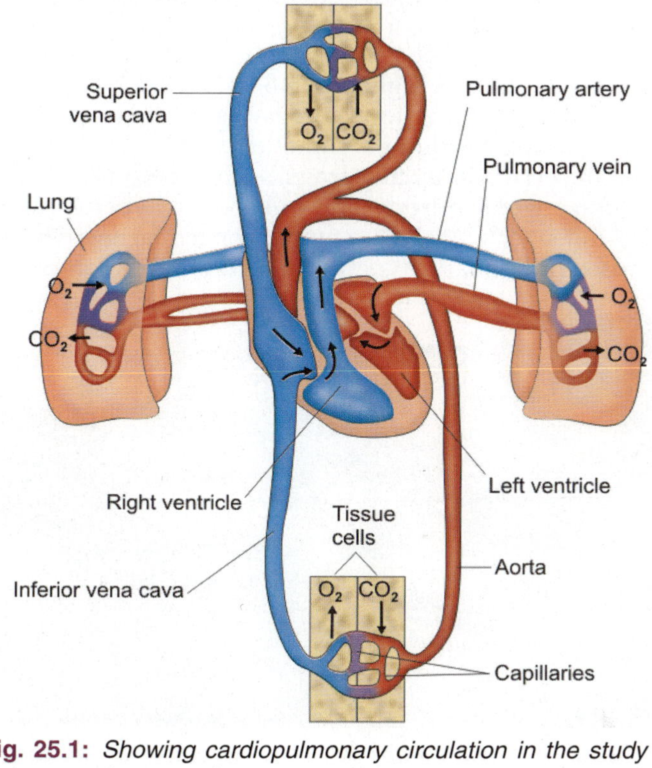

Fig. 25.1: *Showing cardiopulmonary circulation in the study of pulmonary hypertension*

The injury to the pulmonary endothelium causes a tendency to in situ thrombosis in the pulmonary arterial tree, the so-called thrombotic pulmonary arteriopathy. The disease process continues through vascular scarring, endothelial dysfunction and proliferation of smooth muscle cells within the intima and media of the pulmonary arterial tree, causing progressive pulmonary arterial hypertension. This stage is known as plexogenic pulmonary arteriopathy and causes intimal fibrosis replacing normal endothelial structure. This leads to progressive right heart strain due to obliteration of small pulmonary arterial vessels, and eventually right heart failure (Figs 25.1 and 25.2).

Definitions

Pulmonary hypertension (PH) is a haemodynamic and pathophysiological condition defined as an increase in mean pulmonary arterial pressure (PAP) ≥ 25 mmHg at rest as assessed by right heart catheterization.

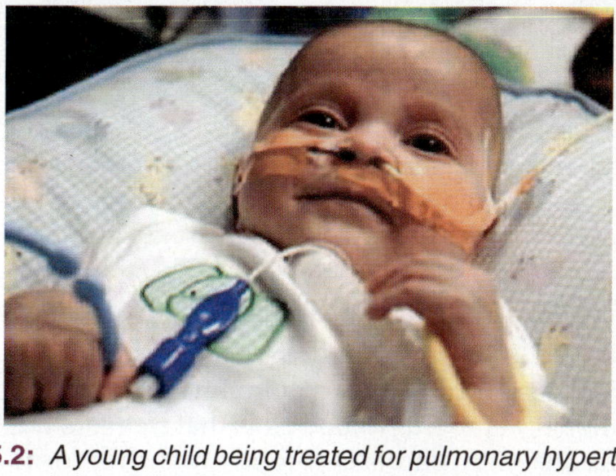

Fig. 25.2: *A young child being treated for pulmonary hypertension with large left to right shunt with heart failure*

Pulmonary arterial hypertension is a clinical condition characterized by the presence of precapillary PH in the absence of other causes of precapillary PH such as PH due to lung diseases, chronic thromboembolic PH, or other rare diseases. PAH includes different forms that share a similar clinical picture and virtually identical pathological changes of the lung microcirculation.

Classification of Pulmonary Hypertension

The WHO Classification of Pulmonary Hypertension

The new WHO classification system attempts to be more specific about the mechanism of pulmonary hypertension, and the expected response to treatment. It is a useful classification system for experts on pulmonary hypertension, but for patients and for many doctors it can be a little confusing.

The WHO classification system divides pulmonary hypertension into five categories (Table 25.1)

Group 1: This group includes disorders in which the pulmonary hypertension is associated with abnormalities in the small branches of the pulmonary artery, the arterioles. Several types of pulmonary hypertension are in Group 1 including idiopathic pulmonary hypertension, and pulmonary hypertension due to several types of infection, connective tissue disorders, and some types of congenital heart disease.

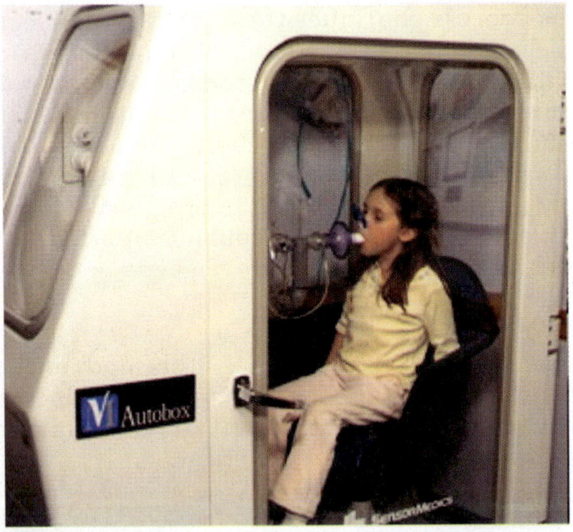

Fig. 25.3: *A child is being tested for pulmonary functions in pulmonary hypertension*

Group 2: This group includes pulmonary hypertension caused by left-sided heart disease, such as cardiomyopathy, diastolic dysfunction, mitral stenosis, mitral regurgitation, aortic stenosis, and aortic regurgitation (Fig. 25.5).

Group 3: This group includes pulmonary hypertension due to lung problems.

Group 4: This group includes pulmonary hypertension due to pulmonary embolus (blood clots that travel to the lungs) or pulmonary thrombosis (blood clots that form in the lungs) (Figs 25.6 to 25.9).

Group 5: This group includes pulmonary hypertension due to other miscellaneous causes, which do not fit into the other four categories.

Etiological Factors

1. Idiopathic Pulmonary Hypertension

When an underlying cause for high blood pressure in the lungs can't be found, the condition is called idiopathic pulmonary hypertension (IPH).

Some people with IPH may have a gene that's a risk factor for developing pulmonary hypertension. But in most people with idiopathic pulmonary hypertension, there is no recognized cause of their pulmonary hypertension.

2. Secondary Pulmonary Hypertension

Pulmonary hypertension that's caused by another medical problem is called secondary pulmonary hypertension. This type of pulmonary hypertension is more common than is idiopathic pulmonary hypertension. Causes of secondary pulmonary hypertension include:

- Blood clots in the lungs (pulmonary emboli)
- Chronic obstructive pulmonary diseases, such as emphysema
- Connective tissue disorders, such as scleroderma or lupus
- Sleep apnea and other sleep disorders
- Heart abnormalities you're born with (congenital heart defects)
- Sickle cell anemia
- Chronic liver disease (cirrhosis)
- AIDS
- Lung diseases such as pulmonary fibrosis, a condition that causes scarring in the tissue between the lungs' air sacs (interstitium)
- Left-sided heart failure
- Living at altitudes higher than 8,000 feet (2,438 meters)
- Climbing or hiking to altitudes higher than 8,000 feet (2,438 meters) without acclimating first
- Use of certain stimulant drugs, such as cocaine
- Eisenmenger syndrome and pulmonary hypertension
- Eisenmenger syndrome, a type of congenital heart defect, causes pulmonary hypertension. It is most commonly

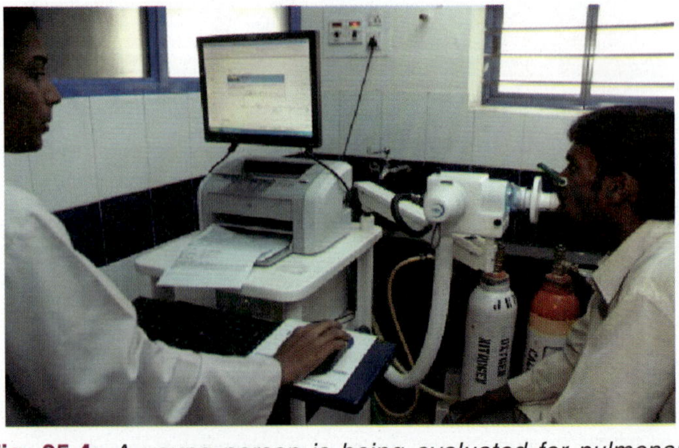

Fig. 25.4: *A young person is being evaluated for pulmonary functions in respiratory laboratory of medical college hospital*

caused by a large hole in your heart between the two lower heart chambers (ventricles), called a ventricular septal defect (VSD). This hole in your heart causes blood to circulate abnormally in your heart. Oxygen-carrying blood (red blood) mixes with oxygen-poor blood (blue blood). The blood then returns to your lungs instead of going to the rest of your body, increasing the pressure in the pulmonary arteries and causing pulmonary hypertension.

Diagnostic Tests

Pulmonary hypertension is hard to diagnose early because it's not often detected in a routine physical examination. Even when the disease is more advanced, its signs and symptoms are similar to those of other heart and lung conditions. Your doctor may do one or more tests to rule out other possible reasons for your condition. The first tests you'll have to diagnose pulmonary hypertension include:

Blood tests: Your doctor may order blood tests to check for certain substances in your blood that may show you have pulmonary hypertension or its complications.

Chest X-ray: This test may be able to check for pulmonary hypertension if your pulmonary arteries or the right ventricle of your heart is enlarged. The X-ray will appear normal in about one-third of people who have pulmonary hypertension (Figs 25.7 and 25.19).

Doppler echocardiogram: Your doctor may first suspect you have pulmonary hypertension based on the results of this test. This noninvasive test uses sound waves that allow your doctor to see your heart without making an incision. During the procedure, a small, plastic instrument called a transducer is placed on your chest. It collects reflected sound waves (echoes) from your heart and transmits them to a machine that uses the sound wave patterns to compose images of your beating heart on a monitor (Figs 25.21 to 25.27).

These images show how well your heart is functioning, and recorded pictures allow your doctor to measure the size and thickness of your heart muscle. Sometimes your doctor will recommend an exercise echocardiogram to help determine how well your heart works under stress. In that case, you'll have an echocardiogram before exercising on a stationary bike or treadmill and another test immediately afterward.

Transesophageal echocardiogram: If it is difficult to get a clear picture of your heart and lungs with a standard echocardiogram, your doctor may recommend a transesophageal echocardiogram. In this procedure, a flexible tube containing a transducer is guided down your throat and into your esophagus after using a numbing spray in the back of your throat. From here, the transducer can get detailed images of your heart.

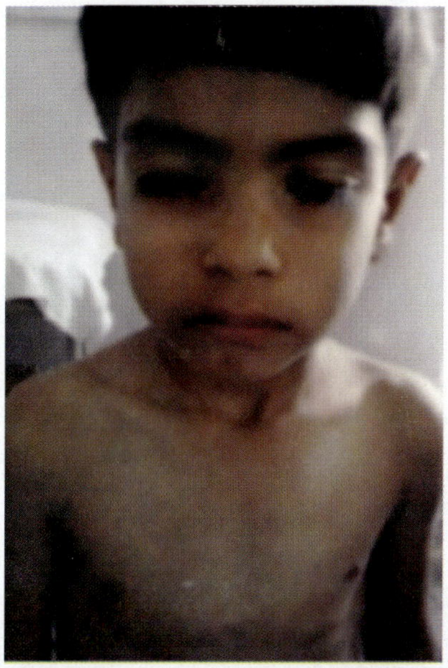

Fig. 25.5: *Photograph of a 7-years-old child who had juvenile rheumatic mitral stenosis (MVA<2.0 cm^2) with severe MR (grade III-IV) TR, enlarged LA with PAH with CCF and on decongestive therapy with digoxin and diuretic*

Right heart catheterization: After you've had an echocardiogram if your doctor thinks you have pulmonary hypertension, you'll likely have a right heart catheterization. This test is often the most reliable way of diagnosing pulmonary hypertension. During the procedure, a cardiologist places a thin, flexible tube (catheter) into a vein in your neck or groin. The catheter is then threaded into

Table 25.1: *Clinical classification of congenital systemic-to-pulmonary shunts associated with PAH*

A. Eisenmenger syndrome	Includes all systemic-to-pulmonary shunts resulting from large defects and leading to a severe increase in PVR and a reversed (pulmonary-to-systemic) or bidirectional shunt; cyanosis, erythrocytosis, and multiple organ involvement are present
B. PAH associated with systemic-to-pulmonary shunts	Includes moderate to large defects; PVR is mildly to moderately increased, systemic-to-pulmonary shunt is still prevalent, and no cyanosis is present at rest
C. PAH with small defects	Small defects (usually ventricular septal defects <1 cm and atrial septal defects <2 cm of effective diameter assessed by echocardiography); clinical picture is very similar to idiopathic PAH
D. PAH after corrective cardiac surgery	Congenital heart disease has been corrected, but PAH is still present immediately after surgery or recurs several months or years after surgery in the absence of significant postoperative residual lesions

PAH, pulmonary arterial hypertension; PVR, pulmonary vascular resistance.

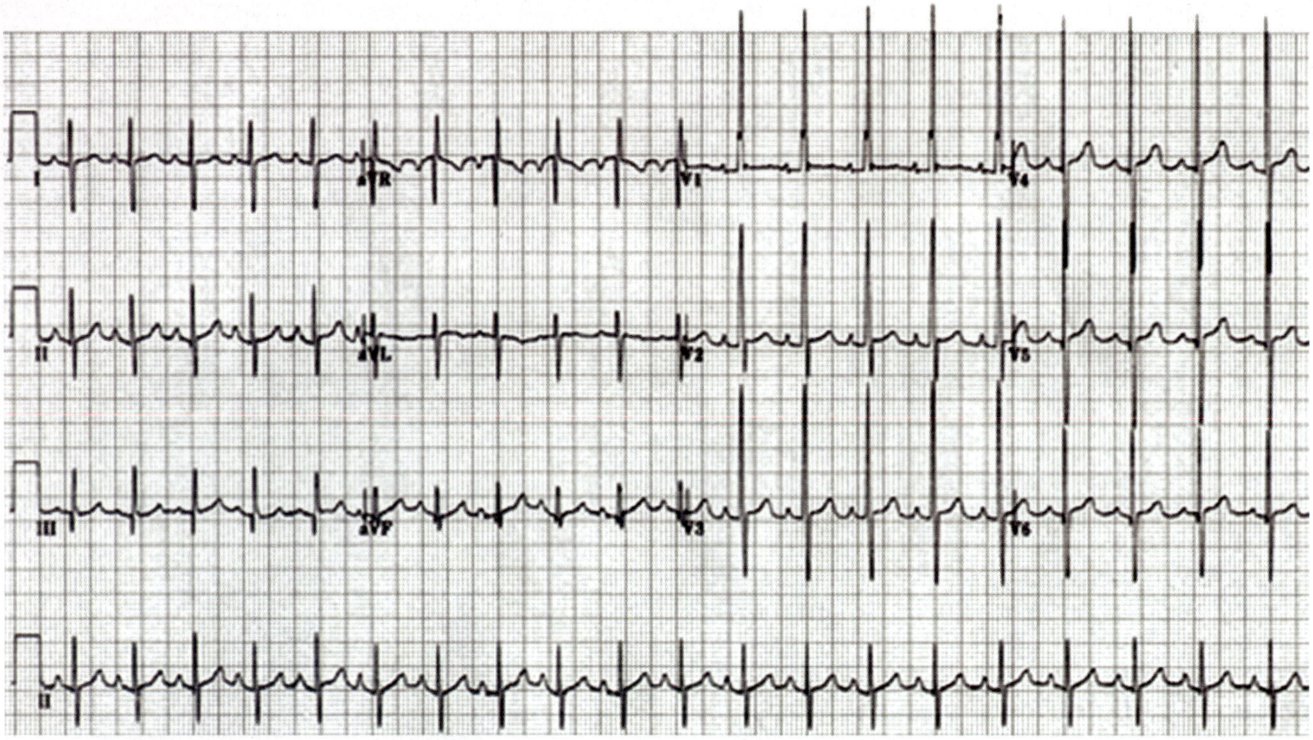

Fig. 25.6: *Leads ECG showing right-axis deviation, tall R waves in V1-V3 with deep 5 waves in left precordial leads (V5-V6) in an adolescent with primary pulmonary hypertension*

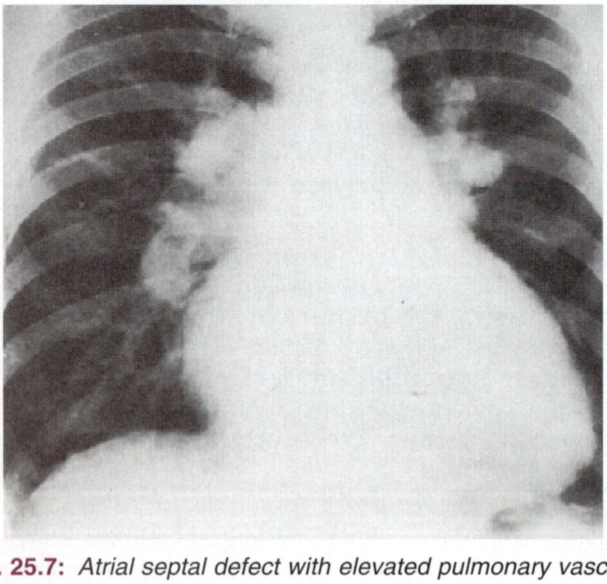

Fig. 25.7: *Atrial septal defect with elevated pulmonary vascular resistance. In secundum atrial septal defect, there is a marked disparity between the size of the hilar arteries and the peripheral pulmonary vessels, indicating an increase in pulmonary vascular resistance. The right ventricle pressure was almost at systemic levels*

your right ventricle and pulmonary artery. Right heart catheterization allows your doctor to directly measure the pressure in the main pulmonary arteries and right ventricle. It's also used to see what effect different medications may have on your pulmonary hypertension.

Right heart catheterization is usually performed during local anesthesia and sedation in a hospital setting. You often can go home soon after the procedure. You'll need someone to drive you home after the test (Figs 25.11, 25.18–25.20, 25.28).

Your doctor may order additional tests to check the condition of your lungs and pulmonary arteries including:

Pulmonary function test: This noninvasive test measures how much air your lungs can hold, and the airflow in and out of your lungs. During the test, you will blow into a simple instrument called a spirometer (Figs 25.3, 25.4, 25.12, 25.15).

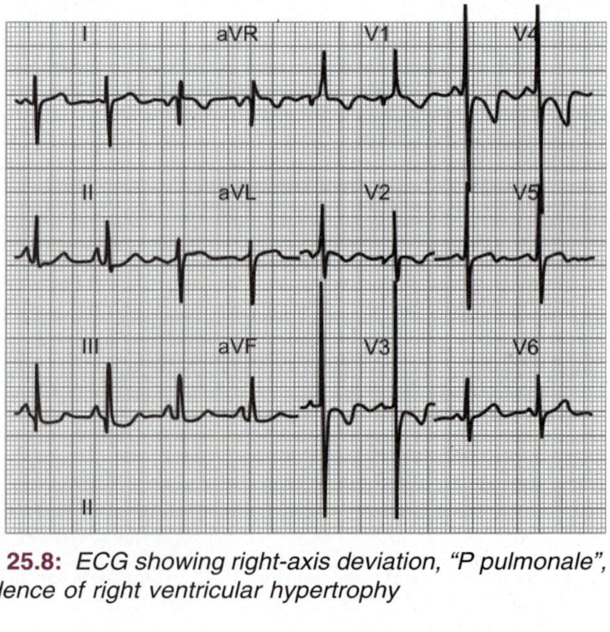

Fig. 25.8: *ECG showing right-axis deviation, "P pulmonale", and evidence of right ventricular hypertrophy*

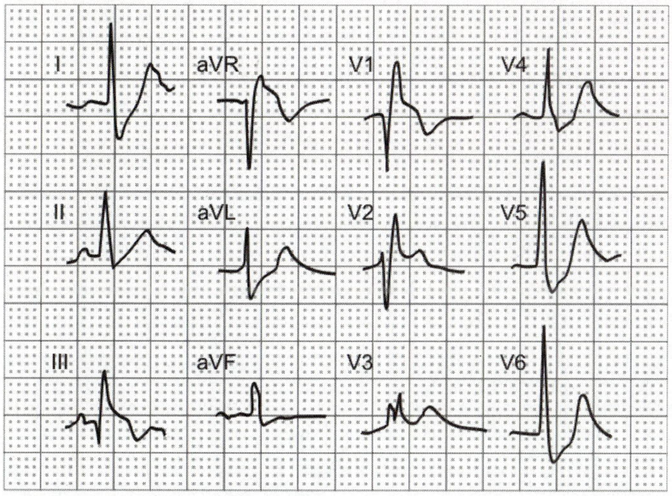

Fig. 25.9: *Graphs shows SI, Q3, T3 pattern right-bundle branch block (incomplete or complete). T wave inversion in the right precordial leads P pulmonale right-axis deviation in patient with acute pulmonary embolism*

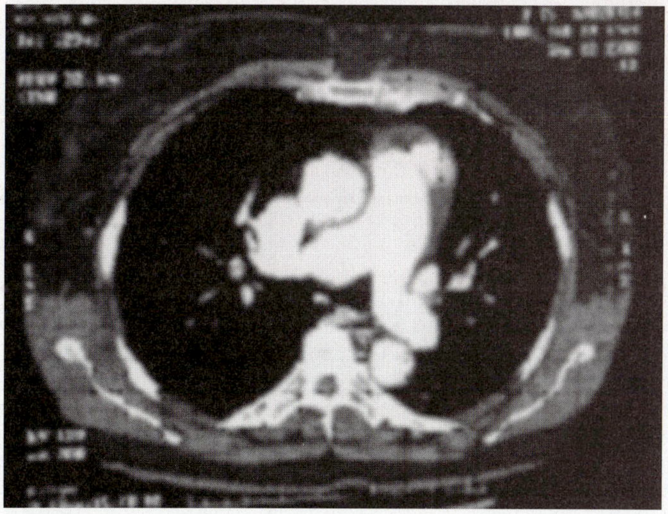

Fig. 25.10: *Pulmonary hypertension. Spiral CT scan in a patient with pulmonary hypertension reveals enlarged pulmonary arteries and an absence of thrombosis*

Cardiopulmonary Exercise Testing (CPET)

CPET is used to tell your specialist how sick you are, and also to see what effects treatments have had upon your condition. In a CPET, you breathe into a mouthpiece (maybe while riding a stationary bicycle or walking on a treadmill) while an ECG is being done. Although not painful, it's not a glamorous procedure. Wear exercise clothes and sneakers. Because your nose is pinched shut and your mouth is clenched around a tube, you may drool a lot. The bicycle seat can be politely described as uncomfortable in spots. Ask for a gel pad if the seat is too hard. If you feel panicky about having to breathe through a mouth tube, try pretending you are snorkeling. If you are feeling tired the day you take exercise tests, you may find them exhausting in more than one sense, and may want to arrange for somebody to drive you home afterwards.

Polysomnogram: This is a combination of tests done if sleep apnea breathing at night. The tests monitor brain wave activity (with an electroencephalogram or EG), the amount of oxygen in your blood (with a pulse oximeter), the movement of air in and out a nostril asou breathe, and the up and down movement of your chest wall. Polysomnography may be used to exclude obstructive sleep apnoea.

Perfusion lung scan: This test uses small amounts of radioactive substances (radioisotopes) to study blood flow (perfusion) in your lungs. The radioisotopes are injected into a vein in your arm. Immediately afterward, a special camera (gamma camera) takes pictures of blood flow in your lungs' blood vessels. A lung scan can then be used to determine whether blood clots are causing symptoms of pulmonary hypertension (Fig. 25.16).

A perfusion lung scan is usually performed with another test, known as a ventilation scan. In this test, you inhale a

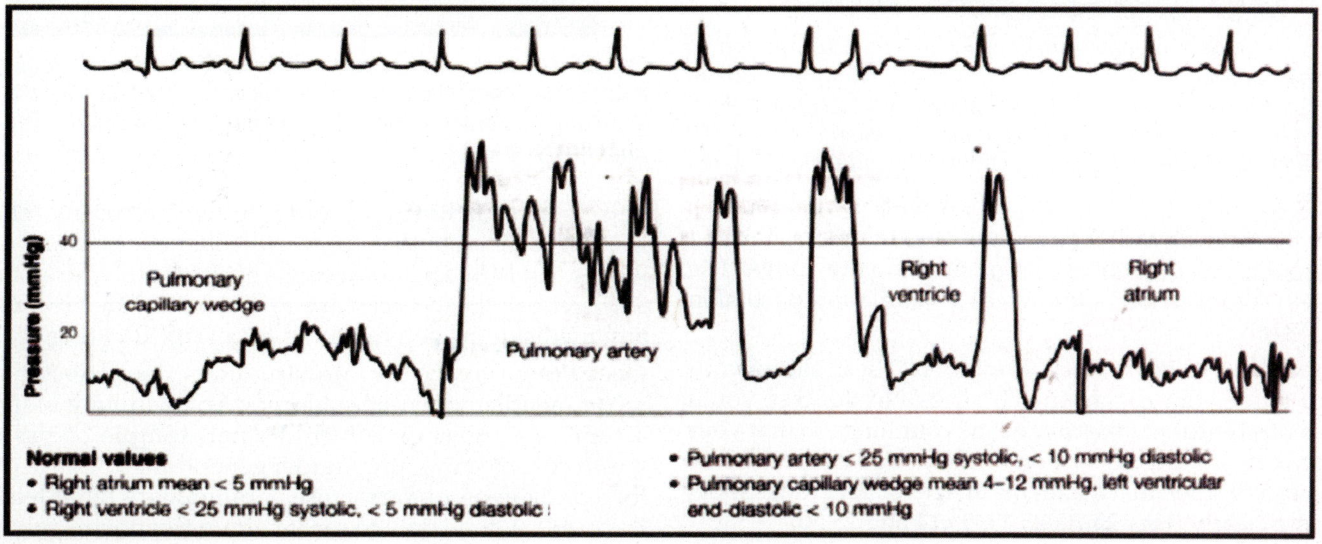

Fig. 25.11: *Showing pull back pressure gradient across pulmonary capillary wedge, main pulmonary artery, right ventricle and right atrium during selective cardiac catheterization in patient with pulmonary artery hypertension*

Normal	Small airway obstruction	Chronic obstruction	Fixed large airway obstruction	Variable extrathoracic	Variable intrathoracic	Restrictive disease
Example	Mild asthma	Moderate COPD	Subglottic stenosis	Croup or obs. sleep anea	Tracheomalacia	Pulmonary fibrosis

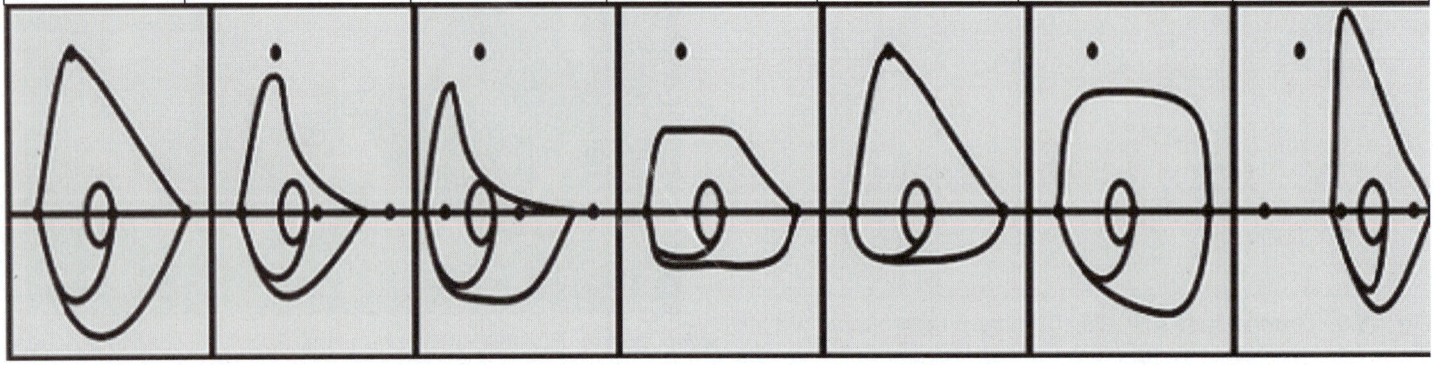

Fig. 25.12: *Flow rates in different respiratory diseases*

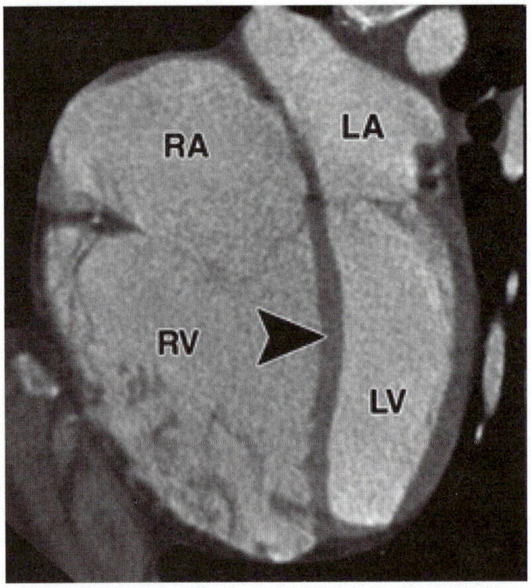

Fig. 25.13: *MDCT revealed sinus venosus type ASD with partial anomalous pulmonary venous return. Four chamber view of MDCT shows right atrium (RA) and right ventricle (RV) dilatation, with interventricular septum (arrow head) bulging toward left ventricular (LV) side, indicating pulmonary hypertension. LA, left atrium*

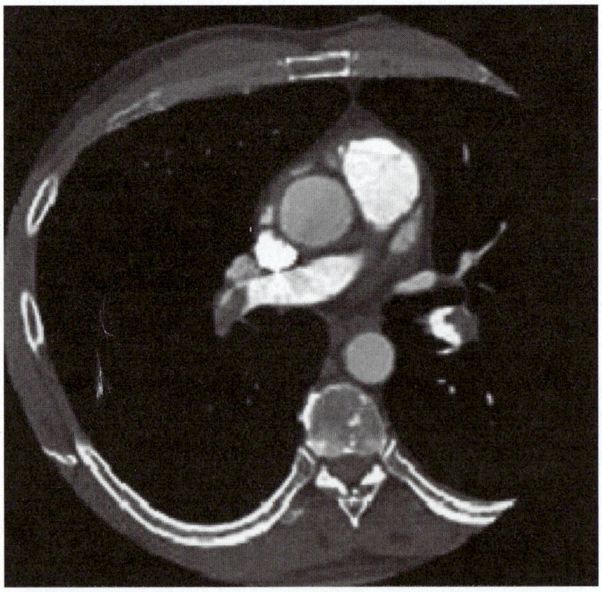

Fig. 25.14: *Pulmonary hypertension. CT pulmonary angiogram in an adolescent who experienced severe chest pain after a long flight. Image demonstrates clots in both the right and the left main pulmonary arteries*

small amount of radioactive substance while a gamma camera records the movement of air into your lungs. The two-test combination is known as a ventilation-perfusion (V/Q) scan.

Computerized tomography (CT) scan: A CT scan allows your doctor to see your organs in 2D "slices". In this test, you'll lie in a machine that takes images of your lungs so that your doctors can see a cross-section of them. You might also be given a medication that makes the images of your lungs show up more clearly (Figs 25.10, 25.13, 25.14 and 25.30).

Magnetic resonance imaging (MRI): This test, which uses no X-rays, is sometimes used to get images of the blood vessels in your lungs. A computer creates tissue "slices" from data generated by a powerful magnetic field and radio waves. An MRI can't, however, measure artery pressure—a procedure that's necessary to check the effectiveness of any medications you're taking to control IPH (Fig. 25.29).

Open-lung biopsy: In rare situations, your doctor may recommend an open-lung biopsy. An open-lung biopsy is a type of surgery in which a small sample of tissue is removed from your lungs under general anesthesia to check for a possible secondary cause of pulmonary hypertension. It would be done only to see if certain treatments might be effective for you, or to allow you to discontinue some medications (Fig. 25.17).

Genetic Tests

If a family member has had pulmonary hypertension, your doctor may screen you for genes that are linked with pulmonary hypertension. If you test positive, your doctor may recommend that other family members be screened for the same genetic mutation.

Pulmonary Hypertension Classifications

Once you've been diagnosed with pulmonary hypertension, your doctor may classify the disease using guidelines developed by the World Health Organization.

Class I: Although you've been diagnosed with pulmonary hypertension, you have no symptoms.
Class II: You don't have symptoms at rest, but you experience fatigue, shortness of breath or chest pain with normal activity.
Class III: You're comfortable at rest, but have symptoms when you're physically active.
Class IV: You have symptoms even at rest.

Epidemiology

In its pure idiopathic form, it is a rare disease with an approximate annual incidence of about 2–6 cases per million population. There is a higher incidence of cases associated with connective tissue disease—about 10% of sufferers of CREST/scleroderma syndromes have the condition.

Risk Factors

Although anyone can develop either type of pulmonary hypertension, older adults are more likely to have secondary pulmonary hypertension, and young people are more likely to have idiopathic pulmonary hypertension. Idiopathic pulmonary hypertension is also more common in women than it is in men.

Another risk factor for pulmonary hypertension is a family history of the disease. Some genes could be linked to idiopathic pulmonary hypertension. These genes might cause an overgrowth of cells in the small arteries of your lungs, making them narrower.

If one of your family members develops idiopathic pulmonary hypertension and tests positive for a gene mutation that can cause pulmonary hypertension, your doctor or genetic counselor may recommend that you or your family members be tested for the mutation.

Sleep Apnea

About 12 million Americans have sleep apnea: they stop breathing several or many times an hour while they sleep. This disease wasn't well known until recently, and most people who have it are unaware that they do. There is much more to be learned about sleep apnea.

To be classified as having sleep apnea you generally have to stop breathing for at least 10 seconds at least 30 times in a 70-hour period (and often over 100 times in an hour!). The condition is found most frequently in very heavy middle-aged men who snore, but it is certainly not limited to them. If you don't breathe often enough, you don't maintain enough oxygen in your blood (the saturation falls below 90% for a significant time). This lack of oxygen can cause pulmonary vasoconstriction and a resulting rise in PAPs.

Those who have the most common kind of sleep apnea, obstructive sleep apnea, keep trying to breathe but can't pull in enough air because of a blockage in the upper airway.

Clinical Presentation

The illness can have a very insidious onset and be hard to notice for both patients and doctors; as it cannot be diagnosed on clinical grounds alone and requires detailed investigation, it is often diagnosed late, when useful therapeutic options may be limited. It may take up to 2 years to diagnose the condition and it can progress very quickly in some cases, so it presents a significant challenge in terms of early detection.

Symptoms

- Dyspnoea
- Generalized weakness and tiredness
- Recurrent syncope or presyncope, often related to exertion.

Signs

- Right ventricular (parasternal) heave may be visible/palpable

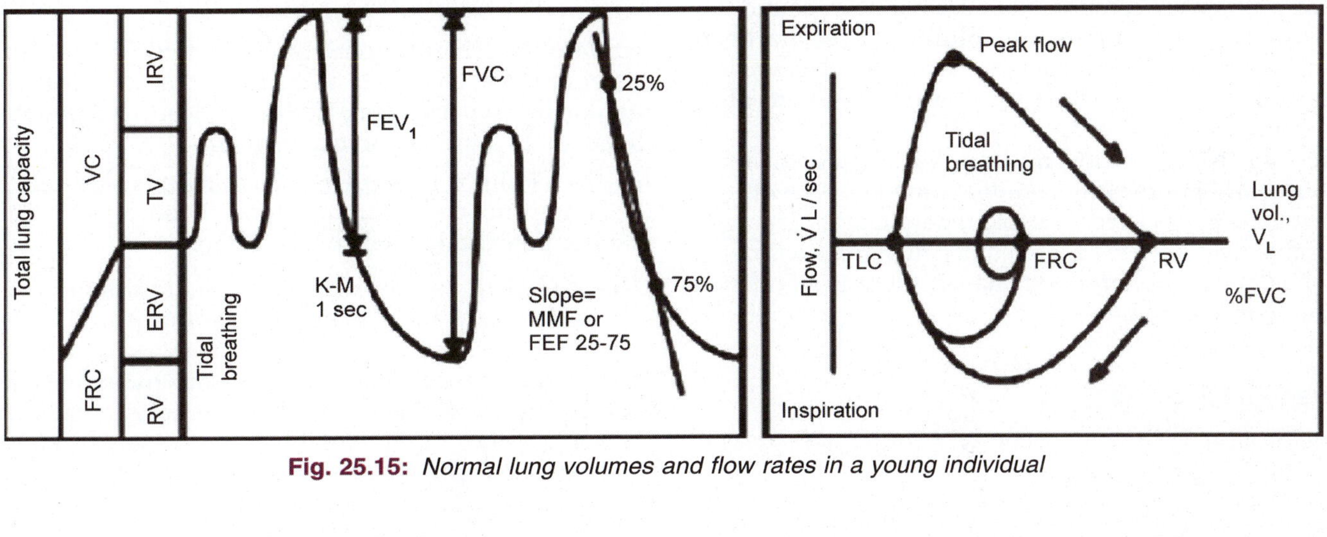

Fig. 25.15: *Normal lung volumes and flow rates in a young individual*

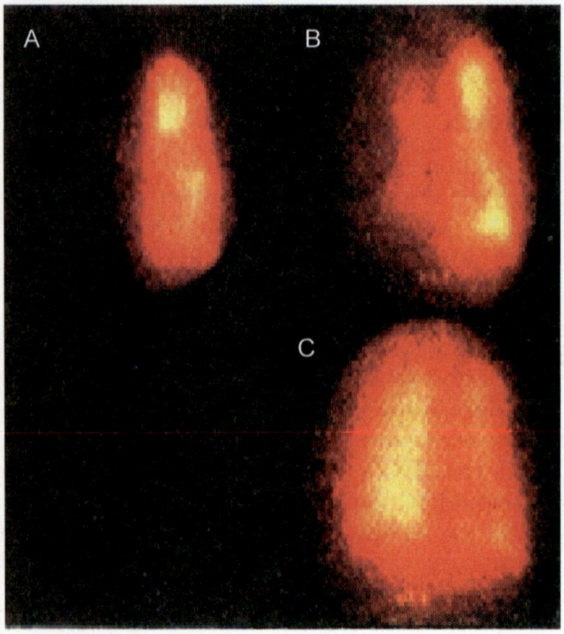

Fig. 25.16: *Perfusion scan shows complete abscence of perfusion of right lung with abnormalities in the left lung*

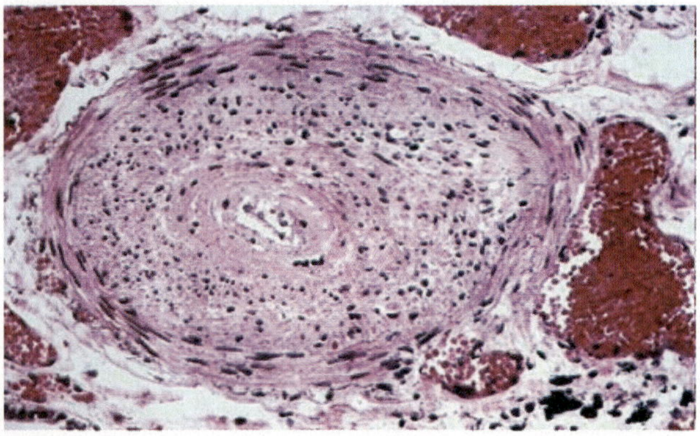

Fig. 25.17 *Cross section of a pulmonary artery revealing intimal proliferation and medial myxomatous change with a mild inflammatory infiltrate emphasizing the heterogeneity of pathologic processes in pulmonary hypertension*

- JVP may be elevated with prominent a and v waves.
- Loud pulmonary component of second heart sound.
- May be fixed or paradoxical splitting of second heart sound-very difficult to detect for most clinicians.
- Murmur of pulmonary regurgitation—Graham Steel murmur.
- Tricuspid regurgitation murmur—if significant right ventricular hypertrophy and dilatation are present.
- If significant associated tricuspid regurgitation—enlarged pulsatile liver with exaggerated hepatojugular reflux.
- Ascites and peripheral oedema—if there is significant right ventricular failure.
- Lung fields are usually clear.

Differential Diagnosis

- Cor pulmonale causing secondary pulmonary hypertension
- Cardiomyopathies
- Primary right ventricular failure—e.g. following myocardial infarction
- Congestive cardiac failure
- Recurrent pulmonary emboli
- Mitral or tricuspid stenosis
- Tricuspid regurgitation
- Pulmonary stenosis
- Portal hypertension
- Obstructive sleep apnoea
- Hypothyroidism
- Sickle cell disease.

Complications

- Deteriorating right heart function and right-sided cardiac failure
- Gross peripheral oedema
- Hepatic congestion and cardiac cirrhosis
- Pleural effusions
- Gross exertional dyspnoea
- Exertional syncope
- Sudden cardiac death
- Problems during childbirth including sudden death.

Pulmonary hypertension can lead to a number of complications including:

Right-sided heart failure (cor pulmonale): In cor pulmonale, your heart's right ventricle becomes enlarged and has to pump harder than usual to move blood through narrowed or blocked pulmonary arteries. At first, the heart tries to compensate by thickening its walls and expanding the chamber of the right ventricle to increase the amount of blood it can hold. But, this thickening and enlarging works only temporarily, and eventually the right ventricle fails from the extra strain.

Blood clots: Clots help stop bleeding after you've been injured. But sometimes, clots form where they're not needed. A number of small clots or just a few large ones dislodge from these veins and travel to the lungs, leading to a form of pulmonary hypertension that is reversible with time and treatment. Having pulmonary hypertension makes it more likely you'll develop clots in the small arteries in your lungs, which is dangerous if you already have narrowed or blocked blood vessels.

Arrhythmia: Irregular heartbeats (arrhythmias) from the upper or lower chambers of the heart are complications of pulmonary hypertension. These can lead to palpitations, dizziness or fainting and can be fatal.

Bleeding: Pulmonary hypertension can lead to bleeding into the lungs and coughing up blood (hemoptysis). This is another potentially fatal complication.

Diastolic heart failure causing pulmonary hypertension and pulmonary hypertension causing diastolic dysfunction?

Left heart disease can cause pulmonary hypertension via multiple mechanisms. In the past, a normal ejection fraction and the absence of left-sided valve disease or congenital heart disease provided reassurance that pulmonary

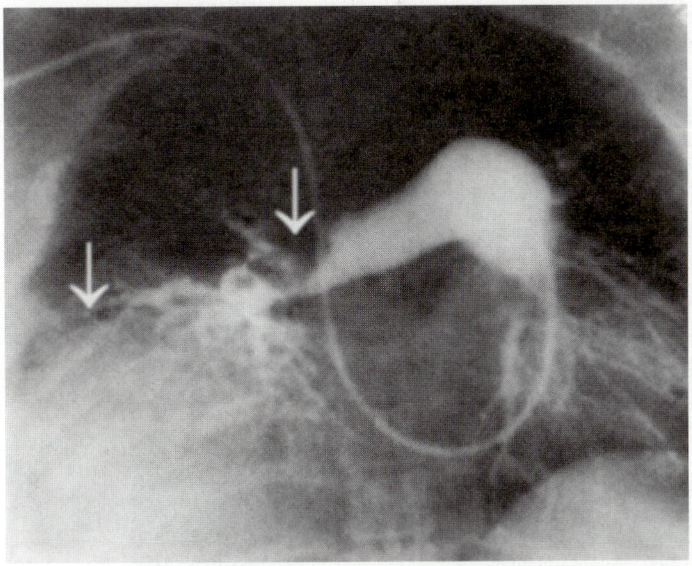

Fig. 25.18: *Pulmonary angiography showing massive thrombus in the right pulmonary artery with almost complete obstruction to the blood flow (arrow). Note also the elevation of right hemidiaphragm (arrow)*

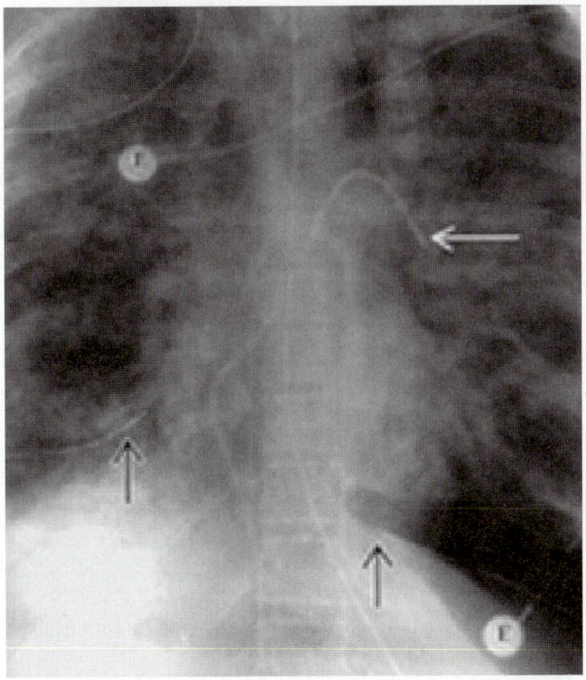

Fig. 25.19: *Frontal chest radiograph shows a Swan-Ganz catheter (white arrow) in the left pulmonary artery via the inferior vena cava. Note also the bilateral chest tubes (black arrows) and ECG leads (E)*

hypertension was not related to left-sided heart disease. However, it is now recognized that patients with clinical heart failure commonly have a normal ejection fraction, a syndrome referred to as diastolic heart failure or heart failure with normal ejection fraction. As reviewed below, the pathophysiologic mechanisms present in patients with diastolic heart failure may be heterogeneous. Although pulmonary hypertension has been reported in patients with

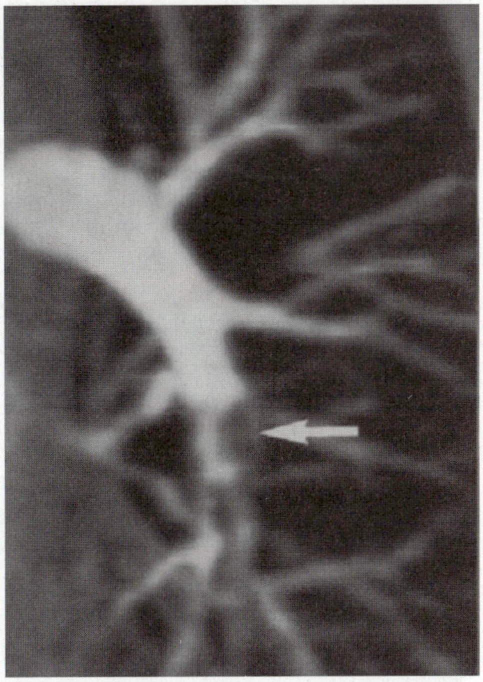

Fig. 25.20: *Anteroposterior view of left lower lobe pulmonary embolus (arrow) on digital subtraction angiogram. The irregular vessels below the embolus (arrow) were considered to represent a change in vessel caliber rather than additional emboli in a patient with pulmonary hypertension*

diastolic heart failure, its prevalence and severity remain poorly defined. Idiopathic pulmonary arterial hypertension (IPAH) has been characterized as a disease of children and young adults, yet increasingly the diagnosis is made in elderly persons. This raises concern that some patients with dyspnea, unexplained pulmonary hypertension, and a normal ejection fraction could have diastolic heart failure with secondary pulmonary hypertension related to chronic pulmonary venous hypertension. However, as reviewed below, chronic right ventricular pressure overload can cause left ventricular diastolic dysfunction. Thus, a diagnostic dilemma arises in elderly dyspneic patients with otherwise unexplained pulmonary hypertension and a normal ejection fraction or when patients with a presumptive diagnosis of IPAH undergo right heart catheterization and are found to have an elevated pulmonary capillary wedge pressure (PCWP). Do these patients have diastolic heart failure with secondary pulmonary hypertension or is it IPAH causing left ventricular diastolic dysfunction and elevated PCWP?

Diastolic Heart Failure

Epidemiologic studies have established that 50% of patients with a clinical diagnosis of heart failure have preserved ejection fraction and this entity has been referred to as diastolic heart failure. Patients with diastolic heart failure are generally elderly but a significant subset are somewhat younger. Although there is a predominance among women, the syndrome also frequently affects men. More recently, the term "heart failure with normal ejection fraction" has

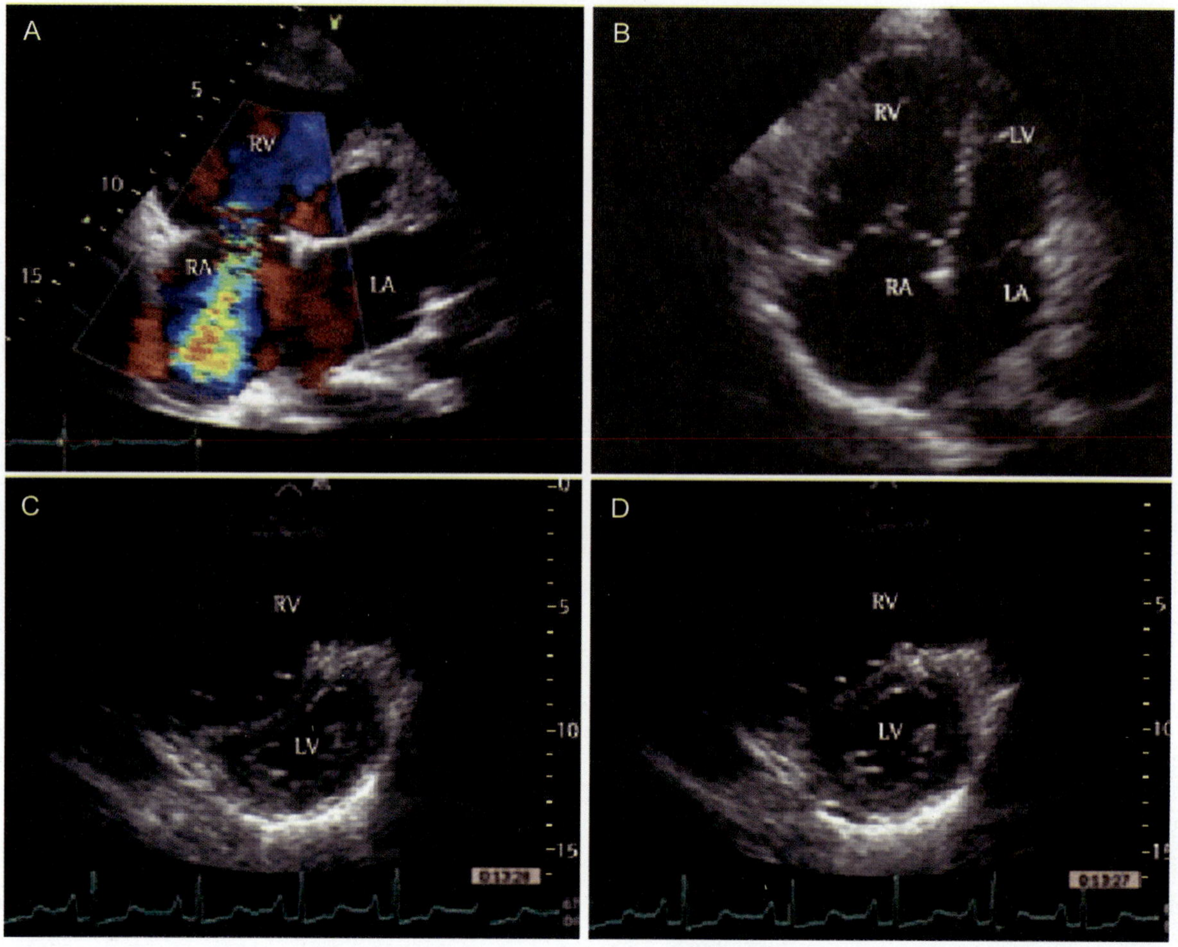

Fig. 25.21: *Echocardiography images. Note the intensity of the continuous wave Doppler signal of the tricuspid regurgitant jet during ventricular systol (A) and the dilated right heart (B). Note the pressure overload in the right ventricle (RV), leading to paradoxical interventricular (IV) septal motion to the left, and reduction in the size of the left ventricle (LV) during diastole (C). During ventricular systole, the IV septrum remians flattened (in D). (Courtesy of Dr Fabio Lario, attending physician in the Department of Echocardiography of the Heart Institute of the University of Sao Paulo School of the Medicine Hospital Das Clinicas.)*

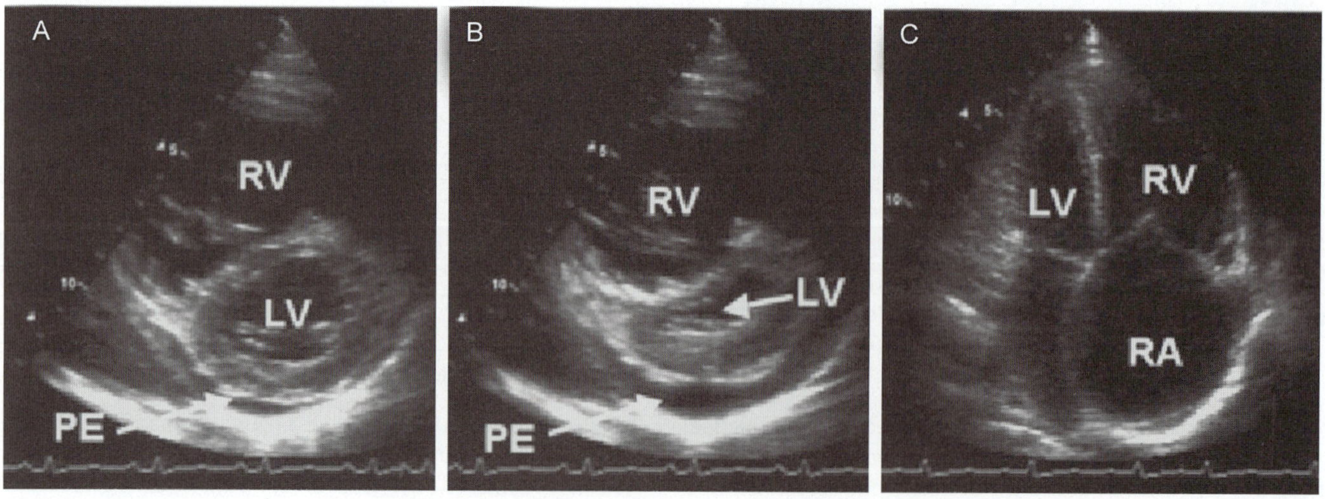

Fig. 25.22: *Doppler echocardiographic findings in an adolescent with severe idiopathic pulmonary arterial hypertension. (A) Short-axis view of the right (RV) and left (LV) ventricles in diastole at the mid-LV level. The RV is markedly enlarged while the LV is normal in size. There is a small pericardial effusion (PE). (B) Short-axis view of the RV and LV in systole. The intraventricular septum is flattened, producing a D-shaped LV. The PE is more apparent in systole. (C) Apical four chamber view demonstrating the marked RV and right atrial (RA) enlargement*

been suggested because of concerns that diastolic dysfunction may not be present in all patients.

Risk factors for diastolic heart failure beyond advanced age and female sex include hypertension, coronary artery disease, and risk factors for coronary artery disease including diabetes. Although classically described in patients with left ventricular hypertrophy, echocardiographic evidence of left ventricular hypertrophy is not uniformly present. Indeed, fewer than 50% of patients have left ventricular hypertrophy in several series of patients with diastolic heart failure.

Although the diagnosis of diastolic heart failure is predicated on the presence of clinical heart failure, a normal ejection fraction, and the absence of significant left-sided valve disease, the proper methods to confirm the presence of diastolic dysfunction remain controversial. To characterize left ventricular diastolic function, invasive assessment of the two primary components of diastolic function, left ventricular relaxation and compliance, is needed.

The degree of impairment in left ventricular relaxation can be quantified by calculating the time constant of isovolumic relaxation (tau) from a high fidelity left ventricular pressure tracing. Impairment in relaxation likely contributes to symptoms of dyspnea with exercise where brisk relaxation is needed to enhance early diastolic filling without increased left atrial pressures. Patients with significantly impaired relaxation are dependent on left ventricular filling during atrial contraction (atrial kick) to maintain filling without increased atrial pressure and thus are prone to develop acute diastolic heart failure associated with the onset of atrial fibrillation. As the speed and extent of left ventricular relaxation are very dependent on afterload, relaxation may become severely impaired with hypertensive episodes and contribute to elevation in mean left atrial pressures, as is likely the case in patients with a normal ejection fraction (hypertensive pulmonary edema). Assessment of alterations in left ventricular compliance depends on demonstration of an upward and leftward shift of the end-diastolic pressure volume relationship (LV-EDPVR) such that the left atrial pressure required to fill the left ventricle to a normal volume is markedly elevated. Marked reduction in left ventricular compliance is clearly present in patients with rare diseases such as infiltrative cardiomyopathy due to amyloidosis, in those with primary restrictive cardiomyopathies, and in some patients with hypertrophic cardiomyopathy. In these patients, blood pressure is low, left ventricular volumes are normal to reduced, and left atrial pressures are chronically elevated. Attempts to lower atrial pressures with diuretic therapy often result in hypotension as left ventricular filling is dependent on markedly elevated filling pressures. Whether the more typical patients with diastolic heart failure (who are often hypertensive) have reduced left ventricular compliance remains somewhat controversial. Demonstration of reduced compliance mandates the need for the instantaneous assessment of left ventricular pressure and volume over a range of pressures and volumes produced by increasing or decreasing preload. Highly accurate instantaneous assessment of left ventricular volume and pressure is very difficult to obtain. In humans, use of the conductance catheter is really the only means of reliably obtaining such data; although some studies have used echocardiography and left ventricular pressure tracings. Further, even once armed with the data defining the LV-EDPVR, the curvilinear nature of the relationship, which is rarely perfectly monoexponential, makes it difficult to derive a single parameter that reflects the steepness and position of the relationship, and advanced analyses are needed.

Comprehensive Doppler echocardiography can be very useful in gaining information regarding diastolic function and filling pressures.

Doppler patterns consistent with impaired relaxation with normal filling pressure (grade I diastolic dysfunction), impaired relaxation with moderate elevation of filling pressures (grade II diastolic dysfunction), impaired relaxation with severe elevation of filling pressures that can be reversed with preload-reducing maneuvers (grade III diastolic dysfunction), or impaired relaxation with severe elevation of filling pressures that can not be reversed with preload reducing maneuvers (grade IV diastolic dysfunction) have been described and validated against invasive assessment of left ventricular relaxation and filling pressures. Equating these Doppler patterns with the severity of diastolic dysfunction makes several assumptions and paramount among these is that the elevation of filling pressures detected by these parameters is mediated by a reduction of left ventricular compliance. Supportive of this assumption is the fact that this grading system has been shown to correlate with worsening prognosis, suggesting that the elevated filling pressures reflected in the Doppler measurements are the result of progressive ventricular remodeling and diastolic dysfunction rather than transient volume overload. Unfortunately, this may not be the case in every patient. Further, diastolic assessment is somewhat difficult to perform, requires informed interpretation, and is limited by atrial fibrillation, tachycardia, conduction defects, and atrial systolic dysfunction. Left atrial enlargement may also be a good indicator of chronic atrial pressure overload and complements the Doppler assessment.

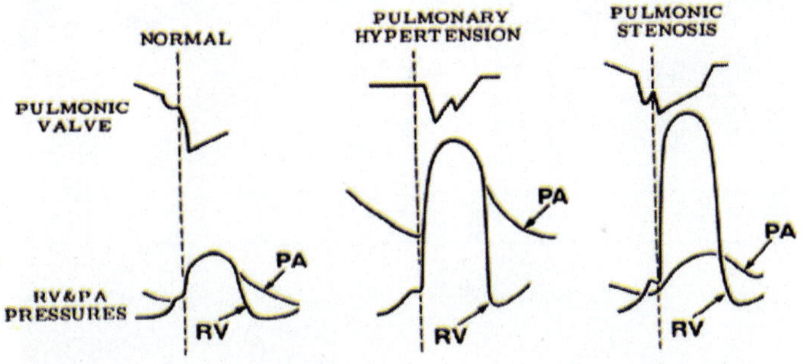

Fig. 25.23: *Graphic representation of relationship between M-mode echocardiographic signatures of normal pulmonary valve, pulmonary arterial hypertension and congenital pulmonic stenosis and their corresponding hemodynamic pressure changes in RV and RA thereby stressing the need of noninvasive echocardiographic evaluation of these disorders*

Unfortunately, no other noninvasive assessment of diastolic function exists. Although less frequently performed in clinical practice, similar Doppler interrogation of the tricuspid inflow and hepatic vein inflow can be performed to gain insight into right ventricular diastolic function.

Given the difficulty in accurately characterizing diastolic function underscored above, few studies have assessed diastolic function in patients with diastolic heart failure. Invasive assessment of impaired ventricular relaxation and reduced ventricular compliance has been demonstrated in a landmark study of patients with heart failure and normal ejection fraction. Another small but elegant invasive study did not demonstrate a significant alteration in either relaxation or compliance as compared to elderly hypertensive patients without heart failure despite the presence of elevated left ventricular diastolic pressures in heart failure patients. However, in these patients blood pressure and left ventricular diastolic pressure increased dramatically in association with marked impairment in relaxation with exercise. In such patients, arterial stiffening, which promotes labile hypertension and load-dependent diastolic dysfunction, may be an important mechanism contributing to diastolic heart failure even if resting diastolic function is not markedly aberrant. Another study that did not characterize diastolic function invasively but used Doppler assessment of left ventricular filling pressures and 3D echocardiography to assess volume suggested that volume expansion with normal systolic and diastolic function may produce the clinical syndrome in some patients. It is quite likely that heart failure with normal ejection fraction is a heterogeneous condition with multiple mechanisms contributing to chronic pulmonary venous hypertension.

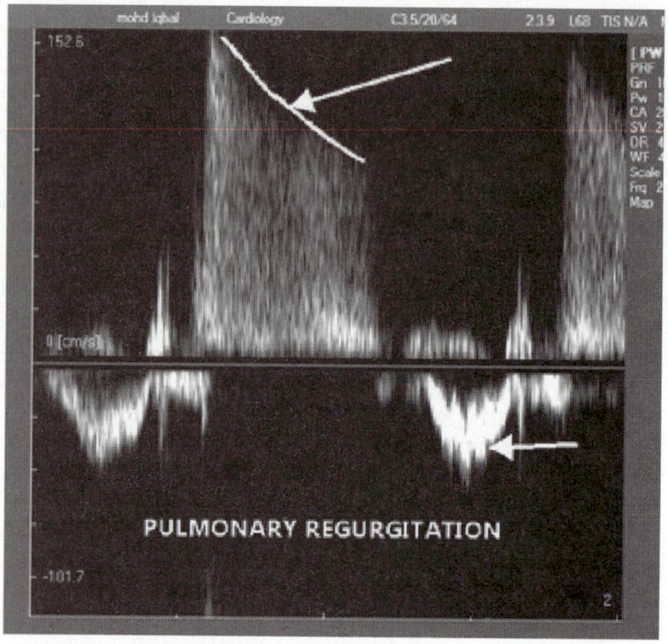

Fig. 25.24: *Doppler pulmonary valve shows moderate pulmonary regurgitation in patient with pulmonary arterial hypertension*

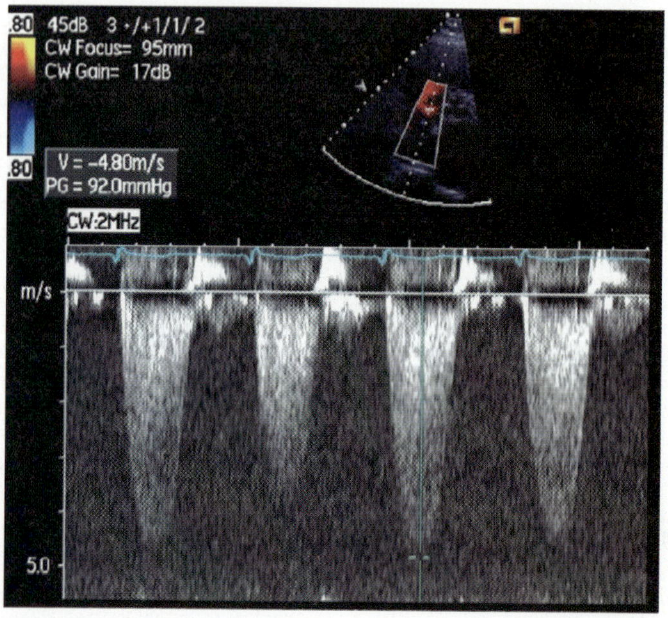

Fig. 25.25: *Doppler estimation of systolic pulmonary artery pressure using two dimensional echocardiography. The peak tricuspid regurgitation (TR) velocity of 4.80 m/s equates to a systolic PAP of 92 mmHg (plus right atrial pressure), indicating severe pulmonary hypertension*

Diastolic Dysfunction Causing Pulmonary Hypertension

That left-sided heart failure is the most common cause of pulmonary hypertension has long been recognized. The passive effect of pulmonary venous hypertension elevates pulmonary artery pressure. However, patients also develop "reactive" pulmonary hypertension with increases in the transpulmonary gradient. This component of pulmonary hypertension may be related to hummoral factors and endothelial dysfunction in chronic heart failure associated with severe systolic dysfunction or mitral stenosis. Finally,

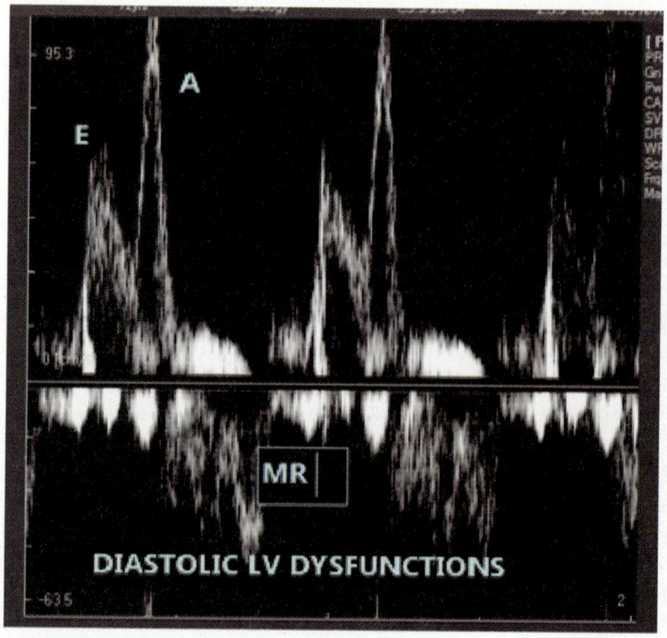

Fig. 25.26: *shows Doppler E/A ratio <1,0 as seen diastolic LV dysfunction*

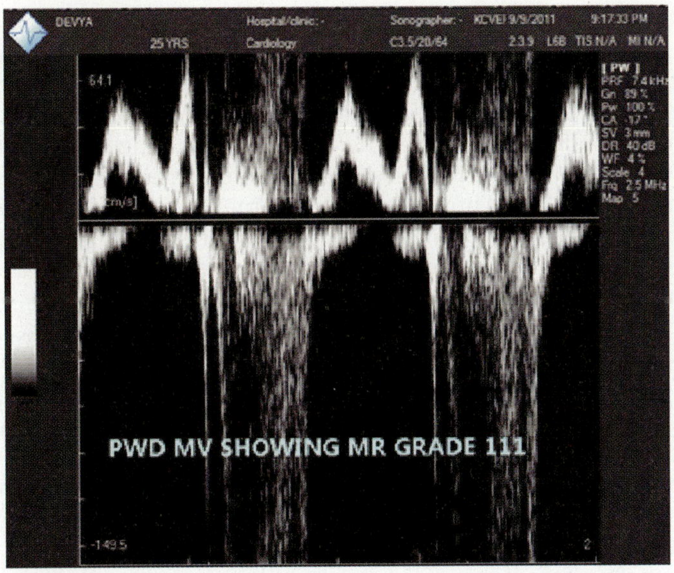

Fig. 25.27: *Doppler E/A ratio <1,0 as seen diastolic LV dysfunction with moderate MR*

chronic pulmonary venous hypertension may lead to congestive pulmonary vasculopathy characterized by pulmonary arteriolar remodeling with medial hyperplasia and intimal fibrosis. Pulmonary hypertension related to reactive pulmonary hypertension and/or congestive pulmonary vasculopathy result in pulmonary hypertension beyond that associated with the passive effects of pulmonary venous hypertension and may not be reversible with acute reduction in pulmonary venous pressures or acute pulmonary vasodilator infusion. Similarly, if medications have normalized resting PCWP or if PCWP primarily becomes elevated with exertion or when blood pressure fluctuates, it may be possible for patients with diastolic heart failure to have elevated pulmonary arterial pressures but a normal PCWP at rest at catheterization and provocative measures may be needed to demonstrate the pulmonary venous hypertension.

Although common in patients with left heart disease, the development of pulmonary hypertension is highly variable. The factors that predispose to development of significant pulmonary hypertension in the presence of chronic pulmonary venous hypertension are not fully understood. As noted above, the presence of humoral activation and endothelial dysfunction likely play a role. Although early case reports described severe pulmonary hypertension in patients with diastolic heart failure, the frequency with which patients with diastolic heart failure develop pulmonary hypertension and its severity remain poorly defined. Klapholz et al described the presence of pulmonary hypertension in patients with diastolic heart failure in a larger series of patients with diastolic heart failure and found that the average right ventricular systolic pressure in patients hospitalized with diastolic heart failure was 47 mmHg using Doppler echocardiography. In patients with aortic stenosis, most of whom had a normal ejection fraction, the severity of diastolic dysfunction rather than the severity of aortic stenosis correlated best with the severity of pulmonary hypertension and a significant number of patients developed severe pulmonary hypertension. Similarly, in patients with heart failure and a reduced ejection fraction (systolic heart failure), it was the severity of concomitant diastolic dysfunction rather than ejection fraction or cardiac output that correlated best with the severity of pulmonary hypertension.

Thus, diastolic dysfunction associated with valvular disease, reduced ejection fraction, or in isolation is the common mediator that results in chronic pulmonary venous hypertension and secondary pulmonary hypertension. It is therefore not unexpected that patients with diastolic heart failure will develop pulmonary hypertension.

It seems reasonable to expect that elderly persons would be more susceptible to the development of pulmonary hypertension as age related systemic vascular stiffening has been consistently reported and age-related pulmonary artery stiffening may well occur. Interestingly, age-related increases in arterial stiffening are worse in women than in men. Thus, the elderly women patients who develop diastolic heart failure may also be more prone to developing pulmonary hypertension in response to chronic pulmonary venous hypertension associated with diastolic heart failure. Alternatively, some patients may have a primary pulmonary arteriopathy of late onset and have concomitant (but unrelated) diastolic dysfunction related to their age.

Atrial compliance is a little studied factor that may contribute to the pathophysiology of diastolic heart failure and predispose to pulmonary hypertension as well. Insight into the role of atrial compliance comes from early hemodynamic studies where large left atrial V waves were described in patients with various cardiac diseases in the

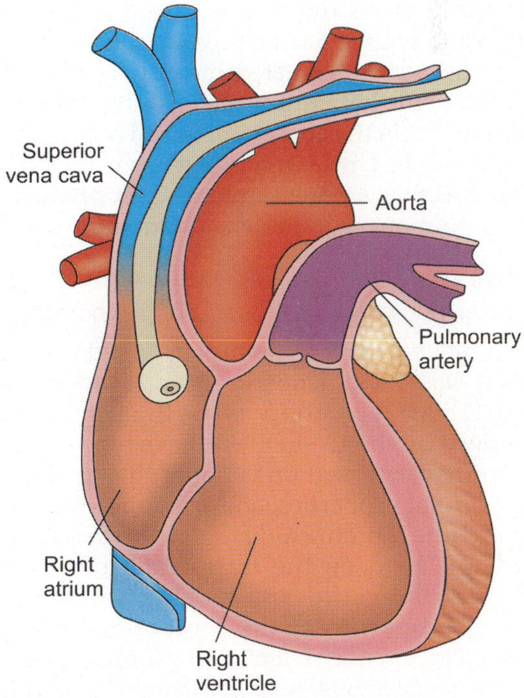

Fig. 25.28: *Placement of Swan-Ganz catheter in the pulmonary artery*

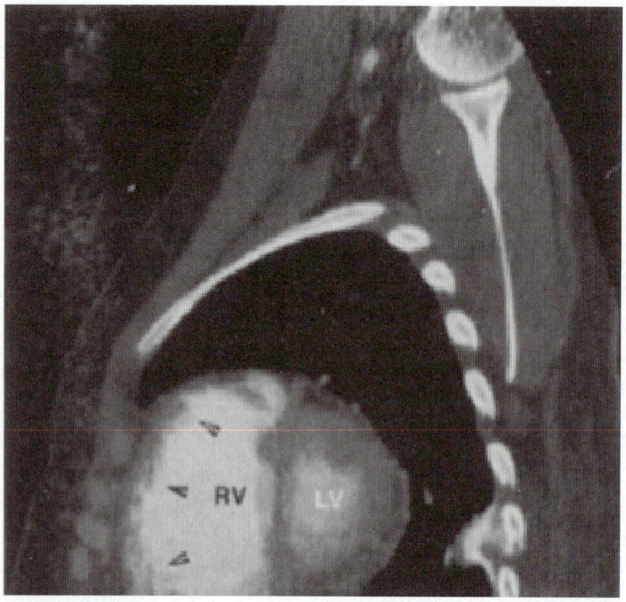

Fig. 25.29: *MRI scan showing reconstruction in short-axis view from a 15-year-old boy with chronic pulmonary hypertension. The right ventricle (RV) is dilated. Notice how flat the interventricular septum appears, causing extrinsic compression of the left ventricle (LV). The thickened right ventricular free wall myocardium is characterized by prominent intracavitary trabeculations (arrow heads)*

absence of mitral regurgitation. The large V wave represents large increases in left atrial pressure in response to the atrial filling that occurs during ventricular systole (closed mitral valve), and thus reflects reduced atrial compliance. Although much focus is placed on left ventricular diastolic pressures in mediating chronic pulmonary venous hypertension, it is mean left atrial pressure that reflects the degree of pulmonary vascular congestion and high left atrial pressure during ventricular systole contributes to elevated mean left atrial pressure. Indeed, in patients with mitral stenosis, two recent studies demonstrate that in the absence of mitral regurgitation, the presence of reduced atrial compliance as reflected by large atrial V waves was a potent independent predictor of the severity of pulmonary hypertension in mitral stenosis.

Left Ventricular Diastolic Dysfunction in Chronic Right Ventricular Pressure Overload

Chronic right ventricular pressure overload can affect left ventricular diastolic function in several ways. Changes in left ventricular relaxation as well as in compliance (characterized by the LV-EDPVR) have been described.

Left ventricular relaxation is under the triple control of load, myocardial properties, and the uniformity of load in space and time. In chronic right ventricular pressure overload, the load on the intraventricular septum is dramatically increased and as it hypertrophies, the myocardial properties of the septum are altered. The motion of the intraventricular septum in systole and diastole is asynchronous. All these factors could contribute to impairment in global left ventricular relaxation. In Doppler echocardiographic studies of IPAH, impaired relaxation with decreased E/A ratio and increased isovolumic relaxation time and deceleration time have been consistently reported. An "impaired relaxation" pattern (grade I diastolic dysfunction) is usually associated with normal left ventricular filling pressures and indeed, patients with severe IPAH entered into clinical trials must have normal PCWP. Thus, based on Doppler echocardiographic studies, the effect of chronic right ventricular pressure overload on relaxation appears unassociated with increases in left ventricular filling pressure.

While patients must have normal PCWP to be diagnosed with IPAH, there is considerable evidence that chronic right ventricular pressure overload can cause reduced left ventricular compliance. The external forces affecting the LV-EDPVR include right ventricular pressure and pericardial pressure. The effect of right ventricular pressures on the LV-EDPVR is termed "ventricular interdependence" and is accentuated in the presence of an intact pericardium. Visner et al used both acute and chronic canine pulmonary banding models and showed that the LV-EDPVR was shifted leftward (decreased compliance) by acute or chronic right ventricular pressure overload. The shift in the LV-EDPVR with acute right ventricular pressure overload was related to ventricular interdependence with decreases in left ventricular volume related to leftward shift

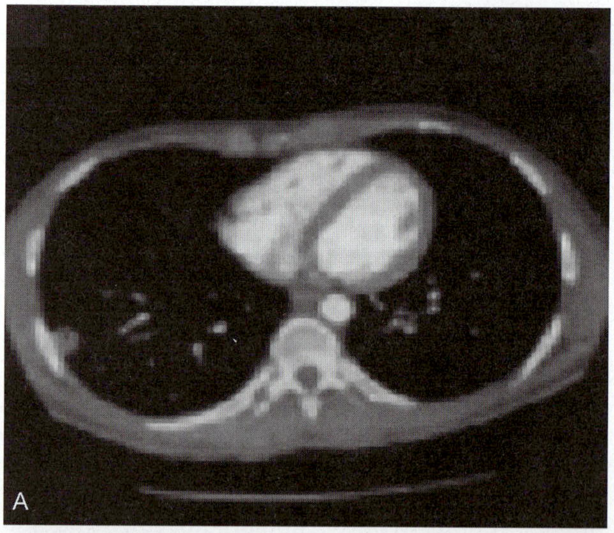

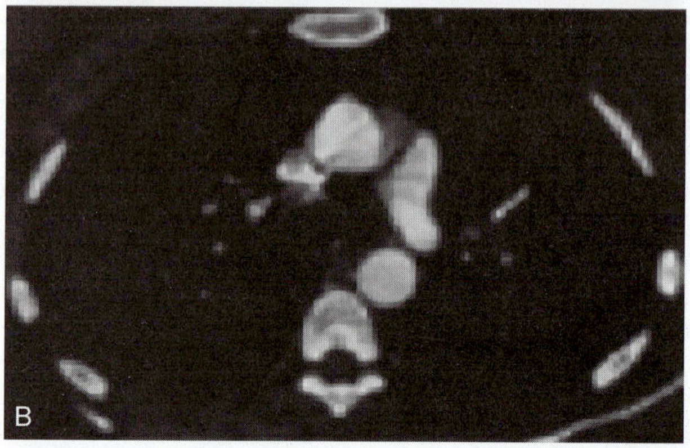

Fig. 25.30: *(A) CT scan showing septic emboli in both lungs. (B) Pulmonary embolism is also observed in left upper lobe (arrow)*

of the intraventricular septum as right ventricular pressures increased. These effects were also apparent in chronic right ventricular pressure overload, but a decrease in myocardial compliance (as assessed by the stress-strain relationship) was also seen. This effect, not seen in acute right ventricular pressure overload, suggests that chronic right ventricular pressure overload alters intrinsic left ventricular myocardial properties. Whether this effect is wholly mediated by the altered intraventricular system or whether the left ventricular free wall myocardium also becomes abnormal is unclear. However, Little et al showed that the effect of right ventricular pressures on the LV-EDPVR was attenuated in the presence of chronic right ventricular pressure overload produced by pulmonary artery banding in the dog. Consistent with concepts introduced by Sunagawa et al., Little's study showed that when the stiffness of the septum was greater than the stiffness of the left ventricular free wall, right ventricular pressures had less effect on the LV-EDPVR. Although this study was performed in the absence of the pericardium, Blanchard et al showed that the pericardium remodels in chronic right ventricular pressure overload and that pericardiotomy did not alter right or left ventricular filling pressures or cardiac output.

Although these animal studies and limited studies in the human confirm adverse effects of right ventricular pressure overload on left ventricular diastolic function, the clinical significance of left ventricular diastolic dysfunction associated with chronic right ventricular pressure overload is difficult to appreciate. In the studies of Little and Visner, dogs with acute and chronic right ventricular pressure overload had left ventricular diastolic pressures that were not different from those of control dogs. Although the compliance of the left ventricle was reduced, it was not reduced enough to result in elevated left ventricular filling pressures. Similarly, in humans with chronic pulmonary hypertension related to thromboembolic disease, indices of left ventricular diastolic compliance were reduced and improved after thrombectomy, but PCWP was normal both before and after surgery. Lastly, patients entered into IPAH trials have severe pulmonary hypertension, often with severe right ventricular remodeling and dysfunction and yet have normal PCWP. These studies would suggest that while left ventricular diastolic function is altered in IPAH, it is not perturbed enough to result in elevated PCWP. However, as most studies describing hemodynamics in IPAH were performed in the context of a drug trial (where patients with elevated PCWP are excluded), the frequency of left ventricular diastolic dysfunction severe enough to result in elevated filling pressures in patients with IPAH may be under recognized.

Strategies for Diagnosing Diastolic Heart Failure in the Setting of Pulmonary Hypertension

It is likely that diastolic heart failure is an under recognized cause of pulmonary hypertension and that otherwise unexplained dyspnea and pulmonary hypertension in elderly patients with a normal ejection fraction and normal valves should prompt consideration of diastolic heart failure as well as IPAH. Yet, distinguishing between diastolic heart failure with secondary pulmonary hypertension and IPAH with secondary diastolic dysfunction can be quite challenging.

Echocardiography may be helpful and evidence of left ventricular hypertrophy, left atrial enlargement, and Doppler evidence of advanced diastolic dysfunction (grades II–IV) may favor the diagnosis of diastolic heart failure. However, not all patients with diastolic heart failure have echocardiographic evidence of left ventricular hypertrophy and not all echocardiographic laboratories perform a comprehensive diastolic assessment nor measure left atrial volume.

All patients with significant pulmonary hypertension should undergo right heart catheterization and if the PCWP is elevated (greater than or equal to 15 mmHg), a diagnosis of isolated pulmonary arteriopathy cannot be made even if there is a significant transpulmonary gradient. In patients with an elevated PCWP, one should look for evidence of systemic hypertension and if present, use of a systemic vasodilator to lower arterial pressures should be considered. Prompt reduction in PCWP with normalization of blood pressure supports the diagnosis of diastolic heart failure. Provocative testing with exercise in elderly patients with pulmonary hypertension in whom diastolic heart failure is suspected may be useful. Marked elevation in PCWP and blood pressure with exercise would support the diagnosis of diastolic heart failure that could be causing the patients' symptoms and their pulmonary hypertension. Patients with severe IPAH should not experience increases in PCWP during exercise . Additionally, one should look for evidence of reduced atrial compliance (large V waves in the PCWP tracing). Exercise testing may also be helpful and if associated with marked increases in PCWP, a diagnosis of diastolic heart failure would be supported. Finally, if diastolic heart failure is strongly suspected, care should be taken with use of vasodilators that are very selective for the pulmonary vasculature (such as inhaled nitric oxide) as increases in right heart output in the presence of a noncompliant left ventricle may result in further increases in left atrial pressure and pulmonary edema.

Management of the Pulmonary Hypertension in Children

In patients with PPH treated with chronic vasodilator therapy the most important determinants of survival are:

1. Age, with a 5-year survival of 88% in children of less than 6 years of age, as compared with 25% for older children
2. The acute response to prostacyclin, the 5-year survival being 86%, as compared with 33% for nonresponders. In congenital heart disease, symptoms and signs reflect the natural history of pulmonary vascular disease with and without surgery in the different anomalies. Lessons learned in the management of children with PPH are now being applied to other forms of pulmonary hypertension in childhood. PPH Treatment for PPH is

lifelong. The therapeutic regimen has to be individualized and adjusted according to changes in clinical and hemodynamic status. Children need close monitoring of the clinical course to ensure a satisfactory and sustained response to treatment, with recatheterization if necessary. Optimizing the management of these patients markedly improves quality of life and survival.

The principles of management are:

- Children with a positive response to acute vasodilator testing are given **calcium channel blockers,** usually nifedipine. Actuarial survival is increased in adults treated with this drug. But, the magnitude of response that predicts long-term survival is unknown in the young, and repeat cardiac catheterization is necessary after several months to detect any deterioration. Loss of acute responsiveness demands urgent revision of therapy. Children unresponsive to acute vasodilator testing are not treated with calcium channel blockers, which can have adverse effects and precipitate or worsen right-heart failure. Older, compliant children in NYHA class II can take **nebulized iloprost**, which has a similar molecular structure to epoprostenol. Regular, effective dosing (6–12 times a day) is difficult in young children.
- **The dual endothelin receptor antagonist**
- Tracleer **(bosentan)**, efficacious in adults, is now being studied in children.
- The **oral prostacyclin analogue beraprost sodium** is efficacious in adults but recommended only for those with less severe pulmonary hypertension and is largely untested in children.
- The **subcutaneous analogue of prostacyclin, treprostinil** (Remodulin), is too painful for use in young children.
- **The phosphodiesterase inhibitor sildenafil** is untested, but its effect appears to be relatively short-lived in sick children.
- **The proven treatment of choice for the very sick child is long-term intravenous epoprostenol (flolan)**. The dose is titrated according to clinical response, subjective and objective. Children generally need much higher doses of epoprostenol than adults and can become very tolerant of the drug, requiring constant, aggressive, upward adjustment of their dosage. Despite the obvious logistical problems, infants and young children can be managed satisfactorily. The side effects experienced by children are similar to those seen in adults.
- **Supplemental domiciliary oxygen** provides symptomatic improvement for those with systemic arterial desaturation.
- **Anticoagulation:** Warfarin rather than aspirin or dipyridamole is recommended to prevent thrombosis in situ, although aspirin is more tolerable in early infancy.
- *Supportive medical therapy:* Diuretics are indicated to control the fluid retention of right-heart failure but should be administered cautiously in very sick children, who need a high preload. Digoxin may be helpful in the treatment of right-heart failure.
- **Atrial septostomy/septectomy** if indicated.

Organization of care in the community and contact with patients' support groups is essential.

- *Screening and genetic testing:* All first-degree relatives are screened in FPPH. It is thought that an individual in a family with FPPH has a 5–10% lifetime risk of developing PPH. Genetic testing entails DNA sequencing because mutations in the BMPR2 gene appear to be "private" to each family.
- *Congenital heart disease:* Correlating the physiological findings with structural observations in different types of intracardiac abnormality has improved the accuracy with which immediate and long-term outcome can be predicted with and without corrective surgery. But, prediction is still more difficult in younger children. The most crucial factor in determining late outcome is the age at which repair is carried out. Most children operated on by 9 months of age have a normal pulmonary vascular resistance 1 year after repair. After 2 years of age-resistance may fall, but not to a normal level. These observations indicate vessel wall remodeling toward normality, continued growth, and a demonstrable improvement in endothelial function. Repairing an intracardiac abnormality in the presence of established disease accelerates the progression of disease and the onset of right ventricular failure and death. If there is doubt about the likely outcome of surgical repair, then an open lung biopsy should clarify the position. Current pulmonary vascular therapies appear to exert their actions on the pulmonary circulation by mechanisms that remain poorly defined. Clearly, the magnitude of the pulmonary vasodilator actions of prostanoids and endothelin antagonists do not account for the degree of clinical benefit observed with these drugs. Rather, additional effects on the endothelial health of the pulmonary circulation and on the inhibition of pathologic intimal fibrosis and smooth muscle proliferation are likely to be the predominant mechanisms involved in the treatment responses.

PHARMACOTHERAPY IN PULMONARY HYPERTENSION

Parenteral Vasodilators

For patients in whom CCBs fail to respond or with an inability to tolerate CCBs with NYHA types III and IV right-sided heart failure.

Epoprostenol (Flolan)

Description: An analogue of PGI_2 that was approved by the FDA in 1995 for use in patients with PPH. It has potent vasodilatory properties, an immediate onset of action, and a half-life of approximately 5 min. In addition to its vasodilator properties, also contributes to inhibition of platelet aggregation and plays a role in inhibition of smooth muscle proliferation. Latter effect may have implications for beneficial remodeling of pulmonary vascular bed. EPO is only FDA-approved medication for treatment of PPH.

Adult dose: Continuous IV infusion via permanent indwelling central venous catheter using a small, battery-powered infusion pump worn at the hip or carried in a backpack. Beginning dose: 2–4 ng/kg/min IV; depending on initial response; initiate under close observation in the ICU with right-sided heart flotation catheter in place.

Subsequent dose: Titrate based on follow-up outpatient evaluation; currently, no upper limit has been defined; most patients derive optimal benefit with doses of 25–40 ng/kg/min; doses exceeding 40 ng/kg/min after 1 year of therapy are not uncommon.

Pediatric dose: Administer as in adults.

Treprostinil (Remodulin)

Description: Used to treat PAH. Structurally very similar to EPO but stable at room temperature and has much longer half-life; therefore, can be given as an SC continuous infusion via a much smaller pump. Elicits direct vasodilation of pulmonary and systemic arterial vessels and inhibits platelet aggregation. Vasodilation reduces right and left ventricular afterload and increases cardiac output and stroke volume. Recently, FDA approved for IV use as a bioequivalent of subcutaneous treprostinil, using same delivery pump used for epoprostenol. Dosing is similar to SC delivery.

Adult dose: 1.25 ng/kg/min SC via continuous infusion initially; may increase by 1.25 ng/kg/min qwk for 4 wk, then may increase by 2.5 ng/kg/min qwk; if initial dose not tolerated, decrease to 0.625 ng/kg/min, then slowly titrate upward; must slowly taper if discontinued (potential for severe rebound pulmonary hypertension and death).

Subsequent dose: Titrate based on follow-up outpatient evaluation; currently, no upper limit defined; most patients derive optimal benefit with 25–40 ng/kg/min; doses exceeding 40 ng/kg/min after 1 y of therapy are not uncommon; IV dosing is similar to that used in SC delivery.

Pediatric dose: Not established; dosing is based on body weight.

Phosphodiesterase (type 5) Enzyme Inhibitor

The antiproliferative effects of the phosphodiesterase type 5 pathway, which regulates cyclic guanosine monophosphate hydrolysis, may be significant in the long-term treatment of pulmonary hypertension with PDE5 inhibitors such as sildenafil.

Sildenafil (Revatio)

Description: It promotes selective smooth muscle relaxation in lung vasculature, possibly by inhibiting phosphodiesterase type 5 (PDE5). This results in subsequent reduction of blood pressure in pulmonary arteries and increase in cardiac output.

Adult dose: 20 mg PO tid

Pediatric dose: Not established

Inhaled vasodilators: Inhaled PGI_2 synthetic analogues are an alternative to parenteral administration and an attempt to limit systemic adverse effects.

Iloprost (Ventavis)

Description: Synthetic analogue of prostacyclin PGI_2 that dilates systemic and pulmonary arterial vascular beds. Indicated for pulmonary arterial hypertension (WHO class I) in patients with NYHA class III or IV symptoms to improve exercise tolerance and symptoms and to delay deterioration.

Adult dose: Initial: 2.5 mcg via nebulizer. Maintenance: if first dose tolerated, increase to 5 mcg/dose via nebulizer 6–9 times/d; do not administer more frequently than q2h. Note: Administration studied only with prodose AAD system nebulizer.

Pediatric dose: Not established.

Oral pulmonary hypertension agents: ERAs are alternative therapy to parenteral prostacyclin agents. Given PO. Competitively bind to ET-1 receptors endothelin-A and endothelin-B, causing reduction in PAP, PVR, and mean RAP. Indicated for treatment of PAH in patients with WHO class III or IV symptoms to improve exercise ability and decrease rate of clinical deterioration.

Bosentan (Tracleer)

Description: First PO PPH therapy to be approved in United States. A mixed endothelin-A and endothelin-B receptor antagonist indicated for PAH including PPH. In clinical trials, improved exercise capacity, decreased rate of clinical deterioration, improved functional class, and improved hemodynamics. Improves pulmonary arterial hemodynamics by competitively binding to ET-1 receptors endothelin-A and endothelin-B in pulmonary vascular endothelium and pulmonary vascular smooth muscle. This leads to a significant increase in CI associated with a significant reduction in PAP, PVR, and mean RAP. These changes result in an improvement in exercise capacity (as measured by the 6-min walk test) and improved PPH symptoms. Because drug has teratogenic potential and because of need for careful scrutiny in choosing appropriate candidates for ERA therapy.

Adult dose: Starting dose: 62.5 mg PO bid for 4 weeks, followed by 125 mg PO bid indefinitely.

Pediatric dose: Not established; 62.5 mg PO bid recommended if < 40 kg or > 12 years; not to exceed 125 mg/d.

Ambrisentan (Letairis)

Description: Endothelin receptor antagonist indicated for pulmonary arterial hypertension in patients with WHO class II or III symptoms. Improves exercise ability and decreases progression of clinical symptoms. Inhibits vessel constriction and elevation of blood pressure by competitively binding to endothelin-1 receptors ET_A and ET_B in endothelium and vascular smooth muscle. This leads to significant increase in cardiac index associated with significant reduction in pulmonary artery pressure, pulmonary vascular resistance, and mean right atrial pressure. Because of the risks of hepatic injury and teratogenic potential, only available through the Letairis Education and Access Program (LEAP). Prescribers and pharmacies must register with LEAP in order to prescribe and dispense.

Adult dose: 5 mg PO qd initially; may increase to 10 mg PO qd if 5 mg/d tolerated; do not chew, crush, or split tab.

Pediatric dose: Not established.

Dipyridamole is thought to reduce platelet aggregation but may also have a beneficial vasodilatory effect as a phosphodiesterase inhibitor. Anticoagulation is recommended.

Phlebotomy with plasma dilution in those with a high hematocrit is not used routinely but may afford symptomatic relief to some patients. Frequent phlebotomy causing iron deficiency can increase the risk of cerebrovascular accidents.

Treatment with prostacyclin is tempting, but its efficacy is not proved in patients with classic Eisenmenger syndrome and it can cause systemic hypotension in the presence of pulmonary-systemic communication.

Endothelin receptor antagonists are promising but still unproved therapies. Long-term administration of L-arginine might be helpful if it could be shown conclusively that these patients have a relative substrate deficiency of NO production. Calcium channel blockers are not used.

Transplantation: Single/double-lung or cardiopulmonary transplantation may be considered in some severe cases. With pulmonary protection and immunosuppression, the long-term prognosis after lung and heart-lung transplant is good.

Prognosis: For untreated PPH, the estimated 3-year survival rate is approximately 41%. One study of long-term continuous intravenous prostacyclin therapy found that 3-year survival increased to approximately 63%. One meta-analysis showed a reduction in mortality of 43% in response to active treatment. The advent of pulmonary vasodilators has improved the outlook for children. Patients who do not respond to medical therapy tend to develop progressive right-sided heart failure if transplantation cannot be carried out, provide feedback.

BIBLIOGRAPHY

1. Rich S. Primary Pulmonary Hypertension: Executive Summary from the World Symposium on Primary Pulmonary Hypertension 1998, Evian, France, 6–10 September 1998. Rich, S. 2002.
2. Haworth SG. Pulmonary hypertension in the young. Heart 2002;88:658–64.
3. Rich S, Dantzker DR, Ayres SM, et al. Primary pulmonary hypertension: a national prospective study. Ann Intern Med 1987;107:216–23.
4. Loyd JE, Butler MG, Foroud TM, et al. Genetic anticipation and abnormal gender ratio at birth in familial primary pulmonary hypertension. Am Respir Crit Care Med 1995;152:93–7.
5. The International PPH Consortium, Lane KB, Machado RD, Pauciulo MW, Thompson JR, Phillips III JA, et al. Heterozygous germline mutations in a TGF-β-receptor, BMPR2, are the cause of familial primary pulmonary hypertension. Genetics 2000;26:81–4.
6. Johnson DW, Berg JN, Baldwin MA, et al. Mutations in the activin receptor-like kinase 1 gene in hereditary haemorrhagic telangiectasia type 2. Nat Genet 1996;13:189–95.
7. Thompson JR, Machado RD, Pauciulo MW. Sporadic primary pulmonary hypertension is associated with germline mutations of the geneencoding BMPR-II, a receptor member of the TGF-B family. J Med Genet 2000;37:741–5.
8. Lee S-D, Shroyer KR, Markham NE, et al. Monoclonal endothelial cell proliferation is present in primary pulmonary but not secondary pulmonary hypertension. J Clin Invest 1997;101:927–34.
9. Christman BW, McPherson CD, Newman JH, et al. An imbalance between the excretion of thromboxane and prostacyclin metabolites in pulmonary hypertension. N Engl J Med 1992;327:70–5.
10. Barst RJ, Rubin LJ, Long WA, et al. A comparison of continuous intravenous epoprostenol (prostacyclin) with conventional treatment for primary pulmonary hypertension. N Engl J Med 1996;334:296–301.
11. Rubin LJ, Badesch DB, Barst RJ, et al. Bosentan therapy for pulmonary arterial hypertension. N Engl J Med 2002;346:896–903.
12. Barst, RJ. Treatment of primary pulmonary hypertension with continuous intravenous prostacyclin. Heart 1997;77, 299–301.
13. Cui Y, Tran S, Tinker A, Clapp LH. The molecular composition of K(ATP) channels in human pulmonary artery smooth muscle cells and their modulation by growth. Am J Respir Cell Mol Biol 2002;26:135–43.
14. Eddahibi S, Humbert M, Fadel E, et al. Serotonin transporter overexpression is responsible for pulmonary artery smooth muscle hyperplasia in primary pulmonary hypertension. J Clin Invest 2001;108:1141–50.
15. Haworth SG. Pathobiology of pulmonary hypertension in infants and children. Prog Ped Cardiol 2001;12:249–69.
16. Tulloh RMR, Hislop AA, Boels PJ, et al. Chronic hypoxia inhibits postnatal maturation of porcine intrapulmonary artery relaxation. Am J Physiol 1997;272:H2436–H2445.
17. Noguchi Y, Hislop AA, Evans, J, et al. Increased plasma endothelin levels and endothelin receptor binding sites in neonatal pulmonary hypertensive pigs. Am J Resp Crit Care Med 1995;151:A517.
18. Adatia I, Barrow SE, Stratton PD, et al. Thromboxane A2 and prosta-cyclinbiosynthesis in children and adolescents with pulmonary vascular disease. Circulation 1993;88:2117–22.
19. Ku DD, Zaleski JK, Liu S, et al. Vascular endothelial growth factor induces EDRF-dependent relaxation in coronary arteries. Am J Physiol 1993;265:H586–H592.
20. Resnick N, Gimbrone MAJr. Hemodynamic forces are complex regulators of endothelial gene expression. FASEB J 1995;9:874–82.
21. Walpola PL, Gotlieb AI, Cybulsky MI, et al. Expression of ICAM-1 and VCAM-1 and monocyte adherence in arteries exposed to altered shear stress. Arterioscler Thromb Vasc Biol 1995;15:3–20.
22. Cowan KN, Heilbut A, Humpl T, et al. Complete reversal of fatal pulmonary hypertension in rats by a serine elastase inhibitor. Nat Med 2000;6:698–702.
23. Geraci MW, Gao B, Shepherd DC, et al. Pulmonary prostacyclin synthase overexpression in transgenic mice protects against development of hypoxic pulmonary hypertension. J Clin Invest 1999;103:1509–15.